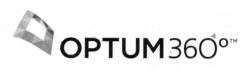

www.optumcoding.com

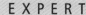

D1405229

Current Procedural Coding Expert

CPT® codes with Medicare essentials
enhanced for accuracy

Supports HIPAA Compliance

2016

ICD-10

A full suite of resources including the latest code set,
mapping products, and expert training to help you make
a smooth transition. **www.optumcoding.com/ICD10**

Acknowledgments

Marianne Randall, CPC, *Product Manager*
Karen Schmidt, BSN, *Technical Director*
Stacy Perry, *Manager, Desktop Publishing*
Lisa Singley, *Project Manager*
Karen H. Kachur, RN, CPC, *Clinical/Technical Editor*
Anita Schmidt, BS, RHIT, *Clinical/Technical Editor*
Elizabeth Leibold, RHIT, *Clinical/Technical Editor*
Anne Kenney, BA, MBA, CCA, CCS, *Clinical/Technical Editor*
Tracy Betzler, *Senior Desktop Publishing Specialist*
Hope M. Dunn, *Senior Desktop Publishing Specialist*
Katie Russell, *Desktop Publishing Specialist*
Kate Holden, *Editor*

About the Contributors

Karen H. Kachur, RN, CPC

Ms. Kachur is a clinical/technical editor for Optum360 with expertise in CPT/HCPCS and ICD-9-CM coding, in addition to physician billing, compliance, and fraud and abuse. Prior to joining Optum360, she worked for many years as a staff RN in a variety of clinical settings, including medicine, surgery, intensive care, and psychiatry. In addition to her clinical background, Ms. Kachur served as assistant director of a hospital utilization management and quality assurance department and has extensive experience as a nurse reviewer for Blue Cross/Blue Shield. She is an active member of the American Academy of Professional Coders.

Elizabeth Leibold, RHIT

Ms. Leibold has expertise in hospital outpatient coding and compliance. Her experience includes conducting coding audits and providing staff education to both tenured and new coding staff. She has a background in professional component coding, with CPT expertise in interventional procedures. Most recently Ms. Leibold was responsible for outpatient coding audits and compliance for a health information management services company. She is an active member of the American Health Information Management Association (AHIMA).

Anne Kenney, BA, MBA, CCA, CCS

Ms. Kenney has expertise in ICD-9-CM, DRG, and CPT coding. Her experience in a major teaching hospital includes assignment of ICD-9-CM codes and DRGs, CPT code assignments, and determining physician evaluation and management levels for inpatient, emergency department, and observation cases. She worked as a volunteer with AHIMA to validate requirements of a Certified Coding Associate (CCA) and assisted in the development of CCA certification exams. Ms. Kenney has completed an AHIMA-approved ICD-10-CM/PCS educational program, and is an active member of the American Health Information Management Association (AHIMA) and the Minnesota Health Information Management Association.

Anita Schmidt, BS, RHIT

Ms. Schmidt has expertise in Level I Adult and Pediatric Trauma hospital coding, specializing in ICD-9-CM, DRG, and CPT coding. Her experience includes analyzing medical record documentation and assigning ICD-9-CM codes and DRGs, as well as CPT codes for same-day surgery cases. She has conducted coding training and auditing, including DRG validation, conducted electronic health record training, and worked with clinical documentation specialists to identify documentation needs and potential areas for physician education. Ms. Schmidt is an active member of the American Health Information Management Association (AHIMA) and the Minnesota Health Information Management Association (MNHIMA).

OPTUM360°™

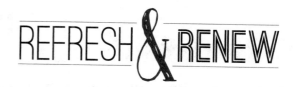

SAVE UP TO 25%*

when you renew your coding essentials.

- Buy 1–2 items, save 15%
- Buy 3–5 items, save 20%
- Buy 6+ items, save 25%

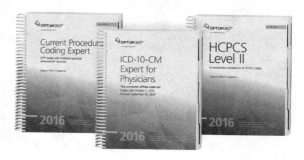

TITLE INDICATE THE ITEMS YOU WISH TO PURCHASE	QUANTITY	PRICE PER PRODUCT	TOTAL
Subtotal			
(AK, DE, HI, MT, NH & OR are exempt) Sales Tax			
1 item $10.95 • 2–4 items $12.95 • 5+ CALL Shipping & Handling			
TOTAL AMOUNT ENCLOSED			

Save up to 25% when you renew.

 Visit **optumcoding.com** and enter the promo code below.

Call

Mail this order form with payment and/or purchase order to:
Optum360, PO Box 88050, Chicago, IL 60680-9920.
Optum360 no longer accepts credit cards by mail.

Name _____

Address _____

_____

Customer Number _____   Contact Number _____

○ CHECK ENCLOSED (PAYABLE TO OPTUM360)

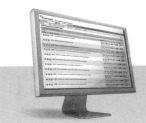
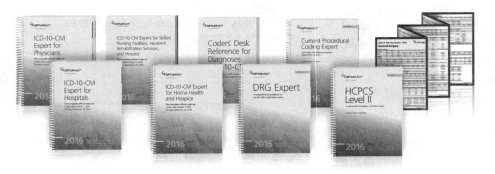

ESSENTIALS CODING, BILLING & COMPLIANCE CONFERENCE

VISIT OPTUMCODING.COM/ESSENTIALS

Only Optum360™ delivers high quality, continuing education and industry-leading content matter at this level and price.

Whether you're looking for daily tips to help make your job just a little easier, or you want to keep your skills current and relevant in this ever-changing world of coding, billing and compliance, Optum360 Essentials is truly, well, essential.

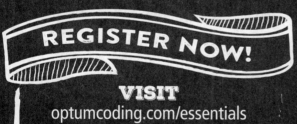

REGISTER NOW!

VISIT
optumcoding.com/essentials

CALL
1-510-463-6073

EMAIL

WHY ATTEND?

- Choose from up to 40 educational sessions, all created to be timely and relevant with what's currently happening in the industry.

- Earn as many as 16 CEUs approved by both AAPC and AHIMA.

- Learn from nationally recognized experts on medical coding, billing and compliance.

- Learn about the CPT® code updates firsthand.

- Stay current with updates on ICD-10-CM/PCS, HCPCS, DRG codes, HCC, PQRS, IPPS and OPPS.

- Focus on ICD-10 with specialty sessions dedicated to your practice.

- Attend vetted presentations that are reviewed and approved by legal and clinical experts.

- Network with a wide spectrum of medical professionals, from entry-level to expert understanding.

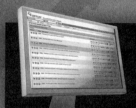
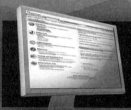

OPTUM 360°™

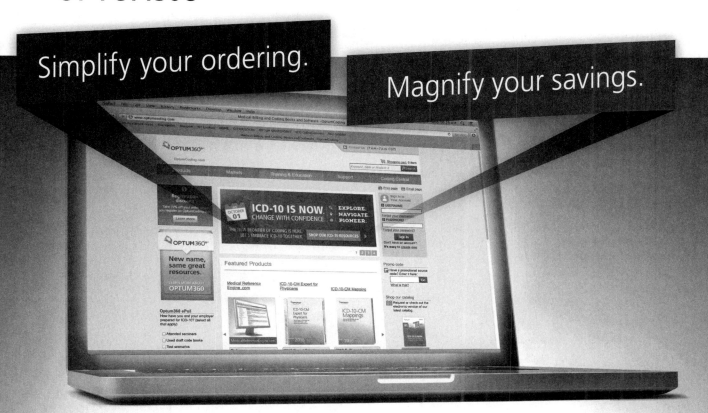

Simplify your ordering.

Magnify your savings.

① Click.

Visit optumcoding.com

- Find the products you need quickly and easily.
- View all available formats and edition years on the same page.
- Chat live with a customer service representative.
- Visit Coding Central for expert resources including articles,

② Register.

By registering, you'll be able to:

- Enjoy special promotions, discounts and automatic rewards.
- Get recommendations based on your order history.
- Check on shipment status and tracking.
- View order and payment history.
- Pay invoices.

③ Save.

Get 15% off your next order

Register for an account and receive a coupon via email for 15% off your next order.

Plus, save even more with our no-cost eRewards program.

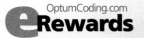

Contents

Introduction

Welcome to Optum360's *Current Procedural Coding Expert*, an exciting Medicare coding and reimbursement tool and definitive procedure coding source that combines the work of the Centers for Medicare and Medicaid Services, American Medical Association, and Optum360 experts with the technical components you need for proper reimbursement and coding accuracy.

This approach to CPT® Medicare coding utilizes innovative and intuitive ways of communicating the information you need to code claims accurately and efficiently. *Includes* and *Excludes* notes, similar to those found in ICD-9-CM and ICD-10-CM manuals, help determine what services are related to the codes you are reporting. Icons help you crosswalk the code you are reporting to laboratory and radiology procedures necessary for proper reimbursement. CMS-mandated icons and relative value units (RVUs) help you determine which codes are most appropriate for the service you are reporting. In addition, icons denoting codes that apply to Physician Quality Reporting System (PQRS) quality indicators are included. Add to that additional information identifying age and sex edits, ambulatory surgery center (ASC) and ambulatory payment classification (APC) indicators, and Medicare coverage and payment rule citations, and *Current Procedural Coding Expert* provides the best in Medicare procedure reporting.

Current Procedural Coding Expert includes the information needed to submit claims to federal contractors and most commercial payers, and is correct at the time of printing. However, CMS, federal contractors, and commercial payers may change payment rules at any time throughout the year. *Current Procedural Coding Expert* includes effective codes that will not be published in the AMA's Physicians' Current Procedural Terminology (CPT®) book until the following year. Commercial payers will announce changes through monthly news or information posted on their websites. CMS will post changes in policy on its website at http://www.cms.gov/transmittals. National and local coverage determinations (NCDs and LCDs) provide universal and individual contractor guidelines for specific services. The existence of a procedure code does not imply coverage under any given insurance plan.

Current Procedural Coding Expert is based on the AMA's Physicians' Current Procedural Terminology coding system, which is copyrighted and owned by the physician organization. The CPT codes are the nation's official, Health Information Portability and Accountability Act (HIPAA) compliant code set for procedures and services provided by physicians, ambulatory surgery centers (ASCs), and hospital outpatient services, as well as laboratories, imaging centers, physical therapy clinics, urgent care centers, and others.

In the 2016 update, the AMA made official changes to the following codes but did not identify them with a change icon or in appendix B. These codes were either first in a series under which other codes were indented, or were previously indented under another code that was deleted. When the nonindented, main code was deleted, its descriptor was incorporated into that of each previously indented code under it, and the semicolon was changed to a comma. Conversely, when a single indented code was deleted, and the code under which it was deleted became an individual stand-alone code, the semicolon was changed to a comma.

Below are the codes for which the semicolon was revised:

32400	Biopsy, pleura, percutaneous needle
43325	Esophagogastric fundoplasty, with fundic patch (Thal-Nissen procedure)
47135	Liver allotransplantation, orthotopic, partial or whole, from cadaver or living donor, any age
47562	Laparoscopy, surgical; cholecystectomy
69801	Labyrinthotomy, with perfusion of vestibuloactive drug(s), transcanal
77078	Computed tomography, bone mineral density study, 1 or more sites, axial skeleton (eg, hips, pelvis, spine)
77778	Interstitial radiation source application, complex, includes supervision, handling, loading of radiation source, when performed
78264	Gastric emptying imaging study (eg, solid, liquid, or both);
81275	*KRAS (v-Ki-ras2 Kirsten rat sarcoma viral oncogene) (eg, carcinoma) gene analysis; variants in exon 2 (eg, codons 12 and 13)*
99174	Instrument-based ocular screening (eg photoscreening, automated-refraction), bilateral; with remote analysis and report

Getting Started with *Current Procedural Coding Expert*

Current Procedural Coding Expert is an exciting tool combining the most current material at publication time from the AMA's *CPT 2016*, CMS's online manual system, the Correct Coding Initiative (CCI), CMS fee schedules, official Medicare guidelines for reimbursement and coverage, and Optum's own coding expertise.

Note: The AMA releases code changes quarterly. *Current Procedural Coding Expert* contains the most current information from the AMA, including new, changed, and deleted codes that are released on its website for future inclusion in the CPT book. Some of these changes will not appear in the AMA's CPT book until the following year.

Another feature of *Current Procedural Coding Expert* that differs from the official CPT book is appendix L, "Glossary." The glossary includes the definition of terms used throughout the manual.

Material is presented in a logical fashion for those billing Medicare, Medicaid, and many private payers. The format, based on customer comments, better addresses what customers tell us they need in a comprehensive Medicare procedure coding guide.

Designed to be easy to use and full of information, this product is an excellent companion to your AMA CPT manual and to Medicare, Optum, or other resources.

General Conventions
Sources of information in this book can be determined by color:

- Information compiled by Optum360 experts from official sources and based on coding knowledge is in blue text.

- Medicare-derived information is in red text.

- Codes, descriptions, and evaluation and management (E/M) guidelines from the American Medical Association are in black text.

Note: Icon colors and icon text do not necessarily follow the black, blue and red text.

Guidelines

Coding guidelines have been incorporated into more specific section notes, code notes, icons, and the glossary. Section notes are listed under a range of codes and apply to all the codes in that range. Code notes are found under individual codes and apply to the single code.

Resequencing of CPT Codes

The American Medical Association (AMA) uses a numbering methodology of resequencing, which is the practice of displaying codes outside of their numerical order according to the description relationship. According to the AMA, there are instances in which a new code is needed within an existing grouping of codes but an unused code number is not available. In these situations, the AMA will resequence the codes. In other words, it will assign a code that is not in numeric sequence with the related codes. However, the code and description will appear in the CPT manual with the other related codes.

An example of resequencing from *Current Procedural Coding Expert* follows:

21555	Excision, tumor, soft tissue of neck or anterior thorax, subcutaneous; less than 3 cm
# 21552	3 cm or greater
21556	Excision, tumor, soft tissue of neck or anterior thorax, subfascial (eg, intramuscular); less than 5 cm
# 21554	5 cm or greater

Note that codes 21552 and 21554 are out of numeric sequence. However, as they are indented codes, they are in the correct place.

In *Current Procedural Coding Expert* the resequenced codes are listed twice. They appear in their resequenced position as shown above as well as in their original numeric position with a note indicating that the code is out of numerical sequence and where it can be found. (See example below.)

51797   Resequenced code. See code following 51729.

This differs from the AMA CPT book, in which the coder is directed to a code range that contains the resequenced code and description, rather than to a specific location.

Resequenced codes will appear in brackets in the headers, section notes, and code ranges. For example:

82286-82308 [82652] Chemistry: Bradykinin-Calcitonin
Code [82652] is included in section 82286-82308 Chemistry: Bradykinin-Calcitonin in its resequenced position.

Code also toxoid/vaccine (90476-90749 [90620, 90621, 90625, 90630, 90644, 90672, 90673])

This shows codes 90620, 90621, 90625, 90630, 90644, 90672, and 90673 are resequenced in this range of codes.

Appendix D identifies all resequenced CPT codes. Optum360 will display the resequenced coding as assigned by the AMA in its CPT products so that the user may understand the code description relationships.

Code Ranges for Medicare Billing

Each particular group of CPT codes in *Current Procedural Coding Expert* is organized in a more intuitive fashion for Medicare billing, being grouped by the Medicare rules and regulations as found in the official CMS online manuals, that govern payment of these particular procedures and services, as in this example:

99221-99233 Inpatient Hospital Visits: Initial and Subsequent

CMS: 100-4,11,40.1.3 Independent Attending Physician Services; 100-4,12,100.1.1 Teaching Physicians E/M Services; 100-4,12,30.6.10 Consultation Services; 100-4,12,30.6.15.1 Prolonged Services With Direct Face-to-Face Patient Contact; 100-4,12,30.6.4 Services Furnished Incident to Physician's Service; 100-4,12,30.6.9 Hospital Visit and Critical Care on Same Day

Icons

- **New Codes**
  Codes that have been added since the last edition of the book was printed.

△ **Revised Codes**
  Codes that have been revised since the last edition of the book was printed.

Resequenced Codes
  Codes that are out of numeric order but apply to the appropriate category.

○ **Reinstated Code**
  Codes that have been reinstated since the last edition of the book was printed.

Pink Color Bar—Not Covered by Medicare
Services and procedures identified by this color bar are never covered benefits under Medicare. Services and procedures that are not covered may be billed directly to the patient at the time of the service.

Yellow Color Bar—Unlisted Procedure
Unlisted CPT codes report procedures that have not been assigned a specific code number. An unlisted code delays payment due to the extra time necessary for review.

Green Color Bar—Resequenced Codes
Resequenced codes are codes that are out of numeric sequence—they are indicated with a green color bar. They are listed twice, in their resequenced position as well as in their original numeric position with a note that the code is out of numerical sequence and where the resequenced code and description can be found.

INCLUDES **Includes notes**
Includes notes identify procedures and services that would be bundled in the procedure code. These are derived from AMA, CMS, CCI, and Optum360 coding guidelines. This is not meant to be an all-inclusive list.

EXCLUDES **Excludes notes**
Excludes notes may lead the user to other codes. They may identify services that are not bundled and may be separately reported, OR may lead the user to another more appropriate code. These are derived from AMA, CMS, CCI, and Optum360 coding guidelines.

Code Also This note identifies an additional code that should be reported with the service and may relate to another CPT code or an appropriate HCPCS code(s) that should be reported along with the CPT code when appropriate.

Code First Found under add-on codes, this note identifies codes for primary procedures that should be reported first, with the add-on code reported as a secondary code.

Do Not Report Indicates when a service is not separately reportable.

⬛ **Laboratory/Pathology Crosswalk**
This icon denotes CPT codes in the laboratory and pathology section of CPT that may be reported separately with the primary CPT code.

⬛ **Radiology Crosswalk**
This icon denotes codes in the radiology section that may be used with the primary CPT code being reported.

TC **Technical Component Only**
Codes with this icon represent only the technical component (staff and equipment costs) of a procedure or service. Do not use either modifier 26 (physician component) or TC (technical component) with these codes.

26 **Professional Component**
Only codes with this icon represent the physician's work or professional component of a procedure or service. Do not use either modifier 26 (physician component) or TC (technical component) with these codes.

FUD **Follow up days**
Defines the number of days included in the global surgical package for the code, which includes all services usually provided by the surgeon before, during, and after a procedure.

50 **Bilateral Procedure**
This icon identifies codes that can be reported bilaterally when the same surgeon provides the service for the same patient on the same date. Medicare allows payment for both procedures at 150 percent of the usual amount for one procedure. The modifier does not apply to bilateral procedures inclusive to one code.

80 **Assist-at-Surgery Allowed**
Services noted by this icon are allowed an assistant at surgery with a Medicare payment equal to 16 percent of the allowed amount for the global surgery for that procedure. No documentation is required.

80 **Assist-at-Surgery Allowed with Documentation**
Services noted by this icon are allowed an assistant at surgery with a Medicare payment equal to 16 percent of the allowed amount for the global surgery for that procedure. Documentation is required.

+ **Add-on Codes**
This icon identifies procedures reported in addition to the primary procedure. The icon "+" denotes add-on codes. An add-on code is neither a stand-alone code nor subject to multiple procedure rules since it describes work in addition to the primary procedure.

According to Medicare guidelines, add-on codes may be identified in the following ways:

- The code is found on Change Request (CR) 7501 or successive CRs as a Type I, Type II, or Type III add-on code.
- The add-on code most often has a global period of "ZZZ" in the Medicare Physician Fee Schedule Database.
- The code is found in the CPT book with the icon "+" appended. Add-on code descriptors typically include the phrases "each additional" or "(List separately in addition to primary procedure)."

⊘ **Modifier 51 Exempt**
Codes identified by this icon indicate that the procedure should not be reported with modifier 51 (Multiple procedures). In the 2016 edition of *Current Procedural Coding Expert*, this icon was moved from a position to the left of the code to the list of applicable icons found with the Relative Value Units under the code descriptor.

(51) **Optum Modifier 51 Exempt**
Codes identified by this Optum icon indicate that the procedure should not be reported with modifier 51 (Multiple procedures). Any code with this icon is backed by official AMA guidelines but was not identified by the AMA with their modifier 51 exempt icon. In the 2016 edition of *Current Procedural Coding Expert*, this icon was moved from a position to the left of the code to the list of applicable icons found with the Relative Value Units under the code descriptor.

Correct Coding Initiative (CCI)
Current Procedural Coding Expert identifies those codes with corresponding CCI edits. The CCI edits define correct coding practices that serve as the basis of the national Medicare policy for paying claims. The code noted is the major service/procedure. The code may represent a column 1 code within the column 1/column 2 correct coding edits table or a code pair that is mutually exclusive of each other.

CLIA Waived Test
This symbol is used to distinguish those laboratory tests that can be performed using test systems that are waived from regulatory oversight established by the Clinical Laboratory Improvement Amendments of 1988 (CLIA). The applicable CPT code for a CLIA waived test may be reported by providers who perform the testing but do not hold a CLIA license.

(63) **Modifier 63 Exempt**
This icon identifies procedures performed on infants that weigh less than 4 kg. Due to the complexity of performing procedures on infants less than 4 kg, modifier 63 may be added to the surgery codes to inform the payers of the special circumstances involved.

A2–Z3 **ASC Payment Indicators**
This icon identifies ASC status payment indicators. They indicate how the ASC payment rate was derived and/or how the procedure, item, or service is treated under the revised ASC payment system. For more information about these indicators and how they affect billing, consult Optum's *Outpatient Billing Editor*.

- A2 Surgical procedure on ASC list in calendar year (CY) 2007; payment based on OPPS relative payment weight.
- B5 Alternative code may be available; no payment made
- D5 Deleted/discontinued code; no payment made.
- F4 Corneal tissue acquisition; hepatitis B vaccine; paid at reasonable cost.
- G2 Non-office-based surgical procedure added in CY 2008 or later; payment based on outpatient prospective payment system (OPPS) relative payment weight.
- H2 Brachytherapy source paid separately when provided integral to a surgical procedure on ASC list; payment based on OPPS rate.
- J7 OPPS pass-through device paid separately when provided integral to a surgical procedure on ASC list; payment contractor-priced.
- J8 Device-intensive procedure; paid at adjusted rate.
- K2 Drugs and biologicals paid separately when provided integral to a surgical procedure on ASC list; payment based on OPPS rate.
- K7 Unclassified drugs and biologicals; payment contractor-priced.
- L1 Influenza vaccine; pneumococcal vaccine. Packaged item/service; no separate payment made.
- L6 New technology intraocular lens (NTIOL); special payment.
- N1 Packaged service/item; no separate payment made.
- P2 Office-based surgical procedure added to ASC list in CY 2008 or later with Medicare physician fee schedule (MPFS) nonfacility practice expense (PE) RVUs; payment based on OPPS relative payment weight.
- P3 Office-based surgical procedure added to ASC list in CY 2008 or later with MPFS nonfacility PE RVUs; payment based on MPFS nonfacility PE RVUs.
- R2 Office-based surgical procedure added to ASC list in CY 2008 or later without MPFS nonfacility PE RVUs; payment based on OPPS relative payment weight.
- Z2 Radiology or diagnostic service paid separately when provided integral to a surgical procedure on ASC list; payment based on OPPS relative payment weight.
- Z3 Radiology or diagnostic service paid separately when provided integral to a surgical procedure on ASC list; payment based on MPFS nonfacility PE RVUs.

⊙ **Moderate Sedation**
This icon identifies procedures that include moderate sedation. Moderate sedation codes should not be reported separately with these procedures. In the 2016 edition of *Current Procedural Coding Expert*, this icon was moved from a position to the left of the code to the list of applicable icons found with the Relative Value Units under the code descriptor.

A **Age Edit**
This icon denotes codes intended for use with a specific age group, such as neonate, newborn, pediatric, and adult. This edit is based on CMS I/OCE designations or age specifications in the CPT code descriptors. Carefully review the code description to ensure the code you report most appropriately reflects the patient's age.

M   **Maternity**
This icon identifies procedures that by definition should be used only for maternity patients generally between 12 and 55 years of age.

♀   **Female Only**
This icon identifies procedures designated by CMS for females only based on CMS I/OCE designations.

♂   **Male Only**
This icon identifies procedures designated by CMS for males only based on CMS I/OCE designations.

Facility RVU
This icon precedes the facility RVU from CMS's 2015 physician fee schedule (PFS). It can be found under the code description.

New codes include no RVU information.

Nonfacility RVU
This icon precedes the nonfacility RVU from CMS's 2015 PFS. It can be found under the code description.

New codes include no RVU information.

FUD: Global days are sometimes referred to as "follow-up days" or FUDs. The global period is the time following surgery during which routine care by the physician is considered postoperative and included in the surgical fee. Office visits or other routine care related to the original surgery cannot be separately reported if provided during the global period. The statuses are:

000   No follow-up care included in this procedure

010   Normal postoperative care is included in this procedure for ten days

090   Normal postoperative care is included in the procedure for 90 days

MMM   Maternity codes; usual global period does not apply

XXX   The global concept does not apply to the code

YYY   The carrier is to determine whether the global concept applies and establishes postoperative period, if appropriate, at time of pricing

ZZZ   The code is related to another service and is always included in the global period of the other service

CMS: This notation indicates that there is a specific CMS guideline pertaining to this code in the CMS Online Manual System which includes the internet-only manual (IOM) *National Coverage Determinations Manual* (NCD). These CMS sources present the rules for submitting these services to the federal government or its contractors and are included in appendix F of this book.

AMA: This indicates discussion of the code in the American Medical Association's *CPT Assistant* newsletter. Use the citation to find the correct issue. This includes citations for the current year and the preceding six years. In the event no citations can be found during this time period, the most recent citations that can be found are used.

Drug Not Approved by FDA
The AMA CPT Editorial Panel is publishing new vaccine product codes prior to Food and Drug Administration approval. This symbol indicates which of these codes are pending FDA approval at press time.

Physician Quality Reporting System (PQRS)
This icon denotes CPT codes that specifically address one or more of the CMS-determined quality measures. See appendix K for a list of denominators that apply to those codes.

OPPS Status Indicators (OPSI)
Status indicators identify how individual CPT codes are paid or not paid under the latest available hospital outpatient prospective payment system (OPPS). The same status indicator is assigned to all the codes within an ambulatory payment classification (APC). Consult your payer or other resource to learn which CPT codes fall within various APCs.

A   Services furnished to a hospital outpatient that are paid under a fee schedule or payment system other than OPPS

B   Codes that are not recognized by OPPS when submitted on an outpatient hospital Part B bill type (12x and 13x).

C   Inpatient procedures

D   Discontinued codes

E   Items, codes, and services:
- For which pricing information is not available
- Not covered by any Medicare outpatient benefit category
- Statutorily excluded by Medicare
- Not reasonable and necessary

F   Corneal tissue acquisition; certain CRNA services and hepatitis B vaccines

G   Pass-through drugs and biologicals

H   Pass-through device categories

J1   Hospital Part B services paid through a comprehensive APC

J2   Hospital Part B services that may be paid through a comprehensive APC

K   Nonpass-through drugs and nonimplantable biologicals, including therapeutic radiopharmaceuticals

L   Influenza vaccine; pneumococcal pneumonia vaccine

M   Items and services not billable to the MAC

N   Items and services packaged into APC rates

P   Partial hospitalization

Q1   STV-packaged codes

Q2   T-packaged codes

Q3   Codes that may be paid through a composite APC

Q4   Conditionally packaged laboratory tests

R   Blood and blood products

S   Procedure or service, not discounted when multiple

T   Procedure or service, multiple procedure reduction applies

U   Brachytherapy sources

V   Clinic or emergency department visit

Y   Nonimplantable durable medical equipment

Appendixes

Appendix A: Modifiers—This appendix identifies modifiers. A modifier is a two-position alpha or numeric code that is appended to a CPT or HCPCS code to clarify the services being billed. Modifiers provide a means by which a service can be altered without changing the procedure code. They add more information, such as anatomical site, to the code. In addition, they help eliminate the appearance of duplicate billing and unbundling. Modifiers are used to increase the accuracy in reimbursement and coding consistency, ease editing, and capture payment data.

Appendix B: New, Changed, and Deleted Codes—This is a list of new, changed, and deleted CPT codes for the current year.

Appendix C: Crosswalk of Deleted Codes—This appendix is a cross-reference from a deleted CPT code to an active code when one is available. The deleted code cross-reference will also appear under the deleted code description in the tabular section of the book.

Appendix D: Resequenced Codes—This appendix contains a list of codes that are not in numeric order in the book. AMA resequenced some of the code numbers to relocate codes in the same category but not in numeric sequence.

Appendix E: Add-on, Modifier 51 Exempt, Optum Modifier 51 Exempt, Modifier 63 Exempt, and Moderate Sedation Codes—This list includes add-on codes that cannot be reported alone, codes that are exempt from modifier 51, codes that should not be reported with modifier 63, and codes that include moderate sedation.

Appendix F: Pub. 100 References—This appendix contains a verbatim printout of the Medicare Internet Only Manual references that pertain to specific codes. The reference, when available, is listed after the header in the CPT section. For example:

93784-93790 Ambulatory Blood Pressure Monitoring

CMS: 100-3,20.19 Ambulatory Blood Pressure Monitoring (20.19); 100-4,32,10.1 Ambulatory Blood Pressure Monitoring Billing Requirements

Since appendix F contains these references from the *Medicare National Coverage Determinations (NCD) Manual*, Pub 100-3, chapter 20, section 20.19, and the *Medicare Claims Processing Manual*, Pub 100-4, chapter 32, section 10.1, there is no need to search the Medicare website for the applicable reference.

Appendix G: Physician Quality Reporting System (PQRS)—Lists the numerators and denominators applicable to Medicare PQRS. Appendix G contains the most recent information available at press time. Due to the large volume of information for some measures, space constraints do not allow for all codes to be listed in the printed copy of the *Current Procedural Coding Expert*. However, the full list of numerators and denominators associated with each individual measure can be found at www.OptumCoding.com/Product/Updates/PQRS16. It is anticipated this information will be available online effective February 2016.

Appendix H: Medically Unlikely Edits—This appendix contains the published medically unlikely edits (MUEs). These edits establish maximum daily allowable units of service. The edits will be applied to the services provided to the same patient, for the same CPT code, on the same date of service when billed by the same provider. Included are the physician and facility edits.

Appendix I: Inpatient-Only Procedures—This appendix identifies services with the status indicator "C." Medicare will not pay an OPPS hospital or ASC when these procedures are performed on a Medicare patient as an outpatient. Physicians should refer to this list when scheduling Medicare patients for surgical procedures. CMS updates this list quarterly.

Appendix J: Place of Service and Type of Service—This appendix contains lists of place-of-service codes that should be used on professional claims and type-of-service codes used by the Medicare Common Working File.

Appendix K: Multianalyte Assays with Algorithmic Analyses—This appendix lists the administrative codes for multianalyte assays with algorithmic analyses. The AMA updates this list three times a year.

Appendix L: Glossary—This appendix contains general terms and definitions as well as those that would apply to or be helpful for billing and reimbursement.

Appendix M: Listing of Sensory, Motor, and Mixed Nerves—This appendix lists a summary of each sensory, motor, and mixed nerve with its appropriate nerve conduction study code.

Appendix N: Vascular Families—Appendix J contains a table of vascular families starting with the aorta. Additional information can be found in the interventional radiology illustrations located behind the index.

For more information about ongoing development of the CPT coding system, consult the AMA website at URL http://www.ama-assn.org/.

Appendix O: Interventional Radiology Illustrations—This appendix contains illustrations specific to interventional radiology procedures.

Note: All data current as of November 8, 2015.

Anatomical Illustrations

Body Planes and Movements

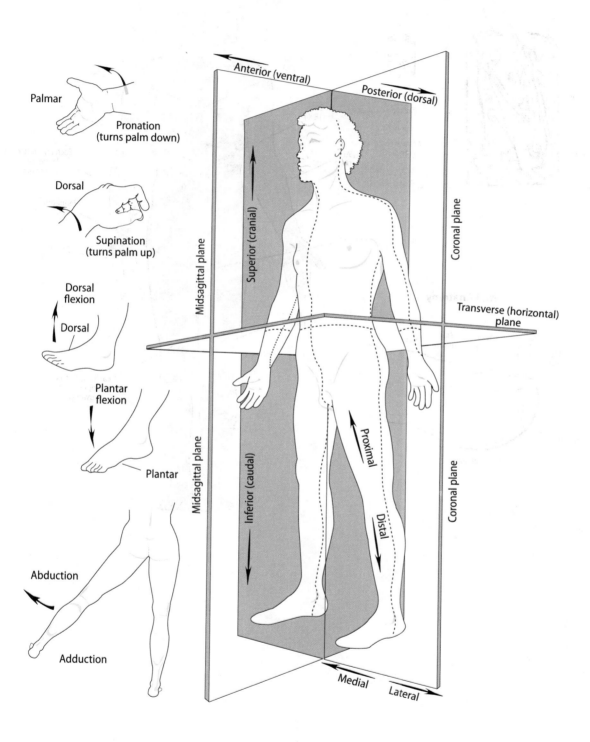

Integumentary System

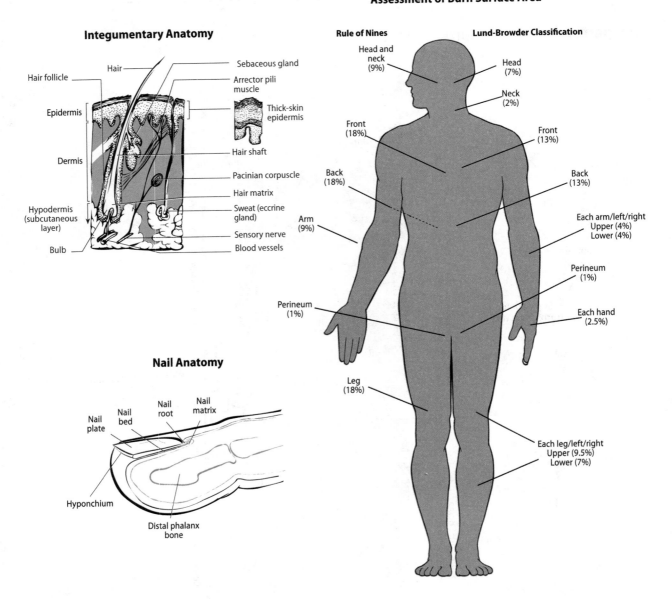

Integumentary Anatomy

- Hair follicle
- Hair
- Sebaceous gland
- Arrector pili muscle
- Epidermis
- Thick-skin epidermis
- Hair shaft
- Dermis
- Pacinian corpuscle
- Hair matrix
- Sweat (eccrine gland)
- Hypodermis (subcutaneous layer)
- Sensory nerve
- Bulb
- Blood vessels

Nail Anatomy

- Nail plate
- Nail bed
- Nail root
- Nail matrix
- Hyponchium
- Distal phalanx bone

Assessment of Burn Surface Area

Rule of Nines

- Head and neck (9%)
- Front (18%)
- Back (18%)
- Arm (9%)
- Perineum (1%)
- Leg (18%)

Lund-Browder Classification

- Head (7%)
- Neck (2%)
- Front (13%)
- Back (13%)
- Each arm/left/right Upper (4%) Lower (4%)
- Perineum (1%)
- Each hand (2.5%)
- Each leg/left/right Upper (9.5%) Lower (7%)

Musculoskeletal System

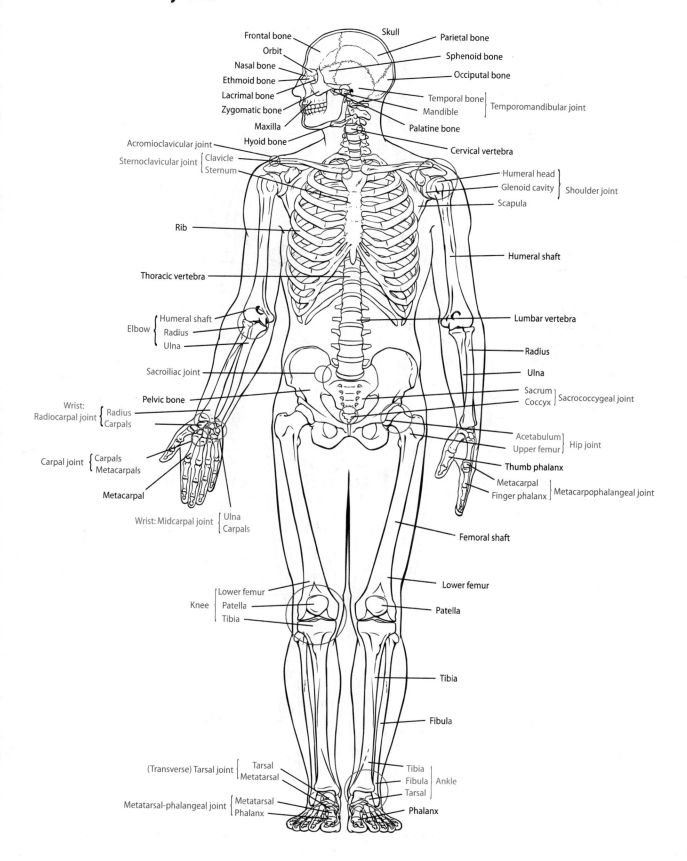

Musculoskeletal System

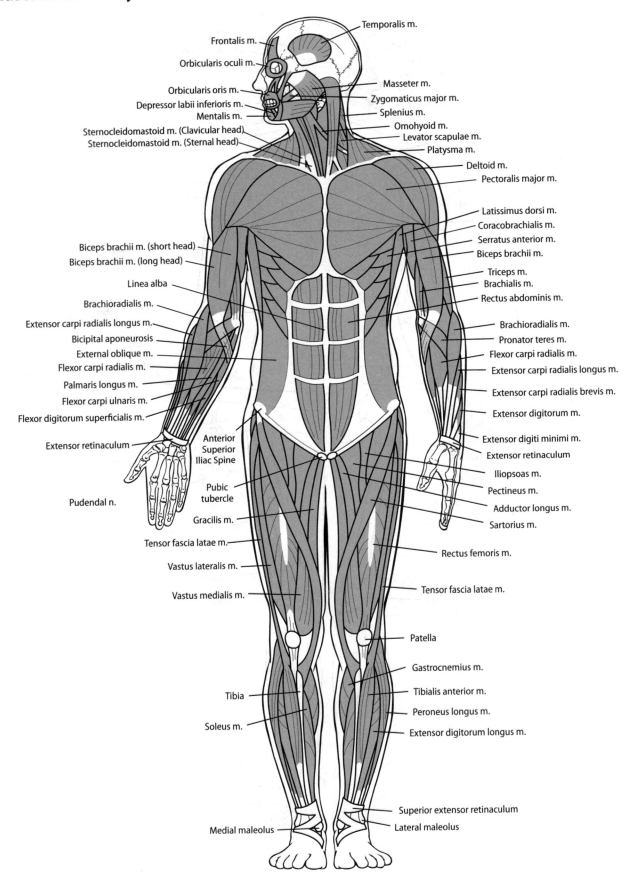

Musculoskeletal System

Shoulder (Anterior View)

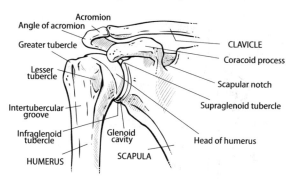

- Angle of acromion
- Acromion
- Greater tubercle
- Lesser tubercle
- Intertubercular groove
- Infraglenoid tubercle
- HUMERUS
- CLAVICLE
- Coracoid process
- Scapular notch
- Supraglenoid tubercle
- Glenoid cavity
- Head of humerus
- SCAPULA

Shoulder (Posterior View)

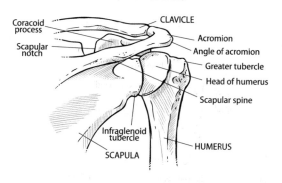

- Coracoid process
- Scapular notch
- CLAVICLE
- Acromion
- Angle of acromion
- Greater tubercle
- Head of humerus
- Scapular spine
- Infraglenoid tubercle
- SCAPULA
- HUMERUS

Skull

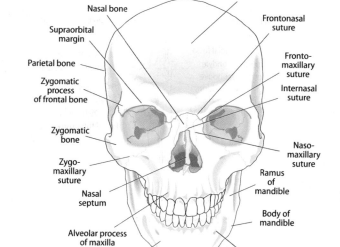

- Nasal bone
- Supraorbital margin
- Parietal bone
- Zygomatic process of frontal bone
- Zygomatic bone
- Zygo-maxillary suture
- Nasal septum
- Alveolar process of maxilla
- Mandible
- Frontal bone
- Frontonasal suture
- Fronto-maxillary suture
- Internasal suture
- Naso-maxillary suture
- Ramus of mandible
- Body of mandible
- Mental foramen

Upper Arm Muscles

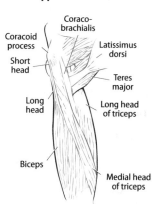

- Coracoid process
- Short head
- Long head
- Biceps
- Coraco-brachialis
- Latissimus dorsi
- Teres major
- Long head of triceps
- Medial head of triceps

Shoulder Muscles

Section of left shoulder (anterior view)

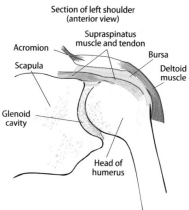

- Acromion
- Scapula
- Glenoid cavity
- Supraspinatus muscle and tendon
- Bursa
- Deltoid muscle
- Head of humerus

Posterior view

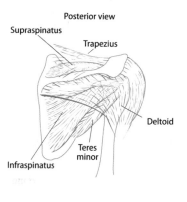

- Supraspinatus
- Infraspinatus
- Trapezius
- Teres minor
- Deltoid

Musculoskeletal System

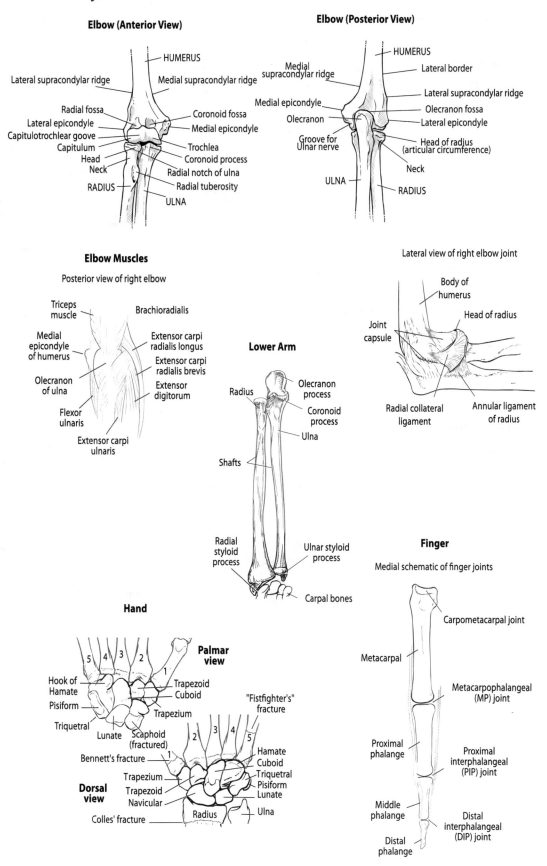

Elbow (Anterior View)

HUMERUS
Lateral supracondylar ridge
Medial supracondylar ridge
Radial fossa
Coronoid fossa
Lateral epicondyle
Capitulotrochlear goove
Medial epicondyle
Capitulum
Trochlea
Head
Coronoid process
Neck
Radial notch of ulna
RADIUS
Radial tuberosity
ULNA

Elbow (Posterior View)

HUMERUS
Medial supracondylar ridge
Lateral border
Lateral supracondylar ridge
Medial epicondyle
Olecranon fossa
Olecranon
Lateral epicondyle
Groove for Ulnar nerve
Head of radius (articular circumference)
Neck
ULNA
RADIUS

Elbow Muscles

Posterior view of right elbow

Triceps muscle
Brachioradialis
Medial epicondyle of humerus
Extensor carpi radialis longus
Olecranon of ulna
Extensor carpi radialis brevis
Extensor digitorum
Flexor ulnaris
Extensor carpi ulnaris

Lateral view of right elbow joint

Body of humerus
Head of radius
Joint capsule
Radial collateral ligament
Annular ligament of radius

Lower Arm

Radius
Olecranon process
Coronoid process
Ulna
Shafts
Radial styloid process
Ulnar styloid process
Carpal bones

Finger

Medial schematic of finger joints

Carpometacarpal joint
Metacarpal
Metacarpophalangeal (MP) joint
Proximal phalange
Proximal interphalangeal (PIP) joint
Middle phalange
Distal interphalangeal (DIP) joint
Distal phalange

Hand

Palmar view
5 4 3 2 1
Hook of Hamate
Trapezoid
Cuboid
Pisiform
Trapezium
Triquetral
Lunate
Scaphoid (fractured)
Bennett's fracture
"Fistfighter's" fracture
2 3 4 5
1
Hamate
Cuboid
Trapezium
Triquetral
Trapezoid
Pisiform
Navicular
Lunate
Dorsal view
Colles' fracture
Radius
Ulna

Musculoskeletal System

Hip (Anterior View)

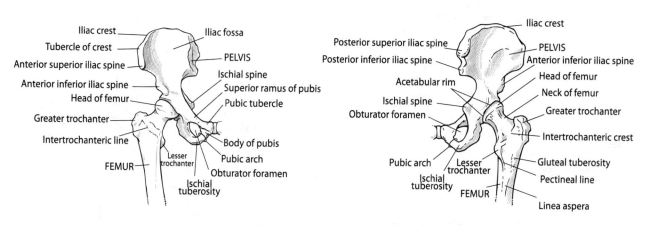

Iliac crest
Tubercle of crest
Anterior superior iliac spine
Anterior inferior iliac spine
Head of femur
Greater trochanter
Intertrochanteric line
FEMUR
Lesser trochanter
Iliac fossa
PELVIS
Ischial spine
Superior ramus of pubis
Pubic tubercle
Body of pubis
Pubic arch
Obturator foramen
Ischial tuberosity

Hip (Posterior View)

Posterior superior iliac spine
Posterior inferior iliac spine
Acetabular rim
Ischial spine
Obturator foramen
Pubic arch
Ischial tuberosity
Lesser trochanter
FEMUR
Iliac crest
PELVIS
Anterior inferior iliac spine
Head of femur
Neck of femur
Greater trochanter
Intertrochanteric crest
Gluteal tuberosity
Pectineal line
Linea aspera

Knee (Anterior View)

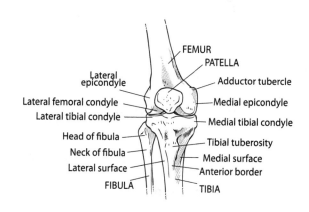

Lateral epicondyle
Lateral femoral condyle
Lateral tibial condyle
Head of fibula
Neck of fibula
Lateral surface
FIBULA
FEMUR
PATELLA
Adductor tubercle
Medial epicondyle
Medial tibial condyle
Tibial tuberosity
Medial surface
Anterior border
TIBIA

Knee (Posterior View)

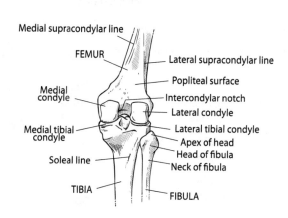

Medial supracondylar line
FEMUR
Medial condyle
Medial tibial condyle
Soleal line
TIBIA
Lateral supracondylar line
Popliteal surface
Intercondylar notch
Lateral condyle
Lateral tibial condyle
Apex of head
Head of fibula
Neck of fibula
FIBULA

Lower Leg

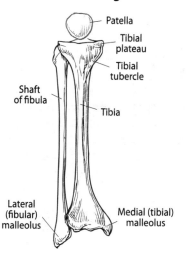

Patella
Tibial plateau
Tibial tubercle
Shaft of fibula
Tibia
Lateral (fibular) malleolus
Medial (tibial) malleolus

Knee

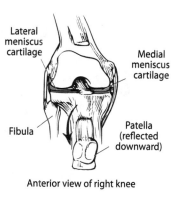

Lateral meniscus cartilage
Medial meniscus cartilage
Fibula
Patella (reflected downward)

Anterior view of right knee

Musculoskeletal System

Ankle

Lateral and posterior views of right ankle

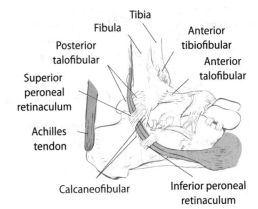

Tibia

Fibula

Posterior talofibular

Anterior tibiofibular

Superior peroneal retinaculum

Anterior talofibular

Achilles tendon

Calcaneofibular

Inferior peroneal retinaculum

Achilles tendon not shown

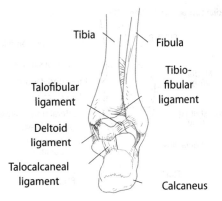

Tibia

Fibula

Talofibular ligament

Tibio-fibular ligament

Deltoid ligament

Talocalcaneal ligament

Calcaneus

Foot

Select extensors of the foot

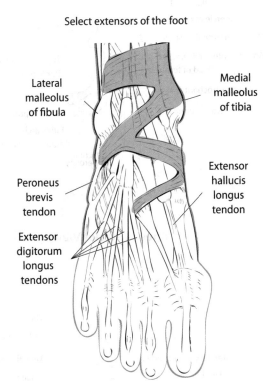

Lateral malleolus of fibula

Medial malleolus of tibia

Peroneus brevis tendon

Extensor hallucis longus tendon

Extensor digitorum longus tendons

Right Foot

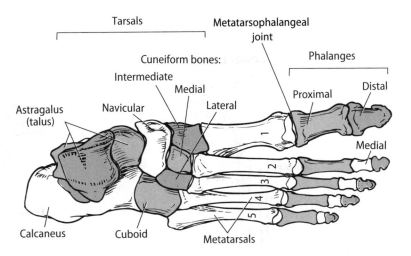

Tarsals

Metatarsophalangeal joint

Cuneiform bones:

Phalanges

Intermediate

Medial

Proximal

Distal

Astragalus (talus)

Navicular

Lateral

Medial

Calcaneus

Cuboid

Metatarsals

Respiratory System

Nose

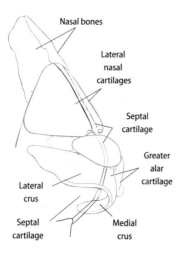

Nasal bones
Lateral nasal cartilages
Septal cartilage
Greater alar cartilage
Lateral crus
Septal cartilage
Medial crus

Pharynx

Nasal cavity
Auditory tube
Nasopharynx region
Epiglottis
Oropharynx region
Larynx
Trachea
Hypopharynx region
Vocal cord

Respiratory

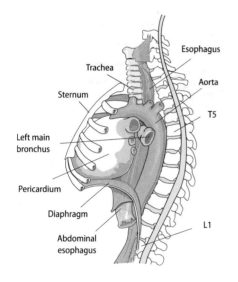

Esophagus
Trachea
Aorta
Sternum
T5
Left main bronchus
Pericardium
Diaphragm
L1
Abdominal esophagus

Bronchi

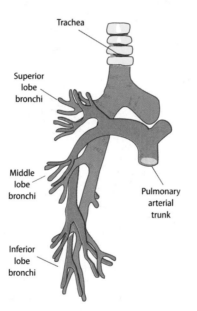

Trachea
Superior lobe bronchi
Middle lobe bronchi
Pulmonary arterial trunk
Inferior lobe bronchi

Nasal Turbinates

Mid frontal cutaway view

Ethmoid air cells (sinus)
Superior turbinate
Middle turbinate
Inferior turbinate
Eye orbit
Maxillary sinus

Paranasal Sinuses

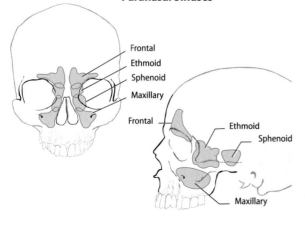

Frontal
Ethmoid
Sphenoid
Maxillary
Frontal
Ethmoid
Sphenoid
Maxillary

Lungs

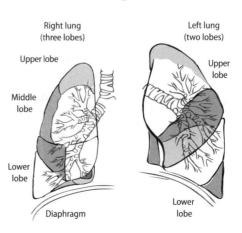

Right lung (three lobes)
Upper lobe
Middle lobe
Lower lobe
Diaphragm
Left lung (two lobes)
Upper lobe
Lower lobe

Arterial System

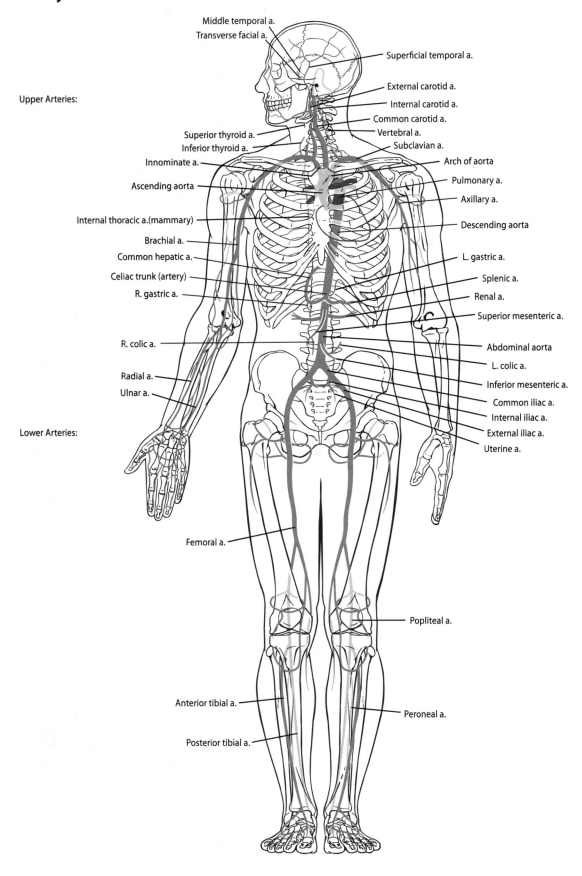

Arterial System

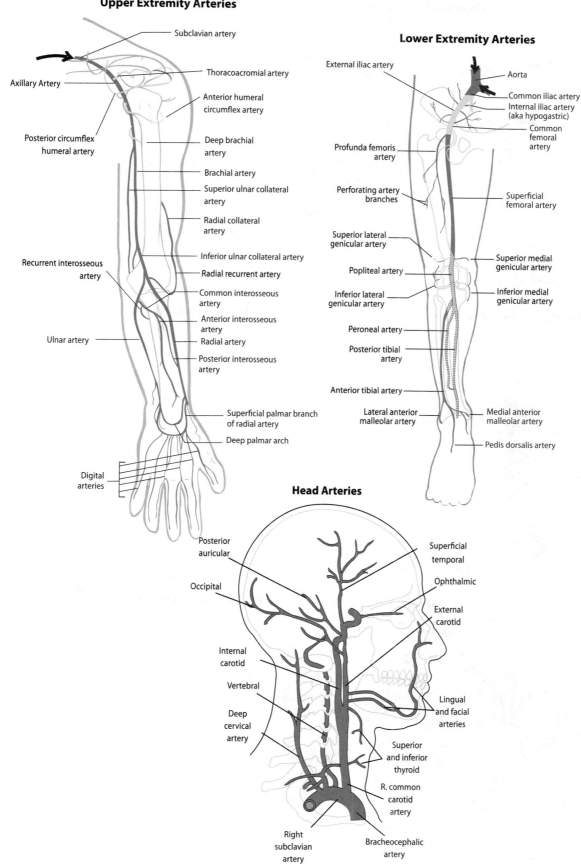

Upper Extremity Arteries

- Subclavian artery
- Thoracoacromial artery
- Axillary Artery
- Anterior humeral circumflex artery
- Deep brachial artery
- Posterior circumflex humeral artery
- Brachial artery
- Superior ulnar collateral artery
- Radial collateral artery
- Inferior ulnar collateral artery
- Recurrent interosseous artery
- Radial recurrent artery
- Common interosseous artery
- Anterior interosseous artery
- Ulnar artery
- Radial artery
- Posterior interosseous artery
- Superficial palmar branch of radial artery
- Deep palmar arch
- Digital arteries

Lower Extremity Arteries

- External iliac artery
- Aorta
- Common iliac artery
- Internal iliac artery (aka hypogastric)
- Common femoral artery
- Profunda femoris artery
- Superficial femoral artery
- Perforating artery branches
- Superior lateral genicular artery
- Superior medial genicular artery
- Popliteal artery
- Inferior lateral genicular artery
- Inferior medial genicular artery
- Peroneal artery
- Posterior tibial artery
- Anterior tibial artery
- Lateral anterior malleolar artery
- Medial anterior malleolar artery
- Pedis dorsalis artery

Head Arteries

- Posterior auricular
- Superficial temporal
- Occipital
- Ophthalmic
- External carotid
- Internal carotid
- Vertebral
- Lingual and facial arteries
- Deep cervical artery
- Superior and inferior thyroid
- R. common carotid artery
- Right subclavian artery
- Bracheocephalic artery

Arterial System

Cerebrovascular Arteries

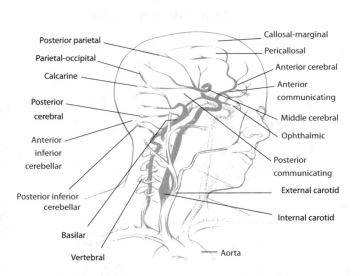

Posterior parietal
Parietal-occipital
Calcarine
Posterior cerebral
Anterior inferior cerebellar
Posterior inferior cerebellar
Basilar
Vertebral

Callosal-marginal
Pericallosal
Anterior cerebral
Anterior communicating
Middle cerebral
Ophthalmic
Posterior communicating
External carotid
Internal carotid
Aorta

Capillary Bed

Schematic of a capillary bed containing arterioles, the smallest type of artery

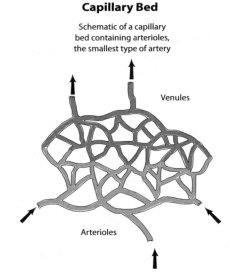

Venules

Arterioles

Branches of Abdominal Aorta

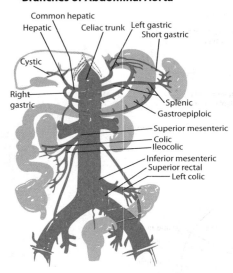

Common hepatic
Hepatic
Celiac trunk
Left gastric
Short gastric
Cystic
Right gastric
Splenic
Gastroepiploic
Superior mesenteric
Colic
Ileocolic
Inferior mesenteric
Superior rectal
Left colic

Arteries of Heart

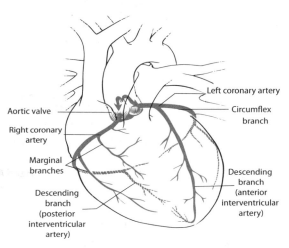

Aortic valve
Right coronary artery
Marginal branches
Descending branch (posterior interventricular artery)
Left coronary artery
Circumflex branch
Descending branch (anterior interventricular artery)

Heart Valves

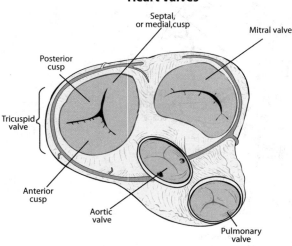

Septal, or medial, cusp
Posterior cusp
Tricuspid valve
Anterior cusp
Aortic valve
Mitral valve
Pulmonary valve

Cardiac Arterial Blood Flow

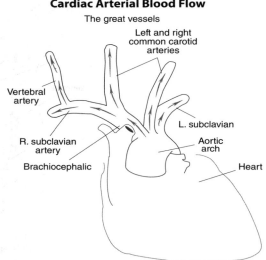

The great vessels
Left and right common carotid arteries
Vertebral artery
R. subclavian artery
Brachiocephalic
L. subclavian
Aortic arch
Heart

Venous System

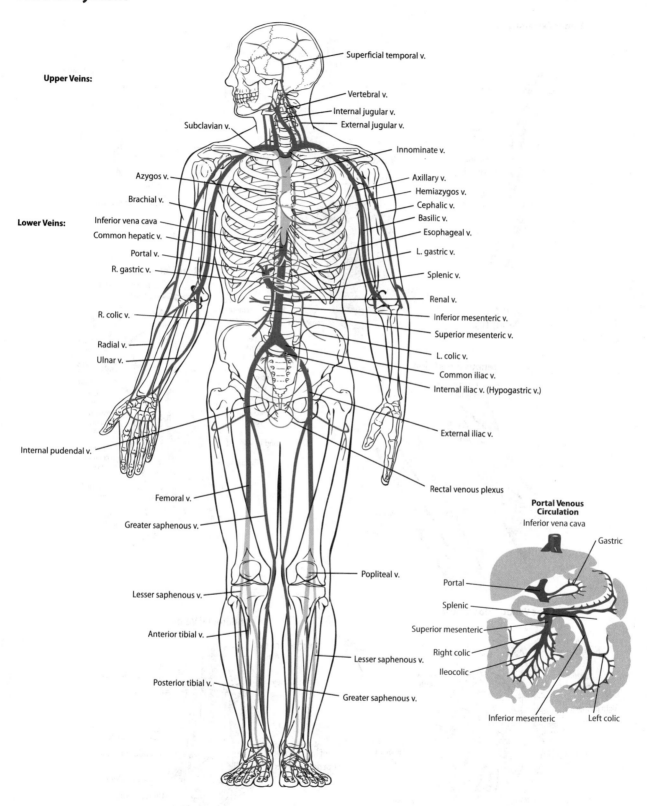

Upper Veins:

Superficial temporal v.

Vertebral v.

Internal jugular v.

External jugular v.

Subclavian v.

Innominate v.

Azygos v.

Axillary v.

Hemiazygos v.

Brachial v.

Cephalic v.

Basilic v.

Lower Veins:

Inferior vena cava

Esophageal v.

Common hepatic v.

L. gastric v.

Portal v.

R. gastric v.

Splenic v.

Renal v.

R. colic v.

Inferior mesenteric v.

Superior mesenteric v.

Radial v.

L. colic v.

Ulnar v.

Common iliac v.

Internal iliac v. (Hypogastric v.)

External iliac v.

Internal pudendal v.

Rectal venous plexus

Femoral v.

Greater saphenous v.

**Portal Venous
Circulation**

Inferior vena cava

Gastric

Portal

Popliteal v.

Splenic

Lesser saphenous v.

Superior mesenteric

Right colic

Anterior tibial v.

Ileocolic

Lesser saphenous v.

Posterior tibial v.

Greater saphenous v.

Inferior mesenteric

Left colic

Venous System

Upper Extremity Veins

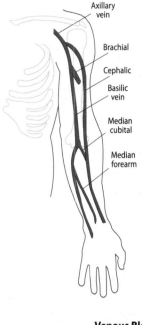

- Axillary vein
- Brachial
- Cephalic
- Basilic vein
- Median cubital
- Median forearm

Venae Comitantes

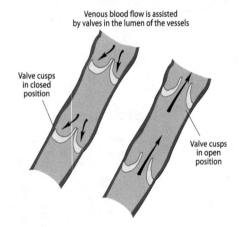

- Artery
- Venae comitantes

Heart Veins

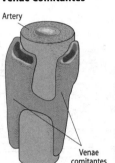

- Superior vena cava vein
- Anterior cardiac veins
- Coronary sinus
- Great cardiac vein
- Small cardiac vein
- Middle cardiac vein

Venous Blood Flow

Venous blood flow is assisted by valves in the lumen of the vessels

- Valve cusps in closed position
- Valve cusps in open position

Head Veins

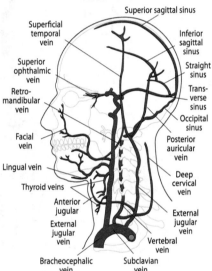

- Superior sagittal sinus
- Superficial temporal vein
- Inferior sagittal sinus
- Superior ophthalmic vein
- Straight sinus
- Retro-mandibular vein
- Transverse sinus
- Occipital sinus
- Facial vein
- Posterior auricular vein
- Lingual vein
- Deep cervical vein
- Thyroid veins
- Anterior jugular
- External jugular vein
- External jugular vein
- Vertebral vein
- Bracheocephalic vein
- Subclavian vein

Cardiac Venous Blood Flow

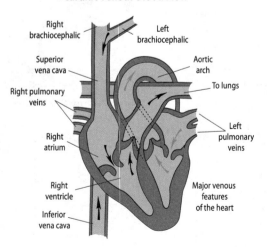

- Right brachiocephalic
- Left brachiocephalic
- Superior vena cava
- Aortic arch
- Right pulmonary veins
- To lungs
- Right atrium
- Left pulmonary veins
- Right ventricle
- Inferior vena cava
- Major venous features of the heart

Abdominal Veins

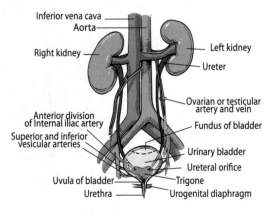

- Inferior vena cava
- Aorta
- Right kidney
- Left kidney
- Ureter
- Ovarian or testicular artery and vein
- Anterior division of internal iliac artery
- Fundus of bladder
- Superior and inferior vesicular arteries
- Urinary bladder
- Ureteral orifice
- Uvula of bladder
- Trigone
- Urethra
- Urogenital diaphragm

Lymphatic System

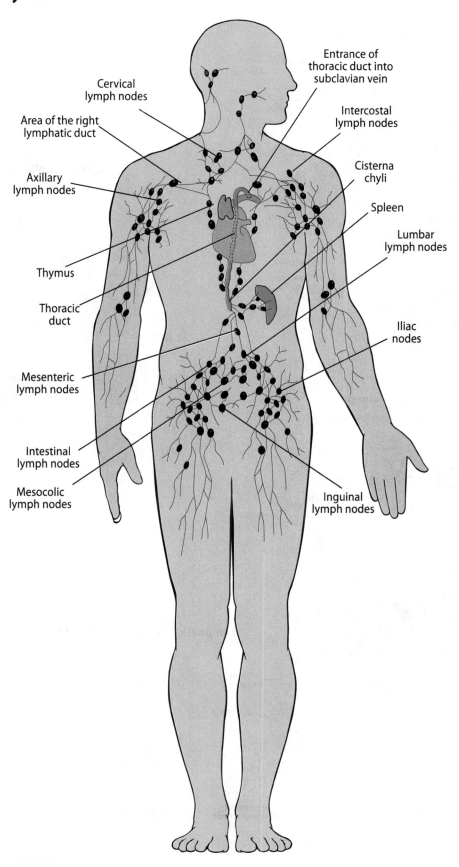

Cervical lymph nodes

Area of the right lymphatic duct

Axillary lymph nodes

Thymus

Thoracic duct

Mesenteric lymph nodes

Intestinal lymph nodes

Mesocolic lymph nodes

Entrance of thoracic duct into subclavian vein

Intercostal lymph nodes

Cisterna chyli

Spleen

Lumbar lymph nodes

Iliac nodes

Inguinal lymph nodes

Anatomical Illustrations

Lymphatic System

Axillary Lymph Nodes

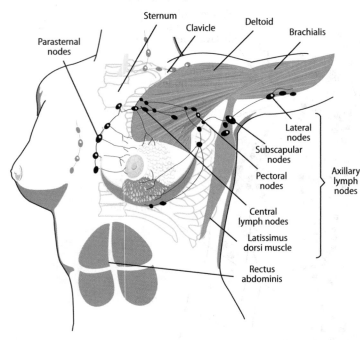

Parasternal nodes
Sternum
Clavicle
Deltoid
Brachialis
Lateral nodes
Subscapular nodes
Pectoral nodes
Axillary lymph nodes
Central lymph nodes
Latissimus dorsi muscle
Rectus abdominis

Lymphatic Capillaries

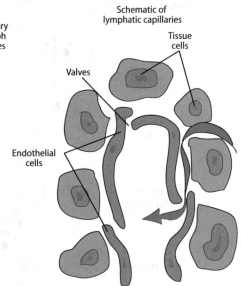

Schematic of lymphatic capillaries

Tissue cells
Valves
Endothelial cells

Fluids and particles can enter the capillary through overlapping valves

Lymphatic Drainage

Lymphatic drainage of the colon follows blood supply

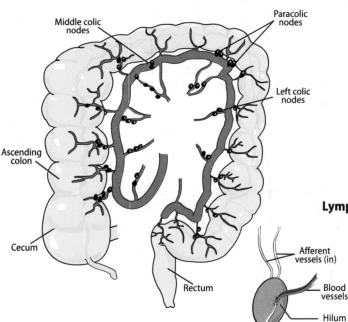

Middle colic nodes
Paracolic nodes
Left colic nodes
Ascending colon
Cecum
Rectum

Afferent vessels (in)
Blood vessels
Hilum
Efferent vessel (out)

Schematic of lymph node

Lymphatic System of Head and Neck

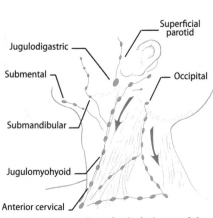

Superficial parotid
Jugulodigastric
Submental
Occipital
Submandibular
Jugulomyohyoid
Anterior cervical

Lymphatic drainage of the head, neck, and face

Digestive System

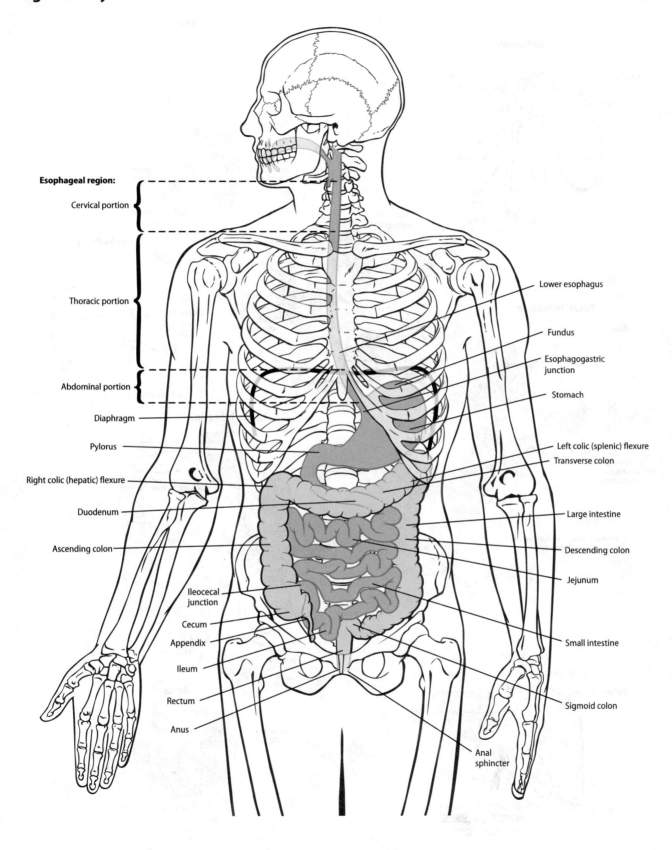

Esophageal region:

Cervical portion

Thoracic portion

Abdominal portion

Diaphragm

Pylorus

Right colic (hepatic) flexure

Duodenum

Ascending colon

Ileocecal junction

Cecum

Appendix

Ileum

Rectum

Anus

Lower esophagus

Fundus

Esophagogastric junction

Stomach

Left colic (splenic) flexure

Transverse colon

Large intestine

Descending colon

Jejunum

Small intestine

Sigmoid colon

Anal sphincter

Digestive System

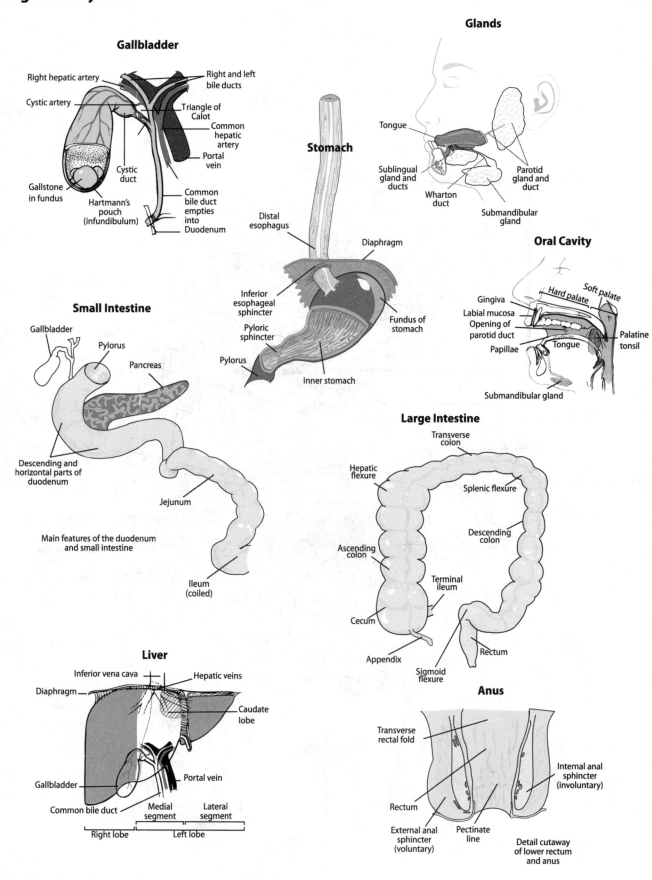

Gallbladder

Right hepatic artery
Cystic artery
Gallstone in fundus
Hartmann's pouch (infundibulum)
Right and left bile ducts
Triangle of Calot
Common hepatic artery
Portal vein
Cystic duct
Common bile duct empties into Duodenum

Glands

Tongue
Sublingual gland and ducts
Wharton duct
Submandibular gland
Parotid gland and duct

Stomach

Distal esophagus
Inferior esophageal sphincter
Pyloric sphincter
Pylorus
Diaphragm
Fundus of stomach
Inner stomach

Oral Cavity

Gingiva
Labial mucosa
Opening of parotid duct
Papillae
Hard palate
Soft palate
Tongue
Palatine tonsil
Submandibular gland

Small Intestine

Gallbladder
Pylorus
Pancreas
Descending and horizontal parts of duodenum
Jejunum
Main features of the duodenum and small intestine
Ileum (coiled)

Large Intestine

Transverse colon
Hepatic flexure
Splenic flexure
Ascending colon
Descending colon
Cecum
Terminal ileum
Appendix
Sigmoid flexure
Rectum

Liver

Inferior vena cava
Diaphragm
Hepatic veins
Caudate lobe
Gallbladder
Portal vein
Common bile duct
Medial segment
Lateral segment
Right lobe
Left lobe

Anus

Transverse rectal fold
Rectum
External anal sphincter (voluntary)
Pectinate line
Internal anal sphincter (involuntary)
Detail cutaway of lower rectum and anus

Genitourinary System

Kidney

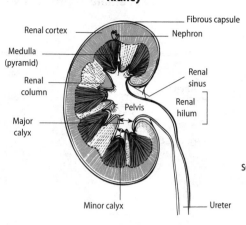

- Fibrous capsule
- Renal cortex
- Nephron
- Medulla (pyramid)
- Renal column
- Renal sinus
- Pelvis
- Renal hilum
- Major calyx
- Minor calyx
- Ureter

Urinary System

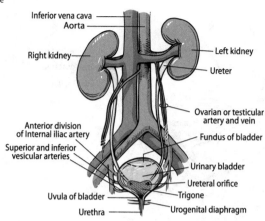

- Inferior vena cava
- Aorta
- Right kidney
- Left kidney
- Ureter
- Ovarian or testicular artery and vein
- Anterior division of Internal iliac artery
- Fundus of bladder
- Superior and inferior vesicular arteries
- Urinary bladder
- Ureteral orifice
- Uvula of bladder
- Trigone
- Urethra
- Urogenital diaphragm

Nephron

Schematic of nephron, the tiny filtering mechanism of the kidney

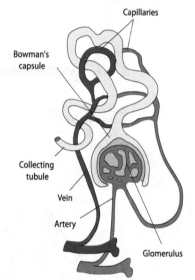

- Capillaries
- Bowman's capsule
- Collecting tubule
- Vein
- Artery
- Glomerulus

Male Genitourinary

Posterior view of male bladder and prostate

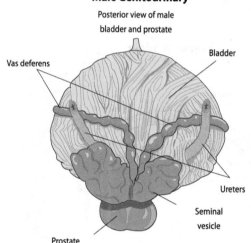

- Vas deferens
- Bladder
- Ureters
- Seminal vesicle
- Prostate

Urinary

Posterior view showing location of kidneys and ureters

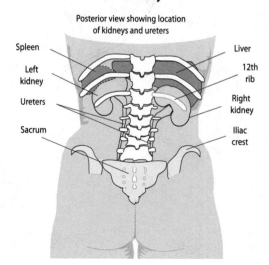

- Spleen
- Liver
- Left kidney
- 12th rib
- Ureters
- Right kidney
- Sacrum
- Iliac crest

Male Genitourinary System

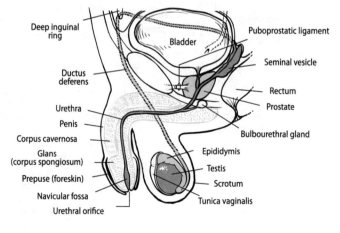

- Deep inguinal ring
- Bladder
- Puboprostatic ligament
- Ductus deferens
- Seminal vesicle
- Urethra
- Rectum
- Penis
- Prostate
- Corpus cavernosa
- Glans (corpus spongiosum)
- Bulbourethral gland
- Prepuse (foreskin)
- Epididymis
- Navicular fossa
- Testis
- Urethral orifice
- Scrotum
- Tunica vaginalis

Genitourinary System

Female Genitourinary

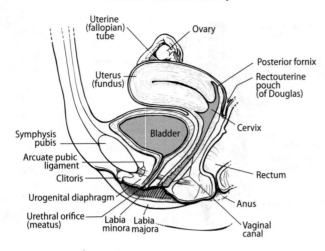

- Uterine (fallopian) tube
- Ovary
- Uterus (fundus)
- Posterior fornix
- Rectouterine pouch (of Douglas)
- Cervix
- Symphysis pubis
- Bladder
- Arcuate pubic ligament
- Clitoris
- Rectum
- Urogenital diaphragm
- Anus
- Urethral orifice (meatus)
- Labia minora
- Labia majora
- Vaginal canal

Female Reproductive

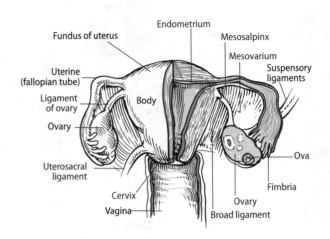

- Fundus of uterus
- Endometrium
- Mesosalpinx
- Mesovarium
- Suspensory ligaments
- Uterine (fallopian tube)
- Body
- Ligament of ovary
- Ovary
- Ova
- Uterosacral ligament
- Fimbria
- Cervix
- Ovary
- Vagina
- Broad ligament

Female Bladder

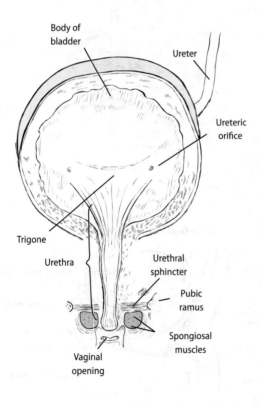

- Body of bladder
- Ureter
- Ureteric orifice
- Trigone
- Urethra
- Urethral sphincter
- Pubic ramus
- Spongiosal muscles
- Vaginal opening

Female Reproductive

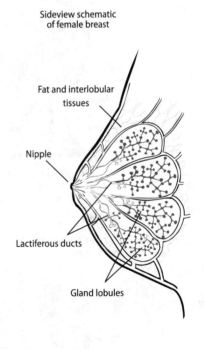

- Sideview schematic of female breast
- Fat and interlobular tissues
- Nipple
- Lactiferous ducts
- Gland lobules

Endocrine System

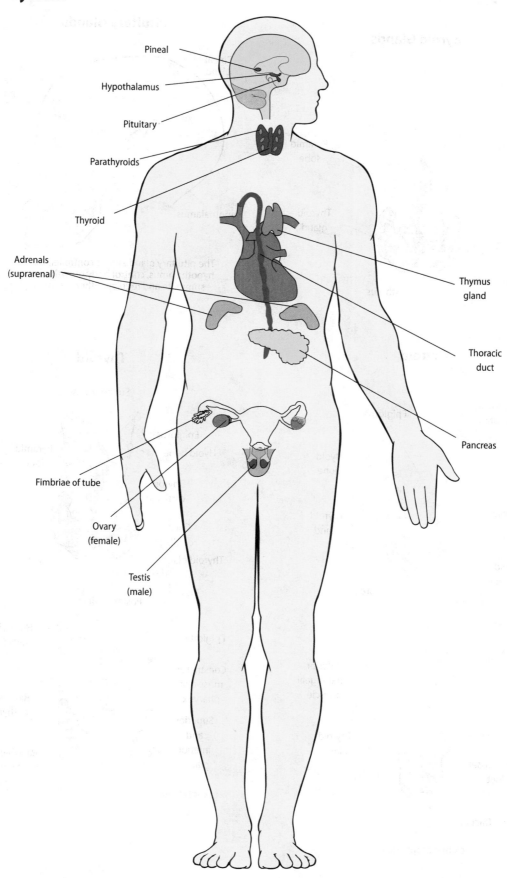

Pineal

Hypothalamus

Pituitary

Parathyroids

Thyroid

Adrenals
(suprarenal)

Thymus
gland

Thoracic
duct

Pancreas

Fimbriae of tube

Ovary
(female)

Testis
(male)

Endocrine System

Thyroid Glands

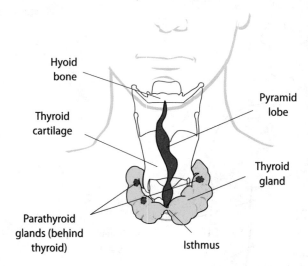

- Hyoid bone
- Thyroid cartilage
- Parathyroid glands (behind thyroid)
- Pyramid lobe
- Thyroid gland
- Isthmus

Pituitary Glands

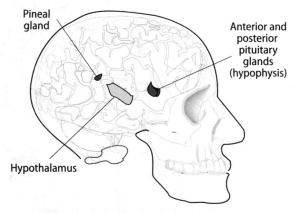

- Pineal gland
- Anterior and posterior pituitary glands (hypophysis)
- Hypothalamus

The pituitary gland and its controller, the hypothalamus, control body growth and stimulate and regulate other glands

Thyroid

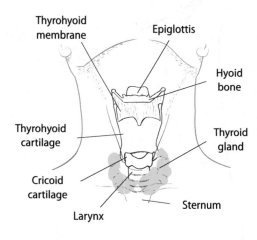

- Thyrohyoid membrane
- Epiglottis
- Hyoid bone
- Thyrohyoid cartilage
- Thyroid gland
- Cricoid cartilage
- Sternum
- Larynx

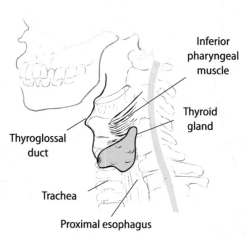

- Inferior pharyngeal muscle
- Thyroid gland
- Thyroglossal duct
- Trachea
- Proximal esophagus

Thyroid

Superior view

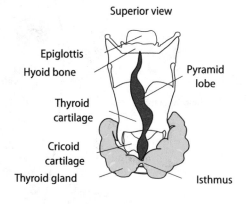

- Epiglottis
- Hyoid bone
- Thyroid cartilage
- Cricoid cartilage
- Thyroid gland
- Pyramid lobe
- Isthmus

Posterior view

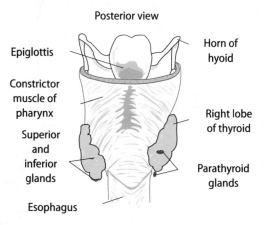

- Epiglottis
- Constrictor muscle of pharynx
- Superior and inferior glands
- Esophagus
- Horn of hyoid
- Right lobe of thyroid
- Parathyroid glands

Nervous System

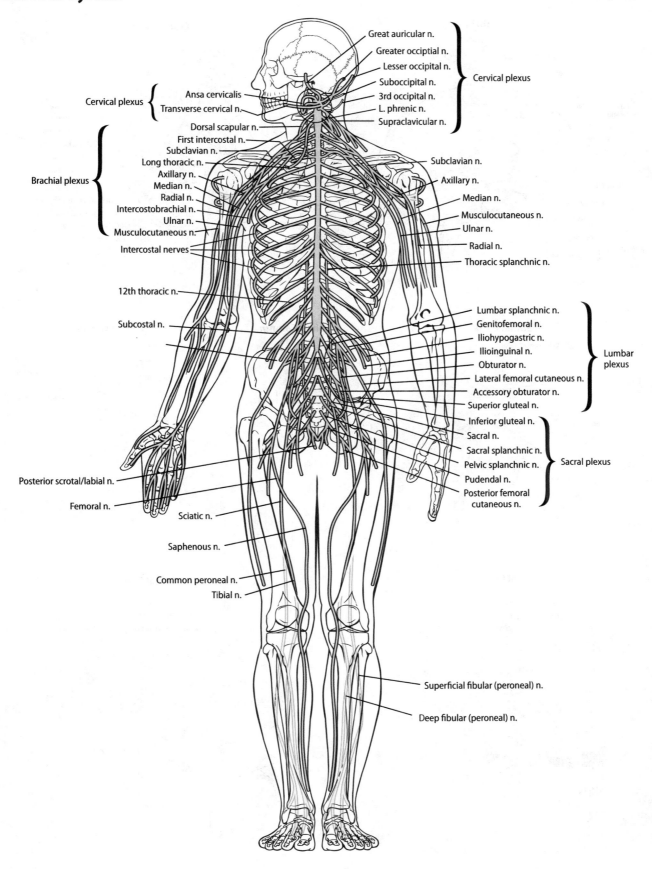

Great auricular n.
Greater occipital n.
Lesser occipital n.
Suboccipital n.
3rd occipital n.
L. phrenic n.
Supraclavicular n.
Cervical plexus

Cervical plexus
Ansa cervicalis
Transverse cervical n.
Dorsal scapular n.
First intercostal n.
Subclavian n.
Long thoracic n.
Axillary n.
Median n.
Radial n.
Intercostobrachial n.
Ulnar n.
Musculocutaneous n.
Intercostal nerves

Brachial plexus

Subclavian n.
Axillary n.
Median n.
Musculocutaneous n.
Ulnar n.
Radial n.
Thoracic splanchnic n.

12th thoracic n.

Subcostal n.

Lumbar splanchnic n.
Genitofemoral n.
Iliohypogastric n.
Ilioinguinal n.
Obturator n.
Lateral femoral cutaneous n.
Accessory obturator n.
Superior gluteal n.

Lumbar plexus

Inferior gluteal n.
Sacral n.
Sacral splanchnic n.
Pelvic splanchnic n.
Pudendal n.
Posterior femoral cutaneous n.

Sacral plexus

Posterior scrotal/labial n.
Femoral n.
Sciatic n.
Saphenous n.
Common peroneal n.
Tibial n.

Superficial fibular (peroneal) n.

Deep fibular (peroneal) n.

Nervous System

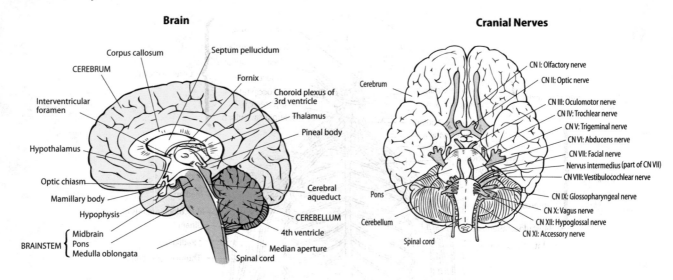

Brain

Cranial Nerves

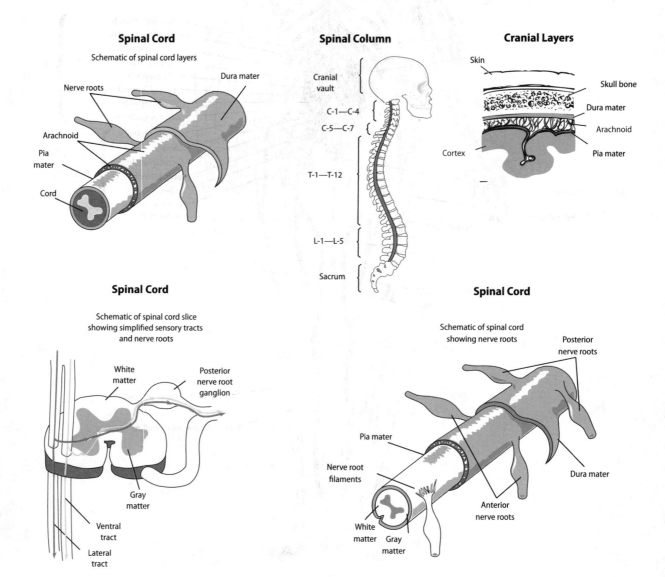

Spinal Cord

Spinal Column

Cranial Layers

Spinal Cord

Spinal Cord

Eye

Eye

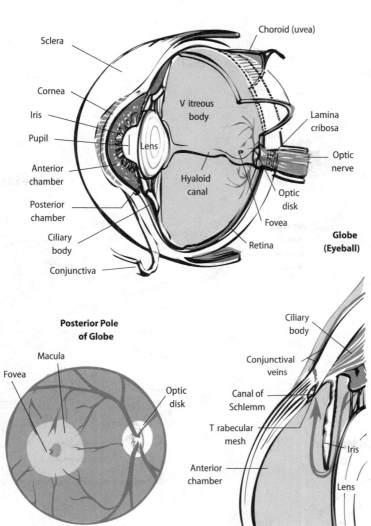

Sclera

Choroid (uvea)

Cornea

Iris

Pupil

Vitreous body

Lamina cribosa

Lens

Optic nerve

Anterior chamber

Posterior chamber

Hyaloid canal

Optic disk

Ciliary body

Optic nerve

Conjunctiva

Fovea

Retina

Globe (Eyeball)

Posterior Pole of Globe

Macula

Fovea

Optic disk

Ciliary body

Conjunctival veins

Canal of Schlemm

Trabecular mesh

Anterior chamber

Iris

Lens

Flow of Aqueous Humor

Muscles of the Eye

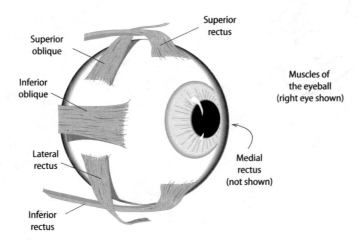

Superior rectus

Superior oblique

Inferior oblique

Muscles of the eyeball (right eye shown)

Lateral rectus

Medial rectus (not shown)

Inferior rectus

Ear and Lacrimal System

Lacrimal System

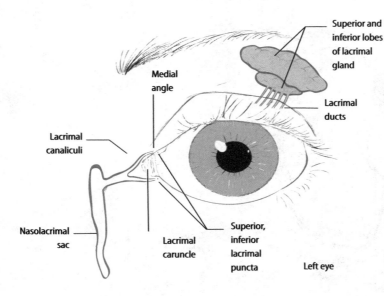

Superior and inferior lobes of lacrimal gland

Medial angle

Lacrimal ducts

Lacrimal canaliculi

Nasolacrimal sac

Lacrimal caruncle

Superior, inferior lacrimal puncta

Left eye

Middle Ear

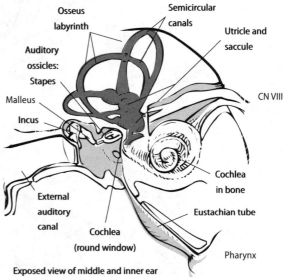

Osseus labyrinth

Semicircular canals

Utricle and saccule

Auditory ossicles:

Stapes

Malleus

Incus

CN VIII

Cochlea in bone

External auditory canal

Cochlea (round window)

Eustachian tube

Pharynx

Exposed view of middle and inner ear

Ear and Mastoid

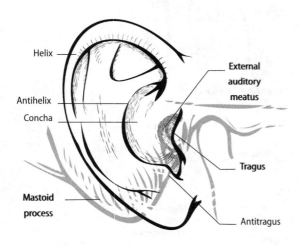

Helix

External auditory meatus

Antihelix

Concha

Tragus

Mastoid process

Antitragus

[Resequenced]

[Resequenced]

[Resequenced]

Assessment — Bacillus Calmette Guerin Vaccine

© 2015 Optum360, LLC
CPT © 2015 American Medical Association. All Rights Reserved.
[Resequenced]
Index — 19

Index
Biopsy — Bladder

Bone, Temporal
See Temporal, Bone
BOOSTRIX, 90715
Bordetella
Antibody, 86615
Antigen Detection
Direct Fluorescent Antibody, 87265
Borrelia (relapsing fever), 86619
Borrelia burgdorferi ab, 86617-86618
Borreliosis, Lyme, 86617-86618
Antigen/infectious agent, 87475-87477
Bost Fusion
Arthrodesis, Wrist, 25800-25810
Bosworth Operation, 23550, 23552
Bottle Type Procedure, 55060
Botulinum Toxin
Chemodenervation
Extraocular Muscle, 67345
Facial Muscle, 64612
Larynx, 64617
Neck Muscle, 64616
Boutonniere Deformity, 26426, 26428
Bowel
See Intestine(s)
Bower's Arthroplasty, 25332
Bowleg Repair, 27455, 27457
Boxer's Fracture Treatment, 26600-26615
Boyce Operation, 50040, 50045
Boyd Amputation, 27880-27889
Boyd Hip Disarticulation, 27590
Brace
See Cast
for Leg Cast, 29358
Vertebral Fracture, 22310, 22315
Brachial Arteries
See Artery, Brachial
Brachial Plexus
Decompression, 64713
Injection
Anesthetic, 64415, 64416
Neuroplasty, 64713
Release, 64713
Repair
Suture, 64861
Brachiocephalic Artery
See Artery, Brachiocephalic
Brachycephaly, 21175
Brachytherapy, 77761-77772, 77789
Dose Plan, 77316-77318
High Dose Electronic, 0394T-0395T
Heyman Capsule, 58346
Intracavitary, 77761-77763, 77770-77772
Placement of Device
Breast, 19296-19298
Genitalia, 55920
Head, 41019
Intraocular, 0190T
Neck, 41019
Pelvis, 55920
Uterus, 57155
Vagina, 57155-57156
Planning
Isodose Plan, 77316-77318
Prostate Volume Study, 76873
Radioelement Solution, 77750
Remote Afterloading
Intracavitary/Interstitial
1 Channel, 77770
2-12 Channels, 77771
Over 12 Channels, 77772
Skin Surface, 77767-77768
Surface Application, 77789-77790
Unlisted Services and Procedures, 77799
Vagina
Insertion
Afterloading Device, 57156
Ovoid, 57155
Tandem, 57155
Bradykinin
Blood or Urine, 82286
BRAF (B-Raf proto-oncogene, serine/threonine kinase), 81210, 81406
Brain
Abscess
Drainage, 61150, 61151
Excision, 61514, 61522

Brain — continued
Abscess — continued
Incision and Drainage, 61320, 61321
Adhesions
Lysis, 62161
Anesthesia, 00210-00218, 00220-00222
Angiography, 36100, 70496
Biopsy, 61140
Stereotactic, 61750, 61751
Catheter
Insertion, 61210
Irrigation, 62194, 62225
Replacement, 62160, 62194, 62225
Catheter Placement
for Chemotherapy, 0169T
for Radiation Source, 61770
Cisternography, 70015
Computer Assisted Procedure, 61781-61782
Cortex
Magnetic Stimulation, 0310T, 90867-90869
Mapping, 90867, 96020
Motor Function, 0310T
Coverings
Tumor
Excision, 61512, 61519
Craniopharyngioma, 61545
Excision, 61545
CT Scan, 0042T, 70450-70470, 70496
Cyst
Drainage, 61150, 61151, 62161, 62162
Excision, 61516, 61524, 62162
Death Determination, 95824
Debridement, 62010
Doppler Transcranial, 93886-93893
Electrocorticography, 61536, 61538, 61539
Electroencephalography
Cerebral Death Evaluation, 95824
Monitored, 95812-95813
Recorded, 95816, 95819, 95822, 95827
Epileptogenic Focus
Excision, 61534, 61536
Monitoring, 61531, 61533, 61535, 61760
Excision
Amygdala, 61566
Choroid Plexus, 61544
Craniopharyngioma, 61545
Hemisphere, 61543
Hemispherectomy, 61543
Hippocampus, 61566
Meningioma, 61512, 61519
Other Lobe, 61323, 61539, 61540
Temporal Lobe, 61537, 61538
Exploration
Infratentorial, 61305
Supratentorial, 61304
Hematoma
Drainage, 61154
Incision and Drainage, 61312-61315
Implantation
Chemotherapeutic Agent, 61517
Electrode, 61210, 61850-61870
Pulse Generator, 61885, 61886
Receiver, 61885, 61886
Reservoir, 61210, 61215
Thermal Perfusion Probe, 61107, 61210
Incision
Corpus Callosum, 61541
Mesencephalic Tract, 61480
Subpial, 61567
Infusion, 0169T, 95990-95991
Insertion
Catheter, 61210
Electrode, 61531, 61533, 61850-61870
Pulse Generator, 61885, 61886
Receiver, 61885, 61886
Reservoir, 61210, 61215
Lesion
Aspiration, Stereotactic, 61750, 61751
Excision, 61534, 61536, 61600-61608, 61615, 61616
Lobectomy, 61537-61540
Magnetic Resonance Imaging (MRI), 70551-70555
Intraoperative, 0398T
Magnetic Stimulation
Transcranial, 90867-90869

Brain — continued
Magnetoencephalography, 95965-95967
Mapping, 90867-90869, 95961-95962, 96020
Meningioma
Excision, 61512, 61519
Myelography, 70010
Neurostimulation
Analysis, 95970-95982
Electrode
Implantation, 61210, 61850, 61860, 61863-61864, 61870
Removal, 61880
Revision, 61880
Pulse Generator
Insertion, 61885-61886
Removal, 61880
Revision, 61880
Nuclear Medicine
Blood Flow, 78610
Cerebrospinal Fluid, 78630-78650
Imaging, 78600-78607
Vascular Flow, 78610
Shunt Evaluation, 78645
Perfusion Analysis, 0042T
Positron Emission Tomography (PET), 78608, 78609
Radiosurgery
for Lesion, 61796-61800
Radiation Treatment Delivery, 77371-77373
Removal
Electrode, 61535, 61880
Foreign Body, 61570, 62163
Pulse Generator, 61888
Receiver, 61888
Shunt, 62256, 62258
Repair
Dura, 61618
Wound, 61571
Shunt
Creation, 62180-62192, 62200-62223
Removal, 62256, 62258
Replacement, 62160, 62194, 62225-62258
Reprogramming, 62252
Skull
Transcochlear Approach, 61596
Transcondylar Approach, 61597
Transpetrosal Approach, 61598
Transtemporal Approach, 61595
Skull Base
Craniofacial Approach, 61580-61585
Infratemporal Approach, 61590, 61591
Orbitocranial Zygomatic Approach, 61592
Stem Auditory Evoked Potential, 92585-92586
Stereotactic
Aspiration, 61750, 61751
Biopsy, 61750, 61751
Catheter Placement, 0169T
Computer Assisted Navigation, 61781-61782
Create Lesion, 61720, 61735, 61790, 61791
Localization for Placement Therapy Fields, 61770
Navigation, 61781-61782
Procedure, 61781-61782
Radiation Treatment, 77432
Radiosurgery, 61796-61800, 63620-63621, 77371-77373, 77435
Trigeminal Tract, 61791
Surface Electrode
Stimulation, 95961-95962
Transcranial Magnetic Stimulation (TMS), 90867-90869
Transection
Subpial, 61541, 61567
Tumor
Excision, 61510, 61518, 61520, 61521, 61526, 61530, 61545, 62164
Ventriculocisternostomy, 62200-62201
Torkildsen Type, 62180
X–ray with Contrast, 70010, 70015
Brainstem (Brain Stem)
See Brain
Auditory Implant, 92640
Biopsy, 61575, 61576
Decompression, 61575, 61576
Evoked Potentials, 92585, 92586

Brainstem (Brain Stem) — continued
Lesion
Excision, 61575, 61576
Branched-Chain Keto Acid Dehydrogenase E1, Beta Polypeptide Gene Analysis, 81205
Branchial Cleft
Cyst
Excision, 42810, 42815
Branchioma
See Branchial Cleft, Cyst
Braun Procedure, 23405-23406
BRCA1, 81214-81215
BRCA1, BRCA 2, 81211-81213, 81432-81433, [81162]
BRCA2, 81216-81217
Breast
Ablation
Cryosurgery, 19105
Fibroadenoma, 19105
Abscess
Incision and Drainage, 19020
Augmentation, 19324, 19325
Biopsy, 19100-19101
with Localization Device Placement, 19081-19086
MRI Guided, 19085-19086
Stereotactic Guided, 19081-19082
Ultrasound Guided, 19083-19084
with Specimen Imaging, 19085-19086
ABBI, 19081-19086
Cancer Gene Analysis, 81211-81217, 81402, 81406, 81432-81433, [81162]
Catheter Placement
for Interstitial Radioelement Application, 19296-19298, 20555, 41019
Catheter Placement for Application Interstitial Radioelement, 19296-19298
Cryosurgical Ablation, 19105
Cyst
Excision, 19120
Puncture Aspiration, 19000, 19001
Excision
Biopsy, 19100-19101
Capsules, 19371
Chest Wall Tumor, 19260-19272
Cyst, 19120
Lactiferous Duct Fistula, 19112
Lesion, 19120-19126
Needle Localization, 19125-19126
Mastectomy, 19300-19307
Nipple Exploration, 19110
Tumors, 19120, 19260, 19271-19272
Exploration
Abscess, 19020
Nipple, 19110
Implants
Insertion, 19325, 19340, 19342
Preparation of Moulage, 19396
Removal, 19328, 19330
Soft Tissue Reinforcement, 15777
Supply, 19396
Incision
Capsules, 19370
Injection
Radiologic, 19030
Magnetic Resonance Imaging (MRI), 77058-77059
with Computer-aided Detection, 0159T
Mammography, 77051-77057
Computer-Aided Detection, 77051-77052
Ductogram, 77053-77054
Galactogram, 77053-77054
Injection, 19030
Results Documented and Reviewed, 3014F
Screening, 3014F, 77057
Mammoplasty
Augmentation, 19324, 19325
Reduction, 19318
Mastectomy
Complete, 19303
Gynecomastia, 19300
Modified Radical, 19307
Partial, 19301-19302
Radical, 19303-19306
Subcutaneous, 19304

Cerebrospinal Fluid Shunt — *continued*
- Replacement, 62160, 62258, 63744
  - Catheter, 62194, 62225, 62230
  - Valve, 62230
- Reprogramming, 62252
- Torkildsen Operation, 62180
- Ventriculocisternostomy, 62180, 62200-62201

Ceruloplasmin, 82390

Cerumen
- Removal, 69209-69210

Cervical Canal
- Instrumental Dilation of, 57800

Cervical Cap, 57170

Cervical Cerclage
- Abdominal Approach, 59325
- Removal under Anesthesia, 59871
- Vaginal Approach, 59320

Cervical Lymphadenectomy, 38720, 38724

Cervical Mucus Penetration Test, 89330

Cervical Plexus
- Injection
  - Anesthetic, 64413

Cervical Pregnancy, 59140

Cervical Puncture, 61050, 61055

Cervical Smears, 88141, 88155, 88164-88167, 88174-88175
- *See* Cytopathology

Cervical Spine
- *See* Vertebra, Cervical

Cervical Stump
- Dilation and Curettage of, 57558

Cervical Sympathectomy
- *See* Sympathectomy, Cervical

Cervicectomy
- Amputation Cervix, 57530
- Pelvic Exenteration, 45126, 58240

Cervicoplasty, 15819

Cervicothoracic Ganglia
- *See* Stellate Ganglion

Cervix
- *See* Cytopathology
- Amputation
  - Total, 57530
- Biopsy, 57500, 57520
  - Colposcopy, 57454, 57455, 57460
- Cauterization, 57522
  - Cryocautery, 57511
  - Electro or Thermal, 57510
  - Laser Ablation, 57513
- Cerclage, 57700
  - Abdominal, 59325
  - Removal under Anesthesia, 59871
  - Vaginal, 59320
- Colposcopy, 57452-57461
- Conization, 57461, 57520, 57522
- Curettage
  - Endocervical, 57454, 57456, 57505
- Dilation
  - Canal, 57800
  - Stump, 57558
- Dilation and Curettage, 57520, 57558
- Ectopic Pregnancy, 59140
- Excision
  - Electrode, 57460
  - Radical, 57531
  - Stump
    - Abdominal Approach, 57540, 57545
    - Vaginal Approach, 57550-57556
  - Total, 57530
- Exploration
  - Endoscopy, 57452
- Insertion
  - Dilation, 59200
  - Laminaria, 59200
  - Prostaglandin, 59200
- Repair
  - Cerclage, 57700
    - Abdominal, 59325
    - Vaginal, 59320
  - Suture, 57720
  - Stump, 57558
  - Suture, 57720
- Unlisted Services and Procedures, 58999

Cesarean Delivery
- with Hysterectomy, 59525
- Antepartum Care, 59610, 59618

Cesarean Delivery — *continued*
- Delivery
  - After Attempted Vaginal Delivery, 59618
    - Delivery Only, 59620
    - Postpartum Care, 59622
    - Routine Care, 59618
  - Routine Care, 59610
- Delivery Only, 59514
- Postpartum Care, 59515
- Routine Care, 59510
- Tubal Ligation at Time of, 58611
- Vaginal after Prior Cesarean
  - Delivery and Postpartum Care, 59614
  - Delivery Only, 59612
  - Routine Care, 59610

CFH/ARMS2, 81401

CFTR, 81220-81224, 81412

CGM (Continuous Glucose Monitoring System), 95250-95251

Chalazion
- Excision, 67800-67808
  - Multiple
    - Different Lids, 67805
    - Same Lids, 67801
  - Single, 67800
  - Under Anesthesia, 67808

Challenge Tests
- Bronchial Inhalation, 95070-95071
- Cholinesterase Inhibitor, 95857
- Ingestion, 95076, 95079

Chambers Procedure, 28300

Change
- Catheter
  - Percutaneous with Contrast, 75984
- Fetal Position
  - by Manipulation, 59412
- Stent
  - (Endoscopic), Bile or Pancreatic Duct, [43275, 43276]
  - Ureteral, 50688
- Tube
  - Gastrostomy, 43760
  - Percutaneous, with Contrast Monitoring, 75984
  - Tracheotomy, 31502
  - Ureterostomy, 50688

Change, Gastrostomy Tube
- *See* Gastrostomy Tube, Change of

Change of, Dressing
- *See* Dressings, Change

CHCT (Caffeine Halothane Contracture Test), 89049

CHD7, 81407

Cheek
- Bone
  - Excision, 21030, 21034
  - Fracture
    - Closed Treatment with Manipulation, 21355
    - Open Treatment, 21360-21366
    - Reconstruction, 21270
- Fascia Graft, 15840
- Muscle Graft, 15841-15845
- Muscle Transfer, 15845
- Rhytidectomy, 15828
- Skin Graft
  - Delay of Flap, 15620
  - Full Thickness, 15240, 15241
  - Pedicle Flap, 15574
  - Split, 15120-15121
- Tissue Transfer, Adjacent, 14040, 14041
- Wound Repair, 13131-13133

Cheekbone
- Fracture
  - Closed Treatment Manipulation, 21355
  - Open Treatment, 21360-21366
  - Reconstruction, 21270

Cheilectomy
- Metatarsophalangeal Joint Release, 28289

Cheiloplasty
- *See* Lip, Repair

Cheiloschisis
- *See* Cleft, Lip

Cheilotomy
- *See* Incision, Lip

Chemical
- Cauterization
  - Corneal Epithelium, 65435-65436
  - Granulation Tissue, 17250
- Exfoliation, 15788-15793, 17360
- Peel, 15788-15793, 17360

Chemiluminescent Assay, 82397

Chemistry Tests
- Organ or Disease Oriented Panel
  - Electrolyte, 80051
  - General Health Panel, 80050
  - Hepatic Function Panel, 80076
  - Hepatitis Panel, Acute, 80074
  - Lipid Panel, 80061
  - Metabolic
    - Basic, 80047-80048
    - Calcium
      - Ionized, 80047
      - Total, 80048
    - Comprehensive, 80053
  - Obstetric Panel, 80055, [80081]
- Unlisted Services and Procedures, 84999

Chemocauterization
- Corneal Epithelium, 65435
  - with Chelating Agent, 65436

Chemodenervation
- Anal Sphincter, 46505
- Bladder, 52287
- Eccrine Glands, 64650, 64653
- Electrical Stimulation for Guidance, 64617, 95873
- Extraocular Muscle, 67345
- Extremity Muscle, 64642-64645
- Facial Muscle, 64612, 64615
- Gland
  - Eccrine, 64650, 64653
  - Parotid, 64611
  - Salivary, 64611
  - Submandibular, 64611
- Internal Anal Sphincter, 46505
- Larynx, 64617
- Muscle
  - Extraocular, 67345
  - Extremity, 64642-64645
  - Facial, 64612
  - Larynx, 64617
  - Neck, 64616
  - Trunk, 64646-64647
- Neck Muscle, 64615-64616
- Needle Electromyography Guidance, 95874
- Salivary Glands, 64611
- Trunk Muscle, 64646-64647

Chemonucleolysis, 62292

Chemosurgery
- Destruction
  - Benign Lesion, 17110-17111
  - Malignant Lesion, 17260-17266, 17270-17286
  - Premalignant Lesion, 17000-17004
- Mohs Technique, 17311-17315

Chemotaxis Assay, 86155

Chemotherapy
- Arterial Catheterization, 36640
- Bladder Instillation, 51720
- Brain, 61517
- Cannulation, 36823
- Central Nervous System, 61517, 96450
- Extracorporeal Circulation Membrane Oxygenation
  - Isolated with Chemotherapy Perfusion, 36823
- Home Infusion Procedures, 99601, 99602
- Intra–Arterial
  - Cannulation, 36823
  - Catheterization, 36640
  - Infusion, 96422-96423, 96425
  - Infusion Pump Insertion, 36260
  - Push Technique, 96420
- Intralesional, 96405, 96406
- Intramuscular, 96401-96402
- Intravenous, 96409-96417
- Kidney Instillation, 50391
- Peritoneal Cavity, 96446
  - Catheterization, 49418
- Pleural Cavity, 96440

Chemotherapy — *continued*
- Pump Services
  - Implantable, 96522
  - Initiation, 96416
  - Maintenance, 95990-95991, 96521-96522
  - Portable, 96521
- Reservoir Filling, 96542
- Subcutaneous, 96401-96402
- Unlisted Services and Procedures, 96549
- Ureteral Instillation, 50391

Chest
- *See* Mediastinum; Thorax
- Angiography, 71275
- Artery
  - Ligation, 37616
- Cavity
  - Bypass Graft, 35905
  - Thoracoscopy
    - Exploration, 32601-32606
    - Surgical, 32650-32665
    - Therapeutic, 32654-32665
- CT Scan, 71250-71275
- Diagnostic Imaging
  - Angiography, 71275
  - CT, 71250, 71260, 71270
  - CT Angiography, 71275
  - Magnetic Resonance Angiography, 71555
  - Magnetic Resonance Imaging (MRI), 71550-71552
  - PET, 78811, 78814
  - Ultrasound, 76604
- Exploration
  - Blood Vessel, 35820
  - Penetrating Wound, 20101
  - Postoperative
    - Hemorrhage, 35820
    - Infection, 35820
    - Thrombosis, 35820
- Flail, 21899
- Funnel
  - Anesthesia, 00474
  - Reconstructive Repair, 21740-21742
    - with Thoracoscopy, 21743
- Magnetic Resonance Imaging (MRI), 71550-71552
- Repair
  - Blood Vessel, 35211, 35216
    - with Other Graft, 35271, 35276
    - with Vein Graft, 35241, 35246
- Tube, 32551
- Ultrasound, 76604
- Wound Exploration
  - Penetrating, 20101
- X–ray, 71010-71035
  - with Computer-aided Detection, 0174T-0175T
  - Complete (four views) with Fluoroscopy, 71034
  - Partial (two views) with Fluoroscopy, 71023
  - Stereo, 71015

Chest Wall
- Debridement, 11044, 11047
- Manipulation, 94667-94669
- Mechanical Oscillation, 94669
- Reconstruction, 49904
  - Lung Tumor Resection, 32504
  - Trauma, 32820
- Repair, 32905
  - Closure, 32810
  - Fistula, 32906
  - Lung Hernia, 32800
- Resection, 32503
- Tumor
  - Ablation, 32998
  - Excision, 19260-19272
- Unlisted Services and Procedures, 32999

Chevron Procedure, 28296

Chiari Osteotomy of the Pelvis
- *See* Osteotomy, Pelvis

Chicken Pox (Varicella)
- Immunization, 90716

Child Procedure, 48146
- *See also* Excision, Pancreas, Partial

Chimerism (Engraftment) Analysis, 81267-81268

Chin
- Cartilage Graft, 21230

Colon — continued
Reduction — continued
Volvulus, 44050
Removal
Foreign Body, 44025, 44390, 45379
Polyp, 44392, 44394, 45384-45385
Tumor, 44392, 44394, 45384-45385
Repair
Diverticula, 44605
Fistula, 44650-44661
Hernia, 44050
Intussusception, 44050
Malrotation, 44055
Obstruction, 44050
Ulcer, 44605
Volvulus, 44050
Wound, 44605
Splenic Flexure Mobilization
Laparoscopic, 44213
Open, 44139
Stoma Closure, 44620, 44625-44626
Suture
Diverticula, 44605
Fistula, 44650-44661
Injury, 44604-44605
Plication, 44680
Rupture, 44604-44605
Stoma, 44620, 44625
Ulcer, 44605
Wound, 44604-44605
Tumor
Ablation, [44401], [45388]
Destruction, [44401], [45388]
Removal, 44392, 44394, 45384-45385
Ultrasound
Endoscopic, 45391-45392
via Colotomy, [45399]
via Stoma, 44388-44408 [44401]
Unlisted Services and Procedures, 44799
X-ray with Contrast
Barium Enema, 74270, 74280
Colonna Procedure, 27120
Acetabulum, Reconstruction, 27120
with Resection, Femoral Head, 27122
Colonography
CT Scan
Diagnostic, 74261-74262
Screening, 74263
Colonoscopy
Ablation Lesions/Polyps/Tumors, [45388]
Band Ligation, [45398]
Biopsy, 45380, 45392
Collection of Specimen, 45378
via Colotomy, [45399]
Decompression, 45393
Destruction
Lesion, [45388]
Tumor, [45388]
Diagnostic, 45378
Dilation, 45386
Hemorrhage Control, 45382
Injection, Submucosal, 45381
Mucosal Resection, [45390]
Placement
Stent, 45389
Removal
Foreign Body, 45379
Polyp, 45384-45385
Tumor, 45384-45385
Surveillance Intervals, 0528F-0529F
Transabdominal, [45399]
Ultrasound, 45391-45392
via Stoma
Biopsy, 44389, 44407
Decompression, 44408
Destruction
Polyp, [44401]
Tumor, [44401]
Dilation, 44405
Exploration, 44388
Hemorrhage, 44391
Injection, Submucosal, 44404
Mucosal Resection, 44403
Placement
Stent, 44402

Colonoscopy — continued
via Stoma — continued
Removal
Foreign Body, 44390
Polyp, 44392, 44394
Tumor, 44392, 44394
Ultrasound, 44406-44407
Virtual, 74261-74263
Colon–Sigmoid
Biopsy
Endoscopy, 45331
Decompression, 45378
Volvulus, 45337
Dilation, 45340
Endoscopy
Ablation
Polyp, [45346]
Tumor, [45346]
Biopsy, 45331
Dilation, 45340
Exploration, 45330, 45335
Hemorrhage, 45334
Needle Biopsy, 45342
Placement
Stent, 45327, 45347
Removal
Foreign Body, 45332
Polyp, 45333, 45338
Tumor, 45333, 45338
Ultrasound, 45341, 45342
Volvulus, 45337
Exploration
Endoscopy, 45330, 45335
Hemorrhage
Endoscopy, 45334
Needle Biopsy
Endoscopy, 45342
Reconstruction Bladder Using Sigmoid, 50810
Removal
Foreign Body, 45332
Repair
Volvulus
Endoscopy, 45337
Ultrasound
Endoscopy, 45341, 45342
Colorrhaphy, 44604
Color Vision Examination, 92283
Colostomy
with Colorrhaphy, 44605
with Partial Colectomy, 44141, 44143-44144, 44146
Hartmann Type, 44143
Laparoscopic, 44206, 44208
with Pelvic Exenteration, 45126, 51597, 58240
with Proctectomy, 45110
Laparoscopic, 45395
with Rectal Repair, 45563, 45805, 45825
Abdominal
with Closure Rectovaginal Fistula, 57307
with Creation Sigmoid Bladder, 50810
Abdominoperineal, 51597, 58240
Delayed Opening, 44799
External Fistulization, 44320
Paracolostomy Hernia, 44346
Revision, 44340
Home Visit, 99505
Ileocolostomy, 44160, 44205
Intestine, Large
with Suture, 44605
Laparoscopic, 44188, 44206, 44208
Perineal, 50810
Revision, 44340
Paracolostomy Hernia, 44345, 44346
Colotomy, 44025
Colpectomy
with Hysterectomy, 58275
with Repair of Enterocele, 58280
Partial, 57106
Total, 57110
Colpoceliocentesis
See Colpocentesis
Colpocentesis, 57020
Colpocleisis, 57120
Colpocleisis Complete
See Vagina, Closure

Colpohysterectomies
See Excision, Uterus, Vaginal
Colpoperineorrhaphy, 57210
Colpopexy, 57280
Laparoscopic, 57425
Open, 57280
Vaginal, 57282-57283
Colpoplasty
See Repair, Vagina
Colporrhaphy
Anterior, 57240, 57289
with Insertion of Mesh, 57267
with Insertion of Prosthesis, 57267
Anteroposterior, 57260, 57265
with Enterocele Repair, 57265
with Insertion of Mesh, 57267
with Insertion of Prosthesis, 57267
Manchester, 58400
Nonobstetrical, 57200
Posterior, 57250
with Insertion of Mesh, 57267
with Insertion of Prosthesis, 57267
Colposcopy
Biopsy, 56821, 57421, 57454-57455, 57460
Endometrial, 58110
Cervix, 57420-57421, 57452-57461
Endometrium, 58110
Exploration, 57452
Loop Electrode Biopsy, 57460
Loop Electrode Conization, 57461
Perineum, 99170
Vagina, 57420-57421, 57452
Vulva, 56820
Biopsy, 56821
Colpotomy
Drainage
Abscess, 57010
Exploration, 57000
Colpo–Urethrocystopexy, 58152, 58267, 58293
Marshall–Marchetti–Krantz procedure, 58152, 58267, 58293
Pereyra Procedure, 58267, 58293
Colprosterone
See Progesterone
Columna Vertebralis
See Spine
Column Chromatography/Mass Spectrometry, 82542
Combined Heart–Lung Transplantation
See Transplantation, Heart–Lung
Combined Right and Left Heart Cardiac Catheterization
See Cardiac Catheterization, Combined Left and Right Heart
Combined Vaccine, 90710
Comedones
Opening or Removal of (Incision and Drainage)
Acne Surgery, 10040
Commando–Type Procedure, 41155
Commissurotomy
Right Ventricular, 33476, 33478
Common Sensory Nerve
Repair, Suture, 64834
Common Truncus
See Truncus, Arteriosus
Communication Device
Non–speech–generating, 92605-92606 [92618]
Speech–generating, 92607-92609
Community/Work Reintegration
See Physical Medicine/Therapy/ Occupational Therapy
Training, 97537
Comparative Analysis Using STR Markers, 81265-81266
Compatibility Test
Blood, 86920
Electronic, 86923
Specimen Pretreatment, 86970-86972
Complement
Antigen, 86160
Fixation Test, 86171
Functional Activity, 86161
Hemolytic
Total, 86162
Total, 86162
Complete Blood Count, 85025-85027

Complete Colectomy
See Colectomy, Total
Complete Pneumonectomy
See Pneumonectomy, Completion
Complete Transposition of Great Vessels
See Transposition, Great Arteries
Complex Chronic Care Management Services, 99487, 99489, [99490]
Complex, Factor IX
See Christmas Factor
Complex, Vitamin B
See B Complex Vitamins
Component Removal, Blood
See Apheresis
Composite Graft, 15760, 15770
Vein, 35681-35683
Autogenous
Three or More Segments
Two Locations, 35683
Two Segments
Two Locations, 35682
Compound B
See Corticosterone
Compound F
See Cortisol
Compression, Nerve, Median
See Carpal Tunnel Syndrome
Compression System Application, 29581-29584
Computed Tomographic Angiography
Abdomen, 74174-74175
Abdominal Aorta, 75635
Arm, 73206
Chest, 71275
Head, 70496
Heart, 75574
Leg, 73706
Neck, 70498
Pelvis, 72191, 74174
Computed Tomographic Scintigraphy
See Emission Computerized Tomography
Computed Tomography (CT Scan)
with Contrast
Abdomen, 74160, 74175
Arm, 73201, 73206
Brain, 70460
Cardiac Structure and Morphology, 75572-75573
Chest, 71275
Ear, 70481
Face, 70487
Head, 70460, 70496
Heart, 75572-75574
Leg, 73701, 73706
Maxilla, 70487
Neck, 70491, 70498
Orbit, 70481
Pelvis, 72191, 72193
Sella Turcica, 70481
Spine
Cervical, 72126
Lumbar, 72132
Thoracic, 72129
Thorax, 71260
without Contrast
Abdomen, 74150
Arm, 73200
Brain, 70450
Ear, 70480
Face, 70486
Head, 70450
Heart, 75571
Leg, 73700
Maxilla, 70486
Neck, 70490
Orbit, 70480
Pelvis, 72192
Sella Turcica, 70480
Spine, Cervical, 72125
Spine, Lumbar, 72131
Spine, Thoracic, 72128
Thorax, 71250
without Contrast, followed by Contrast
Abdomen, 74170
Arm, 73202
Brain, 70470
Ear, 70482

Computed Tomography (CT Scan) — *continued*
without Contrast, followed by Contrast — *continued*
Face, 70488
Leg, 73702
Maxilla, 70488
Neck, 70492
Orbit, 70482
Pelvis, 72194
Sella Turcica, 70482
Spine
Cervical, 72127
Lumbar, 72133
Thoracic, 72130
Thorax, 71270
Bone
Density Study, 77078
Colon
Colonography, 74261-74263
Diagnostic, 74261-74262
Screening, 74263
Virtual Colonoscopy, 74261-74263
Drainage, 75898
Follow–up Study, 76380
Guidance
3D Rendering, 76376-76377
Cyst Aspiration, 77012
Localization, 77011
Needle Biopsy, 77012
Radiation Therapy, 77014
Heart, 75571-75574
Computer
Aided Animation and Analysis Retinal Images, 0380T
Aided Detection
Chest Radiograph, 0174T-0175T
Mammography
Diagnostic, 77051
Magnetic Resonance Imaging (MRI), 0159T
Screening, 77052
Analysis
Cardiac Electrical Data, 0206T
Electrocardiographic Data, 93228
Heart Sounds, Acoustic Recording, 93799
Motion Analysis, 96000-96004
Pediatric Home Apnea Monitor, 94776
Probability Assessment
Patient Specific Findings, 99199
Stored Data, 99090
Assisted Navigation
Orthopedic Surgery, 20985, 0054T-0055T
Assisted Testing
Cytopathology, 88121
Morphometric Analysis, 88121
Neuropsychological, 96120
Psychological, 96103
Urinary Tract Specimen, 88121
Computerized Emission Tomography
See Emission Computerized Tomography
COMVAX, 90748
Concentration, Hydrogen–Ion
See pH
Concentration, Minimum Inhibitory
See Minimum Inhibitory Concentration
Concentration of Specimen
Cytopathology, 88108
Electrophoretic Fractionation and Quantitation, 84166
Immunoelectrophoresis, 86325
Immunofixation Electrophoresis, 86335
Infectious Agent, 87015
Ova and Parasites, 87177
Concentric Procedure, 28296
Concha Bullosa Resection
with Nasal/Sinus Endoscopy, 31240
Conchae Nasale
See Nasal Turbinate
Conduction, Nerve
See Nerve Conduction
Conduit, Ileal
See Ileal Conduit
Condyle
Femur
Arthroplasty, 27442-27443, 27446-27447

Condyle — *continued*
Femur — *continued*
Fracture
Closed, 27508, 27510
Open, 27514
Percutaneous, 27509
Humerus
Fracture
Closed Treatment, 24576, 24577
Open Treatment, 24579
Percutaneous, 24582
Mandible, Reconstruction, 21247
Metatarsal
Excision, 28288
Phalanges
Toe
Excision, 28126
Resection, 28153
Condylectomy
with Skull Base Surgery, 61596, 61597
Metatarsal Head, 28288
Temporomandibular Joint, 21050
Condyle, Mandibular
See Mandibular Condyle
Condyloma
Destruction
Anal, 46900-46924
Penis, 54050-54065
Vagina, 57061, 57065
Vulva, 56501, 56515
Conference
Interactive Videoconference, 0188T-0189T
Medical
with Interdisciplinary Team, 99366-99368
Confirmation
Drug, [80320, 80321, 80322, 80323, 80324, 80325, 80326, 80327, 80328, 80329, 80330, 80331, 80332, 80333, 80334, 80335, 80336, 80337, 80338, 80339, 80340, 80341, 80342, 80343, 80344, 80345, 80346, 80347, 80348, 80349, 80350, 80351, 80352, 80353, 80354, 80355, 80356, 80357, 80358, 80359, 80360, 80361, 80362, 80363, 80364, 80365, 80366, 80367, 80368, 80369, 80370, 80371, 80372, 80373, 80374, 80375, 80376, 80377, 83992]
Confocal Microscopy, 96931-96936
Congenital Arteriovenous Malformation
See Arteriovenous Malformation
Congenital Elevation of Scapula
See Sprengal's Deformity
Congenital Heart Anomaly
Catheterization, 93530-93533
Injection, 93563-93564
Closure
Interatrial Communication, 93580
Ventricular Septal Defect, 93581
Echocardiography
Congenital Anomalies
Transesophageal, 93315
Transthoracic, 93303-93304
Fetal, 76825-76826
Doppler, 76827-76828
Guidance for Intracardiac or Great Vessel Intervention, 93355
Treatment Ventricular Ectopy, 93654
Congenital Heart Septum Defect
See Septal Defect
Congenital Kidney Abnormality
Nephrolithotomy, 50070
Pyeloplasty, 50405
Pyelotomy, 50135
Congenital Laryngocele
See Laryngocele
Congenital Vascular Anomaly
See Vascular Malformation
Conisation
See Cervix, Conization
Conization
Cervix, 57461, 57520, 57522
Conjoint Psychotherapy, 90847
Conjunctiva
Biopsy, 68100
Cyst
Incision and Drainage, 68020

Conjunctiva — *continued*
Excision of Lesion, 68110, 68115
with Adjacent Sclera, 68130
Expression of Follicles, 68040
Fistulize for Drainage
with Tube, 68750
without Tube, 68745
Foreign Body Removal, 65205, 65210
Graft, 65782
Harvesting, 68371
Insertion, 65150, 65782
Injection, 68200
Insertion Stent, 68750
Lesion
Destruction, 68135
Excision, 68110-68130
with Adjacent Sclera, 68130
over 1 cm, 68115
Reconstruction, 68320-68335
with Flap
Bridge or Partial, 68360
Total, 68362
Symblepharon
with Graft, 68335
without Graft, 68330
Total, 68362
Repair
Symblepharon
with Graft, 68335
without Graft, 68330
Division, 68340
Wound
with Eyelid Repair, 67961, 67966
with Wound Repair, 65270, 65272-65273, 67930, 67935
Direct Closure, 65270
Mobilization and Rearrangement, 65272, 65273
Unlisted Services and Procedure, 68399
Conjunctivocystorhinostomy
See Conjunctivorhinostomy
Conjunctivodacryocystostomy
See Conjunctivorhinostomy
Conjunctivoplasty, 68320-68330
with Extensive Rearrangement, 68320
with Graft, 68320
Buccal Mucous Membrane, 68325
Reconstruction Cul–de–Sac
with Extensive Rearrangement, 68326
with Graft, 68328
Buccal Mucous Membrane, 68328
Repair Symblepharon, 68330, 68335, 68340
Conjunctivorhinostomy
with Tube, 68750
without Tube, 68745
Conjunctivo–Tarso–Levator
Resection, 67908
Conjunctivo–Tarso–Muller Resection, 67908
Conscious Sedation
See Sedation
Construction
Apical-Aortic Conduit, 33404
Arterial
Conduit, 33608, 33920
Tunnel, 33505
Bladder from Sigmoid Colon, 50810
Eye Adhesions, 67880
Finger
Toe to Hand Transfer, 26551-26556
Gastric Tube, 43832
IMRT Device, 77332-77334
Multi-leaf Collimator (MLC) Device, 77338
Neobladder, 51596
Tracheoesophageal Fistula, 31611
Vagina
with Graft, 57292
without Graft, 57291
Consultation
See Second Opinion; Third Opinion
Clinical Pathology, 80500, 80502
Initial Inpatient
New or Established Patient, 99251-99255
Interprofessional Via Telephone or Internet, 99446-99449
Office and/or Other Outpatient
New or Established Patient, 99241-99245

Consultation — *continued*
Pathology
During Surgery, 88333-88334
Psychiatric, with Family, 90887
Radiation Therapy
Radiation Physics, 77336, 77370
Surgical Pathology, 88321-88325
Intraoperation, 88329-88334
X–ray, 76140
Consumption Test, Antiglobulin
See Coombs Test
Contact Lens Services
Fitting/Prescription, 92071-92072, 92310-92313
Modification, 92325
Prescription, 92314-92317
Replacement, 92326
Continuous Epidural Analgesia, 01967-01969
Continuous Glucose Monitoring System (CGMS), 95250-95251
Continuous Negative Pressure Breathing (CNPB), 94662
Continuous Positive Airway Pressure (CPAP), 94660
Intermittent Positive Pressure Breathing, 94660
Contouring
Cranial
Bones, 21181
Sutures, 61559
Forehead, 21137-21138
Frontal Sinus Wall, 21139
Septoplasty, 30520
Silicone Injections, 11950-11954
Tumor
Facial Bone, 21029
Contraception
Cervical Cap
Fitting, 57170
Diaphragm
Fitting, 57170
Intrauterine Device (IUD)
Insertion, 58300
Removal, 58301
Contraceptive Capsules, Implantable
Insertion, 11981
Removal, 11976
Contraceptive Device, Intrauterine
See Intrauterine Device (IUD)
Contracture
Bladder Neck Resection, 52640
Elbow
Release with Radical Resection of Capsule, 24149
Finger Cast, 29086
Palm
Release, 26121-26125
Shoulder Capsule Release, 23020
Thumb
Release, 26508
Volkmann, 25315
Wrist Capsulotomy, 25085
Contracture of Palmar Fascia
See Dupuytren's Contracture
Contralateral Ligament
Repair, Knee, 27405
Contrast Aortogram
See Aortography
Contrast Bath Therapy, 97034
See Physical Medicine/ Therapy/Occupational Therapy
Contrast Material
Colonic Tube
Insertion, 49440-49442
Radiological Evaluation, 49465
Removal of Obstruction, 49460
Replacement, 49446, 49450-49452
Cranial
for Ventricular Puncture, 61120
Dacryocystography, 68850
Injection
Arteriovenous Dialysis Shunt, 36147
Central Venous Access Device, 36598
Gastrostomy, Duodenostomy, Jejunostomy, Gastro-jejunostomy, or Cecostomy Tube, Percutaneous, 49465
via Peritoneal Catheter, 49424

Craniectomy — continued
  Craniosynostosis, 61558, 61559
    Multiple Sutures, 61552, 61558-61559
    Single Suture, 61550
  Decompression, 61322-61323, 61340-61343
    Cranial Nerves, 61458
    Sensory Root Gasserian Ganglion, 61450
  Drainage of Abscess, 61320-61321
  Electrode Placement
    Cortical, 61860, 61870
    Subcortical, 61863-61864, 61867-61868
  Excision
    for Osteomyelitis, 61501
    of Lesion or Tumor, 61500
  Exploratory, 61304-61305, 61458
  Section, 61450, 61460
  Stenosis Release, 61550-61552
  Surgical, 61312-61315, 61320-61323, 61450-61480, 61500-61522
  Tractotomy, 61480
  Wound Treatment, 61571
Craniofacial and Maxillofacial
  Unlisted Services and Procedures, 21299
Craniofacial Procedures
  Unlisted Services and Procedures, 21299
Craniofacial Separation
  Bone Graft, 21436
  Closed Treatment, 21431
  External Fixation, 21435
  Open Treatment, 21432-21436
  Wire Fixation, 21431-21432
Craniomegalic Skull
  Reduction, 62115-62117
Craniopharyngioma
  Excision, 61545
Cranioplasty, 62120
  with Autograft, 62146, 62147
  with Bone Graft, 61316, 62146, 62147
  Bone Graft Retrieval, 62148
  Encephalocele Repair, 62120
  for Defect, 62140, 62141, 62145
Craniostenosis
  See Craniosynostosis
Craniosynostosis
  Bifrontal Craniotomy, 61557
  Extensive Craniectomy, 61558, 61559
  Frontal, 61556
  Multiple Sutures, 61552
  Parietal, 61556
  Single Suture, 61550
Craniotomy
  with Bone Flap, 61510-61516, 61526, 61530, 61533-61545, 61566-61567
    for Bone Lesion, 61500
  Abscess Drainage
    Infratentorial, 61321
    Supratentorial, 61320
  Anesthesia, 00211
  Barrel–Stave Procedure, 61559
  Bifrontal Bone Flap, 61557
  Cloverleaf Skull, 61558
  Craniosynostosis, 61556-61557
  Decompression, 61322-61323
    Orbit Only, 61330
    Other, Supratentorial, 61340
    Posterior Fossa, 61345
  Encephalocele, 62121
  Excision Brain Tumor
    Benign of Cranial Bone, 61563
      with Optic Nerve Decompression, 61564
    Cerebellopontine Angle Tumor, 61520
    Cyst, Supratentorial, 61516
    Infratentorial or posterior fossa, 61518
    Meningioma, 61519
    Midline at Skull Base, 61521
    Supratentorial, 61510
  Excision Epileptogenic Focus
    with Electrocorticography, 61536
    without Electrocorticography, 61534
  Exploratory, 61304, 61305
    Orbit with Biopsy, 61332
    Removal
      Lesion, 61333
  Foreign Body, 61570
  Frontal Bone Flap, 61556

Craniotomy — continued
  Hematoma, 61312-61315
  Implantation Electrodes, 61531, 61533
    Stereotactic, 61760
  Implant of Neurostimulator, 61850-61870
  Lobectomy
    with Electrocorticography, 61538
  Meningioma, 61519
  Mesencephalic Tractotomy or Pedunculotomy, 61480
  Multiple Osteotomies and Bone Autografts, 61559
  Neurostimulators, 61850-61870
  Osteomyelitis, 61501
  Parietal Bone Flap, 61556
  Penetrating Wound, 61571
  Pituitary Tumor, 61546
  Recontouring, 61559
  Removal of Electrode Array, 61535
  Suboccipital
    with Cervical Laminectomy, 61343
    for Cranial Nerves, 61458
    Subtemporal, 61450
  Surgery, 61312-61323, 61546, 61570-61571, 61582-61583, 61590, 61592, 61760, 62120
  Transoral Approach, 61575
    requiring Splitting Tongue and/or Mandible, 61576
Cranium
  See Skull
Craterization
  Calcaneus, 28120
  Clavicle, 23180
  Femur, 27070, 27071, 27360
  Fibula, 27360, 27641
  Hip, 27070, 27071
  Humerus, 23184, 24140
  Ileum, 27070, 27071
  Metacarpal, 26230
  Metatarsal, 28122
  Olecranon Process, 24147
  Phalanges
    Finger, 26235, 26236
    Toe, 28124
  Pubis, 27070, 27071
  Radius, 24145, 25151
  Scapula, 23182
  Talus, 28120
  Tarsal, 28122
  Tibia, 27360, 27640
  Ulna, 24147, 25150
CRB1, 81406, 81434
C–Reactive Protein, 86140, 86141
Creatine, 82553-82554
  Blood or Urine, 82540
Creatine Kinase (Total), 82550
Creatine Phosphokinase
  Blood, 82552
  Total, 82550
Creatinine
  Blood, 82565
  Clearance, 82575
  Other Source, 82570
  Urine, 82570, 82575
Creation
  Arteriovenous
    Fistula, 35686, 36825, 36830
  Catheter Exit Site, 49436
  Cavopulmonary Anastomosis, 33622
  Colonic Reservoir, 45119
  Complete Heart Block, 93650
  Cutaneoperitoneal Fistula, 49999
  Defect, 40720
  Ileal Reservoir, 44158, 44211, 45113
  Iliac Artery Conduit, 34833
  Lesion
    Gasserian Ganglion, 61790
    Globus Pallidus, 61720
    Other Subcortical Structure, 61735
    Spinal Cord, 63600
    Thalamus, 61720
    Trigeminal Tract, 61791
  Mucofistula, 44144
  Pericardial Window, 32659, 33025
  Recipient Site, 15002-15003, 15004-15005

Creation — continued
  Shunt
    Cerebrospinal Fluid, 62200
    Subarachnoid
      Lumbar–Peritoneal, 63740
      Subarachnoid–Subdural, 62190
      Ventriculo, 62220
    Sigmoid Bladder, 50810
  Speech Prosthesis, 31611
  Stoma
    Bladder, 51980
    Kidney, 50395
    Renal Pelvis, 50395
    Tympanic Membrane, 69433, 69436
    Ureter, 50860
  Ventral Hernia, 39503
CREBBP, 81406-81407
CRF, 80412
CRH (Corticotropic Releasing Hormone), 80412
Cricoid Cartilage Split, 31587
Cricothyroid Membrane
  Incision, 31605
Cristobalite
  See Silica
CRIT, 85013
Critical Care Services
  Cardiopulmonary Resuscitation, 92950
  Evaluation and Management, 99291-99292, 99466-99476
  Interfacility Transport, 99466-99467 [99485] [99486]
  Ipecac Administration for Poison, 99175
  Neonatal
    Initial, 99468
    Intensive, 99477
    Low Birth Weight Infant, 99478-99479
    Subsequent, 99469
  Pediatric
    Initial, 99471, 99475
    Interfacility Transport, 99466-99467 [99485, 99486]
    Supervision, [99485, 99486]
    Subsequent, 99472, 99476
  Remote Interactive Videoconferenced, 0188T-0189T
Cross Finger Flap, 15574
Crossmatch, 86825-86826, 86920-86923
Crossmatching, Tissue
  See Tissue Typing
CRP, 86140
Cruciate Ligament
  Arthroscopic Repair, 29888-29889
  Repair, 27407, 27409
    Knee with Collateral Ligament, 27409
CRX, 81404
Cryoablation
  See Cryosurgery
Cryofibrinogen, 82585
Cryofixation
  Cells, 38207-38209, 88240-88241
  Embryo, 89258
  for Transplantation, 32850, 33930, 33940, 44132, 47133, 47140, 48550, 50300-50320, 50547
  Freezing and Storage, 38207, 88240
  Oocyte, 89240
  Ovarian Tissue, 89240
  Sperm, 89259
  Testes, 89335
  Thawing
    Embryo, 89352
    Oocytes, 89353
    Reproductive Tissue, 89354
    Sperm, 89356
Cryoglobulin, 82595
Cryopreservation
  Bone Marrow, 38207-38209
  Cells, 38207-38208, 88240, 88241
  Embryo, 89258, 89352
  for Transplantation, 32850, 33930, 33940, 44132-44133, 47140, 48550, 50300-50320, 50547
  Freezing and Storage
    Cells, 88240
    Embryo, 89258

Cryopreservation — continued
  Freezing and Storage — continued
    Reproductive Tissue
      Oocyte(s), 89337, [0357T]
      Ovarian, 0058T
      Sperm, 89259
      Testicular, 89335
      Stem Cells, 38207
    Oocyte, 89337, [0357T]
    Ovarian Tissue, 0058T
    Sperm, 89259
    Testes, 89335
      Embryo, 89352
      Oocytes, 89353
      Reproductive Tissue, 89354
      Sperm, 89356
  Thawing
    Cells, 88241
    Embryo, 89352
    Oocytes, 89356
    Reproductive Tissue, 89354
    Sperm, 89353
Cryosurgery, 17000-17286, 47371, 47381
  See Destruction
  Cervix, 57511
  Fibroadenoma
    Breast, 19105
  Lesion
    Anus, 46916, 46924
    Bladder, 51030, 52224
      Tumor(s), 52234-52235, 52240
    Ear, 17280-17284, 17286
    Eyelid, 17280-17284, 17286
    Face, 17280-17284, 17286
    Kidney, 50250
    Lips, 17280-17284, 17286
    Liver, 47371, 47381
    Mouth, 17280-17284, 17286, 40820
    Nose, 17280-17284, 17286
    Penis, 54056, 54065
    Skin
      Benign, 17000-17004, 17110-17111
      Malignant, 17260-17286
      Premalignant, 17000-17004
      Vascular Proliferative, 17106-17108
    Urethra, 52224
    Vagina, 57061-57065
    Vulva, 56501-56515
  Prostate, 52214, 55873
  Trichiasis, 67825
  Tumor
    Bladder, 52234-52235, 52240
    Rectum, 45190
  Warts, flat, 17110, 17111
Cryotherapy
  Ablation
    Renal Tumor, 50593
    Uterine Fibroid, Transcervical, 0404T
  Acne, 17340
  Destruction
    Bronchial Tumor, 31641
    Ciliary body, 66720
    Retinopathy, 67227
  Lesion
    Cornea, 65450
    Retina, 67208, 67227
  Renal Tumor, 50593
  Retinal Detachment
    Prophylaxis, 67141
    Repair, 67101, 67107-67108, 67113
  Retinopathy, 67229
    Destruction, 67227
    Preterm Infant, 67229
  Trichiasis
    Correction, 67825
Crypectomy, 46999
Cryptococcus
  Antibody, 86641
  Antigen Detection
    Enzyme Immunoassay, 87327
Cryptococcus Neoformans
  Antigen Detection
    Enzyme Immunoassay, 87327
Cryptorchism
  See Testis, Undescended

Device — *continued*
- Venous Access — *continued*
    - Insertion — *continued*
        - Obstruction Clearance, 36595, 36596
        - Peripheral, 36570, 36571
        - Removal, 36590
        - Repair, 36576
        - Replacement, 36582, 36583, 36585
    - Irrigation, 96523
    - Obstruction Clearance, 36595-36596
        - Imaging, 75901-75902
    - Removal, 36590
    - Repair, 36576
    - Replacement, 36582-36583, 36585
        - Catheter, 36578
- Ventricular Assist, 33975-33983, 33990-33993

Device, Orthotic
- *See* Orthotics

Dexamethasone
- Suppression Test, 80420

DFNB59, 81405

D Galactose
- *See* Galactose

D Glucose
- *See* Glucose

DGUOK, 81405

DHA Sulfate
- *See* Dehydroepiandrosterone Sulfate

DHCR7, 81405

DHEA (Dehydroepiandrosterone), 82626

DHEAS, 82627

DHT (Dihydrotestosterone), *[80327, 80328]*

Diagnosis, Psychiatric
- *See* Psychiatric Diagnosis

Diagnostic Amniocentesis
- *See* Amniocentesis

Diagnostic Aspiration of Anterior Chamber of Eye
- *See* Eye, Paracentesis, Anterior Chamber, with Diagnostic Aspiration of Aqueous

Dialysis
- Arteriovenous Fistula
    - Revision
        - without Thrombectomy, 36832
        - Thrombectomy, 36831
- Arteriovenous Shunt, 36147-36148, 75791
    - Revision
        - with Thrombectomy, 36833
        - Thrombectomy, 36831
- Documentation of Nephropathy Treatment, 3066F
- End Stage Renal Disease, 90951-90953, 90963, 90967
- Hemodialysis, 90935, 90937
    - Blood Flow Study, 90940
    - Plan of Care Documented, 0505F
- Hemoperfusion, 90997
- Hepatitis B Vaccine, 90740, 90747
- Kt/V Level, 3082F-3084F
- Patient Training
    - Completed Course, 90989
    - Per Session, 90993
- Peritoneal, 4055F, 90945, 90947
    - Catheter Insertion, 49418-49421
    - Catheter Removal, 49422
    - Home Infusion, 99601-99602
    - Plan of Care Documented, 0507F
- Unlisted Procedures, 90999

Dl–Amphetamine
- *See* Amphetamine

Diaphragm
- Anesthesia, 00540
    - Hernia Repair, 00756
- Assessment, 58943, 58960
- Imbrication for Eventration, 39545
- Repair
    - Esophageal Hiatal, 43280-43282, 43325
    - for Eventration, 39545
    - Hernia, 39503-39541
        - Neonatal, 39503
    - Laceration, 39501
- Resection, 39560, 39561
- Unlisted Procedures, 39599
- Vagina
    - Fitting, 57170

Diaphragm Contraception, 57170

Diaphysectomy
- Calcaneus, 28120
- Clavicle, 23180
- Femur, 27360
- Fibula, 27360, 27641
- Humerus, 23184, 24140
- Metacarpal, 26230
- Metatarsal, 28122
- Olecranon Process, 24147
- Phalanges
    - Finger, 26235, 26236
    - Toe, 28124
- Radius, 24145, 25151
- Scapula, 23182
- Talus, 28120
- Tarsal, 28122
- Tibia, 27360, 27640
- Ulna, 24147, 25150

Diastase
- *See* Amylase

Diastasis
- *See* Separation

Diathermy, 97024
- *See* Physical Medicine/ Therapy/Occupational
- Destruction
    - Ciliary Body, 66700
    - Lesion
        - Retina, 67208, 67227
    - Retinal Detachment
        - Prophylaxis, 67141
        - Repair, 67101
    - Treatment, 97024

Diathermy, Surgical
- *See* Electrocautery

Dibucaine Number, 82638

Dichloride, Methylene
- *See* Dichloromethane

Dichlorides, Ethylene
- *See* Dichloroethane

Dichloroethane, 82441

Dichloromethane, 82441

Diethylamide, Lysergic Acid
- *See* Lysergic Acid Diethylamide

Differential Count
- White Blood Cell Count, 85007, 85009, 85540

Differentiation Reversal Factor
- *See* Prothrombin

Diffusing Capacity, 94729

Diffusion Test, Gel
- *See* Immunodiffusion

Digestive Tract
- *See* Gastrointestinal Tract

Digit(s)
- *See also* Finger, Toe
- Nerve
    - Destruction, 64632
    - Injection, 64455
- Pinch Graft, 15050
- Replantation, 20816, 20822
- Skin Graft
    - Split, 15120, 15121

Digital Artery Sympathectomy, 64820

Digital Slit–Beam Radiograph
- *See* Scanogram

Digoxin
- Assay, 80162-80163
- Blood or Urine, 80162

Dihydrocodeinone
- Definitive Testing, *[80361]*
- Screen, *[80300, 80301, 80302, 80303, 80304]*

Dihydrohydroxycodeinone
- *See* Oxycodone

Dihydromorphinone, *[80361]*
- Screen, *[80300, 80301, 80302, 80303, 80304]*

Dihydrotestosterone, *[80327, 80328]*

Dihydroxyethanes
- *See* Ethylene Glycol

Dihydroxyvitamin D, *[82652]*

Dilation
- *See* Dilation and Curettage
- Anal
    - Endoscopic, 46604
    - Sphincter, 45905, 46940
- Aortic Valve, 33403
- Aqueous Outflow Canal, 66174-66175

Dilation — *continued*
- Bile Duct
    - Endoscopic, 47555, 47556, *[43277]*
    - Percutaneous, 74363
    - Stricture, 74363
- Bladder
    - Cystourethroscopy, 52260, 52265
- Bronchi
    - Endoscopy, 31630, 31636-31638
- Cerebral Vessels
    - Intracranial Vasospasm, 61640-61642
- Cervix
    - Canal, 57800
    - Stump, 57558
- Colon
    - Endoscopy, 45386
- Colon–Sigmoid
    - Endoscopy, 45340
- Curettage, 57558
- Enterostomy Stoma, 44799
- Esophagus, 43450, 43453
    - Endoscopic Balloon, 43195, 43220, 43249, *[43213, 43214], [43233]*
    - Endoscopy, 43195-43196, 43220, 43226, 43248-43249, *[43213, 43214], [43233]*
    - Surgical, 43510
- Frontonasal Duct, 30999
- Gastric/Duodenal Stricture, 43245
    - Open, 43510
- Intestines, Small
    - Endoscopy, 44370
    - Open, 44615
    - Stent Placement, 44379
- Intracranial Vasospasm, 61640-61642
- Kidney, 50080-50081, 50395
    - Intra–Renal Stricture, 52343, 52346
- Lacrimal Punctum, 68801
- Larynx
    - Endoscopy, 31528, 31529
- Nasolacrimal Duct
    - Balloon Catheter, 68816
- Nose
    - Balloon, 31295-31297
- Pancreatic Duct
    - Endoscopy, *[43277]*
- Rectum
    - Endoscopy, 45303
    - Sphincter, 45910
- Salivary Duct, 42650, 42660
- Sinus Ostium, 31295-31297
- Trachea
    - Endoscopic, 31630, 31631, 31636-31638
- Transluminal
    - Aqueous Outflow Canal, 66174-66175
- Ureter, 50395, 50706, 52341-52342, 52344-52346
    - Endoscopic, 50553, 50572, 50575, 50953, 50972
- Urethra, 52260, 52265
    - with Prostatectomy, 55801, 55821
    - with Prostate Resection, 52601, 52630, 52647-52649
    - Female Urethral Syndrome, 52285
    - General, 53665
    - Suppository and/or Instillation, 53660-53661
- Urethral
    - Stenosis, 52281
    - Stricture, 52281, 53600-53621
- Vagina, 57400

Dilation and Curettage
- *See* Curettage; Dilation
- Cervical Stump, 57558
- Cervix, 57520, 57522, 57558, 57800
- Corpus Uteri, 58120
- Hysteroscopy, 58558
- Induced Abortion, 59840
    - with Amniotic Injections, 59851
    - with Vaginal Suppositories, 59856
- Postpartum, 59160

Dilation and Evacuation, 59841
- with Amniotic Injections, 59851
- with Vaginal Suppository, 59856

Dimethadione, *[80339, 80340, 80341]*

Dioxide, Carbon
- *See* Carbon Dioxide

Dioxide Silicon
- *See* Silica

Dipeptidyl Peptidase A
- *See* Angiotensin Converting Enzyme (ACE)

Diphenylhydantoin
- *See* Phenytoin

Diphosphate, Adenosine
- *See* Adenosine Diphosphate

Diphtheria
- Antibody, 86648
- Immunization, 90696-90698, 90700-90702, 90714-90715, 90723

Dipropylacetic Acid
- Assay, 80164
    - *See Also* Valproic Acid

Direct Pedicle Flap
- Formation, 15570-15576
- Transfer, 15570-15576, 15650

Disability Evaluation Services
- Basic Life and/or Disability Evaluation, 99450
- Work–Related or Medical Disability Evaluation, 99455, 99456

Disarticulation
- Ankle, 27889
- Elbow, 20999
- Hip, 27295
- Knee, 27598
- Mandible, 61590
- Shoulder, 23920, 23921
- Wrist, 25920, 25924
    - Revision, 25922

Disarticulation of Shoulder
- *See* Shoulder, Disarticulation

Disc Chemolyses, Intervertebral
- *See* Chemonucleolysis

Discectomies
- *See* Discectomy

Discectomies, Percutaneous
- *See* Discectomy, Percutaneous

Discectomy
- with Endplate Preparation, 22856
    - with Osteophytectomy, 22856
- Additional Segment, 22226
- Anterior with Decompression
    - Cervical Interspace, 63075
        - Each Additional, 63076
    - Thoracic Interspace, 63077
        - Each Additional, 63078
- Arthrodesis
    - Additional Interspace, 22534, 22585, 22634
    - Cervical, 0375T, 22551-22552, 22554, 22585, 22856, 63075-63076
    - Lumbar, 0163T-0164T, 0195T-0196T, 0309T, 22533, 22558, 22585, 22630, 22633-22634, 22857
    - Sacral, 0195T, 22586
    - Thoracic, 22532, 22534, 22556, 22585, 63077-63078
- Vertebra
    - Cervical, 22554
- Cervical, 22220
- Lumbar, 22224, 22630
- Percutaneous, 0274T-0275T
- Sacral, 0195T, 22586
- Thoracic, 22222
    - Additional Segment, 22226

Discharge, Body Substance
- *See* Drainage

Discharge Instructions
- Heart Failure, 4014F

Discharge Services
- *See* Hospital Services
- Hospital, 99238, 99239
- Newborn, 99463
- Nursing Facility, 99315, 99316
- Observation Care, 99217, 99234-99236

Disc, Intervertebral
- *See* Intervertebral Disc

Discission
- Cataract
    - Laser Surgery, 66821
    - Stab Incision, 66820
- Hyaloid Membrane, 65810
- Vitreous Strands, 67030

ECLS (Extracorporeal Life Support Services) —
continued
  Cannulization — *continued*
    Removal, *[33965, 33966, 33969, 33984, 33985, 33986]*
    Repositioning, 33957-33959 *[33962, 33963, 33964]*
  Creation Graft Conduit, *[33987]*
  Daily Management, 33948-33949
  Initiation, 33946-33947
  Left Heart Vent Insertion, *[33988]*
  Left Heart Vent Removal, *[33989]*
ECMO (Extracorporeal Membrane Oxygenation)
  Cannulization
    Insertion, 33951-33956
    Isolated with Chemotherapy Perfusion, 36823
    Removal, *[33965, 33966, 33969, 33984, 33985, 33986]*
    Repositioning, 33957-33959 *[33962, 33963, 33964]*
  Creation Graft Conduit, *[33987]*
  Daily Management, 33948-33949
  Initiation, 33946-33947
  Left Heart Vent Insertion, *[33988]*
  Left Heart Vent Removal, *[33989]*
ECS
  See Emission Computerized Tomography
ECSF (Erythrocyte Colony Stimulating Factor)
  See Erythropoietin
ECT (Emission Computerized Tomography), 78607
ECT (Electroconvulsive Therapy), 90870
Ectasia
  See Dilation
Ectopic Pregnancy
  See Obstetrical Care
  Abdominal, 59130
  Cervix, 59140
  Interstitial
    Partial Resection Uterus, 59136
    Total Hysterectomy, 59135
  Laparoscopy, 59150
    with Salpingectomy and/or Oophorectomy, 59151
  Ovarian
    with Salpingectomy and/or Oophorectomy, 59120
    without Salpingectomy and/or Oophorectomy, 59121
  Tubal
    with Salpingectomy and/or Oophorectomy, 59120
    without Salpingectomy and/or Oophorectomy, 59121
  Uterine
    with Hysterectomy, 59135
    with Partial Uterine Resection, 59136
Ectropion
  Repair
    Blepharoplasty
      Excision Tarsal Wedge, 67916
      Extensive, 67917
    Suture, 67914
    Thermocauterization, 67915
ED, 99281-99288
Education, 99078
  Patient
    Heart Failure, 4003F
    Pediatric Gastroenteritis to Caregiver, 4058F
    Self-management by Nonphysician, 98960-98962
  Services (Group), 99078
  Supplies, 99071
EEG, 95812-95827, 95830, 95950-95953, 95955-95958
  See also Electroencephalography
EFHC1, 81406
EGD, 43235-43255 *[43233]*, 43257, 43259, *[43233]*, *[43266]*, *[43270]*
EGFR, 81235
Egg
  See Ova
Eggers Procedure, 27100
EGR2, 81404

Ehrlichia, 86666
EIF2B2, 81405
EIF2B3, 81405-81406
EIF2B4, 81406
EIF2B5, 81406
EKG, 93000-93010
  64-Lead or Greater, 0178T-0180T
  External, 0295T-0298T, 93224-93272
  Rhythm Strips, 93040-93042
  Routine, 93000-93010
  Signal Averaged, 93278
Elastase, 82656
Elastography
  Liver, 91200
  Ultrasound, 0346T
Elbow
  See Humerus; Radius; Ulna
  Abscess
    Incision and Drainage, 23930, 23935
  Anesthesia, 00400, 01710-01782
  Arthrectomy, 24155
  Arthrocentesis, 20605-20606
  Arthrodesis, 24800, 24802
  Arthrography, 73085
    Contrast Injection, 24220
  Arthroplasty, 24360
    with Implant, 24361-24362
    Removal Prosthesis, 24160, 24164
    Revision, 24370-24371
    Total Replacement, 24363
  Arthroscopy
    Diagnostic, 29830
    Surgical, 29834-29838
  Arthrotomy, 24000
    with Joint Exploration, 24000, 24101
    with Synovectomy, 24102
    with Synovial Biopsy, 24100, 29830
    Capsular Release, 24006
    Drainage, 24000
    Foreign Body Removal, 24000
  Biopsy, 24065-24066, 24101
  Bone Cortex Incision, 23935
  Bursa
    Incision and Drainage, 23931
  Capsule
    Excision, 24006
    Radical Resection, 24149
  Contracture Release, 24149
  Dislocation
    Closed Treatment, 24600, 24605, 24640
    Nursemaid Elbow, 24640
    Open Treatment, 24615
    Partial, 24640
    Subluxate, 24640
  Epicondylitis
    Debridement, 24358-24359
    Percutaneous, 24357
  Excision, 24155
    Bursa, 24105
    Synovium, 24102, 29835-29836
    Tumor
      Soft Tissue, 24077-24079
      Subcutaneous, 24075, *[24071]*
      Subfascial, 24076, *[24073]*
  Exploration, 24000-24101 *[24071, 24073]*
  Fracture
    Monteggia, 24620, 24635
    Open Treatment, 24586, 24587
  Hematoma
    Incision and Drainage, 23930
  Incision and Drainage
    Abscess, Deep, 23930
    Bursa, 23931
    Hematoma, 23930
  Injection
    Arthrography (Radiologic), 24220
  Magnetic Resonance Imaging (MRI), 73221
  Manipulation, 24300
  Prosthesis
    Removal, 24160-24164
  Radical Resection
    Bone Tumor, 24150, 24152
    Capsule, Soft Tissue and Bone with Contracture Release, 24149
    Soft Tissue Tumor, 24077-24079

Elbow — *continued*
  Removal
    Foreign Body, 24000, 24101, 24200, 24201, 29834
    Implant, 24160-24164
    Loose Body, 24101, 29834
    Prosthesis, 24160
  Repair
    Advancement, 24330-24331
    Epicondylitis, 24357-24359
    Fasciotomy, 24357-24359
    Flexorplasty, 24330
    Graft, 24320
    Hemiepiphyseal Arrest, 24470
    Ligament, 24343-24346
    Muscle, 24341
    Muscle Transfer, 24301, 24320
    Tendon, 24340-24342
      Lengthening, 24305
      Release
        Debridement, 24358-24359
        Percutaneous, 24357
        Repair, 24359
      Repair, 24341, 24359
      Tenodesis, 24340
      Tenotomy, 24310, 24357-24359
    Tennis Elbow, 24357-24359
    Seddon-Brookes Procedure, 24320
    Steindler Advancement, 24330
  Strapping, 29260
  Tenotomy, 24357-24359
  Tumor
    Excision, 24075-24076 *[24071]*
    Radical Resection, 24077-24079
  Ulnar Neuroplasty, 64718
  Unlisted Services and Procedures, 24999
  X-ray, 73070, 73080
    with Contrast, 73085
Elbow, Golfer, 24357-24359
Elbow, Tennis, 24357-24359
Electrical Stimulation
  Acupuncture, 97813-97814
  Bone Healing
    Invasive, 20975
    Noninvasive, 20974
  Brain Surface, 95961, 95962
  Cardiac, 93623
    Induction of Arrhythmia, 93618
  Guidance
    Chemodenervation, 95873
  Physical Therapy
    Attended, Manual, 97032
    Unattended, 97014
  Spine, 63650, 63655, 63661-63664, 63685, 63688
Electric Countershock
  See Cardioversion
Electric Modulation Pain Reprocessing
  Transcutaneous, 0278T
Electrocardiogram, 93000-93010
  64-Lead or Greater, 0178T-0180T
  See Electrocardiography
  External, 0295T-0298T, 93224-93272
  Rhythm Strips, 93040-93042
    with Interpretation and Report, 93040
    Interpretation and Report Only, 93042
    Tracing Only Without Interpretation and Report, 93041
  Routine 12-Lead, 93000-93010
  Signal-Averaged, 93278
Electrocardiography
  12-Lead ECG, 3120F, 93000
  24–hour Monitoring, 93224-93272
  48 Hours up to 21 Days, 0295T-0298T
  64 Leads or Greater, 0178T-0180T
    with Interpretation and Report, 0178T
    Interpretation and Report Only, 0180T
    Tracing and Graphics Only without Interpretation and Report, 0179T
  Evaluation, 0178T-0180T, 93000, 93010
  Event Monitors, 93268-93272
  External Recording
    48-Hours Duration, 93224-93229
    Auto Activated, 93268, 93270-93272
    Interpretation, 0295T, 0298T, 93272

Electrocardiography — *continued*
  External Recording — *continued*
    Mobile
      Greater than 24 Hours, 93228-93229
      Patient Activated, 93268, 93270-93272
      Transmission and Evaluation, 93268, 93270-93271
      Up to 30 Days Download, 93268, 93270-93272
    Holter Monitors, 93224-93227
    Microvolt T-Wave Alternans, 93025
    Mobile Telemetry, 93228-93229
    Monitoring
      with Attended Surveillance
        Cardiovascular Telemetry with Physician Review and Report, 93228
        Technical Support, 93229
    Recording, 93224-93272
    Rhythm, 93040
      1-3 Leads, 93040
      Evaluation, 93042
      Interpretation and Report Only, 93042
      Microvolt T-Wave Alternans, 93025
      Recording, 0295T-0296T
      Scanning Analysis with Report, 0295T, 0297T
      Tracing and Evaluation, 93040
      Tracing Only without Interpretation and Report, 93005, 93041
    Routine; at Least 12 Leads, 93000-93010
      with Interpretation and Report, 93000
      Interpretation and Report Only, 93010
      Tracing Only, without Interpretation and Report, 93005
    Signal Averaged, 93278
    Symptom-Related Memory Loop, 93268, 93270-93272
    Tracing, 93005
Electrocautery, 17000-17286
  See Destruction
  Inferior Turbinates, 30801-30802
  Prostate Resection, 52601
  Ureteral Stricture, 52341-52346
Electrochemistry
  See Electrolysis
Electroconvulsive Therapy, 90870
Electrocorticogram
  Intraoperative, 61536, 61538, 95829
Electrode
  Array
    Intracranial, 61850-61868, 61885-61886, 64568-64570
    Peripheral Nerve, 64555, 64575
    Retinal, 0100T
    Spinal, 63650-63655
  Depth Electrode Implantation, 61760
Electrodesiccation, 17000-17286
  Lesion
    Penis, 54055
Electroejaculation, 55870
Electroencephalography (EEG)
  Brain Death, 95824
  Coma, 95822
  Digital Analysis, 95957
  Electrode Placement, 95830
  Intraoperative, 95955
  Monitoring, 95812, 95813, 95950-95953, 95956
    with Drug Activation, 95954
    with Physical Activation, 95954
    with WADA Activation, 95958
  Sleep, 95819, 95822, 95827
  Standard, 95816, 95819
Electrogastrography, 91132, 91133
Electrogram, Atrial
  Esophageal Recording, 93615, 93616
Electro–Hydraulic Procedure, 52325
Electrolysis, 17380
Electromyographs
  See Electromyography, Needle
Electromyography
  Anus
    Biofeedback, 90911
  Extremity, 95860-95872 *[95885, 95886]*
  Fine Wire, 96004
    Dynamic, 96004
  Guidance, 95874

Electromyography — *continued*
    Guidance — *continued*
        Chemodenervation, 95874
        Hemidiaphragm, 95866
    Larynx, 95865
    Needle
        Extremities, 95861-95872 *[95885, 95886, 95887]*
        Extremity, 95860
        Face and Neck Muscles, 95867, 95868
        Guidance
            Chemodenervation, 64617, 95874
            Hemidiaphragm, 95866
            Larynx, 95865
            Muscle Supplied by Cranial Nerve, 95867-95868
            Non-extremity, *[95887]*
            Ocular, 92265
            Other than Thoracic Paraspinal, 95870
            Single Fiber Electrode, 95872
            Thoracic Paraspinal Muscles, 95869
    Nonextremity, *[95887]*
    Rectum
        Biofeedback, 90911
    Sphincter Muscles
        Anus, 51784-51785
            Needle, 51785
        Urethra, 51784, 51785
            Needle, 51785
    Surface
        Dynamic, 96002-96004
Electronic Analysis
    Cardioverter-Defibrillator
        with Reprogramming, 93282-93284, 93287, 93642, 93644
        without Reprogramming, 93289, 93292, 93295, 93640-93641
        Evaluation
            in Person, 93289, 93640, 93642
            Remote, 93295-93296
    Data Analysis, 93289
    Defibrillator, 93282, 93289, 93292, 93295
    Drug Infusion Pump, 62367-62370, 95990-95991
    Loop Recorder System Implantable, 93285, 93291, 93298
        Data Analysis, 93291, 93298-93299
        Evaluation of Programming, 93285, 93291, 93298-93299
    Neurostimulator Pulse Generator, 95970-95975, 95978-95982
    Pulse Generator, 95970-95979
        Field Stimulation, 0285T
        Gastric Neurostimulator, 95980-95982
Electron Microscopy, 88348
Electro-oculography, 92270
Electrophoresis
    Counterimmuno-, 86185
    Hemoglobin, 83020
    High Resolution, 83701
    Immuno-, 86320-86327
    Immunofixation, 86334-86335
    Protein, 84165-84166
    Unlisted Services and Procedures, 82664
Electrophysiology Procedure, 93600-93660
Electroretinography, 92275
Electrostimulation, Analgesic Cutaneous
    See Application, Neurostimulation
Electrosurgery
    Anal, 46924
    Penile, 54065
    Rectal Tumor, 45190
    Skin Lesion, 17000-17111, 17260-17286
    Skin Tags, 11200-11201
    Trichiasis
        Correction, 67825
    Vaginal, 57061, 57065
    Vulva, 56501, 56515
Electroversion, Cardiac
    See Cardioversion
Elevation, Scapula, Congenital
    See Sprengel's Deformity
Elliot Operation, 66130
    Excision, Lesion, Sclera, 66130
Eloesser Procedure, 32035, 32036
Eloesser Thoracoplasty, 32905

Embolectomy
    Aortoiliac Artery, 34151, 34201
    Axillary Artery, 34101
    Brachial Artery, 34101
    Carotid Artery, 34001
    Celiac Artery, 34151
    Femoral, 34201
    Iliac, 34151, 34201
    Innominate Artery, 34001-34101
    Mesentery Artery, 34151
    Peroneal Artery, 34203
    Popliteal Artery, 34201, 34203
    Pulmonary Artery, 33910-33916
    Radial Artery, 34111
    Renal Artery, 34151
    Subclavian Artery, 34001-34101
    Tibial Artery, 34203
    Ulnar Artery, 34111
Embolization
    Arterial (not hemorrhage or tumor), 37242
    Hemorrhage
        Arterial, 37244
        Venous, 37244
    Infarction, 37243
    Leiomyomata, 37243
    Lymphatic Extravasation, 37244
    Organ Ischemia, 37243
    Tumors, 37243
    Ureter, 50705
    Venous Malformations, 37241
Embryo
    Biopsy, 89290, 89291
    Carcinoembryonic Antigen, 82378
    Cryopreservation, 89258
    Cryopreserved
        Preparation/Thawing, 89352
    Culture, 89250
        with Co-Culture Oocyte, 89251
        Extended Culture, 89272
    Hatching
        Assisted Microtechnique, 89253
    Preparation for Transfer, 89255
    Storage, 89342
Embryo/Fetus Monitoring
    See Monitoring, Fetal
Embryo Implantation
    See Implantation
Embryonated Eggs
    Inoculation, 87250
Embryo Transfer
    In Vitro Fertilization, 58970, 58974, 58976
        Intrafallopian Transfer, 58976
        Intrauterine Transfer, 58974
        Preparation for Transfer, 89255
EMD, 81404-81405
Emergency Department Services, 99281-99288
    See Critical Care; Emergency Department
    Anesthesia, 99140
        in Office, 99058
    Physician Direction of Advanced Life Support, 99288
Emesis Induction, 99175
EMG (Electromyography, Needle), 51784, 51785, 92265, 95860-95872 *[95885, 95886, 95887]*
EMI Scan
    See CT Scan
Emission Computerized Tomography, 78607, 78647
Emission Computerized Tomography, Single-Photon
    See SPECT
EML4/ALK, 81401
Emmet Operation, 57720
Empyema
    Closure
        Chest Wall, 32810
        Empyemectomy, 32540
        Enucleation, 32540
        Thoracostomy, 32035, 32036, 32551
Empyemectomy, 32540
EMS, 99288
Encephalitis
    Antibody, 86651-86654
Encephalitis Virus Vaccine, 90738
Encephalocele
    Repair, 62120

Encephalocele — *continued*
    Repair — *continued*
        Craniotomy, 62121
Encephalography, A-Mode, 76506
Encephalon
    See Brain
Endarterectomy
    Coronary Artery, 33572
        Anomaly, 33500-33507
    Pulmonary, 33916
Endemic Flea-Borne Typhus
    See Murine Typhus
End-Expiratory Pressure, Positive
    See Pressure Breathing, Positive
Endobronchial Challenge Tests
    See Bronchial Challenge Test
Endocavitary Fulguration
    See Electrocautery
Endocrine, Pancreas
    See Islet Cell
Endocrine System
    Unlisted Services and Procedures, 60699, 78099
Endocrinology (Type 2 Diabetes) Biochemical Assays, 81506
Endolaser Photocoagulation
    Focal, 67039
    Panretinal, 67040
Endolymphatic Sac
    Exploration
        with Shunt, 69806
        without Shunt, 69805
Endometrial Ablation, 0404T, 58353, 58356, 58563
    Curettage, 58356
    Exploration via Hysteroscopy, 58563
Endometrioma
    Abdomen
        Destruction, 49203-49205
        Excision, 49203-49205
    Mesenteric
        Destruction, 49203-49205
        Excision, 49203-49205
    Peritoneal
        Destruction, 49203-49205
        Excision, 49203-49205
    Retroperitoneal
        Destruction, 49203-49205
        Excision, 49203-49205
Endometriosis, Adhesive
    See Adhesions, Intrauterine
Endometrium
    Ablation, 0404T, 58353, 58356, 58563
    Biopsy, 58100, 58110, 58558
    Curettage, 58356
Endomyocardial
    Biopsy, 93505
Endonuclease, DNA
    See DNAse
Endopyelotomy, 50575
Endorectal Pull-Through
    Proctectomy, Total, 45110, 45112, 45120, 45121
Endoscopic Retrograde Cannulation of Pancreatic Duct (ERCP)
    See Cholangiopancreatography
Endoscopic Retrograde Cholangiopancreatography
    with Optical Endomicroscopy, 0397T
    Ablation Lesion/Polyp/Tumor, *[43278]*
    Balloon Dilation, *[43277]*
    Destruction of Calculi, 43265
    Diagnostic, 43260
    Measure Pressure Sphincter of Oddi, 43263
    Placement
        Stent, *[43274]*
            with Removal and Replacement, *[43276]*
    Removal
        Calculi or Debris, 43264
        Foreign Body, *[43275]*
        Stent, *[43275]*
            with Stent Exchange, *[43276]*
    Removal Calculi or Debris, 43264
Endoscopies, Pleural
    See Thoracoscopy
Endoscopy
    See Arthroscopy; Thoracoscopy

Endoscopy — *continued*
    Adrenal Gland
        Biopsy, 60650
        Excision, 60650
    Anal
        Ablation
            Polyp, 46615
            Tumor, 46615
        Biopsy, 46606, 46607
        Collection of Specimen, 46600-46601
        Diagnostic, 46600-46601
        Dilation, 46604
        Exploration, 46600
        Hemorrhage, 46614
        High Resolution, 46601, 46607
        Removal
            Foreign Body, 46608
            Polyp, 46610, 46612
            Tumor, 46610, 46612
    Atria, 33265-33266
    Bile Duct
        Biopsy, 47553
        Cannulation, 43273
        Catheterization, 74328, 74330
        Destruction
            Calculi (Stone), 43265
            Tumor, *[43278]*
        Diagnostic, 47552
        Dilation, 47555, 47556, *[43277]*
        Exchange
            Stent, *[43276]*
        Exploration, 47552
        Intraoperative, 47550
        Percutaneous, 47552-47556
        Removal
            Calculi (Stone), 43264, 47554
            Foreign Body, *[43275]*
            Stent, *[43275]*
        Specimen Collection, 43260
        Sphincterotomy, 43262, *[43274]*
        Sphincter Pressure, 43263
        Stent Placement, *[43274]*
    Bladder
        Biopsy, 52204, 52250, 52354
        Catheterization, 52005, 52010
        Destruction, 52354
            with Fulguration, 52214
            Lesion, 52400
            Polyps, 52285
        Diagnostic, 52000
        Dilation, 52260, 52265
        Evacuation
            Clot, 52001
        Excision
            Tumor, 52355
        Exploration, 52351
        Insertion
            Radioactive Substance, 52250
            Stent, 52282, 53855
        Instillation, 52010
        Irrigation, 52010
        Lesion, 52224, 52234-52235, 52240, 52400
        Litholapaxy, 52317-52318
        Lithotripsy, 52353
        Neck, 51715
        Removal
            Calculus, 52310, 52315, 52352
            Urethral Stent, 52310, 52315
    Bladder Neck
        Injection of Implant Material, 51715
    Brain
        Catheterization, 62160
        Dissection
            Adhesions, 62161
            Cyst, 62162
        Drainage, 62162
        Excision
            Brain Tumor, 62164
            Cyst, 62162
            Pituitary Tumor, 62165
        Removal Foreign Body, 62163
        Shunt Creation, 62201
    Bronchi
        Aspiration, 31645-31646
        Biopsy, 31625, 31632, 31633
        Computer-assisted Image Guidance, 31627

CPT © 2015 American Medical Association. All Rights Reserved.

Excision — Excision

                                                       Heart

GRN, 81406
Groin Area
Repair
Hernia, 49550-49557
Gross Type Procedure, 49610, 49611
Group Health Education, 99078
Grouping, Blood
See Blood Typing
Growth Factors, Insulin–Like
See Somatomedin
Growth Hormone, 83003
with Arginine Tolerance Test, 80428
Human, 80418, 80428, 80430, 86277
Growth Hormone Release Inhibiting Factor
See Somatostatin
Growth Stimulation Expressed Gene, 83006
GTT, 82951, 82952
Guaiac Test
Blood in Feces, 82270
Guanylic Acids
See Guanosine Monophosphate
Guard Stain, 88313
Gullet
See Esophagus
Gums
Abscess
Incision and Drainage, 41800
Alveolus
Excision, 41830
Cyst
Incision and Drainage, 41800
Excision
Gingiva, 41820
Operculum, 41821
Graft
Mucosa, 41870
Hematoma
Incision and Drainage, 41800
Lesion
Destruction, 41850
Excision, 41822-41828
Mucosa
Excision, 41828
Reconstruction
Alveolus, 41874
Gingiva, 41872
Removal
Foreign Body, 41805
Tumor
Excision, 41825-41827
Unlisted Services and Procedures, 41899
Gunning–Lieben Test, 82009, 82010
Gunther Tulip Filter Insertion, 37191
Guthrie Test, 84030
GYPA, 81403
GYPB, 81403
GYPE, 81403

H

H19, 81401
HAA (Hepatitis Associated Antigen), 87340-87380, 87515-87527
See Hepatitis Antigen, B Surface
HAAb (Antibody, Hepatitis), 86708, 86709
HADHA, 81406
HADHB, 81406
Haemoglobin F
See Fetal Hemoglobin
Haemorrhage
See Hemorrhage
Haemorrhage Rectum
See Hemorrhage, Rectum
Hageman Factor, 85280
Clotting Factor, 85210-85293
Haglund's Deformity Repair, 28119
HAI (Hemagglutination Inhibition Test), 86280
Hair
Electrolysis, 17380
KOH Examination, 87220
Microscopic Evaluation, 96902
Transplant
Punch Graft, 15775, 15776
Strip Graft, 15220, 15221
Hair Removal
See Removal, Hair

Hallux
See Great Toe
Hallux Rigidus
Correction with Cheilectomy, 28289
Halo
Body Cast, 29000
Cranial, 20661
for Thin Skull Osteology, 20664
Femur, 20663
Maxillofacial, 21100
Pelvic, 20662
Removal, 20665
Haloperidol
Assay, 80173
Halstead-Reitan Neuropsychological Battery, 96118
Halsted Mastectomy, 19305
Halsted Repair
Hernia, 49495
Hammertoe Repair, 28285, 28286
Hamster Penetration Test, 89329
Ham Test
Hemolysins, 85475
with Agglutinins, 86940, 86941
Hand
See Carpometacarpal Joint; Intercarpal Joint
Abscess, 26034
Amputation
at Metacarpal, 25927
at Wrist, 25920
Revision, 25922
Revision, 25924, 25929, 25931
Arthrodesis
Carpometacarpal Joint, 26843, 26844
Intercarpal Joint, 25820, 25825
Bone
Incision and Drainage, 26034
Cast, 29085
Decompression, 26035, 26037
Dislocation
Carpal
Closed, 25690
Open, 25695
Carpometacarpal
Closed, 26670, 26675
Open, 26685-26686
Percutaneous, 26676
Interphalangeal
Closed, 26770, 26775
Open, 26785
Percutaneous, 26776
Lunate
Closed, 25690
Open, 25695
Metacarpalphalangeal
Closed, 26700-26705
Open, 26715
Percutaneous, 26706
Radiocarpal
Closed, 25660
Open, 25670
Thumb
See Dislocation Thumb
Wrist
See Dislocation, Wrist
Dupuytren's Contracture(s)
Fasciotomy
Open Partial, 26045
Percutaneous, 26040
Injection
Enzyme, 20527
Manipulation, 26341
Palmar Fascial Cord
Injection
Enzyme, 20527
Manipulation, 26341
Excision
Excess Skin, 15837
Fracture
Carpometacarpal, 26641-26650
Interphalangeal, 26740-26746
Metacarpal, 26600
Metacarpophalangeal, 26740-26746
Phalangeal, 26720-26735, 26750-26765
Implantation
Removal, 26320

Hand — continued
Implantation — continued
Removal — continued
Tube/Rod, 26392, 26416
Tube/Rod, 26390
Insertion
Tendon Graft, 26392
Magnetic Resonance Imaging (MRI), 73218-73223
Reconstruction
Tendon Pulley, 26500-26502
Removal
Implant, 26320
Repair
Blood Vessel, 35207
Cleft Hand, 26580
Muscle, 26591, 26593
Release, 26593
Tendon
Extensor, 26410-26416, 26426, 26428, 26433-26437
Flexor, 26350-26358, 26440
Profundus, 26370-26373
Replantation, 20808
Skin Graft
Delay of Flap, 15620
Full Thickness, 15240, 15241
Pedicle Flap, 15574
Split, 15100, 15101
Strapping, 29280
Tendon
Excision, 26390
Extensor, 26415
Tenotomy, 26450, 26460
Tissue Transfer, Adjacent, 14040, 14041
Tumor
Excision, 26115 [26111]
Radical Resection, 26116-26118 [26113], 26250
Unlisted Services and Procedures, 26989
X–ray, 73120, 73130
Handling
Device, 99002
Radioelement, 77790
Specimen, 99000, 99001
Hand Phalange
See Finger, Bone
Hanganutziu Deicher Antibodies
See Antibody, Heterophile
Haptoglobin, 83010, 83012
Hard Palate
See Palate
Harelip Operation
See Cleft Lip, Repair
Harrington Rod
Insertion, 22840
Removal, 22850
Hartley-Krause, 61450
Hartmann Procedure, 44143
Laparoscopy
Partial Colectomy with Colostomy, 44206
Open, 44143
Harvesting
Bone Graft, 20900, 20902
Bone Marrow
Allogeneic, 38230
Autologous, 38232
Cartilage, 20910, 20912
Conjunctival Graft, 68371
Eggs for In Vitro Fertilization, 58970
Endoscopic
Vein for Bypass Graft, 33508
Fascia Lata Graft, 20920, 20922
Intestines, 44132, 44133
Kidney, 50300, 50320, 50547
Liver, 47133, 47140-47142
Lower Extremity Vein for Vascular Reconstruction, 35572
Skin, 15040
Stem Cell, 38205, 38206
Tendon Graft, 20924
Tissue Grafts, 20926
Upper Extremity Artery
for Coronary Artery Bypass Graft, 35600
Upper Extremity Vein
for Bypass Graft, 35500

Hauser Procedure
Reconstruction, Patella, for Instability, 27420
HAVRIX, 90632-90634
Hayem's Elementary Corpuscle
See Blood, Platelet
Haygroves Procedure, 27120, 27122
HBA1/HBA2, 81257, 81404-81405
HBB, 81401, 81403-81404
Hb Bart Hydrops Fetalis Syndrome, 81257
HBcAb, 86704, 86705
HBeAb, 86707
HBeAg, 87350
HbH Disease, 81257
HBsAb, 86706
HBsAg (Hepatitis B Surface Antigen), 87340
HCG, 84702-84704
HCO3
See Bicarbonate
Hct, 85013, 85014
HCV Antibodies
See Antibody, Hepatitis C
HD, 27295
HDL (High Density Lipoprotein), 83718
Head
Angiography, 70496, 70544-70546
CT Scan, 70450-70470, 70496
Excision, 21015-21070
Fracture and/or Dislocation, 21310-21497
Incision, 21010, 61316, 62148
Introduction, 21076-21116
Lipectomy, Suction Assisted, 15876
Magnetic Resonance Angiography (MRA), 70544-70546
Nerve
Graft, 64885, 64886
Other Procedures, 21299, 21499
Repair
Revision and/or Reconstruction, 21120-21296
Ultrasound Examination, 76506, 76536
Unlisted Services and Procedures, 21499
X–ray, 70350
Head Brace
Application, 21100
Removal, 20661
Head Rings, Stereotactic
See Stereotactic Frame
Heaf Test
TB Test, 86580
Health Behavior
Alcohol and/or Substance Abuse, 99408-99409
Assessment, 96150
Family Intervention, 96154-96155
Group Intervention, 0403T, 96153
Individual Intervention, 96152
Re-assessment, 96151
Smoking and Tobacco Cessation, 99406-99407
Health Risk Assessment Instrument, 99420
Hearing Aid
Bone Conduction
Implant, 69710
Removal, 69711
Repair, 69711
Replace, 69710
Check, 92592, 92593
Hearing Aid Services
Electroacoustic Test, 92594, 92595
Examination, 92590, 92591
Hearing Tests
See Audiologic Function Tests; Hearing Evaluation
Hearing Therapy, 92507, 92601-92604
Heart
Ablation
Arrhythmogenic Focus
Intracardiac Catheter, 93650-93657
Open, 33250-33261
Ventricular Septum
Transcatheter Alcohol Septal Ablation, 93583
Acoustic Cardiography with Computer Analysis, 93799
Allograft Preparation, 33933, 33944
Angiography, 93454-93461
Injection, 93563-93568

[Resequenced]

INS, 81404

Insemination
Artificial, 58321, 58322, 89268

Insertion
See Implantation; Intubation; Transplantation
Aqueous Drainage Device, 0191T, 66179-66185
Balloon
Intra–Aortic, 33967, 33973
Breast
Implants, 19340, 19342
Cannula
Arteriovenous, 36810, 36815
Extracorporeal Circulation for Regional Chemotherapy of Extremity, 36823
Thoracic Duct, 38794
Vein to Vein, 36800
Catheter
Abdomen, 49324, 49419-49421, 49435
Abdominal Artery, 36245-36248
Aorta, 36200
Bile Duct
Percutaneous, 47533-47536
Bladder, 51045, 51701-51703
Brachiocephalic Artery, 36215-36218
Brain, 0169T, 61210, 61770
Breast
for Interstitial Radioelement Application, 19296-19298, 20555
Bronchi, 31717
Bronchus
for Intracavitary Radioelement Application, 31643
Cardiac
See Catheterization, Cardiac
Flow Directed, 93503
Dialysis, 49421
Flow Directed, 93503
Gastrointestinal, Upper, 43241
Head and/or Neck, 41019
Intraperitoneal, 49418
Jejunum, 44015
Lower Extremity Artery, 36245-36248
Nasotracheal, 31720
Pelvic Artery, 36245-36248
Pelvic Organs and/or Genitalia, 55920
Pleural Cavity, 32550
Portal Vein, 36481
Prostate, 55875
Pulmonary Artery, 36013-36015
Renal Artery, 36251-36254
Right Heart, 36013
Skull, 61107
Spinal Cord, 62350, 62351
Suprapubic, 51102
Thoracic Artery, 36215-36218
Tracheobronchial, 31725
Transthoracic, 33621
Urethra, 51701-51703
Vena Cava, 36010
Venous, 36011, 36012, 36400-36425, 36500, 36510, 36555-36558, 36568-36569
Cecostomy Tube, 49442
Cervical Dilator, 59200
Cochlear Device, 69930
Colonic Tube, 49442
Defibrillator
Heart, 33212, 33213
Leads, 33216, 33217
Pulse Generator Only, 33240
Drug Delivery Implant, 11981, 11983
Drug-Eluting Implant Lacrimal Canaliculus, 0356T
Electrode
Brain, 61531, 61533, 61760, 61850-61870
Heart, 33202-33203, 33210-33217 *[33221]*, 33224-33225, 93620-93622
Nerve, 64553-64581
Retina, 0100T
Sphenoidal, 95830
Spinal Cord, 63650, 63655
Stomach
Laparoscopic
Gastric neurostimulator, 43647

Insertion — *continued*
Electrode — *continued*
Stomach — *continued*
Open
Gastric neurostimulator
Antrum, 43881
Lesser curvature, 43999
Endotracheal Tube
Emergency Intubation, 31500
Filiform
Urethra, 53620
Gastrostomy Tube
Laparoscopic, 43653
Percutaneous, 43246, 49440
Graft
Aorta, 33330-33335
Heart Vessel, 33330-33335
Guide
Kidney, Pelvis, 50395
Guide Wire
Endoscopy, 43248
Esophagoscopy, 43248
with Dilation, 43226
Hemodynamic Monitor, 0293T-0294T
Heyman Capsule
Uterus
for Brachytherapy, 58346
Iliac Artery
Occlusion Device, 34808
Implant
Bone
for External Speech Processor/Cochlear Stimulator, 69714-69718
Implantable Defibrillator
Leads, 33216-33220, 33224-33225
Pulse Generator Only, 33240 *[33230, 33231]*
Infusion Pump
Intraarterial, 36260
Intravenous, 36563
Spinal Cord, 62361, 62362
Intracardiac Ischemia Monitoring System, 0302T
Device Only, 0304T
Electrode Only, 0303T
Intracatheter/Needle
Aorta, 36160
Arteriovenous Shunt, 36147-36148
Intraarterial, 36100-36140
Intravenous, 36000
Venous, 36000
Intraocular Lens, 66983
Manual or Mechanical Technique, 66982, 66984
Not Associated with Concurrent Cataract Removal, 66985
Intrauterine Device (IUD), 58300
Ischemia Monitoring System, 0302T
IVC Filter, 37191
Jejunostomy Tube
Endoscopy, 44372
Percutaneous, 49441
Keel
Laryngoplasty, 31580
Laminaria, 59200
Localization device soft tissue, 10035-10036
Mesh
Pelvic Floor, 57267
Needle
Bone, 36680
Head and/or Neck, 41019
Intraosseous, 36680
Pelvic Organs and/or Genitalia, 55920
Prostate, 55875
Needle Wire Dilator
Stent
Trachea, 31730
Transtracheal for Oxygen, 31720
Neurostimulator
Pulse Generator, 64590
Receiver, 64590
Nose
Septal Prosthesis, 30220
Obturator/Larynx, 31527
Ocular Implant
with Foreign Material, 65155
with or without Conjunctival Graft, 65150
in Scleral Shell, 65130, 67550
Muscles Attached, 65140

Insertion — *continued*
Ocular Implant — *continued*
Muscles Not Attached, 65135
Telescope Prosthesis, 0308T
Orbital Transplant, 67550
Oviduct
Chromotubation, 58350
Hydrotubation, 58350
Ovoid
Vagina
for Brachytherapy, 57155
Pacemaker
Heart, 33206-33208, 33212, 33213, *[33221]*
Packing
Vagina, 57180
Penile Prosthesis Inflatable
See Penile Prosthesis, Insertion, Inflatable
Pessary
Vagina, 57160
PICC Line, 36568-36569
Pin
Skeletal Traction, 20650
Port, 49419
Posterior Spinous Process Distraction Devices, 0171T-0172T
Probe
Brain, 61770
Prostaglandin, 59200
Prostate
Radioactive Substance, 55860
Transprostatic Implant, 52441-52442
Prosthesis
Knee, 27438, 27445
Nasal Septal, 30220
Palate, 42281
Pelvic Floor, 57267
Penis
Inflatable, 54401-54405
Non–inflatable, 54400
Speech, 31611
Testis, 54660
Urethral Sphincter, 53444-53445
Pulse Generator
Brain, 61885, 61886
Heart, 33212, 33213
Spinal Cord, 63685
Radiation Afterloading Apparatus, 57156
Radioactive Material
Bladder, 51020
Cystourethroscopy, 52250
High Dose Electronic Brachytherapy, 0394T-0395T
Interstitial Brachytherapy, 77770-77772
Intracavitary Brachytherapy, 77761-77763, 77770-77772
Intraocular, 0190T
Prostate, 55860, 55875
Remote Afterloading Brachytherapy, 77767-77768, 77770-77772
Receiver
Brain, 61885, 61886
Spinal Cord, 63685
Reservoir
Brain, 61210, 61215
Spinal Cord, 62360
Shunt, 36835
Abdomen
Vein, 49425
Venous, 49426
Intrahepatic Portosystemic, 37182
Spinal Instrument, 22849
Spinous Process, 0171T-0172T, 22841
Spinal Instrumentation
Anterior, 22845-22847
Internal Spinal Fixation, 22841
Pelvic Fixation, 22848
Posterior Non–segmental
Harrington Rod Technique, 22840
Posterior Segmental, 22842-22844
Prosthetic Device, 22851
Stent
Bile Duct, 47801, *[43274]*
Bladder, 51045
Conjunctiva, 68750
Esophagus, *[43212]*
Gastrointestinal, Upper, *[43266]*

Insertion — *continued*
Stent — *continued*
Indwelling, 50605
Lacrimal Canaliculus, Drug-Eluting, 0356T
Lacrimal Duct, 68810-68815
Pancreatic Duct, *[43274]*
Small Intestines, 44370, 44379
Ureteral, 50688, 50693-50695, 50947, 52332
Urethral, 52282, 53855
Tamponade
Esophagus, 43460
Tandem
Uterus
for Brachytherapy, 57155
Tendon Graft
Finger, 26392
Hand, 26392
Testicular Prosthesis
See Prosthesis, Testicular, Insertion
Tissue Expanders, Skin, 11960-11971
Tube
Cecostomy, 49442
Duodenostomy or Jejunostomy, 49441
Esophagus, 43510
Gastrointestinal, Upper, 43241
Gastrostomy, 49440
Small Intestines, 44379
Trachea, 31730
Ureter, 50688, 50693-50695
Urethral
Catheter, 51701-51703
Guide Wire, 52344
Implant Material, 51715
Suppository, 53660-53661
Vascular Pedicle
Carpal Bone, 25430
Venous Access Device
Central, 36560-36566
Peripheral, 36570, 36571
Venous Shunt
Abdomen, 49425
Ventilating Tube, 69433
Ventricular Assist Device, 33975
Wire
Skeletal Traction, 20650

In Situ Hybridization
See Nucleic Acid Probe, Cytogenic Studies, Morphometric Analysis

Inspiratory Positive Pressure Breathing
See Intermittent Positive Pressure Breathing (IPPB)

Instillation
Agent for Pleurodesis, 32560-32562
Drugs
Bladder, 51720
Kidney, 50391
Ureter, 50391

Instillation, Bladder
See Bladder, Instillation

Instrumentation
See Application; Bone; Fixation; Spinal Instrumentation
Spinal
Insertion, 22840-22848, 22851
Reinsertion, 22849
Removal, 22850, 22852, 22855

Insufflation, Eustachian Tube
See Eustachian Tube, Inflation

Insulin, 80422, 80432-80435
Antibody, 86337
Blood, 83525
Free, 83527

Insulin C–Peptide Measurement
See C–Peptide

Insulin Like Growth Factors
See Somatomedin

Insurance
Basic Life and/or Disability Evaluation Services, 99450
Examination, 99450-99456

Integumentary System
Ablation
Breast, 19105
Biopsy, 11100, 11101

Integumentary System — continued

Breast
Ablation, 19105
Excision, 19100-19272
Incision, 19000-19030
Localization Device, 19281-19288
with Biopsy, 19081-19086
Reconstruction, 19316-19396
Repair, 19316-19396
Unlisted Services and Procedures, 19499
Burns, 15002-15003, 15005, 16000-16036
Debridement, 11000-11006, 11010-11044
[11045, 11046]
Destruction
See Dermatology
Actinotherapy, 96900
Benign Lesion, 17000-17004
by Photodynamic Therapy, 96567
Chemical Exfoliation, 17360
Cryotherapy, 17340
Electrolysis Epilation, 17380
Malignant Lesion, 17260-17286
by Photodynamic Therapy, 96567
Mohs Micrographic Surgery, 17311-17315
Photodynamic Therapy, 96567, 96570, 96571
Premalignant Lesion, 17000-17004
Unlisted Services and Procedures, 17999
Drainage, 10040-10180
Excision
Benign Lesion, 11400-11471
Debridement, 11000-11006, 11010-11044
[11045, 11046]
Malignant Lesion, 11600-11646
Graft, 14000-14350, 15002-15278
Autograft, 15040-15157
Skin Substitute, 15271-15278
Surgical Preparation, 15002-15005
Tissue Transfer or Rearrangement, 14000-14350
Implantation Biologic Implant, 15777
Incision, 10040-10180
Introduction
Drug Delivery Implant, 11981, 11983
Nails, 11719-11765
Paring, 11055-11057
Photography, 96904
Pressure Ulcers, 15920-15999
Removal
Drug Delivery Implant, 11982, 11983
Repair
Adjacent Tissue Transfer
Rearrangement, 14000-14350
Complex, 13100-13160
Flaps, 15740-15776
Free Skin Grafts, 15002-15005, 15050-15136, 15200-15261
Implantation Acellular Dermal Matrix, 15777
Intermediate, 12031-12057
Other Procedures, 15780-15879
Simple, 12001-12021
Skin and/or Deep Tissue, 15570-15738
Skin Substitute, 15271-15278
Shaving of Epidermal or Dermal Lesion, 11300-11313
Skin Tags
Removal, 11200, 11201

Integumentum Commune
See Integumentary System

Intelligence Test
Computer-Assisted, 96103
Psychiatric Diagnosis, Psychological Testing, 96101-96103

Intensity Modulated Radiation Therapy (IMRT)
Complex, [77386]
Plan, 77301
Simple, [77385]

Intensive Care
Low Birth Weight Infant, 99478-99479
Neonatal
Initial Care, 99479
Subsequent Care, 99478

Intercarpal Joint
Arthrodesis, 25820, 25825

Intercarpal Joint — continued

Dislocation
Closed Treatment, 25660
Repair, 25447

Intercostal Nerve
Destruction, 64620
Injection
Anesthetic, 64420, 64421
Neurolytic Agent, 64620

Intercranial Arterial Perfusion
Thrombolysis, 61624

Interdental Fixation
without Fracture, 21497
Device
Application, 21110
Mandibular Fracture
Closed Treatment, 21453
Open Treatment, 21462

Interdental Papilla
See Gums

Interdental Wire Fixation
Closed Treatment
Craniofacial Separation, 21431

Interferometry
Eye
Biometry, 92136

Intermediate Care Facility (ICF) Visits, 99304-99318

Intermittent Positive Pressure Breathing (IPPB)
See Continuous Negative Pressure Breathing (CNPB); Continuous Positive Airway Pressure (CPAP)

Internal Breast Prostheses
See Breast, Implants

Internal Ear
See Ear, Inner

Internal Rigid Fixation
Reconstruction
Mandibular Rami, 21196

International Normalized Ratio
Test Review, 99363-99364

Internet E/M Service
Nonphysician, 98969
Physician, 99444

Interphalangeal Joint
Arthrodesis, 26860-26863
Arthroplasty, 26535, 26536
Arthrotomy, 26080, 28054
Biopsy
Synovium, 26110
Capsule
Excision, 26525
Incision, 26525
Dislocation
with Manipulation, 26340
Closed Treatment, 26770
Fingers/Hand
with Manipulation, 26340
Closed Treatment, 26770, 26775
Open Treatment, 26785
Percutaneous Fixation, 26776
Open Treatment, 26785
Percutaneous Fixation, 26776
Toes/Foot
Closed Treatment, 28660, 28665
Open Treatment, 28675
Percutaneous Fixation, 28666
Excision, 28160
Exploration, 26080, 28024
Fracture
with Manipulation, 26742
Closed Treatment, 26740
Open Treatment, 26746
Fusion, 26860-26863
Great Toe
Arthrodesis, 28755
with Tendon Transfer, 28760
Fusion, 28755
with Tendon Transfer, 28760
Removal
Foreign Body, 26080
Loose Body, 28024
Repair
Collateral Ligament, 26545
Volar Plate, 26548
Synovectomy, 26140

Interphalangeal Joint — continued

Synovial
Biopsy, 28054
Toe, 28272
Arthrotomy, 28024
Biopsy
Synovial, 28054
Dislocation, 28660-28665, 28675
Percutaneous Fixation, 28666
Excision, 28160
Exploration, 28024
Removal
Foreign Body, 28024
Loose Body, 28024
Synovial
Biopsy, 28054

Interrogation
Cardio-Defibrillator, 93289, 93292, 93295
Cardiovascular Monitoring System, 93290, 93297, 93299
Carotid Sinus Baroreflex Activation Device, 0272T-0273T
Intracardiac Ischemia Monitoring System, 0306T
Loop Recorder, 93291, 93298-93299
Pacemaker, 93288, 93294, 93296
Ventricular Assist Device, 93750

Interruption
Vein
Femoral, 37650
Iliac, 37660

Intersex State
Clitoroplasty, 56805
Vaginoplasty, 57335

Intersex Surgery
Female to Male, 55980
Male to Female, 55970

Interstitial Cell Stimulating Hormone
See Luteinizing Hormone (LH)
Cystitides, Chronic
See Cystitis, Interstitial
Cystitis
See Cystitis, Interstitial
Fluid Pressure
Monitoring, 20950

Intertarsal Joint
Arthrotomy, 28020, 28050
Biopsy
Synovial, 28050
Exploration, 28020
Removal
Foreign Body, 28020
Loose Body, 28020
Synovial
Biopsy, 28050
Excision, 28070

Interthoracoscapular Amputation
See Amputation, Interthoracoscapular

Intertrochanteric Femur Fracture
See Femur, Fracture, Intertrochanteric

Intervertebral Chemonucleolysis
See Chemonucleolysis

Intervertebral Disc
Annuloplasty, 22526-22527
Arthroplasty
Cervical Interspace, 22856
Each Additional Interspace, 0375T, [22858]
Lumbar Interspace, 0163T, 22857-22865
Removal, 0095T, 0164T
Removal, 0095T
Revision, 0098T, 0165T
Discography
Cervical, 72285
Lumbar, 72295
Thoracic, 72285
Excision
Decompression, 63075-63078
Herniated, 63020-63044, 63055-63066
Injection
Chemonucleolysis Agent, 62292
X-ray, 62290, 62291
X-ray with Contrast
Cervical, 72285
Lumbar, 72295

Intestinal Anastomosis
See Anastomosis, Intestines

Intestinal Invagination
See Intussusception

Intestinal Peptide, Vasoconstrictive
See Vasoactive Intestinal Peptide

Intestine(s)
Allotransplantation, 44135, 44136
Removal, 44137
Anastomosis, 44625, 44626
Laparoscopic, 44227
Biopsy, 44100
Closure
Enterostomy
Large or Small, 44625, 44626
Stoma, 44620, 44625
Excision
Donor, 44132, 44133
Exclusion, 44700
Laparoscopic Resection with Anastomosis, 44202, 44203, 44207, 44208
Lesion
Excision, 44110, 44111
Lysis of Adhesions
Laparoscopic, 44180
Nuclear Medicine
Imaging, 78290
Reconstruction
Bladder, 50820
Colonic Reservoir, 45119
Repair
Diverticula, 44605
Obstruction, 44615
Ulcer, 44605
Wound, 44605
Resection, 44227
Suture
Diverticula, 44605
Stoma, 44620, 44625
Ulcer, 44605
Wound, 44605
Transplantation
Allograft Preparation, 44715-44721
Donor Enterectomy, 44132, 44133
Removal of Allograft, 44137
Unlisted Laparoscopic Procedure, 44238

Intestines, Large
See Anus; Cecum; Colon; Rectum

Intestines, Small
Anastomosis, 43845, 44130
Biopsy, 44020, 44100
Endoscopy, 44361
Catheterization
Jejunum, 44015
Closure
Stoma, 44620, 44625
Decompression, 44021
Destruction
Lesion, 44369
Tumor, 44369
Endoscopy, 44360
Biopsy, 44361, 44377
Control of Bleeding, 44366, 44378
via Stoma, 44382
Destruction
Lesion, 44369
Tumor, 44369
Diagnostic, 44376
Exploration, 44360
Hemorrhage, 44366
Insertion
Stent, 44370, 44379
Tube, 44379
Pelvic Pouch, 44385, 44386
Place Tube, 44372
Removal
Foreign Body, 44363
Lesion, 44365
Polyp, 44364, 44365
Tumor, 44364, 44365
Tube Placement, 44372
Tube Revision, 44373
via Stoma, 44380-44384 [44381]
Enterostomy, 44620-44626
Tube Placement, 44300
Excision, 44120-44128
Partial with Anastomosis, 44140
Exclusion, 44700

Lung — *continued*
Decortication — *continued*
Endoscopic, 32651, 32652
Partial, 32225
Total, 32220
Empyema
Excision, 32540
Excision
Bronchus Resection, 32486
Completion, 32488
Donor, 33930
Heart Lung, 33930
Lung, 32850
Emphysematous, 32491
Empyema, 32540
Lobe, 32480, 32482
Segment, 32484
Total, 32440-32445
Tumor, 32503-32504
Wedge Resection, 32505-32507
Endoscopic, 32666-32668
Foreign Body
Removal, 32151
Hemorrhage, 32110
Injection
Radiologic, 93568
Lavage
Bronchial, 31624
Total, 32997
Lysis
Adhesions, 32124
Needle Biopsy, 32405
Nuclear Medicine
Imaging, Perfusion, 78580-78598
Imaging, Ventilation, 78579, 78582, 78598
Unlisted Services and Procedures, 78599
Pneumolysis, 32940
Pneumothorax, 32960
Removal
Bilobectomy, 32482
Bronchoplasty, 32501
Completion Pneumonectomy, 32488
Extrapleural, 32445
Single Lobe, 32480
Single Segment, 32484
Sleeve Lobectomy, 32486
Sleeve Pneumonectomy, 32442
Total Pneumonectomy, 32440-32445
Two Lobes, 32482
Volume Reduction, 32491
Wedge Resection, 32505-32507
Repair
Hernia, 32800
Segmentectomy, 32484
Tear
Repair, 32110
Thoracotomy, 32110-32160
with Excision–Plication of Bullae, 32141
with Open Intrapleural Pneumonolysis, 32124
Biopsy, 32096-32098
Cardiac Massage, 32160
for Post–Operative Complications, 32120
Removal
Bullae, 32141
Cyst, 32140
Intrapleural Foreign Body, 32150
Intrapulmonary Foreign Body, 32151
Repair, 32110
Transplantation, 32851-32854, 33935
Allograft Preparation, 32855-32856, 33933
Donor Pneumonectomy
Heart–Lung, 33930
Lung, 32850
Tumor
Removal, 32503-32504
Unlisted Services and Procedures, 32999
Volume Reduction
Emphysematous, 32491
Lung Function Tests
See Pulmonology, Diagnostic
Lupus Anticoagulant Assay, 85705
Lupus Band Test
Immunofluorescence, 88346, *[88350]*
Luschke Procedure, 45120
LUSCS, 59514-59515, 59618, 59620, 59622

LUSS (Liver Ultrasound Scan), 76705
Luteinizing Hormone (LH), 80418, 80426, 83002
Luteinizing Release Factor, 83727
Luteotropic Hormone, 80418, 84146
Luteotropin, 80418, 84146
Luteotropin Placental, 83632
Lutrepulse Injection, 11980
LVRS, 32491
Lyme Disease, 86617, 86618
Lyme Disease ab, 86617
Lymphadenectomy
Abdominal, 38747
Bilateral Inguinofemoral, 54130, 56632, 56637
Bilateral Pelvic, 51575, 51585, 51595, 54135, 55845, 55865
Total, 38571, 38572, 57531, 58210
Diaphragmatic Assessment, 58960
Gastric, 38747
Inguinofemoral, 38760, 38765
Inguinofemoral, Iliac and Pelvic, 56640
Injection
Sentinel Node, 38792
Limited, for Staging
Para–Aortic, 38562
Pelvic, 38562
Retroperitoneal, 38564
Limited Para–Aortic, Resection of Ovarian Malignancy, 58951
Limited Pelvic, 55842, 55862, 58954
Malignancy, 58951, 58954
Mediastinal, 21632, 32674
Para-Aortic, 58958
Pelvic, 58958
Peripancreatic, 38747
Portal, 38747
Radical
Axillary, 38740, 38745
Cervical, 38720, 38724
Groin Area, 38760, 38765
Pelvic, 54135, 55845, 58548
Suprahyoid, 38700
Retroperitoneal Transabdominal, 38780
Thoracic, 38746
Unilateral Inguinofemoral, 56631, 56634
Lymphadenitis
Incision and Drainage, 38300, 38305
Lymphadenopathy Associated Antibodies
See Antibody, HIV
Lymphadenopathy Associated Virus
See HIV
Lymphangiogram, Abdominal
See Lymphangiography, Abdomen
Lymphangiography
Abdomen, 75805, 75807
Arm, 75801, 75803
Injection, 38790
Leg, 75801, 75803
Pelvis, 75805, 75807
Lymphangioma, Cystic
See Hygroma
Lymphangiotomy, 38308
Lymphatic Channels
Incision, 38308
Lymphatic Cyst
Drainage
Laparoscopic, 49323
Open, 49062
Lymphatic System
Anesthesia, 00320
Unlisted Procedure, 38999
Lymph Duct
Injection, 38790
Lymph Node(s)
Abscess
Incision and Drainage, 38300, 38305
Biopsy, 38500, 38510-38530, 38570
Needle, 38505
Dissection, 38542
Excision, 38500, 38510-38530
Abdominal, 38747
Inguinofemoral, 38760, 38765
Laparoscopic, 38571, 38572
Limited, for Staging
Para–Aortic, 38562
Pelvic, 38562
Retroperitoneal, 38564

Lymph Node(s) — *continued*
Excision — *continued*
Pelvic, 38770
Radical
Axillary, 38740, 38745
Cervical, 38720, 38724
Suprahyoid, 38720, 38724
Retroperitoneal Transabdominal, 38780
Thoracic, 38746
Exploration, 38542
Hygroma, Cystic
Axillary
Cervical
Excision, 38550, 38555
Nuclear Medicine
Imaging, 78195
Removal
Abdominal, 38747
Inguinofemoral, 38760, 38765
Pelvic, 38747, 38770
Retroperitoneal Transabdominal, 38780
Thoracic, 38746
Lymphoblast Transformation
See Blastogenesis
Lymphocele
Drainage
Laparoscopic, 49323
Extraperitoneal
Open Drainage, 49062
Lymphocyte
Culture, 86821, 86822
Toxicity Assay, 86805, 86806
Transformation, 86353
Lymphocytes, CD4
See CD4
Lymphocytes, CD8
See CD8
Lymphocyte, Thymus–Dependent
See T–Cells
Lymphocytic Choriomeningitis
Antibody, 86727
Lymphocytotoxicity, 86805, 86806
Lymphogranuloma Venereum
Antibody, 86729
Lymphoma Virus, Burkitt
See Epstein–Barr Virus
Lymph Vessels
Imaging
Lymphangiography
Abdomen, 75805-75807
Arm, 75801-75803
Leg, 75801-75803
Pelvis, 75805-75807
Nuclear Medicine, 78195
Incision, 38308
Lynch Procedure, 31075
Lysergic Acid Diethylamide, 80299, *[80300, 80301, 80302, 80303, 80304]*
Lysergide, 80299, *[80300, 80301, 80302, 80303, 80304]*
Lysis
Adhesions
Bladder
Intraluminal, 53899
Corneovitreal, 65880
Epidural, 62263, 62264
Fallopian Tube, 58740
Foreskin, 54450
Intestinal, 44005
Labial, 56441
Lung, 32124
Nose, 30560
Ovary, 58740
Oviduct, 58740
Penile
Post–circumcision, 54162
Spermatic Cord, 54699, 55899
Tongue, 41599
Ureter, 50715-50725
Intraluminal, 53899
Urethra, 53500
Uterus, 58559
Euglobulin, 85360
Eye
Goniosynechiae, 65865

Lysis — *continued*
Eye — *continued*
Synechiae
Anterior, 65870
Posterior, 65875
Labial
Adhesions, 56441
Nose
Intranasal Synechia, 30560
Transurethral
Adhesions, 53899
Lysozyme, 85549

M

MacEwen Operation
Hernia Repair, Inguinal, 49495-49500, 49505
Incarcerated, 49496, 49501, 49507, 49521
Laparoscopic, 49650, 49651
Recurrent, 49520
Sliding, 49525
Machado Test
Complement, Fixation Test, 86171
MacLean–De Wesselow Test
Clearance, Urea Nitrogen, 84540, 84545
Macrodactylia
Repair, 26590
Macroscopic Examination and Tissue Preparation, 88387
Intraoperative, 88388
Maculopathy, 67208-67218
Madlener Operation, 58600
Magnesium, 83735
Magnetic Resonance Angiography (MRA)
Abdomen, 74185
Arm, 73225
Chest, 71555
Fetal, 74712-74713
Head, 70544-70546
Leg, 73725
Neck, 70547-70549
Pelvis, 72198
Spine, 72159
Magnetic Resonance Spectroscopy, 76390
Magnetic Stimulation
Transcranial, 90867-90869
Magnetoencephalography (MEG), 95965-95967
Magnet Operation
Eye, Removal of Foreign Body
Conjunctival Embedded, 65210
Conjunctival Superficial, 65205
Corneal without Slit Lamp, 65220
Corneal with Slit Lamp, 65222
Intraocular, 65235-65265
Magnuson Procedure, 23450
MAGPI Operation, 54322
Magpi Procedure, 54322
Major Vestibular Gland
See Bartholin's Gland
Malar Area
Augmentation, 21270
Bone Graft, 21210
Fracture
with Bone Grafting, 21366
with Manipulation, 21355
Open Treatment, 21360-21366
Reconstruction, 21270
Malar Bone
See Cheekbone
Malaria Antibody, 86750
Malaria Smear, 87207
Malate Dehydrogenase, 83775
Maldescent, Testis
See Testis, Undescended
Male Circumcision
See Circumcision
Malformation, Arteriovenous
See Arteriovenous Malformation
Malic Dehydrogenase
See Malate Dehydrogenase
Malignant Hyperthermia Susceptibility
Caffeine Halothane Contracture Test (CHCT), 89049
Malleolus
See Ankle; Fibula; Leg, Lower; Tibia; Tibiofibular Joint
Metatarsophalangeal Joint, 27889

MT-ND6, 81401
MT-RNR1, 81401, 81403
MT-TK, 81401
MT-TL1, 81401
MT-TS1, 81401, 81403
MTWA (Microvolt T-Wave Alternans), 93025
Mucin
　Synovial Fluid, 83872
Mucocele
　Sinusotomy
　　Frontal, 31075
Mucolipin 1, 81290
Mucopolysaccharides, 83864
Mucormycoses
　See Mucormycosis
Mucormycosis
　Antibody, 86732
Mucosa
　Cautery, 30801-30802
　Destruction
　　Cautery, 30801-30802
　　Photodynamic Therapy, 96567
　Ectopic Gastric Imaging, 78290
　Excision of Lesion
　　Alveolar, Hyperplastic, 41828
　　Vestibule of Mouth, 40810-40818
　　via Esophagoscopy, 43229
　　via Small Intestinal Endoscopy, 44369
　　via Upper GI Endoscopy, [43270]
　Periodontal Grafting, 41870
　Urethra, Mucosal Advancement, 53450
　Vaginal Biopsy, 57100, 57105
Mucosa, Buccal
　See Mouth, Mucosa
Mucosectomy
　Rectal, 44799, 45113
Mucous Cyst
　Hand or finger, 26160
Mucous Membrane
　See Mouth, Mucosa
　Cutaneous
　　Biopsy, 11100, 11101
　　Excision
　　　Benign Lesion, 11440-11446
　　　Malignant, 11640-11646
　　Layer Closure, Wounds, 12051-12057
　　Simple Repair, Wounds, 12011-12018
　　Excision
　　　Sphenoid Sinus, 31288
　　Lid Margin
　　　Correction of Trichiasis, 67835
　　　Nasal Test, 95065
　　　Ophthalmic Test, 95060
　　Rectum
　　　Proctoplasty for Prolapse, 45505
Mucus Cyst
　See Mucous Cyst
MUGA (Multiple Gated Acquisition), 78453, 78454, 78472-78473, 78483
Muller Procedure
　Attended, 95806
　Unattended, 95807
Multianalyte Assays with Algorithmic Analyses, 0001M-0004M, 0006M-0010M, 81500, 81503-81504, 81506-81512, 81599
Multifetal Pregnancy Reduction, 59866
Multiple Sleep Latency Testing (MSLT), 95805
Multiple Valve Procedures
　See Valvuloplasty
Mumford Operation, 29824
Mumford Procedure, 23120, 29824
Mumps
　Antibody, 86735
　Immunization, 90707, 90710
　Vaccine
　　MMR, 90707
　　MMRV, 90710
Muramidase, 85549
Murine Typhus, 86000
Muscle(s)
　See Specific Muscle
　Abdomen
　　See Abdominal Wall
　Biofeedback Training, 90911
　Biopsy, 20200-20206

Muscle(s) — continued
　Chemodenervation
　　Extremity, 64642-64645
　　Larynx, 64617
　　Neck, 64616
　　Trunk, 64646-64647
　Debridement
　　Infected, 11004-11006
　Heart
　　See Myocardium
　Neck
　　See Neck Muscle
　Removal
　　Foreign Body, 20520, 20525
　Repair
　　Extraocular, 65290
　　Forearm, 25260-25274
　　Wrist, 25260-25274
　Revision
　　Arm, Upper, 24330, 24331
　　Elbow, 24301
　Transfer
　　Arm, Upper, 24301, 24320
　　Elbow, 24301
　　Femur, 27110
　　Hip, 27100-27105, 27111
　　Shoulder, 23395, 23397, 24301, 24320
Muscle Compartment Syndrome
　Detection, 20950
Muscle Denervation
　See Chemodenervation
Muscle Division
　Scalenus Anticus, 21700, 21705
　Sternocleidomastoid, 21720, 21725
Muscle Flaps, 15731-15738
　Free, 15756
Muscle Grafts, 15841-15845
Muscle, Oculomotor
　See Eye Muscles
Muscle Testing
　Dynamometry, Eye, 92260
　Extraocular Multiple Muscles, 92265
　Manual, 95831-95834
Musculoplasty
　See Muscle, Repair
Musculoskeletal System
　Computer Assisted Surgical Navigational Procedure, 0054T-0055T, 20985
　Unlisted Services and Procedures, 20999, 21499, 24999, 25999, 26989, 27299, 27599, 27899
　Unlisted Services and Procedures, Head, 21499
Musculotendinous (Rotator) Cuff
　Repair, 23410, 23412
Mustard Procedure, 33774-33777
　See Repair, Great Arteries, Revision
MUT, 81406
MutL Homolog 1, Colon Cancer, Nonpolyposis Type 2 Gene Analysis, 81292-81294
MutS Homolog 2, Colon Cancer, Nonpolyposis Type 1 Gene Analysis, 81295-81297
MutS Homolog 6 (E. Coli) Gene Analysis, 81298-81300
MUTYH, 81401, 81406, 81435
MVD (Microvascular Decompression), 61450
MVR, 33430
Myasthenia Gravis
　Cholinesterase Inhibitor Challenge Test, 95857
Myasthenic, Gravis
　See Myasthenia Gravis
MYBPC3, 81407
Mycobacteria
　Culture, 87116
　　Identification, 87118
　Detection, 87550-87562
　Sensitivity Studies, 87190
Mycophenolate
　Assay, 80180
Mycoplasma
　Antibody, 86738
　Culture, 87109
　Detection, 87580-87582
Mycota
　See Fungus
Myectomy, Anorectal
　See Myomectomy, Anorectal

Myelencephalon
　See Medulla
Myelin Basic Protein
　Cerebrospinal Fluid, 83873
Myelography
　Brain, 70010
　Spine
　　Cervical, 62302, 72240
　　Lumbosacral, 62304, 72265
　　Thoracic, 62303, 72255
　　Two or More Regions, 62305, 72270
Myelomeningocele
　Repair, 63704, 63706
　Stereotaxis
　　Creation Lesion, 63600
Myeloperoxidase, 83876
Myelotomy, 63170
MYH11, 81408, 81410-81411
MYH6, 81407
MYH7, 81407
MYL2, 81405
MYL3, 81405
MYO15A, 81430
MYO7A, 81430
Myocardial
　Imaging, 0331T-0332T, 0399T, 78466, 78468, 78469
　Perfusion Imaging, 78451-78454
　　See Nuclear Medicine
　Positron Emission Tomography (PET), 78459, 78491, 78492
　Repair
　　Postinfarction, 33542
Myocardium, 33140-33141
Myocutaneous Flaps, 15732-15738, 15756
Myofascial Pain Dysfunction Syndrome
　See Temporomandibular Joint (TMJ)
Myofascial Release, 97140
Myofibroma
　Embolization, 37243
　Removal, 58140, 58545-58546, 58561
Myoglobin, 83874
Myomectomy
　Anorectal, 45108
　Uterus, 58140-58146, 58545, 58546
Myoplasty
　Extraocular, 65290, 67346
MYOT, 81405
Myotomy
　Esophagus, 43030
　Hyoid, 21685
　Sigmoid Colon
　　Intestine, 44799
　　Rectum, 45999
Myringoplasty, 69620
Myringostomy, 69420-69421
Myringotomy, 69420, 69421
Myxoid Cyst
　Aspiration/Injection, 20612
　Drainage, 20612
　Wrist
　　Excision, 25111-25112

N

Na, 84295
Nabi-HIB, 90371
Naffziger Operation, 61330
Nagel Test, 92283
Nail Bed
　Reconstruction, 11762
　Repair, 11760
Nail Fold
　Excision
　　Wedge, 11765
Nail Plate Separation
　See Onychia
Nails
　Avulsion, 11730, 11732
　Biopsy, 11755
　Debridement, 11720, 11721
　Drainage, 10060-10061
　Evacuation
　　Hematoma, Subungual, 11740
　Excision, 11750, 11752
　KOH Examination, 87220
　Removal, 11730, 11732, 11750, 11752

Nails — continued
　Trimming, 11719
Narcoanalysis, 90865
Narcosynthesis
　Diagnostic and Therapeutic, 90865
Nasal
　Abscess, 30000-30020
　Bleeding, 30901-30906, 31238
　Bone
　　Fracture
　　　with Manipulation, 21315, 21320
　　　without Manipulation, 21310
　　　Closed Treatment, 21310-21320
　　　Open Treatment, 21325-21335
　　X-ray, 70160
　Deformity Repair, 40700-40761
　Function Study, 92512
　Polyp
　　Excision
　　　Extensive, 30115
　　　Simple, 30110
　Prosthesis
　　Impression, 21087
　Septum
　　Abscess
　　　Incision and Drainage, 30020
　　Fracture
　　　Closed Treatment, 21337
　　　Open Treatment, 21336
　　Hematoma
　　　Incision and Drainage, 30020
　　Repair, 30630
　　Submucous Resection, 30520
　Sinuses
　　See Sinus; Sinuses
　Smear
　　Eosinophils, 89190
　Turbinate
　　Fracture
　　　Therapeutic, 30930
Nasoethmoid Complex
　Fracture
　　Open Treatment, 21338, 21339
　　Percutaneous Treatment, 21340
　Reconstruction, 21182-21184
Nasogastric Tube
　Placement, 43752
Nasolacrimal Duct
　Exploration, 68810
　　with Anesthesia, 68811
　Insertion
　　Stent, 68815
　Probing, 68816
　X-ray
　　with Contrast, 70170
Nasomaxillary
　Fracture
　　with Bone Grafting, 21348
　　Closed Treatment, 21345
　　Open Treatment, 21346-21348
Nasopharynges
　See Nasopharynx
Nasopharyngoscopy, 92511
Nasopharynx
　See Pharynx
　Biopsy, 42804, 42806
　Hemorrhage, 42970-42972
　Unlisted Services and Procedures, 42999
Natriuretic Peptide, 83880
Natural Killer Cells (NK)
　Total Count, 86357
Natural Ostium
　Sinus
　　Maxillary, 31000
　　Sphenoid, 31002
Navicular
　Arthroplasty
　　with Implant, 25443
　Fracture
　　with Manipulation, 25624
　　Closed Treatment, 25622
　　Open Treatment, 25628
　Repair, 25440
Navigation
　Computer Assisted, 20985, 61781-61783
NDP, 81403-81404

[Resequenced]

NDUFA1, 81404
NDUFAF2, 81404
NDUFS1, 81406
NDUFS4, 81404
NDUFS7, 81405
NDUFS8, 81405
NDUFV1, 81405
Near-Infrared
    Guidance for Vascular Access, 0287T
    Wound Spectroscopy Studies, 0286T
NEB, 81400, 81408
Neck
    Angiography, 70498, 70547-70549
    Artery
        Ligation, 37615
    Biopsy, 21550
    Bypass Graft, 35901
    CT Scan, 70490-70492, 70498
    Dissection, Radical
        See Radical Neck Dissection
    Exploration
        Blood Vessels, 35800
        Lymph Nodes, 38542
    Incision and Drainage
        Abscess, 21501, 21502
        Hematoma, 21501, 21502
    Lipectomy, Suction Assisted, 15876
    Magnetic Resonance Angiography (MRA), 70547-70549
    Magnetic Resonance Imaging (MRI), 70540-70543
    Nerve
        Graft, 64885, 64886
    Repair
        with Other Graft, 35261
        with Vein Graft, 35231
        Blood Vessel, 35201
    Rhytidectomy, 15825, 15828
    Skin
        Revision, 15819
    Skin Graft
        Delay of Flap, 15620
        Full Thickness, 15240, 15241
        Pedicle Flap, 15574
        Split, 15120, 15121
    Surgery, Unlisted, 21899
    Tissue Transfer, Adjacent, 14040, 14041
    Tumor, 21555-21558 *[21552, 21554]*
    Ultrasound Exam, 76536
    Unlisted Services and Procedures, 21899
    Urinary Bladder
        See Bladder, Neck
    Wound Exploration
        Penetrating, 20100
        X-ray, 70360
Neck, Humerus
    Fracture
        with Shoulder Dislocation
            Closed Treatment, 23680
            Open Treatment, 23675
Neck Muscle
    Division, Scalenus Anticus, 21700, 21705
    Sternocleidomastoid, 21720-21725
Necropsy
    Coroner Examination, 88045
    Forensic Examination, 88040
    Gross and Microscopic Examination, 88020-88029
    Gross Examination, 88000-88016
    Organ, 88037
    Regional, 88036
    Unlisted Services and Procedures, 88099
Needle Biopsy
    See Biopsy
    Abdomen Mass, 49180
    Bone, 20220, 20225
    Bone Marrow, 38221
    Breast, 19100
    Colon
        Endoscopy, 45392
    Colon Sigmoid
        Endoscopy, 45342
    CT Scan Guidance, 77012
    Epididymis, 54800
    Esophagus
        Endoscopy, 43232, 43238

Needle Biopsy — *continued*
    Fluoroscopic Guidance, 77002
    Gastrointestinal, Upper
        Endoscopy, 43238, 43242
    Kidney, 50200
    Liver, 47000, 47001
    Lung, 32405
    Lymph Node, 38505
    Mediastinum, 32405
    Muscle, 20206
    Pancreas, 48102
    Pleura, 32400
    Prostate, 55700
    Retroperitoneal Mass, 49180
    Salivary Gland, 42400
    Spinal Cord, 62269
    Testis, 54500
    Thyroid Gland, 60100
    Transbronchial, 31629, 31633
Needle Localization
    Breast
        with Biopsy, 19081-19086
        with Lesion Excision, 19125, 19126
        Placement, 19281-19288
    Magnetic Resonance Guidance, 77021
Needle Manometer Technique, 20950
Needle Wire
    Introduction
        Trachea, 31730
    Placement
        Breast, 19281-19288
Neer Procedure, 23470
NEFL, 81405
Negative Pressure Wound Therapy (NPWT), 97605-97608
Neisseria Gonorrhoeae, 87590-87592, 87850
Neisseria Meningitidis
    Antibody, 86741
Neobladder
    Construction, 51596
Neonatal Critical Care, 99468-99469
Neonatal Intensive Care
    See Newborn Care
    Initial, 99477-99480
    Subsequent, 99478-99480
Neoplasm
    See Tumor
Neoplastic Growth
    See Tumor
Nephelometry, 83883
Nephrectomy
    with Ureters, 50220-50236, 50546, 50548
    Donor, 50300, 50320, 50547
    Laparoscopic, 50545-50548
    Partial, 50240
        Laparoscopic, 50543
    Recipient, 50340
Nephrolith
    See Calculus, Removal, Kidney
Nephrolithotomy, 50060-50075
Nephropexy, 50400, 50405
Nephroplasty
    See Kidney, Repair
Nephropyeloplasty, 50400-50405, 50544
Nephrorrhaphy, 50500
Nephroscopy
    See Endoscopy, Kidney
Nephrostogram, *[50430, 50431]*
Nephrostolithotomy
    Percutaneous, 50080, 50081
Nephrostomy
    Change Tube, *[50435]*
        with Drainage, 50400
    Closure, 53899
    Endoscopic, 50562-50570
        with Exploration, 50045
    Percutaneous, 52334
    X-ray with Contrast
        to Guide Dilation, 74485
Nephrostomy Tract
    Establishment, 50395
Nephrotomogram
    See Nephrotomography
Nephrotomography, 74415
Nephrotomy, 50040, 50045
    with Exploration, 50045

Nerve
    Cranial
        See Cranial Nerve
    Facial
        See Facial Nerve
    Foot
        Incision, 28035
    Intercostal
        See Intercostal Nerve
    Median
        See Median Nerve
    Obturator
        See Obturator Nerve
    Peripheral
        See Peripheral Nerve
    Phrenic
        See Phrenic Nerve
    Sciatic
        See Sciatic Nerve
    Spinal
        See Spinal Nerve
    Tibial
        See Tibial Nerve
    Ulnar
        See Ulnar Nerve
    Vestibular
        See Vestibular Nerve
Nerve Conduction
    Motor and/or Sensory, 95905-95913
Nerve II, Cranial
    See Optic Nerve
Nerve Root
    See Cauda Equina; Spinal Cord
    Decompression, 63020-63048, 63055-63103
    Incision, 63185, 63190
    Section, 63185, 63190
Nerves
    Anastomosis
        Facial to Hypoglossal, 64868
        Facial to Spinal Accessory, 64866
    Avulsion, 64732-64772
    Biopsy, 64795
    Decompression, 64702-64727
    Destruction, 64600-64681 *[64633, 64634, 64635, 64636]*
        Laryngeal, Recurrent, 31595
        Paravertebral Facet Joint, *[64633, 64634, 64635, 64636]*
    Foot
        Excision, 28055
        Incision, 28035
    Graft, 64885-64907
    Implantation
        Electrode, 64553-64581
        to Bone, 64787
        to Muscle, 64787
    Incision, 43640, 43641, 64732-64772
    Injection
        Anesthetic, 01991-01992, 64400-64530
        Neurolytic Agent, 64600-64681 *[64633, 64634, 64635, 64636]*
    Insertion
        Electrode, 64553-64581
    Lesion
        Excision, 64774-64792
    Neurofibroma
        Excision, 64788-64792
    Neurolemmoma
        Excision, 64788-64792
    Neurolytic
        Internal, 64727
    Neuroma
        Excision, 64774-64786
    Neuroplasty, 64702-64721
    Nuclear Medicine
        Unlisted Services and Procedures, 78699
    Removal
        Electrode, 64585
    Repair
        Graft, 64885-64911
        Microdissection
            with Surgical Microscope, 69990
        Suture, 64831-64876
    Spinal Accessory
        Incision, 63191
        Section, 63191

Nerves — *continued*
    Suture, 64831-64876
    Sympathectomy
        Excision, 64802-64818
    Transection, 43640, 43641, 64732-64772
    Transposition, 64718-64721
    Unlisted Services and Procedures, 64999
Nerve Stimulation, Transcutaneous
    See Application, Neurostimulation
Nerve Teasing, 88362
Nerve V, Cranial
    See Trigeminal Nerve
Nerve VII, Cranial
    See Facial Nerve
Nerve X, Cranial
    See Vagus Nerve
Nerve XI, Cranial
    See Accessory Nerve
Nerve XII, Cranial
    See Hypoglossal Nerve
Nervous System
    Nuclear Medicine
        Unlisted Services and Procedures, 78699
Nesidioblast
    See Islet Cell
Neurectasis, 64999
Neurectomy
    Foot, 28055
    Gastrocnemius, 27326
    Hamstring Muscle, 27325
    Leg, Lower, 27326
    Leg, Upper, 27325
    Popliteal, 27326
    Tympanic, 69676
Neuroendoscopy
    Intracranial, 62160-62165
Neurofibroma
    Cutaneous Nerve
        Excision, 64788
    Extensive
        Excision, 64792
    Peripheral Nerve
        Excision, 64790
Neurolemmoma
    Cutaneous Nerve
        Excision, 64788
    Extensive
        Excision, 64792
    Peripheral Nerve
        Excision, 64790
Neurologic System
    See Nervous System
Neurology
    Brain
        Cortex Magnetic Stimulation, 90867-90869
        Mapping, 96020
        Surface Electrode Stimulation, 95961-95962
    Central Motor
        Electrocorticogram
            Intraoperative, 95829
        Electroencephalogram (EEG)
            Brain Death, 95824
            Electrode Placement, 95830
            Intraoperative, 95955
            Monitoring, 95812, 95813, 95950-95953, 95956
            Physical or Drug Activation, 95954
            Sleep, 95808, 95810, 95822, 95827
                Attended, 95806, 95807
                Standard, 95819
            WADA activation, 95958
        Electroencephalography (EEG)
            Digital Analysis, 95957
        Electromyography
            See Electromyography
            Fine Wire
                Dynamic, 96004
            Ischemic Limb Exercise Test, 95875
            Needle, 51785, 95860-95872
            Surface
                Dynamic, 96002-96004
    Higher Cerebral Function
        Aphasia Test, 96105
        Cognitive Function Tests, 96116
        Developmental Tests, 96110, 96111

Neurology — *continued*
- Central Motor — *continued*
  - Magnetoencephalography (MEG), 95965-95967
  - Motion Analysis
    - by Video and 3–D Kinematics, 96000, 96004
    - Computer–based, 96000, 96004
  - Muscle Testing
    - Manual, 95831-95834
  - Nerve Conduction
    - Motor and Sensory Nerve, 95905-95913
  - Neuromuscular Junction Tests, 95937
  - Neurophysiological Testing, 95921-95924
  - Neuropsychological Testing, 96118-96120
  - Plantar Pressure Measurements
    - Dynamic, 96001, 96004
  - Polysomnography, 95808-95811
  - Range of Motion Test, 95851, 95852
  - Reflex
    - H–Reflex, 95907-95913
  - Reflex Test
    - Blink Reflex, 95933
  - Sleep Study, 95808, 95810
    - Attended, 95806
    - Unattended, 95807
  - Somatosensory Testing, 95925-95927 [95938]
  - Transcranial Motor Stimulation, 95928-95929
  - Unlisted Services and Procedures, 95999
  - Urethral Sphincter, 51785
  - Visual Evoked Potential, CNS, 95930
- Cognitive Performance, 96125
- Diagnostic
  - Anal Sphincter, 51785
  - Autonomic Nervous Function
    - Heart Rate Response, 95921-95923
    - Pseudomotor Response, 95921-95923
    - Sympathetic Function, 95921-95923
  - Brain Surface Electrode Stimulation, 95961, 95962

Neurolysis
- Nerve, 64704, 64708
  - Internal, 64727

Neuroma
- Acoustic
  - *See* Brain, Tumor, Excision
- Cutaneous Nerve
  - Excision, 64774
- Digital Nerve
  - Excision, 64776, 64778
- Excision, 64774
- Foot Nerve
  - Excision, 28080, 64782, 64783
- Hand Nerve
  - Excision, 64782, 64783
- Interdigital, 28080
- Peripheral Nerve
  - Excision, 64784
- Sciatic Nerve
  - Excision, 64786

Neuromuscular Junction Tests, 95937
Neuromuscular Pedicle
- Reinnervation
  - Larynx, 31590

Neuromuscular Reeducation, 97112
- *See* Physical Medicine/Therapy/Occupational Therapy

Neurophysiological Testing
- Autonomic Nervous Function
  - Combined Parasympathetic and Sympathetic, 95924
  - Heart Rate Response, 95921-95923
  - Pseudomotor Response, 95921-95923
  - Sympathetic Function, 95921-95923

Neuroplasty, 64712
- Cranial Nerve, 64716
- Digital Nerve, 64702, 64704
- Peripheral Nerve, 64708-64714, 64718-64721

Neuropsychological Testing, 96118-96120
- Computer Assisted, 96120

Neurorrhaphy, 64831-64876
- Peripheral Nerve
  - with Graft, 64885-64907

Neurorrhaphy — *continued*
- Peripheral Nerve — *continued*
  - Conduit, 64910-64911

Neurostimulation
- Application, 64550
- Tibial, 64566

Neurostimulator
- Analysis, 95970-95982, 0317T
- Implantation
  - Electrodes
    - Incision, 64568, 64575-64581
    - Laparoscopic, 0312T
    - Percutaneous, 64553-64565
  - Insertion
    - Pulse Generator, 61885-61886, 64568, 64590
    - Receiver, 61885-61886, 64590
  - Removal
    - Electrodes, 61880, 63661-63662, 64570, 64585, 0314T
    - Pulse Generator, 61888, 64595, 0314T-0315T
    - Receiver, 61888, 64595
  - Replacement
    - Electrodes, 43647, 43881, 63663-63664, 64569, 0313T
    - Pulse Generator, 61885-61886, 63685, 64590, 0316T
    - Receiver, 61885-61886, 63685, 64590
  - Revision
    - Electrode, 61880, 63663-63664, 64569, 64585, 0313T
    - Pulse Generator, 61888, 63688, 64595
    - Receiver, 61888, 63688, 64595

Neurotomy, Sympathetic
- *See* Gasserian Ganglion, Sensory Root, Decompression

Neurovascular Interventional Procedures
- Balloon Angioplasty, 61630
- Intracranial Balloon Dilatation, 61640-61642
- Occlusion
  - Balloon, 61623
  - Balloon Dilatation, 61640-61642
  - Transcatheter, 61624
    - Non-central nervous system, 61626
- Placement Intravascular Stent, 61635
- Vascular Catheterization, 61630, 61635

Neurovascular Pedicle Flaps, 15750
Neutralization Test
- Virus, 86382

Newborn Care, 99460-99465, 99502
- Attendance at Delivery, 99464
- Birthing Room, 99460-99463
- Blood Transfusion, 36450
  - *See* Neonatal Intensive Care
- Circumcision
  - Clamp or Other Device, 54150
  - Surgical Excision, 54160
- Laryngoscopy, 31520
- Normal, 99460-99463
- Prepuce Slitting, 54000
- Preventive
  - Office, 99461
- Resuscitation, 99465
- Standby for C–Section, 99360
- Subsequent Hospital Care, 99462
- Umbilical Artery Catheterization, 36660

New Patient
- Domiciliary or Rest Home Visit, 99324-99328
- Emergency Department Services, 99281-99288
- Home Services, 99341-99345
- Hospital Inpatient Services, 99221-99239
- Hospital Observation Services, 99217-99220
- Initial Inpatient Consultations, 99251-99255
- Initial Office Visit, 99201-99205
  - *See* Evaluation and Management, Office and Other Outpatient
- Office and/or Other Outpatient Consultations, 99241-99245
- Outpatient Visit, 99211-99215

NF1, 81408
NF2, 81405-81406
NHLRC1, 81403
Nickel, 83885
Nicolas–Durand–Favre Disease
- *See* Lymphogranuloma Venerum

Nicotine, [80323]
Nidation
- *See* Implantation
Nikaidoh Procedure, 33782-33783
NIPA1, 81404
Nipples
- *See* Breast
- Inverted, 19355
- Reconstruction, 19350
Nissen Operation
- *See* Fundoplasty, Esophagogastric
Nitrate Reduction Test
- Urinalysis, 81000-81099
Nitric Oxide, 95012
Nitroblue Tetrazolium Dye Test, 86384
Nitrogen, Blood Urea
- *See* Blood Urea Nitrogen
NLGN3, 81405
NLGN4X, 81404-81405
N. Meningitidis, 86741
NMP22, 86386
NMR Imaging
- *See* Magnetic Resonance Spectroscopy
NMR Spectroscopies
- *See* Magnetic Resonance Spectroscopy
Noble Procedure, 44680
Nocardia
- Antibody, 86744
Nocturnal Penile Rigidity Test, 54250
Nocturnal Penile Tumescence Test, 54250
NOD2, 81401
Node Dissection, Lymph, 38542
Node, Lymph
- *See* Lymph Nodes
Nodes
- *See* Lymph Nodes
No Man's Land
- Tendon Repair, 26356-26358
Non-Invasive Arterial Pressure, 93050
Non-Invasive Vascular Imaging
- *See* Vascular Studies
Non–Office Medical Services, 99056
- Emergency Care, 99060
Non–Stress Test, Fetal, 59025
Nonunion Repair
- Femur
  - with Graft, 27472
  - without Graft, 27470
- Fibula, 27726
- Metatarsal, 28322
- Tarsal Joint, 28320
Noonan Spectrum Disorders (Noonan/Noonan-like Syndrome), 81442
Noradrenalin
- Blood, 82383, 82384
- Urine, 82382
Norchlorimipramine
- *See* Imipramine
Norepinephrine
- *See* Catecholamines
- Blood, 82383, 82384
- Urine, 82382
Nortriptyline
- Assay, [80335, 80336, 80337]
Norwood Procedure, 33619, 33622
Nose
- Abscess
  - Incision and Drainage, 30000, 30020
- Artery
  - Incision, 30915, 30920
- Biopsy
  - Intranasal, 30100
- Dermoid Cyst
  - Excision
    - Complex, 30125
    - Simple, 30124
- Displacement Therapy, 30210
- Endoscopy
  - Diagnostic, 31231-31235
  - Surgical, 31237-31294
- Excision
  - Rhinectomy, 30150, 30160
- Fracture
  - with Fixation, 21330, 21340, 21345-21347
  - Closed Treatment, 21345

Nose — *continued*
- Fracture — *continued*
  - Open Treatment, 21325-21336, 21338, 21339, 21346, 21347
  - Percutaneous Treatment, 21340
- Hematoma
  - Hemorrhage
    - Cauterization, 30901-30906
  - Incision and Drainage, 30000, 30020
- Insertion
  - Septal Prosthesis, 30220
- Intranasal
  - Lesion
    - External Approach, 30118
    - Internal Approach, 30117
- Lysis of Adhesions, 30560
- Polyp
  - Excision
    - Extensive, 30115
    - Simple, 30110
- Reconstruction
  - Cleft Lip
    - Cleft Palate, 30460, 30462
  - Dermatoplasty, 30620
  - Primary, 30400-30420
  - Secondary, 30430-30450
  - Septum, 30520
- Removal
  - Foreign Body, 30300
    - with Anesthesia, 30310
    - by Lateral Rhinotomy, 30320
- Repair
  - Adhesions, 30560
  - Cleft Lip, 40700-40761
  - Fistula, 30580, 30600, 42260
  - Rhinophyma, 30120
  - Septum, 30540, 30545, 30630
  - Synechia, 30560
  - Vestibular Stenosis, 30465
- Skin
  - Excision, 30120
  - Surgical Planing, 30120
- Skin Graft
  - Delay of Flap, 15630
  - Full Thickness, 15260, 15261
  - Pedicle Flap, 15576
- Submucous Resection Turbinate
  - Excision, 30140
- Tissue Transfer, Adjacent, 14060, 14061
- Turbinate
  - Excision, 30130, 30140
  - Fracture, 30930
  - Injection, 30200
- Turbinate Mucosa
  - Cauterization, 30801, 30802
- Unlisted Services and Procedures, 30999
Nose Bleed, 30901-30906
- *See* Hemorrhage, Nasal
NOTCH1, 81407
NOTCH3, 81406
NPC1, 81406
NPC2, 81404
NPHP1, 81405-81406
NPHS1, 81407
NPHS2, 81405
NPM1/ALK (t(2;5)), 81401
NPWT (Negative Pressure Wound Therapy), 97605-97608
NRAS, 81311
NROB1, 81404
NSD1, 81405-81406
NST, 59025
NSVD, 59400-59410, 59610-59614
NTD (Nitroblue Tetrazolium Dye Test), 86384
Nuclear Antigen
- Antibody, 86235
Nuclear Imaging
- *See* Nuclear Medicine
Nuclear Magnetic Resonance Imaging
- *See* Magnetic Resonance Imaging (MRI)
Nuclear Magnetic Resonance Spectroscopy
- *See* Magnetic Resonance Spectroscopy
Nuclear Matrix Protein 22 (NMP22), 86386
Nuclear Medicine
- Abscess Localization, 78805, 78806, 78807
- Adrenal Gland Imaging, 78075

© 2015 Optum360, LLC

CPT © 2015 American Medical Association. All Rights Reserved.

[Resequenced]

Index — 89

Index

Orbit — ORIF

Osteoplasty — *continued*
Femur — *continued*
Shortening, 27465, 27468
Fibula
Lengthening, 27715
Humerus, 24420
Metacarpal, 26568
Phalanges
Finger, 26568
Toe, 28299, 28310-28312
Radius, 25390-25393
Tibia
Lengthening, 27715
Ulna, 25390-25393
Vertebra
Cervicothoracic, 22510, 22512
Lumbosacral, 22511-22512
Osteotomy
with Graft
Reconstruction
Periorbital Region, 21267-21268
Blount, 27455, 27475-27485
Calcaneus, 28300
Chin, 21121-21123
Clavicle, 23480-23485
Femur
with Fixation, 27165
with Open Reduction of Hip, 27156
with Realignment, 27454
without Fixation, 27448-27450
Femoral Neck, 27161
for Slipped Epiphysis, 27181
Greater Trochanter, 27140
Fibula, 27707-27712
Hip, 27146-27156
Femoral
with Open Reduction, 27156
Femur, 27151
Humerus, 24400-24410
Mandible, 21198-21199
Extra-oral, 21047
Intra-oral, 21046
Maxilla, 21206
Extra-oral, 21049
Intra-oral, 21048
Metacarpal, 26565
Metatarsal, 28306-28309
Orbit Reconstruction, 21256
Patella
Wedge, 27448
Pelvis, 27158
Pemberton, 27147
Periorbital
Orbital Hypertelorism, 21260-21263
Osteotomy with Graft, 21267-21268
Phalanges
Finger, 26567
Toe, 28299, 28310-28312
Radius
and Ulna, 25365, 25375
Distal Third, 25350
Middle or Proximal Third, 25355
Multiple, 25370
Salter, 27146
Skull Base, 61582-61585, 61592
Spine
Anterior, 22220-22226
Posterior/Posterolateral, 22210-22214
Cervical, 22210
Each Additional Vertebral Segment, 22208, 22216
Lumbar, 22207, 22214
Thoracic, 22206, 22212
Three-Column, 22206-22208
Talus, 28302
Tarsal, 28304-28305
Tibia, 27455-27457, 27705, 27709-27712
Ulna, 25360
and Radius, 25365, 25375
Multiple, 25370
Vertebra
Additional Segment
Anterior Approach, 22226
Posterior/Posterolateral Approach, 22208, 22216

Osteotomy — *continued*
Vertebra — *continued*
Cervical
Anterior Approach, 22220
Posterior/Posterolateral Approach, 22210
Lumbar
Anterior Approach, 22224
Posterior/Posterolateral Approach, 22214
Thoracic
Anterior Approach, 22222
Posterior/Posterolateral Approach, 22212
OTC, 81405
Other Nonoperative Measurements and Examinations
Acid Perfusion
Esophagus, 91013, 91030
Acid Reflux
Esophagus, 91034-91035, 91037-91038
Attenuation Measurements
Ear Protector, 92596
Bernstein Test, 91030
Breath Hydrogen, 91065
Bronchial Challenge Testing, 95070-95071
Gastric Motility (Manometric) Studies, 91020
Information
Analysis of Data, 99090
Iontophoresis, 97033
Laryngeal Function Studies, 92520
Manometry
Anorectal, 91122
Esophageal, 91010
Photography
Anterior Segment, 92286
External Ocular, 92285
Provocative Testing
for Glaucoma, 92140
Otoacoustic Emission Evaluation, 92587-92588
Otolaryngology
Diagnostic
Exam under Anesthesia, 92502
Otomy
See Incision
Otoplasty, 69300
Otorhinolaryngology
Diagnostic
Otolaryngology Exam, 92502
Unlisted Services and Procedures, 92700
Ouchterlony Immunodiffusion, 86331
Outer Ear
CT Scan, 70480-70482
Outpatient Visit, 99201-99215
Output, Cardiac
by Indicator Dilution, 93561-93562
Ova
Smear, 87177
Oval Window
Repair Fistula, 69666
Oval Window Fistula
Repair, 69666
Ovarian Cyst
Excision, 58925
Incision and Drainage, 58800-58805
Ovarian Vein Syndrome
Uterolysis, 50722
Ovariectomies, 58940-58943
with Hysterectomy, 58262-58263, 58291-58292, 58542, 58544, 58552, 58554, 58571, 58573
for Ectopic Pregnancy, 59120, 59151
Ovariolysis, 58740
Ovary
Abscess
Incision and Drainage, 58820-58822
Abdominal Approach, 58822
Vaginal Approach, 58820
Biopsy, 58900
Cryopreservation, 88240
Cyst
Incision and Drainage, 58800-58805
Ovarian, 58805
Excision, 58662, 58720
Cyst, 58925

Ovary — *continued*
Excision — *continued*
Partial
Oophorectomy, 58661, 58940
Ovarian Malignancy, 58943
Peritoneal Malignancy, 58943
Tubal Malignancy, 58943
Wedge Resection, 58920
Total, 58940-58943
Laparoscopy, 58660-58662, 58679
Lysis
Adhesions, 58660, 58740
Radical Resection, 58950-58952
Transposition, 58825
Tumor
Resection, 58950-58958
Unlisted Services and Procedures, 58679, 58999
Wedge Resection, 58920
Oviduct
Anastomosis, 58750
Chromotubation, 58350
Ectopic Pregnancy, 59120-59121
Excision, 58700-58720
Fulguration
Laparoscopic, 58670
Hysterosalpingography, 74740
Laparoscopy, 58679
Ligation, 58600-58611
Lysis
Adhesions, 58740
Occlusion, 58615
Laparoscopic, 58671
Repair, 58752
Anastomosis, 58750
Create Stoma, 58770
Unlisted Services and Procedures, 58679, 58999
X-ray with Contrast, 74740
Ovocyte
See Oocyte
Ovulation Tests, 84830
Ovum Implantation, 58976
Ovum Transfer Surgery, 58976
Oxalate, 83945
Oxcarbazepine
Assay, 80183
Oxidase, Ceruloplasmin, 82390
Oxidoreductase, Alcohol-Nad+, 84588
Oximetry (Noninvasive)
See Also Pulmonology, Diagnostic
Blood O2 Saturation
Ear or Pulse, 94760-94762
Oxoisomerase, 84087
Oxosteroids, 83586-83593
Oxycodinone, *[80300, 80301, 80302, 80303, 80304]*, *[80361, 80362, 80363, 80364]*
Oxygen Saturation, 82805-82810
Ear Oximetry, 94760-94762
Pulse Oximetry, 94760-94762
Oxyproline, 83500-83505
Oxytocin Stress Test, Fetal, 59020

P

PABPN1, 81401
Pacemaker, Heart
See Also Cardiology, Defibrillator, Heart
Conversion, 33214
Electronic Analysis
Antitachycardia System, 93724
Electrophysiologic Evaluation, 93640-93642
Evaluation, 93279-93281, 93286, 93288, 93293-93294, 93296
Insertion, 33206-33208
Electrode(s), 33202-33203, 33210-33211, 33216-33217, 33224-33225
Pulse Generator, 33212-33213, 33240
Interrogation, 93294, 93296
Permanent Leadless, Ventricular
Device Evaluation, 0389T-0391T
Insertion, 0387T
Removal, 0388T
Replacement, 0387T
Programming, 93279-93281
Relocation
Skin Pocket, 33222-33223
Removal, 33236-33237

Pacemaker, Heart — *continued*
Removal — *continued*
Electrodes, 33234-33235, 33238, 33243-33244
Pulse Generator
Implantable Defibrillator, 33241
Pacemaker, 33233
Repair
Electrode(s), 33218-33220
Leads, 33218-33220
Replacement, 33206-33208
Catheter, 33210
Electrode(s), 33210-33211
Leads, 33210-33211
Pulse Generator, 33212-33213
Repositioning
Electrodes, 33215, 33226, 33249
Telephonic Analysis, 93293
Upgrade, 33214
P-Acetamidophenol, *[80329, 80330, 80331]*
Pachymetry
Eye, 76514
Packing
Nasal Hemorrhage, 30901-30906
PAFAH1B1, 81405-81406
PAH, 81406
Pain Management
Epidural, 62350-62351, 62360-62362, 99601-99602
Intrathecal, 62350-62351, 62360-62362, 99601-99602
Intravenous Therapy, 96360-96368, 96374-96376
Pain Therapy, 0278T, 62350-62365
Palatal Augmentation Prosthesis, 21082
Palatal Lift Prosthesis, 21083
Palate
Abscess
Incision and Drainage, 42000
Biopsy, 42100
Excision, 42120, 42145
Fracture
Closed Treatment, 21421
Open Treatment, 21422-21423
Lesion
Destruction, 42160
Excision, 42104-42120
Prosthesis
Augmentation, 21082
Impression, 42280
Insertion, 42281
Lift, 21089
Reconstruction
Lengthening, 42226-42227
Repair
Cleft Palate, 42200-42225
Laceration, 42180-42182
Vomer Flap, 42235
Unlisted Services and Procedures, 42299
Palate, Cleft
Repair, 42200-42225
Rhinoplasty, 30460-30462
Palatopharyngoplasty, 42145
Palatoplasty, 42200-42225
Palatoschisis, 42200-42225
PALB2, 81406, 81432
Palm
Bursa
Incision and Drainage, 26025-26030
Fasciectomy, 26121-26125
Fasciotomy, 26040-26045
Tendon
Excision, 26170
Tendon Sheath
Excision, 26145
Incision and Drainage, 26020
Palsy, Seventh Nerve
Graft/Repair, 15840-15845
PAMG-1, 84112
P&P, 85230
Pancoast Tumor Resection, 32503-32504
Pancreas
Anastomosis
with Intestines, 48520-48540, 48548
Anesthesia, 00794
Biopsy, 48100

        [Resequenced]

Index

Physician Quality Reporting System (PQRS) — Pineal Gland

Proctosigmoidoscopy — *continued*
  Exploration, 45300
  Hemorrhage Control, 45317
  Placement
    Stent, 45327
  Removal
    Foreign Body, 45307
    Polyp, 45308-45315
    Tumor, 45315
  Stoma
    through Artificial, 45999
  Volvulus Repair, 45321
Proctostomy
  Closure, 45999
Proctotomy, 45160
Products, Gene
  See Protein
Proetz Therapy, 30210
Profibrinolysin, 85420-85421
Progenitor Cell
  See Stem Cell
Progesterone, 84144
Progesterone Receptors, 84234
Progestin Receptors, 84234
Programming
  Defibrillator System, 93282-93284, 93287
  Intracardiac Ischemia Monitoring System, 0305T
  Loop Recorder, 93285
  Pacemaker, 93279-93281, 93286
Proinsulin, 84206
Pro-Insulin C Peptide
  See C-Peptide
Projective Test, 96101-96103
Prokallikrein, 85292
Prokallikrein, Plasma, 85292
Prokinogenase, 85292
Prolactin, 80418, 84146
Prolapse
  Anus, 46750-46751
  Proctopexy, 45400-45402, 45540-45541, 45550
  Proctoplasty, 45505, 45520
  Rectum, 45130-45135, 45900, 46753
  Urethra, 53275
Prolastin
  See Alpha-1 Antitrypsin
Prolonged Services
  with Direct Patient Contact, 99354-99355
  Before or After Direct Patient Contact, 99358, 99359
  Inpatient or Observation, 99356-99357
  Physician Standby Services, 99360
PROM, 95851, 95852, 97110, 97530
Pronuclear Stage Tube Transfer (PROST), 58976
PROP1, 81404
Prophylactic Treatment
  See Also Preventive Medicine
  Antibiotic Documentation, 4042F-4043F, 4045F-4049F
  Antimicrobial Documentation, 4041F
  Clavicle, 23490
  Femoral Neck and Proximal Femur
    Nailing, 27187
    Pinning, 27187
    Wiring, 27187
  Femur, 27495
    Nailing, 27495
    Pinning, 27495
    Wiring, 27495
  Humerus, 23491
    Pinning, Wiring, 24498
  Radius, 25490, 25492
    Nailing, 25490, 25492
    Pinning, 25490, 25492
    Plating, 25490, 25492
    Wiring, 25490, 25492
  Shoulder
    Clavicle, 23490
    Humerus, 23491
  Tibia, 27745
  Ulna, 25491, 25492
    Nailing, 25491, 25492
    Pinning, 25491, 25492
    Plating, 25491, 25492
    Wiring, 25491, 25492
  Venous Thromboembolism (VTE), 4044F

Prophylaxis
  Anticoagulant Therapy, 4075F
  Deep Vein Thrombosis (DVT), 4070F
  Retinal Detachment
    Cryotherapy, 67141
      Cryotherapy, Diathermy, 67141
      Photocoagulation, 67145
    Diathermy, 67141
    Photocoagulation, 67145
ProQuad, 90710
PROST (Pronuclear Stage Tube Transfer), 58976
Prostaglandin, 84150
  Insertion, 59200
Prostanoids
  See Prostaglandin
Prostate
  Ablation
    Cryosurgery, 55873
  Abscess
    Drainage, 52700
    Incision and Drainage, 55720, 55725
  Biopsy, 55700, 55705, 55706
  Brachytherapy
    Needle Insertion, 55875
  Coagulation
    Laser, 52647
  Destruction
    Cryosurgery, 55873
    Thermotherapy, 53850
      Microwave, 53850
      Radio Frequency, 53852
  Enucleation, Laser, 52649
  Excision
    Partial, 55801, 55821, 55831
    Perineal, 55801-55815
    Radical, 55810-55815, 55840-55845
    Retropubic, 55831-55845
    Suprapubic, 55821
    Transurethral, 52402, 52601
  Exploration
    with Nodes, 55862, 55865
    Exposure, 55860
  Incision
    Exposure, 55860-55865
    Transurethral, 52450
  Insertion
    Catheter, 55875
    Needle, 55875
    Radioactive Substance, 55860
  Needle Biopsy, 55700, 55706
  Placement
    Catheter, 55875
    Dosimeter, 55876
    Fiducial Marker, 55876
    Interstitial Device, 55876
    Needle, 55875
  Thermotherapy
    Transurethral, 53850
  Ultrasound, 76872, 76873
  Unlisted Services and Procedures, 54699, 55899
    Urinary System, 53899
  Urethra
    Stent Insertion, 53855
  Vaporization
    Laser, 52648
Prostatectomy, 52601
  Laparoscopic, 55866
  Perineal
    Partial, 55801
    Radical, 55810, 55815
  Retropubic
    Partial, 55831
    Radical, 55840-55845, 55866
  Suprapubic
    Partial, 55821
  Transurethral, 52601
  Walsh Modified Radical, 55810
Prostate Specific Antigen
  Complexed, 84152
  Free, 84154
  Total, 84153
Prostatic Abscess
  Incision and Drainage, 55720, 55725
    Prostatotomy, 55720, 55725
    Transurethral, 52700
Prostatotomy, 55720, 55725

Prosthesis
  Augmentation
    Mandibular Body, 21125
  Auricular, 21086
  Breast
    Insertion, 19340, 19342
    Removal, 19328, 19330
    Supply, 19396
  Check-Out, 97762
    See Physical Medicine/Therapy/ Occupational Therapy
  Cornea, 65770
  Elbow
    Removal, 24160-24164
  Endovascular
    Thoracic Aorta, 33883-33886
  Facial, 21088
  Hernia
    Mesh, 49568
  Hip
    Removal, 27090, 27091
  Impression and Custom Preparation (by Physician)
    Auricular, 21086
    Facial, 21088
    Mandibular Resection, 21081
    Nasal, 21087
    Obturator
      Definitive, 21080
      Interim, 21079
      Surgical, 21076
    Oral Surgical Splint, 21085
    Orbital, 21077
    Palatal
      Augmentation, 21082
      Lift, 21083
    Speech Aid, 21084
  Intestines, 44700
  Knee
    Insertion, 27438, 27445
  Lens
    Insertion, 66982-66985
    Manual or Mechanical Technique, 66982-66984
    not Associated with Concurrent Cataract Removal, 66985
  Mandibular Resection, 21081
  Nasal, 21087
  Nasal Septum
    Insertion, 30220
  Obturator, 21076
    Definitive, 21080
    Interim, 21079
  Ocular, 21077, 65770, 66982-66985, 92358
    Fitting and Prescription, 92002-92014
    Loan, 92358
    Prescription, 92002-92014
  Orbital, 21077
  Orthotic
    Check-Out, 97762
    Training, 97761
  Ossicular Chain
    Partial or Total, 69633, 69637
  Palatal Augmentation, 21082
  Palatal Lift, 21083
  Palate, 42280, 42281
  Penile
    Fitting, 54699, 55899
    Insertion, 54400-54405
    Removal, 54406, 54410-54417
    Repair, 54408
    Replacement, 54410, 54411, 54416, 54417
  Perineum
    Removal, 53442
  Removal
    Elbow, 24160-24164
    Hip, 27090-27091
    Knee, 27488
    Shoulder, 23334-23335
    Wrist, 25250-25251
  Shoulder
    Removal, 23334-23335
  Skull Plate
    Removal, 62142
    Replacement, 62143

Prosthesis — *continued*
  Spectacle
    Fitting, 92352, 92353
    Repair, 92371
  Speech Aid, 21084
  Spinal
    Insertion, 22851
  Synthetic, 69633, 69637
  Temporomandibular Joint
    Arthroplasty, 21243
  Testicular
    Insertion, 54660
    Training, 97761
  Urethral Sphincter
    Insertion, 53444, 53445
    Removal, 53446, 53447
    Repair, 53449
    Replacement, 53448
  Vagina
    Insertion, 57267
  Wrist
    Removal, 25250, 25251
Protease F, 85400
Protein
  A, Plasma (PAPP-A), 84163
  C-Reactive, 86140-86141
  Electrophoresis, 84165-84166
  Glycated, 82985
  Myelin Basic, 83873
  Osteocalcin, 83937
  Other Fluids, 84166
  Other Source, 84157
  Prealbumin, 84134
  Serum, 84155, 84165
  Total, 84155-84160
  Urine, 84156
    by Dipstick, 81000-81003
  Western Blot, 84181, 84182, 88372
Protein Analysis, Tissue
  Western Blot, 88371-88372
Protein Blotting, 84181-84182
Protein C Activator, 85337
Protein C Antigen, 85302
Protein C Assay, 85303
Protein C Resistance Assay, 85307
Protein S
  Assay, 85306
  Total, 85305
Prothrombase, 85260
Prothrombin, 85210
  Coagulation Factor II Gene Analysis, 81240
  Time, 85610, 85611
Prothrombinase
  Inhibition, 85705
  Inhibition Test, 85347
  Partial Time, 85730, 85732
Prothrombokinase, 85230
Protime, 85610-85611
Proton Treatment Delivery
  Complex, 77525
  Intermediate, 77523
  Simple, 77520, 77522
Protoporphyrin, 84202, 84203
Protozoa
  Antibody, 86753
Provitamin A, 84590
Provocation Test
  for Glaucoma, 92140
Prower Factor, 85260
PRP, 67040
PRPF31, 81434
PRPH2, 81404, 81434
PRSS1, 81401, 81404
PRX, 81405
PSA, 84152
  Free, 84154
  Total, 84153
PSEN1, 81405
PSEN2, 81406
Pseudocyst, Pancreas
  Drainage
    Open, 48510
PSG, 95808-95811
Psoriasis Treatment, 96910-96922

Index

Psychiatric Diagnosis — Quantitative Sensory Testing (QST)

Quantitative Sensory Testing (QST) —
  continued
  Using Other Stimuli, 0110T
  Using Touch Pressure Stimuli, 0106T
  Using Vibration Stimuli, 0107T
Quick Test
  Prothrombin Time, 85610, 85611
Quinidine
  Assay, 80194
Quinine, 84228

R

RAB7A, 81405
RabAvert, 90675
Rabies
  Immune Globulin, 90375-90376
  Vaccine, 90675-90676
Rachicentesis, 62270-62272
Radial Arteries
  Aneurysm, 35045
  Embolectomy, 34111
  Sympathectomy, 64821
  Thrombectomy, 34111
Radial Head, Subluxation, 24640
Radial Keratotomy, 65771
Radiation
  Blood Products, 86945
Radiation Physics
  Consultation, 77336-77370
  Unlisted Services and Procedures, 77399
Radiation Therapy
  Consultation
    Radiation Physics, 77336-77370
  CT Scan Guidance, 77014
  Dose Plan, 77300, 77306-77331
    Brachytherapy, 77316-77318
    High-Dose Electronic Brachytherapy,
      0394T-0395T
    Intensity Modulation, 77301
    Teletherapy, 77306-77321
  Field Set-Up, 77280-77290
  Guidance for Localization, [77387]
  Intraoperative, 77469, [77424, 77425]
  Localization of Patient Movement, [77387]
  Multi-leaf Collimator Device Design and Con-
    struction, 77338
  Planning, 77261-77290, 77293-77331 [77295]
  Special, 77470
  Stereotactic, 77371-77373, 77432
    Body, 77373
    Cranial Lesion, 77371-77372, 77432
  Treatment Delivery
    =>1MeV Complex, 77412
    =>1MeV Intermediate, 77407
    =>1MeV Simple, 77402
    Beam Modulation, [77385]
    Guidance for Localization, [77387]
    High Energy Neutron, 77422-77423
    Intensity Modulated Radiation (IMRT)
      Complex, [77386]
      Simple, [77385]
    Intraoperative, [77424, 77425]
    Proton Beam, 77520-77525
    Single, 77402
    Stereotactic
      Body, 77373
      Cranial Lesion(s), 77371-77372
    Superficial, 77401
    Three or More Areas, 77412
    Two Areas, 77407
    Weekly, 77427
  Treatment Device, 77332-77334
  Treatment Management
    Intraoperative, 77469
    One or Two Fractions Only, 77431
    Stereotactic
      Body, 77435
      Cerebral, 77432
    Unlisted Services and Procedures, 77499
    Weekly, 77427
Radiation X
  See X-Ray
Radical Excision of Lymph Nodes
  Axillary, 38740-38745
  Cervical, 38720-38724
  Suprahyoid, 38700

Radical Mastectomies, Modified, 19307
Radical Neck Dissection
  with Auditory Canal Surgery, 69155
  with Thyroidectomy, 60254
  with Tongue Excision, 41135, 41145, 41153,
    41155
  Laryngectomy, 31365-31368
  Pharyngolaryngectomy, 31390, 31395
Radical Vaginal Hysterectomy, 58285
Radical Vulvectomy, 56630-56640
Radioactive Colloid Therapy, 79300
Radioactive Substance
  Insertion
    Prostate, 55860
Radiocarpal Joint
  Arthrotomy, 25040
  Dislocation
    Closed Treatment, 25660
Radiocinematographies
  Esophagus, 74230
  Pharynx, 70371, 74230
  Speech Evaluation, 70371
  Swallowing Evaluation, 74230
  Unlisted Services and Procedures, 76120-76125
Radio-Cobalt B12 Schilling Test
  Vitamin B12 Absorption Study, 78270-78272
Radioelement
  Application, 77761-77772
    with Ultrasound, 76965
    Surface, 77789
  Handling, 77790
  Infusion, 77750
  Placement *See* Radioelement Substance
Radioelement Substance
  Catheterization, 55875
  Catheter Placement
    Breast, 19296-19298
    Bronchus, 31643
    Head and/or Neck, 41019
    Muscle and/or Soft Tissue, 20555
    Pelvic Organs or Genitalia, 55920
    Prostate, 55875
  Needle Placement
    Head and/or Neck, 41019
    Muscle and/or Soft Tissue, 20555
    Pelvic Organs and Genitalia, 55920
    Prostate, 55875
Radiography
  See Radiology, Diagnostic; X-Ray
Radioimmunosorbent Test
  Gammaglobulin, Blood, 82784-82785
Radioisotope Brachytherapy
  See Brachytherapy
Radioisotope Scan
  See Nuclear Medicine
Radiological Marker
  Preoperative Placement
    Excision of Breast Lesion, 19125, 19126
Radiology
  See Also Nuclear Medicine, Radiation Therapy,
    X-Ray, Ultrasound
  Diagnostic
    Unlisted Services and Procedures, 76499
  Examination, 70030
    Stress Views, 77071
  Joint Survey, 77077
  Therapeutic
    Field Set-Up, 77280-77290
    Planning, 77261-77263, 77299
    Port Film, 77417
Radionuclide Therapy
  Heart, 79440
  Interstitial, 79300
  Intra-arterial, 79445
  Intra-articular, 79440
  Intracavitary, 79200
  Intravascular, 79101
  Intravenous, 79101, 79403
  Intravenous Infusion, 79101, 79403
  Oral, 79005
  Remote Afterloading, 77767-77768, 77770-
    77772
  Unlisted Services and Procedures, 79999
**Radionuclide Tomography, Single-Photon
  Emission-Computed**
  Abscess Localization, 78807

**Radionuclide Tomography, Single-Photon
  Emission-Computed** — *continued*
  Bone, 78320
  Brain, 78607
  Cerebrospinal Fluid, 78647
  Heart, 78451-78454
  Joint, 78320
  Kidney, 78710
  Liver, 78205
  Tumor Localization, 78803
Radiopharmaceutical Therapy
  Heart, 79440
  Interstitial, 79300
    Colloid Administration, 79300
  Intra-arterial Particulate, 79445
  Intra-articular, 79440
  Intracavitary, 79200
  Intravascular, 79101
  Intravenous, 78808, 79101, 79403
  Oral, 79005
  Unlisted Services and Procedures, 79999
Radiostereometic Analysis
  Lower Extremity, 0350T
  Placement Interstitial Device, 0347T
  Spine, 0348T
  Upper Extremity, 0349T
Radiosurgery
  Cranial Lesion, 61796-61799
  Spinal Lesion, 63620-63621
Radiotherapeutic
  See Radiation Therapy
Radiotherapies
  See Irradiation
Radiotherapy
  Afterloading, 77767-77768, 77770-77772
    Catheter Insertion, 19296-19298
    Planning, 77316-77318
Radiotherapy, Surface, 77789
Radioulnar Joint
  Arthrodesis
    with Ulnar Resection, 25830
  Dislocation
    Closed Treatment, 25525, 25675
    Open Treatment, 25676
    Percutaneous Fixation, 25671
Radius
  See Also Arm, Lower; Elbow; Ulna
  Arthroplasty, 24365
    with Implant, 24366, 25441
  Craterization, 24145, 25151
  Cyst
    Excision, 24125, 24126, 25120-25126
  Diaphysectomy, 24145, 25151
  Dislocation
    with Fracture
      Closed Treatment, 24620
      Open Treatment, 24635
    Partial, 24640
    Subluxate, 24640
  Excision, 24130, 24136, 24145, 24152
    Epiphyseal Bar, 20150
    Partial, 25145
    Styloid Process, 25230
  Fracture, 25605
    with Ulna, 25560, 25565
      Open Treatment, 25575
    Closed Treatment, 25500, 25505, 25520,
      25600, 25605
      with Manipulation, 25605
      without Manipulation, 25600
    Colles, 25600, 25605
    Distal, 25600-25609
      Closed Treatment, 25600-25605
      Open Treatment, 25607-25609
    Head/Neck
      Closed Treatment, 24650, 24655
      Open Treatment, 24665, 24666
    Open Treatment, 25515, 25525, 25526,
      25574
    Percutaneous Fixation, 25606
    Shaft, 25500-25526
      Open Treatment, 25515, 25574-25575
  Implant
    Removal, 24164
  Incision and Drainage, 25035
  Osteomyelitis, 24136, 24145

Radius — *continued*
  Osteoplasty, 25390-25393
  Prophylactic Treatment, 25490, 25492
  Repair
    with Graft, 25405, 25420-25426
    Epiphyseal Arrest, 25450, 25455
    Epiphyseal Separation
      Closed, 25600
      Closed with Manipulation, 25605
      Open Treatment, 25607, 25608-25609
      Percutaneous Fixation, 25606
    Malunion or Nonunion, 25400, 25415
    Osteotomy, 25350, 25355, 25370, 25375
      and Ulna, 25365
  Saucerization, 24145, 25151
  Sequestrectomy, 24136, 25145
  Subluxation, 24640
  Tumor
    Cyst, 24120
    Excision, 24125, 24126, 25120-25126,
      25170
RAF1, 81404, 81406
RA Factor
  Qualitative, 86430
  Quantitative, 86431
RAI1, 81405
Ramstedt Operation
  Pyloromyotomy, 43520
Ramus Anterior, Nervus Thoracicus
  Destruction, 64620
  Injection
    Anesthetic, 64420-64421
    Neurolytic, 64620
Range of Motion Test
  Extremities, 95851
  Eye, 92018, 92019
  Hand, 95852
  Rectum
    Biofeedback, 90911
  Trunk, 97530
Ranula
  Treatment of, 42408
Rapid Heart Rate
  Heart
    Recording, 93609
Rapid Plasma Reagin Test, 86592, 86593
Rapid Test for Infection, 86308, 86403, 86406
  Monospot Test, 86308
Rapoport Test, 52005
Raskind Procedure, 33735-33737
Rastelli Procedure, 33786
Rathke Pouch Tumor
  Excision, 61545
Rat Typhus, 86000
Rays, Roentgen
  See X-Ray
Raz Procedure, 51845
RBC, 78120, 78121, 78130-78140, 85007, 85014,
  85041, 85547, 85555, 85557, 85651-85660,
  86850-86870, 86970-86978
RBC ab, 86850-86870
RBL (Rubber Band Ligation)
  Hemorrhoids, 46221
  Skin Tags, 11200-11201
RCM, 96931-96936
RDH12,, 81434
Reaction
  Lip
    without Reconstruction, 40530
Realignment
  Femur, with Osteotomy, 27454
  Knee, Extensor, 27422
  Muscle, 20999
    Hand, 26989
  Tendon, Extensor, 26437
Reattachment
  Muscle, 20999
  Thigh, 27599
Receptor
  Antibody, 86243
  CD4, 86360
  Estrogen, 84233
  FC, 86243
  Progesterone, 84234
  Progestin, 84234

Receptor Assay
  Endocrine, 84235
  Estrogen, 84233
  Immunoglobulin, 86243
  Non–Hormone, 84238
  Progesterone, 84234

Recession
  Gastrocnemius
    Leg, Lower, 27687
  Tendon
    Hand, 26989

RECOMBIVAX HB, 90740, 90743–90744, 90746

Reconstruction
  See Also Revision
  Abdominal Wall
    Omental Flap, 49905
  Acetabulum, 27120, 27122
  Anal
    with Implant, 46762
    Congenital Absence, 46730–46740
    Fistula, 46742
    Graft, 46753
    Sphincter, 46750, 46751, 46760–46762
  Ankle, 27700–27703
  Apical–Aortic Conduit, 33404
  Atrial, 33254–33259
    Endoscopic, 33265–33266
    Open, 33254–33259
  Auditory Canal, External, 69310, 69320
  Bile Duct
    Anastomosis, 47800
  Bladder
    with Urethra, 51800, 51820
    from Colon, 50810
    from Intestines, 50820, 51960
  Breast
    with Free Flap, 19364
    with Latissimus Dorsi Flap, 19361
    with Other Techniques, 19366
    with Tissue Expander, 19357
    Augmentation, 19324, 19325
    Mammoplasty, 19318–19325
      Biesenberger, 19318
    Nipple, 19350, 19355
    Revision, 19380
    Transverse Rectus Abdominis Myocutaneous Flap, 19367–19369
  Bronchi
    with Lobectomy, 32501
    with Segmentectomy, 32501
    Graft Repair, 31770
    Stenosis, 31775
  Canthus, 67950
  Cardiac Anomaly, 33622
  Carpal, 25443
  Carpal Bone, 25394, 25430
  Cheekbone, 21270
  Chest Wall
    Omental Flap, 49905
    Trauma, 32820
  Cleft Palate, 42200–42225
  Conduit
    Apical–Aortic, 33404
  Conjunctiva, 68320–68335
    with Flap
      Bridge or Partial, 68360
      Total, 68362
  Cranial Bone
    Extracranial, 21181–21184
  Ear, Middle
    Tympanoplasty with Antrotomy or Mastoidectomy
      with Ossicular Chain Reconstruction, 69636, 69637
    Tympanoplasty with Mastoidectomy, 69641
      with Intact or Reconstructed Wall, 69643, 69644
      with Ossicular Chain Reconstruction, 69642
      Radical or Complete, 69644, 69645
    Tympanoplasty without Mastoidectomy, 69631
      with Ossicular Chain Reconstruction, 69632, 69633
  Elbow, 24360
    with Implant, 24361, 24362

Reconstruction — *continued*
  Elbow — *continued*
    Total Replacement, 24363
  Esophagus, 43300, 43310, 43313
    Creation
      Stoma, 43351–43352
    Esophagostomy, 43351–43352
    Fistula, 43305, 43312, 43314
    Gastrointestinal, 43360–43361
  Eye
    Graft
      Conjunctiva, 65782
      Stem Cell, 65781
    Transplantation
      Amniotic Membrane, 65780
  Eyelid
    Canthus, 67950
    Second Stage, 67975
    Total, 67973–67975
    Total Eyelid
      Lower, One Stage, 67973
      Upper, One Stage, 67974
    Transfer Tarsoconjunctival Flap from Opposing Eyelid, 67971
  Facial Bones
    Secondary, 21275
  Fallopian Tube, 58673, 58750–58752, 58770
  Femur
    Knee, 27442, 27443
    Lengthening, 27466, 27468
    Shortening, 27465, 27468
  Fibula
    Lengthening, 27715
  Finger
    Polydactylous, 26587
  Foot
    Cleft, 28360
  Forehead, 21172–21180, 21182–21184
  Glenoid Fossa, 21255
  Gums
    Alveolus, 41874
    Gingiva, 41872
  Hand
    Tendon Pulley, 26500–26502
    Toe to Finger Transfer, 26551–26556
  Heart
    Atrial, 33254–33259
      Endoscopic, 33265–33266
      Open, 33254–33259
    Atrial Septum, 33735–33737
    Pulmonary Artery Shunt, 33924
    Vena Cava, 34502
  Hip
    Replacement, 27130, 27132
    Secondary, 27134–27138
  Hip Joint
    with Prosthesis, 27125
  Interphalangeal Joint, 26535, 26536
    Collateral Ligament, 26545
  Intestines, Small
    Anastomosis, 44130
  Knee, 27437, 27438
    with Implantation, 27445
    with Prosthesis, 27438, 27445
    Femur, 27442, 27443, 27446
    Instability, 27420, 27424
    Ligament, 27427–27429
    Replacement, 27447
    Revision, 27486, 27487
    Tibia
      Plateau, 27440–27443, 27446
  Kneecap
    Instability, 27420–27424
  Larynx
    Burns, 31588
    Cricoid Split, 31587
    Other, 31545–31546, 31588
    Stenosis, 31582
    Web, 31580
  Lip, 40525, 40527, 40761
  Lunate, 25444
  Malar Augmentation
    with Bone Graft, 21210
    Prosthetic Material, 21270
  Mandible
    with Implant, 21244–21246, 21248, 21249

Reconstruction — *continued*
  Mandibular Condyle, 21247
  Mandibular Rami
    with Bone Graft, 21194
    with Internal Rigid Fixation, 21196
    without Bone Graft, 21193
    without Internal Rigid Fixation, 21195
  Maxilla
    with Implant, 21245, 21246, 21248, 21249
  Metacarpophalangeal Joint, 26530, 26531
  Midface, 21188
    with Bone Graft, 21145–21160, 21188
    with Internal Rigid Fixation, 21196
    without Bone Graft, 21141–21143
    without Internal Rigid Fixation, 21195
    Forehead Advancement, 21159, 21160
  Mouth, 40840–40845
  Nail Bed, 11762
  Nasoethmoid Complex, 21182–21184
  Navicular, 25443
  Nose
    Cleft Lip
      Cleft Palate, 30460, 30462
    Dermatoplasty, 30620
    Primary, 30400–30420
    Secondary, 30430–30462
    Septum, 30520
  Orbit, 21256
  Orbital Rim, 21172–21180
  Orbital Walls, 21182–21184
  Orbit Area
    Secondary, 21275
  Orbitocraniofacial
    Secondary Revision, 21275
  Orbit, with Bone Grafting, 21182–21184
  Oviduct
    Fimbrioplasty, 58760
  Palate
    Cleft Palate, 42200–42225
    Lengthening, 42226, 42227
  Parotid Duct
    Diversion, 42507–42510
  Patella, 27437, 27438
    Instability, 27420–27424
  Penis
    Angulation, 54360
    Chordee, 54300, 54304
    Complications, 54340–54348
    Epispadias, 54380–54390
    Hypospadias, 54332, 54352
      One Stage Distal with Urethroplasty, 54324–54328
      One Stage Perineal, 54336
  Periorbital Region
    Osteotomy with Graft, 21267, 21268
  Pharynx, 42950
  Pyloric Sphincter, 43800
  Radius, 24365, 25390–25393, 25441
    Arthroplasty
      with Implant, 24366
  Shoulder Joint
    with Implant, 23470, 23472
  Skull, 21172–21180
    Defect, 62140, 62141, 62145
  Sternum, 21740–21742
    with Thoracoscopy, 21743
  Stomach
    with Duodenum, 43810, 43850, 43855, 43865
    with Jejunum, 43820, 43825, 43860
    for Obesity, 43644–43645, 43845–43848
    Gastric Bypass, 43644–43846
    Roux–en–Y, 43644, 43846
  Superior–Lateral Orbital Rim and Forehead, 21172, 21175
  Supraorbital Rim and Forehead, 21179, 21180
  Symblepharon, 68335
  Temporomandibular Joint
    Arthroplasty, 21240–21243
  Throat, 42950
  Thumb
    from Finger, 26550
    Opponensplasty, 26490–26496
  Tibia
    Lengthening, 27715
    Tubercle, 27418

Reconstruction — *continued*
  Toe
    Angle Deformity, 28313
    Extra, 28344
    Hammertoe, 28285, 28286
    Macrodactyly, 28340, 28341
    Polydactylous, 26587
    Syndactyly, 28345
    Webbed Toe, 28345
  Tongue
    Frenum, 41520
  Trachea
    Carina, 31766
    Cervical, 31750
    Fistula, 31755
    Graft Repair, 31770
    Intrathoracic, 31760
  Trapezium, 25445
  Tympanic Membrane, 69620
  Ulna, 25390–25393, 25442
    Radioulnar, 25337
  Ureter, 50700
    with Intestines, 50840
  Urethra, 53410–53440, 53445
    Complications, 54340–54348
    Hypospadias
      Meatus, 53450, 53460
      One Stage Distal with Meatal Advancement, 54322
      One Stage Distal with Urethroplasty, 54324–54328
      Suture to Bladder, 51840, 51841
      Urethroplasty for Second Stage, 54308–54316
      Urethroplasty for Third Stage, 54318
  Uterus, 58540
  Vas Deferens, 55400
  Vena Cava, 34502
    with Resection, 37799
  Wound Repair, 13100–13160
  Wrist, 25332
    Capsulectomy, 25320
    Capsulorrhaphy, 25320
    Realign, 25335
  Zygomatic Arch, 21255

Recording
  Tremor, 95999

Rectal Bleeding
  Endoscopic Control, 45317

Rectal Packing, 45999

Rectal Prolapse
  Excision, 45130–45135
  Repair, 45900

Rectal Sphincter
  Dilation, 45910

Rectocele
  Repair, 45560

Rectopexy
  Laparoscopic, 45400–45402
  Open, 45540–45550

Rectoplasty, 45500–45505

Rectorrhaphy, 45540–45541, 45800–45825

Rectovaginal Fistula
  See Fistula, Rectovaginal

Rectovaginal Hernia
  See Rectocele

Rectum
  See Also Anus
  Abscess
    Incision and Drainage, 45005, 45020, 46040, 46060
  Biopsy, 45100
  Dilation
    Endoscopy, 45303
  Endoscopy
    Destruction
      Tumor, 45320
    Dilation, 45303
    Exploration, 45300
    Hemorrhage, 45317
    Removal
      Foreign Body, 45307
      Polyp, 45308–45315
      Tumor, 45308–45315
    Volvulus, 45321

Repair — Repair

Rotator Cuff
    Repair, 23410-23420
Rotavirus
    Antibody, 86759
    Antigen Detection
        Enzyme Immunoassay, 87425
Rotavirus Vaccine, 90680-90681
Round Window
    Repair Fistula, 69667
Round Window Fistula, 69667
Roux–en–Y Procedures
    Biliary Tract, 47740-47741, 47780-47785
    Pancreas, 48540
    Stomach, 43621, 43633, 43644, 43846
        Laparoscopic, 43644
RP1, 81404, 81434
RP2, 81434
RPE65, 81406, 81434
RPGR, 81434
RPP (Radical Perineal Prostatectomy), 55810-55815
RPR, 86592-86593
RPS19, 81405
RRM2B, 81405
RRP (Radical Retropubic Prostatectomy), 55840-55845
RSV
    Antibody, 86756
    Antigen Detection
        Direct Fluorescent Antibody, 87280
        Enzyme Immunoassay, 87420
        Recombinant, 90378
RT3, 84482
Rubber Band Ligation
    Hemorrhoids, 46221
    Skin Tags, 11200-11201
Rubella
    Antibody, 86762
    Vaccine, 90707-90710
Rubella HI Test
    Hemagglutination Inhibition Test, 86280
Rubella Immunization
    MMR, 90707
    MMRV, 90710
Rubeola
    Antibody, 86765
    Antigen Detection
        Immunofluorescence, 87283
Ruiz–Mora Procedure, 28286
RUNX1/RUNX1T1, 81401
Russell Viper Venom Time, 85612-85613
RYR1, 81406, 81408
RYR2, 81408

S

Saccomanno Technique, 88108
Sac, Endolymphatic
    Exploration, 69805-69806
Sacral Nerve
    Implantation
        Electrode, 64561, 64581
    Insertion
        Electrode, 64561, 64581
Sacroiliac Joint
    Arthrodesis, 27280
    Arthrotomy, 27050
    Biopsy, 27050
    Dislocation
        Open Treatment, 27218
    Fusion, 27280
    Injection for Arthrography, 27096
    Stabilization for Arthrodesis, 27279
    X–ray, 72200-72202, 73525
Sacroplasty, 0200T-0201T
Sacrum
    Augmentation, 0200T-0201T
    Pressure Ulcer, 15931-15937
    Tumor
        Excision, 49215
    X–ray, 72220
SAECG, 93278
SAH, 61566
Salabrasion, 15780-15787
Salicylate
    Assay, *[80329, 80330, 80331]*
Saline–Solution Abortion, 59850-59851

Salivary Duct
    Catheterization, 42660
    Dilation, 42650-42660
    Ligation, 42665
    Repair, 42500-42505
        Fistula, 42600
Salivary Glands
    Abscess
        Incision and Drainage, 42310-42320
    Biopsy, 42405
    Calculi (Stone)
        Excision, 42330-42340
    Cyst
        Drainage, 42409
        Excision, 42408
    Injection
        X–ray, 42550
    Needle Biopsy, 42400
    Nuclear Medicine
        Function Study, 78232
        Imaging, 78230-78231
    Parotid
        Abscess, 42300-42305
    Unlisted Services and Procedures, 42699
    X–ray, 70380-70390
        with Contrast, 70390
Salivary Gland Virus
    Antibody, 86644-86645
    Antigen Detection
        Direct Fluorescence, 87271
        Enzyme Immunoassay, 87332
        Nucleic Acid, 87495-87497
Salmonella
    Antibody, 86768
Salpingectomy, 58262-58263, 58291-58292, 58552, 58554, 58661, 58700
    Ectopic Pregnancy
        Laparoscopic Treatment, 59151
        Surgical Treatment, 59120
    Oophorectomy, 58943
Salpingohysterostomy, 58752
Salpingolysis, 58740
Salpingoneostomy, 58673, 58770
Salpingo–Oophorectomy, 58720
    Resection Ovarian Malignancy, 58950-58956
    Resection Peritoneal Malignancy, 58950-58956
    Resection Tubal Malignancy, 58950-58956
Salpingostomy, 58673, 58770
    Laparoscopic, 58673
SALT, 84460
Salter Osteotomy of the Pelvis, 27146
Sampling
    See Biopsy; Brush Biopsy; Needle Biopsy
Sang–Park Procedure
    Septectomy, Atrial, 33735-33737
        Balloon (Rashkind Type), 92992
        Blade Method (Park), 92993
Sao Paulo Typhus, 86000
SAST, 84450
Saucerization
    Calcaneus, 28120
    Clavicle, 23180
    Femur, 27070, 27360
    Fibula, 27360, 27641
    Hip, 27070
    Humerus, 23184, 24140
    Ileum, 27070
    Metacarpal, 26230
    Metatarsal, 28122
    Olecranon Process, 24147
    Phalanges
        Finger, 26235-26236
        Toe, 28124
    Pubis, 27070
    Radius, 24145, 25151
    Scapula, 23182
    Talus, 28120
    Tarsal, 28122
    Tibia, 27360, 27640
    Ulna, 24147, 25150
Saundby Test, 82270, 82272
Sauve–Kapandji Procedure
    Arthrodesis, Distal Radioulnar Joint, 25830
SAVER (Surgical Anterior Ventricular Endocardial Restoration), 33548
SBFT, 74249

SBRT (Stereotactic Body Radiation Therapy), 77373
Scabies, 87220
Scalenotomy, 21700-21705
Scalenus Anticus
    Division, 21700-21705
Scaling
    Chemical for Acne, 17360
Scalp
    Skin Graft
        Delay of Flap, 15610
        Full Thickness, 15220-15221
        Pedicle Flap, 15572
        Split, 15100-15101
    Tissue Transfer, Adjacent, 14020-14021
    Tumor Excision, 21011-21016
Scalp Blood Sampling, 59030
Scan
    See Also Specific Site; Nuclear Medicine
    Abdomen
        Computed Tomography, 74150-74175, 75635
    Computerized
        Ophthalmic, 92132-92134
    CT
        See CT Scan
    MRI
        See Magnetic Resonance Imaging
    PET
        With Computed Tomography (CT)
            Limited, 78814
            Skull Base to Mid-thigh, 78815
            Whole Body, 78816
        Brain, 78608-78609
        Heart, 78459
        Limited Area, 78811
        Myocardial Imaging Perfusion Study, 78491-78492
        Skull Base to Mid-Thigh, 78812
        Whole Body, 78813
    Radionuclide, Brain, 78607
Scanning Radioiosotope
    See Nuclear Medicine
Scanogram, 77073
Scaphoid
    Fracture
        with Manipulation, 25624
        Closed Treatment, 25622
        Open Treatment, 25628
Scapula
    Craterization, 23182
    Cyst
        Excision, 23140
            with Allograft, 23146
            with Autograft, 23145
    Diaphysectomy, 23182
    Excision, 23172, 23190
        Partial, 23182
    Fracture
        Closed Treatment
            with Manipulation, 23575
            without Manipulation, 23570
        Open Treatment, 23585
    Ostectomy, 23190
    Repair
        Fixation, 23400
        Scapulopexy, 23400
    Saucerization, 23182
    Sequestrectomy, 23172
    Tumor
        Excision, 23140, 23210
            with Allograft, 23146
            with Autograft, 23145
        Radical Resection, 23210
    X–ray, 73010
Scapulopexy, 23400
Scarification
    Pleural, 32215
Scarification of Pleura
    Agent for Pleurodesis, 32560
    Endoscopic, 32650
SCBE (Single Contrast Barium Enema), 74270
Schanz Operation, 27448
Schauta Operation, 58285
Schede Procedure, 32905-32906
Scheie Procedure, 66155

Schilling Test, 78270-78272
Schlatter Operation, 43620
Schlemm's Canal Dilation, 66174-66175
Schlicter Test, 87197
Schocket Procedure, 66180
Schuchard Procedure
    Osteotomy
        Maxilla, 21206
Schwannoma, Acoustic
    See Brain, Tumor, Excision
Sciatic Nerve
    Decompression, 64712
    Injection
        Anesthetic, 64445-64446
    Lesion
        Excision, 64786
    Neuroma
        Excision, 64786
    Neuroplasty, 64712
    Release, 64712
    Repair
        Suture, 64858
Scintigraphy
    See Emission Computerized Tomography
    See Nuclear Medicine
Scissoring
    Skin Tags, 11200-11201
Sclera
    Excision, 66130
        Sclerectomy with Punch or Scissors, 66160
    Fistulization
        Sclerectomy with Punch or Scissors with Iridectomy, 66160
        Thermocauterization with Iridectomy, 66155
        Trabeculectomy ab Externo in Absence of Previous Surgery, 66170
        Trephination with Iridectomy, 66150
    Incision (Fistulization)
        Sclerectomy with Punch or Scissors with Iridectomy, 66160
        Thermocauterization with Iridectomy, 66155
        Trabeculectomy ab Externo in Absence of Previous Surgery, 66170
        Trephination with Iridectomy, 66150
    Lesion
        Excision, 66130
    Repair
        with Glue, 65286
        Reinforcement
            with Graft, 67255
            without Graft, 67250
        Staphyloma
            with Graft, 66225
            without Graft, 66220
        Wound (Operative), 66250
        Tissue Glue, 65286
Scleral Buckling Operation
    Retina, Repair, Detachment, 67107-67108, 67113
Scleral Ectasia
    Repair, 66220
        with Graft, 66225
Sclerectomy, 66160
Sclerotherapy
    Percutaneous (Cyst, Lymphocele, Seroma), 49185
    Venous, 36468-36471
Sclerotomy, 66150-66170
SCN1A, 81407
SCN1B, 81404
SCN4A, 81406
SCN5A, 81407
SCNN1A, 81406
SCNN1B, 81406
SCNN1G, 81406
SCO1, 81405
SCO2, 81404
Scoliosis Evaluation, Radiologic, 72081-72084
Scrambler Therapy, 0278T
Screening
    Developmental, 96110
    Drug
        Alcohol and/or Substance Abuse, 99408-99409

[Resequenced]

Skin — Skull Base Surgery

Index

Subcutaneous Implantable Defibrillator Device — Suture

Suture — continued
  Vein
    Femoral, 37650
    Iliac, 37660
    Vena Cava, 37619
  Wound, 44604-44605
    Skin
      Complex, 13100-13160
      Intermediate, 12031-12057
      Simple, 12020-12021
SUZI (Sub-Zonal Insemination), 89280
SVR (Surgical Ventricular Restoration), 33548
Swallowing
  Cine, 74230
  Evaluation, 92610-92613, 92616-92617
  Therapy, 92526
  Video, 74230
Swan-Ganz Catheter Insertion, 93503
Swanson Procedure
  Repair, Metatarsal, 28322
  Osteotomy, 28306-28309
Sweat Collection
  Iontophoresis, 89230
Sweat Glands
  Excision
    Axillary, 11450, 11451
    Inguinal, 11462, 11463
    Perianal, 11470, 11471
    Perineal, 11470, 11471
    Umbilical, 11470, 11471
Sweat Test
  Chloride, Blood, 82435
Swenson Procedure, 45120
Syme Procedure, 27888
Sympathectomy
  with Rib Excision, 21616
  Artery
    Digital, 64820
    Radial, 64821
    Superficial Palmar Arch, 64823
    Ulnar, 64822
  Cervical, 64802
  Cervicothoracic, 64804
  Digital Artery with Magnification, 64820
  Lumbar, 64818
  Presacral, 58410
  Renal, 0338T-0339T
  Thoracic, 32664
  Thoracolumbar, 64809
Sympathetic Nerve
  Excision, 64802-64818
  Injection
    Anesthetic, 64508, 64520-64530
Sympathins, 80424, 82382-82384
Symphysiotomy
  Horseshoe Kidney, 50540
Symphysis, Pubic, 27282
Synagis, 90378
Syncytial Virus, Respiratory
  Antibody, 86756
  Antigen Detection
    Direct Fluorescence, 87280
    Direct Optical Observation, 87807
    Enzyme Immunoassay, 87420
Syndactylism, Toes, 28280
Syndactyly
  Repair, 26560-26562
Syndesmotomy
  Coracoacromial
    Arthroscopic, 29826
    Open, 23130, 23415
  Lateral Retinacular
    Endoscopic, 29873
    Open, 27425
  Transverse Carpal, 29848
Syndrome
  Adrenogenital, 56805, 57335
  Ataxia–Telangiectasia
    Chromosome Analysis, 88248
  Bloom
    Chromosome Analysis, 88245
    Genomic Sequence Analysis, 81412
  Carpal Tunnel
    Decompression, 64721
  Costen's
    See Temporomandibular Joint (TMJ)

Syndrome — continued
  Erb–Goldflam, 95857
  Ovarian Vein
    Ureterolysis, 50722
  Synechiae, Intrauterine
    Lysis, 58559
  Treacher Collins
    Midface Reconstruction, 21150-21151
  Urethral
    Cystourethroscopy, 52285
Syngesterone, 84144
Synostosis (Cranial)
  Bifrontal Craniotomy, 61557
  Extensive Craniectomy, 61558-61559
  Frontal Craniotomy, 61556
  Parietal Craniotomy, 61556
Synovectomy
  Arthrotomy with
    Glenohumeral Joint, 23105
    Sternoclavicular Joint, 23106
  Elbow, 24102
  Excision
    Carpometacarpal Joint, 26130
    Finger Joint, 26135-26140
    Hip Joint, 27054
    Interphalangeal Joint, 26140
    Knee Joint, 27334-27335
    Metacarpophalangeal Joint, 26135
    Palm, 26145
  Wrist, 25105, 25115-25119
    Radical, 25115-25116
Synovial
  Bursa
    See Also Bursa
    Joint Aspiration, 20600-20611
  Cyst
    See Also Ganglion
    Aspiration, 20612
  Membrane
    See Synovium
  Popliteal Space, 27345
Synovium
  Biopsy
    Carpometacarpal Joint, 26100
    Interphalangeal Joint, 26110
    Knee Joint, 27330
    Metacarpophalangeal Joint
      with Synovial Biopsy, 26105
  Excision
    Carpometacarpal Joint, 26130
    Finger Joint, 26135-26140
    Hip Joint, 27054
    Interphalangeal Joint, 26140
    Knee Joint, 27334-27335
Syphilis Nontreponemal Antibody, 86592-86593
Syphilis Test, 86592, 86593
Syrinx
  Spinal Cord
    Aspiration, 62268
System
  Auditory, 69000-69979
  Cardiovascular, 33010-37799 [33221, 33227,
    33228, 33229, 33230, 33231, 33262,
    33263, 33264, 33270, 33271, 33272,
    33273, 33962, 33963, 33964, 33965,
    33966, 33969, 33984, 33985, 33986,
    33987, 33988, 33989, 37211, 37212,
    37213, 37214]
  Digestive, 40490-49999 [43211, 43212, 43213,
    43214, 43233, 43266, 43270, 43274,
    43275, 43276, 43277, 43278, 44381,
    44401, 45346, 45388, 45390, 45398,
    45399, 46220, 46320, 46945, 46946,
    46947]
  Endocrine, 60000-60699
  Eye/Ocular Adnexa, 65091-68899 [67810]
  Genital
    Female, 56405-58999
    Male, 54000-55899
  Hemic/Lymphatic, 38100-38999
  Integumentary, 10040-19499 [11045, 11046]
  Mediastinum/Diaphragm, 39000-39599

System — continued
  Musculoskeletal, 20005-29999 [21552, 21554,
    22858, 23071, 23073, 24071, 24073,
    25071, 25073, 26111, 26113, 27043,
    27045, 27059, 27329, 27337, 27339,
    27632, 27634, 28039, 28041, 29914,
    29915, 29916]
  Nervous, 61000-64999 [64633, 64634, 64635,
    64636]
  Respiratory, 30000-32999 [31651]
  Urinary, 50010-53899 [51797, 52356]

T–3, 84480
T3 Free, 84481
T–4
  T Cells, 86360-86361
  Thyroxine, 84436-84439
T4 Molecule, 86360
T4 Total, 84436
T–7 Index
  Thyroxine, Total, 84436
  Triiodothyronine, 84480-84482
T–8, 86360
Taarnhoj Procedure
  Decompression, Gasserian Ganglion, Sensory
    Root, 61450
Tachycardia
  Heart
    Recording, 93609
TACO1, 81404
Tacrolimus
  Assay, 80197
Tag
  Anus, 46230 [46220]
  Skin Removal, 11200-11201
TAH, 51925, 58150, 58152, 58200-58240, 58951,
  59525
TAHBSO, 58150, 58152, 58200-58240, 58951
Tail Bone
  Excision, 27080
  Fracture, 27200, 27202
Takeuchi Procedure, 33505
Talectomy, 28130
Talotarsal Joint
  Dislocation, 28570, 28575, 28585
  Percutaneous Fixation, 28576
Talus
  Arthrodesis
    Pantalar, 28705
    Subtalar, 28725
    Triple, 28715
  Arthroscopy
    Surgical, 29891, 29892
  Craterization, 28120
  Cyst
    Excision, 28100-28103
  Diaphysectomy, 28120
  Excision, 28120, 28130
  Fracture
    with Manipulation, 28435, 28436
    without Manipulation, 28430
    Open Treatment, 28445
    Percutaneous Fixation, 28436
  Osteochondral Graft, 28446
  Repair
    Osteochondritis Dissecans, 29892
    Osteotomy, 28302
  Saucerization, 28120
  Tumor
    Excision, 27647, 28100-28103
Tap
  Cisternal, 61050-61055
  Lumbar Diagnostic, 62270
TARDBP, 81405
Tarsal
  Fracture
    Percutaneous Fixation, 28456
Tarsal Bone
  See Ankle Bone
Tarsal Joint
  See Also Foot
  Arthrodesis, 28730, 28735, 28740
    with Advancement, 28737
    with Lengthening, 28737
  Craterization, 28122

Tarsal Joint — continued
  Cyst
    Excision, 28104-28107
  Diaphysectomy, 28122
  Dislocation, 28540, 28545, 28555
    Percutaneous Fixation, 28545, 28546
  Excision, 28116, 28122
  Fracture
    with Manipulation, 28455, 28456
    without Manipulation, 28450
    Open Treatment, 28465
  Fusion, 28730, 28735, 28740
    with Advancement, 28737
    with Lengthening, 28737
  Repair, 28320
    Osteotomy, 28304, 28305
  Saucerization, 28122
  Tumor
    Excision, 28104-28107, 28171
Tarsal Strip Procedure, 67917, 67924
Tarsal Tunnel Release, 28035
Tarsal Wedge Procedure, 67916, 67923
Tarsometatarsal Joint
  Arthrodesis, 28730, 28735, 28740
  Arthrotomy, 28020, 28050
  Biopsy
    Synovial, 28050, 28052
  Dislocation, 28600, 28605, 28615
    Percutaneous Fixation, 28606
  Exploration, 28020
  Fusion, 28730, 28735, 28740
  Removal
    Foreign Body, 28020
    Loose Body, 28020
  Synovial
    Biopsy, 28050
    Excision, 28070
Tarsorrhaphy, 67875
  Median, 67880
  Severing, 67710
    with Transposition of Tarsal Plate, 67882
Tattoo
  Cornea, 65600
  Skin, 11920-11922
Tay-Sachs Disease
  Genomic Sequence Analysis, 81412
TAZ, 81406
TB, 87015, 87116, 87190
TBG, 84442
TBNA (Transbronchial Needle Aspiration), 31629,
  31633
TBP, 81401
TBS, 88164, 88166
TB Test
  Antigen Response, 86480
  Cell Mediated Immunity Measurement, 86480-
    86481
  Skin Test, 86580
TBX5, 81405
TCD (Transcranial Doppler), 93886-93893
TCD@, 81402
T Cell
  Antigen Receptor
    Beta Gene Rearrangement Analysis, 81340-
      81341
    Gamma Gene Rearrangement Analysis,
      81342
  Leukemia Lymphoma Virus I, 86687, 86689
  Leukemia Lymphoma Virus II, 86688
T–Cell T8 Antigens, 86360
TCF4, 81405-81406
TCT, 85670
Tear Duct
  See Lacrimal Gland
Tear Film Imaging, 0330T
Tear Gland
  See Lacrimal Gland
Technique
  Pericardial Window, 33015
TEE, 93312-93318
Teeth
  X–ray, 70300-70320
Telangiectasia
  Chromosome Analysis, 88248
  Injection, 36468

Tumor — Ultrasonography

[Resequenced]

X–ray — *continued*
Chest — *continued*
Partial (two views)
with Fluoroscopy, 71023
Stereo, 71015
Clavicle, 73000
Coccyx, 72220
Consultation, 76140
Duodenum, 74260
Elbow, 73070, 73080
Esophagus, 74220
Eye, 70030
Facial Bones, 70140, 70150
Fallopian Tube, 74742
Femur, 73551-73552
Fibula, 73590
Fingers, 73140
Fistula, 76080
Foot, 73620, 73630
Gastrointestinal Tract, 74240-74245
Guide Dilation, 74360
Guide Intubation, 49440, 74340
Upper, 3142F, 3200F
Hand, 73120, 73130
Head, 70350
Heel, 73650
Hip, 73501-73503, 73521-73523
Humerus, 73060
Intestines, Small, 74245, 74249-74251
Guide Intubation, 74355

X–ray — *continued*
Jaws, 70355
Joint
Stress Views, 77071
Knee, 73560-73564, 73580
Bilateral, 73565
Larynx, 70370
Leg, 73592
Lumen Dilator, 74360
Mandible, 70100, 70110
Mastoids, 70120, 70130
Nasal Bones, 70160
Neck, 70360
Nose to Rectum
Foreign Body
Child, 76010
Orbit, 70190, 70200
Pelvis, 72170, 72190
Manometry, 74710
Peritoneum, 74190
Pharynx, 70370, 74210
Ribs, 71100-71111
Sacroiliac Joint, 72200, 72202
Sacrum, 72220
Salivary Gland, 70380
Scapula, 73010
Sella Turcica, 70240
Shoulder, 73020, 73030, 73050
Sinuses, 70210, 70220
Sinus Tract, 76080

X–ray — *continued*
Skull, 70250, 70260
Specimen
Surgical, 76098
Spine, 72020
Cervical, 72040-72052
Lumbosacral, 72100-72120
Thoracic, 72070-72074
Thoracolumbar, 72080, 72084
Thoracolumbar Junction, 72080
Sternum, 71120, 71130
Teeth, 70300-70320
Tibia, 73590
Toe, 73660
Total Body
Foreign Body, 76010
Unlisted Services and Procedures, 76120, 76125
Upper Gastrointestinal Series (Upper GI Series),
3142F, 3200F
Wrist, 73100, 73110
X–Ray Tomography, Computed
See CT Scan
Xylose Absorption Test
Blood, 84620
Urine, 84620

Yacoub Procedure, 33864
YAG, 66821

Yeast
Culture, 87106
Yellow Fever Vaccine, 90717
Yersinia
Antibody, 86793
YF-VAX, 90717
Y–Plasty, 51800

ZEB2, 81404-81405
Ziegler Procedure
Discission Secondary Membranous Cataract,
66820
ZIFT, 58976
Zinc, 84630
Zinc Manganese Leucine Aminopeptidase, 83670
ZNF41, 81404
Zonisamide
Assay, 80203
ZOSTAVAX, 90736
Z–Plasty, 26121-26125, 41520
Zygoma
Fracture Treatment, 21355-21366
Reconstruction, 21270
Zygomatic Arch
Fracture
with Manipulation, 21355
Open Treatment, 21356-21366
Reconstruction, 21255

00100-00126 Anesthesia for Cleft Lip, Ear, ECT, Eyelid, and Salivary Gland Procedures

CMS: 100-4,12,140.1 Qualified Nonphysician Anesthetists; 100-4,12,140.3 Payment for Qualified Nonphysician Anesthetists; 100-4,12,140.3.3 Billing Modifiers; 100-4,12,140.3.4 General Billing Instructions; 100-4,12,140.4.1 Anesthesiologist/Qualified Nonphysican Anesthetist; 100-4,12,140.4.2 Anesthetist and Anesthesiologist in a Single Procedure; 100-4,12,140.4.3 Payment for Medical /Surgical Services by CRNAs; 100-4,12,140.4.4 Conversion Factors for Anesthesia Services; 100-4,4,250.3.2 Anesthesia in a Hospital Outpatient Setting

00100 **Anesthesia for procedures on salivary glands, including biopsy**
0.00   0.00   **FUD** XXX   N ☐ PQ
AMA: 2015,Jan,16; 2014,Aug,5; 2014,Jan,11; 2012,Jul,12-14; 2012,Jan,15-42; 2011,Oct,3-4; 2011,Jul,16-17; 2011,Jan,11

00102 **Anesthesia for procedures involving plastic repair of cleft lip**
0.00   0.00   **FUD** XXX   N ☐ PQ
AMA: 2015,Jan,16; 2014,Aug,5; 2014,Jan,11; 2012,Jul,12-14; 2012,Jan,15-42; 2011,Oct,3-4; 2011,Jul,16-17; 2011,Jan,11

00103 **Anesthesia for reconstructive procedures of eyelid (eg, blepharoplasty, ptosis surgery)**
0.00   0.00   **FUD** XXX   N ☐ PQ
AMA: 2015,Jan,16; 2014,Aug,5; 2014,Jan,11; 2012,Jul,12-14; 2012,Jan,15-42; 2011,Oct,3-4; 2011,Jul,16-17; 2011,Jan,11

00104 **Anesthesia for electroconvulsive therapy**
0.00   0.00   **FUD** XXX   N ☐ PQ
AMA: 2015,Jan,16; 2014,Aug,5; 2014,Jan,11; 2012,Jul,12-14; 2012,Jan,15-42; 2011,Oct,3-4; 2011,Jul,16-17; 2011,Jan,11; 2010,Mar,6-8

00120 **Anesthesia for procedures on external, middle, and inner ear including biopsy; not otherwise specified**
0.00   0.00   **FUD** XXX   N ☐ PQ
AMA: 2015,Jan,16; 2014,Aug,5; 2014,Jan,11; 2012,Jul,12-14; 2012,Jan,15-42; 2011,Oct,3-4; 2011,Jul,16-17; 2011,Jan,11

00124 **otoscopy**
0.00   0.00   **FUD** XXX   N ☐ PQ
AMA: 2015,Jan,16; 2014,Aug,5; 2014,Jan,11; 2012,Jul,12-14; 2012,Jan,15-42; 2011,Oct,3-4; 2011,Jul,16-17; 2011,Jan,11

00126 **tympanotomy**
0.00   0.00   **FUD** XXX   N ☐ PQ
AMA: 2015,Jan,16; 2014,Aug,5; 2014,Jan,11; 2012,Jul,12-14; 2012,Jan,15-42; 2011,Oct,3-4; 2011,Jul,16-17; 2011,Jan,11

00140-00148 Anesthesia for Eye Procedures

CMS: 100-4,12,140.1 Qualified Nonphysician Anesthetists; 100-4,12,140.3 Payment for Qualified Nonphysician Anesthetists; 100-4,12,140.3.3 Billing Modifiers; 100-4,12,140.3.4 General Billing Instructions; 100-4,12,140.4.1 Anesthesiologist/Qualified Nonphysican Anesthetist; 100-4,12,140.4.2 Anesthetist and Anesthesiologist in a Single Procedure; 100-4,12,140.4.3 Payment for Medical /Surgical Services by CRNAs; 100-4,12,140.4.4 Conversion Factors for Anesthesia Services; 100-4,4,250.3.2 Anesthesia in a Hospital Outpatient Setting

00140 **Anesthesia for procedures on eye; not otherwise specified**
0.00   0.00   **FUD** XXX   N ☐ PQ
AMA: 2015,Jan,16; 2014,Aug,5; 2014,Jan,11; 2012,Jul,12-14; 2012,Jan,15-42; 2011,Oct,3-4; 2011,Jul,16-17; 2011,Jan,11

00142 **lens surgery**
0.00   0.00   **FUD** XXX   N ☐ PQ
AMA: 2015,Jan,16; 2014,Aug,5; 2014,Jan,11; 2012,Jul,12-14; 2012,Jan,15-42; 2011,Oct,3-4; 2011,Jul,16-17; 2011,Jan,11

00144 **corneal transplant**
0.00   0.00   **FUD** XXX   N ☐ PQ
AMA: 2015,Jan,16; 2014,Aug,5; 2014,Jan,11; 2012,Jul,12-14; 2012,Jan,15-42; 2011,Oct,3-4; 2011,Jul,16-17; 2011,Jan,11

00145 **vitreoretinal surgery**
0.00   0.00   **FUD** XXX   N ☐ PQ
AMA: 2015,Jan,16; 2014,Aug,5; 2014,Jan,11; 2012,Jul,12-14; 2012,Jan,15-42; 2011,Oct,3-4; 2011,Jul,16-17; 2011,Jan,11

00147 **iridectomy**
0.00   0.00   **FUD** XXX   N ☐ PQ
AMA: 2015,Jan,16; 2014,Aug,5; 2014,Jan,11; 2012,Jul,12-14; 2012,Jan,15-42; 2011,Oct,3-4; 2011,Jul,16-17; 2011,Jan,11

00148 **ophthalmoscopy**
0.00   0.00   **FUD** XXX   N ☐ PQ
AMA: 2015,Jan,16; 2014,Aug,5; 2014,Jan,11; 2012,Jul,12-14; 2012,Jan,15-42; 2011,Oct,3-4; 2011,Jul,16-17; 2011,Jan,11

00160-00326 Anesthesia for Face and Head Procedures

CMS: 100-4,12,140.1 Qualified Nonphysician Anesthetists; 100-4,12,140.3 Payment for Qualified Nonphysician Anesthetists; 100-4,12,140.3.3 Billing Modifiers; 100-4,12,140.3.4 General Billing Instructions; 100-4,12,140.4.1 Anesthesiologist/Qualified Nonphysican Anesthetist; 100-4,12,140.4.2 Anesthetist and Anesthesiologist in a Single Procedure; 100-4,12,140.4.4 Conversion Factors for Anesthesia Services; 100-4,4,250.3.2 Anesthesia in a Hospital Outpatient Setting

00160 **Anesthesia for procedures on nose and accessory sinuses; not otherwise specified**
0.00   0.00   **FUD** XXX   N ☐ PQ
AMA: 2015,Jan,16; 2014,Aug,5; 2014,Jan,11; 2012,Jul,12-14; 2012,Jan,15-42; 2011,Oct,3-4; 2011,Jul,16-17; 2011,Jan,11

00162 **radical surgery**
0.00   0.00   **FUD** XXX   N ☐ PQ
AMA: 2015,Jan,16; 2014,Aug,5; 2014,Jan,11; 2012,Jul,12-14; 2012,Jan,15-42; 2011,Oct,3-4; 2011,Jul,16-17; 2011,Jan,11

00164 **biopsy, soft tissue**
0.00   0.00   **FUD** XXX   N ☐ PQ
AMA: 2015,Jan,16; 2014,Aug,5; 2014,Jan,11; 2012,Jul,12-14; 2012,Jan,15-42; 2011,Oct,3-4; 2011,Jul,16-17; 2011,Jan,11

00170 **Anesthesia for intraoral procedures, including biopsy; not otherwise specified**
0.00   0.00   **FUD** XXX   N ☐ PQ
AMA: 2015,Jan,16; 2014,Aug,5; 2014,Jan,11; 2012,Jul,12-14; 2012,Jan,15-42; 2011,Oct,3-4; 2011,Jul,16-17; 2011,Jan,11

00172 **repair of cleft palate**
0.00   0.00   **FUD** XXX   N ☐ PQ
AMA: 2015,Jan,16; 2014,Aug,5; 2014,Jan,11; 2012,Jul,12-14; 2012,Jan,15-42; 2011,Oct,3-4; 2011,Jul,16-17; 2011,Jan,11

00174 **excision of retropharyngeal tumor**
0.00   0.00   **FUD** XXX   N ☐ PQ
AMA: 2015,Jan,16; 2014,Aug,5; 2014,Jan,11; 2012,Jul,12-14; 2012,Jan,15-42; 2011,Oct,3-4; 2011,Jul,16-17; 2011,Jan,11

00176 **radical surgery**
0.00   0.00   **FUD** XXX   C ☐ PQ
AMA: 2015,Jan,16; 2014,Aug,5; 2014,Jan,11; 2012,Jul,12-14; 2012,Jan,15-42; 2011,Oct,3-4; 2011,Jul,16-17; 2011,Jan,11

00190 **Anesthesia for procedures on facial bones or skull; not otherwise specified**
0.00   0.00   **FUD** XXX   N ☐ PQ
AMA: 2015,Jan,16; 2014,Aug,5; 2014,Jan,11; 2012,Jul,12-14; 2012,Jan,15-42; 2011,Oct,3-4; 2011,Jul,16-17; 2011,Jan,11

00192 **radical surgery (including prognathism)**
0.00   0.00   **FUD** XXX   C ☐ PQ
AMA: 2015,Jan,16; 2014,Aug,5; 2014,Jan,11; 2012,Jul,12-14; 2012,Jan,15-42; 2011,Oct,3-4; 2011,Jul,16-17; 2011,Jan,11

00210 **Anesthesia for intracranial procedures; not otherwise specified**
0.00   0.00   **FUD** XXX   N ☐ PQ
AMA: 2015,Jan,16; 2014,Aug,5; 2014,Jan,11; 2012,Jul,12-14; 2012,Jan,15-42; 2011,Oct,3-4; 2011,Jul,16-17; 2011,Jan,11

00211 **craniotomy or craniectomy for evacuation of hematoma**
0.00   0.00   **FUD** XXX   C PQ
AMA: 2015,Jan,16; 2014,Aug,5; 2014,Jan,11; 2012,Jul,12-14; 2012,Jan,15-42; 2011,Oct,3-4; 2011,Jul,16-17; 2011,Jan,11

00212 **subdural taps**
0.00   0.00   **FUD** XXX   N ☐ PQ
AMA: 2015,Jan,16; 2014,Aug,5; 2014,Jan,11; 2012,Jul,12-14; 2012,Jan,15-42; 2011,Oct,3-4; 2011,Jul,16-17; 2011,Jan,11

00214 **burr holes, including ventriculography**
0.00   0.00   **FUD** XXX   C ☐ PQ
AMA: 2015,Jan,16; 2014,Aug,5; 2014,Jan,11; 2012,Jul,12-14; 2012,Jan,15-42; 2011,Oct,3-4; 2011,Jul,16-17; 2011,Jan,11

Anesthesia

00215 — 00522

00215	**cranioplasty or elevation of depressed skull fracture, extradural (simple or compound)** 📷 0.00 ⚕ 0.00 **FUD** XXX ⊂ ▭ P̄Q̄ **AMA:** 2015,Jan,16; 2014,Aug,5; 2014,Jan,11; 2012,Jul,12-14; 2012,Jan,15-42; 2011,Oct,3-4; 2011,Jul,16-17; 2011,Jan,11
00216	**vascular procedures** 📷 0.00 ⚕ 0.00 **FUD** XXX N̄ ▭ P̄Q̄ **AMA:** 2015,Jan,16; 2014,Aug,5; 2014,Jan,11; 2012,Jul,12-14; 2012,Jan,15-42; 2011,Oct,3-4; 2011,Jul,16-17; 2011,Jan,11
00218	**procedures in sitting position** 📷 0.00 ⚕ 0.00 **FUD** XXX N̄ ▭ P̄Q̄ **AMA:** 2015,Jan,16; 2014,Aug,5; 2014,Jan,11; 2012,Jul,12-14; 2012,Jan,15-42; 2011,Oct,3-4; 2011,Jul,16-17; 2011,Jan,11
00220	**cerebrospinal fluid shunting procedures** 📷 0.00 ⚕ 0.00 **FUD** XXX N̄ ▭ P̄Q̄ **AMA:** 2015,Jan,16; 2014,Aug,5; 2014,Jan,11; 2012,Jul,12-14; 2012,Jan,15-42; 2011,Oct,3-4; 2011,Jul,16-17; 2011,Jan,11
00222	**electrocoagulation of intracranial nerve** 📷 0.00 ⚕ 0.00 **FUD** XXX N̄ ▭ P̄Q̄ **AMA:** 2015,Jan,16; 2014,Aug,5; 2014,Jan,11; 2012,Jul,12-14; 2012,Jan,15-42; 2011,Oct,3-4; 2011,Jul,16-17; 2011,Jan,11
00300	**Anesthesia for all procedures on the integumentary system, muscles and nerves of head, neck, and posterior trunk, not otherwise specified** 📷 0.00 ⚕ 0.00 **FUD** XXX N̄ ▭ P̄Q̄ **AMA:** 2015,Jan,16; 2014,Aug,5; 2014,Jan,11; 2012,Jul,12-14; 2012,Jan,15-42; 2011,Oct,3-4; 2011,Jul,16-17; 2011,Jan,11
00320	**Anesthesia for all procedures on esophagus, thyroid, larynx, trachea and lymphatic system of neck; not otherwise specified, age 1 year or older** 📷 0.00 ⚕ 0.00 **FUD** XXX N̄ ▭ P̄Q̄ **AMA:** 2015,Jan,16; 2014,Aug,5; 2014,Jan,11; 2012,Jul,12-14; 2012,Jan,15-42; 2011,Oct,3-4; 2011,Jul,16-17; 2011,Jan,11
00322	**needle biopsy of thyroid** **EXCLUDES** *Cervical spine and spinal cord procedures (00600, 00604, 00670)* 📷 0.00 ⚕ 0.00 **FUD** XXX N̄ ▭ P̄Q̄ **AMA:** 2015,Jan,16; 2014,Aug,5; 2014,Jan,11; 2012,Jul,12-14; 2012,Jan,15-42; 2011,Oct,3-4; 2011,Jul,16-17; 2011,Jan,11
00326	**Anesthesia for all procedures on the larynx and trachea in children younger than 1 year of age** A Do not report with (99100) 📷 0.00 ⚕ 0.00 **FUD** XXX N̄ ▭ P̄Q̄ **AMA:** 2015,Jan,16; 2014,Aug,5; 2014,Jan,11; 2012,Jul,12-14; 2012,Jan,15-42; 2011,Oct,3-4; 2011,Jul,16-17; 2011,Jan,11

00350-00352 Anesthesia for Neck Vessel Procedures

CMS: 100-4,12,140.1 Qualified Nonphysician Anesthetists; 100-4,12,140.3 Payment for Qualified Nonphysician Anesthetists; 100-4,12,140.3.3 Billing Modifiers; 100-4,12,140.3.4 General Billing Instructions; 100-4,12,140.4.1 Anesthesiologist/Qualified Nonphysician Anesthetist; 100-4,12,140.4.2 Anesthetist and Anesthesiologist in a Single Procedure; 100-4,12,140.4.3 Payment for Medical /Surgical Services by CRNAs; 100-4,12,140.4.4 Conversion Factors for Anesthesia Services; 100-4,4,250.3.2 Anesthesia in a Hospital Outpatient Setting

EXCLUDES *Arteriography (01916)*

00350	**Anesthesia for procedures on major vessels of neck; not otherwise specified** 📷 0.00 ⚕ 0.00 **FUD** XXX N̄ ▭ P̄Q̄ **AMA:** 2015,Jan,16; 2014,Aug,5; 2014,Jan,11; 2012,Jul,12-14; 2012,Jan,15-42; 2011,Oct,3-4; 2011,Jul,16-17; 2011,Jan,11
00352	**simple ligation** 📷 0.00 ⚕ 0.00 **FUD** XXX N̄ ▭ P̄Q̄ **AMA:** 2015,Jan,16; 2014,Aug,5; 2014,Jan,11; 2012,Jul,12-14; 2012,Jan,15-42; 2011,Oct,3-4; 2011,Jul,16-17; 2011,Jan,11

00400-00529 Anesthesia for Chest/Pectoral Girdle Procedures

CMS: 100-4,12,140.1 Qualified Nonphysician Anesthetists; 100-4,12,140.3 Payment for Qualified Nonphysician Anesthetists; 100-4,12,140.3.3 Billing Modifiers; 100-4,12,140.3.4 General Billing Instructions; 100-4,12,140.4.1 Anesthesiologist/Qualified Nonphysican Anesthetist; 100-4,12,140.4.2 Anesthetist and Anesthesiologist in a Single Procedure; 100-4,12,140.4.3 Payment for Medical /Surgical Services by CRNAs; 100-4,12,140.4.4 Conversion Factors for Anesthesia Services; 100-4,4,250.3.2 Anesthesia in a Hospital Outpatient Setting

00400	**Anesthesia for procedures on the integumentary system on the extremities, anterior trunk and perineum; not otherwise specified** 📷 0.00 ⚕ 0.00 **FUD** XXX N̄ ▭ P̄Q̄ **AMA:** 2015,Jan,16; 2014,Aug,5; 2014,Jan,11; 2012,Jul,12-14; 2012,Jan,15-42; 2011,Oct,3-4; 2011,Jul,16-17; 2011,Jan,11
00402	**reconstructive procedures on breast (eg, reduction or augmentation mammoplasty, muscle flaps)** 📷 0.00 ⚕ 0.00 **FUD** XXX N̄ ▭ P̄Q̄ **AMA:** 2015,Jan,16; 2014,Aug,5; 2014,Jan,11; 2012,Jul,12-14; 2012,Jan,15-42; 2011,Oct,3-4; 2011,Jul,16-17; 2011,Jan,11
00404	**radical or modified radical procedures on breast** 📷 0.00 ⚕ 0.00 **FUD** XXX N̄ ▭ P̄Q̄ **AMA:** 2015,Jan,16; 2014,Aug,5; 2014,Jan,11; 2012,Jul,12-14; 2012,Jan,15-42; 2011,Oct,3-4; 2011,Jul,16-17; 2011,Jan,11
00406	**radical or modified radical procedures on breast with internal mammary node dissection** 📷 0.00 ⚕ 0.00 **FUD** XXX N̄ ▭ P̄Q̄ **AMA:** 2015,Jan,16; 2014,Aug,5; 2014,Jan,11; 2012,Jul,12-14; 2012,Jan,15-42; 2011,Oct,3-4; 2011,Jul,16-17; 2011,Jan,11
00410	**electrical conversion of arrhythmias** 📷 0.00 ⚕ 0.00 **FUD** XXX N̄ ▭ P̄Q̄ **AMA:** 2015,Jan,16; 2014,Aug,5; 2014,Jan,11; 2012,Jul,12-14; 2012,Jan,15-42; 2011,Oct,3-4; 2011,Jul,16-17; 2011,Jan,11
00450	**Anesthesia for procedures on clavicle and scapula; not otherwise specified** 📷 0.00 ⚕ 0.00 **FUD** XXX N̄ ▭ P̄Q̄ **AMA:** 2015,Jan,16; 2014,Aug,5; 2014,Jan,11; 2012,Jul,12-14; 2012,Jan,15-42; 2011,Oct,3-4; 2011,Jul,16-17; 2011,Jan,11
00454	**biopsy of clavicle** 📷 0.00 ⚕ 0.00 **FUD** XXX N̄ ▭ P̄Q̄ **AMA:** 2015,Jan,16; 2014,Aug,5; 2014,Jan,11; 2012,Jul,12-14; 2012,Jan,15-42; 2011,Oct,3-4; 2011,Jul,16-17; 2011,Jan,11
00470	**Anesthesia for partial rib resection; not otherwise specified** 📷 0.00 ⚕ 0.00 **FUD** XXX N̄ ▭ P̄Q̄ **AMA:** 2015,Jan,16; 2014,Aug,5; 2014,Jan,11; 2012,Jul,12-14; 2012,Jan,15-42; 2011,Oct,3-4; 2011,Jul,16-17; 2011,Jan,11
00472	**thoracoplasty (any type)** 📷 0.00 ⚕ 0.00 **FUD** XXX N̄ ▭ P̄Q̄ **AMA:** 2015,Jan,16; 2014,Aug,5; 2014,Jan,11; 2012,Jul,12-14; 2012,Jan,15-42; 2011,Oct,3-4; 2011,Jul,16-17; 2011,Jan,11
00474	**radical procedures (eg, pectus excavatum)** 📷 0.00 ⚕ 0.00 **FUD** XXX ⊂ ▭ P̄Q̄ **AMA:** 2015,Jan,16; 2014,Aug,5; 2014,Jan,11; 2012,Jul,12-14; 2012,Jan,15-42; 2011,Oct,3-4; 2011,Jul,16-17; 2011,Jan,11
00500	**Anesthesia for all procedures on esophagus** 📷 0.00 ⚕ 0.00 **FUD** XXX N̄ ▭ P̄Q̄ **AMA:** 2015,Jan,16; 2014,Aug,5; 2014,Jan,11; 2012,Jul,12-14; 2012,Jan,15-42; 2011,Oct,3-4; 2011,Jul,16-17; 2011,Jan,11
00520	**Anesthesia for closed chest procedures; (including bronchoscopy) not otherwise specified** 📷 0.00 ⚕ 0.00 **FUD** XXX N̄ ▭ P̄Q̄ **AMA:** 2015,Jan,16; 2014,Aug,5; 2014,Jan,11; 2012,Jul,12-14; 2012,Jan,15-42; 2011,Oct,3-4; 2011,Jul,16-17; 2011,Jan,11
00522	**needle biopsy of pleura** 📷 0.00 ⚕ 0.00 **FUD** XXX N̄ ▭ P̄Q̄ **AMA:** 2015,Jan,16; 2014,Aug,5; 2014,Jan,11; 2012,Jul,12-14; 2012,Jan,15-42; 2011,Oct,3-4; 2011,Jul,16-17; 2011,Jan,11

00524 pneumocentesis
🔲 0.00 🔪 0.00 **FUD** XXX C PQ

AMA: 2015,Jan,16; 2014,Aug,5; 2014,Jan,11; 2012,Jul,12-14; 2012,Jan,15-42; 2011,Oct,3-4; 2011,Jul,16-17; 2011,Jan,11

00528 mediastinoscopy and diagnostic thoracoscopy not utilizing 1 lung ventilation
EXCLUDES Tracheobronchial reconstruction (00539)
🔲 0.00 🔪 0.00 **FUD** XXX N PQ

AMA: 2015,Jan,16; 2014,Aug,5; 2014,Jan,11; 2012,Jul,12-14; 2012,Jan,15-42; 2011,Oct,3-4; 2011,Jul,16-17; 2011,Jan,11

00529 mediastinoscopy and diagnostic thoracoscopy utilizing 1 lung ventilation
🔲 0.00 🔪 0.00 **FUD** XXX N PQ

AMA: 2015,Jan,16; 2014,Aug,5; 2014,Jan,11; 2012,Jul,12-14; 2012,Jan,15-42; 2011,Oct,3-4; 2011,Jul,16-17; 2011,Jan,11

00530 Anesthesia for Cardiac Pacemaker Procedure

CMS: 100-3,10.6 Anesthesia in Cardiac Pacemaker Surgery; 100-4,12,140.1 Qualified Nonphysician Anesthetists; 100-4,12,140.3 Payment for Qualified Nonphysician Anesthetists; 100-4,12,140.3.3 Billing Modifiers; 100-4,12,140.3.4 General Billing Instructions; 100-4,12,140.4.1 Anesthesiologist/Qualified Nonphysican Anesthetist; 100-4,12,140.4.2 Anesthetist and Anesthesiologist in a Single Procedure; 100-4,12,140.4.3 Payment for Medical /Surgical Services by CRNAs; 100-4,12,140.4.4 Conversion Factors for Anesthesia Services; 100-4,4,250.3.2 Anesthesia in a Hospital Outpatient Setting

00530 Anesthesia for permanent transvenous pacemaker insertion
🔲 0.00 🔪 0.00 **FUD** XXX N PQ

AMA: 2015,Jan,16; 2014,Aug,5; 2014,Jan,11; 2012,Jul,12-14; 2012,Jan,15-42; 2011,Oct,3-4; 2011,Jul,16-17; 2011,Jan,11

00532-00550 Anesthesia for Heart and Lung Procedures

CMS: 100-4,12,140.1 Qualified Nonphysician Anesthetists; 100-4,12,140.3 Payment for Qualified Nonphysician Anesthetists; 100-4,12,140.3.3 Billing Modifiers; 100-4,12,140.3.4 General Billing Instructions; 100-4,12,140.4.1 Anesthesiologist/Qualified Nonphysician Anesthetist; 100-4,12,140.4.2 Anesthetist and Anesthesiologist in a Single Procedure; 100-4,12,140.4.3 Payment for Medical /Surgical Services by CRNAs; 100-4,12,140.4.4 Conversion Factors for Anesthesia Services; 100-4,4,250.3.2 Anesthesia in a Hospital Outpatient Setting

00532 Anesthesia for access to central venous circulation
🔲 0.00 🔪 0.00 **FUD** XXX N PQ

AMA: 2015,Jan,16; 2014,Aug,5; 2014,Jan,11; 2012,Jul,12-14; 2012,Jan,15-42; 2011,Oct,3-4; 2011,Jul,16-17; 2011,Jan,11

00534 Anesthesia for transvenous insertion or replacement of pacing cardioverter-defibrillator
EXCLUDES Transthoracic approach (00560)
🔲 0.00 🔪 0.00 **FUD** XXX N PQ

AMA: 2015,Jan,16; 2014,Aug,5; 2014,Jan,11; 2012,Jul,12-14; 2012,Jan,15-42; 2011,Oct,3-4; 2011,Jul,16-17; 2011,Jan,11

00537 Anesthesia for cardiac electrophysiologic procedures including radiofrequency ablation
🔲 0.00 🔪 0.00 **FUD** XXX N PQ

AMA: 2015,Jan,16; 2014,Aug,5; 2014,Jan,11; 2012,Jul,12-14; 2012,Jan,15-42; 2011,Oct,3-4; 2011,Jul,16-17; 2011,Jan,11

00539 Anesthesia for tracheobronchial reconstruction
🔲 0.00 🔪 0.00 **FUD** XXX N PQ

AMA: 2015,Jan,16; 2014,Aug,5; 2014,Jan,11; 2012,Jul,12-14; 2012,Jan,15-42; 2011,Oct,3-4; 2011,Jul,16-17; 2011,Jan,11

00540 Anesthesia for thoracotomy procedures involving lungs, pleura, diaphragm, and mediastinum (including surgical thoracoscopy); not otherwise specified
EXCLUDES Thoracic spine and spinal cord procedures via anterior transthoracic approach (00625-00626)
🔲 0.00 🔪 0.00 **FUD** XXX C PQ

AMA: 2015,Jan,16; 2014,Aug,5; 2014,Jan,11; 2012,Jul,12-14; 2012,Jan,15-42; 2011,Oct,3-4; 2011,Jul,16-17; 2011,Jan,11

00541 utilizing 1 lung ventilation
EXCLUDES Thoracic spine and spinal cord procedures via anterior transthoracic approach (00625-00626)
🔲 0.00 🔪 0.00 **FUD** XXX N PQ

AMA: 2015,Jan,16; 2014,Aug,5; 2014,Jan,11; 2012,Jul,12-14; 2012,Jan,15-42; 2011,Oct,3-4; 2011,Jul,16-17; 2011,Jan,11

00542 decortication
🔲 0.00 🔪 0.00 **FUD** XXX C PQ

AMA: 2015,Jan,16; 2014,Aug,5; 2014,Jan,11; 2012,Jul,12-14; 2012,Jan,15-42; 2011,Oct,3-4; 2011,Jul,16-17; 2011,Jan,11

00546 pulmonary resection with thoracoplasty
🔲 0.00 🔪 0.00 **FUD** XXX C PQ

AMA: 2015,Jan,16; 2014,Aug,5; 2014,Jan,11; 2012,Jul,12-14; 2012,Jan,15-42; 2011,Oct,3-4; 2011,Jul,16-17; 2011,Jan,11

00548 intrathoracic procedures on the trachea and bronchi
🔲 0.00 🔪 0.00 **FUD** XXX C PQ

AMA: 2015,Jan,16; 2014,Aug,5; 2014,Jan,11; 2012,Jul,12-14; 2012,Jan,15-42; 2011,Oct,3-4; 2011,Jul,16-17; 2011,Jan,11

00550 Anesthesia for sternal debridement
🔲 0.00 🔪 0.00 **FUD** XXX N PQ

AMA: 2015,Jan,16; 2014,Aug,5; 2014,Jan,11; 2012,Jul,12-14; 2012,Jan,15-42; 2011,Oct,3-4; 2011,Jul,16-17; 2011,Jan,11

00560-00580 Anesthesia for Open Heart Procedures

CMS: 100-4,12,140.1 Qualified Nonphysician Anesthetists; 100-4,12,140.3 Payment for Qualified Nonphysician Anesthetists; 100-4,12,140.3.3 Billing Modifiers; 100-4,12,140.3.4 General Billing Instructions; 100-4,12,140.4.1 Anesthesiologist/Qualified Nonphysican Anesthetist; 100-4,12,140.4.2 Anesthetist and Anesthesiologist in a Single Procedure; 100-4,12,140.4.3 Payment for Medical /Surgical Services by CRNAs; 100-4,12,140.4.4 Conversion Factors for Anesthesia Services; 100-4,4,250.3.2 Anesthesia in a Hospital Outpatient Setting

00560 Anesthesia for procedures on heart, pericardial sac, and great vessels of chest; without pump oxygenator
🔲 0.00 🔪 0.00 **FUD** XXX C PQ

AMA: 2015,Jan,16; 2014,Aug,5; 2014,Jan,11; 2012,Jul,12-14; 2012,Jan,15-42; 2011,Oct,3-4; 2011,Jul,16-17; 2011,Jan,11

00561 with pump oxygenator, younger than 1 year of age A
Do not report with (99100, 99116, 99135)
🔲 0.00 🔪 0.00 **FUD** XXX C PQ

AMA: 2015,Jan,16; 2014,Aug,5; 2014,Jan,11; 2012,Jul,12-14; 2012,Jan,15-42; 2011,Oct,3-4; 2011,Jul,16-17; 2011,Jan,11

00562 with pump oxygenator, age 1 year or older, for all noncoronary bypass procedures (eg, valve procedures) or for re-operation for coronary bypass more than 1 month after original operation A
🔲 0.00 🔪 0.00 **FUD** XXX C PQ

AMA: 2015,Jan,16; 2014,Aug,5; 2014,Jan,11; 2012,Jul,12-14; 2012,Jan,15-42; 2011,Oct,3-4; 2011,Jul,16-17; 2011,Jan,11

00563 with pump oxygenator with hypothermic circulatory arrest
🔲 0.00 🔪 0.00 **FUD** XXX N PQ

AMA: 2015,Jan,16; 2014,Aug,5; 2014,Jan,11; 2012,Jul,12-14; 2012,Jan,15-42; 2011,Oct,3-4; 2011,Jul,16-17; 2011,Jan,11

00566 Anesthesia for direct coronary artery bypass grafting; without pump oxygenator
🔲 0.00 🔪 0.00 **FUD** XXX N PQ

AMA: 2015,Jan,16; 2014,Aug,5; 2014,Jan,11; 2012,Jul,12-14; 2012,Jan,15-42; 2011,Oct,3-4; 2011,Jul,16-17; 2011,Jan,11

00567 with pump oxygenator
🔲 0.00 🔪 0.00 **FUD** XXX C PQ

AMA: 2015,Jan,16; 2014,Aug,5; 2014,Jan,11; 2012,Jul,12-14; 2012,Jan,15-42; 2011,Oct,3-4; 2011,Jul,16-17; 2011,Jan,11

00580 Anesthesia for heart transplant or heart/lung transplant
🔲 0.00 🔪 0.00 **FUD** XXX C PQ

AMA: 2015,Jan,16; 2014,Aug,5; 2014,Jan,11; 2012,Jul,12-14; 2012,Jan,15-42; 2011,Oct,3-4; 2011,Jul,16-17; 2011,Jan,11

00600-00670 Anesthesia for Spinal Procedures

CMS: 100-4,12,140.1 Qualified Nonphysician Anesthetists; 100-4,12,140.3 Payment for Qualified Nonphysician Anesthetists; 100-4,12,140.3.3 Billing Modifiers; 100-4,12,140.3.4 General Billing Instructions; 100-4,12,140.4.1 Anesthesiologist/Qualified Nonphysican Anesthetist; 100-4,12,140.4.2 Anesthetist and Anesthesiologist in a Single Procedure; 100-4,12,140.4.3 Payment for Medical /Surgical Services by CRNAs; 100-4,12,140.4.4 Conversion Factors for Anesthesia Services; 100-4,4,250.3.2 Anesthesia in a Hospital Outpatient Setting

00600 Anesthesia for procedures on cervical spine and cord; not otherwise specified

> **EXCLUDES** *Percutaneous image-guided spine and spinal cord anesthesia services (01935-01936)*

🔲 0.00   ♒ 0.00   **FUD** XXX   Ⓝ ▣ 🄿🄾

AMA: 2015,Jan,16; 2014,Aug,5; 2014,Jan,11; 2012,Jul,12-14; 2012,Jan,15-42; 2011,Oct,3-4; 2011,Jul,16-17; 2011,Jan,11

00604 procedures with patient in the sitting position

🔲 0.00   ♒ 0.00   **FUD** XXX   Ⓒ ▣ 🄿🄾

AMA: 2015,Jan,16; 2014,Aug,5; 2014,Jan,11; 2012,Jul,12-14; 2012,Jan,15-42; 2011,Oct,3-4; 2011,Jul,16-17; 2011,Jan,11

00620 Anesthesia for procedures on thoracic spine and cord, not otherwise specified

🔲 0.00   ♒ 0.00   **FUD** XXX   Ⓝ ▣ 🄿🄾

AMA: 2015,Jan,16; 2014,Aug,5; 2014,Jan,11; 2012,Jul,12-14; 2012,Jan,15-42; 2011,Oct,3-4; 2011,Jul,16-17; 2011,Jan,11

00625 Anesthesia for procedures on the thoracic spine and cord, via an anterior transthoracic approach; not utilizing 1 lung ventilation

> **EXCLUDES** *Anesthesia services for thoracotomy procedures other than spine (00540-00541)*

🔲 0.00   ♒ 0.00   **FUD** XXX   Ⓝ 🄿🄾

AMA: 2015,Jan,16; 2014,Aug,5; 2014,Jan,11; 2012,Jul,12-14; 2012,Jan,15-42; 2011,Oct,3-4; 2011,Jul,16-17; 2011,Jan,11

00626 utilizing 1 lung ventilation

> **EXCLUDES** *Anesthesia services for thoracotomy procedures other than spine (00540-00541)*

🔲 0.00   ♒ 0.00   **FUD** XXX   Ⓝ 🄿🄾

AMA: 2015,Jan,16; 2014,Aug,5; 2014,Jan,11; 2012,Jul,12-14; 2012,Jan,15-42; 2011,Oct,3-4; 2011,Jul,16-17; 2011,Jan,11

00630 Anesthesia for procedures in lumbar region; not otherwise specified

🔲 0.00   ♒ 0.00   **FUD** XXX   Ⓝ ▣ 🄿🄾

AMA: 2015,Jan,16; 2014,Aug,5; 2014,Jan,11; 2012,Jul,12-14; 2012,Jan,15-42; 2011,Oct,3-4; 2011,Jul,16-17; 2011,Jan,11

00632 lumbar sympathectomy

🔲 0.00   ♒ 0.00   **FUD** XXX   Ⓒ ▣ 🄿🄾

AMA: 2015,Jan,16; 2014,Aug,5; 2014,Jan,11; 2012,Jul,12-14; 2012,Jan,15-42; 2011,Oct,3-4; 2011,Jul,16-17; 2011,Jan,11

00635 diagnostic or therapeutic lumbar puncture

🔲 0.00   ♒ 0.00   **FUD** XXX   Ⓝ ▣ 🄿🄾

AMA: 2015,Jan,16; 2014,Aug,5; 2014,Jan,11; 2012,Jul,12-14; 2012,Jan,15-42; 2011,Oct,3-4; 2011,Jul,16-17; 2011,Jan,11

00640 Anesthesia for manipulation of the spine or for closed procedures on the cervical, thoracic or lumbar spine

🔲 0.00   ♒ 0.00   **FUD** XXX   Ⓝ ▣ 🄿🄾

AMA: 2015,Jan,16; 2014,Aug,5; 2014,Jan,11; 2012,Jul,12-14; 2012,Jan,15-42; 2011,Oct,3-4; 2011,Jul,16-17; 2011,Jan,11

00670 Anesthesia for extensive spine and spinal cord procedures (eg, spinal instrumentation or vascular procedures)

🔲 0.00   ♒ 0.00   **FUD** XXX   Ⓒ ▣ 🄿🄾

AMA: 2015,Jan,16; 2014,Aug,5; 2014,Jan,11; 2012,Jul,12-14; 2012,Jan,15-42; 2011,Oct,3-4; 2011,Jul,16-17; 2011,Jan,11

00700-00882 Anesthesia for Abdominal Procedures

CMS: 100-4,12,140.1 Qualified Nonphysician Anesthetists; 100-4,12,140.3 Payment for Qualified Nonphysician Anesthetists; 100-4,12,140.3.3 Billing Modifiers; 100-4,12,140.3.4 General Billing Instructions; 100-4,12,140.4.1 Anesthesiologist/Qualified Nonphysican Anesthetist; 100-4,12,140.4.2 Anesthetist and Anesthesiologist in a Single Procedure; 100-4,12,140.4.3 Payment for Medical /Surgical Services by CRNAs; 100-4,12,140.4.4 Conversion Factors for Anesthesia Services; 100-4,4,250.3.2 Anesthesia in a Hospital Outpatient Setting

00700 Anesthesia for procedures on upper anterior abdominal wall; not otherwise specified

🔲 0.00   ♒ 0.00   **FUD** XXX   Ⓝ ▣ 🄿🄾

AMA: 2015,Jan,16; 2014,Aug,5; 2014,Jan,11; 2012,Jul,12-14; 2012,Jan,15-42; 2011,Oct,3-4; 2011,Jul,16-17; 2011,Jan,11

00702 percutaneous liver biopsy

🔲 0.00   ♒ 0.00   **FUD** XXX   Ⓝ ▣ 🄿🄾

AMA: 2015,Jan,16; 2014,Aug,5; 2014,Jan,11; 2012,Jul,12-14; 2012,Jan,15-42; 2011,Oct,3-4; 2011,Jul,16-17; 2011,Jan,11

00730 Anesthesia for procedures on upper posterior abdominal wall

🔲 0.00   ♒ 0.00   **FUD** XXX   Ⓝ ▣ 🄿🄾

AMA: 2015,Jan,16; 2014,Aug,5; 2014,Jan,11; 2012,Jul,12-14; 2012,Jan,15-42; 2011,Oct,3-4; 2011,Jul,16-17; 2011,Jan,11

00740 Anesthesia for upper gastrointestinal endoscopic procedures, endoscope introduced proximal to duodenum

🔲 0.00   ♒ 0.00   **FUD** XXX   Ⓝ ▣ 🄿🄾

AMA: 2015,Jan,16; 2014,Aug,5; 2014,Jan,11; 2012,Jul,12-14; 2012,Jan,15-42; 2011,Oct,3-4; 2011,Jul,16-17; 2011,Jan,11

00750 Anesthesia for hernia repairs in upper abdomen; not otherwise specified

🔲 0.00   ♒ 0.00   **FUD** XXX   Ⓝ ▣ 🄿🄾

AMA: 2015,Jan,16; 2014,Aug,5; 2014,Jan,11; 2012,Jul,12-14; 2012,Jan,15-42; 2011,Oct,3-4; 2011,Jul,16-17; 2011,Jan,11

00752 lumbar and ventral (incisional) hernias and/or wound dehiscence

🔲 0.00   ♒ 0.00   **FUD** XXX   Ⓝ ▣ 🄿🄾

AMA: 2015,Jan,16; 2014,Aug,5; 2014,Jan,11; 2012,Jul,12-14; 2012,Jan,15-42; 2011,Oct,3-4; 2011,Jul,16-17; 2011,Jan,11

00754 omphalocele

🔲 0.00   ♒ 0.00   **FUD** XXX   Ⓝ ▣ 🄿🄾

AMA: 2015,Jan,16; 2014,Aug,5; 2014,Jan,11; 2012,Jul,12-14; 2012,Jan,15-42; 2011,Oct,3-4; 2011,Jul,16-17; 2011,Jan,11

00756 transabdominal repair of diaphragmatic hernia

🔲 0.00   ♒ 0.00   **FUD** XXX   Ⓝ ▣ 🄿🄾

AMA: 2015,Jan,16; 2014,Aug,5; 2014,Jan,11; 2012,Jul,12-14; 2012,Jan,15-42; 2011,Oct,3-4; 2011,Jul,16-17; 2011,Jan,11

00770 Anesthesia for all procedures on major abdominal blood vessels

🔲 0.00   ♒ 0.00   **FUD** XXX   Ⓝ ▣ 🄿🄾

AMA: 2015,Jan,16; 2014,Aug,5; 2014,Jan,11; 2012,Jul,12-14; 2012,Jan,15-42; 2011,Oct,3-4; 2011,Jul,16-17; 2011,Jan,11

00790 Anesthesia for intraperitoneal procedures in upper abdomen including laparoscopy; not otherwise specified

🔲 0.00   ♒ 0.00   **FUD** XXX   Ⓝ ▣ 🄿🄾

AMA: 2015,Jan,16; 2014,Aug,5; 2014,Jan,11; 2012,Jul,12-14; 2012,Jan,15-42; 2011,Oct,3-4; 2011,Jul,16-17; 2011,Jan,11

00792 partial hepatectomy or management of liver hemorrhage (excluding liver biopsy)

🔲 0.00   ♒ 0.00   **FUD** XXX   Ⓒ ▣ 🄿🄾

AMA: 2015,Jan,16; 2014,Aug,5; 2014,Jan,11; 2012,Jul,12-14; 2012,Jan,15-42; 2011,Oct,3-4; 2011,Jul,16-17; 2011,Jan,11

00794 pancreatectomy, partial or total (eg, Whipple procedure)

🔲 0.00   ♒ 0.00   **FUD** XXX   Ⓒ ▣ 🄿🄾

AMA: 2015,Jan,16; 2014,Aug,5; 2014,Jan,11; 2012,Jul,12-14; 2012,Jan,15-42; 2011,Oct,3-4; 2011,Jul,16-17; 2011,Jan,11

00796 liver transplant (recipient)

> **EXCLUDES** *Physiological support during liver harvest (01990)*

🔲 0.00   ♒ 0.00   **FUD** XXX   Ⓒ ▣ 🄿🄾

AMA: 2015,Jan,16; 2014,Aug,5; 2014,Jan,11; 2012,Jul,12-14; 2012,Jan,15-42; 2011,Oct,3-4; 2011,Jul,16-17; 2011,Jan,11

00797 gastric restrictive procedure for morbid obesity

🔲 0.00   ♒ 0.00   **FUD** XXX   Ⓝ ▣ 🄿🄾

AMA: 2015,Jan,16; 2014,Aug,5; 2014,Jan,11; 2012,Jul,12-14; 2012,Jan,15-42; 2011,Oct,3-4; 2011,Jul,16-17; 2011,Jan,11

00800 Anesthesia for procedures on lower anterior abdominal wall; not otherwise specified

🔲 0.00   ♒ 0.00   **FUD** XXX   Ⓝ ▣ 🄿🄾

AMA: 2015,Jan,16; 2014,Aug,5; 2014,Jan,11; 2012,Jul,12-14; 2012,Jan,15-42; 2011,Oct,3-4; 2011,Jul,16-17; 2011,Jan,11

00802 panniculectomy

🔲 0.00   ♒ 0.00   **FUD** XXX   Ⓒ ▣ 🄿🄾

AMA: 2015,Jan,16; 2014,Aug,5; 2014,Jan,11; 2012,Jul,12-14; 2012,Jan,15-42; 2011,Oct,3-4; 2011,Jul,16-17; 2011,Jan,11

00810	**Anesthesia for lower intestinal endoscopic procedures, endoscope introduced distal to duodenum**
	💲 0.00 ♨ 0.00 **FUD** XXX N 🖼 P0
	AMA: 2015,Jan,16; 2014,Aug,5; 2014,Jan,11; 2012,Jul,12-14; 2012,Jan,15-42; 2011,Oct,3-4; 2011,Jul,16-17; 2011,Jan,11

00820	**Anesthesia for procedures on lower posterior abdominal wall**
	💲 0.00 ♨ 0.00 **FUD** XXX N 🖼 P0
	AMA: 2015,Jan,16; 2014,Aug,5; 2014,Jan,11; 2012,Jul,12-14; 2012,Jan,15-42; 2011,Oct,3-4; 2011,Jul,16-17; 2011,Jan,11

00830	**Anesthesia for hernia repairs in lower abdomen; not otherwise specified**
	EXCLUDES Anesthesia for hernia repairs on infants one year old or less (00834, 00836)
	💲 0.00 ♨ 0.00 **FUD** XXX N 🖼 P0
	AMA: 2015,Jan,16; 2014,Aug,5; 2014,Jan,11; 2012,Jul,12-14; 2012,Jan,15-42; 2011,Oct,3-4; 2011,Jul,16-17; 2011,Jan,11

00832	**ventral and incisional hernias**
	EXCLUDES Anesthesia for hernia repairs on infants one year old or less (00834, 00836)
	💲 0.00 ♨ 0.00 **FUD** XXX N 🖼 P0
	AMA: 2015,Jan,16; 2014,Aug,5; 2014,Jan,11; 2012,Jul,12-14; 2012,Jan,15-42; 2011,Oct,3-4; 2011,Jul,16-17; 2011,Jan,11

00834	**Anesthesia for hernia repairs in the lower abdomen not otherwise specified, younger than 1 year of age** 🅐
	Do not report with (99100)
	💲 0.00 ♨ 0.00 **FUD** XXX N 🖼 P0
	AMA: 2015,Jan,16; 2014,Aug,5; 2014,Jan,11; 2012,Jul,12-14; 2012,Jan,15-42; 2011,Oct,3-4; 2011,Jul,16-17; 2011,Jan,11

00836	**Anesthesia for hernia repairs in the lower abdomen not otherwise specified, infants younger than 37 weeks gestational age at birth and younger than 50 weeks gestational age at time of surgery** 🅐
	Do not report with (99100)
	💲 0.00 ♨ 0.00 **FUD** XXX N 🖼 P0
	AMA: 2015,Jan,16; 2014,Aug,5; 2014,Jan,11; 2012,Jul,12-14; 2012,Jan,15-42; 2011,Oct,3-4; 2011,Jul,16-17; 2011,Jan,11

00840	**Anesthesia for intraperitoneal procedures in lower abdomen including laparoscopy; not otherwise specified**
	💲 0.00 ♨ 0.00 **FUD** XXX N 🖼 P0
	AMA: 2015,Jan,16; 2014,Aug,5; 2014,Jan,11; 2012,Jul,12-14; 2012,Jan,15-42; 2011,Oct,3-4; 2011,Jul,16-17; 2011,Jan,11

00842	**amniocentesis** 🅜 ♀
	💲 0.00 ♨ 0.00 **FUD** XXX N 🖼 P0
	AMA: 2015,Jan,16; 2014,Aug,5; 2014,Jan,11; 2012,Jul,12-14; 2012,Jan,15-42; 2011,Oct,3-4; 2011,Jul,16-17; 2011,Jan,11

00844	**abdominoperineal resection**
	💲 0.00 ♨ 0.00 **FUD** XXX C 🖼 P0
	AMA: 2015,Jan,16; 2014,Aug,5; 2014,Jan,11; 2012,Jul,12-14; 2012,Jan,15-42; 2011,Oct,3-4; 2011,Jul,16-17; 2011,Jan,11

00846	**radical hysterectomy** ♀
	💲 0.00 ♨ 0.00 **FUD** XXX C 🖼 P0
	AMA: 2015,Jan,16; 2014,Aug,5; 2014,Jan,11; 2012,Jul,12-14; 2012,Jan,15-42; 2011,Oct,3-4; 2011,Jul,16-17; 2011,Jan,11

00848	**pelvic exenteration**
	💲 0.00 ♨ 0.00 **FUD** XXX C 🖼 P0
	AMA: 2015,Jan,16; 2014,Aug,5; 2014,Jan,11; 2012,Jul,12-14; 2012,Jan,15-42; 2011,Oct,3-4; 2011,Jul,16-17; 2011,Jan,11

00851	**tubal ligation/transection** ♀
	💲 0.00 ♨ 0.00 **FUD** XXX N 🖼 P0
	AMA: 2015,Jan,16; 2014,Oct,14; 2014,Aug,5; 2014,Jan,11; 2012,Jul,12-14; 2012,Jan,15-42; 2011,Oct,3-4; 2011,Jul,16-17; 2011,Jan,11

00860	**Anesthesia for extraperitoneal procedures in lower abdomen, including urinary tract; not otherwise specified**
	💲 0.00 ♨ 0.00 **FUD** XXX N 🖼 P0
	AMA: 2015,Jan,16; 2014,Aug,5; 2014,Jan,11; 2012,Jul,12-14; 2012,Jan,15-42; 2011,Oct,3-4; 2011,Jul,16-17; 2011,Jan,11

00862	**renal procedures, including upper one-third of ureter, or donor nephrectomy**
	💲 0.00 ♨ 0.00 **FUD** XXX N 🖼 P0
	AMA: 2015,Jan,16; 2014,Aug,5; 2014,Jan,11; 2012,Jul,12-14; 2012,Jan,15-42; 2011,Oct,3-4; 2011,Jul,16-17; 2011,Jan,11

00864	**total cystectomy**
	💲 0.00 ♨ 0.00 **FUD** XXX C 🖼 P0
	AMA: 2015,Jan,16; 2014,Aug,5; 2014,Jan,11; 2012,Jul,12-14; 2012,Jan,15-42; 2011,Oct,3-4; 2011,Jul,16-17; 2011,Jan,11

00865	**radical prostatectomy (suprapubic, retropubic)** ♂
	💲 0.00 ♨ 0.00 **FUD** XXX C 🖼 P0
	AMA: 2015,Jan,16; 2014,Aug,5; 2014,Jan,11; 2012,Jul,12-14; 2012,Jan,15-42; 2011,Oct,3-4; 2011,Jul,16-17; 2011,Jan,11

00866	**adrenalectomy**
	💲 0.00 ♨ 0.00 **FUD** XXX C 🖼 P0
	AMA: 2015,Jan,16; 2014,Aug,5; 2014,Jan,11; 2012,Jul,12-14; 2012,Jan,15-42; 2011,Oct,3-4; 2011,Jul,16-17; 2011,Jan,11

00868	**renal transplant (recipient)**
	EXCLUDES Anesthesia for donor nephrectomy (00862) Physiological support during kidney harvest (01990)
	💲 0.00 ♨ 0.00 **FUD** XXX C 🖼 P0
	AMA: 2015,Jan,16; 2014,Aug,5; 2014,Jan,11; 2012,Jul,12-14; 2012,Jan,15-42; 2011,Oct,3-4; 2011,Jul,16-17; 2011,Jan,11

00870	**cystolithotomy**
	💲 0.00 ♨ 0.00 **FUD** XXX N 🖼 P0
	AMA: 2015,Jan,16; 2014,Aug,5; 2014,Jan,11; 2012,Jul,12-14; 2012,Jan,15-42; 2011,Oct,3-4; 2011,Jul,16-17; 2011,Jan,11

00872	**Anesthesia for lithotripsy, extracorporeal shock wave; with water bath**
	💲 0.00 ♨ 0.00 **FUD** XXX N 🖼 P0
	AMA: 2015,Jan,16; 2014,Aug,5; 2014,Jan,11; 2012,Jul,12-14; 2012,Jan,15-42; 2011,Oct,3-4; 2011,Jul,16-17; 2011,Jan,11

00873	**without water bath**
	💲 0.00 ♨ 0.00 **FUD** XXX N 🖼 P0
	AMA: 2015,Jan,16; 2014,Aug,5; 2014,Jan,11; 2012,Jul,12-14; 2012,Jan,15-42; 2011,Oct,3-4; 2011,Jul,16-17; 2011,Jan,11

00880	**Anesthesia for procedures on major lower abdominal vessels; not otherwise specified**
	💲 0.00 ♨ 0.00 **FUD** XXX N 🖼 P0
	AMA: 2015,Jan,16; 2014,Aug,5; 2014,Jan,11; 2012,Jul,12-14; 2012,Jan,15-42; 2011,Oct,3-4; 2011,Jul,16-17; 2011,Jan,11

00882	**inferior vena cava ligation**
	💲 0.00 ♨ 0.00 **FUD** XXX C 🖼 P0
	AMA: 2015,Jan,16; 2014,Aug,5; 2014,Jan,11; 2012,Jul,12-14; 2012,Jan,15-42; 2011,Oct,3-4; 2011,Jul,16-17; 2011,Jan,11

00902-00952 Anesthesia for Genitourinary Procedures

CMS: 100-4,12,140.1 Qualified Nonphysician Anesthetists; 100-4,12,140.3 Payment for Qualified Nonphysician Anesthetists; 100-4,12,140.3.3 Billing Modifiers; 100-4,12,140.3.4 General Billing Instructions; 100-4,12,140.4.1 Anesthesiologist/Qualified Nonphysican Anesthetist; 100-4,12,140.4.2 Anesthetist and Anesthesiologist in a Single Procedure; 100-4,12,140.4.3 Payment for Medical/Surgical Services by CRNAs; 100-4,12,140.4.4 Conversion Factors for Anesthesia Services; 100-4,4,250.3.2 Anesthesia in a Hospital Outpatient Setting

EXCLUDES Perineal procedures on skin, muscles, and nerves (00300, 00400)

00902	**Anesthesia for; anorectal procedure**
	💲 0.00 ♨ 0.00 **FUD** XXX N 🖼 P0
	AMA: 2015,Jan,16; 2014,Aug,5; 2014,Jan,11; 2012,Jul,12-14; 2012,Jan,15-42; 2011,Oct,3-4; 2011,Jul,16-17; 2011,Jan,11

00904	**radical perineal procedure**
	💲 0.00 ♨ 0.00 **FUD** XXX C 🖼 P0
	AMA: 2015,Jan,16; 2014,Aug,5; 2014,Jan,11; 2012,Jul,12-14; 2012,Jan,15-42; 2011,Oct,3-4; 2011,Jul,16-17; 2011,Jan,11

00906	**vulvectomy** ♀
	💲 0.00 ♨ 0.00 **FUD** XXX N 🖼 P0
	AMA: 2015,Jan,16; 2014,Aug,5; 2014,Jan,11; 2012,Jul,12-14; 2012,Jan,15-42; 2011,Oct,3-4; 2011,Jul,16-17; 2011,Jan,11

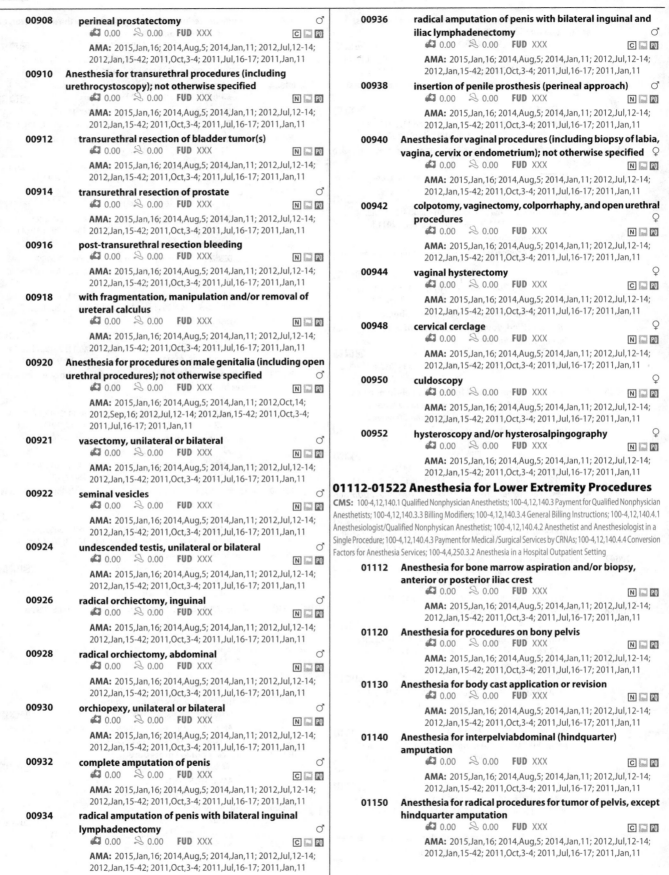

00908 perineal prostatectomy ♂

📋 0.00 ⚕ 0.00 **FUD** XXX C 🖵 P0

AMA: 2015,Jan,16; 2014,Aug,5; 2014,Jan,11; 2012,Jul,12-14; 2012,Jan,15-42; 2011,Oct,3-4; 2011,Jul,16-17; 2011,Jan,11

00910 Anesthesia for transurethral procedures (including urethrocystoscopy); not otherwise specified

📋 0.00 ⚕ 0.00 **FUD** XXX N 🖵 P0

AMA: 2015,Jan,16; 2014,Aug,5; 2014,Jan,11; 2012,Jul,12-14; 2012,Jan,15-42; 2011,Oct,3-4; 2011,Jul,16-17; 2011,Jan,11

00912 transurethral resection of bladder tumor(s)

📋 0.00 ⚕ 0.00 **FUD** XXX N 🖵 P0

AMA: 2015,Jan,16; 2014,Aug,5; 2014,Jan,11; 2012,Jul,12-14; 2012,Jan,15-42; 2011,Oct,3-4; 2011,Jul,16-17; 2011,Jan,11

00914 transurethral resection of prostate ♂

📋 0.00 ⚕ 0.00 **FUD** XXX N 🖵 P0

AMA: 2015,Jan,16; 2014,Aug,5; 2014,Jan,11; 2012,Jul,12-14; 2012,Jan,15-42; 2011,Oct,3-4; 2011,Jul,16-17; 2011,Jan,11

00916 post-transurethral resection bleeding

📋 0.00 ⚕ 0.00 **FUD** XXX N 🖵 P0

AMA: 2015,Jan,16; 2014,Aug,5; 2014,Jan,11; 2012,Jul,12-14; 2012,Jan,15-42; 2011,Oct,3-4; 2011,Jul,16-17; 2011,Jan,11

00918 with fragmentation, manipulation and/or removal of ureteral calculus

📋 0.00 ⚕ 0.00 **FUD** XXX N 🖵 P0

AMA: 2015,Jan,16; 2014,Aug,5; 2014,Jan,11; 2012,Jul,12-14; 2012,Jan,15-42; 2011,Oct,3-4; 2011,Jul,16-17; 2011,Jan,11

00920 Anesthesia for procedures on male genitalia (including open urethral procedures); not otherwise specified ♂

📋 0.00 ⚕ 0.00 **FUD** XXX N 🖵 P0

AMA: 2015,Jan,16; 2014,Aug,5; 2014,Jan,11; 2012,Oct,14; 2012,Sep,16; 2012,Jul,12-14; 2012,Jan,15-42; 2011,Oct,3-4; 2011,Jul,16-17; 2011,Jan,11

00921 vasectomy, unilateral or bilateral ♂

📋 0.00 ⚕ 0.00 **FUD** XXX N 🖵 P0

AMA: 2015,Jan,16; 2014,Aug,5; 2014,Jan,11; 2012,Jul,12-14; 2012,Jan,15-42; 2011,Oct,3-4; 2011,Jul,16-17; 2011,Jan,11

00922 seminal vesicles ♂

📋 0.00 ⚕ 0.00 **FUD** XXX N 🖵 P0

AMA: 2015,Jan,16; 2014,Aug,5; 2014,Jan,11; 2012,Jul,12-14; 2012,Jan,15-42; 2011,Oct,3-4; 2011,Jul,16-17; 2011,Jan,11

00924 undescended testis, unilateral or bilateral ♂

📋 0.00 ⚕ 0.00 **FUD** XXX N 🖵 P0

AMA: 2015,Jan,16; 2014,Aug,5; 2014,Jan,11; 2012,Jul,12-14; 2012,Jan,15-42; 2011,Oct,3-4; 2011,Jul,16-17; 2011,Jan,11

00926 radical orchiectomy, inguinal ♂

📋 0.00 ⚕ 0.00 **FUD** XXX N 🖵 P0

AMA: 2015,Jan,16; 2014,Aug,5; 2014,Jan,11; 2012,Jul,12-14; 2012,Jan,15-42; 2011,Oct,3-4; 2011,Jul,16-17; 2011,Jan,11

00928 radical orchiectomy, abdominal ♂

📋 0.00 ⚕ 0.00 **FUD** XXX N 🖵 P0

AMA: 2015,Jan,16; 2014,Aug,5; 2014,Jan,11; 2012,Jul,12-14; 2012,Jan,15-42; 2011,Oct,3-4; 2011,Jul,16-17; 2011,Jan,11

00930 orchiopexy, unilateral or bilateral ♂

📋 0.00 ⚕ 0.00 **FUD** XXX N 🖵 P0

AMA: 2015,Jan,16; 2014,Aug,5; 2014,Jan,11; 2012,Jul,12-14; 2012,Jan,15-42; 2011,Oct,3-4; 2011,Jul,16-17; 2011,Jan,11

00932 complete amputation of penis ♂

📋 0.00 ⚕ 0.00 **FUD** XXX C 🖵 P0

AMA: 2015,Jan,16; 2014,Aug,5; 2014,Jan,11; 2012,Jul,12-14; 2012,Jan,15-42; 2011,Oct,3-4; 2011,Jul,16-17; 2011,Jan,11

00934 radical amputation of penis with bilateral inguinal lymphadenectomy ♂

📋 0.00 ⚕ 0.00 **FUD** XXX C 🖵 P0

AMA: 2015,Jan,16; 2014,Aug,5; 2014,Jan,11; 2012,Jul,12-14; 2012,Jan,15-42; 2011,Oct,3-4; 2011,Jul,16-17; 2011,Jan,11

00936 radical amputation of penis with bilateral inguinal and iliac lymphadenectomy ♂

📋 0.00 ⚕ 0.00 **FUD** XXX C 🖵 P0

AMA: 2015,Jan,16; 2014,Aug,5; 2014,Jan,11; 2012,Jul,12-14; 2012,Jan,15-42; 2011,Oct,3-4; 2011,Jul,16-17; 2011,Jan,11

00938 insertion of penile prosthesis (perineal approach) ♂

📋 0.00 ⚕ 0.00 **FUD** XXX N 🖵 P0

AMA: 2015,Jan,16; 2014,Aug,5; 2014,Jan,11; 2012,Jul,12-14; 2012,Jan,15-42; 2011,Oct,3-4; 2011,Jul,16-17; 2011,Jan,11

00940 Anesthesia for vaginal procedures (including biopsy of labia, vagina, cervix or endometrium); not otherwise specified ♀

📋 0.00 ⚕ 0.00 **FUD** XXX N 🖵 P0

AMA: 2015,Jan,16; 2014,Aug,5; 2014,Jan,11; 2012,Jul,12-14; 2012,Jan,15-42; 2011,Oct,3-4; 2011,Jul,16-17; 2011,Jan,11

00942 colpotomy, vaginectomy, colporrhaphy, and open urethral procedures ♀

📋 0.00 ⚕ 0.00 **FUD** XXX N 🖵 P0

AMA: 2015,Jan,16; 2014,Aug,5; 2014,Jan,11; 2012,Jul,12-14; 2012,Jan,15-42; 2011,Oct,3-4; 2011,Jul,16-17; 2011,Jan,11

00944 vaginal hysterectomy ♀

📋 0.00 ⚕ 0.00 **FUD** XXX C 🖵 P0

AMA: 2015,Jan,16; 2014,Aug,5; 2014,Jan,11; 2012,Jul,12-14; 2012,Jan,15-42; 2011,Oct,3-4; 2011,Jul,16-17; 2011,Jan,11

00948 cervical cerclage ♀

📋 0.00 ⚕ 0.00 **FUD** XXX N 🖵 P0

AMA: 2015,Jan,16; 2014,Aug,5; 2014,Jan,11; 2012,Jul,12-14; 2012,Jan,15-42; 2011,Oct,3-4; 2011,Jul,16-17; 2011,Jan,11

00950 culdoscopy ♀

📋 0.00 ⚕ 0.00 **FUD** XXX N 🖵 P0

AMA: 2015,Jan,16; 2014,Aug,5; 2014,Jan,11; 2012,Jul,12-14; 2012,Jan,15-42; 2011,Oct,3-4; 2011,Jul,16-17; 2011,Jan,11

00952 hysteroscopy and/or hysterosalpingography ♀

📋 0.00 ⚕ 0.00 **FUD** XXX N 🖵 P0

AMA: 2015,Jan,16; 2014,Aug,5; 2014,Jan,11; 2012,Jul,12-14; 2012,Jan,15-42; 2011,Oct,3-4; 2011,Jul,16-17; 2011,Jan,11

01112-01522 Anesthesia for Lower Extremity Procedures

CMS: 100-4,12,140.1 Qualified Nonphysician Anesthetists; 100-4,12,140.3 Payment for Qualified Nonphysician Anesthetists; 100-4,12,140.3.3 Billing Modifiers; 100-4,12,140.3.4 General Billing Instructions; 100-4,12,140.4.1 Anesthesiologist/Qualified Nonphysican Anesthetist; 100-4,12,140.4.2 Anesthetist and Anesthesiologist in a Single Procedure; 100-4,12,140.4.3 Payment for Medical /Surgical Services by CRNAs; 100-4,12,140.4.4 Conversion Factors for Anesthesia Services; 100-4,4,250.3.2 Anesthesia in a Hospital Outpatient Setting

01112 Anesthesia for bone marrow aspiration and/or biopsy, anterior or posterior iliac crest

📋 0.00 ⚕ 0.00 **FUD** XXX N 🖵 P0

AMA: 2015,Jan,16; 2014,Aug,5; 2014,Jan,11; 2012,Jul,12-14; 2012,Jan,15-42; 2011,Oct,3-4; 2011,Jul,16-17; 2011,Jan,11

01120 Anesthesia for procedures on bony pelvis

📋 0.00 ⚕ 0.00 **FUD** XXX N 🖵 P0

AMA: 2015,Jan,16; 2014,Aug,5; 2014,Jan,11; 2012,Jul,12-14; 2012,Jan,15-42; 2011,Oct,3-4; 2011,Jul,16-17; 2011,Jan,11

01130 Anesthesia for body cast application or revision

📋 0.00 ⚕ 0.00 **FUD** XXX N 🖵 P0

AMA: 2015,Jan,16; 2014,Aug,5; 2014,Jan,11; 2012,Jul,12-14; 2012,Jan,15-42; 2011,Oct,3-4; 2011,Jul,16-17; 2011,Jan,11

01140 Anesthesia for interpelviabdominal (hindquarter) amputation

📋 0.00 ⚕ 0.00 **FUD** XXX C 🖵 P0

AMA: 2015,Jan,16; 2014,Aug,5; 2014,Jan,11; 2012,Jul,12-14; 2012,Jan,15-42; 2011,Oct,3-4; 2011,Jul,16-17; 2011,Jan,11

01150 Anesthesia for radical procedures for tumor of pelvis, except hindquarter amputation

📋 0.00 ⚕ 0.00 **FUD** XXX C 🖵 P0

AMA: 2015,Jan,16; 2014,Aug,5; 2014,Jan,11; 2012,Jul,12-14; 2012,Jan,15-42; 2011,Oct,3-4; 2011,Jul,16-17; 2011,Jan,11

01160 Anesthesia for closed procedures involving symphysis pubis or sacroiliac joint

⏱ 0.00   ⚕ 0.00   **FUD** XXX   N ▢ PQ

AMA: 2015,Jan,16; 2014,Aug,5; 2014,Jan,11; 2012,Jul,12-14; 2012,Jan,15-42; 2011,Oct,3-4; 2011,Jul,16-17; 2011,Jan,11

01170 Anesthesia for open procedures involving symphysis pubis or sacroiliac joint

⏱ 0.00   ⚕ 0.00   **FUD** XXX   N ▢ PQ

AMA: 2015,Jan,16; 2014,Aug,5; 2014,Jan,11; 2012,Jul,12-14; 2012,Jan,15-42; 2011,Oct,3-4; 2011,Jul,16-17; 2011,Jan,11

01173 Anesthesia for open repair of fracture disruption of pelvis or column fracture involving acetabulum

⏱ 0.00   ⚕ 0.00   **FUD** XXX   N ▢ PQ

AMA: 2015,Jan,16; 2014,Aug,5; 2014,Jan,11; 2012,Jul,12-14; 2012,Jan,15-42; 2011,Oct,3-4; 2011,Jul,16-17; 2011,Jan,11

01180 Anesthesia for obturator neurectomy; extrapelvic

⏱ 0.00   ⚕ 0.00   **FUD** XXX   N ▢ PQ

AMA: 2015,Jan,16; 2014,Aug,5; 2014,Jan,11; 2012,Jul,12-14; 2012,Jan,15-42; 2011,Oct,3-4; 2011,Jul,16-17; 2011,Jan,11

01190 intrapelvic

⏱ 0.00   ⚕ 0.00   **FUD** XXX   N ▢ PQ

AMA: 2015,Jan,16; 2014,Aug,5; 2014,Jan,11; 2012,Jul,12-14; 2012,Jan,15-42; 2011,Oct,3-4; 2011,Jul,16-17; 2011,Jan,11

01200 Anesthesia for all closed procedures involving hip joint

⏱ 0.00   ⚕ 0.00   **FUD** XXX   N ▢ PQ

AMA: 2015,Jan,16; 2014,Aug,5; 2014,Jan,11; 2012,Jul,12-14; 2012,Jan,15-42; 2011,Oct,3-4; 2011,Jul,16-17; 2011,Jan,11

01202 Anesthesia for arthroscopic procedures of hip joint

⏱ 0.00   ⚕ 0.00   **FUD** XXX   N ▢ PQ

AMA: 2015,Jan,16; 2014,Aug,5; 2014,Jan,11; 2012,Jul,12-14; 2012,Jan,15-42; 2011,Oct,3-4; 2011,Jul,16-17; 2011,Jan,11

01210 Anesthesia for open procedures involving hip joint; not otherwise specified

⏱ 0.00   ⚕ 0.00   **FUD** XXX   N ▢ PQ

AMA: 2015,Jan,16; 2014,Aug,5; 2014,Jan,11; 2012,Jul,12-14; 2012,Jan,15-42; 2011,Oct,3-4; 2011,Jul,16-17; 2011,Jan,11

01212 hip disarticulation

⏱ 0.00   ⚕ 0.00   **FUD** XXX   C ▢ PQ

AMA: 2015,Jan,16; 2014,Aug,5; 2014,Jan,11; 2012,Jul,12-14; 2012,Jan,15-42; 2011,Oct,3-4; 2011,Jul,16-17; 2011,Jan,11

01214 total hip arthroplasty

⏱ 0.00   ⚕ 0.00   **FUD** XXX   C ▢ PQ

AMA: 2015,Jan,16; 2014,Aug,5; 2014,Jan,11; 2012,Jul,12-14; 2012,Jan,15-42; 2011,Oct,3-4; 2011,Jul,16-17; 2011,Jan,11

01215 revision of total hip arthroplasty

⏱ 0.00   ⚕ 0.00   **FUD** XXX   N ▢ PQ

AMA: 2015,Jan,16; 2014,Aug,5; 2014,Jan,11; 2012,Jul,12-14; 2012,Jan,15-42; 2011,Oct,3-4; 2011,Jul,16-17; 2011,Jan,11

01220 Anesthesia for all closed procedures involving upper two-thirds of femur

⏱ 0.00   ⚕ 0.00   **FUD** XXX   N ▢ PQ

AMA: 2015,Jan,16; 2014,Aug,5; 2014,Jan,11; 2012,Jul,12-14; 2012,Jan,15-42; 2011,Oct,3-4; 2011,Jul,16-17; 2011,Jan,11

01230 Anesthesia for open procedures involving upper two-thirds of femur; not otherwise specified

⏱ 0.00   ⚕ 0.00   **FUD** XXX   N ▢ PQ

AMA: 2015,Jan,16; 2014,Aug,5; 2014,Jan,11; 2012,Jul,12-14; 2012,Jan,15-42; 2011,Oct,3-4; 2011,Jul,16-17; 2011,Jan,11

01232 amputation

⏱ 0.00   ⚕ 0.00   **FUD** XXX   C ▢ PQ

AMA: 2015,Jan,16; 2014,Aug,5; 2014,Jan,11; 2012,Jul,12-14; 2012,Jan,15-42; 2011,Oct,3-4; 2011,Jul,16-17; 2011,Jan,11

01234 radical resection

⏱ 0.00   ⚕ 0.00   **FUD** XXX   C ▢ PQ

AMA: 2015,Jan,16; 2014,Aug,5; 2014,Jan,11; 2012,Jul,12-14; 2012,Jan,15-42; 2011,Oct,3-4; 2011,Jul,16-17; 2011,Jan,11

01250 Anesthesia for all procedures on nerves, muscles, tendons, fascia, and bursae of upper leg

⏱ 0.00   ⚕ 0.00   **FUD** XXX   N ▢ PQ

AMA: 2015,Jan,16; 2014,Aug,5; 2014,Jan,11; 2012,Jul,12-14; 2012,Jan,15-42; 2011,Oct,3-4; 2011,Jul,16-17; 2011,Jan,11

01260 Anesthesia for all procedures involving veins of upper leg, including exploration

⏱ 0.00   ⚕ 0.00   **FUD** XXX   N ▢ PQ

AMA: 2015,Jan,16; 2014,Aug,5; 2014,Jan,11; 2012,Jul,12-14; 2012,Jan,15-42; 2011,Oct,3-4; 2011,Jul,16-17; 2011,Jan,11

01270 Anesthesia for procedures involving arteries of upper leg, including bypass graft; not otherwise specified

⏱ 0.00   ⚕ 0.00   **FUD** XXX   N ▢ PQ

AMA: 2015,Jan,16; 2014,Aug,5; 2014,Jan,11; 2012,Jul,12-14; 2012,Jan,15-42; 2011,Oct,3-4; 2011,Jul,16-17; 2011,Jan,11

01272 femoral artery ligation

⏱ 0.00   ⚕ 0.00   **FUD** XXX   C ▢ PQ

AMA: 2015,Jan,16; 2014,Aug,5; 2014,Jan,11; 2012,Jul,12-14; 2012,Jan,15-42; 2011,Oct,3-4; 2011,Jul,16-17; 2011,Jan,11

01274 femoral artery embolectomy

⏱ 0.00   ⚕ 0.00   **FUD** XXX   C ▢ PQ

AMA: 2015,Jan,16; 2014,Aug,5; 2014,Jan,11; 2012,Jul,12-14; 2012,Jan,15-42; 2011,Oct,3-4; 2011,Jul,16-17; 2011,Jan,11

01320 Anesthesia for all procedures on nerves, muscles, tendons, fascia, and bursae of knee and/or popliteal area

⏱ 0.00   ⚕ 0.00   **FUD** XXX   N ▢ PQ

AMA: 2015,Jan,16; 2014,Aug,5; 2014,Jan,11; 2012,Jul,12-14; 2012,Jan,15-42; 2011,Oct,3-4; 2011,Jul,16-17; 2011,Jan,11

01340 Anesthesia for all closed procedures on lower one-third of femur

⏱ 0.00   ⚕ 0.00   **FUD** XXX   N ▢ PQ

AMA: 2015,Jan,16; 2014,Aug,5; 2014,Jan,11; 2012,Jul,12-14; 2012,Jan,15-42; 2011,Oct,3-4; 2011,Jul,16-17; 2011,Jan,11

01360 Anesthesia for all open procedures on lower one-third of femur

⏱ 0.00   ⚕ 0.00   **FUD** XXX   N ▢ PQ

AMA: 2015,Jan,16; 2014,Aug,5; 2014,Jan,11; 2012,Jul,12-14; 2012,Jan,15-42; 2011,Oct,3-4; 2011,Jul,16-17; 2011,Jan,11

01380 Anesthesia for all closed procedures on knee joint

⏱ 0.00   ⚕ 0.00   **FUD** XXX   N ▢ PQ

AMA: 2015,Jan,16; 2014,Aug,5; 2014,Jan,11; 2012,Jul,12-14; 2012,Jan,15-42; 2011,Oct,3-4; 2011,Jul,16-17; 2011,Jan,11

01382 Anesthesia for diagnostic arthroscopic procedures of knee joint

⏱ 0.00   ⚕ 0.00   **FUD** XXX   N ▢ PQ

AMA: 2015,Jan,16; 2014,Aug,5; 2014,Jan,11; 2012,Jul,12-14; 2012,Jan,15-42; 2011,Oct,3-4; 2011,Jul,16-17; 2011,Jan,11

01390 Anesthesia for all closed procedures on upper ends of tibia, fibula, and/or patella

⏱ 0.00   ⚕ 0.00   **FUD** XXX   N ▢ PQ

AMA: 2015,Jan,16; 2014,Aug,5; 2014,Jan,11; 2012,Jul,12-14; 2012,Jan,15-42; 2011,Oct,3-4; 2011,Jul,16-17; 2011,Jan,11

01392 Anesthesia for all open procedures on upper ends of tibia, fibula, and/or patella

⏱ 0.00   ⚕ 0.00   **FUD** XXX   N ▢ PQ

AMA: 2015,Jan,16; 2014,Aug,5; 2014,Jan,11; 2012,Jul,12-14; 2012,Jan,15-42; 2011,Oct,3-4; 2011,Jul,16-17; 2011,Jan,11

01400 Anesthesia for open or surgical arthroscopic procedures on knee joint; not otherwise specified

⏱ 0.00   ⚕ 0.00   **FUD** XXX   N ▢ PQ

AMA: 2015,Jan,16; 2014,Aug,5; 2014,Jan,11; 2012,Jul,12-14; 2012,Jan,15-42; 2011,Oct,3-4; 2011,Jul,16-17; 2011,Jan,11

01402 total knee arthroplasty

⏱ 0.00   ⚕ 0.00   **FUD** XXX   C ▢ PQ

AMA: 2015,Jan,16; 2014,Aug,5; 2014,Jan,11; 2012,Jul,12-14; 2012,Jan,15-42; 2011,Oct,3-4; 2011,Jul,16-17; 2011,Jan,11

01404   disarticulation at knee

   🖨 0.00   ⚗ 0.00   **FUD** XXX   C P0

AMA: 2015,Jan,16; 2014,Aug,5; 2014,Jan,11; 2012,Jul,12-14; 2012,Jan,15-42; 2011,Oct,3-4; 2011,Jul,16-17; 2011,Jan,11

01420   Anesthesia for all cast applications, removal, or repair involving knee joint

   🖨 0.00   ⚗ 0.00   **FUD** XXX   N P0

AMA: 2015,Jan,16; 2014,Aug,5; 2014,Jan,11; 2012,Jul,12-14; 2012,Jan,15-42; 2011,Oct,3-4; 2011,Jul,16-17; 2011,Jan,11

01430   Anesthesia for procedures on veins of knee and popliteal area; not otherwise specified

   🖨 0.00   ⚗ 0.00   **FUD** XXX   N P0

AMA: 2015,Jan,16; 2014,Aug,5; 2014,Jan,11; 2012,Jul,12-14; 2012,Jan,15-42; 2011,Oct,3-4; 2011,Jul,16-17; 2011,Jan,11

01432   arteriovenous fistula

   🖨 0.00   ⚗ 0.00   **FUD** XXX   N P0

AMA: 2015,Jan,16; 2014,Aug,5; 2014,Jan,11; 2012,Jul,12-14; 2012,Jan,15-42; 2011,Oct,3-4; 2011,Jul,16-17; 2011,Jan,11

01440   Anesthesia for procedures on arteries of knee and popliteal area; not otherwise specified

   🖨 0.00   ⚗ 0.00   **FUD** XXX   N P0

AMA: 2015,Jan,16; 2014,Aug,5; 2014,Jan,11; 2012,Jul,12-14; 2012,Jan,15-42; 2011,Oct,3-4; 2011,Jul,16-17; 2011,Jan,11

01442   popliteal thromboendarterectomy, with or without patch graft

   🖨 0.00   ⚗ 0.00   **FUD** XXX   C P0

AMA: 2015,Jan,16; 2014,Aug,5; 2014,Jan,11; 2012,Jul,12-14; 2012,Jan,15-42; 2011,Oct,3-4; 2011,Jul,16-17; 2011,Jan,11

01444   popliteal excision and graft or repair for occlusion or aneurysm

   🖨 0.00   ⚗ 0.00   **FUD** XXX   C P0

AMA: 2015,Jan,16; 2014,Aug,5; 2014,Jan,11; 2012,Jul,12-14; 2012,Jan,15-42; 2011,Oct,3-4; 2011,Jul,16-17; 2011,Jan,11

01462   Anesthesia for all closed procedures on lower leg, ankle, and foot

   🖨 0.00   ⚗ 0.00   **FUD** XXX   N P0

AMA: 2015,Jan,16; 2014,Aug,5; 2014,Jan,11; 2012,Jul,12-14; 2012,Jan,15-42; 2011,Oct,3-4; 2011,Jul,16-17; 2011,Jan,11

01464   Anesthesia for arthroscopic procedures of ankle and/or foot

   🖨 0.00   ⚗ 0.00   **FUD** XXX   N P0

AMA: 2015,Jan,16; 2014,Aug,5; 2014,Jan,11; 2012,Jul,12-14; 2012,Jan,15-42; 2011,Oct,3-4; 2011,Jul,16-17; 2011,Jan,11

01470   Anesthesia for procedures on nerves, muscles, tendons, and fascia of lower leg, ankle, and foot; not otherwise specified

   🖨 0.00   ⚗ 0.00   **FUD** XXX   N P0

AMA: 2015,Jan,16; 2014,Aug,5; 2014,Jan,11; 2012,Jul,12-14; 2012,Jan,15-42; 2011,Oct,3-4; 2011,Jul,16-17; 2011,Jan,11

01472   repair of ruptured Achilles tendon, with or without graft

   🖨 0.00   ⚗ 0.00   **FUD** XXX   N P0

AMA: 2015,Jan,16; 2014,Aug,5; 2014,Jan,11; 2012,Jul,12-14; 2012,Jan,15-42; 2011,Oct,3-4; 2011,Jul,16-17; 2011,Jan,11

01474   gastrocnemius recession (eg, Strayer procedure)

   🖨 0.00   ⚗ 0.00   **FUD** XXX   N P0

AMA: 2015,Jan,16; 2014,Aug,5; 2014,Jan,11; 2012,Jul,12-14; 2012,Jan,15-42; 2011,Oct,3-4; 2011,Jul,16-17; 2011,Jan,11

01480   Anesthesia for open procedures on bones of lower leg, ankle, and foot; not otherwise specified

   🖨 0.00   ⚗ 0.00   **FUD** XXX   N P0

AMA: 2015,Jan,16; 2014,Aug,5; 2014,Jan,11; 2012,Jul,12-14; 2012,Jan,15-42; 2011,Oct,3-4; 2011,Jul,16-17; 2011,Jan,11

01482   radical resection (including below knee amputation)

   🖨 0.00   ⚗ 0.00   **FUD** XXX   N P0

AMA: 2015,Jan,16; 2014,Aug,5; 2014,Jan,11; 2012,Jul,12-14; 2012,Jan,15-42; 2011,Oct,3-4; 2011,Jul,16-17; 2011,Jan,11

01484   osteotomy or osteoplasty of tibia and/or fibula

   🖨 0.00   ⚗ 0.00   **FUD** XXX   N P0

AMA: 2015,Jan,16; 2014,Aug,5; 2014,Jan,11; 2012,Jul,12-14; 2012,Jan,15-42; 2011,Oct,3-4; 2011,Jul,16-17; 2011,Jan,11

01486   total ankle replacement

   🖨 0.00   ⚗ 0.00   **FUD** XXX   C P0

AMA: 2015,Jan,16; 2014,Aug,5; 2014,Jan,11; 2012,Jul,12-14; 2012,Jan,15-42; 2011,Oct,3-4; 2011,Jul,16-17; 2011,Jan,11

01490   Anesthesia for lower leg cast application, removal, or repair

   🖨 0.00   ⚗ 0.00   **FUD** XXX   N P0

AMA: 2015,Jan,16; 2014,Aug,5; 2014,Jan,11; 2012,Jul,12-14; 2012,Jan,15-42; 2011,Oct,3-4; 2011,Jul,16-17; 2011,Jan,11

01500   Anesthesia for procedures on arteries of lower leg, including bypass graft; not otherwise specified

   🖨 0.00   ⚗ 0.00   **FUD** XXX   N P0

AMA: 2015,Jan,16; 2014,Aug,5; 2014,Jan,11; 2012,Jul,12-14; 2012,Jan,15-42; 2011,Oct,3-4; 2011,Jul,16-17; 2011,Jan,11

01502   embolectomy, direct or with catheter

   🖨 0.00   ⚗ 0.00   **FUD** XXX   C P0

AMA: 2015,Jan,16; 2014,Aug,5; 2014,Jan,11; 2012,Jul,12-14; 2012,Jan,15-42; 2011,Oct,3-4; 2011,Jul,16-17; 2011,Jan,11

01520   Anesthesia for procedures on veins of lower leg; not otherwise specified

   🖨 0.00   ⚗ 0.00   **FUD** XXX   N P0

AMA: 2015,Jan,16; 2014,Aug,5; 2014,Jan,11; 2012,Jul,12-14; 2012,Jan,15-42; 2011,Oct,3-4; 2011,Jul,16-17; 2011,Jan,11

01522   venous thrombectomy, direct or with catheter

   🖨 0.00   ⚗ 0.00   **FUD** XXX   N P0

AMA: 2015,Jan,16; 2014,Aug,5; 2014,Jan,11; 2012,Jul,12-14; 2012,Jan,15-42; 2011,Oct,3-4; 2011,Jul,16-17; 2011,Jan,11

01610-01682 Anesthesia for Shoulder Procedures

CMS: 100-4,12,140.1 Qualified Nonphysician Anesthetists; 100-4,12,140.3 Payment for Qualified Nonphysician Anesthetists; 100-4,12,140.3.3 Billing Modifiers; 100-4,12,140.3.4 General Billing Instructions; 100-4,12,140.4.1 Anesthesiologist/Qualified Nonphysican Anesthetist; 100-4,12,140.4.2 Anesthetist and Anesthesiologist in a Single Procedure; 100-4,12,140.4.3 Payment for Medical /Surgical Services by CRNAs; 100-4,12,140.4.4 Conversion Factors for Anesthesia Services; 100-4,4,250.3.2 Anesthesia in a Hospital Outpatient Setting

INCLUDES   Acromioclavicular joint
    Humeral head and neck
    Shoulder joint
    Sternoclavicular joint

01610   Anesthesia for all procedures on nerves, muscles, tendons, fascia, and bursae of shoulder and axilla

   🖨 0.00   ⚗ 0.00   **FUD** XXX   N P0

AMA: 2015,Jan,16; 2014,Aug,5; 2014,Jan,11; 2012,Jul,12-14; 2012,Jan,15-42; 2011,Oct,3-4; 2011,Jul,16-17; 2011,Jan,11

01620   Anesthesia for all closed procedures on humeral head and neck, sternoclavicular joint, acromioclavicular joint, and shoulder joint

   🖨 0.00   ⚗ 0.00   **FUD** XXX   N P0

AMA: 2015,Jan,16; 2014,Aug,5; 2014,Jan,11; 2012,Jul,12-14; 2012,Jan,15-42; 2011,Oct,3-4; 2011,Jul,16-17; 2011,Jan,11

01622   Anesthesia for diagnostic arthroscopic procedures of shoulder joint

   🖨 0.00   ⚗ 0.00   **FUD** XXX   N P0

AMA: 2015,Jan,16; 2014,Aug,5; 2014,Jan,11; 2012,Jul,12-14; 2012,Jan,15-42; 2011,Oct,3-4; 2011,Jul,16-17; 2011,Jan,11

01630   Anesthesia for open or surgical arthroscopic procedures on humeral head and neck, sternoclavicular joint, acromioclavicular joint, and shoulder joint; not otherwise specified

   🖨 0.00   ⚗ 0.00   **FUD** XXX   N P0

AMA: 2015,Jan,16; 2014,Aug,5; 2014,Jan,11; 2012,Jul,12-14; 2012,Jan,15-42; 2011,Oct,3-4; 2011,Jul,16-17; 2011,Jan,11

01634   shoulder disarticulation

   🖨 0.00   ⚗ 0.00   **FUD** XXX   C P0

AMA: 2015,Jan,16; 2014,Aug,5; 2014,Jan,11; 2012,Jul,12-14; 2012,Jan,15-42; 2011,Oct,3-4; 2011,Jul,16-17; 2011,Jan,11

26/TC PC/TC Component Only   A2-Z3 ASC Pmt   50 Bilateral   ♂ Male Only   ♀ Female Only   🖨 Facility RVU   ⚗ Non-Facility RVU
AMA: CPT Asst   **CMS:** Pub 100   A-Y OPPSI   80/80 Surg Assist Allowed / w/Doc   🔲 Lab Crosswalk   🔳 Radiology Crosswalk

8   Medicare (Red Text)   CPT © 2015 American Medical Association. All Rights Reserved. (Black Text)   © 2015 Optum360, LLC (Blue Text)

01636	**interthoracoscapular (forequarter) amputation**

🔲 0.00 🔲 0.00 **FUD** XXX `C` `🔲` `PQ`

AMA: 2015,Jan,16; 2014,Aug,5; 2014,Jan,11; 2012,Jul,12-14; 2012,Jan,15-42; 2011,Oct,3-4; 2011,Jul,16-17; 2011,Jan,11

01638 **total shoulder replacement**

🔲 0.00 🔲 0.00 **FUD** XXX `C` `🔲` `PQ`

AMA: 2015,Jan,16; 2014,Aug,5; 2014,Jan,11; 2012,Jul,12-14; 2012,Jan,15-42; 2011,Oct,3-4; 2011,Jul,16-17; 2011,Jan,11

01650 **Anesthesia for procedures on arteries of shoulder and axilla; not otherwise specified**

🔲 0.00 🔲 0.00 **FUD** XXX `N` `🔲` `PQ`

AMA: 2015,Jan,16; 2014,Aug,5; 2014,Jan,11; 2012,Jul,12-14; 2012,Jan,15-42; 2011,Oct,3-4; 2011,Jul,16-17; 2011,Jan,11

01652 **axillary-brachial aneurysm**

🔲 0.00 🔲 0.00 **FUD** XXX `C` `🔲` `PQ`

AMA: 2015,Jan,16; 2014,Aug,5; 2014,Jan,11; 2012,Jul,12-14; 2012,Jan,15-42; 2011,Oct,3-4; 2011,Jul,16-17; 2011,Jan,11

01654 **bypass graft**

🔲 0.00 🔲 0.00 **FUD** XXX `C` `🔲` `PQ`

AMA: 2015,Jan,16; 2014,Aug,5; 2014,Jan,11; 2012,Jul,12-14; 2012,Jan,15-42; 2011,Oct,3-4; 2011,Jul,16-17; 2011,Jan,11

01656 **axillary-femoral bypass graft**

🔲 0.00 🔲 0.00 **FUD** XXX `C` `🔲` `PQ`

AMA: 2015,Jan,16; 2014,Aug,5; 2014,Jan,11; 2012,Jul,12-14; 2012,Jan,15-42; 2011,Oct,3-4; 2011,Jul,16-17; 2011,Jan,11

01670 **Anesthesia for all procedures on veins of shoulder and axilla**

🔲 0.00 🔲 0.00 **FUD** XXX `N` `🔲` `PQ`

AMA: 2015,Jan,16; 2014,Aug,5; 2014,Jan,11; 2012,Jul,12-14; 2012,Jan,15-42; 2011,Oct,3-4; 2011,Jul,16-17; 2011,Jan,11

01680 **Anesthesia for shoulder cast application, removal or repair; not otherwise specified**

🔲 0.00 🔲 0.00 **FUD** XXX `N` `🔲` `PQ`

AMA: 2015,Jan,16; 2014,Aug,5; 2014,Jan,11; 2012,Jul,12-14; 2012,Jan,15-42; 2011,Oct,3-4; 2011,Jul,16-17; 2011,Jan,11

01682 **shoulder spica**

🔲 0.00 🔲 0.00 **FUD** XXX `N` `🔲` `PQ`

AMA: 2015,Jan,16; 2014,Aug,5; 2014,Jan,11; 2012,Jul,12-14; 2012,Jan,15-42; 2011,Oct,3-4; 2011,Jul,16-17; 2011,Jan,11

01710-01860 Anesthesia for Upper Extremity Procedures

CMS: 100-4,12,140.1 Qualified Nonphysician Anesthetists; 100-4,12,140.3 Payment for Qualified Nonphysician Anesthetists; 100-4,12,140.3.3 Billing Modifiers; 100-4,12,140.3.4 General Billing Instructions; 100-4,12,140.4.1 Anesthesiologist/Qualified Nonphysican Anesthetist; 100-4,12,140.4.2 Anesthetist and Anesthesiologist in a Single Procedure; 100-4,12,140.4.3 Payment for Medical /Surgical Services by CRNAs; 100-4,12,140.4.4 Conversion Factors for Anesthesia Services; 100-4,4,250.3.2 Anesthesia in a Hospital Outpatient Setting

01710 **Anesthesia for procedures on nerves, muscles, tendons, fascia, and bursae of upper arm and elbow; not otherwise specified**

🔲 0.00 🔲 0.00 **FUD** XXX `N` `🔲` `PQ`

AMA: 2015,Jan,16; 2014,Aug,5; 2014,Jan,11; 2012,Jul,12-14; 2012,Jan,15-42; 2011,Oct,3-4; 2011,Jul,16-17; 2011,Jan,11

01712 **tenotomy, elbow to shoulder, open**

🔲 0.00 🔲 0.00 **FUD** XXX `N` `🔲` `PQ`

AMA: 2015,Jan,16; 2014,Aug,5; 2014,Jan,11; 2012,Jul,12-14; 2012,Jan,15-42; 2011,Oct,3-4; 2011,Jul,16-17; 2011,Jan,11

01714 **tenoplasty, elbow to shoulder**

🔲 0.00 🔲 0.00 **FUD** XXX `N` `🔲` `PQ`

AMA: 2015,Jan,16; 2014,Aug,5; 2014,Jan,11; 2012,Jul,12-14; 2012,Jan,15-42; 2011,Oct,3-4; 2011,Jul,16-17; 2011,Jan,11

01716 **tenodesis, rupture of long tendon of biceps**

🔲 0.00 🔲 0.00 **FUD** XXX `N` `🔲` `PQ`

AMA: 2015,Jan,16; 2014,Aug,5; 2014,Jan,11; 2012,Jul,12-14; 2012,Jan,15-42; 2011,Oct,3-4; 2011,Jul,16-17; 2011,Jan,11

01730 **Anesthesia for all closed procedures on humerus and elbow**

🔲 0.00 🔲 0.00 **FUD** XXX `N` `🔲` `PQ`

AMA: 2015,Jan,16; 2014,Aug,5; 2014,Jan,11; 2012,Jul,12-14; 2012,Jan,15-42; 2011,Oct,3-4; 2011,Jul,16-17; 2011,Jan,11

01732 **Anesthesia for diagnostic arthroscopic procedures of elbow joint**

🔲 0.00 🔲 0.00 **FUD** XXX `N` `🔲` `PQ`

AMA: 2015,Jan,16; 2014,Aug,5; 2014,Jan,11; 2012,Jul,12-14; 2012,Jan,15-42; 2011,Oct,3-4; 2011,Jul,16-17; 2011,Jan,11

01740 **Anesthesia for open or surgical arthroscopic procedures of the elbow; not otherwise specified**

🔲 0.00 🔲 0.00 **FUD** XXX `N` `🔲` `PQ`

AMA: 2015,Jan,16; 2014,Aug,5; 2014,Jan,11; 2012,Jul,12-14; 2012,Jan,15-42; 2011,Oct,3-4; 2011,Jul,16-17; 2011,Jan,11

01742 **osteotomy of humerus**

🔲 0.00 🔲 0.00 **FUD** XXX `N` `🔲` `PQ`

AMA: 2015,Jan,16; 2014,Aug,5; 2014,Jan,11; 2012,Jul,12-14; 2012,Jan,15-42; 2011,Oct,3-4; 2011,Jul,16-17; 2011,Jan,11

01744 **repair of nonunion or malunion of humerus**

🔲 0.00 🔲 0.00 **FUD** XXX `N` `🔲` `PQ`

AMA: 2015,Jan,16; 2014,Aug,5; 2014,Jan,11; 2012,Jul,12-14; 2012,Jan,15-42; 2011,Oct,3-4; 2011,Jul,16-17; 2011,Jan,11

01756 **radical procedures**

🔲 0.00 🔲 0.00 **FUD** XXX `C` `🔲` `PQ`

AMA: 2015,Jan,16; 2014,Aug,5; 2014,Jan,11; 2012,Jul,12-14; 2012,Jan,15-42; 2011,Oct,3-4; 2011,Jul,16-17; 2011,Jan,11

01758 **excision of cyst or tumor of humerus**

🔲 0.00 🔲 0.00 **FUD** XXX `N` `🔲` `PQ`

AMA: 2015,Jan,16; 2014,Aug,5; 2014,Jan,11; 2012,Jul,12-14; 2012,Jan,15-42; 2011,Oct,3-4; 2011,Jul,16-17; 2011,Jan,11

01760 **total elbow replacement**

🔲 0.00 🔲 0.00 **FUD** XXX `N` `🔲` `PQ`

AMA: 2015,Jan,16; 2014,Aug,5; 2014,Jan,11; 2012,Jul,12-14; 2012,Jan,15-42; 2011,Oct,3-4; 2011,Jul,16-17; 2011,Jan,11

01770 **Anesthesia for procedures on arteries of upper arm and elbow; not otherwise specified**

🔲 0.00 🔲 0.00 **FUD** XXX `N` `🔲` `PQ`

AMA: 2015,Jan,16; 2014,Aug,5; 2014,Jan,11; 2012,Jul,12-14; 2012,Jan,15-42; 2011,Oct,3-4; 2011,Jul,16-17; 2011,Jan,11

01772 **embolectomy**

🔲 0.00 🔲 0.00 **FUD** XXX `N` `🔲` `PQ`

AMA: 2015,Jan,16; 2014,Aug,5; 2014,Jan,11; 2012,Jul,12-14; 2012,Jan,15-42; 2011,Oct,3-4; 2011,Jul,16-17; 2011,Jan,11

01780 **Anesthesia for procedures on veins of upper arm and elbow; not otherwise specified**

🔲 0.00 🔲 0.00 **FUD** XXX `N` `🔲` `PQ`

AMA: 2015,Jan,16; 2014,Aug,5; 2014,Jan,11; 2012,Jul,12-14; 2012,Jan,15-42; 2011,Oct,3-4; 2011,Jul,16-17; 2011,Jan,11

01782 **phleborrhaphy**

🔲 0.00 🔲 0.00 **FUD** XXX `N` `🔲` `PQ`

AMA: 2015,Jan,16; 2014,Aug,5; 2014,Jan,11; 2012,Jul,12-14; 2012,Jan,15-42; 2011,Oct,3-4; 2011,Jul,16-17; 2011,Jan,11

01810 **Anesthesia for all procedures on nerves, muscles, tendons, fascia, and bursae of forearm, wrist, and hand**

🔲 0.00 🔲 0.00 **FUD** XXX `N` `🔲` `PQ`

AMA: 2015,Jan,16; 2014,Aug,5; 2014,Jan,11; 2012,Jul,12-14; 2012,Jan,15-42; 2011,Oct,3-4; 2011,Jul,16-17; 2011,Jan,11

01820 **Anesthesia for all closed procedures on radius, ulna, wrist, or hand bones**

🔲 0.00 🔲 0.00 **FUD** XXX `N` `🔲` `PQ`

AMA: 2015,Jan,16; 2014,Aug,5; 2014,Jan,11; 2012,Jul,12-14; 2012,Jan,15-42; 2011,Oct,3-4; 2011,Jul,16-17; 2011,Jan,11

01829 **Anesthesia for diagnostic arthroscopic procedures on the wrist**

🔲 0.00 🔲 0.00 **FUD** XXX `N` `🔲` `PQ`

AMA: 2015,Jan,16; 2014,Aug,5; 2014,Jan,11; 2012,Jul,12-14; 2012,Jan,15-42; 2011,Oct,3-4; 2011,Jul,16-17; 2011,Jan,11

● New Code   ▲ Revised Code   ○ Reinstated   Ⓜ Maternity   Ⓐ Age Edit   Unlisted   Not Covered   # Resequenced
Ⓢ AMA Mod 51 Exempt   ⑤ Optum Mod 51 Exempt   ⑥ Mod 63 Exempt   ⊙ Mod Sedation   + Add-on   🔲 CCI   `PQ` PQRS   **FUD** Follow-up Days

01830 Anesthesia for open or surgical arthroscopic/endoscopic procedures on distal radius, distal ulna, wrist, or hand joints; not otherwise specified

    0.00   0.00   **FUD** XXX   N ▢ PQ

    AMA: 2015,Jan,16; 2014,Aug,5; 2014,Jan,11; 2012,Jul,12-14; 2012,Jan,15-42; 2011,Oct,3-4; 2011,Jul,16-17; 2011,Jan,11

01832 total wrist replacement

    0.00   0.00   **FUD** XXX   N ▢ PQ

    AMA: 2015,Jan,16; 2014,Aug,5; 2014,Jan,11; 2012,Jul,12-14; 2012,Jan,15-42; 2011,Oct,3-4; 2011,Jul,16-17; 2011,Jan,11

01840 Anesthesia for procedures on arteries of forearm, wrist, and hand; not otherwise specified

    0.00   0.00   **FUD** XXX   N ▢ PQ

    AMA: 2015,Jan,16; 2014,Aug,5; 2014,Jan,11; 2012,Jul,12-14; 2012,Jan,15-42; 2011,Oct,3-4; 2011,Jul,16-17; 2011,Jan,11

01842 embolectomy

    0.00   0.00   **FUD** XXX   N ▢ PQ

    AMA: 2015,Jan,16; 2014,Aug,5; 2014,Jan,11; 2012,Jul,12-14; 2012,Jan,15-42; 2011,Oct,3-4; 2011,Jul,16-17; 2011,Jan,11

01844 Anesthesia for vascular shunt, or shunt revision, any type (eg, dialysis)

    0.00   0.00   **FUD** XXX   N ▢ PQ

    AMA: 2015,Jan,16; 2014,Aug,5; 2014,Jan,11; 2012,Jul,12-14; 2012,Jan,15-42; 2011,Oct,3-4; 2011,Jul,16-17; 2011,Jan,11

01850 Anesthesia for procedures on veins of forearm, wrist, and hand; not otherwise specified

    0.00   0.00   **FUD** XXX   N ▢ PQ

    AMA: 2015,Jan,16; 2014,Aug,5; 2014,Jan,11; 2012,Jul,12-14; 2012,Jan,15-42; 2011,Oct,3-4; 2011,Jul,16-17; 2011,Jan,11

01852 phleborrhaphy

    0.00   0.00   **FUD** XXX   N ▢ PQ

    AMA: 2015,Jan,16; 2014,Aug,5; 2014,Jan,11; 2012,Jul,12-14; 2012,Jan,15-42; 2011,Oct,3-4; 2011,Jul,16-17; 2011,Jan,11

01860 Anesthesia for forearm, wrist, or hand cast application, removal, or repair

    0.00   0.00   **FUD** XXX   N ▢ PQ

    AMA: 2015,Jan,16; 2014,Aug,5; 2014,Jan,11; 2012,Jul,12-14; 2012,Jan,15-42; 2011,Oct,3-4; 2011,Jul,16-17; 2011,Jan,11

01916-01936 Anesthesia for Interventional Radiology Procedures

CMS: 100-4,12,140.1 Qualified Nonphysician Anesthetists; 100-4,12,140.3 Payment for Qualified Nonphysician Anesthetists; 100-4,12,140.3.3 Billing Modifiers; 100-4,12,140.3.4 General Billing Instructions; 100-4,12,140.4.1 Anesthesiologist/Qualified Nonphysican Anesthetist; 100-4,12,140.4.2 Anesthetist and Anesthesiologist in a Single Procedure; 100-4,12,140.4.3 Payment for Medical /Surgical Services by CRNAs; 100-4,12,140.4.4 Conversion Factors for Anesthesia Services; 100-4,4,250.3.2 Anesthesia in a Hospital Outpatient Setting

01916 Anesthesia for diagnostic arteriography/venography

    Do not report with (01924-01926, 01930-01933)

    0.00   0.00   **FUD** XXX   N ▢

    AMA: 2015,Jan,16; 2014,Aug,5; 2014,Jan,11; 2012,Jul,12-14; 2012,Jan,15-42; 2011,Oct,3-4; 2011,Jul,16-17; 2011,Jan,11

01920 Anesthesia for cardiac catheterization including coronary angiography and ventriculography (not to include Swan-Ganz catheter)

    0.00   0.00   **FUD** XXX   N ▢

    AMA: 2015,Jan,16; 2014,Aug,5; 2014,Jan,11; 2012,Jul,12-14; 2012,Jan,15-42; 2011,Oct,3-4; 2011,Jul,16-17; 2011,Jan,11

01922 Anesthesia for non-invasive imaging or radiation therapy

    0.00   0.00   **FUD** XXX   N ▢

    AMA: 2015,Jan,16; 2014,Aug,5; 2014,Jan,11; 2012,Jul,12-14; 2012,Jan,15-42; 2011,Oct,3-4; 2011,Jul,16-17; 2011,Jan,11

01924 Anesthesia for therapeutic interventional radiological procedures involving the arterial system; not otherwise specified

    0.00   0.00   **FUD** XXX   N ▢ PQ

    AMA: 2015,Jan,16; 2014,Aug,5; 2014,Jan,11; 2012,Jul,12-14; 2012,Jan,15-42; 2011,Oct,3-4; 2011,Jul,16-17; 2011,Jan,11

01925 carotid or coronary

    0.00   0.00   **FUD** XXX   N ▢ PQ

    AMA: 2015,Jan,16; 2014,Aug,5; 2014,Jan,11; 2012,Jul,12-14; 2012,Jan,15-42; 2011,Oct,3-4; 2011,Jul,16-17; 2011,Jan,11

01926 intracranial, intracardiac, or aortic

    0.00   0.00   **FUD** XXX   N ▢ PQ

    AMA: 2015,Jan,16; 2014,Aug,5; 2014,Jan,11; 2012,Jul,12-14; 2012,Jan,15-42; 2011,Oct,3-4; 2011,Jul,16-17; 2011,Jan,11

01930 Anesthesia for therapeutic interventional radiological procedures involving the venous/lymphatic system (not to include access to the central circulation); not otherwise specified

    0.00   0.00   **FUD** XXX   N ▢ PQ

    AMA: 2015,Jan,16; 2014,Aug,5; 2014,Jan,11; 2012,Jul,12-14; 2012,Jan,15-42; 2011,Oct,3-4; 2011,Jul,16-17; 2011,Jan,11

01931 intrahepatic or portal circulation (eg, transvenous intrahepatic portosystemic shunt[s] [TIPS])

    0.00   0.00   **FUD** XXX   N ▢ PQ

    AMA: 2015,Jan,16; 2014,Aug,5; 2014,Jan,11; 2012,Jul,12-14; 2012,Jan,15-42; 2011,Oct,3-4; 2011,Jul,16-17; 2011,Jan,11

01932 intrathoracic or jugular

    0.00   0.00   **FUD** XXX   N ▢ PQ

    AMA: 2015,Jan,16; 2014,Aug,5; 2014,Jan,11; 2012,Jul,12-14; 2012,Jan,15-42; 2011,Oct,3-4; 2011,Jul,16-17; 2011,Jan,11

01933 intracranial

    0.00   0.00   **FUD** XXX   N ▢ PQ

    AMA: 2015,Jan,16; 2014,Aug,5; 2014,Jan,11; 2012,Jul,12-14; 2012,Jan,15-42; 2011,Oct,3-4; 2011,Jul,16-17; 2011,Jan,11

01935 Anesthesia for percutaneous image guided procedures on the spine and spinal cord; diagnostic

    0.00   0.00   **FUD** XXX   N PQ

    AMA: 2015,Jan,16; 2014,Aug,5; 2014,Jan,11; 2012,Jul,12-14; 2012,Jan,15-42; 2011,Oct,3-4; 2011,Jul,16-17; 2011,Jan,11

01936 therapeutic

    0.00   0.00   **FUD** XXX   N PQ

    AMA: 2015,Jan,16; 2014,Aug,5; 2014,Jan,11; 2012,Jul,12-14; 2012,Jan,15-42; 2011,Oct,3-4; 2011,Jul,16-17; 2011,Jan,11

01951-01953 Anesthesia for Burn Procedures

CMS: 100-4,12,140.1 Qualified Nonphysician Anesthetists; 100-4,12,140.3 Payment for Qualified Nonphysician Anesthetists; 100-4,12,140.3.3 Billing Modifiers; 100-4,12,140.3.4 General Billing Instructions; 100-4,12,140.4.1 Anesthesiologist/Qualified Nonphysican Anesthetist; 100-4,12,140.4.2 Anesthetist and Anesthesiologist in a Single Procedure; 100-4,12,140.4.3 Payment for Medical /Surgical Services by CRNAs; 100-4,12,140.4.4 Conversion Factors for Anesthesia Services; 100-4,4,250.3.2 Anesthesia in a Hospital Outpatient Setting

01951 Anesthesia for second- and third-degree burn excision or debridement with or without skin grafting, any site, for total body surface area (TBSA) treated during anesthesia and surgery; less than 4% total body surface area

    0.00   0.00   **FUD** XXX   N ▢ PQ

    AMA: 2015,Jan,16; 2014,Aug,5; 2014,Jan,11; 2012,Jul,12-14; 2012,Jan,15-42; 2011,Oct,3-4; 2011,Jul,16-17; 2011,Jan,11

01952 between 4% and 9% of total body surface area

    0.00   0.00   **FUD** XXX   N ▢ PQ

    AMA: 2015,Jan,16; 2014,Aug,5; 2014,Jan,11; 2012,Jul,12-14; 2012,Jan,15-42; 2011,Oct,3-4; 2011,Jul,16-17; 2011,Jan,11

+ **01953** each additional 9% total body surface area or part thereof (List separately in addition to code for primary procedure)

    Code first (01952)

    0.00   0.00   **FUD** XXX   N ▢ PQ

    AMA: 2015,Jan,16; 2014,Aug,5; 2014,Jan,11; 2012,Jul,12-14; 2012,Jan,15-42; 2011,Oct,3-4; 2011,Jul,16-17; 2011,Jun,13; 2011,Jan,11

01958-01969 Anesthesia for Obstetric Procedures

CMS: 100-4,12,140.1 Qualified Nonphysician Anesthetists; 100-4,12,140.3 Payment for Qualified Nonphysician Anesthetists; 100-4,12,140.3.3 Billing Modifiers; 100-4,12,140.3.4 General Billing Instructions; 100-4,12,140.4.1 Anesthesiologist/Qualified Nonphysican Anesthetist; 100-4,12,140.4.2 Anesthetist and Anesthesiologist in a Single Procedure; 100-4,12,140.4.3 Payment for Medical /Surgical Services by CRNAs; 100-4,12,140.4.4 Conversion Factors for Anesthesia Services; 100-4,4,250.3.2 Anesthesia in a Hospital Outpatient Setting

01958 Anesthesia for external cephalic version procedure Ⓜ☐
 ⛨ 0.00 ⚕ 0.00 **FUD** XXX Ⓝ☐
 AMA: 2015,Jan,16; 2014,Aug,5; 2014,Jan,11; 2012,Jul,12-14; 2012,Jan,15-42; 2011,Oct,3-4; 2011,Jul,16-17; 2011,Jan,11

01960 Anesthesia for vaginal delivery only Ⓜ♀
 ⛨ 0.00 ⚕ 0.00 **FUD** XXX Ⓝ☐
 AMA: 2015,Jan,16; 2014,Aug,5; 2014,Jan,11; 2012,Jul,12-14; 2012,Jan,15-42; 2011,Oct,3-4; 2011,Jul,16-17; 2011,Jan,11

01961 Anesthesia for cesarean delivery only Ⓜ♀
 ⛨ 0.00 ⚕ 0.00 **FUD** XXX Ⓝ☐Ⓟ
 AMA: 2015,Jan,16; 2014,Aug,5; 2014,Jan,11; 2012,Jul,12-14; 2012,Jan,15-42; 2011,Oct,3-4; 2011,Jul,16-17; 2011,Jan,11

01962 Anesthesia for urgent hysterectomy following delivery Ⓜ♀
 ⛨ 0.00 ⚕ 0.00 **FUD** XXX Ⓝ☐Ⓟ
 AMA: 2015,Jan,16; 2014,Aug,5; 2014,Jan,11; 2012,Jul,12-14; 2012,Jan,15-42; 2011,Oct,3-4; 2011,Jul,16-17; 2011,Jan,11

01963 Anesthesia for cesarean hysterectomy without any labor analgesia/anesthesia care Ⓜ♀
 ⛨ 0.00 ⚕ 0.00 **FUD** XXX Ⓝ☐Ⓟ
 AMA: 2015,Jan,16; 2014,Aug,5; 2014,Jan,11; 2012,Jul,12-14; 2012,Jan,15-42; 2011,Oct,3-4; 2011,Jul,16-17; 2011,Jan,11

01965 Anesthesia for incomplete or missed abortion procedures Ⓜ♀
 ⛨ 0.00 ⚕ 0.00 **FUD** XXX ⓃⓅ
 AMA: 2015,Jan,16; 2014,Aug,5; 2014,Jan,11; 2012,Jul,12-14; 2012,Jan,15-42; 2011,Oct,3-4; 2011,Jul,16-17; 2011,Jan,11

01966 Anesthesia for induced abortion procedures Ⓜ♀
 ⛨ 0.00 ⚕ 0.00 **FUD** XXX ⓃⓅ
 AMA: 2015,Jan,16; 2014,Aug,5; 2014,Jan,11; 2012,Jul,12-14; 2012,Jan,15-42; 2011,Oct,3-4; 2011,Jul,16-17; 2011,Jan,11

01967 Neuraxial labor analgesia/anesthesia for planned vaginal delivery (this includes any repeat subarachnoid needle placement and drug injection and/or any necessary replacement of an epidural catheter during labor) Ⓜ♀
 ⛨ 0.00 ⚕ 0.00 **FUD** XXX Ⓝ☐
 AMA: 2015,Jan,16; 2014,Oct,14; 2014,Aug,5; 2014,Jan,11; 2012,Jul,12-14; 2012,Jan,15-42; 2011,Oct,3-4; 2011,Jul,16-17; 2011,Jan,11

+ 01968 Anesthesia for cesarean delivery following neuraxial labor analgesia/anesthesia (List separately in addition to code for primary procedure performed) Ⓜ♀
 Code first (01967)
 ⛨ 0.00 ⚕ 0.00 **FUD** XXX Ⓝ☐Ⓟ
 AMA: 2015,Jan,16; 2014,Oct,14; 2014,Aug,5; 2014,Jan,11; 2012,Jul,12-14; 2012,Jan,15-42; 2011,Oct,3-4; 2011,Jun,13; 2011,Jul,16-17; 2011,Jan,11

+ 01969 Anesthesia for cesarean hysterectomy following neuraxial labor analgesia/anesthesia (List separately in addition to code for primary procedure performed) Ⓜ♀
 Code first (01967)
 ⛨ 0.00 ⚕ 0.00 **FUD** XXX Ⓝ☐Ⓟ
 AMA: 2015,Jan,16; 2014,Aug,5; 2014,Jan,11; 2012,Jul,12-14; 2012,Jan,15-42; 2011,Oct,3-4; 2011,Jun,13; 2011,Jul,16-17; 2011,Jan,11

01990-01999 Anesthesia Miscellaneous

CMS: 100-4,12,140.1 Qualified Nonphysician Anesthetists; 100-4,12,140.3 Payment for Qualified Nonphysician Anesthetists; 100-4,12,140.3.3 Billing Modifiers; 100-4,12,140.3.4 General Billing Instructions; 100-4,12,140.4.1 Anesthesiologist/Qualified Nonphysican Anesthetist; 100-4,12,140.4.2 Anesthetist and Anesthesiologist in a Single Procedure; 100-4,12,140.4.3 Payment for Medical /Surgical Services by CRNAs; 100-4,12,140.4.4 Conversion Factors for Anesthesia Services; 100-4,4,250.3.2 Anesthesia in a Hospital Outpatient Setting

01990 Physiological support for harvesting of organ(s) from brain-dead patient
 ⛨ 0.00 ⚕ 0.00 **FUD** XXX Ⓒ☐
 AMA: 2015,Jan,16; 2014,Aug,5; 2014,Jan,11; 2012,Jul,12-14; 2012,Jan,15-42; 2011,Oct,3-4; 2011,Jul,16-17; 2011,Jan,11

01991 Anesthesia for diagnostic or therapeutic nerve blocks and injections (when block or injection is performed by a different physician or other qualified health care professional); other than the prone position
 EXCLUDES Bier block for pain management (64999)
 Pain management via intra-arterial or IV therapy (96373-96374)
 Regional or local anesthesia of arms or legs for surgical procedure
 Do not report with (99143-99150)
 ⛨ 0.00 ⚕ 0.00 **FUD** XXX Ⓝ☐
 AMA: 2015,Jan,16; 2014,Aug,5; 2014,Jan,11; 2012,Jul,12-14; 2012,Jan,15-42; 2011,Oct,3-4; 2011,Jul,16-17; 2011,Jan,11

01992 prone position
 EXCLUDES Bier block for pain management (64999)
 Pain management via intra-arterial or IV therapy (96373-96374)
 Regional or local anesthesia of arms or legs for surgical procedure
 Do not report with (99143-99150)
 ⛨ 0.00 ⚕ 0.00 **FUD** XXX Ⓝ☐
 AMA: 2015,Jan,16; 2014,Aug,5; 2014,Jan,11; 2012,Jul,12-14; 2012,Jan,15-42; 2011,Oct,3-4; 2011,Jul,16-17; 2011,Jan,11

01996 Daily hospital management of epidural or subarachnoid continuous drug administration
 INCLUDES Continuous epidural or subarachnoid drug services performed after insertion of an epidural or subarachnoid catheter
 ⛨ 0.00 ⚕ 0.00 **FUD** XXX Ⓝ☐
 AMA: 2015,May,10; 2015,Jan,16; 2014,Aug,5; 2014,Jan,11; 2012,Oct,14; 2012,Jul,3-6; 2012,Jul,12-14; 2012,Jan,15-42; 2011,Oct,3-4; 2011,Jul,16-17; 2011,Jan,11

01999 Unlisted anesthesia procedure(s)
 ⛨ 0.00 ⚕ 0.00 **FUD** XXX Ⓝ
 AMA: 2015,May,10; 2015,Jan,16; 2014,Aug,5; 2014,Aug,14; 2014,Jan,11; 2012,Jul,12-14; 2012,Jan,15-42; 2011,Oct,3-4; 2011,Jul,16-17; 2011,Jan,11

10021-10022 Fine Needle Aspiration

EXCLUDES *Percutaneous localization clip placement during breast biopsy (19081-19086)*
Percutaneous needle biopsy of:
Abdominal or retroperitoneal mass (49180)
Bone (20220, 20225)
Bone marrow (38220-38221)
Breast (19081-19086)
Epididymis (54800)
Kidney (50200)
Liver (47000)
Lung or mediastinum (32405)
Lymph node (38505)
Muscle (20206)
Nucleus pulposus, paravertebral tissue, intervertebral disc (62267)
Pancreas (48102)
Pleura (32400)
Prostate (55700, 55706)
Salivary gland (42400)
Spinal cord (62269)
Testis (54500)
Thyroid (60100)
Soft tissue percutaneous fluid drainage by catheter using image guidance (10030)

10021 **Fine needle aspiration; without imaging guidance**
🔲 (88172-88173)
📖 2.00 ⚖ 4.23 **FUD** XXX ⬜ T P3 80 ▭
AMA: 2015,Jan,16; 2014,Jan,11; 2012,Jan,15-42; 2011,Jan,11

10022 **with imaging guidance**
🔲 (76942, 77002, 77012, 77021)
🔲 (88172-88173)
📖 1.90 ⚖ 4.02 **FUD** XXX ⬜ T P3 80 ▭
AMA: 2015,Jan,16; 2014,Jan,11; 2012,Jan,15-42; 2011,Jan,11

10030-10180 Treatment of Lesions: Skin and Subcutaneous Tissues

EXCLUDES *Excision benign lesion (11400-11471)*

10030 **Image-guided fluid collection drainage by catheter (eg, abscess, hematoma, seroma, lymphocele, cyst), soft tissue (eg, extremity, abdominal wall, neck), percutaneous**
EXCLUDES *Percutaneous drainage with imaging guidance of:*
Peritoneal or retroperitoneal collections (49406)
Visceral collections (49405)
Transvaginal or transrectal drainage with imaging guidance of:
Peritoneal or retroperitoneal collections (49407)
Code also every instance of fluid collection drained using a separate catheter (10030)
Do not report with (75989, 76942, 77002-77003, 77012, 77021)
📖 4.47 ⚖ 22.0 **FUD** XXX ⊙ T P2 80
AMA: 2015,Jan,16; 2014,May,9; 2014,May,3; 2013,Nov,9

● **10035** **Placement of soft tissue localization device(s) (eg, clip, metallic pellet, wire/needle, radioactive seeds), percutaneous, including imaging guidance; first lesion**
Code also each additional target on the same or opposite side (10036)
Do not report for a site with a more specific code descriptor, such as the breast
Do not report more than once per site, regardless of the number of markers used
Do not report with (76942, 77002, 77012, 77021)
📖 0.00 ⚖ 0.00 **FUD** 000

● + **10036** **each additional lesion (List separately in addition to code for primary procedure)**
📖 0.00 ⚖ 0.00 **FUD** 000
Code first (10035)

10040 **Acne surgery (eg, marsupialization, opening or removal of multiple milia, comedones, cysts, pustules)**
📖 2.50 ⚖ 2.86 **FUD** 010 Q1 N1 ▭
AMA: 2015,Jan,16; 2014,Jan,11; 2012,Jan,15-42; 2011,Jan,11

10060 **Incision and drainage of abscess (eg, carbuncle, suppurative hidradenitis, cutaneous or subcutaneous abscess, cyst, furuncle, or paronychia); simple or single**
📖 2.76 ⚖ 3.31 **FUD** 010 T P3 ▭
AMA: 2015,Jan,16; 2014,Jan,11; 2012,Oct,12; 2012,Sep,10; 2012,Jan,15-42; 2011,Jan,11; 2010,Apr,10

10061 **complicated or multiple**
📖 5.13 ⚖ 5.85 **FUD** 010 T P2 ▭
AMA: 2015,Jan,16; 2014,Jan,11; 2012,Oct,12; 2012,Sep,10

10080 **Incision and drainage of pilonidal cyst; simple**
📖 2.95 ⚖ 5.08 **FUD** 010 T P2 ▭
AMA: 2015,Jan,16; 2014,Jan,11

10081 **complicated**
EXCLUDES *Excision of pilonidal cyst (11770-11772)*
📖 4.86 ⚖ 7.61 **FUD** 010 T P3 ▭
AMA: 2015,Jan,16; 2014,Jan,11

10120 **Incision and removal of foreign body, subcutaneous tissues; simple**
📖 2.96 ⚖ 4.32 **FUD** 010 T P3 ▭
AMA: 2015,Jan,16; 2014,Jan,11; 2013,Dec,16; 2013,Apr,10-11; 2012,Oct,12; 2012,Sep,10

10121 **complicated**
EXCLUDES *Debridement associated with a fracture or dislocation (11010-11012)*
Exploration penetrating wound (20100-20103)
📖 5.31 ⚖ 7.75 **FUD** 010 T A2 ▭
AMA: 2015,Jan,16; 2014,Jan,11; 2013,Dec,16; 2012,Oct,12; 2012,Sep,10

10140 **Incision and drainage of hematoma, seroma or fluid collection**
🔲 (76942, 77012, 77021)
📖 3.38 ⚖ 4.62 **FUD** 010 T P3 ▭
AMA: 2015,Jan,16; 2014,Nov,5; 2014,Jan,11; 2012,Jan,15-42; 2011,Jan,11

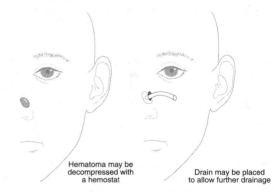

Hematoma may be decompressed with a hemostat

Drain may be placed to allow further drainage

10160 **Puncture aspiration of abscess, hematoma, bulla, or cyst**
🔲 (76942, 77012, 77021)
📖 2.74 ⚖ 3.69 **FUD** 010 T P3 ▭
AMA: 2015,Jan,16; 2014,Jan,11; 2012,Jan,15-42; 2010,Apr,10

10180 **Incision and drainage, complex, postoperative wound infection**
EXCLUDES *Wound dehiscence (12020-12021, 13160)*
📖 5.13 ⚖ 6.99 **FUD** 010 T A2 ▭
AMA: 2015,Jan,16; 2014,Nov,5; 2014,Jan,11; 2012,Jan,15-42; 2011,Jan,11

11000-11012 Removal of Foreign Substances and Infected/Devitalized Tissue

EXCLUDES *Debridement of:*
Burns (16000-16030)
Deeper tissue (11042-11047 [11045, 11046])
Nails (11720-11721)
Skin only (97597-97598)
Wounds (11042-11047 [11045, 11046])
Dermabrasions (15780-15783)
Pressure ulcer excision (15920-15999)

11000   **Debridement of extensive eczematous or infected skin; up to 10% of body surface**

EXCLUDES   *Necrotizing soft tissue infection of:*
Abdominal wall (11005-11006)
External genitalia and perineum (11004, 11006)

📷 0.82   ✂ 1.54   **FUD** 000   [T] [P3] ▢

AMA: 2015,Jan,16; 2014,Jan,11; 2012,Oct,3-8; 2011,May,3-5

+ 11001   **each additional 10% of the body surface, or part thereof (List separately in addition to code for primary procedure)**

EXCLUDES   *Necrotizing soft tissue infection of:*
Abdominal wall (11005-11006)
External genitalia and perineum (11004, 11006)

Code first (11000)

📷 0.40   ✂ 0.59   **FUD** ZZZ   [N] [N1]

AMA: 2015,Jan,16; 2014,Jan,11; 2012,Oct,3-8; 2011,May,3-5

11004   **Debridement of skin, subcutaneous tissue, muscle and fascia for necrotizing soft tissue infection; external genitalia and perineum**

EXCLUDES   *Skin grafts or flaps (14000-14350, 15040-15770)*

📷 16.7   ✂ 16.7   **FUD** 000   [C] ▢

AMA: 2015,Jan,16; 2014,Jan,11; 2013,Oct,15; 2012,Oct,3-8; 2012,Jan,6-10; 2011,May,3-5

11005   **abdominal wall, with or without fascial closure**

EXCLUDES   *Skin grafts or flaps (14000-14350, 15040-15770)*

📷 22.6   ✂ 22.6   **FUD** 000   [C] [80] ▢

AMA: 2015,Jan,16; 2014,Jan,11; 2013,Oct,15; 2012,Oct,3-8; 2012,Jan,6-10; 2011,May,3-5

11006   **external genitalia, perineum and abdominal wall, with or without fascial closure**

EXCLUDES   *Orchiectomy (54520)*
Skin grafts or flaps (14000-14350, 15040-15770)
Testicular transplant (54680)

📷 20.2   ✂ 20.2   **FUD** 000   [C] ▢

AMA: 2015,Jan,16; 2014,Jan,11; 2013,Oct,15; 2012,Oct,3-8; 2012,Jan,6-10; 2011,May,3-5

+ 11008   **Removal of prosthetic material or mesh, abdominal wall for infection (eg, for chronic or recurrent mesh infection or necrotizing soft tissue infection) (List separately in addition to code for primary procedure)**

EXCLUDES   *Insertion of mesh (49568)*
Skin grafts or flaps (14000-14350, 15040-15770)

Code first (10180, 11004-11006)
Do not report with (11000-11001, 11010-11044 [11045, 11046])

📷 7.96   ✂ 7.96   **FUD** ZZZ   [C] [80]

AMA: 2015,Jan,16; 2014,Jan,11; 2012,Oct,3-8; 2012,Jan,6-10; 2011,May,3-5

11010   **Debridement including removal of foreign material at the site of an open fracture and/or an open dislocation (eg, excisional debridement); skin and subcutaneous tissues**

📷 8.04   ✂ 13.9   **FUD** 010   [T] [A2] ▢

AMA: 2015,Jan,16; 2014,Jan,11; 2012,Oct,3-8; 2012,Oct,13; 2012,Jan,15-42; 2011,May,3-5; 2011,Jan,11

11011   **skin, subcutaneous tissue, muscle fascia, and muscle**

📷 8.56   ✂ 14.9   **FUD** 000   [T] [A2] ▢

AMA: 2015,Jan,16; 2014,Jan,11; 2012,Oct,3-8; 2012,Oct,13; 2011,May,3-5

11012   **skin, subcutaneous tissue, muscle fascia, muscle, and bone**

📷 12.2   ✂ 20.1   **FUD** 000   [T] [A2] ▢

AMA: 2015,Jan,16; 2014,Jan,11; 2012,Oct,3-8; 2012,Oct,13; 2012,Jan,15-42; 2011,May,3-5; 2011,Jan,11

11042-11047 [11045, 11046] Removal of Infected/Devitalized Tissue

INCLUDES   Debridement reported by the size and depth
Debridement reported for multiple wounds by adding the total surface area of wounds of the same depth
Injuries, wounds, chronic ulcers, infections

EXCLUDES   *Debridement of:*
Burn (16020-16030)
Dermis/epidermis only (97597-97598)
Eczematous or infected skin (11000-11001)
Nails (11720-11721)
Necrotizing soft tissue infection of external genitalia, perineum, or abdominal wall (11004-11006)
Dermabrasions (15780-15783)
Excision of pressure ulcers (15920-15999)

Code also each additional single wound of different depths
Code also modifier 59 for additional wound debridement
Code also multiple wound groups of different depths
Do not report with active care and management of same wound (97597-97602)

11042   **Debridement, subcutaneous tissue (includes epidermis and dermis, if performed); first 20 sq cm or less**

📷 1.77   ✂ 3.31   **FUD** 000   [T] [A2] ▢ [P0]

AMA: 2015,Jan,16; 2014,Nov,5; 2014,Jan,11; 2013,Oct,15; 2013,Sep,17; 2013,Feb,16-17; 2012,Oct,13; 2012,Oct,3-8; 2012,Mar,3; 2012,Jan,15-42; 2012,Jan,6-10; 2011,Sep,11-12; 2011,May,3-5; 2010,Nov,8

+ # 11045   **each additional 20 sq cm, or part thereof (List separately in addition to code for primary procedure)**

📷 0.75   ✂ 1.17   **FUD** ZZZ   [N] [N1] [80]

AMA: 2015,Jan,16; 2014,Nov,5; 2014,Jan,11; 2013,Feb,16-17; 2012,Oct,13; 2012,Oct,3-8; 2012,Mar,3; 2012,Jan,6-10; 2011,Sep,11-12; 2011,May,3-5

11043   **Debridement, muscle and/or fascia (includes epidermis, dermis, and subcutaneous tissue, if performed); first 20 sq cm or less**

📷 4.47   ✂ 6.48   **FUD** 000   [T] [A2] ▢ [P0]

AMA: 2015,Jan,16; 2014,Nov,5; 2014,Jan,11; 2013,Feb,16-17; 2012,Oct,3-8; 2012,Oct,13; 2012,Mar,3; 2012,Jan,15-42; 2012,Jan,6-10; 2011,Sep,11-12; 2011,May,3-5; 2011,Jan,11; 2010,Nov,8

+ # 11046   **each additional 20 sq cm, or part thereof (List separately in addition to code for primary procedure)**

Code first (11043)

📷 1.60   ✂ 2.07   **FUD** ZZZ   [N] [N1] [80]

AMA: 2015,Jan,16; 2014,Nov,5; 2014,Jan,11; 2013,Feb,16-17; 2012,Oct,13; 2012,Oct,3-8; 2012,Mar,3; 2012,Jan,6-10; 2011,Sep,11-12; 2011,May,3-5

11044   **Debridement, bone (includes epidermis, dermis, subcutaneous tissue, muscle and/or fascia, if performed); first 20 sq cm or less**

📷 6.68   ✂ 8.96   **FUD** 000   [T] [A2] ▢ [P0]

AMA: 2015,Jan,16; 2014,Nov,5; 2014,Jan,11; 2013,Feb,16-17; 2012,Oct,3-8; 2012,Oct,13; 2012,Mar,3; 2012,Jan,15-42; 2012,Jan,6-10; 2011,Sep,11-12; 2011,May,3-5; 2011,Jan,11; 2010,Nov,8

11045   **Resequenced code. See code following 11042.**

11046   **Resequenced code. See code following 11043.**

+ 11047   **each additional 20 sq cm, or part thereof (List separately in addition to code for primary procedure)**

Code first (11044)

📷 2.86   ✂ 3.53   **FUD** ZZZ   [N] [N1] [80]

AMA: 2015,Jan,16; 2014,Nov,5; 2014,Jan,11; 2012,Oct,3-8; 2012,Oct,13; 2012,Mar,3; 2012,Jan,15-42; 2012,Jan,6-10; 2011,Sep,11-12; 2011,May,3-5

Integumentary System

11055 — 11401

11055-11057 Excision Benign Hypertrophic Skin Lesions

CMS: 100-4,32,80.8 CSF Edits: Routine Foot Care

EXCLUDES Destruction (17000-17004)

11055 Paring or cutting of benign hyperkeratotic lesion (eg, corn or callus); single lesion

🔲 0.46   🔾 1.35   **FUD** 000   Q1 N1 ▭ P0

AMA: 2015,Jan,16; 2014,Jan,11; 2012,Jan,15-42; 2011,Jan,11

11056 2 to 4 lesions

🔲 0.65   🔾 1.65   **FUD** 000   T P3 ▭ P0

AMA: 2015,Jan,16; 2014,Jan,11; 2012,Jan,15-42; 2011,Jan,11; 2010,Sep,9

11057 more than 4 lesions

🔲 0.85   🔾 1.85   **FUD** 000   T P3 ▭ P0

AMA: 2015,Jan,16; 2014,Jan,11

11100-11101 Surgical Biopsy Skin and Mucous Membranes

INCLUDES Attaining tissue for pathologic exam

EXCLUDES Biopsy of:
Conjunctiva (68100)
Eyelid ([67810])
Do not report with related procedures

11100 Biopsy of skin, subcutaneous tissue and/or mucous membrane (including simple closure), unless otherwise listed; single lesion

🔲 1.39   🔾 2.92   **FUD** 000   T P3 ▭ P0

AMA: 2015,Jan,16; 2014,Jan,11; 2013,Mar,6-7; 2013,Feb,16-17

+ 11101 each separate/additional lesion (List separately in addition to code for primary procedure)
Code first (11100)

🔲 0.71   🔾 0.92   **FUD** ZZZ   N N1

AMA: 2015,Jan,16; 2014,Jan,11; 2013,Mar,6-7; 2013,Feb,16-17

11200-11201 Skin Tag Removal - All Techniques

INCLUDES Chemical destruction
Electrocauterization
Electrosurgical destruction
Ligature strangulation
Local anesthesia when used
Removal with or without local anesthesia
Sharp excision or scissoring

EXCLUDES Extensive or complicated secondary wound closure (13160)

11200 Removal of skin tags, multiple fibrocutaneous tags, any area; up to and including 15 lesions

🔲 2.09   🔾 2.49   **FUD** 010   Q1 N1 ▭

AMA: 2015,Jan,16; 2014,Jan,11; 2012,Jan,15-42; 2011,Jun,13; 2011,Jan,11

+ 11201 each additional 10 lesions, or part thereof (List separately in addition to code for primary procedure)
Code first (11200)

🔲 0.47   🔾 0.53   **FUD** ZZZ   N N1

AMA: 2015,Jan,16; 2014,Jan,11; 2012,Jan,15-42; 2011,Jun,13

11300-11313 Skin Lesion Removal: Shaving

INCLUDES Local anesthesia
Partial thickness excision by horizontal slicing
Wound cauterization

11300 Shaving of epidermal or dermal lesion, single lesion, trunk, arms or legs; lesion diameter 0.5 cm or less

🔲 1.00   🔾 2.74   **FUD** 000   T P3 80 ▭

AMA: 2015,Jan,16; 2014,Jan,11; 2012,Jan,15-42; 2011,Jan,11

Shave excision of an elevated lesion; technique also used to biopsy

Elliptical excision is often used when tissue removal is larger than 4 mm or when deep pathology is suspected

A punch biopsy cuts a core of tissue as the tool is twisted downward

11301 lesion diameter 0.6 to 1.0 cm

🔲 1.53   🔾 3.38   **FUD** 000   T P2 80 ▭

AMA: 2015,Jan,16; 2014,Jan,11; 2012,Jan,15-42; 2011,Jan,11

11302 lesion diameter 1.1 to 2.0 cm

🔲 1.80   🔾 3.98   **FUD** 000   T P2 80 ▭

AMA: 2015,Jan,16; 2014,Jan,11; 2012,Jan,15-42; 2011,Jan,11

11303 lesion diameter over 2.0 cm

🔲 2.12   🔾 4.39   **FUD** 000   T P2 80 ▭

AMA: 2015,Jan,16; 2014,Jan,11; 2012,Jan,15-42; 2011,Jan,11

11305 Shaving of epidermal or dermal lesion, single lesion, scalp, neck, hands, feet, genitalia; lesion diameter 0.5 cm or less

🔲 1.11   🔾 2.78   **FUD** 000   Q1 N1 80 ▭

AMA: 2015,Jan,16; 2014,Jan,11; 2012,Jan,15-42; 2011,Jan,11

11306 lesion diameter 0.6 to 1.0 cm

🔲 1.48   🔾 3.43   **FUD** 000   T P2 80 ▭

AMA: 2015,Jan,16; 2014,Jan,11; 2012,Jan,15-42; 2011,Jan,11

11307 lesion diameter 1.1 to 2.0 cm

🔲 1.90   🔾 4.05   **FUD** 000   T P2 80 ▭

AMA: 2015,Jan,16; 2014,Jan,11; 2012,Jan,15-42; 2011,Jan,11

11308 lesion diameter over 2.0 cm

🔲 2.11   🔾 4.26   **FUD** 000   T P2 80 ▭

AMA: 2015,Jan,16; 2014,Jan,11; 2012,Jan,15-42; 2011,Jan,11

11310 Shaving of epidermal or dermal lesion, single lesion, face, ears, eyelids, nose, lips, mucous membrane; lesion diameter 0.5 cm or less

🔲 1.35   🔾 3.20   **FUD** 000   T P2 80 ▭

AMA: 2015,Jan,16; 2014,Jan,11; 2013,Mar,6-7; 2013,Feb,16-17; 2012,Jan,15-42; 2011,Jan,11

11311 lesion diameter 0.6 to 1.0 cm

🔲 1.88   🔾 3.14   **FUD** 000   T P3 80 ▭

AMA: 2015,Jan,16; 2014,Jan,11; 2013,Mar,6-7; 2013,Feb,16-17; 2012,Jan,15-42; 2011,Jan,11

11312 lesion diameter 1.1 to 2.0 cm

🔲 2.23   🔾 4.52   **FUD** 000   T P2 80 ▭

AMA: 2015,Jan,16; 2014,Jan,11; 2013,Mar,6-7; 2013,Feb,16-17; 2012,Jan,15-42; 2011,Jan,11

11313 lesion diameter over 2.0 cm

🔲 2.87   🔾 5.23   **FUD** 000   T P2 80 ▭

AMA: 2015,Jan,16; 2014,Jan,11; 2013,Mar,6-7; 2013,Feb,16-17; 2012,Jan,15-42; 2011,Jan,11

11400-11446 Skin Lesion Removal: Benign

INCLUDES Biopsy on same lesion
Full thickness removal including margins
Lesion measurement before excision at largest diameter plus margin
Local anesthesia
Simple, nonlayered closure

EXCLUDES Biopsy of eyelid ([67810])
Destruction of eyelid lesion (67850)
Excision and reconstruction of eyelid (67961-67975)
Excision of chalazion (67800-67808)
Eyelid procedures involving more than skin (67800 and subsequent codes)
Shave removal (11300-11313)
Code also complex closure (13100-13153)
Code also each separate lesion
Code also intermediate closure (12031-12057)
Code also modifier 22 if excision is complicated or unusual
Code also reconstruction (15002-15261, 15570-15770)
Do not report with adjacent tissue transfer (14000-14302)

11400 Excision, benign lesion including margins, except skin tag (unless listed elsewhere), trunk, arms or legs; excised diameter 0.5 cm or less

🔲 2.29   🔾 3.51   **FUD** 010   T P3 ▭

AMA: 2015,Jan,16; 2014,Mar,4; 2014,Mar,12; 2014,Jan,11; 2012,May,13; 2012,Jan,15-42; 2011,Jan,11; 2011,Jan,9-10; 2010,Oct,9; 2010,Jul,10; 2010,Apr,3-4

11401 excised diameter 0.6 to 1.0 cm

🔲 2.96   🔾 4.21   **FUD** 010   T P3 ▭

AMA: 2015,Jan,16; 2014,Mar,4; 2014,Mar,12; 2014,Jan,11; 2012,May,13; 2012,Jan,15-42; 2011,Jan,9-10; 2011,Jan,11; 2010,Oct,9; 2010,Jul,10; 2010,Apr,3-4

 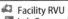

11402 **excised diameter 1.1 to 2.0 cm**
🚗 3.26   ⚖ 4.68   **FUD** 010   T P3 ▭
AMA: 2015,Jan,16; 2014,Mar,4; 2014,Mar,12; 2014,Jan,11; 2012,May,13; 2012,Jan,15-42; 2011,Jan,9-10; 2011,Jan,11; 2010,Oct,9; 2010,Jul,10; 2010,Apr,3-4

11403 **excised diameter 2.1 to 3.0 cm**
🚗 4.22   ⚖ 5.42   **FUD** 010   T P3 ▭
AMA: 2015,Jan,16; 2014,Mar,12; 2014,Mar,4; 2014,Jan,11; 2012,May,13; 2011,Jan,11; 2011,Jan,9-10; 2010,Oct,9; 2010,Jul,10; 2010,Apr,3-4

11404 **excised diameter 3.1 to 4.0 cm**
🚗 4.64   ⚖ 6.14   **FUD** 010   T A2 ▭
AMA: 2015,Jan,16; 2014,Mar,4; 2014,Mar,12; 2014,Jan,11; 2012,May,13; 2012,Jan,15-42; 2011,Jan,9-10; 2011,Jan,11; 2010,Oct,9; 2010,Jul,10; 2010,Apr,3-4

11406 **excised diameter over 4.0 cm**
🚗 7.07   ⚖ 8.88   **FUD** 010   T A2 ▭
AMA: 2015,Jan,16; 2014,Mar,4; 2014,Mar,12; 2014,Jan,11; 2012,May,13; 2012,Jan,15-42; 2011,Jan,9-10; 2011,Jan,11; 2010,Oct,9; 2010,Jul,10; 2010,Apr,3-4

11420 **Excision, benign lesion including margins, except skin tag (unless listed elsewhere), scalp, neck, hands, feet, genitalia; excised diameter 0.5 cm or less**
🚗 2.32   ⚖ 3.46   **FUD** 010   T P3 ▭
AMA: 2015,Jan,16; 2014,Mar,4; 2014,Mar,12; 2014,Jan,11; 2013,Jan,15-16; 2012,May,13; 2012,Jan,15-42; 2011,Jan,11; 2010,Oct,9; 2010,Jul,10; 2010,Apr,3-4

11421 **excised diameter 0.6 to 1.0 cm**
🚗 3.14   ⚖ 4.44   **FUD** 010   T P3 ▭
AMA: 2015,Jan,16; 2014,Mar,4; 2014,Mar,12; 2014,Jan,11; 2013,Jan,15-16; 2012,May,13; 2011,Jan,11; 2010,Oct,9; 2010,Jul,10; 2010,Apr,3-4

11422 **excised diameter 1.1 to 2.0 cm**
🚗 3.87   ⚖ 4.96   **FUD** 010   T P3 ▭
AMA: 2015,Jan,16; 2014,Mar,4; 2014,Mar,12; 2014,Jan,11; 2013,Jan,15-16; 2012,May,13; 2012,Mar,4-7; 2011,Jan,11; 2010,Oct,9; 2010,Jul,10; 2010,Apr,3-4

11423 **excised diameter 2.1 to 3.0 cm**
🚗 4.51   ⚖ 5.72   **FUD** 010   T P3 ▭
AMA: 2015,Jan,16; 2014,Mar,4; 2014,Mar,12; 2014,Jan,11; 2013,Jan,15-16; 2012,May,13; 2011,Jan,11; 2010,Oct,9; 2010,Jul,10; 2010,Apr,3-4

11424 **excised diameter 3.1 to 4.0 cm**
🚗 5.16   ⚖ 6.61   **FUD** 010   T A2 ▭
AMA: 2015,Jan,16; 2014,Mar,4; 2014,Mar,12; 2014,Jan,11; 2013,Jan,15-16; 2012,May,13; 2011,Jan,11; 2010,Oct,9; 2010,Jul,10; 2010,Apr,3-4

11426 **excised diameter over 4.0 cm**
🚗 7.88   ⚖ 9.45   **FUD** 010   T A2 ▭
AMA: 2015,Jan,16; 2014,Mar,4; 2014,Mar,12; 2014,Jan,11; 2013,Jan,15-16; 2012,May,13; 2011,Jan,11; 2010,Oct,9; 2010,Jul,10; 2010,Apr,3-4

11440 **Excision, other benign lesion including margins, except skin tag (unless listed elsewhere), face, ears, eyelids, nose, lips, mucous membrane; excised diameter 0.5 cm or less**
🚗 2.93   ⚖ 3.80   **FUD** 010   T P3 ▭
AMA: 2015,Jan,16; 2014,Mar,4; 2014,Mar,12; 2014,Jan,11; 2012,May,13; 2012,Jan,15-42; 2011,Jan,11; 2010,Oct,9; 2010,Jul,10; 2010,Apr,3-4

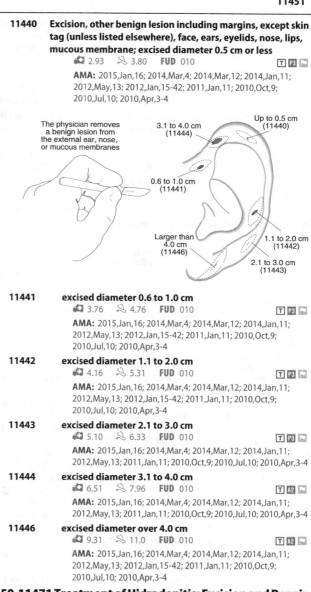

The physician removes a benign lesion from the external ear, nose, or mucous membranes

3.1 to 4.0 cm (11444)
Up to 0.5 cm (11440)
0.6 to 1.0 cm (11441)
Larger than 4.0 cm (11446)
1.1 to 2.0 cm (11442)
2.1 to 3.0 cm (11443)

11441 **excised diameter 0.6 to 1.0 cm**
🚗 3.76   ⚖ 4.76   **FUD** 010   T P3 ▭
AMA: 2015,Jan,16; 2014,Mar,4; 2014,Mar,12; 2014,Jan,11; 2012,May,13; 2012,Jan,15-42; 2011,Jan,11; 2010,Oct,9; 2010,Jul,10; 2010,Apr,3-4

11442 **excised diameter 1.1 to 2.0 cm**
🚗 4.16   ⚖ 5.31   **FUD** 010   T P3 ▭
AMA: 2015,Jan,16; 2014,Mar,4; 2014,Mar,12; 2014,Jan,11; 2012,May,13; 2012,Jan,15-42; 2011,Jan,11; 2010,Oct,9; 2010,Jul,10; 2010,Apr,3-4

11443 **excised diameter 2.1 to 3.0 cm**
🚗 5.10   ⚖ 6.33   **FUD** 010   T P3 ▭
AMA: 2015,Jan,16; 2014,Mar,4; 2014,Mar,12; 2014,Jan,11; 2012,May,13; 2011,Jan,11; 2010,Oct,9; 2010,Jul,10; 2010,Apr,3-4

11444 **excised diameter 3.1 to 4.0 cm**
🚗 6.51   ⚖ 7.96   **FUD** 010   T A2 ▭
AMA: 2015,Jan,16; 2014,Mar,4; 2014,Mar,12; 2014,Jan,11; 2012,May,13; 2011,Jan,11; 2010,Oct,9; 2010,Jul,10; 2010,Apr,3-4

11446 **excised diameter over 4.0 cm**
🚗 9.31   ⚖ 11.0   **FUD** 010   T A2 ▭
AMA: 2015,Jan,16; 2014,Mar,4; 2014,Mar,12; 2014,Jan,11; 2012,May,13; 2012,Jan,15-42; 2011,Jan,11; 2010,Oct,9; 2010,Jul,10; 2010,Apr,3-4

11450-11471 Treatment of Hidradenitis: Excision and Repair
Code also closure by skin graft or flap (14000-14350, 15040-15770)

11450 **Excision of skin and subcutaneous tissue for hidradenitis, axillary; with simple or intermediate repair**
🚗 7.24   ⚖ 10.8   **FUD** 090   T A2 50 ▭
AMA: 2015,Jan,16; 2014,Jan,11; 2012,May,13; 2010,Apr,3-4

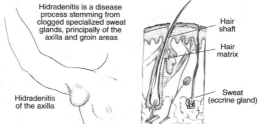

Hidradenitis is a disease process stemming from clogged specialized sweat glands, principally of the axilla and groin areas

Hair shaft
Hair matrix
Sweat (eccrine gland)

Hidradenitis of the axilla

11451 **with complex repair**
🚗 9.27   ⚖ 13.7   **FUD** 090   T A2 80 50 ▭
AMA: 2015,Jan,16; 2014,Jan,11; 2012,May,13; 2010,Apr,3-4

11462 Excision of skin and subcutaneous tissue for hidradenitis, inguinal; with simple or intermediate repair

🔲 6.88   ⚖ 10.5   **FUD** 090   [T] [A2] [80] [50] ▢

AMA: 2015,Jan,16; 2014,Jan,11; 2012,May,13; 2010,Apr,3-4

11463 with complex repair

🔲 9.35   ⚖ 14.0   **FUD** 090   [T] [A2] [80] [50] ▢

AMA: 2015,Jan,16; 2014,Jan,11; 2012,May,13; 2010,Apr,3-4

11470 Excision of skin and subcutaneous tissue for hidradenitis, perianal, perineal, or umbilical; with simple or intermediate repair

🔲 8.02   ⚖ 11.6   **FUD** 090   [T] [A2] ▢

AMA: 2015,Jan,16; 2014,Jan,11; 2012,May,13; 2010,Apr,3-4

11471 with complex repair

🔲 9.89   ⚖ 14.3   **FUD** 090   [T] [A2] [80] ▢

AMA: 2015,Jan,16; 2014,Jan,11; 2012,May,13; 2010,Apr,3-4

11600-11646 Skin Lesion Removal: Malignant

INCLUDES   Biopsy on same lesion
Excision of additional margin at same operative session
Full thickness removal including margins
Lesion measurement before excision at largest diameter plus margin
Local anesthesia
Simple, nonlayered closure

EXCLUDES   Destruction (17260-17286)
Excision of additional margin at subsequent operative session (11600-11646)
Code also complex closure (13100-13153)
Code also each separate lesion
Code also intermediate closure (12031-12057)
Code also modifier 58 if re-excision is performed during postoperative period
Code also reconstruction (15002-15261, 15570-15770)
Do not report with adjacent tissue transfer. Report only adjacent tissue transfer code. (14000-14302)

11600 Excision, malignant lesion including margins, trunk, arms, or legs; excised diameter 0.5 cm or less

🔲 3.42   ⚖ 5.43   **FUD** 010   [T] [P3] ▢ [PQ]

AMA: 2015,Jan,16; 2014,Mar,4; 2014,Mar,12; 2014,Jan,11; 2012,Jul,12-14; 2012,May,13; 2012,Jan,15-42; 2011,Jan,11; 2010,Apr,3-4; 2010,Jan,3-5

11601 excised diameter 0.6 to 1.0 cm

🔲 4.26   ⚖ 6.45   **FUD** 010   [T] [P3] ▢ [PQ]

AMA: 2015,Jan,16; 2014,Mar,12; 2014,Mar,4; 2014,Jan,11; 2012,Jul,12-14; 2012,May,13; 2012,Mar,4-7; 2010,Apr,3-4; 2010,Jan,3-5

11602 excised diameter 1.1 to 2.0 cm

🔲 4.67   ⚖ 6.98   **FUD** 010   [T] [P3] ▢ [PQ]

AMA: 2015,Jan,16; 2014,Mar,12; 2014,Mar,4; 2014,Jan,11; 2012,Jul,12-14; 2012,May,13; 2010,Apr,3-4; 2010,Jan,3-5

11603 excised diameter 2.1 to 3.0 cm

🔲 5.60   ⚖ 7.99   **FUD** 010   [T] [P3] ▢ [PQ]

AMA: 2015,Jan,16; 2014,Mar,12; 2014,Mar,4; 2014,Jan,11; 2012,Jul,12-14; 2012,May,13; 2010,Apr,3-4; 2010,Jan,3-5

11604 excised diameter 3.1 to 4.0 cm

🔲 6.17   ⚖ 8.89   **FUD** 010   [T] [A2] ▢ [PQ]

AMA: 2015,Jan,16; 2014,Mar,12; 2014,Mar,4; 2014,Jan,11; 2012,Jul,12-14; 2012,May,13; 2010,Apr,3-4; 2010,Jan,3-5

11606 excised diameter over 4.0 cm

🔲 9.16   ⚖ 12.7   **FUD** 010   [T] [A2] ▢ [PQ]

AMA: 2015,Jan,16; 2014,Mar,4; 2014,Mar,12; 2014,Jan,11; 2012,Jul,12-14; 2012,May,13; 2010,Apr,3-4; 2010,Jan,3-5

11620 Excision, malignant lesion including margins, scalp, neck, hands, feet, genitalia; excised diameter 0.5 cm or less

🔲 3.46   ⚖ 5.49   **FUD** 010   [T] [P3] ▢ [PQ]

AMA: 2015,Jan,16; 2014,Mar,4; 2014,Mar,12; 2014,Jan,11; 2012,Jul,12-14; 2012,May,13; 2010,Apr,3-4

11621 excised diameter 0.6 to 1.0 cm

🔲 4.30   ⚖ 6.49   **FUD** 010   [T] [P3] ▢ [PQ]

AMA: 2015,Jan,16; 2014,Mar,4; 2014,Mar,12; 2014,Jan,11; 2012,May,13; 2010,Apr,3-4; 2010,Jan,3-5

11622 excised diameter 1.1 to 2.0 cm

🔲 4.91   ⚖ 7.23   **FUD** 010   [T] [P3] ▢ [PQ]

AMA: 2015,Jan,16; 2014,Mar,4; 2014,Mar,12; 2014,Jan,11; 2012,May,13; 2010,Apr,3-4; 2010,Jan,3-5

11623 excised diameter 2.1 to 3.0 cm

🔲 6.08   ⚖ 8.49   **FUD** 010   [T] [P3] ▢ [PQ]

AMA: 2015,Jan,16; 2014,Mar,4; 2014,Mar,12; 2014,Jan,11; 2012,May,13; 2010,Apr,3-4; 2010,Jan,3-5

11624 excised diameter 3.1 to 4.0 cm

🔲 6.88   ⚖ 9.57   **FUD** 010   [T] [A2] ▢ [PQ]

AMA: 2015,Jan,16; 2014,Mar,4; 2014,Mar,12; 2014,Jan,11; 2012,May,13; 2010,Apr,3-4; 2010,Jan,3-5

11626 excised diameter over 4.0 cm

🔲 8.47   ⚖ 11.5   **FUD** 010   [T] [A2] ▢ [PQ]

AMA: 2015,Jan,16; 2014,Mar,4; 2014,Mar,12; 2014,Jan,11; 2012,May,13; 2010,Apr,3-4; 2010,Jan,3-5

11640 Excision, malignant lesion including margins, face, ears, eyelids, nose, lips; excised diameter 0.5 cm or less

EXCLUDES   Eyelid excision involving more than skin (67800-67808, 67840-67850, 67961-67966)

🔲 3.58   ⚖ 5.65   **FUD** 010   [T] [P3] ▢ [PQ]

AMA: 2015,Jan,16; 2014,Mar,4; 2014,Mar,12; 2014,Jan,11; 2012,May,13; 2010,Apr,3-4; 2010,Jan,3-5

11641 excised diameter 0.6 to 1.0 cm

EXCLUDES   Eyelid excision involving more than skin (67800-67808, 67840-67850, 67961-67966)

🔲 4.47   ⚖ 6.71   **FUD** 010   [T] [P3] ▢ [PQ]

AMA: 2015,Jan,16; 2014,Mar,4; 2014,Mar,12; 2014,Jan,11; 2012,May,13; 2010,Apr,3-4; 2010,Jan,3-5

11642 excised diameter 1.1 to 2.0 cm

EXCLUDES   Eyelid excision involving more than skin (67800-67808, 67840-67850, 67961-67966)

🔲 5.27   ⚖ 7.65   **FUD** 010   [T] [P3] ▢ [PQ]

AMA: 2015,Jan,16; 2014,Mar,4; 2014,Mar,12; 2014,Jan,11; 2012,May,13; 2010,Apr,3-4; 2010,Jan,3-5

11643 excised diameter 2.1 to 3.0 cm

EXCLUDES   Eyelid excision involving more than skin (67800-67808, 67840-67850, 67961-67966)

🔲 6.61   ⚖ 9.04   **FUD** 010   [T] [P3] ▢ [PQ]

AMA: 2015,Jan,16; 2014,Mar,4; 2014,Mar,12; 2014,Jan,11; 2012,May,13; 2010,Apr,3-4; 2010,Jan,3-5

11644 excised diameter 3.1 to 4.0 cm

EXCLUDES   Eyelid excision involving more than skin (67800-67808, 67840-67850, 67961-67966)

🔲 8.17   ⚖ 11.1   **FUD** 010   [T] [A2] ▢ [PQ]

AMA: 2015,Jan,16; 2014,Mar,4; 2014,Mar,12; 2014,Jan,11; 2012,May,13; 2010,Apr,3-4; 2010,Jan,3-5

11646 excised diameter over 4.0 cm

EXCLUDES   Eyelid excision involving more than skin (67800-67808, 67840-67850, 67961-67966)

🔲 11.3   ⚖ 14.6   **FUD** 010   [T] [A2] ▢ [PQ]

AMA: 2015,Jan,16; 2014,Mar,4; 2014,Mar,12; 2014,Jan,11; 2012,May,13; 2012,Jan,15-42; 2011,Jan,11; 2010,Apr,3-4; 2010,Jan,3-5

11719-11765 Nails and Supporting Structures

CMS: 100-02,15,290 Foot Care

EXCLUDES   Drainage of paronychia or onychia (10060-10061)

11719 Trimming of nondystrophic nails, any number

🔲 0.22   ⚖ 0.39   **FUD** 000   [Q1] [N1] ▢ [PQ]

AMA: 2015,Jan,16; 2014,Jan,11

11720 Debridement of nail(s) by any method(s); 1 to 5

🔲 0.42   ⚖ 0.91   **FUD** 000   [Q1] [N1] ▢ [PQ]

AMA: 2015,Jan,16; 2014,Jan,11

11721 6 or more

🔲 0.70   ⚖ 1.26   **FUD** 000   [Q1] [N1] ▢ [PQ]

AMA: 2015,Jan,16; 2014,Jan,11

| [26]/[TC] PC/TC Comp Only | [A2]-[Z3] ASC Pmt | [50] Bilateral | ♂ Male Only | ♀ Female Only | 🔲 Facility RVU | ⚖ Non-Facility RVU |
| **AMA:** CPT Asst | **CMS:** Pub 100 | [A]-[Y] OPPSI | [80]/[80] Surg Assist Allowed / w/Doc | | ▣ Lab Crosswalk | ▣ Radiology Crosswalk |

16   Medicare (Red Text)   CPT © 2015 American Medical Association. All Rights Reserved. (Black Text)   © 2015 Optum360, LLC (Blue Text)

11730 Avulsion of nail plate, partial or complete, simple; single
🔧 1.44 ✂ 2.79 **FUD** 000
T P3 🔲 P0
AMA: 2015,Jan,16; 2014,Jan,11; 2012,Jan,15-42; 2011,Jan,11

+ 11732 each additional nail plate (List separately in addition to code for primary procedure)
Code first (11730)
🔧 0.58 ✂ 1.01 **FUD** ZZZ
N N1 🔲
AMA: 2015,Jan,16; 2014,Jan,11

11740 Evacuation of subungual hematoma
🔧 0.93 ✂ 1.40 **FUD** 000
01 N1 🔲 P0
AMA: 2015,Jan,16; 2014,Jan,11

11750 Excision of nail and nail matrix, partial or complete (eg, ingrown or deformed nail), for permanent removal;
EXCLUDES Skin graft (15050)
🔧 4.95 ✂ 6.31 **FUD** 010
T P3 🔲
AMA: 2015,Jan,16; 2014,Jan,11

11752 with amputation of tuft of distal phalanx
EXCLUDES Skin graft (15050)
🔧 7.52 ✂ 9.21 **FUD** 010
T P3 🔲
AMA: 2015,Jan,16; 2014,Jan,11

11755 Biopsy of nail unit (eg, plate, bed, matrix, hyponychium, proximal and lateral nail folds) (separate procedure)
🔧 2.22 ✂ 3.77 **FUD** 000
T P3 80 🔲 P0
AMA: 2015,Jan,16; 2014,Jan,11; 2012,Jan,15-42; 2011,Jan,11

11760 Repair of nail bed
🔧 3.76 ✂ 6.47 **FUD** 010
T G2 🔲
AMA: 2015,Jan,16; 2014,Jan,11

11762 Reconstruction of nail bed with graft
🔧 5.31 ✂ 8.00 **FUD** 010
T P3 🔲
AMA: 2015,Jan,16; 2014,Jan,11

11765 Wedge excision of skin of nail fold (eg, for ingrown toenail)
INCLUDES Cotting's operation
🔧 2.68 ✂ 4.73 **FUD** 010
T P2 🔲
AMA: 2015,Jan,16; 2014,Jan,11

11770-11772 Treatment Pilonidal Cyst: Excision
EXCLUDES Incision of pilonidal cyst (10080-10081)

11770 Excision of pilonidal cyst or sinus; simple
🔧 5.30 ✂ 7.84 **FUD** 010
T A2 🔲

11771 extensive
🔧 12.4 ✂ 16.2 **FUD** 090
T A2 🔲

11772 complicated
🔧 16.5 ✂ 19.8 **FUD** 090
T A2 🔲

11900-11901 Treatment of Lesions: Injection
EXCLUDES Injection of veins (36470-36471)
Intralesional chemotherapy (96405, 96406)
Do not report for injection of local anesthesia performed preoperatively

11900 Injection, intralesional; up to and including 7 lesions
🔧 0.89 ✂ 1.56 **FUD** 000
01 N1 🔲
AMA: 2015,Jan,16; 2014,Jan,11; 2013,Nov,14; 2012,Jan,15-42; 2011,Jan,11

11901 more than 7 lesions
🔧 1.37 ✂ 1.96 **FUD** 000
01 N1 🔲
AMA: 2015,Jan,16; 2014,Jan,11; 2012,Jan,15-42; 2011,Jan,11

11920-11971 Tattoos, Tissue Expanders, and Dermal Fillers
CMS: 100-2,16,10 Exclusions from Coverage; 100-2,16,120 Cosmetic Procedures; 100-2,16,180 Services Related to Noncovered Procedures

11920 Tattooing, intradermal introduction of insoluble opaque pigments to correct color defects of skin, including micropigmentation; 6.0 sq cm or less
🔧 3.27 ✂ 4.84 **FUD** 000
T P3 80 🔲

11921 6.1 to 20.0 sq cm
🔧 3.85 ✂ 5.60 **FUD** 000
T P3 80 🔲

+ 11922 each additional 20.0 sq cm, or part thereof (List separately in addition to code for primary procedure)
🔧 0.85 ✂ 1.73 **FUD** ZZZ
N N1 80
Code first (11921)

11950 Subcutaneous injection of filling material (eg, collagen); 1 cc or less
🔧 1.53 ✂ 2.21 **FUD** 000
T P3 80 🔲
AMA: 2015,Jan,16; 2014,Jan,11; 2012,Jun,15-16

11951 1.1 to 5.0 cc
🔧 2.15 ✂ 3.01 **FUD** 000
T P3 80 🔲
AMA: 2015,Jan,16; 2014,Jan,11; 2012,Jun,15-16

11952 5.1 to 10.0 cc
🔧 2.75 ✂ 3.66 **FUD** 000
T P3 80 🔲
AMA: 2015,Jan,16; 2014,Jan,11; 2012,Jun,15-16

11954 over 10.0 cc
🔧 3.31 ✂ 4.50 **FUD** 000
T P3 80 🔲
AMA: 2015,Jan,16; 2014,Jan,11; 2012,Jun,15-16

11960 Insertion of tissue expander(s) for other than breast, including subsequent expansion
EXCLUDES Breast reconstruction with tissue expander(s) (19357)
🔧 26.9 ✂ 26.9 **FUD** 090
T A2 🔲
AMA: 1991,Win,1

11970 Replacement of tissue expander with permanent prosthesis
🔧 17.4 ✂ 17.4 **FUD** 090
T A2 50 🔲
AMA: 2015,Jan,16; 2014,Jan,11; 2013,Jan,15-16

11971 Removal of tissue expander(s) without insertion of prosthesis
🔧 9.09 ✂ 13.3 **FUD** 090
Q2 A2 80 50 🔲
AMA: 2015,Jan,16; 2014,Jan,11; 2012,Jan,15-42; 2011,Jan,11

11976-11983 Drug Implantation

11976 Removal, implantable contraceptive capsules
♀
🔧 2.70 ✂ 4.05 **FUD** 000
Q2 P3 80 🔲
AMA: 1992,Win,1; 1991,Win,1

11980 Subcutaneous hormone pellet implantation (implantation of estradiol and/or testosterone pellets beneath the skin)
🔧 1.61 ✂ 2.66 **FUD** 000
01 N1 🔲
AMA: 2015,Jan,16; 2014,Jan,11

11981 Insertion, non-biodegradable drug delivery implant
🔧 2.39 ✂ 4.01 **FUD** XXX
01 N1 80 🔲
AMA: 2015,Jan,16; 2014,Jan,11; 2012,Jan,15-42; 2011,Apr,12; 2011,Jan,11

11982 Removal, non-biodegradable drug delivery implant
🔧 2.89 ✂ 4.54 **FUD** XXX
01 N1 80 🔲

11983 Removal with reinsertion, non-biodegradable drug delivery implant
🔧 5.00 ✂ 6.32 **FUD** XXX
01 N1 80 🔲

12001-12021 Suturing of Superficial Wounds

INCLUDES Administration of local anesthesia
Cauterization without closure
Simple:
 Exploration nerves, blood vessels, tendons
 Vessel ligation, in wound
Simple repair that involves:
 Routine debridement and decontamination
 Simple one layer closure
 Superficial tissues
 Sutures, staples, tissue adhesives
 Total length of several repairs in same code category

EXCLUDES *Adhesive strips only, see appropriate evaluation and management service*
Complex repair nerves, blood vessels, tendons (see appropriate anatomical section)
Debridement:
 Performed separately, no closure (11042-11047 [11045, 11046])
 That requires:
  Comprehensive cleaning
  Removal of significant tissue
  Removal soft tissue and/or bone, no fracture/dislocation (11042-11047 [11045, 11046])
  Removal soft tissue and/or bone with open fracture/dislocation (11010-11012)
Deep tissue repair (12031-13153)
Major exploration (20100-20103)
Repair of nerves, blood vessels, tendons (See appropriate anatomical section. These repairs include simple and intermediate closure. Report complex closure with modifier 59.)
Secondary closure/dehiscence (13160)
Code also modifier 59 added to the less complicated procedure code if reporting more than one classification of wound repair

12001   **Simple repair of superficial wounds of scalp, neck, axillae, external genitalia, trunk and/or extremities (including hands and feet); 2.5 cm or less**
        🚑 1.27   ⚕ 2.53   **FUD** 000   Q1 N1 ⬜
        AMA: 2015,Jan,16; 2014,Jan,11; 2012,Mar,4-7; 2012,Jan,15-42; 2011,Jan,11

12002   **2.6 cm to 7.5 cm**
        🚑 1.68   ⚕ 3.09   **FUD** 000   Q1 N1 ⬜
        AMA: 2015,Jan,16; 2014,Oct,14; 2014,Jan,11; 2012,Jan,15-42; 2011,Jan,11

12004   **7.6 cm to 12.5 cm**
        🚑 2.10   ⚕ 3.64   **FUD** 000   Q1 N1 ⬜
        AMA: 2015,Jan,16; 2014,Jan,11; 2012,Jan,15-42; 2011,Jan,11

12005   **12.6 cm to 20.0 cm**
        🚑 2.84   ⚕ 4.72   **FUD** 000   T A2 ⬜
        AMA: 2015,Jan,16; 2014,Jan,11; 2012,Jan,15-42; 2011,Jan,11

12006   **20.1 cm to 30.0 cm**
        🚑 3.45   ⚕ 5.64   **FUD** 000   T A2 ⬜
        AMA: 2015,Jan,16; 2014,Jan,11; 2012,Jan,15-42; 2011,Jan,11

12007   **over 30.0 cm**
        🚑 4.30   ⚕ 6.56   **FUD** 000   T A2 ⬜
        AMA: 2015,Jan,16; 2014,Jan,11; 2012,Jan,15-42; 2011,Jan,11

12011   **Simple repair of superficial wounds of face, ears, eyelids, nose, lips and/or mucous membranes; 2.5 cm or less**
        🚑 1.58   ⚕ 3.10   **FUD** 000   Q1 N1 ⬜
        AMA: 2015,Jan,16; 2014,Jan,11; 2012,Jan,15-42; 2011,Jan,11

12013   **2.6 cm to 5.0 cm**
        🚑 1.78   ⚕ 3.40   **FUD** 000   Q1 N1 ⬜
        AMA: 2015,Jan,16; 2014,Jan,11; 2012,Jan,15-42; 2011,Jan,11

12014   **5.1 cm to 7.5 cm**
        🚑 2.26   ⚕ 4.02   **FUD** 000   Q1 N1 ⬜
        AMA: 2015,Jan,16; 2014,Jan,11; 2012,Jan,15-42; 2011,Jan,11

12015   **7.6 cm to 12.5 cm**
        🚑 2.82   ⚕ 4.86   **FUD** 000   T G2 ⬜
        AMA: 2015,Jan,16; 2014,Jan,11; 2012,Jan,15-42; 2011,Jan,11

12016   **12.6 cm to 20.0 cm**
        🚑 3.82   ⚕ 6.04   **FUD** 000   T A2 ⬜
        AMA: 2015,Jan,16; 2014,Jan,11; 2012,Jan,15-42; 2011,Jan,11

12017   **20.1 cm to 30.0 cm**
        🚑 4.42   ⚕ 4.42   **FUD** 000   T A2 80 ⬜
        AMA: 2015,Jan,16; 2014,Jan,11; 2012,Jan,15-42; 2011,Jan,11

12018   **over 30.0 cm**
        🚑 5.02   ⚕ 5.02   **FUD** 000   T A2 80 ⬜
        AMA: 2015,Jan,16; 2014,Jan,11; 2012,Jan,15-42; 2011,Jan,11

12020   **Treatment of superficial wound dehiscence; simple closure**
        EXCLUDES *Secondary closure major/complex wound or dehiscence (13160)*
        🚑 5.41   ⚕ 7.95   **FUD** 010   T A2 ⬜
        AMA: 2015,Jan,16; 2014,Jan,11; 2012,Jan,15-42; 2011,Jan,11

12021   **with packing**
        EXCLUDES *Secondary closure major/complex wound or dehiscence (13160)*
        🚑 3.98   ⚕ 4.65   **FUD** 010   T A2 ⬜
        AMA: 2015,Jan,16; 2014,Jan,11; 2012,Jan,15-42; 2011,Jan,11

12031-12057 Suturing of Intermediate Wounds

INCLUDES Administration of local anesthesia
Intermediate repair that involves:
 Closure of contaminated single layer wound
 Layer closure (e.g., subcutaneous tissue, superficial fascia)
 Removal foreign material (e.g. gravel, glass)
 Routine debridement and decontamination
Simple:
 Exploration nerves, blood vessels, tendons in wound
 Vessel ligation, in wound
Total length of several repairs in same code category

EXCLUDES *Debridement:*
 Performed separately, no closure (11042-11047 [11045, 11046])
 That requires:
  Removal soft tissue and/or bone, no fracture/dislocation (11042-11047 [11045, 11046])
  Removal soft tissue/bone due to open fracture/dislocation (11010-11012)
Major exploration (20100-20103)
Repair of nerves, blood vessels, tendons (See appropriate anatomical section. These repairs include simple and intermediate closure. Report complex closure with modifier 59.)
Secondary closure major/complex wound or dehiscence (13160)
Wound repair involving more than layer closure
Code also modifier 59 added to the less complicated procedure code if reporting more than one classification of wound repair

12031   **Repair, intermediate, wounds of scalp, axillae, trunk and/or extremities (excluding hands and feet); 2.5 cm or less**
        🚑 4.38   ⚕ 6.68   **FUD** 010   T P2 ⬜
        AMA: 2015,Jan,16; 2014,Jan,11; 2012,Jan,15-42; 2011,Jan,11; 2010,Apr,3-4

12032   **2.6 cm to 7.5 cm**
        🚑 5.58   ⚕ 8.54   **FUD** 010   T P2 ⬜
        AMA: 2015,Jan,16; 2014,Jan,11; 2012,Jan,15-42; 2011,Jan,11; 2010,Apr,3-4

12034   **7.6 cm to 12.5 cm**
        🚑 5.93   ⚕ 8.80   **FUD** 010   T A2 ⬜
        AMA: 2015,Jan,16; 2014,Jan,11; 2012,Jan,15-42; 2011,Jan,11; 2010,Apr,3-4

12035   **12.6 cm to 20.0 cm**
        🚑 6.90   ⚕ 10.8   **FUD** 010   T A2 ⬜
        AMA: 2015,Jan,16; 2014,Jan,11; 2012,Jan,15-42; 2011,Jan,11; 2010,Apr,3-4

12036   **20.1 cm to 30.0 cm**
        🚑 8.00   ⚕ 11.8   **FUD** 010   T A2 ⬜
        AMA: 2015,Jan,16; 2014,Jan,11; 2012,Jan,15-42; 2011,Jan,11; 2010,Apr,3-4

12037   **over 30.0 cm**
        🚑 9.45   ⚕ 13.6   **FUD** 010   T A2 80 ⬜
        AMA: 2015,Jan,16; 2014,Jan,11; 2012,Jan,15-42; 2011,Jan,11; 2010,Apr,3-4

12041   **Repair, intermediate, wounds of neck, hands, feet and/or external genitalia; 2.5 cm or less**
        🚑 4.49   ⚕ 6.82   **FUD** 010   T P2 ⬜
        AMA: 2015,Jan,16; 2014,Jan,11; 2013,Jan,15-16; 2012,Jan,15-42; 2011,Jan,11; 2010,Apr,3-4

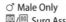

12042   **2.6 cm to 7.5 cm**
🚗 5.73   ⚕ 8.14   **FUD** 010   T P2 ▢
AMA: 2015,Jan,16; 2014,Jan,11; 2013,Jan,15-16; 2012,Jan,15-42; 2011,Jan,11; 2010,Apr,3-4

12044   **7.6 cm to 12.5 cm**
🚗 6.18   ⚕ 10.1   **FUD** 010   T A2 ▢
AMA: 2015,Jan,16; 2014,Jan,11; 2013,Jan,15-16; 2012,Jan,15-42; 2011,Jan,11; 2010,Apr,3-4

12045   **12.6 cm to 20.0 cm**
🚗 7.81   ⚕ 11.4   **FUD** 010   T A2 ▢
AMA: 2015,Jan,16; 2014,Jan,11; 2013,Jan,15-16; 2012,Jan,15-42; 2011,Jan,11; 2010,Apr,3-4

12046   **20.1 cm to 30.0 cm**
🚗 8.95   ⚕ 13.6   **FUD** 010   T A2 80 ▢
AMA: 2015,Jan,16; 2014,Jan,11; 2013,Jan,15-16; 2012,Jan,15-42; 2011,Jan,11; 2010,Apr,3-4

12047   **over 30.0 cm**
🚗 10.8   ⚕ 15.8   **FUD** 010   T A2 80 ▢
AMA: 2015,Jan,16; 2014,Jan,11; 2013,Jan,15-16; 2012,Jan,15-42; 2011,Jan,11; 2010,Apr,3-4

12051   **Repair, intermediate, wounds of face, ears, eyelids, nose, lips and/or mucous membranes; 2.5 cm or less**
🚗 4.91   ⚕ 7.27   **FUD** 010   T P2 ▢
AMA: 2015,Jan,16; 2014,Jan,11; 2012,Jan,15-42; 2011,Jan,11; 2010,Apr,3-4

12052   **2.6 cm to 5.0 cm**
🚗 5.84   ⚕ 8.29   **FUD** 010   T P2 ▢
AMA: 2015,Jan,16; 2014,Jan,11; 2012,Jan,15-42; 2011,Jan,11; 2010,Apr,3-4

12053   **5.1 cm to 7.5 cm**
🚗 6.24   ⚕ 9.75   **FUD** 010   T P2 ▢
AMA: 2015,Jan,16; 2014,Jan,11; 2012,Jan,15-42; 2011,Jan,11; 2010,Apr,3-4

12054   **7.6 cm to 12.5 cm**
🚗 6.53   ⚕ 10.3   **FUD** 010   T A2 ▢
AMA: 2015,Jan,16; 2014,Jan,11; 2012,Jan,15-42; 2011,Jan,11; 2010,Apr,3-4

12055   **12.6 cm to 20.0 cm**
🚗 8.66   ⚕ 13.4   **FUD** 010   T A2 ▢
AMA: 2015,Jan,16; 2014,Jan,11; 2012,Jan,15-42; 2011,Jan,11; 2010,Apr,3-4

12056   **20.1 cm to 30.0 cm**
🚗 10.0   ⚕ 14.1   **FUD** 010   T A2 80 ▢
AMA: 2015,Jan,16; 2014,Jan,11; 2012,Jan,15-42; 2011,Jan,11; 2010,Apr,3-4

12057   **over 30.0 cm**
🚗 10.8   ⚕ 16.4   **FUD** 010   T A2 80 ▢
AMA: 2015,Jan,16; 2014,Jan,11; 2012,Jan,15-42; 2011,Jan,11; 2010,Apr,3-4

13100-13160 Suturing of Complicated Wounds

INCLUDES   Creation of a limited defect for repair
Debridement complicated wounds/avulsions
More complicated than layered closure
Simple:
    Exploration nerves, vessels, tendons in wound
    Vessel ligation in wound
Total length of several repairs in same code category
Undermining, stents, retention sutures

EXCLUDES   Complex/secondary wound closure or dehiscence 13160
Debridement of open fracture/dislocation (15002-15005)
Excision:
    Benign lesions (11400-11446)
    Malignant lesions (11600-11646)
Extensive exploration (20100-20103)
Repair of nerves, blood vessel, tendons (See appropriate anatomical section. These repairs include simple and intermediate closure. Report complex closure with modifier 59.)
Surgical preparation of a wound bed (15002-15005)
Code also modifier 59 added to the less complicated procedure code if reporting more than one classification of wound repair

13100   **Repair, complex, trunk; 1.1 cm to 2.5 cm**
EXCLUDES   Complex repair 1.0 cm or less (12001, 12031)
🚗 5.91   ⚕ 9.44   **FUD** 010   T A2 ▢
AMA: 2015,Jan,16; 2014,Jan,11; 2012,Dec,6-8; 2012,Jan,15-42; 2012,Jan,6-10; 2011,May,3-5; 2011,Jan,11; 2010,Apr,3-4; 2010,Jan,3-5

13101   **2.6 cm to 7.5 cm**
🚗 7.24   ⚕ 11.1   **FUD** 010   T A2 ▢
AMA: 2015,Jan,16; 2014,Jan,11; 2012,Dec,6-8; 2012,Jan,6-10; 2012,Jan,15-42; 2011,May,6; 2011,May,3-5; 2011,Jan,11; 2010,Apr,3-4; 2010,Jan,3-5

+ 13102   **each additional 5 cm or less (List separately in addition to code for primary procedure)**
Code first (13101)
🚗 2.14   ⚕ 3.45   **FUD** ZZZ   N N1 ▢
AMA: 2015,Jan,16; 2014,Jan,11; 2012,Dec,6-8; 2012,Jan,6-10; 2012,Jan,15-42; 2011,May,6; 2011,May,3-5; 2011,Jan,11; 2010,Apr,3-4; 2010,Jan,3-5

13120   **Repair, complex, scalp, arms, and/or legs; 1.1 cm to 2.5 cm**
EXCLUDES   Complex repair 1.0 cm or less (12001, 12031)
🚗 6.77   ⚕ 9.87   **FUD** 010   T A2 ▢
AMA: 2015,Jan,16; 2014,Jan,11; 2012,Dec,6-8; 2012,Jan,6-10; 2012,Jan,15-42; 2011,May,3-5; 2011,Jan,11; 2010,Apr,3-4; 2010,Jan,3-5

13121   **2.6 cm to 7.5 cm**
🚗 7.65   ⚕ 12.0   **FUD** 010   T A2 ▢
AMA: 2015,Jan,16; 2014,Jan,11; 2012,Dec,6-8; 2012,Jan,6-10; 2012,Jan,15-42; 2011,May,6; 2011,May,3-5; 2011,Jan,11; 2010,Apr,3-4; 2010,Jan,3-5

+ 13122   **each additional 5 cm or less (List separately in addition to code for primary procedure)**
Code first (13121)
🚗 2.46   ⚕ 3.78   **FUD** ZZZ   N N1 ▢
AMA: 2015,Jan,16; 2014,Jan,11; 2012,Dec,6-8; 2012,Jan,6-10; 2012,Jan,15-42; 2011,May,3-5; 2011,Jan,11; 2010,Apr,3-4; 2010,Jan,3-5

13131   **Repair, complex, forehead, cheeks, chin, mouth, neck, axillae, genitalia, hands and/or feet; 1.1 cm to 2.5 cm**
EXCLUDES   Complex repair 1.0 cm or less (12001, 12011, 12031, 12041, 12051)
🚗 7.17   ⚕ 10.8   **FUD** 010   T A2 ▢
AMA: 2015,Jan,16; 2014,Jan,11; 2013,Jan,15-16; 2012,Dec,6-8; 2012,Jan,6-10; 2012,Jan,15-42; 2011,May,6; 2011,May,3-5; 2011,Jan,11; 2010,Apr,3-4; 2010,Jan,3-5

13132   **2.6 cm to 7.5 cm**
🚗 9.00   ⚕ 13.4   **FUD** 010   T A2 ▢
AMA: 2015,Jan,16; 2014,Oct,14; 2014,Jan,11; 2013,Jan,15-16; 2012,Dec,6-8; 2012,Jan,6-10; 2012,Jan,15-42; 2011,May,6; 2011,Jan,11; 2010,Apr,3-4; 2010,Jan,3-5

+ 13133   **each additional 5 cm or less (List separately in addition to code for primary procedure)**
Code first (13132)
🚗 3.77   ⚕ 5.06   **FUD** ZZZ   N N1 ▢
AMA: 2015,Jan,16; 2014,Jan,11; 2013,Jan,15-16; 2012,Dec,6-8; 2012,Jan,6-10; 2012,Jan,15-42; 2011,May,3-5; 2011,Jan,11; 2010,Apr,3-4; 2010,Jan,3-5

13151   **Repair, complex, eyelids, nose, ears and/or lips; 1.1 cm to 2.5 cm**
EXCLUDES   Complex repair 1.0 cm or less (12011, 12051)
🚗 8.23   ⚕ 11.9   **FUD** 010   T A2 ▢
AMA: 2015,Jan,16; 2014,May,3; 2014,Mar,12; 2014,Jan,11; 2012,Dec,6-8; 2012,Jan,6-10; 2012,Jan,15-42; 2011,May,3-5; 2011,Jan,11; 2010,Apr,3-4; 2010,Jan,3-5

13152   **2.6 cm to 7.5 cm**
🚗 9.96   ⚕ 14.3   **FUD** 010   T A2 ▢
AMA: 2015,Jan,16; 2014,Oct,14; 2014,May,3; 2014,Mar,12; 2014,Jan,11; 2012,Dec,6-8; 2012,Jan,6-10; 2012,Jan,15-42; 2011,May,3-5; 2011,Jan,11; 2010,Apr,3-4; 2010,Jan,3-5

● New Code   ▲ Revised Code   ○ Reinstated   M Maternity   A Age Edit   Unlisted   Not Covered   # Resequenced
⊘ AMA Mod 51 Exempt   ⑤ Optum Mod 51 Exempt   ⊛ Mod 63 Exempt   ⊙ Mod Sedation   + Add-on   ▢ CCI   PQ PQRS   FUD Follow-up Days

+ 13153   **each additional 5 cm or less (List separately in addition to code for primary procedure)**
Code first (13152)
🔧 4.07   ✂ 5.50   **FUD** ZZZ   N N1 ▭
AMA: 2015,Jan,16; 2014,May,3; 2014,Mar,12; 2014,Jan,11; 2012,Dec,6-8; 2012,Jan,6-10; 2012,Jan,15-42; 2011,May,3-5; 2011,Jan,11; 2010,Apr,3-4; 2010,Jan,3-5

13160   **Secondary closure of surgical wound or dehiscence, extensive or complicated**
EXCLUDES *Packing or simple secondary wound closure (12020-12021)*
🔧 23.1   ✂ 23.1   **FUD** 090   T A2 ▭
AMA: 2015,Jan,16; 2014,Jan,11; 2012,Dec,6-8; 2012,Jan,15-42; 2011,May,3-5; 2011,Jan,11

14000-14350 Reposition Contiguous Tissue

INCLUDES Excision of lesion with repair by adjacent tissue transfer or tissue rearrangement
Size of defect includes primary (due to excision) and secondary (due to flap design)
Z-plasty, W-plasty, VY-plasty, rotation flap, advancement flap, double pedicle flap, random island flap
EXCLUDES *Closure of wounds by undermining surrounding tissue without additional incisions (13100-13160)*
Full thickness closure of:
Eyelid (67930-67935, 67961-67975)
Lip (40650-40654)
Code also skin graft necessary to repair secondary defect (15040-15731)

14000   **Adjacent tissue transfer or rearrangement, trunk; defect 10 sq cm or less**
INCLUDES Burrow's operation
Do not report with (11400-11446, 11600-11646)
🔧 14.3   ✂ 17.6   **FUD** 090   T A2 ▭ P0
AMA: 2015,Feb,10; 2015,Jan,16; 2014,Apr,10; 2014,Jan,11; 2012,Dec,6-8; 2012,Nov,13-14; 2012,May,13; 2012,Jan,15-42; 2012,Jan,6-10; 2011,Jan,11; 2010,Apr,3-4; 2010,Mar,4-5

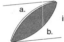
Example of common Z-plasty. Lesion is removed with oval-shaped incision

Two additional incisions (a. and b.) intersect the area

Skin of each incision is reflected back

The flaps are then transposed and the repair is closed

An adjacent flap, or other rearrangement flap, is performed to repair a defect of 10 sq cm or less (14000); a larger defect (up to 30 sq cm) is coded 14001

14001   **defect 10.1 sq cm to 30.0 sq cm**
Do not report with (11400-11446, 11600-11646)
🔧 18.7   ✂ 22.6   **FUD** 090   T A2 ▭ P0
AMA: 2015,Feb,10; 2015,Jan,16; 2014,Apr,10; 2014,Jan,11; 2012,Dec,6-8; 2012,Nov,13-14; 2012,May,13; 2012,Jan,15-42; 2012,Jan,6-10; 2011,Jan,11; 2010,Apr,3-4; 2010,Mar,4-5

14020   **Adjacent tissue transfer or rearrangement, scalp, arms and/or legs; defect 10 sq cm or less**
Do not report with (11400-11446, 11600-11646)
🔧 16.2   ✂ 19.7   **FUD** 090   T A2 ▭ P0
AMA: 2015,Jan,16; 2014,Jan,11; 2012,Dec,6-8; 2012,Nov,13-14; 2012,May,13; 2012,Jan,6-10; 2012,Jan,15-42; 2011,Jan,11; 2010,Apr,3-4; 2010,Mar,4-5

14021   **defect 10.1 sq cm to 30.0 sq cm**
Do not report with (11400-11446, 11600-11646)
🔧 20.5   ✂ 24.6   **FUD** 090   T A2 ▭ P0
AMA: 2015,Jan,16; 2014,Jan,11; 2012,Dec,6-8; 2012,Nov,13-14; 2012,May,13; 2012,Jan,6-10; 2012,Jan,15-42; 2011,Jan,11; 2010,Apr,3-4; 2010,Mar,4-5

14040   **Adjacent tissue transfer or rearrangement, forehead, cheeks, chin, mouth, neck, axillae, genitalia, hands and/or feet; defect 10 sq cm or less**
INCLUDES Krimer's palatoplasty
Do not report with (11400-11446, 11600-11646)
🔧 18.1   ✂ 21.5   **FUD** 090   T A2 ▭ P0
AMA: 2015,Jan,16; 2014,Jan,11; 2012,Dec,6-8; 2012,Nov,13-14; 2012,May,13; 2012,Jan,6-10; 2012,Jan,15-42; 2011,Jan,11; 2010,Apr,3-4; 2010,Mar,4-5

14041   **defect 10.1 sq cm to 30.0 sq cm**
Do not report with (11400-11446, 11600-11646)
🔧 22.2   ✂ 26.6   **FUD** 090   T A2 ▭ P0
AMA: 2015,Jan,16; 2014,Jan,11; 2012,Dec,6-8; 2012,Nov,13-14; 2012,May,13; 2012,Jan,6-10; 2012,Jan,15-42; 2011,Jan,11; 2010,Apr,3-4; 2010,Mar,4-5

14060   **Adjacent tissue transfer or rearrangement, eyelids, nose, ears and/or lips; defect 10 sq cm or less**
INCLUDES Denonvillier's operation
EXCLUDES *Eyelid, full thickness (67961-67966)*
Do not report with (11400-11446, 11600-11646)
🔧 19.2   ✂ 22.0   **FUD** 090   T A2 ▭ P0
AMA: 2015,Jan,16; 2014,Jan,11; 2012,Dec,6-8; 2012,Nov,13-14; 2012,Aug,13-14; 2012,May,13; 2012,Jan,15-42; 2012,Jan,6-10; 2011,Jan,11; 2010,Apr,3-4; 2010,Mar,4-5

14061   **defect 10.1 sq cm to 30.0 sq cm**
EXCLUDES *Eyelid, full thickness (67961 and subsequent codes)*
Do not report with (11400-11446, 11600-11646)
🔧 23.8   ✂ 28.7   **FUD** 090   T A2 ▭ P0
AMA: 2015,Jan,16; 2014,Jan,11; 2012,Dec,6-8; 2012,Nov,13-14; 2012,May,13; 2012,Jan,6-10; 2012,Jan,15-42; 2011,Jan,11; 2010,Apr,3-4; 2010,Mar,4-5

14301   **Adjacent tissue transfer or rearrangement, any area; defect 30.1 sq cm to 60.0 sq cm**
Do not report with (11400-11446, 11600-11646)
🔧 25.2   ✂ 30.5   **FUD** 090   T 62 80 P0
AMA: 2015,Jan,16; 2014,Jan,11; 2012,Dec,6-8; 2012,Nov,13-14; 2012,May,13; 2010,Apr,3-4; 2010,Mar,4-5

+ 14302   **each additional 30.0 sq cm, or part thereof (List separately in addition to code for primary procedure)**
Code first (14301)
Do not report with (11400-11446, 11600-11646)
🔧 6.38   ✂ 6.38   **FUD** ZZZ   N N1 80 P0
AMA: 2015,Jan,16; 2014,Jan,11; 2012,Dec,6-8; 2012,Nov,13-14; 2012,May,13; 2010,Apr,3-4; 2010,Mar,4-5

14350   **Filleted finger or toe flap, including preparation of recipient site**
🔧 19.8   ✂ 19.8   **FUD** 090   T A2 80 ▭
AMA: 2015,Jan,16; 2014,Jan,11; 2012,Dec,6-8; 2012,May,13; 2012,Jan,15-42; 2011,Jan,11; 2010,Mar,4-5

15002-15005 Development of Base for Tissue Grafting

INCLUDES
Add together the surface area of multiple wounds in the same anatomical locations as indicated in the code descriptor groups, such as face and scalp. Do not add together multiple wounds at different anatomical site groups such as trunk and face
Ankle or wrist if code description describes leg or arm
Cleaning and preparing a viable wound surface for grafting or negative pressure wound therapy used to heal the wound primarily
Code selection based on the defect size and location
Percentage applies to children younger than age 10
Removal of nonviable tissue in nonchronic wounds for primary healing
Square centimeters applies to children and adults age 10 or older

EXCLUDES
Chronic wound management on wounds left to heal by secondary intention (11042-11047 [11045, 11046], 97597-97598)
Necrotizing soft tissue infections for specific anatomical locations (11004-11008)

15002
Surgical preparation or creation of recipient site by excision of open wounds, burn eschar, or scar (including subcutaneous tissues), or incisional release of scar contracture, trunk, arms, legs; first 100 sq cm or 1% of body area of infants and children

> EXCLUDES *Linear scar revision (13100-13153)*
>
> 6.53 9.85 **FUD** 000 T A2 80
>
> **AMA:** 2015,Jan,16; 2014,Mar,12; 2014,Jan,11; 2013,Feb,16-17; 2012,Dec,6-8; 2012,Oct,3-8; 2012,Oct,13; 2012,Jan,15-42; 2012,Jan,6-10; 2011,Jan,11; 2010,Apr,3-4; 2010,Jan,12-15

+ **15003**
each additional 100 sq cm, or part thereof, or each additional 1% of body area of infants and children (List separately in addition to code for primary procedure)

> Code first (15002)
>
> 1.32 2.16 **FUD** ZZZ N N1
>
> **AMA:** 2015,Jan,16; 2014,Mar,12; 2014,Jan,11; 2013,Feb,16-17; 2012,Oct,3-8; 2012,Oct,13; 2012,Jan,15-42; 2012,Jan,6-10; 2011,Jan,11; 2010,Apr,3-4

15004
Surgical preparation or creation of recipient site by excision of open wounds, burn eschar, or scar (including subcutaneous tissues), or incisional release of scar contracture, face, scalp, eyelids, mouth, neck, ears, orbits, genitalia, hands, feet and/or multiple digits; first 100 sq cm or 1% of body area of infants and children

> 7.81 11.4 **FUD** 000 T A2 80
>
> **AMA:** 2015,Jan,16; 2014,Mar,12; 2014,Jan,11; 2013,Feb,16-17; 2012,Oct,3-8; 2012,Oct,13; 2012,Jan,15-42; 2012,Jan,6-10; 2011,Jan,11; 2010,Apr,3-4; 2010,Jan,12-15

+ **15005**
each additional 100 sq cm, or part thereof, or each additional 1% of body area of infants and children (List separately in addition to code for primary procedure)

> Code first (15004)
>
> 2.62 3.55 **FUD** ZZZ N N1 80
>
> **AMA:** 2015,Jan,16; 2014,Mar,12; 2014,Jan,11; 2013,Feb,16-17; 2012,Oct,3-8; 2012,Oct,13; 2012,Jan,15-42; 2012,Jan,6-10; 2011,Jan,11; 2010,Apr,3-4

15040 Obtain Autograft

INCLUDES
Ankle or wrist if code description describes leg or arm
Percentage applies to children younger than age 10
Square centimeters applies to children and adults age 10 or older

15040
Harvest of skin for tissue cultured skin autograft, 100 sq cm or less

> 3.67 7.21 **FUD** 000 T A2
>
> **AMA:** 2015,Jan,16; 2014,Jan,11; 2012,Jan,6-10; 2012,Jan,15-42; 2011,Jan,11; 2010,Apr,3-4

15050 Pinch Graft

INCLUDES
Autologous skin graft harvest and application
Current graft removal
Fixation and anchoring skin graft
Simple cleaning
Code also graft or flap necessary to repair donor site
Do not report with (97602)

15050
Pinch graft, single or multiple, to cover small ulcer, tip of digit, or other minimal open area (except on face), up to defect size 2 cm diameter

> 12.8 16.1 **FUD** 090 T A2
>
> **AMA:** 2015,Jan,16; 2014,Jan,11; 2012,Jan,6-10; 2012,Jan,15-42; 2011,Mar,9; 2011,Jan,11; 2010,Apr,3-4

15100-15261 Skin Grafts and Replacements

INCLUDES
Add together the surface area of multiple wounds in the same anatomical locations as indicated in the code description groups, such as face and scalp. Do not add together multiple wounds at different anatomical site groups such as trunk and face
Ankle or wrist if code description describes leg or arm
Autologous skin graft harvest and application
Code selection based on recipient site location and size and type of graft
Current graft removal
Fixation and anchoring skin graft
Percentage applies to children younger than age 10
Simple cleaning
Simple tissue debridement
Square centimeters applies to children and adults age 10 or older

EXCLUDES
Debridement without immediate primary closure, when wound is grossly contaminated and extensive cleaning is needed, or when necrotic or contaminated tissue is removed (11042-11047 [11045, 11046], 97597-97598)
Code also graft or flap necessary to repair donor site
Code also primary procedure requiring skin graft for definitive closure
Do not report with (97602)

15100
Split-thickness autograft, trunk, arms, legs; first 100 sq cm or less, or 1% of body area of infants and children (except 15050)

> 20.5 24.4 **FUD** 090 T A2
>
> **AMA:** 2015,Jan,16; 2014,Jan,11; 2012,Oct,3-8; 2012,Jan,6-10; 2012,Jan,15-42; 2011,Mar,9; 2011,Jan,11; 2010,Apr,3-4

+ **15101**
each additional 100 sq cm, or each additional 1% of body area of infants and children, or part thereof (List separately in addition to code for primary procedure)

> Code first (15100)
>
> 3.20 5.29 **FUD** ZZZ N N1
>
> **AMA:** 2015,Jan,16; 2014,Jan,11; 2012,Oct,3-8; 2012,Jan,6-10; 2012,Jan,15-42; 2011,Mar,9; 2011,Jan,11; 2010,Apr,3-4

15110
Epidermal autograft, trunk, arms, legs; first 100 sq cm or less, or 1% of body area of infants and children

> 20.3 23.2 **FUD** 090 T A2
>
> **AMA:** 2015,Jan,16; 2014,Jan,11; 2012,Oct,3-8; 2012,Jan,6-10; 2012,Jan,15-42; 2011,Mar,9; 2011,Jan,11; 2010,Apr,3-4

+ **15111**
each additional 100 sq cm, or each additional 1% of body area of infants and children, or part thereof (List separately in addition to code for primary procedure)

> Code first (15110)
>
> 3.00 3.32 **FUD** ZZZ N N1
>
> **AMA:** 2015,Jan,16; 2014,Jan,11; 2012,Oct,3-8; 2012,Jan,6-10; 2012,Jan,15-42; 2011,Mar,9; 2011,Jan,11; 2010,Apr,3-4

15115
Epidermal autograft, face, scalp, eyelids, mouth, neck, ears, orbits, genitalia, hands, feet, and/or multiple digits; first 100 sq cm or less, or 1% of body area of infants and children

> 20.6 23.5 **FUD** 090 T A2
>
> **AMA:** 2015,Jan,16; 2014,Jan,11; 2012,Oct,3-8; 2012,Jan,6-10; 2012,Jan,15-42; 2011,Mar,9; 2011,Jan,11; 2010,Apr,3-4

+ **15116**
each additional 100 sq cm, or each additional 1% of body area of infants and children, or part thereof (List separately in addition to code for primary procedure)

> Code first (15115)
>
> 4.39 4.81 **FUD** ZZZ N N1
>
> **AMA:** 2015,Jan,16; 2014,Jan,11; 2012,Oct,3-8; 2012,Jan,6-10; 2012,Jan,15-42; 2011,Mar,9; 2011,Jan,11; 2010,Apr,3-4

Integumentary System

15120   Split-thickness autograft, face, scalp, eyelids, mouth, neck, ears, orbits, genitalia, hands, feet, and/or multiple digits; first 100 sq cm or less, or 1% of body area of infants and children (except 15050)

EXCLUDES   *Other eyelid repair (67961-67975)*

🚑 20.0   ✂ 24.1   **FUD** 090   T A2 ▯

AMA: 2015,Jan,16; 2014,Jan,11; 2012,Oct,3-8; 2012,Jan,6-10; 2012,Jan,15-42; 2011,Mar,9; 2011,Jan,11; 2010,Apr,3-4

+ 15121   each additional 100 sq cm, or each additional 1% of body area of infants and children, or part thereof (List separately in addition to code for primary procedure)

EXCLUDES   *Other eyelid repair (67961-67975)*

Code first (15120)

🚑 3.83   ✂ 5.92   **FUD** ZZZ   N N1

AMA: 2015,Jan,16; 2014,Jan,11; 2012,Oct,3-8; 2012,Jan,6-10; 2012,Jan,15-42; 2011,Mar,9; 2011,Jan,11; 2010,Apr,3-4

15130   Dermal autograft, trunk, arms, legs; first 100 sq cm or less, or 1% of body area of infants and children

🚑 16.3   ✂ 19.3   **FUD** 090   T A2

AMA: 2015,Jan,16; 2014,Jan,11; 2012,Oct,3-8; 2012,Jan,6-10; 2012,Jan,15-42; 2011,Mar,9; 2011,Jan,11; 2010,Apr,3-4

+ 15131   each additional 100 sq cm, or each additional 1% of body area of infants and children, or part thereof (List separately in addition to code for primary procedure)

Code first (15130)

🚑 2.40   ✂ 2.62   **FUD** ZZZ   N N1

AMA: 2015,Jan,16; 2014,Jan,11; 2012,Oct,3-8; 2012,Jan,6-10; 2012,Jan,15-42; 2011,Mar,9; 2011,Jan,11; 2010,Apr,3-4

15135   Dermal autograft, face, scalp, eyelids, mouth, neck, ears, orbits, genitalia, hands, feet, and/or multiple digits; first 100 sq cm or less, or 1% of body area of infants and children

🚑 21.0   ✂ 23.9   **FUD** 090   T A2

AMA: 2015,Jan,16; 2014,Jan,11; 2012,Oct,3-8; 2012,Jan,6-10; 2012,Jan,15-42; 2011,Mar,9; 2011,Jan,11; 2010,Apr,3-4

+ 15136   each additional 100 sq cm, or each additional 1% of body area of infants and children, or part thereof (List separately in addition to code for primary procedure)

Code first (15135)

🚑 2.54   ✂ 2.72   **FUD** ZZZ   N N1

AMA: 2015,Jan,16; 2014,Jan,11; 2012,Oct,3-8; 2012,Jan,6-10; 2012,Jan,15-42; 2011,Mar,9; 2011,Jan,11; 2010,Apr,3-4

15150   Tissue cultured skin autograft, trunk, arms, legs; first 25 sq cm or less

🚑 18.2   ✂ 19.9   **FUD** 090   T A2

AMA: 2015,Jan,16; 2014,Jan,11; 2012,Oct,3-8; 2012,Jan,6-10; 2012,Jan,15-42; 2011,Mar,9; 2011,Jan,11; 2010,Apr,3-4

+ 15151   additional 1 sq cm to 75 sq cm (List separately in addition to code for primary procedure)

EXCLUDES   *Grafts over 75 sq cm (15152)*

Code first (15150)

Do not report more than one time per session

🚑 3.20   ✂ 3.46   **FUD** ZZZ   N N1

AMA: 2015,Jan,16; 2014,Jan,11; 2012,Oct,3-8; 2012,Jan,6-10; 2012,Jan,15-42; 2011,Mar,9; 2011,Jan,11; 2010,Apr,3-4

+ 15152   each additional 100 sq cm, or each additional 1% of body area of infants and children, or part thereof (List separately in addition to code for primary procedure)

Code first (15151)

🚑 4.01   ✂ 4.27   **FUD** ZZZ   N N1

AMA: 2015,Jan,16; 2014,Jan,11; 2012,Oct,3-8; 2012,Jan,6-10; 2012,Jan,15-42; 2011,Mar,9; 2011,Jan,11; 2010,Apr,3-4

15155   Tissue cultured skin autograft, face, scalp, eyelids, mouth, neck, ears, orbits, genitalia, hands, feet, and/or multiple digits; first 25 sq cm or less

🚑 18.1   ✂ 19.6   **FUD** 090   T A2

AMA: 2015,Jan,16; 2014,Jan,11; 2012,Oct,3-8; 2012,Jan,6-10; 2012,Jan,15-42; 2011,Mar,9; 2011,Jan,11; 2010,Apr,3-4

+ 15156   additional 1 sq cm to 75 sq cm (List separately in addition to code for primary procedure)

EXCLUDES   *Grafts over 75 sq cm (15157)*

Code first (15155)

Do not report more than one time per session

🚑 4.42   ✂ 4.67   **FUD** ZZZ   N N1

AMA: 2015,Jan,16; 2014,Jan,11; 2012,Oct,3-8; 2012,Jan,6-10; 2012,Jan,15-42; 2011,Mar,9; 2011,Jan,11; 2010,Apr,3-4

+ 15157   each additional 100 sq cm, or each additional 1% of body area of infants and children, or part thereof (List separately in addition to code for primary procedure)

Code first (15156)

🚑 4.16   ✂ 4.47   **FUD** ZZZ   N N1

AMA: 2015,Jan,16; 2014,Jan,11; 2012,Oct,3-8; 2012,Jan,6-10; 2012,Jan,15-42; 2011,Mar,9; 2011,Jan,11; 2010,Apr,3-4

15200   Full thickness graft, free, including direct closure of donor site, trunk; 20 sq cm or less

🚑 19.2   ✂ 23.5   **FUD** 090   T A2 ▯

AMA: 2015,Jan,16; 2014,Jan,11; 2012,Oct,3-8; 2012,Jan,6-10; 2012,Jan,15-42; 2011,Jan,11; 2010,Apr,3-4

+ 15201   each additional 20 sq cm, or part thereof (List separately in addition to code for primary procedure)

Code first (15200)

🚑 2.27   ✂ 4.20   **FUD** ZZZ   N N1

AMA: 2015,Jan,16; 2014,Jan,11; 2012,Oct,3-8; 2012,Jan,6-10; 2012,Jan,15-42; 2011,Jan,11; 2010,Apr,3-4

15220   Full thickness graft, free, including direct closure of donor site, scalp, arms, and/or legs; 20 sq cm or less

🚑 17.6   ✂ 21.8   **FUD** 090   T A2 ▯

AMA: 2015,Jan,16; 2014,Jan,11; 2012,Oct,3-8; 2012,Jan,6-10; 2012,Jan,15-42; 2011,Jan,11; 2010,Apr,3-4

+ 15221   each additional 20 sq cm, or part thereof (List separately in addition to code for primary procedure)

Code first (15220)

🚑 2.06   ✂ 3.89   **FUD** ZZZ   N N1

AMA: 2015,Jan,16; 2014,Jan,11; 2012,Oct,3-8; 2012,Jan,6-10; 2012,Jan,15-42; 2011,Jan,11; 2010,Apr,3-4

15240   Full thickness graft, free, including direct closure of donor site, forehead, cheeks, chin, mouth, neck, axillae, genitalia, hands, and/or feet; 20 sq cm or less

EXCLUDES   *Fingertip graft (15050)*
            Syndactyly repair fingers (26560-26562)

🚑 22.9   ✂ 26.4   **FUD** 090   T A2 ▯

AMA: 2015,Jan,16; 2014,Jan,11; 2012,Oct,3-8; 2012,Jan,6-10; 2012,Jan,15-42; 2011,Jan,11; 2010,Apr,3-4

+ 15241   each additional 20 sq cm, or part thereof (List separately in addition to code for primary procedure)

Code first (15240)

🚑 3.21   ✂ 5.26   **FUD** ZZZ   N N1

AMA: 2015,Jan,16; 2014,Jan,11; 2012,Oct,3-8; 2012,Jan,6-10; 2012,Jan,15-42; 2011,Jan,11; 2010,Apr,3-4

15260   Full thickness graft, free, including direct closure of donor site, nose, ears, eyelids, and/or lips; 20 sq cm or less

EXCLUDES   *Other eyelid repair (67961-67975)*

🚑 24.5   ✂ 28.6   **FUD** 090   T A2 ▯

AMA: 2015,Jan,16; 2014,Jan,11; 2012,Oct,3-8; 2012,Jan,6-10; 2012,Jan,15-42; 2011,Jan,11; 2010,Apr,3-4

+ 15261   each additional 20 sq cm, or part thereof (List separately in addition to code for primary procedure)

EXCLUDES   *Other eyelid repair (67961-67975)*

Code first (15260)

🚑 4.03   ✂ 6.09   **FUD** ZZZ   N N1

AMA: 2015,Jan,16; 2014,Jan,11; 2012,Oct,3-8; 2012,Jan,6-10; 2012,Jan,15-42; 2011,Jan,11; 2010,Apr,3-4

15271-15278 Skin Substitute Graft Application

INCLUDES Add together the surface area of multiple wounds in the same anatomical locations as indicated in the code description groups, such as face and scalp. Do not add together multiple wounds at different anatomical site groups such as trunk and face.
Ankle or wrist if code description describes leg or arm
Code selection based on defect site location and size
Fixation and anchoring skin graft
Graft types include:
 Biological material used for scaffolding for growing skin
 Nonautologous human skin such as:
  Dermal
  Epidermal
  Cellular
  Acellular
  Allograft
  Homograft
 Nonhuman grafts
Percentage applies to children younger than age 10
Removing current graft
Simple cleaning
Simple tissue debridement
Square centimeters applies to children and adults age 10 or older
Code also biologic implant for soft tissue reinforcement (15777)
Code also primary procedure requiring skin graft for definitive closure
Code also supply of skin substitute product
Do not report for application of nongraft dressing
Do not report for injected skin substitutes
Do not report with (97602)

15271 **Application of skin substitute graft to trunk, arms, legs, total wound surface area up to 100 sq cm; first 25 sq cm or less wound surface area**

EXCLUDES *Total wound area greater than or equal to 100 sq cm (15273-15274)*
Do not report with (15273-15274)
2.44   4.00   **FUD** 000   T G2

AMA: 2015,Jan,16; 2014,Jun,14; 2014,Jan,11; 2013,Oct,15; 2012,Oct,3-8; 2012,Jan,6-10; 2012,Jan,15-42

+ 15272 **each additional 25 sq cm wound surface area, or part thereof (List separately in addition to code for primary procedure)**

EXCLUDES *Total wound area greater than or equal to 100 sq cm (15273-15274)*
Code first (15271)
Do not report with (15273-15274)
0.50   0.77   **FUD** ZZZ   N N1

AMA: 2015,Jan,16; 2014,Jun,14; 2014,Jan,11; 2013,Oct,15; 2012,Oct,3-8; 2012,Jan,6-10; 2012,Jan,15-42

15273 **Application of skin substitute graft to trunk, arms, legs, total wound surface area greater than or equal to 100 sq cm; first 100 sq cm wound surface area, or 1% of body area of infants and children**

EXCLUDES *Total wound surface area up to 100 cm (15271-15272)*
Do not report with (15271-15272)
5.84   8.45   **FUD** 000   T G2

AMA: 2015,Jan,16; 2014,Jun,14; 2014,Jan,11; 2013,Oct,15; 2013,Nov,14; 2012,Oct,3-8; 2012,Jan,6-10; 2012,Jan,15-42

+ 15274 **each additional 100 sq cm wound surface area, or part thereof, or each additional 1% of body area of infants and children, or part thereof (List separately in addition to code for primary procedure)**

EXCLUDES *Total wound surface area up to 100 cm (15271-15272)*
Code first (15273)
1.32   2.02   **FUD** ZZZ   N N1

AMA: 2015,Jan,16; 2014,Jun,14; 2014,Jan,11; 2013,Oct,15; 2013,Nov,14; 2012,Oct,3-8; 2012,Jan,6-10; 2012,Jan,15-42

15275 **Application of skin substitute graft to face, scalp, eyelids, mouth, neck, ears, orbits, genitalia, hands, feet, and/or multiple digits, total wound surface area up to 100 sq cm; first 25 sq cm or less wound surface area**

EXCLUDES *Total wound area greater than or equal to 100 sq cm (15277-15278)*
Do not report with (15277-15278)
2.77   4.24   **FUD** 000   T G2

AMA: 2015,Jan,16; 2014,Jun,14; 2014,Jan,11; 2013,Oct,15; 2012,Oct,3-8; 2012,Jan,6-10; 2012,Jan,15-42

+ 15276 **each additional 25 sq cm wound surface area, or part thereof (List separately in addition to code for primary procedure)**

EXCLUDES *Total wound area greater than or equal to 100 sq cm (15277-15278)*
Code first (15275)
Do not report with (15277-15278)
0.71   0.97   **FUD** ZZZ   N N1

AMA: 2015,Jan,16; 2014,Jun,14; 2014,Jan,11; 2013,Oct,15; 2012,Oct,3-8; 2012,Jan,6-10; 2012,Jan,15-42

15277 **Application of skin substitute graft to face, scalp, eyelids, mouth, neck, ears, orbits, genitalia, hands, feet, and/or multiple digits, total wound surface area greater than or equal to 100 sq cm; first 100 sq cm wound surface area, or 1% of body area of infants and children**

EXCLUDES *Total surface area up to 100 sq cm (15275-15276)*
Do not report with (15275-15276)
6.51   9.20   **FUD** 000   T G2

AMA: 2015,Jan,16; 2014,Jun,14; 2014,Jan,11; 2013,Oct,15; 2013,Nov,14; 2012,Oct,3-8; 2012,Jan,6-10; 2012,Jan,15-42

+ 15278 **each additional 100 sq cm wound surface area, or part thereof, or each additional 1% of body area of infants and children, or part thereof (List separately in addition to code for primary procedure)**

EXCLUDES *Total surface area up to 100 sq cm (15275-15276)*
Code first (15277)
Do not report with (15275-15276)
1.65   2.42   **FUD** ZZZ   N N1

AMA: 2015,Jan,16; 2014,Jun,14; 2014,Jan,11; 2013,Oct,15; 2013,Nov,14; 2012,Oct,3-8; 2012,Jan,6-10; 2012,Jan,15-42

15570-15731 Wound Reconstruction: Skin Flaps

INCLUDES Ankle or wrist if code description describes leg or arm
Code based on recipient site when the flap is attached in the transfer or to a final site and is based on donor site when a tube is created for transfer later or when the flap is delayed prior to transfer
Fixation and anchoring skin graft
Simple tissue debridement
Tube formation for later transfer

EXCLUDES *Contiguous tissue transfer flaps (14000-14302)*
Debridement without immediate primary closure (11042-11047 [11045, 11046], 97597-97598)
Excision of:
 Benign lesion (11400-11471)
 Burn eschar or scar (15002-15005)
 Malignant lesion (11600-11646)
Microvascular repair (15756-15758)
Primary procedure such as radical mastectomy, extensive tumor removal, orbitectomy (see appropriate anatomical site)
Code also application of extensive immobilization apparatus
Code also repair of donor site with skin grafts or flaps

15570 Formation of direct or tubed pedicle, with or without transfer; trunk

INCLUDES Flaps without a vascular pedicle

🔾 21.0 ⚖ 25.9 **FUD** 090 T A2 ▣

AMA: 2015,Jan,16; 2014,Jan,11; 2012,Dec,6-8; 2012,Jan,15-42; 2011,Jan,11; 2010,Apr,3-4; 2010,Mar,4-5

Pedicle Flap

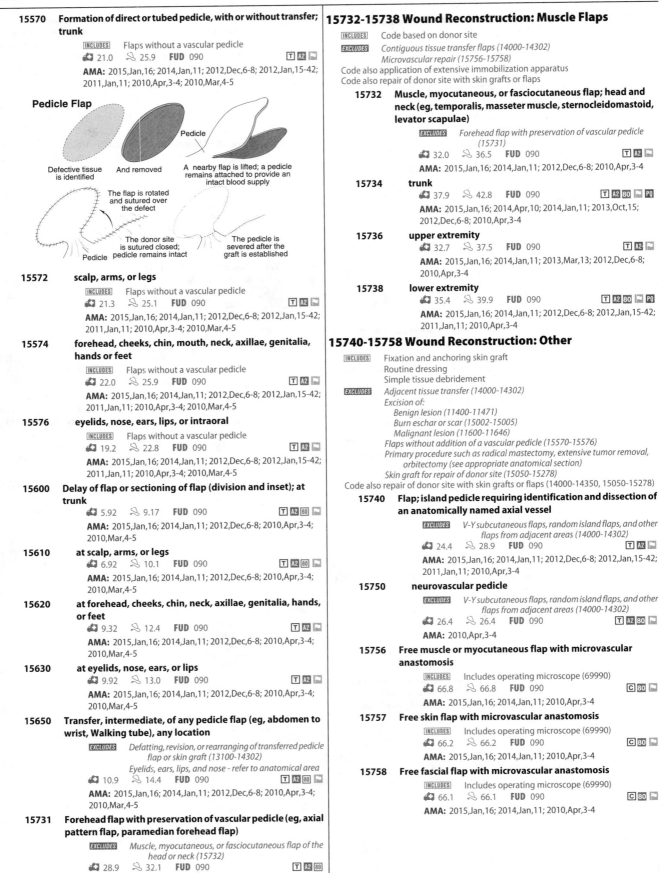

Defective tissue is identified

And removed

A nearby flap is lifted; a pedicle remains attached to provide an intact blood supply

Pedicle

The flap is rotated and sutured over the defect

The donor site is sutured closed; pedicle remains intact

Pedicle

The pedicle is severed after the graft is established

15572 scalp, arms, or legs

INCLUDES Flaps without a vascular pedicle

🔾 21.3 ⚖ 25.1 **FUD** 090 T A2 ▣

AMA: 2015,Jan,16; 2014,Jan,11; 2012,Dec,6-8; 2012,Jan,15-42; 2011,Jan,11; 2010,Apr,3-4; 2010,Mar,4-5

15574 forehead, cheeks, chin, mouth, neck, axillae, genitalia, hands or feet

INCLUDES Flaps without a vascular pedicle

🔾 22.0 ⚖ 25.9 **FUD** 090 T A2 ▣

AMA: 2015,Jan,16; 2014,Jan,11; 2012,Dec,6-8; 2012,Jan,15-42; 2011,Jan,11; 2010,Apr,3-4; 2010,Mar,4-5

15576 eyelids, nose, ears, lips, or intraoral

INCLUDES Flaps without a vascular pedicle

🔾 19.2 ⚖ 22.8 **FUD** 090 T A2 ▣

AMA: 2015,Jan,16; 2014,Jan,11; 2012,Dec,6-8; 2012,Jan,15-42; 2011,Jan,11; 2010,Apr,3-4; 2010,Mar,4-5

15600 Delay of flap or sectioning of flap (division and inset); at trunk

🔾 5.92 ⚖ 9.17 **FUD** 090 T A2 80 ▣

AMA: 2015,Jan,16; 2014,Jan,11; 2012,Dec,6-8; 2010,Apr,3-4; 2010,Mar,4-5

15610 at scalp, arms, or legs

🔾 6.92 ⚖ 10.1 **FUD** 090 T A2 80 ▣

AMA: 2015,Jan,16; 2014,Jan,11; 2012,Dec,6-8; 2010,Apr,3-4; 2010,Mar,4-5

15620 at forehead, cheeks, chin, neck, axillae, genitalia, hands, or feet

🔾 9.32 ⚖ 12.4 **FUD** 090 T A2 ▣

AMA: 2015,Jan,16; 2014,Jan,11; 2012,Dec,6-8; 2010,Apr,3-4; 2010,Mar,4-5

15630 at eyelids, nose, ears, or lips

🔾 9.92 ⚖ 13.0 **FUD** 090 T A2 ▣

AMA: 2015,Jan,16; 2014,Jan,11; 2012,Dec,6-8; 2010,Apr,3-4; 2010,Mar,4-5

15650 Transfer, intermediate, of any pedicle flap (eg, abdomen to wrist, Walking tube), any location

EXCLUDES Defatting, revision, or rearranging of transferred pedicle flap or skin graft (13100-14302)

Eyelids, ears, lips, and nose - refer to anatomical area

🔾 10.9 ⚖ 14.4 **FUD** 090 T A2 80 ▣

AMA: 2015,Jan,16; 2014,Jan,11; 2012,Dec,6-8; 2010,Apr,3-4; 2010,Mar,4-5

15731 Forehead flap with preservation of vascular pedicle (eg, axial pattern flap, paramedian forehead flap)

EXCLUDES Muscle, myocutaneous, or fasciocutaneous flap of the head or neck (15732)

🔾 28.9 ⚖ 32.1 **FUD** 090 T A2 80

AMA: 2015,Jan,16; 2014,Jan,11; 2012,Dec,6-8; 2010,Apr,3-4

15732-15738 Wound Reconstruction: Muscle Flaps

INCLUDES Code based on donor site

EXCLUDES Contiguous tissue transfer flaps (14000-14302)
Microvascular repair (15756-15758)

Code also application of extensive immobilization apparatus

Code also repair of donor site with skin grafts or flaps

15732 Muscle, myocutaneous, or fasciocutaneous flap; head and neck (eg, temporalis, masseter muscle, sternocleidomastoid, levator scapulae)

EXCLUDES Forehead flap with preservation of vascular pedicle (15731)

🔾 32.0 ⚖ 36.5 **FUD** 090 T A2 ▣

AMA: 2015,Jan,16; 2014,Jan,11; 2012,Dec,6-8; 2010,Apr,3-4

15734 trunk

🔾 37.9 ⚖ 42.8 **FUD** 090 T A2 80 ▣ P0

AMA: 2015,Jan,16; 2014,Apr,10; 2014,Jan,11; 2013,Oct,15; 2012,Dec,6-8; 2010,Apr,3-4

15736 upper extremity

🔾 32.7 ⚖ 37.5 **FUD** 090 T A2 ▣

AMA: 2015,Jan,16; 2014,Jan,11; 2013,Mar,13; 2012,Dec,6-8; 2010,Apr,3-4

15738 lower extremity

🔾 35.4 ⚖ 39.9 **FUD** 090 T A2 80 ▣ P0

AMA: 2015,Jan,16; 2014,Jan,11; 2012,Dec,6-8; 2012,Jan,15-42; 2011,Jan,11; 2010,Apr,3-4

15740-15758 Wound Reconstruction: Other

INCLUDES Fixation and anchoring skin graft
Routine dressing
Simple tissue debridement

EXCLUDES Adjacent tissue transfer (14000-14302)
Excision of:
Benign lesion (11400-11471)
Burn eschar or scar (15002-15005)
Malignant lesion (11600-11646)
Flaps without addition of a vascular pedicle (15570-15576)
Primary procedure such as radical mastectomy, extensive tumor removal, orbitectomy (see appropriate anatomical section)
Skin graft for repair of donor site (15050-15278)

Code also repair of donor site with skin grafts or flaps (14000-14350, 15050-15278)

15740 Flap; island pedicle requiring identification and dissection of an anatomically named axial vessel

EXCLUDES V-Y subcutaneous flaps, random island flaps, and other flaps from adjacent areas (14000-14302)

🔾 24.4 ⚖ 28.9 **FUD** 090 T A2 ▣

AMA: 2015,Jan,16; 2014,Jan,11; 2012,Dec,6-8; 2012,Jan,15-42; 2011,Jan,11; 2010,Apr,3-4

15750 neurovascular pedicle

EXCLUDES V-Y subcutaneous flaps, random island flaps, and other flaps from adjacent areas (14000-14302)

🔾 26.4 ⚖ 26.4 **FUD** 090 T A2 80 ▣

AMA: 2010,Apr,3-4

15756 Free muscle or myocutaneous flap with microvascular anastomosis

INCLUDES Includes operating microscope (69990)

🔾 66.8 ⚖ 66.8 **FUD** 090 C 80 ▣

AMA: 2015,Jan,16; 2014,Jan,11; 2010,Apr,3-4

15757 Free skin flap with microvascular anastomosis

INCLUDES Includes operating microscope (69990)

🔾 66.2 ⚖ 66.2 **FUD** 090 C 80 ▣

AMA: 2015,Jan,16; 2014,Jan,11; 2010,Apr,3-4

15758 Free fascial flap with microvascular anastomosis

INCLUDES Includes operating microscope (69990)

🔾 66.1 ⚖ 66.1 **FUD** 090 C 80 ▣

AMA: 2015,Jan,16; 2014,Jan,11; 2010,Apr,3-4

15760-15770 Grafts Comprising Multiple Tissue Types

INCLUDES   Fixation and anchoring skin graft
Routine dressing
Simple tissue debridement

EXCLUDES   Adjacent tissue transfer (14000-14302)
Excision of:
    Benign lesion (11400-11471)
    Burn eschar or scar (15002-15005)
    Malignant lesion (11600-11646)
Flaps without addition of vascular pedicle (15570-15576)
Microvascular repair (15756-15758)
Primary procedure such as extensive tumor removal (see appropriate anatomical site)
Repair of donor site with skin grafts or flaps (14000-14350, 15050-15278)
Skin graft (15050-15278)

15760   **Graft; composite (eg, full thickness of external ear or nasal ala), including primary closure, donor area**
    20.3   24.2   **FUD** 090   T A2
    AMA: 2015,Jan,16; 2014,Jan,11; 2010,Apr,3-4

15770   **derma-fat-fascia**
    19.2   19.2   **FUD** 090   T A2 80
    AMA: 2015,Jan,16; 2014,Jan,11; 2010,Apr,3-4

15775-15839 Plastic, Reconstructive, and Aesthetic Surgery

CMS: 100-2,16,10 Exclusions from Coverage; 100-2,16,120 Cosmetic Procedures; 100-2,16,180 Services Related to Noncovered Procedures

15775   **Punch graft for hair transplant; 1 to 15 punch grafts**
    EXCLUDES   Strip transplant (15220)
    6.16   8.29   **FUD** 000   T A2 80
    AMA: 2015,Jan,16; 2014,Jan,11

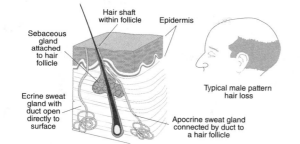

Hair shaft within follicle
Epidermis
Sebaceous gland attached to hair follicle
Ecrine sweat gland with duct open directly to surface
Apocrine sweat gland connected by duct to a hair follicle
Typical male pattern hair loss

15776   **more than 15 punch grafts**
    EXCLUDES   Strip transplant (15220)
    9.89   13.5   **FUD** 000   T A2 80
    AMA: 2015,Jan,16; 2014,Jan,11

+ **15777**   **Implantation of biologic implant (eg, acellular dermal matrix) for soft tissue reinforcement (ie, breast, trunk) (List separately in addition to code for primary procedure)**
    EXCLUDES   Application of skin substitute to an external wound (15271-15278)
      Mesh implantation for:
        Open repair of ventral or incisional hernia (49568)
        Repair of devitalized soft tissue infection (49568)
        Repair of pelvic floor (57267)
       Repair anorectal fistula with plug (46707)
      Soft tissue reinforcement with biologic implants other than in the breast or trunk (17999)
    Code also supply of biologic implant
    Code first primary procedure   *17999.14*
    6.16   6.16   **FUD** ZZZ   N N1 50
    AMA: 2015,Jan,16; 2014,Jan,11; 2013,Oct,15; 2012,Jan,6-10

15780   **Dermabrasion; total face (eg, for acne scarring, fine wrinkling, rhytids, general keratosis)**
    18.3   24.1   **FUD** 090   T P3 80
    AMA: 2015,Jan,16; 2014,Jan,11; 2012,Jan,15-42; 2011,Jan,11

15781   **segmental, face**
    12.3   15.6   **FUD** 090   T P3
    AMA: 1997,Nov,1

15782   **regional, other than face**
    12.8   18.1   **FUD** 090   T P2 80
    AMA: 1997,Nov,1

15783   **superficial, any site (eg, tattoo removal)**
    10.6   13.7   **FUD** 090   T P2 80
    AMA: 2015,Jan,16; 2014,Jan,11

15786   **Abrasion; single lesion (eg, keratosis, scar)**
    3.85   6.86   **FUD** 010   Q1 N1
    AMA: 1997,Nov,1

+ **15787**   **each additional 4 lesions or less (List separately in addition to code for primary procedure)**
    Code first (15786)
    0.49   1.38   **FUD** ZZZ   N N1
    AMA: 1997,Nov,1

15788   **Chemical peel, facial; epidermal**
    7.02   13.0   **FUD** 090   Q1 N1
    AMA: 1997,Nov,1; 1993,Win,1

15789   **dermal**
    12.1   15.7   **FUD** 090   T P2
    AMA: 1997,Nov,1; 1993,Win,1

15792   **Chemical peel, nonfacial; epidermal**
    7.29   12.2   **FUD** 090   Q1 N1 80
    AMA: 1997,Nov,1; 1993,Win,1

15793   **dermal**
    10.4   13.9   **FUD** 090   Q1 N1 80
    AMA: 1997,Nov,1; 1993,Win,1

15819   **Cervicoplasty**
    22.6   22.6   **FUD** 090   T G2 80
    AMA: 1997,Nov,1

15820   **Blepharoplasty, lower eyelid;**
    14.5   16.1   **FUD** 090   T A2 80 50
    AMA: 2015,Jan,16; 2014,Jan,11; 2012,Jan,15-42; 2011,Jan,11

15821   **with extensive herniated fat pad**
    15.4   17.1   **FUD** 090   T A2 80 50
    AMA: 2015,Jan,16; 2014,Jan,11

15822   **Blepharoplasty, upper eyelid;**
    11.0   12.6   **FUD** 090   T A2 50
    AMA: 2015,Jan,16; 2014,Jan,11

15823   **with excessive skin weighting down lid**
    15.4   17.1   **FUD** 090   T A2 50
    AMA: 2015,Jan,16; 2014,Jan,11; 2011,Aug,8

15824   **Rhytidectomy; forehead**
    EXCLUDES   Repair of brow ptosis (67900)
    0.00   0.00   **FUD** 000   T A2 80 50
    AMA: 1997,Nov,1

Frontalis (elevates brow)
Forehead rhytidectomy incision (15824)
A rhytidectomy is an excision to eliminate wrinkles. This procedure in the forehead region typically involves an incision just inside the scalp line. Skin and underlying tissues are then manipulated to eliminate wrinkles in the forehead
Procerus (wrinkles nose)
Corrugators (move brows medially)

15825   **neck with platysmal tightening (platysmal flap, P-flap)**
    0.00   0.00   **FUD** 000   T A2 80 50
    AMA: 1997,Nov,1

15826   **glabellar frown lines**
    0.00   0.00   **FUD** 000   T A2 80 50
    AMA: 1997,Nov,1

15828 cheek, chin, and neck
🔲 0.00 ⚓ 0.00 **FUD** 000 [T] [A2] [80] [50] [□]
AMA: 1997,Nov,1

15829 superficial musculoaponeurotic system (SMAS) flap
🔲 0.00 ⚓ 0.00 **FUD** 000 [T] [A2] [80] [50] [□]
AMA: 1997,Nov,1

15830 Excision, excessive skin and subcutaneous tissue (includes lipectomy); abdomen, infraumbilical panniculectomy
🔲 33.6 ⚓ 33.6 **FUD** 090 [T] [A2] [80] [□]
EXCLUDES Other abdominoplasty (17999)
Code also (15847)
Do not report with (12031-12032, 12034-12037, 13100-13102, 14000-14001, 14302)

15832 thigh
🔲 26.1 ⚓ 26.1 **FUD** 090 [T] [A2] [80] [50] [□]
AMA: 1997,Nov,1

15833 leg
🔲 24.9 ⚓ 24.9 **FUD** 090 [T] [A2] [80] [50] [□]
AMA: 1997,Nov,1

15834 hip
🔲 25.4 ⚓ 25.4 **FUD** 090 [T] [A2] [80] [50] [□]
AMA: 1997,Nov,1

15835 buttock
🔲 26.8 ⚓ 26.8 **FUD** 090 [T] [A2] [80] [□]
AMA: 1997,Nov,1

15836 arm
🔲 22.5 ⚓ 22.5 **FUD** 090 [T] [A2] [80] [50] [□]
AMA: 1997,Nov,1

15837 forearm or hand
🔲 21.3 ⚓ 25.2 **FUD** 090 [T] [G2] [80] [□]
AMA: 1997,Nov,1

15838 submental fat pad
🔲 16.3 ⚓ 16.3 **FUD** 090 [T] [G2] [80] [□]
AMA: 1998,Feb,1; 1997,Nov,1

15839 other area
🔲 21.1 ⚓ 25.1 **FUD** 090 [T] [A2] [80] [□]
AMA: 1997,Nov,1

15840-15845 Reanimation of the Paralyzed Face

INCLUDES Routine dressing and supplies
EXCLUDES Intravenous fluorescein evaluation of blood flow in graft or flap (15860)
Nerve:
  Decompression (69720, 69725, 69955)
  Pedicle transfer (64905, 64907)
  Suture (64831-64876, 69740, 69745)
Code also repair of donor site with skin grafts or flaps

15840 Graft for facial nerve paralysis; free fascia graft (including obtaining fascia)
🔲 28.8 ⚓ 28.8 **FUD** 090 [T] [A2] [□]
AMA: 1997,Nov,1

15841 free muscle graft (including obtaining graft)
🔲 46.0 ⚓ 46.0 **FUD** 090 [T] [A2] [80] [□]
AMA: 1997,Nov,1

15842 free muscle flap by microsurgical technique
INCLUDES Operating microscope (69990)
🔲 70.2 ⚓ 70.2 **FUD** 090 [T] [G2] [80] [□]
AMA: 1997,Nov,1

15845 regional muscle transfer
🔲 28.6 ⚓ 28.6 **FUD** 090 [T] [A2] [80] [□]
AMA: 1998,Feb,1; 1997,Nov,1

15847 Removal of Excess Abdominal Tissue Add-on

CMS: 100-2,16,10 Exclusions from Coverage; 100-2,16,120 Cosmetic Procedures; 100-2,16,180 Services Related to Noncovered Procedures

+ **15847** Excision, excessive skin and subcutaneous tissue (includes lipectomy), abdomen (eg, abdominoplasty) (includes umbilical transposition and fascial plication) (List separately in addition to code for primary procedure)
🔲 0.00 ⚓ 0.00 **FUD** YYY [N] [N1] [80]
EXCLUDES Abdominal wall hernia repair (49491-49587)
Other abdominoplasty (17999)
Code first (15830)

15850-15852 Suture Removal/Dressing Change: Anesthesia Required

15850 Removal of sutures under anesthesia (other than local), same surgeon
🔲 1.13 ⚓ 2.46 **FUD** XXX [T] [G2]
AMA: 2015,Jan,16; 2014,Jan,11

15851 Removal of sutures under anesthesia (other than local), other surgeon
🔲 1.31 ⚓ 2.80 **FUD** 000 [T] [P3]
AMA: 2015,Jan,16; 2014,Jan,11

15852 Dressing change (for other than burns) under anesthesia (other than local)
EXCLUDES Dressing change for burns (16020-16030)
🔲 1.36 ⚓ 1.36 **FUD** 000 [Q1] [N1]
AMA: 1997,Nov,1

15860 Injection for Vascular Flow Determination

15860 Intravenous injection of agent (eg, fluorescein) to test vascular flow in flap or graft
🔲 3.20 ⚓ 3.20 **FUD** 000 [Q1] [N1] [80] [□]
AMA: 2002,May,7; 1997,Nov,1

15876-15879 Liposuction

CMS: 100-2,16,10 Exclusions from Coverage; 100-2,16,120 Cosmetic Procedures; 100-2,16,180 Services Related to Noncovered Procedures

15876 Suction assisted lipectomy; head and neck
🔲 0.00 ⚓ 0.00 **FUD** 000 [T] [A2] [80] [□]
AMA: 1997,Nov,1

Cannula typically inserted through incision in front of ear

15877 trunk
🔲 0.00 ⚓ 0.00 **FUD** 000 [T] [A2] [80] [□]
AMA: 2015,Jan,16; 2014,Jan,11; 2012,Jan,15-42; 2011,Jan,11

15878 upper extremity
🔲 0.00 ⚓ 0.00 **FUD** 000 [T] [A2] [80] [50] [□]
AMA: 1997,Nov,1

15879 lower extremity
🔲 0.00 ⚓ 0.00 **FUD** 000 [T] [A2] [80] [50] [□]
AMA: 1997,Nov,1

15920-15999 Treatment of Decubitus Ulcers

Code also free skin graft to repair ulcer or donor site

15920 Excision, coccygeal pressure ulcer, with coccygectomy; with primary suture
🔲 17.2 ⚓ 17.2 **FUD** 090 [T] [A2] [80] [□]
AMA: 2011,May,3-5

15922 with flap closure
🔲 22.3 ⚓ 22.3 **FUD** 090 [T] [A2] [80] [□]
AMA: 2011,May,3-5

| [26]/[10] PC/TC Comp Only | [A2]-[Z3] ASC Pmt | [50] Bilateral | ♂ Male Only | ♀ Female Only | 🔲 Facility RVU | ⚓ Non-Facility RVU |
| **AMA:** CPT Asst | **CMS:** Pub 100 | [A]-[Y] OPPSI | [80]/[80] Surg Assist Allowed / w/Doc | | [▪] Lab Crosswalk | [▪] Radiology Crosswalk |

26   Medicare (Red Text)   CPT © 2015 American Medical Association. All Rights Reserved. (Black Text)   © 2015 Optum360, LLC (Blue Text)

15931 Excision, sacral pressure ulcer, with primary suture;
🚑 19.7　🔪 19.7　**FUD** 090　　T A2 📄
AMA: 2011,May,3-5

15933 with ostectomy
🚑 24.3　🔪 24.3　**FUD** 090　　T A2 80 📄
AMA: 2011,May,3-5

15934 Excision, sacral pressure ulcer, with skin flap closure;
🚑 26.7　🔪 26.7　**FUD** 090　　T A2 📄
AMA: 2011,May,3-5

15935 with ostectomy
🚑 31.5　🔪 31.5　**FUD** 090　　T A2 80 📄
AMA: 2011,May,3-5

15936 Excision, sacral pressure ulcer, in preparation for muscle or myocutaneous flap or skin graft closure;
Code also any defect repair with:
Muscle or myocutaneous flap (15734, 15738)
Split skin graft (15100-15101)
🚑 25.4　🔪 25.4　**FUD** 090　　T A2 📄
AMA: 2011,May,3-5

15937 with ostectomy
Code also any defect repair with:
Muscle or myocutaneous flap (15734, 15738)
Split skin graft (15100-15101)
🚑 29.4　🔪 29.4　**FUD** 090　　T A2 📄
AMA: 2011,May,3-5

15940 Excision, ischial pressure ulcer, with primary suture;
🚑 20.0　🔪 20.0　**FUD** 090　　T A2 📄
AMA: 2011,May,3-5

15941 with ostectomy (ischiectomy)
🚑 25.8　🔪 25.8　**FUD** 090　　T A2 80 📄
AMA: 2011,May,3-5

15944 Excision, ischial pressure ulcer, with skin flap closure;
🚑 25.6　🔪 25.6　**FUD** 090　　T A2 80 📄
AMA: 2011,May,3-5

15945 with ostectomy
🚑 27.9　🔪 27.9　**FUD** 090　　T A2 80 📄
AMA: 2011,May,3-5

15946 Excision, ischial pressure ulcer, with ostectomy, in preparation for muscle or myocutaneous flap or skin graft closure
Code also any defect repair with:
Muscle or myocutaneous flap (15734, 15738)
Split skin graft (15100-15101)
🚑 46.8　🔪 46.8　**FUD** 090　　T A2 📄
AMA: 2015,Jan,16; 2014,Jan,11; 2012,Jan,15-42; 2011,May,3-5; 2011,Jan,11

15950 Excision, trochanteric pressure ulcer, with primary suture;
🚑 16.9　🔪 16.9　**FUD** 090　　T A2 📄
AMA: 2011,May,3-5

15951 with ostectomy
🚑 25.1　🔪 25.1　**FUD** 090　　T A2 80 📄
AMA: 2011,May,3-5

15952 Excision, trochanteric pressure ulcer, with skin flap closure;
🚑 25.8　🔪 25.8　**FUD** 090　　T A2 80 📄
AMA: 2011,May,3-5

15953 with ostectomy
🚑 28.4　🔪 28.4　**FUD** 090　　T A2 📄
AMA: 2011,May,3-5

15956 Excision, trochanteric pressure ulcer, in preparation for muscle or myocutaneous flap or skin graft closure;
Code also any defect repair with:
Muscle or myocutaneous flap (15734, 15738)
Split skin graft (15100-15101)
🚑 32.9　🔪 32.9　**FUD** 090　　T A2 📄
AMA: 2011,May,3-5

15958 with ostectomy
Code also any defect repair with:
Muscle or myocutaneous flap (15734-15738)
Split skin graft (15100-15101)
🚑 33.6　🔪 33.6　**FUD** 090　　T A2 📄
AMA: 2011,May,3-5

15999 Unlisted procedure, excision pressure ulcer
🚑 0.00　🔪 0.00　**FUD** YYY　　T 80
AMA: 2011,May,3-5

16000-16036 Burn Care

INCLUDES Local care of burn surface only

EXCLUDES *Application of skin grafts including all services described in the following codes (15100-15777)*
Evaluation and management services
Flaps (15570-15650)

16000 Initial treatment, first degree burn, when no more than local treatment is required
🚑 1.32　🔪 1.95　**FUD** 000　　Q1 N1 📄
AMA: 2015,Jan,16; 2014,Jan,11; 2012,Oct,3-8

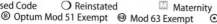

Head and neck 9%
Each arm 9%
Posterior trunk 18%
Anterior trunk 18%
Genitalia 1%
Posterior leg 9%
Anterior leg 9%

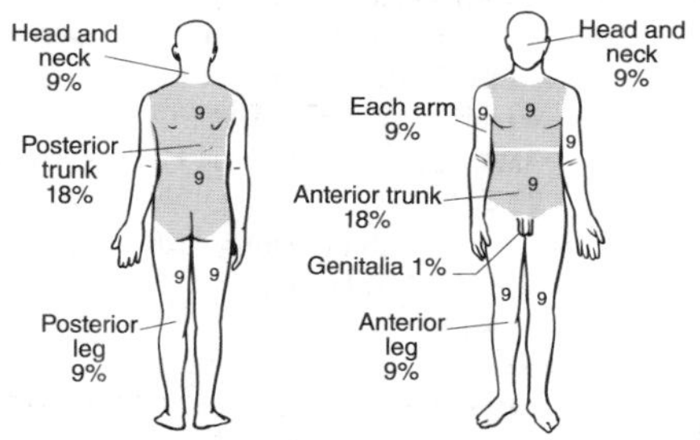

16020 Dressings and/or debridement of partial-thickness burns, initial or subsequent; small (less than 5% total body surface area)
INCLUDES Wound coverage other than skin graft
🚑 1.55　🔪 2.32　**FUD** 000　　T P3 📄
AMA: 2015,Jan,16; 2014,Jan,11; 2012,Oct,3-8

16025 medium (eg, whole face or whole extremity, or 5% to 10% total body surface area)
INCLUDES Wound coverage other than skin graft
🚑 3.21　🔪 4.21　**FUD** 000　　T A2 📄
AMA: 2015,Jan,16; 2014,Jan,11; 2012,Oct,3-8; 2012,Jan,15-42; 2011,Jan,11

16030 large (eg, more than 1 extremity, or greater than 10% total body surface area)
INCLUDES Wound coverage other than skin graft
🚑 3.79　🔪 5.19　**FUD** 000　　T A2 📄
AMA: 2015,Jan,16; 2014,Jan,11; 2012,Oct,3-8; 2012,Jan,15-42; 2011,Jan,11

16035 Escharotomy; initial incision
EXCLUDES *Debridement or scraping of burn (16020-16030)*
🚑 5.59　🔪 5.59　**FUD** 000　　T G2 📄
AMA: 2015,Jan,16; 2014,Jan,11; 2012,Oct,3-8

+ 16036 each additional incision (List separately in addition to code for primary procedure)
EXCLUDES *Debridement or scraping of burn (16020-16030)*
Code first (16035)
🚑 2.34　🔪 2.34　**FUD** ZZZ　　C
AMA: 2015,Jan,16; 2014,Jan,11; 2012,Oct,3-8

● New Code　▲ Revised Code　○ Reinstated　Ⓜ Maternity　Ⓐ Age Edit　Unlisted　　# Resequenced
⊘ AMA Mod 51 Exempt　⑤ Optum Mod 51 Exempt　⑥ Mod 63 Exempt　⊙ Mod Sedation　+ Add-on　　Not Covered　FUD Follow-up Days
　　　　　　　　　　　　　　　　　　　　　　　CCI　ⓅⓆ PQRS

17000-17004 Destruction Any Method: Premalignant Lesion

CMS: 100-3,140.5 Laser Procedures

EXCLUDES   *Cryotherapy acne (17340)*
Destruction of:
  Benign lesions other than cutaneous vascular proliferative lesions (17110-17111)
  Cutaneous vascular proliferative lesions (17106-17108)
  Malignant lesions (17260-17286)
  Plantar warts (17110-17111)
Destruction of lesion of:
  Anus (46900-46917, 46924)
  Conjunctiva (68135)
  Eyelid (67850)
  Penis (54050-54057, 54065)
  Vagina (57061, 57065)
  Vestibule of mouth (40820)
  Vulva (56501, 56515)
Destruction or excision of skin tags (11200-11201)
Localized chemotherapy treatment see appropriate office visit service code
Paring or excision of benign hyperkeratotic lesion (11055-11057)
Shaving skin lesions (11300-11313)
Treatment of inflammatory skin disease via laser (96920-96922)

17000   **Destruction (eg, laser surgery, electrosurgery, cryosurgery, chemosurgery, surgical curettement), premalignant lesions (eg, actinic keratoses); first lesion**
  🔧 1.50   ⚕ 1.87   **FUD** 010   T P3 ▭
  AMA: 2015,Jan,16; 2014,Jan,11; 2012,May,13; 2012,Mar,4-7; 2012,Jan,15-42; 2011,Jan,11; 2010,Oct,9; 2010,Mar,9-11

+ 17003   **second through 14 lesions, each (List separately in addition to code for first lesion)**
  Code first (17000)
  🔧 0.07   ⚕ 0.16   **FUD** ZZZ   N N1
  AMA: 2015,Jan,16; 2014,Jan,11; 2012,May,13; 2012,Jan,15-42; 2011,Jan,11; 2010,Mar,9-11

17004   **Destruction (eg, laser surgery, electrosurgery, cryosurgery, chemosurgery, surgical curettement), premalignant lesions (eg, actinic keratoses), 15 or more lesions**
  Do not report with (17000-17003)
  🔧 2.83   ⚕ 4.23   **FUD** 010   ⊘ T P3 ▭
  AMA: 2015,Jan,16; 2014,Jan,11; 2012,May,13; 2012,Jan,15-42; 2011,Jan,11; 2010,Mar,9-11

17106-17250 Destruction Any Method: Vascular Proliferative Lesion

CMS: 100-2,16,10 Exclusions from Coverage; 100-2,16,120 Cosmetic Procedures

EXCLUDES   *Destruction of lesion of:*
  Anus (46900-46917, 46924)
  Conjunctiva (68135)
  Eyelid (67850)
  Penis (54050-54057, 54065)
  Vagina (57061, 57065)
  Vestibule of mouth (40820)
  Vulva (56501, 56515)
Treatment of inflammatory skin disease via laser (96920-96922)

17106   **Destruction of cutaneous vascular proliferative lesions (eg, laser technique); less than 10 sq cm**
  🔧 7.86   ⚕ 9.67   **FUD** 090   T P2 ▭
  AMA: 2015,Jan,16; 2014,Jan,11; 2012,May,13; 2012,Jan,15-42; 2011,Jan,11; 2010,Oct,9

17107   **10.0 to 50.0 sq cm**
  🔧 9.83   ⚕ 12.2   **FUD** 090   T P2 ▭
  AMA: 2015,Jan,16; 2014,Jan,11; 2012,May,13; 2012,Jan,15-42; 2011,Jan,11; 2010,Oct,9

17108   **over 50.0 sq cm**
  🔧 15.0   ⚕ 18.1   **FUD** 090   T P2 80 ▭
  AMA: 2015,Jan,16; 2014,Jan,11; 2012,May,13; 2012,Jan,15-42; 2011,Jan,11; 2010,Oct,9

17110   **Destruction (eg, laser surgery, electrosurgery, cryosurgery, chemosurgery, surgical curettement), of benign lesions other than skin tags or cutaneous vascular proliferative lesions; up to 14 lesions**
  🔧 1.97   ⚕ 3.12   **FUD** 010   Q1 N1 ▭
  AMA: 2015,Jan,16; 2014,Jan,11; 2012,May,13; 2012,Jan,15-42; 2011,Jan,11; 2010,Oct,9

17111   **15 or more lesions**
  🔧 2.43   ⚕ 3.70   **FUD** 010   T P2 ▭
  AMA: 2015,Jan,16; 2014,Jan,11; 2012,May,13; 2012,Jan,15-42; 2011,Jan,11; 2010,Oct,9

17250   **Chemical cauterization of granulation tissue (proud flesh, sinus or fistula)**
  Do not report with excision/removal codes for the same lesion
  🔧 1.05   ⚕ 2.24   **FUD** 000   T P3 ▭
  AMA: 2015,Jan,16; 2014,Jan,11; 2012,Dec,12; 2012,May,13; 2012,Jan,15-42; 2011,Jan,11; 2010,Oct,9

17260-17286 Destruction, Any Method: Malignant Lesion

CMS: 100-3,140.5 Laser Procedures

EXCLUDES   *Destruction of lesion of:*
  Anus (46900-46917, 46924)
  Conjunctiva (68135)
  Eyelid (67850)
  Penis (54050-54057, 54065)
  Vestibule of mouth (40820)
  Vulva (56501-56515)
Localized chemotherapy treatment see appropriate office visit service code
Shaving skin lesion (11300-11313)
Treatment of inflammatory skin disease via laser (96920-96922)

17260   **Destruction, malignant lesion (eg, laser surgery, electrosurgery, cryosurgery, chemosurgery, surgical curettement), trunk, arms or legs; lesion diameter 0.5 cm or less**
  🔧 1.99   ⚕ 2.67   **FUD** 010   T P3 ▭
  AMA: 2015,Jan,16; 2014,Jan,11; 2012,May,13

17261   **lesion diameter 0.6 to 1.0 cm**
  🔧 2.61   ⚕ 4.05   **FUD** 010   T P2 ▭
  AMA: 2015,Jan,16; 2014,Jan,11; 2012,May,13

17262   **lesion diameter 1.1 to 2.0 cm**
  🔧 3.32   ⚕ 4.93   **FUD** 010   T P2 ▭
  AMA: 2015,Jan,16; 2014,Jan,11; 2012,May,13

17263   **lesion diameter 2.1 to 3.0 cm**
  🔧 3.68   ⚕ 5.38   **FUD** 010   T P2 ▭
  AMA: 2015,Jan,16; 2014,Jan,11; 2012,May,13

17264   **lesion diameter 3.1 to 4.0 cm**
  🔧 3.94   ⚕ 5.79   **FUD** 010   T P2 ▭
  AMA: 2015,Jan,16; 2014,Jan,11; 2012,May,13

17266   **lesion diameter over 4.0 cm**
  🔧 4.62   ⚕ 6.55   **FUD** 010   T P3 ▭
  AMA: 2015,Jan,16; 2014,Jan,11; 2012,May,13

17270   **Destruction, malignant lesion (eg, laser surgery, electrosurgery, cryosurgery, chemosurgery, surgical curettement), scalp, neck, hands, feet, genitalia; lesion diameter 0.5 cm or less**
  🔧 2.85   ⚕ 4.25   **FUD** 010   T P2 ▭
  AMA: 2015,Jan,16; 2014,Jan,11; 2012,May,13

17271   **lesion diameter 0.6 to 1.0 cm**
  🔧 3.17   ⚕ 4.61   **FUD** 010   T P2 ▭
  AMA: 2015,Jan,16; 2014,Jan,11; 2012,May,13

17272   **lesion diameter 1.1 to 2.0 cm**
  🔧 3.65   ⚕ 5.24   **FUD** 010   T P2 ▭
  AMA: 2015,Jan,16; 2014,Jan,11; 2012,May,13

17273   **lesion diameter 2.1 to 3.0 cm**
  🔧 4.13   ⚕ 5.86   **FUD** 010   T P3 ▭
  AMA: 2015,Jan,16; 2014,Jan,11; 2012,May,13

17274   **lesion diameter 3.1 to 4.0 cm**
  🔧 5.03   ⚕ 6.90   **FUD** 010   T P3 ▭
  AMA: 2015,Jan,16; 2014,Jan,11; 2012,May,13

26/TC PC/TC Comp Only   A2-Z3 ASC Pmt   50 Bilateral   ♂ Male Only   ♀ Female Only   🔧 Facility RVU   ⚕ Non-Facility RVU
AMA: CPT Asst   **CMS:** Pub 100   A-Y OPPSI   80/80 Surg Assist Allowed / w/Doc   🔲 Lab Crosswalk   ✚ Radiology Crosswalk

28   Medicare (Red Text)   CPT © 2015 American Medical Association. All Rights Reserved. (Black Text)   © 2015 Optum360, LLC (Blue Text)

17276   lesion diameter over 4.0 cm
     6.03   7.98   **FUD** 010   T P2
     AMA: 2015,Jan,16; 2014,Jan,11; 2012,May,13

17280   **Destruction, malignant lesion (eg, laser surgery, electrosurgery, cryosurgery, chemosurgery, surgical curettement); face, ears, eyelids, nose, lips, mucous membrane; lesion diameter 0.5 cm or less**
     2.59   3.97   **FUD** 010   T P2
     AMA: 2015,Jan,16; 2014,Jan,11; 2012,May,13

17281   lesion diameter 0.6 to 1.0 cm
     3.56   5.01   **FUD** 010   T P2
     AMA: 2015,Jan,16; 2014,Jan,11; 2012,May,13

17282   lesion diameter 1.1 to 2.0 cm
     4.12   5.76   **FUD** 010   T P3
     AMA: 2015,Jan,16; 2014,Jan,11; 2012,May,13

17283   lesion diameter 2.1 to 3.0 cm
     5.13   6.88   **FUD** 010   T P3
     AMA: 2015,Jan,16; 2014,Jan,11; 2012,May,13

17284   lesion diameter 3.1 to 4.0 cm
     6.01   7.88   **FUD** 010   T P3
     AMA: 2015,Jan,16; 2014,Jan,11; 2012,May,13

17286   lesion diameter over 4.0 cm
     8.10   10.1   **FUD** 010   T P2
     AMA: 2015,Jan,16; 2014,Jan,11; 2012,May,13

17311-17315 Mohs Surgery

INCLUDES   The following surgical/pathology services performed by the same physician or other qualified health care provider:
   Evaluation of skin margins by surgeon
   Pathology exam on Mohs surgery specimen (88302-88309)
   Routine frozen section stain (88314)
   Tumor removal, mapping, preparation, and examination of lesion

EXCLUDES   *Frozen section if no prior diagnosis determination has been performed (88331)*
Code also any special histochemical stain on a frozen section, nonroutine (with modifier 59) (88311-88314, 88342)
Code also biopsy (with modifier 59) if no prior diagnosis determination has been performed, if biopsy is indeterminate, or performed more than 90 days preoperatively (11100-11101)
Code also complex repair (13100-13160)
Code also flaps or grafts (14000-14350, 15050-15770)
Code also intermediate repair (12031-12057)
Code also simple repair (12001-12021)

17311   **Mohs micrographic technique, including removal of all gross tumor, surgical excision of tissue specimens, mapping, color coding of specimens, microscopic examination of specimens by the surgeon, and histopathologic preparation including routine stain(s) (eg, hematoxylin and eosin, toluidine blue), head, neck, hands, feet, genitalia, or any location with surgery directly involving muscle, cartilage, bone, tendon, major nerves, or vessels; first stage, up to 5 tissue blocks**
     10.7   18.6   **FUD** 000   T P2 P0
     AMA: 2015,Jan,16; 2014,Oct,14; 2014,Feb,10; 2012,May,13

+ **17312**   **each additional stage after the first stage, up to 5 tissue blocks (List separately in addition to code for primary procedure)**
     Code first (17311)
     5.76   10.9   **FUD** ZZZ   N N1
     AMA: 2015,Jan,16; 2014,Oct,14; 2014,Feb,10; 2012,May,13

17313   **Mohs micrographic technique, including removal of all gross tumor, surgical excision of tissue specimens, mapping, color coding of specimens, microscopic examination of specimens by the surgeon, and histopathologic preparation including routine stain(s) (eg, hematoxylin and eosin, toluidine blue), of the trunk, arms, or legs; first stage, up to 5 tissue blocks**
     9.69   17.4   **FUD** 000   T P2 P0
     AMA: 2015,Jan,16; 2014,Oct,14; 2014,Feb,10; 2012,May,13

+ **17314**   **each additional stage after the first stage, up to 5 tissue blocks (List separately in addition to code for primary procedure)**
     Code first (17313)
     5.33   10.5   **FUD** ZZZ   N N1
     AMA: 2015,Jan,16; 2014,Oct,14; 2014,Feb,10; 2012,May,13

+ **17315**   **Mohs micrographic technique, including removal of all gross tumor, surgical excision of tissue specimens, mapping, color coding of specimens, microscopic examination of specimens by the surgeon, and histopathologic preparation including routine stain(s) (eg, hematoxylin and eosin, toluidine blue), each additional block after the first 5 tissue blocks, any stage (List separately in addition to code for primary procedure)**
     Code first (17311-17314)
     1.51   2.25   **FUD** ZZZ   N N1
     AMA: 2015,Jan,16; 2014,Oct,14; 2014,Feb,10; 2014,Jan,11; 2012,May,13

17340-17999 Treatment for Active Acne and Permanent Hair Removal

CMS: 100-2,16,10 Exclusions from Coverage; 100-2,16,120 Cosmetic Procedures

17340   **Cryotherapy (CO2 slush, liquid N2) for acne**
     1.40   1.47   **FUD** 010   Q1 N1
     AMA: 2015,Jan,16; 2014,Jan,11; 2012,May,13

17360   **Chemical exfoliation for acne (eg, acne paste, acid)**
     2.80   3.63   **FUD** 010   T P3
     AMA: 2015,Jan,16; 2014,Jan,11; 2012,May,13

17380   **Electrolysis epilation, each 30 minutes**
     EXCLUDES   *Actinotherapy (96900)*
     0.00   0.00   **FUD** 000   T R2 80
     AMA: 2015,Jan,16; 2014,Jan,11; 2012,May,13

17999   **Unlisted procedure, skin, mucous membrane and subcutaneous tissue**

17999.14 Bio implant (handwritten)

     0.00   0.00   **FUD** YYY   Q1 80
     AMA: 2015,Jan,16; 2014,Jan,11; 2013,Oct,15; 2012,May,13; 2012,Jan,15-42; 2011,Mar,9; 2011,Jan,11

19000-19030 Treatment of Breast Abscess and Cyst with Injection, Aspiration, Incision

19000   **Puncture aspiration of cyst of breast;**
     (76942, 77021)
     1.26   3.21   **FUD** 000   T P3
     AMA: 2015,Jan,16; 2014,Jan,11; 2013,Dec,16

+ **19001**   **each additional cyst (List separately in addition to code for primary procedure)**
     Code first (19000)
     (76942, 77021)
     0.63   0.77   **FUD** ZZZ   N N1
     AMA: 2015,Jan,16; 2014,Jan,11; 2013,Dec,16

19020   **Mastotomy with exploration or drainage of abscess, deep**
     8.72   13.4   **FUD** 090   T A2 50
     AMA: 2015,Jan,16; 2014,Dec,16; 2014,Dec,16; 2014,Jan,11

19030   **Injection procedure only for mammary ductogram or galactogram**
     (77053-77054)
     2.26   4.71   **FUD** 000   N N1 50
     AMA: 2015,Jan,16; 2014,Jan,11

19081-19086 Breast Biopsy with Imaging Guidance

CMS: 100-3,220.13 Percutaneous Image-guided Breast Biopsy; 100-4,12,40.7 Bilateral Procedures; 100-4,13,80.1 Physician Presence; 100-4,13,80.2 S&I Multiple Procedure Reduction

INCLUDES Breast biopsy with placement of localization devices

EXCLUDES *Biopsy of breast without imaging guidance (19100-19101)*
Lesion removal without concentration on surgical margins (19110-19126)
Open biopsy after placement of localization device (19101, 19281-19288)
Partial mastectomy (19301-19302)
Placement of localization devices only (19281-19288)
Total mastectomy (19303-19307)
Code also additional biopsies performed with different imaging modalities
Do not report for same lesion with (19281-19288, 76098, 76942, 77002, 77021)

19081 **Biopsy, breast, with placement of breast localization device(s) (eg, clip, metallic pellet), when performed, and imaging of the biopsy specimen, when performed, percutaneous; first lesion, including stereotactic guidance**
🔲 4.84   ⚕ 18.8   **FUD** 000   T G2 80 50
AMA: 2015,May,8; 2015,Mar,5; 2015,Jan,16; 2014,Jun,14; 2014,May,3

+ 19082 **each additional lesion, including stereotactic guidance (List separately in addition to code for primary procedure)**
Code first (19081)
🔲 2.42   ⚕ 15.4   **FUD** ZZZ   N N1 80
AMA: 2015,May,8; 2015,Mar,5; 2015,Jan,16; 2014,Jun,14; 2014,May,3

19083 **Biopsy, breast, with placement of breast localization device(s) (eg, clip, metallic pellet), when performed, and imaging of the biopsy specimen, when performed, percutaneous; first lesion, including ultrasound guidance**
🔲 4.77   ⚕ 18.4   **FUD** 000   T G2 80 50
AMA: 2015,May,8; 2015,Mar,5; 2015,Jan,16; 2014,Jun,14; 2014,May,3

+ 19084 **each additional lesion, including ultrasound guidance (List separately in addition to code for primary procedure)**
Code first (19083)
🔲 2.28   ⚕ 14.8   **FUD** ZZZ   N N1 80
AMA: 2015,May,8; 2015,Mar,5; 2015,Jan,16; 2014,Jun,14; 2014,May,3

19085 **Biopsy, breast, with placement of breast localization device(s) (eg, clip, metallic pellet), when performed, and imaging of the biopsy specimen, when performed, percutaneous; first lesion, including magnetic resonance guidance**
🔲 5.80   ⚕ 29.1   **FUD** 000   T G2 80 50
AMA: 2015,May,8; 2015,Mar,5; 2015,Jan,16; 2014,Jun,14; 2014,May,3

+ 19086 **each additional lesion, including magnetic resonance guidance (List separately in addition to code for primary procedure)**
Code first (19085)
🔲 2.73   ⚕ 23.2   **FUD** ZZZ   N N1 80
AMA: 2015,May,8; 2015,Mar,5; 2015,Jan,16; 2014,Jun,14; 2014,May,3

19100-19101 Breast Biopsy Without Imaging Guidance

EXCLUDES *Biopsy of breast with imaging guidance (19081-19086)*
Lesion removal without concentration on surgical margins (19110-19126)
Partial mastectomy (19301-19302)
Total mastectomy (19303-19307)

19100 **Biopsy of breast; percutaneous, needle core, not using imaging guidance (separate procedure)**
EXCLUDES *Fine needle aspiration:*
With imaging guidance (10022)
Without imaging guidance (10021)
🔲 2.03   ⚕ 4.31   **FUD** 000   T A2 50 ▦ PQ
AMA: 2015,Jan,16; 2014,May,3; 2014,Jan,11; 2012,Jan,15-42; 2011,Jan,11

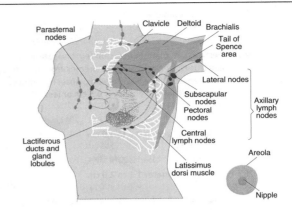

19101 **open, incisional**
Code also placement of localization device with imaging guidance (19281-19288)
🔲 6.37   ⚕ 9.70   **FUD** 010   T A2 50 ▦ PQ
AMA: 2015,Jan,16; 2014,May,3; 2014,Jan,11; 2012,Jan,15-42; 2011,Jan,11

19105 Treatment of Fibroadenoma: Cryoablation

CMS: 100-4,13,80.1 Physician Presence; 100-4,13,80.2 S&I Multiple Procedure Reduction

INCLUDES Adjacent lesions treated with one cryoprobe
Ultrasound guidance

19105 **Ablation, cryosurgical, of fibroadenoma, including ultrasound guidance, each fibroadenoma**
Do not report with (76940, 76942)
🔲 5.88   ⚕ 70.8   **FUD** 000   T P2 50
AMA: 2007,Mar,7-8

19110-19126 Excisional Procedures: Breast

INCLUDES Open removal of breast mass without concentration on surgical margins

19110 **Nipple exploration, with or without excision of a solitary lactiferous duct or a papilloma lactiferous duct**
🔲 9.78   ⚕ 13.7   **FUD** 090   T A2 50 ▦
AMA: 2015,Jan,16; 2014,Jan,11

19112 **Excision of lactiferous duct fistula**
🔲 8.96   ⚕ 13.1   **FUD** 090   T A2 80 50 ▦
AMA: 2015,Jan,16; 2014,Jan,11

19120 **Excision of cyst, fibroadenoma, or other benign or malignant tumor, aberrant breast tissue, duct lesion, nipple or areolar lesion (except 19300), open, male or female, 1 or more lesions**
🔲 11.8   ⚕ 14.0   **FUD** 090   T A2 50 ▦
AMA: 2015,Mar,5; 2015,Jan,16; 2014,Mar,13; 2014,Jan,11; 2012,Jan,15-42; 2011,Jan,11

26/TC PC/TC Comp Only	A2-Z1 ASC Pmt	50 Bilateral	♂ Male Only	♀ Female Only	🔲 Facility RVU	⚕ Non-Facility RVU
AMA: CPT Asst						

CMS: Pub 100   A-Y OPPSI   80/80 Surg Assist Allowed / w/Doc   ▦ Lab Crosswalk   ▦ Radiology Crosswalk

30   Medicare (Red Text)   CPT © 2015 American Medical Association. All Rights Reserved. (Black Text)   © 2015 Optum360, LLC (Blue Text)

19125 **Excision of breast lesion identified by preoperative placement of radiological marker, open; single lesion**
13.1　15.6　**FUD** 090　T A2 50 ▢ PQ
AMA: 2015,Mar,5; 2015,Jan,16; 2014,Jan,11; 2012,Jan,15-42; 2011,Jan,11

\+ 19126 **each additional lesion separately identified by a preoperative radiological marker (List separately in addition to code for primary procedure)**
Code first (19125)
4.68　4.68　**FUD** ZZZ　N N1 ▢
AMA: 2015,Jan,16; 2014,Jan,11; 2012,Jan,15-42; 2011,Jan,11

19260-19272 Excisional Procedures: Chest Wall
Do not report with (32100, 32503-32504, 32551, 32554-32555)

19260 **Excision of chest wall tumor including ribs**
34.6　34.6　**FUD** 090　T 80 ▢ PQ
AMA: 2015,Jan,16; 2014,Jan,11; 2012,Oct,9-11; 2012,Sep,3-8; 2010,Apr,3-4

19271 **Excision of chest wall tumor involving ribs, with plastic reconstruction; without mediastinal lymphadenectomy**
46.8　46.8　**FUD** 090　C 80 ▢ PQ
AMA: 2015,Jan,16; 2014,Jan,11; 2012,Oct,9-11; 2012,Sep,3-8

19272 **with mediastinal lymphadenectomy**
51.4　51.4　**FUD** 090　C 80 ▢ PQ
AMA: 2015,Jan,16; 2014,Jan,11; 2012,Oct,9-11; 2012,Sep,3-8

19281-19288 Placement of Localization Markers
INCLUDES Placement of localization devices only
EXCLUDES *Biopsy of breast without imaging guidance (19100-19101)*
Localization device placement with biopsy of breast (19081-19086)
Code also open incisional breast biopsy when performed after localization device placement (19101)
Code also radiography of surgical specimen (76098)
Do not report for same lesion with (19081-19086, 76942, 77002, 77021)

19281 **Placement of breast localization device(s) (eg, clip, metallic pellet, wire/needle, radioactive seeds), percutaneous; first lesion, including mammographic guidance**
2.94　6.80　**FUD** 000　Q1 N1 80 50
AMA: 2015,May,8; 2015,Jan,16; 2014,Jun,14; 2014,May,3

\+ 19282 **each additional lesion, including mammographic guidance (List separately in addition to code for primary procedure)**
Code first (19281)
1.49　4.76　**FUD** ZZZ　N N1 80
AMA: 2015,May,8; 2015,Jan,16; 2014,Jun,14; 2014,May,3

19283 **Placement of breast localization device(s) (eg, clip, metallic pellet, wire/needle, radioactive seeds), percutaneous; first lesion, including stereotactic guidance**
2.95　7.75　**FUD** 000　Q1 N1 80 50
AMA: 2015,May,8; 2015,Jan,16; 2014,May,3

\+ 19284 **each additional lesion, including stereotactic guidance (List separately in addition to code for primary procedure)**
Code first (19283)
1.50　5.73　**FUD** ZZZ　N N1 80
AMA: 2015,May,8; 2015,Jan,16; 2014,May,3

19285 **Placement of breast localization device(s) (eg, clip, metallic pellet, wire/needle, radioactive seeds), percutaneous; first lesion, including ultrasound guidance**
2.51　12.6　**FUD** 000　Q1 N1 80 50
AMA: 2015,May,8; 2015,Jan,16; 2014,May,3

\+ 19286 **each additional lesion, including ultrasound guidance (List separately in addition to code for primary procedure)**
Code first (19285)
1.27　10.7　**FUD** ZZZ　N N1 80
AMA: 2015,May,8; 2015,Jan,16; 2014,May,3

19287 **Placement of breast localization device(s) (eg clip, metallic pellet, wire/needle, radioactive seeds), percutaneous; first lesion, including magnetic resonance guidance**
3.96　24.7　**FUD** 000　Q1 N1 80 50
AMA: 2015,Jan,16; 2014,May,3

\+ 19288 **each additional lesion, including magnetic resonance guidance (List separately in addition to code for primary procedure)**
Code first (19287)
1.93　19.8　**FUD** ZZZ　N N1 80
AMA: 2015,Jan,16; 2014,May,3

19296-19298 Insertion Radiotherapy Afterloading Catheters
CMS: 100-4,12,40.7 Bilateral Procedures

19296 **Placement of radiotherapy afterloading expandable catheter (single or multichannel) into the breast for interstitial radioelement application following partial mastectomy, includes imaging guidance; on date separate from partial mastectomy**
6.08　110.　**FUD** 000　J P2 80 50 ▢
AMA: 2015,Jan,16; 2014,Jan,11; 2012,Jan,15-42; 2011,Jan,11; 2010,Mar,9-11

\+ 19297 **concurrent with partial mastectomy (List separately in addition to code for primary procedure)**
Code first (19301-19302)
2.74　2.74　**FUD** ZZZ　N N1 80 ▢
AMA: 2015,Jan,16; 2014,Jan,11; 2012,Jan,15-42; 2010,Mar,9-11

19298 **Placement of radiotherapy afterloading brachytherapy catheters (multiple tube and button type) into the breast for interstitial radioelement application following (at the time of or subsequent to) partial mastectomy, includes imaging guidance**
9.39　29.6　**FUD** 000　⊙ J J8 80 50 ▢
AMA: 2015,Jan,16; 2014,Jan,11

19300-19307 Mastectomies: Partial, Simple, Radical
CMS: 100-4,12,40.7 Bilateral Procedures
EXCLUDES *Insertion of prosthesis (19340, 19342)*

19300 **Mastectomy for gynecomastia**　♂
11.8　14.9　**FUD** 090　T A2 50
AMA: 2015,Jan,16; 2014,Mar,13; 2014,Jan,11

19301 **Mastectomy, partial (eg, lumpectomy, tylectomy, quadrantectomy, segmentectomy);**
EXCLUDES *Insertion of radiotherapy afterloading balloon or brachytherapy catheters (19296-19298)*
18.7　18.7　**FUD** 090　T A2 80 50 PQ
AMA: 2015,Mar,5; 2015,Jan,16; 2014,Jan,11; 2013,Nov,14; 2012,Jan,15-42; 2011,Jan,11; 2010,Mar,9-11

19302 **with axillary lymphadenectomy**
EXCLUDES *Insertion of radiotherapy afterloading balloon or brachytherapy catheters (19296-19298)*
25.8　25.8　**FUD** 090　T A2 80 50 PQ
AMA: 2015,Mar,5; 2015,Jan,16; 2014,Jan,11; 2012,Jan,15-42; 2011,Jan,11; 2010,Mar,9-11

19303 **Mastectomy, simple, complete**
EXCLUDES *Gynecomastia (19300)*
29.0　29.0　**FUD** 090　T A2 80 50 PQ
AMA: 2015,Mar,5; 2015,Jan,16; 2014,Jan,11

19304 **Mastectomy, subcutaneous**
16.4　16.4　**FUD** 090　T A2 80 50 PQ
AMA: 2015,Jan,16; 2014,Jan,11; 2012,Jan,15-42; 2011,Jan,11

19305 **Mastectomy, radical, including pectoral muscles, axillary lymph nodes**
32.3　32.3　**FUD** 090　C 80 50 PQ
AMA: 2015,Jan,16; 2014,Jan,11

19306 **Mastectomy, radical, including pectoral muscles, axillary and internal mammary lymph nodes (Urban type operation)**
34.4　34.4　**FUD** 090　C 80 50 PQ
AMA: 2015,Jan,16; 2014,Jan,11

Integumentary System

19307 — 19499

19307 **Mastectomy, modified radical, including axillary lymph nodes, with or without pectoralis minor muscle, but excluding pectoralis major muscle**
🚑 34.3 ⚅ 34.3 **FUD** 090 Ⓣ 80 50 P0
AMA: 2015,Mar,5; 2015,Jan,16; 2014,Jan,11

19316-19499 Plastic, Reconstructive, and Aesthetic Breast Procedures

CMS: 100-3,140.2 Breast Reconstruction Following Mastectomy; 100-4,12,40.7 Bilateral Procedures
Code also biologic implant for tissue reinforcement (15777)

19316 **Mastopexy**
🚑 22.0 ⚅ 22.0 **FUD** 090 Ⓣ A2 80 50 P0
AMA: 2015,Jan,16; 2014,Jan,11; 2012,Feb,11

19318 **Reduction mammaplasty**
INCLUDES   Aries-Pitanguy mammaplasty
Biesenberger mammaplasty
🚑 31.5 ⚅ 31.5 **FUD** 090 Ⓣ A2 80 50 P0
AMA: 2015,Jan,16; 2014,Apr,10; 2014,Jan,11; 2012,Jan,15-42; 2011,Jan,11

19324 **Mammaplasty, augmentation; without prosthetic implant**
🚑 14.0 ⚅ 14.0 **FUD** 090 Ⓣ A2 80 50 P0
AMA: 2015,Jan,16; 2014,Jan,11

19325 **with prosthetic implant**
EXCLUDES   Flap or graft (15100-15650)
🚑 18.3 ⚅ 18.3 **FUD** 090 Ⓙ J8 80 50 P0
AMA: 2015,Jan,16; 2014,Jan,11

19328 **Removal of intact mammary implant**
🚑 14.1 ⚅ 14.1 **FUD** 090 02 A2 50 P0
AMA: 2015,Jan,16; 2014,Jan,11

19330 **Removal of mammary implant material**
🚑 18.1 ⚅ 18.1 **FUD** 090 02 A2 50 P0
AMA: 2015,Jan,16; 2014,Jan,11; 2012,Jan,15-42; 2011,Jan,11

19340 **Immediate insertion of breast prosthesis following mastopexy, mastectomy or in reconstruction**
EXCLUDES   Supply of prosthetic implant (99070, L8030, L8039, L8600)
🚑 28.7 ⚅ 28.7 **FUD** 090 Ⓣ A2 50
AMA: 2015,Jan,16; 2014,Jan,11; 2012,Jan,15-42; 2010,Mar,9-11

19342 **Delayed insertion of breast prosthesis following mastopexy, mastectomy or in reconstruction**
EXCLUDES   Preparation of moulage for custom breast implant (19396)
🚑 26.4 ⚅ 26.4 **FUD** 090 Ⓙ J8 80 50 P0
AMA: 2015,Jan,16; 2014,Jan,11; 2013,Jan,15-16

19350 **Nipple/areola reconstruction**
🚑 19.2 ⚅ 23.4 **FUD** 090 Ⓣ A2 50 P0
AMA: 2015,Jan,16; 2014,Jan,11; 2013,Jan,15-16; 2012,Jan,15-42; 2011,Jan,11

19355 **Correction of inverted nipples**
🚑 16.4 ⚅ 20.0 **FUD** 090 Ⓣ A2 80 50 P0
AMA: 2015,Jan,16; 2014,Jan,11

19357 **Breast reconstruction, immediate or delayed, with tissue expander, including subsequent expansion**
🚑 43.0 ⚅ 43.0 **FUD** 090 Ⓙ J8 80 50 P0
AMA: 2015,Feb,10; 2015,Jan,16; 2014,Jan,11; 2013,Oct,15; 2012,Jan,15-42; 2010,Mar,9-11

19361 **Breast reconstruction with latissimus dorsi flap, without prosthetic implant**
EXCLUDES   Implant of prosthesis (19340)
🚑 45.1 ⚅ 45.1 **FUD** 090 Ⓒ 80 50 P0
AMA: 2015,Feb,10; 2015,Jan,16; 2014,Jan,11; 2010,Mar,9-11

19364 **Breast reconstruction with free flap**
INCLUDES   Closure of donor site
Harvesting of skin graft
Inset shaping of flap into breast
Microvascular repair
Operating microscope (69990)
🚑 79.1 ⚅ 79.1 **FUD** 090 Ⓒ 80 50 P0
AMA: 2015,Feb,10; 2015,Jan,16; 2014,Apr,10; 2014,Jan,11; 2013,Mar,13; 2012,Jul,12-14; 2012,Jan,15-42; 2011,Dec,14-18; 2011,Jan,11; 2010,Jun,8

19366 **Breast reconstruction with other technique**
EXCLUDES   Operating microscope (69990)
Code also implant of prosthesis if appropriate (19340, 19342)
🚑 40.4 ⚅ 40.4 **FUD** 090 Ⓣ A2 80 50 P0
AMA: 2015,Feb,10; 2015,Jan,16; 2014,Apr,10; 2014,Jan,11; 2012,Jan,15-42; 2011,Dec,14-18

19367 **Breast reconstruction with transverse rectus abdominis myocutaneous flap (TRAM), single pedicle, including closure of donor site;**
🚑 51.4 ⚅ 51.4 **FUD** 090 Ⓒ 80 50 P0
AMA: 2015,Feb,10; 2015,Jan,16; 2014,Jan,11

19368 **with microvascular anastomosis (supercharging)**
INCLUDES   Operating microscope (69990)
🚑 63.2 ⚅ 63.2 **FUD** 090 Ⓒ 80 50 P0
AMA: 2015,Feb,10; 2015,Jan,16; 2014,Jan,11

19369 **Breast reconstruction with transverse rectus abdominis myocutaneous flap (TRAM), double pedicle, including closure of donor site**
🚑 58.6 ⚅ 58.6 **FUD** 090 Ⓒ 80 50 P0
AMA: 2015,Feb,10; 2015,Jan,16; 2014,Jan,11

19370 **Open periprosthetic capsulotomy, breast**
🚑 19.6 ⚅ 19.6 **FUD** 090 Ⓣ A2 50 P0
AMA: 2015,Jan,16; 2014,Jan,11

19371 **Periprosthetic capsulectomy, breast**
🚑 22.4 ⚅ 22.4 **FUD** 090 Ⓣ A2 50 P0
AMA: 2015,Jan,16; 2014,Jan,11; 2013,Jan,15-16; 2012,Jan,15-42; 2011,Jan,11

19380 **Revision of reconstructed breast**
🚑 22.1 ⚅ 22.1 **FUD** 090 Ⓣ A2 50 P0
AMA: 2015,Jan,16; 2014,Jan,11

19396 **Preparation of moulage for custom breast implant**
🚑 4.19 ⚅ 8.29 **FUD** 000 Ⓣ 62 80 50
AMA: 2015,Jan,16; 2014,Jan,11

19499 **Unlisted procedure, breast**
🚑 0.00 ⚅ 0.00 **FUD** YYY Ⓣ 80 50
AMA: 2015,Mar,5; 2015,Jan,16; 2014,Dec,16; 2014,Dec,16; 2014,Jan,11; 2013,Nov,14; 2012,Jan,15-42; 2011,Jan,11

20005 Incisional Treatment Soft Tissue Abscess

EXCLUDES *Superficial incision and drainage (10040-10160)*

20005 **Incision and drainage of soft tissue abscess, subfascial (ie, involves the soft tissue below the deep fascia)**
🔲 6.69 ⚕ 8.76 **FUD** 010 [T][G2][▭]

20100-20103 Exploratory Surgery of Traumatic Wound

INCLUDES Debridement
Expanded dissection of wound for exploration
Extraction of foreign material
Open examination
Tying or coagulation of small vessels

EXCLUDES *Cutaneous/subcutaneous incision and drainage procedures (10060-10061)*
Laparotomy (49000-49010)
Repair of major vessels of:
Abdomen (35221, 35251, 35281)
Chest (35211, 35216, 35241, 35246, 35271, 35276)
Extremity (35206-35207, 35226, 35236, 35256, 35266, 35286)
Neck (35201, 35231, 35261)
Thoracotomy (32100-32160)

20100 **Exploration of penetrating wound (separate procedure); neck**
🔲 17.5 ⚕ 17.5 **FUD** 010 [T][80][50][▭]
AMA: 2015,Jan,16; 2014,Jan,11; 2012,Jan,15-42; 2011,Jan,11

20101 **chest**
🔲 6.04 ⚕ 12.8 **FUD** 010 [T][▭]
AMA: 2015,Jan,16; 2014,Jan,11; 2012,Jan,15-42; 2011,Jan,11

20102 **abdomen/flank/back**
🔲 7.36 ⚕ 13.9 **FUD** 010 [T][▭]
AMA: 2015,Jan,16; 2014,Jan,11; 2012,Jan,15-42; 2011,Jan,11

20103 **extremity**
🔲 9.98 ⚕ 16.5 **FUD** 010 [T][G2][80][▭]
AMA: 2015,Jan,16; 2014,Jan,11; 2012,Jan,15-42; 2011,Jan,11

20150 Epiphyseal Bar Resection

EXCLUDES *Bone marrow aspiration (38220)*

20150 **Excision of epiphyseal bar, with or without autogenous soft tissue graft obtained through same fascial incision**
🔲 26.0 ⚕ 26.0 **FUD** 090 [T][G2][80][50][▭]
AMA: 1996,Nov,1

20200-20206 Muscle Biopsy

EXCLUDES *Removal of muscle tumor (see appropriate anatomic section)*

20200 **Biopsy, muscle; superficial**
🔲 2.76 ⚕ 5.91 **FUD** 000 [T][A2][▭][PQ]

20205 **deep**
🔲 4.51 ⚕ 8.24 **FUD** 000 [T][A2][▭][PQ]

20206 **Biopsy, muscle, percutaneous needle**
INCLUDES Fluoroscopic guidance (77002)
EXCLUDES *Fine needle aspiration (10021-10022)*
🔳 (76942, 77012, 77021)
🔳 (88172-88173)
🔲 1.71 ⚕ 6.71 **FUD** 000 [T][A2][▭][PQ]
AMA: 2001,Jan,8

20220-20225 Percutaneous Bone Biopsy

EXCLUDES *Bone marrow biopsy (38221)*

20220 **Biopsy, bone, trocar, or needle; superficial (eg, ilium, sternum, spinous process, ribs)**
🔳 (77002, 77012, 77021)
🔲 2.10 ⚕ 4.79 **FUD** 000 [T][A2][▭][PQ]
AMA: 2015,Jan,16; 2014,Jan,11

20225 **deep (eg, vertebral body, femur)**
Do not report at same level as (22510-22515, 0200T-0201T)
🔳 (77002, 77012, 77021)
🔲 3.16 ⚕ 14.9 **FUD** 000 [T][A2][▭][PQ]
AMA: 2015,Jan,16; 2015,Jan,8; 2014,Jan,11; 2012,Jun,10-11

20240-20251 Open Bone Biopsy

EXCLUDES *Sequestrectomy or incision and drainage of bone abscess of:*
Calcaneus (28120)
Carpal bone (25145)
Clavicle (23170)
Humeral head (23174)
Humerus (24134)
Olecranon process (24138)
Radius (24136, 25145)
Scapula (23172)
Skull (61501)
Talus (28120)
Ulna (24138, 24145)

20240 **Biopsy, bone, open; superficial (eg, ilium, sternum, spinous process, ribs, trochanter of femur)**
🔲 6.23 ⚕ 6.23 **FUD** 010 [T][A2][▭][PQ]
AMA: 2015,Jan,16; 2014,Jan,11; 2012,Jan,15-42; 2011,Jan,11

20245 **deep (eg, humerus, ischium, femur)**
🔲 17.7 ⚕ 17.7 **FUD** 010 [T][A2][▭][PQ]
AMA: 2015,Jan,16; 2014,Jan,11

20250 **Biopsy, vertebral body, open; thoracic**
🔲 11.3 ⚕ 11.3 **FUD** 010 [T][A2][▭][PQ]
AMA: 2015,Jan,16; 2014,Jan,11

20251 **lumbar or cervical**
🔲 12.1 ⚕ 12.1 **FUD** 010 [T][A2][80][▭][PQ]
AMA: 2015,Jan,16; 2014,Jan,11

20500-20501 Injection Fistula/Sinus Tract

EXCLUDES *Arthrography injection of:*
Ankle (27648)
Elbow (24220)
Hip (27093, 27095)
Knee (27370)
Sacroiliac joint (27096)
Shoulder (23350)
Temporomandibular joint (TMJ) (21116)
Wrist (25246)

20500 **Injection of sinus tract; therapeutic (separate procedure)**
🔲 2.44 ⚕ 2.98 **FUD** 010 [T][P3][▭]
🔳 (76080)

20501 **diagnostic (sinogram)**
🔲 1.10 ⚕ 3.36 **FUD** 000 [N][N1][▭]
EXCLUDES *Contrast injection or injections for radiological evaluation of existing gastrostomy, duodenostomy, jejunostomy, gastro-jejunostomy, or cecostomy (or other colonic) tube from percutaneous approach (49465)*
🔳 (76080)

20520-20525 Foreign Body Removal

20520 **Removal of foreign body in muscle or tendon sheath; simple**
🔲 4.21 ⚕ 5.79 **FUD** 010 [T][P3][▭]

20525 **deep or complicated**
🔲 7.18 ⚕ 13.7 **FUD** 010 [T][A2][▭]

20526-20553 Therapeutic Injections: Tendons, Trigger Points

EXCLUDES *Platelet rich plasma (PRP) injections (0232T)*

20526 **Injection, therapeutic (eg, local anesthetic, corticosteroid), carpal tunnel**
🔲 1.66 ⚕ 2.20 **FUD** 000 [T][P3][50][▭]
AMA: 2015,Jan,16; 2014,Jan,11; 2012,Jan,15-42; 2011,Jan,11

20527 **Injection, enzyme (eg, collagenase), palmar fascial cord (ie, Dupuytren's contracture)**
EXCLUDES *Post injection palmar fascial cord manipulation (26341)*
🔲 1.91 ⚕ 2.40 **FUD** 000 [T][P3][50]
AMA: 2015,Jan,16; 2014,Jan,11; 2012,Jul,8

Musculoskeletal System

20550 — 20690

20550 Injection(s); single tendon sheath, or ligament, aponeurosis (eg, plantar "fascia")

　　EXCLUDES Morton's neuroma (64455, 64632)

　　Do not report with (0232T)

　　🔅 (76942, 77002, 77021)

　　🏥 1.20　🔻 1.68　**FUD** 000　　T P3 50 ▭

　　AMA: 2015,Jan,16; 2014,Oct,9; 2014,Jan,11; 2012,Jul,8; 2012,Jan,15-42; 2011,Jan,11

20551 single tendon origin/insertion

　　EXCLUDES Platelet rich plasma injection (0232T)

　　Do not report with (0232T)

　　🔅 (76942, 77002, 77021)

　　🏥 1.23　🔻 1.72　**FUD** 000　　T P3 ▭

　　AMA: 2015,Jan,16; 2014,Oct,9; 2014,Jan,11; 2012,Jan,15-42; 2011,Jan,11

20552 Injection(s); single or multiple trigger point(s), 1 or 2 muscle(s)

　　🔅 (76942, 77002, 77021)

　　🏥 1.08　🔻 1.56　**FUD** 000　　T P3 ▭

　　AMA: 2015,Jan,16; 2014,Oct,9; 2014,Jan,11; 2012,Apr,19; 2012,Jan,15-42; 2011,Jul,16-17; 2011,Feb,4-5; 2011,Jan,11; 2010,Jan,9-11

20553 single or multiple trigger point(s), 3 or more muscles

　　🔅 (76942, 77002, 77021)

　　🏥 1.23　🔻 1.81　**FUD** 000　　T P3 ▭

　　AMA: 2015,Jan,16; 2014,Oct,9; 2014,Jan,11; 2012,Jan,15-42; 2011,Jul,16-17; 2011,Feb,4-5; 2011,Jan,11; 2010,Jan,9-11

20555 Placement of Catheters/Needles for Brachytherapy

CMS: 100-4,13,70.4 Clinical Brachytherapy

Code also interstitial radioelement application (77770-77772, 77778)

Do not report with (0232T)

20555 Placement of needles or catheters into muscle and/or soft tissue for subsequent interstitial radioelement application (at the time of or subsequent to the procedure)

　　EXCLUDES Interstitial radioelement:

　　　　Devices placed into the breast (19296-19298)

　　　　Placement of needle, catheters, or devices into muscle or soft tissue of the head and neck (41019)

　　　　Placement of needles or catheters into pelvic organs or genitalia (55920)

　　　　Placement of needles or catheters into prostate (55875)

　　🔅 (76942, 77002, 77012, 77021)

　　🏥 9.56　🔻 9.56　**FUD** 000　　T B2 80 ▭

　　AMA: 2015,Jan,16; 2014,Jan,11; 2012,Jan,15-42; 2011,Jan,11

20600-20611 Aspiration and/or Injection of Joint

CMS: 100-3,150.7 Prolotherapy, Joint Sclerotherapy, and Ligamentous Injections with Sclerosing Agents

20600 Arthrocentesis, aspiration and/or injection, small joint or bursa (eg, fingers, toes); without ultrasound guidance

　　Do not report with (76942)

　　🔅 (77002, 77012, 77021)

　　🏥 1.02　🔻 1.35　**FUD** 000　　T P3 50 ▭

　　AMA: 2015,Feb,6; 2015,Jan,16; 2014,Jan,11

20604 with ultrasound guidance, with permanent recording and reporting

　　Do not report with (76942)

　　🔅 (77002, 77012, 77021)

　　🏥 1.32　🔻 2.05　**FUD** 000　　T P3 50 ▭

　　AMA: 2015,Jul,10; 2015,Feb,6

20605 Arthrocentesis, aspiration and/or injection, intermediate joint or bursa (eg, temporomandibular, acromioclavicular, wrist, elbow or ankle, olecranon bursa); without ultrasound guidance

　　Do not report with (76942)

　　🔅 (77002, 77012, 77021)

　　🏥 1.06　🔻 1.41　**FUD** 000　　T P3 50 ▭

　　AMA: 2015,Feb,6; 2015,Jan,16; 2014,Jan,11

20606 with ultrasound guidance, with permanent recording and reporting

　　Do not report with (76942)

　　🔅 (77002, 77012, 77021)

　　🏥 1.51　🔻 2.27　**FUD** 000　　T P3 50 ▭

　　AMA: 2015,Jul,10; 2015,Feb,6

20610 Arthrocentesis, aspiration and/or injection, major joint or bursa (eg, shoulder, hip, knee, subacromial bursa); without ultrasound guidance

　　Do not report with (27370, 76942)

　　🔅 (77002, 77012, 77021)

　　🏥 1.32　🔻 1.71　**FUD** 000　　T P3 50 ▭

　　AMA: 2015,Aug,6; 2015,Feb,6; 2015,Jan,16; 2014,Dec,18; 2014,Jan,11; 2012,Jun,14; 2012,Mar,4-7; 2012,Jan,15-42; 2011,Jan,11

20611 with ultrasound guidance, with permanent recording and reporting

　　Do not report with (27370, 76942)

　　🔅 (77002, 77012, 77021)

　　🏥 1.78　🔻 2.62　**FUD** 000　　T P3 50 ▭

　　AMA: 2015,Aug,6; 2015,Jul,10; 2015,Feb,6

20612-20615 Aspiration and/or Injection of Cyst

20612 Aspiration and/or injection of ganglion cyst(s) any location

　　🏥 1.20　🔻 1.73　**FUD** 000　　T P3 ▭

　　Code also modifier 59 for multiple major joint aspirations or injections

20615 Aspiration and injection for treatment of bone cyst

　　🏥 4.74　🔻 7.03　**FUD** 010　　T P3 ▭

20650-20697 Procedures Related to Bony Fixation

20650 Insertion of wire or pin with application of skeletal traction, including removal (separate procedure)

　　🏥 4.48　🔻 5.87　**FUD** 010　　T A2 ▭

20660 Application of cranial tongs, caliper, or stereotactic frame, including removal (separate procedure)

　　🏥 7.19　🔻 7.19　**FUD** 000　　02 ▭

　　AMA: 2015,Jan,16; 2014,Jan,11; 2012,Aug,14; 2012,Apr,13; 2012,Apr,11-13; 2012,Jan,15-42; 2011,Jan,11

20661 Application of halo, including removal; cranial

　　🏥 14.6　🔻 14.6　**FUD** 090　　C ▭

　　AMA: 2015,Jan,16; 2014,Jan,11; 2012,Aug,14

20662 pelvic

　　🏥 13.3　🔻 13.3　**FUD** 090　　T B2 80 ▭

20663 femoral

　　🏥 11.3　🔻 11.3　**FUD** 090　　T B2 80 50 ▭

20664 Application of halo, including removal, cranial, 6 or more pins placed, for thin skull osteology (eg, pediatric patients, hydrocephalus, osteogenesis imperfecta)

　　🏥 25.5　🔻 25.5　**FUD** 090　　C ▭

　　AMA: 2015,Jan,16; 2014,Jan,11; 2013,Aug,12; 2012,Aug,14

20665 Removal of tongs or halo applied by another individual

　　🏥 2.57　🔻 2.98　**FUD** 010　　01 B2 80 ▭

　　AMA: 2015,Jan,16; 2014,Jan,11; 2012,Apr,11-13

20670 Removal of implant; superficial (eg, buried wire, pin or rod) (separate procedure)

　　🏥 4.24　🔻 10.8　**FUD** 010　　02 A2 ▭

　　AMA: 2015,Jan,16; 2014,Jan,11; 2012,Apr,17-18; 2012,Jan,15-42; 2011,Jan,11

20680 deep (eg, buried wire, pin, screw, metal band, nail, rod or plate)

　　🏥 12.1　🔻 17.6　**FUD** 090　　02 A2 80 ▭

　　AMA: 2015,Jan,16; 2014,Mar,4; 2014,Jan,11; 2012,Oct,14; 2012,Sep,16; 2012,Jan,15-42; 2011,Jan,11

20690 Application of a uniplane (pins or wires in 1 plane), unilateral, external fixation system

　　🏥 17.1　🔻 17.1　**FUD** 090　　T A2 ▭

　　AMA: 2015,Jan,16; 2014,Jan,11; 2012,Jan,15-42; 2011,Jan,11

| 26/TC PC/TC Comp Only | A2-Z1 ASC Pmt | 50 Bilateral | ♂ Male Only | ♀ Female Only | 🏥 Facility RVU | 🔻 Non-Facility RVU |
| **AMA:** CPT Asst | **CMS:** Pub 100 | A-Y OPPSI | 80/80 Surg Assist Allowed / w/Doc | | 🔅 Lab Crosswalk | 🔅 Radiology Crosswalk |

34　　　　Medicare (Red Text)　　　　CPT © 2015 American Medical Association. All Rights Reserved. (Black Text)　　　© 2015 Optum360, LLC (Blue Text)

20692 Application of a multiplane (pins or wires in more than 1 plane), unilateral, external fixation system (eg, Ilizarov, Monticelli type)
🖐 32.1   ⚖ 32.1   **FUD** 090   T A2 80 ▭
AMA: 2015,Jan,16; 2014,Jan,11; 2012,Jan,15-42; 2011,Jan,11

20693 Adjustment or revision of external fixation system requiring anesthesia (eg, new pin[s] or wire[s] and/or new ring[s] or bar[s])
🖐 12.8   ⚖ 12.8   **FUD** 090   T A2 ▭
AMA: 2015,Jan,16; 2014,Jan,11; 2012,Jan,15-42; 2011,Jan,11

20694 Removal, under anesthesia, of external fixation system
🖐 9.70   ⚖ 12.1   **FUD** 090   02 A2 ▭
AMA: 2015,Jan,16; 2014,Jan,11; 2012,Jan,15-42; 2011,Jan,11

20696 Application of multiplane (pins or wires in more than 1 plane), unilateral, external fixation with stereotactic computer-assisted adjustment (eg, spatial frame), including imaging; initial and subsequent alignment(s), assessment(s), and computation(s) of adjustment schedule(s)
Do not report with (20692, 20697)
🖐 34.8   ⚖ 34.8   **FUD** 090   T 62 80
AMA: 2015,Jan,16; 2014,Jan,11

20697 exchange (ie, removal and replacement) of strut, each
Do not report with (20692, 20696)
🖐 59.9   ⚖ 59.9   **FUD** 000   ⊘ T P2 80 IC
AMA: 2015,Jan,16; 2014,Jan,11

20802-20838 Reimplantation Procedures

EXCLUDES *Repair of incomplete amputation (see individual repair codes for bone(s), ligament(s), tendon(s), nerve(s), or blood vessel(s) and append modifier 52)*

20802 Replantation, arm (includes surgical neck of humerus through elbow joint), complete amputation
🖐 79.8   ⚖ 79.8   **FUD** 090   C 80 50 ▭
AMA: 1997,Apr,4

20805 Replantation, forearm (includes radius and ulna to radial carpal joint), complete amputation
🖐 94.6   ⚖ 94.6   **FUD** 090   C 80 50 ▭
AMA: 1997,Apr,4

20808 Replantation, hand (includes hand through metacarpophalangeal joints), complete amputation
🖐 114.   ⚖ 114.   **FUD** 090   C 80 50 ▭
AMA: 1997,Apr,4

20816 Replantation, digit, excluding thumb (includes metacarpophalangeal joint to insertion of flexor sublimis tendon), complete amputation
🖐 60.5   ⚖ 60.5   **FUD** 090   C 80 ▭
AMA: 2015,Jan,16; 2014,Jan,11; 2012,Jan,15-42; 2011,Jan,11

20822 Replantation, digit, excluding thumb (includes distal tip to sublimis tendon insertion), complete amputation
🖐 51.7   ⚖ 51.7   **FUD** 090   T 62 80 ▭
AMA: 1997,Apr,4

20824 Replantation, thumb (includes carpometacarpal joint to MP joint), complete amputation
🖐 58.5   ⚖ 58.5   **FUD** 090   C 80 50 ▭
AMA: 1997,Apr,4

20827 Replantation, thumb (includes distal tip to MP joint), complete amputation
🖐 53.1   ⚖ 53.1   **FUD** 090   C 80 50 ▭
AMA: 1997,Apr,4

20838 Replantation, foot, complete amputation
🖐 62.2   ⚖ 62.2   **FUD** 090   C 80 50 ▭
AMA: 1997,Apr,4

20900-20926 Bone and Tissue Autografts

EXCLUDES *Acquisition of autogenous bone graft, cartilage, tendon, fascia lata through distinct incision unless included in the code description*
Bone graft procedures on the spine (20930-20938)

20900 Bone graft, any donor area; minor or small (eg, dowel or button)
🖐 5.49   ⚖ 11.9   **FUD** 000   T A2 80 ▭
AMA: 2015,Jan,16; 2014,Jan,11; 2012,Jan,15-42; 2011,Jul,16-17; 2011,Jan,11

20902 major or large
🖐 8.28   ⚖ 8.28   **FUD** 000   T A2 80 ▭
AMA: 2015,Jan,16; 2014,Jan,11; 2012,Jan,15-42; 2011,Jul,16-17; 2011,Jan,11

20910 Cartilage graft; costochondral
EXCLUDES *Graft with ear cartilage (21235)*
🖐 13.1   ⚖ 13.1   **FUD** 090   T A2 80 ▭
AMA: 2015,Jan,16; 2014,Jan,11; 2013,Jan,15-16

20912 nasal septum
EXCLUDES *Graft with ear cartilage (21235)*
🖐 13.7   ⚖ 13.7   **FUD** 090   T A2 80 ▭
AMA: 2002,Apr,13; 1999,Aug,5

20920 Fascia lata graft; by stripper
🖐 11.3   ⚖ 11.3   **FUD** 090   T A2 ▭
AMA: 2015,Jan,16; 2014,Jan,11

20922 by incision and area exposure, complex or sheet
🖐 14.3   ⚖ 17.3   **FUD** 090   T A2 80 ▭
AMA: 2015,Jan,16; 2014,Jan,11

20924 Tendon graft, from a distance (eg, palmaris, toe extensor, plantaris)
🖐 14.6   ⚖ 14.6   **FUD** 090   T A2 80 ▭
AMA: 2005,Jan,7-13; 2002,Apr,13

20926 Tissue grafts, other (eg, paratenon, fat, dermis)
Do not report with (0232T)
🖐 12.3   ⚖ 12.3   **FUD** 090   T A2 ▭
AMA: 2015,Jan,16; 2014,Jan,11; 2012,Jun,15-16; 2012,Apr,14-16; 2012,Jan,15-42; 2011,Jan,11

20930-20938 Bone Allograft and Autograft of Spine

EXCLUDES *Bone marrow aspiration for bone grafting (38220)*

+ **20930** Allograft, morselized, or placement of osteopromotive material, for spine surgery only (List separately in addition to code for primary procedure)
Code first (22319, 22532-22533, 22548-22558, 22590-22612, 22630, 22633-22634, 22800-22812)
🖐 0.00   ⚖ 0.00   **FUD** XXX   N N1
AMA: 2015,Jan,16; 2014,Jan,11; 2013,Jul,3-5; 2012,Jun,10-11; 2012,Apr,14-16; 2012,Jan,15-42; 2011,Dec,14-18; 2011,Jul,16-17; 2011,Jan,11; 2010,Nov,8

+ **20931** Allograft, structural, for spine surgery only (List separately in addition to code for primary procedure)
Code first (22319, 22532-22533, 22548-22558, 22590-22612, 22630, 22633-22634, 22800-22812)
🖐 3.31   ⚖ 3.31   **FUD** ZZZ   N N1
AMA: 2015,Jan,16; 2014,Jan,11; 2013,Jul,3-5; 2012,Jun,10-11; 2012,Apr,14-16; 2012,Jan,15-42; 2011,Dec,14-18; 2011,Sep,11-12; 2011,Jul,16-17; 2011,Jan,11; 2010,Nov,8

+ **20936** Autograft for spine surgery only (includes harvesting the graft); local (eg, ribs, spinous process, or laminar fragments) obtained from same incision (List separately in addition to code for primary procedure)
Code first (22319, 22532-22533, 22548-22558, 22590-22612, 22630, 22633-22634, 22800-22812)
🖐 0.00   ⚖ 0.00   **FUD** XXX   C
AMA: 2015,Jan,16; 2014,Jan,11; 2013,Jul,3-5; 2012,Jun,10-11; 2012,Apr,14-16; 2012,Jan,15-42; 2011,Dec,14-18; 2011,Jan,11

+ **20937** morselized (through separate skin or fascial incision) (List separately in addition to code for primary procedure)
Code first (22319, 22532-22533, 22548-22558, 22590-22612, 22630, 22633-22634, 22800-22812)
🖐 4.91   ⚖ 4.91   **FUD** ZZZ   C 80 ▭
AMA: 2015,Jan,16; 2014,Jan,11; 2013,Jul,3-5; 2012,Jun,10-11; 2012,Apr,14-16; 2012,Jan,15-42; 2011,Dec,14-18; 2011,Jul,16-17; 2011,Jan,11

+ 20938 structural, bicortical or tricortical (through separate skin or fascial incision) (List separately in addition to code for primary procedure)

Code first (22319, 22532-22533, 22548-22558, 22590-22612, 22630, 22633-22634, 22800-22812)

📓 5.44 ✂ 5.44 **FUD** ZZZ 　C 80 ▣

AMA: 2015,Jan,16; 2014,Jan,11; 2013,Jul,3-5; 2012,May,11-12; 2012,Jun,10-11; 2012,Apr,14-16; 2012,Apr,11-13; 2012,Jan,15-42; 2011,Dec,14-18; 2011,Jul,16-17; 2011,Jan,11

20950 Measurement of Intracompartmental Pressure

20950 Monitoring of interstitial fluid pressure (includes insertion of device, eg, wick catheter technique, needle manometer technique) in detection of muscle compartment syndrome

📓 2.61 ✂ 7.02 **FUD** 000 　T 62 80 ▣

AMA: 2015,Jan,16; 2014,Jan,11; 2012,Jan,15-42; 2011,Jan,11

20955-20973 Bone and Osteocutaneous Grafts

INCLUDES　Operating microscope (69990)

20955 Bone graft with microvascular anastomosis; fibula

📓 72.7 ✂ 72.7 **FUD** 090 　C 80 ▣

AMA: 2015,Jan,16; 2014,Jan,11

20956 iliac crest

📓 76.7 ✂ 76.7 **FUD** 090 　C 80 ▣

AMA: 2015,Jan,16; 2014,Jan,11

20957 metatarsal

📓 60.6 ✂ 60.6 **FUD** 090 　C 80 ▣

AMA: 2015,Jan,16; 2014,Jan,11

20962 other than fibula, iliac crest, or metatarsal

📓 58.3 ✂ 58.3 **FUD** 090 　C 80 ▣

AMA: 2002,Apr,13; 1998,Nov,1

20969 Free osteocutaneous flap with microvascular anastomosis; other than iliac crest, metatarsal, or great toe

📓 79.5 ✂ 79.5 **FUD** 090 　C 80 ▣

AMA: 2015,Jan,16; 2014,Jan,11

20970 iliac crest

📓 83.0 ✂ 83.0 **FUD** 090 　C 80 ▣

AMA: 2015,Jan,16; 2014,Jan,11

20972 metatarsal

📓 66.1 ✂ 66.1 **FUD** 090 　T 62 80 ▣

AMA: 2015,Jan,16; 2014,Jan,11

20973 great toe with web space

EXCLUDES　Wrap-around repair (26551)

📓 72.9 ✂ 72.9 **FUD** 090 　T R2 80 50 ▣

AMA: 2015,Jan,16; 2014,Jan,11

20974-20979 Osteogenic Stimulation

CMS: 100-3,150.2 Osteogenic Stimulation

20974 Electrical stimulation to aid bone healing; noninvasive (nonoperative)

📓 1.45 ✂ 2.19 **FUD** 000 　⊘ A ▣

AMA: 2015,Jan,16; 2014,Jan,11; 2012,Jan,15-42; 2011,Jan,11

20975 invasive (operative)

📓 5.19 ✂ 5.19 **FUD** 000 　⊘ N N1 80 ▣

AMA: 2002,Apr,13; 2000,Nov,8

20979 Low intensity ultrasound stimulation to aid bone healing, noninvasive (nonoperative)

📓 0.92 ✂ 1.47 **FUD** 000 　Q1 N1 ▣

AMA: 2015,Jan,16; 2014,Jan,11; 2012,Jan,15-42; 2011,Jan,11

20982-20999 General Musculoskeletal Procedures

20982 Ablation therapy for reduction or eradication of 1 or more bone tumors (eg, metastasis) including adjacent soft tissue when involved by tumor extension, percutaneous, including imaging guidance when performed; radiofrequency

Do not report with (76940, 77002, 77013, 77022)

📓 11.0 ✂ 106. **FUD** 000 　⊙ T 62 50 ▣

AMA: 2015,Jul,8

20983 cryoablation

Do not report with (76940, 77002, 77013, 77022)

📓 11.4 ✂ 196. **FUD** 000 　⊙ T 62 50

AMA: 2015,Jul,8

+ 20985 Computer-assisted surgical navigational procedure for musculoskeletal procedures, image-less (List separately in addition to code for primary procedure)

EXCLUDES　Image guidance derived from intraoperative and preoperative obtained images (0054T-0055T)

Code first primary procedure

Do not report with (61781-61783)

📓 4.27 ✂ 4.27 **FUD** ZZZ 　N N1 80

AMA: 2015,Jan,16; 2014,Jan,11; 2011,Jul,12-13

20999 Unlisted procedure, musculoskeletal system, general

📓 0.00 ✂ 0.00 **FUD** YYY 　T 80

AMA: 2015,Jul,8; 2015,Jan,16; 2014,Oct,9; 2014,Jan,11

21010 Temporomandibular Joint Arthrotomy

21010 Arthrotomy, temporomandibular joint

EXCLUDES　Excision of foreign body from dentoalveolar site (41805-41806)

Soft tissue (subfascial) abscess drainage (20005)

Superficial abscess and hematoma drainage (10060-10061)

📓 21.9 ✂ 21.9 **FUD** 090 　T A2 80 50 ▣

AMA: 2002,Apr,13

21011-21016 Excision Soft Tissue Tumors Face and Scalp

INCLUDES　Any necessary elevation of tissue planes or dissection

Measurement of tumor and necessary margin at greatest diameter prior to excision

Simple and intermediate repairs

Types of excision:

Fascial or subfascial soft tissue tumors: simple and marginal resection of tumors found either in or below the deep fascia, not including bone or excision of a substantial amount of normal tissue; primarily benign and intramuscular tumors

Radical resection soft tissue tumor: wide resection of tumor involving substantial margins of normal tissue and may include tissue removal from one or more layers; most often malignant or aggressive benign

Subcutaneous: simple and marginal resection of tumors in the subcutaneous tissue above the deep fascia; most often benign

EXCLUDES　Complex repair

Excision of benign cutaneous lesions (eg, sebaceous cyst) (11420-11426)

Radical resection of cutaneous tumors (eg, melanoma) (11620-11646)

Significant exploration of vessels or neuroplasty

21011 Excision, tumor, soft tissue of face or scalp, subcutaneous; less than 2 cm

📓 7.42 ✂ 9.93 **FUD** 090 　T P3 80

AMA: 2015,Jan,16; 2014,Jan,11; 2010,Apr,3-4; 2010,Jan,3-5

21012 2 cm or greater

📓 9.70 ✂ 9.70 **FUD** 090 　T R2 80

AMA: 2015,Jan,16; 2014,Jan,11; 2010,Apr,3-4; 2010,Jan,3-5

21013 Excision, tumor, soft tissue of face and scalp, subfascial (eg, subgaleal, intramuscular); less than 2 cm

📓 11.5 ✂ 14.8 **FUD** 090 　T P3 80

AMA: 2015,Jan,16; 2014,Jan,11; 2010,Apr,3-4; 2010,Jan,3-5

21014 2 cm or greater

📓 14.9 ✂ 14.9 **FUD** 090 　T R2 80

AMA: 2015,Jan,16; 2014,Jan,11; 2010,Apr,3-4; 2010,Jan,3-5

21015 Radical resection of tumor (eg, sarcoma), soft tissue of face or scalp; less than 2 cm

EXCLUDES　Removal of cranial tumor for osteomyelitis (61501)

📓 20.3 ✂ 20.3 **FUD** 090 　T 62 ▣

AMA: 2015,Jan,16; 2014,Jan,11; 2010,Apr,3-4; 2010,Jan,3-5

21016 2 cm or greater

📓 29.3 ✂ 29.3 **FUD** 090 　T 62 80

AMA: 2015,Jan,16; 2014,Jan,11; 2010,Apr,3-4; 2010,Jan,3-5

| 26/TC PC/TC Comp Only | A2-Z3 ASC Pmt | 50 Bilateral | ♂ Male Only | ♀ Female Only | 📓 Facility RVU | ✂ Non-Facility RVU |
| AMA: CPT Asst | CMS: Pub 100 | A-Y OPPSI | 80/80 Surg Assist Allowed / w/Doc | | ▣ Lab Crosswalk | 🔲 Radiology Crosswalk |

36　　Medicare (Red Text)　CPT © 2015 American Medical Association. All Rights Reserved. (Black Text)　© 2015 Optum360, LLC (Blue Text)

21025-21070 Procedures of Cranial and Facial Bones

INCLUDES Any necessary elevation of tissue planes or dissection
Measurement of tumor and necessary margins prior to excision
Radical resection of bone tumor involves resection of the tumor (may include entire bone) and wide margins of normal tissue primarily for malignant or aggressive benign tumors
Simple and intermediate repairs

EXCLUDES *Complex repair*
Radical resection of cutaneous tumors (e.g., melanoma) (11620-11646)
Significant exploration of vessels, neuroplasty, reconstruction, or complex bone repair

Do not report excision of soft tissue codes when adjacent soft tissue is removed during the bone tumor resection (21011-21016)

21025 **Excision of bone (eg, for osteomyelitis or bone abscess); mandible**

🔧 21.8   ✂ 25.7   **FUD** 090   T A2 ▱

AMA: 2015,Jan,16; 2014,Jan,11; 2012,Jan,15-42; 2011,Oct,10

21026 **facial bone(s)**

🔧 14.4   ✂ 17.8   **FUD** 090   T A2 ▱

AMA: 2002,Apr,13

21029 **Removal by contouring of benign tumor of facial bone (eg, fibrous dysplasia)**

🔧 18.3   ✂ 21.9   **FUD** 090   T A2 80 ▱

AMA: 2002,Apr,13

Vestibular incision

Burs, files, and osteotomes used to remove bone   Area of benign bone growth

21030 **Excision of benign tumor or cyst of maxilla or zygoma by enucleation and curettage**

🔧 12.0   ✂ 14.9   **FUD** 090   T P3 50 ▱

AMA: 2015,Jan,16; 2014,Jan,11

21031 **Excision of torus mandibularis**

🔧 8.55   ✂ 11.4   **FUD** 090   T P3 50 ▱

AMA: 2002,Apr,13

21032 **Excision of maxillary torus palatinus**

🔧 8.46   ✂ 11.5   **FUD** 090   T P3 ▱

AMA: 2002,Apr,13

21034 **Excision of malignant tumor of maxilla or zygoma**

🔧 33.6   ✂ 38.0   **FUD** 090   T A2 80 ▱

AMA: 2015,Jan,16; 2014,Jan,11

21040 **Excision of benign tumor or cyst of mandible, by enucleation and/or curettage**

INCLUDES Removal of benign tumor or cyst without osteotomy
EXCLUDES *Removal of benign tumor or cyst with osteotomy (21046-21047)*

🔧 12.1   ✂ 15.1   **FUD** 090   T A2 ▱

AMA: 2015,Jan,16; 2014,Jan,11

21044 **Excision of malignant tumor of mandible;**

🔧 25.4   ✂ 25.4   **FUD** 090   T A2 80 ▱

AMA: 2002,Apr,13

21045 **radical resection**

Code also bone graft procedure (21215)

🔧 35.4   ✂ 35.4   **FUD** 090   C 80 ▱

AMA: 2002,Apr,13

21046 **Excision of benign tumor or cyst of mandible; requiring intra-oral osteotomy (eg, locally aggressive or destructive lesion[s])**

🔧 32.4   ✂ 32.4   **FUD** 090   T A2 80 ▱

AMA: 2015,Jan,16; 2014,Jan,11

21047 **requiring extra-oral osteotomy and partial mandibulectomy (eg, locally aggressive or destructive lesion[s])**

🔧 38.2   ✂ 38.2   **FUD** 090   T A2 80 ▱

AMA: 2015,Jan,16; 2014,Jan,11

21048 **Excision of benign tumor or cyst of maxilla; requiring intra-oral osteotomy (eg, locally aggressive or destructive lesion[s])**

🔧 33.3   ✂ 33.3   **FUD** 090   T R2 80 ▱

AMA: 2015,Jan,16; 2014,Jan,11

21049 **requiring extra-oral osteotomy and partial maxillectomy (eg, locally aggressive or destructive lesion[s])**

🔧 35.0   ✂ 35.0   **FUD** 090   T 80 ▱

AMA: 2015,Jan,16; 2014,Jan,11

21050 **Condylectomy, temporomandibular joint (separate procedure)**

🔧 24.2   ✂ 24.2   **FUD** 090   T A2 80 50 ▱

AMA: 2002,Apr,13

21060 **Meniscectomy, partial or complete, temporomandibular joint (separate procedure)**

🔧 23.4   ✂ 23.4   **FUD** 090   T A2 80 50 ▱

AMA: 2002,Apr,13

21070 **Coronoidectomy (separate procedure)**

🔧 17.8   ✂ 17.8   **FUD** 090   T A2 80 50 ▱

AMA: 2002,Apr,13

21073 Temporomandibular Joint Manipulation with Anesthesia

21073 **Manipulation of temporomandibular joint(s) (TMJ), therapeutic, requiring an anesthesia service (ie, general or monitored anesthesia care)**

EXCLUDES *Closed treatment of TMJ dislocation (21480, 21485)*
Manipulation of TMJ without general or MAC anesthesia (97140, 98925-98929, 98943)

🔧 7.35   ✂ 11.3   **FUD** 090   T P3 80 50 ▱

AMA: 2015,Jan,16; 2014,Jan,11; 2012,Jan,15-42; 2011,Jan,11

21076-21089 Medical Impressions for Fabrication Maxillofacial Prosthesis

INCLUDES Design, preparation, and professional services rendered by a physician or other qualified health care professional
EXCLUDES *Application or removal of caliper or tongs (20660, 20665)*
Professional services rendered for outside laboratory designed and prepared prosthesis

21076 **Impression and custom preparation; surgical obturator prosthesis**

🔧 24.4   ✂ 29.0   **FUD** 010   T P3 80 ▱

AMA: 2015,Jan,16; 2014,Jan,11; 2012,Jan,15-42; 2011,Jan,11

21077 **orbital prosthesis**

🔧 61.6   ✂ 73.0   **FUD** 090   T P3 80 50 ▱

AMA: 2015,Jan,16; 2014,Jan,11

21079 **interim obturator prosthesis**

🔧 40.8   ✂ 49.1   **FUD** 090   T P3 ▱

AMA: 2015,Jan,16; 2014,Jan,11

21080 **definitive obturator prosthesis**

🔧 45.2   ✂ 54.9   **FUD** 090   T P3 ▱

AMA: 2015,Jan,16; 2014,Jan,11

21081 **mandibular resection prosthesis**

🔧 41.8   ✂ 50.8   **FUD** 090   T P3 80 ▱

AMA: 2015,Jan,16; 2014,Jan,11

21082 **palatal augmentation prosthesis**

🔧 39.3   ✂ 48.2   **FUD** 090   T P3 80 ▱

AMA: 2015,Jan,16; 2014,Jan,11

21083   **palatal lift prosthesis**
🔹 36.5   ⚕ 45.9   **FUD** 090   T P3 80 ▦
AMA: 2015,Jan,16; 2014,Jan,11

21084   **speech aid prosthesis**
🔹 42.2   ⚕ 52.5   **FUD** 090   T P3 80 ▦
AMA: 2015,Jan,16; 2014,Jan,11

21085   **oral surgical splint**
🔹 16.5   ⚕ 22.0   **FUD** 010   T P2 80 ▦
AMA: 2015,Jan,16; 2014,Jan,11

21086   **auricular prosthesis**
🔹 45.4   ⚕ 54.2   **FUD** 090   T P3 80 50 ▦
AMA: 2015,Jan,16; 2014,Jan,11

21087   **nasal prosthesis**
🔹 45.4   ⚕ 54.2   **FUD** 090   T P3 80 ▦
AMA: 2015,Jan,16; 2014,Jan,11

21088   **facial prosthesis**
🔹 0.00   ⚕ 0.00   **FUD** 090   T R2 80 ▦
AMA: 2015,Jan,16; 2014,Jan,11

21089   **Unlisted maxillofacial prosthetic procedure**
🔹 0.00   ⚕ 0.00   **FUD** YYY   T
AMA: 2015,Jan,16; 2014,Jan,11; 2012,Jan,15-42; 2011,Jan,11

21100-21110 Application Fixation Device

21100   **Application of halo type appliance for maxillofacial fixation, includes removal (separate procedure)**
🔹 15.0   ⚕ 33.1   **FUD** 090   T A2 80 ▦
AMA: 2002,Apr,13

21110   **Application of interdental fixation device for conditions other than fracture or dislocation, includes removal**
EXCLUDES   *Removal of interdental fixation by another individual (20670-20680)*
🔹 19.5   ⚕ 23.3   **FUD** 090   02 P2 ▦
AMA: 2015,Jan,16; 2014,Jan,11; 2013,Dec,16; 2012,Jan,15-42; 2011,Jan,11

21116 Injection for TMJ Arthrogram

CMS: 100-2,15,150.1 Treatment of Temporomandibular Joint (TMJ) Syndrome; 100-4,13,80.1 Physician Presence; 100-4,13,80.2 S&I Multiple Procedure Reduction

21116   **Injection procedure for temporomandibular joint arthrography**
📷 (70332)
🔹 1.28   ⚕ 4.23   **FUD** 000   N N1 50 ▦
AMA: 2015,Aug,6

21120-21299 Repair/Reconstruction Craniofacial Bones

EXCLUDES   *Cranioplasty (21179-21180, 62120, 62140-62147)*

21120   **Genioplasty; augmentation (autograft, allograft, prosthetic material)**
🔹 13.8   ⚕ 17.2   **FUD** 090   T A2
AMA: 2002,Apr,13

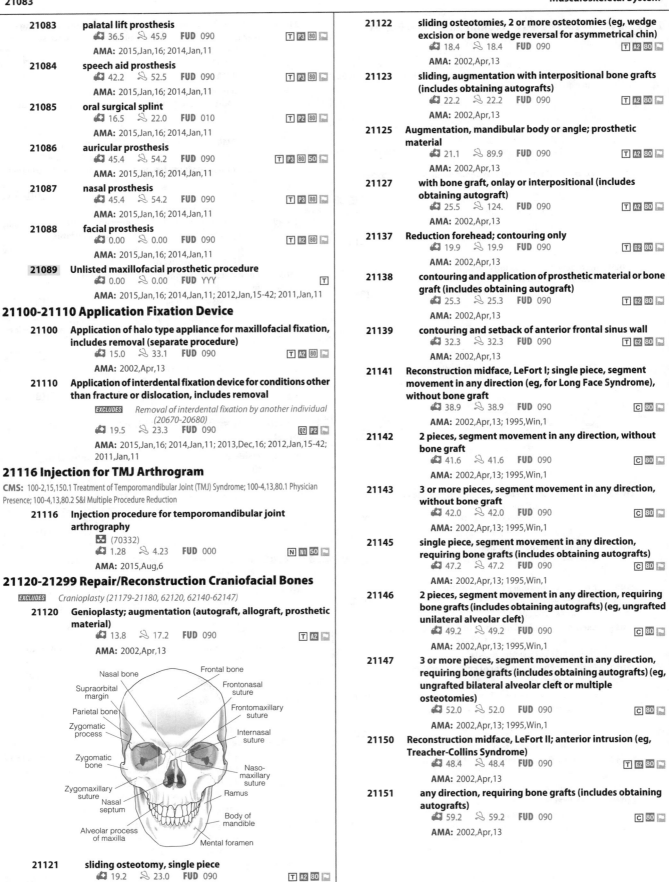

Nasal bone — Frontal bone — Frontonasal suture — Supraorbital margin — Frontomaxillary suture — Parietal bone — Internasal suture — Zygomatic process — Zygomatic bone — Naso-maxillary suture — Zygomaxillary suture — Ramus — Nasal septum — Body of mandible — Alveolar process of maxilla — Mental foramen

21121   **sliding osteotomy, single piece**
🔹 19.2   ⚕ 23.0   **FUD** 090   T A2 80 ▦
AMA: 2002,Apr,13

21122   **sliding osteotomies, 2 or more osteotomies (eg, wedge excision or bone wedge reversal for asymmetrical chin)**
🔹 18.4   ⚕ 18.4   **FUD** 090   T A2 80 ▦
AMA: 2002,Apr,13

21123   **sliding, augmentation with interpositional bone grafts (includes obtaining autografts)**
🔹 22.2   ⚕ 22.2   **FUD** 090   T A2 80 ▦
AMA: 2002,Apr,13

21125   **Augmentation, mandibular body or angle; prosthetic material**
🔹 21.1   ⚕ 89.9   **FUD** 090   T A2 80 ▦
AMA: 2002,Apr,13

21127   **with bone graft, onlay or interpositional (includes obtaining autograft)**
🔹 25.5   ⚕ 124.   **FUD** 090   T A2 80 ▦
AMA: 2002,Apr,13

21137   **Reduction forehead; contouring only**
🔹 19.9   ⚕ 19.9   **FUD** 090   T G2 80 ▦
AMA: 2002,Apr,13

21138   **contouring and application of prosthetic material or bone graft (includes obtaining autograft)**
🔹 25.3   ⚕ 25.3   **FUD** 090   T G2 80 ▦
AMA: 2002,Apr,13

21139   **contouring and setback of anterior frontal sinus wall**
🔹 32.3   ⚕ 32.3   **FUD** 090   T G2 80 ▦
AMA: 2002,Apr,13

21141   **Reconstruction midface, LeFort I; single piece, segment movement in any direction (eg, for Long Face Syndrome), without bone graft**
🔹 38.9   ⚕ 38.9   **FUD** 090   C 80 ▦
AMA: 2002,Apr,13; 1995,Win,1

21142   **2 pieces, segment movement in any direction, without bone graft**
🔹 41.6   ⚕ 41.6   **FUD** 090   C 80 ▦
AMA: 2002,Apr,13; 1995,Win,1

21143   **3 or more pieces, segment movement in any direction, without bone graft**
🔹 42.0   ⚕ 42.0   **FUD** 090   C 80 ▦
AMA: 2002,Apr,13; 1995,Win,1

21145   **single piece, segment movement in any direction, requiring bone grafts (includes obtaining autografts)**
🔹 47.2   ⚕ 47.2   **FUD** 090   C 80 ▦
AMA: 2002,Apr,13; 1995,Win,1

21146   **2 pieces, segment movement in any direction, requiring bone grafts (includes obtaining autografts) (eg, ungrafted unilateral alveolar cleft)**
🔹 49.2   ⚕ 49.2   **FUD** 090   C 80 ▦
AMA: 2002,Apr,13; 1995,Win,1

21147   **3 or more pieces, segment movement in any direction, requiring bone grafts (includes obtaining autografts) (eg, ungrafted bilateral alveolar cleft or multiple osteotomies)**
🔹 52.0   ⚕ 52.0   **FUD** 090   C 80 ▦
AMA: 2002,Apr,13; 1995,Win,1

21150   **Reconstruction midface, LeFort II; anterior intrusion (eg, Treacher-Collins Syndrome)**
🔹 48.4   ⚕ 48.4   **FUD** 090   T G2 80 ▦
AMA: 2002,Apr,13

21151   **any direction, requiring bone grafts (includes obtaining autografts)**
🔹 59.2   ⚕ 59.2   **FUD** 090   C 80 ▦
AMA: 2002,Apr,13

21154 Reconstruction midface, LeFort III (extracranial), any type, requiring bone grafts (includes obtaining autografts); without LeFort I

🔲 63.7 ✄ 63.7 **FUD** 090

AMA: 2002,Apr,13

C 80 ▢

21155 with LeFort I

🔲 67.8 ✄ 67.8 **FUD** 090

AMA: 2002,Apr,13

C 80 ▢

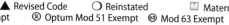

Bicoronal scalp flap
Lower eyelid
Circum-vestibular

Typical transcutaneous and transoral incisions

LeFort III with LeFort I down-fracture

21159 Reconstruction midface, LeFort III (extra and intracranial) with forehead advancement (eg, mono bloc), requiring bone grafts (includes obtaining autografts); without LeFort I

🔲 69.3 ✄ 69.3 **FUD** 090

AMA: 2002,Apr,13

C 80 ▢

21160 with LeFort I

🔲 75.2 ✄ 75.2 **FUD** 090

AMA: 2002,Apr,13

C 80 ▢

21172 Reconstruction superior-lateral orbital rim and lower forehead, advancement or alteration, with or without grafts (includes obtaining autografts)

EXCLUDES *Frontal or parietal craniotomy for craniosynostosis (61556)*

🔲 50.9 ✄ 50.9 **FUD** 090

AMA: 2002,Apr,13

T 80 ▢

21175 Reconstruction, bifrontal, superior-lateral orbital rims and lower forehead, advancement or alteration (eg, plagiocephaly, trigonocephaly, brachycephaly), with or without grafts (includes obtaining autografts)

EXCLUDES *Bifrontal craniotomy for craniosynostosis (61557)*

🔲 66.8 ✄ 66.8 **FUD** 090

AMA: 2002,Apr,13

T 80 ▢

21179 Reconstruction, entire or majority of forehead and/or supraorbital rims; with grafts (allograft or prosthetic material)

EXCLUDES *Extensive craniotomy for numerous suture craniosynostosis (61558-61559)*

🔲 37.6 ✄ 37.6 **FUD** 090

AMA: 2002,Apr,13

C 80 ▢

21180 with autograft (includes obtaining grafts)

EXCLUDES *Extensive craniotomy for numerous suture craniosynostosis (61558-61559)*

🔲 44.1 ✄ 44.1 **FUD** 090

AMA: 2002,Apr,13

C 80 ▢

21181 Reconstruction by contouring of benign tumor of cranial bones (eg, fibrous dysplasia), extracranial

🔲 21.2 ✄ 21.2 **FUD** 090

AMA: 2002,Apr,13

T A2 80 ▢

21182 Reconstruction of orbital walls, rims, forehead, nasoethmoid complex following intra- and extracranial excision of benign tumor of cranial bone (eg, fibrous dysplasia), with multiple autografts (includes obtaining grafts); total area of bone grafting less than 40 sq cm

EXCLUDES *Removal of benign tumor of the skull (61563-61564)*

🔲 55.1 ✄ 55.1 **FUD** 090

AMA: 2002,May,7; 2002,Apr,13

C 80 ▢

21183 total area of bone grafting greater than 40 sq cm but less than 80 sq cm

EXCLUDES *Removal of benign tumor of the skull (61563-61564)*

🔲 64.1 ✄ 64.1 **FUD** 090

AMA: 2002,Apr,13

C 80 ▢

21184 total area of bone grafting greater than 80 sq cm

EXCLUDES *Removal of benign tumor of the skull (61563-61564)*

🔲 69.3 ✄ 69.3 **FUD** 090

AMA: 2002,Apr,13

C 80 ▢

21188 Reconstruction midface, osteotomies (other than LeFort type) and bone grafts (includes obtaining autografts)

🔲 45.0 ✄ 45.0 **FUD** 090

AMA: 2002,Apr,13

C 80 ▢

21193 Reconstruction of mandibular rami, horizontal, vertical, C, or L osteotomy; without bone graft

🔲 34.2 ✄ 34.2 **FUD** 090

AMA: 2015,Jan,16; 2014,Jan,11; 2012,Jan,15-42; 2011,Jan,11

T 80 ▢

21194 with bone graft (includes obtaining graft)

🔲 43.2 ✄ 43.2 **FUD** 090

AMA: 2015,Jan,16; 2014,Jan,11

C 80 ▢

21195 Reconstruction of mandibular rami and/or body, sagittal split; without internal rigid fixation

🔲 38.7 ✄ 38.7 **FUD** 090

AMA: 2015,Jan,16; 2014,Jan,11; 2012,Jan,15-42; 2011,Jan,11

T 80 ▢

21196 with internal rigid fixation

🔲 42.6 ✄ 42.6 **FUD** 090

AMA: 2015,Jan,16; 2014,Jan,11; 2012,Jan,15-42; 2011,Jan,11

C 80 ▢

21198 Osteotomy, mandible, segmental;

EXCLUDES *Total maxillary osteotomy (21141-21160)*

🔲 33.6 ✄ 33.6 **FUD** 090

AMA: 2015,Jan,16; 2014,Jan,11; 2013,Dec,16

T G2 80 ▢

21199 with genioglossus advancement

EXCLUDES *Total maxillary osteotomy (21141-21160)*

🔲 28.9 ✄ 28.9 **FUD** 090

AMA: 2015,Jan,16; 2014,Jan,11

T G2 80 ▢

21206 Osteotomy, maxilla, segmental (eg, Wassmund or Schuchard)

🔲 35.7 ✄ 35.7 **FUD** 090

AMA: 2002,Apr,13

T A2 80 ▢

21208 Osteoplasty, facial bones; augmentation (autograft, allograft, or prosthetic implant)

🔲 24.4 ✄ 54.8 **FUD** 090

AMA: 2002,Apr,13

T A2 80 ▢

21209 reduction

🔲 17.7 ✄ 23.2 **FUD** 090

AMA: 2002,Apr,13

T A2 80 ▢

21210 Graft, bone; nasal, maxillary or malar areas (includes obtaining graft)

EXCLUDES *Cleft palate procedures (42200-42225)*

🔲 25.2 ✄ 66.1 **FUD** 090

AMA: 2002,Apr,13

T A2

21215 mandible (includes obtaining graft)

🔲 26.1 ✄ 118. **FUD** 090

AMA: 2002,Apr,13

T A2 ▢

● New Code ▲ Revised Code ○ Reinstated Ⓜ Maternity Ⓐ Age Edit Unlisted # Resequenced
⊘ AMA Mod 51 Exempt ⑪ Optum Mod 51 Exempt ⑥③ Mod 63 Exempt ⊙ Mod Sedation + Add-on ▢ CCI Ⓟ⓪ PQRS FUD Follow-up Days

21230   **Graft; rib cartilage, autogenous, to face, chin, nose or ear (includes obtaining graft)**
EXCLUDES   *Augmentation of facial bones (21208)*
🔷 21.9   ⚖ 21.9   **FUD** 090   T A2 80 ▣
AMA: 2002,Apr,13

21235   **ear cartilage, autogenous, to nose or ear (includes obtaining graft)**
EXCLUDES   *Augmentation of facial bones (21208)*
🔷 16.3   ⚖ 20.7   **FUD** 090   T A2 ▣
AMA: 2015,Jan,16; 2012,Jan,15-42; 2011,Jan,11

21240   **Arthroplasty, temporomandibular joint, with or without autograft (includes obtaining graft)**
🔷 32.4   ⚖ 32.4   **FUD** 090   T A2 80 50 ▣
AMA: 2002,Apr,13; 1994,Win,1

TMJ syndrome is often related to stress and tooth-grinding; in other cases, arthritis, injury, poorly aligned teeth, or ill-fitting dentures may be the cause

Upper joint space
Lower joint space
Articular disc (meniscus)
Cutaway detail
Condyle
Mandible
Cutaway view of temporomandibular joint (TMJ)
Symptoms include facial pain and chewing problems; TMJ syndrome occurs more frequently in women

21242   **Arthroplasty, temporomandibular joint, with allograft**
🔷 29.7   ⚖ 29.7   **FUD** 090   T A2 80 50 ▣
AMA: 2002,Apr,13

21243   **Arthroplasty, temporomandibular joint, with prosthetic joint replacement**
🔷 49.2   ⚖ 49.2   **FUD** 090   T A2 80 50 ▣
AMA: 2002,Apr,13

21244   **Reconstruction of mandible, extraoral, with transosteal bone plate (eg, mandibular staple bone plate)**
🔷 30.8   ⚖ 30.8   **FUD** 090   T A2 80 ▣
AMA: 2004,Mar,7; 2002,Apr,13

21245   **Reconstruction of mandible or maxilla, subperiosteal implant; partial**
🔷 25.4   ⚖ 31.7   **FUD** 090   T A2 80 ▣
AMA: 2002,Apr,13

21246   **complete**
🔷 25.9   ⚖ 25.9   **FUD** 090   T A2 80 ▣
AMA: 2002,Apr,13

21247   **Reconstruction of mandibular condyle with bone and cartilage autografts (includes obtaining grafts) (eg, for hemifacial microsomia)**
🔷 43.9   ⚖ 43.9   **FUD** 090   C 80 50 ▣
AMA: 2002,Apr,13

21248   **Reconstruction of mandible or maxilla, endosteal implant (eg, blade, cylinder); partial**
EXCLUDES   *Midface reconstruction (21141-21160)*
🔷 26.3   ⚖ 32.1   **FUD** 090   T A2 ▣
AMA: 2002,Apr,13

21249   **complete**
EXCLUDES   *Midface reconstruction (21141-21160)*
🔷 37.5   ⚖ 44.1   **FUD** 090   T A2 80 ▣
AMA: 2002,Apr,13

21255   **Reconstruction of zygomatic arch and glenoid fossa with bone and cartilage (includes obtaining autografts)**
🔷 37.9   ⚖ 37.9   **FUD** 090   C 80 50 ▣
AMA: 2002,Apr,13

21256   **Reconstruction of orbit with osteotomies (extracranial) and with bone grafts (includes obtaining autografts) (eg, micro-ophthalmia)**
🔷 34.3   ⚖ 34.3   **FUD** 090   T 80 50 ▣
AMA: 2002,Apr,13

21260   **Periorbital osteotomies for orbital hypertelorism, with bone grafts; extracranial approach**
🔷 32.9   ⚖ 32.9   **FUD** 090   T 62 80 ▣
AMA: 2002,Apr,13

21261   **combined intra- and extracranial approach**
🔷 58.4   ⚖ 58.4   **FUD** 090   T 80 ▣
AMA: 2002,Apr,13

21263   **with forehead advancement**
🔷 54.0   ⚖ 54.0   **FUD** 090   T 80 ▣
AMA: 2002,Apr,13

Grafts

In 21263, a frontal craniotomy is performed, the brain retracted, and the orbit approached from inside the skull; frontal bone is advanced and secured

Osteotomies are cut 360 degrees around the orbit; portions of nasal and ethmoid bones are removed

Grafts are placed and the bony orbits realigned

21267   **Orbital repositioning, periorbital osteotomies, unilateral, with bone grafts; extracranial approach**
🔷 45.2   ⚖ 45.2   **FUD** 090   T A2 80 50 ▣
AMA: 2002,Apr,13

21268   **combined intra- and extracranial approach**
🔷 53.1   ⚖ 53.1   **FUD** 090   C 80 50 ▣
AMA: 2002,Apr,13

21270   **Malar augmentation, prosthetic material**
EXCLUDES   *Bone graft (21210)*
🔷 20.7   ⚖ 27.6   **FUD** 090   T A2 80 50 ▣
AMA: 2002,Apr,13

21275   **Secondary revision of orbitocraniofacial reconstruction**
🔷 24.0   ⚖ 24.0   **FUD** 090   T A2 80 ▣
AMA: 2002,Apr,13

21280   **Medial canthopexy (separate procedure)**
EXCLUDES   *Reconstruction of canthus (67950)*
🔷 16.2   ⚖ 16.2   **FUD** 090   T A2 80 50 ▣
AMA: 2002,Apr,13

21282   **Lateral canthopexy**
🔷 10.8   ⚖ 10.8   **FUD** 090   T A2 50 ▣
AMA: 2002,Apr,13

21295   **Reduction of masseter muscle and bone (eg, for treatment of benign masseteric hypertrophy); extraoral approach**
🔷 5.41   ⚖ 5.41   **FUD** 090   T A2 80 50 ▣
AMA: 2002,Apr,13

21296   **intraoral approach**
🔷 12.0   ⚖ 12.0   **FUD** 090   T A2 80 50 ▣
AMA: 2002,Apr,13

21299   **Unlisted craniofacial and maxillofacial procedure**
🔷 0.00   ⚖ 0.00   **FUD** YYY   T 80
AMA: 2002,Apr,13; 1995,Win,1

21310-21499 Care of Fractures/Dislocations of the Cranial and Facial Bones

EXCLUDES   Closed treatment of skull fracture, report with appropriate E&M service
Open treatment of skull fracture (62000-62010)

21310   Closed treatment of nasal bone fracture without manipulation
🔧 0.77   ✂ 3.75   FUD 000   T A2 ▢
AMA: 2002,Apr,13

21315   Closed treatment of nasal bone fracture; without stabilization
🔧 4.39   ✂ 7.97   FUD 010   T A2 ▢
AMA: 2002,Apr,13

21320   with stabilization
🔧 3.90   ✂ 7.34   FUD 010   T A2 ▢
AMA: 2002,Apr,13

21325   Open treatment of nasal fracture; uncomplicated
🔧 13.7   ✂ 13.7   FUD 090   T A2 80 ▢
AMA: 2002,Apr,13

21330   complicated, with internal and/or external skeletal fixation
🔧 16.4   ✂ 16.4   FUD 090   T A2 80 ▢
AMA: 2002,Apr,13

21335   with concomitant open treatment of fractured septum
🔧 20.8   ✂ 20.8   FUD 090   T A2 ▢
AMA: 2002,Apr,13

21336   Open treatment of nasal septal fracture, with or without stabilization
🔧 18.5   ✂ 18.5   FUD 090   T A2 80 ▢
AMA: 2002,Apr,13

21337   Closed treatment of nasal septal fracture, with or without stabilization
🔧 8.50   ✂ 11.6   FUD 090   T A2 80 ▢
AMA: 2002,Apr,13

21338   Open treatment of nasoethmoid fracture; without external fixation
🔧 21.6   ✂ 21.6   FUD 090   T A2 80 ▢
AMA: 2002,Apr,13

21339   with external fixation
🔧 24.4   ✂ 24.4   FUD 090   T A2 80 ▢
AMA: 2002,Apr,13

21340   Percutaneous treatment of nasoethmoid complex fracture, with splint, wire or headcap fixation, including repair of canthal ligaments and/or the nasolacrimal apparatus
🔧 22.9   ✂ 22.9   FUD 090   T A2 80 ▢
AMA: 2002,Apr,13

21343   Open treatment of depressed frontal sinus fracture
🔧 34.9   ✂ 34.9   FUD 090   C 80 ▢
AMA: 2002,Apr,13

21344   Open treatment of complicated (eg, comminuted or involving posterior wall) frontal sinus fracture, via coronal or multiple approaches
🔧 40.0   ✂ 40.0   FUD 090   C 80 ▢
AMA: 2002,Apr,13

21345   Closed treatment of nasomaxillary complex fracture (LeFort II type), with interdental wire fixation or fixation of denture or splint
🔧 18.0   ✂ 22.4   FUD 090   T A2 80 ▢
AMA: 2002,Apr,13

21346   Open treatment of nasomaxillary complex fracture (LeFort II type); with wiring and/or local fixation
🔧 26.0   ✂ 26.0   FUD 090   T ▢ PQ
AMA: 2002,Apr,13

21347   requiring multiple open approaches
🔧 32.7   ✂ 32.7   FUD 090   C 80 ▢ PQ
AMA: 2002,Apr,13

21348   with bone grafting (includes obtaining graft)
🔧 34.7   ✂ 34.7   FUD 090   C 80 ▢ PQ
AMA: 2002,Apr,13

21355   Percutaneous treatment of fracture of malar area, including zygomatic arch and malar tripod, with manipulation
🔧 10.3   ✂ 13.8   FUD 010   T A2 80 50 ▢
AMA: 2002,Apr,13

21356   Open treatment of depressed zygomatic arch fracture (eg, Gillies approach)
🔧 10.8   ✂ 14.4   FUD 010   T A2 80 50 ▢
AMA: 2002,Apr,13

21360   Open treatment of depressed malar fracture, including zygomatic arch and malar tripod
🔧 15.4   ✂ 15.4   FUD 090   T 62 80 50 ▢
AMA: 2002,Apr,13

21365   Open treatment of complicated (eg, comminuted or involving cranial nerve foramina) fracture(s) of malar area, including zygomatic arch and malar tripod; with internal fixation and multiple surgical approaches
🔧 32.0   ✂ 32.0   FUD 090   T 80 50 ▢
AMA: 2002,Apr,13

21366   with bone grafting (includes obtaining graft)
🔧 33.3   ✂ 33.3   FUD 090   C 80 50 ▢
AMA: 2002,Apr,13

21385   Open treatment of orbital floor blowout fracture; transantral approach (Caldwell-Luc type operation)
🔧 19.6   ✂ 19.6   FUD 090   T 80 50 ▢
AMA: 2002,Apr,13

21386   periorbital approach
🔧 20.0   ✂ 20.0   FUD 090   T 80 50 ▢
AMA: 2002,Apr,13

21387   combined approach
🔧 20.4   ✂ 20.4   FUD 090   T 80 50 ▢
AMA: 2002,Apr,13

21390   periorbital approach, with alloplastic or other implant
🔧 22.7   ✂ 22.7   FUD 090   T 62 80 50 ▢
AMA: 2003,Jan,1; 2002,Apr,13

21395   periorbital approach with bone graft (includes obtaining graft)
🔧 28.9   ✂ 28.9   FUD 090   T 80 50 ▢
AMA: 2002,Apr,13

21400   Closed treatment of fracture of orbit, except blowout; without manipulation
🔧 4.52   ✂ 5.55   FUD 090   T A2 80 50 ▢
AMA: 2002,Apr,13

21401   with manipulation
🔧 8.82   ✂ 14.1   FUD 090   T A2 80 50 ▢
AMA: 2002,Apr,13

21406   Open treatment of fracture of orbit, except blowout; without implant
🔧 16.4   ✂ 16.4   FUD 090   T 62 80 50 ▢
AMA: 2002,Apr,13

21407   with implant
🔧 18.5   ✂ 18.5   FUD 090   T 62 80 50 ▢
AMA: 2002,Apr,13

21408   with bone grafting (includes obtaining graft)
🔧 25.8   ✂ 25.8   FUD 090   T 80 50 ▢
AMA: 2002,Apr,13

21421   Closed treatment of palatal or maxillary fracture (LeFort I type), with interdental wire fixation or fixation of denture or splint
🔧 20.0   ✂ 24.2   FUD 090   T A2 80 ▢
AMA: 2002,Apr,13

21422   Open treatment of palatal or maxillary fracture (LeFort I type);
🔧 19.4   ✂ 19.4   FUD 090   C 80 ▢ PQ
AMA: 2002,Apr,13

21423   complicated (comminuted or involving cranial nerve foramina), multiple approaches
⚙ 22.7   ✂ 22.7   **FUD** 090   C 80 ▦ P0
AMA: 2002,Apr,13

21431   Closed treatment of craniofacial separation (LeFort III type) using interdental wire fixation of denture or splint
⚙ 22.6   ✂ 22.6   **FUD** 090   C 80 ▦
AMA: 2002,Apr,13

21432   Open treatment of craniofacial separation (LeFort III type); with wiring and/or internal fixation
⚙ 18.4   ✂ 18.4   **FUD** 090   C 80 ▦ P0
AMA: 2002,Apr,13

21433   complicated (eg, comminuted or involving cranial nerve foramina), multiple surgical approaches
⚙ 50.0   ✂ 50.0   **FUD** 090   C 80 ▦ P0
AMA: 2002,Apr,13

21435   complicated, utilizing internal and/or external fixation techniques (eg, head cap, halo device, and/or intermaxillary fixation)
EXCLUDES   *Removal of internal or external fixation (20670)*
⚙ 36.3   ✂ 36.3   **FUD** 090   C 80 ▦ P0
AMA: 2002,Apr,13

21436   complicated, multiple surgical approaches, internal fixation, with bone grafting (includes obtaining graft)
⚙ 58.7   ✂ 58.7   **FUD** 090   C 80 ▦ P0
AMA: 2002,Apr,13

21440   Closed treatment of mandibular or maxillary alveolar ridge fracture (separate procedure)
⚙ 13.5   ✂ 16.6   **FUD** 090   T P3 80 ▦
AMA: 2002,Apr,13

21445   Open treatment of mandibular or maxillary alveolar ridge fracture (separate procedure)
⚙ 18.1   ✂ 22.3   **FUD** 090   T A2 80 ▦
AMA: 2002,Apr,13

21450   Closed treatment of mandibular fracture; without manipulation
⚙ 14.4   ✂ 18.0   **FUD** 090   T A2 80 ▦
AMA: 2002,Apr,13

21451   with manipulation
⚙ 19.5   ✂ 23.7   **FUD** 090   T A2 80 ▦
AMA: 2002,Apr,13

21452   Percutaneous treatment of mandibular fracture, with external fixation
⚙ 9.80   ✂ 16.5   **FUD** 090   T A2 80 ▦
AMA: 2002,Apr,13

In 21452, external fixation is necessary

Comminuted fractures

Metal or acrylic bar

Rods and pins placed in drilled holes

21453   Closed treatment of mandibular fracture with interdental fixation
⚙ 22.6   ✂ 26.4   **FUD** 090   T A2 80 ▦
AMA: 2015,Jan,16; 2014,Jan,11; 2012,Jan,15-42; 2011,Jan,11

21454   Open treatment of mandibular fracture with external fixation
⚙ 16.5   ✂ 16.5   **FUD** 090   T A2 80 ▦ P0
AMA: 2002,Apr,13

21461   Open treatment of mandibular fracture; without interdental fixation
⚙ 27.1   ✂ 61.4   **FUD** 090   T A2 ▦ P0
AMA: 2002,Apr,13

21462   with interdental fixation
⚙ 30.2   ✂ 65.3   **FUD** 090   T A2 80 ▦ P0
AMA: 2002,Apr,13

21465   Open treatment of mandibular condylar fracture
⚙ 26.9   ✂ 26.9   **FUD** 090   T A2 80 50 ▦ P0
AMA: 2002,Apr,13

21470   Open treatment of complicated mandibular fracture by multiple surgical approaches including internal fixation, interdental fixation, and/or wiring of dentures or splints
⚙ 34.9   ✂ 34.9   **FUD** 090   T 80 ▦ P0
AMA: 2015,Jan,16; 2014,Jan,11; 2012,Jan,15-42; 2011,Jan,11

21480   Closed treatment of temporomandibular dislocation; initial or subsequent
⚙ 0.92   ✂ 2.82   **FUD** 000   T A2 50 ▦
AMA: 2002,Apr,13

21485   complicated (eg, recurrent requiring intermaxillary fixation or splinting), initial or subsequent
⚙ 17.0   ✂ 20.3   **FUD** 090   T A2 80 50 ▦
AMA: 2002,Apr,13

21490   Open treatment of temporomandibular dislocation
EXCLUDES   *Interdental wiring (21497)*
⚙ 26.6   ✂ 26.6   **FUD** 090   T A2 80 50 ▦
AMA: 2002,Apr,13

21495   Open treatment of hyoid fracture
EXCLUDES   *Closed treatment of larynx fracture, see appropriate evaluation and management service code*
Laryngoplasty with open fracture repair (31584)
⚙ 18.3   ✂ 18.3   **FUD** 090   T G2 80 ▦
AMA: 2002,Apr,13

21497   Interdental wiring, for condition other than fracture
⚙ 17.6   ✂ 21.2   **FUD** 090   T A2 80 ▦
AMA: 2015,Jan,16; 2014,Jan,11; 2012,Jan,15-42; 2011,Jan,11

21499   Unlisted musculoskeletal procedure, head
EXCLUDES   *Unlisted procedures of craniofacial or maxillofacial areas (21299)*
⚙ 0.00   ✂ 0.00   **FUD** YYY   T 80
AMA: 2002,Apr,13; 1995,Win,1

21501-21510 Surgical Incision for Drainage: Chest and Soft Tissues of Neck

EXCLUDES   *Biopsy of the flank or back (21920-21925)*
Simple incision and drainage of abscess or hematoma (10060, 10140)
Tumor removal of flank or back (21930-21936)

21501   Incision and drainage, deep abscess or hematoma, soft tissues of neck or thorax;
EXCLUDES   *Deep incision and drainage of posterior spine (22010-22015)*
⚙ 9.21   ✂ 12.9   **FUD** 090   T A2 ▦
AMA: 2015,Jan,16; 2014,Dec,16; 2014,Dec,16

21502   with partial rib ostectomy
⚙ 14.6   ✂ 14.6   **FUD** 090   T A2 80 ▦
AMA: 2002,Apr,13

21510   Incision, deep, with opening of bone cortex (eg, for osteomyelitis or bone abscess), thorax
⚙ 12.6   ✂ 12.6   **FUD** 090   C 80 ▦
AMA: 2002,Apr,13

21550 Soft Tissue Biopsy of Chest or Neck

EXCLUDES   *Biopsy of bone (20220-20251)*
Soft tissue needle biopsy (20206)

21550   Biopsy, soft tissue of neck or thorax
⚙ 4.54   ✂ 7.49   **FUD** 010   T G2 ▦ P0
AMA: 2002,Apr,13

26/TC PC/TC Comp Only	A2-Z3 ASC Pmt	50 Bilateral	♂ Male Only	♀ Female Only	⚙ Facility RVU	✂ Non-Facility RVU
AMA: CPT Asst	**CMS:** Pub 100	A-Y OPPSI	80/80 Surg Assist Allowed / w/Doc		▦ Lab Crosswalk	▦ Radiology Crosswalk

42   Medicare (Red Text)   CPT © 2015 American Medical Association. All Rights Reserved. (Black Text)   © 2015 Optum360, LLC (Blue Text)

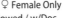

21552-21558 [21552, 21554] Excision Soft Tissue Tumors Chest and Neck

INCLUDES Any necessary elevation of tissue planes or dissection
Measurement of tumor and necessary margin at greatest diameter prior to excision
Resection without removal of significant normal tissue
Simple and intermediate repairs
Types of excision:
    Fascial or subfascial soft tissue tumors: simple and marginal resection of tumors found either in or below the deep fascia, not involving bone or excision of a substantial amount of normal tissue; primarily benign and intramuscular tumors
    Radical resection soft tissue tumor: wide resection of tumor, involving substantial margins of normal tissue and may involve tissue removal from one or more layers; most often malignant or aggressive benign
    Subcutaneous: simple and marginal resection of tumors in the subcutaneous tissue above the deep fascia; most often benign

EXCLUDES *Complex repair*
Excision of benign cutaneous lesions (eg, sebaceous cyst) (11400-11426)
Radical resection of cutaneous tumors (eg, melanoma) (11600-11626)
Significant exploration of the vessels or neuroplasty

21552 Resequenced code. See code following 21555.

21554 Resequenced code. See code following 21556.

21555 Excision, tumor, soft tissue of neck or anterior thorax, subcutaneous; less than 3 cm
    🖐 8.79   ✂ 11.8   **FUD** 090   T G2 🔲
    AMA: 2015,Jan,16; 2014,Jan,11; 2012,Jan,15-42; 2011,Jan,11

\# **21552** 3 cm or greater
    🖐 12.8   ✂ 12.8   **FUD** 090   T G2 80

21556 Excision, tumor, soft tissue of neck or anterior thorax, subfascial (eg, intramuscular); less than 5 cm
    🖐 15.2   ✂ 15.2   **FUD** 090   T G2 🔲
    AMA: 2002,Apr,13

\# **21554** 5 cm or greater
    🖐 21.0   ✂ 21.0   **FUD** 090   T G2 80

21557 Radical resection of tumor (eg, sarcoma), soft tissue of neck or anterior thorax; less than 5 cm
    🖐 27.6   ✂ 27.6   **FUD** 090   T G2 80 🔲
    AMA: 2015,Jan,16; 2014,Jan,11; 2010,Apr,3-4

21558 5 cm or greater
    🖐 38.7   ✂ 38.7   **FUD** 090   T G2 80

21600-21632 Bony Resection Chest and Neck

21600 Excision of rib, partial
    EXCLUDES *Extensive debridement (11044, 11047)*
    Extensive tumor removal (19260)
    🖐 16.0   ✂ 16.0   **FUD** 090   T A2 80 🔲
    AMA: 2015,Jan,16; 2014,Jan,11; 2013,Mar,13; 2012,Jul,12-14

21610 Costotransversectomy (separate procedure)
    🖐 35.4   ✂ 35.4   **FUD** 090   T A2 80 🔲
    AMA: 2002,Apr,13

21615 Excision first and/or cervical rib;
    🖐 18.0   ✂ 18.0   **FUD** 090   C 80 50 🔲
    AMA: 2015,Jan,16; 2014,Mar,13

21616 with sympathectomy
    🖐 21.1   ✂ 21.1   **FUD** 090   C 80 50 🔲
    AMA: 2002,Apr,13

21620 Ostectomy of sternum, partial
    🖐 14.5   ✂ 14.5   **FUD** 090   C 80 🔲
    AMA: 2002,Apr,13

21627 Sternal debridement
    EXCLUDES *Debridement with sternotomy closure (21750)*
    🖐 15.6   ✂ 15.6   **FUD** 090   C 80 🔲 PQ
    AMA: 2015,Jan,16; 2014,Jan,11; 2011,May,3-5

21630 Radical resection of sternum;
    🖐 34.6   ✂ 34.6   **FUD** 090   C 80 🔲
    AMA: 2002,Apr,13; 1994,Win,1

21632 with mediastinal lymphadenectomy
    🖐 34.8   ✂ 34.8   **FUD** 090   C 80 🔲 PQ
    AMA: 2002,Apr,13

21685-21750 Repair/Reconstruction Chest and Soft Tissues Neck

EXCLUDES *Biopsy of chest or neck (21550)*
Repair of simple wounds (12001-12007)
Tumor removal of chest or neck (21552-21558 [21552, 21554])

21685 Hyoid myotomy and suspension
    🖐 28.6   ✂ 28.6   **FUD** 090   T G2 80 🔲
    AMA: 2015,Jan,16; 2014,Jan,11; 2012,Jan,15-42; 2011,Jan,11

21700 Division of scalenus anticus; without resection of cervical rib
    🖐 10.6   ✂ 10.6   **FUD** 090   T A2 80 50 🔲
    AMA: 2002,Apr,13

21705 with resection of cervical rib
    🖐 15.8   ✂ 15.8   **FUD** 090   C 80 50 🔲
    AMA: 2015,Jan,16; 2014,Mar,13

21720 Division of sternocleidomastoid for torticollis, open operation; without cast application
    EXCLUDES *Transection of spinal accessory and cervical nerves (63191, 64722)*
    🖐 13.8   ✂ 13.8   **FUD** 090   T A2 80 🔲
    AMA: 2002,Apr,13

21725 with cast application
    EXCLUDES *Transection of spinal accessory and cervical nerves (63191, 64722)*
    🖐 15.5   ✂ 15.5   **FUD** 090   T A2 80 🔲
    AMA: 2002,Apr,13

21740 Reconstructive repair of pectus excavatum or carinatum; open
    🖐 29.8   ✂ 29.8   **FUD** 090   C 80 🔲 PQ
    AMA: 2002,Apr,13

21742 minimally invasive approach (Nuss procedure), without thoracoscopy
    🖐 0.00   ✂ 0.00   **FUD** 090   T 80 🔲
    AMA: 2002,Apr,13

21743 minimally invasive approach (Nuss procedure), with thoracoscopy
    🖐 0.00   ✂ 0.00   **FUD** 090   T 80 🔲
    AMA: 2002,Apr,13

21750 Closure of median sternotomy separation with or without debridement (separate procedure)
    🖐 19.7   ✂ 19.7   **FUD** 090   C 80 🔲 PQ
    AMA: 2015,Jan,16; 2014,Jan,11; 2011,May,3-5

21805-21825 Fracture Care: Ribs and Sternum

EXCLUDES *Closed treatment uncomplicated rib fractures*

~~**21805** Open treatment of rib fracture without fixation, each~~

21811 Open treatment of rib fracture(s) with internal fixation, includes thoracoscopic visualization when performed, unilateral; 1-3 ribs
    🖐 17.4   ✂ 17.4   **FUD** 000   T 80 50
    AMA: 2015,Aug,3

21812 4-6 ribs
    🖐 20.9   ✂ 20.9   **FUD** 000   T 80 50
    AMA: 2015,Aug,3

21813 7 or more ribs
    🖐 28.5   ✂ 28.5   **FUD** 000   T 80 50
    AMA: 2015,Aug,3

21820 Closed treatment of sternum fracture
    🖐 4.17   ✂ 4.07   **FUD** 090   T A2 🔲
    AMA: 2002,Apr,13

21825   **Open treatment of sternum fracture with or without skeletal fixation**

EXCLUDES *Treatment of sternoclavicular dislocation (23520-23532)*

⏱ 15.6   ✂ 15.6   **FUD** 090   [C] [80] [▭] [P0]

AMA: 2002,Apr,13

21899 Unlisted Procedures of Chest or Neck

CMS: 100-4,4,180.3 Unlisted Service or Procedure

21899   **Unlisted procedure, neck or thorax**

⏱ 0.00   ✂ 0.00   **FUD** YYY   [T] [80]

AMA: 2015,Aug,3

21920-21925 Biopsy Soft Tissue of Back and Flank

EXCLUDES *Soft tissue needle biopsy (20206)*

21920   **Biopsy, soft tissue of back or flank; superficial**

⏱ 4.59   ✂ 7.30   **FUD** 010   [T] [P3] [▭] [P0]

AMA: 2002,Apr,13; 1993,Sum,25

21925   **deep**

⏱ 10.2   ✂ 12.7   **FUD** 090   [T] [A2] [▭] [P0]

AMA: 2002,Apr,13

21930-21936 Excision Soft Tissue Tumors Back or Flank

INCLUDES Any necessary elevation of tissue planes or dissection
Measurement of tumor and necessary margin at greatest diameter prior to excision
Simple and intermediate repairs
Types of excision:
  Fascial or subfascial soft tissue tumors: simple and marginal resection of tumors found either in or below the deep fascia, not involving bone or excision of a substantial amount of normal tissue; most often benign and intramuscular tumors
  Radical resection soft tissue tumor: wide resection of tumor, involving substantial margins of normal tissue and may include tissue removal from one or more layers; most often malignant or aggressive benign
  Subcutaneous: simple and marginal resection of tumors in the subcutaneous tissue above the deep fascia; most often benign

EXCLUDES Complex repair
Excision of benign cutaneous lesions (eg, sebaceous cyst) (11400-11406)
Radical resection of cutaneous tumors (eg, melanoma) (11600-11606)
Significant exploration of the vessels or neuroplasty

21930   **Excision, tumor, soft tissue of back or flank, subcutaneous; less than 3 cm**

⏱ 10.4   ✂ 13.5   **FUD** 090   [T] [G2] [▭]

AMA: 2015,Jan,16; 2014,Jan,11; 2012,Jan,15-42; 2011,Jan,11

21931   **3 cm or greater**

⏱ 13.5   ✂ 13.5   **FUD** 090   [T] [G2] [80]

21932   **Excision, tumor, soft tissue of back or flank, subfascial (eg, intramuscular); less than 5 cm**

⏱ 19.0   ✂ 19.0   **FUD** 090   [T] [G2] [80]

21933   **5 cm or greater**

⏱ 21.2   ✂ 21.2   **FUD** 090   [T] [G2] [80]

21935   **Radical resection of tumor (eg, sarcoma), soft tissue of back or flank; less than 5 cm**

⏱ 29.5   ✂ 29.5   **FUD** 090   [T] [G2] [▭]

AMA: 2002,Apr,13; 1990,Win,4

21936   **5 cm or greater**

⏱ 40.7   ✂ 40.7   **FUD** 090   [T] [G2] [80]

22010-22015 Incision for Drainage of Deep Spinal Abscess

EXCLUDES Incision and drainage of hematoma (10060, 10140)
Injection:
  Chemonucleolysis (62292)
  Discography (62290-62291)
  Facet joint (64490-64495, [64633, 64634, 64635, 64636])
  Myelography (62284)
Needle/trocar biopsy (20220-20225)

22010   **Incision and drainage, open, of deep abscess (subfascial), posterior spine; cervical, thoracic, or cervicothoracic**

⏱ 27.5   ✂ 27.5   **FUD** 090   [C] [80]

22015   **lumbar, sacral, or lumbosacral**

⏱ 26.2   ✂ 26.2   **FUD** 090   [C]

Do not report with (10180, 22010, 22850, 22852)

22100-22103 Partial Resection Vertebral Component

EXCLUDES *Back or flank biopsy (21920-21925)*
Bone biopsy (20220-20251)
Injection:
  Chemonucleolysis (62292)
  Discography (62290-62291)
  Facet joint (64490-64495, [64633, 64634, 64635, 64636])
  Myelography (62284)
Removal of tumor flank or back (21930)
Soft tissue needle biopsy (20206)

22100   **Partial excision of posterior vertebral component (eg, spinous process, lamina or facet) for intrinsic bony lesion, single vertebral segment; cervical**

⏱ 27.2   ✂ 27.2   **FUD** 090   [T] [80] [▭]

AMA: 2015,Jan,16; 2013,Jul,3-5

22101   **thoracic**

⏱ 23.7   ✂ 23.7   **FUD** 090   [T] [80] [▭]

AMA: 2015,Jan,16; 2013,Jul,3-5

22102   **lumbar**

EXCLUDES *Insertion of posterior spinous process distraction devices (0171T-0172T)*

⏱ 23.0   ✂ 23.0   **FUD** 090   [T] [G2] [80] [▭]

AMA: 2015,Jan,16; 2013,Jul,3-5

+   **22103**   **each additional segment (List separately in addition to code for primary procedure)**

Code first (22100-22102)

⏱ 4.10   ✂ 4.10   **FUD** ZZZ   [N] [N1] [80] [▭]

AMA: 2003,Jan,1; 2002,Apr,13

22110-22116 Partial Resection Vertebral Component without Decompression

EXCLUDES *Back or flank biopsy (21920-21925)*
Bone biopsy (20220-20251)
Bone grafting procedures (20930-20938)
Harvest bone graft (20931, 20938)
Injection:
  Chemonucleolysis (62292)
  Discography (62290-62291)
  Facet joint (64490-64495, [64633, 64634, 64635, 64636])
  Myelography (62284)
Osteotomy (22210-22226)
Removal of tumor flank or back (21930)
Restoration after vertebral body resection (22585, 63082, 63086, 63088, 63091)
Spinal restoration with graft:
  Cervical (20931, 20938, 22554, 63081)
  Lumbar (20931, 20938, 22558, 63087, 63090)
  Thoracic (20931, 20938, 22556, 63085, 63087)
Spinal restoration with prosthesis:
  Cervical (20931, 20938, 22554, 22851, 63081)
  Lumbar (20931, 20938, 22558, 22851, 63087, 63090)
  Thoracic (20931, 20938, 22556, 22851, 63085, 63087)
Vertebral corpectomy (63081-63091)

22110   **Partial excision of vertebral body, for intrinsic bony lesion, without decompression of spinal cord or nerve root(s), single vertebral segment; cervical**

⏱ 30.4   ✂ 30.4   **FUD** 090   [C] [80] [▭]

AMA: 2015,Jan,16; 2013,Jul,3-5

22112   **thoracic**

⏱ 33.0   ✂ 33.0   **FUD** 090   [C] [80] [▭]

AMA: 2015,Jan,16; 2013,Jul,3-5

22114   **lumbar**

⏱ 28.7   ✂ 28.7   **FUD** 090   [C] [80] [▭]

AMA: 2015,Jan,16; 2013,Jul,3-5

+   **22116**   **each additional vertebral segment (List separately in addition to code for primary procedure)**

Code first (22110-22114)

⏱ 4.14   ✂ 4.14   **FUD** ZZZ   [C] [80] [▭]

AMA: 2003,Feb,7; 2002,Apr,13

 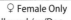

22206-22216 Spinal Osteotomy: Posterior/Posterolateral Approach

CMS: 100-4,12,40.8 Co-surgery and team surgery

EXCLUDES *Decompression of the spinal cord and/or nerve roots (63001-63308)*
Injection:
Chemonucleolysis (62292)
Discography (62290-62292)
Facet joint (64490-64495, [64633, 64634, 64635, 64636])
Myelography (62284)
Repair of vertebral fracture by the anterior approach, see appropriate arthrodesis, bone graft, instrumentation codes, and (63081-63091)
Code also arthrodesis (22590-22632)
Code also bone grafting procedures (20930-20938)
Code also spinal instrumentation (22840-22855)

22206 **Osteotomy of spine, posterior or posterolateral approach, 3 columns, 1 vertebral segment (eg, pedicle/vertebral body subtraction); thoracic**

Do not report with (22207)
Do not report with the following codes if performed at same level (22210-22226, 22830, 63001-63048, 63055-63066, 63075-63091, 63101-63103)

🔧 71.3 ✂ 71.3 **FUD** 090 C 80

AMA: 2015,Jan,16; 2014,Jan,11; 2013,Jul,3-5; 2012,Jan,15-42; 2011,Jan,11

22207 **lumbar**

Do not report with (22206)
Do not report with the following codes if performed at the same level (22210-22226, 22830, 63001-63048, 63055-63066, 63075-63091, 63101-63103)

🔧 69.7 ✂ 69.7 **FUD** 090 C 80

AMA: 2015,Jan,16; 2014,Jan,11; 2013,Jul,3-5; 2012,Jan,15-42; 2011,Jan,11

+ **22208** **each additional vertebral segment (List separately in addition to code for primary procedure)**

Code first (22206, 22207)
Do not report with the following codes if performed at the same level (22210-22226, 22830, 63001-63048, 63055-63066, 63075-63091, 63101-63103)

🔧 16.7 ✂ 16.7 **FUD** ZZZ C 80

AMA: 2015,Jan,16; 2014,Jan,11; 2012,Jan,15-42; 2011,Jan,11

22210 **Osteotomy of spine, posterior or posterolateral approach, 1 vertebral segment; cervical**

🔧 52.1 ✂ 52.1 **FUD** 090 C 80

AMA: 2015,Jan,16; 2013,Jul,3-5

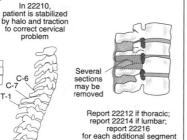

In 22210, patient is stabilized by halo and traction to correct cervical problem

C-6
C-7
T-1

Several sections may be removed

Report 22212 if thoracic; report 22214 if lumbar; report 22216 for each additional segment

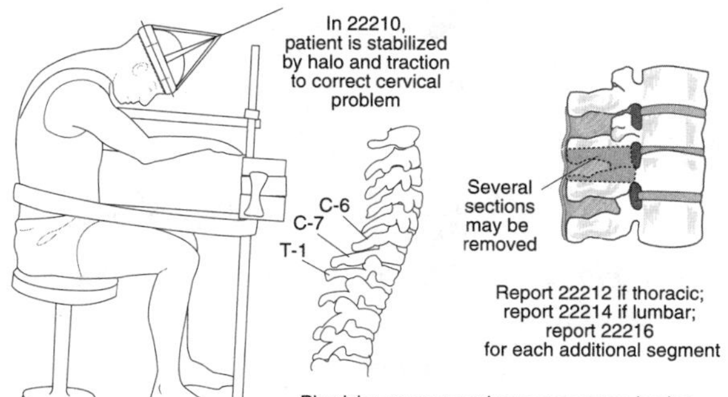

Physician removes spinous processes, lamina

22212 **thoracic**

🔧 43.2 ✂ 43.2 **FUD** 090 C 80

AMA: 2015,Jan,16; 2014,Jan,11; 2013,Jul,3-5

22214 **lumbar**

🔧 43.1 ✂ 43.1 **FUD** 090 C 80

AMA: 2015,Jan,16; 2014,Dec,16; 2014,Dec,16; 2014,Jan,11; 2013,Jul,3-5

+ **22216** **each additional vertebral segment (List separately in addition to primary procedure)**

Code first (22210-22214)

🔧 10.6 ✂ 10.6 **FUD** ZZZ C 80

AMA: 2015,Jan,16; 2014,Jan,11

22220-22226 Spinal Osteotomy: Anterior Approach

CMS: 100-4,12,40.8 Co-surgery and team surgery

EXCLUDES *Corpectomy (63081-63091)*
Decompression of the spinal cord and/or nerve roots (63001-63308)
Injection:
Chemonucleolysis (62292)
Discography (62290-62291)
Facet joint (64490-64495, [64633], [64634], [64635], [64636])
Myelography (62284)
Needle/trocar biopsy (20220-20225)
Repair of vertebral fracture by the anterior approach, see appropriate arthrodesis, bone graft, instrumentation codes, and (63081-63091)
Code also arthrodesis (22590-22632)
Code also bone grafting procedures (20930-20938)
Code also spinal instrumentation (22840-22855)

22220 **Osteotomy of spine, including discectomy, anterior approach, single vertebral segment; cervical**

🔧 46.4 ✂ 46.4 **FUD** 090 C 80

AMA: 2015,Jan,16; 2013,Jul,3-5

22222 **thoracic**

🔧 45.2 ✂ 45.2 **FUD** 090 C 80

AMA: 2015,Jan,16; 2014,Jan,11; 2013,Jul,3-5

22224 **lumbar**

🔧 45.8 ✂ 45.8 **FUD** 090 C 80

AMA: 2015,Jan,16; 2013,Jul,3-5

+ **22226** **each additional vertebral segment (List separately in addition to code for primary procedure)**

Code first (22220-22224)

🔧 10.5 ✂ 10.5 **FUD** ZZZ C 80

AMA: 2002,Feb,4; 2002,Apr,13

22305-22315 Closed Treatment Vertebral Fractures

EXCLUDES *Injection:*
Chemonucleolysis (62292)
Discography (62290-62291)
Facet joint (64490-64495, [64633], [64634], [64635], [64636])
Myelography (62284)
Code also arthrodesis (22590-22632)
Code also bone grafting procedures (20930-20938)
Code also spinal instrumentation (22840-22855)

22305 **Closed treatment of vertebral process fracture(s)**

🔧 4.96 ✂ 5.47 **FUD** 090 T A2 PQ

AMA: 2015,Jan,16; 2013,Jul,3-5

22310 **Closed treatment of vertebral body fracture(s), without manipulation, requiring and including casting or bracing**

Do not report at same level as (22510-22515)

🔧 8.13 ✂ 8.82 **FUD** 090 T A2 PQ

AMA: 2015,Jan,16; 2015,Jan,8; 2014,Jul,8; 2014,Jan,11; 2013,Jul,3-5; 2012,Jun,10-11; 2012,Jan,15-42; 2011,Jan,11

22315 **Closed treatment of vertebral fracture(s) and/or dislocation(s) requiring casting or bracing, with and including casting and/or bracing by manipulation or traction**

EXCLUDES *Spinal manipulation (97140)*

Do not report at the same level as (22510-22515)

🔧 22.3 ✂ 25.5 **FUD** 090 T A2 PQ

AMA: 2015,Jan,16; 2015,Jan,8; 2014,Jan,11; 2013,Jul,3-5; 2012,Jun,10-11; 2012,Apr,11-13

22318-22319 Open Treatment Odontoid Fracture: Anterior Approach

EXCLUDES *Injection:*
Chemonucleolysis (62292)
Discography (62290-62291)
Facet joint (64490-64495, [64633, 64634, 64635, 64636])
Myelography (62284)
Needle/trocar biopsy (20220-20225)
Code also arthrodesis (22590-22632)
Code also bone grafting procedures (20930-20938)
Code also spinal instrumentation (22840-22855)

● New Code ▲ Revised Code ○ Reinstated Ⓜ Maternity Ⓐ Age Edit Unlisted # Resequenced
⊘ AMA Mod 51 Exempt ⑤⓪ Optum Mod 51 Exempt ◎ Mod 63 Exempt ⊙ Mod Sedation + Add-on CCI PQ PQRS FUD Follow-up Days

© 2015 Optum360, LLC (Blue Text) CPT © 2015 American Medical Association. All Rights Reserved. (Black Text) Medicare (Red Text) 45

Musculoskeletal System (side tab)

22318 — 22532 (side tab)

22318   Open treatment and/or reduction of odontoid fracture(s) and or dislocation(s) (including os odontoideum), anterior approach, including placement of internal fixation; without grafting

     48.0   48.0   **FUD** 090   C 80 P0

     AMA: 2015,Jan,16; 2014,Jan,11; 2013,Jul,3-5; 2012,Apr,11-13

22319   with grafting

     54.1   54.1   **FUD** 090   C 80 P0

     AMA: 2015,Jan,16; 2014,Jan,11; 2013,Jul,3-5; 2012,Apr,14-16

22325-22328 Open Treatment Vertebral Fractures: Posterior Approach

EXCLUDES   Corpectomy (63081-63091)
Injection:
    Chemonucleolysis (62292)
    Discography (62290-62291)
    Facet joint (64490-64495, [64633], [64634], [64635], [64636])
    Myelography (62284)
Needle/trocar biopsy (20220-20225)
Spine decompression (63001-63091)
Vertebral fracture care by arthrodesis (22548-22632)
Vertebral fracture care frontal approach (63081-63091)
Code also arthrodesis (22548-22632)
Code also bone grafting procedures (20930-20938)
Code also spinal instrumentation (22840-22855)

22325   Open treatment and/or reduction of vertebral fracture(s) and/or dislocation(s), posterior approach, 1 fractured vertebra or dislocated segment; lumbar

     Do not report at the same level as (22511-22512, 22514-22515)

     41.7   41.7   **FUD** 090   C 80 P0

     AMA: 2015,Jan,16; 2015,Jan,8; 2014,Jan,11; 2013,Jul,3-5; 2012,Jun,10-11

22326   cervical

     Do not report at the same level as (22510, 22512)

     43.7   43.7   **FUD** 090   C 80 P0

     AMA: 2015,Jan,16; 2014,Jan,11; 2013,Jul,3-5

22327   thoracic

     Do not report at the same level as (22510, 22512-22513, 22515)

     43.8   43.8   **FUD** 090   C 80 P0

     AMA: 2015,Jan,16; 2015,Jan,8; 2014,Jan,11; 2013,Jul,3-5; 2012,Jun,10-11

+ **22328**   each additional fractured vertebra or dislocated segment (List separately in addition to code for primary procedure)

     Code first (22325-22327)

     8.33   8.33   **FUD** ZZZ   C 80

     AMA: 2002,Apr,13; 1997,Nov,1

22505 Spinal Manipulation with Anesthesia

EXCLUDES   Manipulation not requiring anesthesia (97140)

22505   Manipulation of spine requiring anesthesia, any region

     3.83   3.83   **FUD** 010   T A2

     AMA: 2015,Jan,16; 2014,Jan,11; 2012,Jan,15-42; 2011,Jan,11

22510-22515 Percutaneous Vertebroplasty/Kyphoplasty

INCLUDES   Bone biopsy when applicable
EXCLUDES   Sacroplasty/augmentation (0200T-0201T)
Do not report sacral procedures more than one time per encounter
Do not report with (20225, 22310, 22315, 22325, 22327)

22510   Percutaneous vertebroplasty (bone biopsy included when performed), 1 vertebral body, unilateral or bilateral injection, inclusive of all imaging guidance; cervicothoracic

     13.1   50.1   **FUD** 010   T G2

     AMA: 2015,Jan,8

22511   lumbosacral

     12.3   49.6   **FUD** 010   T G2

     AMA: 2015,Apr,8; 2015,Jan,8

+ **22512**   each additional cervicothoracic or lumbosacral vertebral body (List separately in addition to code for primary procedure)

     Code first (22510-22511)

     6.12   27.8   **FUD** ZZZ   N M1

     AMA: 2015,Jan,8

22513   Percutaneous vertebral augmentation, including cavity creation (fracture reduction and bone biopsy included when performed) using mechanical device (eg, kyphoplasty), 1 vertebral body, unilateral or bilateral cannulation, inclusive of all imaging guidance; thoracic

     15.6   208.   **FUD** 010   T G2

     AMA: 2015,Jan,8

22514   lumbar

     14.6   207.   **FUD** 010   T G2

     AMA: 2015,Jan,8

+ **22515**   each additional thoracic or lumbar vertebral body (List separately in addition to code for primary procedure)

     Code first (22513-22514)

     6.61   125.   **FUD** ZZZ   N M1

     AMA: 2015,Jan,8

22526-22527 Percutaneous Annuloplasty

CMS: 100-4,32,220.1 Thermal Intradiscal Procedures (TIPS)

EXCLUDES   Needle/trocar biopsy (20220-20225)
Injection:
    Chemonucleolysis (62292)
    Discography (62290-62291)
    Facet joint (64490-64495, [64633], [64634], [64635], [64636])
    Myelography (62284)
    Procedure performed by other methods (22899)
Do not report with (77002, 77003)

22526   Percutaneous intradiscal electrothermal annuloplasty, unilateral or bilateral including fluoroscopic guidance; single level

     INCLUDES   Contrast injection during fluoroscopic guidance/localization (77003)

     EXCLUDES   Percutaneous intradiscal annuloplasty other than electrothermal (22899)

     9.69   67.3   **FUD** 010   E

     AMA: 2015,Jan,16; 2015,Jan,8; 2014,Jan,11; 2012,Jan,15-42; 2011,Jan,8; 2011,Jan,11; 2010,Nov,1; 2010,Nov,3

+ **22527**   1 or more additional levels (List separately in addition to code for primary procedure)

     INCLUDES   Contrast injection during fluoroscopic guidance/localization (77003)

     EXCLUDES   Percutaneous intradiscal annuloplasty other than electrothermal (22899)

     Code first (22526)

     4.40   56.0   **FUD** ZZZ   E

     AMA: 2015,Jan,16; 2015,Jan,8; 2014,Jan,11; 2011,Jan,8; 2010,Nov,1; 2010,Nov,3

22532-22534 Spinal Fusion: Lateral Extracavitary Approach

EXCLUDES   Corpectomy (63101-63103)
Exploration of spinal fusion (22830)
Fracture care (22305-22328)
Injection:
    Chemonucleolysis (62292)
    Discography (62290-62291)
    Facet joint (64490-64495, [64633], [64634], [64635], [64636])
    Myelography (62284)
Laminectomy (63001-63017)
Needle/trocar biopsy (20220-20225)
Osteotomy (22206-22226)
Code also bone grafting procedures (20930-20938)
Code also spinal instrumentation (22840-22855)

22532   Arthrodesis, lateral extracavitary technique, including minimal discectomy to prepare interspace (other than for decompression); thoracic

     51.8   51.8   **FUD** 090   C 80

     AMA: 2015,Jan,16; 2014,Jan,11; 2013,Jul,3-5; 2012,Apr,14-16

22533 **lumbar**
🦴 47.9 ⚕ 47.9 **FUD** 090 C 80 ▢
AMA: 2015,Jan,16; 2014,Jan,11; 2013,Jul,3-5; 2012,Apr,14-16

\+ 22534 **thoracic or lumbar, each additional vertebral segment (List separately in addition to code for primary procedure)**
Code first (22532-22533)
🦴 10.5 ⚕ 10.5 **FUD** ZZZ C 80 ▢
AMA: 2002,Apr,13; 1993,Spr,36

22548-22634 Spinal Fusion: Anterior and Posterior Approach

EXCLUDES Corpectomy (63081-63091)
Exploration of spinal fusion (22830)
Fracture care (22305-22328)
Facet joint arthrodesis (0219T-0222T)
Injection:
  Chemonucleolysis (62292)
  Discography (62290-62291)
  Facet joint (64490-64495, [64633], [64634], [64635], [64636])
  Myelography (62284)
Laminectomy (63001-63017)
Needle/trocar biopsy (20220-20225)
Osteotomy (22206-22216)
Code also bone grafting procedures (20930-20938)
Code also spinal instrumentation (22840-22855)

22548 **Arthrodesis, anterior transoral or extraoral technique, clivus-C1-C2 (atlas-axis), with or without excision of odontoid process**
EXCLUDES Laminectomy or laminotomy with disc removal (63020-63042)
🦴 58.1 ⚕ 58.1 **FUD** 090 C 80 ▢
AMA: 2015,Jan,16; 2014,Jan,11; 2013,Jul,3-5; 2012,Apr,14-16; 2012,Jan,15-42; 2011,Jan,11

22551 **Arthrodesis, anterior interbody, including disc space preparation, discectomy, osteophytectomy and decompression of spinal cord and/or nerve roots; cervical below C2**
INCLUDES Operating microscope (69990)
🦴 50.2 ⚕ 50.2 **FUD** 090 J J8 80
AMA: 2015,Jan,13; 2015,Jan,16; 2014,Jan,11; 2013,Jul,3-5; 2012,Apr,14-16; 2012,Jan,15-42; 2011,Jan,11

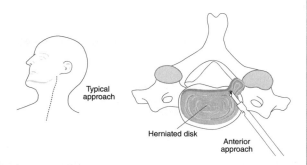

Typical approach

Herniated disk

Anterior approach

\+ 22552 **cervical below C2, each additional interspace (List separately in addition to code for separate procedure)**
INCLUDES Operating microscope (69990)
Code first (22551)
🦴 11.7 ⚕ 11.7 **FUD** ZZZ C 80
AMA: 2015,Jan,16; 2014,Jan,11; 2013,Jul,3-5; 2012,Apr,14-16; 2012,Jan,15-42; 2011,Jan,11

22554 **Arthrodesis, anterior interbody technique, including minimal discectomy to prepare interspace (other than for decompression); cervical below C2**
EXCLUDES Anterior discectomy and interbody fusion during the same operative session (regardless if performed by multiple surgeons) (22551)
Do not report with anterior discectomy (even by separate individual) (63075)
🦴 36.7 ⚕ 36.7 **FUD** 090 J J8 80 ▢ PQ
AMA: 2015,Apr,7; 2015,Jan,16; 2014,Jan,11; 2013,Jul,3-5; 2012,Apr,14-16; 2012,Apr,11-13; 2012,Jan,15-42; 2011,Jan,11

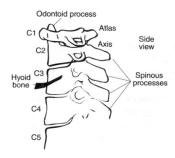

Odontoid process
Atlas
C1
Axis
C2
Side view
C3
Hyoid bone
Spinous processes
C4
C5

22556 **thoracic**
🦴 48.8 ⚕ 48.8 **FUD** 090 C 80 ▢
AMA: 2015,Jan,16; 2014,Jan,11; 2013,Jul,3-5; 2012,Apr,14-16; 2012,Jan,15-42; 2011,Jan,11

22558 **lumbar**
EXCLUDES Arthrodesis using pre-sacral interbody technique (22586, 0195T)
🦴 44.8 ⚕ 44.8 **FUD** 090 C 80 ▢ PQ
AMA: 2015,Mar,9; 2015,Jan,16; 2014,Jan,11; 2013,Jul,3-5; 2012,Apr,14-16; 2012,Jan,15-42; 2011,Jan,11

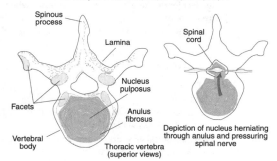

Spinous process
Lamina
Spinal cord
Nucleus pulposus
Facets
Anulus fibrosus
Vertebral body
Thoracic vertebra (superior views)
Depiction of nucleus herniating through anulus and pressuring spinal nerve

\+ 22585 **each additional interspace (List separately in addition to code for primary procedure)**
EXCLUDES Anterior discectomy and interbody fusion during the same operative session (regardless if performed by multiple surgeons) (22552)
Code first (22554-22558)
Do not report with anterior discectomy (even by another individual) (63075)
🦴 9.67 ⚕ 9.67 **FUD** ZZZ C 80 ▢
AMA: 2015,Jan,16; 2014,Jan,11; 2012,Jan,15-42; 2011,Jan,11

22586 **Arthrodesis, pre-sacral interbody technique, including disc space preparation, discectomy, with posterior instrumentation, with image guidance, includes bone graft when performed, L5-S1 interspace**
🦴 59.1 ⚕ 59.1 **FUD** 090 C 80
Do not report with (20930-20938, 22840, 22848, 72275, 77002-77003, 77011-77012)

22590   **Arthrodesis, posterior technique, craniocervical (occiput-C2)**

> EXCLUDES   *Posterior intrafacet implant insertion (0219T-0222T)*
> 🦴 46.2   ⚖ 46.2   **FUD** 090   C 80 ▭
> **AMA:** 2015,Jan,16; 2014,Jan,11; 2013,Jul,3-5; 2012,Apr,14-16

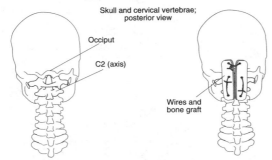

Skull and cervical vertebrae;
posterior view

Occiput

C2 (axis)

Wires and
bone graft

In 22590, the physician fuses skull to C2 (axis) to stabilize cervical
vertebrae; anchor holes are drilled in the occiput of the skull

22595   **Arthrodesis, posterior technique, atlas-axis (C1-C2)**

> EXCLUDES   *Posterior intrafacet implant insertion (0219T-0222T)*
> 🦴 44.2   ⚖ 44.2   **FUD** 090   C 80 ▭
> **AMA:** 2015,Jan,16; 2014,Jan,11; 2013,Jul,3-5; 2012,Apr,14-16; 2012,Apr,11-13

22600   **Arthrodesis, posterior or posterolateral technique, single level; cervical below C2 segment**

> EXCLUDES   *Posterior intrafacet implant insertion (0219T-0222T)*
> 🦴 37.7   ⚖ 37.7   **FUD** 090   C 80 ▭ PQ
> **AMA:** 2015,Jan,16; 2014,Jan,11; 2013,Jul,3-5; 2012,Jun,10-11; 2012,Apr,14-16; 2010,Nov,8

22610   **thoracic (with lateral transverse technique, when performed)**

> EXCLUDES   *Posterior intrafacet implant insertion (0219T-0222T)*
> 🦴 36.8   ⚖ 36.8   **FUD** 090   C 80 ▭
> **AMA:** 2015,Jan,16; 2014,Jan,11; 2013,Jul,3-5; 2012,Jun,10-11; 2012,Apr,14-16; 2010,Nov,8

22612   **lumbar (with lateral transverse technique, when performed)**

> EXCLUDES   *Combined technique at the same interspace and segment (22633)*
> *Posterior intrafacet implant insertion (0219T-0222T)*
> Do not report with the following code when performed at the same interspace and segment (22630)
> 🦴 46.3   ⚖ 46.3   **FUD** 090   J J8 80 ▭ PQ
> **AMA:** 2015,Jan,16; 2014,Jan,11; 2013,Dec,14; 2013,Jul,3-5; 2012,Jun,10-11; 2012,Apr,14-16; 2012,Jan,15-42; 2012,Jan,3-5; 2011,Dec,14-18; 2011,Jan,11; 2010,Nov,8

+   22614   **each additional vertebral segment (List separately in addition to code for primary procedure)**

> INCLUDES   Additional level fusion arthrodesis posterior or posterolateral interbody
> EXCLUDES   *Additional level interbody arthrodesis combined posterolateral or posterior with posterior interbody arthrodesis (22634)*
> *Additional level posterior interbody arthrodesis (22632)*
> *Posterior intrafacet implant insertion (0219T-0222T)*
> Code first (22600, 22610, 22612, 22630, 22633)
> 🦴 11.5   ⚖ 11.5   **FUD** ZZZ   N N1 80 ▭
> **AMA:** 2015,Jan,16; 2014,Jan,11; 2013,Jul,3-5; 2012,Jun,10-11; 2010,Nov,8

22630   **Arthrodesis, posterior interbody technique, including laminectomy and/or discectomy to prepare interspace (other than for decompression), single interspace; lumbar**

> EXCLUDES   *Combined technique at the same interspace and segment (22633)*
> Do not report with the following code at the same interspace and segment (22612)
> 🦴 45.9   ⚖ 45.9   **FUD** 090   C 80 ▭ PQ
> **AMA:** 2015,Jan,16; 2014,Jan,11; 2013,Jul,3-5; 2012,Jun,10-11; 2012,Apr,14-16; 2012,Jan,3-5; 2012,Jan,15-42; 2011,Dec,14-18; 2011,Jan,11

+   22632   **each additional interspace (List separately in addition to code for primary procedure)**

> INCLUDES   Includes posterior interbody fusion arthrodesis, additional level
> EXCLUDES   *Additional level combined technique (22634)*
> *Additional level posterior or posterolateral fusion (22614)*
> Code first (22612, 22630, 22633)
> 🦴 9.46   ⚖ 9.46   **FUD** ZZZ   C 80 ▭
> **AMA:** 2015,Jan,16; 2014,Jan,11; 2013,Jul,3-5; 2012,Jun,10-11

22633   **Arthrodesis, combined posterior or posterolateral technique with posterior interbody technique including laminectomy and/or discectomy sufficient to prepare interspace (other than for decompression), single interspace and segment; lumbar**

> Do not report same level (22612, 22630)
> 🦴 54.1   ⚖ 54.1   **FUD** 090   C 80
> **AMA:** 2015,Jan,16; 2014,Jan,11; 2013,Jul,3-5; 2012,Jun,10-11; 2012,Jan,15-42; 2012,Jan,3-5; 2011,Dec,14-18

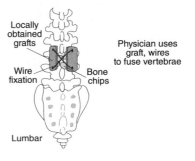

Locally
obtained
grafts

Physician uses
graft, wires
to fuse vertebrae

Wire
fixation

Bone
chips

Lumbar

Using a posterior or posterolateral technique
the vertebral interbody is fused

+   22634   **each additional interspace and segment (List separately in addition to code for primary procedure)**

> Code first (22633)
> 🦴 14.6   ⚖ 14.6   **FUD** ZZZ   C 80
> **AMA:** 2015,Jan,16; 2014,Jan,11; 2013,Jul,3-5; 2012,Jun,10-11; 2012,Jan,15-42; 2011,Dec,14-18

22800-22819 Procedures to Correct Anomalous Spinal Vertebrae

CMS: 100-3,150.2 Osteogenic Stimulation
> EXCLUDES   *Facet injection (64490-64495, [64633, 64634, 64635, 64636])*
> Code also bone grafting procedures (20930-20938)
> Code also spinal instrumentation (22840-22855)

22800   **Arthrodesis, posterior, for spinal deformity, with or without cast; up to 6 vertebral segments**

> 🦴 39.3   ⚖ 39.3   **FUD** 090   C 80 ▭ PQ
> **AMA:** 2015,Jan,16; 2014,Jan,11; 2013,Jul,3-5; 2012,Apr,14-16

22802   **7 to 12 vertebral segments**

> 🦴 61.1   ⚖ 61.1   **FUD** 090   C 80 ▭ PQ
> **AMA:** 2015,Jan,16; 2014,Jan,11; 2013,Jul,3-5; 2012,Apr,14-16; 2012,Jan,15-42; 2011,Jan,11

22804   **13 or more vertebral segments**

🚗 70.8   ⚖ 70.8   **FUD** 090   C 80 ▢ P0

AMA: 2015,Jan,16; 2014,Jan,11; 2013,Jul,3-5; 2012,Apr,14-16

22808   **Arthrodesis, anterior, for spinal deformity, with or without cast; 2 to 3 vertebral segments**

INCLUDES   Smith-Robinson arthrodesis

🚗 53.8   ⚖ 53.8   **FUD** 090   C 80 ▢

AMA: 2015,Jan,16; 2014,Jan,11; 2013,Jul,3-5; 2012,Apr,14-16

22810   **4 to 7 vertebral segments**

🚗 58.9   ⚖ 58.9   **FUD** 090   C 80 ▢

AMA: 2015,Jan,16; 2014,Jan,11; 2013,Jul,3-5; 2012,Apr,14-16; 2012,Jan,15-42; 2011,Jan,11

22812   **8 or more vertebral segments**

🚗 64.1   ⚖ 64.1   **FUD** 090   C 80 ▢

AMA: 2015,Jan,16; 2014,Jan,11; 2013,Jul,3-5; 2012,Apr,14-16

22818   **Kyphectomy, circumferential exposure of spine and resection of vertebral segment(s) (including body and posterior elements); single or 2 segments**

EXCLUDES   *Arthrodesis (22800-22804)*

🚗 63.0   ⚖ 63.0   **FUD** 090   C 80 ▢

AMA: 2002,Apr,13; 1999,Dec,3

22819   **3 or more segments**

EXCLUDES   *Arthrodesis (22800-22804)*

🚗 81.5   ⚖ 81.5   **FUD** 090   C 80 ▢

AMA: 2002,Apr,13; 1999,Dec,3

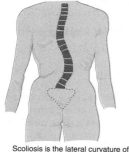
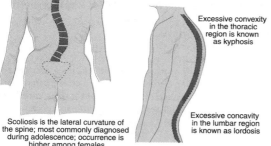

Excessively kyphotic thoracic spine may be caused by Scheuermann's disease or juvenile kyphosis

Excessive convexity in the thoracic region is known as kyphosis

Scoliosis is the lateral curvature of the spine; most commonly diagnosed during adolescence; occurrence is higher among females

Excessive concavity in the lumbar region is known as lordosis

22830 Surgical Exploration Previous Spinal Fusion

CMS: 100-3,150.2 Osteogenic Stimulation

EXCLUDES   *Arthrodesis (22532-22819)*
     Bone grafting procedures (20930-20938)
     Facet injection (64490-64495, [64633, 64634, 64635, 64636])
     Spinal decompression (63001-63103)
Code also spinal instrumentation (22840-22855)

22830   **Exploration of spinal fusion**

Do not report with (22850, 22852, 22855)

🚗 23.6   ⚖ 23.6   **FUD** 090   C 80 ▢

AMA: 2015,Jan,16; 2014,Jan,11; 2012,Jan,15-42; 2011,Jan,11; 2010,Mar,9-11

22840-22848 Posterior, Anterior, Pelvic Spinal Instrumentation

INCLUDES   Removal or revision of previously placed spinal instrumentation during same session as insertion of new instrumentation at levels including all or part of previously instrumented segments

EXCLUDES   *Arthrodesis (22532-22534, 22548-22812)*
     Bone grafting procedures (20930-20938)
     Exploration of spinal fusion (22830)
     Fracture treatment (22325-22328)
Do not report removal or reinsertion in addition to insertion of the new instrumentation (22849, 22850, 22852, 22855)

+ **22840**   **Posterior non-segmental instrumentation (eg, Harrington rod technique, pedicle fixation across 1 interspace, atlantoaxial transarticular screw fixation, sublaminar wiring at C1, facet screw fixation) (List separately in addition to code for primary procedure)**

EXCLUDES   *Insertion of posterior spinous process distraction devices (0171T-0172T)*

Code first (22100-22102, 22110-22114, 22206-22207, 22210-22214, 22220-22224, 22305-22327, 22532-22533, 22548-22558, 22590-22612, 22630, 22633-22634, 22800-22812, 63001-63030, 63040-63042, 63045-63047, 63050-63056, 63064, 63075, 63077, 63081, 63085, 63087, 63090, 63101-63102, 63170-63290, 63300-63307)

🚗 22.3   ⚖ 22.3   **FUD** ZZZ   C 80 ▢

AMA: 2015,Jan,16; 2014,Oct,14; 2014,Jan,11; 2013,Dec,16; 2013,Jul,3-5; 2012,Jun,10-11; 2012,Apr,11-13; 2012,Jan,15-42; 2011,Dec,14-18; 2011,Jan,11; 2011,Jan,9-10; 2010,Nov,8

+ **22841**   **Internal spinal fixation by wiring of spinous processes (List separately in addition to code for primary procedure)**

Code first (22100-22102, 22110-22114, 22206-22207, 22210-22214, 22220-22224, 22305-22327, 22532-22533, 22548-22558, 22590-22612, 22630, 22633-22634, 22800-22812, 63001-63030, 63040-63042, 63045-63047, 63050-63056, 63064, 63075, 63077, 63081, 63085, 63087, 63090, 63101-63102, 63170-63290, 63300-63307)

🚗 0.00   ⚖ 0.00   **FUD** XXX   C

AMA: 2015,Jan,16; 2014,Jan,11; 2013,Jul,3-5; 2012,Jun,10-11

+ **22842**   **Posterior segmental instrumentation (eg, pedicle fixation, dual rods with multiple hooks and sublaminar wires); 3 to 6 vertebral segments (List separately in addition to code for primary procedure)**

Code first (22100-22102, 22110-22114, 22206-22207, 22210-22214, 22220-22224, 22305-22327, 22532-22533, 22548-22558, 22590-22612, 22630, 22633-22634, 22800-22812, 63001-63030, 63040-63042, 63045-63047, 63050-63056, 63064, 63075, 63077, 63081, 63085, 63087, 63090, 63101-63102, 63170-63290, 63300-63307)

🚗 22.4   ⚖ 22.4   **FUD** ZZZ   C 80 ▢

AMA: 2015,Jan,16; 2014,Jan,11; 2013,Jul,3-5; 2012,Jun,10-11; 2011,Dec,14-18

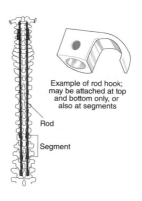

Example of rod hook; may be attached at top and bottom only, or also at segments

Rod

Segment

+ **22843**   **7 to 12 vertebral segments (List separately in addition to code for primary procedure)**

Code first (22100-22102, 22110-22114, 22206-22207, 22210-22214, 22220-22224, 22305-22327, 22532-22533, 22548-22558, 22590-22612, 22630, 22633-22634, 22800-22812, 63001-63030, 63040-63042, 63045-63047, 63050-63056, 63064, 63075, 63077, 63081, 63085, 63087, 63090, 63101-63102, 63170-63290, 63300-63307)

🚗 24.0   ⚖ 24.0   **FUD** ZZZ   C 80 ▢

AMA: 2015,Jan,16; 2014,Jan,11; 2013,Jul,3-5; 2012,Jun,10-11; 2011,Dec,14-18

+ 22844 **13 or more vertebral segments** (List separately in addition to code for primary procedure)

Code first (22100-22102, 22110-22114, 22206-22207, 22210-22214, 22220-22224, 22305-22327, 22532-22533, 22548-22558, 22590-22612, 22630, 22633-22634, 22800-22812, 63001-63030, 63040-63042, 63045-63047, 63050-63056, 63064, 63075, 63077, 63081, 63085, 63087, 63090, 63101-63102, 63170-63290, 63300-63307)

🛏 28.9   ⚕ 28.9   **FUD** ZZZ   [C] [80] 🔲

AMA: 2015,Jan,16; 2014,Jan,11; 2013,Jul,3-5; 2012,Jun,10-11; 2011,Dec,14-18

+ 22845 **Anterior instrumentation; 2 to 3 vertebral segments** (List separately in addition to code for primary procedure)

INCLUDES   Dwyer instrumentation technique

Code first (22100-22102, 22110-22114, 22206-22207, 22210-22214, 22220-22224, 22305-22327, 22532-22533, 22548-22558, 22590-22612, 22630, 22633-22634, 22800-22812, 63001-63030, 63040-63042, 63045-63047, 63050-63056, 63064, 63075, 63077, 63081, 63085, 63087, 63090, 63101-63102, 63170-63290, 63300-63307)

🛏 21.5   ⚕ 21.5   **FUD** ZZZ   [C] [80] 🔲

AMA: 2015,Apr,7; 2015,Mar,9; 2015,Jan,16; 2015,Jan,13; 2014,Nov,14; 2014,Jan,11; 2013,Jul,3-5; 2012,Jun,10-11; 2012,Jan,15-42; 2011,Jan,11

+ 22846 **4 to 7 vertebral segments** (List separately in addition to code for primary procedure)

INCLUDES   Dwyer instrumentation technique

Code first (22100-22102, 22110-22114, 22206-22207, 22210-22214, 22220-22224, 22305-22327, 22532-22533, 22548-22558, 22590-22612, 22630, 22633-22634, 22800-22812, 63001-63030, 63040-63042, 63045-63047, 63050-63056, 63064, 63075, 63077, 63081, 63085, 63087, 63090, 63101-63102, 63170-63290, 63300-63307)

🛏 22.3   ⚕ 22.3   **FUD** ZZZ   [C] [80] 🔲

AMA: 2015,Jan,16; 2014,Jan,11; 2013,Jul,3-5; 2012,Jun,10-11; 2012,Jan,15-42; 2011,Jan,11

+ 22847 **8 or more vertebral segments** (List separately in addition to code for primary procedure)

INCLUDES   Dwyer instrumentation technique

Code first (22100-22102, 22110-22114, 22206-22207, 22210-22214, 22220-22224, 22305-22327, 22532-22533, 22548-22558, 22590-22612, 22630, 22633-22634, 22800-22812, 63001-63030, 63040-63042, 63045-63047, 63050-63056, 63064, 63075, 63077, 63081, 63085, 63087, 63090, 63101-63102, 63170-63290, 63300-63307)

🛏 23.3   ⚕ 23.3   **FUD** ZZZ   [C] [80] 🔲

AMA: 2015,Jan,16; 2014,Jan,11; 2013,Jul,3-5; 2012,Jun,10-11; 2012,Jan,15-42; 2011,Jan,11

+ 22848 **Pelvic fixation (attachment of caudal end of instrumentation to pelvic bony structures) other than sacrum** (List separately in addition to code for primary procedure)

Code first (22100-22102, 22110-22114, 22206-22207, 22210-22214, 22220-22224, 22305-22327, 22532-22533, 22548-22558, 22590-22612, 22630, 22633-22634, 22800-22812, 63001-63030, 63040-63042, 63045-63047, 63050-63056, 63064, 63075, 63077, 63081, 63085, 63087, 63090, 63101-63102, 63170-63290, 63300-63307)

🛏 10.5   ⚕ 10.5   **FUD** ZZZ   [C] [80] 🔲

AMA: 2015,Jan,16; 2014,Jan,11; 2013,Jul,3-5; 2012,Jun,10-11

22849-22855 Miscellaneous Spinal Instrumentation

EXCLUDES   Arthrodesis (22532-22534, 22548-22812)
Bone grafting procedures (20930-20938)
Exploration of spinal fusion (22830)
Facet injection (64490-64495, [64633], [64634], [64635], [64636])
Fracture treatment (22325-22328)

22849 **Reinsertion of spinal fixation device**

Do not report with removal of instrumentation at the same level (22850, 22852, 22855)

🛏 37.9   ⚕ 37.9   **FUD** 090   [C] [80] 🔲

AMA: 2015,Jan,16; 2014,Jan,11; 2013,Jul,3-5; 2012,Jun,10-11; 2012,Jan,15-42; 2011,Oct,10

22850 **Removal of posterior nonsegmental instrumentation (eg, Harrington rod)**

🛏 21.0   ⚕ 21.0   **FUD** 090   [C] [80] 🔲

AMA: 2015,Jan,16; 2014,Jan,11; 2013,Jul,3-5; 2012,Jun,10-11

+ 22851 **Application of intervertebral biomechanical device(s) (eg, synthetic cage(s), methylmethacrylate) to vertebral defect or interspace** (List separately in addition to code for primary procedure)

EXCLUDES   Application of intervertebral bone device/graft (20930-20938)
Insertion of posterior spinous process distraction devices (0171T-0172T)

Code first (22100-22102, 22110-22114, 22206-22207, 22210-22214, 22220-22224, 22305-22327, 22532-22533, 22548-22558, 22590-22612, 22630, 22633-22634, 22800-22812, 63001-63030, 63040-63042, 63045-63047, 63050-63056, 63064, 63075, 63077, 63081, 63085, 63087, 63090, 63101-63102, 63170-63290, 63300-63307)

🛏 11.9   ⚕ 11.9   **FUD** ZZZ   [N] [80] 🔲

AMA: 2015,Apr,7; 2015,Mar,9; 2015,Jan,13; 2015,Jan,16; 2014,Nov,14; 2014,Jan,11; 2013,Jul,3-5; 2012,Jun,10-11; 2012,Jan,15-42; 2011,Dec,14-18; 2011,Oct,10; 2011,Jan,11; 2010,Nov,8

22852 **Removal of posterior segmental instrumentation**

🛏 20.1   ⚕ 20.1   **FUD** 090   [C] [80] 🔲

AMA: 2015,Jan,16; 2014,Jan,11; 2012,Jun,10-11; 2012,Jan,15-42; 2011,Jan,11

22855 **Removal of anterior instrumentation**

🛏 32.3   ⚕ 32.3   **FUD** 090   [C] [80] 🔲

AMA: 2015,Jan,16; 2014,Jan,11; 2012,Jun,10-11

22856-22899 [22858] Artificial Disc Replacement

CMS: 100-3,150.10 Lumbar Artificial Disc Replacement (LADR)

INCLUDES   Fluoroscopy (76000-76001)
EXCLUDES   Facet injection (64490-64495, [64633], [64634], [64635], [64636])
Spinal decompression (63001-63048)

22856 **Total disc arthroplasty (artificial disc), anterior approach, including discectomy with end plate preparation (includes osteophytectomy for nerve root or spinal cord decompression and microdissection); single interspace, cervical**

INCLUDES   Operating microscope (69990)
EXCLUDES   Cervical total disc arthroplasty, 3 or more levels (0375T)
Code also ([22858])
Do not report at same level as (22554, 22845, 22851, 63075, 0375T)

🛏 46.4   ⚕ 46.4   **FUD** 090   [J] [80]

AMA: 2015,Apr,7

+ # 22858 **second level, cervical** (List separately in addition to code for primary procedure)

🛏 14.5   ⚕ 14.5   **FUD** ZZZ   [C] [80]

AMA: 2015,Apr,7

22857 **Total disc arthroplasty (artificial disc), anterior approach, including discectomy to prepare interspace (other than for decompression), single interspace, lumbar**

INCLUDES   Operating microscope (69990)
EXCLUDES   Arthroplasty more than one interspace (0163T)
Do not report at same level (22558, 22845, 22851, 49010)

🛏 51.5   ⚕ 51.5   **FUD** 090   [C] [80]

AMA: 2007,Jun,1-3

22858 **Resequenced code. See code following 22856.**

22861 **Revision including replacement of total disc arthroplasty (artificial disc), anterior approach, single interspace; cervical**

🛏 55.9   ⚕ 55.9   **FUD** 090   [C] [80]

INCLUDES   Operating microscope (69990)
EXCLUDES   Removal of artificial disc (22864)
Revision of additional cervical arthroplasty (0098T)
Do not report at same level (22845, 22851, 22864, 63075)

 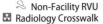

22862 **lumbar**

EXCLUDES Arthroplasty revision more than one interspace (0165T)
Do not report at same level (22558, 22845, 22851, 22864, 49010)
🔧 50.7 ✂ 50.7 **FUD** 090 [C] [80]
AMA: 2015,Jan,16; 2014,Jan,11

22864 **Removal of total disc arthroplasty (artificial disc), anterior approach, single interspace; cervical**

🔧 61.6 ✂ 61.6 **FUD** 090 [C] [80]

INCLUDES Operating microscope (69990)
EXCLUDES Cervical total disc arthroplasty with additional interspace removal (0095T)
Do not report with (22861)

22865 **lumbar**

EXCLUDES Arthroplasty more than one level (0164T)
Do not report with (49010)
🔧 59.4 ✂ 59.4 **FUD** 090 [C] [80]
AMA: 2015,Jan,16; 2014,Jan,11

22899 **Unlisted procedure, spine**

🔧 0.00 ✂ 0.00 **FUD** YYY [T] [80]
AMA: 2015,Jan,16; 2015,Jan,8; 2014,Oct,14; 2014,Jan,11; 2013,Dec,14; 2013,Dec,16; 2012,Dec,12; 2012,Oct,14; 2012,Sep,16; 2012,Jan,15-42; 2012,Jan,13-14; 2011,Jan,11; 2010,Nov,4; 2010,Jan,12-15

22900-22999 Musculoskeletal Procedures of Abdomen

INCLUDES Any necessary elevation of tissue planes or dissection
Measurement of tumor and necessary margin at greatest diameter prior to excision
Simple and intermediate repairs
Types of excision:
Fascial or subfascial soft tissue tumors: simple and marginal resection of tumors found either in or below the deep fascia, not involving bone or excision of a substantial amount of normal tissue; primarily benign and intramuscular tumors
Radical resection soft tissue tumor: wide resection of tumor involving substantial margins of normal tissue and may include tissue removal from one or more layers; most often malignant or aggressive benign
Subcutaneous: simple and marginal resection of tumors in the subcutaneous tissue above the deep fascia; most often benign
EXCLUDES Complex repair
Excision of benign cutaneous lesions (eg, sebaceous cyst) (11400-11406)
Radical resection of cutaneous tumors (eg, melanoma) (11600-11606)
Significant exploration of the vessels or neuroplasty

22900 **Excision, tumor, soft tissue of abdominal wall, subfascial (eg, intramuscular); less than 5 cm**

🔧 16.2 ✂ 16.2 **FUD** 090 [T] [62] [80] ⌐
AMA: 2002,Apr,13

22901 **5 cm or greater**

🔧 19.1 ✂ 19.1 **FUD** 090 [T] [62] [80]

22902 **Excision, tumor, soft tissue of abdominal wall, subcutaneous; less than 3 cm**

🔧 9.50 ✂ 12.5 **FUD** 090 [T] [62] [80]

22903 **3 cm or greater**

🔧 12.6 ✂ 12.6 **FUD** 090 [T] [62] [80]

22904 **Radical resection of tumor (eg, sarcoma), soft tissue of abdominal wall; less than 5 cm**

🔧 30.3 ✂ 30.3 **FUD** 090 [T] [62] [80]

22905 **5 cm or greater**

🔧 38.3 ✂ 38.3 **FUD** 090 [T] [62] [80]

22999 **Unlisted procedure, abdomen, musculoskeletal system**

🔧 0.00 ✂ 0.00 **FUD** YYY [T] [80]
AMA: 2002,Apr,13

23000-23044 Surgical Incision Shoulder: Drainage, Foreign Body Removal, Contracture Release

23000 **Removal of subdeltoid calcareous deposits, open**

EXCLUDES Arthroscopic removal calcium deposits of bursa (29999)
🔧 10.7 ✂ 16.8 **FUD** 090 [T] [A2] [80] [50] ⌐
AMA: 2002,Apr,13

23020 **Capsular contracture release (eg, Sever type procedure)**

EXCLUDES Simple incision and drainage (10040-10160)
🔧 19.8 ✂ 19.8 **FUD** 090 [T] [A2] [80] [50] ⌐
AMA: 2002,Apr,13; 1998,Nov,1

23030 **Incision and drainage, shoulder area; deep abscess or hematoma**

🔧 7.36 ✂ 12.6 **FUD** 010 [T] [A2] ⌐
AMA: 2002,Apr,13

23031 **infected bursa**

🔧 6.33 ✂ 12.2 **FUD** 010 [T] [A2] [50] ⌐
AMA: 2002,Apr,13

Supraspinatus muscle and tendon
Acromion
Scapula
Bursa
Head of humerus
Acromion
Clavicle
Glenoid cavity
Deltoid muscle
Coracoid process
Teres major muscle
Humerus
Scapula
Triceps

Section of left shoulder

The fibrous capsule enclosing the shoulder is thin and loose to allow freedom of movement; four rotator cuff muscles (supraspinatus, infraspinatus, teres minor, and scapularis) work together to hold the head of the humerus in the glenoid cavity

23035 **Incision, bone cortex (eg, osteomyelitis or bone abscess), shoulder area**

🔧 19.5 ✂ 19.5 **FUD** 090 [T] [A2] [80] [50] ⌐
AMA: 2003,Jan,1; 2002,Apr,13

23040 **Arthrotomy, glenohumeral joint, including exploration, drainage, or removal of foreign body**

🔧 20.7 ✂ 20.7 **FUD** 090 [T] [A2] [80] [50] ⌐
AMA: 2002,Apr,13; 1998,Nov,1

23044 **Arthrotomy, acromioclavicular, sternoclavicular joint, including exploration, drainage, or removal of foreign body**

🔧 16.4 ✂ 16.4 **FUD** 090 [T] [A2] [50] ⌐
AMA: 2002,Apr,13; 1998,Nov,1

23065-23066 Shoulder Biopsy

EXCLUDES Soft tissue needle biopsy (20206)

23065 **Biopsy, soft tissue of shoulder area; superficial**

🔧 4.79 ✂ 6.16 **FUD** 010 [T] [P3] [50] ⌐ [P0]
AMA: 2002,Apr,13

23066 **deep**

🔧 10.2 ✂ 15.9 **FUD** 090 [T] [A2] [50] ⌐ [P0]
AMA: 2002,Apr,13

23071-23078 [23071, 23073] Excision Soft Tissue Tumors of Shoulder

INCLUDES Any necessary elevation of tissue planes or dissection
Measurement of tumor and necessary margin at greatest diameter prior to excision
Simple and intermediate repairs
Types of excision:
Fascial or subfascial soft tissue tumors: simple and marginal resection of tumors found either in or below the deep fascia, not involving bone or excision of a substantial amount of normal tissue; primarily benign and intramuscular tumors
Radical resection soft tissue tumor: wide resection of tumor, involving substantial margins of normal tissue and may involve tissue removal from one or more layers; most often malignant or aggressive benign
Subcutaneous: simple and marginal resection of tumors in the subcutaneous tissue above the deep fascia; most often benign
EXCLUDES Complex repair
Excision of benign cutaneous lesions (eg, sebaceous cyst) (11400-11406)
Radical resection of cutaneous tumors (eg, melanoma) (11600-11606)
Significant exploration of the vessels or neuroplasty

23071 **Resequenced code. See code following 23075.**

Musculoskeletal System

23073 — 23210

	23073	Resequenced code. See code following 23076.				

23075 Excision, tumor, soft tissue of shoulder area, subcutaneous; less than 3 cm
🔹 9.37 ✂ 13.3 **FUD** 090 T G2 50 ▢
AMA: 2015,Jan,16; 2014,Jan,11

\# **23071** 3 cm or greater
🔹 12.0 ✂ 12.0 **FUD** 090 T G2 80 50 ▢
AMA: 2009,Oct,7,8&13

23076 Excision, tumor, soft tissue of shoulder area, subfascial (eg, intramuscular); less than 5 cm
🔹 15.5 ✂ 15.5 **FUD** 090 T G2 50 ▢
AMA: 2015,Jan,16; 2014,Jan,11

\# **23073** 5 cm or greater
🔹 19.9 ✂ 19.9 **FUD** 090 T G2 80 50 ▢
AMA: 2009,Oct,7,8&13

23077 Radical resection of tumor (eg, sarcoma), soft tissue of shoulder area; less than 5 cm
🔹 32.8 ✂ 32.8 **FUD** 090 T G2 80 50 ▢
AMA: 2002,Apr,13; 1990,Win,4

23078 5 cm or greater
🔹 41.2 ✂ 41.2 **FUD** 090 T G2 80 50

23100-23195 Bone and Joint Procedures of Shoulder

INCLUDES Acromioclavicular joint
Clavicle
Head and neck of humerus
Scapula
Shoulder joint
Sternoclavicular joint

23100 Arthrotomy, glenohumeral joint, including biopsy
🔹 14.3 ✂ 14.3 **FUD** 090 T A2 80 50 ▢ PQ
AMA: 2002,Apr,13; 1998,Nov,1

23101 Arthrotomy, acromioclavicular joint or sternoclavicular joint, including biopsy and/or excision of torn cartilage
🔹 12.9 ✂ 12.9 **FUD** 090 T A2 50 ▢ PQ
AMA: 2002,Apr,13; 1998,Nov,1

23105 Arthrotomy; glenohumeral joint, with synovectomy, with or without biopsy
🔹 18.3 ✂ 18.3 **FUD** 090 T A2 80 50 ▢
AMA: 2002,Apr,13; 1998,Nov,1

23106 sternoclavicular joint, with synovectomy, with or without biopsy
🔹 14.2 ✂ 14.2 **FUD** 090 T A2 50 ▢
AMA: 2002,Apr,13; 1998,Nov,1

23107 Arthrotomy, glenohumeral joint, with joint exploration, with or without removal of loose or foreign body
🔹 18.9 ✂ 18.9 **FUD** 090 T A2 80 50 ▢
AMA: 2002,Apr,13

23120 Claviculectomy; partial
INCLUDES Mumford operation
EXCLUDES Arthroscopic claviculectomy (29824)
🔹 16.8 ✂ 16.8 **FUD** 090 T A2 80 50 ▢
AMA: 2015,Jan,16; 2014,Jan,11; 2012,Oct,14; 2012,Sep,16

23125 total
🔹 20.4 ✂ 20.4 **FUD** 090 T A2 80 50 ▢
AMA: 2003,Jan,1; 2002,Apr,13

23130 Acromioplasty or acromionectomy, partial, with or without coracoacromial ligament release
🔹 17.5 ✂ 17.5 **FUD** 090 T A2 50 ▢
AMA: 2015,Mar,7; 2015,Feb,10; 2015,Jan,16; 2014,Jan,11; 2012,Jan,15-42; 2011,Jan,11

23140 Excision or curettage of bone cyst or benign tumor of clavicle or scapula;
🔹 15.1 ✂ 15.1 **FUD** 090 T A2 50 ▢
AMA: 2002,Apr,13

23145 with autograft (includes obtaining graft)
🔹 20.0 ✂ 20.0 **FUD** 090 T A2 80 50 ▢
AMA: 2002,Apr,13

23146 with allograft
🔹 17.8 ✂ 17.8 **FUD** 090 T A2 80 50 ▢
AMA: 2002,Apr,13

23150 Excision or curettage of bone cyst or benign tumor of proximal humerus;
🔹 19.0 ✂ 19.0 **FUD** 090 T A2 80 50 ▢
AMA: 2002,Apr,13

23155 with autograft (includes obtaining graft)
🔹 22.8 ✂ 22.8 **FUD** 090 T A2 80 50 ▢
AMA: 2002,Apr,13

23156 with allograft
🔹 19.5 ✂ 19.5 **FUD** 090 T A2 80 50 ▢
AMA: 2002,Apr,13

23170 Sequestrectomy (eg, for osteomyelitis or bone abscess), clavicle
🔹 16.1 ✂ 16.1 **FUD** 090 T A2 50 ▢
AMA: 2002,Apr,13

23172 Sequestrectomy (eg, for osteomyelitis or bone abscess), scapula
🔹 16.2 ✂ 16.2 **FUD** 090 T A2 80 50 ▢
AMA: 2002,Apr,13

23174 Sequestrectomy (eg, for osteomyelitis or bone abscess), humeral head to surgical neck
🔹 21.8 ✂ 21.8 **FUD** 090 T A2 80 50 ▢
AMA: 2002,Apr,13

23180 Partial excision (craterization, saucerization, or diaphysectomy) bone (eg, osteomyelitis), clavicle
🔹 19.2 ✂ 19.2 **FUD** 090 T A2 50 ▢
AMA: 2002,Apr,13; 1998,Nov,1

23182 Partial excision (craterization, saucerization, or diaphysectomy) bone (eg, osteomyelitis), scapula
🔹 18.9 ✂ 18.9 **FUD** 090 T A2 80 50 ▢
AMA: 2002,Apr,13; 1998,Nov,1

23184 Partial excision (craterization, saucerization, or diaphysectomy) bone (eg, osteomyelitis), proximal humerus
🔹 21.1 ✂ 21.1 **FUD** 090 T A2 80 50 ▢
AMA: 2002,Apr,13; 1998,Nov,1

23190 Ostectomy of scapula, partial (eg, superior medial angle)
🔹 16.4 ✂ 16.4 **FUD** 090 T A2 80 50 ▢
AMA: 2002,Apr,13

23195 Resection, humeral head
EXCLUDES Arthroplasty with replacement with implant (23470)
🔹 21.7 ✂ 21.7 **FUD** 090 T A2 80 50 ▢
AMA: 2003,Jan,1; 2002,Apr,13

23200-23220 Radical Resection of Bone Tumors of Shoulder

INCLUDES Any necessary elevation of tissue planes or dissection
Measurement of tumor and necessary margin at greatest diameter prior to excision
Radical resection of cutaneous tumors (e.g., melanoma)
Resection of the tumor (may include entire bone) and wide margins of normal tissues primarily for malignant or aggressive benign tumors
Simple and intermediate repairs
EXCLUDES Complex repair
Significant exploration of vessels, neuroplasty, reconstruction, or complex bone repair
Do not report excision of soft tissue codes when adjacent soft tissue is removed during the bone tumor resection (23071-23078 [23071, 23073])

23200 Radical resection of tumor; clavicle
🔹 43.8 ✂ 43.8 **FUD** 090 C 80 50 ▢
AMA: 2002,Apr,13

23210 scapula
🔹 51.5 ✂ 51.5 **FUD** 090 C 80 50 ▢
AMA: 2002,Apr,13

23220 Radical resection of tumor, proximal humerus

      🔲 56.5   ⚕ 56.5   **FUD** 090   C 80 50 ▯

       AMA: 2002,Apr,13; 1998,Nov,1

23330-23335 Removal Implant/Foreign Body from Shoulder

EXCLUDES   Bursal arthrocentesis or needling (20610)
          K-wire or pin insertion (20650)
          K-wire or pin removal (20670, 20680)

23330 Removal of foreign body, shoulder; subcutaneous

       🔲 4.40   ⚕ 6.88   **FUD** 010   T A2 80 50 ▯

       AMA: 2015,Jan,16; 2014,Mar,4; 2014,Jan,11

23333 deep (subfascial or intramuscular)

       🔲 13.0   ⚕ 13.0   **FUD** 090   T 62 80 50

       AMA: 2015,Jan,16; 2014,Mar,4

23334 Removal of prosthesis, includes debridement and synovectomy when performed; humeral or glenoid component

       EXCLUDES   Foreign body removal (23330, 23333)
              Hardware removal other than prosthesis (20680)
       Do not report with prosthesis removal and replacement in same shoulder (eg, glenoid and/or humeral components) (23473-23474)

       🔲 30.8   ⚕ 30.8   **FUD** 090   T 62 50

       AMA: 2015,Jan,16; 2014,Mar,4

23335 humeral and glenoid components (eg, total shoulder)

       EXCLUDES   Foreign body removal (23330, 23333)
              Hardware removal other than prosthesis (20680)
       Do not report with prosthesis removal and replacement in same shoulder (eg, glenoid and/or humeral components) (23473-23474)

       🔲 36.7   ⚕ 36.7   **FUD** 090   C 50

       AMA: 2015,Jan,16; 2014,Mar,4

23350 Injection for Shoulder Arthrogram

23350 Injection procedure for shoulder arthrography or enhanced CT/MRI shoulder arthrography

       EXCLUDES   Shoulder biopsy (29805-29826)
       🔁 (73040, 73201-73202, 73222-73223, 77002)
       🔲 1.48   ⚕ 3.73   **FUD** 000   N M1 50 ▯

       AMA: 2015,Aug,6; 2015,Jan,16; 2014,Jan,11

23395-23491 Repair/Reconstruction of Shoulder

23395 Muscle transfer, any type, shoulder or upper arm; single

       🔲 37.0   ⚕ 37.0   **FUD** 090   T A2 80 ▯

       AMA: 2003,Jan,1; 2002,Apr,13

23397 multiple

       🔲 32.9   ⚕ 32.9   **FUD** 090   T A2 80 ▯

       AMA: 2003,Jan,1; 2002,Apr,13

23400 Scapulopexy (eg, Sprengels deformity or for paralysis)

       🔲 28.0   ⚕ 28.0   **FUD** 090   T A2 80 50 ▯

       AMA: 2003,Jan,1; 2002,Apr,13

23405 Tenotomy, shoulder area; single tendon

       🔲 17.9   ⚕ 17.9   **FUD** 090   T A2 80 ▯

       AMA: 2002,Apr,13; 1998,Nov,1

23406 multiple tendons through same incision

       🔲 22.1   ⚕ 22.1   **FUD** 090   T A2 80 ▯

       AMA: 2002,Apr,13; 1998,Nov,1

23410 Repair of ruptured musculotendinous cuff (eg, rotator cuff) open; acute

       EXCLUDES   Arthroscopic repair (29827)
       🔲 23.6   ⚕ 23.6   **FUD** 090   T A2 80 50 ▯

       AMA: 2015,Jan,16; 2014,Jan,11; 2012,Jan,15-42; 2011,Jan,11

23412 chronic

       EXCLUDES   Arthroscopic repair (29827)
       🔲 24.5   ⚕ 24.5   **FUD** 090   T A2 80 50 ▯

       AMA: 2015,Jun,10; 2015,Feb,10; 2015,Jan,16; 2014,Jan,11; 2012,Oct,14; 2012,Sep,16; 2012,Jan,15-42; 2011,Jan,11

23415 Coracoacromial ligament release, with or without acromioplasty

       EXCLUDES   Arthroscopic repair (29826)
       🔲 20.0   ⚕ 20.0   **FUD** 090   T A2 50 ▯

       AMA: 2015,Mar,7

23420 Reconstruction of complete shoulder (rotator) cuff avulsion, chronic (includes acromioplasty)

       🔲 27.8   ⚕ 27.8   **FUD** 090   T A2 80 50 ▯

       AMA: 2015,Jan,16; 2014,Jan,11; 2012,Jan,15-42; 2011,Jan,11

23430 Tenodesis of long tendon of biceps

       EXCLUDES   Arthroscopic biceps tenodesis (29828)
       🔲 21.4   ⚕ 21.4   **FUD** 090   T A2 80 50 ▯

       AMA: 2002,Apr,13; 1994,Win,1

23440 Resection or transplantation of long tendon of biceps

       🔲 21.7   ⚕ 21.7   **FUD** 090   T A2 80 50 ▯

       AMA: 2002,Apr,13; 1994,Win,1

23450 Capsulorrhaphy, anterior; Putti-Platt procedure or Magnuson type operation

       EXCLUDES   Arthroscopic thermal capsulorrhaphy (29999)
       🔲 27.3   ⚕ 27.3   **FUD** 090   T A2 80 50 ▯

       AMA: 2002,Apr,13; 1998,Nov,1

23455 with labral repair (eg, Bankart procedure)

       EXCLUDES   Arthroscopic repair (29806)
       🔲 28.8   ⚕ 28.8   **FUD** 090   T A2 80 50 ▯

       AMA: 2002,Apr,13; 1998,Nov,1

23460 Capsulorrhaphy, anterior, any type; with bone block

       INCLUDES   Bristow procedure
       🔲 31.4   ⚕ 31.4   **FUD** 090   T A2 80 50 ▯

       AMA: 2002,Apr,13; 1994,Win,1

23462 with coracoid process transfer

       EXCLUDES   Open thermal capsulorrhaphy (23929)
       🔲 30.7   ⚕ 30.7   **FUD** 090   T A2 80 50 ▯

       AMA: 2002,Apr,13

23465 Capsulorrhaphy, glenohumeral joint, posterior, with or without bone block

       EXCLUDES   Sternoclavicular and acromioclavicular joint repair (23530, 23550)
       🔲 32.3   ⚕ 32.3   **FUD** 090   T A2 80 50 ▯

       AMA: 2002,Apr,13; 1998,Nov,1

23466 Capsulorrhaphy, glenohumeral joint, any type multi-directional instability

       🔲 32.3   ⚕ 32.3   **FUD** 090   T A2 80 50 ▯

       AMA: 2002,Apr,13; 1998,Nov,1

23470 Arthroplasty, glenohumeral joint; hemiarthroplasty

       🔲 34.7   ⚕ 34.7   **FUD** 090   J 80 50 ▯

       AMA: 2015,Jan,16; 2014,Mar,4

23472 total shoulder (glenoid and proximal humeral replacement (eg, total shoulder))

       EXCLUDES   Proximal humerus osteotomy (24400)
              Removal of total shoulder components (23334-23335)
       🔲 42.0   ⚕ 42.0   **FUD** 090   C 80 50 ▯

       AMA: 2015,Jan,16; 2014,Mar,4; 2014,Jan,11; 2013,Mar,12; 2012,Jan,15-42; 2011,Jan,11

23473 Revision of total shoulder arthroplasty, including allograft when performed; humeral or glenoid component

       Do not report with removal of prosthesis only (glenoid and/or humeral component) (23334-23335)
       🔲 46.9   ⚕ 46.9   **FUD** 090   T 80 50

       AMA: 2015,Jan,16; 2014,Mar,4; 2014,Jan,11; 2013,Mar,12; 2013,Feb,11-12

23474 humeral and glenoid component

       Do not report with removal of prosthesis only (glenoid and/or humeral component) (23334-23335)
       🔲 50.8   ⚕ 50.8   **FUD** 090   C 80 50

       AMA: 2015,Jan,16; 2014,Mar,4; 2014,Jan,11; 2013,Mar,12; 2013,Feb,11-12

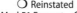

● New Code   ▲ Revised Code   ○ Reinstated   M Maternity   A Age Edit   Unlisted   Not Covered   # Resequenced
⊘ AMA Mod 51 Exempt   51 Optum Mod 51 Exempt   63 Mod 63 Exempt   ⦿ Mod Sedation   + Add-on   ▯ CCI   PQ PQRS   **FUD** Follow-up Days

23480 Osteotomy, clavicle, with or without internal fixation;
🔶 23.6 ✂ 23.6 **FUD** 090   T A2 80 50 ▭
AMA: 2002,Apr,13

23485 with bone graft for nonunion or malunion (includes obtaining graft and/or necessary fixation)
🔶 27.4 ✂ 27.4 **FUD** 090   T A2 80 50 ▭
AMA: 2002,Apr,13

23490 Prophylactic treatment (nailing, pinning, plating or wiring) with or without methylmethacrylate; clavicle
🔶 24.8 ✂ 24.8 **FUD** 090   T A2 80 50 ▭
AMA: 2002,Apr,13

23491 proximal humerus
🔶 29.2 ✂ 29.2 **FUD** 090   T A2 80 50 ▭
AMA: 2002,Apr,13; 1998,Nov,1

23500-23680 Treatment of Shoulder Fracture/Dislocation

23500 Closed treatment of clavicular fracture; without manipulation
🔶 6.30 ✂ 6.20 **FUD** 090   T A2 50 ▭
AMA: 2002,Apr,13

23505 with manipulation
🔶 9.50 ✂ 10.0 **FUD** 090   T A2 50 ▭
AMA: 2002,Apr,13

23515 Open treatment of clavicular fracture, includes internal fixation, when performed
🔶 20.7 ✂ 20.7 **FUD** 090   T J8 80 50 ▭
AMA: 2015,Jan,16; 2014,Jan,11

23520 Closed treatment of sternoclavicular dislocation; without manipulation
🔶 6.70 ✂ 6.61 **FUD** 090   T A2 80 50 ▭
AMA: 2002,Apr,13

23525 with manipulation
🔶 10.1 ✂ 11.0 **FUD** 090   T A2 80 50 ▭
AMA: 2002,Apr,13

23530 Open treatment of sternoclavicular dislocation, acute or chronic;
🔶 16.4 ✂ 16.4 **FUD** 090   T A2 80 50 ▭
AMA: 2002,Apr,13

23532 with fascial graft (includes obtaining graft)
🔶 17.9 ✂ 17.9 **FUD** 090   T A2 80 50 ▭
AMA: 2002,Apr,13

23540 Closed treatment of acromioclavicular dislocation; without manipulation
🔶 6.51 ✂ 6.41 **FUD** 090   T A2 50 ▭
AMA: 2002,Apr,13

23545 with manipulation
🔶 8.81 ✂ 9.70 **FUD** 090   T A2 80 50 ▭
AMA: 2002,Apr,13

23550 Open treatment of acromioclavicular dislocation, acute or chronic;
🔶 16.2 ✂ 16.2 **FUD** 090   T A2 80 50 ▭
AMA: 2002,Apr,13

23552 with fascial graft (includes obtaining graft)
🔶 18.7 ✂ 18.7 **FUD** 090   T A2 80 50 ▭
AMA: 2002,Apr,13

23570 Closed treatment of scapular fracture; without manipulation
🔶 6.81 ✂ 6.61 **FUD** 090   T A2 50 ▭
AMA: 2002,Apr,13

23575 with manipulation, with or without skeletal traction (with or without shoulder joint involvement)
🔶 10.7 ✂ 11.4 **FUD** 090   T A2 80 50 ▭
AMA: 2002,Apr,13

23585 Open treatment of scapular fracture (body, glenoid or acromion) includes internal fixation, when performed
🔶 28.2 ✂ 28.2 **FUD** 090   T J8 80 50 ▭
AMA: 2015,Jan,16; 2014,Jan,11; 2012,Jan,15-42; 2011,Jan,11

23600 Closed treatment of proximal humeral (surgical or anatomical neck) fracture; without manipulation
🔶 8.74 ✂ 9.28 **FUD** 090   T P2 50 ▭
AMA: 2002,Apr,13

23605 with manipulation, with or without skeletal traction
🔶 12.1 ✂ 13.2 **FUD** 090   T A2 50 ▭
AMA: 2002,Apr,13

23615 Open treatment of proximal humeral (surgical or anatomical neck) fracture, includes internal fixation, when performed, includes repair of tuberosity(s), when performed;
🔶 25.4 ✂ 25.4 **FUD** 090   T J8 80 50 ▭
AMA: 2015,Jan,16; 2014,Jan,11

23616 with proximal humeral prosthetic replacement
🔶 35.8 ✂ 35.8 **FUD** 090   T J8 80 50 ▭
AMA: 2002,Apr,13

23620 Closed treatment of greater humeral tuberosity fracture; without manipulation
🔶 7.32 ✂ 7.69 **FUD** 090   T P2 50 ▭
AMA: 2002,Apr,13; 1998,Nov,1

23625 with manipulation
🔶 10.1 ✂ 10.8 **FUD** 090   T A2 50 ▭
AMA: 2002,Apr,13

23630 Open treatment of greater humeral tuberosity fracture, includes internal fixation, when performed
🔶 22.4 ✂ 22.4 **FUD** 090   T J8 80 50 ▭
AMA: 2002,Apr,13; 1998,Nov,1

23650 Closed treatment of shoulder dislocation, with manipulation; without anesthesia
🔶 8.18 ✂ 8.92 **FUD** 090   T A2 50 ▭
AMA: 2002,Apr,13

23655 requiring anesthesia
🔶 11.4 ✂ 11.4 **FUD** 090   T A2 50 ▭
AMA: 2002,Apr,13

23660 Open treatment of acute shoulder dislocation
EXCLUDES   Chronic dislocation repair (23450-23466)
🔶 16.6 ✂ 16.6 **FUD** 090   T A2 80 50 ▭
AMA: 2015,Jan,16; 2014,Jan,11

23665 Closed treatment of shoulder dislocation, with fracture of greater humeral tuberosity, with manipulation
🔶 11.2 ✂ 12.1 **FUD** 090   T A2 50 ▭
AMA: 2002,Apr,13; 1998,Nov,1

23670 Open treatment of shoulder dislocation, with fracture of greater humeral tuberosity, includes internal fixation, when performed
🔶 25.2 ✂ 25.2 **FUD** 090   T J8 80 50 ▭
AMA: 2002,Apr,13; 1998,Nov,1

23675 Closed treatment of shoulder dislocation, with surgical or anatomical neck fracture, with manipulation
🔶 14.4 ✂ 15.8 **FUD** 090   T A2 50 ▭
AMA: 2002,Apr,13

23680 Open treatment of shoulder dislocation, with surgical or anatomical neck fracture, includes internal fixation, when performed
🔶 26.7 ✂ 26.7 **FUD** 090   T A2 80 50 ▭
AMA: 2002,Apr,13

23700-23929 Other/Unlisted Shoulder Procedures

23700 Manipulation under anesthesia, shoulder joint, including application of fixation apparatus (dislocation excluded)
🔶 5.66 ✂ 5.66 **FUD** 010   T A2 50 ▭
AMA: 2015,Jun,10; 2015,Jan,16; 2014,Jan,11; 2012,Jan,15-42; 2011,Jan,11

Musculoskeletal System

23480 — 23700

23800 **Arthrodesis, glenohumeral joint;**
🔧 29.6 ⚖ 29.6 **FUD** 090 T A2 80 50 ▢
AMA: 2002,Apr,13; 1998,Nov,1

23802 **with autogenous graft (includes obtaining graft)**
🔧 37.1 ⚖ 37.1 **FUD** 090 T A2 80 50 ▢
AMA: 2002,Apr,13; 1998,Nov,1

23900 **Interthoracoscapular amputation (forequarter)**
🔧 40.1 ⚖ 40.1 **FUD** 090 C 80
AMA: 2002,Apr,13

23920 **Disarticulation of shoulder;**
🔧 32.5 ⚖ 32.5 **FUD** 090 C 80 50 ▢
AMA: 2002,Apr,13

23921 **secondary closure or scar revision**
🔧 13.1 ⚖ 13.1 **FUD** 090 T A2 50 ▢
AMA: 2002,Apr,13

23929 **Unlisted procedure, shoulder**
🔧 0.00 ⚖ 0.00 **FUD** YYY T 80
AMA: 2002,Apr,13

23930-24006 Surgical Incision Elbow/Upper Arm

EXCLUDES *Simple incision and drainage procedures (10040-10160)*

23930 **Incision and drainage, upper arm or elbow area; deep abscess or hematoma**
🔧 6.19 ⚖ 10.0 **FUD** 010 T A2 50 ▢
AMA: 2002,Apr,13

23931 **bursa**
🔧 4.59 ⚖ 8.17 **FUD** 010 T A2 50 ▢
AMA: 2002,Apr,13; 1998,Nov,1

23935 **Incision, deep, with opening of bone cortex (eg, for osteomyelitis or bone abscess), humerus or elbow**
🔧 14.5 ⚖ 14.5 **FUD** 090 T A2 80 50 ▢
AMA: 2002,Apr,13

24000 **Arthrotomy, elbow, including exploration, drainage, or removal of foreign body**
🔧 13.7 ⚖ 13.7 **FUD** 090 T A2 80 50 ▢
AMA: 2002,Apr,13; 1998,Nov,1

24006 **Arthrotomy of the elbow, with capsular excision for capsular release (separate procedure)**
🔧 20.4 ⚖ 20.4 **FUD** 090 T A2 80 50 ▢
AMA: 2002,Apr,13; 1996,Nov,1

24065-24066 Biopsy of Elbow/Upper Arm

EXCLUDES *Soft tissue needle biopsy (20206)*

24065 **Biopsy, soft tissue of upper arm or elbow area; superficial**
🔧 4.81 ⚖ 7.28 **FUD** 010 T P3 50 ▢ PQ
AMA: 2002,Apr,13

24066 **deep (subfascial or intramuscular)**
🔧 11.9 ⚖ 17.8 **FUD** 090 T A2 50 ▢ PQ
AMA: 2002,Apr,13; 1998,Nov,1

24071-24079 [24071, 24073] Excision Soft Tissue Tumors Elbow/Upper Arm

INCLUDES Any necessary elevation of tissue planes or dissection
Measurement of tumor and necessary margin at greatest diameter prior to excision
Types of excision:
  Fascial or subfascial soft tissue tumors: simple and marginal resection of tumors found either in or below the deep fascia, not involving bone or excision of a substantial amount of normal tissue; primarily benign and intramuscular tumors
  Radical resection of soft tissue tumor: wide resection of tumor involving substantial margins of normal tissue and may involve tissue removal from one or more layers; most often malignant or aggressive benign
  Subcutaneous: simple and marginal resection of tumors found in the subcutaneous tissue above the deep fascia; most often benign
EXCLUDES *Complex repair*
  Excision of benign cutaneous lesion (eg, sebaceous cyst) (11400-11406)
  Radical resection of cutaneous tumors (eg, melanoma) (11600-11606)
  Significant exploration of vessels or neuroplasty

24071 Resequenced code. See code following 24075

24073 **Resequenced code. See code following 24076.**

24075 **Excision, tumor, soft tissue of upper arm or elbow area, subcutaneous; less than 3 cm**
🔧 9.44 ⚖ 13.9 **FUD** 090 T G2 50 ▢

\# *24071* **3 cm or greater**
🔧 11.6 ⚖ 11.6 **FUD** 090 T G2 80 50

24076 **Excision, tumor, soft tissue of upper arm or elbow area, subfascial (eg, intramuscular); less than 5 cm**
🔧 15.5 ⚖ 15.5 **FUD** 090 T G2 50 ▢
AMA: 2002,Apr,13

\# *24073* **5 cm or greater**
🔧 19.9 ⚖ 19.9 **FUD** 090 T G2 80 50

24077 **Radical resection of tumor (eg, sarcoma), soft tissue of upper arm or elbow area; less than 5 cm**
🔧 29.7 ⚖ 29.7 **FUD** 090 T G2 50 ▢
AMA: 2002,Apr,13; 1990,Win,4

24079 **5 cm or greater**
🔧 38.2 ⚖ 38.2 **FUD** 090 T G2 80 50

24100-24149 Bone/Joint Procedures Upper Arm/Elbow

24100 **Arthrotomy, elbow; with synovial biopsy only**
🔧 12.0 ⚖ 12.0 **FUD** 090 T A2 80 50 ▢ PQ
AMA: 2002,Apr,13; 1994,Win,1

24101 **with joint exploration, with or without biopsy, with or without removal of loose or foreign body**
🔧 14.3 ⚖ 14.3 **FUD** 090 T A2 80 50 ▢ PQ
AMA: 2002,Apr,13

24102 **with synovectomy**
🔧 17.6 ⚖ 17.6 **FUD** 090 T A2 80 50 ▢
AMA: 2002,Apr,13; 1994,Win,1

24105 **Excision, olecranon bursa**
🔧 10.0 ⚖ 10.0 **FUD** 090 T A2 50 ▢
AMA: 2002,Apr,13

24110 **Excision or curettage of bone cyst or benign tumor, humerus;**
🔧 16.9 ⚖ 16.9 **FUD** 090 T A2 50 ▢
AMA: 2002,Apr,13

24115 **with autograft (includes obtaining graft)**
🔧 21.2 ⚖ 21.2 **FUD** 090 T A2 80 50 ▢
AMA: 2002,Apr,13

24116 **with allograft**
🔧 24.8 ⚖ 24.8 **FUD** 090 T A2 80 50 ▢
AMA: 2002,Apr,13

24120 **Excision or curettage of bone cyst or benign tumor of head or neck of radius or olecranon process;**
🔧 15.1 ⚖ 15.1 **FUD** 090 T A2 80 50 ▢
AMA: 2002,Apr,13

24125 **with autograft (includes obtaining graft)**
🔧 17.8 ⚖ 17.8 **FUD** 090 T A2 80 50 ▢
AMA: 2002,Apr,13

24126 **with allograft**
🔧 18.6 ⚖ 18.6 **FUD** 090 T A2 80 50 ▢
AMA: 2002,Apr,13

24130 **Excision, radial head**
EXCLUDES *Radial head arthroplasty with implant (24366)*
🔧 14.5 ⚖ 14.5 **FUD** 090 T A2 50 ▢
AMA: 2002,Apr,13

24134 **Sequestrectomy (eg, for osteomyelitis or bone abscess), shaft or distal humerus**
🔧 21.5 ⚖ 21.5 **FUD** 090 T A2 80 50 ▢
AMA: 2002,Apr,13

Musculoskeletal System

24136 — 24344

24136   Sequestrectomy (eg, for osteomyelitis or bone abscess), radial head or neck
     ⚙ 16.6   ✂ 16.6   **FUD** 090   T A2 50 ▭
     AMA: 2002,Apr,13

24138   Sequestrectomy (eg, for osteomyelitis or bone abscess), olecranon process
     ⚙ 19.4   ✂ 19.4   **FUD** 090   T A2 80 50 ▭
     AMA: 2002,Apr,13

24140   Partial excision (craterization, saucerization, or diaphysectomy) bone (eg, osteomyelitis), humerus
     ⚙ 20.2   ✂ 20.2   **FUD** 090   T A2 80 50 ▭
     AMA: 2002,Apr,13; 1998,Nov,1

24145   Partial excision (craterization, saucerization, or diaphysectomy) bone (eg, osteomyelitis), radial head or neck
     ⚙ 17.0   ✂ 17.0   **FUD** 090   T A2 50 ▭
     AMA: 2002,Apr,13; 1998,Nov,1

24147   Partial excision (craterization, saucerization, or diaphysectomy) bone (eg, osteomyelitis), olecranon process
     ⚙ 17.9   ✂ 17.9   **FUD** 090   T A2 50 ▭
     AMA: 2002,Apr,13; 1998,Nov,1

24149   Radical resection of capsule, soft tissue, and heterotopic bone, elbow, with contracture release (separate procedure)
     EXCLUDES   *Capsular and soft tissue release (24006)*
     ⚙ 33.7   ✂ 33.7   **FUD** 090   T G2 80 50 ▭
     AMA: 2002,Apr,13; 1996,Nov,1

24150-24152 Radical Resection Bone Tumor Upper Arm

INCLUDES   Any necessary elevation of tissue planes or dissection
     Measurement of tumor and necessary margin at greatest diameter prior to excision
     Resection of the tumor (may include entire bone) and wide margins of normal tissue primarily for malignant or aggressive benign tumors
     Simple and intermediate repairs
EXCLUDES   *Complex repair*
     Significant exploration of vessels, neuroplasty, reconstruction, or complex bone repair
Do not report excision of soft tissue codes when adjacent soft tissue is removed during the bone tumor resection (24071-24079 [24071, 24073])

24150   Radical resection of tumor, shaft or distal humerus
     ⚙ 45.0   ✂ 45.0   **FUD** 090   T 80 50 ▭
     AMA: 2003,Jan,1; 2002,Apr,13

24152   Radical resection of tumor, radial head or neck
     ⚙ 39.1   ✂ 39.1   **FUD** 090   T G2 80 50 ▭
     AMA: 2003,Jan,1; 2002,Apr,13

24155 Elbow Arthrectomy

24155   Resection of elbow joint (arthrectomy)
     ⚙ 24.6   ✂ 24.6   **FUD** 090   T A2 80 50 ▭
     AMA: 2002,Apr,13; 1996,Nov,1

24160-24201 Removal Implant/Foreign Body from Elbow/Upper Arm

EXCLUDES   *Bursal or joint arthrocentesis or needling (20605)*
     K-wire or pin insertion (20650)
     K-wire or pin removal (20670, 20680)

24160   Removal of prosthesis, includes debridement and synovectomy when performed; humeral and ulnar components
     EXCLUDES   *Foreign body removal (24200-24201)*
        Hardware removal other than prosthesis (20680)
     Do not report with prosthesis removal and replacement in same elbow (eg, humeral and/or ulnar component(s)) (24370-24371)
     ⚙ 36.3   ✂ 36.3   **FUD** 090   02 A2 50 ▭
     AMA: 2015,Jan,16; 2014,Mar,4; 2014,Jan,11; 2013,Feb,11-12

24164   radial head
     EXCLUDES   *Foreign body removal (24200-24201)*
        Hardware removal other than prosthesis (20680)
     ⚙ 20.9   ✂ 20.9   **FUD** 090   02 A2 50 ▭
     AMA: 2015,Jan,16; 2014,Mar,4

24200   Removal of foreign body, upper arm or elbow area; subcutaneous
     ⚙ 4.03   ✂ 5.91   **FUD** 010   T P3 80 50 ▭
     AMA: 2015,Jan,16; 2014,Mar,4

24201   deep (subfascial or intramuscular)
     ⚙ 10.5   ✂ 15.9   **FUD** 090   T A2 50 ▭
     AMA: 2015,Jan,16; 2014,Mar,4

24220 Injection for Elbow Arthrogram

24220   Injection procedure for elbow arthrography
     EXCLUDES   *Injection tennis elbow (20550)*
     ☒ (73085)
     ⚙ 1.99   ✂ 4.57   **FUD** 000   N N1 80 50 ▭
     AMA: 2015,Aug,6

24300-24498 Repair/Reconstruction of Elbow/Upper Arm

24300   Manipulation, elbow, under anesthesia
     EXCLUDES   *External fixation (20690, 20692)*
     ⚙ 11.9   ✂ 11.9   **FUD** 090   T G2 50 ▭
     AMA: 2002,Apr,13

24301   Muscle or tendon transfer, any type, upper arm or elbow, single (excluding 24320-24331)
     ⚙ 21.4   ✂ 21.4   **FUD** 090   T A2 80 ▭
     AMA: 2002,Apr,13

24305   Tendon lengthening, upper arm or elbow, each tendon
     ⚙ 16.4   ✂ 16.4   **FUD** 090   T A2 80 ▭
     AMA: 2002,Apr,13; 1998,Nov,1

24310   Tenotomy, open, elbow to shoulder, each tendon
     ⚙ 13.5   ✂ 13.5   **FUD** 090   T A2 80 ▭
     AMA: 2002,Apr,13; 1998,Nov,1

24320   Tenoplasty, with muscle transfer, with or without free graft, elbow to shoulder, single (Seddon-Brookes type procedure)
     ⚙ 22.5   ✂ 22.5   **FUD** 090   T A2 80 ▭
     AMA: 2002,Apr,13

24330   Flexor-plasty, elbow (eg, Steindler type advancement);
     ⚙ 20.6   ✂ 20.6   **FUD** 090   T A2 80 50 ▭
     AMA: 2002,Apr,13

24331   with extensor advancement
     ⚙ 22.6   ✂ 22.6   **FUD** 090   T A2 80 50 ▭
     AMA: 2002,Apr,13

24332   Tenolysis, triceps
     ⚙ 17.6   ✂ 17.6   **FUD** 090   T G2 50 ▭
     AMA: 2002,Apr,13

24340   Tenodesis of biceps tendon at elbow (separate procedure)
     ⚙ 17.5   ✂ 17.5   **FUD** 090   T A2 80 50 ▭
     AMA: 2002,Apr,13; 1994,Win,1

24341   Repair, tendon or muscle, upper arm or elbow, each tendon or muscle, primary or secondary (excludes rotator cuff)
     ⚙ 21.4   ✂ 21.4   **FUD** 090   T A2 80 50 ▭
     AMA: 2002,Apr,13; 1996,Nov,1

24342   Reinsertion of ruptured biceps or triceps tendon, distal, with or without tendon graft
     ⚙ 22.3   ✂ 22.3   **FUD** 090   T A2 80 50 ▭
     AMA: 2002,Apr,13; 1996,Nov,1

24343   Repair lateral collateral ligament, elbow, with local tissue
     ⚙ 20.2   ✂ 20.2   **FUD** 090   T G2 80 50 ▭
     AMA: 2002,Apr,13

24344   Reconstruction lateral collateral ligament, elbow, with tendon graft (includes harvesting of graft)
     ⚙ 31.6   ✂ 31.6   **FUD** 090   T G2 80 50 ▭
     AMA: 2002,Apr,13

24345 **Repair medial collateral ligament, elbow, with local tissue**
20.3 20.3 **FUD** 090 T A2 80 50 CCI
AMA: 2002,Apr,13

24346 **Reconstruction medial collateral ligament, elbow, with tendon graft (includes harvesting of graft)**
31.6 31.6 **FUD** 090 T G2 80 50 CCI
AMA: 2002,Apr,13

24357 **Tenotomy, elbow, lateral or medial (eg, epicondylitis, tennis elbow, golfer's elbow); percutaneous**
Do not report with (29837-29838)
12.3 12.3 **FUD** 090 T G2 80 50
AMA: 2015,Jan,16; 2014,Jan,11

24358 **debridement, soft tissue and/or bone, open**
Do not report with (29837-29838)
14.9 14.9 **FUD** 090 T G2 80 50
AMA: 2015,Jan,16; 2014,Jan,11

24359 **debridement, soft tissue and/or bone, open with tendon repair or reattachment**
Do not report with (29837-29838)
18.9 18.9 **FUD** 090 T G2 80 50
AMA: 2015,Jan,16; 2014,Jan,11

24360 **Arthroplasty, elbow; with membrane (eg, fascial)**
25.9 25.9 **FUD** 090 T A2 80 50 CCI
AMA: 2002,Apr,13; 1998,Nov,1

24361 **with distal humeral prosthetic replacement**
29.0 29.0 **FUD** 090 J J8 80 50 CCI
AMA: 2002,Apr,13

24362 **with implant and fascia lata ligament reconstruction**
30.5 30.5 **FUD** 090 T A2 80 50 CCI
AMA: 2002,Apr,13

24363 **with distal humerus and proximal ulnar prosthetic replacement (eg, total elbow)**
EXCLUDES Total elbow implant revision (24370-24371)
41.9 41.9 **FUD** 090 J J8 80 50 CCI
AMA: 2015,Jan,16; 2014,Jan,11; 2013,Feb,11-12

24365 **Arthroplasty, radial head;**
18.4 18.4 **FUD** 090 J J8 80 50 CCI
AMA: 2002,Apr,13

24366 **with implant**
19.5 19.5 **FUD** 090 J J8 80 50 CCI
AMA: 2002,Apr,13

24370 **Revision of total elbow arthroplasty, including allograft when performed; humeral or ulnar component**
Do not report with prosthesis removal without replacement (eg, humeral or ulnar component/s) (24160)
44.7 44.7 **FUD** 090 J J8 80 50
AMA: 2015,Jan,16; 2014,Mar,4; 2013,Feb,11-12

24371 **humeral and ulnar component**
Do not report with prosthesis removal without replacement (eg, humeral and/or ulnar component/s) (24160)
51.8 51.8 **FUD** 090 J J8 80 50
AMA: 2015,Jan,16; 2014,Mar,4; 2013,Feb,11-12

24400 **Osteotomy, humerus, with or without internal fixation**
23.5 23.5 **FUD** 090 T A2 80 50 CCI
AMA: 2015,Jan,16; 2014,Mar,4

24410 **Multiple osteotomies with realignment on intramedullary rod, humeral shaft (Sofield type procedure)**
30.5 30.5 **FUD** 090 T A2 80 50 CCI
AMA: 2002,Apr,13

24420 **Osteoplasty, humerus (eg, shortening or lengthening) (excluding 64876)**
28.6 28.6 **FUD** 090 T A2 80 50 CCI
AMA: 2002,Apr,13

24430 **Repair of nonunion or malunion, humerus; without graft (eg, compression technique)**
30.4 30.4 **FUD** 090 T A2 80 50 CCI
AMA: 2002,Apr,13

24435 **with iliac or other autograft (includes obtaining graft)**
31.0 31.0 **FUD** 090 J J8 80 50 CCI
AMA: 2002,Apr,13

24470 **Hemiepiphyseal arrest (eg, cubitus varus or valgus, distal humerus)**
19.3 19.3 **FUD** 090 T A2 80 50 CCI
AMA: 2002,Apr,13; 1998,Nov,1

24495 **Decompression fasciotomy, forearm, with brachial artery exploration**
15.4 15.4 **FUD** 090 T A2 80 50 CCI
AMA: 2002,Apr,13

24498 **Prophylactic treatment (nailing, pinning, plating or wiring), with or without methylmethacrylate, humeral shaft**
25.0 25.0 **FUD** 090 J J8 80 50 CCI
AMA: 2002,Apr,13; 1998,Nov,1

24500-24685 Treatment of Fracture/Dislocation of Elbow/Upper Arm

INCLUDES Treatment for either closed or open fractures or dislocations

24500 **Closed treatment of humeral shaft fracture; without manipulation**
9.30 10.2 **FUD** 090 T A2 50 CCI
AMA: 2002,Apr,13

24505 **with manipulation, with or without skeletal traction**
12.9 14.2 **FUD** 090 T A2 50 CCI
AMA: 2002,Apr,13

24515 **Open treatment of humeral shaft fracture with plate/screws, with or without cerclage**
25.2 25.2 **FUD** 090 T J8 80 50 CCI
AMA: 2002,Apr,13

24516 **Treatment of humeral shaft fracture, with insertion of intramedullary implant, with or without cerclage and/or locking screws**
24.7 24.7 **FUD** 090 T J8 80 50 CCI
AMA: 2015,Jan,16; 2014,Jan,11

24530 **Closed treatment of supracondylar or transcondylar humeral fracture, with or without intercondylar extension; without manipulation**
9.81 10.8 **FUD** 090 T A2 50 CCI
AMA: 2002,Apr,13

24535 **with manipulation, with or without skin or skeletal traction**
16.2 17.5 **FUD** 090 T A2 50 CCI
AMA: 2002,Apr,13

24538 **Percutaneous skeletal fixation of supracondylar or transcondylar humeral fracture, with or without intercondylar extension**
21.4 21.4 **FUD** 090 T A2 50 CCI
AMA: 2015,Jan,16; 2014,Jan,11

24545 **Open treatment of humeral supracondylar or transcondylar fracture, includes internal fixation, when performed; without intercondylar extension**
26.7 26.7 **FUD** 090 T J8 80 50 CCI
AMA: 2002,Apr,13

24546 **with intercondylar extension**
29.9 29.9 **FUD** 090 T J8 80 50 CCI
AMA: 2002,Apr,13

24560 **Closed treatment of humeral epicondylar fracture, medial or lateral; without manipulation**
8.15 9.11 **FUD** 090 T A2 50 CCI
AMA: 2002,Apr,13

24565 **with manipulation**
14.0 15.2 **FUD** 090 T A2 50 CCI
AMA: 2002,Apr,13

24566 **Percutaneous skeletal fixation of humeral epicondylar fracture, medial or lateral, with manipulation**
20.6 20.6 **FUD** 090 T A2 50 CCI
AMA: 2002,Apr,13; 1993,Win,1

24575 Open treatment of humeral epicondylar fracture, medial or lateral, includes internal fixation, when performed
⏱ 21.1 ✂ 21.1 **FUD** 090 [T] [J8] [80] [50] ▢
AMA: 2002,Apr,13

24576 Closed treatment of humeral condylar fracture, medial or lateral; without manipulation
⏱ 8.71 ✂ 9.70 **FUD** 090 [T] [A2] [50] ▢
AMA: 2002,Apr,13

24577 with manipulation
⏱ 14.4 ✂ 15.7 **FUD** 090 [T] [A2] [50] ▢
AMA: 2002,Apr,13

24579 Open treatment of humeral condylar fracture, medial or lateral, includes internal fixation, when performed
> EXCLUDES Closed treatment without manipulation (24530, 24560, 24576, 24650, 24670)
> Repair with manipulation (24535, 24565, 24577, 24675)
⏱ 24.0 ✂ 24.0 **FUD** 090 [T] [J8] [80] [50] ▢
AMA: 2002,Apr,13

24582 Percutaneous skeletal fixation of humeral condylar fracture, medial or lateral, with manipulation
⏱ 23.2 ✂ 23.2 **FUD** 090 [T] [A2] [50] ▢
AMA: 2002,Apr,13; 1993,Win,1

24586 Open treatment of periarticular fracture and/or dislocation of the elbow (fracture distal humerus and proximal ulna and/or proximal radius);
⏱ 31.2 ✂ 31.2 **FUD** 090 [T] [J8] [80] [50] ▢
AMA: 2002,Apr,13

24587 with implant arthroplasty
> EXCLUDES Distal humerus arthroplasty with implant (24361)
⏱ 31.4 ✂ 31.4 **FUD** 090 [T] [J8] [80] [50] ▢
AMA: 2002,Apr,13

24600 Treatment of closed elbow dislocation; without anesthesia
⏱ 9.49 ✂ 10.3 **FUD** 090 [T] [A2] [50] ▢
AMA: 2002,Apr,13

24605 requiring anesthesia
⏱ 13.4 ✂ 13.4 **FUD** 090 [T] [A2] [50] ▢
AMA: 2002,Apr,13

24615 Open treatment of acute or chronic elbow dislocation
⏱ 20.4 ✂ 20.4 **FUD** 090 [T] [J8] [80] [50] ▢
AMA: 2002,Apr,13

24620 Closed treatment of Monteggia type of fracture dislocation at elbow (fracture proximal end of ulna with dislocation of radial head), with manipulation
⏱ 15.6 ✂ 15.6 **FUD** 090 [T] [A2] [80] [50] ▢
AMA: 2002,Apr,13

24635 Open treatment of Monteggia type of fracture dislocation at elbow (fracture proximal end of ulna with dislocation of radial head), includes internal fixation, when performed
⏱ 19.3 ✂ 19.3 **FUD** 090 [T] [J8] [80] [50] ▢
AMA: 2002,Apr,13

24640 Closed treatment of radial head subluxation in child, nursemaid elbow, with manipulation [A]
⏱ 2.70 ✂ 3.98 **FUD** 010 [T] [P3] [80] [50] ▢
AMA: 2002,Apr,13

24650 Closed treatment of radial head or neck fracture; without manipulation
⏱ 6.82 ✂ 7.43 **FUD** 090 [T] [P2] [50] ▢
AMA: 2002,Apr,13

24655 with manipulation
⏱ 11.2 ✂ 12.3 **FUD** 090 [T] [A2] [50] ▢
AMA: 2002,Apr,13

24665 Open treatment of radial head or neck fracture, includes internal fixation or radial head excision, when performed;
⏱ 18.7 ✂ 18.7 **FUD** 090 [T] [A2] [80] [50] ▢
AMA: 2002,Apr,13

24666 with radial head prosthetic replacement
⏱ 21.0 ✂ 21.0 **FUD** 090 [T] [J8] [80] [50] ▢
AMA: 2002,Apr,13

24670 Closed treatment of ulnar fracture, proximal end (eg, olecranon or coronoid process[es]); without manipulation
⏱ 7.47 ✂ 8.29 **FUD** 090 [T] [A2] [50] ▢
AMA: 2002,Apr,13

24675 with manipulation
⏱ 11.8 ✂ 13.0 **FUD** 090 [T] [A2] [50] ▢
AMA: 2002,Apr,13

24685 Open treatment of ulnar fracture, proximal end (eg, olecranon or coronoid process[es]), includes internal fixation, when performed
Do not report with (24100-24102)
⏱ 18.7 ✂ 18.7 **FUD** 090 [T] [A2] [80] [50] ▢
AMA: 2002,Apr,13

24800-24999 Other/Unlisted Elbow/Upper Arm Procedures

24800 Arthrodesis, elbow joint; local
⏱ 23.9 ✂ 23.9 **FUD** 090 [T] [A2] [80] [50] ▢
AMA: 2002,Apr,13; 1998,Nov,1

24802 with autogenous graft (includes obtaining graft)
⏱ 28.8 ✂ 28.8 **FUD** 090 [T] [A2] [80] [50] ▢
AMA: 2002,Apr,13; 1998,Nov,1

24900 Amputation, arm through humerus; with primary closure
⏱ 20.8 ✂ 20.8 **FUD** 090 [C] [80] [50] ▢
AMA: 2002,Apr,13

24920 open, circular (guillotine)
⏱ 21.1 ✂ 21.1 **FUD** 090 [C] [80] [50] ▢
AMA: 2002,Apr,13

24925 secondary closure or scar revision
⏱ 14.6 ✂ 14.6 **FUD** 090 [T] [A2] [80] [50] ▢
AMA: 2002,Apr,13

24930 re-amputation
⏱ 22.3 ✂ 22.3 **FUD** 090 [C] [80] [50] ▢
AMA: 2002,Apr,13

24931 with implant
⏱ 22.1 ✂ 22.1 **FUD** 090 [C] [80] [50] ▢
AMA: 2002,Apr,13

24935 Stump elongation, upper extremity
⏱ 26.0 ✂ 26.0 **FUD** 090 [T] [80] [50] ▢
AMA: 2002,Apr,13

24940 Cineplasty, upper extremity, complete procedure
⏱ 0.00 ✂ 0.00 **FUD** 090 [C] [80] [50] ▢
AMA: 2002,Apr,13

24999 Unlisted procedure, humerus or elbow
⏱ 0.00 ✂ 0.00 **FUD** YYY [T] [80] [50]
AMA: 2002,Apr,13

25000-25001 Incision Tendon Sheath of Wrist

25000 Incision, extensor tendon sheath, wrist (eg, deQuervains disease)
> EXCLUDES Carpal tunnel release (64721)
⏱ 9.61 ✂ 9.61 **FUD** 090 [T] [A2] [50] ▢
AMA: 2002,Apr,13; 1998,Nov,1

25001 Incision, flexor tendon sheath, wrist (eg, flexor carpi radialis)
⏱ 9.83 ✂ 9.83 **FUD** 090 [T] [02] [50] ▢
AMA: 2002,Apr,13

25020-25025 Decompression Fasciotomy Forearm/Wrist

25020 Decompression fasciotomy, forearm and/or wrist, flexor OR extensor compartment; without debridement of nonviable muscle and/or nerve
> EXCLUDES Brachial artery exploration (24495)
> Superficial incision and drainage (10060-10160)
⏱ 16.4 ✂ 16.4 **FUD** 090 [T] [A2] [50] ▢
AMA: 2002,Apr,13

25023   **with debridement of nonviable muscle and/or nerve**

EXCLUDES   Debridement (11000-11044 [11045, 11046])
Decompression fasciotomy with exploration brachial
    artery exploration (24495)
Superficial incision and drainage (10060-10160)

🖑 31.5   🔪 31.5   **FUD** 090   T A2 80 50 🔲

AMA: 2002,Apr,13

25024   **Decompression fasciotomy, forearm and/or wrist, flexor AND extensor compartment; without debridement of nonviable muscle and/or nerve**

🖑 22.3   🔪 22.3   **FUD** 090   T A2 50 🔲

AMA: 2002,Apr,13

25025   **with debridement of nonviable muscle and/or nerve**

🖑 35.4   🔪 35.4   **FUD** 090   T A2 80 50 🔲

AMA: 2002,Apr,13

25028-25040 Incision for Drainage/Foreign Body Removal

25028   **Incision and drainage, forearm and/or wrist; deep abscess or hematoma**

🖑 14.9   🔪 14.9   **FUD** 090   T A2 50 🔲

AMA: 2002,Apr,13

25031   **bursa**

🖑 10.4   🔪 10.4   **FUD** 090   T A2 80 50 🔲

AMA: 2002,Apr,13; 1998,Nov,1

25035   **Incision, deep, bone cortex, forearm and/or wrist (eg, osteomyelitis or bone abscess)**

🖑 16.7   🔪 16.7   **FUD** 090   T A2 80 50 🔲

AMA: 2002,Apr,13; 1998,Nov,1

25040   **Arthrotomy, radiocarpal or midcarpal joint, with exploration, drainage, or removal of foreign body**

🖑 16.1   🔪 16.1   **FUD** 090   T A2 80 50 🔲

AMA: 2002,Apr,13; 1994,Win,1

25065-25066 Biopsy Forearm/Wrist

EXCLUDES   Soft tissue needle biopsy (20206)

25065   **Biopsy, soft tissue of forearm and/or wrist; superficial**

🖑 4.70   🔪 7.24   **FUD** 010   T P3 50 🔲 PQ

AMA: 2002,Apr,13

25066   **deep (subfascial or intramuscular)**

🖑 10.3   🔪 10.3   **FUD** 090   T A2 50 🔲 PQ

AMA: 2002,Apr,13; 1998,Nov,1

25071-25078 [25071, 25073] Excision Soft Tissue Tumors Forearm/Wrist

INCLUDES   Any necessary elevation of tissue planes or dissection
Measurement of tumor and necessary margin at greatest diameter prior
    to excision
Simple and intermediate repairs
Types of excision:
    Fascial or subfascial soft tissue tumors: simple and marginal resection
      of tumors found either in or below the deep fascia, not involving
      bone or excision of a substantial amount of normal tissue; primarily
      benign and intramuscular tumors
    Radical resection soft tissue tumor: wide resection of tumor involving
      substantial margins of normal tissue and may include tissue
      removal from one or more layers; most often malignant or
      aggressive benign
    Subcutaneous: simple and marginal resection of tumors in the
      subcutaneous tissue above the deep fascia; most often benign

EXCLUDES   Complex repair
Excision of benign cutaneous lesions (eg, sebaceous cyst) (11400-11406)
Radical resection of cutaneous tumors (eg, melanoma) (11600-11606)
Significant exploration of vessels or neuroplasty

25071   **Resequenced code. See code following 25075.**

25073   **Resequenced code. See code following 25076.**

25075   **Excision, tumor, soft tissue of forearm and/or wrist area, subcutaneous; less than 3 cm**

🖑 9.04   🔪 13.6   **FUD** 090   T 62 50 🔲

AMA: 2002,Apr,13

\#   **25071**   **3 cm or greater**

🖑 12.2   🔪 12.2   **FUD** 090   T 62 80 50 🔲

25076   **Excision, tumor, soft tissue of forearm and/or wrist area, subfascial (eg, intramuscular); less than 3 cm**

🖑 14.8   🔪 14.8   **FUD** 090   T 62 50 🔲

AMA: 2002,Apr,13

\#   **25073**   **3 cm or greater**

🖑 15.2   🔪 15.2   **FUD** 090   T 62 80 50 🔲

25077   **Radical resection of tumor (eg, sarcoma), soft tissue of forearm and/or wrist area; less than 3 cm**

🖑 25.4   🔪 25.4   **FUD** 090   T 62 50 🔲

AMA: 2002,Apr,13; 1990,Win,4

25078   **3 cm or greater**

🖑 33.5   🔪 33.5   **FUD** 090   T 62 80 50 🔲

25085-25240 Procedures of Bones/Joints Lower Arm/Wrist

25085   **Capsulotomy, wrist (eg, contracture)**

🖑 12.9   🔪 12.9   **FUD** 090   T A2 80 50 🔲

AMA: 2002,Apr,13; 1998,Nov,1

25100   **Arthrotomy, wrist joint; with biopsy**

🖑 9.92   🔪 9.92   **FUD** 090   T A2 80 50 🔲 PQ

AMA: 2002,Apr,13; 2000,Dec,12

25101   **with joint exploration, with or without biopsy, with or without removal of loose or foreign body**

🖑 11.5   🔪 11.5   **FUD** 090   T A2 80 50 🔲 PQ

AMA: 2002,Apr,13

25105   **with synovectomy**

🖑 13.7   🔪 13.7   **FUD** 090   T A2 80 50 🔲

AMA: 2002,Apr,13; 2000,Dec,12

25107   **Arthrotomy, distal radioulnar joint including repair of triangular cartilage, complex**

🖑 17.6   🔪 17.6   **FUD** 090   T A2 80 50 🔲

AMA: 2002,Apr,13; 1998,Nov,1

25109   **Excision of tendon, forearm and/or wrist, flexor or extensor, each**

🖑 15.3   🔪 15.3   **FUD** 090   T 62 50

25110   **Excision, lesion of tendon sheath, forearm and/or wrist**

🖑 9.75   🔪 9.75   **FUD** 090   T A2 50 🔲

AMA: 2002,Apr,13

25111   **Excision of ganglion, wrist (dorsal or volar); primary**

EXCLUDES   Excision of ganglion hand or finger (26160)

🖑 9.15   🔪 9.15   **FUD** 090   T A2 50 🔲

AMA: 2002,Apr,13

Synovial sheaths (blue) of the dorsum of right wrist, containing extensor tendons

Ganglion

Anatomical "snuffbox"

Anatomical "snuffbox"

Typical location of ganglion

Ganglions are round cystic swellings usually appearing on the dorsum of the wrist or hand; these swellings often communicate with the synovial sheath

25112   **recurrent**

EXCLUDES   Excision of ganglion hand or finger (26160)

🖑 11.0   🔪 11.0   **FUD** 090   T A2 50 🔲

AMA: 2002,Apr,13

Musculoskeletal System

25115 — 25260

25115   **Radical excision of bursa, synovia of wrist, or forearm tendon sheaths (eg, tenosynovitis, fungus, Tbc, or other granulomas, rheumatoid arthritis); flexors**

> *EXCLUDES*   *Finger synovectomy (26145)*
>
> 🔧 21.7   ✂ 21.7   **FUD** 090   T A2 50 ▣
>
> **AMA:** 2015,Jan,16; 2012,Jun,15-16

25116   **extensors, with or without transposition of dorsal retinaculum**

> *EXCLUDES*   *Finger synovectomy (26145)*
>
> 🔧 17.1   ✂ 17.1   **FUD** 090   T A2 80 50 ▣
>
> **AMA:** 2002,Apr,13

25118   **Synovectomy, extensor tendon sheath, wrist, single compartment;**

> *EXCLUDES*   *Finger synovectomy (26145)*
>
> 🔧 10.8   ✂ 10.8   **FUD** 090   T A2 50 ▣
>
> **AMA:** 2015,Jun,10; 2015,Jan,16; 2014,Jan,11; 2012,Apr,17-18

25119   **with resection of distal ulna**

> *EXCLUDES*   *Finger synovectomy (26145)*
>
> 🔧 14.3   ✂ 14.3   **FUD** 090   T A2 80 50 ▣
>
> **AMA:** 2002,Apr,13

25120   **Excision or curettage of bone cyst or benign tumor of radius or ulna (excluding head or neck of radius and olecranon process);**

> *EXCLUDES*   *Removal of bone cyst or tumor of radial head, neck, or olecranon process (24120-24126)*
>
> 🔧 14.2   ✂ 14.2   **FUD** 090   T A2 80 50 ▣
>
> **AMA:** 2002,Apr,13

25125   **with autograft (includes obtaining graft)**

> 🔧 17.2   ✂ 17.2   **FUD** 090   T A2 80 50 ▣
>
> **AMA:** 2002,Apr,13

25126   **with allograft**

> 🔧 17.1   ✂ 17.1   **FUD** 090   T A2 80 50 ▣
>
> **AMA:** 2002,Apr,13

25130   **Excision or curettage of bone cyst or benign tumor of carpal bones;**

> 🔧 12.7   ✂ 12.7   **FUD** 090   T A2 80 50 ▣
>
> **AMA:** 2002,Apr,13

25135   **with autograft (includes obtaining graft)**

> 🔧 16.0   ✂ 16.0   **FUD** 090   T A2 80 50 ▣
>
> **AMA:** 2002,Apr,13

25136   **with allograft**

> 🔧 14.1   ✂ 14.1   **FUD** 090   T A2 80 50 ▣
>
> **AMA:** 2002,Apr,13

25145   **Sequestrectomy (eg, for osteomyelitis or bone abscess), forearm and/or wrist**

> 🔧 14.8   ✂ 14.8   **FUD** 090   T A2 80 50 ▣
>
> **AMA:** 2002,Apr,13

25150   **Partial excision (craterization, saucerization, or diaphysectomy) of bone (eg, for osteomyelitis); ulna**

> 🔧 16.3   ✂ 16.3   **FUD** 090   T A2 50 ▣
>
> **AMA:** 2002,Apr,13

25151   **radius**

> *EXCLUDES*   *Partial removal of radial head, neck, or olecranon process (24145, 24147)*
>
> 🔧 16.8   ✂ 16.8   **FUD** 090   T A2 80 50 ▣
>
> **AMA:** 2002,Apr,13

25170   **Radical resection of tumor, radius or ulna**

> *INCLUDES*   Any necessary elevation of tissue planes or dissection
>
> Measurement of tumor and necessary margin at greatest diameter prior to excision
>
> Resection of the tumor (may include entire bone) and wide margins of normal tissue primarily for malignant or aggressive benign tumors
>
> Resection without removal of significant normal tissue
>
> Simple and intermediate repairs
>
> *EXCLUDES*   *Complex repair*
>
> *Radical resection of cutaneous tumors (e.g., melanoma) (11600-11646)*
>
> *Significant exploration of vessels, neuroplasty, reconstruction, or complex bone repair*
>
> Do not report radical excision of soft tissue codes when adjacent soft tissue is removed during the bone tumor resection (25071-25078 [25071, 25073])
>
> 🔧 42.7   ✂ 42.7   **FUD** 090   T 80 50 ▣
>
> **AMA:** 2003,Jan,1; 2002,Apr,13

25210   **Carpectomy; 1 bone**

> *EXCLUDES*   *Carpectomy with insertion of implant (25441-25445)*
>
> 🔧 13.9   ✂ 13.9   **FUD** 090   T A2 80 ▣
>
> **AMA:** 2002,Apr,13

25215   **all bones of proximal row**

> 🔧 17.6   ✂ 17.6   **FUD** 090   T A2 80 50 ▣
>
> **AMA:** 2002,Apr,13

25230   **Radial styloidectomy (separate procedure)**

> 🔧 12.3   ✂ 12.3   **FUD** 090   T A2 50 ▣
>
> **AMA:** 2002,Apr,13

25240   **Excision distal ulna partial or complete (eg, Darrach type or matched resection)**

> *EXCLUDES*   *Acquisition of fascia for interposition (20920, 20922)*
>
> *Implant replacement (25442)*
>
> 🔧 12.2   ✂ 12.2   **FUD** 090   T A2 80 50 ▣
>
> **AMA:** 2002,Apr,13; 1994,Win,1

25246 Injection for Wrist Arthrogram

25246   **Injection procedure for wrist arthrography**

> *EXCLUDES*   *Excision of superficial foreign body (20520)*
>
> 📷 (73115)
>
> 🔧 2.18   ✂ 4.62   **FUD** 000   N N1 50 ▣
>
> **AMA:** 2015,Aug,6

25248-25251 Removal Foreign Body of Wrist

> *EXCLUDES*   *Excision of superficial foreign body (20520)*
>
> *K-wire, pin, or rod insertion (20650)*
>
> *K-wire, pin, or rod removal (20670, 20680)*

25248   **Exploration with removal of deep foreign body, forearm or wrist**

> 🔧 11.8   ✂ 11.8   **FUD** 090   T A2 50 ▣
>
> **AMA:** 2002,Apr,13; 1994,Win,1

25250   **Removal of wrist prosthesis; (separate procedure)**

> 🔧 15.2   ✂ 15.2   **FUD** 090   02 A2 80 50 ▣
>
> **AMA:** 2002,Apr,13

25251   **complicated, including total wrist**

> 🔧 20.3   ✂ 20.3   **FUD** 090   02 A2 80 50 ▣
>
> **AMA:** 2002,Apr,13

25259 Manipulation of Wrist with Anesthesia

25259   **Manipulation, wrist, under anesthesia**

> *EXCLUDES*   *Application external fixation (20690, 20692)*
>
> 🔧 11.9   ✂ 11.9   **FUD** 090   T G2 50 ▣
>
> **AMA:** 2015,Jan,16; 2014,Jan,11; 2012,Jan,15-42; 2011,Jan,11

25260-25492 Repair/Reconstruction of Forearm/Wrist

25260   **Repair, tendon or muscle, flexor, forearm and/or wrist; primary, single, each tendon or muscle**

> 🔧 18.0   ✂ 18.0   **FUD** 090   T A2
>
> **AMA:** 2002,Apr,13; 1996,Nov,1

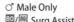
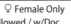
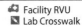

25263   secondary, single, each tendon or muscle
  ⏲ 18.0   ⏳ 18.0   **FUD** 090   T A2 80 ▣
  AMA: 2002,Apr,13; 1996,Nov,1

25265   secondary, with free graft (includes obtaining graft), each tendon or muscle
  ⏲ 21.5   ⏳ 21.5   **FUD** 090   T A2 80 ▣
  AMA: 2002,Apr,13; 1996,Nov,1

25270   Repair, tendon or muscle, extensor, forearm and/or wrist; primary, single, each tendon or muscle
  ⏲ 14.0   ⏳ 14.0   **FUD** 090   T A2 80 ▣
  AMA: 2002,Apr,13; 1996,Nov,1

25272   secondary, single, each tendon or muscle
  ⏲ 15.9   ⏳ 15.9   **FUD** 090   T A2 80 ▣
  AMA: 2002,Apr,13; 1996,Nov,1

25274   secondary, with free graft (includes obtaining graft), each tendon or muscle
  ⏲ 19.3   ⏳ 19.3   **FUD** 090   T A2 80 ▣
  AMA: 2002,Apr,13; 1996,Nov,1

25275   Repair, tendon sheath, extensor, forearm and/or wrist, with free graft (includes obtaining graft) (eg, for extensor carpi ulnaris subluxation)
  ⏲ 19.2   ⏳ 19.2   **FUD** 090   T A2 80 50 ▣
  AMA: 2002,Apr,13

25280   Lengthening or shortening of flexor or extensor tendon, forearm and/or wrist, single, each tendon
  ⏲ 16.0   ⏳ 16.0   **FUD** 090   T A2 80 ▣
  AMA: 2002,Apr,13

25290   Tenotomy, open, flexor or extensor tendon, forearm and/or wrist, single, each tendon
  ⏲ 12.4   ⏳ 12.4   **FUD** 090   T A2 ▣
  AMA: 2002,Apr,13

25295   Tenolysis, flexor or extensor tendon, forearm and/or wrist, single, each tendon
  ⏲ 14.9   ⏳ 14.9   **FUD** 090   T A2 ▣
  AMA: 2015,Jan,16; 2014,Jan,11; 2012,Jan,15-42; 2011,Jan,11

25300   Tenodesis at wrist; flexors of fingers
  ⏲ 19.7   ⏳ 19.7   **FUD** 090   T A2 80 50 ▣
  AMA: 2002,Apr,13

25301   extensors of fingers
  ⏲ 18.4   ⏳ 18.4   **FUD** 090   T A2 80 50 ▣
  AMA: 2002,Apr,13

25310   Tendon transplantation or transfer, flexor or extensor, forearm and/or wrist, single; each tendon
  ⏲ 17.7   ⏳ 17.7   **FUD** 090   T A2 80 ▣
  AMA: 2015,Jan,16; 2014,Jan,11; 2012,Jan,15-42; 2011,Jan,11

25312   with tendon graft(s) (includes obtaining graft), each tendon
  ⏲ 20.5   ⏳ 20.5   **FUD** 090   T A2 80 ▣
  AMA: 2002,Apr,13

25315   Flexor origin slide (eg, for cerebral palsy, Volkmann contracture), forearm and/or wrist;
  ⏲ 22.2   ⏳ 22.2   **FUD** 090   T A2 80 50 ▣
  AMA: 2002,Apr,13; 1994,Win,1

25316   with tendon(s) transfer
  ⏲ 26.3   ⏳ 26.3   **FUD** 090   T A2 80 50 ▣
  AMA: 2002,Apr,13; 1994,Win,1

25320   Capsulorrhaphy or reconstruction, wrist, open (eg, capsulodesis, ligament repair, tendon transfer or graft) (includes synovectomy, capsulotomy and open reduction) for carpal instability
  ⏲ 28.2   ⏳ 28.2   **FUD** 090   T A2 80 50 ▣
  AMA: 2002,Apr,13; 1994,Win,1

25332   Arthroplasty, wrist, with or without interposition, with or without external or internal fixation
  EXCLUDES   *Acquiring fascia for interposition (20920, 20922)*
      Arthroplasty with prosthesis (25441-25446)
  ⏲ 24.0   ⏳ 24.0   **FUD** 090   T A2 80 50 ▣
  AMA: 2015,Jan,16; 2014,Jan,11

25335   Centralization of wrist on ulna (eg, radial club hand)
  ⏲ 27.1   ⏳ 27.1   **FUD** 090   T A2 80 50 ▣
  AMA: 2002,Apr,13

25337   Reconstruction for stabilization of unstable distal ulna or distal radioulnar joint, secondary by soft tissue stabilization (eg, tendon transfer, tendon graft or weave, or tenodesis) with or without open reduction of distal radioulnar joint
  EXCLUDES   *Acquiring fascia lata graft (20920, 20922)*
  ⏲ 25.4   ⏳ 25.4   **FUD** 090   T A2 50 ▣
  AMA: 2002,Apr,13; 1994,Win,1

25350   Osteotomy, radius; distal third
  ⏲ 19.3   ⏳ 19.3   **FUD** 090   T A2 80 50 ▣
  AMA: 2002,Apr,13

25355   middle or proximal third
  ⏲ 22.0   ⏳ 22.0   **FUD** 090   T A2 80 50 ▣
  AMA: 2002,Apr,13

25360   Osteotomy; ulna
  ⏲ 18.7   ⏳ 18.7   **FUD** 090   T A2 80 50 ▣
  AMA: 2002,Apr,13

25365   radius AND ulna
  ⏲ 26.3   ⏳ 26.3   **FUD** 090   T A2 80 50 ▣
  AMA: 2002,Apr,13

25370   Multiple osteotomies, with realignment on intramedullary rod (Sofield type procedure); radius OR ulna
  ⏲ 29.0   ⏳ 29.0   **FUD** 090   T A2 80 50 ▣
  AMA: 2002,Apr,13

25375   radius AND ulna
  ⏲ 27.4   ⏳ 27.4   **FUD** 090   T A2 80 50 ▣
  AMA: 2002,Apr,13

25390   Osteoplasty, radius OR ulna; shortening
  ⏲ 22.0   ⏳ 22.0   **FUD** 090   T A2 80 50 ▣
  AMA: 2003,Jan,1; 2002,Apr,13

25391   lengthening with autograft
  ⏲ 28.7   ⏳ 28.7   **FUD** 090   T A2 80 50 ▣
  AMA: 2003,Jan,1; 2002,Apr,13

25392   Osteoplasty, radius AND ulna; shortening (excluding 64876)
  ⏲ 28.9   ⏳ 28.9   **FUD** 090   T A2 80 50 ▣
  AMA: 2003,Jan,1; 2002,Apr,13

25393   lengthening with autograft
  ⏲ 32.3   ⏳ 32.3   **FUD** 090   T A2 80 50 ▣
  AMA: 2003,Jan,1; 2002,Apr,13

25394   Osteoplasty, carpal bone, shortening
  ⏲ 22.9   ⏳ 22.9   **FUD** 090   T G2 80 50 ▣
  AMA: 2002,Apr,13

25400   Repair of nonunion or malunion, radius OR ulna; without graft (eg, compression technique)
  ⏲ 23.0   ⏳ 23.0   **FUD** 090   T A2 80 50 ▣
  AMA: 2002,Apr,13

25405   with autograft (includes obtaining graft)
  ⏲ 29.7   ⏳ 29.7   **FUD** 090   T A2 80 50 ▣
  AMA: 2002,Apr,13

25415   Repair of nonunion or malunion, radius AND ulna; without graft (eg, compression technique)
  ⏲ 27.9   ⏳ 27.9   **FUD** 090   T A2 80 50 ▣
  AMA: 2002,Apr,13

25420   with autograft (includes obtaining graft)
  ⏲ 33.7   ⏳ 33.7   **FUD** 090   T A2 80 50 ▣
  AMA: 2003,Jan,1; 2002,Apr,13

25425 Repair of defect with autograft; radius OR ulna
27.7 ≋ 27.7 **FUD** 090 [T] [A2] [80] [50] ▣
AMA: 2002,Apr,13

25426 radius AND ulna
32.4 ≋ 32.4 **FUD** 090 [T] [A2] [80] [50] ▣
AMA: 2002,Apr,13

25430 Insertion of vascular pedicle into carpal bone (eg, Hori procedure)
21.0 ≋ 21.0 **FUD** 090 [T] [62] [50] ▣
AMA: 2002,Apr,13

25431 Repair of nonunion of carpal bone (excluding carpal scaphoid (navicular)) (includes obtaining graft and necessary fixation), each bone
22.4 ≋ 22.4 **FUD** 090 [T] [62] [80] [50] ▣
AMA: 2002,Apr,13

25440 Repair of nonunion, scaphoid carpal (navicular) bone, with or without radial styloidectomy (includes obtaining graft and necessary fixation)
22.0 ≋ 22.0 **FUD** 090 [T] [A2] [80] [50] ▣
AMA: 2002,May,7; 2002,Apr,13

25441 Arthroplasty with prosthetic replacement; distal radius
26.7 ≋ 26.7 **FUD** 090 [J] [J8] [80] [50] ▣
AMA: 2015,Jan,16; 2014,Jan,11

25442 distal ulna
22.8 ≋ 22.8 **FUD** 090 [J] [J8] [80] [50] ▣
AMA: 2015,Jan,16; 2014,Jan,11

25443 scaphoid carpal (navicular)
22.5 ≋ 22.5 **FUD** 090 [T] [A2] [80] [50] ▣
AMA: 2015,Jan,16; 2014,Jan,11

25444 lunate
23.7 ≋ 23.7 **FUD** 090 [J] [J8] [80] [50] ▣
AMA: 2015,Jan,16; 2014,Jan,11

25445 trapezium
20.7 ≋ 20.7 **FUD** 090 [T] [A2] [50] ▣
AMA: 2015,Jan,16; 2014,Jan,11

25446 distal radius and partial or entire carpus (total wrist)
33.6 ≋ 33.6 **FUD** 090 [J] [J8] [80] [50] ▣
AMA: 2015,Jan,16; 2014,Jan,11

25447 Arthroplasty, interposition, intercarpal or carpometacarpal joints
EXCLUDES *Wrist arthroplasty (25332)*
23.7 ≋ 23.7 **FUD** 090 [T] [A2] [80] [50] ▣
AMA: 2015,Jan,16; 2014,Jan,11

25449 Revision of arthroplasty, including removal of implant, wrist joint
29.5 ≋ 29.5 **FUD** 090 [T] [A2] [80] [50] ▣
AMA: 2002,Apr,13

25450 Epiphyseal arrest by epiphysiodesis or stapling; distal radius OR ulna
14.2 ≋ 14.2 **FUD** 090 [T] [A2] [50] ▣
AMA: 2002,Apr,13

25455 distal radius AND ulna
16.9 ≋ 16.9 **FUD** 090 [T] [A2] [50] ▣
AMA: 2002,Apr,13

25490 Prophylactic treatment (nailing, pinning, plating or wiring) with or without methylmethacrylate; radius
19.0 ≋ 19.0 **FUD** 090 [T] [A2] [80] [50] ▣
AMA: 2002,Apr,13

25491 ulna
21.3 ≋ 21.3 **FUD** 090 [T] [A2] [80] [50] ▣
AMA: 2002,Apr,13

25492 radius AND ulna
26.0 ≋ 26.0 **FUD** 090 [T] [A2] [80] [50] ▣
AMA: 2002,Apr,13

25500-25695 Treatment of Fracture/Dislocation of Forearm/Wrist
Code also external fixation (20690)

25500 Closed treatment of radial shaft fracture; without manipulation
7.11 ≋ 7.75 **FUD** 090 [T] [P2] [50] ▣
AMA: 2002,Apr,13

25505 with manipulation
13.1 ≋ 14.3 **FUD** 090 [T] [A2] [50] ▣
AMA: 2003,May,7; 2002,Apr,13

25515 Open treatment of radial shaft fracture, includes internal fixation, when performed
19.2 ≋ 19.2 **FUD** 090 [T] [A2] [80] [50] ▣
AMA: 2002,Apr,13

25520 Closed treatment of radial shaft fracture and closed treatment of dislocation of distal radioulnar joint (Galeazzi fracture/dislocation)
15.4 ≋ 16.2 **FUD** 090 [T] [A2] [50] ▣
AMA: 2002,Apr,13

25525 Open treatment of radial shaft fracture, includes internal fixation, when performed, and closed treatment of distal radioulnar joint dislocation (Galeazzi fracture/ dislocation), includes percutaneous skeletal fixation, when performed
22.5 ≋ 22.5 **FUD** 090 [T] [A2] [80] [50] ▣
AMA: 2002,Apr,13

25526 Open treatment of radial shaft fracture, includes internal fixation, when performed, and open treatment of distal radioulnar joint dislocation (Galeazzi fracture/ dislocation), includes internal fixation, when performed, includes repair of triangular fibrocartilage complex
27.5 ≋ 27.5 **FUD** 090 [T] [A2] [80] [50] ▣
AMA: 2002,Apr,13

25530 Closed treatment of ulnar shaft fracture; without manipulation
6.74 ≋ 7.46 **FUD** 090 [T] [P2] [50] ▣
AMA: 2002,Apr,13

25535 with manipulation
12.9 ≋ 13.9 **FUD** 090 [T] [A2] [50] ▣
AMA: 2010,Sep,6-7

25545 Open treatment of ulnar shaft fracture, includes internal fixation, when performed
17.8 ≋ 17.8 **FUD** 090 [T] [A2] [80] [50] ▣
AMA: 2015,Jan,16; 2014,Jan,11

25560 Closed treatment of radial and ulnar shaft fractures; without manipulation
7.13 ≋ 7.89 **FUD** 090 [T] [P2] [50] ▣
AMA: 2002,Apr,13

25565 with manipulation
13.4 ≋ 14.8 **FUD** 090 [T] [A2] [50] ▣
AMA: 2002,Apr,13

25574 Open treatment of radial AND ulnar shaft fractures, with internal fixation, when performed; of radius OR ulna
19.3 ≋ 19.3 **FUD** 090 [T] [J8] [80] [50] ▣
AMA: 2015,Jan,16; 2014,Jan,11

25575 of radius AND ulna
25.8 ≋ 25.8 **FUD** 090 [T] [J8] [80] [50] ▣
AMA: 2002,Apr,13

25600 Closed treatment of distal radial fracture (eg, Colles or Smith type) or epiphyseal separation, includes closed treatment of fracture of ulnar styloid, when performed; without manipulation
Do not report with (25650)
8.82 ≋ 9.33 **FUD** 090 [T] [P2] [50] ▣ [P0]
AMA: 2015,Jan,16; 2014,Jan,11; 2013,Apr,10-11

 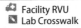

25605	with manipulation

Do not report with (25650)

🔧 14.6 ✂ 15.5 **FUD** 090 　 T A2 50 ▣ PQ

AMA: 2015,Jan,16; 2014,Jan,11; 2013,Apr,10-11

25606	Percutaneous skeletal fixation of distal radial fracture or epiphyseal separation

EXCLUDES *Open repair of ulnar styloid fracture (25652)*
Percutaneous repair of ulnar styloid fracture (25651)

Do not report with (25650)

🔧 19.0 ✂ 19.0 **FUD** 090 　 T A2 50 PQ

AMA: 2007,Oct,7-10

25607	Open treatment of distal radial extra-articular fracture or epiphyseal separation, with internal fixation

EXCLUDES *Open repair of ulnar styloid fracture (25652)*
Percutaneous repair of ulnar styloid fracture (25651)

Do not report with (25650)

🔧 21.0 ✂ 21.0 **FUD** 090 　 T J8 80 50 PQ

AMA: 2015,Jan,16; 2014,Jan,11; 2012,Nov,13-14

25608	Open treatment of distal radial intra-articular fracture or epiphyseal separation; with internal fixation of 2 fragments

EXCLUDES *Open repair of ulnar styloid fracture (25652)*
Percutaneous repair of ulnar styloid fracture (25651)

Do not report with (25609, 25650)

🔧 23.6 ✂ 23.6 **FUD** 090 　 T J8 80 50 PQ

AMA: 2015,Jan,16; 2014,Jan,11

25609	with internal fixation of 3 or more fragments

EXCLUDES *Open repair of ulnar styloid fracture (25652)*
Percutaneous repair of ulnar styloid fracture (25651)

Do not report with (25650)

🔧 30.0 ✂ 30.0 **FUD** 090 　 T J8 80 50 PQ

AMA: 2015,Jan,16; 2014,Jan,11; 2013,Dec,14; 2013,Mar,13

25622	Closed treatment of carpal scaphoid (navicular) fracture; without manipulation

🔧 7.86 ✂ 8.63 **FUD** 090 　 T P2 50 ▣

AMA: 2002,Apr,13

25624	with manipulation

🔧 12.4 ✂ 13.6 **FUD** 090 　 T A2 80 50 ▣

AMA: 2002,Apr,13

25628	Open treatment of carpal scaphoid (navicular) fracture, includes internal fixation, when performed

🔧 20.6 ✂ 20.6 **FUD** 090 　 T A2 80 50 ▣

AMA: 2002,Apr,13

25630	Closed treatment of carpal bone fracture (excluding carpal scaphoid [navicular]); without manipulation, each bone

🔧 7.97 ✂ 8.68 **FUD** 090 　 T P2 50 ▣

AMA: 2002,Apr,13

25635	with manipulation, each bone

🔧 11.3 ✂ 12.7 **FUD** 090 　 T A2 80 50 ▣

AMA: 2002,Apr,13

25645	Open treatment of carpal bone fracture (other than carpal scaphoid [navicular]), each bone

🔧 16.3 ✂ 16.3 **FUD** 090 　 T A2 80 50 ▣

AMA: 2002,Apr,13

25650	Closed treatment of ulnar styloid fracture

Do not report with (25600, 25605, 25607-25609)

🔧 8.52 ✂ 9.08 **FUD** 090 　 T P2 50 ▣

AMA: 2015,Jan,16; 2014,Jan,11; 2013,Apr,10-11

25651	Percutaneous skeletal fixation of ulnar styloid fracture

🔧 13.8 ✂ 13.8 **FUD** 090 　 T 62 80 50 ▣ PQ

AMA: 2007,Oct,7-10; 2002,Apr,13

25652	Open treatment of ulnar styloid fracture

🔧 17.9 ✂ 17.9 **FUD** 090 　 T 62 50 ▣

AMA: 2015,Jan,16; 2014,Jan,11

25660	Closed treatment of radiocarpal or intercarpal dislocation, 1 or more bones, with manipulation

🔧 11.6 ✂ 11.6 **FUD** 090 　 T A2 80 50

AMA: 2002,Apr,13

25670	Open treatment of radiocarpal or intercarpal dislocation, 1 or more bones

🔧 17.3 ✂ 17.3 **FUD** 090 　 T A2 80 50 ▣

AMA: 2002,Apr,13

25671	Percutaneous skeletal fixation of distal radioulnar dislocation

🔧 15.2 ✂ 15.2 **FUD** 090 　 T A2 50 ▣

AMA: 2002,Apr,13

25675	Closed treatment of distal radioulnar dislocation with manipulation

🔧 11.3 ✂ 12.4 **FUD** 090 　 T A2 80 50 ▣

AMA: 2002,Apr,13

25676	Open treatment of distal radioulnar dislocation, acute or chronic

🔧 18.0 ✂ 18.0 **FUD** 090 　 T A2 80 50 ▣

AMA: 2002,Apr,13

25680	Closed treatment of trans-scaphoperilunar type of fracture dislocation, with manipulation

🔧 13.3 ✂ 13.3 **FUD** 090 　 T A2 80 50 ▣

AMA: 2002,Apr,13

25685	Open treatment of trans-scaphoperilunar type of fracture dislocation

🔧 21.2 ✂ 21.2 **FUD** 090 　 T A2 80 50 ▣

AMA: 2002,Apr,13

25690	Closed treatment of lunate dislocation, with manipulation

🔧 13.8 ✂ 13.8 **FUD** 090 　 T A2 80 50 ▣

AMA: 2002,Apr,13

25695	Open treatment of lunate dislocation

🔧 18.2 ✂ 18.2 **FUD** 090 　 T A2 80 50 ▣

AMA: 2002,Apr,13

25800-25830 Wrist Fusion

25800	Arthrodesis, wrist; complete, without bone graft (includes radiocarpal and/or intercarpal and/or carpometacarpal joints)

🔧 20.9 ✂ 20.9 **FUD** 090 　 T A2 80 50 ▣

AMA: 2002,Apr,13; 1998,Nov,1

25805	with sliding graft

🔧 24.3 ✂ 24.3 **FUD** 090 　 T A2 80 50 ▣

AMA: 2002,Apr,13

25810	with iliac or other autograft (includes obtaining graft)

🔧 24.8 ✂ 24.8 **FUD** 090 　 T A2 80 50 ▣

AMA: 2002,Apr,13

25820	Arthrodesis, wrist; limited, without bone graft (eg, intercarpal or radiocarpal)

🔧 17.6 ✂ 17.6 **FUD** 090 　 T A2 80 50 ▣

AMA: 2002,Apr,13; 1998,Nov,1

25825	with autograft (includes obtaining graft)

🔧 21.6 ✂ 21.6 **FUD** 090 　 T A2 80 50 ▣

AMA: 2015,Jan,16; 2014,Jan,11; 2012,Jul,12-14

25830	Arthrodesis, distal radioulnar joint with segmental resection of ulna, with or without bone graft (eg, Sauve-Kapandji procedure)

🔧 27.3 ✂ 27.3 **FUD** 090 　 T A2 80 50 ▣

AMA: 2002,Apr,13; 1998,Nov,1

25900-25999 Amputation Through Forearm/Wrist

25900	Amputation, forearm, through radius and ulna;

🔧 20.2 ✂ 20.2 **FUD** 090 　 C 80 50 ▣

AMA: 2002,Apr,13

25905	open, circular (guillotine)

🔧 20.2 ✂ 20.2 **FUD** 090 　 C 80 50 ▣

AMA: 2002,Apr,13

● New Code　▲ Revised Code　○ Reinstated　Ⓜ Maternity　🅰 Age Edit　Unlisted　Not Covered　# Resequenced
🚫 AMA Mod 51 Exempt　⑧ Optum Mod 51 Exempt　⑥⑧ Mod 63 Exempt　⊙ Mod Sedation　+ Add-on　▣ CCI　PQ PQRS　**FUD** Follow-up Days

© 2015 Optum360, LLC (Blue Text)　　CPT © 2015 American Medical Association. All Rights Reserved. (Black Text)　　Medicare (Red Text)　　**63**

25907 secondary closure or scar revision
⛭ 17.6 ⚗ 17.6 **FUD** 090   T A2 80 50 ▢
AMA: 2002,Apr,13

25909 re-amputation
⛭ 19.7 ⚗ 19.7 **FUD** 090   T 80 50 ▢
AMA: 2002,Apr,13

25915 **Krukenberg procedure**
⛭ 27.9 ⚗ 27.9 **FUD** 090   C 80 50 ▢
AMA: 2002,Apr,13

25920 **Disarticulation through wrist;**
⛭ 20.0 ⚗ 20.0 **FUD** 090   C 80 50 ▢
AMA: 2002,Apr,13

25922 secondary closure or scar revision
⛭ 17.5 ⚗ 17.5 **FUD** 090   T A2 80 50 ▢
AMA: 2002,Apr,13

25924 re-amputation
⛭ 19.5 ⚗ 19.5 **FUD** 090   C 80 50 ▢
AMA: 2002,Apr,13

25927 **Transmetacarpal amputation;**
⛭ 23.2 ⚗ 23.2 **FUD** 090   C 80 50 ▢
AMA: 2002,Apr,13

25929 secondary closure or scar revision
⛭ 15.7 ⚗ 15.7 **FUD** 090   T A2 80 50 ▢
AMA: 2002,Apr,13

25931 re-amputation
⛭ 21.3 ⚗ 21.3 **FUD** 090   T G2 50 ▢
AMA: 2002,Apr,13

25999 **Unlisted procedure, forearm or wrist**
⛭ 0.00 ⚗ 0.00 **FUD** YYY   T 80 50
AMA: 2002,Apr,13

26010-26037 Incision Hand/Fingers

26010 **Drainage of finger abscess; simple**
⛭ 3.93 ⚗ 7.49 **FUD** 010   T P2 ▢
AMA: 2003,May,7; 2003,Sep,3

The six synovial sheaths (blue) of the dorsum of the wrist branch into nine extensor tendons

Extensor pollicis longus

Anatomical "snuffbox"

Extensor digitorum (five tendons)

Extensor retinaculum

Head of ulna

Fibrous sheaths

Synovium

Flexor tendons

Tendons typically join in a common synovial sheath

26011 complicated (eg, felon)
⛭ 5.30 ⚗ 11.0 **FUD** 010   T A2 ▢
AMA: 2002,Apr,13

26020 **Drainage of tendon sheath, digit and/or palm, each**
⛭ 12.4 ⚗ 12.4 **FUD** 090   T A2 ▢
AMA: 2002,Apr,13; 1998,Nov,1

26025 **Drainage of palmar bursa; single, bursa**
⛭ 12.0 ⚗ 12.0 **FUD** 090   T A2 80 50 ▢
AMA: 2002,Apr,13; 1998,Nov,1

26030 multiple bursa
⛭ 14.0 ⚗ 14.0 **FUD** 090   T A2 80 50 ▢
AMA: 2002,Apr,13; 1998,Nov,1

26034 **Incision, bone cortex, hand or finger (eg, osteomyelitis or bone abscess)**
⛭ 15.4 ⚗ 15.4 **FUD** 090   T A2 ▢
AMA: 2002,Apr,13; 1998,Nov,1

26035 **Decompression fingers and/or hand, injection injury (eg, grease gun)**
⛭ 24.6 ⚗ 24.6 **FUD** 090   T G2 80 ▢
AMA: 2002,Apr,13

26037 **Decompressive fasciotomy, hand (excludes 26035)**
EXCLUDES Injection injury (26035)
⛭ 16.1 ⚗ 16.1 **FUD** 090   T G2 80 50 ▢
AMA: 2002,Apr,13

26040-26045 Incision Palmar Fascia

EXCLUDES Enzyme injection fasciotomy (20527, 26341)
Fasciectomy (26121, 26123, 26125)

26040 **Fasciotomy, palmar (eg, Dupuytren's contracture); percutaneous**
⛭ 8.88 ⚗ 8.88 **FUD** 090   T A2 50 ▢
AMA: 2015,Jan,16; 2014,Jan,11; 2012,Jan,15-42; 2011,Jun,13; 2011,Jan,11; 2010,Oct,9; 2010,Apr,10

26045 open, partial
⛭ 13.4 ⚗ 13.4 **FUD** 090   T A2 50 ▢
AMA: 2015,Jan,16; 2014,Jan,11; 2012,Jan,15-42; 2011,Jun,13

26055-26080 Incision Tendon/Joint of Fingers/Hand

26055 **Tendon sheath incision (eg, for trigger finger)**
⛭ 8.85 ⚗ 15.8 **FUD** 090   T A2
AMA: 2002,Apr,13; 1994,Win,1

26060 **Tenotomy, percutaneous, single, each digit**
EXCLUDES Arthrocentesis (20610)
⛭ 7.49 ⚗ 7.49 **FUD** 090   T A2 80
AMA: 2002,Apr,13; 1996,Nov,1

26070 **Arthrotomy, with exploration, drainage, or removal of loose or foreign body; carpometacarpal joint**
⛭ 9.03 ⚗ 9.03 **FUD** 090   T A2 50 ▢
AMA: 2002,Apr,13; 1998,Nov,1

26075 metacarpophalangeal joint, each
⛭ 9.53 ⚗ 9.53 **FUD** 090   T A2 50 ▢
AMA: 2015,Jan,16; 2014,Jan,11; 2012,Oct,12; 2012,Sep,10

26080 interphalangeal joint, each
⛭ 11.1 ⚗ 11.1 **FUD** 090   T A2
AMA: 2015,Jan,16; 2014,Jan,11; 2012,Oct,12; 2012,Sep,10

26100-26110 Arthrotomy with Biopsy of Joint Hand/Fingers

26100 **Arthrotomy with biopsy; carpometacarpal joint, each**
⛭ 9.61 ⚗ 9.61 **FUD** 090   T A2 80 50 ▢ PQ
AMA: 2002,Apr,13; 1998,Nov,1

26105 metacarpophalangeal joint, each
⛭ 9.67 ⚗ 9.67 **FUD** 090   T A2 80 50 ▢ PQ
AMA: 2002,Apr,13; 1998,Nov,1

26110 interphalangeal joint, each
⛭ 9.17 ⚗ 9.17 **FUD** 090   T A2 ▢ PQ
AMA: 2002,Apr,13; 1994,Win,1

26111-26118 [26111, 26113] Excision Soft Tissue Tumors Fingers and Hand

INCLUDES Any necessary elevation of tissue planes or dissection
Measurement of tumor and necessary margin at greatest diameter prior to excision
Simple and intermediate repairs
Types of excision:
    Fascial or subfascial soft tissue tumors: simple and marginal resection of tumors found either in or below the deep fascia, not involving bone or excision of a substantial amount of normal tissue; primarily benign and intramuscular tumors
    Tumors of fingers and toes involving joint capsules, tendons and tendon sheaths
    Radical resection soft tissue tumor: wide resection of tumor, involving substantial margins of normal tissue and may include tissue removal from one or more layers; most often malignant or aggressive benign
    Tumors of fingers and toes adjacent to joints, tendons and tendon sheaths
    Subcutaneous: simple and marginal resection of tumors found in the subcutaneous tissue above the deep fascia; most often benign

EXCLUDES Complex repair
Excision of benign cutaneous lesions (eg, sebaceous cyst) (11420-11426)
Radical resection of cutaneous tumors (eg, melanoma) (11620-11626)
Significant exploration of the vessels or neuroplasty

26111 Resequenced code. See code following 26115.

26113 Resequenced code. See code following 26116.

26115 Excision, tumor or vascular malformation, soft tissue of hand or finger, subcutaneous; less than 1.5 cm
    9.51   14.3   **FUD** 090   T 62
    AMA: 2002,Apr,13

\# **26111** 1.5 cm or greater
    11.9   11.9   **FUD** 090   T 62 80

26116 Excision, tumor, soft tissue, or vascular malformation, of hand or finger, subfascial (eg, intramuscular); less than 1.5 cm
    15.0   15.0   **FUD** 090   T 62
    AMA: 2015,Jan,16; 2014,Jan,11; 2010,Apr,3-4

\# **26113** 1.5 cm or greater
    15.6   15.6   **FUD** 090   T 62 80

26117 Radical resection of tumor (eg, sarcoma), soft tissue of hand or finger; less than 3 cm
    21.3   21.3   **FUD** 090   T 62
    AMA: 2002,Apr,13; 1990,Win,4

26118 3 cm or greater
    30.3   30.3   **FUD** 090   T 62 80

26121-26236 Procedures of Bones, Fascia, Joints and Tendons Hands and Fingers

26121 Fasciectomy, palm only, with or without Z-plasty, other local tissue rearrangement, or skin grafting (includes obtaining graft)
    EXCLUDES Enzyme injection fasciotomy (20527, 26341)
        Fasciotomy (26040, 26045)
    17.1   17.1   **FUD** 090   T A2 50
    AMA: 2015,Jan,16; 2014,Jan,11; 2012,Jan,15-42; 2011,Jun,13; 2010,Oct,9

26123 Fasciectomy, partial palmar with release of single digit including proximal interphalangeal joint, with or without Z-plasty, other local tissue rearrangement, or skin grafting (includes obtaining graft);
    EXCLUDES Enzyme injection fasciotomy (20527, 26341)
        Fasciotomy (26040, 26045)
    23.8   23.8   **FUD** 090   T A2 50
    AMA: 2015,Jan,16; 2014,Jan,11; 2012,Jan,15-42; 2011,Jun,13; 2010,Oct,9

\+ **26125** each additional digit (List separately in addition to code for primary procedure)
    EXCLUDES Enzyme injection fasciotomy (20527, 26341)
        Fasciotomy (26040, 26045)
    Code first (26123)
    7.91   7.91   **FUD** ZZZ   N N1
    AMA: 2015,Jan,16; 2014,Jan,11; 2012,Jan,15-42; 2011,Jun,13; 2010,Oct,9

26130 Synovectomy, carpometacarpal joint
    13.2   13.2   **FUD** 090   T A2 50
    AMA: 2002,Apr,13

26135 Synovectomy, metacarpophalangeal joint including intrinsic release and extensor hood reconstruction, each digit
    15.6   15.6   **FUD** 090   T A2 80
    AMA: 2002,Apr,13

26140 Synovectomy, proximal interphalangeal joint, including extensor reconstruction, each interphalangeal joint
    14.4   14.4   **FUD** 090   T A2
    AMA: 2002,Apr,13

26145 Synovectomy, tendon sheath, radical (tenosynovectomy), flexor tendon, palm and/or finger, each tendon
    EXCLUDES Wrist synovectomy (25115-25116)
    14.6   14.6   **FUD** 090   T A2
    AMA: 2002,Apr,13; 1998,Nov,1

26160 Excision of lesion of tendon sheath or joint capsule (eg, cyst, mucous cyst, or ganglion), hand or finger
    EXCLUDES Trigger finger (26055)
        Wrist ganglion removal (25111-25112)
    9.52   16.3   **FUD** 090   T A2
    AMA: 2002,Apr,13

26170 Excision of tendon, palm, flexor or extensor, single, each tendon
    Do not report with (26390, 26415)
    11.6   11.6   **FUD** 090   T A2 80
    AMA: 2015,Jan,16; 2013,Jun,13

26180 Excision of tendon, finger, flexor or extensor, each tendon
    Do not report with (26390, 26415)
    12.6   12.6   **FUD** 090   T A2 80
    AMA: 2002,Apr,13; 1998,Nov,1

26185 Sesamoidectomy, thumb or finger (separate procedure)
    15.4   15.4   **FUD** 090   T A2 80 50
    AMA: 2002,Apr,13; 1996,Nov,1

26200 Excision or curettage of bone cyst or benign tumor of metacarpal;
    12.8   12.8   **FUD** 090   T A2 80
    AMA: 2002,Apr,13

26205 with autograft (includes obtaining graft)
    17.3   17.3   **FUD** 090   T A2
    AMA: 2002,Apr,13

26210 Excision or curettage of bone cyst or benign tumor of proximal, middle, or distal phalanx of finger;
    12.6   12.6   **FUD** 090   T A2
    AMA: 2002,Apr,13

26215 with autograft (includes obtaining graft)
    16.1   16.1   **FUD** 090   T A2
    AMA: 2002,Apr,13

26230 Partial excision (craterization, saucerization, or diaphysectomy) bone (eg, osteomyelitis); metacarpal
    14.2   14.2   **FUD** 090   T A2 80
    AMA: 2002,Apr,13; 1998,Nov,1

26235 proximal or middle phalanx of finger
    14.1   14.1   **FUD** 090   T A2 80
    AMA: 2002,Apr,13

26236 distal phalanx of finger
    12.5   12.5   **FUD** 090   T A2
    AMA: 2002,Apr,13

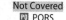

26250-26262 Radical Resection Bone Tumor of Hand/Finger

INCLUDES Any necessary elevation of tissue planes or dissection
Measurement of tumor and necessary margin at greatest diameter prior to excision
Resection of the tumor (may include entire bone) and wide margins of normal tissue primarily for malignant or aggressive benign tumors
Simple and intermediate repairs

EXCLUDES Complex repair
Significant exploration of vessels, neuroplasty, reconstruction, or complex bone repair

Do not report radical excision of soft tissue codes when adjacent soft tissue is removed during the bone tumor resection (26111-26118 [26111, 26113])

26250 **Radical resection of tumor, metacarpal**
🔢 30.8　⚕ 30.8　**FUD** 090　　　T A2 80 ▭
AMA: 2002,Apr,13; 1998,Nov,1

26260 **Radical resection of tumor, proximal or middle phalanx of finger**
🔢 23.1　⚕ 23.1　**FUD** 090　　　T A2 80 ▭
AMA: 2002,Apr,13; 1998,Nov,1

26262 **Radical resection of tumor, distal phalanx of finger**
🔢 18.2　⚕ 18.2　**FUD** 090　　　T A2 80 ▭
AMA: 2002,Apr,13; 1998,Nov,1

26320 Implant Removal Hand/Finger

26320 **Removal of implant from finger or hand**
EXCLUDES Excision of foreign body (20520, 20525)
🔢 9.89　⚕ 9.89　**FUD** 090　　　Q2 A2 ▭
AMA: 2002,Apr,13

26340-26548 Repair/Reconstruction of Fingers and Hand

26340 **Manipulation, finger joint, under anesthesia, each joint**
EXCLUDES Application external fixation (20690, 20692)
🔢 9.49　⚕ 9.49　**FUD** 090　　　T 62 50 ▭
AMA: 2015,Jan,16; 2014,Jan,11; 2012,Jan,15-42; 2011,Jan,11

26341 **Manipulation, palmar fascial cord (ie, Dupuytren's cord), post enzyme injection (eg, collagenase), single cord**
EXCLUDES Enzyme injection fasciotomy (20527)
Code also custom orthotic fabrication and/or fitting
🔢 2.15　⚕ 2.82　**FUD** 010　　　T P3 50
AMA: 2015,Jan,16; 2014,Jan,11; 2012,Jul,8

26350 **Repair or advancement, flexor tendon, not in zone 2 digital flexor tendon sheath (eg, no man's land); primary or secondary without free graft, each tendon**
🔢 20.0　⚕ 20.0　**FUD** 090　　　T A2 ▭
AMA: 2002,Apr,13; 1998,Nov,1

26352 **secondary with free graft (includes obtaining graft), each tendon**
🔢 22.8　⚕ 22.8　**FUD** 090　　　T A2 80 ▭
AMA: 2002,Apr,13

26356 **Repair or advancement, flexor tendon, in zone 2 digital flexor tendon sheath (eg, no man's land); primary, without free graft, each tendon**
🔢 30.8　⚕ 30.8　**FUD** 090　　　T A2 ▭
AMA: 2015,Jan,16; 2014,Sep,13; 2014,Jan,11; 2012,Jan,15-42; 2011,Jan,11

26357 **secondary, without free graft, each tendon**
🔢 24.6　⚕ 24.6　**FUD** 090　　　T A2 80 ▭
AMA: 2002,Apr,13

26358 **secondary, with free graft (includes obtaining graft), each tendon**
🔢 25.3　⚕ 25.3　**FUD** 090　　　T A2 80 ▭
AMA: 2002,Apr,13

26370 **Repair or advancement of profundus tendon, with intact superficialis tendon; primary, each tendon**
🔢 21.3　⚕ 21.3　**FUD** 090　　　T A2 80 ▭
AMA: 2015,Jan,16; 2014,Jan,11; 2012,Jan,15-42

26372 **secondary with free graft (includes obtaining graft), each tendon**
🔢 25.1　⚕ 25.1　**FUD** 090　　　T A2 80 ▭
AMA: 2002,Apr,13; 1998,Nov,1

26373 **secondary without free graft, each tendon**
🔢 23.3　⚕ 23.3　**FUD** 090　　　T A2 80 ▭
AMA: 2002,Apr,13; 1998,Nov,1

26390 **Excision flexor tendon, with implantation of synthetic rod for delayed tendon graft, hand or finger, each rod**
🔢 23.7　⚕ 23.7　**FUD** 090　　　T A2 80 ▭
AMA: 2002,Apr,13; 1998,Nov,1

26392 **Removal of synthetic rod and insertion of flexor tendon graft, hand or finger (includes obtaining graft), each rod**
🔢 27.6　⚕ 27.6　**FUD** 090　　　T A2 80 ▭
AMA: 2002,Apr,13; 1998,Nov,1

26410 **Repair, extensor tendon, hand, primary or secondary; without free graft, each tendon**
🔢 15.8　⚕ 15.8　**FUD** 090　　　T A2 ▭
AMA: 2002,Apr,13; 1998,Nov,1

26412 **with free graft (includes obtaining graft), each tendon**
🔢 19.5　⚕ 19.5　**FUD** 090　　　T A2 80 ▭
AMA: 2002,Apr,13; 1998,Nov,1

26415 **Excision of extensor tendon, with implantation of synthetic rod for delayed tendon graft, hand or finger, each rod**
🔢 19.2　⚕ 19.2　**FUD** 090　　　T A2 80 ▭
AMA: 2002,Apr,13; 1998,Nov,1

26416 **Removal of synthetic rod and insertion of extensor tendon graft (includes obtaining graft), hand or finger, each rod**
🔢 25.1　⚕ 25.1　**FUD** 090　　　T A2 ▭
AMA: 2015,Jan,16; 2014,Jan,11

26418 **Repair, extensor tendon, finger, primary or secondary; without free graft, each tendon**
🔢 16.2　⚕ 16.2　**FUD** 090　　　T A2 ▭
AMA: 2015,Jan,16; 2014,Jan,11; 2012,Jan,15-42; 2011,Jan,11

26420 **with free graft (includes obtaining graft) each tendon**
🔢 19.9　⚕ 19.9　**FUD** 090　　　T A2 80 ▭
AMA: 2002,Apr,13

26426 **Repair of extensor tendon, central slip, secondary (eg, boutonniere deformity); using local tissue(s), including lateral band(s), each finger**
🔢 14.3　⚕ 14.3　**FUD** 090　　　T A2 ▭
AMA: 2002,Apr,13; 1998,Nov,1

26428 **with free graft (includes obtaining graft), each finger**
🔢 20.8　⚕ 20.8　**FUD** 090　　　T A2 80 ▭
AMA: 2002,Apr,13; 1998,Nov,1

26432 **Closed treatment of distal extensor tendon insertion, with or without percutaneous pinning (eg, mallet finger)**
🔢 14.0　⚕ 14.0　**FUD** 090　　　T A2 ▭
AMA: 2002,Apr,13; 1998,Nov,1

26433 **Repair of extensor tendon, distal insertion, primary or secondary; without graft (eg, mallet finger)**
EXCLUDES Trigger finger (26055)
🔢 14.9　⚕ 14.9　**FUD** 090　　　T A2 ▭
AMA: 2002,Apr,13; 1998,Nov,1

26434 **with free graft (includes obtaining graft)**
EXCLUDES Trigger finger (26055)
🔢 18.3　⚕ 18.3　**FUD** 090　　　T A2 80 ▭
AMA: 2002,Apr,13

26437 **Realignment of extensor tendon, hand, each tendon**
🔢 17.5　⚕ 17.5　**FUD** 090　　　T A2 ▭
AMA: 2002,Apr,13; 1998,Nov,1

26440 **Tenolysis, flexor tendon; palm OR finger, each tendon**
🔢 17.3　⚕ 17.3　**FUD** 090　　　T A2 ▭
AMA: 2015,Jun,10; 2015,Jan,16; 2014,Jan,11; 2012,Jan,15-42; 2011,Jan,11

26442 palm AND finger, each tendon
🔧 27.1 ✂ 27.1 **FUD** 090
T A2
AMA: 2002,Apr,13

26445 Tenolysis, extensor tendon, hand OR finger, each tendon
🔧 16.1 ✂ 16.1 **FUD** 090
T A2
AMA: 2015,Jan,16; 2014,Jan,11; 2012,Jan,15-42; 2011,Jan,11

26449 Tenolysis, complex, extensor tendon, finger, including forearm, each tendon
🔧 19.8 ✂ 19.8 **FUD** 090
T A2 80
AMA: 2002,Apr,13; 1998,Nov,1

26450 Tenotomy, flexor, palm, open, each tendon
🔧 11.4 ✂ 11.4 **FUD** 090
T A2 80
AMA: 2002,Apr,13; 1998,Nov,1

26455 Tenotomy, flexor, finger, open, each tendon
🔧 11.3 ✂ 11.3 **FUD** 090
T A2 80
AMA: 2002,Apr,13; 1998,Nov,1

26460 Tenotomy, extensor, hand or finger, open, each tendon
🔧 11.0 ✂ 11.0 **FUD** 090
T A2
AMA: 2002,Apr,13; 1998,Nov,1

26471 Tenodesis; of proximal interphalangeal joint, each joint
🔧 17.2 ✂ 17.2 **FUD** 090
T A2 80
AMA: 2002,Apr,13; 1998,Nov,1

26474 of distal joint, each joint
🔧 17.0 ✂ 17.0 **FUD** 090
T A2 80
AMA: 2002,Apr,13; 1998,Nov,1

26476 Lengthening of tendon, extensor, hand or finger, each tendon
🔧 16.5 ✂ 16.5 **FUD** 090
T A2
AMA: 2002,Apr,13; 1998,Nov,1

26477 Shortening of tendon, extensor, hand or finger, each tendon
🔧 16.1 ✂ 16.1 **FUD** 090
T A2
AMA: 2002,Apr,13; 1998,Nov,1

26478 Lengthening of tendon, flexor, hand or finger, each tendon
🔧 17.3 ✂ 17.3 **FUD** 090
T A2 80
AMA: 2015,Jan,16; 2014,Jan,11; 2013,Dec,16

26479 Shortening of tendon, flexor, hand or finger, each tendon
🔧 17.1 ✂ 17.1 **FUD** 090
T A2 80
AMA: 2002,Apr,13; 1998,Nov,1

26480 Transfer or transplant of tendon, carpometacarpal area or dorsum of hand; without free graft, each tendon
🔧 21.1 ✂ 21.1 **FUD** 090
T A2 80
AMA: 2015,Jan,16; 2014,Jan,11; 2013,Dec,16

26483 with free tendon graft (includes obtaining graft), each tendon
🔧 23.7 ✂ 23.7 **FUD** 090
T A2 80
AMA: 2002,Apr,13

26485 Transfer or transplant of tendon, palmar; without free tendon graft, each tendon
🔧 22.7 ✂ 22.7 **FUD** 090
T A2 80
AMA: 2002,Apr,13; 1998,Nov,1

26489 with free tendon graft (includes obtaining graft), each tendon
🔧 26.5 ✂ 26.5 **FUD** 090
T A2 80
AMA: 2002,Apr,13

26490 Opponensplasty; superficialis tendon transfer type, each tendon
EXCLUDES *Thumb fusion (26820)*
🔧 22.5 ✂ 22.5 **FUD** 090
T A2 80
AMA: 2002,Apr,13; 1998,Nov,1

26492 tendon transfer with graft (includes obtaining graft), each tendon
EXCLUDES *Thumb fusion (26820)*
🔧 25.0 ✂ 25.0 **FUD** 090
T A2 80
AMA: 2002,Apr,13; 1998,Nov,1

26494 hypothenar muscle transfer
EXCLUDES *Thumb fusion (26820)*
🔧 21.9 ✂ 21.9 **FUD** 090
T A2 80
AMA: 2002,Apr,13

26496 other methods
EXCLUDES *Thumb fusion (26820)*
🔧 24.0 ✂ 24.0 **FUD** 090
T A2 80
AMA: 2002,Apr,13

26497 Transfer of tendon to restore intrinsic function; ring and small finger
🔧 24.5 ✂ 24.5 **FUD** 090
T A2 80
AMA: 2002,Apr,13; 1998,Nov,1

26498 all 4 fingers
🔧 32.7 ✂ 32.7 **FUD** 090
T A2 80
AMA: 2002,Apr,13

26499 Correction claw finger, other methods
🔧 23.0 ✂ 23.0 **FUD** 090
T A2 80
AMA: 2002,Apr,13

26500 Reconstruction of tendon pulley, each tendon; with local tissues (separate procedure)
🔧 17.5 ✂ 17.5 **FUD** 090
T A2 80
AMA: 2002,Apr,13; 1998,Nov,1

26502 with tendon or fascial graft (includes obtaining graft) (separate procedure)
🔧 20.1 ✂ 20.1 **FUD** 090
T A2 80
AMA: 2002,Apr,13

26508 Release of thenar muscle(s) (eg, thumb contracture)
🔧 17.7 ✂ 17.7 **FUD** 090
T A2 80 50
AMA: 2002,Apr,13; 1998,Nov,1

26510 Cross intrinsic transfer, each tendon
🔧 16.6 ✂ 16.6 **FUD** 090
T A2 80
AMA: 2002,Apr,13

26516 Capsulodesis, metacarpophalangeal joint; single digit
🔧 19.6 ✂ 19.6 **FUD** 090
T A2 80 50
AMA: 2002,Apr,13; 1998,Nov,1

26517 2 digits
🔧 23.4 ✂ 23.4 **FUD** 090
T A2 80 50
AMA: 2002,Apr,13

26518 3 or 4 digits
🔧 23.2 ✂ 23.2 **FUD** 090
T A2 80 50
AMA: 2002,Apr,13

26520 Capsulectomy or capsulotomy; metacarpophalangeal joint, each joint
EXCLUDES *Carpometacarpal joint arthroplasty (25447)*
🔧 18.2 ✂ 18.2 **FUD** 090
T A2
AMA: 2002,Apr,13; 1998,Nov,1

26525 interphalangeal joint, each joint
EXCLUDES *Carpometacarpal joint arthroplasty (25447)*
🔧 18.2 ✂ 18.2 **FUD** 090
T A2
AMA: 2015,Jun,10; 2015,Jan,16; 2014,Jan,11; 2012,Jan,15-42; 2011,Jan,11

26530 Arthroplasty, metacarpophalangeal joint; each joint
EXCLUDES *Carpometacarpal joint arthroplasty (25447)*
🔧 15.3 ✂ 15.3 **FUD** 090
T A2 80
AMA: 2002,Apr,13; 1998,Nov,1

26531 with prosthetic implant, each joint
EXCLUDES *Carpometacarpal joint arthroplasty (25447)*
🔧 17.8 ✂ 17.8 **FUD** 090
T A2 80
AMA: 2015,Jan,16; 2014,Jan,11; 2012,Jan,15-42; 2011,Sep,11-12

26535 Arthroplasty, interphalangeal joint; each joint
EXCLUDES *Carpometacarpal joint arthroplasty (25447)*
🔧 12.0 ✂ 12.0 **FUD** 090
T A2
AMA: 2002,Apr,13; 1998,Nov,1

26536 with prosthetic implant, each joint
EXCLUDES Carpometacarpal joint arthroplasty (25447)
🦴 19.9 ⚖ 19.9 **FUD** 090 T A2 80 ▭
AMA: 2002,Apr,13; 1998,Nov,1

26540 Repair of collateral ligament, metacarpophalangeal or interphalangeal joint
🦴 18.4 ⚖ 18.4 **FUD** 090 T A2 80 ▭
AMA: 2002,Apr,13; 1996,Nov,1

26541 Reconstruction, collateral ligament, metacarpophalangeal joint, single; with tendon or fascial graft (includes obtaining graft)
🦴 22.5 ⚖ 22.5 **FUD** 090 T A2 80 ▭
AMA: 2015,Jan,16; 2014,Jan,11

26542 with local tissue (eg, adductor advancement)
🦴 19.1 ⚖ 19.1 **FUD** 090 T A2 80 ▭
AMA: 2015,Jan,16; 2014,Jan,11

26545 Reconstruction, collateral ligament, interphalangeal joint, single, including graft, each joint
🦴 20.0 ⚖ 20.0 **FUD** 090 T A2 80 ▭
AMA: 2002,Apr,13

26546 Repair non-union, metacarpal or phalanx (includes obtaining bone graft with or without external or internal fixation)
🦴 28.1 ⚖ 28.1 **FUD** 090 T A2 80 50 ▭
AMA: 2002,Apr,13; 1996,Nov,1

26548 Repair and reconstruction, finger, volar plate, interphalangeal joint
🦴 21.3 ⚖ 21.3 **FUD** 090 T A2 80 ▭
AMA: 2002,Apr,13

26550-26556 Reconstruction Procedures with Finger and Toe Transplants

26550 Pollicization of a digit
🦴 47.0 ⚖ 47.0 **FUD** 090 T A2 80 50 ▭
AMA: 2002,Apr,13

26551 Transfer, toe-to-hand with microvascular anastomosis; great toe wrap-around with bone graft
INCLUDES Operating microscope (69990)
EXCLUDES Big toe with web space (20973)
🦴 94.8 ⚖ 94.8 **FUD** 090 C 80 50 ▭
AMA: 2015,Jan,16; 2014,Jan,11

26553 other than great toe, single
INCLUDES Operating microscope (69990)
🦴 77.6 ⚖ 77.6 **FUD** 090 C 80 50 ▭
AMA: 2015,Jan,16; 2014,Jan,11

26554 other than great toe, double
INCLUDES Operating microscope (69990)
🦴 90.8 ⚖ 90.8 **FUD** 090 C 80 50 ▭
AMA: 2015,Jan,16; 2014,Jan,11

26555 Transfer, finger to another position without microvascular anastomosis
🦴 39.1 ⚖ 39.1 **FUD** 090 T A2 80 ▭
AMA: 2002,Apr,13; 1998,Nov,1

26556 Transfer, free toe joint, with microvascular anastomosis
INCLUDES Operating microscope (69990)
EXCLUDES Big toe to hand transfer (20973)
🦴 81.1 ⚖ 81.1 **FUD** 090 C 80 ▭
AMA: 2015,Jan,16; 2014,Jan,11

26560-26596 Repair of Other Deformities of the Fingers/Hand

26560 Repair of syndactyly (web finger) each web space; with skin flaps
🦴 16.7 ⚖ 16.7 **FUD** 090 T A2 80 ▭
AMA: 2002,Apr,13

26561 with skin flaps and grafts
🦴 26.2 ⚖ 26.2 **FUD** 090 T A2 80 ▭
AMA: 2002,Apr,13

26562 complex (eg, involving bone, nails)
🦴 37.6 ⚖ 37.6 **FUD** 090 T A2 80 ▭
AMA: 2002,Apr,13

26565 Osteotomy; metacarpal, each
🦴 19.2 ⚖ 19.2 **FUD** 090 T A2 80 ▭
AMA: 2002,Apr,13; 1998,Nov,1

26567 phalanx of finger, each
🦴 19.1 ⚖ 19.1 **FUD** 090 T A2 80 ▭
AMA: 2015,Jan,16; 2014,Jan,11; 2012,Apr,17-18

26568 Osteoplasty, lengthening, metacarpal or phalanx
🦴 25.5 ⚖ 25.5 **FUD** 090 T A2 80 ▭
AMA: 2002,Apr,13; 1998,Nov,1

26580 Repair cleft hand
INCLUDES Barsky's procedure
🦴 43.1 ⚖ 43.1 **FUD** 090 T A2 80 50 ▭
AMA: 2002,Apr,13

26587 Reconstruction of polydactylous digit, soft tissue and bone
EXCLUDES Soft tissue removal only (11200)
🦴 27.5 ⚖ 27.5 **FUD** 090 T A2 80 ▭
AMA: 2015,Jan,16; 2014,Jan,11; 2012,Jan,15-42; 2011,Jan,11

26590 Repair macrodactylia, each digit
🦴 40.2 ⚖ 40.2 **FUD** 090 T A2 80 ▭
AMA: 2015,Jan,16; 2014,Jan,11; 2012,Jan,15-42; 2011,Jan,11

26591 Repair, intrinsic muscles of hand, each muscle
🦴 12.1 ⚖ 12.1 **FUD** 090 T A2 80 ▭
AMA: 2015,Jan,16; 2014,Jan,11; 2012,Jan,15-42; 2011,Jan,11

26593 Release, intrinsic muscles of hand, each muscle
🦴 16.8 ⚖ 16.8 **FUD** 090 T A2
AMA: 2002,Apr,13; 1998,Nov,1

26596 Excision of constricting ring of finger, with multiple Z-plasties
EXCLUDES Graft repair or scar contracture release (11042, 14040-14041, 15120, 15240)
🦴 21.2 ⚖ 21.2 **FUD** 090 T A2 80 ▭
AMA: 2002,Apr,13

26600-26785 Treatment of Fracture/Dislocation of Fingers and Hand

INCLUDES Closed, percutaneous, and open treatment of fractures or dislocations

26600 Closed treatment of metacarpal fracture, single; without manipulation, each bone
🦴 7.86 ⚖ 8.35 **FUD** 090 T P2 ▭
AMA: 2002,Apr,13

26605 with manipulation, each bone
🦴 8.34 ⚖ 9.16 **FUD** 090 T A2 ▭
AMA: 2002,Apr,13

26607 Closed treatment of metacarpal fracture, with manipulation, with external fixation, each bone
🦴 13.1 ⚖ 13.1 **FUD** 090 T A2 80 ▭
AMA: 2002,Apr,13

26608 Percutaneous skeletal fixation of metacarpal fracture, each bone
🦴 13.6 ⚖ 13.6 **FUD** 090 T A2 80 ▭ P0
AMA: 2002,Apr,13

26615 Open treatment of metacarpal fracture, single, includes internal fixation, when performed, each bone
🦴 16.5 ⚖ 16.5 **FUD** 090 T A2 ▭
AMA: 2002,Apr,13

26641 Closed treatment of carpometacarpal dislocation, thumb, with manipulation
🦴 9.78 ⚖ 10.7 **FUD** 090 T P2 80 50 ▭
AMA: 2002,Apr,13

| 26/TC PC/TC Comp Only | A2-Z3 ASC Pmt | 50 Bilateral | ♂ Male Only | ♀ Female Only | 🦴 Facility RVU | ⚖ Non-Facility RVU |
| AMA: CPT Asst | CMS: Pub 100 | A-Y OPPSI | 80/80 Surg Assist Allowed / w/Doc | | 🔬 Lab Crosswalk | ☢ Radiology Crosswalk |

68 Medicare (Red Text) CPT © 2015 American Medical Association. All Rights Reserved. (Black Text) © 2015 Optum360, LLC (Blue Text)

26645 Closed treatment of carpometacarpal fracture dislocation, thumb (Bennett fracture), with manipulation
🔧 11.2 🔪 12.2 **FUD** 090 T A2 80 50 ▣
AMA: 2002,Apr,13

26650 Percutaneous skeletal fixation of carpometacarpal fracture dislocation, thumb (Bennett fracture), with manipulation
🔧 13.6 🔪 13.6 **FUD** 090 T A2 50 ▣ PQ
AMA: 2002,Apr,13

26665 Open treatment of carpometacarpal fracture dislocation, thumb (Bennett fracture), includes internal fixation, when performed
🔧 18.0 🔪 18.0 **FUD** 090 T A2 50 ▣
AMA: 2002,Apr,13

26670 Closed treatment of carpometacarpal dislocation, other than thumb, with manipulation, each joint; without anesthesia
🔧 8.71 🔪 9.58 **FUD** 090 T P2 80 ▣
AMA: 2002,Apr,13

26675 requiring anesthesia
🔧 11.9 🔪 13.0 **FUD** 090 T A2 80 ▣
AMA: 2002,Apr,13

26676 Percutaneous skeletal fixation of carpometacarpal dislocation, other than thumb, with manipulation, each joint
🔧 14.3 🔪 14.3 **FUD** 090 T A2 ▣ PQ
AMA: 2002,Apr,13

26685 Open treatment of carpometacarpal dislocation, other than thumb; includes internal fixation, when performed, each joint
🔧 16.5 🔪 16.5 **FUD** 090 T A2 ▣
AMA: 2002,Apr,13

26686 complex, multiple, or delayed reduction
🔧 17.9 🔪 17.9 **FUD** 090 T J8 80 ▣
AMA: 2002,Apr,13

26700 Closed treatment of metacarpophalangeal dislocation, single, with manipulation; without anesthesia
🔧 8.57 🔪 9.14 **FUD** 090 T P2 ▣
AMA: 2002,Apr,13

26705 requiring anesthesia
🔧 10.9 🔪 11.8 **FUD** 090 T A2 80 ▣
AMA: 2002,Apr,13

26706 Percutaneous skeletal fixation of metacarpophalangeal dislocation, single, with manipulation
🔧 12.4 🔪 12.4 **FUD** 090 T A2 ▣ PQ
AMA: 2002,Apr,13

26715 Open treatment of metacarpophalangeal dislocation, single, includes internal fixation, when performed
🔧 16.3 🔪 16.3 **FUD** 090 T A2 80 ▣
AMA: 2002,Apr,13

26720 Closed treatment of phalangeal shaft fracture, proximal or middle phalanx, finger or thumb; without manipulation, each
🔧 5.23 🔪 5.62 **FUD** 090 T P2 ▣
AMA: 2002,Apr,13

26725 with manipulation, with or without skin or skeletal traction, each
🔧 8.64 🔪 9.58 **FUD** 090 T P2 ▣
AMA: 2002,Apr,13

26727 Percutaneous skeletal fixation of unstable phalangeal shaft fracture, proximal or middle phalanx, finger or thumb, with manipulation, each
🔧 13.4 🔪 13.4 **FUD** 090 T A2 ▣ PQ
AMA: 2002,Apr,13

26735 Open treatment of phalangeal shaft fracture, proximal or middle phalanx, finger or thumb, includes internal fixation, when performed, each
🔧 17.0 🔪 17.0 **FUD** 090 T A2 ▣
AMA: 2002,Apr,13

26740 Closed treatment of articular fracture, involving metacarpophalangeal or interphalangeal joint; without manipulation, each
🔧 6.11 🔪 6.51 **FUD** 090 T P2 ▣
AMA: 2002,Apr,13

26742 with manipulation, each
🔧 9.45 🔪 10.4 **FUD** 090 T A2 ▣
AMA: 2002,Apr,13

26746 Open treatment of articular fracture, involving metacarpophalangeal or interphalangeal joint, includes internal fixation, when performed, each
🔧 21.2 🔪 21.2 **FUD** 090 T A2 ▣
AMA: 2002,Apr,13

26750 Closed treatment of distal phalangeal fracture, finger or thumb; without manipulation, each
🔧 5.23 🔪 5.22 **FUD** 090 T P2 ▣
AMA: 2002,Apr,13

26755 with manipulation, each
🔧 7.75 🔪 8.92 **FUD** 090 T G2 ▣
AMA: 2002,Apr,13

26756 Percutaneous skeletal fixation of distal phalangeal fracture, finger or thumb, each
🔧 11.8 🔪 11.8 **FUD** 090 T A2 80 ▣
AMA: 2002,Apr,13

26765 Open treatment of distal phalangeal fracture, finger or thumb, includes internal fixation, when performed, each
🔧 14.3 🔪 14.3 **FUD** 090 T A2 ▣
AMA: 2002,Apr,13

26770 Closed treatment of interphalangeal joint dislocation, single, with manipulation; without anesthesia
🔧 7.23 🔪 7.81 **FUD** 090 T G2 ▣
AMA: 2002,Apr,13

26775 requiring anesthesia
🔧 9.87 🔪 10.9 **FUD** 090 S P2 ▣
AMA: 2002,Apr,13

26776 Percutaneous skeletal fixation of interphalangeal joint dislocation, single, with manipulation
🔧 12.6 🔪 12.6 **FUD** 090 T A2 ▣
AMA: 2002,Apr,13

26785 Open treatment of interphalangeal joint dislocation, includes internal fixation, when performed, single
🔧 15.6 🔪 15.6 **FUD** 090 T A2 ▣
AMA: 2002,Apr,13

26820-26863 Fusion of Joint(s) of Fingers or Hand

26820 Fusion in opposition, thumb, with autogenous graft (includes obtaining graft)
🔧 22.3 🔪 22.3 **FUD** 090 T A2 80 50 ▣
AMA: 2002,Apr,13

26841 Arthrodesis, carpometacarpal joint, thumb, with or without internal fixation;
🔧 20.4 🔪 20.4 **FUD** 090 T A2 80 50 ▣
AMA: 2002,Apr,13

26842 with autograft (includes obtaining graft)
🔧 22.1 🔪 22.1 **FUD** 090 T A2 80 50 ▣
AMA: 2002,Apr,13

26843 Arthrodesis, carpometacarpal joint, digit, other than thumb, each;
🔧 20.9 🔪 20.9 **FUD** 090 T A2 80 ▣
AMA: 2015,Jan,16; 2014,Jan,11; 2012,Jan,15-42; 2011,Jan,11

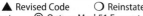

26844 with autograft (includes obtaining graft)
🖪 22.7　⚕ 22.7　**FUD** 090　　　　T A2 80 ▣
AMA: 2002,Apr,13

26850 Arthrodesis, metacarpophalangeal joint, with or without internal fixation;
🖪 19.4　⚕ 19.4　**FUD** 090　　　　T A2 80 ▣
AMA: 2002,Apr,13

26852 with autograft (includes obtaining graft)
🖪 22.3　⚕ 22.3　**FUD** 090　　　　T A2 80 ▣
AMA: 2002,Apr,13

26860 Arthrodesis, interphalangeal joint, with or without internal fixation;
🖪 15.8　⚕ 15.8　**FUD** 090　　　　T A2 ▣
AMA: 2015,Jan,16; 2014,Jan,11; 2012,Jan,15-42; 2011,Jan,11

+ 26861 each additional interphalangeal joint (List separately in addition to code for primary procedure)
Code first (26860)
🖪 2.99　⚕ 2.99　**FUD** ZZZ　　　　N N1 ▣
AMA: 2015,Jan,16; 2014,Jan,11; 2012,Jan,15-42; 2011,Jan,11

26862 with autograft (includes obtaining graft)
🖪 20.4　⚕ 20.4　**FUD** 090　　　　T A2 80 ▣
AMA: 2002,Apr,13

+ 26863 with autograft (includes obtaining graft), each additional joint (List separately in addition to code for primary procedure)
Code first (26862)
🖪 6.61　⚕ 6.61　**FUD** ZZZ　　　　N N1 80 ▣
AMA: 2002,Apr,13

26910-26989 Amputations and Unlisted Procedures Finger/Hand

26910 Amputation, metacarpal, with finger or thumb (ray amputation), single, with or without interosseous transfer
EXCLUDES　Repositioning (26550, 26555)
　　　　　　Transmetacarpal amputation of hand (25927)
🖪 20.2　⚕ 20.2　**FUD** 090　　　　T A2 ▣
AMA: 2002,Apr,13

26951 Amputation, finger or thumb, primary or secondary, any joint or phalanx, single, including neurectomies; with direct closure
EXCLUDES　Repair necessitating flaps or grafts (15050-15758)
　　　　　　Transmetacarpal amputation of hand (25927)
🖪 18.3　⚕ 18.3　**FUD** 090　　　　T A2 ▣
AMA: 2002,Apr,13

26952 with local advancement flaps (V-Y, hood)
EXCLUDES　Repair necessitating flaps or grafts (15050-15758)
　　　　　　Transmetacarpal amputation of hand (25927)
🖪 18.1　⚕ 18.1　**FUD** 090　　　　T A2 ▣
AMA: 2002,Apr,13

26989 Unlisted procedure, hands or fingers
🖪 0.00　⚕ 0.00　**FUD** YYY　　　　T
AMA: 2002,Apr,13

26990-26992 Incision for Drainage of Pelvis or Hip

EXCLUDES　Simple incision and drainage procedures (10040-10160)

26990 Incision and drainage, pelvis or hip joint area; deep abscess or hematoma
🖪 17.9　⚕ 17.9　**FUD** 090　　　　T A2 ▣
AMA: 2002,Apr,13

26991 infected bursa
🖪 14.9　⚕ 20.0　**FUD** 090　　　　T A2 80 ▣
AMA: 2002,Apr,13

26992 Incision, bone cortex, pelvis and/or hip joint (eg, osteomyelitis or bone abscess)
🖪 27.5　⚕ 27.5　**FUD** 090　　　　C 80 ▣
AMA: 2015,Jan,16; 2014,Jan,11; 2012,Oct,14; 2012,Jan,15-42; 2011,Jan,11

27000-27006 Tenotomy Procedures of Hip

27000 Tenotomy, adductor of hip, percutaneous (separate procedure)
🖪 11.9　⚕ 11.9　**FUD** 090　　　　T A2 50 ▣
AMA: 2002,Apr,13; 1998,Nov,1

27001 Tenotomy, adductor of hip, open
🖪 15.5　⚕ 15.5　**FUD** 090　　　　T A2 80 50 ▣
AMA: 2002,Apr,13; 1998,Nov,1

27003 Tenotomy, adductor, subcutaneous, open, with obturator neurectomy
🖪 17.1　⚕ 17.1　**FUD** 090　　　　T A2 80 50 ▣
AMA: 2002,Apr,13

27005 Tenotomy, hip flexor(s), open (separate procedure)
🖪 20.8　⚕ 20.8　**FUD** 090　　　　C 80 50 ▣
AMA: 2002,Apr,13; 1998,Nov,1

27006 Tenotomy, abductors and/or extensor(s) of hip, open (separate procedure)
🖪 21.1　⚕ 21.1　**FUD** 090　　　　T 80 50 ▣
AMA: 2002,Apr,13; 1998,Nov,1

27025-27036 Surgical Incision of Hip

27025 Fasciotomy, hip or thigh, any type
🖪 26.2　⚕ 26.2　**FUD** 090　　　　C 80 50 ▣
AMA: 2002,Apr,13

27027 Decompression fasciotomy(ies), pelvic (buttock) compartment(s) (eg, gluteus medius-minimus, gluteus maximus, iliopsoas, and/or tensor fascia lata muscle), unilateral
🖪 25.5　⚕ 25.5　**FUD** 090　　　　T 80 50
AMA: 2002,Apr,13

27030 Arthrotomy, hip, with drainage (eg, infection)
🖪 27.0　⚕ 27.0　**FUD** 090　　　　C 80 50 ▣
AMA: 2002,Apr,13; 1998,Nov,1

27033 Arthrotomy, hip, including exploration or removal of loose or foreign body
🖪 28.0　⚕ 28.0　**FUD** 090　　　　T A2 80 50 ▣
AMA: 2015,Jan,16; 2014,Jan,11

27035 Denervation, hip joint, intrapelvic or extrapelvic intra-articular branches of sciatic, femoral, or obturator nerves
EXCLUDES　Transection of obturator nerve (64763, 64766)
🖪 30.8　⚕ 30.8　**FUD** 090　　　　T A2 80 50 ▣
AMA: 2015,Jan,16; 2014,Mar,13

27036 Capsulectomy or capsulotomy, hip, with or without excision of heterotopic bone, with release of hip flexor muscles (ie, gluteus medius, gluteus minimus, tensor fascia latae, rectus femoris, sartorius, iliopsoas)
🖪 29.1　⚕ 29.1　**FUD** 090　　　　C 80 50 ▣
AMA: 2002,Apr,13; 1996,Nov,1

27040-27041 Biopsy of Hip/Pelvis

EXCLUDES　Soft tissue needle biopsy (20206)

27040 Biopsy, soft tissue of pelvis and hip area; superficial
🖪 5.75　⚕ 9.83　**FUD** 010　　　　T A2 50 ▣ PQ
AMA: 2002,Apr,13

27041 deep, subfascial or intramuscular
🖪 19.7　⚕ 19.7　**FUD** 090　　　　T A2 50 ▣ PQ
AMA: 2002,Apr,13; 1998,Nov,1

27043-27049 [27043, 27045, 27059] Excision Soft Tissue Tumors Hip/ Pelvis

INCLUDES Any necessary elevation of tissue planes or dissection
Measurement of tumor and necessary margin at greatest diameter prior to excision
Simple and intermediate repairs
Types of excision:
 Fascial or subfascial soft tissue tumors: simple and marginal resection of tumors found either in or below the deep fascia, not involving bone or excision of a substantial amount of normal tissue; primarily benign and intramuscular tumors
 Radical resection of soft tissue tumor: wide resection of tumor involving substantial margins of normal tissue and may involve tissue removal from one or more layers; mostly malignant or aggressive benign,
 Subcutaneous: simple and marginal resection of tumors found in the subcutaneous tissue above the deep fascia; most often benign

EXCLUDES Complex repair
Excision of benign cutaneous lesions (eg, sebaceous cyst) (11400-11406)
Radical resection of cutaneous tumors (eg, melanoma) (11600-11606)
Significant exploration of vessels, neuroplasty, reconstruction, or complex bone repair

27043 Resequenced code. See code following 27047.

27045 Resequenced code. See code following 27048.

27047 **Excision, tumor, soft tissue of pelvis and hip area, subcutaneous; less than 3 cm**
  10.4 13.4 **FUD** 090 T G2 50
  AMA: 2002,Apr,13; 1998,Nov,1

\# **27043** **3 cm or greater**
  13.5 13.5 **FUD** 090 T G2 50

27048 **Excision, tumor, soft tissue of pelvis and hip area, subfascial (eg, intramuscular); less than 5 cm**
  17.5 17.5 **FUD** 090 T G2 80 50
  AMA: 2002,Apr,13

\# **27045** **5 cm or greater**
  21.5 21.5 **FUD** 090 T G2 80 50

27049 **Radical resection of tumor (eg, sarcoma), soft tissue of pelvis and hip area; less than 5 cm**
  38.5 38.5 **FUD** 090 T G2 80 50
  AMA: 2002,Apr,13; 1998,Nov,1

\# **27059** **5 cm or greater**
  52.5 52.5 **FUD** 090 T G2 80 50

27050-27071 Procedures of Bones and Joints of Hip and Pelvis

27050 **Arthrotomy, with biopsy; sacroiliac joint**
  11.5 11.5 **FUD** 090 T A2 80 50 PQ
  AMA: 2002,Apr,13; 1994,Win,1

27052 **hip joint**
  16.6 16.6 **FUD** 090 T A2 80 50 PQ
  AMA: 2002,Apr,13

27054 **Arthrotomy with synovectomy, hip joint**
  19.6 19.6 **FUD** 090 C 80 50
  AMA: 2002,Apr,13; 1994,Win,1

27057 **Decompression fasciotomy(ies), pelvic (buttock) compartment(s) (eg, gluteus medius-minimus, gluteus maximus, iliopsoas, and/or tensor fascia lata muscle) with debridement of nonviable muscle, unilateral**
  29.2 29.2 **FUD** 090 T 80 50

27059 Resequenced code. See code following 27049.

27060 **Excision; ischial bursa**
  13.3 13.3 **FUD** 090 T A2 50
  AMA: 2002,Apr,13

27062 **trochanteric bursa or calcification**
  EXCLUDES *Arthrocentesis (20610)*
  13.1 13.1 **FUD** 090 T A2 50
  AMA: 2002,Apr,13

27065 **Excision of bone cyst or benign tumor, wing of ilium, symphysis pubis, or greater trochanter of femur; superficial, includes autograft, when performed**
  14.8 14.8 **FUD** 090 T A2 80 50
  AMA: 2002,Apr,13

27066 **deep (subfascial), includes autograft, when performed**
  23.4 23.4 **FUD** 090 T A2 80 50
  AMA: 2002,Apr,13

27067 **with autograft requiring separate incision**
  29.8 29.8 **FUD** 090 T A2 80 50
  AMA: 2002,Apr,13

27070 **Partial excision, wing of ilium, symphysis pubis, or greater trochanter of femur, (craterization, saucerization) (eg, osteomyelitis or bone abscess); superficial**
  24.4 24.4 **FUD** 090 C 80 50
  AMA: 2002,Apr,13; 1998,Nov,1

27071 **deep (subfascial or intramuscular)**
  26.3 26.3 **FUD** 090 C 80 50
  AMA: 2002,Apr,13

27075-27078 Radical Resection Bone Tumor of Hip/Pelvis

INCLUDES Any necessary elevation of tissue planes or dissection
Measurement of tumor and necessary margin at greatest diameter prior to excision
Resection of the tumor (may include entire bone) and wide margins of normal tissue primarily for malignant or aggressive benign tumors
Simple and intermediate repairs

EXCLUDES Complex repair
Significant exploration of vessels, neuroplasty, reconstruction, or complex bone repair

Do not report radical excision of soft tissue codes when adjacent soft tissue is removed during the bone tumor resection (27043-27049 [27043, 27045, 27059])

27075 **Radical resection of tumor; wing of ilium, 1 pubic or ischial ramus or symphysis pubis**
  60.8 60.8 **FUD** 090 C 80
  AMA: 2002,Apr,13; 1994,Win,1

27076 **ilium, including acetabulum, both pubic rami, or ischium and acetabulum**
  73.7 73.7 **FUD** 090 C 80
  AMA: 2002,Apr,13

27077 **innominate bone, total**
  82.3 82.3 **FUD** 090 C 80
  AMA: 2002,Apr,13

27078 **ischial tuberosity and greater trochanter of femur**
  60.0 60.0 **FUD** 090 C 80 50
  AMA: 2002,Apr,13

27080 Excision of Coccyx

EXCLUDES *Surgical excision of decubitus ulcers (15920, 15922, 15931-15958)*

27080 **Coccygectomy, primary**
  14.7 14.7 **FUD** 090 T A2 80
  AMA: 2002,Apr,13

27086-27091 Removal Foreign Body or Hip Prosthesis

27086 **Removal of foreign body, pelvis or hip; subcutaneous tissue**
  4.84 8.43 **FUD** 010 T A2 80 50
  AMA: 2015,Jan,16; 2014,Jan,11

27087   **deep (subfascial or intramuscular)**
🦴 17.9   ⚗ 17.9   **FUD** 090   T A2 80 50 ▭
AMA: 2002,Apr,13; 1998,Nov,1

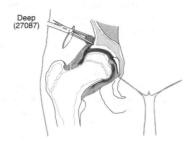

Deep
(27087)

A foreign body is removed
from the pelvis or hip

27090   **Removal of hip prosthesis; (separate procedure)**
🦴 23.8   ⚗ 23.8   **FUD** 090   C 80 50 ▭
AMA: 2002,Apr,13

27091   **complicated, including total hip prosthesis, methylmethacrylate with or without insertion of spacer**
🦴 46.1   ⚗ 46.1   **FUD** 090   C 80 50 ▭
AMA: 2015,Jan,16; 2014,Jan,11

27093-27096 Injection for Arthrogram Hip/Sacroiliac Joint

27093   **Injection procedure for hip arthrography; without anesthesia**
🔬 (73525)
🦴 2.03   ⚗ 5.33   **FUD** 000   N N1 50 ▭
AMA: 2015,Aug,6; 2015,Jan,16; 2014,Jan,11; 2012,Jun,14

27095   **with anesthesia**
🔬 (73525)
🦴 2.39   ⚗ 6.87   **FUD** 000   N N1 50 ▭
AMA: 2015,Aug,6; 2015,Jan,16; 2014,Jan,11; 2012,Jun,14

27096   **Injection procedure for sacroiliac joint, anesthetic/steroid, with image guidance (fluoroscopy or CT) including arthrography when performed**
> INCLUDES   Confirmation of intra-articular needle placement with CT or fluoroscopy
> EXCLUDES   *Procedure performed without fluoroscopy or CT guidance (20552)*
> Do not report with (77002-77003)
🦴 2.42   ⚗ 4.56   **FUD** 000   B 50 ▭
AMA: 2015,Aug,6; 2015,Jan,16; 2014,Jan,11; 2012,Jan,3-5; 2012,Jan,15-42; 2011,Jan,11

27097-27187 Revision/Reconstruction Hip and Pelvis

> INCLUDES   Closed, open and percutaneous treatment of fractures and dislocations

27097   **Release or recession, hamstring, proximal**
🦴 19.6   ⚗ 19.6   **FUD** 090   T A2 80 50 ▭
AMA: 2002,Apr,13; 1998,Nov,1

27098   **Transfer, adductor to ischium**
🦴 20.0   ⚗ 20.0   **FUD** 090   T A2 80 50 ▭
AMA: 2002,Apr,13; 1998,Nov,1

27100   **Transfer external oblique muscle to greater trochanter including fascial or tendon extension (graft)**
> INCLUDES   Eggers procedure
🦴 23.8   ⚗ 23.8   **FUD** 090   T A2 80 50 ▭
AMA: 2002,Apr,13

27105   **Transfer paraspinal muscle to hip (includes fascial or tendon extension graft)**
🦴 24.9   ⚗ 24.9   **FUD** 090   T A2 80 50 ▭
AMA: 2002,Apr,13

27110   **Transfer iliopsoas; to greater trochanter of femur**
🦴 27.9   ⚗ 27.9   **FUD** 090   T A2 80 50 ▭
AMA: 2002,May,7; 2002,Apr,13

27111   **to femoral neck**
🦴 25.9   ⚗ 25.9   **FUD** 090   T A2 80 50 ▭
AMA: 2002,Apr,13

27120   **Acetabuloplasty; (eg, Whitman, Colonna, Haygroves, or cup type)**
🦴 37.6   ⚗ 37.6   **FUD** 090   C 80 50 ▭
AMA: 2002,Apr,13

27122   **resection, femoral head (eg, Girdlestone procedure)**
🦴 31.6   ⚗ 31.6   **FUD** 090   C 80 50 ▭
AMA: 2002,Apr,13; 1998,Nov,1

27125   **Hemiarthroplasty, hip, partial (eg, femoral stem prosthesis, bipolar arthroplasty)**
> EXCLUDES   *Hip replacement following hip fracture (27236)*
🦴 32.7   ⚗ 32.7   **FUD** 090   C 80 50 ▭ P0
AMA: 2015,Jan,16; 2014,Jan,11; 2012,Jan,15-42; 2011,Jan,11

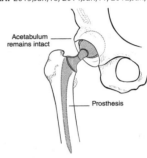

Acetabulum
remains intact

Prosthesis

27130   **Arthroplasty, acetabular and proximal femoral prosthetic replacement (total hip arthroplasty), with or without autograft or allograft**
🦴 39.1   ⚗ 39.1   **FUD** 090   C 80 50 ▭ P0
AMA: 2015,Jan,16; 2014,Jan,11; 2012,Jan,15-42; 2011,Dec,14-18

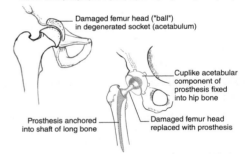

Damaged femur head ("ball") in degenerated socket (acetabulum)

Cuplike acetabular component of prosthesis fixed into hip bone

Prosthesis anchored into shaft of long bone

Damaged femur head replaced with prosthesis

27132   **Conversion of previous hip surgery to total hip arthroplasty, with or without autograft or allograft**
🦴 48.4   ⚗ 48.4   **FUD** 090   C 80 50 ▭ P0
AMA: 2015,Jan,16; 2014,Jan,11

27134   **Revision of total hip arthroplasty; both components, with or without autograft or allograft**
🦴 55.3   ⚗ 55.3   **FUD** 090   C 80 50 ▭ P0
AMA: 2015,Jan,16; 2014,Jan,11

27137   **acetabular component only, with or without autograft or allograft**
🦴 42.5   ⚗ 42.5   **FUD** 090   C 80 50 ▭ P0
AMA: 2015,Jan,16; 2014,Jan,11

27138   **femoral component only, with or without allograft**
🦴 44.2   ⚗ 44.2   **FUD** 090   C 80 50 ▭ P0
AMA: 2015,Jan,16; 2014,Jan,11

27140   **Osteotomy and transfer of greater trochanter of femur (separate procedure)**
🦴 25.8   ⚗ 25.8   **FUD** 090   C 80 50 ▭
AMA: 2008,Dec,3-4; 2002,Apr,13

27146 Osteotomy, iliac, acetabular or innominate bone;

INCLUDES Salter osteotomy

🦴 37.0 ✂ 37.0 **FUD** 090 C 80 50 ▣

AMA: 2015,Jan,16; 2014,Jan,11; 2012,Jan,15-42; 2011,Jan,11

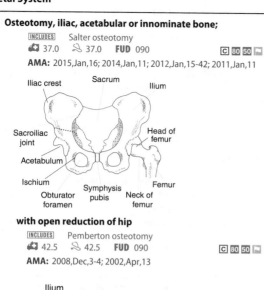

Iliac crest — Sacrum — Ilium
Sacroiliac joint — Head of femur
Acetabulum
Ischium — Femur
Obturator foramen — Symphysis pubis — Neck of femur

27147 with open reduction of hip

INCLUDES Pemberton osteotomy

🦴 42.5 ✂ 42.5 **FUD** 090 C 80 50 ▣

AMA: 2008,Dec,3-4; 2002,Apr,13

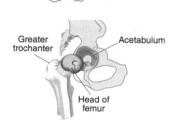

Ilium
Example of innominate osteotomy

Greater trochanter — Acetabulum
Head of femur

Femoral head is reduced into the acetabulum

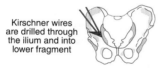

Kirschner wires are drilled through the ilium and into lower fragment

27151 with femoral osteotomy

🦴 46.0 ✂ 46.0 **FUD** 090 C 80 50 ▣

AMA: 2008,Dec,3-4; 2002,Apr,13

27156 with femoral osteotomy and with open reduction of hip

INCLUDES Chiari osteotomy

🦴 49.6 ✂ 49.6 **FUD** 090 C 80 50 ▣

AMA: 2008,Dec,3-4; 2002,Apr,13

27158 Osteotomy, pelvis, bilateral (eg, congenital malformation)

🦴 40.5 ✂ 40.5 **FUD** 090 C 80 ▣

AMA: 2008,Dec,3-4; 2002,Apr,13

27161 Osteotomy, femoral neck (separate procedure)

🦴 35.1 ✂ 35.1 **FUD** 090 C 80 50 ▣

AMA: 2008,Dec,3-4; 2002,Apr,13

27165 Osteotomy, intertrochanteric or subtrochanteric including internal or external fixation and/or cast

🦴 39.5 ✂ 39.5 **FUD** 090 C 80 50 ▣

AMA: 2015,Jan,16; 2014,Jan,11

27170 Bone graft, femoral head, neck, intertrochanteric or subtrochanteric area (includes obtaining bone graft)

🦴 34.0 ✂ 34.0 **FUD** 090 C 80 50 ▣

AMA: 2015,Jan,16; 2014,Jan,11

27175 Treatment of slipped femoral epiphysis; by traction, without reduction

🦴 19.2 ✂ 19.2 **FUD** 090 C 80 50 ▣

AMA: 2008,Dec,3-4; 2002,Apr,13

27176 by single or multiple pinning, in situ

🦴 26.4 ✂ 26.4 **FUD** 090 C 80 50 ▣

AMA: 2008,Dec,3-4; 2002,Apr,13

27177 Open treatment of slipped femoral epiphysis; single or multiple pinning or bone graft (includes obtaining graft)

🦴 32.1 ✂ 32.1 **FUD** 090 C 80 50 ▣

AMA: 2008,Dec,3-4; 2002,Apr,13

27178 closed manipulation with single or multiple pinning

🦴 26.4 ✂ 26.4 **FUD** 090 C 80 50 ▣

AMA: 2008,Dec,3-4; 2002,Apr,13

27179 osteoplasty of femoral neck (Heyman type procedure)

🦴 28.1 ✂ 28.1 **FUD** 090 T 80 50 ▣

AMA: 2008,Dec,3-4; 2002,Apr,13

27181 osteotomy and internal fixation

🦴 32.4 ✂ 32.4 **FUD** 090 C 80 50 ▣

AMA: 2008,Dec,3-4; 2002,Apr,13

27185 Epiphyseal arrest by epiphysiodesis or stapling, greater trochanter of femur

🦴 16.8 ✂ 16.8 **FUD** 090 C 50 ▣

AMA: 2008,Dec,3-4; 2002,Apr,13

27187 Prophylactic treatment (nailing, pinning, plating or wiring) with or without methylmethacrylate, femoral neck and proximal femur

🦴 28.6 ✂ 28.6 **FUD** 090 C 80 50 ▣

AMA: 2015,Jan,16; 2014,Jan,11

27193-27269 Treatment of Fracture/Dislocation Hip/Pelvis

27193 Closed treatment of pelvic ring fracture, dislocation, diastasis or subluxation; without manipulation

🦴 13.6 ✂ 13.5 **FUD** 090 T A2 ▣

AMA: 2015,Jan,16; 2014,Jan,11

27194 with manipulation, requiring more than local anesthesia

🦴 20.5 ✂ 20.5 **FUD** 090 T A2 80 ▣

AMA: 2008,Dec,3-4; 2002,Apr,13

27200 Closed treatment of coccygeal fracture

🦴 5.38 ✂ 5.16 **FUD** 090 T P2 ▣

AMA: 2008,Dec,3-4; 2002,Apr,13

27202 Open treatment of coccygeal fracture

🦴 15.3 ✂ 15.3 **FUD** 090 T A2 80 ▣

AMA: 2008,Dec,3-4; 2002,Apr,13

27215 Open treatment of iliac spine(s), tuberosity avulsion, or iliac wing fracture(s), unilateral, for pelvic bone fracture patterns that do not disrupt the pelvic ring, includes internal fixation, when performed

🦴 17.2 ✂ 17.2 **FUD** 090 E ▣

AMA: 2008,Dec,3-4; 2002,Apr,13

27216 Percutaneous skeletal fixation of posterior pelvic bone fracture and/or dislocation, for fracture patterns that disrupt the pelvic ring, unilateral (includes ipsilateral ilium, sacroiliac joint and/or sacrum)

EXCLUDES Sacroiliac joint arthrodesis without fracture and/or dislocation, percutaneous or minimally invasive (27279)

🦴 25.5 ✂ 25.5 **FUD** 090 E ▣

AMA: 2015,Jan,16; 2014,Mar,4; 2013,Sep,17

27217 Open treatment of anterior pelvic bone fracture and/or dislocation for fracture patterns that disrupt the pelvic ring, unilateral, includes internal fixation, when performed (includes pubic symphysis and/or ipsilateral superior/inferior rami)

🦴 23.9 ✂ 23.9 **FUD** 090 E ▣

AMA: 2008,Dec,3-4; 2002,Apr,13

27218 Open treatment of posterior pelvic bone fracture and/or dislocation, for fracture patterns that disrupt the pelvic ring, unilateral, includes internal fixation, when performed (includes ipsilateral ilium, sacroiliac joint and/or sacrum)

EXCLUDES *Sacroiliac joint arthrodesis without fracture and/or dislocation, percutaneous or minimally invasive (27279)*

🔲 33.0   ⚖ 33.0   **FUD** 090   E 🔲

AMA: 2015,Jan,16; 2014,Mar,4

27220 Closed treatment of acetabulum (hip socket) fracture(s); without manipulation

🔲 15.0   ⚖ 15.2   **FUD** 090   T G2 50 🔲

AMA: 2008,Dec,3-4; 2002,Apr,13

27222   with manipulation, with or without skeletal traction

🔲 28.2   ⚖ 28.2   **FUD** 090   C 50 🔲

AMA: 2008,Dec,3-4; 2002,Apr,13

27226 Open treatment of posterior or anterior acetabular wall fracture, with internal fixation

🔲 30.5   ⚖ 30.5   **FUD** 090   C 80 50 🔲

AMA: 2008,Dec,3-4; 2002,Apr,13

27227 Open treatment of acetabular fracture(s) involving anterior or posterior (one) column, or a fracture running transversely across the acetabulum, with internal fixation

🔲 47.9   ⚖ 47.9   **FUD** 090   C 80 50 🔲

AMA: 2008,Dec,3-4; 2002,Apr,13

27228 Open treatment of acetabular fracture(s) involving anterior and posterior (two) columns, includes T-fracture and both column fracture with complete articular detachment, or single column or transverse fracture with associated acetabular wall fracture, with internal fixation

🔲 54.7   ⚖ 54.7   **FUD** 090   C 80 50 🔲

AMA: 2008,Dec,3-4; 2002,Apr,13

27230 Closed treatment of femoral fracture, proximal end, neck; without manipulation

🔲 13.5   ⚖ 13.6   **FUD** 090   T A2 50 🔲 P0

AMA: 2008,Dec,3-4; 2002,Apr,13

27232   with manipulation, with or without skeletal traction

🔲 21.7   ⚖ 21.7   **FUD** 090   C 50 🔲 P0

AMA: 2008,Dec,3-4; 2002,Apr,13

27235 Percutaneous skeletal fixation of femoral fracture, proximal end, neck

🔲 26.2   ⚖ 26.2   **FUD** 090   T 50 🔲 P0

AMA: 2015,Jan,16; 2014,Jan,11

27236 Open treatment of femoral fracture, proximal end, neck, internal fixation or prosthetic replacement

🔲 34.5   ⚖ 34.5   **FUD** 090   C 80 50 🔲 P0

AMA: 2015,Jan,16; 2014,Jan,11; 2012,Jan,15-42; 2011,Jan,11

27238 Closed treatment of intertrochanteric, peritrochanteric, or subtrochanteric femoral fracture; without manipulation

🔲 13.2   ⚖ 13.2   **FUD** 090   T A2 50 🔲 P0

AMA: 2015,Jan,16; 2014,Jan,11

27240   with manipulation, with or without skin or skeletal traction

🔲 27.6   ⚖ 27.6   **FUD** 090   C 50 🔲 P0

AMA: 2015,Jan,16; 2014,Jan,11

27244 Treatment of intertrochanteric, peritrochanteric, or subtrochanteric femoral fracture; with plate/screw type implant, with or without cerclage

🔲 35.5   ⚖ 35.5   **FUD** 090   C 80 50 🔲 P0

AMA: 2015,Jan,16; 2014,Jan,11

27245   with intramedullary implant, with or without interlocking screws and/or cerclage

🔲 35.5   ⚖ 35.5   **FUD** 090   C 80 50 🔲 P0

AMA: 2015,Jan,16; 2014,Jan,11; 2013,Sep,17

27246 Closed treatment of greater trochanteric fracture, without manipulation

🔲 11.0   ⚖ 11.0   **FUD** 090   T A2 50 🔲 P0

AMA: 2008,Dec,3-4; 2002,Apr,13

27248 Open treatment of greater trochanteric fracture, includes internal fixation, when performed

🔲 21.4   ⚖ 21.4   **FUD** 090   C 80 50 🔲 P0

AMA: 2008,Dec,3-4; 2002,Apr,13

27250 Closed treatment of hip dislocation, traumatic; without anesthesia

🔲 5.23   ⚖ 5.23   **FUD** 000   T A2 50 🔲

AMA: 2008,Dec,3-4; 2002,Apr,13

27252   requiring anesthesia

🔲 21.9   ⚖ 21.9   **FUD** 090   T A2 50 🔲

AMA: 2008,Dec,3-4; 2002,Apr,13

27253 Open treatment of hip dislocation, traumatic, without internal fixation

🔲 27.1   ⚖ 27.1   **FUD** 090   C 80 50 🔲

AMA: 2008,Dec,3-4; 2002,Apr,13

27254 Open treatment of hip dislocation, traumatic, with acetabular wall and femoral head fracture, with or without internal or external fixation

EXCLUDES *Acetabular fracture treatment (27226-27227)*

🔲 36.7   ⚖ 36.7   **FUD** 090   C 80 50 🔲

AMA: 2008,Dec,3-4; 2002,Apr,13

27256 Treatment of spontaneous hip dislocation (developmental, including congenital or pathological), by abduction, splint or traction; without anesthesia, without manipulation

🔲 6.78   ⚖ 8.65   **FUD** 010   T G2 80 50 🔲

AMA: 2008,Dec,3-4; 2002,Apr,13

27257   with manipulation, requiring anesthesia

🔲 9.85   ⚖ 9.85   **FUD** 010   T A2 80 50 🔲

AMA: 2008,Dec,3-4; 2002,Apr,13

27258 Open treatment of spontaneous hip dislocation (developmental, including congenital or pathological), replacement of femoral head in acetabulum (including tenotomy, etc);

INCLUDES Lorenz's operation

🔲 32.0   ⚖ 32.0   **FUD** 090   C 80 50 🔲

AMA: 2008,Dec,3-4; 2002,Apr,13

27259   with femoral shaft shortening

🔲 44.9   ⚖ 44.9   **FUD** 090   C 80 50 🔲

AMA: 2008,Dec,3-4; 2002,Apr,13

27265 Closed treatment of post hip arthroplasty dislocation; without anesthesia

🔲 11.3   ⚖ 11.3   **FUD** 090   T A2 50 🔲

AMA: 2008,Dec,3-4; 2002,Apr,13

27266   requiring regional or general anesthesia

🔲 16.7   ⚖ 16.7   **FUD** 090   T A2 50 🔲

AMA: 2008,Dec,3-4; 2002,Apr,13

27267 Closed treatment of femoral fracture, proximal end, head; without manipulation

🔲 12.4   ⚖ 12.4   **FUD** 090   T G2 80 50

AMA: 2015,Jan,16; 2014,Jan,11

27268   with manipulation

🔲 15.5   ⚖ 15.5   **FUD** 090   C 80 50

AMA: 2015,Jan,16; 2014,Jan,11

27269 Open treatment of femoral fracture, proximal end, head, includes internal fixation, when performed

Do not report with (27033, 27253)

🔲 35.9   ⚖ 35.9   **FUD** 090   C 80 50 🔲

AMA: 2015,Jan,16; 2014,Jan,11

27275 Hip Manipulation with Anesthesia

27275   Manipulation, hip joint, requiring general anesthesia

🔲 5.25   ⚖ 5.25   **FUD** 010   T A2

AMA: 2015,Jan,16; 2014,Jan,11

| 26/TC PC/TC Comp Only | A2-Z3 ASC Pmt | 50 Bilateral | ♂ Male Only | ♀ Female Only | 🔲 Facility RVU | ⚖ Non-Facility RVU |
| AMA: CPT Asst | CMS: Pub 100 | A-Y OPPSI | 80/80 Surg Assist Allowed / w/Doc | | 🔲 Lab Crosswalk | 🔲 Radiology Crosswalk |

74   Medicare (Red Text)   CPT © 2015 American Medical Association. All Rights Reserved. (Black Text)   © 2015 Optum360, LLC (Blue Text)

27279-27286 Arthrodesis of Hip and Pelvis

27279 **Arthrodesis, sacroiliac joint, percutaneous or minimally invasive (indirect visualization), with image guidance, includes obtaining bone graft when performed, and placement of transfixing device**
🔧 16.0   ⚕ 16.0   **FUD** 090
J J8 80 50

27280 **Arthrodesis, open, sacroiliac joint, including obtaining bone graft, including instrumentation, when performed**
EXCLUDES *Sacroiliac joint arthrodesis without fracture and/or dislocation, percutaneous or minimally invasive (27279)*
🔧 31.1   ⚕ 31.1   **FUD** 090
C 80 50
AMA: 2015,Jan,16; 2014,Mar,4; 2014,Jan,11; 2013,Sep,17

27282 **Arthrodesis, symphysis pubis (including obtaining graft)**
🔧 21.5   ⚕ 21.5   **FUD** 090
C 80
AMA: 2008,Dec,3-4; 2002,Apr,13

27284 **Arthrodesis, hip joint (including obtaining graft);**
🔧 44.1   ⚕ 44.1   **FUD** 090
C 80 50
AMA: 2008,Dec,3-4; 2002,Apr,13

27286 **with subtrochanteric osteotomy**
🔧 47.8   ⚕ 47.8   **FUD** 090
C 80 50
AMA: 2015,Jan,16; 2014,Jan,11

27290-27299 Amputations and Unlisted Procedures of Hip and Pelvis

27290 **Interpelviabdominal amputation (hindquarter amputation)**
INCLUDES Pean's amputation
🔧 47.0   ⚕ 47.0   **FUD** 090
C 80
AMA: 2015,Jan,16; 2014,Jan,11

27295 **Disarticulation of hip**
🔧 36.3   ⚕ 36.3   **FUD** 090
C 80 50
AMA: 2015,Jan,16; 2014,Jan,11

27299 **Unlisted procedure, pelvis or hip joint**
🔧 0.00   ⚕ 0.00   **FUD** YYY
T 80 50
AMA: 2015,Jan,16; 2014,Mar,13; 2014,Jan,11; 2012,Nov,13-14; 2012,Oct,14; 2012,Jan,15-42; 2011,Jan,11

27301-27310 Incisional Procedures Femur or Knee

EXCLUDES *Superficial incision and drainage (10040-10160)*

27301 **Incision and drainage, deep abscess, bursa, or hematoma, thigh or knee region**
🔧 14.2   ⚕ 18.9   **FUD** 090
T A2 50
AMA: 2015,Jan,16; 2014,Jan,11

27303 **Incision, deep, with opening of bone cortex, femur or knee (eg, osteomyelitis or bone abscess)**
🔧 18.3   ⚕ 18.3   **FUD** 090
C 80 50
AMA: 2008,Dec,3-4; 2002,Apr,13

27305 **Fasciotomy, iliotibial (tenotomy), open**
EXCLUDES *Ober-Yount (gluteal-iliotibial) fasciotomy (27025)*
🔧 13.8   ⚕ 13.8   **FUD** 090
T A2 80 50
AMA: 2008,Dec,3-4; 2002,Apr,13

27306 **Tenotomy, percutaneous, adductor or hamstring; single tendon (separate procedure)**
🔧 10.3   ⚕ 10.3   **FUD** 090
T A2 80 50
AMA: 2008,Dec,3-4; 2002,Apr,13

27307 **multiple tendons**
🔧 13.8   ⚕ 13.8   **FUD** 090
T A2 80 50
AMA: 2008,Dec,3-4; 2002,Apr,13

27310 **Arthrotomy, knee, with exploration, drainage, or removal of foreign body (eg, infection)**
🔧 21.0   ⚕ 21.0   **FUD** 090
T A2 80 50
AMA: 2015,Jan,16; 2014,Jan,11

27323-27324 Biopsy Femur or Knee

EXCLUDES *Soft tissue needle biopsy (20206)*

27323 **Biopsy, soft tissue of thigh or knee area; superficial**
🔧 5.09   ⚕ 7.68   **FUD** 010
T A2 50 PQ
AMA: 2015,Jan,16; 2014,Jan,11

27324 **deep (subfascial or intramuscular)**
🔧 11.3   ⚕ 11.3   **FUD** 090
T A2 50 PQ
AMA: 2015,Jan,16; 2014,Jan,11

27325-27326 Neurectomy

27325 **Neurectomy, hamstring muscle**
🔧 14.6   ⚕ 14.6   **FUD** 090
T A2 80 50

27326 **Neurectomy, popliteal (gastrocnemius)**
🔧 14.7   ⚕ 14.7   **FUD** 090
T A2 80 50

27327-27329 [27337, 27339] Excision Soft Tissue Tumors Femur/ Knee

INCLUDES Any necessary elevation of tissue planes or dissection
Measurement of tumor and necessary margin at greatest diameter prior to excision
Simple and intermediate repairs
Types of excision:
Fascial or subfascial soft tissue tumors: simple and marginal resection of tumors found either in or below the deep fascia, not including bone or excision of a substantial amount of normal tissue; primarily benign and intramuscular tumors
Radical resection of soft tissue tumor: wide resection of tumor involving substantial margins of normal tissue and may involve tissue removal from one or more layers; most often malignant or aggressive benign
Subcutaneous: simple and marginal resection of tumors in the subcutaneous tissue above the deep fascia; most often benign

EXCLUDES *Complex repair*
Excision of benign cutaneous lesions (eg, sebaceous cyst) (11400-11406)
Radical resection of cutaneous tumors (eg, melanoma) (11600-11606)
Significant exploration of vessels or neuroplasty

\# **27327** **Excision, tumor, soft tissue of thigh or knee area, subcutaneous; less than 3 cm**
🔧 9.00   ⚕ 13.1   **FUD** 090
T 62 50
AMA: 2002,Apr,13

27337 **3 cm or greater**
🔧 12.0   ⚕ 12.0   **FUD** 090
T 62 80 50

\# **27328** **Excision, tumor, soft tissue of thigh or knee area, subfascial (eg, intramuscular); less than 5 cm**
🔧 17.8   ⚕ 17.8   **FUD** 090
T 62 50
AMA: 2002,Apr,13

27339 **5 cm or greater**
🔧 21.7   ⚕ 21.7   **FUD** 090
T 62 80 50

27329 **Resequenced code. See code following 27360.**

27330-27360 Resection Procedures Thigh/Knee

27330 **Arthrotomy, knee; with synovial biopsy only**
🔧 11.9   ⚕ 11.9   **FUD** 090
T A2 50 PQ
AMA: 2015,Jan,16; 2014,Jan,11; 2012,Mar,9-10

27331 **including joint exploration, biopsy, or removal of loose or foreign bodies**
🔧 13.6   ⚕ 13.6   **FUD** 090
T A2 80 50 PQ
AMA: 2015,Jan,16; 2014,Jan,11; 2012,Nov,13-14

Musculoskeletal System

27332 — 27392

27332 Arthrotomy, with excision of semilunar cartilage (meniscectomy) knee; medial OR lateral
🔪 18.5   🔪 18.5   **FUD** 090   T A2 80 50 ▣
AMA: 2002,Apr,13; 1998,Nov,1

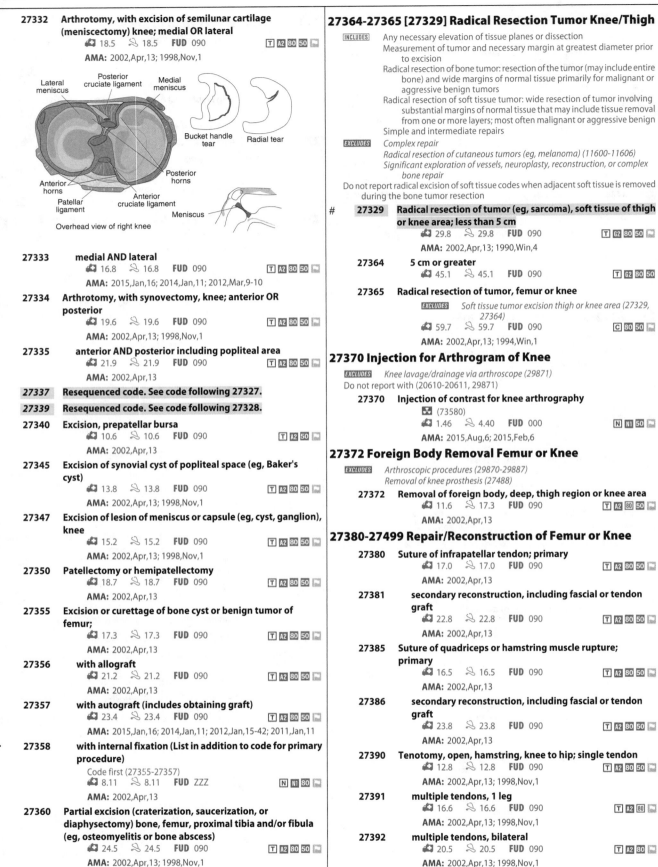

Overhead view of right knee

27333 medial AND lateral
🔪 16.8   🔪 16.8   **FUD** 090   T A2 80 50 ▣
AMA: 2015,Jan,16; 2014,Jan,11; 2012,Mar,9-10

27334 Arthrotomy, with synovectomy, knee; anterior OR posterior
🔪 19.6   🔪 19.6   **FUD** 090   T A2 80 50 ▣
AMA: 2002,Apr,13; 1998,Nov,1

27335 anterior AND posterior including popliteal area
🔪 21.9   🔪 21.9   **FUD** 090   T A2 80 50 ▣
AMA: 2002,Apr,13

27337 Resequenced code. See code following 27327.

27339 Resequenced code. See code following 27328.

27340 Excision, prepatellar bursa
🔪 10.6   🔪 10.6   **FUD** 090   T A2 50 ▣
AMA: 2002,Apr,13

27345 Excision of synovial cyst of popliteal space (eg, Baker's cyst)
🔪 13.8   🔪 13.8   **FUD** 090   T A2 80 50 ▣
AMA: 2002,Apr,13; 1998,Nov,1

27347 Excision of lesion of meniscus or capsule (eg, cyst, ganglion), knee
🔪 15.2   🔪 15.2   **FUD** 090   T A2 80 50 ▣
AMA: 2002,Apr,13; 1998,Nov,1

27350 Patellectomy or hemipatellectomy
🔪 18.7   🔪 18.7   **FUD** 090   T A2 80 50 ▣
AMA: 2002,Apr,13

27355 Excision or curettage of bone cyst or benign tumor of femur;
🔪 17.3   🔪 17.3   **FUD** 090   T A2 80 50 ▣
AMA: 2002,Apr,13

27356 with allograft
🔪 21.2   🔪 21.2   **FUD** 090   T A2 80 50 ▣
AMA: 2002,Apr,13

27357 with autograft (includes obtaining graft)
🔪 23.4   🔪 23.4   **FUD** 090   T A2 80 50 ▣
AMA: 2015,Jan,16; 2014,Jan,11; 2012,Jan,15-42; 2011,Jan,11

+ 27358 with internal fixation (List in addition to code for primary procedure)
Code first (27355-27357)
🔪 8.11   🔪 8.11   **FUD** ZZZ   N N1 80 ▣
AMA: 2002,Apr,13

27360 Partial excision (craterization, saucerization, or diaphysectomy) bone, femur, proximal tibia and/or fibula (eg, osteomyelitis or bone abscess)
🔪 24.5   🔪 24.5   **FUD** 090   T A2 80 50 ▣
AMA: 2002,Apr,13; 1998,Nov,1

27364-27365 [27329] Radical Resection Tumor Knee/Thigh

INCLUDES   Any necessary elevation of tissue planes or dissection
Measurement of tumor and necessary margin at greatest diameter prior to excision
Radical resection of bone tumor: resection of the tumor (may include entire bone) and wide margins of normal tissue primarily for malignant or aggressive benign tumors
Radical resection of soft tissue tumor: wide resection of tumor involving substantial margins of normal tissue that may include tissue removal from one or more layers; most often malignant or aggressive benign
Simple and intermediate repairs
EXCLUDES   *Complex repair*
Radical resection of cutaneous tumors (eg, melanoma) (11600-11606)
Significant exploration of vessels, neuroplasty, reconstruction, or complex bone repair
Do not report radical excision of soft tissue codes when adjacent soft tissue is removed during the bone tumor resection

 # 27329 Radical resection of tumor (eg, sarcoma), soft tissue of thigh or knee area; less than 5 cm
🔪 29.8   🔪 29.8   **FUD** 090   T G2 80 50 ▣
AMA: 2002,Apr,13; 1990,Win,4

27364 5 cm or greater
🔪 45.1   🔪 45.1   **FUD** 090   T G2 80 50
AMA: 2002,Apr,13; 1994,Win,1

27365 Radical resection of tumor, femur or knee
EXCLUDES   *Soft tissue tumor excision thigh or knee area (27329, 27364)*
🔪 59.7   🔪 59.7   **FUD** 090   C 80 50 ▣
AMA: 2002,Apr,13; 1994,Win,1

27370 Injection for Arthrogram of Knee

EXCLUDES   *Knee lavage/drainage via arthroscope (29871)*
Do not report with (20610-20611, 29871)

27370 Injection of contrast for knee arthrography
🔬 (73580)
🔪 1.46   🔪 4.40   **FUD** 000   N N1 50 ▣
AMA: 2015,Aug,6; 2015,Feb,6

27372 Foreign Body Removal Femur or Knee

EXCLUDES   *Arthroscopic procedures (29870-29887)*
Removal of knee prosthesis (27488)

27372 Removal of foreign body, deep, thigh region or knee area
🔪 11.6   🔪 17.3   **FUD** 090   T A2 80 50 ▣
AMA: 2002,Apr,13

27380-27499 Repair/Reconstruction of Femur or Knee

27380 Suture of infrapatellar tendon; primary
🔪 17.0   🔪 17.0   **FUD** 090   T A2 80 50 ▣
AMA: 2002,Apr,13

27381 secondary reconstruction, including fascial or tendon graft
🔪 22.8   🔪 22.8   **FUD** 090   T A2 80 50 ▣
AMA: 2002,Apr,13

27385 Suture of quadriceps or hamstring muscle rupture; primary
🔪 16.5   🔪 16.5   **FUD** 090   T A2 80 50 ▣
AMA: 2002,Apr,13

27386 secondary reconstruction, including fascial or tendon graft
🔪 23.8   🔪 23.8   **FUD** 090   T A2 80 50 ▣
AMA: 2002,Apr,13

27390 Tenotomy, open, hamstring, knee to hip; single tendon
🔪 12.8   🔪 12.8   **FUD** 090   T A2 80 50 ▣
AMA: 2002,Apr,13; 1998,Nov,1

27391 multiple tendons, 1 leg
🔪 16.6   🔪 16.6   **FUD** 090   T A2 80
AMA: 2002,Apr,13; 1998,Nov,1

27392 multiple tendons, bilateral
🔪 20.5   🔪 20.5   **FUD** 090   T A2 80
AMA: 2002,Apr,13; 1998,Nov,1

27393	**Lengthening of hamstring tendon; single tendon**

🔧 14.6   ✂ 14.6   **FUD** 090   T A2 80 50 ▣

AMA: 2002,Apr,13; 1998,Nov,1

27394   **multiple tendons, 1 leg**

🔧 18.7   ✂ 18.7   **FUD** 090   T A2 80 ▣

AMA: 2002,Apr,13; 1998,Nov,1

27395   **multiple tendons, bilateral**

🔧 25.3   ✂ 25.3   **FUD** 090   T A2 80 ▣

AMA: 2002,Apr,13; 1998,Nov,1

27396   **Transplant or transfer (with muscle redirection or rerouting), thigh (eg, extensor to flexor); single tendon**

🔧 17.7   ✂ 17.7   **FUD** 090   T A2 80 50 ▣

AMA: 2002,Apr,13; 1998,Nov,1

27397   **multiple tendons**

🔧 26.4   ✂ 26.4   **FUD** 090   T A2 80 50 ▣

AMA: 2002,Apr,13; 1998,Nov,1

27400   **Transfer, tendon or muscle, hamstrings to femur (eg, Egger's type procedure)**

🔧 20.0   ✂ 20.0   **FUD** 090   T A2 80 50 ▣

AMA: 2002,Apr,13; 1998,Nov,1

27403   **Arthrotomy with meniscus repair, knee**

EXCLUDES   *Arthroscopic treatment (29882)*

🔧 18.4   ✂ 18.4   **FUD** 090   T A2 80 50 ▣

AMA: 2002,Apr,13; 1998,Nov,1

27405   **Repair, primary, torn ligament and/or capsule, knee; collateral**

🔧 19.4   ✂ 19.4   **FUD** 090   T A2 80 50 ▣

AMA: 2015,Jan,16; 2014,Jan,11; 2012,Dec,12

27407   **cruciate**

EXCLUDES   *Reconstruction (27427)*

🔧 22.8   ✂ 22.8   **FUD** 090   T A2 80 50 ▣

AMA: 2002,Apr,13; 1999,Nov,1

27409   **collateral and cruciate ligaments**

EXCLUDES   *Reconstruction (27427-27429)*

🔧 27.8   ✂ 27.8   **FUD** 090   T A2 80 50 ▣

AMA: 2002,Apr,13; 1999,Nov,1

27412   **Autologous chondrocyte implantation, knee**

EXCLUDES   *Obtaining chondrocytes (29870)*

Do not report with (20926, 27331, 27570)

🔧 47.8   ✂ 47.8   **FUD** 090   J 80 50 ▣

AMA: 2002,Apr,13

27415   **Osteochondral allograft, knee, open**

EXCLUDES   *Arthroscopic procedure (29867)*

Do not report with (27416)

🔧 39.7   ✂ 39.7   **FUD** 090   J J8 80 50 ▣

AMA: 2015,Jan,16; 2014,Jan,11; 2012,Jan,15-42; 2011,Jan,11

27416   **Osteochondral autograft(s), knee, open (eg, mosaicplasty) (includes harvesting of autograft[s])**

EXCLUDES   *Surgical arthroscopy of the knee with osteochondral autograft(s) (29866)*

Do not report with the following procedures in the same compartment (29874, 29877, 29879, 29885-29887)

Do not report with the following procedures performed at the same surgical session (27415, 29870-29871, 29875, 29884)

🔧 28.3   ✂ 28.3   **FUD** 090   T 62 80 50

AMA: 2015,Jan,16; 2014,Jan,11

27418   **Anterior tibial tubercleplasty (eg, Maquet type procedure)**

🔧 23.8   ✂ 23.8   **FUD** 090   T A2 80 50 ▣

AMA: 2015,Jan,16; 2014,Jan,11; 2012,Jan,15-42; 2011,Jan,11; 2010,Jan,12-15

27420   **Reconstruction of dislocating patella; (eg, Hauser type procedure)**

🔧 21.2   ✂ 21.2   **FUD** 090   T A2 80 50 ▣

AMA: 2015,Jan,16; 2014,Jan,11; 2012,Nov,13-14

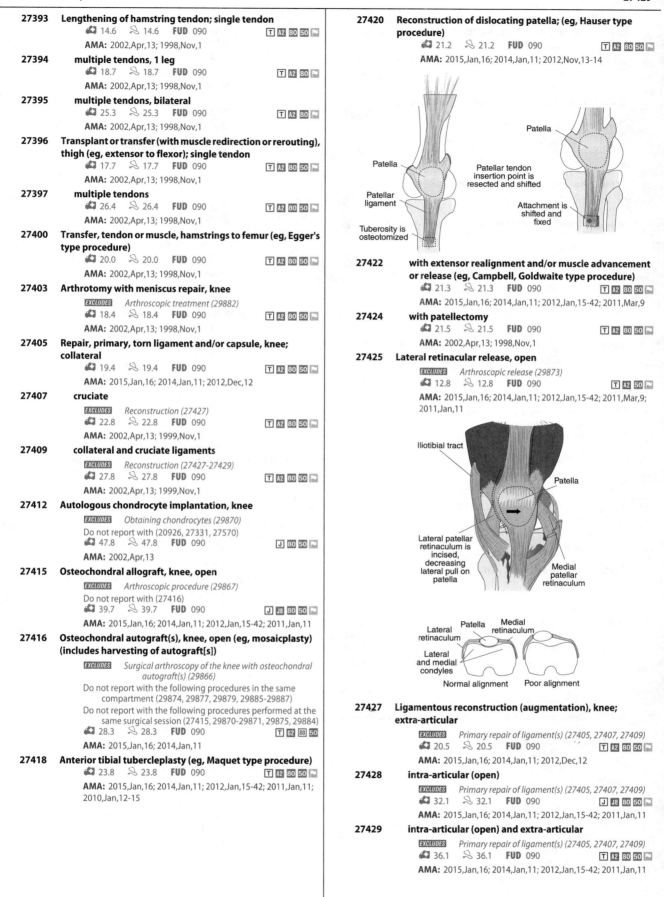

Patella

Patella

Patellar tendon insertion point is resected and shifted

Patellar ligament

Attachment is shifted and fixed

Tuberosity is osteotomized

27422   **with extensor realignment and/or muscle advancement or release (eg, Campbell, Goldwaite type procedure)**

🔧 21.3   ✂ 21.3   **FUD** 090   T A2 80 50 ▣

AMA: 2015,Jan,16; 2014,Jan,11; 2012,Jan,15-42; 2011,Mar,9

27424   **with patellectomy**

🔧 21.5   ✂ 21.5   **FUD** 090   T A2 80 50 ▣

AMA: 2002,Apr,13; 1998,Nov,1

27425   **Lateral retinacular release, open**

EXCLUDES   *Arthroscopic release (29873)*

🔧 12.8   ✂ 12.8   **FUD** 090   T A2 50 ▣

AMA: 2015,Jan,16; 2014,Jan,11; 2012,Jan,15-42; 2011,Mar,9; 2011,Jan,11

Iliotibial tract

Patella

Lateral patellar retinaculum is incised, decreasing lateral pull on patella

Medial patellar retinaculum

Lateral retinaculum

Patella

Medial retinaculum

Lateral and medial condyles

Normal alignment

Poor alignment

27427   **Ligamentous reconstruction (augmentation), knee; extra-articular**

EXCLUDES   *Primary repair of ligament(s) (27405, 27407, 27409)*

🔧 20.5   ✂ 20.5   **FUD** 090   T A2 80 50 ▣

AMA: 2015,Jan,16; 2014,Jan,11; 2012,Dec,12

27428   **intra-articular (open)**

EXCLUDES   *Primary repair of ligament(s) (27405, 27407, 27409)*

🔧 32.1   ✂ 32.1   **FUD** 090   J J8 80 50 ▣

AMA: 2015,Jan,16; 2014,Jan,11; 2012,Jan,15-42; 2011,Jan,11

27429   **intra-articular (open) and extra-articular**

EXCLUDES   *Primary repair of ligament(s) (27405, 27407, 27409)*

🔧 36.1   ✂ 36.1   **FUD** 090   T A2 80 50 ▣

AMA: 2015,Jan,16; 2014,Jan,11; 2012,Jan,15-42; 2011,Jan,11

27430   Quadricepsplasty (eg, Bennett or Thompson type)
    🛏 21.2   ✂ 21.2   **FUD** 090   T A2 80 50 ▣
    AMA: 2002,Apr,13; 1998,Nov,1

27435   Capsulotomy, posterior capsular release, knee
    🛏 23.1   ✂ 23.1   **FUD** 090   T A2 80 50 ▣
    AMA: 2002,Apr,13; 1998,Nov,1

27437   Arthroplasty, patella; without prosthesis
    🛏 19.0   ✂ 19.0   **FUD** 090   T A2 50 ▣
    AMA: 2002,Apr,13

27438   with prosthesis
    🛏 24.2   ✂ 24.2   **FUD** 090   J J8 80 50 ▣
    AMA: 2002,Apr,13

27440   Arthroplasty, knee, tibial plateau;
    🛏 23.0   ✂ 23.0   **FUD** 090   J J8 80 50 ▣ P0
    AMA: 2002,Apr,13

27441   with debridement and partial synovectomy
    🛏 23.7   ✂ 23.7   **FUD** 090   T A2 80 50 ▣ P0
    AMA: 2002,Apr,13

27442   Arthroplasty, femoral condyles or tibial plateau(s), knee;
    🛏 25.0   ✂ 25.0   **FUD** 090   J J8 80 50 ▣ P0
    AMA: 2002,Apr,13; 1999,Nov,1

27443   with debridement and partial synovectomy
    🛏 23.5   ✂ 23.5   **FUD** 090   J J8 80 50 ▣ P0
    AMA: 2002,Apr,13

27445   Arthroplasty, knee, hinge prosthesis (eg, Walldius type)
    EXCLUDES   *Removal knee prosthesis (27488)*
           Revision knee arthroplasty (27487)
    🛏 36.1   ✂ 36.1   **FUD** 090   C 80 50 ▣ P0
    AMA: 2002,Apr,13; 1998,Nov,1

27446   Arthroplasty, knee, condyle and plateau; medial OR lateral compartment
    EXCLUDES   *Removal knee prosthesis (27488)*
           Revision knee arthroplasty (27487)
    🛏 33.4   ✂ 33.4   **FUD** 090   J J8 80 50 ▣ P0
    AMA: 2002,Apr,13

27447   medial AND lateral compartments with or without patella resurfacing (total knee arthroplasty)
    EXCLUDES   *Removal knee prosthesis (27488)*
           Revision knee arthroplasty (27487)
    🛏 39.1   ✂ 39.1   **FUD** 090   C 80 50 ▣ P0
    AMA: 2015,Jan,16; 2014,Jan,11

27448   Osteotomy, femur, shaft or supracondylar; without fixation
    🛏 22.0   ✂ 22.0   **FUD** 090   C 80 50 ▣
    AMA: 2002,Apr,13

27450   with fixation
    🛏 29.0   ✂ 29.0   **FUD** 090   C 80 50 ▣
    AMA: 2002,Apr,13

27454   Osteotomy, multiple, with realignment on intramedullary rod, femoral shaft (eg, Sofield type procedure)
    🛏 37.5   ✂ 37.5   **FUD** 090   C 80 50 ▣
    AMA: 2002,Apr,13; 1998,Nov,1

27455   Osteotomy, proximal tibia, including fibular excision or osteotomy (includes correction of genu varus [bowleg] or genu valgus [knock-knee]); before epiphyseal closure
    🛏 27.2   ✂ 27.2   **FUD** 090   C 80 50 ▣
    AMA: 2002,Apr,13

27457   after epiphyseal closure
    🛏 27.7   ✂ 27.7   **FUD** 090   C 80 50 ▣
    AMA: 2002,Apr,13

27465   Osteoplasty, femur; shortening (excluding 64876)
    🛏 36.0   ✂ 36.0   **FUD** 090   C 80 50 ▣
    AMA: 2002,Apr,13

27466   lengthening
    🛏 34.2   ✂ 34.2   **FUD** 090   C 80 50 ▣
    AMA: 2002,Apr,13

27468   combined, lengthening and shortening with femoral segment transfer
    🛏 38.8   ✂ 38.8   **FUD** 090   C 80 50 ▣
    AMA: 2002,Apr,13

27470   Repair, nonunion or malunion, femur, distal to head and neck; without graft (eg, compression technique)
    🛏 33.9   ✂ 33.9   **FUD** 090   C 80 50 ▣
    AMA: 2002,Apr,13

27472   with iliac or other autogenous bone graft (includes obtaining graft)
    🛏 36.5   ✂ 36.5   **FUD** 090   C 80 50 ▣
    AMA: 2002,Apr,13

27475   Arrest, epiphyseal, any method (eg, epiphysiodesis); distal femur
    🛏 19.0   ✂ 19.0   **FUD** 090   T G2 50 ▣
    AMA: 2002,Apr,13; 2002,May,7

27477   tibia and fibula, proximal
    🛏 21.1   ✂ 21.1   **FUD** 090   C 50 ▣
    AMA: 2002,May,7; 2002,Apr,13

27479   combined distal femur, proximal tibia and fibula
    🛏 26.5   ✂ 26.5   **FUD** 090   T G2 80 50 ▣
    AMA: 2002,May,7; 2002,Apr,13

27485   Arrest, hemiepiphyseal, distal femur or proximal tibia or fibula (eg, genu varus or valgus)
    🛏 19.3   ✂ 19.3   **FUD** 090   C 50 ▣
    AMA: 2002,Apr,13; 1998,Nov,1

27486   Revision of total knee arthroplasty, with or without allograft; 1 component
    🛏 40.6   ✂ 40.6   **FUD** 090   C 80 50 ▣
    AMA: 2015,Jul,10; 2015,Jan,16; 2014,Jan,11; 2013,Dec,16

27487   femoral and entire tibial component
    🛏 50.7   ✂ 50.7   **FUD** 090   C 80 50 ▣
    AMA: 2015,Jan,16; 2013,Jul,6

27488   Removal of prosthesis, including total knee prosthesis, methylmethacrylate with or without insertion of spacer, knee
    🛏 34.6   ✂ 34.6   **FUD** 090   C 80 50 ▣
    AMA: 2015,Jan,16; 2013,Jul,6

27495   Prophylactic treatment (nailing, pinning, plating, or wiring) with or without methylmethacrylate, femur
    🛏 32.5   ✂ 32.5   **FUD** 090   C 80 50 ▣
    AMA: 2002,Apr,13

27496   Decompression fasciotomy, thigh and/or knee, 1 compartment (flexor or extensor or adductor);
    🛏 15.6   ✂ 15.6   **FUD** 090   T A2 50 ▣
    AMA: 2002,Apr,13

27497   with debridement of nonviable muscle and/or nerve
    🛏 17.0   ✂ 17.0   **FUD** 090   T A2 80 50 ▣
    AMA: 2002,Apr,13

27498   Decompression fasciotomy, thigh and/or knee, multiple compartments;
    🛏 18.8   ✂ 18.8   **FUD** 090   T A2 80 50 ▣
    AMA: 2002,Apr,13

27499   with debridement of nonviable muscle and/or nerve
    🛏 20.1   ✂ 20.1   **FUD** 090   T A2 80 50 ▣
    AMA: 2002,Apr,13

27500-27566 Treatment of Fracture/Dislocation of Femur/Knee

    INCLUDES   Closed, percutaneous, and open treatment of fractures and dislocations

27500   Closed treatment of femoral shaft fracture, without manipulation
    🛏 13.8   ✂ 14.9   **FUD** 090   T A2 50 ▣
    AMA: 2002,Apr,13

27501 Closed treatment of supracondylar or transcondylar femoral fracture with or without intercondylar extension, without manipulation
  14.3 14.4 **FUD** 090 T A2 80 50 ▢
  AMA: 2002,Apr,13

27502 Closed treatment of femoral shaft fracture, with manipulation, with or without skin or skeletal traction
  22.0 22.0 **FUD** 090 T A2 50 ▢
  AMA: 2015,Jan,16; 2014,Jan,11

27503 Closed treatment of supracondylar or transcondylar femoral fracture with or without intercondylar extension, with manipulation, with or without skin or skeletal traction
  23.1 23.1 **FUD** 090 T A2 80 50 ▢
  AMA: 2002,Apr,13

27506 Open treatment of femoral shaft fracture, with or without external fixation, with insertion of intramedullary implant, with or without cerclage and/or locking screws
  38.6 38.6 **FUD** 090 C 80 50 ▢
  AMA: 2015,Jan,16; 2014,Jan,11

27507 Open treatment of femoral shaft fracture with plate/screws, with or without cerclage
  28.0 28.0 **FUD** 090 C 80 50 ▢
  AMA: 2002,Apr,13

27508 Closed treatment of femoral fracture, distal end, medial or lateral condyle, without manipulation
  14.1 15.0 **FUD** 090 T A2 50 ▢
  AMA: 2002,Apr,13

27509 Percutaneous skeletal fixation of femoral fracture, distal end, medial or lateral condyle, or supracondylar or transcondylar, with or without intercondylar extension, or distal femoral epiphyseal separation
  18.5 18.5 **FUD** 090 T A2 80 50 ▢ PQ
  AMA: 2002,Apr,13; 1993,Win,1

Pins are placed percutaneously

27510 Closed treatment of femoral fracture, distal end, medial or lateral condyle, with manipulation
  19.6 19.6 **FUD** 090 T A2 50 ▢
  AMA: 2002,Apr,13

27511 Open treatment of femoral supracondylar or transcondylar fracture without intercondylar extension, includes internal fixation, when performed
  28.7 28.7 **FUD** 090 C 80 50 ▢
  AMA: 2002,Apr,13; 1996,May,6

27513 Open treatment of femoral supracondylar or transcondylar fracture with intercondylar extension, includes internal fixation, when performed
  35.8 35.8 **FUD** 090 C 80 50 ▢
  AMA: 2002,Apr,13

27514 Open treatment of femoral fracture, distal end, medial or lateral condyle, includes internal fixation, when performed
  27.9 27.9 **FUD** 090 C 80 50 ▢
  AMA: 2002,Apr,13

27516 Closed treatment of distal femoral epiphyseal separation; without manipulation
  13.7 14.6 **FUD** 090 T A2 50 ▢
  AMA: 2002,Apr,13

27517 with manipulation, with or without skin or skeletal traction
  19.7 19.7 **FUD** 090 T A2 80 50 ▢
  AMA: 2002,Apr,13

27519 Open treatment of distal femoral epiphyseal separation, includes internal fixation, when performed
  25.7 25.7 **FUD** 090 C 80 50 ▢
  AMA: 2002,Apr,13

27520 Closed treatment of patellar fracture, without manipulation
  8.41 9.22 **FUD** 090 T A2 50 ▢
  AMA: 2002,Apr,13

27524 Open treatment of patellar fracture, with internal fixation and/or partial or complete patellectomy and soft tissue repair
  21.7 21.7 **FUD** 090 T 62 80 50 ▢
  AMA: 2002,Apr,13

27530 Closed treatment of tibial fracture, proximal (plateau); without manipulation
  EXCLUDES *Arthroscopic repair (29855-29856)*
  7.99 8.62 **FUD** 090 T A2 50 ▢
  AMA: 2002,Apr,13

27532 with or without manipulation, with skeletal traction
  EXCLUDES *Arthroscopic repair (29855-29856)*
  16.6 17.7 **FUD** 090 T A2 50 ▢
  AMA: 2002,Apr,13

27535 Open treatment of tibial fracture, proximal (plateau); unicondylar, includes internal fixation, when performed
  EXCLUDES *Arthroscopic repair (29855-29856)*
  25.8 25.8 **FUD** 090 C 80 50 ▢
  AMA: 2002,Apr,13

27536 bicondylar, with or without internal fixation
  EXCLUDES *Arthroscopic repair (29855-29856)*
  34.3 34.3 **FUD** 090 C 80 50 ▢
  AMA: 2002,Apr,13

27538 Closed treatment of intercondylar spine(s) and/or tuberosity fracture(s) of knee, with or without manipulation
  EXCLUDES *Arthroscopic repair (29850-29851)*
  12.7 13.5 **FUD** 090 T A2 80 50 ▢
  AMA: 2002,Apr,13

27540 Open treatment of intercondylar spine(s) and/or tuberosity fracture(s) of the knee, includes internal fixation, when performed
  23.3 23.3 **FUD** 090 C 80 50 ▢
  AMA: 2002,Apr,13

27550 Closed treatment of knee dislocation; without anesthesia
  13.3 14.4 **FUD** 090 T A2 80 50 ▢
  AMA: 2002,Apr,13

27552 requiring anesthesia
  17.9 17.9 **FUD** 090 T A2 80 50 ▢
  AMA: 2002,Apr,13

27556 Open treatment of knee dislocation, includes internal fixation, when performed; without primary ligamentous repair or augmentation/reconstruction
  25.3 25.3 **FUD** 090 C 80 50 ▢
  AMA: 2002,Apr,13

Musculoskeletal System

27557 — 27615

27557   **with primary ligamentous repair**
🖪 30.3   ✄ 30.3   **FUD** 090   C 80 50 ▢
AMA: 2002,Apr,13

27558   **with primary ligamentous repair, with augmentation/reconstruction**
🖪 34.5   ✄ 34.5   **FUD** 090   C 80 50 ▢
AMA: 2002,Apr,13

27560   **Closed treatment of patellar dislocation; without anesthesia**
     EXCLUDES   *Recurrent dislocation (27420-27424)*
🖪 9.47   ✄ 10.2   **FUD** 090   T A2 50 ▢
AMA: 2002,Apr,13

27562   **requiring anesthesia**
     EXCLUDES   *Recurrent dislocation (27420-27424)*
🖪 13.9   ✄ 13.9   **FUD** 090   T A2 80 50 ▢
AMA: 2002,Apr,13

27566   **Open treatment of patellar dislocation, with or without partial or total patellectomy**
     EXCLUDES   *Recurrent dislocation (27420-27424)*
🖪 25.7   ✄ 25.7   **FUD** 090   T A2 80 50 ▢
AMA: 2002,Apr,13

27570 Knee Manipulation with Anesthesia

27570   **Manipulation of knee joint under general anesthesia (includes application of traction or other fixation devices)**
🖪 4.35   ✄ 4.35   **FUD** 010   T A2 50 ▢
AMA: 2015,Jan,16; 2014,Jan,11; 2012,Jan,15-42; 2011,Mar,9

27580 Knee Arthrodesis

27580   **Arthrodesis, knee, any technique**
     INCLUDES   Albert's operation
🖪 41.4   ✄ 41.4   **FUD** 090   C 80 50 ▢
AMA: 2002,Apr,13

27590-27599 Amputations and Unlisted Procedures at Femur or Knee

27590   **Amputation, thigh, through femur, any level;**
🖪 23.4   ✄ 23.4   **FUD** 090   C 80 50 ▢
AMA: 2002,Apr,13

27591   **immediate fitting technique including first cast**
🖪 27.9   ✄ 27.9   **FUD** 090   C 80 50 ▢
AMA: 2002,Apr,13

27592   **open, circular (guillotine)**
🖪 19.9   ✄ 19.9   **FUD** 090   C 80 50 ▢
AMA: 2002,Apr,13

27594   **secondary closure or scar revision**
🖪 14.6   ✄ 14.6   **FUD** 090   T A2 50 ▢
AMA: 2002,Apr,13

27596   **re-amputation**
🖪 20.9   ✄ 20.9   **FUD** 090   C 50 ▢
AMA: 2002,Apr,13

27598   **Disarticulation at knee**
     INCLUDES   Batch-Spittler-McFaddin operation
                 Callandar knee disarticulation
                  Gritti amputation
🖪 20.8   ✄ 20.8   **FUD** 090   C 80 50 ▢
AMA: 2002,Apr,13

27599   **Unlisted procedure, femur or knee**
🖪 0.00   ✄ 0.00   **FUD** YYY   T 80 50
AMA: 2015,Jan,13; 2015,Jan,16; 2014,Jan,9; 2014,Jan,11; 2012,Dec,12; 2012,Jan,15-42; 2011,Jan,11

27600-27602 Decompression Fasciotomy of Leg

     EXCLUDES   *Fasciotomy with debridement (27892-27894)*
                 Simple incision and drainage (10140-10160)

27600   **Decompression fasciotomy, leg; anterior and/or lateral compartments only**
🖪 11.9   ✄ 11.9   **FUD** 090   T A2 50 ▢
AMA: 2002,Apr,13

27601   **posterior compartment(s) only**
🖪 12.9   ✄ 12.9   **FUD** 090   T A2 50 ▢
AMA: 2002,Apr,13

27602   **anterior and/or lateral, and posterior compartment(s)**
🖪 14.2   ✄ 14.2   **FUD** 090   T A2 80 50 ▢
AMA: 2002,Apr,13

27603-27612 Incisional Procedures Lower Leg and Ankle

27603   **Incision and drainage, leg or ankle; deep abscess or hematoma**
🖪 11.1   ✄ 15.1   **FUD** 090   T A2 50 ▢
AMA: 2002,Apr,13

27604   **infected bursa**
🖪 9.87   ✄ 14.0   **FUD** 090   T A2 80 50 ▢
AMA: 2002,Apr,13

27605   **Tenotomy, percutaneous, Achilles tendon (separate procedure); local anesthesia**
🖪 5.30   ✄ 9.72   **FUD** 010   T A2 80 50 ▢
AMA: 2002,Apr,13; 1998,Nov,1

27606   **general anesthesia**
🖪 8.22   ✄ 8.22   **FUD** 010   T A2 50 ▢
AMA: 2002,Apr,13

27607   **Incision (eg, osteomyelitis or bone abscess), leg or ankle**
🖪 17.5   ✄ 17.5   **FUD** 090   T A2 50 ▢
AMA: 2002,Apr,13; 1998,Nov,1

27610   **Arthrotomy, ankle, including exploration, drainage, or removal of foreign body**
🖪 18.7   ✄ 18.7   **FUD** 090   T A2 50 ▢
AMA: 2002,Apr,13; 1998,Nov,1

27612   **Arthrotomy, posterior capsular release, ankle, with or without Achilles tendon lengthening**
     EXCLUDES   *Lengthening or shortening tendon (27685)*
🖪 16.2   ✄ 16.2   **FUD** 090   T A2 80 50 ▢
AMA: 2002,Apr,13; 1998,Nov,1

27613-27614 Biopsy Lower Leg and Ankle

     EXCLUDES   *Needle biopsy (20206)*

27613   **Biopsy, soft tissue of leg or ankle area; superficial**
🖪 4.65   ✄ 7.14   **FUD** 010   T P3 50 ▢ P0
AMA: 2002,Apr,13

27614   **deep (subfascial or intramuscular)**
🖪 11.5   ✄ 16.3   **FUD** 090   T A2 50 ▢ P0
AMA: 2002,Apr,13; 1998,Nov,1

27615-27619 [27632, 27634] Excision Soft Tissue Tumors Lower Leg/Ankle

     INCLUDES   Any necessary elevation of tissue planes or dissection
                 Measurement of tumor and necessary margin at greatest diameter prior to excision
                 Resection without removal of significant normal tissue
                 Simple and intermediate repairs
                 Types of excision:
                   Fascial or subfascial soft tissue tumors: simple and marginal resection of most often benign and intramuscular tumors found either in or below the deep fascia, not involving bone
                   Resection of the tumor (may include entire bone) and wide margins of normal tissue primarily for malignant or aggressive benign tumors
                   Subcutaneous: simple and marginal resection of most often benign tumors found in the subcutaneous tissue above the deep fascia
     EXCLUDES   *Complex repair*
                 Excision of benign cutaneous lesions (eg, sebaceous cyst) (11400-11406)
                 Radical resection of cutaneous tumors (eg, melanoma) (11600-11606)
                 Significant exploration of vessels or neuroplasty

27615   **Radical resection of tumor (eg, sarcoma), soft tissue of leg or ankle area; less than 5 cm**
🖪 29.4   ✄ 29.4   **FUD** 090   T 62 80 50 ▢
AMA: 2002,Apr,13; 1990,Win,4

27616	**5 cm or greater**

🔧 36.5   ⚙ 36.5   **FUD** 090   T G2 80 50

27618	**Excision, tumor, soft tissue of leg or ankle area, subcutaneous; less than 3 cm**

🔧 8.83   ⚙ 12.8   **FUD** 090   T G2 50

AMA: 2015,Jan,16; 2014,Jan,11; 2010,Apr,3-4

# 27632	**3 cm or greater**

🔧 11.9   ⚙ 11.9   **FUD** 090   T G2 80 50

27619	**Excision, tumor, soft tissue of leg or ankle area, subfascial (eg, intramuscular); less than 5 cm**

🔧 13.5   ⚙ 13.5   **FUD** 090   T G2 50

AMA: 2002,Apr,13

# 27634	**5 cm or greater**

🔧 19.7   ⚙ 19.7   **FUD** 090   T G2 80 50

27620-27641 Bone and Joint Procedures Ankle/Leg

27620	**Arthrotomy, ankle, with joint exploration, with or without biopsy, with or without removal of loose or foreign body**

🔧 13.1   ⚙ 13.1   **FUD** 090   T A2 80 50 PQ

AMA: 2002,Apr,13

27625	**Arthrotomy, with synovectomy, ankle;**

🔧 16.8   ⚙ 16.8   **FUD** 090   T A2 80 50

AMA: 2002,Apr,13; 1998,Nov,1

27626	**including tenosynovectomy**

🔧 17.7   ⚙ 17.7   **FUD** 090   T A2 80 50

AMA: 2002,Apr,13

27630	**Excision of lesion of tendon sheath or capsule (eg, cyst or ganglion), leg and/or ankle**

🔧 10.4   ⚙ 16.0   **FUD** 090   T A2 50

AMA: 2002,Apr,13

27632	Resequenced code. See code following 27618.
27634	Resequenced code. See code following 27619.

27635	**Excision or curettage of bone cyst or benign tumor, tibia or fibula;**

🔧 16.9   ⚙ 16.9   **FUD** 090   T A2 50

AMA: 2015,Jan,16; 2014,Jan,11; 2012,Apr,17-18

27637	**with autograft (includes obtaining graft)**

🔧 22.0   ⚙ 22.0   **FUD** 090   T A2 80 50

AMA: 2002,Apr,13

27638	**with allograft**

🔧 22.4   ⚙ 22.4   **FUD** 090   T A2 80 50

AMA: 2002,Apr,13

27640	**Partial excision (craterization, saucerization, or diaphysectomy), bone (eg, osteomyelitis); tibia**

EXCLUDES Excision of exostosis (27635)

🔧 24.1   ⚙ 24.1   **FUD** 090   T A2 50

AMA: 2015,Jan,16; 2014,Jan,11; 2012,Apr,17-18

27641	**fibula**

EXCLUDES Excision of exostosis (27635)

🔧 19.2   ⚙ 19.2   **FUD** 090   T A2 50

AMA: 2002,Apr,13

27645-27647 Radical Resection Bone Tumor Ankle/Leg

INCLUDES Any necessary elevation of tissue planes or dissection
Measurement of tumor and necessary margin at greatest diameter prior to excision
Resection of the tumor (may include entire bone) and wide margins of normal tissue primarily for malignant or aggressive benign tumors
Simple and intermediate repairs

EXCLUDES Complex repair
Significant exploration of vessels, neuroplasty, reconstruction, or complex bone repair
Do not report radical excision of soft tissue codes when adjacent soft tissue is removed during the bone tumor resection (27615-27619 [27632, 27634])

27645	**Radical resection of tumor; tibia**

🔧 51.5   ⚙ 51.5   **FUD** 090   C 80 50

AMA: 2002,Apr,13; 1994,Win,1

27646	**fibula**

🔧 44.7   ⚙ 44.7   **FUD** 090   C 80 50

AMA: 2002,Apr,13; 1994,Win,1

27647	**talus or calcaneus**

🔧 29.5   ⚙ 29.5   **FUD** 090   T A2 80 50

AMA: 2002,Apr,13; 1994,Win,1

27648 Injection for Ankle Arthrogram

EXCLUDES   Arthroscopy (29894-29898)

27648	**Injection procedure for ankle arthrography**

🔼 (73615)

🔧 1.50   ⚙ 4.62   **FUD** 000   N N1 80 50

AMA: 2015,Aug,6

27650-27745 Repair/Reconstruction Lower Leg/Ankle

27650	**Repair, primary, open or percutaneous, ruptured Achilles tendon;**

🔧 18.9   ⚙ 18.9   **FUD** 090   T A2 80 50

AMA: 2015,Jan,16; 2014,Jul,5

27652	**with graft (includes obtaining graft)**

🔧 19.7   ⚙ 19.7   **FUD** 090   T A2 50

AMA: 2015,Jan,16; 2014,Jul,5

27654	**Repair, secondary, Achilles tendon, with or without graft**

🔧 20.3   ⚙ 20.3   **FUD** 090   T A2 80 50

AMA: 2015,Jan,16; 2014,Jul,5

27656	**Repair, fascial defect of leg**

🔧 11.4   ⚙ 18.2   **FUD** 090   T A2 80 50

AMA: 2002,Apr,13

27658	**Repair, flexor tendon, leg; primary, without graft, each tendon**

🔧 10.7   ⚙ 10.7   **FUD** 090   T A2 80

AMA: 2002,Apr,13; 1998,Nov,1

27659	**secondary, with or without graft, each tendon**

🔧 13.7   ⚙ 13.7   **FUD** 090   T A2 80

AMA: 2015,Jan,13

27664	**Repair, extensor tendon, leg; primary, without graft, each tendon**

🔧 10.4   ⚙ 10.4   **FUD** 090   T A2 80

AMA: 2015,Jan,13

27665	**secondary, with or without graft, each tendon**

🔧 11.7   ⚙ 11.7   **FUD** 090   T A2 80

AMA: 2002,Apr,13; 1998,Nov,1

27675	**Repair, dislocating peroneal tendons; without fibular osteotomy**

🔧 13.8   ⚙ 13.8   **FUD** 090   T A2 80 50

AMA: 2002,Apr,13; 1998,Nov,1

27676	**with fibular osteotomy**

🔧 17.0   ⚙ 17.0   **FUD** 090   T A2 80 50

AMA: 2002,Apr,13

27680	**Tenolysis, flexor or extensor tendon, leg and/or ankle; single, each tendon**

🔧 12.3   ⚙ 12.3   **FUD** 090   T A2

AMA: 2015,Jan,16; 2014,Jan,11

27681	**multiple tendons (through separate incision[s])**

🔧 15.7   ⚙ 15.7   **FUD** 090   T A2 50

AMA: 2002,Apr,13; 1998,Nov,1

27685	**Lengthening or shortening of tendon, leg or ankle; single tendon (separate procedure)**

🔧 13.3   ⚙ 19.0   **FUD** 090   T A2 80 50

AMA: 2015,Jan,16; 2014,Jan,11; 2012,Jan,15-42; 2011,Jan,11

27686	**multiple tendons (through same incision), each**

🔧 16.2   ⚙ 16.2   **FUD** 090   T A2 50

AMA: 2015,Jan,16; 2014,Jan,11; 2012,Jan,15-42; 2011,Jan,11

27687	**Gastrocnemius recession (eg, Strayer procedure)**

🔧 13.1   ⚙ 13.1   **FUD** 090   T A2 80 50

AMA: 2002,Apr,13

27690 Transfer or transplant of single tendon (with muscle redirection or rerouting); superficial (eg, anterior tibial extensors into midfoot)

INCLUDES Toe extensors considered a single tendon with transplant into midfoot

🔷 18.0 ⚕ 18.0 **FUD** 090 T A2 80 50 ▢

AMA: 2002,Apr,13; 1995,Win,1

27691 deep (eg, anterior tibial or posterior tibial through interosseous space, flexor digitorum longus, flexor hallucis longus, or peroneal tendon to midfoot or hindfoot)

INCLUDES Barr procedure
Toe extensors considered a single tendon with transplant into midfoot

🔷 21.6 ⚕ 21.6 **FUD** 090 T A2 80 50 ▢

AMA: 2002,Apr,13; 1995,Win,1

+ **27692** each additional tendon (List separately in addition to code for primary procedure)

INCLUDES Toe extensors considered a single tendon with transplant into midfoot

Code first (27690-27691)

🔷 3.01 ⚕ 3.01 **FUD** ZZZ N N1 80

AMA: 2003,Feb,7; 2002,Apr,13

27695 Repair, primary, disrupted ligament, ankle; collateral

🔷 13.7 ⚕ 13.7 **FUD** 090 T A2 50 ▢

AMA: 2015,Jan,16; 2014,Mar,13; 2014,Jan,11

Tibia
Fibula
Anterior talofibular
Posterior talofibular
Lateral view of right ankle showing components of the collateral ligament
Calcaneus
Calcaneofibular

27696 both collateral ligaments

🔷 15.8 ⚕ 15.8 **FUD** 090 T A2 50 ▢

AMA: 2015,Jan,16; 2014,Mar,13

27698 Repair, secondary, disrupted ligament, ankle, collateral (eg, Watson-Jones procedure)

🔷 18.3 ⚕ 18.3 **FUD** 090 T A2 80 50 ▢

AMA: 2015,Jan,16; 2014,Mar,13

27700 Arthroplasty, ankle;

🔷 16.7 ⚕ 16.7 **FUD** 090 T A2 80 50 ▢

AMA: 2002,Apr,13

27702 with implant (total ankle)

🔷 27.9 ⚕ 27.9 **FUD** 090 C 80 50 ▢ P0

AMA: 2002,Apr,13

27703 revision, total ankle

🔷 32.0 ⚕ 32.0 **FUD** 090 C 80 50 ▢ P0

AMA: 2002,Apr,13; 1998,Nov,1

27704 Removal of ankle implant

🔷 16.5 ⚕ 16.5 **FUD** 090 02 A2 50 ▢ P0

AMA: 2002,Apr,13

27705 Osteotomy; tibia

EXCLUDES Genu varus or genu valgus repair (27455-27457)

🔷 21.6 ⚕ 21.6 **FUD** 090 T A2 80 50 ▢

AMA: 2002,Apr,13

27707 fibula

EXCLUDES Genu varus or genu valgus repair (27455-27457)

🔷 11.5 ⚕ 11.5 **FUD** 090 T A2 50 ▢

AMA: 2002,Apr,13

27709 tibia and fibula

EXCLUDES Genu varus or genu valgus repair (27455-27457)

🔷 33.8 ⚕ 33.8 **FUD** 090 T A2 80 50 ▢

AMA: 2002,Apr,13

27712 multiple, with realignment on intramedullary rod (eg, Sofield type procedure)

EXCLUDES Genu varus or genu valgus repair (27455-27457)

🔷 31.9 ⚕ 31.9 **FUD** 090 C 80 50 ▢

AMA: 2002,Apr,13; 1998,Nov,1

27715 Osteoplasty, tibia and fibula, lengthening or shortening

INCLUDES Anderson tibial lengthening

🔷 30.3 ⚕ 30.3 **FUD** 090 C 80 50 ▢

AMA: 2002,Apr,13; 1998,Nov,1

27720 Repair of nonunion or malunion, tibia; without graft, (eg, compression technique)

🔷 25.2 ⚕ 25.2 **FUD** 090 T 62 80 50 ▢

AMA: 2002,Apr,13

27722 with sliding graft

🔷 25.7 ⚕ 25.7 **FUD** 090 T 80 50 ▢

AMA: 2002,Apr,13

27724 with iliac or other autograft (includes obtaining graft)

🔷 36.5 ⚕ 36.5 **FUD** 090 C 80 50 ▢

AMA: 2015,Jan,16; 2014,Jan,11; 2012,May,11-12

27725 by synostosis, with fibula, any method

🔷 35.2 ⚕ 35.2 **FUD** 090 C 80 50 ▢

AMA: 2002,Apr,13

27726 Repair of fibula nonunion and/or malunion with internal fixation

Do not report with (27707)

🔷 27.8 ⚕ 27.8 **FUD** 090 T 62 50

AMA: 2015,Jan,16; 2014,Jan,11; 2012,Jan,15-42; 2011,Jan,11

27727 Repair of congenital pseudarthrosis, tibia

🔷 24.5 ⚕ 24.5 **FUD** 090 C 80 50 ▢

AMA: 2002,Apr,13

27730 Arrest, epiphyseal (epiphysiodesis), open; distal tibia

🔷 16.8 ⚕ 16.8 **FUD** 090 T A2 50 ▢

AMA: 2002,Apr,13; 1998,Nov,1

27732 distal fibula

🔷 12.8 ⚕ 12.8 **FUD** 090 T A2 50 ▢

AMA: 2002,Apr,13

27734 distal tibia and fibula

🔷 18.9 ⚕ 18.9 **FUD** 090 T A2 50 ▢

AMA: 2002,Apr,13

27740 Arrest, epiphyseal (epiphysiodesis), any method, combined, proximal and distal tibia and fibula;

EXCLUDES Epiphyseal arrest of proximal tibia and fibula (27477)

🔷 20.4 ⚕ 20.4 **FUD** 090 T A2 80 50 ▢

AMA: 2002,Apr,13; 1998,Nov,1

27742 and distal femur

EXCLUDES Epiphyseal arrest of proximal tibia and fibula (27477)

🔷 22.4 ⚕ 22.4 **FUD** 090 T A2 80 50 ▢

AMA: 2002,Apr,13

27745 Prophylactic treatment (nailing, pinning, plating or wiring) with or without methylmethacrylate, tibia

🔷 21.8 ⚕ 21.8 **FUD** 090 J J8 80 50 ▢

AMA: 2002,Apr,13

27750-27848 Treatment of Fracture/Dislocation Lower Leg/Ankle

INCLUDES Treatment of open or closed fracture or dislocation

27750 Closed treatment of tibial shaft fracture (with or without fibular fracture); without manipulation

🔷 9.09 ⚕ 9.90 **FUD** 090 T A2 50 ▢

AMA: 2015,Jan,16; 2014,Jan,11; 2012,Jan,15-42; 2011,Jan,11

27752 **with manipulation, with or without skeletal traction**
  14.2   15.3   **FUD** 090   T A2 50
  AMA: 2015,Jan,16; 2014,Jan,11

27756 **Percutaneous skeletal fixation of tibial shaft fracture (with or without fibular fracture) (eg, pins or screws)**
  16.6   16.6   **FUD** 090   T A2 80 50 PQ
  AMA: 2015,Jan,16; 2014,Jan,11

27758 **Open treatment of tibial shaft fracture (with or without fibular fracture), with plate/screws, with or without cerclage**
  25.7   25.7   **FUD** 090   T A2 80 50 PQ
  AMA: 2015,Jan,16; 2014,Jan,11; 2012,Jan,15-42; 2011,Jan,11

27759 **Treatment of tibial shaft fracture (with or without fibular fracture) by intramedullary implant, with or without interlocking screws and/or cerclage**
  28.8   28.8   **FUD** 090   T J8 80 50 PQ
  AMA: 2015,Jan,16; 2014,Jan,11

27760 **Closed treatment of medial malleolus fracture; without manipulation**
  8.67   9.51   **FUD** 090   T A2 50
  AMA: 2002,Apr,13; 1994,Sum,29

27762 **with manipulation, with or without skin or skeletal traction**
  12.3   13.5   **FUD** 090   T A2 50
  AMA: 2002,Apr,13; 1994,Sum,29

27766 **Open treatment of medial malleolus fracture, includes internal fixation, when performed**
  17.6   17.6   **FUD** 090   T A2 50 PQ
  AMA: 2002,Apr,13; 1994,Sum,29

27767 **Closed treatment of posterior malleolus fracture; without manipulation**
  8.08   8.04   **FUD** 090   T P2 50
  Do not report with (27808-27823)

27768 **with manipulation**
  12.6   12.6   **FUD** 090   T 62 50
  Do not report with (27808-27823)

27769 **Open treatment of posterior malleolus fracture, includes internal fixation, when performed**
  20.9   20.9   **FUD** 090   T 62 50 PQ
  Do not report with (27808-27823)

27780 **Closed treatment of proximal fibula or shaft fracture; without manipulation**
  7.92   8.72   **FUD** 090   T A2 50
  AMA: 2015,Jan,16; 2014,Jan,11

27781 **with manipulation**
  11.2   12.1   **FUD** 090   T A2 50
  AMA: 2002,Apr,13

27784 **Open treatment of proximal fibula or shaft fracture, includes internal fixation, when performed**
  20.6   20.6   **FUD** 090   T A2 50
  AMA: 2015,Jan,16; 2014,Jan,11; 2012,Jan,15-42; 2011,Jan,11

27786 **Closed treatment of distal fibular fracture (lateral malleolus); without manipulation**
  8.16   9.03   **FUD** 090   T A2 50
  AMA: 2002,Apr,13

27788 **with manipulation**
  11.0   12.0   **FUD** 090   T A2 50
  AMA: 2002,Apr,13

27792 **Open treatment of distal fibular fracture (lateral malleolus), includes internal fixation, when performed**
  EXCLUDES *Repair of tibia and fibula shaft fracture (27750-27759)*
  18.8   18.8   **FUD** 090   T A2 50 PQ
  AMA: 2015,Jan,16; 2014,Jan,11

27808 **Closed treatment of bimalleolar ankle fracture (eg, lateral and medial malleoli, or lateral and posterior malleoli or medial and posterior malleoli); without manipulation**
  8.57   9.53   **FUD** 090   T A2 50
  AMA: 2002,Apr,13

27810 **with manipulation**
  12.1   13.3   **FUD** 090   T A2 50
  AMA: 2002,Apr,13

27814 **Open treatment of bimalleolar ankle fracture (eg, lateral and medial malleoli, or lateral and posterior malleoli, or medial and posterior malleoli), includes internal fixation, when performed**
  22.2   22.2   **FUD** 090   T A2 80 50 PQ
  AMA: 2002,Apr,13

27816 **Closed treatment of trimalleolar ankle fracture; without manipulation**
  8.21   9.16   **FUD** 090   T A2 50
  AMA: 2002,Apr,13

27818 **with manipulation**
  12.4   13.8   **FUD** 090   T A2 50
  AMA: 2002,Apr,13

27822 **Open treatment of trimalleolar ankle fracture, includes internal fixation, when performed, medial and/or lateral malleolus; without fixation of posterior lip**
  24.1   24.1   **FUD** 090   T A2 80 50
  AMA: 2002,Apr,13

27823 **with fixation of posterior lip**
  27.5   27.5   **FUD** 090   T J8 80 50
  AMA: 2002,Apr,13

27824 **Closed treatment of fracture of weight bearing articular portion of distal tibia (eg, pilon or tibial plafond), with or without anesthesia; without manipulation**
  8.66   8.92   **FUD** 090   T A2 50
  AMA: 2002,Apr,13

27825 **with skeletal traction and/or requiring manipulation**
  14.2   15.6   **FUD** 090   T A2 80 50
  AMA: 2002,Apr,13

27826 **Open treatment of fracture of weight bearing articular surface/portion of distal tibia (eg, pilon or tibial plafond), with internal fixation, when performed; of fibula only**
  23.9   23.9   **FUD** 090   T A2 80 50
  AMA: 2002,Apr,13

27827 **of tibia only**
  31.1   31.1   **FUD** 090   T J8 80 50
  AMA: 2002,Apr,13

27828 **of both tibia and fibula**
  37.3   37.3   **FUD** 090   T J8 80 50
  AMA: 2015,Jan,16; 2014,Apr,10

27829 **Open treatment of distal tibiofibular joint (syndesmosis) disruption, includes internal fixation, when performed**
  19.7   19.7   **FUD** 090   T A2 80 50
  AMA: 2015,Jan,16; 2014,Jan,11; 2012,Jan,15-42; 2011,Jan,11

27830 **Closed treatment of proximal tibiofibular joint dislocation; without anesthesia**
  10.0   10.7   **FUD** 090   T A2 80 50
  AMA: 2002,Apr,13

27831 **requiring anesthesia**
  11.4   11.4   **FUD** 090   T A2 80 50
  AMA: 2002,Apr,13

27832 **Open treatment of proximal tibiofibular joint dislocation, includes internal fixation, when performed, or with excision of proximal fibula**
  21.8   21.8   **FUD** 090   T A2 80 50
  AMA: 2002,Apr,13

27840 Closed treatment of ankle dislocation; without anesthesia
🔲 10.5 ⚕ 10.5 **FUD** 090 [T] [A2] [50] 🔳
AMA: 2002,Apr,13

27842 requiring anesthesia, with or without percutaneous skeletal fixation
🔲 14.2 ⚕ 14.2 **FUD** 090 [T] [A2] [50] 🔳
AMA: 2002,Apr,13

27846 Open treatment of ankle dislocation, with or without percutaneous skeletal fixation; without repair or internal fixation
[EXCLUDES] *Arthroscopy (29894-29898)*
🔲 21.1 ⚕ 21.1 **FUD** 090 [T] [A2] [80] [50] 🔳
AMA: 2002,Apr,13

27848 with repair or internal or external fixation
[EXCLUDES] *Arthroscopy (29894-29898)*
🔲 23.4 ⚕ 23.4 **FUD** 090 [T] [A2] [80] [50] 🔳
AMA: 2002,Apr,13

27860 Ankle Manipulation with Anesthesia

27860 Manipulation of ankle under general anesthesia (includes application of traction or other fixation apparatus)
🔲 4.99 ⚕ 4.99 **FUD** 010 [T] [A2] [80] [50] 🔳
AMA: 2002,Apr,13

27870-27871 Arthrodesis Lower Leg/Ankle

27870 Arthrodesis, ankle, open
[EXCLUDES] *Arthroscopic arthrodesis of ankle (29899)*
🔲 29.7 ⚕ 29.7 **FUD** 090 [T] [A2] [80] [50] 🔳
AMA: 2002,Apr,13; 2001,Dec,3

27871 Arthrodesis, tibiofibular joint, proximal or distal
🔲 19.7 ⚕ 19.7 **FUD** 090 [T] [A2] [80] [50] 🔳
AMA: 2002,Apr,13

27880-27889 Amputations of Lower Leg/Ankle

27880 Amputation, leg, through tibia and fibula;
[INCLUDES] *Burgess amputation*
🔲 26.8 ⚕ 26.8 **FUD** 090 [C] [80] [50] 🔳
AMA: 2002,Apr,13

27881 with immediate fitting technique including application of first cast
🔲 25.1 ⚕ 25.1 **FUD** 090 [C] [80] [50] 🔳
AMA: 2002,Apr,13

27882 open, circular (guillotine)
🔲 17.5 ⚕ 17.5 **FUD** 090 [C] [80] [50] 🔳
AMA: 2002,Apr,13

27884 secondary closure or scar revision
🔲 16.7 ⚕ 16.7 **FUD** 090 [T] [A2] [50] 🔳
AMA: 2002,Apr,13

27886 re-amputation
🔲 19.2 ⚕ 19.2 **FUD** 090 [C] [50] 🔳
AMA: 2002,Apr,13

27888 Amputation, ankle, through malleoli of tibia and fibula (eg, Syme, Pirogoff type procedures), with plastic closure and resection of nerves
🔲 19.9 ⚕ 19.9 **FUD** 090 [C] [80] [50] 🔳
AMA: 2002,Apr,13; 1998,Nov,1

27889 Ankle disarticulation
🔲 18.8 ⚕ 18.8 **FUD** 090 [T] [A2] [50] 🔳
AMA: 2002,Apr,13

27892-27899 Decompression Fasciotomy Lower Leg

[EXCLUDES] *Decompression fasciotomy without debridement (27600-27602)*

27892 Decompression fasciotomy, leg; anterior and/or lateral compartments only, with debridement of nonviable muscle and/or nerve
🔲 15.7 ⚕ 15.7 **FUD** 090 [T] [A2] [80] [50] 🔳
AMA: 2002,Apr,13

27893 posterior compartment(s) only, with debridement of nonviable muscle and/or nerve
🔲 17.5 ⚕ 17.5 **FUD** 090 [T] [A2] [80] [50] 🔳
AMA: 2002,Apr,13

27894 anterior and/or lateral, and posterior compartment(s), with debridement of nonviable muscle and/or nerve
🔲 24.9 ⚕ 24.9 **FUD** 090 [T] [A2] [80] [50] 🔳
AMA: 2002,Apr,13

27899 Unlisted procedure, leg or ankle
🔲 0.00 ⚕ 0.00 **FUD** YYY [T] [80] [50]
AMA: 2015,Jan,16; 2014,Jan,11; 2012,Jan,15-42; 2011,Jan,11

28001-28008 Surgical Incision Foot/Toe

[EXCLUDES] *Simple incision and drainage (10060-10160)*

28001 Incision and drainage, bursa, foot
🔲 4.96 ⚕ 8.07 **FUD** 010 [T] [P3] 🔳
AMA: 2002,Apr,13; 1998,Nov,1

28002 Incision and drainage below fascia, with or without tendon sheath involvement, foot; single bursal space
🔲 9.15 ⚕ 12.7 **FUD** 010 [T] [A2] 🔳
AMA: 2002,Apr,13; 1998,Nov,1

28003 multiple areas
🔲 16.2 ⚕ 20.3 **FUD** 090 [T] [A2] 🔳
AMA: 2002,Apr,13; 1998,Nov,1

28005 Incision, bone cortex (eg, osteomyelitis or bone abscess), foot
🔲 16.6 ⚕ 16.6 **FUD** 090 [T] [A2] 🔳
AMA: 2002,Apr,13; 1998,Nov,1

28008 Fasciotomy, foot and/or toe
[EXCLUDES] *Plantar fascia division (28250)*
Plantar fasciectomy (28060, 28062)
🔲 8.45 ⚕ 12.4 **FUD** 090 [T] [A2] [50] 🔳
AMA: 2002,Apr,13

28010-28011 Tenotomy/Toe

[EXCLUDES] *Open tenotomy (28230-28234)*
Simple incision and drainage (10140-10160)

28010 Tenotomy, percutaneous, toe; single tendon
🔲 6.02 ⚕ 6.67 **FUD** 090 [T] [P3] 🔳
AMA: 2002,Apr,13; 1998,Nov,1

28011 multiple tendons
🔲 8.28 ⚕ 9.28 **FUD** 090 [T] [A2] 🔳
AMA: 2002,Apr,13; 1998,Nov,1

28020-28024 Arthrotomy Foot/Toe

[EXCLUDES] *Simple incision and drainage (10140-10160)*

28020 Arthrotomy, including exploration, drainage, or removal of loose or foreign body; intertarsal or tarsometatarsal joint
🔲 10.4 ⚕ 15.7 **FUD** 090 [T] [A2] 🔳
AMA: 2002,Apr,13; 1998,Nov,1

28022 metatarsophalangeal joint
🔲 9.37 ⚕ 14.1 **FUD** 090 [T] [A2] 🔳
AMA: 2002,Apr,13

28024 interphalangeal joint
🔲 8.80 ⚕ 13.3 **FUD** 090 [T] [A2] 🔳
AMA: 2002,Apr,13

28035 Tarsal Tunnel Release

[EXCLUDES] *Other nerve decompression (64722)*
Other neuroplasty (64704)

28035 Release, tarsal tunnel (posterior tibial nerve decompression)
🔲 10.2 ⚕ 15.2 **FUD** 090 [T] [A2] [50] 🔳
AMA: 2002,Apr,13; 1998,Nov,1

[26]/[TC] PC/TC Comp Only   [A2]-[Z3] ASC Pmt   [50] Bilateral   ♂ Male Only   ♀ Female Only   🔲 Facility RVU   ⚕ Non-Facility RVU
AMA: CPT Asst   **CMS:** Pub 100   [A]-[Y] OPPSI   [80]/[80] Surg Assist Allowed / w/Doc   🔳 Lab Crosswalk   🔳 Radiology Crosswalk

84   Medicare (Red Text)   CPT © 2015 American Medical Association. All Rights Reserved. (Black Text)   © 2015 Optum360, LLC (Blue Text)

28039-28047 [28039, 28041] Excision Soft Tissue Tumors Foot/Toe

INCLUDES Any necessary elevation of tissue planes or dissection
Measurement of tumor and necessary margin at greatest diameter prior to excision
Simple and intermediate repairs
Types of excision:
Fascial or subfascial soft tissue tumors: simple and marginal resection of tumors found either in or below the deep fascia, not involving bone or excision of a substantial amount of normal tissue; primarily benign and intramuscular tumors
Tumors of fingers and toes involving joint capsules, tendons and tendon sheaths
Radical resection soft tissue tumor: wide resection of tumor, involving substantial margins of normal tissue and may involve tissue removal from one or more layers; most often malignant or aggressive benign
Tumors of fingers and toes adjacent to joints, tendons and tendon sheaths
Subcutaneous: simple and marginal resection of tumors in the subcutaneous tissue above the deep fascia; most often benign

EXCLUDES Complex repair
Excision of benign cutaneous lesions (eg, sebaceous cyst) (11420-11426)
Radical resection of cutaneous tumors (eg, melanoma) (11620-11626)
Significant exploration of vessels, neuroplasty, or reconstruction

28039 Resequenced code. See code following 28043.

28041 Resequenced code. See code following 28045.

28043 Excision, tumor, soft tissue of foot or toe, subcutaneous; less than 1.5 cm
🔷 7.54   ⚖ 11.5   **FUD** 090   T G2 50
AMA: 2002,Apr,13; 1998,Nov,1

**28039** 1.5 cm or greater
🔷 10.0   ⚖ 14.6   **FUD** 090   T G2 80 50

28045 Excision, tumor, soft tissue of foot or toe, subfascial (eg, intramuscular); less than 1.5 cm
🔷 9.97   ⚖ 14.2   **FUD** 090   T G2 80 50
AMA: 2002,Apr,13

**28041** 1.5 cm or greater
🔷 13.1   ⚖ 13.1   **FUD** 090   T G2 80 50

28046 Radical resection of tumor (eg, sarcoma), soft tissue of foot or toe; less than 3 cm
🔷 21.0   ⚖ 21.0   **FUD** 090   T G2 50
AMA: 2002,Apr,13; 1990,Win,4

28047 3 cm or greater
🔷 31.0   ⚖ 31.0   **FUD** 090   T G2 80 50

28050-28160 Resection Procedures Foot/Toes

28050 Arthrotomy with biopsy; intertarsal or tarsometatarsal joint
🔷 8.89   ⚖ 13.8   **FUD** 090   T A2 50 PQ
AMA: 2002,Apr,13; 1998,Nov,1

28052 metatarsophalangeal joint
🔷 8.00   ⚖ 12.6   **FUD** 090   T A2 50 PQ
AMA: 2002,Apr,13

28054 interphalangeal joint
🔷 6.79   ⚖ 10.8   **FUD** 090   T A2 80 50 PQ
AMA: 2002,Apr,13

28055 Neurectomy, intrinsic musculature of foot
🔷 10.8   ⚖ 10.8   **FUD** 090   T A2 80 50

28060 Fasciectomy, plantar fascia; partial (separate procedure)
EXCLUDES Plantar fasciotomy (28008, 28250)
🔷 10.2   ⚖ 14.9   **FUD** 090   T A2 50
AMA: 2015,Jan,16; 2014,Jan,11; 2012,Jan,15-42; 2011,Jan,11

28062 radical (separate procedure)
EXCLUDES Plantar fasciotomy (28008, 28250)
🔷 11.6   ⚖ 16.8   **FUD** 090   T A2 50
AMA: 2002,Apr,13

28070 Synovectomy; intertarsal or tarsometatarsal joint, each
🔷 10.1   ⚖ 15.2   **FUD** 090   T A2
AMA: 2002,Apr,13

28072 metatarsophalangeal joint, each
🔷 9.69   ⚖ 14.9   **FUD** 090   T A2
AMA: 2002,Apr,13

28080 Excision, interdigital (Morton) neuroma, single, each
🔷 10.5   ⚖ 15.2   **FUD** 090   T A2 80
AMA: 2015,Jan,16; 2014,Jan,11

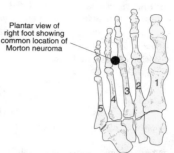

Plantar view of right foot showing common location of Morton neuroma

Morton neuroma is a chronic inflammation or irritation of the nerves in the web space between the heads of the metatarsals and phalanges

28086 Synovectomy, tendon sheath, foot; flexor
🔷 10.4   ⚖ 15.9   **FUD** 090   T A2 80 50
AMA: 2002,Apr,13

28088 extensor
🔷 7.89   ⚖ 12.6   **FUD** 090   T A2 80 50
AMA: 2002,Apr,13

28090 Excision of lesion, tendon, tendon sheath, or capsule (including synovectomy) (eg, cyst or ganglion); foot
🔷 8.87   ⚖ 13.6   **FUD** 090   T A2 50
AMA: 2002,Apr,13; 1998,Nov,1

28092 toe(s), each
🔷 7.72   ⚖ 12.2   **FUD** 090   T A2
AMA: 2002,Apr,13; 1998,Nov,1

28100 Excision or curettage of bone cyst or benign tumor, talus or calcaneus;
🔷 11.9   ⚖ 17.6   **FUD** 090   T A2 80 50
AMA: 2002,Apr,13

28102 with iliac or other autograft (includes obtaining graft)
🔷 17.4   ⚖ 17.4   **FUD** 090   T A2 80 50
AMA: 2002,Apr,13

28103 with allograft
🔷 11.2   ⚖ 11.2   **FUD** 090   T A2 80 50
AMA: 2002,Apr,13

28104 Excision or curettage of bone cyst or benign tumor, tarsal or metatarsal, except talus or calcaneus;
🔷 10.2   ⚖ 15.3   **FUD** 090   T A2 80
AMA: 2002,May,7; 2002,Apr,13

28106 with iliac or other autograft (includes obtaining graft)
🔷 12.3   ⚖ 12.3   **FUD** 090   T A2 80
AMA: 2002,May,7; 2002,Apr,13

28107 with allograft
🔷 10.0   ⚖ 14.9   **FUD** 090   T A2 80
AMA: 2002,May,7; 2002,Apr,13

28108 Excision or curettage of bone cyst or benign tumor, phalanges of foot
EXCLUDES Hallux valgus (28290)
🔷 8.33   ⚖ 12.8   **FUD** 090   T A2
AMA: 2002,Apr,13

28110 Ostectomy, partial excision, fifth metatarsal head (bunionette) (separate procedure)   *Tailor's Bunionectomy*
🔷 8.33   ⚖ 13.4   **FUD** 090   T A2 50
AMA: 2015,Jan,16; 2014,Jan,11; 2012,Jan,15-42; 2011,Jan,11; 2010,Dec,12

28111 Ostectomy, complete excision; first metatarsal head
🔹 9.42 ⚕ 14.3 **FUD** 090   T A2 50 ▣
AMA: 2002,Apr,13

28112 other metatarsal head (second, third or fourth)
🔹 9.03 ⚕ 14.2 **FUD** 090   T A2 50 ▣
AMA: 2002,Apr,13

28113 fifth metatarsal head
🔹 12.3 ⚕ 17.1 **FUD** 090   T A2 80 50 ▣
AMA: 2002,Apr,13

28114 all metatarsal heads, with partial proximal phalangectomy, excluding first metatarsal (eg, Clayton type procedure)
🔹 24.2 ⚕ 31.2 **FUD** 090   T A2 80 50 ▣
AMA: 2002,Apr,13; 1998,Nov,1

28116 Ostectomy, excision of tarsal coalition
🔹 16.4 ⚕ 21.8 **FUD** 090   T A2 50 ▣
AMA: 2002,Apr,13

28118 Ostectomy, calcaneus;
🔹 11.8 ⚕ 17.1 **FUD** 090   T A2 80 50 ▣
AMA: 2015,Jan,13; 2015,Jan,16; 2014,Jan,11; 2012,Jan,15-42; 2011,May,9

28119 for spur, with or without plantar fascial release
🔹 10.3 ⚕ 15.1 **FUD** 090   T A2 50 ▣
AMA: 2015,Jan,16; 2014,Jan,11; 2012,Jan,15-42; 2011,May,9

28120 Partial excision (craterization, saucerization, sequestrectomy, or diaphysectomy) bone (eg, osteomyelitis or bossing); talus or calcaneus
INCLUDES Barker operation
🔹 14.3 ⚕ 19.5 **FUD** 090   T A2 50 ▣
AMA: 2015,Jan,16; 2014,Jan,11; 2012,Jan,15-42; 2011,May,9

28122 tarsal or metatarsal bone, except talus or calcaneus
EXCLUDES Hallux rigidus cheilectomy (28289)
Partial removal of talus or calcaneus (28120)
🔹 12.6 ⚕ 17.3 **FUD** 090   T A2 80 50 ▣
AMA: 2002,Apr,13; 1998,Nov,1

28124 phalanx of toe
🔹 9.48 ⚕ 13.7 **FUD** 090   T P3 50 ▣
AMA: 2002,Apr,13

28126 Resection, partial or complete, phalangeal base, each toe
🔹 7.14 ⚕ 11.4 **FUD** 090   T A2 ▣
AMA: 2015,Mar,9

28130 Talectomy (astragalectomy)
INCLUDES Whitman astragalectomy
EXCLUDES Calcanectomy (28118)
🔹 17.5 ⚕ 17.5 **FUD** 090   T A2 80 50 ▣
AMA: 2002,Apr,13

28140 Metatarsectomy
🔹 12.6 ⚕ 17.2 **FUD** 090   T A2 ▣
AMA: 2002,Apr,13

28150 Phalangectomy, toe, each toe
🔹 8.10 ⚕ 12.3 **FUD** 090   T A2 ▣
AMA: 2002,Apr,13; 1998,Nov,1

28153 Resection, condyle(s), distal end of phalanx, each toe
🔹 7.60 ⚕ 11.9 **FUD** 090   T A2 ▣
AMA: 2015,Jan,16; 2014,Jan,11; 2012,Jan,15-42; 2011,Dec,14-18

28160 Hemiphalangectomy or interphalangeal joint excision, toe, proximal end of phalanx, each
🔹 7.78 ⚕ 12.2 **FUD** 090   T A2 ▣
AMA: 2002,Apr,13; 1998,Nov,1

28171-28175 Radical Resection Bone Tumor Foot/Toes

INCLUDES Any necessary elevation of tissue planes or dissection
Measurement of tumor and necessary margin at greatest diameter prior to excision
Resection of the tumor (may include entire bone) and wide margins of normal tissue primarily for malignant or aggressive benign tumors
Simple and intermediate repairs

EXCLUDES Complex repair
Significant exploration of vessels, neuroplasty, reconstruction, or complex bone repair

Do not report radical excision of soft tissue codes when adjacent soft tissue is removed during the bone tumor resection (28039-28047 [28039, 28041])

28171 Radical resection of tumor; tarsal (except talus or calcaneus)
EXCLUDES Talus or calcaneus resection (27647)
🔹 24.4 ⚕ 24.4 **FUD** 090   T A2 80 ▣
AMA: 2002,Apr,13; 1994,Win,1

28173 metatarsal
EXCLUDES Talus or calcaneus resection (27647)
🔹 21.9 ⚕ 21.9 **FUD** 090   T A2 ▣
AMA: 2002,Apr,13; 1994,Win,1

28175 phalanx of toe
EXCLUDES Talus or calcaneus resection (27647)
🔹 14.0 ⚕ 14.0 **FUD** 090   T A2 ▣
AMA: 2002,Apr,13

28190-28193 Foreign Body Removal: Foot

28190 Removal of foreign body, foot; subcutaneous
🔹 3.85 ⚕ 7.40 **FUD** 010   T P3 50 ▣
AMA: 2015,Jan,16; 2014,Jan,11; 2013,Dec,16

28192 deep
🔹 9.02 ⚕ 13.5 **FUD** 090   T A2 50 ▣ P0
AMA: 2015,Jan,16; 2014,Jan,11; 2013,Dec,16

28193 complicated
🔹 10.6 ⚕ 15.4 **FUD** 090   T A2 50 ▣ P0
AMA: 2002,Apr,13

28200-28360 Repair/Reconstruction of Foot/Toe

INCLUDES Closed, open and percutaneous treatment of fractures and dislocations

28200 Repair, tendon, flexor, foot; primary or secondary, without free graft, each tendon
🔹 9.22 ⚕ 14.1 **FUD** 090   T A2 ▣
AMA: 2015,Jan,16; 2014,Jul,5; 2014,Jan,11; 2012,Jan,15-42; 2011,May,9

28202 secondary with free graft, each tendon (includes obtaining graft)
🔹 12.1 ⚕ 17.1 **FUD** 090   T A2 80 ▣
AMA: 2002,Apr,13

28208 Repair, tendon, extensor, foot; primary or secondary, each tendon
🔹 8.98 ⚕ 13.7 **FUD** 090   T A2 ▣
AMA: 2002,Apr,13; 1998,Nov,1

28210 secondary with free graft, each tendon (includes obtaining graft)
🔹 11.8 ⚕ 16.8 **FUD** 090   T A2 80 ▣
AMA: 2002,Apr,13

28220 Tenolysis, flexor, foot; single tendon
🔹 8.69 ⚕ 13.0 **FUD** 090   T P3 50 ▣
AMA: 2002,Apr,13; 1998,Nov,1

28222 multiple tendons
🔹 9.97 ⚕ 14.5 **FUD** 090   T A2 50 ▣
AMA: 2002,Apr,13; 1998,Nov,1

28225 Tenolysis, extensor, foot; single tendon
🔹 7.42 ⚕ 11.7 **FUD** 090   T A2 50 ▣
AMA: 2002,Apr,13; 1998,Nov,1

28226 multiple tendons
🔹 8.41 ⚕ 12.7 **FUD** 090   T A2 50 ▣
AMA: 2002,Apr,13; 1998,Nov,1

28230 Tenotomy, open, tendon flexor; foot, single or multiple tendon(s) (separate procedure)
8.19 ⚖ 12.6 **FUD** 090 〔T〕〔P3〕〔50〕▭
AMA: 2002,Apr,13; 1998,Nov,1

28232 toe, single tendon (separate procedure)
7.00 ⚖ 11.2 **FUD** 090 〔T〕〔P3〕▭
AMA: 2015,Mar,9

28234 Tenotomy, open, extensor, foot or toe, each tendon
EXCLUDES Tendon transfer (27690-27691)
7.60 ⚖ 11.8 **FUD** 090 〔T〕〔A2〕▭
AMA: 2015,Jan,16; 2014,Jan,11; 2011,Jan,11; 2010,Sep,9

28238 Reconstruction (advancement), posterior tibial tendon with excision of accessory tarsal navicular bone (eg, Kidner type procedure)
EXCLUDES Extensor hallucis longus transfer with big toe fusion (28760)
Jones procedure (28760)
Subcutaneous tenotomy (28010-28011)
Transfer or transplant of tendon with muscle redirection or rerouting (27690-27692)
14.1 ⚖ 19.5 **FUD** 090 〔T〕〔A2〕〔80〕〔50〕▭
AMA: 2002,Apr,13; 2002,May,7

28240 Tenotomy, lengthening, or release, abductor hallucis muscle
8.34 ⚖ 12.7 **FUD** 090 〔T〕〔A2〕〔50〕▭
AMA: 2002,Apr,13

28250 Division of plantar fascia and muscle (eg, Steindler stripping) (separate procedure)
11.6 ⚖ 16.7 **FUD** 090 〔T〕〔A2〕〔80〕〔50〕▭
AMA: 2002,Apr,13; 1998,Nov,1

28260 Capsulotomy, midfoot; medial release only (separate procedure)
14.7 ⚖ 19.8 **FUD** 090 〔T〕〔A2〕〔80〕〔50〕▭
AMA: 2002,Apr,13

28261 with tendon lengthening
22.7 ⚖ 28.8 **FUD** 090 〔T〕〔A2〕〔80〕〔50〕▭
AMA: 2002,Apr,13

28262 extensive, including posterior talotibial capsulotomy and tendon(s) lengthening (eg, resistant clubfoot deformity)
34.2 ⚖ 42.5 **FUD** 090 〔T〕〔A2〕〔80〕〔50〕▭
AMA: 2002,Apr,13; 1998,Nov,1

28264 Capsulotomy, midtarsal (eg, Heyman type procedure)
18.5 ⚖ 24.3 **FUD** 090 〔T〕〔A2〕〔80〕〔50〕▭
AMA: 2002,Apr,13; 1998,Nov,1

28270 Capsulotomy; metatarsophalangeal joint, with or without tenorrhaphy, each joint (separate procedure)
9.60 ⚖ 14.2 **FUD** 090 〔T〕〔A2〕〔50〕▭
AMA: 2015,Jan,16; 2014,Sep,13; 2014,Jan,11; 2012,Jan,15-42; 2011,Sep,11-12; 2011,Jan,11; 2010,Sep,9

28272 interphalangeal joint, each joint (separate procedure)
7.34 ⚖ 11.4 **FUD** 090 〔T〕〔P3〕〔50〕▭
AMA: 2015,Jan,16; 2014,Jan,11; 2012,Jan,15-42; 2011,Jan,11

28280 Syndactylization, toes (eg, webbing or Kelikian type procedure)
9.99 ⚖ 14.8 **FUD** 090 〔T〕〔A2〕〔80〕〔50〕▭
AMA: 2002,Apr,13; 1998,Nov,1

28285 Correction, hammertoe (eg, interphalangeal fusion, partial or total phalangectomy)
10.8 ⚖ 15.4 **FUD** 090 〔T〕〔A2〕〔50〕▭
AMA: 2015,Mar,9; 2015,Jan,16; 2014,Jan,11; 2012,Jan,15-42; 2011,Sep,11-12; 2011,Jan,11; 2010,Sep,9

28286 Correction, cock-up fifth toe, with plastic skin closure (eg, Ruiz-Mora type procedure)
8.57 ⚖ 12.9 **FUD** 090 〔T〕〔A2〕〔50〕▭
AMA: 2002,Apr,13; 1998,Nov,1

28288 Ostectomy, partial, exostectomy or condylectomy, metatarsal head, each metatarsal head
12.3 ⚖ 17.4 **FUD** 090 〔T〕〔A2〕▭
AMA: 2002,Apr,13; 1998,Nov,1

28289 Hallux rigidus correction with cheilectomy, debridement and capsular release of the first metatarsophalangeal joint
15.7 ⚖ 21.1 **FUD** 090 〔T〕〔A2〕〔80〕〔50〕▭
AMA: 2015,Jan,16; 2014,Jan,11; 2011,May,3-5

28290 Correction, hallux valgus (bunion), with or without sesamoidectomy; simple exostectomy (eg, Silver type procedure)
11.4 ⚖ 17.1 **FUD** 090 〔T〕〔A2〕〔50〕▭
AMA: 2015,Jan,16; 2014,Jan,11; 2012,Jan,15-42; 2011,Jan,11

Hallux valgus bunion

Base of proximal phalanx is resected

Kirshner wires stabilize the osteotomy

Keller type approach

Medial eminence of metatarsal bone

A portion of the metatarsal head is resected

Prosthetic implant placed in the joint

Right foot

Correction of hallux valgus bunion by resection of joint

28292 Keller, McBride, or Mayo type procedure
17.3 ⚖ 22.8 **FUD** 090 〔T〕〔A2〕〔80〕〔50〕▭
AMA: 2015,Jan,16; 2014,Jan,11; 2012,Jan,15-42; 2011,Jan,11; 2010,Dec,12

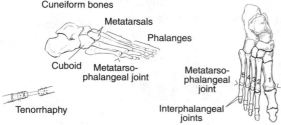

Cuneiform bones

Metatarsals

Phalanges

Cuboid

Metatarso-phalangeal joint

Metatarso-phalangeal joint

Tenorrhaphy

Interphalangeal joints

28293   **resection of joint with implant**
📖 20.4   ✂ 30.1   **FUD** 090   T A2 80 50 ▢ PQ
AMA: 2015,Jan,16; 2014,Jan,11

28294   **with tendon transplants (eg, Joplin type procedure)**
📖 15.5   ✂ 22.0   **FUD** 090   T A2 80 50 ▢
AMA: 2015,Jan,16; 2014,Jan,11

28296   **with metatarsal osteotomy (eg, Mitchell, Chevron, or concentric type procedures)**
📖 15.0   ✂ 20.6   **FUD** 090   T A2 80 50 ▢
AMA: 2015,Jan,16; 2014,Jan,11; 2013,Sep,17; 2012,Jan,15-42; 2011,Jan,11; 2010,Dec,12

28297   **Lapidus-type procedure**
📖 16.7   ✂ 23.4   **FUD** 090   T A2 80 50 ▢
AMA: 2015,Jan,16; 2014,Jan,11

28298   **by phalanx osteotomy**
INCLUDES   Akin procedure
📖 14.5   ✂ 20.7   **FUD** 090   T A2 80 50 ▢
AMA: 2015,Jan,16; 2014,Jan,11; 2013,Oct,18

28299   **by double osteotomy**
📖 19.5   ✂ 25.9   **FUD** 090   T A2 80 50 ▢
AMA: 2015,Jan,16; 2014,Jan,11; 2013,Oct,18; 2013,Sep,17; 2012,Jan,15-42; 2011,Jan,11

Medial eminence of metatarsal bone

Hallux valgus bunion

Kirshner wires stabilize the osteotomies

A portion of the metatarsal head is resected

A wedge of the proximal phalanx is resected

28300   **Osteotomy; calcaneus (eg, Dwyer or Chambers type procedure), with or without internal fixation**
📖 18.8   ✂ 18.8   **FUD** 090   T A2 80 50 ▢
AMA: 2002,Apr,13; 1998,Nov,1

28302   **talus**
📖 20.6   ✂ 20.6   **FUD** 090   T A2 80 50 ▢
AMA: 2002,Apr,13

28304   **Osteotomy, tarsal bones, other than calcaneus or talus;**
📖 17.5   ✂ 23.9   **FUD** 090   T A2 80 50 ▢
AMA: 2002,Apr,13; 1998,Nov,1

28305   **with autograft (includes obtaining graft) (eg, Fowler type)**
📖 18.7   ✂ 18.7   **FUD** 090   T A2 80 50 ▢
AMA: 2002,Apr,13; 1998,Nov,1

28306   **Osteotomy, with or without lengthening, shortening or angular correction, metatarsal; first metatarsal**
📖 11.6   ✂ 17.7   **FUD** 090   T A2 80 50 ▢
AMA: 2015,Jan,16; 2014,Jan,11; 2012,Jan,15-42; 2010,Dec,12

28307   **first metatarsal with autograft (other than first toe)**
📖 13.6   ✂ 20.5   **FUD** 090   T A2 80 50 ▢
AMA: 2002,Apr,13; 1998,Nov,1

28308   **other than first metatarsal, each**
📖 10.8   ✂ 16.3   **FUD** 090   T A2 80 50 ▢
AMA: 2002,Apr,13; 1998,Nov,1

28309   **multiple (eg, Swanson type cavus foot procedure)**
📖 26.2   ✂ 26.2   **FUD** 090   T A2 80 50 ▢
AMA: 2015,Jan,16; 2014,Jan,11

28310   **Osteotomy, shortening, angular or rotational correction; proximal phalanx, first toe (separate procedure)**
📖 10.3   ✂ 15.8   **FUD** 090   T A2 50 ▢
AMA: 2015,Jan,16; 2013,Sep,17

28312   **other phalanges, any toe**
📖 9.32   ✂ 14.9   **FUD** 090   T A2 ▢
AMA: 2002,Apr,13

28313   **Reconstruction, angular deformity of toe, soft tissue procedures only (eg, overlapping second toe, fifth toe, curly toes)**
📖 10.3   ✂ 15.3   **FUD** 090   T A2 ▢
AMA: 2002,Apr,13; 1998,Nov,1

28315   **Sesamoidectomy, first toe (separate procedure)**
📖 9.38   ✂ 13.9   **FUD** 090   T A2 50 ▢
AMA: 2002,Apr,13

28320   **Repair, nonunion or malunion; tarsal bones**
📖 17.5   ✂ 17.5   **FUD** 090   T A2 80 50 ▢
AMA: 2002,Apr,13; 1998,Nov,1

28322   **metatarsal, with or without bone graft (includes obtaining graft)**
📖 16.6   ✂ 22.8   **FUD** 090   T A2 80 ▢
AMA: 2002,Apr,13

28340   **Reconstruction, toe, macrodactyly; soft tissue resection**
📖 11.8   ✂ 16.7   **FUD** 090   T A2 ▢
AMA: 2002,Apr,13

28341   **requiring bone resection**
📖 14.1   ✂ 19.3   **FUD** 090   T A2 ▢
AMA: 2002,Apr,13

28344   **Reconstruction, toe(s); polydactyly**
📖 10.3   ✂ 16.0   **FUD** 090   T A2 50 ▢
AMA: 2002,Apr,13

28345   **syndactyly, with or without skin graft(s), each web**
📖 10.4   ✂ 15.1   **FUD** 090   T A2 80 ▢
AMA: 2002,Apr,13

28360   **Reconstruction, cleft foot**
📖 23.5   ✂ 23.5   **FUD** 090   T 80 50 ▢
AMA: 2002,Apr,13

28400-28675 Treatment of Fracture/Dislocation of Foot/Toe

28400   **Closed treatment of calcaneal fracture; without manipulation**
📖 6.51   ✂ 7.12   **FUD** 090   T A2 50 ▢
AMA: 2002,Apr,13

28405   **with manipulation**
INCLUDES   Bohler reduction
📖 10.3   ✂ 11.4   **FUD** 090   T A2 80 50 ▢
AMA: 2002,Apr,13

28406 Percutaneous skeletal fixation of calcaneal fracture, with manipulation
🔧 15.1   ⚕ 15.1   **FUD** 090   T A2 80 50 ▭ PQ
AMA: 2002,Apr,13

28415 Open treatment of calcaneal fracture, includes internal fixation, when performed;
🔧 31.9   ⚕ 31.9   **FUD** 090   T J8 80 50 ▭ PQ
AMA: 2002,Apr,13

28420 with primary iliac or other autogenous bone graft (includes obtaining graft)
🔧 36.2   ⚕ 36.2   **FUD** 090   T A2 80 50 ▭ PQ
AMA: 2002,Apr,13

28430 Closed treatment of talus fracture; without manipulation
🔧 6.03   ⚕ 6.79   **FUD** 090   T P2 50 ▭
AMA: 2002,Apr,13

28435 with manipulation
🔧 8.32   ⚕ 9.28   **FUD** 090   T A2 80 50 ▭
AMA: 2002,Apr,13

28436 Percutaneous skeletal fixation of talus fracture, with manipulation
🔧 12.9   ⚕ 12.9   **FUD** 090   T A2 50 ▭ PQ
AMA: 2002,Apr,13

28445 Open treatment of talus fracture, includes internal fixation, when performed
🔧 30.8   ⚕ 30.8   **FUD** 090   T A2 80 50 ▭ PQ
AMA: 2002,Apr,13

28446 Open osteochondral autograft, talus (includes obtaining graft[s])
EXCLUDES   *Arthroscopically aided osteochondral talus graft (29892)*
Open osteochondral allograft or repairs with industrial grafts (28899)
Do not report with (27705-27707)
🔧 35.4   ⚕ 35.4   **FUD** 090   T 62 80 50
AMA: 2015,Jan,16; 2014,Jan,11

28450 Treatment of tarsal bone fracture (except talus and calcaneus); without manipulation, each
🔧 5.51   ⚕ 6.18   **FUD** 090   T P2 ▭
AMA: 2015,Jan,16; 2014,Jan,11; 2012,Jan,15-42; 2011,Jan,11

28455 with manipulation, each
🔧 7.43   ⚕ 8.27   **FUD** 090   T P2 80 ▭
AMA: 2002,Apr,13

28456 Percutaneous skeletal fixation of tarsal bone fracture (except talus and calcaneus), with manipulation, each
🔧 9.18   ⚕ 9.18   **FUD** 090   T A2 ▭ PQ
AMA: 2002,Apr,13

28465 Open treatment of tarsal bone fracture (except talus and calcaneus), includes internal fixation, when performed, each
🔧 17.7   ⚕ 17.7   **FUD** 090   T A2 ▭ PQ
AMA: 2002,Apr,13

28470 Closed treatment of metatarsal fracture; without manipulation, each
🔧 5.86   ⚕ 6.28   **FUD** 090   T P2 ▭
AMA: 2002,Apr,13

28475 with manipulation, each
🔧 6.53   ⚕ 7.35   **FUD** 090   T P2 ▭
AMA: 2002,Apr,13

28476 Percutaneous skeletal fixation of metatarsal fracture, with manipulation, each
🔧 10.0   ⚕ 10.0   **FUD** 090   T A2 80 ▭ PQ
AMA: 2002,Apr,13

28485 Open treatment of metatarsal fracture, includes internal fixation, when performed, each
🔧 15.1   ⚕ 15.1   **FUD** 090   T A2 ▭ PQ
AMA: 2002,Apr,13

28490 Closed treatment of fracture great toe, phalanx or phalanges; without manipulation
🔧 3.60   ⚕ 4.18   **FUD** 090   T P2 50 ▭
AMA: 2002,Apr,13

28495 with manipulation
🔧 4.35   ⚕ 5.16   **FUD** 090   T P2 50 ▭
AMA: 2002,Apr,13

28496 Percutaneous skeletal fixation of fracture great toe, phalanx or phalanges, with manipulation
🔧 6.85   ⚕ 12.7   **FUD** 090   T A2 50 ▭
AMA: 2002,Apr,13

28505 Open treatment of fracture, great toe, phalanx or phalanges, includes internal fixation, when performed
🔧 14.5   ⚕ 19.5   **FUD** 090   T A2 50 ▭ PQ
AMA: 2002,Apr,13

28510 Closed treatment of fracture, phalanx or phalanges, other than great toe; without manipulation, each
🔧 3.47   ⚕ 3.56   **FUD** 090   T P3 ▭
AMA: 2002,Apr,13

28515 with manipulation, each
🔧 4.12   ⚕ 4.67   **FUD** 090   T P3 ▭
AMA: 2002,Apr,13

28525 Open treatment of fracture, phalanx or phalanges, other than great toe, includes internal fixation, when performed, each
🔧 11.3   ⚕ 16.1   **FUD** 090   T A2 80 ▭ PQ
AMA: 2002,Apr,13

28530 Closed treatment of sesamoid fracture
🔧 2.94   ⚕ 3.31   **FUD** 090   T P3 80 50 ▭
AMA: 2002,Apr,13

28531 Open treatment of sesamoid fracture, with or without internal fixation
🔧 5.24   ⚕ 9.88   **FUD** 090   T A2 50 ▭ PQ
AMA: 2002,Apr,13

28540 Closed treatment of tarsal bone dislocation, other than talotarsal; without anesthesia
🔧 4.99   ⚕ 5.52   **FUD** 090   T P2 80 50 ▭
AMA: 2002,Apr,13

28545 requiring anesthesia
🔧 7.52   ⚕ 8.50   **FUD** 090   T A2 80 50 ▭
AMA: 2002,Apr,13

28546 Percutaneous skeletal fixation of tarsal bone dislocation, other than talotarsal, with manipulation
🔧 9.77   ⚕ 16.6   **FUD** 090   T A2 80 50 ▭
AMA: 2002,Apr,13

28555 Open treatment of tarsal bone dislocation, includes internal fixation, when performed
🔧 19.3   ⚕ 25.4   **FUD** 090   T A2 80 50 ▭ PQ
AMA: 2002,Apr,13

28570 Closed treatment of talotarsal joint dislocation; without anesthesia
🔧 4.24   ⚕ 4.91   **FUD** 090   T P3 80 50 ▭
AMA: 2002,Apr,13

28575 requiring anesthesia
🔧 9.42   ⚕ 10.4   **FUD** 090   T A2 80 50 ▭
AMA: 2002,Apr,13

28576 Percutaneous skeletal fixation of talotarsal joint dislocation, with manipulation
🔧 11.4   ⚕ 11.4   **FUD** 090   T A2 80 50 ▭
AMA: 2002,Apr,13

28585 Open treatment of talotarsal joint dislocation, includes internal fixation, when performed
🔧 19.2   ⚕ 24.6   **FUD** 090   T A2 80 50 ▭ PQ
AMA: 2015,Jan,16; 2014,Jan,11; 2012,Jan,15-42; 2011,Sep,11-12

28600 Closed treatment of tarsometatarsal joint dislocation; without anesthesia
     5.37   6.22   **FUD** 090   T P2 80
     AMA: 2002,Apr,13

28605 requiring anesthesia
     8.46   9.41   **FUD** 090   T A2 80
     AMA: 2002,Apr,13

28606 Percutaneous skeletal fixation of tarsometatarsal joint dislocation, with manipulation
     11.3   11.3   **FUD** 090   T A2
     AMA: 2002,Apr,13

28615 Open treatment of tarsometatarsal joint dislocation, includes internal fixation, when performed
     22.7   22.7   **FUD** 090   T A2 80 P0
     AMA: 2002,Apr,13

28630 Closed treatment of metatarsophalangeal joint dislocation; without anesthesia
     3.14   4.49   **FUD** 010   T P3 80
     AMA: 2002,Apr,13

28635 requiring anesthesia
     3.72   4.93   **FUD** 010   T A2 80
     AMA: 2002,Apr,13

28636 Percutaneous skeletal fixation of metatarsophalangeal joint dislocation, with manipulation
     6.47   10.1   **FUD** 010   T A2
     AMA: 2002,Apr,13

28645 Open treatment of metatarsophalangeal joint dislocation, includes internal fixation, when performed
     13.9   18.9   **FUD** 090   T A2 P0
     AMA: 2015,Jan,16; 2014,Sep,13

28660 Closed treatment of interphalangeal joint dislocation; without anesthesia
     2.55   3.35   **FUD** 010   T P3
     AMA: 2002,Apr,13

28665 requiring anesthesia
     3.79   4.45   **FUD** 010   S A2 80
     AMA: 2002,Apr,13

28666 Percutaneous skeletal fixation of interphalangeal joint dislocation, with manipulation
     5.53   5.53   **FUD** 010   T A2
     AMA: 2002,Apr,13

28675 Open treatment of interphalangeal joint dislocation, includes internal fixation, when performed
     11.9   17.0   **FUD** 090   T A2 P0
     AMA: 2002,Apr,13

28705-28760 Arthrodesis of Foot/Toe

28705 Arthrodesis; pantalar
     36.2   36.2   **FUD** 090   T A2 80 50 P0
     AMA: 2002,Apr,13

28715 triple
     27.0   27.0   **FUD** 090   J J8 80 50 P0
     AMA: 2002,Apr,13; 1998,Nov,1

28725 subtalar
     INCLUDES   Dunn arthrodesis
               Grice arthrosis
     22.4   22.4   **FUD** 090   T A2 80 50 P0
     AMA: 2015,Jan,16; 2014,Jan,11; 2012,Jan,15-42; 2011,Sep,11-12

28730 Arthrodesis, midtarsal or tarsometatarsal, multiple or transverse;
     INCLUDES   Lambrinudi arthrodesis
     21.0   21.0   **FUD** 090   T A2 80 50 P0
     AMA: 2002,Apr,13

28735 with osteotomy (eg, flatfoot correction)
     22.5   22.5   **FUD** 090   T A2 80 50 P0
     AMA: 2002,Apr,13; 1998,Nov,1

28737 Arthrodesis, with tendon lengthening and advancement, midtarsal, tarsal navicular-cuneiform (eg, Miller type procedure)
     19.9   19.9   **FUD** 090   T A2 80 50 P0
     AMA: 2002,Apr,13; 2002,May,7

28740 Arthrodesis, midtarsal or tarsometatarsal, single joint
     17.9   24.4   **FUD** 090   T A2 80
     AMA: 2015,Jan,16; 2014,Jan,11; 2012,Jan,15-42; 2011,Jan,11; 2010,Jan,11-12

28750 Arthrodesis, great toe; metatarsophalangeal joint
     17.0   23.5   **FUD** 090   T A2 80 50
     AMA: 2015,Jan,16; 2014,Jan,11

28755 interphalangeal joint
     9.49   14.6   **FUD** 090   T A2 50
     AMA: 2002,Apr,13

28760 Arthrodesis, with extensor hallucis longus transfer to first metatarsal neck, great toe, interphalangeal joint (eg, Jones type procedure)
     EXCLUDES   Hammer toe repair or interphalangeal fusion (28285)
     16.6   22.8   **FUD** 090   T A2 80 50
     AMA: 2002,Apr,13; 1998,Nov,1

28800-28825 Amputation Foot/Toe

28800 Amputation, foot; midtarsal (eg, Chopart type procedure)
     15.7   15.7   **FUD** 090   C 80 50
     AMA: 2002,Apr,13; 1998,Nov,1

28805 transmetatarsal
     21.1   21.1   **FUD** 090   T 80 50
     AMA: 2002,Apr,13; 1997,May,4

28810 Amputation, metatarsal, with toe, single
     EXCLUDES   Removal of tuft of distal phalanx (11752)
     12.4   12.4   **FUD** 090   T A2 80
     AMA: 2002,Apr,13

28820 Amputation, toe; metatarsophalangeal joint
     EXCLUDES   Removal of tuft of distal phalanx (11752)
     11.4   16.3   **FUD** 090   T A2
     AMA: 2002,Apr,13; 1997,May,4

28825 interphalangeal joint
     EXCLUDES   Removal of tuft of distal phalanx (11752)
     10.7   15.6   **FUD** 090   T A2
     AMA: 2002,Apr,13

28890-28899 Other/Unlisted Procedures Foot/Toe

28890 Extracorporeal shock wave, high energy, performed by a physician or other qualified health care professional, requiring anesthesia other than local, including ultrasound guidance, involving the plantar fascia
     EXCLUDES   Extracorporeal shock wave therapy of integumentary system not otherwise specified (0299T-0300T)
               Extracorporeal shock wave therapy of musculoskeletal system not otherwise specified (0019T, 0101T, 0102T)
     Do not report with treatment of same area (0299T-0300T)
     6.48   9.33   **FUD** 090   T P3 50
     AMA: 2015,Jan,16; 2014,Jan,11; 2012,Jan,15-42; 2011,Jan,11

28899 Unlisted procedure, foot or toes
     0.00   0.00   **FUD** YYY   T 80
     AMA: 2015,Jan,16; 2014,Jan,11; 2012,Jan,15-42; 2011,Sep,11-12; 2011,Jan,11; 2010,Oct,9

29000-29086 Casting: Arm/Shoulder/Torso

[INCLUDES] Application of cast or strapping when provided as:
An initial service to stabilize the fracture or injury without restorative treatment
A replacement procedure
Removal of cast

[EXCLUDES] *Cast or splint material*
Evaluation and management services provided as part of the initial service when restorative treatment is not provided
Orthotic supervision and training (97760-97762)

Do not report with restorative procedures that include application and removal of the initial cast

29000 Application of halo type body cast (see 20661-20663 for insertion)
5.40 8.72 **FUD** 000 [S] [G2] [80] ⚑
AMA: 2015,Jan,16; 2014,Jan,11

29010 Application of Risser jacket, localizer, body; only
4.06 6.33 **FUD** 000 [S] [P2] [80] ⚑
AMA: 2015,Jan,16; 2014,Jan,11

29015 including head
5.07 7.91 **FUD** 000 [S] [P2] [80] ⚑
AMA: 2015,Jan,16; 2014,Jan,11

29035 Application of body cast, shoulder to hips;
3.84 6.40 **FUD** 000 [S] [P2] [80] ⚑
AMA: 2015,Jan,16; 2014,Jan,11

29040 including head, Minerva type
4.05 6.29 **FUD** 000 [S] [G2] [80] ⚑
AMA: 2015,Jan,16; 2014,Jan,11

29044 including 1 thigh
4.50 7.40 **FUD** 000 [S] [P2] [80] ⚑
AMA: 2015,Jan,16; 2014,Jan,11

29046 including both thighs
4.40 6.78 **FUD** 000 [S] [G2] [80] ⚑
AMA: 2015,Jan,16; 2014,Jan,11

29049 Application, cast; figure-of-eight
1.64 2.10 **FUD** 000 [S] [P3] [80] ⚑
AMA: 2015,Jan,16; 2014,Jan,11

29055 shoulder spica
4.01 6.38 **FUD** 000 [S] [P2] [80] ⚑
AMA: 2015,Jan,16; 2014,Jan,11

29058 plaster Velpeau
2.75 3.58 **FUD** 000 [S] [P3] [80] ⚑
AMA: 2015,Jan,16; 2014,Jan,11

29065 shoulder to hand (long arm)
1.97 2.76 **FUD** 000 [S] [P3] [50] ⚑
AMA: 2015,Jan,16; 2014,Jan,11

29075 elbow to finger (short arm)
1.80 2.49 **FUD** 000 [S] [P3] [50] ⚑
AMA: 2015,Jan,16; 2014,Jan,11

29085 hand and lower forearm (gauntlet)
1.95 2.74 **FUD** 000 [S] [P3] [50] ⚑
AMA: 2015,Jan,16; 2014,Jan,11; 2012,Jan,15-42; 2011,Jan,11

29086 finger (eg, contracture)
1.44 2.21 **FUD** 000 [S] [P3] [50] ⚑
AMA: 2015,Jan,16; 2014,Jan,11

29105-29280 Splinting and Strapping: Torso/Upper Extremities

[INCLUDES] Application of splint or strapping when provided as:
An initial service to stabilize the fracture or dislocation
A replacement procedure

[EXCLUDES] *Evaluation and management services provided as part of the initial service when restorative treatment is not provided*
Orthotic supervision and training (97760-97762)
Splinting and strapping material

Do not report with restorative procedures that included application and removal of the initial splint or strap

29105 Application of long arm splint (shoulder to hand)
1.72 2.53 **FUD** 000 [S] [P3] [50] ⚑
AMA: 2015,Jan,16; 2014,Jan,11; 2012,Jan,15-42; 2011,Jan,11

29125 Application of short arm splint (forearm to hand); static
1.12 1.83 **FUD** 000 [Q1] [N1] [50] ⚑
AMA: 2015,Jan,16; 2014,Jan,11

29126 dynamic
1.40 2.21 **FUD** 000 [Q1] [N1] [50] ⚑
AMA: 2015,Jan,16; 2014,Jan,11

29130 Application of finger splint; static
0.81 1.16 **FUD** 000 [Q1] [N1] [50] ⚑
AMA: 2015,Jan,16; 2014,Jan,11

29131 dynamic
0.95 1.46 **FUD** 000 [Q1] [N1] [50] ⚑
AMA: 2015,Jan,16; 2014,Jan,11

29200 Strapping; thorax
[EXCLUDES] *Strapping of low back (29799)*
0.52 0.85 **FUD** 000 [S] [P3] ⚑
AMA: 2015,Jan,16; 2014,Jan,11

29240 shoulder (eg, Velpeau)
0.53 0.82 **FUD** 000 [Q1] [N1] [50] ⚑
AMA: 2015,Jan,16; 2014,Jan,11; 2011,Jan,11; 2010,Jun,8

29260 elbow or wrist
0.55 0.82 **FUD** 000 [Q1] [N1] [50] ⚑
AMA: 2015,Jan,16; 2014,Jan,11

29280 hand or finger
0.56 0.83 **FUD** 000 [Q1] [N1] [50] ⚑
AMA: 2015,Jan,16; 2014,Jan,11

29305-29450 Casting: Legs

[INCLUDES] Application of cast when provided as:
An initial service to stabilize the fracture or injury without restorative treatment
A replacement procedure
Removal of cast

[EXCLUDES] *Cast or splint materials*
Evaluation and management services provided as part of the initial service when restorative treatment is not provided
Orthotic supervision and training (97760-97762)

Do not report with restorative procedures that include application and removal of the initial cast

29305 Application of hip spica cast; 1 leg
[EXCLUDES] *Hip spica cast thighs only (29046)*
4.62 7.10 **FUD** 000 [S] [P2] [80] ⚑
AMA: 2015,Jan,16; 2014,Jan,11

29325 1 and one-half spica or both legs
[EXCLUDES] *Hip spica cast thighs only (29046)*
5.18 7.86 **FUD** 000 [S] [P2] [80] ⚑
AMA: 2015,Jan,16; 2014,Jan,11

29345 Application of long leg cast (thigh to toes);
2.92 3.92 **FUD** 000 [S] [P3] [50] ⚑
AMA: 2015,Jan,16; 2014,Jan,11; 2011,Sep,11-12

29355 walker or ambulatory type
3.07 4.04 **FUD** 000 [S] [P3] [50] ⚑
AMA: 2015,Jan,16; 2014,Jan,11; 2011,Sep,11-12

29358 Application of long leg cast brace
3.01 4.62 **FUD** 000 [S] [P3] [50] ⚑
AMA: 2015,Jan,16; 2014,Jan,11; 2011,Sep,11-12

29365 Application of cylinder cast (thigh to ankle)
2.52 3.52 **FUD** 000 [S] [P3] [50] ⚑
AMA: 2015,Jan,16; 2014,Jan,11; 2011,Sep,11-12

29405 Application of short leg cast (below knee to toes);
1.73 2.34 **FUD** 000 [S] [P3] [50] ⚑
AMA: 2015,Jan,16; 2014,Jan,11; 2011,Sep,11-12

29425 walking or ambulatory type
1.63 2.24 **FUD** 000 [S] [P3] [50] ⚑
AMA: 2015,Jan,16; 2014,Jan,11; 2011,Sep,11-12

29435 **Application of patellar tendon bearing (PTB) cast**
  🖫 2.41   ⚖ 3.39   **FUD** 000   S P3 50 ▢
  AMA: 2015,Jan,16; 2014,Jan,11; 2011,Sep,11-12

29440 **Adding walker to previously applied cast**
  🖫 0.83   ⚖ 1.25   **FUD** 000   S P3 50 ▢
  AMA: 2015,Jan,16; 2014,Jan,11

29445 **Application of rigid total contact leg cast**
  🖫 3.02   ⚖ 3.89   **FUD** 000   S P3 50 ▢
  AMA: 2015,Jan,16; 2014,Jan,11; 2012,Jan,15-42; 2011,Sep,11-12

29450 **Application of clubfoot cast with molding or manipulation, long or short leg**
  🖫 3.24   ⚖ 4.12   **FUD** 000   S P3 50 ▢
  AMA: 2015,Jan,16; 2014,Jan,11

29505-29584 Splinting and Strapping Ankle/Foot/Leg/Toes

INCLUDES   Application of splinting and strapping when provided as:
       An initial service to stabilize the fracture or injury without restorative treatment
       A replacement procedure
EXCLUDES   *Evaluation and management services provided as part of the initial service when restorative treatment is not provided*
       Orthotic supervision and training (97760-97762)
Do not report with restorative procedures that include application and removal of the initial cast

29505 **Application of long leg splint (thigh to ankle or toes)**
  🖫 1.43   ⚖ 2.38   **FUD** 000   S P3 50 ▢
  AMA: 2015,Jan,16; 2014,Jan,11; 2012,Jan,15-42; 2011,Jan,11

29515 **Application of short leg splint (calf to foot)**
  🖫 1.42   ⚖ 2.05   **FUD** 000   S P3 50 ▢
  AMA: 2015,Jan,16; 2014,Jan,11

29520 **Strapping; hip**
  🖫 0.53   ⚖ 0.88   **FUD** 000   01 N1 80 50 ▢
  AMA: 2015,Jan,16; 2014,Jan,11

29530 **knee**
  🖫 0.52   ⚖ 0.80   **FUD** 000   01 N1 50 ▢
  AMA: 2015,Jan,16; 2014,Jan,11; 2010,Aug,12; 2010,Aug,12

29540 **ankle and/or foot**
  Do not report with (29581, 29582)
  🖫 0.51   ⚖ 0.73   **FUD** 000   S P3 50 ▢
  AMA: 2015,Jan,16; 2014,Mar,4; 2014,Jan,11; 2012,Oct,14; 2012,Sep,16; 2012,Jan,15-42; 2011,Jan,11; 2010,Aug,12; 2010,Aug,12; 2010,Jun,8

29550 **toes**
  🖫 0.33   ⚖ 0.54   **FUD** 000   01 N1 50 ▢
  AMA: 2015,Jan,16; 2014,Jan,11

29580 **Unna boot**
  Do not report with (29581-29582)
  🖫 1.01   ⚖ 1.49   **FUD** 000   S P3 50 ▢ P0
  AMA: 2015,Jan,16; 2014,Mar,4; 2014,Jan,11; 2012,Oct,14; 2012,Sep,16; 2012,Jan,15-42; 2011,Jan,11

29581 **Application of multi-layer compression system; leg (below knee), including ankle and foot**
  Do not report with (29540, 29580, 29582, 36475-36476, 36478-36479)
  🖫 0.38   ⚖ 1.77   **FUD** 000   S P3 80 50 ▢ P0
  AMA: 2015,Mar,9; 2015,Jan,16; 2014,Oct,6; 2014,Mar,4; 2014,Jan,11; 2013,Sep,17; 2012,Oct,14; 2012,Sep,16; 2011,May,3-5

29582 **thigh and leg, including ankle and foot, when performed**
  Do not report with (29540, 29580-29581, 36475-36476, 36478-36479)
  🖫 0.47   ⚖ 2.01   **FUD** 000   S P3 80 50
  AMA: 2015,Mar,9; 2015,Jan,16; 2014,Oct,6; 2014,Mar,4

29583 **upper arm and forearm**
  Do not report with (29584)
  🖫 0.34   ⚖ 1.26   **FUD** 000   S P3 80 50
  AMA: 2015,Mar,9

29584 **upper arm, forearm, hand, and fingers**
  Do not report with (29583)
  🖫 0.47   ⚖ 2.01   **FUD** 000   S P3 80 50
  AMA: 2015,Mar,9

29700-29799 Casting Services Other Than Application

INCLUDES   Casts applied by treating individual
Do not report removal of casts applied by treating individual

29700 **Removal or bivalving; gauntlet, boot or body cast**
  🖫 0.96   ⚖ 1.75   **FUD** 000   S P3 ▢
  AMA: 2015,Jan,16; 2014,Jan,11

29705 **full arm or full leg cast**
  🖫 1.37   ⚖ 1.93   **FUD** 000   S P3 50 ▢
  AMA: 2015,Jan,16; 2014,Jan,11

29710 **shoulder or hip spica, Minerva, or Risser jacket, etc.**
  🖫 2.44   ⚖ 3.57   **FUD** 000   S P3 80 50 ▢
  AMA: 2015,Jan,16; 2014,Jan,11

29720 **Repair of spica, body cast or jacket**
  🖫 1.29   ⚖ 2.45   **FUD** 000   S P3 ▢
  AMA: 2015,Jan,16; 2014,Jan,11

29730 **Windowing of cast**
  🖫 1.28   ⚖ 1.83   **FUD** 000   S P3 ▢
  AMA: 2015,Jan,16; 2014,Jan,11

29740 **Wedging of cast (except clubfoot casts)**
  🖫 2.04   ⚖ 2.86   **FUD** 000   S P3 ▢
  AMA: 2015,Jan,16; 2014,Jan,11

29750 **Wedging of clubfoot cast**
  🖫 2.11   ⚖ 2.74   **FUD** 000   S P3 80 50 ▢
  AMA: 2015,Jan,16; 2014,Jan,11

29799 **Unlisted procedure, casting or strapping**
  🖫 0.00   ⚖ 0.00   **FUD** YYY   S 80
  AMA: 2015,Jan,16; 2014,Jan,11; 2012,Oct,14; 2012,Sep,16

29800-29999 [29914, 29915, 29916] Arthroscopic Procedures

INCLUDES   Diagnostic arthroscopy with surgical arthroscopy
Code also modifier 51 if arthroscopy is performed with arthrotomy

29800 **Arthroscopy, temporomandibular joint, diagnostic, with or without synovial biopsy (separate procedure)**
  🖫 14.9   ⚖ 14.9   **FUD** 090   T A2 80 50
  AMA: 2015,Jan,16; 2013,May,12

29804 **Arthroscopy, temporomandibular joint, surgical**
  EXCLUDES   *Open surgery (21010)*
  🖫 18.4   ⚖ 18.4   **FUD** 090   T A2 80 50 ▢
  AMA: 2015,Jan,16; 2013,May,12

29805 **Arthroscopy, shoulder, diagnostic, with or without synovial biopsy (separate procedure)**
  EXCLUDES   *Open surgery (23065-23066, 23100-23101)*
  🖫 13.6   ⚖ 13.6   **FUD** 090   T A2 50 ▢
  AMA: 2015,Jun,10; 2015,Jan,16; 2013,May,12

29806 **Arthroscopy, shoulder, surgical; capsulorrhaphy**
  EXCLUDES   *Open surgery (23450-23466)*
          Thermal capsulorrhaphy (29999)
  🖫 30.6   ⚖ 30.6   **FUD** 090   T A2 50 ▢
  AMA: 2015,Jul,10; 2015,Mar,7; 2015,Jan,16; 2013,May,12

29807 **repair of SLAP lesion**
  🖫 29.9   ⚖ 29.9   **FUD** 090   T A2 50 ▢
  AMA: 2015,Mar,7; 2015,Jan,16; 2013,May,12

29819 **with removal of loose body or foreign body**
  EXCLUDES   *Open surgery (23040-23044, 23107)*
  🖫 16.9   ⚖ 16.9   **FUD** 090   T A2 50 ▢
  AMA: 2015,Mar,7; 2015,Jan,16; 2013,May,12

29820 **synovectomy, partial**
  EXCLUDES   *Open surgery (23105)*
  🖫 15.3   ⚖ 15.3   **FUD** 090   T A2 80 50 ▢
  AMA: 2015,Mar,7; 2015,Jan,16; 2013,Jun,13; 2013,May,12

29821 synovectomy, complete

EXCLUDES   Open surgery (23105)

🗐 16.7   ⚕ 16.7   **FUD** 090   T A2 80 50 ▭

AMA: 2015,Mar,7; 2015,Jan,16; 2013,Jun,13; 2013,May,12

29822 debridement, limited

EXCLUDES   Open surgery (see specific shoulder section)

🗐 16.2   ⚕ 16.2   **FUD** 090   T A2 80 50 ▭

AMA: 2015,Mar,7; 2015,Jan,16; 2014,Jan,11; 2013,May,12;
2012,Oct,14; 2012,Sep,16; 2012,Apr,17-18

29823 debridement, extensive

EXCLUDES   Open surgery (see specific shoulder section)

🗐 17.7   ⚕ 17.7   **FUD** 090   T A2 80 50 ▭

AMA: 2015,Mar,7; 2015,Jan,16; 2014,Jan,11; 2013,May,12;
2012,Oct,14; 2012,Sep,16; 2012,Apr,17-18

29824 distal claviculectomy including distal articular surface
(Mumford procedure)

INCLUDES   Mumford procedure

EXCLUDES   Open surgery (23120)

🗐 19.1   ⚕ 19.1   **FUD** 090   T A2 80 50 ▭

AMA: 2015,Mar,7; 2015,Jan,16; 2013,May,12

29825 with lysis and resection of adhesions, with or without
manipulation

EXCLUDES   Open surgery (see specific shoulder section)

🗐 16.6   ⚕ 16.6   **FUD** 090   T A2 80 50 ▭

AMA: 2015,Mar,7; 2015,Jan,16; 2013,May,12

+ 29826 decompression of subacromial space with partial
acromioplasty, with coracoacromial ligament (ie, arch)
release, when performed (List separately in addition to
code for primary procedure)

EXCLUDES   Open surgery (23130, 23415)

Code also modifier 51 when performed arthroscopically during
the same session (29824, 29826)
Code first (29806-29825, 29827-29828)

🗐 5.10   ⚕ 5.10   **FUD** ZZZ   N N1 80 50 ▭

AMA: 2015,Mar,7; 2015,Jan,16; 2014,Jan,11; 2013,May,12;
2012,Oct,14; 2012,Sep,16

29827 with rotator cuff repair

EXCLUDES   Distal clavicle excision (29824)
Open surgery or mini open repair (23412)
Subacromial decompression (29826)

🗐 30.3   ⚕ 30.3   **FUD** 090   T A2 80 50 ▭

AMA: 2015,Mar,7; 2015,Jan,16; 2014,Jan,11; 2013,May,12;
2012,Jan,15-42; 2011,Jan,11

29828 biceps tenodesis

EXCLUDES   Tenodesis of long tendon of biceps (23430)

Do not report with (29805, 29820, 29822)

🗐 26.1   ⚕ 26.1   **FUD** 090   T 62 80 50

AMA: 2015,Mar,7; 2015,Jan,16; 2014,Jan,11; 2013,May,12;
2012,Jan,15-42; 2011,Jan,11

29830 Arthroscopy, elbow, diagnostic, with or without synovial
biopsy (separate procedure)

🗐 13.1   ⚕ 13.1   **FUD** 090   T A2 50 ▭

AMA: 2015,Jan,16; 2013,May,12

29834 Arthroscopy, elbow, surgical; with removal of loose body or
foreign body

🗐 13.9   ⚕ 13.9   **FUD** 090   T A2 80 50 ▭

AMA: 2015,Jan,16; 2013,May,12

29835 synovectomy, partial

🗐 14.5   ⚕ 14.5   **FUD** 090   T A2 80 50 ▭

AMA: 2015,Jan,16; 2013,May,12

29836 synovectomy, complete

🗐 16.6   ⚕ 16.6   **FUD** 090   T A2 80 50 ▭

AMA: 2015,Jan,16; 2013,May,12

29837 debridement, limited

🗐 15.0   ⚕ 15.0   **FUD** 090   T A2 80 50 ▭

AMA: 2015,Jan,16; 2013,May,12

29838 debridement, extensive

🗐 16.8   ⚕ 16.8   **FUD** 090   T A2 80 50 ▭

AMA: 2015,Jan,16; 2013,May,12

29840 Arthroscopy, wrist, diagnostic, with or without synovial
biopsy (separate procedure)

🗐 13.0   ⚕ 13.0   **FUD** 090   T A2 80 50 ▭

AMA: 2015,Jan,16; 2013,May,12

29843 Arthroscopy, wrist, surgical; for infection, lavage and
drainage

🗐 13.9   ⚕ 13.9   **FUD** 090   T A2 80 50 ▭

AMA: 2015,Jan,16; 2013,May,12

29844 synovectomy, partial

🗐 14.1   ⚕ 14.1   **FUD** 090   T A2 80 50 ▭

AMA: 2015,Jan,16; 2013,May,12

29845 synovectomy, complete

🗐 16.5   ⚕ 16.5   **FUD** 090   T A2 80 50 ▭

AMA: 2015,Jan,16; 2014,Jan,11; 2013,May,12; 2012,Jan,15-42;
2011,Jan,11

29846 excision and/or repair of triangular fibrocartilage and/or
joint debridement

🗐 14.9   ⚕ 14.9   **FUD** 090   T A2 80 50 ▭

AMA: 2015,Jan,16; 2014,Jan,11; 2013,May,12; 2012,Jan,15-42;
2011,Jan,11

29847 internal fixation for fracture or instability

🗐 15.6   ⚕ 15.6   **FUD** 090   T A2 80 50 ▭

AMA: 2015,Jan,16; 2013,May,12

29848 Endoscopy, wrist, surgical, with release of transverse carpal
ligament

EXCLUDES   Open surgery (64721)

🗐 14.6   ⚕ 14.6   **FUD** 090   T A2 50 ▭

AMA: 2015,Jul,10; 2015,Jan,16; 2014,Jan,11; 2013,May,12

29850 Arthroscopically aided treatment of intercondylar spine(s)
and/or tuberosity fracture(s) of the knee, with or without
manipulation; without internal or external fixation (includes
arthroscopy)

🗐 18.0   ⚕ 18.0   **FUD** 090   T A2 80 50 ▭

AMA: 2015,Jan,16; 2013,May,12

29851 with internal or external fixation (includes arthroscopy)

EXCLUDES   Bone graft (20900, 20902)

🗐 26.9   ⚕ 26.9   **FUD** 090   T A2 80 50 ▭

AMA: 2015,Jan,16; 2013,May,12

29855 Arthroscopically aided treatment of tibial fracture, proximal
(plateau); unicondylar, includes internal fixation, when
performed (includes arthroscopy)

🗐 22.6   ⚕ 22.6   **FUD** 090   T A2 80 50 ▭

AMA: 2015,Jan,16; 2013,May,12

29856 bicondylar, includes internal fixation, when performed
(includes arthroscopy)

EXCLUDES   Bone graft (20900, 20902)

🗐 28.8   ⚕ 28.8   **FUD** 090   T A2 80 50 ▭

AMA: 2015,Jan,16; 2013,May,12

29860 Arthroscopy, hip, diagnostic with or without synovial biopsy
(separate procedure)

🗐 19.2   ⚕ 19.2   **FUD** 090   T A2 80 50 ▭

AMA: 2015,Jan,16; 2014,Jan,11; 2013,May,12; 2011,Sep,5-7

29861 Arthroscopy, hip, surgical; with removal of loose body or
foreign body

🗐 20.6   ⚕ 20.6   **FUD** 090   T A2 80 50 ▭

AMA: 2015,Jan,16; 2014,Jan,11; 2013,May,12; 2011,Sep,5-7

29862 with debridement/shaving of articular cartilage
(chondroplasty), abrasion arthroplasty, and/or resection
of labrum

🗐 23.1   ⚕ 23.1   **FUD** 090   T A2 80 50 ▭

AMA: 2015,Jan,16; 2014,Jan,11; 2013,May,12; 2011,Sep,5-7

● New Code   ▲ Revised Code   ○ Reinstated   M Maternity   A Age Edit   Unlisted   Not Covered   # Resequenced
⊘ AMA Mod 51 Exempt   ⑨ Optum Mod 51 Exempt   ⓑ Mod 63 Exempt   ⊙ Mod Sedation   + Add-on   ▭ CCI   P0 PQRS   FUD Follow-up Days

© 2015 Optum360, LLC (Blue Text)   CPT © 2015 American Medical Association. All Rights Reserved. (Black Text)   Medicare (Red Text)   93

29863 with synovectomy
🔪 23.1 ✂ 23.1 **FUD** 090 T A2 80 50 ▣
AMA: 2015,Jan,16; 2014,Jan,11; 2013,May,12; 2011,Sep,5-7

\# **29914** with femoroplasty (ie, treatment of cam lesion)
Do not report with (29862-29863)
🔪 28.5 ✂ 28.5 **FUD** 090 T 62 80 50 ▣
AMA: 2015,Jan,16; 2014,Jan,11; 2012,Jan,15-42; 2011,Sep,5-7

\# **29915** with acetabuloplasty (ie, treatment of pincer lesion)
🔪 29.0 ✂ 29.0 **FUD** 090 T 62 80 50 ▣
AMA: 2015,Jan,16; 2014,Jan,11; 2012,Jan,15-42; 2011,Sep,5-7

\# **29916** with labral repair
EXCLUDES Labral repair secondary to acetabuloplasty
Do not report with (29862-29863, [29915])
🔪 29.1 ✂ 29.1 **FUD** 090 T 62 80 50 ▣
AMA: 2015,Jan,16; 2014,Jan,11; 2012,Jan,15-42; 2011,Sep,5-7

29866 Arthroscopy, knee, surgical; osteochondral autograft(s) (eg, mosaicplasty) (includes harvesting of the autograft[s])
EXCLUDES Open osteochondral autograft of the knee (27416)
Do not report with procedure performed at the same surgical session (29870, 29871, 29875, 29884)
Do not report with procedure performed in the same compartment (29874, 29877, 29879, 29885-29887)
🔪 30.3 ✂ 30.3 **FUD** 090 T 62 80 50 ▣
AMA: 2015,Jan,16; 2013,May,12

Cylindrical plugs of healthy bone are harvested, usually from a non-weight bearing area of the femur

The technique employs arthroscopy

Recipient holes are drilled and the grafts tamped into position

29867 osteochondral allograft (eg, mosaicplasty)
Do not report with procedures performed at the same surgical session (27415, 27570, 29870-29871, 29875, 29884)
Do not report with procedures performed in the same compartment (29874, 29877, 29879, 29885-29887)
🔪 37.0 ✂ 37.0 **FUD** 090 T 80 50 ▣
AMA: 2015,Jan,16; 2014,Jan,11; 2013,May,12; 2012,Jan,15-42

29868 meniscal transplantation (includes arthrotomy for meniscal insertion), medial or lateral
Do not report with procedures performed at same surgical session (29870-29871, 29875, 29880, 29883-29884)
Do not report with procedure performed in same compartment (29874, 29877, 29881-29882)
🔪 48.4 ✂ 48.4 **FUD** 090 T 80 50 ▣
AMA: 2015,Jan,16; 2013,May,12

29870 Arthroscopy, knee, diagnostic, with or without synovial biopsy (separate procedure)
EXCLUDES Open procedure (27412)
🔪 11.8 ✂ 16.7 **FUD** 090 T A2 50 ▣
AMA: 2015,Jan,16; 2014,Jan,11; 2013,May,12; 2012,Jan,15-42; 2011,Mar,9; 2011,Jan,11

29871 Arthroscopy, knee, surgical; for infection, lavage and drainage
EXCLUDES Osteochondral graft (27412, 27415, 29866-29867)
Do not report with (27370)
🔪 14.8 ✂ 14.8 **FUD** 090 T A2 50 ▣
AMA: 2015,Aug,6; 2015,Jan,16; 2014,Jan,11; 2013,May,12

29873 with lateral release
EXCLUDES Open procedure (27425)
🔪 15.1 ✂ 15.1 **FUD** 090 T A2 50 ▣
AMA: 2015,Jan,16; 2014,Jan,11; 2013,May,12; 2012,Jan,15-42; 2011,Jan,11

29874 for removal of loose body or foreign body (eg, osteochondritis dissecans fragmentation, chondral fragmentation)
🔪 15.4 ✂ 15.4 **FUD** 090 T A2 80 50 ▣
AMA: 2015,Jan,16; 2014,Jan,11; 2013,May,12

29875 synovectomy, limited (eg, plica or shelf resection) (separate procedure)
🔪 14.2 ✂ 14.2 **FUD** 090 T A2 80 50 ▣
AMA: 2015,Jan,16; 2014,May,10; 2014,Jan,11; 2013,May,12

29876 synovectomy, major, 2 or more compartments (eg, medial or lateral)
🔪 18.9 ✂ 18.9 **FUD** 090 T A2 50 ▣
AMA: 2015,Jan,16; 2014,Jan,11; 2013,May,12

29877 debridement/shaving of articular cartilage (chondroplasty)
Do not report when arthroscopic meniscectomy is also performed (29880-29881)
🔪 17.9 ✂ 17.9 **FUD** 090 T A2 80 50 ▣
AMA: 2015,Jan,16; 2014,Jan,11; 2013,May,12; 2012,Jan,15-42; 2011,Jan,11

29879 abrasion arthroplasty (includes chondroplasty where necessary) or multiple drilling or microfracture
🔪 19.1 ✂ 19.1 **FUD** 090 T A2 80 50 ▣
AMA: 2015,Jan,16; 2014,Jan,11; 2013,May,12

29880 with meniscectomy (medial AND lateral, including any meniscal shaving) including debridement/shaving of articular cartilage (chondroplasty), same or separate compartment(s), when performed
🔪 16.2 ✂ 16.2 **FUD** 090 T A2 80 50 ▣
AMA: 2015,Jan,16; 2014,Jan,11; 2013,May,12; 2012,Jan,3-5

29881 with meniscectomy (medial OR lateral, including any meniscal shaving) including debridement/shaving of articular cartilage (chondroplasty), same or separate compartment(s), when performed
🔪 15.5 ✂ 15.5 **FUD** 090 T A2 80 50 ▣
AMA: 2015,Jan,16; 2014,May,10; 2014,Jan,11; 2013,May,12; 2012,Jan,3-5; 2012,Jan,15-42; 2011,Jan,11

29882 with meniscus repair (medial OR lateral)
EXCLUDES Meniscus transplant (29868)
🔪 20.2 ✂ 20.2 **FUD** 090 T A2 50 ▣
AMA: 2015,Jan,16; 2014,Jan,11; 2013,May,12; 2012,Jan,15-42; 2011,Dec,14-18; 2011,Jan,11

29883 with meniscus repair (medial AND lateral)
EXCLUDES Meniscus transplant (29868)
🔪 24.3 ✂ 24.3 **FUD** 090 T A2 80 50 ▣
AMA: 2015,Jan,16; 2014,Jan,11; 2013,May,12; 2012,Jan,15-42; 2011,Dec,14-18; 2011,Jan,11

29884 with lysis of adhesions, with or without manipulation (separate procedure)
🔪 17.6 ✂ 17.6 **FUD** 090 T A2 80 50 ▣
AMA: 2015,Jan,16; 2014,Jan,11; 2013,May,12; 2012,Jan,15-42; 2011,Mar,9

29885 drilling for osteochondritis dissecans with bone grafting, with or without internal fixation (including debridement of base of lesion)
🔪 21.7 ✂ 21.7 **FUD** 090 T A2 80 50 ▣
AMA: 2015,Jan,16; 2014,Jan,11; 2013,May,12

29886 drilling for intact osteochondritis dissecans lesion
🔪 18.3 ✂ 18.3 **FUD** 090 T A2 50 ▣
AMA: 2015,Jan,16; 2014,Jan,11; 2013,May,12

| 26/TC PC/TC Comp Only | A2-Z4 ASC Pmt | 50 Bilateral | ♂ Male Only | ♀ Female Only | 🔪 Facility RVU | ✂ Non-Facility RVU |
| AMA: CPT Asst | CMS: Pub 100 | A-Y OPPSI | 80/80 Surg Assist Allowed / w/Doc | | ▣ Lab Crosswalk | ▣ Radiology Crosswalk |

94   Medicare (Red Text)   CPT © 2015 American Medical Association. All Rights Reserved. (Black Text)   © 2015 Optum360, LLC (Blue Text)

29887	drilling for intact osteochondritis dissecans lesion with internal fixation

🦴 21.5   ✂ 21.5   **FUD** 090   T A2 80 50 ▭

AMA: 2015,Jan,16; 2014,Jan,11; 2013,May,12

29888   Arthroscopically aided anterior cruciate ligament repair/augmentation or reconstruction

Do not report with ligamentous reconstruction (27427-27429)

🦴 28.4   ✂ 28.4   **FUD** 090   T A2 80 50 ▭

AMA: 2015,Jan,16; 2014,Jan,11; 2013,May,12; 2012,Jan,15-42; 2011,Jan,11

29889   Arthroscopically aided posterior cruciate ligament repair/augmentation or reconstruction

Do not report with ligamentous reconstruction (27427-27429)

🦴 35.3   ✂ 35.3   **FUD** 090   T A2 80 50 ▭

AMA: 2015,Jan,16; 2014,Jan,11; 2013,May,12; 2012,Jan,15-42; 2011,Jan,11

29891   Arthroscopy, ankle, surgical, excision of osteochondral defect of talus and/or tibia, including drilling of the defect

🦴 19.5   ✂ 19.5   **FUD** 090   T A2 80 50 ▭

AMA: 2015,Jan,16; 2013,May,12

29892   Arthroscopically aided repair of large osteochondritis dissecans lesion, talar dome fracture, or tibial plafond fracture, with or without internal fixation (includes arthroscopy)

🦴 18.0   ✂ 18.0   **FUD** 090   T A2 80 50 ▭

AMA: 2015,Jan,16; 2014,Jan,11; 2013,May,12

29893   Endoscopic plantar fasciotomy

🦴 12.3   ✂ 17.6   **FUD** 090   T A2 50 ▭

AMA: 2015,Jan,16; 2013,May,12

29894   Arthroscopy, ankle (tibiotalar and fibulotalar joints), surgical; with removal of loose body or foreign body

🦴 14.4   ✂ 14.4   **FUD** 090   T A2 80 50 ▭

AMA: 2015,Jan,16; 2013,May,12

29895   synovectomy, partial

🦴 13.9   ✂ 13.9   **FUD** 090   T A2 80 50 ▭

AMA: 2015,Jan,16; 2014,Jan,11; 2013,May,12; 2012,Jan,15-42

29897   debridement, limited

🦴 14.6   ✂ 14.6   **FUD** 090   T A2 80 50 ▭

AMA: 2015,Jan,16; 2013,May,12

29898   debridement, extensive

🦴 16.3   ✂ 16.3   **FUD** 090   T A2 80 50 ▭

AMA: 2015,Jan,16; 2013,May,12

29899   with ankle arthrodesis

EXCLUDES   Open procedure (27870)

🦴 30.1   ✂ 30.1   **FUD** 090   T A2 80 50 ▭

AMA: 2015,Jan,16; 2013,May,12

29900   Arthroscopy, metacarpophalangeal joint, diagnostic, includes synovial biopsy

Do not report with (29901-29902)

🦴 12.0   ✂ 12.0   **FUD** 090   T A2 80 50 ▭

AMA: 2015,Jan,16; 2013,May,12

29901   Arthroscopy, metacarpophalangeal joint, surgical; with debridement

🦴 15.0   ✂ 15.0   **FUD** 090   T A2 80 50 ▭

AMA: 2015,Jan,16; 2013,May,12

29902   with reduction of displaced ulnar collateral ligament (eg, Stenar lesion)

🦴 13.9   ✂ 13.9   **FUD** 090   T A2 80 50 ▭

AMA: 2015,Jan,16; 2013,May,12

29904   Arthroscopy, subtalar joint, surgical; with removal of loose body or foreign body

🦴 18.4   ✂ 18.4   **FUD** 090   T 62 80 50

AMA: 2015,Jan,16; 2013,May,12

29905   with synovectomy

🦴 18.7   ✂ 18.7   **FUD** 090   T 62 80 50

AMA: 2015,Jan,16; 2013,May,12

29906   with debridement

🦴 20.4   ✂ 20.4   **FUD** 090   T 62 80 50

AMA: 2015,Jan,16; 2013,May,12

29907   with subtalar arthrodesis

🦴 25.3   ✂ 25.3   **FUD** 090   T 62 80 50

AMA: 2015,Jan,16; 2013,May,12

29914   **Resequenced code. See code following 29863.**

29915   **Resequenced code. See code following 29863.**

29916   **Resequenced code. See code before 29866.**

29999   Unlisted procedure, arthroscopy

🦴 0.00   ✂ 0.00   **FUD** YYY   T 80 50 ▭

AMA: 2015,Jan,16; 2014,Jan,11; 2013,May,12; 2012,Apr,17-18; 2012,Jan,15-42; 2011,Dec,14-18; 2011,Jan,11

30000-30115 I&D, Biopsy, Excision Procedures of the Nose

30000   **Drainage abscess or hematoma, nasal, internal approach**

EXCLUDES   *Incision and drainage (10060, 10140)*

🚑 3.39   ⚕ 6.56   **FUD** 010   T P2 80

AMA: 2005,May,13-14; 1994,Spr,24

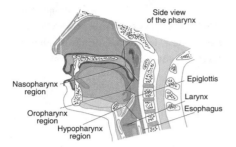

Side view of the pharynx

The nasopharynx is the membranous passage above the level of the soft palate; the oropharynx is the region between the soft palate and the upper edge of the epiglottis; the hypopharynx is the region of the epiglottis to the juncture of the larynx and esophagus; the three regions are collectively known as the pharynx

30020   **Drainage abscess or hematoma, nasal septum**

🚑 3.42   ⚕ 6.64   **FUD** 010   T P3

EXCLUDES   *Lateral rhinotomy incision (30118, 30320)*

30100   **Biopsy, intranasal**

🚑 1.99   ⚕ 4.04   **FUD** 000   T P3 P0

EXCLUDES   *Superficial biopsy of nose (11100-11101)*

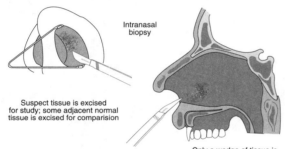

Intranasal biopsy

Suspect tissue is excised for study; some adjacent normal tissue is excised for comparision

Only a wedge of tissue is removed for larger lesions

30110   **Excision, nasal polyp(s), simple**

🚑 3.75   ⚕ 6.58   **FUD** 010   T P3 50

30115   **Excision, nasal polyp(s), extensive**

🚑 12.3   ⚕ 12.3   **FUD** 090   T A2 50

30117-30118 Destruction Procedures Nose

CMS: 100-3,140.5 Laser Procedures

30117   **Excision or destruction (eg, laser), intranasal lesion; internal approach**

🚑 9.72   ⚕ 24.9   **FUD** 090   T A2

AMA: 1990,Win,4

30118   **external approach (lateral rhinotomy)**

🚑 21.8   ⚕ 21.8   **FUD** 090   T A2

30120-30140 Excision Procedures Nose, Turbinate

30120   **Excision or surgical planing of skin of nose for rhinophyma**

🚑 12.4   ⚕ 14.7   **FUD** 090   T A2

AMA: 2015,Jan,16; 2014,Jan,11; 2012,Jan,15-42; 2011,Jan,11

30124   **Excision dermoid cyst, nose; simple, skin, subcutaneous**

🚑 8.13   ⚕ 8.13   **FUD** 090   T R2

30125   **complex, under bone or cartilage**

🚑 17.3   ⚕ 17.3   **FUD** 090   T A2 80

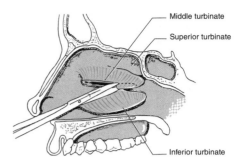

Middle turbinate
Superior turbinate
Inferior turbinate

30130   **Excision inferior turbinate, partial or complete, any method**

EXCLUDES   *Excision middle/superior turbinate(s) (30999)*

Do not report with (30801, 30802, 30930)

🚑 10.8   ⚕ 10.8   **FUD** 090   T A2 50

AMA: 2015,Jan,16; 2014,Jan,11; 2012,Jan,15-42; 2011,Jan,11

30140   **Submucous resection inferior turbinate, partial or complete, any method**

EXCLUDES   *Endoscopic resection of concha bullosa of middle turbinate (31240)*
Submucous resection:
Nasal septum (30520)
Superior or middle turbinate (30999)

Do not report with (30801, 30802, 30930)

🚑 12.5   ⚕ 12.5   **FUD** 090   T A2 50

AMA: 2015,Jan,16; 2014,Jan,11; 2012,Jan,15-42; 2011,Jan,11

30150-30160 Surgical Removal: Nose

EXCLUDES   *Reconstruction and/or closure (primary or delayed primary intention) (13151-13160, 14060-14302, 15120-15121, 15260-15261, 15760, 20900-20912)*

30150   **Rhinectomy; partial**

🚑 21.9   ⚕ 21.9   **FUD** 090   T A2

30160   **total**

🚑 22.0   ⚕ 22.0   **FUD** 090   T A2 80

30200-30320 Turbinate Injection, Removal Foreign Substance in the Nose

30200   **Injection into turbinate(s), therapeutic**

🚑 1.71   ⚕ 3.24   **FUD** 000   T P3

AMA: 2015,Jan,16; 2014,Jan,11; 2012,Jan,15-42; 2011,Jan,11

30210   **Displacement therapy (Proetz type)**

🚑 2.85   ⚕ 4.29   **FUD** 010   T P3

AMA: 2015,Jan,16; 2014,Jan,11; 2012,Jan,15-42; 2011,Jan,11

30220   **Insertion, nasal septal prosthesis (button)**

🚑 3.58   ⚕ 8.62   **FUD** 010   T A2

30300   **Removal foreign body, intranasal; office type procedure**

🚑 3.61   ⚕ 6.57   **FUD** 010   Q1 N1

AMA: 2015,Jan,16; 2014,Jan,11; 2012,Jan,13-14

30310   **requiring general anesthesia**

🚑 5.85   ⚕ 5.85   **FUD** 010   T A2 80

30320   **by lateral rhinotomy**

🚑 12.9   ⚕ 12.9   **FUD** 090   T A2 80

30400-30630 Reconstruction or Repair of Nose

EXCLUDES *Bone/tissue grafts (20900-20926, 21210)*

30400 Rhinoplasty, primary; lateral and alar cartilages and/or elevation of nasal tip

🚗 28.6   ✂ 28.6   **FUD** 090   T A2 80 ▭

INCLUDES Carpue's operation

EXCLUDES *Reconstruction of columella (13151-13153)*

30410 complete, external parts including bony pyramid, lateral and alar cartilages, and/or elevation of nasal tip

🚗 33.6   ✂ 33.6   **FUD** 090   T A2 80 ▭

30420 including major septal repair

🚗 39.1   ✂ 39.1   **FUD** 090   T A2 ▭

30430 Rhinoplasty, secondary; minor revision (small amount of nasal tip work)

🚗 24.6   ✂ 24.6   **FUD** 090   T A2 80 ▭

30435 intermediate revision (bony work with osteotomies)

🚗 35.5   ✂ 35.5   **FUD** 090   T A2 80 ▭

30450 major revision (nasal tip work and osteotomies)

🚗 42.6   ✂ 42.6   **FUD** 090   T A2 80 ▭

30460 Rhinoplasty for nasal deformity secondary to congenital cleft lip and/or palate, including columellar lengthening; tip only

🚗 23.2   ✂ 23.2   **FUD** 090   T A2 80 ▭

AMA: 2015,Jan,16; 2014,Dec,18

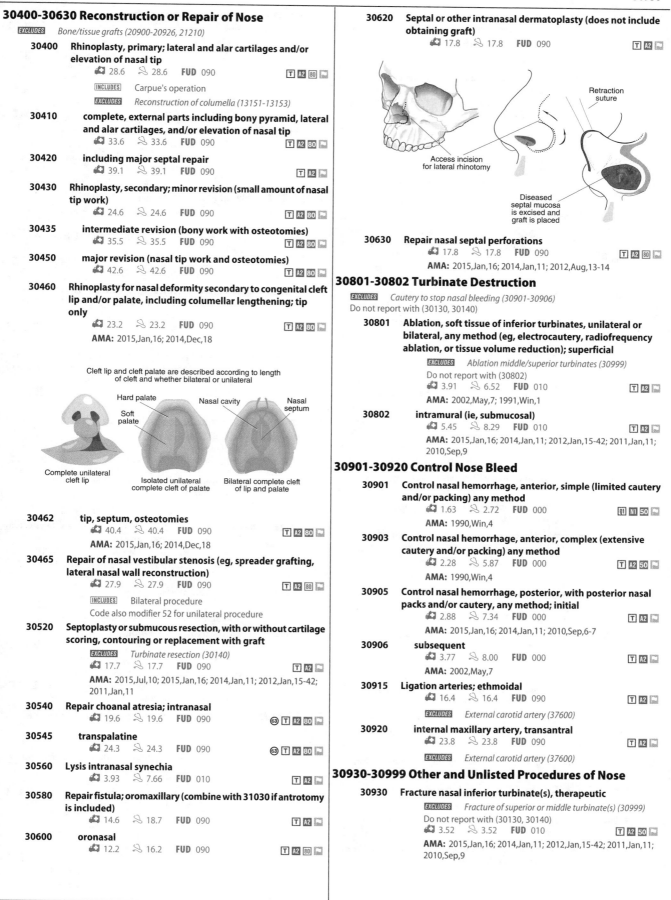

Cleft lip and cleft palate are described according to length of cleft and whether bilateral or unilateral

Hard palate

Nasal cavity

Nasal septum

Soft palate

Complete unilateral cleft lip

Isolated unilateral complete cleft of palate

Bilateral complete cleft of lip and palate

30462 tip, septum, osteotomies

🚗 40.4   ✂ 40.4   **FUD** 090   T A2 80 ▭

AMA: 2015,Jan,16; 2014,Dec,18

30465 Repair of nasal vestibular stenosis (eg, spreader grafting, lateral nasal wall reconstruction)

🚗 27.9   ✂ 27.9   **FUD** 090   T A2 80 ▭

INCLUDES Bilateral procedure

Code also modifier 52 for unilateral procedure

30520 Septoplasty or submucous resection, with or without cartilage scoring, contouring or replacement with graft

EXCLUDES *Turbinate resection (30140)*

🚗 17.7   ✂ 17.7   **FUD** 090   T A2 ▭

AMA: 2015,Jul,10; 2015,Jan,16; 2014,Jan,11; 2012,Jan,15-42; 2011,Jan,11

30540 Repair choanal atresia; intranasal

🚗 19.6   ✂ 19.6   **FUD** 090   63 T A2 80 ▭

30545 transpalatine

🚗 24.3   ✂ 24.3   **FUD** 090   63 T A2 80 ▭

30560 Lysis intranasal synechia

🚗 3.93   ✂ 7.66   **FUD** 010   T A2 ▭

30580 Repair fistula; oromaxillary (combine with 31030 if antrotomy is included)

🚗 14.6   ✂ 18.7   **FUD** 090   T A2 ▭

30600 oronasal

🚗 12.2   ✂ 16.2   **FUD** 090   T A2 80 ▭

30620 Septal or other intranasal dermatoplasty (does not include obtaining graft)

🚗 17.8   ✂ 17.8   **FUD** 090   T A2 ▭

Retraction suture

Access incision for lateral rhinotomy

Diseased septal mucosa is excised and graft is placed

30630 Repair nasal septal perforations

🚗 17.8   ✂ 17.8   **FUD** 090   T A2 80 ▭

AMA: 2015,Jan,16; 2014,Jan,11; 2012,Aug,13-14

30801-30802 Turbinate Destruction

EXCLUDES *Cautery to stop nasal bleeding (30901-30906)*

Do not report with (30130, 30140)

30801 Ablation, soft tissue of inferior turbinates, unilateral or bilateral, any method (eg, electrocautery, radiofrequency ablation, or tissue volume reduction); superficial

EXCLUDES *Ablation middle/superior turbinates (30999)*

Do not report with (30802)

🚗 3.91   ✂ 6.52   **FUD** 010   T A2 ▭

AMA: 2002,May,7; 1991,Win,1

30802 intramural (ie, submucosal)

🚗 5.45   ✂ 8.29   **FUD** 010   T A2 ▭

AMA: 2015,Jan,16; 2014,Jan,11; 2012,Jan,15-42; 2011,Jan,11; 2010,Sep,9

30901-30920 Control Nose Bleed

30901 Control nasal hemorrhage, anterior, simple (limited cautery and/or packing) any method

🚗 1.63   ✂ 2.72   **FUD** 000   01 M1 50 ▭

AMA: 1990,Win,4

30903 Control nasal hemorrhage, anterior, complex (extensive cautery and/or packing) any method

🚗 2.28   ✂ 5.87   **FUD** 000   T A2 50 ▭

AMA: 1990,Win,4

30905 Control nasal hemorrhage, posterior, with posterior nasal packs and/or cautery, any method; initial

🚗 2.88   ✂ 7.34   **FUD** 000   T A2 ▭

AMA: 2015,Jan,16; 2014,Jan,11; 2010,Sep,6-7

30906 subsequent

🚗 3.77   ✂ 8.00   **FUD** 000   T A2 ▭

AMA: 2002,May,7

30915 Ligation arteries; ethmoidal

🚗 16.4   ✂ 16.4   **FUD** 090   T A2 ▭

EXCLUDES *External carotid artery (37600)*

30920 internal maxillary artery, transantral

🚗 23.8   ✂ 23.8   **FUD** 090   T A2 ▭

EXCLUDES *External carotid artery (37600)*

30930-30999 Other and Unlisted Procedures of Nose

30930 Fracture nasal inferior turbinate(s), therapeutic

EXCLUDES *Fracture of superior or middle turbinate(s) (30999)*

Do not report with (30130, 30140)

🚗 3.52   ✂ 3.52   **FUD** 010   T A2 50 ▭

AMA: 2015,Jan,16; 2014,Jan,11; 2012,Jan,15-42; 2011,Jan,11; 2010,Sep,9

Respiratory System

30999 — 31254

30999 Unlisted procedure, nose
    0.00   0.00   **FUD** YYY   T 80
    AMA: 2015,Jan,16; 2013,Feb,13

31000-31230 Opening Sinuses

31000 Lavage by cannulation; maxillary sinus (antrum puncture or natural ostium)
    3.04   5.24   **FUD** 010   T P3 50
    AMA: 2015,Jan,16; 2014,Apr,10

Frontal sinus
Crista galli
Ethmoidal cells
Orbital cavity
Superior, middle, and inferior conchae
Maxillary sinus
Caldwell-Luc approach

Frontal sinus
Posterior ethmoidal cells
Sphenoid sinus
Nostril
Conchae (nasal cavity)
Hard palate
Schematic showing lateral wall of the nasal cavity (above) and coronal section showing nasal and paranasal sinuses (left)

31002 sphenoid sinus
    5.51   5.51   **FUD** 010   T R2 80 50

31020 Sinusotomy, maxillary (antrotomy); intranasal
    10.3   13.8   **FUD** 090   T A2 50

31030 radical (Caldwell-Luc) without removal of antrochoanal polyps
    15.1   19.7   **FUD** 090   T A2 50

31032 radical (Caldwell-Luc) with removal of antrochoanal polyps
    16.4   16.4   **FUD** 090   T A2 50

31040 Pterygomaxillary fossa surgery, any approach
    21.9   21.9   **FUD** 090   T R2 50
    EXCLUDES Transantral ligation internal maxillary artery (30920)

31050 Sinusotomy, sphenoid, with or without biopsy;
    13.8   13.8   **FUD** 090   T A2 50 P0

31051 with mucosal stripping or removal of polyp(s)
    18.3   18.3   **FUD** 090   T A2 50 P0

31070 Sinusotomy frontal; external, simple (trephine operation)
    12.5   12.5   **FUD** 090   T A2 50
    INCLUDES Killian operation
    EXCLUDES Intranasal frontal sinusotomy (31276)

31075 transorbital, unilateral (for mucocele or osteoma, Lynch type)
    22.2   22.2   **FUD** 090   T A2 80 50

31080 obliterative without osteoplastic flap, brow incision (includes ablation)
    29.3   29.3   **FUD** 090   T A2 80 50
    INCLUDES Ridell sinusotomy

31081 obliterative, without osteoplastic flap, coronal incision (includes ablation)
    43.6   43.6   **FUD** 090   T A2 80 50

31084 obliterative, with osteoplastic flap, brow incision
    32.8   32.8   **FUD** 090   T A2 80 50

31085 obliterative, with osteoplastic flap, coronal incision
    41.9   41.9   **FUD** 090   T A2 80 50

31086 nonobliterative, with osteoplastic flap, brow incision
    31.9   31.9   **FUD** 090   T A2 80 50

31087 nonobliterative, with osteoplastic flap, coronal incision
    30.8   30.8   **FUD** 090   T A2 80 50

31090 Sinusotomy, unilateral, 3 or more paranasal sinuses (frontal, maxillary, ethmoid, sphenoid)
    29.1   29.1   **FUD** 090   T A2 50
    AMA: 1998,Nov,1; 1997,Nov,1

31200 Ethmoidectomy; intranasal, anterior
    16.1   16.1   **FUD** 090   T A2 50

31201 intranasal, total
    21.1   21.1   **FUD** 090   T A2 50

31205 extranasal, total
    25.4   25.4   **FUD** 090   T A2 80 50

31225 Maxillectomy; without orbital exenteration
    53.6   53.6   **FUD** 090   C 80 50

31230 with orbital exenteration (en bloc)
    59.3   59.3   **FUD** 090   C 80 50
    EXCLUDES Orbital exenteration without maxillectomy (65110-65114)
                Skin grafts (15120-15121)

31231-31235 Nasal Endoscopy, Diagnostic

INCLUDES Complete sinus exam (e.g., nasal cavity, turbinates, sphenoethmoidal recess)

31231 Nasal endoscopy, diagnostic, unilateral or bilateral (separate procedure)
    1.88   5.97   **FUD** 000   T P2
    AMA: 2015,Jan,16; 2014,Jan,11

31233 Nasal/sinus endoscopy, diagnostic with maxillary sinusoscopy (via inferior meatus or canine fossa puncture)
    Do not report for same sinus with (31295)
    3.94   7.49   **FUD** 000   T A2 80 50
    AMA: 2015,Jan,16; 2014,Jan,11; 2011,Jun,11-12

31235 Nasal/sinus endoscopy, diagnostic with sphenoid sinusoscopy (via puncture of sphenoidal face or cannulation of ostium)
    Do not report for same sinus with (31297)
    4.66   8.53   **FUD** 000   T A2 80 50
    AMA: 2015,Jan,16; 2014,Jan,11; 2011,Jun,11-12

31237-31240 Nasal Endoscopy, Surgical

INCLUDES Diagnostic nasal/sinus endoscopy
          Unilateral procedure
EXCLUDES Frontal sinus exploration (31276)
          Maxillary antrostomy (31256)
          Osteomeatal complex (OMC) resection and/or partial (anterior) ethmoidectomy (31254)
          Removal of maxillary sinus tissue (31267)
          Total (anterior and posterior) ethmoidectomy (31255)

31237 Nasal/sinus endoscopy, surgical; with biopsy, polypectomy or debridement (separate procedure)
    4.64   7.37   **FUD** 000   T A2 50 P0
    AMA: 2015,Jan,13; 2015,Jan,16; 2014,Jan,11; 2012,Jan,15-42; 2011,Dec,13; 2011,Jun,11-12; 2011,Jan,11

31238 with control of nasal hemorrhage
    4.87   7.36   **FUD** 000   T A2 80 50
    AMA: 2015,Jan,16; 2014,Jan,11; 2011,Jun,11-12

31239 with dacryocystorhinostomy
    17.5   17.5   **FUD** 010   T A2 80 50
    AMA: 2015,Jan,16; 2014,Jan,11; 2011,Jun,11-12

31240 with concha bullosa resection
    4.63   4.63   **FUD** 000   T A2 80 50
    AMA: 2015,Jan,16; 2014,Jan,11; 2011,Jun,11-12

31254-31255 Nasal Endoscopy with Ethmoid Removal

INCLUDES Diagnostic nasal/sinus endoscopy
          Sinusotomy, when applicable

31254 Nasal/sinus endoscopy, surgical; with ethmoidectomy, partial (anterior)
    Code also any combination of the following endoscopic procedures when performed in conjunction with partial (anterior) ethmoidectomy and/or osteomeatal complex (OMC) resection, regardless of whether polyps are removed:
       Antrostomy, with or without removal of maxillary sinus tissue; either (31256, 31267)
       Frontal sinus exploration (31276)
    7.87   7.87   **FUD** 000   T A2 50
    AMA: 2015,Jan,16; 2014,Jan,11; 2012,Jan,15-42; 2011,Jun,11-12; 2011,Jan,11

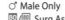

26/TC PC/TC Comp Only   A2-Z3 ASC Pmt   50 Bilateral   ♂ Male Only   ♀ Female Only   Facility RVU   Non-Facility RVU
AMA: CPT Asst   CMS: Pub 100   A-Y OPPSI   80/80 Surg Assist Allowed / w/Doc   Lab Crosswalk   Radiology Crosswalk

98   Medicare (Red Text)   CPT © 2015 American Medical Association. All Rights Reserved. (Black Text)   © 2015 Optum360, LLC (Blue Text)

31255   **with ethmoidectomy, total (anterior and posterior)**

Code also any combination of the following endoscopic procedures when performed in conjunction with total (anterior and posterior) ethmoidectomy, regardless of whether polyps are removed:

Antrostomy, with or without removal of maxillary sinus tissue; either (31256, 31267)

Frontal sinus exploration (31276)

Sphenoidotomy, with or without removal of tissue; either (31287, 31288)

🖭 11.5   ⚖ 11.5   **FUD** 000   T A2 50 ▢

AMA: 2015,Jan,16; 2014,Jan,11; 2012,Jan,15-42; 2011,Jun,11-12; 2011,Jan,11

31256-31267 Nasal Endoscopy with Maxillary Procedures

INCLUDES   Diagnostic nasal/sinus endoscopy
Sinusotomy, when applicable

Do not report with (31295)

31256   **Nasal/sinus endoscopy, surgical, with maxillary antrostomy;**

Code also any combination of the following endoscopic procedures when performed in conjunction with maxillary antrostomy, regardless if polyps are removed:

Frontal sinus exploration (31276)

Sphenoidotomy, with or without removal of tissue; either (31287, 31288)

Total (anterior and posterior) ethmoidectomy (31255)

🖭 5.71   ⚖ 5.71   **FUD** 000   T A2 50 ▢

AMA: 2015,Jan,16; 2014,Jan,11; 2013,Jun,13; 2011,Jun,11-12

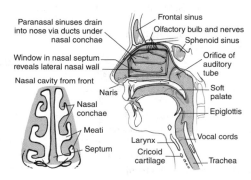

Paranasal sinuses drain into nose via ducts under nasal conchae

Frontal sinus
Olfactory bulb and nerves
Sphenoid sinus

Window in nasal septum reveals lateral nasal wall

Orifice of auditory tube

Nasal cavity from front

Naris

Nasal conchae

Soft palate

Meati

Epiglottis

Larynx

Vocal cords

Septum

Cricoid cartilage

Trachea

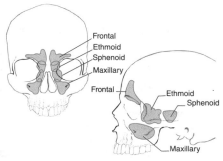

Frontal
Ethmoid
Sphenoid
Maxillary

Frontal

Ethmoid
Sphenoid

Maxillary

31267   **with removal of tissue from maxillary sinus**

Code also any combination of the following endoscopic procedures when performed in conjunction with maxillary antrostomy with removal of maxillary sinus tissue, regardless of whether polyps are removed:

Frontal sinus exploration (31276)

Sphenoidotomy, with or without removal of tissue; either (31287, 31288)

Total (anterior and posterior) ethmoidectomy (31255)

🖭 9.16   ⚖ 9.16   **FUD** 000   T A2 50 ▢

AMA: 2015,Jan,16; 2014,Jan,11; 2012,Jan,15-42; 2011,Jun,11-12; 2011,Jan,11

31276 Nasal Endoscopy with Frontal Sinus Examination

INCLUDES   Diagnostic nasal/sinus endoscopy
Sinusotomy, when applicable
Unilateral procedure

EXCLUDES   *Unilateral endoscopy two or more sinuses (31231-31235)*

Code also any combination of the following endoscopic procedures when performed in conjunction with frontal sinus exploration, regardless of whether polyps are removed:

Antrostomy, with or without removal of maxillary sinus tissue; either (31256, 31267)

Sphenoidotomy, with or without removal of tissue; either (31287, 31288)

Total (anterior and posterior) ethmoidectomy (31255)

Do not report with (31296)

31276   **Nasal/sinus endoscopy, surgical with frontal sinus exploration, with or without removal of tissue from frontal sinus**

🖭 14.5   ⚖ 14.5   **FUD** 000   T A2 50 ▢

AMA: 2015,Jan,16; 2014,Jan,11; 2012,Jan,15-42; 2011,Jun,11-12; 2011,Jan,11; 2010,Jan,11-12

31287-31288 Nasal Endoscopy with Sphenoid Procedures

Do not report with (31297)

31287   **Nasal/sinus endoscopy, surgical, with sphenoidotomy;**

🖭 6.69   ⚖ 6.69   **FUD** 000   T A2 80 50 ▢

AMA: 2015,Jan,16; 2014,Jan,11; 2011,Jun,11-12

31288   **with removal of tissue from the sphenoid sinus**

🖭 7.76   ⚖ 7.76   **FUD** 000   T A2 80 50 ▢

AMA: 2015,Jan,16; 2014,Jan,11; 2011,Jun,11-12

31290-31294 Nasal Endoscopy with Repair and Decompression

INCLUDES   Diagnostic nasal/sinus endoscopy
Sinusotomy, when applicable

31290   **Nasal/sinus endoscopy, surgical, with repair of cerebrospinal fluid leak; ethmoid region**

🖭 33.3   ⚖ 33.3   **FUD** 010   C 80 50 ▢

AMA: 2015,Jan,16; 2014,Jan,11; 2011,Jun,11-12

31291   **sphenoid region**

🖭 35.5   ⚖ 35.5   **FUD** 010   C 80 50 ▢

AMA: 2015,Jan,16; 2014,Jan,11; 2011,Jun,11-12

31292   **Nasal/sinus endoscopy, surgical; with medial or inferior orbital wall decompression**

🖭 28.6   ⚖ 28.6   **FUD** 010   T 80 50 ▢

AMA: 2015,Jan,16; 2014,Jan,11; 2011,Jun,11-12

31293   **with medial orbital wall and inferior orbital wall decompression**

🖭 31.1   ⚖ 31.1   **FUD** 010   T 80 50 ▢

AMA: 2015,Jan,16; 2014,Jan,11; 2011,Jun,11-12

31294   **with optic nerve decompression**

🖭 35.6   ⚖ 35.6   **FUD** 010   T 80 50 ▢

AMA: 2015,Jan,16; 2014,Jan,11; 2011,Jun,11-12

31295-31297 Nasal Endoscopy with Sinus Ostia Dilation

INCLUDES   Any method of tissue displacement
Fluoroscopy, when performed

31295   **Nasal/sinus endoscopy, surgical; with dilation of maxillary sinus ostium (eg, balloon dilation), transnasal or via canine fossa**

Do not report with (31233, 31256, 31267)

🖭 4.82   ⚖ 58.3   **FUD** 000   T P2 80 50

AMA: 2015,Jan,16; 2014,Jan,11; 2011,Jun,11-12

31296   **with dilation of frontal sinus ostium (eg, balloon dilation)**

Do not report with (31276)

🖭 5.75   ⚖ 59.1   **FUD** 000   T P2 80 50

AMA: 2015,Jan,16; 2014,Jan,11; 2011,Jun,11-12

31297   **with dilation of sphenoid sinus ostium (eg, balloon dilation)**

Do not report with (31235, 31287, 31288)

🖭 4.71   ⚖ 58.1   **FUD** 000   T P2 80 50

AMA: 2015,Jan,16; 2014,Jan,11; 2011,Jun,11-12

31299 Unlisted Procedures of Accessory Sinuses

CMS: 100-4,4,180.3 Unlisted Service or Procedure

EXCLUDES   Hypophysectomy (61546, 61548)

31299   **Unlisted procedure, accessory sinuses**
    0.00   0.00   **FUD** YYY   T 80

     AMA: 2015,Jul,10; 2015,Jan,16; 2014,Jan,11; 2013,Jun,13; 2012,Jan,15-42; 2011,Jun,11-12; 2010,Jan,11-12

31300-31502 Procedures of the Larynx

31300   **Laryngotomy (thyrotomy, laryngofissure); with removal of tumor or laryngocele, cordectomy**
    36.1   36.1   **FUD** 090   T A2 80

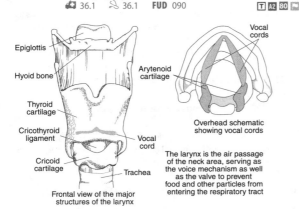

Epiglottis
Hyoid bone
Thyroid cartilage
Cricothyroid ligament
Cricoid cartilage
Vocal cords
Arytenoid cartilage
Vocal cord
Trachea

Frontal view of the major structures of the larynx

Overhead schematic showing vocal cords

The larynx is the air passage of the neck area, serving as the voice mechanism as well as the valve to prevent food and other particles from entering the respiratory tract

31320   **diagnostic**
    18.7   18.7   **FUD** 090   T A2 80

31360   **Laryngectomy; total, without radical neck dissection**
    59.6   59.6   **FUD** 090   C 80 PQ

     AMA: 2015,Jan,16; 2014,Jan,11; 2010,Aug,3-7; 2010,Aug,3-7

31365   **total, with radical neck dissection**
    73.7   73.7   **FUD** 090   C 80 PQ

     AMA: 2015,Jan,16; 2014,Jan,11; 2012,Jan,15-42; 2011,Jan,11; 2010,Aug,3-7; 2010,Aug,3-7

31367   **subtotal supraglottic, without radical neck dissection**
    63.1   63.1   **FUD** 090   C 80 PQ

     AMA: 2015,Jan,16; 2014,Jan,11; 2010,Aug,3-7; 2010,Aug,3-7

31368   **subtotal supraglottic, with radical neck dissection**
    70.0   70.0   **FUD** 090   C 80 PQ

31370   **Partial laryngectomy (hemilaryngectomy); horizontal**
    59.3   59.3   **FUD** 090   C 80 PQ

31375   **laterovertical**
    56.3   56.3   **FUD** 090   C 80 PQ

31380   **anterovertical**
    55.5   55.5   **FUD** 090   C 80 PQ

31382   **antero-latero-vertical**
    60.8   60.8   **FUD** 090   C 80 PQ

31390   **Pharyngolaryngectomy, with radical neck dissection; without reconstruction**
    81.7   81.7   **FUD** 090   C 80 PQ

31395   **with reconstruction**
    86.0   86.0   **FUD** 090   C 80 PQ

31400   **Arytenoidectomy or arytenoidopexy, external approach**
    28.5   28.5   **FUD** 090   T A2 80

     EXCLUDES   Endoscopic arytenoidectomy (31560)

31420   **Epiglottidectomy**
    23.8   23.8   **FUD** 090   T A2 80

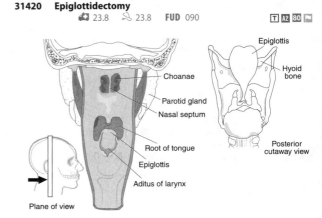

Epiglottis
Hyoid bone
Choanae
Parotid gland
Nasal septum
Root of tongue
Epiglottis
Aditus of larynx
Posterior cutaway view
Plane of view

31500   **Intubation, endotracheal, emergency procedure**
    3.17   3.17   **FUD** 000   ⊘ T 62

     AMA: 2015,Jan,16; 2014,Jan,11; 2012,Jan,15-42; 2011,Jan,11

31502   **Tracheotomy tube change prior to establishment of fistula tract**
    1.00   1.00   **FUD** 000   T 62

     AMA: 1990,Win,4

31505-31541 Endoscopy of the Larynx

31505   **Laryngoscopy, indirect; diagnostic (separate procedure)**
    1.40   2.36   **FUD** 000   T P3

     AMA: 2015,Jan,16; 2014,Jan,11

31510   **with biopsy**
    3.54   6.06   **FUD** 000   T A2 80 PQ

     AMA: 2015,Jan,16; 2014,Jan,11

31511   **with removal of foreign body**
    3.74   6.04   **FUD** 000   T A2

     AMA: 2015,Jan,16; 2014,Jan,11

31512   **with removal of lesion**
    3.77   5.92   **FUD** 000   T A2 80

     AMA: 2015,Jan,16; 2014,Jan,11

31513   **with vocal cord injection**
    3.83   3.83   **FUD** 000   T A2 80

     AMA: 2015,Jan,16; 2014,Jan,11

31515   **Laryngoscopy direct, with or without tracheoscopy; for aspiration**
    3.21   5.92   **FUD** 000   T A2

     AMA: 1998,Nov,1; 1997,Nov,1

31520   **diagnostic, newborn**
    4.54   4.54   **FUD** 000   63 T 62 80

     AMA: 1998,Nov,1; 1997,Nov,1

31525   **diagnostic, except newborn**
    4.63   7.23   **FUD** 000   T A2

     AMA: 2015,Jan,16; 2014,Jan,11; 2010,Aug,3-7; 2010,Aug,3-7

31526   **diagnostic, with operating microscope or telescope**
     INCLUDES   Operating microscope (69990)
    4.55   4.55   **FUD** 000   T A2

     AMA: 1999,Nov,1; 1998,Nov,1

31527   **with insertion of obturator**
    5.68   5.68   **FUD** 000   T A2 80

     AMA: 1998,Nov,1; 1997,Nov,1

31528   **with dilation, initial**
    4.19   4.19   **FUD** 000   T A2 80

     AMA: 2002,May,7; 1998,Nov,1

31529   **with dilation, subsequent**
    4.70   4.70   **FUD** 000   T A2 80

     AMA: 2002,May,7; 1998,Nov,1

26/TC PC/TC Comp Only	A2-Z3 ASC Pmt	50 Bilateral	♂ Male Only	♀ Female Only	Facility RVU	Non-Facility RVU
AMA: CPT Asst	**CMS:** Pub 100	A-Y OPPSI	80/80 Surg Assist Allowed / w/Doc		Lab Crosswalk	Radiology Crosswalk

100   Medicare (Red Text)   CPT © 2015 American Medical Association. All Rights Reserved. (Black Text)   © 2015 Optum360, LLC (Blue Text)

31530 Laryngoscopy, direct, operative, with foreign body removal;
5.70   5.70   **FUD** 000   T A2 ▭
AMA: 1998,Nov,1; 1997,Nov,1

31531 with operating microscope or telescope
INCLUDES   Operating microscope (69990)
6.17   6.17   **FUD** 000   T A2 80 ▭
AMA: 1999,Nov,1; 1998,Nov,1

31535 Laryngoscopy, direct, operative, with biopsy;
5.51   5.51   **FUD** 000   T A2 ▭
AMA: 1998,Nov,1; 1997,Nov,1

31536 with operating microscope or telescope
INCLUDES   Operating microscope (69990)
6.12   6.12   **FUD** 000   T A2 ▭
AMA: 1999,Nov,1; 1998,Nov,1

31540 Laryngoscopy, direct, operative, with excision of tumor and/or stripping of vocal cords or epiglottis;
7.03   7.03   **FUD** 000   T A2 ▭
AMA: 1998,Nov,1; 1997,Nov,1

31541 with operating microscope or telescope
INCLUDES   Operating microscope (69990)
7.68   7.68   **FUD** 000   T A2 ▭
AMA: 1999,Nov,1; 1998,Nov,1

31545-31546 Endoscopy of Larynx with Reconstruction

INCLUDES   Operating microscope (69990)
EXCLUDES   *Vocal cord reconstruction with allograft (31599)*
Do not report with (31540, 31541)

31545 Laryngoscopy, direct, operative, with operating microscope or telescope, with submucosal removal of non-neoplastic lesion(s) of vocal cord; reconstruction with local tissue flap(s)
10.5   10.5   **FUD** 000   T A2 50 ▭
AMA: 1998,Nov,1; 1997,Nov,1

31546 reconstruction with graft(s) (includes obtaining autograft)
Do not report with (20926)
15.9   15.9   **FUD** 000   T A2 50 ▭
AMA: 2015,Jan,16; 2014,Jan,11; 2012,Jan,15-42; 2011,Jan,11

31560-31571 Endoscopy of Larynx with Arytenoid Removal, Vocal Cord Injection

31560 Laryngoscopy, direct, operative, with arytenoidectomy;
9.11   9.11   **FUD** 000   T A2 80 ▭
AMA: 1998,Nov,1; 1997,Nov,1

31561 with operating microscope or telescope
INCLUDES   Operating microscope (69990)
9.96   9.96   **FUD** 000   T A2 80 ▭
AMA: 1999,Nov,1; 1998,Nov,1

31570 Laryngoscopy, direct, with injection into vocal cord(s), therapeutic;
6.68   9.73   **FUD** 000   T A2 ▭
AMA: 2015,Jan,16; 2014,Jan,6

31571 with operating microscope or telescope
INCLUDES   Operating microscope (69990)
7.26   7.26   **FUD** 000   T A2 ▭
AMA: 2015,Jan,16; 2014,Jan,6; 2014,Jan,11; 2012,Nov,13-14

31575-31579 Endoscopy of Larynx, Flexible Fiberoptic

EXCLUDES   *Evaluation by flexible fiberoptic endoscope:*
Sensory assessment (92614-92615)
Swallowing (92612-92613)
Swallowing and sensory assessment (92616-92617)
Flexible fiberoptic endoscopic examination/testing by cine or video recording (92612-92617)

31575 Laryngoscopy, flexible fiberoptic; diagnostic
Do not report with (43197-43198)
2.21   3.27   **FUD** 000   T P3 ▭
AMA: 1999,Nov,1; 1997,Nov,1

31576 with biopsy
3.58   6.39   **FUD** 000   T A2 ▭ PQ
AMA: 1997,Nov,1

31577 with removal of foreign body
4.35   6.92   **FUD** 000   T A2 80 ▭
AMA: 1997,Nov,1

31578 with removal of lesion
4.97   7.95   **FUD** 000   T A2 80 ▭
AMA: 1997,Nov,1

31579 Laryngoscopy, flexible or rigid fiberoptic, with stroboscopy
4.08   6.02   **FUD** 000   T P3 ▭
AMA: 1997,Nov,1; 1995,Win,1

31580-31599 Larynx Reconstruction

31580 Laryngoplasty; for laryngeal web, 2-stage, with keel insertion and removal
34.9   34.9   **FUD** 090   T A2 80 ▭

31582 for laryngeal stenosis, with graft or core mold, including tracheotomy
54.3   54.3   **FUD** 090   T A2 ▭
AMA: 2003,Jan,1

31584 with open reduction of fracture
43.2   43.2   **FUD** 090   C 80 ▭

31587 Laryngoplasty, cricoid split
28.7   28.7   **FUD** 090   C 80 ▭

31588 Laryngoplasty, not otherwise specified (eg, for burns, reconstruction after partial laryngectomy)
32.6   32.6   **FUD** 090   T A2 80 ▭
AMA: 2015,Jan,16; 2014,Jan,11; 2012,Jan,15-42; 2011,Jan,11

31590 Laryngeal reinnervation by neuromuscular pedicle
25.4   25.4   **FUD** 090   T A2 80 ▭

31595 Section recurrent laryngeal nerve, therapeutic (separate procedure), unilateral
21.8   21.8   **FUD** 090   T A2 80 50 ▭

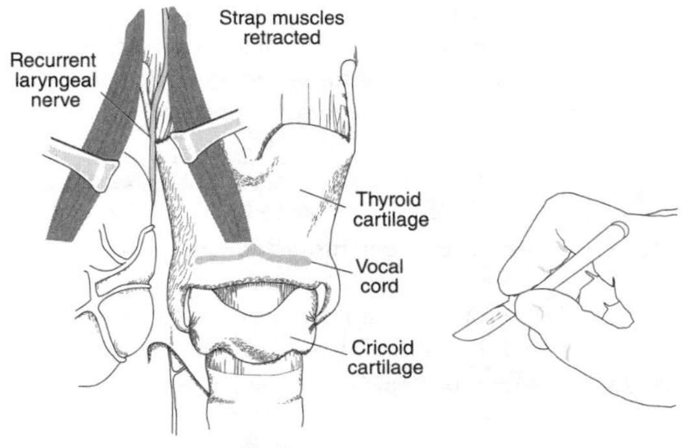

Strap muscles retracted
Recurrent laryngeal nerve
Thyroid cartilage
Vocal cord
Cricoid cartilage

31599 Unlisted procedure, larynx
0.00   0.00   **FUD** YYY   T 80
AMA: 2015,Jan,16; 2014,Jan,11; 2012,Nov,13-14

31600-31610 Stoma Creation: Trachea

EXCLUDES   *Aspiration of trachea, direct vision (31515)*
Endotracheal intubation (31500)

31600 Tracheostomy, planned (separate procedure);
11.4   11.4   **FUD** 000   T ▭
AMA: 2010,Aug,3-7; 2010,Aug,3-7

31601 younger than 2 years
7.91   7.91   **FUD** 000   T 80 ▭

31603 Tracheostomy, emergency procedure; transtracheal
6.46   6.46   **FUD** 000   T A2 ▭

31605 cricothyroid membrane
5.32   5.32   **FUD** 000   T 62 ▭

● New Code   ▲ Revised Code   ○ Reinstated   M Maternity   A Age Edit   Unlisted   Not Covered   # Resequenced
⊘ AMA Mod 51 Exempt   ⑤ Optum Mod 51 Exempt   ⑬ Mod 63 Exempt   ⊙ Mod Sedation   + Add-on   CCI   PQ PQRS   FUD Follow-up Days

31610   **Tracheostomy, fenestration procedure with skin flaps**
          🚗 20.5   ⚕ 20.5   **FUD** 090   T 🔲

31611-31614 Procedures of the Trachea

31611   **Construction of tracheoesophageal fistula and subsequent insertion of an alaryngeal speech prosthesis (eg, voice button, Blom-Singer prosthesis)**
          🚗 15.4   ⚕ 15.4   **FUD** 090   T A2 80 🔲

31612   **Tracheal puncture, percutaneous with transtracheal aspiration and/or injection**
          EXCLUDES   *Tracheal aspiration under direct vision (31515)*
          🚗 1.46   ⚕ 2.47   **FUD** 000   T A2 80 🔲
          AMA: 1994,Win,1

31613   **Tracheostoma revision; simple, without flap rotation**
          🚗 13.0   ⚕ 13.0   **FUD** 090   T A2 🔲

31614   **complex, with flap rotation**
          🚗 21.6   ⚕ 21.6   **FUD** 090   T A2 🔲

31615 Endoscopy Through Tracheostomy

INCLUDES   Diagnostic bronchoscopy
EXCLUDES   *Endobronchial ultrasound [EBUS] guided biopsies of mediastinal or hilar lymph nodes (31652-31653)*
          Tracheoscopy (31515-31578)
Code also endobronchial ultrasound [EBUS] during diagnostic/therapeutic peripheral lesion intervention (31654)

31615   **Tracheobronchoscopy through established tracheostomy incision**
          🚗 3.71   ⚕ 5.20   **FUD** 000   ⊙ T A2 🔲
          AMA: 2015,Jan,16; 2014,Jan,11; 2013,Mar,8-9; 2012,Nov,13-14; 2010,Apr,5; 2010,Jan,6

31620 Endobronchial Ultrasound (EBUS)

~~31620~~   ~~Endobronchial ultrasound (EBUS) during bronchoscopic diagnostic or therapeutic intervention(s) (List separately in addition to code for primary procedure[s])~~
          To report, see ~31652-31654

31622-31654 [31651] Endoscopy of Lung

INCLUDES   Diagnostic bronchoscopy with surgical bronchoscopy procedures
          Fluoroscopic imaging guidance, when performed

31622   **Bronchoscopy, rigid or flexible, including fluoroscopic guidance, when performed; diagnostic, with cell washing, when performed (separate procedure)**
          🚗 4.20   ⚕ 8.92   **FUD** 000   ⊙ T A2 🔲
          AMA: 2015,Jan,16; 2014,Jan,11; 2013,Mar,8-9; 2012,Jan,15-42; 2011,Feb,8-9; 2011,Jan,11; 2011,Jan,6-7; 2010,Apr,5; 2010,Jan,6

31623   **with brushing or protected brushings**
          🚗 4.23   ⚕ 9.43   **FUD** 000   ⊙ T A2 🔲
          AMA: 2015,Jan,16; 2014,Jan,11; 2013,Mar,8-9; 2012,Jan,15-42; 2011,Jan,11; 2011,Jan,6-7; 2010,Apr,5; 2010,Jan,6

31624   **with bronchial alveolar lavage**
          🚗 4.27   ⚕ 8.93   **FUD** 000   ⊙ T A2 🔲
          AMA: 2015,Jan,16; 2014,Jan,11; 2013,Mar,8-9; 2012,Jan,15-42; 2011,Jan,11; 2011,Jan,6-7; 2010,Apr,5; 2010,Jan,6

31625   **with bronchial or endobronchial biopsy(s), single or multiple sites**
          🚗 4.92   ⚕ 9.49   **FUD** 000   ⊙ T A2 🔲 P0
          AMA: 2015,Jan,16; 2014,Jan,11; 2013,Mar,8-9; 2012,Jan,15-42; 2011,Jan,11; 2011,Jan,6-7; 2010,Apr,5; 2010,Jan,6

31626   **with placement of fiducial markers, single or multiple**
          Code also device
          🚗 6.14   ⚕ 12.7   **FUD** 000   ⊙ T G2 80
          AMA: 2015,Jun,6; 2015,Jan,16; 2014,Jan,11; 2013,Mar,8-9; 2011,Jan,6-7; 2010,Apr,5; 2010,Jan,6

+ **31627**   **with computer-assisted, image-guided navigation (List separately in addition to code for primary procedure[s])**
          INCLUDES   3D reconstruction
          Code first (31615, 31622-31626, 31628-31631, 31635-31636, 31638-31643)
          Do not report with (76376-76377)
          🚗 2.81   ⚕ 40.1   **FUD** ZZZ   ⊙ N N1 80
          AMA: 2015,Jan,16; 2014,Jan,11; 2013,Mar,8-9; 2011,Jan,6-7; 2010,Apr,5; 2010,Jan,6

31628   **with transbronchial lung biopsy(s), single lobe**
          INCLUDES   All biopsies taken from lobe
          EXCLUDES   *Transbronchial biopsies by needle aspiration (31629, 31633)*
          Code also transbronchial biopsies of additional lobe(s) (31632)
          🚗 5.48   ⚕ 10.6   **FUD** 000   ⊙ T A2 🔲 P0
          AMA: 2015,Jan,16; 2014,Jan,11; 2013,Mar,8-9; 2012,Jan,15-42; 2011,Jan,11; 2011,Jan,6-7; 2010,Apr,5; 2010,Jan,6

31629   **with transbronchial needle aspiration biopsy(s), trachea, main stem and/or lobar bronchus(i)**
          INCLUDES   All biopsies from same lobe or upper airway
          EXCLUDES   *Transbronchial biopsies of lung (31628, 31632)*
          Code also transbronchial needle biopsies of additional lobe(s) (31633)
          🚗 5.91   ⚕ 16.7   **FUD** 000   ⊙ T A2 🔲 P0
          AMA: 2015,Jan,16; 2014,Jan,11; 2013,Mar,8-9; 2012,Jan,15-42; 2011,Apr,12; 2011,Jan,11; 2011,Jan,6-7; 2010,Apr,5; 2010,Jan,6

31630   **with tracheal/bronchial dilation or closed reduction of fracture**
          🚗 5.79   ⚕ 5.79   **FUD** 000   T A2 🔲
          AMA: 2015,Jan,16; 2014,Jan,11; 2013,Mar,8-9; 2011,Jan,6-7; 2010,Apr,5; 2010,Jan,6

31631   **with placement of tracheal stent(s) (includes tracheal/bronchial dilation as required)**
          EXCLUDES   *Bronchial stent placement (31636-31637)*
          Revision bronchial or tracheal stent (31638)
          🚗 6.70   ⚕ 6.70   **FUD** 000   T A2 🔲
          AMA: 2015,Jan,16; 2014,Jan,11; 2013,Mar,8-9; 2011,Jan,6-7; 2010,Apr,5; 2010,Jan,6

▲ + **31632**   **with transbronchial lung biopsy(s), each additional lobe (List separately in addition to code for primary procedure)**
          INCLUDES   All biopsies of additional lobe of lung
          Code first (31628)
          🚗 1.41   ⚕ 2.03   **FUD** ZZZ   ⊙ N N1 🔲
          AMA: 2015,Jan,16; 2014,Jan,11; 2013,Mar,8-9

▲ + **31633**   **with transbronchial needle aspiration biopsy(s), each additional lobe (List separately in addition to code for primary procedure)**
          INCLUDES   All needle biopsies from another lobe or from trachea
          Code first (31629)
          🚗 1.83   ⚕ 2.51   **FUD** ZZZ   ⊙ N N1 🔲
          AMA: 2015,Jan,16; 2014,Jan,11; 2013,Mar,8-9; 2012,Jan,15-42; 2011,Apr,12; 2011,Jan,11

31634   **with balloon occlusion, with assessment of air leak, with administration of occlusive substance (eg, fibrin glue), if performed**
          Do not report with (31647, [31651])
          🚗 5.99   ⚕ 53.5   **FUD** 000   ⊙ T G2 80
          AMA: 2015,Jan,16; 2014,Jan,11; 2013,Mar,8-9; 2011,Jan,6-7

31635   **with removal of foreign body**
          EXCLUDES   *Removal implanted bronchial valves (31648-31649)*
          🚗 5.45   ⚕ 9.97   **FUD** 000   ⊙ T A2 🔲
          AMA: 2015,Jan,16; 2014,Jan,11; 2013,Mar,8-9; 2012,Jan,15-42; 2011,Jan,11; 2011,Jan,6-7; 2010,Apr,5; 2010,Jan,6

31636 with placement of bronchial stent(s) (includes tracheal/bronchial dilation as required), initial bronchus
🚗 6.41 ⚖ 6.41 **FUD** 000   T A2 ▭
AMA: 2015,Jan,16; 2014,Jan,11; 2013,Mar,8-9; 2011,Jan,6-7; 2010,Apr,5; 2010,Jan,6

+ 31637 each additional major bronchus stented (List separately in addition to code for primary procedure)
Code first (31636)
🚗 2.14 ⚖ 2.14 **FUD** ZZZ   N N1
AMA: 2015,Jan,16; 2014,Jan,11; 2013,Mar,8-9

31638 with revision of tracheal or bronchial stent inserted at previous session (includes tracheal/bronchial dilation as required)
🚗 7.34 ⚖ 7.34 **FUD** 000   T A2 ▭
AMA: 2015,Jan,16; 2014,Jan,11; 2013,Mar,8-9; 2011,Jan,6-7; 2010,Apr,5; 2010,Jan,6

31640 with excision of tumor
🚗 7.36 ⚖ 7.36 **FUD** 000   T A2 ▭
AMA: 2015,Jan,16; 2014,Jan,11; 2013,Mar,8-9; 2011,Jan,6-7; 2010,Apr,5; 2010,Jan,6

31641 with destruction of tumor or relief of stenosis by any method other than excision (eg, laser therapy, cryotherapy)
Code also any photodynamic therapy via bronchoscopy (96570-96571)
🚗 7.44 ⚖ 7.44 **FUD** 000   T A2 ▭
AMA: 2015,Jan,16; 2014,Jan,11; 2013,Apr,8-9; 2013,Mar,8-9; 2011,Oct,3-4; 2011,Jan,6-7; 2010,Apr,5; 2010,Jan,6

31643 with placement of catheter(s) for intracavitary radioelement application
Code also if appropriate (77761-77763, 77770-77772)
🚗 5.10 ⚖ 5.10 **FUD** 000   T A2 ▭
AMA: 2015,Jan,16; 2014,Jan,11; 2013,Mar,8-9; 2011,Jan,6-7; 2010,Apr,5; 2010,Jan,6

31645 with therapeutic aspiration of tracheobronchial tree, initial (eg, drainage of lung abscess)
EXCLUDES Bedside aspiration of trachea, bronchi (31725)
🚗 4.66 ⚖ 9.22 **FUD** 000   ⊙ T A2 ▭
AMA: 2015,Jan,16; 2014,Jan,11; 2013,Mar,8-9; 2011,Jan,6-7

31646 with therapeutic aspiration of tracheobronchial tree, subsequent
EXCLUDES Bedside aspiration of trachea, bronchi (31725)
🚗 4.04 ⚖ 8.29 **FUD** 000   ⊙ T A2 ▭
AMA: 2015,Jan,16; 2014,Jan,11; 2013,Mar,8-9; 2011,Jan,6-7

31647 with balloon occlusion, when performed, assessment of air leak, airway sizing, and insertion of bronchial valve(s), initial lobe
🚗 6.44 ⚖ 6.44 **FUD** 000   ⊙ T G2
AMA: 2015,Jan,16; 2014,Jan,11; 2013,Mar,8-9

+ # 31651 with balloon occlusion, when performed, assessment of air leak, airway sizing, and insertion of bronchial valve(s), each additional lobe (List separately in addition to code for primary procedure[s])
Code first (31647)
🚗 2.14 ⚖ 2.14 **FUD** ZZZ   ⊙ N N1
AMA: 2015,Jan,16; 2014,Jan,11; 2013,Mar,8-9

31648 with removal of bronchial valve(s), initial lobe
EXCLUDES Removal with reinsertion bronchial valve during same session (31647 and 31648) and ([31651])
🚗 5.86 ⚖ 5.86 **FUD** 000   ⊙ T G2
AMA: 2015,Jan,16; 2014,Jan,11; 2013,Mar,8-9

+ 31649 with removal of bronchial valve(s), each additional lobe (List separately in addition to code for primary procedure)
Code first (31648)
🚗 1.96 ⚖ 1.96 **FUD** ZZZ   ⊙ 02 G2
AMA: 2015,Jan,16; 2014,Jan,11; 2013,Mar,8-9

31651   Resequenced code. See code following 31647.

● **31652** with endobronchial ultrasound (EBUS) guided transtracheal and/or transbronchial sampling (eg, aspiration[s]/biopsy[ies]), one or two mediastinal and/or hilar lymph node stations or structures
Do not report more than one time per session   ⊙
🚗 0.00 ⚖ 0.00 **FUD** 000

● **31653** with endobronchial ultrasound (EBUS) guided transtracheal and/or transbronchial sampling (eg, aspiration[s]/biopsy[ies]), 3 or more mediastinal and/or hilar lymph node stations or structures
Do not report more than one time per session   ⊙
🚗 0.00 ⚖ 0.00 **FUD** 000

● + **31654** with transendoscopic endobronchial ultrasound (EBUS) during bronchoscopic diagnostic or therapeutic intervention(s) for peripheral lesion(s) (List separately in addition to code for primary procedure[s])
EXCLUDES Endobronchial ultrasound [EBUS] for mediastinal/ ⊙ hilar lymph node station/adjacent structure access (31652-31653)
Code first (31622-31629, 31640, 31643-31646)
Do not report more than one time per session
🚗 0.00 ⚖ 0.00 **FUD** 000

31660-31661 Bronchial Thermoplasty

INCLUDES Fluoroscopic imaging guidance, when performed

31660 Bronchoscopy, rigid or flexible, including fluoroscopic guidance, when performed; with bronchial thermoplasty, 1 lobe
🚗 6.02 ⚖ 6.02 **FUD** 000   ⊙ T
AMA: 2015,Jan,16; 2014,Jan,11; 2013,Mar,8-9

31661 with bronchial thermoplasty, 2 or more lobes
🚗 6.30 ⚖ 6.30 **FUD** 000   ⊙ T
AMA: 2015,Jan,16; 2014,Jan,11; 2013,Mar,8-9

31717-31899 Respiratory Procedures

EXCLUDES Endotracheal intubation (31500)
Tracheal aspiration under direct vision (31515)

31717 Catheterization with bronchial brush biopsy
🚗 3.12 ⚖ 7.44 **FUD** 000   T A2 ▭ PQ
AMA: 2015,Jan,16; 2014,Jan,11; 2012,Jan,15-42; 2011,Jan,11

31720 Catheter aspiration (separate procedure); nasotracheal
🚗 1.47 ⚖ 1.47 **FUD** 000   01 N1 ▭
AMA: 1994,Win,1

31725 tracheobronchial with fiberscope, bedside
🚗 2.57 ⚖ 2.57 **FUD** 000   ⊙ C ▭

31730 Transtracheal (percutaneous) introduction of needle wire dilator/stent or indwelling tube for oxygen therapy
🚗 4.30 ⚖ 34.8 **FUD** 000   T A2 ▭
AMA: 1992,Win,1

31750 Tracheoplasty; cervical
🚗 39.4 ⚖ 39.4 **FUD** 090   T A2 80 ▭

31755 tracheopharyngeal fistulization, each stage
🚗 49.3 ⚖ 49.3 **FUD** 090   T A2 80 ▭

31760 intrathoracic
🚗 40.0 ⚖ 40.0 **FUD** 090   C 80 ▭ PQ

31766 Carinal reconstruction
🚗 48.9 ⚖ 48.9 **FUD** 090   C 80 ▭ PQ

31770 Bronchoplasty; graft repair
🚗 38.8 ⚖ 38.8 **FUD** 090   C 80 ▭ PQ
EXCLUDES Bronchoplasty done with lobectomy (32501)

31775 excision stenosis and anastomosis
🚗 35.6 ⚖ 35.6 **FUD** 090   C 80 ▭ PQ
EXCLUDES Bronchoplasty done with lobectomy (32501)

31780 Excision tracheal stenosis and anastomosis; cervical
🚗 34.2 ⚖ 34.2 **FUD** 090   C 80 ▭

31781   cervicothoracic
🚗 40.4   ⚕ 40.4   **FUD** 090   C 80 💬

31785   Excision of tracheal tumor or carcinoma; cervical
🚗 30.9   ⚕ 30.9   **FUD** 090   T 80 💬
AMA: 2003,Jan,1

31786   thoracic
🚗 45.8   ⚕ 45.8   **FUD** 090   C 80 💬 PQ

31800   Suture of tracheal wound or injury; cervical
🚗 20.4   ⚕ 20.4   **FUD** 090   C 80 💬
AMA: 1994,Win,1

31805   intrathoracic
🚗 23.7   ⚕ 23.7   **FUD** 090   C 80 💬 PQ

31820   Surgical closure tracheostomy or fistula; without plastic repair
🚗 9.40   ⚕ 12.4   **FUD** 090   T A2 80 💬
EXCLUDES   Tracheoesophageal fistula repair (43305, 43312)

31825   with plastic repair
🚗 13.8   ⚕ 17.2   **FUD** 090   T A2 80 💬
EXCLUDES   Tracheoesophageal fistula repair (43305, 43312)

31830   Revision of tracheostomy scar
🚗 9.84   ⚕ 12.6   **FUD** 090   T A2 80 💬

Any of a wide variety of scar revision techniques may be employed. A Z-plasty may be used to lengthen or irregularize the scar line. Revision also serves to neutralize contractures that occur along the scar line

Thyroid cartilage

Cricoid cartilage

Tracheostomies typically enter at the second, third, or fourth ring

1st ring
2nd ring
3rd ring

Example of a common Z-plasty where flaps are rotated to break scar line

A tracheostomy closure scar is revised, usually to make the scar less noticeable (31830)

31899   Unlisted procedure, trachea, bronchi
🚗 0.00   ⚕ 0.00   **FUD** YYY   T 80
AMA: 2015,Jan,16; 2014,May,10; 2014,Jan,11; 2013,Mar,8-9; 2012,Jan,15-42; 2011,Jan,11; 2010,Jan,11-12

32035-32036 Procedures for Empyema

32035   Thoracostomy; with rib resection for empyema
🚗 21.0   ⚕ 21.0   **FUD** 090   C 80 50 💬

32036   with open flap drainage for empyema
🚗 22.5   ⚕ 22.5   **FUD** 090   C 80 50 💬
EXCLUDES   Wound exploration due to penetrating trauma without thoracotomy (20101)

32096-32098 Open Biopsy of Chest and Pleura

INCLUDES   Varying amounts of lung tissue excised for analysis
Wedge technique with tissue obtained without precise consideration of margins
EXCLUDES   Percutaneous needle biopsy of pleura, lung, and mediastinum (32400, 32405)
Thoracoscopy with biopsy (32607-32609)
Thoracoscopy with diagnostic wedge resection resulting in anatomic lung resection (32668)
Thoracotomy with diagnostic wedge resection resulting in anatomic lung resection (32507)

32096   Thoracotomy, with diagnostic biopsy(ies) of lung infiltrate(s) (eg, wedge, incisional), unilateral
Code also appropriate add-on code for the more extensive procedure at the same location if diagnostic wedge resection results in the need for further surgery (32507, 32668)
Do not report more than one time per lung
Do not report with (32440-32445, 32488)
🚗 23.3   ⚕ 23.3   **FUD** 090   C 80
AMA: 2015,Jan,16; 2014,Jan,11; 2012,Oct,9-11; 2012,Sep,3-8

32097   Thoracotomy, with diagnostic biopsy(ies) of lung nodule(s) or mass(es) (eg, wedge, incisional), unilateral
Code also appropriate add-on code for the more extensive procedure in the same location if diagnostic wedge resection results in the need for further surgery (32507, 32668)
Do not report more than one time per lung
Do not report with (32440-32445, 32488)
🚗 23.3   ⚕ 23.3   **FUD** 090   C 80
AMA: 2015,Jan,16; 2014,Jan,11; 2012,Oct,9-11; 2012,Sep,3-8

Trachea
Right lung
R. main bronchus
L. main bronchus
Upper bronchial lobe
Carini
Middle bronchial lobe
Mass
Lower bronchial lobe

32098   Thoracotomy, with biopsy(ies) of pleura
🚗 22.1   ⚕ 22.1   **FUD** 090   C 80
AMA: 2015,Jan,16; 2014,Jan,11

32100-32160 Open Procedures: Chest

INCLUDES   Exploration of penetrating wound of chest
EXCLUDES   Lung resection (32480-32504)
Wound exploration without thoracotomy for penetrating wound of chest (20101)

32100   Thoracotomy; with exploration
Do not report with (19260, 19271-19272, 32503-32504, 33955-33957, [33963, 33964])
🚗 23.4   ⚕ 23.4   **FUD** 090   C 80 💬 PQ
AMA: 2015,Jul,3; 2015,Jan,16; 2014,Jan,11; 2013,Jan,6-8

32110   with control of traumatic hemorrhage and/or repair of lung tear
🚗 42.4   ⚕ 42.4   **FUD** 090   C 80 💬 PQ
AMA: 2015,Jan,16; 2014,Jan,11

32120   for postoperative complications
🚗 25.2   ⚕ 25.2   **FUD** 090   C 80 💬 PQ

32124   with open intrapleural pneumonolysis
🚗 26.9   ⚕ 26.9   **FUD** 090   C 80 💬 PQ
AMA: 2015,Jan,16; 2014,Jan,11

32140   with cyst(s) removal, includes pleural procedure when performed
🚗 28.9   ⚕ 28.9   **FUD** 090   C 80 💬 PQ
AMA: 2015,Jan,16; 2014,Jan,11

32141   with resection-plication of bullae, includes any pleural procedure when performed
EXCLUDES   Lung volume reduction (32491)
🚗 44.2   ⚕ 44.2   **FUD** 090   C 80 💬 PQ
AMA: 2015,Jan,16; 2014,Jan,11

32150 with removal of intrapleural foreign body or fibrin deposit
🔲 29.2 ⚖ 29.2 **FUD** 090   C 80 ▢ PQ
AMA: 2015,Jan,16; 2014,Jan,11

32151 with removal of intrapulmonary foreign body
🔲 29.3 ⚖ 29.3 **FUD** 090   C 80 ▢

32160 with cardiac massage
🔲 22.8 ⚖ 22.8 **FUD** 090   C 80 ▢

32200-32320 Open Procedures: Lung

32200 Pneumonostomy, with open drainage of abscess or cyst
EXCLUDES   Image-guided, percutaneous drainage (eg, abscess, cyst) of lungs/mediastinum via catheter (49405)
🔀 (75989)
🔲 33.2 ⚖ 33.2 **FUD** 090   C 80 ▢
AMA: 2013,Nov,9

32215 Pleural scarification for repeat pneumothorax
🔲 23.2 ⚖ 23.2 **FUD** 090   C 80 50 ▢ PQ

32220 Decortication, pulmonary (separate procedure); total
🔲 45.9 ⚖ 45.9 **FUD** 090   C 80 50 ▢ PQ

32225 partial
🔲 28.8 ⚖ 28.8 **FUD** 090   C 80 50 ▢ PQ

32310 Pleurectomy, parietal (separate procedure)
🔲 26.2 ⚖ 26.2 **FUD** 090   C 80 ▢ PQ
AMA: 1994,Win,1

32320 Decortication and parietal pleurectomy
🔲 46.4 ⚖ 46.4 **FUD** 090   C 80 ▢ PQ
AMA: 1994,Fall,1

32400-32405 Lung Biopsy

EXCLUDES   Open lung biopsy (32096-32097)
Open mediastinal biopsy (39000-39010)
Thoracoscopic (VATS) biopsy of lung, pericardium, pleural or mediastinal space (32604-32609)

32400 Biopsy, pleura, percutaneous needle
EXCLUDES   Fine needle aspiration (10021-10022)
🔀 (76942, 77002, 77012, 77021)
🔲 2.54 ⚖ 4.34 **FUD** 000   T A2 ▢ PQ
AMA: 2015,Jan,16; 2014,Jan,11

32405 Biopsy, lung or mediastinum, percutaneous needle
EXCLUDES   Fine needle aspiration (10022)
🔀 (76942, 77002, 77012, 77021)
🔲 3.02 ⚖ 12.8 **FUD** 000   ⊙ T A2 ▢ PQ
AMA: 2015,Jan,16; 2014,Jan,11; 2012,Jan,15-42; 2011,Jan,11

32440-32501 Lung Resection

32440 Removal of lung, pneumonectomy;
Code also excision of chest wall tumor (19260-19272)
🔲 45.4 ⚖ 45.4 **FUD** 090   C 80 ▢ PQ
AMA: 2015,Jan,16; 2014,Jan,11; 2012,Oct,9-11; 2012,Sep,3-8

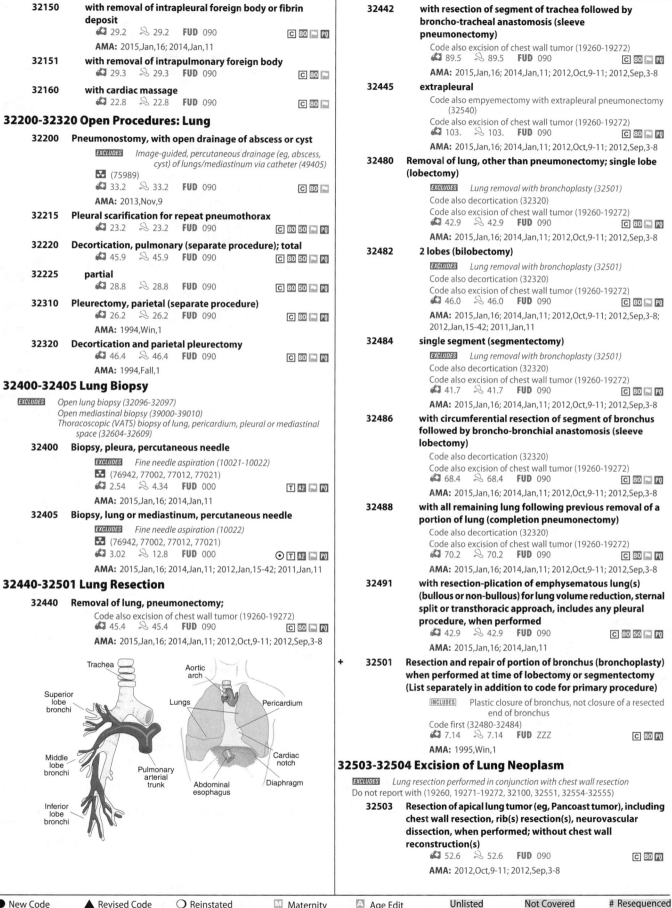

Trachea
Aortic arch
Superior lobe bronchi
Lungs
Pericardium
Middle lobe bronchi
Pulmonary arterial trunk
Cardiac notch
Abdominal esophagus
Diaphragm
Inferior lobe bronchi

32442 with resection of segment of trachea followed by broncho-tracheal anastomosis (sleeve pneumonectomy)
Code also excision of chest wall tumor (19260-19272)
🔲 89.5 ⚖ 89.5 **FUD** 090   C 80 ▢ PQ
AMA: 2015,Jan,16; 2014,Jan,11; 2012,Oct,9-11; 2012,Sep,3-8

32445 extrapleural
Code also empyemectomy with extrapleural pneumonectomy (32540)
Code also excision of chest wall tumor (19260-19272)
🔲 103. ⚖ 103. **FUD** 090   C 80 ▢ PQ
AMA: 2015,Jan,16; 2014,Jan,11; 2012,Oct,9-11; 2012,Sep,3-8

32480 Removal of lung, other than pneumonectomy; single lobe (lobectomy)
EXCLUDES   Lung removal with bronchoplasty (32501)
Code also decortication (32320)
Code also excision of chest wall tumor (19260-19272)
🔲 42.9 ⚖ 42.9 **FUD** 090   C 80 ▢ PQ
AMA: 2015,Jan,16; 2014,Jan,11; 2012,Oct,9-11; 2012,Sep,3-8

32482 2 lobes (bilobectomy)
EXCLUDES   Lung removal with bronchoplasty (32501)
Code also decortication (32320)
Code also excision of chest wall tumor (19260-19272)
🔲 46.0 ⚖ 46.0 **FUD** 090   C 80 ▢ PQ
AMA: 2015,Jan,16; 2014,Jan,11; 2012,Oct,9-11; 2012,Sep,3-8; 2012,Jan,15-42; 2011,Jan,11

32484 single segment (segmentectomy)
EXCLUDES   Lung removal with bronchoplasty (32501)
Code also decortication (32320)
Code also excision of chest wall tumor (19260-19272)
🔲 41.7 ⚖ 41.7 **FUD** 090   C 80 ▢ PQ
AMA: 2015,Jan,16; 2014,Jan,11; 2012,Oct,9-11; 2012,Sep,3-8

32486 with circumferential resection of segment of bronchus followed by broncho-bronchial anastomosis (sleeve lobectomy)
Code also decortication (32320)
Code also excision of chest wall tumor (19260-19272)
🔲 68.4 ⚖ 68.4 **FUD** 090   C 80 ▢ PQ
AMA: 2015,Jan,16; 2014,Jan,11; 2012,Oct,9-11; 2012,Sep,3-8

32488 with all remaining lung following previous removal of a portion of lung (completion pneumonectomy)
Code also decortication (32320)
Code also excision of chest wall tumor (19260-19272)
🔲 70.2 ⚖ 70.2 **FUD** 090   C 80 ▢ PQ
AMA: 2015,Jan,16; 2014,Jan,11; 2012,Oct,9-11; 2012,Sep,3-8

32491 with resection-plication of emphysematous lung(s) (bullous or non-bullous) for lung volume reduction, sternal split or transthoracic approach, includes any pleural procedure, when performed
🔲 42.9 ⚖ 42.9 **FUD** 090   C 80 50 ▢ PQ
AMA: 2015,Jan,16; 2014,Jan,11

+ **32501** Resection and repair of portion of bronchus (bronchoplasty) when performed at time of lobectomy or segmentectomy (List separately in addition to code for primary procedure)
INCLUDES   Plastic closure of bronchus, not closure of a resected end of bronchus
Code first (32480-32484)
🔲 7.14 ⚖ 7.14 **FUD** ZZZ   C 80 PQ
AMA: 1995,Win,1

32503-32504 Excision of Lung Neoplasm

EXCLUDES   Lung resection performed in conjunction with chest wall resection
Do not report with (19260, 19271-19272, 32100, 32551, 32554-32555)

32503 Resection of apical lung tumor (eg, Pancoast tumor), including chest wall resection, rib(s) resection(s), neurovascular dissection, when performed; without chest wall reconstruction(s)
🔲 52.6 ⚖ 52.6 **FUD** 090   C 80 PQ
AMA: 2012,Oct,9-11; 2012,Sep,3-8

32504 with chest wall reconstruction

🔲 60.4 ⚕ 60.4 **FUD** 090   C 80 P0

AMA: 2012,Oct,9-11; 2012,Sep,3-8

32505-32507 Thoracotomy with Wedge Resection

INCLUDES Wedge technique with tissue obtained with precise consideration of margins and complete resection
Code also resection of chest wall tumor with lung resection when performed (19260-19272)

32505 Thoracotomy; with therapeutic wedge resection (eg, mass, nodule), initial

Code also a more extensive procedure of the lung when performed on the contralateral lung or different lobe with modifier 59 regardless of intraoperative pathology consultation
Do not report with (32440, 32442, 32445, 32488)

🔲 27.0 ⚕ 27.0 **FUD** 090   C 80 P0

AMA: 2015,Jan,16; 2014,Jan,11; 2012,Oct,9-11; 2012,Sep,3-8

+ 32506 with therapeutic wedge resection (eg, mass or nodule), each additional resection, ipsilateral (List separately in addition to code for primary procedure)

Code also a more extensive procedure of the lung when performed on the contralateral lung or different lobe with modifier 59
Code first (32505)

🔲 4.58 ⚕ 4.58 **FUD** ZZZ   C 80

AMA: 2015,Jan,16; 2014,Jan,11; 2012,Oct,9-11; 2012,Sep,3-8

+ 32507 with diagnostic wedge resection followed by anatomic lung resection (List separately in addition to code for primary procedure)

INCLUDES Classification as a diagnostic wedge resection if intraoperative pathology consultation dictates more extensive resection in the same anatomical area
EXCLUDES Diagnostic wedge resection by thoracoscopy (32668)
Therapeutic wedge resection (32505-32506, 32666-32667)
Code first (32440, 32442, 32445, 32480-32488, 32503-32504)

🔲 4.57 ⚕ 4.57 **FUD** ZZZ   C 80

AMA: 2015,Jan,16; 2014,Jan,11; 2012,Oct,9-11; 2012,Sep,3-8

32540 Removal of Empyema

32540 Extrapleural enucleation of empyema (empyemectomy)

EXCLUDES Lung removal code when empyemectomy is performed with lobectomy (see appropriate lung removal code)
Code also appropriate removal of lung code when done with lobectomy (32480-32488)

🔲 50.3 ⚕ 50.3 **FUD** 090   C 80 🔲

AMA: 1994,Fall,1

32550-32552 Chest Tube/Catheter

32550 Insertion of indwelling tunneled pleural catheter with cuff

Do not report on same side of chest with (32554-32557)
🔳 (75989)

🔲 6.47 ⚕ 22.3 **FUD** 000   ⊙ T G2

AMA: 2015,Jan,16; 2014,May,3; 2014,Mar,13; 2014,Jan,11; 2012,Nov,3-5; 2012,Jan,15-42; 2011,Jan,11; 2010,Jul,10; 2010,Jan,6

32551 Tube thoracostomy, includes connection to drainage system (eg, water seal), when performed, open (separate procedure)

🔲 4.93 ⚕ 4.93 **FUD** 000   ⊙ T 50

AMA: 2015,Jan,16; 2014,May,3; 2014,Jan,11; 2012,Nov,3-5; 2011,Aug,3-5; 2010,Sep,6-7; 2010,Jan,6

32552 Removal of indwelling tunneled pleural catheter with cuff

🔲 4.63 ⚕ 5.34 **FUD** 010   02 G2 80

AMA: 2015,Jan,16; 2014,Jan,11; 2012,Nov,3-5; 2012,Jan,15-42; 2011,Jan,11; 2010,Jan,6

32553 Intrathoracic Placement Radiation Therapy Devices

EXCLUDES Percutaneous placement of interstitial device(s) for radiation therapy guidance: intra-abdominal, intrapelvic, and/or retroperitoneal (49411)
Code also device

32553 Placement of interstitial device(s) for radiation therapy guidance (eg, fiducial markers, dosimeter), percutaneous, intra-thoracic, single or multiple

🔳 (76942, 77002, 77012, 77021)

🔲 5.64 ⚕ 16.8 **FUD** 000   ⊙ S G2 80

AMA: 2015,Jun,6; 2015,Jan,16; 2014,Jan,11; 2010,Jan,6; 2010,Jan,7-8

32554-32557 Pleural Aspiration and Drainage

EXCLUDES Open tube thoracostomy (32551)
Placement of indwelling tunneled pleural drainage catheter (cuffed) (32550)
Do not report for same side of chest with (32550-32551)
Do not report with (75989, 76942, 77002, 77012, 77021)

32554 Thoracentesis, needle or catheter, aspiration of the pleural space; without imaging guidance

🔲 2.58 ⚕ 5.71 **FUD** 000   T G2 50

AMA: 2015,Jan,16; 2014,Jan,11; 2013,Nov,9; 2012,Nov,3-5

32555 with imaging guidance

🔲 3.27 ⚕ 8.21 **FUD** 000   T G2 50

AMA: 2015,Jan,16; 2014,Jan,11; 2013,Nov,9; 2012,Nov,3-5

32556 Pleural drainage, percutaneous, with insertion of indwelling catheter; without imaging guidance

🔲 3.57 ⚕ 15.7 **FUD** 000   T G2 50

AMA: 2015,Jan,16; 2014,Jan,11; 2013,Nov,9; 2012,Nov,3-5

32557 with imaging guidance

🔲 4.47 ⚕ 14.5 **FUD** 000   T G2 50

AMA: 2015,Jan,16; 2014,May,3; 2014,Jan,11; 2013,Nov,9; 2012,Nov,3-5

32560-32562 Instillation Drug/Chemical by Chest Tube

EXCLUDES Insertion of chest tube (32551)

32560 Instillation, via chest tube/catheter, agent for pleurodesis (eg, talc for recurrent or persistent pneumothorax)

🔲 2.27 ⚕ 6.94 **FUD** 000   T

AMA: 2015,Jan,16; 2014,Jan,11; 2010,Jan,6

32561 Instillation(s), via chest tube/catheter, agent for fibrinolysis (eg, fibrinolytic agent for break up of multiloculated effusion); initial day

Do not report more than one time on the date of initial treatment
🔲 1.99 ⚕ 2.66 **FUD** 000   T 80

AMA: 2015,Jan,16; 2014,Jan,11; 2010,Jan,6

32562 subsequent day

Do not report more than one time on each day of subsequent treatment
🔲 1.80 ⚕ 2.41 **FUD** 000   T 80

AMA: 2015,Jan,16; 2014,Jan,11; 2010,Jan,6

32601-32674 Thoracic Surgery: Video-Assisted (VATS)

INCLUDES Diagnostic thoracoscopy in surgical thoracoscopy

32601 Thoracoscopy, diagnostic (separate procedure); lungs, pericardial sac, mediastinal or pleural space, without biopsy

🔲 8.96 ⚕ 8.96 **FUD** 000   T 80 🔲

AMA: 2015,Jan,16; 2014,Jan,11; 2013,Aug,13; 2012,Oct,9-11; 2012,Sep,3-8

32604 pericardial sac, with biopsy

EXCLUDES Open biopsy of pericardium (39010)
🔲 14.0 ⚕ 14.0 **FUD** 000   T 80 🔲

AMA: 2015,Jan,16; 2014,Jan,11; 2013,Aug,13; 2012,Oct,9-11; 2012,Sep,3-8

32606 mediastinal space, with biopsy

🔲 13.4 ⚕ 13.4 **FUD** 000   T 80 🔲

AMA: 2015,Jan,16; 2014,Jan,11; 2013,Aug,13; 2012,Oct,9-11; 2012,Sep,3-8

26/TC PC/TC Comp Only	A2-Z3 ASC Pmt	50 Bilateral	♂ Male Only	♀ Female Only	🔲 Facility RVU	⚕ Non-Facility RVU
AMA: CPT Asst	CMS: Pub 100	A-Y OPPSI		80/80 Surg Assist Allowed / w/Doc	🔲 Lab Crosswalk	🔳 Radiology Crosswalk

106   Medicare (Red Text)   CPT © 2015 American Medical Association. All Rights Reserved. (Black Text)   © 2015 Optum360, LLC (Blue Text)

32607 **Thoracoscopy; with diagnostic biopsy(ies) of lung infiltrate(s) (eg, wedge, incisional), unilateral**

Do not report more than one time per lung
Do not report with (32440-32445, 32488, 32671)

🚑 8.98   ⚕ 8.98   **FUD** 000   T 80

AMA: 2015,Jan,16; 2014,Jan,11; 2013,Aug,13; 2012,Oct,9-11; 2012,Sep,3-8

32608 **with diagnostic biopsy(ies) of lung nodule(s) or mass(es) (eg, wedge, incisional), unilateral**

Do not report more than one time per lung
Do not report with (32440-32445, 32488, 32671)

🚑 11.0   ⚕ 11.0   **FUD** 000   T 80

AMA: 2015,Jan,16; 2014,Jan,11; 2013,Aug,13; 2012,Oct,9-11; 2012,Sep,3-8

32609 **with biopsy(ies) of pleura**

🚑 7.54   ⚕ 7.54   **FUD** 000   T 80

AMA: 2015,Jan,16; 2014,Jan,11; 2013,Aug,13; 2012,Oct,9-11; 2012,Sep,3-8

32650 **Thoracoscopy, surgical; with pleurodesis (eg, mechanical or chemical)**

🚑 19.3   ⚕ 19.3   **FUD** 090   C 80 50 ▭

AMA: 2015,Jan,16; 2014,Jan,11; 2013,Aug,13

32651 **with partial pulmonary decortication**

🚑 31.8   ⚕ 31.8   **FUD** 090   C 80 50 ▭

AMA: 2015,Jan,16; 2014,Jan,11; 2013,Aug,13

32652 **with total pulmonary decortication, including intrapleural pneumonolysis**

🚑 48.2   ⚕ 48.2   **FUD** 090   C 80 50 ▭

AMA: 2015,Jan,16; 2014,Jan,11; 2013,Aug,13

32653 **with removal of intrapleural foreign body or fibrin deposit**

🚑 30.7   ⚕ 30.7   **FUD** 090   C 80 ▭

AMA: 2015,Jan,16; 2014,Jan,11; 2013,Aug,13

32654 **with control of traumatic hemorrhage**

🚑 33.2   ⚕ 33.2   **FUD** 090   C 80 50 ▭

AMA: 2015,Jan,16; 2014,Jan,11; 2013,Aug,13

32655 **with resection-plication of bullae, includes any pleural procedure when performed**

EXCLUDES   *Thoracoscopic lung volume reduction surgery (32672)*

🚑 27.7   ⚕ 27.7   **FUD** 090   C 80 50 ▭

AMA: 2015,Jan,16; 2014,Jan,11; 2013,Aug,13; 2012,Jan,15-42; 2011,Jan,11

32656 **with parietal pleurectomy**

🚑 23.3   ⚕ 23.3   **FUD** 090   C 80 50 ▭

AMA: 2015,Jan,16; 2014,Jan,11; 2013,Aug,13

32658 **with removal of clot or foreign body from pericardial sac**

🚑 20.8   ⚕ 20.8   **FUD** 090   C 80 ▭

AMA: 2015,Jan,16; 2014,Jan,11; 2013,Aug,13

32659 **with creation of pericardial window or partial resection of pericardial sac for drainage**

🚑 21.2   ⚕ 21.2   **FUD** 090   C 80 ▭

AMA: 2015,Jan,16; 2014,Jan,11; 2013,Aug,13

32661 **with excision of pericardial cyst, tumor, or mass**

🚑 23.2   ⚕ 23.2   **FUD** 090   C 80 ▭

AMA: 2015,Jan,16; 2014,Jan,11; 2013,Aug,13

32662 **with excision of mediastinal cyst, tumor, or mass**

🚑 25.9   ⚕ 25.9   **FUD** 090   C 80 ▭

AMA: 2015,Jan,16; 2014,Jan,11; 2013,Aug,13; 2012,Jan,15-42; 2011,Jan,11

32663 **with lobectomy (single lobe)**

EXCLUDES   *Thoracoscopic segmentectomy (32669)*

🚑 40.7   ⚕ 40.7   **FUD** 090   C 80 ▭ PQ

AMA: 2015,Jan,16; 2014,Jan,11; 2013,Aug,13; 2012,Oct,9-11; 2012,Sep,3-8

32664 **with thoracic sympathectomy**

🚑 24.7   ⚕ 24.7   **FUD** 090   C 80 50 ▭

AMA: 2015,Jan,16; 2014,Jan,11; 2013,Aug,13; 2012,Jan,15-42; 2011,Jan,11

32665 **with esophagomyotomy (Heller type)**

EXCLUDES   *Exploratory thoracoscopy with and without biopsy (32601-32609)*

🚑 36.0   ⚕ 36.0   **FUD** 090   C 80 ▭

AMA: 2015,Jan,16; 2014,Jan,11; 2013,Aug,13

32666 **with therapeutic wedge resection (eg, mass, nodule), initial unilateral**

Code also a more extensive procedure of the lung when performed on the contralateral lung or different lobe with modifier 59 regardless of pathology consultation
Do not report with (32440-32445, 32488, 32671)

🚑 25.3   ⚕ 25.3   **FUD** 090   C 80 PQ

AMA: 2015,Jan,16; 2014,Jan,11; 2013,Aug,13; 2012,Oct,9-11; 2012,Sep,3-8

+ **32667** **with therapeutic wedge resection (eg, mass or nodule), each additional resection, ipsilateral (List separately in addition to code for primary procedure)**

Code also a more extensive procedure of the lung when performed on the contralateral lung or different lobe with modifier 59 regardless of intraoperative pathology consultation
Code first (32666)
Do not report with (32440-32445, 32488, 32671)

🚑 4.59   ⚕ 4.59   **FUD** ZZZ   C 80

AMA: 2015,Jan,16; 2014,Jan,11; 2013,Aug,13; 2012,Oct,9-11; 2012,Sep,3-8

+ **32668** **with diagnostic wedge resection followed by anatomic lung resection (List separately in addition to code for primary procedure)**

INCLUDES   Classification as a diagnostic wedge resection if intraoperative pathology consultation dictates more extensive resection in the same anatomical area
Code first (32440-32488, 32503-32504, 32663, 32669-32671)

🚑 4.58   ⚕ 4.58   **FUD** ZZZ   C 80

AMA: 2015,Jan,16; 2014,Jan,11; 2013,Aug,13; 2012,Oct,9-11; 2012,Sep,3-8

32669 **with removal of a single lung segment (segmentectomy)**

🚑 39.1   ⚕ 39.1   **FUD** 090   C 80 PQ

AMA: 2015,Jan,16; 2014,Jan,11; 2013,Aug,13; 2012,Oct,9-11; 2012,Sep,3-8

Upper lobe   Left lung (two lobes)
Middle lobe
Lower lobe
Diaphragm

32670 **with removal of two lobes (bilobectomy)**

🚑 46.6   ⚕ 46.6   **FUD** 090   C 80 PQ

AMA: 2015,Jan,16; 2014,Jan,11; 2013,Aug,13; 2012,Oct,9-11; 2012,Sep,3-8

32671 **with removal of lung (pneumonectomy)**

🚑 51.9   ⚕ 51.9   **FUD** 090   C 80 PQ

AMA: 2015,Jan,16; 2014,Jan,11; 2013,Aug,13; 2012,Oct,9-11; 2012,Sep,3-8

Respiratory System

32672   32672 — 32997

32672   **with resection-plication for emphysematous lung (bullous or non-bullous) for lung volume reduction (LVRS), unilateral includes any pleural procedure, when performed**
  📷 44.2   ⚷ 44.2   **FUD** 090   C 80 PQ
  AMA: 2015,Jan,16; 2014,Jan,11; 2013,Aug,13; 2012,Oct,9-11; 2012,Sep,3-8

32673   **with resection of thymus, unilateral or bilateral**
  EXCLUDES   *Exploratory thoracoscopy with and without biopsy (32601-32609)*
  Open excision mediastinal cyst (39200)
  Open excision mediastinal tumor (39220)
  Open thymectomy (60520-60522)
  📷 35.4   ⚷ 35.4   **FUD** 090   C 80 PQ
  AMA: 2015,Jan,16; 2014,Jan,11; 2013,Aug,13; 2012,Oct,9-11; 2012,Sep,3-8

+   **32674**   **with mediastinal and regional lymphadenectomy (List separately in addition to code for primary procedure)**
  INCLUDES   Mediastinal lymph nodes:
      Left side:
        Aortopulmonary window
        Inferior pulmonary ligament
        Paraesophageal
        Subcarinal
      Right side:
        Inferior pulmonary ligament
        Paraesophageal
        Paratracheal
        Subcarinal
  EXCLUDES   *Mediastinal and regional lymphadenectomy by thoracotomy (38746)*
  Code first (19260, 31760, 31766, 31786, 32096-32200, 32220-32320, 32440-32491, 32503-32505, 32601-32663, 32666, 32669-32673, 32815, 33025, 33030, 33050-33130, 39200-39220, 39560-39561, 43101, 43112, 43117-43118, 43122-43123, 43351, 60270, 60505)
  📷 6.30   ⚷ 6.30   **FUD** ZZZ   C 80
  AMA: 2015,Jan,16; 2014,May,3; 2014,Jan,11; 2013,Aug,13; 2012,Oct,9-11; 2012,Sep,3-8

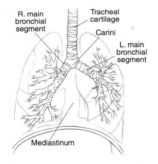

R. main bronchial segment   Tracheal cartilage
Carini
L. main bronchial segment
Mediastinum

32701 Target Delineation for Stereotactic Radiation Therapy

  INCLUDES   Collaboration between the radiation oncologist and surgeon
      Correlation of tumor and contiguous body structures
      Determination of borders and volume of tumor
      Identification of fiducial markers
      Verification of target when fiducial markers are not used
  EXCLUDES   *Fiducial marker insertion (31626, 32553)*
      Radiation oncology services (77295, 77331, 77370, 77373, 77435)
  Do not report when performed by same physician as radiation treatment management (77427-77499)
  Do not report with (77261-77799 [77295, 77385, 77386, 77387, 77424, 77425])

32701   **Thoracic target(s) delineation for stereotactic body radiation therapy (SRS/SBRT), (photon or particle beam), entire course of treatment**
  📷 6.23   ⚷ 6.23   **FUD** XXX   B 80 26
  AMA: 2015,Jun,6

32800-32820 Chest Repair and Reconstruction Procedures

32800   **Repair lung hernia through chest wall**
  📷 27.7   ⚷ 27.7   **FUD** 090   C 80 PQ

32810   **Closure of chest wall following open flap drainage for empyema (Clagett type procedure)**
  📷 26.3   ⚷ 26.3   **FUD** 090   C 80 PQ

32815   **Open closure of major bronchial fistula**
  📷 81.5   ⚷ 81.5   **FUD** 090   C 80 PQ

32820   **Major reconstruction, chest wall (posttraumatic)**
  📷 40.7   ⚷ 40.7   **FUD** 090   C 80

32850-32856 Lung Transplant Procedures

  INCLUDES   Harvesting donor lung(s), cold preservation, preparation of donor lung(s), transplantation into recipient
  EXCLUDES   *Repairs or resection of donor lung(s) (32491, 32505-32507, 35216, 35276)*

32850   **Donor pneumonectomy(s) (including cold preservation), from cadaver donor**
  📷 0.00   ⚷ 0.00   **FUD** XXX   C
  AMA: 1993,Win,1

32851   **Lung transplant, single; without cardiopulmonary bypass**
  📷 95.8   ⚷ 95.8   **FUD** 090   C 80
  AMA: 1993,Win,1

32852   **with cardiopulmonary bypass**
  📷 105.   ⚷ 105.   **FUD** 090   C 80
  AMA: 1993,Win,1

32853   **Lung transplant, double (bilateral sequential or en bloc); without cardiopulmonary bypass**
  📷 133.   ⚷ 133.   **FUD** 090   C 80
  AMA: 1993,Win,1

32854   **with cardiopulmonary bypass**
  📷 142.   ⚷ 142.   **FUD** 090   C 80
  AMA: 1993,Win,1

32855   **Backbench standard preparation of cadaver donor lung allograft prior to transplantation, including dissection of allograft from surrounding soft tissues to prepare pulmonary venous/atrial cuff, pulmonary artery, and bronchus; unilateral**
  📷 0.00   ⚷ 0.00   **FUD** XXX   C 80

32856   **bilateral**
  📷 0.00   ⚷ 0.00   **FUD** XXX   C 80

32900-32997 Chest and Respiratory Procedures

32900   **Resection of ribs, extrapleural, all stages**
  📷 41.4   ⚷ 41.4   **FUD** 090   C 80 PQ

32905   **Thoracoplasty, Schede type or extrapleural (all stages);**
  📷 39.0   ⚷ 39.0   **FUD** 090   C 80 PQ

32906   **with closure of bronchopleural fistula**
  📷 48.2   ⚷ 48.2   **FUD** 090   C 80 PQ
  EXCLUDES   *Open closure of bronchial fistula (32815)*
      Resection first rib for thoracic compression (21615-21616)

32940   **Pneumonolysis, extraperiosteal, including filling or packing procedures**
  📷 36.0   ⚷ 36.0   **FUD** 090   C 80 PQ

32960   **Pneumothorax, therapeutic, intrapleural injection of air**
  📷 2.64   ⚷ 3.61   **FUD** 000   T 62

32997   **Total lung lavage (unilateral)**
  EXCLUDES   *Broncho-alveolar lavage by bronchoscopy (31624)*
  📷 9.87   ⚷ 9.87   **FUD** 000   C 50
  AMA: 2015,Jan,16; 2014,Jan,11

32998-32999 Destruction of Lung Neoplasm

32998   **Ablation therapy for reduction or eradication of 1 or more pulmonary tumor(s) including pleura or chest wall when involved by tumor extension, percutaneous, radiofrequency, unilateral**

    8.31   84.0   **FUD** 000   T 62 80 50

    (76940, 77013, 77022)

32999   **Unlisted procedure, lungs and pleura**

    0.00   0.00   **FUD** YYY   T

    AMA: 2015,Jun,6; 2015,Jan,16; 2014,Jan,11; 2012,Jan,15-42; 2011,Aug,9-10; 2011,Jan,11; 2010,Apr,10

Cardiovascular System

33010 — 33206

33010-33050 Procedures of the Pericardial Sac

> EXCLUDES Surgical thoracoscopy (video-assisted thoracic surgery [VATS]) procedures of pericardium (32601, 32604, 32658-32659, 32661)

33010 **Pericardiocentesis; initial**
☒ (76930)
🔧 3.49   ⚕ 3.49   **FUD** 000
⊙ T A2 ▱
AMA: 2015,Feb,10

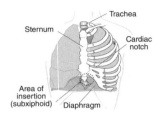

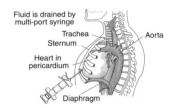

A centesis syringe is inserted into the pericardial sac, either under fluoroscopic guidance or by use of anatomical landmarks, and excess fluid is removed

33011 **subsequent**
☒ (76930)
🔧 3.52   ⚕ 3.52   **FUD** 000
⊙ T A2 80 ▱
AMA: 2015,Feb,10; 2015,Jan,16; 2014,Jan,11; 2010,Sep,6-7

33015 **Tube pericardiostomy**
🔧 14.7   ⚕ 14.7   **FUD** 090
C ▱
AMA: 2015,Jan,16; 2014,Aug,14

33020 **Pericardiotomy for removal of clot or foreign body (primary procedure)**
🔧 25.6   ⚕ 25.6   **FUD** 090
C 80 ▱ PQ
AMA: 1997,Nov,1

33025 **Creation of pericardial window or partial resection for drainage**
> EXCLUDES Surgical thoracoscopy (video-assisted thoracic surgery [VATS]) creation of pericardial window (32659)

🔧 23.2   ⚕ 23.2   **FUD** 090
C 80 ▱ PQ
AMA: 1997,Nov,1

33030 **Pericardiectomy, subtotal or complete; without cardiopulmonary bypass**
> INCLUDES Delorme pericardiectomy

🔧 58.2   ⚕ 58.2   **FUD** 090
C 80 ▱ PQ
AMA: 1997,Nov,1; 1994,Win,1

33031 **with cardiopulmonary bypass**
🔧 71.7   ⚕ 71.7   **FUD** 090
C 80 ▱ PQ
AMA: 1997,Nov,1; 1994,Win,1

33050 **Resection of pericardial cyst or tumor**
> EXCLUDES Open biopsy of pericardium (39010)
> Surgical thoracoscopy (video-assisted thoracic surgery [VATS]) resection of cyst, mass, or tumor of pericardium (32661)

🔧 29.2   ⚕ 29.2   **FUD** 090
C 80 ▱ PQ
AMA: 1997,Nov,1

33120-33130 Neoplasms of Heart

Code also removal of thrombus through a separate heart incision, when performed (33310-33315); append modifier 59 to (33315)

33120 **Excision of intracardiac tumor, resection with cardiopulmonary bypass**
🔧 61.0   ⚕ 61.0   **FUD** 090
C 80 ▱ PQ
AMA: 2015,Jan,16; 2014,Jan,11

33130 **Resection of external cardiac tumor**
🔧 40.3   ⚕ 40.3   **FUD** 090
C 80 ▱ PQ
AMA: 2015,Jan,16; 2014,Jan,11

33140-33141 Transmyocardial Revascularization

33140 **Transmyocardial laser revascularization, by thoracotomy; (separate procedure)**
🔧 46.1   ⚕ 46.1   **FUD** 090
C 80 ▱ PQ
AMA: 2015,Jan,16; 2014,Jan,11; 2012,Jan,15-42; 2011,Jan,11

+ **33141** **performed at the time of other open cardiac procedure(s) (List separately in addition to code for primary procedure)**
Code first (33400-33496, 33510-33536, 33542)
🔧 3.82   ⚕ 3.82   **FUD** ZZZ
C 80 PQ
AMA: 2015,Jan,16; 2014,Jan,11

33202-33203 Placement Epicardial Leads

Code also insertion of pulse generator when performed by same physician/same surgical session (33212-33213, [33221], 33230-33231, 33240)

33202 **Insertion of epicardial electrode(s); open incision (eg, thoracotomy, median sternotomy, subxiphoid approach)**
🔧 22.5   ⚕ 22.5   **FUD** 090
C PQ
AMA: 2015,May,3; 2015,Jan,16; 2014,Nov,5; 2014,Jan,11; 2012,Jun,3-9

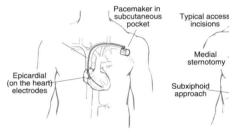

Epicardial electrodes are placed on the outside of the heart in an open procedure

33203 **endoscopic approach (eg, thoracoscopy, pericardioscopy)**
🔧 23.4   ⚕ 23.4   **FUD** 090
C PQ
AMA: 2015,May,3; 2015,Jan,16; 2014,Nov,5; 2014,Jan,11; 2012,Jun,3-9

33206-33214 [33221] Pacemakers

> INCLUDES Dual lead: device that paces and senses in two heart chambers
> Multiple lead: device that paces and senses in three or more heart chambers
> Radiological supervision and interpretation for pacemaker procedure
> Single lead: device that paces and senses in one heart chamber
> Skin pocket revision, when performed
> If revision includes incision/drainage of a wound infection or hematoma code also (10140, 10180, 11042-11047 [11045, 11046])

> EXCLUDES Electrode repositioning:
> Left ventricle (33226)
> Pacemaker (33215)
> Insertion of lead for left ventricular (biventricular) pacing (33224-33225)
> Leadless pacemaker systems (0387T-0391T)

Do not report with codes for device evaluation (93279-93299 [93260, 93261])

33206 **Insertion of new or replacement of permanent pacemaker with transvenous electrode(s); atrial**
> INCLUDES Pulse generator insertion/transvenous electrode placement

Code also removal of pacemaker pulse generator and electrodes when removal and replacement of pulse generator and electrodes is performed (33233, 33234, 33235)
Do not report with (33216-33217, 33227-33229)
🔧 13.3   ⚕ 13.3   **FUD** 090
⊙ J J8 ▱ PQ
AMA: 2015,May,3; 2015,Jan,16; 2014,Nov,5; 2014,Jan,11; 2013,Apr,10-11; 2012,Jun,3-9; 2012,Jan,15-42; 2011,Jan,11

33207 ventricular

INCLUDES Pulse generator insertion/transvenous electrode placement

Code also removal of pacemaker pulse generator and electrodes when removal and replacement of pulse generator and electrodes is performed (33224, 33225, 33233)

Do not report with (33216-33217, 33227-33229)

🚑 14.2 ⚕ 14.2 **FUD** 090 ⊙ J J8 ▢ PQ

AMA: 2015,May,3; 2015,Jan,16; 2014,Nov,5; 2014,Jan,11; 2013,Apr,10-11; 2012,Jun,3-9; 2012,Jan,15-42; 2011,Jan,11

33208 atrial and ventricular

INCLUDES Pulse generator insertion/transvenous electrode placement

Code also removal of pacemaker pulse generator and electrodes when removal and replacement of pulse generator and electrodes is performed (33233, 33234, 33235)

Do not report with (33216-33217, 33227-33229)

🚑 15.4 ⚕ 15.4 **FUD** 090 ⊙ J J8 ▢ PQ

AMA: 2015,May,3; 2015,Jan,16; 2014,Nov,5; 2014,Jan,11; 2013,Apr,10-11; 2012,Jun,3-9; 2012,Jan,15-42; 2011,Jan,11

33210 Insertion or replacement of temporary transvenous single chamber cardiac electrode or pacemaker catheter (separate procedure)

🚑 5.19 ⚕ 5.19 **FUD** 000 ⊙ J J8 ▢

AMA: 2015,May,3; 2015,Jan,16; 2014,Nov,5; 2014,Jan,11; 2013,Jan,6-8; 2012,Jun,3-9; 2011,Aug,3-5

33211 Insertion or replacement of temporary transvenous dual chamber pacing electrodes (separate procedure)

🚑 5.29 ⚕ 5.29 **FUD** 000 ⊙ J J8 ▢

AMA: 2015,May,3; 2015,Jan,16; 2014,Nov,5; 2014,Jan,11; 2012,Jun,3-9; 2011,Aug,3-5

33212 Insertion of pacemaker pulse generator only; with existing single lead

EXCLUDES Removal and replacement of pacemaker pulse generator (33227-33229)

Code also placement of epicardial leads by same physician/same surgical session (33202-33203)

Do not report with (33216-33217, 33233)

🚑 9.64 ⚕ 9.64 **FUD** 090 ⊙ J J8 ▢ PQ

AMA: 2015,May,3; 2015,Jan,16; 2014,Nov,5; 2014,Jan,11; 2012,Jun,3-9; 2012,Jan,15-42; 2011,Jan,11

33213 with existing dual leads

EXCLUDES Removal and replacement of pacemaker pulse generator (33227-33229)

Code also placement of epicardial leads by same physician/same surgical session (33202-33203)

Do not report with (33216-33217, 33233)

🚑 10.0 ⚕ 10.0 **FUD** 090 ⊙ J J8 ▢ PQ

AMA: 2015,May,3; 2015,Jan,16; 2014,Nov,5; 2014,Jan,11; 2012,Jun,3-9; 2012,Jan,15-42; 2011,Jan,11

\# **33221** with existing multiple leads

EXCLUDES Removal and replacement of pacemaker pulse generator (33227-33229)

Code also placement of epicardial leads by same physician/same surgical session (33202-33203)

Do not report with (33216-33217, 33233)

🚑 10.7 ⚕ 10.7 **FUD** 090 ⊙ J J8

AMA: 2015,May,3; 2015,Jan,16; 2014,Nov,5; 2014,Jan,11; 2012,Jun,3-9

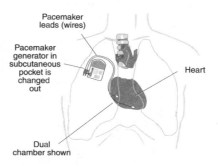

Pacemaker leads (wires)

Pacemaker generator in subcutaneous pocket is changed out

Heart

Dual chamber shown

33214 Upgrade of implanted pacemaker system, conversion of single chamber system to dual chamber system (includes removal of previously placed pulse generator, testing of existing lead, insertion of new lead, insertion of new pulse generator)

Do not report with (33216-33217, 33227-33229)

🚑 14.1 ⚕ 14.1 **FUD** 090 ⊙ J J8 80 ▢ PQ

AMA: 2015,May,3; 2015,Jan,16; 2014,Nov,5; 2014,Jan,11; 2012,Jun,3-9

33215-33249 [33227, 33228, 33229, 33230, 33231, 33262, 33263, 33264] Pacemakers/Implantable Defibrillator/Electrode Insertion/Replacement/Revision/Repair

INCLUDES Dual lead: device that paces and senses in two heart chambers

Multiple lead: device that paces and senses in three or more heart chambers

Radiological supervision and interpretation for pacemaker or pacing cardioverter-defibrillator procedure

Single lead: device that paces and senses in one heart chamber

Skin pocket revision, when performed

If revision includes incision/drainage of a wound infection or hematoma code also (10140, 10180, 11042-11047 [11045, 11046])

EXCLUDES Electrode repositioning:

Left ventricle (33226)

Pacemaker or implantable defibrillator (33215)

Fluoroscopic guidance for lead evaluation without lead change, insertion, or revision (76000)

Insertion of lead for left ventricular (biventricular) pacing (33224-33225)

Removal of leadless pacemaker system (0388T)

Removal of subcutaneous implantable defibrillator electrode ([33272])

Testing of defibrillator threshold (DFT) during follow-up evaluation (93642-93644)

Testing of defibrillator threshold (DFT) during insertion/replacement (93640-93641)

Do not report with codes for device evaluation (93279-93299 [93260, 93261])

33215 Repositioning of previously implanted transvenous pacemaker or implantable defibrillator (right atrial or right ventricular) electrode

🚑 8.97 ⚕ 8.97 **FUD** 090 T G2 ▢ PQ

AMA: 2015,May,3; 2015,Jan,16; 2014,Nov,5; 2014,Jan,11; 2012,Jun,3-9

● New Code ▲ Revised Code ○ Reinstated Ⓜ Maternity ▲ Age Edit Unlisted Not Covered \# Resequenced

⊘ AMA Mod 51 Exempt ⑤⓪ Optum Mod 51 Exempt ⑥③ Mod 63 Exempt ⊙ Mod Sedation + Add-on ▢ CCI PQ PQRS **FUD** Follow-up Days

© 2015 Optum360, LLC (Blue Text) CPT © 2015 American Medical Association. All Rights Reserved. (Black Text) Medicare (Red Text) **111**

33216 **Insertion of a single transvenous electrode, permanent pacemaker or implantable defibrillator**

> EXCLUDES   *Insertion or replacement of a lead for a cardiac venous system (33224-33225)*
> Do not report with (33206-33208, 33212-33213, [33221], 33214, 33227-33229, 33230-33231, 33240, [33262, 33263, 33264], 33249)

🚗 11.0   🔧 11.0   **FUD** 090   ⊙ Ⓙ J8 🖂 P0

AMA: 2015,May,3; 2015,Jan,16; 2014,Nov,5; 2014,Jan,11; 2012,Jun,3-9; 2012,Jan,15-42; 2011,Jan,11

33217 **Insertion of 2 transvenous electrodes, permanent pacemaker or implantable defibrillator**

> EXCLUDES   *Insertion or replacement of a lead for a cardiac venous system (33224-33225)*
> Do not report with (33206-33208, 33212-33213, [33221], 33214, 33227-33229, 33230-33231, 33240, [33262, 33263, 33264], 33249)

🚗 10.8   🔧 10.8   **FUD** 090   ⊙ Ⓙ J8 🖂 P0

AMA: 2015,May,3; 2015,Jan,16; 2014,Nov,5; 2014,Jan,11; 2012,Jun,3-9; 2012,Jan,15-42; 2011,Jan,11

33218 **Repair of single transvenous electrode, permanent pacemaker or implantable defibrillator**

> Code also replacement of implantable defibrillator pulse generator, when performed ([33262, 33263, 33264])
> Code also replacement of pacemaker pulse generator, when performed (33227-33229)

🚗 11.5   🔧 11.5   **FUD** 090   ⊙ Ⓣ 62 🖂 P0

AMA: 2015,May,3; 2015,Jan,16; 2014,Nov,5; 2014,Jan,11; 2012,Jun,3-9; 2012,Jan,15-42; 2011,Jan,11

33220 **Repair of 2 transvenous electrodes for permanent pacemaker or implantable defibrillator**

> Code also modifier 52 Reduced services, when one electrode of a two-chamber system is repaired
> Code also replacement of implantable defibrillator pulse generator, when performed ([33263, 33264])
> Code also replacement of pacemaker pulse generator, when performed (33228-33229)

🚗 11.6   🔧 11.6   **FUD** 090   ⊙ Ⓣ 62 🖂 P0

AMA: 2015,May,3; 2015,Jan,16; 2014,Nov,5; 2014,Jan,11; 2012,Jun,3-9; 2012,Jan,15-42; 2011,Jan,11

33221 **Resequenced code. See code following 33213.**

33222 **Relocation of skin pocket for pacemaker**

> INCLUDES   Formation of the new pocket
> Procedures related to the existing pocket:
> Accessing the pocket
> Incision/drainage of any abscess or hematoma
> Pocket closure
> Code also removal and replacement of an existing generator
> Do not report with (10140, 10180, 11042-11047 [11045, 11046], 13100-13102)

🚗 10.0   🔧 10.0   **FUD** 090   ⊙ Ⓣ A2 🖂 P0

AMA: 2015,May,3; 2015,Jan,16; 2014,Nov,5; 2014,Jan,11; 2012,Jun,3-9

33223 **Relocation of skin pocket for implantable defibrillator**

> INCLUDES   Formation of the new pocket
> Procedures related to the existing pocket:
> Accessing the pocket
> Incision/drainage of any abscess or hematoma
> Pocket closure
> Code also removal and replacement of an existing generator
> Do not report with (10140, 10180, 11042-11047 [11045, 11046], 13100-13102)

🚗 12.1   🔧 12.1   **FUD** 090   ⊙ Ⓣ A2 80 🖂 P0

AMA: 2015,Jan,16; 2014,Nov,5; 2014,Jan,11; 2012,Jun,3-9

33224 **Insertion of pacing electrode, cardiac venous system, for left ventricular pacing, with attachment to previously placed pacemaker or implantable defibrillator pulse generator (including revision of pocket, removal, insertion, and/or replacement of existing generator)**

> Code also placement of epicardial electrode when appropriate (33202-33203)

🚗 14.9   🔧 14.9   **FUD** 000   Ⓙ J8 🖂 P0

AMA: 2015,May,3; 2015,Jan,16; 2014,Nov,5; 2014,Jan,11; 2012,Jun,3-9; 2012,Jan,15-42; 2011,Jan,11

+ **33225** **Insertion of pacing electrode, cardiac venous system, for left ventricular pacing, at time of insertion of implantable defibrillator or pacemaker pulse generator (eg, for upgrade to dual chamber system) (List separately in addition to code for primary procedure)**

> Code first (33206-33208, 33212-33213, [33221], 33214, 33216-33217, 33223, 33228-33229, 33230-33231, 33233, 33234-33235, 33240, [33263, 33264], 33249)
> Code first (33223) for relocation of pocket for implantable defibrillator
> Code first (33222) for relocation of pocket for pacemaker pulse generator

🚗 13.5   🔧 13.5   **FUD** ZZZ   Ⓝ N1 🖂 P0

AMA: 2015,May,3; 2015,Jan,16; 2014,Nov,5; 2014,Jan,11; 2012,Jun,3-9; 2012,Jan,15-42; 2011,Jan,11

33226 **Repositioning of previously implanted cardiac venous system (left ventricular) electrode (including removal, insertion and/or replacement of existing generator)**

🚗 14.3   🔧 14.3   **FUD** 000   Ⓣ 62 🖂 P0

AMA: 2015,May,3; 2015,Jan,16; 2014,Nov,5; 2014,Jan,11; 2012,Jun,3-9

33227 **Resequenced code. See code following 33233.**

33228 **Resequenced code. See code following 33233.**

33229 **Resequenced code. See code before 33234.**

33230 **Resequenced code. See code following 33240.**

33231 **Resequenced code. See code before 33241.**

33233 **Removal of permanent pacemaker pulse generator only**

> EXCLUDES   *Removal and replacement of pacemaker pulse generator and transvenous electrode(s): code 33233 with (33206, 33207, 33208, 33234, 33235)*
> Do not report with (33227-33229)

🚗 7.02   🔧 7.02   **FUD** 090   ⊙ Ⓙ J8 🖂 P0

AMA: 2015,Jan,16; 2014,Nov,5; 2014,Jan,11; 2012,Jun,3-9; 2012,Jan,15-42; 2011,Jan,11

\# **33227** **Removal of permanent pacemaker pulse generator with replacement of pacemaker pulse generator; single lead system**

🚗 10.1   🔧 10.1   **FUD** 090   ⊙ Ⓙ J8

AMA: 2015,Jan,16; 2014,Nov,5; 2014,Jan,11; 2013,Apr,10-11; 2012,Jun,3-9

\# **33228** **dual lead system**

🚗 10.5   🔧 10.5   **FUD** 090   ⊙ Ⓙ J8

AMA: 2015,Jan,16; 2014,Nov,5; 2014,Jan,11; 2013,Apr,10-11; 2012,Jun,3-9

\# **33229** **multiple lead system**

🚗 11.0   🔧 11.0   **FUD** 090   ⊙ Ⓙ J8

AMA: 2015,Jan,16; 2014,Nov,5; 2014,Jan,11; 2013,Apr,10-11; 2012,Jun,3-9

33234 **Removal of transvenous pacemaker electrode(s); single lead system, atrial or ventricular**

EXCLUDES *Removal and replacement of pacemaker pulse generator and transvenous electrode 33234 and 33233 and (33206, 33207, 33208)*
Thoracotomy to remove electrodes (33238, 33243)

Code also pacing electrode insertion in cardiac venous system for pacing of left ventricle during insertion of pulse generator (pacemaker or implantable defibrillator) when performed (33225)

🚑 14.3 ⚗ 14.3 **FUD** 090 ⊙ 02 G2 ▭ PQ

AMA: 2015,Jan,16; 2014,Nov,5; 2014,Jan,11; 2012,Oct,14; 2012,Jun,3-9

33235 **dual lead system**

EXCLUDES *Removal and replacement of pacemaker pulse generator and transvenous electrode(s) 33235 and 33233 and (33206, 33207, 33208, 33233, 33235)*
Thoracotomy to remove electrode(s) (33238, 33243)

Code also pacing electrode insertion in cardiac venous system for pacing of left ventricle during insertion of pulse generator (pacemaker or implantable defibrillator) when performed (33225)

🚑 18.7 ⚗ 18.7 **FUD** 090 ⊙ 02 G2 ▭ PQ

AMA: 2015,Jan,16; 2014,Nov,5; 2014,Jan,11; 2013,Dec,14; 2012,Oct,14; 2012,Jun,3-9

33236 **Removal of permanent epicardial pacemaker and electrodes by thoracotomy; single lead system, atrial or ventricular**

EXCLUDES *Removal of implantable defibrillator electrode(s) by thoracotomy (33243)*
Removal of transvenous electrodes by thoracotomy (33238)
Removal of transvenous pacemaker electrodes, single or dual lead system; without thoracotomy (33234, 33235)

🚑 22.7 ⚗ 22.7 **FUD** 090 C 80 ▭ PQ

AMA: 2015,Jan,16; 2014,Nov,5; 2014,Jan,11; 2012,Jun,3-9

33237 **dual lead system**

EXCLUDES *Removal of implantable defibrillator electrode(s) by thoracotomy (33243)*
Removal of transvenous electrodes by thoracotomy (33238)
Removal of transvenous pacemaker electrodes, single or dual lead system; without thoracotomy (33234, 33235)

🚑 24.4 ⚗ 24.4 **FUD** 090 C 80 ▭ PQ

AMA: 2015,Jan,16; 2014,Nov,5; 2014,Jan,11; 2012,Jun,3-9

33238 **Removal of permanent transvenous electrode(s) by thoracotomy**

EXCLUDES *Removal of implantable defibrillator electrode(s) by thoracotomy (33243)*
Removal of transvenous pacemaker electrodes, single or dual lead system; without thoracotomy (33234, 33235)

🚑 27.1 ⚗ 27.1 **FUD** 090 C 80 ▭ PQ

AMA: 2015,Jan,16; 2014,Nov,5; 2014,Jan,11; 2012,Jun,3-9

33240 **Insertion of implantable defibrillator pulse generator only; with existing single lead**

EXCLUDES *Removal and replacement of implantable defibrillator pulse generator ([33262, 33263, 33264])*

Code also placement of epicardial leads by same physician/same surgical session as generator insertion (33202-33203)
Do not report with (33216-33217, [33271], 93260, 93261)

🚑 10.9 ⚗ 10.9 **FUD** 090 ⊙ J J8 ▭ PQ

AMA: 2015,Jan,16; 2014,Nov,5; 2014,Jan,11; 2012,Jun,3-9; 2012,Jan,15-42; 2011,Jan,11

33230 **with existing dual leads**

EXCLUDES *Removal and replacement of implantable defibrillator pulse generator ([33262, 33263, 33264])*

Code also placement of epicardial leads by same physician/same surgical session as generator insertion (33202-33203)
Do not report with (33216-33217)

🚑 11.4 ⚗ 11.4 **FUD** 090 ⊙ J J8

AMA: 2015,Jan,16; 2014,Nov,5; 2014,Jan,11; 2012,Jun,3-9

33231 **with existing multiple leads**

EXCLUDES *Removal and replacement of implantable defibrillator pulse generator ([33262, 33263, 33264])*

Code also placement of epicardial leads by same physician/same surgical session as generator placement (33202-33203)
Do not report with (33216-33217)

🚑 12.0 ⚗ 12.0 **FUD** 090 ⊙ J J8

AMA: 2015,Jan,16; 2014,Nov,5; 2014,Jan,11; 2012,Jun,3-9

R. atrium — Aorta — L. coronary artery — Right coronary artery — Subclavian vein — Extravascular or vascular electrode leads — Pulse generator (pacemaker) in subcutaneous pocket — Thoracotomy incision — Electrodes on surface of heart

33241 **Removal of implantable defibrillator pulse generator only**

Code also electrode removal by thoracotomy (33243)
Code also insertion of subcutaneous defibrillator system and removal of subcutaneous defibrillator lead, when performed ([33270], [33272])
Code also removal of defibrillator leads and insertion of defibrillator system, when performed (33243, 33244, 33249)
Code also transvenous removal of electrode(s) (33244)
Do not report with (33230-33231, 33240, [33262, 33263, 33264], 93260, 93261)

🚑 6.61 ⚗ 6.61 **FUD** 090 ⊙ 02 G2 ▭ PQ

AMA: 2015,Jan,16; 2014,Nov,5; 2014,Jan,11; 2012,Jun,3-9

33262 **Removal of implantable defibrillator pulse generator with replacement of implantable defibrillator pulse generator; single lead system**

EXCLUDES *Repair of implantable defibrillator pulse generator and/or leads (33218, 33220)*

Code also electrode(s) removal by thoracotomy (33243)
Code also subcutaneous electrode removal ([33272])
Code also transvenous removal of electrode(s) (33244)
Do not report with (33216-33217, 33241, [33271], 93260, 93261)

🚑 11.1 ⚗ 11.1 **FUD** 090 ⊙ J J8

AMA: 2015,Jan,16; 2014,Nov,5; 2014,Jan,11; 2012,Jun,3-9

33263 **dual lead system**

EXCLUDES *Repair of implantable defibrillator pulse generator and/or leads (33218, 33220)*

Code also removal of electrodes by thoracotomy (33243)
Code also subcutaneous electrode removal ([33272])
Code also transvenous removal of electrodes (33244)
Do not report with (33216-33217, 33241)

🚑 11.5 ⚗ 11.5 **FUD** 090 ⊙ J J8

AMA: 2015,Jan,16; 2014,Nov,5; 2014,Jan,11; 2013,Dec,16; 2012,Jun,3-9

33264 **multiple lead system**

EXCLUDES *Repair of implantable defibrillator pulse generator and/or leads (33218, 33220)*

Code also removal of electrodes by thoracotomy (33243)
Code also subcutaneous electrode removal ([33272])
Code also transvenous removal of electrodes (33244)
Do not report with (33216-33217, 33241)

🚑 12.0 ⚗ 12.0 **FUD** 090 ⊙ J J8

AMA: 2015,Jan,16; 2014,Nov,5; 2014,Jan,11; 2013,Dec,16; 2012,Jun,3-9

33243 **Removal of single or dual chamber implantable defibrillator electrode(s); by thoracotomy**

EXCLUDES *Transvenous removal of defibrillator electrode(s) (33244)*

Code also removal of defibrillator generator and insertion/replacement of defibrillator system (generator and leads), when performed (33241, 33249)

🚑 39.8 ⚗ 39.8 **FUD** 090 C 80 ▭ PQ

AMA: 2015,Jan,16; 2014,Nov,5; 2014,Jan,11; 2012,Jun,3-9

33244   **by transvenous extraction**

> EXCLUDES   *Thoracotomy to remove electrodes (33238, 33243)*
>
> Code also removal of defibrillator generator and
>   insertion/replacement of defibrillator system (generator
>   and leads), when performed (33241, 33249)
>
> 💠 25.1   ⚖ 25.1   **FUD** 090   ⊙ 02 🔲 P0
>
> **AMA:** 2015,Jan,16; 2014,Nov,5; 2014,Jan,11; 2012,Jun,3-9

33249   **Insertion or replacement of permanent implantable defibrillator system, with transvenous lead(s), single or dual chamber**

> Code also removal of defibrillator generator and removal of leads
>   (by thoracotomy or transvenous), when performed (33241,
>   33243, 33244)
> Code also removal of defibrillator generator when upgrading
>   from single to dual-chamber system (33241)
> Do not report with (33216-33217)
>
> 💠 26.8   ⚖ 26.8   **FUD** 090   ⊙ J J8 🔲 P0
>
> **AMA:** 2015,Jan,16; 2014,Nov,5; 2014,Jan,11; 2012,Jun,3-9

[33270, 33271, 33272, 33273] Subcutaneous Implantable Defibrillator

> Do not report with (93260, 93261)
> Do not report defibrillation threshold testing (DFT) during subcutaneous defibrillator
>   implant (93640-93641)

33270   **Insertion or replacement of permanent subcutaneous implantable defibrillator system, with subcutaneous electrode, including defibrillation threshold evaluation, induction of arrhythmia, evaluation of sensing for arrhythmia termination, and programming or reprogramming of sensing or therapeutic parameters, when performed**

> Code also removal of defibrillator generator and subcutaneous
>   electrode, when performed (33241, [33272])
> Do not report with ([33271], 93644)
>
> 💠 17.0   ⚖ 17.0   **FUD** 090   J J8
>
> **AMA:** 2015,Jan,16; 2014,Nov,5

33271   **Insertion of subcutaneous implantable defibrillator electrode**

> Do not report with (33240, [33262], [33270])
>
> 💠 14.3   ⚖ 14.3   **FUD** 090   J J8
>
> **AMA:** 2015,Jan,16; 2014,Nov,5

33272   **Removal of subcutaneous implantable defibrillator electrode**

> Code also removal defibrillator generator and
>   insertion/replacement subcutaneous defibrillator system
>   (generator and leads), when performed (33241, [33270])
> Code also removal of defibrillator generator with replacement,
>   when performed ([33262])
> Code also removal of defibrillator generator (without
>   replacement), when performed (33241)
>
> 💠 10.5   ⚖ 10.5   **FUD** 090   02
>
> **AMA:** 2015,Jan,16; 2014,Nov,5

33273   **Repositioning of previously implanted subcutaneous implantable defibrillator electrode**

> 💠 11.6   ⚖ 11.6   **FUD** 090   T 62
>
> **AMA:** 2015,Jan,16; 2014,Nov,5

33250-33251 Surgical Ablation Arrhythmogenic Foci, Supraventricular

> INCLUDES   Procedures using cryotherapy, laser, microwave, radiofrequency, and
>   ultrasound

33250   **Operative ablation of supraventricular arrhythmogenic focus or pathway (eg, Wolff-Parkinson-White, atrioventricular node re-entry), tract(s) and/or focus (foci); without cardiopulmonary bypass**

> EXCLUDES   *Pacing and mapping during surgery by other provider
>   (93631)*
>
> 💠 43.0   ⚖ 43.0   **FUD** 090   C 80 🔲 P0
>
> **AMA:** 2015,Jan,16; 2014,Jan,11

33251   **with cardiopulmonary bypass**

> 💠 47.2   ⚖ 47.2   **FUD** 090   C 80 🔲 P0
>
> **AMA:** 2015,Jan,16; 2014,Jan,11

33254-33256 Surgical Ablation Arrhythmogenic Foci, Atrial (e.g., Maze)

> INCLUDES   Excision or isolation of the left atrial appendage
>   Procedures using cryotherapy, laser, microwave, radiofrequency, and
>   ultrasound
> Do not report with (32100, 32551, 33120, 33130, 33210-33211, 33400-33507,
>   33510-33523, 33533-33548, 33600-33853, 33860-33864, 33910-33920)
> Do not report with any procedure involving median sternotomy or cardiopulmonary
>   bypass

33254   **Operative tissue ablation and reconstruction of atria, limited (eg, modified maze procedure)**

> 💠 39.6   ⚖ 39.6   **FUD** 090   C 80 P0
>
> **AMA:** 2015,Jan,16; 2014,Jan,11

33255   **Operative tissue ablation and reconstruction of atria, extensive (eg, maze procedure); without cardiopulmonary bypass**

> 💠 47.7   ⚖ 47.7   **FUD** 090   C 80 P0
>
> **AMA:** 2015,Jan,16; 2014,Jan,11

33256   **with cardiopulmonary bypass**

> 💠 56.7   ⚖ 56.7   **FUD** 090   C 80 P0
>
> **AMA:** 2015,Jan,16; 2014,Jan,11

33257-33259 Surgical Ablation Arrhythmogenic Foci, Atrial, with Other Heart Procedure(s)

> Do not report with (32551, 33210-33211, 33254-33256, 33265-33266)

+   **33257**   **Operative tissue ablation and reconstruction of atria, performed at the time of other cardiac procedure(s), limited (eg, modified maze procedure) (List separately in addition to code for primary procedure)**

> 💠 16.9   ⚖ 16.9   **FUD** ZZZ   C 80
>
> Code first (33120-33130, 33250-33251, 33261, 33300-33335,
>   33400-33496, 33500-33507, 33510-33516, 33533-33548,
>   33600-33619, 33641-33697, 33702-33732, 33735-33767,
>   33770-33814, 33840-33877, 33910-33922, 33925-33926,
>   33935-33945, 33975-33980)

+   **33258**   **Operative tissue ablation and reconstruction of atria, performed at the time of other cardiac procedure(s), extensive (eg, maze procedure), without cardiopulmonary bypass (List separately in addition to code for primary procedure)**

> 💠 19.1   ⚖ 19.1   **FUD** ZZZ   C 80
>
> Code first (33130, 33250, 33300, 33310, 33320-33321, 33330,
>   33401, 33414-33417, 33420, 33470-33471, 33501-33503,
>   33510-33516, 33533-33536, 33690, 33735, 33737,
>   33800-33813, 33840-33852, 33915, 33925)

+   **33259**   **Operative tissue ablation and reconstruction of atria, performed at the time of other cardiac procedure(s), extensive (eg, maze procedure), with cardiopulmonary bypass (List separately in addition to code for primary procedure)**

> 💠 24.5   ⚖ 24.5   **FUD** ZZZ   C 80
>
> Code first (33120, 33251, 33261, 33305, 33315, 33322, 33335,
>   33400, 33403-33413, 33422-33468, 33474-33478, 33496,
>   33500, 33504-33507, 33510-33516, 33533-33548,
>   33600-33688, 33692-33722, 33730, 33732, 33736,
>   33750-33767, 33770-33781, 33786-33788, 33814, 33853,
>   33860-33877, 33910, 33916-33922, 33926, 33935, 33945,
>   33975-33980)

26/TC PC/TC Comp Only	A2-Z3 ASC Pmt	50 Bilateral	♂ Male Only	♀ Female Only	💠 Facility RVU	⚖ Non-Facility RVU
AMA: CPT Asst	**CMS:** Pub 100	A-Y OPPSI	80/80 Surg Assist Allowed / w/Doc		🔲 Lab Crosswalk	📻 Radiology Crosswalk

114   Medicare (Red Text)   CPT © 2015 American Medical Association. All Rights Reserved. (Black Text)   © 2015 Optum360, LLC (Blue Text)

33261-33264 Surgical Ablation Arrhythmogenic Foci, Ventricular

33261   **Operative ablation of ventricular arrhythmogenic focus with cardiopulmonary bypass**
    🔲 47.2   ⚖ 47.2   **FUD** 090   [C] [80] [▭] [P0]
AMA: 2015,Jan,16; 2014,Jan,11

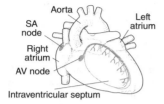

Impulse centers that are causing arrhythmia are treated with ablation

Aorta
SA node
Left atrium
Right atrium
AV node
Intraventricular septum

Bypass schematic

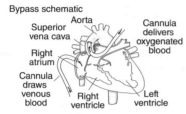

Superior vena cava
Aorta
Cannula delivers oxygenated blood
Right atrium
Cannula draws venous blood
Right ventricle
Left ventricle

33262   Resequenced code. See code following 33241.

33263   Resequenced code. See code following 33241.

33264   Resequenced code. See code before 33243.

33265-33273 Surgical Ablation Arrhythmogenic Foci, Endoscopic

Do not report with (32551, 33210-33211)

33265   **Endoscopy, surgical; operative tissue ablation and reconstruction of atria, limited (eg, modified maze procedure), without cardiopulmonary bypass**
    🔲 39.4   ⚖ 39.4   **FUD** 090   [C] [80]
AMA: 2015,Jan,16; 2014,Jan,11

33266   **operative tissue ablation and reconstruction of atria, extensive (eg, maze procedure), without cardiopulmonary bypass**
    🔲 53.8   ⚖ 53.8   **FUD** 090   [C] [80]
AMA: 2015,Jan,16; 2014,Jan,11

33270   Resequenced code. See code following 33249.

33271   Resequenced code. See code following 33249.

33272   Resequenced code. See code following 33249.

33273   Resequenced code. See code following 33249.

33282-33284 Implantable Loop Recorder

33282   **Implantation of patient-activated cardiac event recorder**
    [INCLUDES]   Initial programming of device
    [EXCLUDES]   Subsequent electronic analysis and/or reprogramming of device (93285, 93291, 93298-93299)
    🔲 6.90   ⚖ 6.90   **FUD** 090   ⊙ [J] [J8] [▭]
AMA: 2015,Jan,16; 2014,Jan,11; 2012,Jan,15-42; 2011,Jan,11

33284   **Removal of an implantable, patient-activated cardiac event recorder**
    🔲 6.12   ⚖ 6.12   **FUD** 090   ⊙ [02] [G2] [▭]
AMA: 2015,Jan,16; 2014,Jan,11

33300-33315 Procedures for Injury of the Heart

[INCLUDES]   Procedures with and without cardiopulmonary bypass
[EXCLUDES]   *Cardiac assist services (33946-33949, 33967-33983, 33990-33993)*

33300   **Repair of cardiac wound; without bypass**
    🔲 71.2   ⚖ 71.2   **FUD** 090   [C] [80] [▭] [P0]
AMA: 1997,Nov,1

33305   **with cardiopulmonary bypass**
    🔲 119.   ⚖ 119.   **FUD** 090   [C] [80] [▭] [P0]
AMA: 1997,Nov,1

33310   **Cardiotomy, exploratory (includes removal of foreign body, atrial or ventricular thrombus); without bypass**
    Do not report with other cardiac procedures unless separate incision into heart is necessary in order to remove thrombus
    🔲 34.8   ⚖ 34.8   **FUD** 090   [C] [80] [▭] [P0]
AMA: 1997,Nov,1

33315   **with cardiopulmonary bypass**
    Code also excision of thrombus with cardiopulmonary bypass and append modifier 59 if separate incision is required with (33120, 33130, 33420-33430, 33460-33468, 33496, 33542, 33545, 33641-33647, 33670, 33681, 33975-33980)
    Do not report with other cardiac procedures unless separate incision into heart is necessary in order to remove thrombus
    🔲 55.7   ⚖ 55.7   **FUD** 090   [C] [80] [▭] [P0]
AMA: 2015,Jan,16; 2014,Jan,11; 2012,Jan,15-42; 2011,Jan,11; 2010,Dec,12

33320-33335 Procedures for Injury of the Aorta/Great Vessels

33320   **Suture repair of aorta or great vessels; without shunt or cardiopulmonary bypass**
    🔲 30.9   ⚖ 30.9   **FUD** 090   [C] [80] [▭] [P0]
AMA: 2015,Jan,16; 2014,Jan,11

33321   **with shunt bypass**
    🔲 35.0   ⚖ 35.0   **FUD** 090   [C] [80] [▭] [P0]
AMA: 1997,Nov,1; 1994,Win,1

33322   **with cardiopulmonary bypass**
    🔲 40.3   ⚖ 40.3   **FUD** 090   [C] [80] [▭] [P0]
AMA: 2015,Jan,16; 2014,Jan,11

33330   **Insertion of graft, aorta or great vessels; without shunt, or cardiopulmonary bypass**
    🔲 41.7   ⚖ 41.7   **FUD** 090   [C] [80] [▭]
AMA: 1997,Nov,1; 1994,Win,1

33335   **with cardiopulmonary bypass**
    🔲 55.0   ⚖ 55.0   **FUD** 090   [C] [80] [▭] [P0]
AMA: 1997,Nov,1

33361-33369 Transcatheter Aortic Valve Replacement

CMS: 100-3,20.32 Transcatheter Aortic Valve Replacement (TAVR); 100-4,32,290.1.1 Coding Requirements for TAVR Services; 100-4,32,290.2 Claims Processing for TAVR/ Professional Claims; 100-4,32,290.3 Claims Processing TAVR Inpatient; 100-4,32,290.4 Payment of TAVR for MA Plan Participants

INCLUDES Access and implantation of the aortic valve (33361-33366)
Access sheath placement
Advancement of valve delivery system
Arteriotomy closure
Balloon aortic valvuloplasty
Cardiac or open arterial approach
Deployment of valve
Percutaneous access
Temporary pacemaker
Valve repositioning when necessary
Radiology procedures:
    Angiography during and after procedure
    Assessment of access site for closure
    Documentation of completion of the intervention
    Guidance for valve placement
    Supervision and interpretation

EXCLUDES *Percutaneous coronary interventional procedures*
Transvascular ventricular support (33967, 33970, 33973, 33975-33976, 33990-33993, 33999)

Code also add-on codes for cardiopulmonary bypass, when appropriate (33367-33369)
Code also cardiac catheterization services for purposes other than TAVR/TAVI
Code also diagnostic coronary angiography at a different session from the interventional procedure
Code also diagnostic coronary angiography at the same time as TAVR/TAVI when:
  A previous study is available, but documentation states the patient's condition has changed since the previous study, visualization of the anatomy/pathology is inadequate, or a change occurs during the procedure warranting additional evaluation of an area outside the current target area
  No previous catheter-based coronary angiography study is available, and a full diagnostic study is performed, with the decision to perform the intervention based on that study
Code also modifier 59 when diagnostic coronary angiography procedures are performed as separate and distinct procedural services on the same day or session as TAVR/TAVI
Code also modifier 62 as all TAVI/TAVR procedures require the work of two physicians
Do not report separately when included in the TAVR/TAVI service (93452-93453, 93458-93461, 93567)

33361   **Transcatheter aortic valve replacement (TAVR/TAVI) with prosthetic valve; percutaneous femoral artery approach**
Code also cardiopulmonary bypass when performed (33367-33369)
🚗 39.5   ✂ 39.5   **FUD** 000   C 80
AMA: 2015,Mar,9; 2015,Jan,16; 2014,Jul,8; 2014,Jan,11; 2014,Jan,5; 2013,Jan,6-8

33362   **open femoral artery approach**
Code also cardiopulmonary bypass when performed (33367-33369)
🚗 43.2   ✂ 43.2   **FUD** 000   C 80
AMA: 2015,Mar,9; 2015,Jan,16; 2014,Jul,8; 2014,Jan,11; 2014,Jan,5; 2013,Jan,6-8

33363   **open axillary artery approach**
Code also cardiopulmonary bypass when performed (33367-33369)
🚗 45.4   ✂ 45.4   **FUD** 000   C 80
AMA: 2015,Mar,9; 2015,Jan,16; 2014,Jul,8; 2014,Jan,11; 2014,Jan,5; 2013,Jan,6-8

33364   **open iliac artery approach**
Code also cardiopulmonary bypass when performed (33367-33369)
🚗 47.0   ✂ 47.0   **FUD** 000   C 80
AMA: 2015,Mar,9; 2015,Jan,16; 2014,Jul,8; 2014,Jan,11; 2014,Jan,5; 2013,Jan,6-8

33365   **transaortic approach (eg, median sternotomy, mediastinotomy)**
Code also cardiopulmonary bypass when performed (33367-33369)
🚗 51.8   ✂ 51.8   **FUD** 000   C 80
AMA: 2015,Mar,9; 2015,Jan,16; 2014,Jul,8; 2014,Jan,11; 2014,Jan,5; 2013,Jan,6-8

33366   **transapical exposure (eg, left thoracotomy)**
Code also cardiopulmonary bypass when performed (33367-33369)
🚗 56.0   ✂ 56.0   **FUD** 000   C 80
AMA: 2015,Mar,9; 2015,Jan,16; 2014,Jul,8; 2014,Jan,5

+ 33367   **cardiopulmonary bypass support with percutaneous peripheral arterial and venous cannulation (eg, femoral vessels) (List separately in addition to code for primary procedure)**
Code first (33361-33366, 33418, 33477)
Do not report with (33368-33369)
🚗 18.1   ✂ 18.1   **FUD** ZZZ   C 80
AMA: 2015,Jan,16; 2013,Jan,6-8

+ 33368   **cardiopulmonary bypass support with open peripheral arterial and venous cannulation (eg, femoral, iliac, axillary vessels) (List separately in addition to code for primary procedure)**
Code first (33361-33366, 33418, 33477)
Do not report with (33367, 33369)
🚗 21.8   ✂ 21.8   **FUD** ZZZ   C 80
AMA: 2015,Jan,16; 2013,Jan,6-8

+ 33369   **cardiopulmonary bypass support with central arterial and venous cannulation (eg, aorta, right atrium, pulmonary artery) (List separately in addition to code for primary procedure)**
Code first (33361-33366, 33418, 33477)
Do not report with (33367-33368)
🚗 28.8   ✂ 28.8   **FUD** ZZZ   C 80
AMA: 2015,Jan,16; 2013,Jan,6-8

33400-33415 Aortic Valve Procedures

33400   **Valvuloplasty, aortic valve; open, with cardiopulmonary bypass**
🚗 66.3   ✂ 66.3   **FUD** 090   C 80 ▭ P0
AMA: 2015,Jan,16; 2014,Jan,11

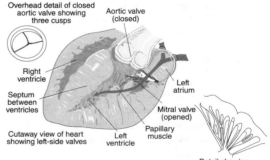

Overhead detail of closed aortic valve showing three cusps
Aortic valve (closed)
Right ventricle
Septum between ventricles
Cutaway view of heart showing left-side valves
Left ventricle
Left atrium
Mitral valve (opened)
Papillary muscle
Detail showing closed valve leaflet and chordae tendineae

33401   **open, with inflow occlusion**
🚗 42.0   ✂ 42.0   **FUD** 090   63 C 80 ▭ P0
AMA: 2015,Jan,16; 2014,Jan,11

33403   **using transventricular dilation, with cardiopulmonary bypass**
🚗 43.1   ✂ 43.1   **FUD** 090   63 C 80 ▭ P0
AMA: 2015,Jan,16; 2014,Jan,11

33404   **Construction of apical-aortic conduit**
🚗 51.6   ✂ 51.6   **FUD** 090   C 80 ▭ P0
AMA: 2015,Jan,16; 2014,Jan,11; 2012,Jan,15-42; 2011,Jan,11

33405   **Replacement, aortic valve, with cardiopulmonary bypass; with prosthetic valve other than homograft or stentless valve**
EXCLUDES *Valvotomy of aortic valve:*
  With cardiopulmonary bypass (33403)
  With inflow occlusion (33401)
🚗 66.0   ✂ 66.0   **FUD** 090   C 80 ▭ P0
AMA: 2015,Jan,16; 2014,Jan,11; 2013,Jan,6-8; 2011,Aug,3-5

33406 **with allograft valve (freehand)**

EXCLUDES *Valvotomy of aortic valve:*
With cardiopulmonary bypass (33403)
With inflow occlusion (33401)

83.6   83.6   **FUD** 090   C 80 🖙 PQ

AMA: 2015,Jan,16; 2014,Jan,11; 2011,Aug,3-5

33410 **with stentless tissue valve**

73.8   73.8   **FUD** 090   C 80 🖙 PQ

AMA: 2015,Jan,16; 2014,Jan,11; 2011,Aug,3-5

33411 **Replacement, aortic valve; with aortic annulus enlargement, noncoronary sinus**

97.6   97.6   **FUD** 090   C 80 🖙 PQ

AMA: 2015,Jan,16; 2014,Jan,11; 2012,Jan,15-42; 2011,Aug,3-5

Replacement valve   19 mm

The aortic valve is replaced

Tricuspid valve
Noncoronary leaflet
Mitral valve
Incision line to widen annulus
R. coronary artery
Incision
Valve annulus
Aortic valve (replaced)
Pulmonary valve
L. coronary artery

Overhead schematic of major heart valves

33412 **with transventricular aortic annulus enlargement (Konno procedure)**

92.5   92.5   **FUD** 090   C 80 🖙 PQ

AMA: 2015,Jan,16; 2014,Jan,11; 2011,Aug,3-5

33413 **by translocation of autologous pulmonary valve with allograft replacement of pulmonary valve (Ross procedure)**

95.4   95.4   **FUD** 090   C 80 🖙 PQ

AMA: 2015,Jan,16; 2014,Jan,11; 2011,Aug,3-5

33414 **Repair of left ventricular outflow tract obstruction by patch enlargement of the outflow tract**

62.5   62.5   **FUD** 090   C 80 🖙 PQ

AMA: 2015,Jan,16; 2014,Jan,11

33415 **Resection or incision of subvalvular tissue for discrete subvalvular aortic stenosis**

59.1   59.1   **FUD** 090   C 80 🖙 PQ

AMA: 2015,Jan,16; 2014,Jan,11

33416 Ventriculectomy

CMS: 100-3,20.26 Partial Ventriculectomy

EXCLUDES *Percutaneous transcatheter septal reduction therapy (93583)*

33416 **Ventriculomyotomy (-myectomy) for idiopathic hypertrophic subaortic stenosis (eg, asymmetric septal hypertrophy)**

59.1   59.1   **FUD** 090   C 80 🖙 PQ

AMA: 2015,Jan,16; 2014,Jan,11

33417 Repair of Supravalvular Stenosis by Aortoplasty

33417 **Aortoplasty (gusset) for supravalvular stenosis**

48.2   48.2   **FUD** 090   C 80 🖙 PQ

AMA: 2015,Jan,16; 2014,Jan,11

33418-33419 Transcatheter Mitral Valve Procedures

INCLUDES Access sheath placement
Advancement of valve delivery system
Deployment of valve
Radiology procedures:
   Angiography during and after procedure
   Documentation of completion of the intervention
   Guidance for valve placement
   Supervision and interpretation
Valve repositioning when necessary

EXCLUDES *Cardiac catheterization services for purposes other than TMVR*
Diagnostic angiography at different session from interventional procedure
Percutaneous coronary interventional procedures

Code also cardiopulmonary bypass:
  Central (33369)
  Open peripheral (33368)
  Percutaneous peripheral (33367)

Code also diagnostic coronary angiography and cardiac catheterization procedures when:
  No previous study available and full diagnostic study performed
  Previous study inadequate or patient's clinical indication for the study changed prior to or during the procedure
  Use modifier 59 with cardiac catheterization procedures when on same day or same session as TMVR

Code also transvascular ventricular support:
  Balloon pump (33967, 33970, 33973)
  Ventricular assist device (33990-33993)

33418 **Transcatheter mitral valve repair, percutaneous approach, including transseptal puncture when performed; initial prosthesis**

54.0   54.0   **FUD** 090   C 80

Code also left heart catheterization when performed by transapical puncture (93462)

+ **33419** **additional prosthesis(es) during same session (List separately in addition to code for primary procedure)**

12.6   12.6   **FUD** ZZZ   N NI 80

EXCLUDES *Percutaneous approach through the coronary sinus for TMVR (0345T)*

Code first (33418)
Do not report more than one time per session

33420-33430 Mitral Valve Procedures

Code also removal of thrombus through a separate heart incision, when performed (33310-33315); append modifier 59 to (33315)

33420 **Valvotomy, mitral valve; closed heart**

41.9   41.9   **FUD** 090   C 🖙 PQ

AMA: 2015,Jan,16; 2014,Jan,11

33422 **open heart, with cardiopulmonary bypass**

48.7   48.7   **FUD** 090   C 80 🖙 PQ

AMA: 2015,Jan,16; 2014,Jan,11

33425 **Valvuloplasty, mitral valve, with cardiopulmonary bypass;**

79.4   79.4   **FUD** 090   C 80 🖙 PQ

AMA: 2015,Jan,16; 2014,Jan,11; 2012,Jan,15-42; 2011,Jan,11

33426 **with prosthetic ring**

69.2   69.2   **FUD** 090   C 80 🖙 PQ

AMA: 2015,Jan,16; 2014,Jan,11

33427 **radical reconstruction, with or without ring**

71.0   71.0   **FUD** 090   C 80 🖙 PQ

AMA: 2015,Jan,16; 2014,Jan,11

33430 **Replacement, mitral valve, with cardiopulmonary bypass**

81.3   81.3   **FUD** 090   C 80 🖙 PQ

AMA: 2015,Jan,16; 2014,Jan,11

33460-33468 Tricuspid Valve Procedures

Code also removal of thrombus through a separate heart incision, when performed (33310-33315); append modifier 59 to (33315)

33460 **Valvectomy, tricuspid valve, with cardiopulmonary bypass**

71.1   71.1   **FUD** 090   C 80 🖙 PQ

AMA: 2015,Jan,16; 2014,Jan,11

33463 **Valvuloplasty, tricuspid valve; without ring insertion**

90.0   90.0   **FUD** 090   C 80 🖙 PQ

AMA: 2015,Jan,16; 2014,Jan,11

● New Code   ▲ Revised Code   ○ Reinstated   M Maternity   A Age Edit   Unlisted   Not Covered   # Resequenced
⊘ AMA Mod 51 Exempt   51 Optum Mod 51 Exempt   63 Mod 63 Exempt   ⊙ Mod Sedation   + Add-on   🖙 CCI   PQ PQRS   FUD Follow-up Days

© 2015 Optum360, LLC (Blue Text)   CPT © 2015 American Medical Association. All Rights Reserved. (Black Text)   Medicare (Red Text)   **117**

33464 with ring insertion
🔳 71.0　✂ 71.0　**FUD** 090
Ⓒ 80 ▢ ℗
AMA: 2015,Jan,16; 2014,Jan,11

33465 Replacement, tricuspid valve, with cardiopulmonary bypass
🔳 80.2　✂ 80.2　**FUD** 090
Ⓒ 80 ▢ ℗
AMA: 2015,Jan,16; 2014,Jan,11

33468 Tricuspid valve repositioning and plication for Ebstein anomaly
🔳 71.3　✂ 71.3　**FUD** 090
Ⓒ 80 ▢ ℗
AMA: 2015,Jan,16; 2014,Jan,11

33470-33474 Pulmonary Valvotomy

INCLUDES　Brock's operation
Code also the concurrent ligation/takedown of a systemic-to-pulmonary artery shunt (33924)

33470 Valvotomy, pulmonary valve, closed heart; transventricular
🔳 35.9　✂ 35.9　**FUD** 090
㉓ Ⓒ 80 ▢ ℗
AMA: 2015,Jan,16; 2014,Jan,11

33471 via pulmonary artery
EXCLUDES　*Percutaneous valvuloplasty of pulmonary valve (92990)*
🔳 40.4　✂ 40.4　**FUD** 090
Ⓒ 80 ▢ ℗
AMA: 2015,Jan,16; 2014,Jan,11

33474 Valvotomy, pulmonary valve, open heart, with cardiopulmonary bypass
🔳 63.3　✂ 63.3　**FUD** 090
Ⓒ 80 ▢ ℗
AMA: 2007,Mar,1-3; 2005,Feb,13-16

33475-33476 Other Procedures Pulmonary Valve

Code also the concurrent ligation/takedown of a systemic-to-pulmonary artery shunt (33924)

33475 Replacement, pulmonary valve
🔳 68.3　✂ 68.3　**FUD** 090
Ⓒ 80 ▢ ℗
AMA: 2015,Jan,16; 2014,Jan,11

33476 Right ventricular resection for infundibular stenosis, with or without commissurotomy
INCLUDES　Brock's operation
🔳 44.4　✂ 44.4　**FUD** 090
Ⓒ 80 ▢ ℗
AMA: 2015,Jan,16; 2014,Jan,11

33477 Transcatheter Pulmonary Valve Implantation

INCLUDES　Cardiac catheterization, contrast injection, angiography, fluoroscopic guidance and the supervision and interpretation for device placement
Percutaneous balloon angioplasty within the treatment area
Valvulopasty or stent insertion in pulmonary valve conduit (37236-37237, 92997-92998)
Pre-, intra-, and post-operative hemodynamic measurements
EXCLUDES　*Balloon pump insertion (33967, 33970, 33973)*
Cardiopulmonary bypass performed in the same session (33367-33369)
Extracorporeal membrane oxygenation (ECMO) (33946-33959 [33962, 33963, 33964, 33965, 33966, 33969, 33984, 33985, 33986, 33987, 33988, 33989])
Percutaneous cardiac intervention procedures, when performed
Ventricular assist device (VAD) (33990-33993)
Do not report more than one time per session
Do not report with (76000-76001, 93451, 93453-93461, 93530-93533, 93563, 93566-93568)

● **33477** Transcatheter pulmonary valve implantation, percutaneous approach, including pre-stenting of the valve delivery site, when performed
🔳 0.00　✂ 0.00　**FUD** 000

33478 Outflow Tract Augmentation

Code also for cavopulmonary anastamosis to a second superior vena cava (33768)

33478 Outflow tract augmentation (gusset), with or without commissurotomy or infundibular resection
🔳 45.6　✂ 45.6　**FUD** 090
Ⓒ 80 ▢ ℗
AMA: 2015,Jan,16; 2014,Jan,11

33496 Prosthetic Valve Repair

Code also removal of thrombus through a separate heart incision, when performed (33310-33315); append modifier 59 to (33315)
Code also reoperation if performed (33530)

33496 Repair of non-structural prosthetic valve dysfunction with cardiopulmonary bypass (separate procedure)
🔳 48.8　✂ 48.8　**FUD** 090
Ⓒ 80 ▢ ℗
AMA: 2015,Jan,16; 2014,Jan,11

33500-33507 Repair Aberrant Coronary Artery Anatomy

INCLUDES　Angioplasty and/or endarterectomy

33500 Repair of coronary arteriovenous or arteriocardiac chamber fistula; with cardiopulmonary bypass
🔳 45.7　✂ 45.7　**FUD** 090
Ⓒ 80 ▢
AMA: 2007,Mar,1-3; 1997,Nov,1

33501 without cardiopulmonary bypass
🔳 32.6　✂ 32.6　**FUD** 090
Ⓒ 80 ▢
AMA: 2007,Mar,1-3; 1997,Nov,1

33502 Repair of anomalous coronary artery from pulmonary artery origin; by ligation
🔳 37.0　✂ 37.0　**FUD** 090
㉓ Ⓒ 80 ▢
AMA: 2007,Mar,1-3; 1997,Nov,1

33503 by graft, without cardiopulmonary bypass
🔳 38.4　✂ 38.4　**FUD** 090
㉓ Ⓒ 80 ▢
AMA: 2007,Mar,1-3; 1997,Nov,1

33504 by graft, with cardiopulmonary bypass
🔳 42.5　✂ 42.5　**FUD** 090
Ⓒ 80 ▢
AMA: 2007,Mar,1-3; 1997,Nov,1

33505 with construction of intrapulmonary artery tunnel (Takeuchi procedure)
🔳 60.0　✂ 60.0　**FUD** 090
㉓ Ⓒ 80 ▢
AMA: 2007,Mar,1-3; 1997,Nov,1

33506 by translocation from pulmonary artery to aorta
🔳 63.0　✂ 63.0　**FUD** 090
㉓ Ⓒ 80 ▢
AMA: 2007,Mar,1-3; 1997,Nov,1

33507 Repair of anomalous (eg, intramural) aortic origin of coronary artery by unroofing or translocation
🔳 50.1　✂ 50.1　**FUD** 090
Ⓒ 80
AMA: 2015,Jan,16; 2014,Jan,11

33508 Endoscopic Harvesting of Venous Graft

INCLUDES　Diagnostic endoscopy
EXCLUDES　*Harvesting of vein of upper extremity (35500)*
Code first (33510-33523)

+ **33508** Endoscopy, surgical, including video-assisted harvest of vein(s) for coronary artery bypass procedure (List separately in addition to code for primary procedure)
🔳 0.46　✂ 0.46　**FUD** ZZZ
Ⓝ Ⓝ① 80 ▢
AMA: 1997,Nov,1

33510-33516 Coronary Artery Bypass: Venous Grafts

INCLUDES　Obtaining saphenous vein grafts
Venous bypass grafting only
EXCLUDES　*Arterial bypass (33533-33536)*
Combined arterial-venous bypass (33517-33523, 33533-33536)
Obtaining vein graft:
Femoropopliteal vein (35572)
Upper extremity vein (35500)
Percutaneous ventricular assist devices (33990-33993)
Code also modifier 80 when assistant at surgery obtains grafts

33510 Coronary artery bypass, vein only; single coronary venous graft
🔳 56.1　✂ 56.1　**FUD** 090
Ⓒ 80 ▢ ℗
AMA: 2015,Jan,16; 2014,Aug,14; 2014,Jan,11; 2012,Apr,3-9; 2012,Jan,15-42; 2011,Jan,11

33511 2 coronary venous grafts
🔳 61.7　✂ 61.7　**FUD** 090
Ⓒ 80 ▢ ℗
AMA: 2015,Jan,16; 2014,Aug,14; 2014,Jan,11; 2012,Apr,3-9

33512 3 coronary venous grafts
🔳 70.2　✂ 70.2　**FUD** 090
Ⓒ 80 ▢ ℗
AMA: 2015,Jan,16; 2014,Aug,14; 2014,Jan,11; 2012,Apr,3-9

33513 **4 coronary venous grafts**
72.2   72.2   **FUD** 090   C 80 PQ
AMA: 2015,Jan,16; 2014,Aug,14; 2014,Jan,11; 2012,Apr,3-9

33514 **5 coronary venous grafts**
76.3   76.3   **FUD** 090   C 80 PQ
AMA: 2015,Jan,16; 2014,Aug,14; 2014,Jan,11; 2012,Apr,3-9

33516 **6 or more coronary venous grafts**
80.0   80.0   **FUD** 090   C 80 PQ
AMA: 2015,Jan,16; 2014,Aug,14; 2014,Jan,11; 2012,Apr,3-9

33517-33523 Coronary Artery Bypass: Venous AND Arterial Grafts

INCLUDES   Obtaining saphenous vein grafts
EXCLUDES   *Obtaining arterial graft:*
    Upper extremity (35600)
  Obtaining vein graft:
    Femoropopliteal vein graft (35572)
    Upper extremity (35500)
  Percutaneous ventricular assist devices (33990-33993)
Code also modifier 80 when assistant at surgery obtains grafts
Code first (33533-33536)

+ **33517** **Coronary artery bypass, using venous graft(s) and arterial graft(s); single vein graft (List separately in addition to code for primary procedure)**
5.46   5.46   **FUD** ZZZ   C 80 PQ
AMA: 2015,Jan,16; 2014,Jan,11; 2012,Apr,3-9

+ **33518** **2 venous grafts (List separately in addition to code for primary procedure)**
12.0   12.0   **FUD** ZZZ   C 80 PQ
AMA: 2015,Jan,16; 2014,Jan,11; 2012,Apr,3-9

+ **33519** **3 venous grafts (List separately in addition to code for primary procedure)**
15.8   15.8   **FUD** ZZZ   C 80 PQ
AMA: 2015,Jan,16; 2014,Jan,11; 2012,Apr,3-9

+ **33521** **4 venous grafts (List separately in addition to code for primary procedure)**
19.0   19.0   **FUD** ZZZ   C 80 PQ
AMA: 2015,Jan,16; 2014,Jan,11; 2012,Apr,3-9

Left subclavian artery, Aortic arch, Arterial graft, Vein graft, Vein graft, Right coronary artery, Circumflex branch

+ **33522** **5 venous grafts (List separately in addition to code for primary procedure)**
21.3   21.3   **FUD** ZZZ   C 80 PQ
AMA: 2015,Jan,16; 2014,Jan,11; 2012,Apr,3-9

+ **33523** **6 or more venous grafts (List separately in addition to code for primary procedure)**
24.4   24.4   **FUD** ZZZ   C 80 PQ
AMA: 2015,Jan,16; 2014,Jan,11; 2012,Apr,3-9

33530 Reoperative Coronary Artery Bypass Graft or Valve Procedure

EXCLUDES   *Percutaneous ventricular assist devices (33990-33993)*
Code first (33400-33496, 33510-33536, 33863)

+ **33530** **Reoperation, coronary artery bypass procedure or valve procedure, more than 1 month after original operation (List separately in addition to code for primary procedure)**
15.3   15.3   **FUD** ZZZ   C 80 PQ
AMA: 2015,Jan,16; 2014,Jan,11; 2012,Apr,3-9; 2012,Jan,15-42; 2011,Feb,8-9; 2011,Jan,11

33533-33536 Coronary Artery Bypass: Arterial Grafts

INCLUDES   Obtaining arterial graft (eg, epigastric, internal mammary, gastroepiploic and others)
EXCLUDES   *Obtaining arterial graft:*
    Upper extremity (35600)
  Obtaining venous graft:
    Femoropopliteal vein (35572)
    Upper extremity (35500)
  Percutaneous ventricular assist devices (33990-33993)
  Venous bypass (33510-33516)
Code also (33517-33523)
Code also modifier 80 when assistant at surgery obtains grafts

33533 **Coronary artery bypass, using arterial graft(s); single arterial graft**
54.3   54.3   **FUD** 090   C 80 PQ
AMA: 2015,Jan,16; 2014,Nov,14; 2014,Jan,11; 2012,Apr,3-9

33534 **2 coronary arterial grafts**
63.9   63.9   **FUD** 090   C 80 PQ
AMA: 2015,Jan,16; 2014,Jan,11; 2012,Apr,3-9

33535 **3 coronary arterial grafts**
71.3   71.3   **FUD** 090   C 80 PQ
AMA: 2015,Jan,16; 2014,Jan,11; 2012,Apr,3-9

33536 **4 or more coronary arterial grafts**
76.9   76.9   **FUD** 090   C 80 PQ
AMA: 2015,Jan,16; 2014,Nov,14; 2014,Jan,11; 2012,Apr,3-9

33542-33548 Ventricular Reconstruction

33542 **Myocardial resection (eg, ventricular aneurysmectomy)**
Code also removal of thrombus through a separate heart incision, when performed (33310-33315); append modifier 59 to (33315)
76.3   76.3   **FUD** 090   C 80 PQ
AMA: 2015,Jan,16; 2014,Jan,11

33545 **Repair of postinfarction ventricular septal defect, with or without myocardial resection**
Code also removal of thrombus through a separate heart incision, when performed (33310-33315); append modifier 59 to (33315)
90.1   90.1   **FUD** 090   C 80 PQ
AMA: 2015,Jan,16; 2014,Jan,11

33548 **Surgical ventricular restoration procedure, includes prosthetic patch, when performed (eg, ventricular remodeling, SVR, SAVER, Dor procedures)**
EXCLUDES   *Batista procedure or pachopexy (33999)*
Do not report with (32551, 33210-33211, 33310, 33315)
86.2   86.2   **FUD** 090   C 80 PQ
AMA: 2015,Jan,16; 2014,Jan,11; 2012,Jan,15-42; 2011,Jan,11

33572 Endarterectomy with CABG (LAD, RCA, Cx)

Code first (33510-33516, 33533-33536)

+ **33572** **Coronary endarterectomy, open, any method, of left anterior descending, circumflex, or right coronary artery performed in conjunction with coronary artery bypass graft procedure, each vessel (List separately in addition to primary procedure)**
6.72   6.72   **FUD** ZZZ   C 80 PQ
AMA: 1997,Nov,1; 1994,Win,1

33600-33622 Repair Aberrant Heart Anatomy

33600 **Closure of atrioventricular valve (mitral or tricuspid) by suture or patch**

Code also the concurrent ligation/takedown of a systemic-to-pulmonary artery shunt (33924)

🔲 50.3   ⚖ 50.3   **FUD** 090   C 80 ▢ P0

AMA: 2015,Jan,16; 2014,Jan,11

33602 **Closure of semilunar valve (aortic or pulmonary) by suture or patch**

Code also the concurrent ligation/takedown of a systemic-to-pulmonary artery shunt (33924)

🔲 48.8   ⚖ 48.8   **FUD** 090   C 80 ▢ P0

AMA: 2007,Mar,1-3; 1997,Nov,1

33606 **Anastomosis of pulmonary artery to aorta (Damus-Kaye-Stansel procedure)**

Code also the concurrent ligation/takedown of a systemic-to-pulmonary artery shunt (33924)

🔲 54.6   ⚖ 54.6   **FUD** 090   C 80 ▢

AMA: 2007,Mar,1-3; 1997,Nov,1

33608 **Repair of complex cardiac anomaly other than pulmonary atresia with ventricular septal defect by construction or replacement of conduit from right or left ventricle to pulmonary artery**

EXCLUDES   Unifocalization of arborization anomalies of pulmonary artery (33925, 33926)

Code also the concurrent ligation/takedown of a systemic-to-pulmonary artery shunt (33924)

🔲 52.2   ⚖ 52.2   **FUD** 090   C 80 ▢

AMA: 2007,Mar,1-3; 1997,Nov,1

33610 **Repair of complex cardiac anomalies (eg, single ventricle with subaortic obstruction) by surgical enlargement of ventricular septal defect**

Code also the concurrent ligation/takedown of a systemic-to-pulmonary artery shunt (33924)

🔲 52.0   ⚖ 52.0   **FUD** 090   63 C 80 ▢

AMA: 2007,Mar,1-3; 2002,May,7

33611 **Repair of double outlet right ventricle with intraventricular tunnel repair;**

Code also the concurrent ligation/takedown of a systemic-to-pulmonary artery shunt (33924)

🔲 60.2   ⚖ 60.2   **FUD** 090   63 C 80 ▢

AMA: 2007,Mar,1-3; 1997,Nov,1

33612 **with repair of right ventricular outflow tract obstruction**

Code also the concurrent ligation/takedown of a systemic-to-pulmonary artery shunt (33924)

🔲 58.2   ⚖ 58.2   **FUD** 090   C 80 ▢

AMA: 2007,Mar,1-3; 1997,Nov,1

33615 **Repair of complex cardiac anomalies (eg, tricuspid atresia) by closure of atrial septal defect and anastomosis of atria or vena cava to pulmonary artery (simple Fontan procedure)**

Code also the concurrent ligation/takedown of a systemic-to-pulmonary artery shunt (33924)

🔲 58.5   ⚖ 58.5   **FUD** 090   C 80 ▢

AMA: 2007,Mar,1-3; 1997,Nov,1

33617 **Repair of complex cardiac anomalies (eg, single ventricle) by modified Fontan procedure**

Code also 33768 for cavopulmonary anastomosis to a second superior vena cava

Code also the concurrent ligation/takedown of a systemic-to-pulmonary artery shunt (33924)

🔲 62.8   ⚖ 62.8   **FUD** 090   C 80 ▢

AMA: 2007,Mar,1-3; 1997,Nov,1

33619 **Repair of single ventricle with aortic outflow obstruction and aortic arch hypoplasia (hypoplastic left heart syndrome) (eg, Norwood procedure)**

Code also the concurrent ligation/takedown of a systemic-to-pulmonary artery shunt (33924)

🔲 83.8   ⚖ 83.8   **FUD** 090   63 C 80 ▢

AMA: 2015,Jan,16; 2014,Jan,11; 2012,May,14-15; 2011,Apr,3-8

33620 **Application of right and left pulmonary artery bands (eg, hybrid approach stage 1)**

EXCLUDES   Banding of main pulmonary artery related to septal defect (33690)

Code also transthoracic insertion of catheter for stent placement with removal of catheter and closure when performed during same session

🔲 44.0   ⚖ 44.0   **FUD** 090   C 80

AMA: 2015,Jan,16; 2014,Jan,11; 2012,May,14-15; 2011,Apr,3-8

33621 **Transthoracic insertion of catheter for stent placement with catheter removal and closure (eg, hybrid approach stage 1)**

Code also application of right and left pulmonary artery bands when performed during same session (33620)

Code also stent placement (37236)

🔲 27.2   ⚖ 27.2   **FUD** 090   C 80

AMA: 2015,Jan,16; 2014,Jan,11; 2012,May,14-15; 2011,Apr,3-8

33622 **Reconstruction of complex cardiac anomaly (eg, single ventricle or hypoplastic left heart) with palliation of single ventricle with aortic outflow obstruction and aortic arch hypoplasia, creation of cavopulmonary anastomosis, and removal of right and left pulmonary bands (eg, hybrid approach stage 2, Norwood, bidirectional Glenn, pulmonary artery debanding)**

Code also anastomosis, cavopulmonary, second superior vena cava for bilateral bidirectional Glenn procedure (33768)

Code also the concurrent ligation/takedown of a systemic-to-pulmonary artery shunt (33924)

Do not report with (33619, 33767, 33822, 33840, 33845, 33851, 33853, 33917)

🔲 98.9   ⚖ 98.9   **FUD** 090   C 80

AMA: 2015,Jan,16; 2014,Jan,11; 2012,May,14-15; 2011,Apr,3-8

33641-33645 Closure of Defect: Atrium

33641 **Repair atrial septal defect, secundum, with cardiopulmonary bypass, with or without patch**

🔲 47.5   ⚖ 47.5   **FUD** 090   C 80 ▢

AMA: 2015,Jan,16; 2014,Jan,11; 2012,Jan,15-42; 2010,Dec,12

33645 **Direct or patch closure, sinus venosus, with or without anomalous pulmonary venous drainage**

Do not report with (33724, 33726)

🔲 50.3   ⚖ 50.3   **FUD** 090   C 80 ▢

AMA: 2007,Mar,1-3; 1997,Nov,1

33647 Closure of Septal Defect: Atrium AND Ventricle

EXCLUDES   Tricuspid atresia repair procedures (33615)

33647 **Repair of atrial septal defect and ventricular septal defect, with direct or patch closure**

🔲 52.8   ⚖ 52.8   **FUD** 090   63 C 80 ▢

AMA: 2007,Mar,1-3; 1997,Nov,1

33660-33670 Closure of Defect: Atrioventricular Canal

33660 **Repair of incomplete or partial atrioventricular canal (ostium primum atrial septal defect), with or without atrioventricular valve repair**

🔲 51.5   ⚖ 51.5   **FUD** 090   C 80 ▢

AMA: 2007,Mar,1-3; 1997,Nov,1

33665 **Repair of intermediate or transitional atrioventricular canal, with or without atrioventricular valve repair**

🔲 55.6   ⚖ 55.6   **FUD** 090   C 80 ▢

AMA: 2007,Mar,1-3; 1997,Nov,1

33670 **Repair of complete atrioventricular canal, with or without prosthetic valve**

Code also removal of thrombus through a separate heart incision, when performed (33310-33315); append modifier 59 to (33315)

🔲 57.8   ⚖ 57.8   **FUD** 090   63 C 80 ▢

AMA: 2007,Mar,1-3; 1997,Nov,1

33675-33677 Closure of Multiple Septal Defects: Ventricle

EXCLUDES Percutaneous closure (93581)
Do not report with (32100, 32551, 32554-32555, 33210, 33681, 33684, 33688)

33675 Closure of multiple ventricular septal defects;
🔲 57.8 ⚖ 57.8 **FUD** 090
C 80
AMA: 2015,Jan,16; 2014,Jan,11

33676 with pulmonary valvotomy or infundibular resection (acyanotic)
🔲 62.5 ⚖ 62.5 **FUD** 090
C 80
AMA: 2015,Jan,16; 2014,Jan,11

33677 with removal of pulmonary artery band, with or without gusset
🔲 64.6 ⚖ 64.6 **FUD** 090
C 80
AMA: 2015,Jan,16; 2014,Jan,11

33681-33688 Closure of Septal Defect: Ventricle

EXCLUDES Repair of pulmonary vein that requires creating an atrial septal defect (33724)

33681 Closure of single ventricular septal defect, with or without patch;
EXCLUDES Code also removal of thrombus through a separate heart incision, when performed (33310-33315); append modifier 59 to (33315)
🔲 53.5 ⚖ 53.5 **FUD** 090
C 80 🖵
AMA: 2015,Jan,16; 2014,Jan,11

33684 with pulmonary valvotomy or infundibular resection (acyanotic)
Code also concurrent ligation/takedown of a systemic-to-pulmonary artery shunt if performed (33924)
🔲 55.4 ⚖ 55.4 **FUD** 090
C 80 🖵
AMA: 2007,Mar,1-3; 1997,Nov,1

33688 with removal of pulmonary artery band, with or without gusset
Code also the concurrent ligation/takedown of a systemic-to-pulmonary artery shunt if performed (33924)
🔲 54.8 ⚖ 54.8 **FUD** 090
C 80 🖵
AMA: 2007,Mar,1-3; 1997,Nov,1

33690 Reduce Pulmonary Overcirculation in Septal Defects

EXCLUDES Left and right pulmonary artery banding in a single ventricle (33620)

33690 Banding of pulmonary artery
🔲 35.1 ⚖ 35.1 **FUD** 090
63 C 80 🖵
AMA: 2015,Jan,16; 2014,Jan,11; 2012,May,14-15; 2011,Apr,3-8

33692-33697 Repair of Defects of Tetralogy of Fallot

Code also the concurrent ligation/takedown of a systemic-to-pulmonary artery shunt (33924)

33692 Complete repair tetralogy of Fallot without pulmonary atresia;
🔲 60.6 ⚖ 60.6 **FUD** 090
C 80 🖵
AMA: 2007,Mar,1-3; 1997,Nov,1

33694 with transannular patch
🔲 56.7 ⚖ 56.7 **FUD** 090
63 C 80 🖵
AMA: 2007,Mar,1-3; 1997,Nov,1

33697 Complete repair tetralogy of Fallot with pulmonary atresia including construction of conduit from right ventricle to pulmonary artery and closure of ventricular septal defect
🔲 61.1 ⚖ 61.1 **FUD** 090
C 80 🖵
AMA: 2015,Jan,16; 2014,Jan,11

33702-33722 Repair Anomalies Sinus of Valsalva

33702 Repair sinus of Valsalva fistula, with cardiopulmonary bypass;
🔲 44.9 ⚖ 44.9 **FUD** 090
C 80 🖵
AMA: 2015,Jan,16; 2014,Jan,11

33710 with repair of ventricular septal defect
🔲 61.0 ⚖ 61.0 **FUD** 090
C 80 🖵
AMA: 2007,Mar,1-3; 1997,Nov,1

33720 Repair sinus of Valsalva aneurysm, with cardiopulmonary bypass
🔲 45.3 ⚖ 45.3 **FUD** 090
C 80 🖵
AMA: 2007,Mar,1-3; 1997,Nov,1

33722 Closure of aortico-left ventricular tunnel
🔲 47.5 ⚖ 47.5 **FUD** 090
C 80 🖵
AMA: 2015,Jan,16; 2014,Jan,11

33724-33732 Repair Aberrant Pulmonary Venous Connection

33724 Repair of isolated partial anomalous pulmonary venous return (eg, Scimitar Syndrome)
Do not report with (32551, 33210-33211)
🔲 44.7 ⚖ 44.7 **FUD** 090
C 80
AMA: 2015,Jan,16; 2014,Jan,11

33726 Repair of pulmonary venous stenosis
Do not report with (32551, 33210-33211)
🔲 59.6 ⚖ 59.6 **FUD** 090
C 80
AMA: 2015,Jan,16; 2014,Jan,11

33730 Complete repair of anomalous pulmonary venous return (supracardiac, intracardiac, or infracardiac types)
EXCLUDES Partial anomalous pulmonary venous return (33724)
Repair of pulmonary venous stenosis (33726)
🔲 58.7 ⚖ 58.7 **FUD** 090
63 C 80 🖵
AMA: 2015,Jan,16; 2014,Jan,11

33732 Repair of cor triatriatum or supravalvular mitral ring by resection of left atrial membrane
🔲 48.2 ⚖ 48.2 **FUD** 090
63 C 80 🖵
AMA: 2015,Jan,16; 2014,Jan,11

33735-33737 33735-33737 Creation of Atrial Septal Defect

Code also the concurrent ligation/takedown of a systemic-to-pulmonary artery shunt (33924)

33735 Atrial septectomy or septostomy; closed heart (Blalock-Hanlon type operation)
🔲 37.9 ⚖ 37.9 **FUD** 090
63 C 80 🖵
AMA: 2015,Jan,16; 2014,Jan,11

33736 open heart with cardiopulmonary bypass
🔲 40.8 ⚖ 40.8 **FUD** 090
63 C 80 🖵
AMA: 2007,Mar,1-3; 1997,Nov,1

33737 open heart, with inflow occlusion
EXCLUDES Atrial septectomy/septostomy:
Blade method (92993)
Transvenous balloon method (92992)
🔲 39.6 ⚖ 39.6 **FUD** 090
C 80 🖵
AMA: 2007,Mar,1-3; 1997,Nov,1

33750-33767 Systemic Vessel to Pulmonary Artery Shunts

Code also the concurrent ligation/takedown of a systemic-to-pulmonary artery shunt (33924)

33750 Shunt; subclavian to pulmonary artery (Blalock-Taussig type operation)
🔲 38.7 ⚖ 38.7 **FUD** 090
63 C 80 🖵
AMA: 2007,Mar,1-3; 1997,Nov,1

33755 ascending aorta to pulmonary artery (Waterston type operation)
🔲 40.0 ⚖ 40.0 **FUD** 090
63 C 80 🖵
AMA: 2007,Mar,1-3; 1997,Nov,1

33762 descending aorta to pulmonary artery (Potts-Smith type operation)
🔲 39.3 ⚖ 39.3 **FUD** 090
63 C 80 🖵
AMA: 2007,Mar,1-3; 1997,Nov,1

33764 central, with prosthetic graft
🔲 40.1 ⚖ 40.1 **FUD** 090
C 80 🖵
AMA: 2007,Mar,1-3; 1997,Nov,1

33766 superior vena cava to pulmonary artery for flow to 1 lung (classical Glenn procedure)
🔲 40.8 ⚖ 40.8 **FUD** 090
C 80 🖵
AMA: 2007,Mar,1-3; 1997,Nov,1

33767 superior vena cava to pulmonary artery for flow to both lungs (bidirectional Glenn procedure)
🔲 41.3 ⚖ 41.3 **FUD** 090
C 80 🖵
AMA: 2011,Apr,3-8

33768 Cavopulmonary Anastomosis to Decrease Volume Load

Code first (33478, 33617, 33622, 33767)
Do not report with (32551, 33210-33211)

+ **33768** **Anastomosis, cavopulmonary, second superior vena cava (List separately in addition to primary procedure)**
🔧 13.0   ⚕ 13.0   **FUD** ZZZ   C 80
AMA: 2015,Jan,16; 2014,Jan,11; 2011,Apr,3-8

33770-33783 Repair Aberrant Anatomy: Transposition Great Vessels

Code also the concurrent ligation/takedown of a systemic-to-pulmonary artery shunt (33924)

33770 **Repair of transposition of the great arteries with ventricular septal defect and subpulmonary stenosis; without surgical enlargement of ventricular septal defect**
🔧 65.5   ⚕ 65.5   **FUD** 090   C 80
AMA: 2015,Jan,16; 2014,Jan,11

33771 **with surgical enlargement of ventricular septal defect**
🔧 67.6   ⚕ 67.6   **FUD** 090   C 80
AMA: 2007,Mar,1-3; 1997,Nov,1

33774 **Repair of transposition of the great arteries, atrial baffle procedure (eg, Mustard or Senning type) with cardiopulmonary bypass;**
🔧 52.7   ⚕ 52.7   **FUD** 090   C 80
AMA: 2007,Mar,1-3; 1997,Nov,1

33775 **with removal of pulmonary band**
🔧 56.9   ⚕ 56.9   **FUD** 090   C 80
AMA: 2007,Mar,1-3; 1997,Nov,1

33776 **with closure of ventricular septal defect**
🔧 60.1   ⚕ 60.1   **FUD** 090   C 80
AMA: 2007,Mar,1-3; 1997,Nov,1

33777 **with repair of subpulmonic obstruction**
🔧 58.3   ⚕ 58.3   **FUD** 090   C 80
AMA: 2007,Mar,1-3; 1997,Nov,1

33778 **Repair of transposition of the great arteries, aortic pulmonary artery reconstruction (eg, Jatene type);**
🔧 72.5   ⚕ 72.5   **FUD** 090   63 C 80
AMA: 2007,Mar,1-3; 1997,Nov,1

33779 **with removal of pulmonary band**
🔧 72.1   ⚕ 72.1   **FUD** 090   C 80
AMA: 2007,Mar,1-3; 1997,Nov,1

33780 **with closure of ventricular septal defect**
🔧 73.4   ⚕ 73.4   **FUD** 090   C 80
AMA: 2007,Mar,1-3; 1997,Nov,1

33781 **with repair of subpulmonic obstruction**
🔧 71.8   ⚕ 71.8   **FUD** 090   C 80
AMA: 2015,Jan,16; 2014,Jan,11

33782 **Aortic root translocation with ventricular septal defect and pulmonary stenosis repair (ie, Nikaidoh procedure); without coronary ostium reimplantation**
🔧 94.6   ⚕ 94.6   **FUD** 090   C 80
Do not report with (33412-33413, 33608, 33681, 33770-33771, 33778, 33780, 33920)

33783 **with reimplantation of 1 or both coronary ostia**
🔧 108.   ⚕ 108.   **FUD** 090   C 80

33786-33788 Repair Aberrant Anatomy: Truncus Arteriosus

33786 **Total repair, truncus arteriosus (Rastelli type operation)**
Code also the concurrent ligation/takedown of a systemic-to-pulmonary artery shunt (33924)
🔧 70.4   ⚕ 70.4   **FUD** 090   63 C 80
AMA: 2015,Jan,16; 2014,Jan,11

33788 **Reimplantation of an anomalous pulmonary artery**
EXCLUDES   Pulmonary artery banding (33690)
🔧 44.9   ⚕ 44.9   **FUD** 090   C 80
AMA: 2015,Jan,16; 2014,Jan,11

33800-33853 Repair Aberrant Anatomy: Aorta

33800 **Aortic suspension (aortopexy) for tracheal decompression (eg, for tracheomalacia) (separate procedure)**
🔧 30.3   ⚕ 30.3   **FUD** 090   C 80
AMA: 2015,Jan,16; 2014,Jan,11

33802 **Division of aberrant vessel (vascular ring);**
🔧 33.3   ⚕ 33.3   **FUD** 090   C 80
AMA: 2007,Mar,1-3; 1997,Nov,1

33803 **with reanastomosis**
🔧 35.2   ⚕ 35.2   **FUD** 090   C 80
AMA: 2007,Mar,1-3; 1997,Nov,1

33813 **Obliteration of aortopulmonary septal defect; without cardiopulmonary bypass**
🔧 37.8   ⚕ 37.8   **FUD** 090   C 80
AMA: 2007,Mar,1-3; 1997,Nov,1

33814 **with cardiopulmonary bypass**
🔧 44.6   ⚕ 44.6   **FUD** 090   C 80
AMA: 2007,Mar,1-3; 1997,Nov,1

33820 **Repair of patent ductus arteriosus; by ligation**
EXCLUDES   Percutaneous transcatheter closure patent ductus arteriosus (93582)
🔧 28.1   ⚕ 28.1   **FUD** 090   C 80
AMA: 2015,Jan,16; 2014,Jan,11

33822 **by division, younger than 18 years**   A
EXCLUDES   Percutaneous transcatheter closure patent ductus arteriosus (93582)
🔧 31.2   ⚕ 31.2   **FUD** 090   C 80
AMA: 2015,Jan,16; 2014,Jan,11; 2011,Apr,3-8

33824 **by division, 18 years and older**
EXCLUDES   Percutaneous closure patent ductus arteriosus (93582)
🔧 34.2   ⚕ 34.2   **FUD** 090   C 80
AMA: 2007,Mar,1-3; 1997,Nov,1

33840 **Excision of coarctation of aorta, with or without associated patent ductus arteriosus; with direct anastomosis**
🔧 37.8   ⚕ 37.8   **FUD** 090   C 80
AMA: 2011,Apr,3-8

33845 **with graft**
🔧 38.7   ⚕ 38.7   **FUD** 090   C 80
AMA: 2011,Apr,3-8

33851 **repair using either left subclavian artery or prosthetic material as gusset for enlargement**
🔧 38.8   ⚕ 38.8   **FUD** 090   C 80
AMA: 2011,Apr,3-8

33852 **Repair of hypoplastic or interrupted aortic arch using autogenous or prosthetic material; without cardiopulmonary bypass**
EXCLUDES   Hypoplastic left heart syndrome repair by excision of coarctation of aorta (33619)
🔧 40.6   ⚕ 40.6   **FUD** 090   C 80
AMA: 2007,Mar,1-3; 1997,Nov,1

33853 **with cardiopulmonary bypass**
EXCLUDES   Hypoplastic left heart syndrome repair by excision of coarctation of aorta (33619)
🔧 53.2   ⚕ 53.2   **FUD** 090   C 80
AMA: 2015,Jan,16; 2014,Jan,11; 2011,Apr,3-8

Aortic valve; Left coronary artery; Left, right atria; Basal; Descending branch (anterior ventricular); Apical; Right coronary artery; Descending branch (posterior interventricular); Posterior wall; Intraventricular septum divides left and right ventricles

33860-33877 Aortic Graft Procedures

33860 **Ascending aorta graft, with cardiopulmonary bypass, includes valve suspension, when performed**
🔧 93.4   ⚲ 93.4   **FUD** 090   [C] [80] ▢
AMA: 2015,Jan,16; 2014,Jan,11; 2011,Aug,3-5

33863 **Ascending aorta graft, with cardiopulmonary bypass, with aortic root replacement using valved conduit and coronary reconstruction (eg, Bentall)**
Do not report with (33405-33406, 33410-33413, 33860)
🔧 91.7   ⚲ 91.7   **FUD** 090   [C] [80] ▢
AMA: 2015,Jan,16; 2014,Jan,11; 2012,Jan,15-42; 2011,Aug,3-5

33864 **Ascending aorta graft, with cardiopulmonary bypass with valve suspension, with coronary reconstruction and valve-sparing aortic root remodeling (eg, David Procedure, Yacoub Procedure)**
Do not report with (33400, 33860-33863)
🔧 94.0   ⚲ 94.0   **FUD** 090   [C] [80]
AMA: 2015,Jan,16; 2014,Jan,11; 2012,Jan,15-42; 2011,Aug,3-5

33870 **Transverse arch graft, with cardiopulmonary bypass**
🔧 73.3   ⚲ 73.3   [C] [80] ▢
AMA: 1997,Nov,1

33875 **Descending thoracic aorta graft, with or without bypass**
🔧 80.0   ⚲ 80.0   **FUD** 090   [C] [80] ▢
AMA: 1997,Nov,1

33877 **Repair of thoracoabdominal aortic aneurysm with graft, with or without cardiopulmonary bypass**
🔧 106.   ⚲ 106.   **FUD** 090   [C] [80] ▢ [PQ]
AMA: 1997,Nov,1

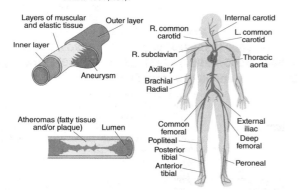

33880-33891 Endovascular Repair Aortic Aneurysm: Thoracic

INCLUDES   Balloon angioplasty
Deployment of stent
Introduction, manipulation, placement, and deployment of the device
EXCLUDES   *Additional interventional procedures provided during the endovascular repair*
Carotid-carotid bypass (33891)
Guidewire and catheter insertion (36140, 36200-36218)
Open exposure of artery/subsequent closure (34812, 34820, 34833-34834)
Study, interpretation, and report of implanted wireless pressure sensor in an aneurysmal sac (93982)
Subclavian to carotid artery transposition (33889)
Substantial artery repair/replacement (35226, 35286)
Transcatheter insertion of wireless physiologic sensor in an aneurysmal sac (34806)

33880 **Endovascular repair of descending thoracic aorta (eg, aneurysm, pseudoaneurysm, dissection, penetrating ulcer, intramural hematoma, or traumatic disruption); involving coverage of left subclavian artery origin, initial endoprosthesis plus descending thoracic aortic extension(s), if required, to level of celiac artery origin**
INCLUDES   Placement of distal extensions in distal thoracic aorta
EXCLUDES   *Proximal extensions*
🔧 (75956)
🔧 52.9   ⚲ 52.9   **FUD** 090   [C] [80] [PQ]
AMA: 2015,Jan,16; 2014,Jan,11

33881 **not involving coverage of left subclavian artery origin, initial endoprosthesis plus descending thoracic aortic extension(s), if required, to level of celiac artery origin**
INCLUDES   Placement of distal extensions in distal thoracic aorta
EXCLUDES   *Proximal extensions*
Do not report if placement of extension includes coverage of left subclavian artery origin
🔧 (75957)
🔧 45.5   ⚲ 45.5   **FUD** 090   [C] [80] [PQ]
AMA: 2015,Jan,16; 2014,Jan,11

33883 **Placement of proximal extension prosthesis for endovascular repair of descending thoracic aorta (eg, aneurysm, pseudoaneurysm, dissection, penetrating ulcer, intramural hematoma, or traumatic disruption); initial extension**
Do not report if placement of extension includes coverage of left subclavian artery origin
🔧 (75958)
🔧 32.9   ⚲ 32.9   **FUD** 090   [C] [80] [PQ]
AMA: 2015,Jan,16; 2014,Jan,11

+ **33884** **each additional proximal extension (List separately in addition to code for primary procedure)**
Code first (33883)
🔧 (75958)
🔧 12.1   ⚲ 12.1   **FUD** ZZZ   [C] [80]
AMA: 2015,Jan,16; 2014,Jan,11

33886 **Placement of distal extension prosthesis(s) delayed after endovascular repair of descending thoracic aorta**
INCLUDES   All modules deployed
Do not report with (33880, 33881)
🔧 (75959)
🔧 28.4   ⚲ 28.4   **FUD** 090   [C] [80] [PQ]
AMA: 2015,Jan,16; 2014,Jan,11

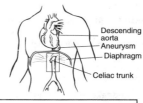

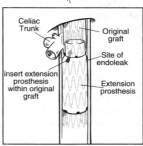

Repair of endoleak in
descending thoracic aorta

33889 **Open subclavian to carotid artery transposition performed in conjunction with endovascular repair of descending thoracic aorta, by neck incision, unilateral**
Do not report with (35694)
🔧 23.3   ⚲ 23.3   **FUD** 000   [C] [80] [50]
AMA: 2015,Jan,16; 2014,Jan,11

Cardiovascular System

33891 — 33949

33891   **Bypass graft, with other than vein, transcervical retropharyngeal carotid-carotid, performed in conjunction with endovascular repair of descending thoracic aorta, by neck incision**

Do not report with (35509, 35601)

🔹 28.6   ⚖ 28.6   **FUD** 000   C 80 50 P0

AMA: 2015,Jan,16; 2014,Jan,11

33910-33926 Surgical Procedures of Pulmonary Artery

33910   **Pulmonary artery embolectomy; with cardiopulmonary bypass**

🔹 76.7   ⚖ 76.7   **FUD** 090   C 80 ▣

AMA: 2015,Jan,16; 2014,Jan,11

33915   **without cardiopulmonary bypass**

🔹 37.3   ⚖ 37.3   **FUD** 090   C 80 ▣

AMA: 2015,Jan,16; 2014,Jan,11

33916   **Pulmonary endarterectomy, with or without embolectomy, with cardiopulmonary bypass**

🔹 122.   ⚖ 122.   **FUD** 090   C 80 ▣

AMA: 2015,Jan,16; 2014,Jan,11

33917   **Repair of pulmonary artery stenosis by reconstruction with patch or graft**

Code also the concurrent ligation/takedown of a systemic-to-pulmonary artery shunt (33924)

🔹 42.6   ⚖ 42.6   **FUD** 090   C 80 ▣

AMA: 2015,Jan,16; 2014,Jan,11; 2011,Apr,3-8

33920   **Repair of pulmonary atresia with ventricular septal defect, by construction or replacement of conduit from right or left ventricle to pulmonary artery**

EXCLUDES   *Repair of complicated cardiac anomalies by creating/replacing conduit from ventricle to pulmonary artery (33608)*

Code also the concurrent ligation/takedown of a systemic-to-pulmonary artery shunt (33924)

🔹 53.0   ⚖ 53.0   **FUD** 090   C 80 ▣

AMA: 2015,Jan,16; 2014,Jan,11

33922   **Transection of pulmonary artery with cardiopulmonary bypass**

Code also the concurrent ligation/takedown of a systemic-to-pulmonary artery shunt (33924)

🔹 40.3   ⚖ 40.3   **FUD** 090   63 C 80 ▣

AMA: 1997,Nov,1; 1995,Win,1

+ 33924   **Ligation and takedown of a systemic-to-pulmonary artery shunt, performed in conjunction with a congenital heart procedure (List separately in addition to code for primary procedure)**

Code first (33470-33478, 33600-33617, 33622, 33684-33688, 33692-33697, 33735-33767, 33770-33783, 33786, 33917, 33920-33922, 33925-33926, 33935, 33945)

🔹 8.33   ⚖ 8.33   **FUD** ZZZ   C 80 ▣

AMA: 1997,Nov,1; 1995,Win,1

33925   **Repair of pulmonary artery arborization anomalies by unifocalization; without cardiopulmonary bypass**

🔹 50.3   ⚖ 50.3   **FUD** 090   C 80

Code also the concurrent ligation/takedown of a systemic-to-pulmonary artery shunt (33924)

33926   **with cardiopulmonary bypass**

🔹 74.0   ⚖ 74.0   **FUD** 090   C 80

Code also the concurrent ligation/takedown of a systemic-to-pulmonary artery shunt (33924)

33930-33945 Heart and Heart-Lung Transplants

CMS: 100-3,260.9 Heart Transplants; 100-4,3,90.2 Heart Transplants

INCLUDES   Backbench work to prepare the donor heart and/or lungs for transplantation (33933, 33944)
Harvesting of donor organs with cold preservation (33930, 33940)
Transplantation of heart and/or lungs into recipient (33935, 33945)

EXCLUDES   *Implantation/repair/replacement of artificial heart or components (0051T-0053T)*
Procedures performed on donor heart (33300, 33310, 33320, 33400, 33463, 33464, 33510, 33641, 35216, 35276, 35685)

33930   **Donor cardiectomy-pneumonectomy (including cold preservation)**

🔹 0.00   ⚖ 0.00   **FUD** XXX   C ▣

AMA: 1997,Nov,1

33933   **Backbench standard preparation of cadaver donor heart/lung allograft prior to transplantation, including dissection of allograft from surrounding soft tissues to prepare aorta, superior vena cava, inferior vena cava, and trachea for implantation**

🔹 0.00   ⚖ 0.00   **FUD** XXX   C 80 ▣

AMA: 1997,Nov,1

33935   **Heart-lung transplant with recipient cardiectomy-pneumonectomy**

Code also the concurrent ligation/takedown of a systemic-to-pulmonary artery shunt (33924)

🔹 144.   ⚖ 144.   **FUD** 090   C 80 ▣ P0

AMA: 1997,Nov,1

33940   **Donor cardiectomy (including cold preservation)**

🔹 0.00   ⚖ 0.00   **FUD** XXX   C ▣

AMA: 2015,Jan,16; 2014,Jan,11

33944   **Backbench standard preparation of cadaver donor heart allograft prior to transplantation, including dissection of allograft from surrounding soft tissues to prepare aorta, superior vena cava, inferior vena cava, pulmonary artery, and left atrium for implantation**

🔹 0.00   ⚖ 0.00   **FUD** XXX   C 80 ▣

AMA: 1997,Nov,1

33945   **Heart transplant, with or without recipient cardiectomy**

Code also the concurrent ligation/takedown of a systemic-to-pulmonary artery shunt (33924)

🔹 141.   ⚖ 141.   **FUD** 090   C 80 ▣ P0

AMA: 1997,May,4; 1997,Nov,1

33946-33959 [33962, 33963, 33964, 33965, 33966, 33969, 33984, 33985, 33986, 33987, 33988, 33989] Extracorporeal Circulatory and Respiratory Support

INCLUDES   Multiple physician and nonphysician team collaboration
Veno-arterial ECMO/ECLS for heart and lung support
Veno-venous ECMO/ECLS for lung support

EXCLUDES   *Overall daily management services needed to manage a patient; report the appropriate observation, hospital inpatient, or critical care E/M codes*

Code also extensive arterial repair/replacement (35266, 35286, 35371, 35665)
Do not report cannula repositioning and cannula insertion performed during same session
Do not report cannula repositioning and initiation of ECMO/ECLS on the same day
Do not report ECMO/ECLS daily management codes with ECMO/ECLS initiation codes

33946   **Extracorporeal membrane oxygenation (ECMO)/extracorporeal life support (ECLS) provided by physician; initiation, veno-venous**

Code also cannula insertion (33951-33956)
Do not report with (33948, 33957-33959 [33962, 33963, 33964])

🔹 8.99   ⚖ 8.99   **FUD** XXX   63 C

AMA: 2015,Jul,3

33947   **initiation, veno-arterial**

Code also cannula insertion (33951-33956)
Do not report with (33949, 33957-33959 [33962, 33963, 33964])

🔹 9.93   ⚖ 9.93   **FUD** XXX   63 C

AMA: 2015,Jul,3

33948   **daily management, each day, veno-venous**

Do not report with (33946)

🔹 7.10   ⚖ 7.10   **FUD** XXX   63 C

AMA: 2015,Jul,3

33949   **daily management, each day, veno-arterial**

Do not report with (33947)

🔹 6.91   ⚖ 6.91   **FUD** XXX   63 C

AMA: 2015,Jul,3

33951 insertion of peripheral (arterial and/or venous) cannula(e), percutaneous, birth through 5 years of age (includes fluoroscopic guidance, when performed) [A]

INCLUDES Cannula replacement in same vessel
Cannula repositioning during same episode of care
Code also cannula removal if new cannula inserted in different vessel with ([33965, 33966, 33969, 33984, 33985, 33986])
Code also ECMO/ECLS initiation or daily management (33946-33947, 33948-33949)
🔲 12.9 🔲 12.9 **FUD** 000 [C] [80]

AMA: 2015,Jul,3

33952 insertion of peripheral (arterial and/or venous) cannula(e), percutaneous, 6 years and older (includes fluoroscopic guidance, when performed) [A]

INCLUDES Cannula replacement in same vessel
Cannula repositioning during same episode of care
Code also cannula removal if new cannula inserted in different vessel with ([33965, 33966, 33969, 33984, 33985, 33986])
Code also ECMO/ECLS initiation or daily management (33946-33947, 33948-33949)
🔲 12.5 🔲 12.5 **FUD** 000 [C] [80]

AMA: 2015,Jul,3

33953 insertion of peripheral (arterial and/or venous) cannula(e), open, birth through 5 years of age [A]

INCLUDES Cannula replacement in same vessel
Cannula repositioning during same episode of care
Code also cannula removal if new cannula inserted in different vessel with ([33965, 33966, 33969, 33984, 33985, 33986])
Code also ECMO/ECLS initiation or daily management (33496-33947, 33948-33949)
Do not report with (34812, 34820, 34834)
🔲 14.3 🔲 14.3 **FUD** 000 [C] [80]

AMA: 2015,Jul,3

33954 insertion of peripheral (arterial and/or venous) cannula(e), open, 6 years and older [A]

INCLUDES Cannula replacement in same vessel
Cannula repositioning during same episode of care
Code also cannula removal if new cannula inserted in different vessel with ([33965, 33966, 33969, 33984, 33985, 33986])
Code also ECMO/ECLS initiation or daily management (33946-33947, 33948-33949)
Do not report with (34812, 34820, 34834)
🔲 14.0 🔲 14.0 **FUD** 000 [C] [80]

AMA: 2015,Jul,3

33955 insertion of central cannula(e) by sternotomy or thoracotomy, birth through 5 years of age [A]

INCLUDES Cannula replacement in same vessel
Cannula repositioning during same episode of care
Code also cannula removal if new cannula inserted in different vessel with ([33965, 33966, 33969, 33984, 33985, 33986])
Code also ECMO/ECLS initiation or daily management (33946-33947, 33948-33949)
Do not report with (32100, 39010)
🔲 25.9 🔲 25.9 **FUD** 000 [C] [80]

AMA: 2015,Jul,3

33956 insertion of central cannula(e) by sternotomy or thoracotomy, 6 years and older [A]

INCLUDES Cannula replacement in same vessel
Cannula repositioning during same episode of care
Code also cannula removal if new cannula inserted in different vessel with ([33965, 33966, 33969, 33984, 33985, 33986])
Code also ECMO/ECLS initiation or daily management (33946-33947, 33948-33949)
Do not report with (32100, 39010)
🔲 24.5 🔲 24.5 **FUD** 000 [C] [80]

AMA: 2015,Jul,3

33957 reposition peripheral (arterial and/or venous) cannula(e), percutaneous, birth through 5 years of age (includes fluoroscopic guidance, when performed) [A]

INCLUDES Fluoroscopic guidance
Do not report when cannula insertion performed during same session
Do not report with (33946-33947, 34812, 34820, 34834)
🔲 5.77 🔲 5.77 **FUD** 000 [C] [80]

AMA: 2015,Jul,3

33958 reposition peripheral (arterial and/or venous) cannula(e), percutaneous, 6 years and older (includes fluoroscopic guidance, when performed) [A]

INCLUDES Fluoroscopic guidance
Do not report when cannula insertion performed during same session
Do not report with (33946-33947, 34812, 34820, 34834)
🔲 5.58 🔲 5.58 **FUD** 000 [C] [80]

AMA: 2015,Jul,3

33959 reposition peripheral (arterial and/or venous) cannula(e), open, birth through 5 years of age (includes fluoroscopic guidance, when performed) [A]

INCLUDES Fluoroscopic guidance
Do not report when cannula insertion performed during same session
Do not report with (33946-33947, 34812, 34820, 34834)
🔲 7.33 🔲 7.33 **FUD** 000 [C] [80]

AMA: 2015,Jul,3

\# **33962** reposition peripheral (arterial and/or venous) cannula(e), open, 6 years and older (includes fluoroscopic guidance, when performed) [A]

INCLUDES Fluoroscopic guidance
Do not report when cannula insertion performed during same session
Do not report with (33946-33947, 34812, 34820, 34834)
🔲 6.88 🔲 6.88 **FUD** 000 [C] [80]

AMA: 2015,Jul,3

\# **33963** reposition of central cannula(e) by sternotomy or thoracotomy, birth through 5 years of age (includes fluoroscopic guidance, when performed) [A]

INCLUDES Fluoroscopic guidance
Do not report when cannula insertion performed during same session
Do not report with (32100, 33946-33947, 39010)
🔲 14.6 🔲 14.6 **FUD** 000 [C] [80]

AMA: 2015,Jul,3

\# **33964** reposition central cannula(e) by sternotomy or thoracotomy, 6 years and older (includes fluoroscopic guidance, when performed) [A]

INCLUDES Fluoroscopic guidance
Do not report when cannula insertion performed during same session
Do not report with (32100, 33946-33947, 39010)
🔲 14.9 🔲 14.9 **FUD** 000 [C] [80]

AMA: 2015,Jul,3

\# **33965** removal of peripheral (arterial and/or venous) cannula(e), percutaneous, birth through 5 years of age [A]

Code also extensive arterial repair/replacement, when performed (35266, 35286, 35371, 35665)
Code also new cannula insertion into different vessel (33951-33956)
🔲 5.77 🔲 5.77 **FUD** 000 [C] [80]

AMA: 2015,Jul,3

\# **33966** removal of peripheral (arterial and/or venous) cannula(e), percutaneous, 6 years and older [A]

Code also new cannula insertion into different vessel (33951-33956)
Code also extensive arterial repair/replacement, when performed (35266, 35286, 35371, 35665)
🔲 6.93 🔲 6.93 **FUD** 000 [C] [80]

AMA: 2015,Jul,3

● New Code   ▲ Revised Code   ○ Reinstated   Ⓜ Maternity   [A] Age Edit   Unlisted   Not Covered   \# Resequenced
⊘ AMA Mod 51 Exempt   ⑤ Optum Mod 51 Exempt   ㊌ Mod 63 Exempt   ⊙ Mod Sedation   + Add-on    CCI   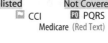 PQRS   **FUD** Follow-up Days

CPT © 2015 American Medical Association. All Rights Reserved. (Black Text)   Medicare (Red Text)

Cardiovascular System

33969 — 33977

\# **33969**   **removal of peripheral (arterial and/or venous) cannula(e), open, birth through 5 years of age**   A

Code also extensive arterial repair/replacement, when performed (35266, 35286, 35371, 35665)
Code also new cannula insertion into different vessel (33951-33956)
Do not report with (34812, 34820, 34834, 35201, 35206, 35211, 35216, 35226)

🔲 8.50   🔳 8.50   **FUD** 000   C 80

AMA: 2015,Jul,3

\# **33984**   **removal of peripheral (arterial and/or venous) cannula(e), open, 6 years and older**   A

Code also extensive arterial repair/replacement, when performed (35266, 35286, 35371, 35665)
Code also new cannula insertion into different vessel (33951-33956)
Do not report with (34812, 34820, 34834, 35201, 35206, 35211, 35216, 35226)

🔲 8.34   🔳 8.34   **FUD** 000   C 80

AMA: 2015,Jul,3

\# **33985**   **removal of central cannula(e) by sternotomy or thoracotomy, birth through 5 years of age**   A

Code also extensive arterial repair/replacement, when performed (35266, 35286, 35371, 35665)
Code also new cannula insertion into different vessel (33951-33956)
Do not report with (35201, 35206, 35211, 35216, 35226)

🔲 16.0   🔳 16.0   **FUD** 000   C 80

AMA: 2015,Jul,3

\# **33986**   **removal of central cannula(e) by sternotomy or thoracotomy, 6 years and older**   A

Code also extensive arterial repair/replacement, when performed (35266, 35286, 35371, 35665)
Code also new cannula insertion into different vessel (33951-33956)
Do not report with (35201, 35206, 35211, 35216, 35226)

🔲 15.2   🔳 15.2   **FUD** 000   C 80

AMA: 2015,Jul,3

+ \# **33987**   **Arterial exposure with creation of graft conduit (eg, chimney graft) to facilitate arterial perfusion for ECMO/ECLS (List separately in addition to code for primary procedure)**

Code first (33953-33956)
Do not report with (34833)

🔲 6.10   🔳 6.10   **FUD** ZZZ   C 80

AMA: 2015,Jul,3

\# **33988**   **Insertion of left heart vent by thoracic incision (eg, sternotomy, thoracotomy) for ECMO/ECLS**

🔲 22.6   🔳 22.6   **FUD** 000   C 80

AMA: 2015,Jul,3

\# **33989**   **Removal of left heart vent by thoracic incision (eg, sternotomy, thoracotomy) for ECMO/ECLS**

🔲 14.4   🔳 14.4   **FUD** 000   C 80

AMA: 2015,Jul,3

33962-33999 Mechanical Circulatory Support

33962   Resequenced code. See code following 33959.
33963   Resequenced code. See code following 33959.
33964   Resequenced code. See code following 33959.
33965   Resequenced code. See code following 33959.
33966   Resequenced code. See code following 33959.

33967   **Insertion of intra-aortic balloon assist device, percutaneous**

🔲 7.55   🔳 7.55   **FUD** 000   C 80

AMA: 2015,Jul,3; 2015,Jan,16; 2014,Jan,11; 2013,Mar,10-11; 2012,Jan,15-42

33968   **Removal of intra-aortic balloon assist device, percutaneous**

🔲 0.97   🔳 0.97   **FUD** 000   C

AMA: 2015,Jul,3; 2015,Jan,16; 2014,Jan,11; 2012,Jan,15-42; 2011,Jan,11

33969   **Resequenced code. See code following 33959.**

33970   **Insertion of intra-aortic balloon assist device through the femoral artery, open approach**

EXCLUDES Percutaneous insertion of intra-aortic balloon assist device (33967)

🔲 10.3   🔳 10.3   **FUD** 000   C 80

AMA: 2015,Jul,3; 2015,Jan,16; 2014,Jan,11; 2013,Mar,10-11

33971   **Removal of intra-aortic balloon assist device including repair of femoral artery, with or without graft**

🔲 20.6   🔳 20.6   **FUD** 090   C

AMA: 2015,Jul,3; 2015,Jan,16; 2014,Jan,11

33973   **Insertion of intra-aortic balloon assist device through the ascending aorta**

🔲 15.0   🔳 15.0   **FUD** 000   C 80

AMA: 2015,Jul,3; 2015,Jan,16; 2014,Jan,11; 2013,Mar,10-11

33974   **Removal of intra-aortic balloon assist device from the ascending aorta, including repair of the ascending aorta, with or without graft**

🔲 26.0   🔳 26.0   **FUD** 090   C

AMA: 2015,Jul,3; 2015,Jan,16; 2014,Jan,11

33975   **Insertion of ventricular assist device; extracorporeal, single ventricle**

INCLUDES Insertion of the new pump with de-airing, connection, and initiation
Removal of the old pump with replacement of the entire ventricular assist device system, including pump(s) and cannulas
Transthoracic approach

EXCLUDES Percutaneous approach (33990-33991)
Replacement percutaneous transseptal approach (33999)

Code also removal of thrombus through a separate heart incision, when performed (33310-33315); append modifier 59 to (33315)

🔲 38.2   🔳 38.2   **FUD** XXX   C 80

AMA: 2015,Jul,3; 2015,Jan,16; 2014,Jan,11; 2013,Mar,10-11; 2012,Jan,15-42; 2011,Jan,11; 2010,Apr,6-8; 2010,Jan,11-12

33976   **extracorporeal, biventricular**

INCLUDES Insertion of the new pump with de-airing, connection, and initiation
Removal with replacement of the entire ventricular assist device system, including pump(s) and cannulas
Transthoracic approach

EXCLUDES Percutaneous approach (33990-33991)
Replacement percutaneous transseptal approach (33999)

Code also removal of thrombus through a separate heart incision, when performed (33310-33315); append modifier 59 to (33315)

🔲 46.6   🔳 46.6   **FUD** XXX   C 80

AMA: 2015,Jul,3; 2015,Jan,16; 2014,Jan,11; 2013,Mar,10-11; 2012,Jan,15-42; 2010,Apr,6-8; 2010,Jan,11-12

33977   **Removal of ventricular assist device; extracorporeal, single ventricle**

INCLUDES Removal of the entire device and the cannulas

EXCLUDES Replacement percutaneous transseptal approach (33999)

Code also removal of thrombus through a separate heart incision, when performed (33310-33315); append modifier 59 to (33315)
Do not report removal of the ventricular assist device when performed at the time of insertion of a new device

🔲 32.9   🔳 32.9   **FUD** XXX   C 80

AMA: 2015,Jul,3; 2015,Jan,16; 2014,Jan,11; 2013,Mar,10-11; 2012,Jan,15-42; 2010,Apr,6-8; 2010,Jan,11-12

| 26 /TC PC/TC Comp Only | A2-Z3 ASC Pmt | 50 Bilateral | ♂ Male Only | ♀ Female Only | 🔲 Facility RVU | 🔳 Non-Facility RVU |
| AMA: CPT Asst | CMS: Pub 100 | A-Y OPPSI | 80 /80 Surg Assist Allowed / w/Doc | | 🔳 Lab Crosswalk | 🔳 Radiology Crosswalk |

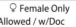 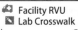 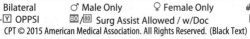

126   Medicare (Red Text)   CPT © 2015 American Medical Association. All Rights Reserved. (Black Text)   © 2015 Optum360, LLC (Blue Text)

33978 extracorporeal, biventricular

> **INCLUDES** Removal of the entire device and the cannulas
>
> **EXCLUDES** *Replacement percutaneous transseptal approach (33999)*
>
> Code also removal of thrombus through a separate heart incision, when performed (33310-33315); append modifier 59 to (33315)
>
> Do not report removal of the ventricular assist device when performed at the time of insertion of a new device
>
> 🚑 39.1   ⚕ 39.1   **FUD** XXX   C 80 ▱
>
> **AMA:** 2015,Jul,3; 2015,Jan,16; 2014,Jan,11; 2013,Mar,10-11; 2012,Jan,15-42; 2010,Apr,6-8; 2010,Jan,11-12

33979 Insertion of ventricular assist device, implantable intracorporeal, single ventricle

> **INCLUDES** New pump insertion with connection, de-airing, and initiation
>
> Removal with replacement of the entire ventricular assist device system, including pump(s) and cannulas
>
> Transthoracic approach
>
> **EXCLUDES** *Percutaneous approach (33990-33991)*
>
> *Replacement percutaneous transseptal approach (33999)*
>
> Code also removal of thrombus through a separate heart incision, when performed (33310-33315); append modifier 59 to (33315)
>
> 🚑 57.0   ⚕ 57.0   **FUD** XXX   C 80 ▱
>
> **AMA:** 2015,Jul,3; 2015,Jan,16; 2014,Jan,11; 2013,Mar,10-11; 2012,Jan,15-42; 2010,Apr,6-8; 2010,Jan,11-12

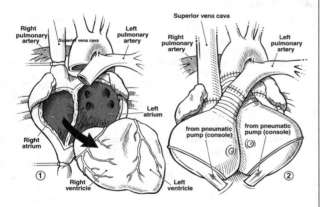

33980 Removal of ventricular assist device, implantable intracorporeal, single ventricle

> **INCLUDES** Removal of the entire device and the cannulas
>
> **EXCLUDES** *Percutaneous transseptal approach (33999)*
>
> Code also removal of thrombus through a separate heart incision, when performed (33310-33315); append modifier 59 to (33315)
>
> Do not report removal of the ventricular assist device when performed at the time of insertion of a new device
>
> 🚑 52.0   ⚕ 52.0   **FUD** XXX   C 80 ▱
>
> **AMA:** 2015,Jul,3; 2015,Jan,16; 2014,Jan,11; 2013,Mar,10-11; 2010,Apr,6-8; 2010,Jan,11-12

33981 Replacement of extracorporeal ventricular assist device, single or biventricular, pump(s), single or each pump

> **INCLUDES** Insertion of the new pump with de-airing, connection, and initiation
>
> Removal of the old pump
>
> **EXCLUDES** *Percutaneous transseptal approach (33999)*
>
> 🚑 24.4   ⚕ 24.4   **FUD** XXX   C 80
>
> **AMA:** 2015,Jul,3; 2015,Jan,16; 2014,Jan,11; 2010,Apr,6-8; 2010,Jan,11-12

33982 Replacement of ventricular assist device pump(s); implantable intracorporeal, single ventricle, without cardiopulmonary bypass

> **INCLUDES** New pump insertion with connection, de-airing, and initiation
>
> Removal of the old pump
>
> **EXCLUDES** *Percutaneous transseptal approach (33999)*
>
> 🚑 57.4   ⚕ 57.4   **FUD** XXX   C 80
>
> **AMA:** 2015,Jul,3; 2015,Jan,16; 2014,Jan,11; 2010,Apr,6-8; 2010,Jan,11-12

33983 implantable intracorporeal, single ventricle, with cardiopulmonary bypass

> **INCLUDES** Insertion of the new pump with de-airing, connection, and initiation
>
> Removal of the old pump
>
> **EXCLUDES** *Percutaneous transseptal approach (33999)*
>
> 🚑 67.7   ⚕ 67.7   **FUD** XXX   C 80
>
> **AMA:** 2015,Jul,3; 2015,Jan,16; 2014,Jan,11; 2010,Apr,6-8; 2010,Jan,11-12

33984 **Resequenced code. See code following 33959.**

33985 **Resequenced code. See code following 33959.**

33986 **Resequenced code. See code following 33959.**

33987 **Resequenced code. See code following 33959.**

33988 **Resequenced code. See code following 33959.**

33989 **Resequenced code. See code following 33959.**

33990 Insertion of ventricular assist device, percutaneous including radiological supervision and interpretation; arterial access only

> **INCLUDES** Initial insertion and replacement of percutaneous ventricular assist device
>
> **EXCLUDES** *Extensive artery repair/replacement (35226, 35286)*
>
> *Open arterial approach to aid insertion of percutaneous ventricular assist device, when used (34812)*
>
> *Transthoracic approach (33975-33976)*
>
> Do not report removal of percutaneous ventricular assist device at time of replacement of the entire system (33992)
>
> 🚑 12.7   ⚕ 12.7   **FUD** XXX   ⊙ C 80
>
> **AMA:** 2015,Jan,16; 2014,Oct,14; 2014,Jan,11; 2013,Mar,10-11

33991 both arterial and venous access, with transseptal puncture

> **INCLUDES** Initial insertion as well as replacement of percutaneous ventricular assist device
>
> **EXCLUDES** *Extensive artery repair/replacement (35226, 35286)*
>
> *Open arterial approach to aid with insertion of percutaneous ventricular assist device, when performed (34812)*
>
> *Transthoracic approach (33975-33976)*
>
> Do not report removal of percutaneous ventricular assist device at time of replacement of the entire system (33992)
>
> 🚑 18.5   ⚕ 18.5   **FUD** XXX   ⊙ C 80
>
> **AMA:** 2015,Jan,16; 2014,Jan,11; 2013,Mar,10-11

33992 Removal of percutaneous ventricular assist device at separate and distinct session from insertion

> **INCLUDES** Removal of device and cannulas
>
> Code also modifier 59 when percutaneous ventricular assist device is removed on the same day as the insertion, but at a different session
>
> 🚑 6.23   ⚕ 6.23   **FUD** XXX   ⊙ C 80
>
> **AMA:** 2015,Jan,16; 2014,Jan,11; 2013,Mar,10-11

33993 **Repositioning of percutaneous ventricular assist device with imaging guidance at separate and distinct session from insertion**

> Code also modifier 59 when percutaneous ventricular assist device is repositioned using imaging guidance on the same day as the insertion, but at a different session
> Do not report repositioning of a percutaneous ventricular assist device without image guidance
> Do not report repositioning of the percutaneous ventricular assist device at the same session as the insertion

🔧 5.49   ✂ 5.49   **FUD** XXX   ⊙ C 80

AMA: 2015,Jan,16; 2014,Jan,11; 2013,Mar,10-11

33999 **Unlisted procedure, cardiac surgery**

🔧 0.00   ✂ 0.00   **FUD** YYY   T 80 P0

AMA: 2015,Jan,16; 2014,Dec,16; 2014,Dec,16; 2014,Jan,11; 2013,Dec,14; 2013,Mar,10-11; 2013,Feb,13; 2012,Jan,15-42; 2011,Jan,11; 2010,Apr,6-8; 2010,Jan,11-12

34001-34530 Surgical Revascularization: Veins and Arteries

INCLUDES   Repair of blood vessel
          Surgeon's component of operative arteriogram

34001 **Embolectomy or thrombectomy, with or without catheter; carotid, subclavian or innominate artery, by neck incision**

🔧 29.1   ✂ 29.1   **FUD** 090   C 80 50 ▢

AMA: 1997,Nov,1

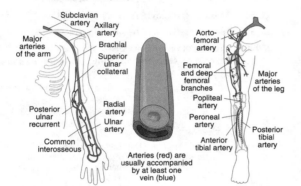

Arteries (red) are usually accompanied by at least one vein (blue)

34051 **innominate, subclavian artery, by thoracic incision**

🔧 26.3   ✂ 26.3   **FUD** 090   C 80 50 ▢ P0

AMA: 1997,Nov,1

34101 **axillary, brachial, innominate, subclavian artery, by arm incision**

🔧 17.7   ✂ 17.7   **FUD** 090   T 80 50 ▢

AMA: 1997,Nov,1

34111 **radial or ulnar artery, by arm incision**

🔧 17.6   ✂ 17.6   **FUD** 090   T 80 50 ▢

AMA: 1997,Nov,1

34151 **renal, celiac, mesentery, aortoiliac artery, by abdominal incision**

🔧 41.4   ✂ 41.4   **FUD** 090   C 80 50 ▢

AMA: 1997,Nov,1

34201 **femoropopliteal, aortoiliac artery, by leg incision**

🔧 30.5   ✂ 30.5   **FUD** 090   T 80 50 ▢

AMA: 2015,Jan,16; 2014,Jan,11; 2012,Jan,15-42; 2011,Aug,9-10

34203 **popliteal-tibio-peroneal artery, by leg incision**

🔧 28.1   ✂ 28.1   **FUD** 090   T 80 50 ▢

AMA: 1997,Nov,1

34401 **Thrombectomy, direct or with catheter; vena cava, iliac vein, by abdominal incision**

🔧 43.0   ✂ 43.0   **FUD** 090   C 80 50 ▢

AMA: 1997,Nov,1

34421 **vena cava, iliac, femoropopliteal vein, by leg incision**

🔧 21.5   ✂ 21.5   **FUD** 090   T 80 50 ▢

AMA: 2015,Jan,16; 2014,Jan,11

34451 **vena cava, iliac, femoropopliteal vein, by abdominal and leg incision**

🔧 48.5   ✂ 48.5   **FUD** 090   C 80 50 ▢

AMA: 1997,Nov,1

34471 **subclavian vein, by neck incision**

🔧 31.9   ✂ 31.9   **FUD** 090   T 50 ▢

AMA: 1997,Nov,1

34490 **axillary and subclavian vein, by arm incision**

🔧 18.0   ✂ 18.0   **FUD** 090   T 62 50 ▢

AMA: 1997,Nov,1

34501 **Valvuloplasty, femoral vein**

🔧 26.4   ✂ 26.4   **FUD** 090   T 80 50 ▢

AMA: 1997,Nov,1

34502 **Reconstruction of vena cava, any method**

🔧 44.9   ✂ 44.9   **FUD** 090   C 80 ▢

AMA: 1997,Nov,1

34510 **Venous valve transposition, any vein donor**

🔧 34.8   ✂ 34.8   **FUD** 090   T 80 50 ▢

AMA: 1997,Nov,1

34520 **Cross-over vein graft to venous system**

🔧 29.3   ✂ 29.3   **FUD** 090   T 80 50 ▢

AMA: 1997,Nov,1

34530 **Saphenopopliteal vein anastomosis**

🔧 32.3   ✂ 32.3   **FUD** 090   T 80 50 ▢

AMA: 1997,Nov,1

34800-34834 Endovascular Stent Grafting for Abdominal Aneurysms

INCLUDES   Balloon angioplasty/stent deployment within the target treatment zone
          Introduction, manipulation, placement, and deployment of the device
          Open exposure of femoral or iliac artery/subsequent closure
          Thromboendarterectomy at site of aneurysm

EXCLUDES   *Additional interventional procedures outside of target treatment zone*
          Guidewire and catheter insertion (36140, 36200, 36245-36248)
          Study, interpretation, and report of implanted wireless pressure sensor in an aneurysmal sac (93982)
          Substantial artery repair/replacement (35226, 35286)
          Transcatheter insertion of wireless physiologic sensor in an aneurysmal sac (34806)

34800 **Endovascular repair of infrarenal abdominal aortic aneurysm or dissection; using aorto-aortic tube prosthesis**

> Code also open arterial exposure as appropriate (34812, 34820, 34833, 34834)
> Do not report with (34841-34848)
> ✚ (75952)

🔧 33.3   ✂ 33.3   **FUD** 090   C 80 50 ▢ P0

AMA: 2015,Jan,16; 2014,Jan,11; 2013,Dec,8; 2012,Apr,3-9; 2012,Jan,15-42; 2011,Jan,11

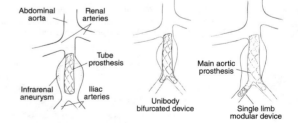

Abdominal aorta   Renal arteries

Infrarenal aneurysm   Iliac arteries   Tube prosthesis

Unibody bifurcated device

Main aortic prosthesis

Single limb modular device

34802 **using modular bifurcated prosthesis (1 docking limb)**

> Code also open arterial exposure as appropriate (34812, 34820, 34833, 34834)
> Do not report with (34841-34848)
> ✚ (75952)

🔧 36.8   ✂ 36.8   **FUD** 090   C 80 ▢ P0

AMA: 2015,Jan,16; 2014,Jan,11; 2013,Dec,8; 2012,Apr,3-9; 2012,Jan,15-42; 2011,Jan,11

34803 **using modular bifurcated prosthesis (2 docking limbs)**
Code also open arterial exposure as appropriate (34812, 34820, 34833, 34834)
Do not report with (34841-34848)
⊠ (75952)
📋 38.0 ⚕ 38.0 **FUD** 090   C 80 ▭ P0
AMA: 2015,Jan,16; 2014,Jan,11; 2013,Dec,8; 2012,Apr,3-9

34804 **using unibody bifurcated prosthesis**
Code also open arterial exposure as appropriate (34812, 34820, 34833, 34834)
Do not report with (34841-34848)
⊠ (75952)
📋 36.8 ⚕ 36.8 **FUD** 090   C 80 ▭ P0
AMA: 2015,Jan,16; 2014,Jan,11; 2013,Dec,8; 2012,Apr,3-9

34805 **using aorto-uniiliac or aorto-unifemoral prosthesis**
Code also open arterial exposure as appropriate (34812, 34820, 34833, 34834)
Do not report with (34841-34848)
⊠ (75952)
📋 35.4 ⚕ 35.4 **FUD** 090   C 80 ▭ P0
AMA: 2015,Jan,16; 2014,Jan,11; 2013,Dec,8; 2012,Apr,3-9; 2012,Jan,15-42; 2011,Jan,11

+ **34806** **Transcatheter placement of wireless physiologic sensor in aneurysmal sac during endovascular repair, including radiological supervision and interpretation, instrument calibration, and collection of pressure data (List separately in addition to code for primary procedure)**
Code also open arterial exposure as appropriate (34812, 34820, 34833-34834)
Code first (33880-33881, 33886, 34800-34805, 34825, 34900)
Do not report with (93982)
📋 2.96 ⚕ 2.96 **FUD** ZZZ   C 80
AMA: 2015,Jan,16; 2014,Jan,11; 2012,Apr,3-9

+ **34808** **Endovascular placement of iliac artery occlusion device (List separately in addition to code for primary procedure)**
Code also open arterial exposure as appropriate (34812, 34820, 34833-34834)
Code first (34800, 34805, 34813, 34825-34826)
📋 6.17 ⚕ 6.17 **FUD** ZZZ   C 80 ▭
AMA: 2015,Jan,16; 2014,Jan,11; 2012,Apr,3-9

34812 **Open femoral artery exposure for delivery of endovascular prosthesis, by groin incision, unilateral**
Code also as appropriate (34800-34808)
Do not report with (33953-33954, 33959, [33962], [33969], [33984])
📋 9.98 ⚕ 9.98 **FUD** 000   C 80 50 ▭
AMA: 2015,Jul,3; 2015,Jan,16; 2014,Jan,11; 2013,Dec,8; 2013,Mar,10-11; 2012,Apr,3-9; 2012,Jan,15-42; 2011,Jan,11

+ **34813** **Placement of femoral-femoral prosthetic graft during endovascular aortic aneurysm repair (List separately in addition to code for primary procedure)**
EXCLUDES *Grafting of femoral artery (35521, 35533, 35539, 35540, 35556, 35558, 35566, 35621, 35646, 35654-35661, 35666, 35700)*
Code first (34812)
📋 7.01 ⚕ 7.01 **FUD** ZZZ   C 80 ▭
AMA: 2015,Jan,16; 2014,Jan,11; 2012,Apr,3-9

34820 **Open iliac artery exposure for delivery of endovascular prosthesis or iliac occlusion during endovascular therapy, by abdominal or retroperitoneal incision, unilateral**
Code also as appropriate (34800-34808)
Do not report with (33953-33954, 33959, [33962], [33969], [33984])
📋 14.5 ⚕ 14.5 **FUD** 000   C 80 50 ▭
AMA: 2015,Jul,3; 2015,Jan,16; 2014,Jan,11; 2012,Apr,3-9; 2012,Jan,15-42; 2011,Jan,11

34825 **Placement of proximal or distal extension prosthesis for endovascular repair of infrarenal abdominal aortic or iliac aneurysm, false aneurysm, or dissection; initial vessel**
Code also as appropriate (34800-34805, 34900)
⊠ (75953)
📋 20.5 ⚕ 20.5 **FUD** 090   C 80 ▭ P0
AMA: 2015,Jan,16; 2014,Jan,11; 2013,Dec,8; 2012,Apr,3-9

+ **34826** **each additional vessel (List separately in addition to code for primary procedure)**
Code also as appropriate (34800-34805, 34900)
Code first (34825)
⊠ (75953)
📋 6.08 ⚕ 6.08 **FUD** ZZZ   C 80 ▭ P0
AMA: 2015,Jan,16; 2014,Jan,11; 2013,Dec,8; 2012,Apr,3-9

34830 **Open repair of infrarenal aortic aneurysm or dissection, plus repair of associated arterial trauma, following unsuccessful endovascular repair; tube prosthesis**
📋 52.3 ⚕ 52.3 **FUD** 090   C 80 ▭ P0
AMA: 2015,Jan,16; 2014,Jan,11; 2012,Jan,15-42; 2011,Jan,11

Abdominal aorta
Renal arteries
Infrarenal aneurysm
Tube prosthesis (34830)
The vessel is opened and repaired
Aorto-bi-iliac prosthesis
Iliac ar
Aorto-bifemoral prosthesis
Prosthesis extends into the femoral arteries

An infrarenal aortic aneurysm or disse[...] treated in an open surgical sessi[...] following an unsuccessful endovasc[...] treatment attempt. A tube prosthesi[...] placed and any associated arteri[...] trauma is repaired

34831 **aorto-bi-iliac prosthesis**
📋 56.2 ⚕ 56.2 **FUD** 090   C 80 ▭ P0
AMA: 2015,Jan,16; 2014,Jan,11; 2012,Jan,15-42; 2011,Jan,11

34832 **aorto-bifemoral prosthesis**
📋 56.2 ⚕ 56.2 **FUD** 090   C 80 ▭ P0
AMA: 2015,Jan,16; 2014,Jan,11; 2012,Jan,15-42; 2011,Jan,11

34833 **Open iliac artery exposure with creation of conduit for delivery of aortic or iliac endovascular prosthesis, by abdominal or retroperitoneal incision, unilateral**
Code also as appropriate (34800-34805)
Do not report with ([33987], 34820)
📋 18.0 ⚕ 18.0 **FUD** 000   C 80 50 ▭
AMA: 2015,Jul,3; 2015,Jan,16; 2014,Jan,11; 2012,Jan,15-42; 2011,Jan,11

34834 **Open brachial artery exposure to assist in the deployment of aortic or iliac endovascular prosthesis by arm incision, unilateral**
Code also as appropriate (34800-34805)
Do not report with (33953-33954, 33959, [33962], [33969], [33984])
📋 8.05 ⚕ 8.05 **FUD** 000   C 80 50 ▭
AMA: 2015,Jul,3; 2015,Jan,16; 2014,Jan,11

34839-34848 Repair Visceral Aorta with Fenestrated Endovascular Grafts

INCLUDES Angiography
Balloon angioplasty before and after deployment of graft
Fluoroscopic guidance
Guidewire and catheter insertion of vessels in the target treatment zone
Radiologic supervision and interpretation
Visceral aorta (34841-34844)
Visceral aorta and associated infrarenal abdominal aorta (34845-34848)

EXCLUDES *Catheterization of:*
Arterial families outside treatment zone
Hypogastric arteries
Distal extension prosthesis terminating in the common femoral, external iliac, or internal iliac artery (34825-34826, 75953, 0254T-0255T)
Interventional procedures outside treatment zone
Open exposure of access vessels (34812)
Repair of abdominal aortic aneurysm without a fenestrated graft (34800-34805)
Substantial artery repair (35226, 35286)
Code also associated endovascular repair of descending thoracic aorta (33880-33886, 75956-75959)
Do not report with placement of bare metal or covered intravascular stents in visceral branches in the target treatment zone (37236-37237)

34839 **Physician planning of a patient-specific fenestrated visceral aortic endograft requiring a minimum of 90 minutes of physician time**

🚑 0.00   ⚖ 0.00   **FUD** YYY   **B** 80

Do not report on day of or day before endovascular repair procedure
Do not report when total planning time is less than 90 minutes
Do not report with (76376-76377)

34841 **Endovascular repair of visceral aorta (eg, aneurysm, pseudoaneurysm, dissection, penetrating ulcer, intramural hematoma, or traumatic disruption) by deployment of a fenestrated visceral aortic endograft and all associated radiological supervision and interpretation, including target zone angioplasty, when performed; including one visceral artery endoprosthesis (superior mesenteric, celiac or renal artery)**

INCLUDES Repairs extending from the visceral aorta to one or more of the four visceral artery origins to the level of the infrarenal aorta

EXCLUDES *Devices extending into the common iliac arteries (34845-34848)*

Do not report with (34800, 34802-34805, 34839, 34845-34848, 35452, 35472, 75952)

🚑 0.00   ⚖ 0.00   **FUD** YYY   **C** 80

AMA: 2015,Jan,16; 2014,Jan,11; 2013,Dec,8

34842 **including two visceral artery endoprostheses (superior mesenteric, celiac and/or renal artery[s])**

INCLUDES Repairs extending from the visceral aorta to one or more of the four visceral artery origins to the level of the infrarenal aorta

EXCLUDES *Devices extending into the common iliac arteries (34845-34848)*

Do not report with (34800, 34802-34805, 34839, 34845-34848, 35452, 35472, 75952)

🚑 0.00   ⚖ 0.00   **FUD** YYY   **C** 80

AMA: 2015,Jan,16; 2014,Jan,11; 2013,Dec,8

34843 **including three visceral artery endoprostheses (superior mesenteric, celiac and/or renal artery[s])**

INCLUDES Repairs extending from the visceral aorta to one or more of the four visceral artery origins to the level of the infrarenal aorta

EXCLUDES *Devices extending into the common iliac arteries (34845-34848)*

Do not report with (34800, 34802-34805, 34839, 34845-34848, 35452, 35472, 75952)

🚑 0.00   ⚖ 0.00   **FUD** YYY   **C** 80

AMA: 2015,Jan,16; 2014,Jan,11; 2013,Dec,8

34844 **including four or more visceral artery endoprostheses (superior mesenteric, celiac and/or renal artery[s])**

INCLUDES Repairs extending from the visceral aorta to one or more of the four visceral artery origins to the level of the infrarenal aorta

EXCLUDES *Devices extending into the common iliac arteries (34845-34848)*

Do not report with (34800, 34802-34805, 34839, 34845-34848, 35452, 35472, 75952)

🚑 0.00   ⚖ 0.00   **FUD** YYY   **C** 80

AMA: 2015,Jan,16; 2014,Jan,11; 2013,Dec,8

34845 **Endovascular repair of visceral aorta and infrarenal abdominal aorta (eg, aneurysm, pseudoaneurysm, dissection, penetrating ulcer, intramural hematoma, or traumatic disruption) with a fenestrated visceral aortic endograft and concomitant unibody or modular infrarenal aortic endograft and all associated radiological supervision and interpretation, including target zone angioplasty, when performed; including one visceral artery endoprosthesis (superior mesenteric, celiac or renal artery)**

INCLUDES Placement of device and extensions into the common iliac arteries
Repairs extending from the visceral aorta into the common iliac arteries

Code also iliac artery revascularization when performed outside zone of target treatment (37220-37223)
Do not report with (34800, 34802-34805, 34839, 34841-34844, 35081, 35102, 35452, 35472, 75952)

🚑 0.00   ⚖ 0.00   **FUD** YYY   **C** 80

AMA: 2015,Jan,16; 2014,Jan,11; 2013,Dec,8

34846 **including two visceral artery endoprostheses (superior mesenteric, celiac and/or renal artery[s])**

INCLUDES Placement of device and extensions into the common iliac arteries
Repairs extending from the visceral aorta into the common iliac arteries

Code also iliac artery revascularization when performed outside zone of target treatment (37220-37223)
Do not report with (34800, 34802-34805, 34839, 34841-34844, 35081, 35102, 35452, 35472, 75952)

🚑 0.00   ⚖ 0.00   **FUD** YYY   **C** 80

AMA: 2015,Jan,16; 2014,Jan,11; 2013,Dec,8

34847 **including three visceral artery endoprostheses (superior mesenteric, celiac and/or renal artery[s])**

INCLUDES Placement of device and extensions into the common iliac arteries
Repairs extending from the visceral aorta into the common iliac arteries

Code also iliac artery revascularization when performed outside zone of target treatment (37220-37223)
Do not report with (34800, 34802-34805, 34839, 34841-34844, 35081, 35102, 35452, 35472, 75952)

🚑 0.00   ⚖ 0.00   **FUD** YYY   **C** 80

AMA: 2015,Jan,16; 2014,Jan,11; 2013,Dec,8

34848 **including four or more visceral artery endoprostheses (superior mesenteric, celiac and/or renal artery[s])**

INCLUDES Placement of device and extensions into the common iliac arteries
Repairs extending from the visceral aorta into the common iliac arteries

Code also iliac artery revascularization when performed outside zone of target treatment (37220-37223)
Do not report with (34800, 34802-34805, 34839, 34841-34844, 35081, 35102, 35452, 35472, 75952)

🚑 0.00   ⚖ 0.00   **FUD** YYY   **C** 80

AMA: 2015,Jan,16; 2014,Jan,11; 2013,Dec,8

34900 Endovascular Stent Grafting Iliac Artery

INCLUDES   Balloon angioplasty/stent deployment within the target treatment zone
Introduction, manipulation, placement, and deployment

EXCLUDES   *Endovascular repair of iliac artery bifurcation (e.g.; aneurysm, arteriovenous malformation, pseudoaneurysm, trauma) using bifurcated endoprosthesis (0254T)*
Insertion guidewires, catheters (36200, 36245-36248)
Open exposure femoral or iliac artery (34812, 34820)
Other concurrent interventional procedures outside of target zone
Placement extension prosthesis (34825-34826)
Substantial artery repair/replacement (35206-35286)

34900   **Endovascular repair of iliac artery (eg, aneurysm, pseudoaneurysm, arteriovenous malformation, trauma) using ilio-iliac tube endoprosthesis**
   (75954)
   26.4   26.4   **FUD** 090   C 80 50 PQ
   AMA: 2015,Jan,16; 2014,Jan,11; 2012,Apr,3-9

35001-35152 Repair Aneurysm, False Aneurysm, Related Arterial Disease

INCLUDES   Endarterectomy procedures

EXCLUDES   *Endovascular repairs of:*
Abdominal aortic aneurysm (34800-34826)
Aneurysm of iliac artery (34900)
Thoracic aortic aneurysm (33880-33891)
Intracranial aneurysms (61697-61710)
Open repairs thoracic aortic aneurysm (33860-33875)
Repairs related to occlusive disease only (35201-35286)

35001   **Direct repair of aneurysm, pseudoaneurysm, or excision (partial or total) and graft insertion, with or without patch graft; for aneurysm and associated occlusive disease, carotid, subclavian artery, by neck incision**
   33.4   33.4   **FUD** 090   C 80 50
   AMA: 2002,May,7; 2000,Dec,1

35002   **for ruptured aneurysm, carotid, subclavian artery, by neck incision**
   33.6   33.6   **FUD** 090   C 80 50
   AMA: 2002,May,7; 1997,Nov,1

35005   **for aneurysm, pseudoaneurysm, and associated occlusive disease, vertebral artery**
   33.9   33.9   **FUD** 090   C 80 50
   AMA: 2002,May,7; 1997,Nov,1

An incision is made in the back of the neck to directly approach an aneurysm or false aneurysm of the vertebral artery. The artery is either repaired directly or excised with a graft

Graft repair

Vertebral artery

Subclavian artery

35011   **for aneurysm and associated occlusive disease, axillary-brachial artery, by arm incision**
   29.6   29.6   **FUD** 090   T 80 50
   AMA: 2002,May,7; 1997,Nov,1

35013   **for ruptured aneurysm, axillary-brachial artery, by arm incision**
   36.8   36.8   **FUD** 090   C 80 50
   AMA: 2002,May,7; 1997,Nov,1

35021   **for aneurysm, pseudoaneurysm, and associated occlusive disease, innominate, subclavian artery, by thoracic incision**
   37.1   37.1   **FUD** 090   C 80 50 PQ
   AMA: 2002,May,7; 1997,Nov,1

35022   **for ruptured aneurysm, innominate, subclavian artery, by thoracic incision**
   42.5   42.5   **FUD** 090   C 80 50
   AMA: 2002,May,7; 1997,Nov,1

35045   **for aneurysm, pseudoaneurysm, and associated occlusive disease, radial or ulnar artery**
   29.3   29.3   **FUD** 090   T 80 50
   AMA: 2002,May,7; 1997,Nov,1

35081   **for aneurysm, pseudoaneurysm, and associated occlusive disease, abdominal aorta**
   51.7   51.7   **FUD** 090   C 80 PQ
   AMA: 2015,Jan,16; 2014,Jan,11; 2013,Dec,8; 2012,Jan,15-42; 2011,Jan,11

35082   **for ruptured aneurysm, abdominal aorta**
   64.9   64.9   **FUD** 090   C 80
   AMA: 2002,May,7; 1997,Nov,1

35091   **for aneurysm, pseudoaneurysm, and associated occlusive disease, abdominal aorta involving visceral vessels (mesenteric, celiac, renal)**
   53.1   53.1   **FUD** 090   C 80 50 PQ
   AMA: 2015,Jan,16; 2014,Jan,11

35092   **for ruptured aneurysm, abdominal aorta involving visceral vessels (mesenteric, celiac, renal)**
   77.3   77.3   **FUD** 090   C 80 50
   AMA: 2002,May,7; 1997,Nov,1

35102   **for aneurysm, pseudoaneurysm, and associated occlusive disease, abdominal aorta involving iliac vessels (common, hypogastric, external)**
   55.9   55.9   **FUD** 090   C 80 50 PQ
   AMA: 2015,Jan,16; 2014,Jan,11; 2013,Dec,8

35103   **for ruptured aneurysm, abdominal aorta involving iliac vessels (common, hypogastric, external)**
   66.7   66.7   **FUD** 090   C 80 50
   AMA: 2002,May,7; 1997,Nov,1

35111   **for aneurysm, pseudoaneurysm, and associated occlusive disease, splenic artery**
   39.3   39.3   **FUD** 090   C 80 50
   AMA: 2002,May,7; 1997,Nov,1

35112   **for ruptured aneurysm, splenic artery**
   55.1   55.1   **FUD** 090   C 80 50
   AMA: 2002,May,7; 1997,Nov,1

35121   **for aneurysm, pseudoaneurysm, and associated occlusive disease, hepatic, celiac, renal, or mesenteric artery**
   48.6   48.6   **FUD** 090   C 80 50
   AMA: 2002,May,7; 1997,Nov,1

35122   **for ruptured aneurysm, hepatic, celiac, renal, or mesenteric artery**
   63.6   63.6   **FUD** 090   C 80 50
   AMA: 2002,May,7; 1997,Nov,1

35131   **for aneurysm, pseudoaneurysm, and associated occlusive disease, iliac artery (common, hypogastric, external)**
   41.1   41.1   **FUD** 090   C 80 50 PQ
   AMA: 2015,Jan,16; 2014,Jan,11

35132   **for ruptured aneurysm, iliac artery (common, hypogastric, external)**
   48.5   48.5   **FUD** 090   C 80 50
   AMA: 2002,May,7; 1997,Nov,1

35141   **for aneurysm, pseudoaneurysm, and associated occlusive disease, common femoral artery (profunda femoris, superficial femoral)**
   32.8   32.8   **FUD** 090   C 80 50 PQ
   AMA: 2002,May,7; 1997,Nov,1

35142   **for ruptured aneurysm, common femoral artery (profunda femoris, superficial femoral)**
   39.0   39.0   **FUD** 090   C 80 50
   AMA: 2002,May,7; 1997,Nov,1

● New Code   ▲ Revised Code   ○ Reinstated   M Maternity   A Age Edit   Unlisted   Not Covered   # Resequenced
◎ AMA Mod 51 Exempt   ⑨ Optum Mod 51 Exempt   63 Mod 63 Exempt   ⊙ Mod Sedation   + Add-on   CCI   PQ PQRS   **FUD** Follow-up Days

35151 **for aneurysm, pseudoaneurysm, and associated occlusive disease, popliteal artery**
   36.8   36.8   **FUD** 090   C 80 50 ▢ P0
   AMA: 2002,May,7; 1997,Nov,1

35152 **for ruptured aneurysm, popliteal artery**
   41.4   41.4   **FUD** 090   C 80 50 ▢
   AMA: 2002,May,7; 1997,Nov,1

35180-35190 Surgical Repair Arteriovenous Fistula

35180 **Repair, congenital arteriovenous fistula; head and neck**
   26.4   26.4   **FUD** 090   T 80 ▢
   AMA: 2015,Jan,16; 2014,Jan,11; 2012,Jan,15-42; 2011,Aug,9-10

35182 **thorax and abdomen**
   47.8   47.8   **FUD** 090   C 80 ▢
   AMA: 2015,Jan,16; 2014,Jan,11; 2012,Jan,15-42; 2011,Aug,9-10

35184 **extremities**
   32.8   32.8   **FUD** 090   T 80 ▢
   AMA: 2015,Jan,16; 2014,Jan,11; 2012,Jan,15-42; 2011,Aug,9-10

35188 **Repair, acquired or traumatic arteriovenous fistula; head and neck**
   31.2   31.2   **FUD** 090   T A2 80 ▢
   AMA: 2015,Jan,16; 2014,Jan,11; 2012,Jan,15-42; 2011,Aug,9-10

35189 **thorax and abdomen**
   44.7   44.7   **FUD** 090   C 80 ▢
   AMA: 2015,Jan,16; 2014,Jan,11; 2012,Jan,15-42; 2011,Aug,9-10

35190 **extremities**
   22.4   22.4   **FUD** 090   T 80 ▢
   AMA: 2015,Jan,16; 2014,Jan,11; 2012,Jan,15-42; 2011,Aug,9-10

35201-35286 Surgical Repair Artery or Vein

EXCLUDES *Arteriovenous fistula repair (35180-35190)*
Do not report with a primary open vascular procedure

35201 **Repair blood vessel, direct; neck**
   Do not report with ([33969, 33984, 33985, 33986])
   28.1   28.1   **FUD** 090   T 80 50 ▢
   AMA: 2015,Jul,3; 2015,Jan,16; 2014,Mar,8

35206 **upper extremity**
   Do not report with ([33969, 33984, 33985, 33986])
   22.8   22.8   **FUD** 090   T 80 50 ▢
   AMA: 2015,Jul,3; 2015,Jan,16; 2014,Apr,10; 2014,Jan,11; 2012,Apr,3-9

35207 **hand, finger**
   21.7   21.7   **FUD** 090   T A2 50 ▢
   AMA: 2012,Apr,3-9

35211 **intrathoracic, with bypass**
   Do not report with ([33969, 33984, 33985, 33986])
   40.2   40.2   **FUD** 090   C 80 50 ▢ P0
   AMA: 2015,Jul,3; 2012,Apr,3-9

35216 **intrathoracic, without bypass**
   Do not report with ([33969, 33984, 33985, 33986])
   59.8   59.8   **FUD** 090   C 80 50 ▢ P0
   AMA: 2015,Jan,16; 2014,Jan,11; 2012,Apr,3-9

35221 **intra-abdominal**
   42.6   42.6   **FUD** 090   C 80 50 ▢
   AMA: 2012,Apr,3-9

35226 **lower extremity**
   Do not report with ([33969, 33984, 33985, 33986])
   24.5   24.5   **FUD** 090   T 80 50 ▢
   AMA: 2015,Jul,3; 2015,Jan,16; 2014,Jan,11; 2013,Dec,8; 2013,Mar,10-11; 2012,Apr,3-9

35231 **Repair blood vessel with vein graft; neck**
   35.9   35.9   **FUD** 090   T 80 50 ▢
   AMA: 2012,Apr,3-9

35236 **upper extremity**
   28.9   28.9   **FUD** 090   T 80 50 ▢
   AMA: 2015,Jan,16; 2014,Jan,11; 2012,Apr,3-9

35241 **intrathoracic, with bypass**
   42.1   42.1   **FUD** 090   C 80 50 ▢ P0
   AMA: 2012,Apr,3-9

35246 **intrathoracic, without bypass**
   46.2   46.2   **FUD** 090   C 80 50 ▢ P0
   AMA: 2012,Apr,3-9

35251 **intra-abdominal**
   50.2   50.2   **FUD** 090   C 80 50 ▢
   AMA: 2012,Apr,3-9

35256 **lower extremity**
   30.0   30.0   **FUD** 090   T 80 50 ▢
   AMA: 2012,Apr,3-9

35261 **Repair blood vessel with graft other than vein; neck**
   31.6   31.6   **FUD** 090   T 80 50 ▢
   AMA: 2012,Apr,3-9

35266 **upper extremity**
   25.5   25.5   **FUD** 090   T 80 50 ▢
   AMA: 2015,Jan,16; 2014,Jan,11; 2012,Apr,3-9

35271 **intrathoracic, with bypass**
   40.4   40.4   **FUD** 090   C 80 50 ▢ P0
   AMA: 2012,Apr,3-9

35276 **intrathoracic, without bypass**
   42.9   42.9   **FUD** 090   C 80 50 ▢ P0
   AMA: 2012,Apr,3-9

35281 **intra-abdominal**
   47.8   47.8   **FUD** 090   C 80 50 ▢
   AMA: 2012,Apr,3-9

35286 **lower extremity**
   27.5   27.5   **FUD** 090   T 80 50 ▢
   AMA: 2015,Jan,16; 2014,Jan,11; 2013,Dec,8; 2013,Mar,10-11; 2012,Apr,3-9

35301-35372 Surgical Thromboendarterectomy Peripheral and Visceral Arteries

INCLUDES Obtaining saphenous or arm vein for graft
Thrombectomy/embolectomy
EXCLUDES *Coronary artery bypass procedures (33510-33536, 33572)*
Thromboendarterectomy for vascular occlusion on a different vessel during the same session

35301 **Thromboendarterectomy, including patch graft, if performed; carotid, vertebral, subclavian, by neck incision**
   33.4   33.4   **FUD** 090   C 80 50 ▢ P0
   AMA: 2015,Jan,16; 2014,Jan,11; 2010,Sep,6-7

Vertebral

Thrombus (blood clot)

External carotid

Carotid artery

Internal carotid

Subclavian artery

Aorta

Plaque

Tool to remove clot and/or plaque

35302 **superficial femoral artery**
   Do not report with (35500, 37225, 37227)
   33.3   33.3   **FUD** 090   C 80 50
   AMA: 2015,Jan,16; 2014,Jan,11

35303 **popliteal artery**
   Do not report with (35500, 37225, 37227)
   36.7   36.7   **FUD** 090   C 80 50
   AMA: 2015,Jan,16; 2014,Jan,11

35304 **tibioperoneal trunk artery**
Do not report with (35500, 37229, 37231, 37233, 37235)
⚙ 38.0 ⚒ 38.0 **FUD** 090
[C] [80] [50]
AMA: 2015,Jan,16; 2014,Jan,11

35305 **tibial or peroneal artery, initial vessel**
Do not report with (35500, 37229, 37231, 37233, 37235)
⚙ 36.2 ⚒ 36.2 **FUD** 090
[C] [80] [50]
AMA: 2015,Jan,16; 2014,Jan,11; 2012,Jan,15-42; 2011,Jan,11

+ **35306** **each additional tibial or peroneal artery (List separately in addition to code for primary procedure)**
Code first (35305)
Do not report with (35500, 37229, 37231, 37233, 37235)
⚙ 13.2 ⚒ 13.2 **FUD** ZZZ
[C] [80]
AMA: 2015,Jan,16; 2014,Jan,11

35311 **subclavian, innominate, by thoracic incision**
⚙ 45.9 ⚒ 45.9 **FUD** 090
[C] [80] [50] [□] [PQ]
AMA: 1997,Nov,1

35321 **axillary-brachial**
⚙ 26.2 ⚒ 26.2 **FUD** 090
[T] [80] [50]
AMA: 1997,Nov,1

35331 **abdominal aorta**
⚙ 43.0 ⚒ 43.0 **FUD** 090
[C] [80] [50] [□]
AMA: 1997,Nov,1

35341 **mesenteric, celiac, or renal**
⚙ 40.2 ⚒ 40.2 **FUD** 090
[C] [80] [50] [□]
AMA: 1997,Nov,1

35351 **iliac**
⚙ 37.9 ⚒ 37.9 **FUD** 090
[C] [80] [50] [□]
AMA: 1997,Nov,1

35355 **iliofemoral**
⚙ 30.6 ⚒ 30.6 **FUD** 090
[C] [80] [50] [□]
AMA: 1997,Nov,1

35361 **combined aortoiliac**
⚙ 45.1 ⚒ 45.1 **FUD** 090
[C] [80] [50] [□]
AMA: 1997,Nov,1

35363 **combined aortoiliofemoral**
⚙ 51.8 ⚒ 51.8 **FUD** 090
[C] [80] [50] [□]
AMA: 1997,Nov,1

35371 **common femoral**
⚙ 24.2 ⚒ 24.2 **FUD** 090
[C] [80] [50] [□]
AMA: 2015,Jan,16; 2014,Jan,11; 2012,Apr,3-9

35372 **deep (profunda) femoral**
⚙ 29.0 ⚒ 29.0 **FUD** 090
[C] [80] [50] [□]
AMA: 2015,Jan,16; 2014,Jan,11

35390 Surgical Thromboendarterectomy: Carotid Reoperation

Code first (35301)

+ **35390** **Reoperation, carotid, thromboendarterectomy, more than 1 month after original operation (List separately in addition to code for primary procedure)**
⚙ 4.73 ⚒ 4.73 **FUD** ZZZ
[C] [80] [□]
AMA: 1997,Nov,1; 1993,Win,1

35400 Endoscopic Visualization of Vessels

Code first the therapeutic intervention

+ **35400** **Angioscopy (noncoronary vessels or grafts) during therapeutic intervention (List separately in addition to code for primary procedure)**
⚙ 4.42 ⚒ 4.42 **FUD** ZZZ
[C] [80] [□]
AMA: 1997,Dec,1; 1997,Nov,1

35450-35460 Transluminal Angioplasty: Open

35450 **Transluminal balloon angioplasty, open; renal or other visceral artery**
(75962-75968, 75978)
⚙ 14.8 ⚒ 14.8 **FUD** 000
[C] [80] [50] [□]
AMA: 2015,Jan,16; 2014,Jan,11

35452 **aortic**
Do not report with (34841-34848)
(75962-75968, 75978)
⚙ 10.1 ⚒ 10.1 **FUD** 000
[C] [80] [50] [□]
AMA: 2015,Jan,16; 2014,Jan,11; 2013,Dec,8

35458 **brachiocephalic trunk or branches, each vessel**
Do not report with transcatheter intravascular stent placement of common carotid or innominate artery on the same side (37217)
(75962-75968, 75978)
⚙ 14.4 ⚒ 14.4 **FUD** 000
[J] [80] [50] [□]
AMA: 2015,Jan,16; 2014,Mar,8; 2014,Jan,11; 2012,Apr,3-9; 2012,Jan,15-42; 2011,Jan,11

35460 **venous**
(75962-75968, 75978)
⚙ 9.26 ⚒ 9.26 **FUD** 000
[J] [62] [50] [□]
AMA: 1997,Feb,1; 1997,Nov,1

35471-35476 Transluminal Angioplasty: Percutaneous

EXCLUDES   Catheter placement
Radiological supervision and interpretation

35471 **Transluminal balloon angioplasty, percutaneous; renal or visceral artery**
(75966, 75968)
⚙ 15.3 ⚒ 72.8 **FUD** 000
⊙ [J] [50] [□]
AMA: 2015,Jan,16; 2014,Jan,11

In 35471, a balloon is delivered into narrowed section of renal or visceral artery. Access is by catheter through femoral artery.

Celiac
Renal

Balloon is inflated in narrowed section of the artery and patency is restored

A balloon angioplasty is performed on the renal or visceral artery in a percutaneous procedure

35472 **aortic**
Do not report with (34841-34848)
(75966, 75968)
⚙ 10.5 ⚒ 53.3 **FUD** 000
⊙ [J] [80] [50] [□]
AMA: 2015,Jan,16; 2014,Jan,11; 2013,Dec,8

35475 **brachiocephalic trunk or branches, each vessel**
INCLUDES   All work performed for AV shunt to treat lesion(s) from the peri-arterial anastomosis through the axillary vein
EXCLUDES   Removal of arterial plug (36870)
(75962)
⚙ 9.78 ⚒ 44.4 **FUD** 000
⊙ [J] [P3] [50] [□]
AMA: 2015,Jan,16; 2014,Jan,11; 2012,Apr,3-9; 2012,Jan,15-42; 2011,Jan,11

35476 **venous**
INCLUDES   All services in an AV shunt segment including treatment of multiple distinct lesions
EXCLUDES   Removal of arterial plug (36870)
Do not report venous interventional codes for stenosis at the arterial anastomosis (peri-anastomotic or juxta-anastomotic region) (35475)
(75978)
⚙ 7.91 ⚒ 40.6 **FUD** 000
⊙ [J] [P3] [50] [□]
AMA: 2015,Jan,16; 2014,Jan,11; 2012,Apr,3-9; 2012,Jan,15-42; 2011,Dec,14-18

35500 Obtain Arm Vein for Graft

EXCLUDES Endoscopic harvest (33508)
          Harvesting of multiple vein segments (35682, 35683)
Code first (33510-33536, 35556, 35566, 35570-35571, 35583-35587)

+ 35500   **Harvest of upper extremity vein, 1 segment, for lower extremity or coronary artery bypass procedure (List separately in addition to code for primary procedure)**
           🚗 9.46   ✂ 9.46   **FUD** ZZZ   N 80 ▭ P0
           AMA: 2015,Jan,16; 2014,Jan,11; 2012,Apr,3-9

35501-35571 Arterial Bypass Using Vein Grafts

INCLUDES Obtaining saphenous vein grafts
EXCLUDES Obtaining multiple vein segments (35682, 35683)
          Obtaining vein grafts, upper extremity or femoropopliteal (35500, 35572)
          Treatment of different sites with different bypass procedures during the same operative session

35501   **Bypass graft, with vein; common carotid-ipsilateral internal carotid**
         🚗 44.5   ✂ 44.5   **FUD** 090   C 80 50 ▭
         AMA: 2015,Jan,16; 2014,Jan,11; 2012,Apr,3-9

35506   **carotid-subclavian or subclavian-carotid**
         🚗 37.8   ✂ 37.8   **FUD** 090   C 80 50 ▭
         AMA: 2015,Jan,16; 2014,Jan,11

35508   **carotid-vertebral**
         INCLUDES Endoscopic procedure
         🚗 39.4   ✂ 39.4   **FUD** 090   C 80 50 ▭
         AMA: 1999,Mar,6; 1999,Apr,11

35509   **carotid-contralateral carotid**
         🚗 41.9   ✂ 41.9   **FUD** 090   C 80 50 ▭
         AMA: 2015,Jan,16; 2014,Jan,11; 2012,Jan,15-42; 2011,Jan,11

35510   **carotid-brachial**
         🚗 36.5   ✂ 36.5   **FUD** 090   C 80 50 ▭
         AMA: 2015,Jan,16; 2014,Jan,11; 2012,Jan,15-42; 2011,Jan,11

35511   **subclavian-subclavian**
         🚗 33.2   ✂ 33.2   **FUD** 090   C 80 50 ▭
         AMA: 2015,Jan,16; 2014,Jan,11

35512   **subclavian-brachial**
         🚗 40.7   ✂ 40.7   **FUD** 090   C 80 50 ▭
         AMA: 2015,Jan,16; 2014,Jan,11

35515   **subclavian-vertebral**
         🚗 45.1   ✂ 45.1   **FUD** 090   C 80 50 ▭
         AMA: 1999,Mar,6; 1999,Apr,11

35516   **subclavian-axillary**
         🚗 36.2   ✂ 36.2   **FUD** 090   C 80 50 ▭
         AMA: 1999,Mar,6; 1999,Apr,11

35518   **axillary-axillary**
         🚗 33.9   ✂ 33.9   **FUD** 090   C 80 50 ▭
         AMA: 2015,Jan,16; 2014,Jan,11

35521   **axillary-femoral**
         EXCLUDES Synthetic graft (35621)
         🚗 36.3   ✂ 36.3   **FUD** 090   C 80 50 ▭
         AMA: 2015,Jan,16; 2014,Jan,11; 2012,Apr,3-9

35522   **axillary-brachial**
         🚗 36.0   ✂ 36.0   **FUD** 090   C 80 50 ▭
         AMA: 2015,Jan,16; 2014,Jan,11

35523   **brachial-ulnar or -radial**
         🚗 38.2   ✂ 38.2   **FUD** 090   C 80 50
         EXCLUDES Bypass graft using synthetic conduit (37799)
         Do not report with (35206, 35500, 35525, 36838)

35525   **brachial-brachial**
         🚗 34.0   ✂ 34.0   **FUD** 090   C 80 50 ▭
         AMA: 2015,Jan,16; 2014,Jan,11

35526   **aortosubclavian, aortoinnominate, or aortocarotid**
         EXCLUDES Synthetic graft (35626)
         🚗 51.1   ✂ 51.1   **FUD** 090   C 80 50 ▭ P0
         AMA: 1999,Mar,6; 1999,Apr,11

35531   **aortoceliac or aortomesenteric**
         🚗 59.9   ✂ 59.9   **FUD** 090   C 80 50 ▭
         AMA: 1999,Mar,6; 1999,Apr,11

35533   **axillary-femoral-femoral**
         EXCLUDES Synthetic graft (35654)
         🚗 44.7   ✂ 44.7   **FUD** 090   C 80 50 ▭
         AMA: 2012,Apr,3-9

35535   **hepatorenal**
         🚗 56.4   ✂ 56.4   **FUD** 090   C 80 50
         Do not report with (35221, 35251, 35281, 35500, 35536, 35560, 35631, 35636)

35536   **splenorenal**
         🚗 50.1   ✂ 50.1   **FUD** 090   C 80 50 ▭
         AMA: 2015,Jan,16; 2014,Jan,11; 2012,Jan,15-42; 2011,Jan,11

35537   **aortoiliac**
         EXCLUDES Synthetic graft (35637)
         Do not report with (35538)
         🚗 70.1   ✂ 70.1   **FUD** 090   C 80
         AMA: 2015,Jan,16; 2014,Jan,11; 2012,Apr,3-9

35538   **aortobi-iliac**
         EXCLUDES Synthetic graft (35638)
         Do not report with (35537)
         🚗 69.2   ✂ 69.2   **FUD** 090   C 80
         AMA: 2015,Jan,16; 2014,Jan,11; 2012,Apr,3-9

35539   **aortofemoral**
         EXCLUDES Synthetic graft (35647)
         Do not report with (35540)
         🚗 65.0   ✂ 65.0   **FUD** 090   C 80 50
         AMA: 2015,Jan,16; 2014,Jan,11; 2012,Apr,3-9

Report 35539 for aortofemoral or 35540 for grafts aortobifemoral

Aorta
Common iliac
Femoral

Blockage in lower aorta
Femoral arteries (bilateral graft shown)

35540   **aortobifemoral**
         EXCLUDES Synthetic graft (35646)
         Do not report with (35539)
         🚗 76.0   ✂ 76.0   **FUD** 090   C 50
         AMA: 2015,Jan,16; 2014,Jan,11; 2012,Apr,3-9

35556   **femoral-popliteal**
         🚗 41.5   ✂ 41.5   **FUD** 090   C 80 50 ▭ P0
         AMA: 2015,Jan,16; 2014,Jan,11; 2012,Apr,3-9

35558   **femoral-femoral**
         🚗 36.3   ✂ 36.3   **FUD** 090   C 80 50 ▭
         AMA: 2012,Apr,3-9

35560   **aortorenal**
         🚗 50.5   ✂ 50.5   **FUD** 090   C 80 50 ▭
         AMA: 2015,Jan,16; 2014,Jan,11; 2012,Jan,15-42; 2011,Jan,11

35563   **ilioiliac**
         🚗 44.8   ✂ 44.8   **FUD** 090   C 80 50 ▭
         AMA: 1999,Mar,6; 1999,Apr,11

35565   **iliofemoral**
         🚗 39.3   ✂ 39.3   **FUD** 090   C 80 50 ▭
         AMA: 2012,Apr,3-9

35566   **femoral-anterior tibial, posterior tibial, peroneal artery or other distal vessels**
         🚗 49.5   ✂ 49.5   **FUD** 090   C 80 50 ▭ P0
         AMA: 2015,Jan,16; 2014,Jan,11; 2012,Apr,3-9

35570 **tibial-tibial, peroneal-tibial, or tibial/peroneal trunk-tibial**
Do not report with (35256, 35286)
🔪 45.0 ⚕ 45.0 **FUD** 090 Ⓒ 80 50
AMA: 2015,Jan,16; 2014,Jan,11; 2012,Apr,3-9

35571 **popliteal-tibial, -peroneal artery or other distal vessels**
🔪 39.4 ⚕ 39.4 **FUD** 090 Ⓒ 80 50 ⬜ PQ
AMA: 2015,Jan,16; 2014,Jan,11; 2012,Apr,3-9

35572 Obtain Femoropopliteal Vein for Graft
Code first (33510-33523, 33533-33536, 34502, 34520, 35001-35002, 35011-35022, 35102-35103, 35121-35152, 35231-35256, 35501-35587, 35879-35907)

+ **35572** **Harvest of femoropopliteal vein, 1 segment, for vascular reconstruction procedure (eg, aortic, vena caval, coronary, peripheral artery) (List separately in addition to code for primary procedure)**
🔪 10.2 ⚕ 10.2 **FUD** ZZZ Ⓝ N1 80 ⬜
AMA: 2015,Jan,16; 2014,Jan,11; 2012,Jan,15-42; 2011,Jan,11

35583-35587 Lower Extremity Revascularization: In-situ Vein Bypass
INCLUDES Obtaining saphenous vein grafts
EXCLUDES Obtaining multiple vein segments (35682, 35683)
Obtaining vein graft, upper extremity or femoropopliteal (35500, 35572)

35583 **In-situ vein bypass; femoral-popliteal**
Code also aortobifemoral bypass graft other than vein for aortobifemoral bypass using synthetic conduit and femoral-popliteal bypass with vein conduit in situ (35646)
Code also concurrent aortofemoral bypass for aortofemoral bypass graft with synthetic conduit and femoral-popliteal bypass with vein conduit in-situ (35647)
Code also concurrent aortofemoral bypass (vein) for an aortofemoral bypass using a vein conduit or a femoral-popliteal bypass with vein conduit in-situ (35539)
🔪 43.0 ⚕ 43.0 **FUD** 090 Ⓒ 80 50 ⬜ PQ
AMA: 2015,Jan,16; 2014,Jan,11; 2012,Apr,3-9

35585 **femoral-anterior tibial, posterior tibial, or peroneal artery**
🔪 49.8 ⚕ 49.8 **FUD** 090 Ⓒ 80 50 ⬜ PQ
AMA: 2015,Jan,16; 2014,Jan,11; 2012,Apr,3-9

35587 **popliteal-tibial, peroneal**
🔪 40.6 ⚕ 40.6 **FUD** 090 Ⓒ 80 50 ⬜ PQ
AMA: 2015,Jan,16; 2014,Jan,11; 2012,Apr,3-9

35600 Obtain Arm Artery for Coronary Bypass
EXCLUDES Transposition and/or reimplantation of arteries (35691-35695)
Code first (33533-33536)

+ **35600** **Harvest of upper extremity artery, 1 segment, for coronary artery bypass procedure (List separately in addition to code for primary procedure)**
🔪 7.47 ⚕ 7.47 **FUD** ZZZ Ⓒ 80 ⬜ PQ
AMA: 2015,Jan,16; 2014,Jan,11; 2012,Jan,15-42; 2011,Jan,11

35601-35671 Arterial Bypass: Grafts Other Than Veins
EXCLUDES Transposition and/or reimplantation of arteries (35691-35695)

35601 **Bypass graft, with other than vein; common carotid-ipsilateral internal carotid**
EXCLUDES Open transcervical common carotid-common carotid bypass with endovascular repair of descending thoracic aorta (33891)
🔪 41.5 ⚕ 41.5 **FUD** 090 Ⓒ 80 50 ⬜ PQ
AMA: 2015,Jan,16; 2014,Jan,11

35606 **carotid-subclavian**
EXCLUDES Open subclavian to carotid artery transposition performed with endovascular thoracic aneurysm repair via neck incision (33889)
🔪 34.9 ⚕ 34.9 **FUD** 090 Ⓒ 80 50 ⬜ PQ
AMA: 1997,Nov,1

35612 **subclavian-subclavian**
🔪 30.9 ⚕ 30.9 **FUD** 090 Ⓒ 80 50 ⬜ PQ
AMA: 1997,Nov,1

35616 **subclavian-axillary**
🔪 32.7 ⚕ 32.7 **FUD** 090 Ⓒ 80 50 ⬜ PQ
AMA: 1997,Nov,1

35621 **axillary-femoral**
🔪 32.6 ⚕ 32.6 **FUD** 090 Ⓒ 80 50 ⬜ PQ
AMA: 2015,Jan,16; 2014,Jan,11; 2012,Apr,3-9

35623 **axillary-popliteal or -tibial**
🔪 38.9 ⚕ 38.9 **FUD** 090 Ⓒ 80 50 ⬜ PQ
AMA: 2012,Apr,3-9

35626 **aortosubclavian, aortoinnominate, or aortocarotid**
🔪 46.4 ⚕ 46.4 **FUD** 090 Ⓒ 80 50 ⬜ PQ
AMA: 1997,Nov,1

35631 **aortoceliac, aortomesenteric, aortorenal**
🔪 54.9 ⚕ 54.9 **FUD** 090 Ⓒ 80 50 ⬜ PQ
AMA: 1997,Nov,1

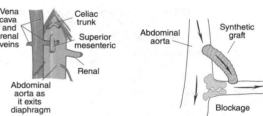

Vena cava and renal veins — Celiac trunk — Superior mesenteric — Renal — Abdominal aorta as it exits diaphragm — Abdominal aorta — Synthetic graft — Blockage

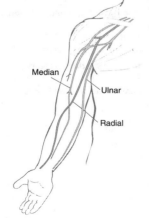

Median — Ulnar — Radial

An upper extremity artery or segment is harvested for a coronary artery bypass procedure

35632 **ilio-celiac**
📇 53.6 ⚗ 53.6 **FUD** 090 C 80 50
Do not report with (35221, 35251, 35281, 35531, 35631)

35633 **ilio-mesenteric**
📇 59.7 ⚗ 59.7 **FUD** 090 C 80 50 P0
Do not report with (35221, 35251, 35281, 35531, 35631)

35634 **iliorenal**
📇 54.3 ⚗ 54.3 **FUD** 090 C 80 50 P0
Do not report with (35221, 35251, 35281, 35536, 35560, 35631)

35636 **splenorenal (splenic to renal arterial anastomosis)**
📇 47.3 ⚗ 47.3 **FUD** 090 C 80 50 P0
AMA: 1997,Nov,1; 1994,Win,1

35637 **aortoiliac**
Do not report with (35638, 35646)
📇 51.6 ⚗ 51.6 **FUD** 090 C 80 P0
AMA: 2015,Jan,16; 2014,Jan,11; 2012,Jan,15-42; 2011,Jan,11

35638 **aortobi-iliac**
EXCLUDES *Open placement of aorto-bi-iliac prosthesis after a failed endovascular repair (34831)*
Do not report with (35637, 35646)
📇 52.3 ⚗ 52.3 **FUD** 090 C 80 P0
AMA: 2015,Jan,16; 2014,Jan,11; 2012,Jan,15-42; 2011,Jan,11

35642 **carotid-vertebral**
📇 33.9 ⚗ 33.9 **FUD** 090 C 80 50 ⬜ P0
AMA: 1997,Nov,1

35645 **subclavian-vertebral**
📇 28.0 ⚗ 28.0 **FUD** 090 C 80 50 ⬜ P0
AMA: 1997,Nov,1

35646 **aortobifemoral**
EXCLUDES *Bypass graft using vein graft (35540)*
Open placement of aortobifemoral prosthesis after a failed endovascular repair (34832)
📇 50.9 ⚗ 50.9 **FUD** 090 C 80 ⬜ P0
AMA: 2015,Jan,16; 2014,Jan,11; 2012,Apr,3-9

35647 **aortofemoral**
EXCLUDES *Bypass graft using vein graft (35539)*
📇 45.9 ⚗ 45.9 **FUD** 090 C 80 50 ⬜ P0
AMA: 2015,Jan,16; 2014,Jan,11

35650 **axillary-axillary**
📇 32.2 ⚗ 32.2 **FUD** 090 C 80 50 ⬜ P0
AMA: 1997,Nov,1

35654 **axillary-femoral-femoral**
📇 40.7 ⚗ 40.7 **FUD** 090 C 80 ⬜ P0
AMA: 2015,Jan,16; 2014,Jan,11; 2012,Apr,3-9

35656 **femoral-popliteal**
📇 32.1 ⚗ 32.1 **FUD** 090 C 80 50 ⬜ P0
AMA: 2015,Jan,16; 2014,Jan,11; 2012,Apr,3-9

35661 **femoral-femoral**
📇 32.1 ⚗ 32.1 **FUD** 090 C 80 50 ⬜ P0
AMA: 2015,Jan,16; 2014,Jan,11; 2012,Apr,3-9

35663 **ilioiliac**
📇 37.4 ⚗ 37.4 **FUD** 090 C 80 50 ⬜ P0
AMA: 1997,Nov,1

35665 **iliofemoral**
📇 34.7 ⚗ 34.7 **FUD** 090 C 80 50 ⬜ P0
AMA: 2015,Jan,16; 2014,Jan,11

35666 **femoral-anterior tibial, posterior tibial, or peroneal artery**
📇 37.4 ⚗ 37.4 **FUD** 090 C 80 50 ⬜ P0
AMA: 2015,Jan,16; 2014,Jan,11; 2012,Apr,3-9

35671 **popliteal-tibial or -peroneal artery**
📇 33.1 ⚗ 33.1 **FUD** 090 C 80 50 ⬜ P0
AMA: 2012,Apr,3-9

35681-35683 Arterial Bypass Using Combination Synthetic and Donor Graft

INCLUDES Acquiring multiple segments of vein from sites other than the extremity for which the arterial bypass is performed
Anastomosis of vein segments to creat bypass graft conduits

+ 35681 **Bypass graft; composite, prosthetic and vein (List separately in addition to code for primary procedure)**
Code first primary procedure
Do not report with (35682, 35683)
📇 2.37 ⚗ 2.37 **FUD** ZZZ C 80 ⬜
AMA: 2015,Jan,16; 2014,Jan,11; 2012,Jan,15-42; 2011,Jan,11

+ 35682 **autogenous composite, 2 segments of veins from 2 locations (List separately in addition to code for primary procedure)**
Code first (35556, 35566, 35570-35571, 35583-35587)
Do not report with (35681, 35683)
📇 10.4 ⚗ 10.4 **FUD** ZZZ C 80 ⬜
AMA: 2015,Jan,16; 2014,Jan,11; 2012,Jan,15-42

+ 35683 **autogenous composite, 3 or more segments of vein from 2 or more locations (List separately in addition to code for primary procedure)**
Code first (35556, 35566, 35570-35571, 35583-35587)
Do not report with (35681, 35682)
📇 12.1 ⚗ 12.1 **FUD** ZZZ C 80 ⬜
AMA: 2015,Jan,16; 2014,Jan,11; 2012,Jan,15-42; 2011,Jan,11

35685-35686 Supplemental Procedures

INCLUDES Additional procedures that may be needed with a bypass graft to increase the patency of the graft
EXCLUDES *Composite grafts (35681-35683)*

+ 35685 **Placement of vein patch or cuff at distal anastomosis of bypass graft, synthetic conduit (List separately in addition to code for primary procedure)**
INCLUDES Connection of a segment of vein (cuff or patch) between the distal portion of the synthetic graft and the native artery
Code first (35656, 35666, 35671)
📇 5.90 ⚗ 5.90 **FUD** ZZZ N 80 ⬜
AMA: 2015,Jan,16; 2014,Jan,11

+ 35686 **Creation of distal arteriovenous fistula during lower extremity bypass surgery (non-hemodialysis) (List separately in addition to code for primary procedure)**
INCLUDES Creation of a fistula between the peroneal or tibial artery and vein at or past the site of the distal anastomosis
Code first (35556, 35566, 35570-35571, 35583-35587, 35623, 35656, 35666, 35671)
📇 4.79 ⚗ 4.79 **FUD** ZZZ N 80 ⬜
AMA: 2015,Jan,16; 2014,Jan,11; 2012,Apr,3-9

35691-35697 Arterial Translocation

CMS: 100-3,160.8 Electroencephalographic Monitoring During Cerebral Vasculature Surgery

35691 **Transposition and/or reimplantation; vertebral to carotid artery**
📇 28.0 ⚗ 28.0 **FUD** 090 C 80 50 ⬜
AMA: 1997,Nov,1; 1993,Win,1

35693 **vertebral to subclavian artery**
📇 24.7 ⚗ 24.7 **FUD** 090 C 80 50 ⬜
AMA: 1997,Nov,1; 1994,Sum,29

35694   **subclavian to carotid artery**

  EXCLUDES   *Subclavian to carotid artery transposition procedure (open) with concurrent repair of descending thoracic aorta (endovascular) (33889)*

  29.2   29.2   **FUD** 090   C 80 50 ▣
  AMA: 1997,Nov,1; 1993,Win,1

35695   **carotid to subclavian artery**

  30.4   30.4   **FUD** 090   C 80 50 ▣
  AMA: 1997,Nov,1; 1993,Win,1

+ **35697**   **Reimplantation, visceral artery to infrarenal aortic prosthesis, each artery (List separately in addition to code for primary procedure)**

  Code first primary procedure
  Do not report with (33877)
  4.38   4.38   **FUD** ZZZ   C 80 ▣
  AMA: 1997,Nov,1

35700 Reoperative Bypass Lower Extremities

Code first (35556, 35566, 35570-35571, 35583, 35585, 35587, 35656, 35666, 35671)

+ **35700**   **Reoperation, femoral-popliteal or femoral (popliteal)-anterior tibial, posterior tibial, peroneal artery, or other distal vessels, more than 1 month after original operation (List separately in addition to code for primary procedure)**

  4.53   4.53   **FUD** ZZZ   C 80 ▣
  AMA: 2015,Jan,16; 2014,Jan,11; 2012,Apr,3-9

35701-35761 Arterial Exploration without Repair

35701   **Exploration (not followed by surgical repair), with or without lysis of artery; carotid artery**

  16.5   16.5   **FUD** 090   C 80 50 ▣
  AMA: 1997,Nov,1

35721   **femoral artery**

  13.4   13.4   **FUD** 090   C 80 50 ▣
  AMA: 2015,Jan,16; 2014,Jan,11

35741   **popliteal artery**

  15.0   15.0   **FUD** 090   C 80 50 ▣
  AMA: 1997,Nov,1

35761   **other vessels**

  11.4   11.4   **FUD** 090   T 62 80 50 ▣
  AMA: 1997,Nov,1

35800-35860 Arterial Exploration for Postoperative Complication

  INCLUDES   Return to the operating room for postoperative hemorrhage

35800   **Exploration for postoperative hemorrhage, thrombosis or infection; neck**

  20.9   20.9   **FUD** 090   C 80 ▣
  AMA: 1997,Nov,1

35820   **chest**

  58.5   58.5   **FUD** 090   C 80 ▣
  AMA: 1997,Nov,1

35840   **abdomen**

  34.6   34.6   **FUD** 090   C 80 ▣
  AMA: 1997,May,4; 1997,Nov,1

35860   **extremity**

  24.7   24.7   **FUD** 090   T 80 ▣
  AMA: 2015,Jan,16; 2014,Apr,10

35870 Repair Secondary Aortoenteric Fistula

35870   **Repair of graft-enteric fistula**

  36.9   36.9   **FUD** 090   C 80 ▣
  AMA: 1997,Nov,1

35875-35876 Removal of Thrombus from Graft

  EXCLUDES   *Thrombectomy dialysis fistula or graft (36831, 36833)*
  Thrombectomy with blood vessel repair, lower extremity, vein graft (35256)
  Thrombectomy with blood vessel repair, lower extremity, with/without patch angioplasty (35226)

35875   **Thrombectomy of arterial or venous graft (other than hemodialysis graft or fistula);**

  17.5   17.5   **FUD** 090   T A2 ▣
  AMA: 2015,Jan,16; 2014,Jan,11; 2012,Jan,15-42; 2011,Jan,11

35876   **with revision of arterial or venous graft**

  27.9   27.9   **FUD** 090   T A2 80 ▣
  AMA: 1999,Mar,6; 1999,Nov,1

35879-35884 Revision Lower Extremity Bypass Graft

  EXCLUDES   *Removal of infected graft (35901-35907)*
  Revascularization following removal of infected graft(s)
  Thrombectomy dialysis fistula or graft (36831, 36833)
  Thrombectomy with blood vessel repair, lower extremity, vein graft (35256)
  Thrombectomy with blood vessel repair, lower extremity, with/without patch angioplasty (35226)
  Thrombectomy with graft revision (35876)

35879   **Revision, lower extremity arterial bypass, without thrombectomy, open; with vein patch angioplasty**

  27.3   27.3   **FUD** 090   T 80 50 ▣
  AMA: 2015,Jan,16; 2014,Jan,11

35881   **with segmental vein interposition**

  EXCLUDES   *Revision of femoral anastomosis of synthetic arterial bypass graft (35883-35884)*

  30.1   30.1   **FUD** 090   T 80 50 ▣
  AMA: 2015,Jan,16; 2014,Jan,11

35883   **Revision, femoral anastomosis of synthetic arterial bypass graft in groin, open; with nonautogenous patch graft (eg, Dacron, ePTFE, bovine pericardium)**

  Do not report with (35700, 35875-35876, 35884)
  35.8   35.8   **FUD** 090   T 80 50
  AMA: 2015,Jan,16; 2014,Jan,11; 2012,Jan,15-42; 2011,Jan,11

35884   **with autogenous vein patch graft**

  Do not report with (35700, 35875-35876, 35883)
  36.8   36.8   **FUD** 090   T 80 50
  AMA: 2015,Jan,16; 2014,Jan,11; 2012,Jan,15-42; 2011,Jan,11

35901-35907 Removal of Infected Graft

35901   **Excision of infected graft; neck**

  14.5   14.5   **FUD** 090   C 80 ▣
  AMA: 1997,Nov,1; 1993,Win,1

Infected graft is removed

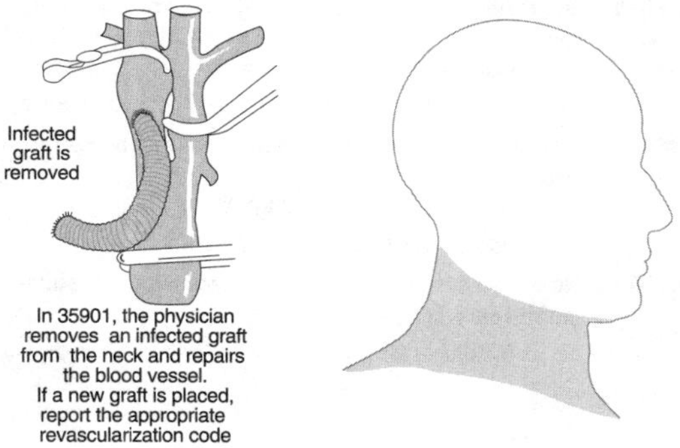

In 35901, the physician removes an infected graft from the neck and repairs the blood vessel. If a new graft is placed, report the appropriate revascularization code

35903   **extremity**

  16.6   16.6   **FUD** 090   T 80 ▣
  AMA: 1997,Nov,1; 1993,Win,1

35905   **thorax**

  52.0   52.0   **FUD** 090   C 80 ▣
  AMA: 1997,Nov,1; 1993,Win,1

35907   **abdomen**

  56.6   56.6   **FUD** 090   C 80 ▣
  AMA: 1997,Nov,1; 1993,Win,1

● New Code   ▲ Revised Code   ○ Reinstated   M Maternity   A Age Edit   Unlisted   Not Covered   # Resequenced
⊘ AMA Mod 51 Exempt   ⑤ Optum Mod 51 Exempt   63 Mod 63 Exempt   ⊙ Mod Sedation   + Add-on   ▣ CCI   P0 PQRS   **FUD** Follow-up Days

36000 Intravenous Access Established

INCLUDES   Venous access for phlebotomy, prophylactic intravenous access, infusion therapy, chemotherapy, hydration, transfusion, drug administration, etc. which is included in the work value of the primary procedure

36000   Introduction of needle or intracatheter, vein

⚕ 0.26   ⚖ 0.72   **FUD** XXX   N N1 ▣

AMA: 2015,Jan,16; 2014,Oct,6; 2014,Sep,13; 2014,May,4; 2014,Jan,11; 2012,Jan,15-42; 2011,Jan,11

36002 Injection Treatment of Pseudoaneurysm

INCLUDES   Insertion of needle or catheter, local anesthesia, injection of contrast, power injections, and all pre- and postinjection care provided

EXCLUDES   *Compression repair pseudoaneurysm, ultrasound guided (76936)*
Medications, contrast material, catheters

Do not report for arteriotomy site sealant

36002   Injection procedures (eg, thrombin) for percutaneous treatment of extremity pseudoaneurysm

▣ (76942, 77002, 77012, 77021)

⚕ 3.12   ⚖ 4.67   **FUD** 000   S 62 50 ▣

AMA: 2015,Jan,16; 2014,Oct,6; 2014,Jan,11; 2013,Nov,6

36005-36015 Insertion Needle or Intracatheter: Venous

INCLUDES   Insertion of needle/catheter, local anesthesia, injection of contrast, power injections, all pre- and postinjection care

EXCLUDES   *Medications, contrast materials, catheters*

Code also catheterization of second order vessels (or higher) supplied by the same first order branch, same vascular family (36012)
Code also each vascular family (e.g., bilateral procedures are separate vascular families)

36005   Injection procedure for extremity venography (including introduction of needle or intracatheter)

▣ (75820, 75822)

⚕ 1.41   ⚖ 9.18   **FUD** 000   N N1 80 50 ▣

AMA: 2015,Jan,16; 2014,Oct,6

36010   Introduction of catheter, superior or inferior vena cava

⚕ 3.58   ⚖ 14.2   **FUD** XXX   ⊙ N N1 50 ▣

AMA: 2015,Jan,16; 2014,Jan,11; 2012,Apr,3-9; 2012,Jan,15-42; 2011,Jan,11

36011   Selective catheter placement, venous system; first order branch (eg, renal vein, jugular vein)

⚕ 4.61   ⚖ 23.7   **FUD** XXX   N N1 50 ▣

AMA: 2015,Jan,16; 2014,Jan,11; 2012,Apr,3-9

36012   second order, or more selective, branch (eg, left adrenal vein, petrosal sinus)

⚕ 5.09   ⚖ 24.5   **FUD** XXX   N N1 50 ▣

AMA: 2015,Jan,16; 2014,Jan,11; 2012,Apr,3-9

36013   Introduction of catheter, right heart or main pulmonary artery

⚕ 3.64   ⚖ 22.2   **FUD** XXX   N N1 ▣

AMA: 2015,Jan,16; 2014,Jan,11; 2012,Jan,15-42; 2011,Jan,11

36014   Selective catheter placement, left or right pulmonary artery

⚕ 4.41   ⚖ 23.1   **FUD** XXX   N N1 50 ▣

AMA: 2015,Jan,16; 2014,Jan,11

36015   Selective catheter placement, segmental or subsegmental pulmonary artery

EXCLUDES   *Placement of Swan Ganz/other flow directed catheter for monitoring (93503)*
Selective blood sampling, specific organs (36500)

⚕ 4.98   ⚖ 24.5   **FUD** XXX   N N1 50 ▣

AMA: 2015,Jan,16; 2014,Jan,11; 2012,Mar,9-10

36100-36218 Insertion Needle or Intracatheter: Arterial

INCLUDES   Introduction of the catheter and catheterization of all lesser order vessels used for the approach
Local anesthesia, placement of catheter/needle, injection of contrast, power injections, all pre- and postinjection care

EXCLUDES   *Angiography (36222-36228, 75600-75774, 75791)*
Angioplasty (35472, 35475)
Chemotherapy injections (96401-96549)
Injection procedures for cardiac catheterizations (93455, 93457, 93459, 93461, 93530-93533, 93564)
Internal mammary artery angiography without left heart catheterization (36216, 36217)
Medications, contrast, catheters
Transcatheter interventions (37200, [37211], [37213, 37214], 37236-37239, 37241-37244, 61624, 61626)

Code also additional first order or higher catheterization for vascular families if the vascular family is supplied by a first order vessel that is different from one already coded
Code also catheterization of second and third order vessels supplied by the same first order branch, same vascular family (36218, 36248)

36100   Introduction of needle or intracatheter, carotid or vertebral artery

⚕ 4.51   ⚖ 13.9   **FUD** XXX   N N1 50 ▣

AMA: 2000,Oct,4; 1998,Apr,1

36120   Introduction of needle or intracatheter; retrograde brachial artery

EXCLUDES   *Arteriovenous cannula insertion (36810-36821)*

⚕ 2.94   ⚖ 11.9   **FUD** XXX   N N1 ▣

AMA: 2015,Jan,16; 2014,Jan,11; 2012,Jan,15-42; 2011,Jan,11

36140   extremity artery

EXCLUDES   *Arteriovenous cannula insertion (36810-36821)*

⚕ 3.00   ⚖ 12.4   **FUD** XXX   ⊙ N N1 ▣

AMA: 2015,Jan,16; 2014,Jan,11; 2012,Jan,15-42; 2011,Jul,3-11; 2011,Jan,11

36147 Introduction of needle and/or catheter, arteriovenous shunt created for dialysis (graft/fistula); initial access with complete radiological evaluation of dialysis access, including fluoroscopy, image documentation and report (includes access of shunt, injection[s] of contrast, and all necessary imaging from the arterial anastomosis and adjacent artery through entire venous outflow including the inferior or superior vena cava)

INCLUDES Access and imaging of the AV shunt
Antegrade and/or retrograde punctures for contrast injection through a needle or catheter for imaging
Catheter manipulation for:
Advancement of the tip of the catheter to the vena cava
Diagnostic imaging of the AV shunt
Visualization of the arterial anastomosis or central veins
Catheterization of all veins in arteriovenous shunt
Diagnostic procedures of all upper and lower arteriovenous fistulae and grafts from the arterial anastomosis to the right atrium
Evaluation of peri-anastomotic portion of the inflow which includes:
Portion of the artery bordering the anastomosis
Portion of the graft or vessel just distal to the anastomosis
Site of the anastomosis

EXCLUDES *Additional catheter work/imaging to evaluate proximal arterial inflow to AV access*
Selective catheter advancement from the AV shunt puncture to the inflow artery (most often AV shunt of upper extremity) (36215)
Ultrasound guidance (76937)
Code also the second shunt catheterization if a need is identified for a therapeutic interventional procedure (36148)
Do not report selective catheterization of inferior/superior vena cava or central veins when performed by direct puncture of the fistula or graft
Do not report with (75791)

🔲 5.44 ⚖ 23.7 **FUD** XXX   ⊙ Ⓣ P2 80 P0

AMA: 2015,Jan,16; 2014,Jan,11; 2012,Apr,3-9; 2012,Jan,15-42; 2011,Dec,14-18; 2011,Jan,11; 2010,Mar,3

+ 36148 additional access for therapeutic intervention (List separately in addition to code for primary procedure)

INCLUDES All interventional procedures performed in a single segment no matter how many lesions are taken care of
Catheterization of all veins in arteriovenous shunt
Interventional procedures in arteriovenous shunts (arteriovenous fistulae and grafts) considered to be primarily venous
Two vessel segments:
First segment (peripheral) extends from peri-arterial anastomosis through the axillary vein or the complete cephalic vein for cephalic venous outflow
Second segment: veins central to the axillary and cephalic veins (eg, subclavian and innominate veins through the vena cava)

EXCLUDES *Arterial intervention with radiological supervision and interpretation in the peri-anastomotic region (35475, 75962)*
Catheterization for intervention in an accessory vein (36011-36012)
Embolization of an accessory vein (37241)
Fistula thrombectomy (36870)
Other venous interventional procedures, as appropriate
Radiological supervision and interpretation for venous angioplasty (75978)
Stent placement for central venous stenosis (37239)
Stent placement from the peri-arterial anastomosis through the axillary and cephalic veins (37236, 37238)
Venous angioplasty, once per vessel only (35476)
Code first (36147)
Do not report selective catheterization of inferior/superior vena cava or central veins when performed by direct puncture of the fistula or graft
Do not report venous interventional codes for stenosis at the arterial anastomosis (peri-anastomotic or juxta-anastomotic region)

🔲 1.44 ⚖ 7.45 **FUD** ZZZ   ⊙ Ⓝ Ⓜ 80

AMA: 2015,Jan,16; 2014,Jan,11; 2012,Apr,3-9; 2012,Jan,15-42; 2011,Jan,11; 2010,Mar,3

36160 Introduction of needle or intracatheter, aortic, translumbar

🔲 3.62 ⚖ 14.1 **FUD** XXX   Ⓝ Ⓜ 🔲

AMA: 2015,Jan,16; 2014,Jan,11

36200 Introduction of catheter, aorta

EXCLUDES *Nonselective angiography of the extracranial carotid and/or cerebral vessels and cervicocerebral arch (36221)*

🔲 4.50 ⚖ 17.8 **FUD** 000   ⊙ Ⓝ Ⓜ 50 🔲

AMA: 2015,Jan,16; 2014,Jan,11; 2013,Feb,16-17; 2012,Apr,3-9; 2012,Jan,15-42; 2011,Oct,9; 2011,Jul,3-11; 2011,Jan,11

36215 Selective catheter placement, arterial system; each first order thoracic or brachiocephalic branch, within a vascular family

INCLUDES Introduction of catheter into the aorta (36200)
EXCLUDES *Placement of catheter for coronary angiography (93454-93461)*

🔲 6.89 ⚖ 32.0 **FUD** XXX   Ⓝ Ⓜ 🔲

AMA: 2015,Jan,16; 2014,Jan,11; 2012,Apr,3-9; 2012,Jan,15-42; 2011,Jan,11

36216 initial second order thoracic or brachiocephalic branch, within a vascular family

🔲 8.00 ⚖ 33.3 **FUD** XXX   Ⓝ Ⓜ 🔲

AMA: 2015,Jan,16; 2014,Jan,11; 2013,Nov,14; 2012,Apr,3-9; 2011,Dec,9-12

36217 initial third order or more selective thoracic or brachiocephalic branch, within a vascular family

🔲 9.49 ⚖ 53.9 **FUD** XXX   Ⓝ Ⓜ 🔲

AMA: 2015,Jan,16; 2014,Jan,11; 2012,Apr,3-9; 2011,Dec,9-12

Cardiovascular System

+ **36218** additional second order, third order, and beyond, thoracic or brachiocephalic branch, within a vascular family (List in addition to code for initial second or third order vessel as appropriate)

Code also transcatheter therapy procedures (37200, [37211], [37213, 37214], 37236-37239, 37241-37244, 61624, 61626)
Code first (36216-36217, 36225-36226)
🔗 1.53 ⚕ 5.25 **FUD** ZZZ [N] [N1] ⬜

AMA: 2015,Jan,16; 2014,Jan,11; 2013,May,3-5; 2012,Apr,3-9

36221-36228 Diagnostic Studies: Aortic Arch/Carotid/Vertebral Arteries

INCLUDES Accessing the vessel
Arterial contrast injection that includes arterial, capillary, and venous phase imaging, when performed
Arteriotomy closure (pressure or closure device)
Catheter placement
Radiologic supervision and interpretation
Reporting of selective catheter placement based on intensity of services in the following hierarchy:
36226>36225
36224>36223>36222
EXCLUDES 3D rendering when performed (76376-76377)
Interventional procedures
Ultrasound guidance (76937)
Code also diagnostic angiography of upper extremities/other vascular beds during the same session, if performed (75774)
Do not report with angiography of cervicocerebral vessels (75774)

36221 Non-selective catheter placement, thoracic aorta, with angiography of the extracranial carotid, vertebral, and/or intracranial vessels, unilateral or bilateral, and all associated radiological supervision and interpretation, includes angiography of the cervicocerebral arch, when performed

Do not report with (36222-36226)
Do not report with transcatheter intravascular stent placement of common carotid or innominate artery on the same side (37217)
🔗 6.29 ⚕ 31.1 **FUD** 000 ⊙ [02] [N1]

AMA: 2015,May,7; 2015,Jan,16; 2014,Mar,8; 2014,Jan,11; 2013,Oct,18; 2013,Jun,12; 2013,May,3-5; 2013,Feb,16-17

36222 Selective catheter placement, common carotid or innominate artery, unilateral, any approach, with angiography of the ipsilateral extracranial carotid circulation and all associated radiological supervision and interpretation, includes angiography of the cervicocerebral arch, when performed

INCLUDES Unilateral catheterization of artery
Code also modifier 59 when different territories on both sides of the body are being studied
Do not report with (37215-37216, 37218)
Do not report with transcatheter intravascular stent placement of common carotid or innominate artery on the same side (37217)
🔗 8.63 ⚕ 36.0 **FUD** 000 ⊙ [02] [N1] [50]

AMA: 2015,May,7; 2015,Jan,16; 2014,Mar,8; 2014,Jan,11; 2013,Oct,18; 2013,Nov,14; 2013,Jun,12; 2013,May,3-5; 2013,Feb,16-17

36223 Selective catheter placement, common carotid or innominate artery, unilateral, any approach, with angiography of the ipsilateral intracranial carotid circulation and all associated radiological supervision and interpretation, includes angiography of the extracranial carotid and cervicocerebral arch, when performed

INCLUDES Unilateral catheterization of artery
Code also modifier 59 when different territories on both sides of the body are being studied
Do not report with (37215-37216, 37218)
Do not report with transcatheter intravascular stent placement of common carotid or innominate artery on the same side (37217)
🔗 9.44 ⚕ 43.2 **FUD** 000 ⊙ [02] [N1] [50]

AMA: 2015,Jan,16; 2014,Mar,8; 2014,Jan,11; 2013,Oct,18; 2013,Jun,12; 2013,May,3-5; 2013,Feb,16-17

36224 Selective catheter placement, internal carotid artery, unilateral, with angiography of the ipsilateral intracranial carotid circulation and all associated radiological supervision and interpretation, includes angiography of the extracranial carotid and cervicocerebral arch, when performed

INCLUDES Unilateral catheterization of artery
Code also modifier 59 when different territories on both sides of the body are being studied
Do not report with (37215-37216, 37218)
Do not report with transcatheter intravascular stent placement of common carotid or innominate artery on the same side (37217)
🔗 10.6 ⚕ 54.0 **FUD** 000 ⊙ [02] [N1] [50]

AMA: 2015,Jan,16; 2014,Mar,8; 2014,Jan,11; 2013,Oct,18; 2013,Jun,12; 2013,May,3-5; 2013,Feb,16-17

36225 Selective catheter placement, subclavian or innominate artery, unilateral, with angiography of the ipsilateral vertebral circulation and all associated radiological supervision and interpretation, includes angiography of the cervicocerebral arch, when performed

Do not report with transcatheter intravascular stent placement of common carotid or innominate artery on the same side (37217)
🔗 9.42 ⚕ 41.7 **FUD** 000 ⊙ [02] [N1] [50]

AMA: 2015,Jan,16; 2014,Mar,8; 2014,Jan,11; 2013,Oct,18; 2013,Nov,14; 2013,Jun,12; 2013,May,3-5

36226 Selective catheter placement, vertebral artery, unilateral, with angiography of the ipsilateral vertebral circulation and all associated radiological supervision and interpretation, includes angiography of the cervicocerebral arch, when performed

Do not report with transcatheter intravascular stent placement of common carotid or innominate artery on the same side (37217)
🔗 10.6 ⚕ 52.7 **FUD** 000 ⊙ [02] [N1] [50]

AMA: 2015,Jan,16; 2014,Mar,8; 2013,Oct,18; 2013,Jun,12; 2013,May,3-5

+ **36227** Selective catheter placement, external carotid artery, unilateral, with angiography of the ipsilateral external carotid circulation and all associated radiological supervision and interpretation (List separately in addition to code for primary procedure)

INCLUDES Unilateral catheter placement/diagnostic imaging of ipsilateral external carotid circulation
Code first (36222-36224)
Do not report with transcatheter intravascular stent placement of common carotid or innominate artery on the same side (37217)
🔗 3.39 ⚕ 7.47 **FUD** ZZZ ⊙ [N] [N1] [50]

AMA: 2015,Jan,16; 2014,Mar,8; 2014,Jan,11; 2013,Oct,18; 2013,Jun,12; 2013,May,3-5; 2013,Feb,16-17

+ **36228** Selective catheter placement, each intracranial branch of the internal carotid or vertebral arteries, unilateral, with angiography of the selected vessel circulation and all associated radiological supervision and interpretation (eg, middle cerebral artery, posterior inferior cerebellar artery) (List separately in addition to code for primary procedure)

INCLUDES Unilateral catheter placement/imaging of initial and each additional intracranial branch of internal carotid or vertebral arteries
Code first (36223-36226)
Do not report more than 2 times per side
Do not report with transcatheter intravascular stent placement of common carotid or innominate artery on the same side (37217)
🔗 6.89 ⚕ 35.9 **FUD** ZZZ ⊙ [N] [N1] [50]

AMA: 2015,Jan,16; 2014,Jan,11; 2013,Oct,18; 2013,Jun,12; 2013,May,3-5; 2013,Feb,16-17

36245-36254 Catheter Placement: Arteries of the Lower Body

INCLUDES Introduction of the catheter and catheterization of all lesser order vessels used for the approach
Local anesthesia, placement of catheter/needle, injection of contrast, power injections

EXCLUDES Angiography (36147, 36222-36228, 75600-75774, 75791)
Angioplasty (35471-35472, 35475)
Chemotherapy injections (96401-96549)
Injection procedures for cardiac catheterizations (93455, 93457, 93459, 93461, 93530-93533, 93564)
Internal mammary artery angiography without left heart catheterization (36216-36217)
Medications, contrast, catheters
Transcatheter procedures (37200, [37211], [37213, 37214], 37236-37239, 37241-37244, 61624, 61626)

Code also additional first order or higher catheterization for vascular families if the vascular family is supplied by a first order vessel that is different from one already coded
Code also catheterization of second and third order vessels supplied by the same first order branch, same vascular family (36218, 36248)
⊠ (75600-75791)

36245 **Selective catheter placement, arterial system; each first order abdominal, pelvic, or lower extremity artery branch, within a vascular family**
🔪 7.38 ⚖ 38.9 **FUD** XXX ⊙ N N1 50 ▢
AMA: 2015,Jan,16; 2014,Jan,11; 2013,Nov,14; 2012,Apr,3-9; 2012,Jan,15-42; 2011,Oct,9; 2011,Jul,3-11; 2011,Jan,11

36246 **initial second order abdominal, pelvic, or lower extremity artery branch, within a vascular family**
🔪 7.88 ⚖ 25.4 **FUD** 000 ⊙ N N1 50 ▢
AMA: 2015,Jan,16; 2014,Jan,11; 2013,Nov,14; 2012,Apr,3-9; 2012,Jan,15-42; 2011,Oct,9; 2011,Jul,3-11; 2011,Jan,11

36247 **initial third order or more selective abdominal, pelvic, or lower extremity artery branch, within a vascular family**
🔪 9.32 ⚖ 44.9 **FUD** 000 ⊙ N N1 50 ▢
AMA: 2015,Jan,16; 2014,Jan,11; 2013,Nov,14; 2012,Apr,3-9; 2012,Jan,15-42; 2011,Jul,3-11; 2011,Jan,11

+ **36248** **additional second order, third order, and beyond, abdominal, pelvic, or lower extremity artery branch, within a vascular family (List in addition to code for initial second or third order vessel as appropriate)**
Code first (36246, 36247)
🔪 1.44 ⚖ 4.35 **FUD** ZZZ ⊙ N N1 ▢
AMA: 2015,Jan,16; 2014,Jan,11; 2012,Apr,3-9; 2012,Jan,15-42; 2011,Jul,3-11; 2011,Jan,11

36251 **Selective catheter placement (first-order), main renal artery and any accessory renal artery(s) for renal angiography, including arterial puncture and catheter placement(s), fluoroscopy, contrast injection(s), image postprocessing, permanent recording of images, and radiological supervision and interpretation, including pressure gradient measurements when performed, and flush aortogram when performed; unilateral**
INCLUDES Closure device placement at vascular access site
Do not report with (0338T-0339T)
🔪 8.24 ⚖ 40.5 **FUD** 000 ⊙ 02 N1
AMA: 2015,Jan,16; 2014,Jan,11; 2013,Nov,14; 2012,Aug,13-14; 2012,Apr,3-9; 2012,Jan,15-42

36252 **bilateral**
INCLUDES Closure device placement at vascular access site
Do not report with (0338T-0339T)
🔪 10.9 ⚖ 43.9 **FUD** 000 ⊙ 02 N1
AMA: 2015,Jan,16; 2014,Jan,11; 2012,Apr,3-9; 2012,Jan,15-42

36253 **Superselective catheter placement (one or more second order or higher renal artery branches) renal artery and any accessory renal artery(s) for renal angiography, including arterial puncture, catheterization, fluoroscopy, contrast injection(s), image postprocessing, permanent recording of images, and radiological supervision and interpretation, including pressure gradient measurements when performed, and flush aortogram when performed; unilateral**
INCLUDES Closure device placement at vascular access site
Do not report for same kidney with (36251)
Do not report with (0338T-0339T)
🔪 11.0 ⚖ 64.5 **FUD** 000 ⊙ 02 N1
AMA: 2015,Jan,16; 2014,Jan,11; 2013,Nov,14; 2012,Aug,13-14; 2012,Apr,3-9; 2012,Jan,15-42

36254 **bilateral**
INCLUDES Closure device placement at vascular access site
Do not report with (36252, 0338T-0339T)
🔪 12.7 ⚖ 62.7 **FUD** 000 ⊙ 02 N1
AMA: 2015,Jan,16; 2014,Jan,11; 2012,Aug,13-14; 2012,Apr,3-9; 2012,Jan,15-42

36260-36299 Implanted Infusion Pumps: Intra-arterial

36260 **Insertion of implantable intra-arterial infusion pump (eg, for chemotherapy of liver)**
🔪 18.7 ⚖ 18.7 **FUD** 090 T A2 ▢
AMA: 2015,Jan,16; 2014,Jan,11

36261 **Revision of implanted intra-arterial infusion pump**
🔪 10.4 ⚖ 10.4 **FUD** 090 T A2 80 ▢
AMA: 2000,Oct,4; 1997,Nov,1

36262 **Removal of implanted intra-arterial infusion pump**
🔪 8.84 ⚖ 8.84 **FUD** 090 02 A2 ▢
AMA: 2000,Oct,4; 1997,Nov,1

36299 **Unlisted procedure, vascular injection**
🔪 0.00 ⚖ 0.00 **FUD** YYY N 80
AMA: 2000,Oct,4; 1997,Nov,1

36400-36425 Specimen Collection: Phlebotomy

EXCLUDES Collection of specimen from:
A completely implantable device (36591)
An established catheter (36592)

36400 **Venipuncture, younger than age 3 years, necessitating the skill of a physician or other qualified health care professional, not to be used for routine venipuncture; femoral or jugular vein** A
🔪 0.55 ⚖ 0.80 **FUD** XXX N N1 ▢
AMA: 2015,Jan,16; 2014,May,4; 2014,Jan,11

36405 **scalp vein** A
🔪 0.46 ⚖ 0.75 **FUD** XXX N N1 ▢
AMA: 2015,Jan,16; 2014,May,4; 2014,Jan,11

36406 **other vein** A
🔪 0.29 ⚖ 0.58 **FUD** XXX N N1 ▢
AMA: 2015,Jan,16; 2014,May,4; 2014,Jan,11

36410 **Venipuncture, age 3 years or older, necessitating the skill of a physician or other qualified health care professional (separate procedure), for diagnostic or therapeutic purposes (not to be used for routine venipuncture)** A
🔪 0.27 ⚖ 0.48 **FUD** XXX N N1 ▢
AMA: 2015,Jan,16; 2014,Oct,6; 2014,Jan,11; 2013,Sep,17; 2012,Jan,15-42; 2011,Jan,11

36415 **Collection of venous blood by venipuncture**
🔪 0.00 ⚖ 0.00 **FUD** XXX 63 N
AMA: 2015,Jan,16; 2014,May,4; 2014,Jan,11; 2012,Jan,15-42; 2011,Jan,11

36416 **Collection of capillary blood specimen (eg, finger, heel, ear stick)**
🔪 0.00 ⚖ 0.00 **FUD** XXX N N1
AMA: 2008,Apr,-9; 2003,Feb,7

36420 **Venipuncture, cutdown; younger than age 1 year** [A]
🏥 1.46 ⚕ 1.46 **FUD** XXX [63] [Q1] [N1] [80] ⚑
AMA: 2015,Jan,16; 2014,Jan,11

36425 **age 1 or over** [A]
Do not report with (36475-36476, 36478-36479)
🏥 1.15 ⚕ 1.15 **FUD** XXX [Q1] [N1] ⚑
AMA: 2015,Jan,16; 2014,Oct,6

36430-36460 Transfusions

CMS: 100-1,3,20.5 Blood Deductibles; 100-3,110.16 Transfusion in Kidney Transplants; 100-3,110.7 Blood Transfusions; 100-3,110.8 Blood Platelet Transfusions

36430 **Transfusion, blood or blood components**
🏥 0.98 ⚕ 0.98 **FUD** XXX [S] [P3] ⚑
AMA: 2015,Jan,16; 2014,Jan,11; 2012,Jan,15-42; 2011,Jan,11

36440 **Push transfusion, blood, 2 years or younger** [A]
🏥 1.62 ⚕ 1.62 **FUD** XXX [S] [R2] [80] ⚑
AMA: 2015,Jan,16; 2014,Jan,11

36450 **Exchange transfusion, blood; newborn** [A]
🏥 3.42 ⚕ 3.42 **FUD** XXX [63] [S] [R2] [80] ⚑
AMA: 2003,Apr,7; 1997,Nov,1

36455 **other than newborn** [A]
🏥 3.72 ⚕ 3.72 **FUD** XXX [S] [R2] ⚑
AMA: 2003,Apr,7; 1997,Nov,1

36460 **Transfusion, intrauterine, fetal** [A] ♀
☢ (76941)
🏥 9.99 ⚕ 9.99 **FUD** XXX [63] [S] [80] ⚑
AMA: 2003,Apr,7; 1997,Nov,1

36468-36479 Destruction of Veins

CMS: 100-2,16,180 Services Related to Noncovered Procedures

36468 **Single or multiple injections of sclerosing solutions, spider veins (telangiectasia), limb or trunk**
Do not report in the same operative field with (37241)
🏥 0.00 ⚕ 0.00 **FUD** 000 [T] [R2] [80] ⚑
AMA: 2015,Apr,10; 2015,Jan,16; 2014,Oct,6; 2014,Aug,14; 2013,Nov,6

36470 **Injection of sclerosing solution; single vein**
[EXCLUDES] *Vascular occlusion and embolization services (37241-37244)*
Do not report in same operative field with (37241)
🏥 2.43 ⚕ 4.27 **FUD** 010 [T] [P3] [50] ⚑
AMA: 2015,Apr,10; 2015,Jan,16; 2014,Oct,6; 2014,Aug,14; 2013,Nov,6

36471 **multiple veins, same leg**
[EXCLUDES] *Vascular occlusion and embolization services (37241-37244)*
Do not report in same operative field with (37241)
🏥 2.91 ⚕ 4.99 **FUD** 010 [T] [P2] [50] ⚑
AMA: 2015,Aug,8; 2015,Apr,10; 2015,Jan,16; 2014,Oct,6; 2014,Aug,14; 2013,Nov,6

36475 **Endovenous ablation therapy of incompetent vein, extremity, inclusive of all imaging guidance and monitoring, percutaneous, radiofrequency; first vein treated**
Do not report in same operative field with (29581-29582, 36000-36005, 36410, 36425, 36478-36479, 37241-37244, 75894, 76000-76001, 76937, 76942, 76998, 77022, 93970-93971)
🏥 8.22 ⚕ 43.6 **FUD** 000 [T] [A2] [50] ⚑
AMA: 2015,Apr,10; 2015,Jan,16; 2014,Oct,6; 2014,Aug,14; 2014,Mar,4; 2014,Jan,11; 2013,Nov,6; 2012,Jan,15-42; 2010,Jul,10

\+ **36476** **second and subsequent veins treated in a single extremity, each through separate access sites (List separately in addition to code for primary procedure)**
Code first (36475)
Do not report in same operative field with (29581-29582, 36000-36005, 36410, 36425, 36478-36479, 37241-37244, 75894, 76000-76001, 76937, 76942, 76998, 77022, 93970-93971)
🏥 3.96 ⚕ 8.45 **FUD** ZZZ [N] [N1] [50]
AMA: 2015,Apr,10; 2015,Jan,16; 2014,Oct,6; 2014,Aug,14; 2014,Mar,4; 2014,Jan,11; 2013,Nov,6; 2012,Jan,15-42; 2010,Jul,10

36478 **Endovenous ablation therapy of incompetent vein, extremity, inclusive of all imaging guidance and monitoring, percutaneous, laser; first vein treated**
Do not report in same operative field with (29581-29582, 36000-36005, 36410, 36425, 36475-36476, 37241, 75894, 76000-76001, 76937, 76942, 76998, 77022, 93970-93971)
🏥 8.17 ⚕ 34.1 **FUD** 000 [T] [A2] [50] ⚑
AMA: 2015,Apr,10; 2015,Jan,16; 2014,Oct,6; 2014,Aug,14; 2014,Mar,4; 2014,Jan,11; 2013,Nov,6; 2012,Jul,12-14

\+ **36479** **second and subsequent veins treated in a single extremity, each through separate access sites (List separately in addition to code for primary procedure)**
Code first (36478)
Do not report in same operative field with (29581-29582, 36000-36005, 36410, 36425, 36475-36476, 37241, 75894, 76000-76001, 76937, 76942, 76998, 77022, 93970-93971)
🏥 3.98 ⚕ 8.78 **FUD** ZZZ [N] [N1] [50]
AMA: 2015,Apr,10; 2015,Jan,16; 2014,Oct,6; 2014,Aug,14; 2014,Mar,4; 2014,Jan,11; 2013,Nov,6; 2012,Jul,12-14; 2012,Jan,15-42; 2010,Jul,10

36481-36510 Other Venous Catheterization Procedures

[EXCLUDES] *Collection of a specimen from:*
A completely implantable device (36591)
An established catheter (36592)

36481 **Percutaneous portal vein catheterization by any method**
☢ (75885, 75887)
🏥 10.2 ⚕ 58.6 **FUD** 000 ⊙ [N] [N1] ⚑
AMA: 2015,Jan,16; 2014,Jan,11; 2012,Jan,15-42; 2011,Jan,11

36500 **Venous catheterization for selective organ blood sampling**
[EXCLUDES] *Inferior or superior vena cava catheterization (36010)*
☢ (75893)
🏥 5.27 ⚕ 5.27 **FUD** 000 [N] [N1] ⚑
AMA: 2014,Jan,11

36510 **Catheterization of umbilical vein for diagnosis or therapy, newborn** [A]
[EXCLUDES] *Collection of a specimen from:*
Capillary blood (36416)
Venipuncture (36415)
🏥 1.67 ⚕ 2.64 **FUD** 000 [63] [N] [N1] [80] ⚑
AMA: 2015,Jan,16; 2014,Jan,11

36511-36516 Apheresis

CMS: 100-3,110.14 Apheresis (Therapeutic Pheresis); 100-4,4,231.9 Billing for Pheresis and Apheresis Services

[EXCLUDES] *Collection of a specimen from:*
A completely implantable device (36591)
An established catheter (36592)
Code also modifier 26 for a professional evaluation

36511 **Therapeutic apheresis; for white blood cells**
🏥 2.65 ⚕ 2.65 **FUD** 000 [S] [R2] ⚑
AMA: 2015,Jan,16; 2014,Jan,11; 2013,Oct,3; 2011,Jan,11

36512 **for red blood cells**
🏥 2.72 ⚕ 2.72 **FUD** 000 [S] [R2] ⚑
AMA: 2015,Jan,16; 2014,Jan,11; 2013,Oct,3; 2011,Jan,11

36513 **for platelets**
🏥 2.79 ⚕ 2.79 **FUD** 000 [S] [R2] ⚑
AMA: 2015,Jan,16; 2014,Jan,11; 2013,Oct,3; 2012,Jan,15-42; 2011,Jan,11

CPT © 2015 American Medical Association. All Rights Reserved. (Black Text) © 2015 Optum360, LLC (Blue Text)

36514 **for plasma pheresis**
 2.67 15.1 **FUD** 000 S 62
AMA: 2015,Jan,16; 2014,Jan,11; 2013,Oct,3; 2011,Jan,11

36515 **with extracorporeal immunoadsorption and plasma reinfusion**
 2.62 58.2 **FUD** 000 S P2
AMA: 2015,Jan,16; 2014,Jan,11; 2013,Oct,3; 2011,Jan,11

36516 **with extracorporeal selective adsorption or selective filtration and plasma reinfusion**
 2.02 58.8 **FUD** 000 S P2
AMA: 2015,Jan,16; 2014,Jan,11; 2013,Oct,3; 2011,Jan,11

36522 Extracorporeal Photopheresis

CMS: 100-3,110.4 Extracorporeal Photopheresis; 100-4,32,190 Billing for Extracorporeal Photopheresis; 100-4,32,190.2 Extracorporeal Photopheresis; 100-4,32,190.3 Medicare Denial Codes; 100-4,4,231.9 Billing for Pheresis and Apheresis Services

36522 **Photopheresis, extracorporeal**
 2.91 39.4 **FUD** 000 S 62
AMA: 2015,Jan,16; 2014,Jan,11; 2013,Oct,3; 2012,Jan,15-42; 2011,Jan,11; 2010,Aug,12; 2010,Aug,12

36555-36571 Placement of Implantable Venous Access Device

INCLUDES Devices accessed by an exposed catheter, or a subcutaneous port or pump
Devices inserted via cutdown or percutaneous access:
Centrally (eg, femoral, jugular, subclavian veins, or inferior vena cava)
Peripherally (eg, basilic or cephalic)
Devices terminating in the brachiocephalic (innominate), iliac, or subclavian veins, vena cava, or right atrium
Venous access obtained by cutdown or percutaneously with any size catheter

EXCLUDES Maintenance/refilling of implantable pump/reservoir (96522)
Code also removal of central venous access device (if code available) when a new device is placed through a separate venous access

36555 **Insertion of non-tunneled centrally inserted central venous catheter; younger than 5 years of age** A
EXCLUDES Peripheral insertion (36568)
 3.38 7.23 **FUD** 000 ⊙ T A2 PQ
AMA: 2015,Jan,16; 2014,Jan,11

Under age 5

Direct CVC

A non-tunneled centrally inserted CVC is inserted. Report 36555 for a patient under age 5 and 36556 for patients older than age 5

Direct CVC

Age 5 and older

36556 **age 5 years or older** A
EXCLUDES Peripheral insertion (36569)
 3.50 6.65 **FUD** 000 T A2 PQ
AMA: 2015,Jan,16; 2014,Jan,11

36557 **Insertion of tunneled centrally inserted central venous catheter, without subcutaneous port or pump; younger than 5 years of age** A
 9.57 29.1 **FUD** 010 ⊙ T A2 80 50 PQ
AMA: 2015,Jan,16; 2014,Jan,11

Under age 5

Age 5 and older

Tunneled portion

Tunneled portion

A tunneled centrally inserted CVC is inserted

36558 **age 5 years or older** A
EXCLUDES Peripheral insertion (36571)
 8.07 22.3 **FUD** 010 ⊙ T A2 80 50 PQ
AMA: 2015,Jan,13; 2015,Jan,16; 2014,Jan,11

36560 **Insertion of tunneled centrally inserted central venous access device, with subcutaneous port; younger than 5 years of age** A
EXCLUDES Peripheral insertion (36570)
 10.2 30.5 **FUD** 010 ⊙ T A2 80 50 PQ
AMA: 2015,Jan,16; 2014,Jan,11; 2012,Jan,15-42; 2011,Jan,11

36561 **age 5 years or older** A
EXCLUDES Peripheral insertion (36571)
 10.2 33.5 **FUD** 010 ⊙ T A2 80 50 PQ
AMA: 2015,Jan,16; 2014,Jan,11; 2012,Jan,15-42; 2011,Jan,11

36563 **Insertion of tunneled centrally inserted central venous access device with subcutaneous pump**
 11.0 38.0 **FUD** 010 ⊙ T A2 80 PQ
AMA: 2015,Jan,16; 2014,Jan,11

36565 **Insertion of tunneled centrally inserted central venous access device, requiring 2 catheters via 2 separate venous access sites; without subcutaneous port or pump (eg, Tesio type catheter)**
 10.1 27.5 **FUD** 010 ⊙ T A2 80 50 PQ
AMA: 2015,Jan,16; 2014,Jan,11

36566 **with subcutaneous port(s)**
 11.2 157. **FUD** 010 ⊙ T A2 80 50 PQ
AMA: 2015,Jan,16; 2014,Jan,11

36568 **Insertion of peripherally inserted central venous catheter (PICC), without subcutaneous port or pump; younger than 5 years of age** A
EXCLUDES Centrally inserted placement (36555)
Do not report removal of PICC lines with codes for removal of tunneled central venous catheters; report appropriate E&M code
 2.87 8.64 **FUD** 000 ⊙ T A2 PQ
AMA: 2015,Jan,16; 2014,Jan,11; 2012,Nov,13-14; 2012,Jan,15-42; 2011,Jan,11

36569 **age 5 years or older** A
EXCLUDES Centrally inserted placement (36556)
Do not report removal of PICC lines with codes for removal of tunneled central venous catheters; report appropriate E&M code
 2.66 7.12 **FUD** 000 T A2 PQ
AMA: 2015,Jan,16; 2014,Sep,13; 2014,Jan,11; 2013,Sep,17; 2012,Nov,13-14; 2012,Jan,15-42; 2011,Jan,11

Cardiovascular System

36570 — 36593

36570 **Insertion of peripherally inserted central venous access device, with subcutaneous port; younger than 5 years of age** Ⓐ

EXCLUDES *Centrally inserted placement (36560)*

📋 8.85 ⚕ 33.8 **FUD** 010 ⊙ T A2 80 50 ▭ PQ

AMA: 2015,Jan,16; 2014,Jan,11; 2012,Jan,15-42

36571 **age 5 years or older** Ⓐ

EXCLUDES *Centrally inserted placement (36561)*

📋 9.40 ⚕ 37.2 **FUD** 010 ⊙ T A2 80 50 ▭ PQ

AMA: 2015,Jan,16; 2014,Jan,11; 2012,Jan,15-42

36575-36590 Repair, Removal, and Replacement Implantable Venous Access Device

EXCLUDES *Mechanical removal obstructive material, pericatheter/intraluminal (36595, 36596)*

Code also a frequency of two for procedures involving both catheters from a multicatheter device

36575 **Repair of tunneled or non-tunneled central venous access catheter, without subcutaneous port or pump, central or peripheral insertion site**

INCLUDES *Repair of the device without replacing any parts*

📋 1.02 ⚕ 4.73 **FUD** 000 T A2 80 ▭

AMA: 2015,Jan,16; 2014,Jan,11

36576 **Repair of central venous access device, with subcutaneous port or pump, central or peripheral insertion site**

INCLUDES *Repair of the device without replacing any parts*

📋 5.76 ⚕ 11.1 **FUD** 010 ⊙ T A2 80 ▭

AMA: 2015,Jan,16; 2014,Jan,11

36578 **Replacement, catheter only, of central venous access device, with subcutaneous port or pump, central or peripheral insertion site**

INCLUDES *Partial replacement (catheter only)*

EXCLUDES *Total replacement of the entire device using the same venous access sites (36582-36583)*

📋 6.31 ⚕ 14.8 **FUD** 010 ⊙ T A2 80 ▭ PQ

AMA: 2015,Jan,16; 2014,Jan,11

36580 **Replacement, complete, of a non-tunneled centrally inserted central venous catheter, without subcutaneous port or pump, through same venous access**

INCLUDES *Complete replacement (replace all components/same access site)*

📋 1.95 ⚕ 6.13 **FUD** 000 T A2 ▭ PQ

AMA: 2015,Jan,16; 2014,Jan,11

36581 **Replacement, complete, of a tunneled centrally inserted central venous catheter, without subcutaneous port or pump, through same venous access**

INCLUDES *Complete replacement (replace all components/same access site)*

EXCLUDES *Removal of old device and insertion of new device using a separate venous access site*

📋 5.72 ⚕ 21.8 **FUD** 010 ⊙ T A2 80 ▭ PQ

AMA: 2015,Jan,16; 2014,Jan,11

36582 **Replacement, complete, of a tunneled centrally inserted central venous access device, with subcutaneous port, through same venous access**

INCLUDES *Complete replacement (replace all components/same access site)*

EXCLUDES *Removal of old device and insertion of new device using a separate venous access site*

📋 8.91 ⚕ 31.2 **FUD** 010 ⊙ T A2 80 ▭ PQ

AMA: 2015,Jan,16; 2014,Jan,11

36583 **Replacement, complete, of a tunneled centrally inserted central venous access device, with subcutaneous pump, through same venous access**

INCLUDES *Complete replacement (replace all components/same access site)*

EXCLUDES *Removal of old device and insertion of new device using a separate venous access site*

📋 9.82 ⚕ 38.9 **FUD** 010 ⊙ T A2 80 ▭ PQ

AMA: 2015,Jan,16; 2014,Jan,11

36584 **Replacement, complete, of a peripherally inserted central venous catheter (PICC), without subcutaneous port or pump, through same venous access**

INCLUDES *Complete replacement (replace all components/same access site)*

📋 1.93 ⚕ 5.82 **FUD** 000 T A2 ▭ PQ

AMA: 2015,Jan,16; 2014,Jan,11

36585 **Replacement, complete, of a peripherally inserted central venous access device, with subcutaneous port, through same venous access**

INCLUDES *Complete replacement (replace all components/same access site)*

📋 8.26 ⚕ 33.0 **FUD** 010 ⊙ T A2 80 ▭ PQ

AMA: 2015,Jan,16; 2014,Jan,11

36589 **Removal of tunneled central venous catheter, without subcutaneous port or pump**

INCLUDES *Complete removal/all components*

EXCLUDES *Non-tunneled central venous catheter removal; report appropriate E&M code*

📋 4.01 ⚕ 4.74 **FUD** 010 02 A2 80 ▭

AMA: 2015,Jan,16; 2014,Jan,11

36590 **Removal of tunneled central venous access device, with subcutaneous port or pump, central or peripheral insertion**

INCLUDES *Complete removal/all components*

EXCLUDES *Non-tunneled central venous catheter removal; report appropriate E&M code*

📋 5.96 ⚕ 8.40 **FUD** 010 ⊙ 02 A2 80 ▭

AMA: 2015,Jan,16; 2014,Jan,11; 2012,Jan,15-42; 2010,Jul,10

36591-36592 Obtain Blood Specimen from Implanted Device or Catheter

Do not report with any other service except laboratory services

36591 **Collection of blood specimen from a completely implantable venous access device**

EXCLUDES *Collection of:*
Capillary blood specimen (36416)
Venous blood specimen by venipuncture (36415)

📋 0.66 ⚕ 0.66 **FUD** XXX 01 N1 80 TC

AMA: 2015,Jan,16; 2014,May,4; 2014,Jan,11; 2012,Jan,15-42; 2011,Jul,16-17

36592 **Collection of blood specimen using established central or peripheral catheter, venous, not otherwise specified**

EXCLUDES *Collection of blood from an established arterial catheter (37799)*

📋 0.74 ⚕ 0.74 **FUD** XXX 01 N1 80 TC

AMA: 2015,Jan,16; 2014,Jan,11; 2012,Jan,15-42; 2011,Jul,16-17

36593-36596 Restore Patency of Occluded Catheter or Device

EXCLUDES *Venous catheterization (36010-36012)*

36593 **Declotting by thrombolytic agent of implanted vascular access device or catheter**

📋 0.87 ⚕ 0.87 **FUD** XXX T P3 80 TC

AMA: 2015,Jan,16; 2014,Jan,11; 2013,Feb,3-6; 2012,Jan,15-42; 2011,Aug,9-10; 2011,Jan,11

36595 Mechanical removal of pericatheter obstructive material (eg, fibrin sheath) from central venous device via separate venous access

Do not report with (36593)

⚒ (75901)

🚗 5.37   ⚖ 16.6   **FUD** 000   T P3 ▯

AMA: 2015,Jan,16; 2014,Jan,11

36596 Mechanical removal of intraluminal (intracatheter) obstructive material from central venous device through device lumen

Do not report with (36593)

⚒ (75902)

🚗 1.30   ⚖ 3.80   **FUD** 000   T G2 ▯

AMA: 2015,Jan,16; 2014,Jan,11

36597-36598 Repositioning or Assessment of In Situ Venous Access Device

36597 Repositioning of previously placed central venous catheter under fluoroscopic guidance

⚒ (76000)

🚗 1.80   ⚖ 3.66   **FUD** 000   T G2 ▯

AMA: 2015,Jan,16; 2014,Sep,5; 2014,Jan,11

36598 Contrast injection(s) for radiologic evaluation of existing central venous access device, including fluoroscopy, image documentation and report

EXCLUDES   Complete venography studies (75820, 75825, 75827)

Do not report with (36595-36596, 76000)

🚗 1.06   ⚖ 3.13   **FUD** 000   T P3 80 50 P0

AMA: 2014,Jan,11

36600-36660 Insertion Needle or Catheter: Artery

36600 Arterial puncture, withdrawal of blood for diagnosis

Do not report with critical care services

🚗 0.44   ⚖ 0.90   **FUD** XXX   03 N1 ▯

AMA: 2015,Jan,16; 2014,May,4; 2014,Jan,11

36620 Arterial catheterization or cannulation for sampling, monitoring or transfusion (separate procedure); percutaneous

🚗 1.47   ⚖ 1.47   **FUD** 000   ⊘ N N1 ▯

AMA: 2015,Jan,16; 2014,Jan,11

36625 cutdown

🚗 2.98   ⚖ 2.98   **FUD** 000   N N1 ▯

AMA: 2015,Jan,16; 2014,Jan,11

36640 Arterial catheterization for prolonged infusion therapy (chemotherapy), cutdown

EXCLUDES   Intraarterial chemotherapy (96420-96425)
Transcatheter embolization (75894)

🚗 3.44   ⚖ 3.44   **FUD** 000   T A2 ▯

AMA: 2015,Jan,16; 2014,Jan,11

36660 Catheterization, umbilical artery, newborn, for diagnosis or therapy   A

🚗 1.75   ⚖ 1.75   **FUD** 000   63 C 80 ▯

AMA: 2015,Jan,16; 2014,Jan,11

36680 Percutaneous Placement of Catheter/Needle into Bone Marrow Cavity

36680 Placement of needle for intraosseous infusion

🚗 1.70   ⚖ 1.70   **FUD** 000   01 N1 80 ▯

AMA: 2015,Jan,16; 2014,Jan,11; 2012,Jan,15-42; 2011,Jan,11

36800-36821 Vascular Access for Hemodialysis

36800 Insertion of cannula for hemodialysis, other purpose (separate procedure); vein to vein

🚗 3.58   ⚖ 3.58   **FUD** 000   T A2 ▯

AMA: 2015,Jan,16; 2014,Jan,11

36810 arteriovenous, external (Scribner type)

🚗 6.24   ⚖ 6.24   **FUD** 000   T A2 ▯

AMA: 2015,Jan,16; 2014,Jan,11

36815 arteriovenous, external revision, or closure

🚗 4.04   ⚖ 4.04   **FUD** 000   T A2 ▯

AMA: 2015,Jan,16; 2014,Jan,11

36818 Arteriovenous anastomosis, open; by upper arm cephalic vein transposition

INCLUDES   Two incisions in the upper arm; a medial incision over the brachial artery and a lateral incision for exposure of a portion of the cephalic vein

Code also modifier 50 or 59, as appropriate, for a bilateral procedure

Do not report with (for unilateral procedure) (36819-36821, 36830)

🚗 20.4   ⚖ 20.4   **FUD** 090   T A2 80 ▯ P0

AMA: 2015,Jan,16; 2014,Jan,11

36819 by upper arm basilic vein transposition

Code also modifier 50 or 59, as appropriate, for bilateral procedure

Do not report with (for unilateral procedure) (36818, 36820-36821, 36830)

🚗 21.6   ⚖ 21.6   **FUD** 090   T A2 80 ▯ P0

AMA: 2015,Jan,16; 2014,Jan,11

36820 by forearm vein transposition

🚗 21.5   ⚖ 21.5   **FUD** 090   T A2 80 50 ▯ P0

AMA: 2015,Jan,16; 2014,Jan,11

36821 direct, any site (eg, Cimino type) (separate procedure)

🚗 19.6   ⚖ 19.6   **FUD** 090   T A2 80 ▯ P0

AMA: 2015,Aug,8; 2015,Jan,16; 2014,Jan,11

36823 Vascular Access for Extracorporeal Circulation

INCLUDES   Chemotherapy perfusion

EXCLUDES   Maintenance for extracorporeal circulation (33946-33949)

Do not report with (96409-96425)

36823 Insertion of arterial and venous cannula(s) for isolated extracorporeal circulation including regional chemotherapy perfusion to an extremity, with or without hyperthermia, with removal of cannula(s) and repair of arteriotomy and venotomy sites

🚗 40.3   ⚖ 40.3   **FUD** 090   C ▯

AMA: 2014,Jan,11

36825-36835 Permanent Vascular Access Procedures

36825 Creation of arteriovenous fistula by other than direct arteriovenous anastomosis (separate procedure); autogenous graft

EXCLUDES   Direct arteriovenous (AV) anastomosis (36821)

🚗 23.6   ⚖ 23.6   **FUD** 090   T A2 80 ▯ P0

AMA: 2015,Jan,16; 2014,Jan,11

In 36825, the artery and vein are connected by a vein graft in an end-to-side manner, creating an arteriovenous fistula

Radial artery

Radial artery

Basilic vein

Graft

Basilic vein

In 36830, the artery and vein are connected by a synthetic graft

36830 nonautogenous graft (eg, biological collagen, thermoplastic graft)

EXCLUDES   Direct arteriovenous (AV) anastomosis (36821)

🚗 19.7   ⚖ 19.7   **FUD** 090   T A2 80 ▯ P0

AMA: 2015,Jan,16; 2015,Jan,13; 2014,Jan,11

36831   Thrombectomy, open, arteriovenous fistula without revision, autogenous or nonautogenous dialysis graft (separate procedure)

     18.2   18.2   **FUD** 090   T A2 80 ▭

     AMA: 2015,Jan,16; 2014,Jan,11; 2012,Jan,15-42; 2011,Jan,11

36832   Revision, open, arteriovenous fistula; without thrombectomy, autogenous or nonautogenous dialysis graft (separate procedure)

     INCLUDES   Revision of an arteriovenous access fistula or graft

     22.3   22.3   **FUD** 090   T A2 80 ▭

     AMA: 2015,Jan,16; 2014,Jan,11; 2012,Jan,15-42; 2011,Jan,11

36833   with thrombectomy, autogenous or nonautogenous dialysis graft (separate procedure)

     23.9   23.9   **FUD** 090   T A2 80 ▭

     AMA: 2015,Jan,16; 2014,Jan,11; 2012,Jan,15-42; 2011,Jan,11

36835   Insertion of Thomas shunt (separate procedure)

     14.6   14.6   **FUD** 090   T A2 ▭

     AMA: 2014,Jan,11

36838 DRIL Procedure for Ischemic Steal Syndrome

Do not report with (35512, 35522-35523, 36832, 37607, 37618)

36838   Distal revascularization and interval ligation (DRIL), upper extremity hemodialysis access (steal syndrome)

     33.8   33.8   **FUD** 090   T 80 50 ▭

     AMA: 2014,Jan,11

36860-36870 Restore Patency of Occluded Cannula or Arteriovenous Fistula

36860   External cannula declotting (separate procedure); without balloon catheter

     (76000)

     3.19   5.92   **FUD** 000   T A2 ▭

     AMA: 2015,Jan,16; 2014,Jan,11

36861   with balloon catheter

     (76000)

     3.85   3.85   **FUD** 000   T A2 ▭

     AMA: 2015,Jan,16; 2014,Jan,11

36870   Thrombectomy, percutaneous, arteriovenous fistula, autogenous or nonautogenous graft (includes mechanical thrombus extraction and intra-graft thrombolysis)

     INCLUDES   Declotting using thrombolytics

           Moving thrombus using a mechanical methodology including using a balloon catheter

     EXCLUDES   Catheterization for arteriovenous (AV) shunt (36147-36148)

     Do not report for removal arterial plug with arterial or venous angioplasty (35475-35476)

     Do not report with (36593)

     (75791)

     8.77   52.1   **FUD** 090   ⊙ J A2 50 ▭

     AMA: 2015,Jan,16; 2014,Jan,11; 2013,Feb,3-6; 2012,Apr,3-9; 2011,Dec,14-18

37140-37181 Open Decompression of Portal Circulation

     EXCLUDES   Peritoneal-venous shunt (49425)

37140   Venous anastomosis, open; portocaval

     67.2   67.2   **FUD** 090   C ▭

     AMA: 2014,Jan,11

37145   renoportal

     62.3   62.3   **FUD** 090   C 80 ▭

     AMA: 2014,Jan,11

37160   caval-mesenteric

     64.0   64.0   **FUD** 090   C 80 ▭

     AMA: 2014,Jan,11

37180   splenorenal, proximal

     61.5   61.5   **FUD** 090   C 80 ▭

     AMA: 2014,Jan,11

37181   splenorenal, distal (selective decompression of esophagogastric varices, any technique)

     EXCLUDES   Percutaneous procedure (37182)

     67.2   67.2   **FUD** 090   C 80 ▭

     AMA: 2014,Jan,11

37182-37183 Transvenous Decompression of Portal Circulation

Do not report with (75885, 75887)

37182   Insertion of transvenous intrahepatic portosystemic shunt(s) (TIPS) (includes venous access, hepatic and portal vein catheterization, portography with hemodynamic evaluation, intrahepatic tract formation/dilatation, stent placement and all associated imaging guidance and documentation)

     EXCLUDES   Open procedure (37140)

     24.4   24.4   **FUD** 000   C 80 ▭ P0

     AMA: 2015,Jan,16; 2014,Jan,11; 2013,Sep,17; 2012,Jan,15-42; 2011,Jan,11

37183   Revision of transvenous intrahepatic portosystemic shunt(s) (TIPS) (includes venous access, hepatic and portal vein catheterization, portography with hemodynamic evaluation, intrahepatic tract recanulization/dilatation, stent placement and all associated imaging guidance and documentation)

     EXCLUDES   Arteriovenous (AV) aneurysm repair (36832)

     11.5   168.   **FUD** 000   ⊙ J 80 ▭ P0

     AMA: 2015,Jan,16; 2014,Jan,11; 2012,Jan,15-42; 2011,Jan,11

37184-37188 Removal of Thrombus from Vessel: Percutaneous

     INCLUDES   Fluoroscopic guidance

           Injection(s) of thrombolytics during the procedure

           Postprocedure evaluation

           Pretreatment planning

     EXCLUDES   Continuous infusion of thrombolytics prior to and after the procedure ([37211, 37212, 37213, 37214])

           Diagnostic studies

           Intracranial arterial mechanical thrombectomy or infusion (61645)

           Mechanical thrombectomy, coronary (92973)

           Other interventions performed percutaneously (e.g., balloon angioplasty)

           Percutaneous thrombectomy of an arteriovenous fistula (36870)

           Placement of catheters

           Radiological supervision/interpretation

▲ **37184**   Primary percutaneous transluminal mechanical thrombectomy, noncoronary, non-intracranial, arterial or arterial bypass graft, including fluoroscopic guidance and intraprocedural pharmacological thrombolytic injection(s); initial vessel

     EXCLUDES   Mechanical thrombectomy for embolus/thrombus complicating another percutaneous interventional procedure (37186)

           Mechanical thrombectomy of another vascular family/separate access site, append modifier 51 to code, as appropriate

     Do not report with (61645, 76000-76001, 96374, 99143-99150)

     13.5   64.7   **FUD** 000   ⊙ T 82 50 P0

     AMA: 2015,Apr,10; 2015,Jan,16; 2014,Jan,11; 2013,Feb,3-6

▲ + 37185   second and all subsequent vessel(s) within the same vascular family (List separately in addition to code for primary mechanical thrombectomy procedure)

> INCLUDES Treatment of second and all succeeding vessel(s) in same vascular family

> EXCLUDES *Intravenous drug injections administered subsequent to an initial service*
> *Mechanical thrombectomy for treating of embolus/thrombus complicating another percutaneous interventional procedure (37186)*
> *Mechanical thrombectomy of another vascular family/separate access site, append modifier 51 to code as appropriate*

Code first (37184)
Do not report with (61645, 76000-76001, 96375)
Do not report with arterial mechanical thrombectomy in the same vascular area (61645)

🔧 4.92   ✂ 20.5   **FUD** ZZZ   ⊙ Ⓝ Ⓝ1

AMA: 2015,Apr,10; 2015,Jan,16; 2014,Jan,11; 2013,Feb,3-6

▲ + 37186   **Secondary percutaneous transluminal thrombectomy (eg, nonprimary mechanical, snare basket, suction technique), noncoronary, non-intracranial, arterial or arterial bypass graft, including fluoroscopic guidance and intraprocedural pharmacological thrombolytic injections, provided in conjunction with another percutaneous intervention other than primary mechanical thrombectomy (List separately in addition to code for primary procedure)**

> INCLUDES Removal of small emboli/thrombi prior to or after another percutaneous procedure

Code first primary procedure
Do not report with (37184-37185, 76000-76001, 96375)
Do not report with arterial mechanical thrombectomy in the same vascular area (61645)

🔧 7.30   ✂ 39.2   **FUD** ZZZ   ⊙ Ⓝ Ⓝ1

AMA: 2015,Jan,16; 2014,Jan,11; 2013,Feb,3-6; 2012,Jan,15-42; 2011,Jul,3-11; 2011,Jan,11

37187   **Percutaneous transluminal mechanical thrombectomy, vein(s), including intraprocedural pharmacological thrombolytic injections and fluoroscopic guidance**

> INCLUDES Secondary or subsequent intravenous injection after another initial service

Do not report with (76000-76001, 96375)

🔧 11.9   ✂ 58.8   **FUD** 000   ⊙ Ⓣ Ⓖ2 Ⓢ0 Ⓟ0

AMA: 2015,Jan,16; 2014,Jan,11; 2013,Feb,3-6

37188   **Percutaneous transluminal mechanical thrombectomy, vein(s), including intraprocedural pharmacological thrombolytic injections and fluoroscopic guidance, repeat treatment on subsequent day during course of thrombolytic therapy**

Do not report with (76000-76001, 96375)

🔧 8.59   ✂ 50.2   **FUD** 000   ⊙ Ⓣ Ⓖ2 Ⓢ0 Ⓟ0

AMA: 2015,Jan,16; 2014,Jan,11; 2013,Feb,3-6

37191-37193 Vena Cava Filters

37191   **Insertion of intravascular vena cava filter, endovascular approach including vascular access, vessel selection, and radiological supervision and interpretation, intraprocedural roadmapping, and imaging guidance (ultrasound and fluoroscopy), when performed**

> EXCLUDES *Open ligation of inferior vena cava via laparotomy or retroperitoneal approach (37619)*

🔧 7.00   ✂ 74.9   **FUD** 000   ⊙ Ⓣ

AMA: 2015,Jan,16; 2014,Jan,11; 2013,Feb,3-6; 2012,Apr,3-9

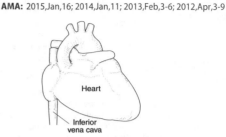

Heart

Inferior vena cava

The inverior vena cava (or IVC) is the major return vessel of the lower body. It extends from the right atrium of the heart down to the bifurcation of the iliac veins

An intravascular "umbrella" device in the IVC. Such devices are intended to entrap clots and prevent clot passage into the pulmonary arteries

37192   **Repositioning of intravascular vena cava filter, endovascular approach including vascular access, vessel selection, and radiological supervision and interpretation, intraprocedural roadmapping, and imaging guidance (ultrasound and fluoroscopy), when performed**

Do not report with (37191)

🔧 10.9   ✂ 47.8   **FUD** 000   ⊙ Ⓣ

AMA: 2015,Jan,16; 2014,Jan,11; 2013,Feb,3-6; 2012,Apr,3-9

37193   **Retrieval (removal) of intravascular vena cava filter, endovascular approach including vascular access, vessel selection, and radiological supervision and interpretation, intraprocedural roadmapping, and imaging guidance (ultrasound and fluoroscopy), when performed**

Do not report with (37197)

🔧 10.7   ✂ 45.6   **FUD** 000   ⊙ Ⓣ

AMA: 2015,Jan,16; 2014,Jan,11; 2013,Feb,3-6; 2012,Apr,3-9

37195 Intravenous Cerebral Thrombolysis

37195   **Thrombolysis, cerebral, by intravenous infusion**

🔧 0.00   ✂ 0.00   **FUD** XXX   Ⓣ Ⓢ0 Ⓜ

AMA: 2014,Jan,11

37197-37214 [37211, 37212, 37213, 37214] Transcatheter Procedures: Infusions, Biopsy, Foreign Body Removal

37197   **Transcatheter retrieval, percutaneous, of intravascular foreign body (eg, fractured venous or arterial catheter), includes radiological supervision and interpretation, and imaging guidance (ultrasound or fluoroscopy), when performed**

> EXCLUDES *Percutaneous vena cava filter retrieval (37193)*
> *Removal leadless pacemaker system (0388T)*

🔧 9.29   ✂ 43.3   **FUD** 000   ⊙ Ⓣ Ⓖ2

AMA: 2015,Jan,16; 2014,Jan,11; 2013,Feb,3-6

37200   **Transcatheter biopsy**

📷 (75970)

🔧 6.45   ✂ 6.45   **FUD** 000   Ⓣ Ⓖ2 Ⓜ Ⓟ0

AMA: 2014,Jan,11

Cardiovascular System

37211 — 37215

▲ # **37211** **Transcatheter therapy, arterial infusion for thrombolysis other than coronary or intracranial, any method, including radiological supervision and interpretation, initial treatment day**

> INCLUDES Catheter exchange or position change
> Evaluation and management services on the day of and related to thrombolysis
> First day of transcatheter thrombolytic infusion
> Fluoroscopic guidance
> Follow-up arteriography or venography
> Radiologic supervision and interpretation
>
> EXCLUDES *Catheter placement*
> *Declotting of implanted catheter or vascular access device by thrombolytic agent (36593)*
> *Diagnostic studies*
> *Iintracranial arterial mechanical thrombectomy or infusion (61645)*
> *Percutaneous interventions*
> *Ultrasound guidance (76937)*
>
> Code also significant, separately identifiable E&M service on the day of thrombolysis using modifier 25
> Do not report more than one time per date of service
> Do not report with (75898)
> 🔹 11.7   ⬦ 11.7   **FUD** 000   ⊙ T 62 50
>
> **AMA:** 2015,Jan,16; 2014,Jan,11; 2013,Feb,3-6

37212 **Transcatheter therapy, venous infusion for thrombolysis, any method, including radiological supervision and interpretation, initial treatment day**

> INCLUDES Catheter position change or exchange
> Evaluation and management services on the day of and related to thrombolysis
> First day of transcatheter thrombolytic infusion
> Fluoroscopic guidance
> Follow-up arteriography or venography
> Initiation and completion of thrombolysis on same date of service
> Radiologic supervision and interpretation
>
> EXCLUDES *Catheter placement*
> *Declotting of implanted catheter or vascular access device by thrombolytic agent (36593)*
> *Diagnostic studies*
> *Percutaneous interventions*
> *Ultrasound guidance (76937)*
>
> Code also significant, separately identifiable E&M service on the same day as thrombolysis using modifier 25
> Do not report more than one time per date of service
> Do not report with (75898)
> 🔹 10.2   ⬦ 10.2   **FUD** 000   ⊙ T 62 50
>
> **AMA:** 2015,Jan,16; 2014,Jan,11; 2013,Feb,3-6

37213 **Transcatheter therapy, arterial or venous infusion for thrombolysis other than coronary, any method, including radiological supervision and interpretation, continued treatment on subsequent day during course of thrombolytic therapy, including follow-up catheter contrast injection, position change, or exchange, when performed;**

> INCLUDES Continued thrombolytic infusions on subsequent days besides the initial and last days of treatment
> Evaluation and management services on the day of and related to the thrombolysis
> Fluoroscopic guidance
> Radiologic supervision and interpretation
>
> EXCLUDES *Catheter placement*
> *Declotting of implanted catheter or vascular access device by thrombolytic agent (36593)*
> *Diagnostic studies*
> *Percutaneous interventions*
> *Ultrasound guidance (76937)*
>
> Code also significant, separately identifiable E&M services not related to the thrombolysis using modifier 25
> Do not report more than one time per date of service
> Do not report with (75898)
> 🔹 7.25   ⬦ 7.25   **FUD** 000   ⊙ T
>
> **AMA:** 2015,Jan,16; 2014,Jan,11; 2013,Feb,3-6

37214   **cessation of thrombolysis including removal of catheter and vessel closure by any method**

> INCLUDES Evaluation and management services on the day of and related to the thrombolysis
> Fluoroscopic guidance
> Last day of transcatheter thrombolytic infusions
> Radiologic supervision and interpretation
>
> EXCLUDES *Catheter placement*
> *Declotting of implanted catheter or vascular access device by thrombolytic agent (36593)*
> *Diagnostic studies*
> *Percutaneous interventions*
> *Ultrasound guidance (76937)*
>
> Code also significant, separately identifiable E&M service not related to thrombolysis using modifier 25
> Do not report more than one time per date of service
> Do not report with (75898)
> 🔹 3.99   ⬦ 3.99   **FUD** 000   ⊙ T
>
> **AMA:** 2015,Jan,16; 2014,Jan,11; 2013,Feb,3-6

37202   ~~Transcatheter therapy, infusion other than for thrombolysis, any type (eg, spasmolytic, vasoconstrictive)~~

> To report, see ~61650-61651

37211   Resequenced code. See code following 37200.

37212   Resequenced code. See code following 37200.

37213   Resequenced code. See code following 37200.

37214   Resequenced code. See code following 37200.

37215-37216 Stenting of Cervical Carotid Artery with/without Insertion Distal Embolic Protection Device

> INCLUDES Carotid stenting, if required
> Ipsilateral cerebral and cervical carotid diagnostic imaging/supervision and interpretation
> Ipsilateral selective carotid catheterization
>
> EXCLUDES *Carotid catheterization and imaging, if carotid stenting not required*
> *Transcatheter placement extracranial vertebral artery stents, open or percutaneous (0075T, 0076T)*
>
> Do not report with (36222-36224)

37215   **Transcatheter placement of intravascular stent(s), cervical carotid artery, open or percutaneous, including angioplasty, when performed, and radiological supervision and interpretation; with distal embolic protection**

> 🔹 31.9   ⬦ 31.9   **FUD** 090   ⊙ C 80 50 ▯
>
> **AMA:** 2015,Jan,16; 2014,Mar,8; 2014,Jan,11; 2013,Feb,3-6

Balloon is advanced to the affected portion of artery

Balloon is inflated, which activates the stent

The catheter is withdrawn

Report 37216 when a clot filtering stent is placed

Temporal artery

External carotid

Internal carotid

Common carotid (cervical)

| 37216 | without distal embolic protection |

🚑 0.00 ✂ 0.00 **FUD** 090 ⊙ Ⓔ ▱

AMA: 2015,Jan,16; 2014,Mar,8; 2014,Jan,11; 2013,Feb,3-6

37217-37218 Stenting of Intrathoracic Carotid Artery/Innominate Artery

INCLUDES
Access to vessel (open)
Arteriotomy closure by suture
Catheterization of the vessel (selective)
Imaging during and after the procedure
Radiological supervision and interpretation

EXCLUDES
Transcatheter insertion extracranial vertebral artery stents, open or percutaneous (0075T-0076T)
Transcatheter insertion intracranial stents (61635)
Transcatheter insertion intravascular cervical carotid artery stents, open or percutaneous (37215-37216)

37217 **Transcatheter placement of intravascular stent(s), intrathoracic common carotid artery or innominate artery by retrograde treatment, open ipsilateral cervical carotid artery exposure, including angioplasty, when performed, and radiological supervision and interpretation**

Code also revascularization of carotid artery, when performed (33891, 35301, 35509-35510, 35601, 35606)
Do not report with the following services performed on the same side (35201, 35458, 36221-36227, 75962)
🚑 32.9 ✂ 32.9 **FUD** 090 Ⓒ 80 50

AMA: 2015,May,7; 2015,Jan,16; 2014,Mar,8; 2014,Jan,11

37218 **Transcatheter placement of intravascular stent(s), intrathoracic common carotid artery or innominate artery, open or percutaneous antegrade approach, including angioplasty, when performed, and radiological supervision and interpretation**

Do not report with (36222-36224)
🚑 24.0 ✂ 24.0 **FUD** 090 ⊙ Ⓒ 80 50

AMA: 2015,May,7

37220-37235 Endovascular Revascularization Lower Extremities

INCLUDES
Percutaneous and open interventional and associated procedures for lower extremity occlusive disease; unilateral
Accessing the vessel
Arteriotomy closure by suturing of puncture or pressure with application of arterial closure device
Atherectomy (e.g., directional, laser, rotational)
Balloon angioplasty (e.g., cryoplasty, cutting balloon, low-profile)
Catheterization of the vessel (selective)
Embolic protection
Imaging once procedure is complete
Radiological supervision and interpretation of intervention(s)
Stenting (e.g., bare metal, balloon-expandable, covered, drug-eluting, self-expanding)
Transversing of the lesion
Reporting the most comprehensive treatment in a given vessel according to the following hierarchy:
1. Stent and atherectomy
2. Atherectomy
3. Stent
4. PTA
Revascularization procedures for three arterial vascular territories:
Femoral/popliteal vascular territory including the common, deep, and superficial femoral arteries, and the popliteal artery (one extremity = a single vessel) (37224-37227)
Iliac vascular territory: common iliac, external iliac, internal iliac (37220-37223)
Tibial/peroneal territory: includes anterior tibial, peroneal artery, posterior tibial (37228-37235)

EXCLUDES
Extensive repair or replacement of artery (35226, 35286)
Mechanical thrombectomy and/or thrombolysis
Code also add-on codes for different vessels, but not different lesions in the same vessel; and for multiple territories in the same leg
Code also modifier 59 for a bilateral procedure
Code first one primary code for the initial service in each leg
Do not report more than one code from this family for each lower extremity vessel treated
Do not report more than one code when multiple vessels are treated in the femoral/popliteal territory (report the most complex service for more than one lesion in the territory); when a contiguous lesion that spans from one territory to another can be opened with a single procedure; or when more than one stent is deployed in the same vessel

37220 **Revascularization, endovascular, open or percutaneous, iliac artery, unilateral, initial vessel; with transluminal angioplasty**

Code also only when transluminal angioplasty is performed outside the treatment target zone of (34802-34805, 34825-34826, 34845-34848, 34900, 0254T)
🚑 12.2 ✂ 89.9 **FUD** 000 ⊙ Ⓙ 62 50 PQ

AMA: 2015,Jan,16; 2014,Jan,11; 2013,Dec,8; 2011,Oct,9; 2011,Jul,3-11

37221 **with transluminal stent placement(s), includes angioplasty within the same vessel, when performed**

Code also only when transluminal angioplasty is performed outside the treatment target zone of (34802-34805, 34825-34826, 34845-34848, 34900, 0254T)
🚑 15.0 ✂ 132. **FUD** 000 ⊙ Ⓙ J8 80 50 PQ

AMA: 2015,Jan,13; 2015,Jan,16; 2014,Jan,11; 2013,Dec,8; 2012,Apr,3-9; 2012,Jan,15-42; 2011,Oct,9; 2011,Jul,16-17; 2011,Jul,3-11

+ **37222** **Revascularization, endovascular, open or percutaneous, iliac artery, each additional ipsilateral iliac vessel; with transluminal angioplasty (List separately in addition to code for primary procedure)**

Code also only when transluminal angioplasty is performed outside the treatment target zone of (34802-34805, 34825-34826, 34845-34848, 34900, 0254T)
Code first (37220-37221)
🚑 5.51 ✂ 25.2 **FUD** ZZZ ⊙ Ⓝ N1 80 50 PQ

AMA: 2015,Jan,16; 2014,Jan,11; 2013,Dec,8; 2011,Oct,9; 2011,Jul,3-11

+ **37223** **with transluminal stent placement(s), includes angioplasty within the same vessel, when performed (List separately in addition to code for primary procedure)**

Code also only when transluminal angioplasty is performed outside the treatment target zone of (34802-34805, 34825-34826, 34845-34848, 34900, 0254T)
Code first (37221)
🚑 6.33 ✂ 73.8 **FUD** ZZZ ⊙ Ⓝ N1 80 50 PQ

AMA: 2015,Jan,16; 2014,Jan,11; 2013,Dec,8; 2012,Apr,3-9; 2011,Oct,9; 2011,Jul,3-11

37224 **Revascularization, endovascular, open or percutaneous, femoral, popliteal artery(s), unilateral; with transluminal angioplasty**

🚑 13.4 ✂ 109. **FUD** 000 ⊙ Ⓙ 62 80 50 PQ

AMA: 2015,Jan,16; 2014,Jan,11; 2012,Jan,15-42; 2011,Dec,14-18; 2011,Oct,9; 2011,Jul,3-11

37225 **with atherectomy, includes angioplasty within the same vessel, when performed**

🚑 18.2 ✂ 313. **FUD** 000 ⊙ Ⓙ J8 80 50 PQ

AMA: 2015,Jan,16; 2014,Jan,11; 2011,Oct,9; 2011,Jul,3-11

37226 **with transluminal stent placement(s), includes angioplasty within the same vessel, when performed**

🚑 15.8 ✂ 258. **FUD** 000 ⊙ Ⓙ J8 80 50 PQ

AMA: 2015,Jan,16; 2014,Jan,11; 2012,Jan,15-42; 2011,Dec,14-18; 2011,Oct,9; 2011,Jul,3-11

37227 **with transluminal stent placement(s) and atherectomy, includes angioplasty within the same vessel, when performed**

🚑 21.9 ✂ 423. **FUD** 000 ⊙ Ⓙ J8 80 50 PQ

AMA: 2015,Jan,16; 2014,Jan,11; 2011,Oct,9; 2011,Jul,3-11

37228 **Revascularization, endovascular, open or percutaneous, tibial, peroneal artery, unilateral, initial vessel; with transluminal angioplasty**

🚑 16.4 ✂ 155. **FUD** 000 ⊙ Ⓙ J8 80 50 PQ

AMA: 2015,Jan,16; 2014,Jan,11; 2011,Oct,9; 2011,Jul,3-11

37229 **with atherectomy, includes angioplasty within the same vessel, when performed**

🚑 21.2 ✂ 309. **FUD** 000 ⊙ Ⓙ J8 80 50 PQ

AMA: 2015,Jan,16; 2014,Jan,11; 2012,Apr,3-9; 2011,Oct,9; 2011,Jul,3-11

37230 **with transluminal stent placement(s), includes angioplasty within the same vessel, when performed**
🏥 20.9 ⚕ 236. **FUD** 000 ⊙ [J] [J8] [80] [50] [PQ]
AMA: 2015,Jan,16; 2014,Jan,11; 2012,Apr,3-9; 2011,Oct,9; 2011,Jul,3-11

37231 **with transluminal stent placement(s) and atherectomy, includes angioplasty within the same vessel, when performed**
🏥 22.7 ⚕ 380. **FUD** 000 ⊙ [J] [J8] [80] [50] [PQ]
AMA: 2015,Jan,16; 2014,Jan,11; 2012,Apr,3-9; 2011,Oct,9; 2011,Jul,3-11

\+ **37232** **Revascularization, endovascular, open or percutaneous, tibial/peroneal artery, unilateral, each additional vessel; with transluminal angioplasty (List separately in addition to code for primary procedure)**
Code first (37228-37231)
🏥 5.97 ⚕ 34.6 **FUD** ZZZ ⊙ [N] [N1] [80] [50] [PQ]
AMA: 2015,Jan,16; 2014,Jan,11; 2012,Apr,3-9; 2011,Oct,9; 2011,Jul,3-11

\+ **37233** **with atherectomy, includes angioplasty within the same vessel, when performed (List separately in addition to code for primary procedure)**
Code first (37229, 37231)
🏥 9.70 ⚕ 41.8 **FUD** ZZZ ⊙ [N] [N1] [80] [50]
AMA: 2015,Jan,16; 2014,Jan,11; 2012,Apr,3-9; 2011,Oct,9; 2011,Jul,3-11

\+ **37234** **with transluminal stent placement(s), includes angioplasty within the same vessel, when performed (List separately in addition to code for primary procedure)**
Code first (37229-37231)
🏥 8.39 ⚕ 110. **FUD** ZZZ ⊙ [N] [N1] [80] [50] [PQ]
AMA: 2015,Jan,16; 2014,Jan,11; 2012,Apr,3-9; 2011,Oct,9; 2011,Jul,3-11

\+ **37235** **with transluminal stent placement(s) and atherectomy, includes angioplasty within the same vessel, when performed (List separately in addition to code for primary procedure)**
Code first (37231)
🏥 11.5 ⚕ 118. **FUD** ZZZ ⊙ [N] [N1] [80] [50] [PQ]
AMA: 2015,Jan,16; 2014,Jan,11; 2011,Oct,9; 2011,Jul,3-11

37236-37239 Endovascular Revascularization Excluding Lower Extremities

[INCLUDES] Arteriotomy closure by suturing of a puncture, pressure or application of arterial closure device
Balloon angioplasty
- Post-dilation after stent deployment
- Predilation performed as primary or secondary angioplasty
- Treatment of lesion inside same vessel but outside of stented portion
- Treatment using different-sized balloons to accomplish the procedure

Endovascular revascularization of arteries and veins other than carotid, coronary, extracranial, intracranial, lower extremities
Imaging once procedure is complete
Radiological supervision and interpretation
Stent placement provided as the only treatment

[EXCLUDES] *Angioplasty in an unrelated vessel*
Extensive repair or replacement of an artery (35226, 35286)
Intravascular ultrasound (37252-37253)
Mechanical thrombectomy (37184-37188)
Selective and nonselective catheterization (36005, 36010-36015, 36200, 36215-36218, 36245-36248)
Stent placement in:
- *Arteries of the lower extremities for occlusive disease (37221, 37223, 37226-37227, 37230-37231, 37234-37235)*
- *Cervical carotid artery (37215-37216)*
- *Extracranial vertebral (0075T-0076T)*
- *Intracoronary (92928-92929, 92933-92934, 92937-92938, 92941, 92943-92944)*
- *Intracranial (61635)*
- *Intrathoracic common carotid or innominate artery, retrograde or antegrade approach (37218)*
- *Visceral arteries with fenestrated aortic repair (34841-34848)*

Thrombolytic therapy ([37211, 37212, 37213, 37214])
Ultrasound guidance (76937)

Code also add-on codes for different vessels treated during the same operative session
Do not report insertion of multiple stents in a single vessel with more than one code
Do not report stent placement when performed with embolization procedure

37236 **Transcatheter placement of an intravascular stent(s) (except lower extremity artery(s) for occlusive disease, cervical carotid, extracranial vertebral or intrathoracic carotid, intracranial, or coronary), open or percutaneous, including radiological supervision and interpretation and including all angioplasty within the same vessel, when performed; initial artery**
Do not report in the same target treatment zone with (34841-34848)
🏥 13.3 ⚕ 118. **FUD** 000 ⊙ [J] [J8] [80] [50]
AMA: 2015,May,7; 2015,Jan,16; 2014,Jan,11; 2013,Dec,8

\+ **37237** **each additional artery (List separately in addition to code for primary procedure)**
Code first (37236)
Do not report in the same target treatment zone with (34841-34848)
🏥 6.34 ⚕ 70.7 **FUD** ZZZ ⊙ [N] [N1] [80] [50]
AMA: 2015,Jan,16; 2014,Jan,11; 2013,Dec,8

37238 **Transcatheter placement of an intravascular stent(s), open or percutaneous, including radiological supervision and interpretation and including angioplasty within the same vessel, when performed; initial vein**
🏥 9.35 ⚕ 117. **FUD** 000 ⊙ [J] [J8] [80] [50]
AMA: 2014,Jan,11

\+ **37239** **each additional vein (List separately in addition to code for primary procedure)**
Code first (37238)
🏥 4.43 ⚕ 57.7 **FUD** ZZZ ⊙ [N] [N1] [80] [50]
AMA: 2014,Jan,11

37241-37244 Therapeutic Vascular Embolization/Occlusion

CMS: 100-3,20.28 Therapeutic Embolization

INCLUDES Embolization or occlusion of arteries, lymphatics, and veins except for head/neck and central nervous system
Imaging once procedure is complete
Intraprocedural guidance
Radiological supervision and interpretation
Roadmapping
Stent placement provided as support for embolization

EXCLUDES Head, neck, or central nervous system embolization (61624, 61626, 61710)
Stent deployment as primary management of aneurysm, pseudoaneurysm, or vascular extravasation

Code also additional embolization procedure(s) and the appropriate modifiers (eg, modifier 59) when embolization procedures are performed in multiple operative fields
Code also diagnostic angiography and catheter placement using modifier 59 when appropriate
Do not report in same operative field with (75894, 75898)
Do not report more than one embolization code per operative field
Do not report multiple codes for indications that overlap, code only the indication needing the most immediate attention

37241 **Vascular embolization or occlusion, inclusive of all radiological supervision and interpretation, intraprocedural roadmapping, and imaging guidance necessary to complete the intervention; venous, other than hemorrhage (eg, congenital or acquired venous malformations, venous and capillary hemangiomas, varices, varicoceles)**

INCLUDES Embolization of side branch(s) of an outflow vein from a hemodialysis access

EXCLUDES Vein destruction (36468-36479)

Do not report in same operative field with (36468, 36470-36471, 36475-36479)

🔪 12.9   ⚕ 130.   **FUD** 000   ⊙ J

AMA: 2015,Aug,8; 2015,Apr,10; 2015,Jan,16; 2014,Oct,6; 2014,Aug,14; 2014,Jan,11; 2013,Nov,6; 2013,Nov,14

37242 **arterial, other than hemorrhage or tumor (eg, congenital or acquired arterial malformations, arteriovenous malformations, arteriovenous fistulas, aneurysms, pseudoaneurysms)**

EXCLUDES Percutaneous treatment of pseudoaneurysm of an extremity (36002)

🔪 14.4   ⚕ 220.   **FUD** 000   ⊙ J

AMA: 2015,Jan,16; 2014,Oct,6; 2014,Jan,11; 2013,Nov,14; 2013,Nov,6

37243 **for tumors, organ ischemia, or infarction**

INCLUDES Embolization of uterine fibroids

Code also chemotherapy when provided with embolization procedure (96420-96425)
Code also injection of radioisotopes when provided with embolization procedure (79445)

🔪 17.2   ⚕ 278.   **FUD** 000   ⊙ J

AMA: 2015,Jan,16; 2014,Oct,6; 2014,Jan,11; 2013,Nov,14; 2013,Nov,6

37244 **for arterial or venous hemorrhage or lymphatic extravasation**

INCLUDES Embolization of uterine arteries for hemorrhage

🔪 20.1   ⚕ 194.   **FUD** 000   ⊙ J

AMA: 2015,Jan,16; 2014,Oct,6; 2014,Aug,14; 2014,Jan,11; 2013,Nov,14; 2013,Nov,6

37250-37253 Intravascular Ultrasound: Noncoronary

INCLUDES Manipulation and repositioning of the transducer prior to and after therapeutic interventional procedures

EXCLUDES Selective or non-selective catheter placement for access (36005-36248)
Transcatheter procedures (37200, 37236-37239, 37241-37244, 61624, 61626)

37250 ~~Intravascular ultrasound (non-coronary vessel) during diagnostic evaluation and/or therapeutic intervention; initial vessel (List separately in addition to code for primary procedure)~~

To report, see ~37252

37251 ~~each additional vessel (List separately in addition to code for primary procedure)~~

To report, see ~37253

● + **37252** **Intravascular ultrasound (noncoronary vessel) during diagnostic evaluation and/or therapeutic intervention, including radiological supervision and interpretation; initial noncoronary vessel (List separately in addition to code for primary procedure)**

🔪 0.00   ⚕ 0.00   **FUD** 000   ⊙

Code first primary procedure
Do not report with (37191-37193, 37197)

● + **37253** **each additional noncoronary vessel (List separately in addition to code for primary procedure)**

🔪 0.00   ⚕ 0.00   **FUD** 000   ⊙

Code first (37252)
Do not report with (37191-37193, 37197)

37500-37501 Vascular Endoscopic Procedures

INCLUDES Diagnostic endoscopy

EXCLUDES Open procedure (37760)

37500 **Vascular endoscopy, surgical, with ligation of perforator veins, subfascial (SEPS)**

🔪 18.8   ⚕ 18.8   **FUD** 090   T A2 50

AMA: 2015,Jan,16; 2014,Jan,11; 2010,Jul,6

37501 **Unlisted vascular endoscopy procedure**

🔪 0.00   ⚕ 0.00   **FUD** YYY   T 50

AMA: 2014,Jan,11

37565-37606 Ligation Procedures: Jugular Vein, Carotid Arteries

CMS: 100-3,160.8 Electroencephalographic Monitoring During Cerebral Vasculature Surgery

EXCLUDES Arterial balloon occlusion, endovascular, temporary (61623)
Suture of arteries and veins (35201-35286)
Transcatheter arterial embolization/occlusion, permanent (61624-61626)
Treatment of intracranial aneurysm (61703)

37565 **Ligation, internal jugular vein**

🔪 21.3   ⚕ 21.3   **FUD** 090   T 80 50

AMA: 2014,Jan,11

37600 **Ligation; external carotid artery**

🔪 21.1   ⚕ 21.1   **FUD** 090   T 80

AMA: 2014,Jan,11

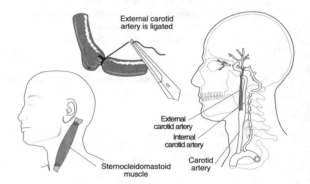

External carotid artery is ligated

External carotid artery

Internal carotid artery

Carotid artery

Sternocleidomastoid muscle

37605 **internal or common carotid artery**

🔪 23.2   ⚕ 23.2   **FUD** 090   T 80

AMA: 2014,Jan,11

37606 **internal or common carotid artery, with gradual occlusion, as with Selverstone or Crutchfield clamp**

🔪 14.2   ⚕ 14.2   **FUD** 090   T 80

AMA: 2014,Jan,11

37607-37609 Ligation Hemodialysis Angioaccess or Temporal Artery

EXCLUDES Suture of arteries and veins (35201-35286)

37607 **Ligation or banding of angioaccess arteriovenous fistula**

🔪 11.0   ⚕ 11.0   **FUD** 090   T A2

AMA: 2014,Jan,11

37609 **Ligation or biopsy, temporal artery**

🔪 6.03   ⚕ 8.91   **FUD** 010   T A2 50 P0

AMA: 2014,Jan,11

● New Code   ▲ Revised Code   ○ Reinstated   M Maternity   A Age Edit   Unlisted   Not Covered   # Resequenced
⊘ AMA Mod 51 Exempt   ⑤① Optum Mod 51 Exempt   ⊚ Mod 63 Exempt   ⊙ Mod Sedation   + Add-on   ▢ CCI   P0 PQRS   FUD Follow-up Days

© 2015 Optum360, LLC (Blue Text)   CPT © 2015 American Medical Association. All Rights Reserved. (Black Text)   Medicare (Red Text)   151

Cardiovascular System *(side tab)*

37615-37618 Arterial Ligation, Major Vessel, for Injury/Rupture

EXCLUDES *Suture of arteries and veins (35201-35286)*

37615 **Ligation, major artery (eg, post-traumatic, rupture); neck**
INCLUDES Touroff ligation
📇 14.7   🔪 14.7   **FUD** 090   T 80 ▭
AMA: 2014,Jan,11

37616 **chest**
INCLUDES Bardenheurer operation
📇 32.2   🔪 32.2   **FUD** 090   C 80 ▭ PQ
AMA: 2014,Jan,11

37617 **abdomen**
📇 39.2   🔪 39.2   **FUD** 090   C 80 ▭
AMA: 2015,Jan,16; 2014,Jan,11; 2013,Aug,13

37618 **extremity**
📇 11.1   🔪 11.1   **FUD** 090   C 80 ▭
AMA: 2014,Jan,11

37619 Ligation Inferior Vena Cava

EXCLUDES *Suture of arteries and veins (35201-35286)*
Endovascular delivery of inferior vena cava filter (37191)

37619 **Ligation of inferior vena cava**
📇 47.7   🔪 47.7   **FUD** 090   T 80
AMA: 2015,Jan,16; 2014,Jan,11; 2012,Apr,3-9

37650-37660 Venous Ligation, Femoral and Common Iliac

EXCLUDES *Suture of arteries and veins (35201-35286)*

37650 **Ligation of femoral vein**
📇 13.6   🔪 13.6   **FUD** 090   T A2 50 ▭
AMA: 2014,Jan,11

37660 **Ligation of common iliac vein**
📇 38.0   🔪 38.0   **FUD** 090   C 80 50 ▭
AMA: 2014,Jan,11

37700-37785 Treatment of Varicose Veins of Legs

EXCLUDES *Suture of arteries and veins (35201-35286)*

37700 **Ligation and division of long saphenous vein at saphenofemoral junction, or distal interruptions**
INCLUDES Babcock operation
Do not report with (37718, 37722)
📇 7.32   🔪 7.32   **FUD** 090   T A2 50 ▭
AMA: 2015,Jan,16; 2014,Jan,11; 2012,Jan,15-42; 2011,Jan,11

37718 **Ligation, division, and stripping, short saphenous vein**
Do not report with (37700, 37735, 37780)
📇 12.8   🔪 12.8   **FUD** 090   T A2 50
AMA: 2014,Jan,11

37722 **Ligation, division, and stripping, long (greater) saphenous veins from saphenofemoral junction to knee or below**
EXCLUDES *Ligation/division/stripping short saphenous vein (37718)*
Do not report with (37700, 37735)
📇 14.0   🔪 14.0   **FUD** 090   T A2 50
AMA: 2014,Jan,11; 2011,Jul,3-11

37735 **Ligation and division and complete stripping of long or short saphenous veins with radical excision of ulcer and skin graft and/or interruption of communicating veins of lower leg, with excision of deep fascia**
Do not report with (37700, 37718, 37722, 37780)
📇 17.2   🔪 17.2   **FUD** 090   T A2 50 ▭
AMA: 2015,Jan,16; 2014,Jan,11; 2011,Jul,3-11

37760 **Ligation of perforator veins, subfascial, radical (Linton type), including skin graft, when performed, open, 1 leg**
EXCLUDES *Ligation of subfascial perforator veins, endoscopic (37500)*
Do not report with (76937, 76942, 76998, 93971)
📇 18.0   🔪 18.0   **FUD** 090   T A2 50 ▭
AMA: 2015,Jan,16; 2014,Jan,11; 2010,Jul,6

37761 **Ligation of perforator vein(s), subfascial, open, including ultrasound guidance, when performed, 1 leg**
EXCLUDES *Ligation of subfascial perforator veins, endoscopic (37500)*
Do not report with (76937, 76942, 76998, 93971)
📇 16.3   🔪 16.3   **FUD** 090   T R2 80 50
AMA: 2015,Jan,16; 2014,Jan,11; 2010,Jul,6

37765 **Stab phlebectomy of varicose veins, 1 extremity; 10-20 stab incisions**
EXCLUDES *Fewer than 10 incisions (37799)*
More than 20 incisions (37766)
📇 13.1   🔪 18.9   **FUD** 090   T P3 50 ▭
AMA: 2015,Jan,16; 2014,Oct,6; 2014,Jan,11; 2010,Nov,8

37766 **more than 20 incisions**
EXCLUDES *Fewer than 10 incisions (37799)*
10-20 incisions (37765)
📇 16.1   🔪 22.4   **FUD** 090   T P3 50 ▭
AMA: 2015,Jan,16; 2014,Oct,6; 2014,Jan,11; 2013,Sep,17

37780 **Ligation and division of short saphenous vein at saphenopopliteal junction (separate procedure)**
📇 7.57   🔪 7.57   **FUD** 090   T A2 50 ▭
AMA: 2015,Jan,16; 2014,Jan,11; 2012,Jan,15-42; 2011,Jan,11

37785 **Ligation, division, and/or excision of varicose vein cluster(s), 1 leg**
📇 7.73   🔪 10.3   **FUD** 090   T A2 50 ▭
AMA: 2015,Jan,16; 2014,Jan,11; 2012,Jan,15-42; 2011,Jan,11; 2010,Nov,8

37788-37790 Treatment of Vascular Disease of the Penis

37788 **Penile revascularization, artery, with or without vein graft** ♂
📇 36.2   🔪 36.2   **FUD** 090   C 80 ▭
AMA: 2014,Jan,11

37790 **Penile venous occlusive procedure**
📇 13.9   🔪 13.9   **FUD** 090   T A2 80 ▭
AMA: 2014,Jan,11

37799 Unlisted Vascular Surgery Procedures

CMS: 100-4,32,161 Intracranial Percutaneous Transluminal Angioplasty (PTA) With Stenting; 100-4,4,180.3 Unlisted Service or Procedure

37799 **Unlisted procedure, vascular surgery**
📇 0.00   🔪 0.00   **FUD** YYY   01 80
AMA: 2015,Apr,10; 2015,Jan,16; 2014,Oct,6; 2014,Aug,14; 2014,Mar,8; 2014,Jan,11; 2013,Nov,14; 2012,Jan,15-42; 2011,Aug,9-10; 2011,Jan,11; 2010,Nov,8

38100-38200 Splenic Procedures

38100 **Splenectomy; total (separate procedure)**
📇 33.3   🔪 33.3   **FUD** 090   C 80 ▭ PQ
AMA: 2015,Jan,16; 2014,Jan,11; 2012,Oct,3-8; 2012,Sep,11-13

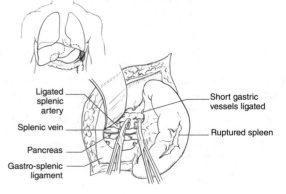

Ligated splenic artery

Splenic vein

Pancreas

Gastro-splenic ligament

Short gastric vessels ligated

Ruptured spleen

38101 **partial (separate procedure)**
📇 33.7   🔪 33.7   **FUD** 090   C 80 ▭ PQ
AMA: 2015,Jan,16; 2014,Jan,11; 2012,Oct,3-8; 2012,Sep,11-13

37615 — 38101 *(side tab)*

+ 38102 **total, en bloc for extensive disease, in conjunction with other procedure (List in addition to code for primary procedure)**

Code first primary procedure

🚑 7.60   🔗 7.60   **FUD** ZZZ   C 80 ▢

AMA: 2015,Jan,16; 2014,Jan,11; 2012,Oct,3-8; 2012,Sep,11-13

38115 **Repair of ruptured spleen (splenorrhaphy) with or without partial splenectomy**

🚑 36.9   🔗 36.9   **FUD** 090   C 80 ▢ PQ

AMA: 2015,Jan,16; 2014,Jan,11; 2012,Oct,3-8; 2012,Sep,11-13

38120 **Laparoscopy, surgical, splenectomy**

INCLUDES Diagnostic laparoscopy (49320)

🚑 30.4   🔗 30.4   **FUD** 090   T 80 ▢ PQ

AMA: 2015,Jan,16; 2014,Jan,11; 2012,Oct,3-8; 2012,Sep,11-13

38129 **Unlisted laparoscopy procedure, spleen**

🚑 0.00   🔗 0.00   **FUD** YYY   T 80

AMA: 2015,Jan,16; 2014,Jan,11; 2012,Oct,3-8; 2012,Sep,11-13

38200 **Injection procedure for splenoportography**

⚡ (75810)

🚑 3.90   🔗 3.90   **FUD** 000   N M1 80 ▢

AMA: 2014,Jan,11

38204-38215 Hematopoietic Stem Cell Preparation

CMS: 100-3,110.8.1 Stem Cell Transplantation; 100-4,3,90.3 Stem Cell Transplantation; 100-4,3,90.3.1 Allogeneic Stem Cell Transplantation; 100-4,3,90.3.3 Billing for Allogeneic Stem Cell Transplants; 100-4,32,90 Billing for Stem Cell Transplantation; 100-4,32,90.2.1 Coding for Stem Cell Transplantation; 100-4,4,231.10 Billing for Autologous Stem Cell Transplants; 100-4,4,231.11 Billing for Allogeneic Stem Cell Transplants

INCLUDES Preservation, preparation, purification of stem cells before transplant or reinfusion

Do not report each code more than one time per day

38204 **Management of recipient hematopoietic progenitor cell donor search and cell acquisition**

🚑 2.91   🔗 2.91   **FUD** XXX   N M1

AMA: 2015,Jan,16; 2014,Jan,11; 2013,Oct,3

38205 **Blood-derived hematopoietic progenitor cell harvesting for transplantation, per collection; allogeneic**

🚑 2.36   🔗 2.36   **FUD** 000   B 80 ▢

AMA: 2015,Jan,16; 2014,Jan,11; 2013,Oct,3

38206 **autologous**

🚑 2.38   🔗 2.38   **FUD** 000   S G2 80 ▢

AMA: 2015,Jan,16; 2014,Jan,11; 2013,Oct,3

38207 **Transplant preparation of hematopoietic progenitor cells; cryopreservation and storage**

Do not report with (88182, 88184-88189)

⚡ (88240)

🚑 1.28   🔗 1.28   **FUD** XXX   S

AMA: 2015,Jan,16; 2014,Jan,11; 2013,Oct,3

38208 **thawing of previously frozen harvest, without washing, per donor**

Do not report with (88182, 88184-88189)

⚡ (88241)

🚑 0.80   🔗 0.80   **FUD** XXX   S

AMA: 2015,Jan,16; 2014,Jan,11; 2013,Oct,3

38209 **thawing of previously frozen harvest, with washing, per donor**

Do not report with (88182, 88184-88189)

🚑 0.34   🔗 0.34   **FUD** XXX   S

AMA: 2015,Jan,16; 2014,Jan,11; 2013,Oct,3

38210 **specific cell depletion within harvest, T-cell depletion**

Do not report with (88182, 88184-88189)

🚑 2.28   🔗 2.28   **FUD** XXX   S

AMA: 2015,Jan,16; 2014,Jan,11; 2013,Oct,3

38211 **tumor cell depletion**

Do not report with (88182, 88184-88189)

🚑 2.06   🔗 2.06   **FUD** XXX   S

AMA: 2015,Jan,16; 2014,Jan,11; 2013,Oct,3

38212 **red blood cell removal**

Do not report with (88182, 88184-88189)

🚑 1.36   🔗 1.36   **FUD** XXX   S

AMA: 2015,Jan,16; 2014,Jan,11; 2013,Oct,3

38213 **platelet depletion**

Do not report with (88182, 88184-88189)

🚑 0.34   🔗 0.34   **FUD** XXX   S

AMA: 2015,Jan,16; 2014,Jan,11; 2013,Oct,3

38214 **plasma (volume) depletion**

Do not report with (88182, 88184-88189)

🚑 1.17   🔗 1.17   **FUD** XXX   S

AMA: 2015,Jan,16; 2014,Jan,11; 2013,Oct,3

38215 **cell concentration in plasma, mononuclear, or buffy coat layer**

Do not report with (88182, 88184-88189)

🚑 1.36   🔗 1.36   **FUD** XXX   S

AMA: 2015,Jan,16; 2014,Jan,11; 2013,Oct,3

38220-38232 Bone Marrow Procedures

CMS: 100-3,110.8.1 Stem Cell Transplantation; 100-4,3,90.3 Stem Cell Transplantation; 100-4,32,90 Billing for Stem Cell Transplantation; 100-4,4,231.11 Billing for Allogeneic Stem Cell Transplants

38220 **Bone marrow; aspiration only**

INCLUDES Bone marrow aspiration for bone graft

EXCLUDES *Bone marrow aspiration for platelet rich stem cell injection (0232T)*

🚑 1.77   🔗 4.67   **FUD** XXX   T P3 80 50 ▢

AMA: 2015,Mar,9; 2015,Jan,16; 2014,Jan,11; 2013,Oct,3; 2012,May,11-12; 2012,Apr,14-16; 2012,Jan,15-42; 2011,Jan,11

38221 **biopsy, needle or trocar**

EXCLUDES *Bone marrow aspiration for platelet rich stem cell injection (0232T)*

⚡ (88305)

🚑 2.16   🔗 4.76   **FUD** XXX   T P3 80 50 ▢ PQ

AMA: 2015,Mar,9; 2014,Jan,11; 2012,May,11-12

38230 **Bone marrow harvesting for transplantation; allogeneic**

EXCLUDES *Bone marrow aspiration for platelet rich stem cell injection (0232T)*

Harvesting of blood-derived hematopoietic progenitor cells for transplant (allogeneic) (38205)

🚑 5.70   🔗 5.70   **FUD** 000   S G2 80 ▢

AMA: 2015,Jan,16; 2014,Jan,11; 2013,Oct,3; 2012,May,11-12

38232 **autologous**

EXCLUDES *Aspiration of bone marrow (38220)*

Harvesting of blood-derived peripheral stem cells for transplant (autologous) (38206)

🚑 5.86   🔗 5.86   **FUD** 000   S G2 80

AMA: 2015,Jan,16; 2014,Jan,11; 2013,Oct,3; 2012,May,11-12

38240-38243 [38243] Hematopoietic Progenitor Cell Transplantation

CMS: 100-3,110.8.1 Stem Cell Transplantation; 100-4,3,90.3 Stem Cell Transplantation; 100-4,3,90.3.1 Allogeneic Stem Cell Transplantation; 100-4,3,90.3.2 Autologous Stem Cell Transplantation (AuSCT); 100-4,3,90.3.3 Billing for Allogeneic Stem Cell Transplants; 100-4,32,90 Billing for Stem Cell Transplantation; 100-4,32,90.2 Allogeneic Stem Cell Transplantation; 100-4,32,90.2.1 Coding for Stem Cell Transplantation; 100-4,32,90.3 Autologous Stem Cell Transplantation; 100-4,32,90.4 Edits Stem Cell Transplant; 100-4,32,90.6 Clinical Trials for Stem Cell Transplant for Myelodysplastic Syndrome (; 100-4,4,231.10 Billing for Autologous Stem Cell Transplants; 100-4,4,231.11 Billing for Allogeneic Stem Cell Transplants

INCLUDES Evaluation of patient prior to, during, and after the infusion
Management of uncomplicated adverse reactions such as hives or nausea
Monitoring of physiological parameters
Physician presence during the infusion
Supervision of clinical staff

EXCLUDES *Cryopreservation, freezing, and storage of hematopoietic progenitor cells for transplant (38207)*
Human leukocyte antigen (HLA) testing (81370-81383, 86812-86822)
Modification, treatment, processing of hematopoietic progenitor cell specimens for transplant (38210-38215)
Thawing and expansion of hematopoietic progenitor cells for transplant (38208-38209)

Code also administration of medications and/or fluids not related to the transplant with modifier 59
Code also evaluation and management service for the treatment of more complicated adverse reactions after the infusion, as appropriate
Code also separately identifiable evaluation and management service on the same date, using modifier 25 as appropriate (99211-99215, 99217-99220, [99224, 99225, 99226], 99221-99223, 99231-99239, 99471-99472, 99475-99476)
Do not report administration of fluids for the transplant or for incidental hydration separately
Do not report concurrent administration of medications with the infusion for the transplant

38240 **Hematopoietic progenitor cell (HPC); allogeneic transplantation per donor**
Do not report on same date of service with ([38243], 38242)
🔷 6.42   ⚖ 6.42   **FUD** XXX   Ⓢ 80 ▱
AMA: 2015,Jan,16; 2014,Jan,11; 2013,Oct,3

38241 **autologous transplantation**
🔷 4.83   ⚖ 4.83   **FUD** XXX   Ⓢ 62 80 ▱
AMA: 2015,Jan,16; 2014,Jan,11; 2013,Oct,3

\# **38243** **HPC boost**
Do not report on same date of service with (38240, 38242)
🔷 3.42   ⚖ 3.42   **FUD** 000   Ⓢ R2 80
AMA: 2015,Feb,10; 2015,Jan,16; 2014,Jan,11; 2013,Oct,3; 2013,Jun,13

38242 **Allogeneic lymphocyte infusions**
EXCLUDES *Aspiration of bone marrow (38220)*
Do not report on same date of service with (38240, [38243])
✎ (81379-81383, 86812-86822)
🔷 3.42   ⚖ 3.42   **FUD** 000   Ⓢ R2 80 ▱
AMA: 2015,Jan,16; 2014,Jan,11; 2013,Oct,3; 2013,Jun,13

38243 **Resequenced code. See code following 38241.**

38300-38382 Incision Lymphatic Vessels

38300 **Drainage of lymph node abscess or lymphadenitis; simple**
🔷 5.31   ⚖ 7.85   **FUD** 010   Ⓣ A2 ▱
AMA: 2014,Jan,11

38305 **extensive**
🔷 13.3   ⚖ 13.3   **FUD** 090   Ⓣ A2 ▱
AMA: 2014,Jan,11

38308 **Lymphangiotomy or other operations on lymphatic channels**
🔷 12.8   ⚖ 12.8   **FUD** 090   Ⓣ A2 80 ▱
AMA: 2014,Jan,11

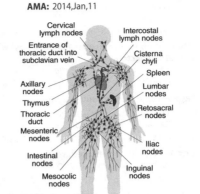

38380 **Suture and/or ligation of thoracic duct; cervical approach**
🔷 16.1   ⚖ 16.1   **FUD** 090   Ⓒ 80 ▱
AMA: 2014,Jan,11

38381 **thoracic approach**
🔷 23.2   ⚖ 23.2   **FUD** 090   Ⓒ 80 ▱ PQ
AMA: 2014,Jan,11

38382 **abdominal approach**
🔷 19.6   ⚖ 19.6   **FUD** 090   Ⓒ 80 ▱
AMA: 2014,Jan,11

38500-38555 Biopsy/Excision Lymphatic Vessels

EXCLUDES *Injection for sentinel node identification (38792)*
Percutaneous needle biopsy retroperitoneal mass (49180)

38500 **Biopsy or excision of lymph node(s); open, superficial**
Do not report with (38700-38780)
🔷 7.34   ⚖ 9.49   **FUD** 010   Ⓣ A2 50 ▱ PQ
AMA: 2015,Jan,16; 2014,Jan,11; 2012,Jun,15-16; 2012,Jan,15-42; 2011,Jan,11

38505 **by needle, superficial (eg, cervical, inguinal, axillary)**
EXCLUDES *Fine needle aspiration (10021-10022)*
✦ (76942, 77012, 77021)
◨ (88173)
🔷 2.07   ⚖ 3.63   **FUD** 000   Ⓣ A2 50 ▱ PQ
AMA: 2015,Jan,16; 2014,Jan,11; 2012,Jan,15-42; 2011,Jan,11

38510 **open, deep cervical node(s)**
🔷 12.1   ⚖ 14.9   **FUD** 010   Ⓣ A2 50 ▱ PQ
AMA: 2015,Jan,16; 2014,Jan,11; 2012,Jun,15-16; 2012,Jan,15-42; 2011,Jan,11

38520 **open, deep cervical node(s) with excision scalene fat pad**
🔷 13.3   ⚖ 13.3   **FUD** 090   Ⓣ A2 50 ▱ PQ
AMA: 2015,Jan,16; 2014,Jan,11; 2012,Jan,15-42; 2011,Jan,11

38525 **open, deep axillary node(s)**
🔷 12.5   ⚖ 12.5   **FUD** 090   Ⓣ A2 50 ▱ PQ
AMA: 2015,Mar,5; 2015,Jan,16; 2014,Apr,10; 2014,Jan,11; 2012,Jan,15-42; 2011,Jan,11

38530 **open, internal mammary node(s)**
EXCLUDES *Fine needle aspiration (10022)*
Do not report with (38720-38746)
🔷 15.7   ⚖ 15.7   **FUD** 090   Ⓣ A2 80 50 ▱ PQ
AMA: 2015,Jan,16; 2014,Apr,10; 2014,Jan,11; 2010,Aug,3-7; 2010,Aug,3-7

38542 **Dissection, deep jugular node(s)**
EXCLUDES *Complete cervical lymphadenectomy (38720)*
🔷 14.9   ⚖ 14.9   **FUD** 090   Ⓣ A2 80 50 ▱ PQ
AMA: 2015,Jan,16; 2014,Jan,11; 2010,Aug,3-7; 2010,Aug,3-7

38550 Excision of cystic hygroma, axillary or cervical; without deep neurovascular dissection
14.6   14.6   **FUD** 090   T A2 80 ▭
AMA: 2014,Jan,11

38555 with deep neurovascular dissection
29.0   29.0   **FUD** 090   T A2 80 ▭
AMA: 2014,Jan,11

38562-38564 Limited Lymphadenectomy: Staging

38562 Limited lymphadenectomy for staging (separate procedure); pelvic and para-aortic
EXCLUDES   *Prostatectomy (55812, 55842)*
Radioactive substance inserted into prostate (55862)
20.3   20.3   **FUD** 090   C 80 ▭
AMA: 2015,Jan,16; 2014,Jan,11; 2012,Jan,15-42; 2011,Jan,11

38564 retroperitoneal (aortic and/or splenic)
20.3   20.3   **FUD** 090   C 80 ▭
AMA: 2014,Jan,11

38570-38589 Laparoscopic Lymph Node Procedures

INCLUDES   Diagnostic laparoscopy (49320)
EXCLUDES   *Laparoscopy with draining of lymphocele to peritoneal cavity (49323)*
Limited lymphadenectomy:
Pelvic (38562)
Retroperitoneal (38564)

38570 Laparoscopy, surgical; with retroperitoneal lymph node sampling (biopsy), single or multiple
15.5   15.5   **FUD** 010   T A2 80 ▭ PQ
AMA: 2015,Jan,16; 2014,Jan,11

38571 with bilateral total pelvic lymphadenectomy
23.0   23.0   **FUD** 010   T A2 80 ▭ PQ
AMA: 2015,Jan,16; 2014,Jan,11

38572 with bilateral total pelvic lymphadenectomy and peri-aortic lymph node sampling (biopsy), single or multiple
28.4   28.4   **FUD** 010   T A2 80 ▭ PQ
AMA: 2015,Jan,13; 2015,Jan,16; 2014,Jan,11

38589 Unlisted laparoscopy procedure, lymphatic system
0.00   0.00   **FUD** YYY   T 80 50
AMA: 2015,Jan,16; 2014,Jan,11

38700-38780 Lymphadenectomy Procedures

INCLUDES   Lymph node biopsy/excision
EXCLUDES   *Excision of lymphedematous skin and subcutaneous tissue (15004-15005)*
Limited lymphadenectomy
Pelvic (38562)
Retroperitoneal (38564)
Repair of lymphademateous skin and tissue (15570-15650)
Do not report with (38500)

38700 Suprahyoid lymphadenectomy
23.2   23.2   **FUD** 090   T 62 80 50 ▭ PQ
AMA: 2015,Jan,16; 2014,Jan,11; 2010,Aug,3-7; 2010,Aug,3-7

38720 Cervical lymphadenectomy (complete)
38.8   38.8   **FUD** 090   T 80 50 ▭ PQ
AMA: 2015,Jan,16; 2014,Jan,11; 2012,Jan,15-42; 2011,Jan,11; 2010,Aug,3-7; 2010,Aug,3-7

38724 Cervical lymphadenectomy (modified radical neck dissection)
42.0   42.0   **FUD** 090   C 80 50 ▭ PQ
AMA: 2015,Jan,16; 2014,Jan,11; 2012,Dec,3-5; 2012,Jan,15-42; 2011,Jan,11; 2010,Aug,3-7; 2010,Aug,3-7

38740 Axillary lymphadenectomy; superficial
20.0   20.0   **FUD** 090   T A2 80 50 ▭ PQ
AMA: 2015,Jan,16; 2014,Apr,10; 2014,Jan,11; 2010,Aug,3-7; 2010,Aug,3-7

38745 complete
25.2   25.2   **FUD** 090   T A2 80 50 ▭ PQ
AMA: 2014,Jan,11; 2010,Aug,3-7; 2010,Aug,3-7

+ **38746** Thoracic lymphadenectomy by thoracotomy, mediastinal and regional lymphadenectomy (List separately in addition to code for primary procedure)
INCLUDES   Left side
    Aortopulmonary window
    Inferior pulmonary ligament
    Paraesophageal
    Subcarinal
   Right side
    Inferior pulmonary ligament
    Paraesophageal
    Paratracheal
    Subcarinal
EXCLUDES   *Thoracoscopic mediastinal and regional lymphadenectomy (32674)*
Code first primary procedure (19260, 31760, 31766, 31786, 32096-32200, 32220-32320, 32440-32491, 32503-32505, 33025, 33030, 33050-33130, 39200-39220, 39560-39561, 43101, 43112, 43117-43118, 43122-43123, 43351, 60270, 60505)
6.28   6.28   **FUD** ZZZ   C 80 ▭ PQ
AMA: 2015,Jan,16; 2014,May,3; 2014,Jan,11; 2012,Oct,9-11; 2012,Sep,3-8; 2010,Aug,3-7; 2010,Aug,3-7

Parasternal nodes

Central nodes

+ **38747** Abdominal lymphadenectomy, regional, including celiac, gastric, portal, peripancreatic, with or without para-aortic and vena caval nodes (List separately in addition to code for primary procedure)
Code first primary procedure
7.75   7.75   **FUD** ZZZ   C 80 ▭ PQ
AMA: 2014,Jan,11

38760 Inguinofemoral lymphadenectomy, superficial, including Cloquets node (separate procedure)
24.3   24.3   **FUD** 090   T A2 80 50 ▭ PQ
AMA: 2015,Jan,16; 2014,Jan,11; 2012,Jan,15-42; 2011,Jan,11

38765 Inguinofemoral lymphadenectomy, superficial, in continuity with pelvic lymphadenectomy, including external iliac, hypogastric, and obturator nodes (separate procedure)
37.3   37.3   **FUD** 090   C 80 50 ▭ PQ
AMA: 2015,Jan,16; 2014,Jan,11; 2012,Jan,15-42; 2011,Jan,11

38770 Pelvic lymphadenectomy, including external iliac, hypogastric, and obturator nodes (separate procedure)
23.2   23.2   **FUD** 090   C 80 50 ▭ PQ
AMA: 2014,Jan,11

38780 Retroperitoneal transabdominal lymphadenectomy, extensive, including pelvic, aortic, and renal nodes (separate procedure)
29.6   29.6   **FUD** 090   C 80 ▭ PQ
AMA: 2014,Jan,11

38790-38999 Cannulation/Injection/Other Procedures

38790 Injection procedure; lymphangiography
(75801-75807)
2.42   2.42   **FUD** 000   N NI 50 ▭
AMA: 2014,Jan,11

38792   radioactive tracer for identification of sentinel node

> EXCLUDES *Sentinel node excision (38500-38542)*
> *Sentinel node(s) identification (mapping) intraoperative with nonradioactive dye injection (38900)*

☒ (78195)

🔧 1.14   ⚒ 1.14   **FUD** 000   [01] [N1] [50] ▢

AMA: 2015,Mar,5; 2015,Jan,16; 2014,Jan,11

38794   **Cannulation, thoracic duct**

🔧 8.70   ⚒ 8.70   **FUD** 090   [N] [N1] [80] ▢

AMA: 2014,Jan,11

+ **38900**   **Intraoperative identification (eg, mapping) of sentinel lymph node(s) includes injection of non-radioactive dye, when performed (List separately in addition to code for primary procedure)**

> EXCLUDES *Injection of tracer for sentinel node identification (38792)*

Code first (19302, 19307, 38500, 38510, 38520, 38525, 38530, 38542, 38740, 38745)

🔧 3.99   ⚒ 3.99   **FUD** ZZZ   [N] [N1] [80] [50] [P0]

AMA: 2015,Mar,5; 2014,Jan,11

38999   **Unlisted procedure, hemic or lymphatic system**

🔧 0.00   ⚒ 0.00   **FUD** YYY   [S] [80]

AMA: 2015,Jan,16; 2014,Jan,11; 2012,Jan,15-42; 2011,Jan,11

39000-39499 Surgical Procedures: Mediastinum

39000   **Mediastinotomy with exploration, drainage, removal of foreign body, or biopsy; cervical approach**

🔧 14.4   ⚒ 14.4   **FUD** 090   [C] [80] ▢ [P0]

AMA: 2014,Jan,11

39010   transthoracic approach, including either transthoracic or median sternotomy

> EXCLUDES *Video-assisted thoracic surgery (VATS) pericardial biopsy (32604)*

Do not report with (33955-33956, [33963, 33964])

🔧 22.8   ⚒ 22.8   **FUD** 090   [C] [80] ▢ [P0]

AMA: 2015,Jul,3; 2015,Jan,16; 2014,Jan,11; 2014,Jan,5; 2013,Jan,6-8

39200   **Resection of mediastinal cyst**

🔧 25.5   ⚒ 25.5   **FUD** 090   [C] [80] ▢ [P0]

AMA: 2014,Jan,11; 2012,Oct,9-11; 2012,Sep,3-8

39220   **Resection of mediastinal tumor**

> EXCLUDES *Thymectomy (60520)*
> *Thyroidectomy, substernal (60270)*
> *Video-assisted thoracic surgery (VATS) resection cyst, mass, or tumor of mediastinum (32662)*

🔧 33.1   ⚒ 33.1   **FUD** 090   [C] [80] ▢ [P0]

AMA: 2014,Jan,11; 2012,Oct,9-11; 2012,Sep,3-8

~~**39400**   **Mediastinoscopy, includes biopsy(ies), when performed**~~

To report, see ~39401-39402

● **39401**   **Mediastinoscopy; includes biopsy(ies) of mediastinal mass (eg, lymphoma), when performed**

🔧 0.00   ⚒ 0.00   **FUD** 000

● **39402**   with lymph node biopsy(ies) (eg, lung cancer staging)

🔧 0.00   ⚒ 0.00   **FUD** 000

39499   **Unlisted procedure, mediastinum**

🔧 0.00   ⚒ 0.00   **FUD** YYY   [C] [80]

AMA: 2014,Jan,11

39501-39599 Surgical Procedures: Diaphragm

> EXCLUDES *Repair of diaphragmatic (esophageal) hernias:*
> *Laparoscopic with fundoplication (43280-43282)*
> *Laparotomy (43332-43333)*
> *Thoracoabdominal (43336-43337)*
> *Thoracotomy (43334-43335)*

39501   **Repair, laceration of diaphragm, any approach**

🔧 24.6   ⚒ 24.6   **FUD** 090   [C] [80] ▢ [P0]

AMA: 2015,Jan,16; 2014,Dec,16; 2014,Dec,16; 2014,Jan,11

39503   **Repair, neonatal diaphragmatic hernia, with or without chest tube insertion and with or without creation of ventral hernia**   [A]

🔧 178.   ⚒ 178.   **FUD** 090   ⊛ [C] [80] ▢ [P0]

AMA: 2015,Jan,16; 2014,Jan,11; 2012,Feb,3-7

Esophagus

Lung

Diaphragm

A defect of the diaphragm can allow abdominal contents to herniate into the thoracic cavity

39540   **Repair, diaphragmatic hernia (other than neonatal), traumatic; acute**

🔧 25.1   ⚒ 25.1   **FUD** 090   [C] [80] ▢ [P0]

AMA: 2015,Jan,16; 2014,Jan,11

39541   chronic

🔧 27.4   ⚒ 27.4   **FUD** 090   [C] [80] ▢ [P0]

AMA: 2015,Jan,16; 2014,Jan,11

39545   **Imbrication of diaphragm for eventration, transthoracic or transabdominal, paralytic or nonparalytic**

🔧 25.9   ⚒ 25.9   **FUD** 090   [C] [80] ▢ [P0]

AMA: 2015,Jan,16; 2014,Jan,11

39560   **Resection, diaphragm; with simple repair (eg, primary suture)**

🔧 23.0   ⚒ 23.0   **FUD** 090   [C] [80] ▢ [P0]

AMA: 2015,Jan,16; 2014,Jan,11

39561   with complex repair (eg, prosthetic material, local muscle flap)

🔧 35.8   ⚒ 35.8   **FUD** 090   [C] [80] ▢ [P0]

AMA: 2015,Jan,16; 2014,Jan,11

39599   **Unlisted procedure, diaphragm**

🔧 0.00   ⚒ 0.00   **FUD** YYY   [C] [80]

AMA: 2014,Jan,11

| [26]/[TC] PC/TC Comp Only | [A2]-[Z3] ASC Pmt | [50] Bilateral | ♂ Male Only | ♀ Female Only | 🔧 Facility RVU | ⚒ Non-Facility RVU |
| **AMA:** CPT Asst | **CMS:** Pub 100 | [A]-[Y] OPPSI | [80]/[80] Surg Assist Allowed / w/Doc | | 📘 Lab Crosswalk | 📕 Radiology Crosswalk |

156   Medicare (Red Text)   CPT © 2015 American Medical Association. All Rights Reserved. (Black Text)   © 2015 Optum360, LLC (Blue Text)

40490-40799 Resection and Repair Procedures of the Lips

EXCLUDES Procedures on the skin of lips (10040-17999 [11045, 11046])

40490 **Biopsy of lip**
🚑 2.11 ⚗ 3.68 **FUD** 000 T P3 ▭ P0
AMA: 2014,Jan,11

40500 **Vermilionectomy (lip shave), with mucosal advancement**
🚑 10.5 ⚗ 14.5 **FUD** 090 T A2 ▭
AMA: 2014,Jan,11

40510 **Excision of lip; transverse wedge excision with primary closure**
EXCLUDES Excision of mucous lesions (40810-40816)
🚑 10.3 ⚗ 13.9 **FUD** 090 T A2 ▭
AMA: 2014,Jan,11

40520 **V-excision with primary direct linear closure**
EXCLUDES Excision of mucous lesions (40810-40816)
🚑 10.4 ⚗ 14.1 **FUD** 090 T A2 ▭
AMA: 2014,Jan,11

40525 **full thickness, reconstruction with local flap (eg, Estlander or fan)**
🚑 15.9 ⚗ 15.9 **FUD** 090 T A2 ▭
AMA: 2014,Jan,11

40527 **full thickness, reconstruction with cross lip flap (Abbe-Estlander)**
INCLUDES Cleft lip repair with cross lip pedicle flap (Abbe-Estlander type), without pedicle sectioning and insertion
EXCLUDES Cleft lip repair with cross lip pedicle flap (Abbe-Estlander type), with pedicle sectioning and insertion (40761)
🚑 17.8 ⚗ 17.8 **FUD** 090 T A2 80 ▭
AMA: 2014,Jan,11

40530 **Resection of lip, more than one-fourth, without reconstruction**
EXCLUDES Reconstruction (13131-13153)
🚑 11.6 ⚗ 15.5 **FUD** 090 T A2 ▭
AMA: 2014,Jan,11

40650 **Repair lip, full thickness; vermilion only**
🚑 8.62 ⚗ 12.5 **FUD** 090 T A2 80 ▭
AMA: 2015,Jan,16; 2014,Jan,11; 2012,Jan,15-42; 2011,Jan,11

40652 **up to half vertical height**
🚑 10.2 ⚗ 14.1 **FUD** 090 T A2 80 ▭
AMA: 2015,Jan,16; 2014,Jan,11; 2012,Jan,15-42; 2011,Jan,11

40654 **over one-half vertical height, or complex**
🚑 12.2 ⚗ 16.3 **FUD** 090 T A2 ▭
AMA: 2014,Jan,11

40700 **Plastic repair of cleft lip/nasal deformity; primary, partial or complete, unilateral**
EXCLUDES Cleft lip repair with cross lip pedicle flap (Abbe-Estlander type):
With pedicle sectioning and insertion (40761)
Without pedicle sectioning and insertion (40527)
Rhinoplasty for nasal deformity secondary to congenital cleft lip (30460, 30462)
🚑 29.0 ⚗ 29.0 **FUD** 090 T A2 80 ▭
AMA: 2015,Jan,16; 2014,Dec,18; 2014,Jan,11

40701 **primary bilateral, 1-stage procedure**
EXCLUDES Cleft lip repair with cross lip pedicle flap (Abbe-Estlander type):
With pedicle sectioning and insertion (40761)
Without pedicle sectioning and insertion (40527)
Rhinoplasty for nasal deformity secondary to congenital cleft lip (30460, 30462)
🚑 28.2 ⚗ 28.2 **FUD** 090 T A2 80 ▭
AMA: 2015,Jan,16; 2014,Dec,18; 2014,Jan,11

Bilateral cleft lip

Cleft margins on both sides are incised

Margins are closed, correcting cleft

40702 **primary bilateral, 1 of 2 stages**
EXCLUDES Cleft lip repair with cross lip pedicle flap (Abbe-Estlander type):
With pedicle sectioning and insertion (40761)
Without pedicle sectioning and insertion (40527)
Rhinoplasty for nasal deformity secondary to congenital cleft lip (30460, 30462)
🚑 27.1 ⚗ 27.1 **FUD** 090 T R2 80 ▭
AMA: 2015,Jan,16; 2014,Dec,18; 2014,Jan,11

40720 **secondary, by recreation of defect and reclosure**
EXCLUDES Cleft lip repair with cross lip pedicle flap (Abbe-Estlander type):
With pedicle sectioning and insertion (40761)
Without pedicle sectioning and insertion (40527)
Rhinoplasty for nasal deformity secondary to congenital cleft lip (30460, 30462)
🚑 29.7 ⚗ 29.7 **FUD** 090 T A2 80 50 ▭
AMA: 2015,Jan,16; 2014,Dec,18; 2014,Jan,11

40761 **with cross lip pedicle flap (Abbe-Estlander type), including sectioning and inserting of pedicle**
EXCLUDES Cleft lip repair with cross lip pedicle flap (Abbe-Estlander type) without sectioning and insertion of pedicle (40527)
Cleft palate repair (42200-42225)
Other reconstructive procedures (14060-14061, 15120-15261, 15574, 15576, 15630)
🚑 28.2 ⚗ 28.2 **FUD** 090 T A2 ▭
AMA: 2014,Jan,11

40799 **Unlisted procedure, lips**
🚑 0.00 ⚗ 0.00 **FUD** YYY T 80
AMA: 2014,Jan,11

40800-40819 Incision and Resection of Buccal Cavity

INCLUDES Mucosal/submucosal tissue of lips/cheeks
Oral cavity outside the dentoalveolar structures

40800 **Drainage of abscess, cyst, hematoma, vestibule of mouth; simple**
🚑 3.87 ⚗ 6.17 **FUD** 010 T P2 ▭
AMA: 2014,Jan,11

40801 **complicated**
🚑 6.54 ⚗ 9.24 **FUD** 010 T A2 ▭
AMA: 2014,Jan,11

40804 **Removal of embedded foreign body, vestibule of mouth; simple**
🚑 3.84 ⚗ 6.17 **FUD** 010 Q1 N1 80 ▭
AMA: 2014,Jan,11

Digestive System

40805 — 41019

40805 complicated
🔲 6.86 ⚕ 9.43 **FUD** 010
AMA: 2014,Jan,11
`T` `P3` `80`

40806 Incision of labial frenum (frenotomy)
🔲 0.97 ⚕ 3.13 **FUD** 000
AMA: 2014,Jan,11
`T` `P3` `80`

40808 Biopsy, vestibule of mouth
🔲 3.19 ⚕ 5.44 **FUD** 010
AMA: 2014,Jan,11
`T` `P3` `PQ`

40810 Excision of lesion of mucosa and submucosa, vestibule of mouth; without repair
🔲 3.76 ⚕ 6.01 **FUD** 010
AMA: 2014,Jan,11
`T` `P3`

40812 with simple repair
🔲 5.81 ⚕ 8.42 **FUD** 010
AMA: 2014,Jan,11
`T` `P3`

40814 with complex repair
🔲 8.96 ⚕ 11.2 **FUD** 090
AMA: 2014,Jan,11
`T` `A2`

40816 complex, with excision of underlying muscle
🔲 9.29 ⚕ 11.7 **FUD** 090
AMA: 2014,Jan,11
`T` `A2`

40818 Excision of mucosa of vestibule of mouth as donor graft
🔲 7.99 ⚕ 10.4 **FUD** 090
AMA: 2014,Jan,11
`T` `A2` `80`

40819 Excision of frenum, labial or buccal (frenumectomy, frenulectomy, frenectomy)
🔲 7.00 ⚕ 9.17 **FUD** 090
AMA: 2014,Jan,11
`T` `A2` `80`

40820 Destruction of Lesion of Buccal Cavity

CMS: 100-3,140.5 Laser Procedures
INCLUDES Mucosal/submucosal tissue of lips/cheeks
Oral cavity outside the dentoalveolar structures

40820 Destruction of lesion or scar of vestibule of mouth by physical methods (eg, laser, thermal, cryo, chemical)
🔲 5.04 ⚕ 7.74 **FUD** 010
AMA: 2014,Jan,11
`T` `P3`

40830-40899 Repair Procedures of the Buccal Cavity

INCLUDES Mucosal/submucosal tissue of lips/cheeks
Oral cavity outside the dentoalveolar structures
EXCLUDES Skin grafts (15002-15630)

40830 Closure of laceration, vestibule of mouth; 2.5 cm or less
🔲 4.87 ⚕ 7.74 **FUD** 010
AMA: 2014,Jan,11
`T` `G2` `80`

40831 over 2.5 cm or complex
🔲 6.56 ⚕ 9.81 **FUD** 010
AMA: 2014,Jan,11
`T` `A2` `80`

40840 Vestibuloplasty; anterior
🔲 18.3 ⚕ 23.6 **FUD** 090
AMA: 2014,Jan,11
`T` `A2` `80`

40842 posterior, unilateral
🔲 19.0 ⚕ 23.8 **FUD** 090
AMA: 2014,Jan,11
`T` `A2` `80`

40843 posterior, bilateral
🔲 25.1 ⚕ 31.6 **FUD** 090
AMA: 2014,Jan,11
`T` `A2` `80`

40844 entire arch
🔲 30.5 ⚕ 37.4 **FUD** 090
AMA: 2014,Jan,11
`T` `A2` `80`

40845 complex (including ridge extension, muscle repositioning)
🔲 35.7 ⚕ 42.5 **FUD** 090
AMA: 2014,Jan,11
`T` `A2` `80`

40899 Unlisted procedure, vestibule of mouth
🔲 0.00 ⚕ 0.00 **FUD** YYY
AMA: 2014,Jan,11
`T` `80`

41000-41018 Surgical Incision of Floor of Mouth or Tongue

EXCLUDES Frenoplasty (41520)

41000 Intraoral incision and drainage of abscess, cyst, or hematoma of tongue or floor of mouth; lingual
🔲 3.30 ⚕ 4.74 **FUD** 010
AMA: 2014,Jan,11
`T` `P3`

Palantine tonsil
Epiglottis
The posterior one-third of the tongue is part of the oropharynx and differs from the oral two-thirds in its nerve supply and mucous membrane; the sulcus terminalis marks the division.
Foramen cecum
Lingual tonsils
Median groove
Sulcus terminalis
Apex (tip) of tongue

41005 sublingual, superficial
🔲 3.66 ⚕ 6.59 **FUD** 010
AMA: 2014,Jan,11
`T` `A2` `80`

41006 sublingual, deep, supramylohyoid
🔲 7.84 ⚕ 11.1 **FUD** 090
AMA: 2014,Jan,11
`T` `A2` `80`

41007 submental space
🔲 7.61 ⚕ 11.0 **FUD** 090
AMA: 2014,Jan,11
`T` `A2` `80`

41008 submandibular space
🔲 7.91 ⚕ 11.0 **FUD** 090
AMA: 2014,Jan,11
`T` `A2` `80`

41009 masticator space
🔲 8.59 ⚕ 11.7 **FUD** 090
AMA: 2014,Jan,11
`T` `A2` `80`

41010 Incision of lingual frenum (frenotomy)
🔲 3.16 ⚕ 5.87 **FUD** 010
AMA: 2014,Jan,11
`T` `A2` `80`

41015 Extraoral incision and drainage of abscess, cyst, or hematoma of floor of mouth; sublingual
🔲 10.2 ⚕ 13.2 **FUD** 090
AMA: 2014,Jan,11
`T` `A2` `80`

41016 submental
🔲 10.3 ⚕ 12.8 **FUD** 090
AMA: 2014,Jan,11
`T` `A2` `80`

41017 submandibular
🔲 10.4 ⚕ 13.0 **FUD** 090
AMA: 2014,Jan,11
`T` `A2` `80`

41018 masticator space
🔲 12.0 ⚕ 14.7 **FUD** 090
AMA: 2014,Jan,11
`T` `A2` `80`

41019 Placement of Devices for Brachytherapy

EXCLUDES Application of interstitial radioelements (77770-77772, 77778)
Intracranial brachytherapy radiation sources with stereotactic insertion (61770)

41019 Placement of needles, catheters, or other device(s) into the head and/or neck region (percutaneous, transoral, or transnasal) for subsequent interstitial radioelement application
⚕ (76942, 77002, 77012, 77021)
🔲 13.3 ⚕ 13.3 **FUD** 000
AMA: 2015,Jan,16; 2014,Jan,11
`T` `G2` `80`

41100-41599 Resection and Repair of the Tongue

41100   **Biopsy of tongue; anterior two-thirds**
   🔧 3.16   ⚕ 4.89   **FUD** 010   T P3 ▣ P0
   AMA: 2014,Jan,11

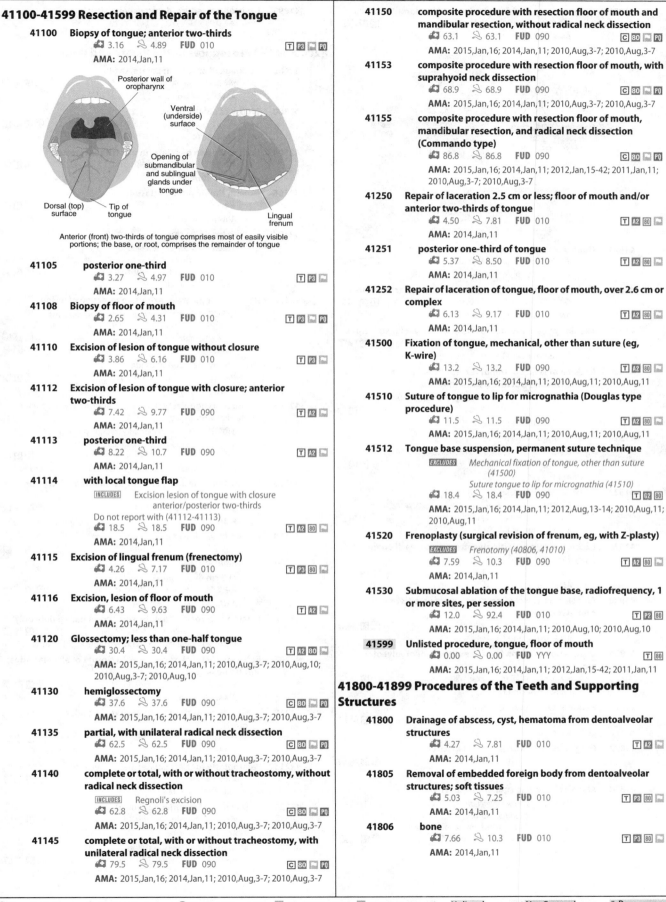

Posterior wall of oropharynx

Ventral (underside) surface

Opening of submandibular and sublingual glands under tongue

Dorsal (top) surface   Tip of tongue

Lingual frenum

Anterior (front) two-thirds of tongue comprises most of easily visible portions; the base, or root, comprises the remainder of tongue

41105   **posterior one-third**
   🔧 3.27   ⚕ 4.97   **FUD** 010   T P3 ▣
   AMA: 2014,Jan,11

41108   **Biopsy of floor of mouth**
   🔧 2.65   ⚕ 4.31   **FUD** 010   T P3 ▣ P0
   AMA: 2014,Jan,11

41110   **Excision of lesion of tongue without closure**
   🔧 3.86   ⚕ 6.16   **FUD** 010   T P3 ▣
   AMA: 2014,Jan,11

41112   **Excision of lesion of tongue with closure; anterior two-thirds**
   🔧 7.42   ⚕ 9.77   **FUD** 090   T A2 ▣
   AMA: 2014,Jan,11

41113   **posterior one-third**
   🔧 8.22   ⚕ 10.7   **FUD** 090   T A2 ▣
   AMA: 2014,Jan,11

41114   **with local tongue flap**
   INCLUDES   Excision lesion of tongue with closure anterior/posterior two-thirds
   Do not report with (41112-41113)
   🔧 18.5   ⚕ 18.5   **FUD** 090   T A2 80 ▣
   AMA: 2014,Jan,11

41115   **Excision of lingual frenum (frenectomy)**
   🔧 4.26   ⚕ 7.17   **FUD** 010   T P3 80 ▣
   AMA: 2014,Jan,11

41116   **Excision, lesion of floor of mouth**
   🔧 6.43   ⚕ 9.63   **FUD** 090   T A2 ▣
   AMA: 2014,Jan,11

41120   **Glossectomy; less than one-half tongue**
   🔧 30.4   ⚕ 30.4   **FUD** 090   T A2 80 ▣
   AMA: 2015,Jan,16; 2014,Jan,11; 2010,Aug,3-7; 2010,Aug,10; 2010,Aug,3-7; 2010,Aug,10

41130   **hemiglossectomy**
   🔧 37.6   ⚕ 37.6   **FUD** 090   C 80 ▣ P0
   AMA: 2015,Jan,16; 2014,Jan,11; 2010,Aug,3-7; 2010,Aug,3-7

41135   **partial, with unilateral radical neck dissection**
   🔧 62.5   ⚕ 62.5   **FUD** 090   C 80 ▣ P0
   AMA: 2015,Jan,16; 2014,Jan,11; 2010,Aug,3-7; 2010,Aug,3-7

41140   **complete or total, with or without tracheostomy, without radical neck dissection**
   INCLUDES   Regnoli's excision
   🔧 62.8   ⚕ 62.8   **FUD** 090   C 80 ▣ P0
   AMA: 2015,Jan,16; 2014,Jan,11; 2010,Aug,3-7; 2010,Aug,3-7

41145   **complete or total, with or without tracheostomy, with unilateral radical neck dissection**
   🔧 79.5   ⚕ 79.5   **FUD** 090   C 80 ▣ P0
   AMA: 2015,Jan,16; 2014,Jan,11; 2010,Aug,3-7; 2010,Aug,3-7

41150   **composite procedure with resection floor of mouth and mandibular resection, without radical neck dissection**
   🔧 63.1   ⚕ 63.1   **FUD** 090   C 80 ▣ P0
   AMA: 2015,Jan,16; 2014,Jan,11; 2010,Aug,3-7; 2010,Aug,3-7

41153   **composite procedure with resection floor of mouth, with suprahyoid neck dissection**
   🔧 68.9   ⚕ 68.9   **FUD** 090   C 80 ▣ P0
   AMA: 2015,Jan,16; 2014,Jan,11; 2010,Aug,3-7; 2010,Aug,3-7

41155   **composite procedure with resection floor of mouth, mandibular resection, and radical neck dissection (Commando type)**
   🔧 86.8   ⚕ 86.8   **FUD** 090   C 80 ▣ P0
   AMA: 2015,Jan,16; 2014,Jan,11; 2012,Jan,15-42; 2011,Jan,11; 2010,Aug,3-7; 2010,Aug,3-7

41250   **Repair of laceration 2.5 cm or less; floor of mouth and/or anterior two-thirds of tongue**
   🔧 4.50   ⚕ 7.81   **FUD** 010   T A2 80 ▣
   AMA: 2014,Jan,11

41251   **posterior one-third of tongue**
   🔧 5.37   ⚕ 8.50   **FUD** 010   T A2 80 ▣
   AMA: 2014,Jan,11

41252   **Repair of laceration of tongue, floor of mouth, over 2.6 cm or complex**
   🔧 6.13   ⚕ 9.17   **FUD** 010   T A2 80 ▣
   AMA: 2014,Jan,11

41500   **Fixation of tongue, mechanical, other than suture (eg, K-wire)**
   🔧 13.2   ⚕ 13.2   **FUD** 090   T A2 80 ▣
   AMA: 2015,Jan,16; 2014,Jan,11; 2010,Aug,11; 2010,Aug,11

41510   **Suture of tongue to lip for micrognathia (Douglas type procedure)**
   🔧 11.5   ⚕ 11.5   **FUD** 090   T A2 80 ▣
   AMA: 2015,Jan,16; 2014,Jan,11; 2010,Aug,11; 2010,Aug,11

41512   **Tongue base suspension, permanent suture technique**
   EXCLUDES   Mechanical fixation of tongue, other than suture (41500)
   Suture tongue to lip for micrognathia (41510)
   🔧 18.4   ⚕ 18.4   **FUD** 090   T 62 80
   AMA: 2015,Jan,16; 2014,Jan,11; 2012,Aug,13-14; 2010,Aug,11; 2010,Aug,11

41520   **Frenoplasty (surgical revision of frenum, eg, with Z-plasty)**
   EXCLUDES   Frenotomy (40806, 41010)
   🔧 7.59   ⚕ 10.3   **FUD** 090   T A2 80 ▣
   AMA: 2014,Jan,11

41530   **Submucosal ablation of the tongue base, radiofrequency, 1 or more sites, per session**
   🔧 12.0   ⚕ 92.4   **FUD** 010   T P2 80 ▣
   AMA: 2015,Jan,16; 2014,Jan,11; 2010,Aug,10; 2010,Aug,10

41599   **Unlisted procedure, tongue, floor of mouth**
   🔧 0.00   ⚕ 0.00   **FUD** YYY   T 80
   AMA: 2015,Jan,16; 2014,Jan,11; 2012,Jan,15-42; 2011,Jan,11

41800-41899 Procedures of the Teeth and Supporting Structures

41800   **Drainage of abscess, cyst, hematoma from dentoalveolar structures**
   🔧 4.27   ⚕ 7.81   **FUD** 010   T A2 ▣
   AMA: 2014,Jan,11

41805   **Removal of embedded foreign body from dentoalveolar structures; soft tissues**
   🔧 5.03   ⚕ 7.25   **FUD** 010   T P3 80 ▣
   AMA: 2014,Jan,11

41806   **bone**
   🔧 7.66   ⚕ 10.3   **FUD** 010   T P3 80 ▣
   AMA: 2014,Jan,11

Digestive System

41820 **Gingivectomy, excision gingiva, each quadrant**
🔷 0.00 🔶 0.00 **FUD** 000 T R2 80 ▣
AMA: 2014,Jan,11

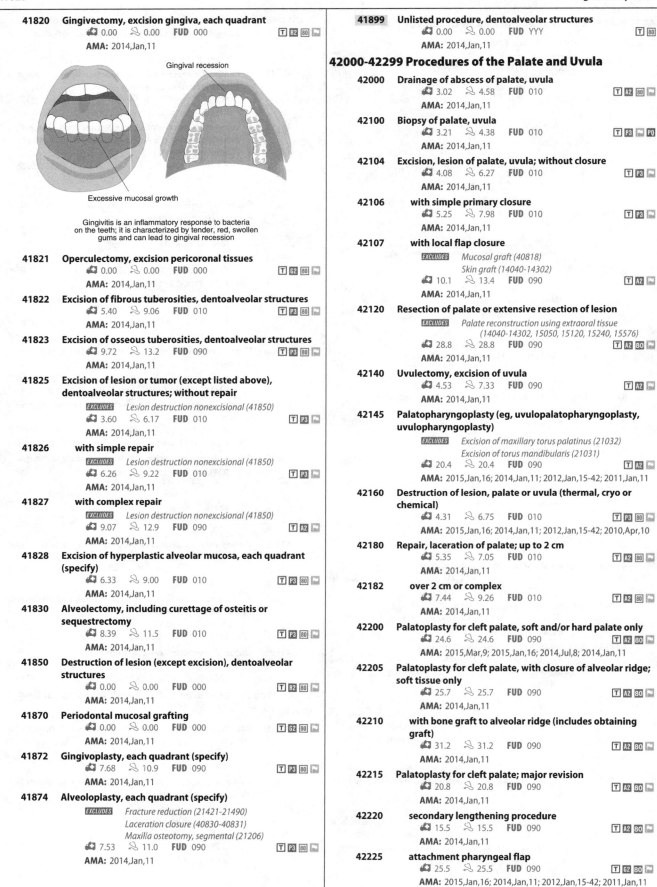

Gingival recession

Excessive mucosal growth

Gingivitis is an inflammatory response to bacteria on the teeth; it is characterized by tender, red, swollen gums and can lead to gingival recession

41821 **Operculectomy, excision pericoronal tissues**
🔷 0.00 🔶 0.00 **FUD** 000 T G2 80 ▣
AMA: 2014,Jan,11

41822 **Excision of fibrous tuberosities, dentoalveolar structures**
🔷 5.40 🔶 9.06 **FUD** 010 T P3 80 ▣
AMA: 2014,Jan,11

41823 **Excision of osseous tuberosities, dentoalveolar structures**
🔷 9.72 🔶 13.2 **FUD** 090 T P3 80 ▣
AMA: 2014,Jan,11

41825 **Excision of lesion or tumor (except listed above), dentoalveolar structures; without repair**
EXCLUDES Lesion destruction nonexcisional (41850)
🔷 3.60 🔶 6.17 **FUD** 010 T P3 ▣
AMA: 2014,Jan,11

41826 **with simple repair**
EXCLUDES Lesion destruction nonexcisional (41850)
🔷 6.26 🔶 9.22 **FUD** 010 T P3 ▣
AMA: 2014,Jan,11

41827 **with complex repair**
EXCLUDES Lesion destruction nonexcisional (41850)
🔷 9.07 🔶 12.9 **FUD** 090 T A2 ▣
AMA: 2014,Jan,11

41828 **Excision of hyperplastic alveolar mucosa, each quadrant (specify)**
🔷 6.33 🔶 9.00 **FUD** 010 T P3 80 ▣
AMA: 2014,Jan,11

41830 **Alveolectomy, including curettage of osteitis or sequestrectomy**
🔷 8.39 🔶 11.5 **FUD** 010 T P3 80 ▣
AMA: 2014,Jan,11

41850 **Destruction of lesion (except excision), dentoalveolar structures**
🔷 0.00 🔶 0.00 **FUD** 000 T R2 80 ▣
AMA: 2014,Jan,11

41870 **Periodontal mucosal grafting**
🔷 0.00 🔶 0.00 **FUD** 000 T G2 80 ▣
AMA: 2014,Jan,11

41872 **Gingivoplasty, each quadrant (specify)**
🔷 7.68 🔶 10.9 **FUD** 090 T P3 80 ▣
AMA: 2014,Jan,11

41874 **Alveoloplasty, each quadrant (specify)**
EXCLUDES Fracture reduction (21421-21490)
         Laceration closure (40830-40831)
         Maxilla osteotomy, segmental (21206)
🔷 7.53 🔶 11.0 **FUD** 090 T P3 80 ▣
AMA: 2014,Jan,11

41899 **Unlisted procedure, dentoalveolar structures**
🔷 0.00 🔶 0.00 **FUD** YYY T 80
AMA: 2014,Jan,11

42000-42299 Procedures of the Palate and Uvula

42000 **Drainage of abscess of palate, uvula**
🔷 3.02 🔶 4.58 **FUD** 010 T A2 80 ▣
AMA: 2014,Jan,11

42100 **Biopsy of palate, uvula**
🔷 3.21 🔶 4.38 **FUD** 010 T P3 ▣ P0
AMA: 2014,Jan,11

42104 **Excision, lesion of palate, uvula; without closure**
🔷 4.08 🔶 6.27 **FUD** 010 T P3 ▣
AMA: 2014,Jan,11

42106 **with simple primary closure**
🔷 5.25 🔶 7.98 **FUD** 010 T P3 ▣
AMA: 2014,Jan,11

42107 **with local flap closure**
EXCLUDES Mucosal graft (40818)
         Skin graft (14040-14302)
🔷 10.1 🔶 13.4 **FUD** 090 T A2 ▣
AMA: 2014,Jan,11

42120 **Resection of palate or extensive resection of lesion**
EXCLUDES Palate reconstruction using extraoral tissue
         (14040-14302, 15050, 15120, 15240, 15576)
🔷 28.8 🔶 28.8 **FUD** 090 T A2 80 ▣
AMA: 2014,Jan,11

42140 **Uvulectomy, excision of uvula**
🔷 4.53 🔶 7.33 **FUD** 090 T A2 ▣
AMA: 2014,Jan,11

42145 **Palatopharyngoplasty (eg, uvulopalatopharyngoplasty, uvulopharyngoplasty)**
EXCLUDES Excision of maxillary torus palatinus (21032)
         Excision of torus mandibularis (21031)
🔷 20.4 🔶 20.4 **FUD** 090 T A2 ▣
AMA: 2015,Jan,16; 2014,Jan,11; 2012,Jan,15-42; 2011,Jan,11

42160 **Destruction of lesion, palate or uvula (thermal, cryo or chemical)**
🔷 4.31 🔶 6.75 **FUD** 010 T P3 80 ▣
AMA: 2015,Jan,16; 2014,Jan,11; 2012,Jan,15-42; 2010,Apr,10

42180 **Repair, laceration of palate; up to 2 cm**
🔷 5.35 🔶 7.05 **FUD** 010 T A2 80 ▣
AMA: 2014,Jan,11

42182 **over 2 cm or complex**
🔷 7.44 🔶 9.26 **FUD** 010 T A2 80 ▣
AMA: 2014,Jan,11

42200 **Palatoplasty for cleft palate, soft and/or hard palate only**
🔷 24.6 🔶 24.6 **FUD** 090 T A2 80 ▣
AMA: 2015,Mar,9; 2015,Jan,16; 2014,Jul,8; 2014,Jan,11

42205 **Palatoplasty for cleft palate, with closure of alveolar ridge; soft tissue only**
🔷 25.7 🔶 25.7 **FUD** 090 T A2 80 ▣
AMA: 2014,Jan,11

42210 **with bone graft to alveolar ridge (includes obtaining graft)**
🔷 31.2 🔶 31.2 **FUD** 090 T A2 80 ▣
AMA: 2014,Jan,11

42215 **Palatoplasty for cleft palate; major revision**
🔷 20.8 🔶 20.8 **FUD** 090 T A2 80 ▣
AMA: 2014,Jan,11

42220 **secondary lengthening procedure**
🔷 15.5 🔶 15.5 **FUD** 090 T A2 80 ▣
AMA: 2014,Jan,11

42225 **attachment pharyngeal flap**
🔷 25.5 🔶 25.5 **FUD** 090 T G2 80 ▣
AMA: 2015,Jan,16; 2014,Jan,11; 2012,Jan,15-42; 2011,Jan,11

42226 Lengthening of palate, and pharyngeal flap
🖐 25.9 ⚕ 25.9 **FUD** 090 　 T A2 80 ▢
AMA: 2014,Jan,11

42227 Lengthening of palate, with island flap
🖐 24.3 ⚕ 24.3 **FUD** 090 　 T G2 80 ▢
AMA: 2014,Jan,11

42235 Repair of anterior palate, including vomer flap
EXCLUDES　Oronasal fistula repair (30600)
🖐 21.3 ⚕ 21.3 **FUD** 090 　 T A2 80 ▢
AMA: 2015,Mar,9; 2015,Jan,16; 2014,Jul,8; 2014,Jan,11

42260 Repair of nasolabial fistula
EXCLUDES　Cleft lip repair (40700-40761)
🖐 20.9 ⚕ 25.0 **FUD** 090 　 T A2 80 ▢
AMA: 2014,Jan,11

42280 Maxillary impression for palatal prosthesis
🖐 3.26 ⚕ 4.80 **FUD** 010 　 T P3 80 ▢
AMA: 2014,Jan,11

42281 Insertion of pin-retained palatal prosthesis
🖐 4.40 ⚕ 5.93 **FUD** 010 　 T G2 80 ▢
AMA: 2014,Jan,11

42299 Unlisted procedure, palate, uvula
🖐 0.00 ⚕ 0.00 **FUD** YYY 　 T 80
AMA: 2015,Jan,16; 2014,Jul,8; 2014,Jan,11; 2012,Jan,15-42; 2011,Jan,11; 2010,Nov,8; 2010,Apr,10

42300-42699 Procedures of the Salivary Ducts and Glands

42300 Drainage of abscess; parotid, simple
🖐 4.45 ⚕ 6.06 **FUD** 010 　 T A2 ▢
AMA: 2014,Jan,11

42305 parotid, complicated
🖐 12.5 ⚕ 12.5 **FUD** 090 　 T A2 80 ▢
AMA: 2014,Jan,11

42310 Drainage of abscess; submaxillary or sublingual, intraoral
🖐 3.62 ⚕ 4.68 **FUD** 010 　 T A2 80 ▢
AMA: 2014,Jan,11

42320 submaxillary, external
🖐 5.11 ⚕ 7.22 **FUD** 010 　 T A2 80 ▢
AMA: 2014,Jan,11

42330 Sialolithotomy; submandibular (submaxillary), sublingual or parotid, uncomplicated, intraoral
🖐 4.82 ⚕ 6.73 **FUD** 010 　 T P3 ▢
AMA: 2014,Jan,11

42335 submandibular (submaxillary), complicated, intraoral
🖐 7.48 ⚕ 10.8 **FUD** 090 　 T P3 ▢
AMA: 2014,Jan,11

42340 parotid, extraoral or complicated intraoral
🖐 9.82 ⚕ 13.5 **FUD** 090 　 T A2 80 50 ▢
AMA: 2014,Jan,11

42400 Biopsy of salivary gland; needle
EXCLUDES　Fine needle aspiration (10021, 10022)
　(76942, 77002, 77012, 77021)
　(88172-88173)
🖐 1.60 ⚕ 3.07 **FUD** 000 　 T P3 ▢ P0
AMA: 2014,Jan,11

42405 incisional
　(76942, 77002, 77012, 77021)
🖐 6.58 ⚕ 8.63 **FUD** 010 　 T A2 ▢ P0
AMA: 2014,Jan,11

42408 Excision of sublingual salivary cyst (ranula)
🖐 9.46 ⚕ 13.1 **FUD** 090 　 T A2 80 ▢
AMA: 2014,Jan,11

42409 Marsupialization of sublingual salivary cyst (ranula)
🖐 6.46 ⚕ 9.65 **FUD** 090 　 A2 80 ▢
AMA: 2014,Jan,11

42410 Excision of parotid tumor or parotid gland; lateral lobe, without nerve dissection
EXCLUDES　Facial nerve suture or graft (64864, 64865, 69740, 69745)
🖐 18.0 ⚕ 18.0 **FUD** 090 　 T A2 80 50 ▢
AMA: 2014,Jan,11

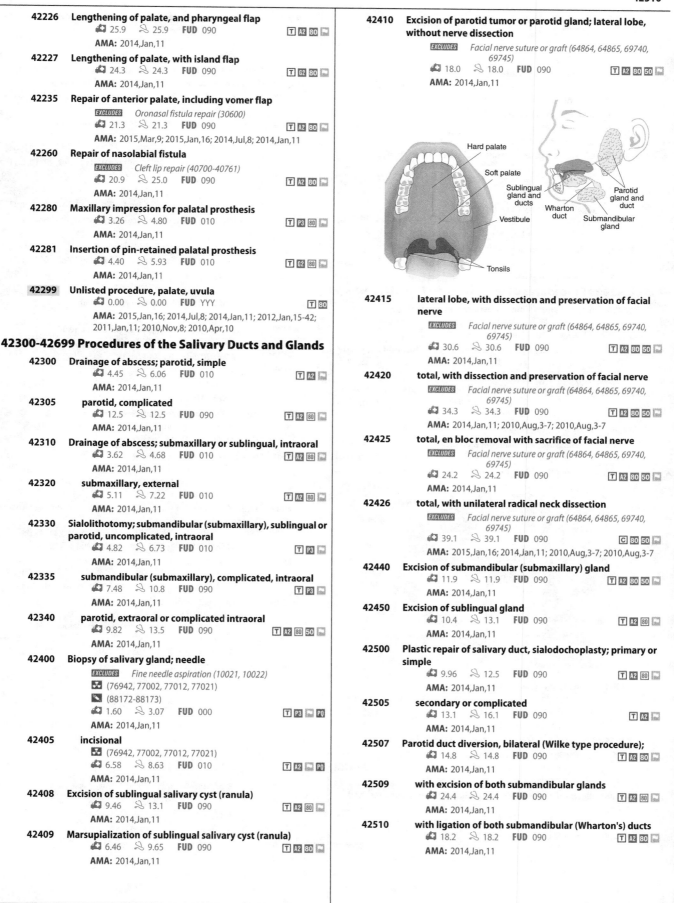

Hard palate
Soft palate
Sublingual gland and ducts
Wharton duct
Vestibule
Tonsils
Parotid gland and duct
Submandibular gland

42415 lateral lobe, with dissection and preservation of facial nerve
EXCLUDES　Facial nerve suture or graft (64864, 64865, 69740, 69745)
🖐 30.6 ⚕ 30.6 **FUD** 090 　 T A2 80 50 ▢
AMA: 2014,Jan,11

42420 total, with dissection and preservation of facial nerve
EXCLUDES　Facial nerve suture or graft (64864, 64865, 69740, 69745)
🖐 34.3 ⚕ 34.3 **FUD** 090 　 T A2 80 50 ▢
AMA: 2014,Jan,11; 2010,Aug,3-7; 2010,Aug,3-7

42425 total, en bloc removal with sacrifice of facial nerve
EXCLUDES　Facial nerve suture or graft (64864, 64865, 69740, 69745)
🖐 24.2 ⚕ 24.2 **FUD** 090 　 T A2 80 50 ▢
AMA: 2014,Jan,11

42426 total, with unilateral radical neck dissection
EXCLUDES　Facial nerve suture or graft (64864, 64865, 69740, 69745)
🖐 39.1 ⚕ 39.1 **FUD** 090 　 C 80 50 ▢
AMA: 2015,Jan,16; 2014,Jan,11; 2010,Aug,3-7; 2010,Aug,3-7

42440 Excision of submandibular (submaxillary) gland
🖐 11.9 ⚕ 11.9 **FUD** 090 　 T A2 80 50 ▢
AMA: 2014,Jan,11

42450 Excision of sublingual gland
🖐 10.4 ⚕ 13.1 **FUD** 090 　 T A2 80 ▢
AMA: 2014,Jan,11

42500 Plastic repair of salivary duct, sialodochoplasty; primary or simple
🖐 9.96 ⚕ 12.5 **FUD** 090 　 T A2 80 ▢
AMA: 2014,Jan,11

42505 secondary or complicated
🖐 13.1 ⚕ 16.1 **FUD** 090 　 T A2 ▢
AMA: 2014,Jan,11

42507 Parotid duct diversion, bilateral (Wilke type procedure);
🖐 14.8 ⚕ 14.8 **FUD** 090 　 T A2 80 ▢
AMA: 2014,Jan,11

42509 with excision of both submandibular glands
🖐 24.4 ⚕ 24.4 **FUD** 090 　 T A2 80 ▢
AMA: 2014,Jan,11

42510 with ligation of both submandibular (Wharton's) ducts
🖐 18.2 ⚕ 18.2 **FUD** 090 　 T A2 80 ▢
AMA: 2014,Jan,11

Digestive System

42550 — 42860

42550 Injection procedure for sialography
📻 (70390)
🔧 1.84 ⚖ 3.88 **FUD** 000   N N1 💻
AMA: 2014,Jan,11

42600 Closure salivary fistula
🔧 10.0 ⚖ 13.8 **FUD** 090   T A2 80 💻
AMA: 2014,Jan,11

42650 Dilation salivary duct
🔧 1.71 ⚖ 2.42 **FUD** 000   T P3 💻
AMA: 2014,Jan,11

42660 Dilation and catheterization of salivary duct, with or without injection
🔧 2.60 ⚖ 3.68 **FUD** 000   T P3 80 💻
AMA: 2014,Jan,11

42665 Ligation salivary duct, intraoral
🔧 5.98 ⚖ 9.01 **FUD** 090   T A2 80 💻
AMA: 2014,Jan,11

42699 Unlisted procedure, salivary glands or ducts
🔧 0.00 ⚖ 0.00 **FUD** YYY   T 80
AMA: 2014,Jan,11

42700-42999 Procedures of the Adenoids/Throat/Tonsils

42700 Incision and drainage abscess; peritonsillar
🔧 3.96 ⚖ 5.50 **FUD** 010   T A2 💻
AMA: 2014,Jan,11

42720 retropharyngeal or parapharyngeal, intraoral approach
🔧 11.3 ⚖ 13.1 **FUD** 010   T A2 80 💻
AMA: 2014,Jan,11

42725 retropharyngeal or parapharyngeal, external approach
🔧 23.7 ⚖ 23.7 **FUD** 090   T A2 80 💻
AMA: 2014,Jan,11

42800 Biopsy; oropharynx
EXCLUDES Laryngoscopy with biopsy (31510, 31535, 31536, 31576)
🔧 3.26 ⚖ 4.60 **FUD** 010   T P3 💻 P0
AMA: 2014,Jan,11

The nasal cavities and paranasal sinuses are lined with a continuous mucous membrane
Nasal cavity
Auditory tube
Epiglottis
Orbit
Nasopharynx region
Ethmoidal cells
Oropharynx region
Maxillary sinus
Hypopharynx region
Middle and inferior meatus
Vocal cord and larynx
Trachea
Frontal coronal section of left side of skull showing sinuses
The pharynx is a transitional zone between the oral cavity and the rest of the digestive canal. It is the common route for both air and food

42804 nasopharynx, visible lesion, simple
EXCLUDES Laryngoscopy with biopsy (31510, 31535, 31536)
🔧 3.29 ⚖ 5.64 **FUD** 010   T A2 💻 P0
AMA: 2014,Jan,11

42806 nasopharynx, survey for unknown primary lesion
EXCLUDES Laryngoscopy with biopsy (31510, 31535, 31536)
🔧 3.83 ⚖ 6.33 **FUD** 010   T A2 💻 P0
AMA: 2014,Jan,11

42808 Excision or destruction of lesion of pharynx, any method
🔧 4.71 ⚖ 6.55 **FUD** 010   T A2 💻
AMA: 2014,Jan,11

42809 Removal of foreign body from pharynx
🔧 3.87 ⚖ 5.02 **FUD** 010   01 N1 💻
AMA: 2014,Jan,11

42810 Excision branchial cleft cyst or vestige, confined to skin and subcutaneous tissues
🔧 8.39 ⚖ 11.2 **FUD** 090   T A2 80 50 💻
AMA: 2014,Jan,11

42815 Excision branchial cleft cyst, vestige, or fistula, extending beneath subcutaneous tissues and/or into pharynx
🔧 16.2 ⚖ 16.2 **FUD** 090   T A2 80 50 💻
AMA: 2014,Jan,11

42820 Tonsillectomy and adenoidectomy; younger than age 12   A
🔧 8.40 ⚖ 8.40 **FUD** 090   T A2 80 💻
AMA: 2015,Jan,16; 2014,Jan,11; 2012,Jan,15-42; 2011,Jan,11

42821 age 12 or over   A
🔧 8.72 ⚖ 8.72 **FUD** 090   T A2 80 💻
AMA: 2015,Jan,16; 2014,Jan,11; 2012,Jan,15-42; 2011,Jan,11

42825 Tonsillectomy, primary or secondary; younger than age 12   A
🔧 7.58 ⚖ 7.58 **FUD** 090   T A2 80 💻
AMA: 2015,Jan,16; 2014,Jan,11; 2012,Jan,15-42; 2011,Jan,11

42826 age 12 or over   A
🔧 7.28 ⚖ 7.28 **FUD** 090   T A2
AMA: 2015,Jan,16; 2014,Jan,11; 2012,Jan,15-42; 2011,Jan,11; 2010,Apr,10

42830 Adenoidectomy, primary; younger than age 12   A
🔧 6.02 ⚖ 6.02 **FUD** 090   T A2 80 💻
AMA: 2015,Jan,16; 2014,Jan,11

42831 age 12 or over   A
🔧 6.47 ⚖ 6.47 **FUD** 090   T A2 80 💻
AMA: 2015,Jan,16; 2014,Jan,11

42835 Adenoidectomy, secondary; younger than age 12   A
🔧 5.60 ⚖ 5.60 **FUD** 090   T A2 80 💻
AMA: 2015,Jan,16; 2014,Jan,11

42836 age 12 or over   A
🔧 6.98 ⚖ 6.98 **FUD** 090   T A2 80 💻
AMA: 2015,Jan,16; 2014,Jan,11; 2012,Jan,15-42; 2011,Jan,11; 2010,Nov,8

42842 Radical resection of tonsil, tonsillar pillars, and/or retromolar trigone; without closure
🔧 28.8 ⚖ 28.8 **FUD** 090   T 80 💻
AMA: 2015,Jan,16; 2014,Jan,11; 2010,Aug,3-7; 2010,Aug,3-7

42844 closure with local flap (eg, tongue, buccal)
🔧 39.6 ⚖ 39.6 **FUD** 090   T 80 💻
AMA: 2015,Jan,16; 2014,Jan,11; 2010,Aug,3-7; 2010,Aug,3-7

42845 closure with other flap
Code also closure with other flap(s)
Code also radical neck dissection when combined (38720)
🔧 64.1 ⚖ 64.1 **FUD** 090   C 80 💻
AMA: 2015,Jan,16; 2014,Jan,11; 2010,Aug,3-7; 2010,Aug,3-7

42860 Excision of tonsil tags
🔧 5.47 ⚖ 5.47 **FUD** 090   T A2 80 💻
AMA: 2014,Jan,11

Tonsillar tags or polyps are removed
Snare
Electrocautery tool

42870 **Excision or destruction lingual tonsil, any method (separate procedure)**

EXCLUDES *Nasopharynx resection (juvenile angiofibroma) by transzygomatic/bicoronal approach (61586, 61600)*

🔧 16.7 ♦ 16.7 **FUD** 090   T A2 80 ▢

AMA: 2014,Jan,11

42890 **Limited pharyngectomy**

Code also radical neck dissection when combined (38720)

🔧 40.8 ♦ 40.8 **FUD** 090   T A2 80 ▢

AMA: 2014,Jan,11; 2010,Aug,3-7; 2010,Aug,3-7

Side view of the pharynx

Nasopharynx region

Epiglottis

Larynx

Esophagus

Oropharynx region

Hypopharynx region

The nasopharynx is the membranous passage above the level of the soft palate; the oropharynx is the region between the soft palate and the upper edge of the epiglottis; the hypopharynx is the region of the epiglottis to the juncture of the larynx and esophagus; the three regions are collectively known as the pharynx

42892 **Resection of lateral pharyngeal wall or pyriform sinus, direct closure by advancement of lateral and posterior pharyngeal walls**

Code also radical neck dissection when combined (38720)

🔧 54.3 ♦ 54.3 **FUD** 090   T A2 80 ▢

AMA: 2015,Jan,16; 2014,Jan,11; 2010,Aug,3-7; 2010,Aug,3-7

42894 **Resection of pharyngeal wall requiring closure with myocutaneous or fasciocutaneous flap or free muscle, skin, or fascial flap with microvascular anastomosis**

EXCLUDES *Flap used for reconstruction (15732, 15734, 15756-15758)*

Code also radical neck dissection when combined (38720)

🔧 68.1 ♦ 68.1 **FUD** 090   C 80 ▢

AMA: 2015,Jan,16; 2014,Jan,11; 2012,Jan,15-42; 2011,Jan,11; 2010,Aug,3-7; 2010,Aug,3-7

42900 **Suture pharynx for wound or injury**

🔧 9.82 ♦ 9.82 **FUD** 010   T A2 80 ▢

AMA: 2014,Jan,11

42950 **Pharyngoplasty (plastic or reconstructive operation on pharynx)**

EXCLUDES *Pharyngeal flap (42225)*

🔧 22.9 ♦ 22.9 **FUD** 090   T A2 80 ▢

AMA: 2014,Jan,11

42953 **Pharyngoesophageal repair**

Code also closure using myocutaneous or other flap

🔧 27.6 ♦ 27.6 **FUD** 090   C 80 ▢

AMA: 2014,Jan,11

42955 **Pharyngostomy (fistulization of pharynx, external for feeding)**

🔧 21.7 ♦ 21.7 **FUD** 090   T A2 80 ▢

AMA: 2014,Jan,11

42960 **Control oropharyngeal hemorrhage, primary or secondary (eg, post-tonsillectomy); simple**

🔧 4.95 ♦ 4.95 **FUD** 010   T A2 80 ▢

AMA: 2014,Jan,11

42961 **complicated, requiring hospitalization**

🔧 12.2 ♦ 12.2 **FUD** 090   C 80 ▢

AMA: 2014,Jan,11

42962 **with secondary surgical intervention**

🔧 15.0 ♦ 15.0 **FUD** 090   T A2 ▢

AMA: 2014,Jan,11

42970 **Control of nasopharyngeal hemorrhage, primary or secondary (eg, postadenoidectomy); simple, with posterior nasal packs, with or without anterior packs and/or cautery**

🔧 12.0 ♦ 12.0 **FUD** 090   T R2 ▢

AMA: 2014,Jan,11

42971 **complicated, requiring hospitalization**

🔧 13.2 ♦ 13.2 **FUD** 090   C 80 ▢

AMA: 2014,Jan,11

42972 **with secondary surgical intervention**

🔧 14.8 ♦ 14.8 **FUD** 090   T A2 80 ▢

AMA: 2014,Jan,11

42999 **Unlisted procedure, pharynx, adenoids, or tonsils**

🔧 0.00 ♦ 0.00 **FUD** YYY   T 80

AMA: 2015,Jan,16; 2014,Feb,11; 2014,Jan,11

43020-43135 Incision/Resection of Esophagus

EXCLUDES *Gastrointestinal reconstruction for previous esophagectomy (43360, 43361)*
Gastrotomy with intraluminal tube insertion (43510)

43020 **Esophagotomy, cervical approach, with removal of foreign body**

EXCLUDES *Laparotomy with esophageal intubation (43510)*

🔧 16.3 ♦ 16.3 **FUD** 090   T 80 ▢ PQ

AMA: 2014,Jan,11

43030 **Cricopharyngeal myotomy**

EXCLUDES *Laparotomy with esophageal intubation (43510)*

🔧 15.0 ♦ 15.0 **FUD** 090   T G2 80 ▢ PQ

AMA: 2014,Jan,11

43045 **Esophagotomy, thoracic approach, with removal of foreign body**

EXCLUDES *Laparotomy with esophageal intubation (43510)*

🔧 37.9 ♦ 37.9 **FUD** 090   C 80 ▢ PQ

AMA: 2014,Jan,11

43100 **Excision of lesion, esophagus, with primary repair; cervical approach**

EXCLUDES *Wide excision of malignant lesion of cervical esophagus, with total laryngectomy:*
With radical neck dissection (31365, 43107, 43116, 43124)
Without radical neck dissection (31360, 43107, 43116, 43124)

🔧 18.1 ♦ 18.1 **FUD** 090   C 80 ▢ PQ

AMA: 2014,Jan,11

43101 **thoracic or abdominal approach**

EXCLUDES *Wide excision of malignant lesion of cervical esophagus with total laryngectomy:*
With radical neck dissection (31365, 43107, 43116, 43124)
Without radical neck dissection (31360, 43107, 43116, 43124)

🔧 30.8 ♦ 30.8 **FUD** 090   C 80 ▢ PQ

AMA: 2015,Jan,16; 2014,Jan,11; 2010,Aug,3-7; 2010,Aug,3-7

43107 **Total or near total esophagectomy, without thoracotomy; with pharyngogastrostomy or cervical esophagogastrostomy, with or without pyloroplasty (transhiatal)**

🔧 74.4 ♦ 74.4 **FUD** 090   C 80 ▢ PQ

AMA: 2014,Jan,11; 2010,Aug,3-7; 2010,Aug,3-7

43108 **with colon interposition or small intestine reconstruction, including intestine mobilization, preparation and anastomosis(es)**

🔧 136. ♦ 136. **FUD** 090   C 80 ▢ PQ

AMA: 2014,Jan,11

43112 **Total or near total esophagectomy, with thoracotomy; with pharyngogastrostomy or cervical esophagogastrostomy, with or without pyloroplasty**

🔧 78.4 ♦ 78.4 **FUD** 090   C 80 ▢ PQ

AMA: 2015,Jan,16; 2014,Jan,11; 2013,Aug,13

● New Code   ▲ Revised Code   ○ Reinstated   M Maternity   A Age Edit   Unlisted   Not Covered   # Resequenced
⊘ AMA Mod 51 Exempt   91 Optum Mod 51 Exempt   63 Mod 63 Exempt   ⊙ Mod Sedation   + Add-on   CCI   PQ PQRS   **FUD** Follow-up Days

© 2015 Optum360, LLC (Blue Text)   CPT © 2015 American Medical Association. All Rights Reserved. (Black Text)   Medicare (Red Text)   **163**

Digestive System

43113 — **43196**

43113   with colon interposition or small intestine reconstruction, including intestine mobilization, preparation, and anastomosis(es)
🔧 127.   ⚕ 127.   **FUD** 090   C 80 ▣ PQ
AMA: 2014,Jan,11

43116   Partial esophagectomy, cervical, with free intestinal graft, including microvascular anastomosis, obtaining the graft and intestinal reconstruction
INCLUDES   Operating microscope (69990)
EXCLUDES   *Free jejunal graft with microvascular anastomosis done by a different physician (43496)*
Code also modifier 52 if intestinal or free jejunal graft with microvascular anastomosis is done by another physician
🔧 151.   ⚕ 151.   **FUD** 090   C 80 ▣ PQ
AMA: 2014,Jan,11; 2010,Aug,3-7; 2010,Aug,3-7

43117   Partial esophagectomy, distal two-thirds, with thoracotomy and separate abdominal incision, with or without proximal gastrectomy; with thoracic esophagogastrostomy, with or without pyloroplasty (Ivor Lewis)
EXCLUDES   *Esophagogastrectomy (lower third) and vagotomy (43122)*
Total esophagectomy with gastropharyngostomy (43107, 43124)
🔧 71.7   ⚕ 71.7   **FUD** 090   C 80 ▣ PQ
AMA: 2014,Jan,11

43118   with colon interposition or small intestine reconstruction, including intestine mobilization, preparation, and anastomosis(es)
EXCLUDES   *Esophagogastrectomy (lower third) and vagotomy (43122)*
Total esophagectomy with gastropharyngostomy (43107, 43124)
🔧 111.   ⚕ 111.   **FUD** 090   C 80 ▣ PQ
AMA: 2014,Jan,11

43121   Partial esophagectomy, distal two-thirds, with thoracotomy only, with or without proximal gastrectomy, with thoracic esophagogastrostomy, with or without pyloroplasty
🔧 83.6   ⚕ 83.6   **FUD** 090   C 80 ▣ PQ
AMA: 2014,Jan,11

43122   Partial esophagectomy, thoracoabdominal or abdominal approach, with or without proximal gastrectomy; with esophagogastrostomy, with or without pyloroplasty
🔧 74.3   ⚕ 74.3   **FUD** 090   C 80 ▣ PQ
AMA: 2014,Jan,11

43123   with colon interposition or small intestine reconstruction, including intestine mobilization, preparation, and anastomosis(es)
🔧 138.   ⚕ 138.   **FUD** 090   C 80 ▣ PQ
AMA: 2014,Jan,11

43124   Total or partial esophagectomy, without reconstruction (any approach), with cervical esophagostomy
🔧 111.   ⚕ 111.   **FUD** 090   C 80 ▣ PQ
AMA: 2015,Jan,16; 2014,Jan,11; 2010,Aug,3-7; 2010,Aug,3-7

43130   Diverticulectomy of hypopharynx or esophagus, with or without myotomy; cervical approach
EXCLUDES   *Diverticulectomy hypopharynx or cervical esophagus, endoscopic (43180)*
🔧 22.8   ⚕ 22.8   **FUD** 090   T G2 80 ▣ PQ
AMA: 2015,Jan,16; 2014,Jan,11; 2012,Jan,15-42; 2011,Jan,11; 2010,Dec,12

43135   thoracic approach
EXCLUDES   *Diverticulectomy hypopharynx or cervical esophagus, endoscopic (43180)*
🔧 43.4   ⚕ 43.4   **FUD** 090   C 80 ▣ PQ
AMA: 2015,Jan,16; 2014,Jan,11; 2012,Jan,15-42; 2011,Jan,11; 2010,Dec,12

43180-43233 [43211, 43212, 43213, 43214] Endoscopic Procedures: Esophagus

INCLUDES   Control of bleeding as result of the endoscopic procedure during same operative session
Diagnostic endoscopy with surgical endoscopy
Examination of upper esophageal sphincter (cricopharyngeus muscle) to/including the gastroesophageal junction
Retroflexion examination of proximal region of stomach

43180   Esophagoscopy, rigid, transoral with diverticulectomy of hypopharynx or cervical esophagus (eg, Zenker's diverticulum), with cricopharyngeal myotomy, includes use of telescope or operating microscope and repair, when performed
🔧 16.1   ⚕ 16.1   **FUD** 090   T G2
INCLUDES   Operating microscope (69990)
EXCLUDES   *Open diverticulectomy hypopharynx or esophagus (43130-43135)*
Do not report with (43210)

43191   Esophagoscopy, rigid, transoral; diagnostic, including collection of specimen(s) by brushing or washing when performed (separate procedure)
EXCLUDES   *Flexible, transnasal (43197-43198)*
Flexible, transoral (43200)
Do not report with (43192-43198, 43210)
🔧 4.45   ⚕ 4.45   **FUD** 000   T G2
AMA: 2015,Jan,16; 2014,Feb,9; 2014,Jan,11; 2013,Dec,3

43192   with directed submucosal injection(s), any substance
EXCLUDES   *Flexible, transoral (43201)*
Injection sclerosis of esophageal varices:
Flexible, transoral (43204)
Rigid, transoral (43499)
Do not report with (43191, 43197-43198)
🔧 4.94   ⚕ 4.94   **FUD** 000   T G2
AMA: 2015,Jan,16; 2014,Feb,9; 2014,Jan,11; 2013,Dec,3

43193   with biopsy, single or multiple
EXCLUDES   *Flexible, transoral (43202)*
Do not report with (43191, 43197-43198)
🔧 4.93   ⚕ 4.93   **FUD** 000   T G2
AMA: 2015,Jan,16; 2014,Feb,9; 2014,Jan,11; 2013,Dec,3

43194   with removal of foreign body(s)
EXCLUDES   *Flexible, transoral (43215)*
Do not report with (43191, 43197-43198)
⬚ (76000)
🔧 5.56   ⚕ 5.56   **FUD** 000   T G2
AMA: 2015,Jan,16; 2014,Feb,9; 2014,Jan,11; 2013,Dec,3

43195   with balloon dilation (less than 30 mm diameter)
EXCLUDES   *Dilation of esophagus:*
Flexible, with balloon diameter 30 mm or larger (43214, 43233)
Flexible, with balloon diameter less than 30 mm (43220)
Without endoscopic visualization (43450-43453)
Do not report with (43191, 43197-43198)
⬚ (74360)
🔧 5.39   ⚕ 5.39   **FUD** 000   T G2
AMA: 2015,Jan,16; 2014,Feb,9; 2014,Jan,11; 2013,Dec,3

43196   with insertion of guide wire followed by dilation over guide wire
EXCLUDES   *Flexible, transoral (43226)*
Do not report with (43191, 43197-43198)
⬚ (74360)
🔧 5.71   ⚕ 5.71   **FUD** 000   T G2
AMA: 2015,Jan,16; 2014,Feb,9; 2014,Jan,11; 2013,Dec,3

43197 **Esophagoscopy, flexible, transnasal; diagnostic, including collection of specimen(s) by brushing or washing, when performed (separate procedure)**

EXCLUDES *Flexible, transoral (43200)*
Rigid, transoral (43191)

Do not report with (31575, 43191-43196, 43198, 43200-43232 [43211, 43212, 43213, 43214], 43235-43259 [43233, 43266, 43270], 92511)

Do not report with diagnostic nasal endoscopy (31231) unless different type of endoscope used

🔧 2.40 ⚖ 5.39 **FUD** 000 T G2

AMA: 2015,Jan,16; 2014,Feb,9; 2014,Jan,11; 2013,Dec,3

43198 **with biopsy, single or multiple**

EXCLUDES *Flexible, transoral (43202)*
Rigid, transoral (43193)

Do not report with (31575, 43191-43197, 43200-43232 [43211, 43212, 43213, 43214], 43235-43259 [43233, 43266, 43270], 92511)

Do not report with diagnostic nasal endoscopy (31231) unless different type of endoscope used

🔧 2.88 ⚖ 6.06 **FUD** 000 T G2

AMA: 2015,Jan,16; 2014,Feb,9; 2014,Jan,11; 2013,Dec,3

43200 **Esophagoscopy, flexible, transoral; diagnostic, including collection of specimen(s) by brushing or washing, when performed (separate procedure)**

EXCLUDES *Flexible, transnasal (43197)*
Rigid, transoral (43191)
Upper gastrointestinal endoscopy (43235)

Do not report with (43197-43198, 43201-43232 [43211, 43212, 43213, 43214])

🔧 2.74 ⚖ 7.75 **FUD** 000 ⊙ T A2 ▣

AMA: 2015,Jan,16; 2014,Feb,9; 2014,Jan,11; 2013,Dec,3; 2013,Feb,16-17; 2013,Jan,11-12; 2012,Jan,15-42; 2011,Jan,11

43201 **with directed submucosal injection(s), any substance**

EXCLUDES *Injection sclerosis of esophageal varices:*
Flexible, transoral (43204)
Rigid, transoral (43192, 43499)

Do not report with (43197-43198, 43200)

Do not report with on same lesion (43204, 43211, 43227)

🔧 3.22 ⚖ 7.92 **FUD** 000 ⊙ T A2 ▣

AMA: 2015,Jan,16; 2014,Feb,9; 2014,Jan,11; 2013,Dec,3; 2013,Jan,11-12; 2010,Jun,4-5

43202 **with biopsy, single or multiple**

EXCLUDES *Flexible, transnasal (43198)*
Rigid, transoral (43193)

Do not report with (43197-43198, 43200)

Do not report with on same lesion (43211)

🔧 3.23 ⚖ 10.4 **FUD** 000 ⊙ T A2 ▣ P0

AMA: 2015,Jan,16; 2014,Feb,9; 2014,Jan,11; 2013,Dec,3; 2013,Jan,11-12

43204 **with injection sclerosis of esophageal varices**

EXCLUDES *Rigid, transoral (43499)*

Do not report with (43197-43198, 43200)

Do not report with on same lesion (43201, 43227)

🔧 4.22 ⚖ 4.22 **FUD** 000 ⊙ T A2 ▣

AMA: 2015,Jan,16; 2014,Feb,9; 2014,Jan,11; 2013,Dec,3; 2013,Jan,11-12; 2010,Jun,4-5

43205 **with band ligation of esophageal varices**

EXCLUDES *Band ligation non-variceal bleeding (43227)*

Do not report with (43197-43198, 43200)

Do not report with on same lesion (43227)

🔧 4.35 ⚖ 4.35 **FUD** 000 ⊙ T A2 ▣

AMA: 2015,Jan,16; 2014,Feb,9; 2014,Jan,11; 2013,Dec,3; 2013,Jan,11-12

43206 **with optical endomicroscopy**

Code also contrast agent

Do not report with (43197-43198, 43200, 88375)

🔧 4.11 ⚖ 9.46 **FUD** 000 ⊙ T G2

AMA: 2015,Jan,16; 2014,Feb,9; 2014,Jan,11; 2013,Dec,3; 2013,Aug,5; 2013,Jan,11-12

43210 Resequenced code. See code following 43259.

43211 Resequenced code. See code following 43217.

43212 Resequenced code. See code following 43217.

43213 Resequenced code. See code following 43220.

43214 Resequenced code. See code following 43220.

43215 **with removal of foreign body(s)**

EXCLUDES *Rigid, transoral (43194)*
Upper gastrointestinal endoscopy (43247)

Do not report with (43197-43198, 43200)

⊠ (76000)

🔧 4.36 ⚖ 11.7 **FUD** 000 ⊙ T A2 ▣

AMA: 2015,Jan,16; 2014,Feb,9; 2014,Jan,11; 2013,Dec,3; 2013,Jan,11-12

43216 **with removal of tumor(s), polyp(s), or other lesion(s) by hot biopsy forceps**

EXCLUDES *Removal by snare technique (43217)*

Do not report with (43197-43198, 43200)

🔧 4.18 ⚖ 12.0 **FUD** 000 ⊙ T A2 ▣

AMA: 2015,Jan,16; 2014,Feb,9; 2014,Jan,11; 2013,Dec,3; 2013,Jan,11-12

43217 **with removal of tumor(s), polyp(s), or other lesion(s) by snare technique**

EXCLUDES *Upper gastrointestinal endoscopy with snare technique (43251)*

Do not report with (43197-43198, 43200)

Do not report with on same lesion (43211)

🔧 4.94 ⚖ 12.8 **FUD** 000 ⊙ T A2 ▣

AMA: 2015,Jan,16; 2014,Feb,9; 2014,Jan,11; 2013,Dec,3; 2013,Jan,11-12

\# **43211** **with endoscopic mucosal resection**

Do not report with (43197-43198, 43200, 43201-43202, 43217)

🔧 7.27 ⚖ 7.27 **FUD** 000 ⊙ T G2

AMA: 2015,Jan,16; 2014,Feb,9; 2014,Jan,11; 2013,Dec,3

\# **43212** **with placement of endoscopic stent (includes pre- and post-dilation and guide wire passage, when performed)**

Do not report with (43197-43198, 43200, 43220, 43226, 43241)

⊠ (74360)

🔧 5.79 ⚖ 5.79 **FUD** 000 ⊙ J G2

AMA: 2015,Jan,16; 2014,Feb,9; 2014,Jan,11; 2013,Dec,3

43220 **with transendoscopic balloon dilation (less than 30 mm diameter)**

EXCLUDES *Dilation of esophagus:*
Rigid, with balloon diameter 30 mm or larger (43214)
Rigid, with balloon diameter less than 30mm (43195)
Without endoscopic visualization (43450, 43453)

Do not report with (43197-43198, 43200, 43212, 43226, 43229)

⊠ (74360)

🔧 3.67 ⚖ 32.4 **FUD** 000 ⊙ T A2 ▣

AMA: 2015,Jan,16; 2014,Feb,9; 2014,Jan,11; 2013,Dec,3; 2013,Jan,11-12; 2012,Jan,15-42; 2011,Jan,11

\# **43213** **with dilation of esophagus, by balloon or dilator, retrograde (includes fluoroscopic guidance, when performed)**

Code also each additional stricture treated in same operative session with modifier 59 and (43213)

Do not report with (43197-43198, 43200, 74360, 76000-76001)

🔧 7.85 ⚖ 35.3 **FUD** 000 ⊙ T G2

AMA: 2015,Jan,16; 2014,Feb,9; 2014,Jan,11; 2013,Dec,3

\# **43214** **with dilation of esophagus with balloon (30 mm diameter or larger) (includes fluoroscopic guidance, when performed)**

Do not report with (43197-43198, 43200, 74360, 76000-76001)

🔧 5.86 ⚖ 5.86 **FUD** 000 ⊙ T G2

AMA: 2015,Jan,16; 2014,Feb,9; 2014,Jan,11; 2013,Dec,3

43226 **with insertion of guide wire followed by passage of dilator(s) over guide wire**

EXCLUDES Rigid, transoral (43196)

Do not report with (43197-43198, 43200, 43212, 43220)

Do not report with on same lesion (43229)

⚕ (74360)

🔧 4.04 ⚗ 10.9 **FUD** 000 ⊙ T A2 ▭

AMA: 2015,Jan,16; 2014,Feb,9; 2014,Jan,11; 2013,Dec,3; 2013,Jan,11-12

43227 **with control of bleeding, any method**

Do not report with (43197-43198, 43200)

Do not report with on same lesion (43201, 43204-43205)

🔧 5.09 ⚗ 11.3 **FUD** 000 ⊙ T A2 ▭

AMA: 2015,Jan,16; 2014,Feb,9; 2014,Feb,11; 2014,Jan,11; 2013,Dec,3; 2013,Jan,11-12; 2010,Jun,4-5

43229 **with ablation of tumor(s), polyp(s), or other lesion(s) (includes pre- and post-dilation and guide wire passage, when performed)**

Code also esophagoscopic photodynamic therapy, when performed (96570-96571)

Do not report with (43197-43198, 43200)

Do not report with on same lesion (43220, 43226)

🔧 6.06 ⚗ 20.8 **FUD** 000 ⊙ T G2

AMA: 2015,Jan,16; 2014,Feb,9; 2014,Jan,11; 2013,Dec,3

43231 **with endoscopic ultrasound examination**

Do not report more than one time per operative session

Do not report with (43197-43198, 43200, 43232, 76975)

🔧 4.94 ⚗ 11.5 **FUD** 000 ⊙ T A2 ▭

AMA: 2015,Jan,16; 2014,Feb,9; 2014,Jan,11; 2013,Dec,3; 2013,Jan,11-12

43232 **with transendoscopic ultrasound-guided intramural or transmural fine needle aspiration/biopsy(s)**

Do not report more than one time per operative session

Do not report with (43197-43198, 43200, 43231, 76942, 76975)

🔧 6.05 ⚗ 13.7 **FUD** 000 ⊙ T A2 ▭

AMA: 2015,Jan,16; 2014,Feb,9; 2014,Jan,11; 2013,Dec,3; 2013,Jan,11-12; 2012,Jan,15-42; 2011,Jan,11

43233 **Resequenced code. See code following 43249.**

43235-43259 [43210, 43233, 43266, 43270] Endoscopic Procedures: Esophagogastroduodenoscopy (EGD)

INCLUDES Control of bleeding as result of the endoscopic procedure during same operative session

Diagnostic endoscopy with surgical endoscopy

EXCLUDES Exam of jejunum distal to the anastomosis in surgically altered stomach, including post-gastroenterostomy (Billroth II) and gastric bypass (43235-43259 [43233, 43266, 43270])

Exam of upper esophageal sphincter (cricopharyngeus muscle) to/including gastroesophageal junction and/or retroflexion exam of proximal region of stomach (43197-43232 [43211, 43212, 43213, 43214])

Code also modifier 52 when duodenum is not examined either deliberately or due to significant issues and repeat procedure will not be performed

Code also modifier 53 when duodenum is not examined either deliberately or due to significant issues and repeat procedure is planned

43235 **Esophagogastroduodenoscopy, flexible, transoral; diagnostic, including collection of specimen(s) by brushing or washing, when performed (separate procedure)**

Do not report with (43197-43198, 43210, 43236-43259 [43233, 43266, 43270], 44360-44379)

🔧 3.82 ⚗ 8.99 **FUD** 000 ⊙ T A2 ▭

AMA: 2015,Jan,16; 2014,Jan,11; 2013,Dec,3; 2013,Jan,11-12; 2012,Jan,15-42; 2011,Jan,11

43236 **with directed submucosal injection(s), any substance**

EXCLUDES Injection sclerosis of varices, esophageal/gastric (43243)

Do not report with (43197-43198, 43235, 44360-44379)

Do not report with on same lesion (43243, 43254-43255)

🔧 4.30 ⚗ 11.2 **FUD** 000 ⊙ T A2 ▭

AMA: 2015,Jan,16; 2014,Jan,11; 2013,Dec,3; 2013,Jan,11-12; 2010,Jun,4-5

43237 **with endoscopic ultrasound examination limited to the esophagus, stomach or duodenum, and adjacent structures**

Do not report more than one time per operative session

Do not report with (43197-43198, 43235, 43238, 43242, 43253, 43259, 44360-44379, 76975)

🔧 6.00 ⚗ 6.00 **FUD** 000 ⊙ T A2 ▭

AMA: 2015,Jan,16; 2014,Jan,11; 2013,Dec,3; 2013,Jan,11-12

43238 **with transendoscopic ultrasound-guided intramural or transmural fine needle aspiration/biopsy(s), (includes endoscopic ultrasound examination limited to the esophagus, stomach or duodenum, and adjacent structures)**

Do not report more than one time per operative session

Do not report with (43197-43198, 43235, 43237, 43242, 44360-44379, 76942, 76975)

🔧 7.14 ⚗ 7.14 **FUD** 000 ⊙ T A2 ▭

AMA: 2015,Jan,16; 2014,Jan,11; 2013,Dec,3; 2013,Jan,11-12

43239 **with biopsy, single or multiple**

Do not report with (43197-43198, 43235, 44360-44379)

Do not report with on same lesion (43254)

🔧 4.29 ⚗ 11.4 **FUD** 000 ⊙ T A2 ▭ P0

AMA: 2015,Jan,16; 2014,Jan,11; 2013,Dec,3; 2013,Jan,11-12; 2012,Jan,15-42; 2011,Jan,11

43240 **with transmural drainage of pseudocyst (includes placement of transmural drainage catheter[s]/stent[s], when performed, and endoscopic ultrasound, when performed)**

EXCLUDES Endoscopic pancreatic necrosectomy (48999)

Do not report more than one time per operative session

Do not report with (43197-43198, 43235, 43242, [43266], 43259, 44360-44379)

Do not report with on same lesion (43253)

🔧 11.8 ⚗ 11.8 **FUD** 000 ⊙ T A2 ▭

AMA: 2015,Jan,16; 2014,Jan,11; 2013,Dec,3; 2013,Jan,11-12

43241 **with insertion of intraluminal tube or catheter**

EXCLUDES Tube placement:

Enteric, non-endoscopic (44500, 74340)

Naso or oro-gastric requiring professional skill and fluoroscopic guidance (43752)

Do not report with (43197-43198, 43212, 43235, [43266], 44360-44379)

🔧 4.40 ⚗ 4.40 **FUD** 000 ⊙ T A2 ▭

AMA: 2015,Jan,16; 2014,Jan,11; 2013,Dec,3; 2013,Jan,11-12

43242 **with transendoscopic ultrasound-guided intramural or transmural fine needle aspiration/biopsy(s) (includes endoscopic ultrasound examination of the esophagus, stomach, and either the duodenum or a surgically altered stomach where the jejunum is examined distal to the anastomosis)**

EXCLUDES Transmural fine needle biopsy/aspiration with ultrasound guidance, transendoscopic, esophagus/stomach/duodenum/neighboring structure (43238)

Do not report more than one time per operative session

Do not report with (43197-43198, 43235, 43237-43238, 43240, 43259, 44360-44379, 76942, 76975)

🔬 88172-88173

🔧 8.05 ⚗ 8.05 **FUD** 000 ⊙ T A2 ▭

AMA: 2015,Jan,16; 2014,Jan,11; 2013,Dec,3; 2013,Jan,11-12

43243 **with injection sclerosis of esophageal/gastric varices**

Do not report with (43197-43198, 43235, 44360-44379)

Do not report with on same lesion (43236, 43255)

🔧 7.25 ⚗ 7.25 **FUD** 000 ⊙ T A2 ▭

AMA: 2015,Jan,16; 2014,Jan,11; 2013,Dec,3; 2013,Jan,11-12; 2010,Jun,4-5

43244 **with band ligation of esophageal/gastric varices**

EXCLUDES   *Band ligation, non-variceal bleeding (43255)*

Do not report with (43197-43198, 43235, 43255, 44360-44379)

📖 7.52   ⚕ 7.52   **FUD** 000   ⊙ T A2 ▭

AMA: 2015,Jan,16; 2014,Jan,11; 2013,Dec,3; 2013,Jan,11-12; 2012,Jan,15-42; 2011,Jun,13

43245 **with dilation of gastric/duodenal stricture(s) (eg, balloon, bougie)**

Do not report with (43197-43198, 43235, [43266], 44360-44379)

⟰ (74360)

📖 5.39   ⚕ 17.6   **FUD** 000

AMA: 2015,Jan,16; 2014,Jan,11; 2013,Dec,3; 2013,Jan,11-12; 2012,Jan,15-42; 2011,Jan,11

43246 **with directed placement of percutaneous gastrostomy tube**

EXCLUDES   *Gastrostomy tube replacement without endoscopy or imaging (43760)*
         Percutaneous insertion of gastrostomy tube, nonendoscopic (49440)

Do not report with (43197-43198, 43235, 44360-44372, 44376-44379)

📖 6.11   ⚕ 6.11   **FUD** 000   ⊙ T A2 80 ▭

AMA: 2015,Jan,16; 2014,Jan,11; 2013,Dec,3; 2013,May,12; 2013,Jan,11-12; 2012,Jan,15-42; 2011,Jan,11; 2010,Mar,9-11

43247 **with removal of foreign body(s)**

Do not report with (43197-43198, 43235, 44360-44379)

⟰ (76000)

📖 5.45   ⚕ 11.7   **FUD** 000   ⊙ T A2 ▭

AMA: 2015,Jan,16; 2014,Jan,11; 2013,Dec,3; 2013,Jan,11-12; 2012,Jan,15-42; 2011,Jan,11

43248 **with insertion of guide wire followed by passage of dilator(s) through esophagus over guide wire**

Do not report with (43197-43198, 43235, [43266], [43270], 44360-44379)

⟰ (74360)

📖 5.14   ⚕ 11.8   **FUD** 000   ⊙ T A2 ▭

AMA: 2015,Jan,16; 2014,Jan,11; 2013,Dec,3; 2013,Jan,11-12; 2012,Jan,15-42; 2011,Jan,11

43249 **with transendoscopic balloon dilation of esophagus (less than 30 mm diameter)**

Do not report with (43197-43198, 43235, [43266], [43270], 44360-44379)

⟰ (74360)

📖 4.75   ⚕ 31.0   **FUD** 000   ⊙ T A2 ▭

AMA: 2015,Jan,16; 2014,Jan,11; 2013,Dec,3; 2013,Jan,11-12

\# **43233** **with dilation of esophagus with balloon (30 mm diameter or larger) (includes fluoroscopic guidance, when performed)**

Do not report with (43197-43198, 43235, 44360-44379, 74360, 76000-76001)

📖 6.91   ⚕ 6.91   **FUD** 000   ⊙ T G2

AMA: 2015,Jan,16; 2014,Jan,11; 2013,Dec,3

43250 **with removal of tumor(s), polyp(s), or other lesion(s) by hot biopsy forceps**

Do not report with (43197-43198, 43235, 44360-44379)

📖 5.22   ⚕ 13.1   **FUD** 000   ⊙ T A2 ▭

AMA: 2015,Jan,16; 2014,Jan,11; 2013,Dec,3; 2013,Jan,11-12; 2012,Jan,15-42; 2011,Jan,11

43251 **with removal of tumor(s), polyp(s), or other lesion(s) by snare technique**

INCLUDES   *Do not report with on same lesion (43254)*
EXCLUDES   *Endoscopic mucosal resection (43254)*

Do not report with (43197-43198, 43235, 44360-44379)

📖 6.02   ⚕ 14.4   **FUD** 000   ⊙ T A2 ▭

AMA: 2015,Jan,16; 2014,Jan,11; 2013,Dec,3; 2013,Jan,11-12; 2012,Jan,15-42; 2011,Jun,13

43252 **with optical endomicroscopy**

Code also contrast agent

Do not report with (43197-43198, 43235, 44360-44379, 88375)

📖 5.21   ⚕ 10.5   **FUD** 000   ⊙ T G2 ▭

AMA: 2015,Jan,16; 2014,Jan,11; 2013,Dec,3; 2013,Aug,5; 2013,Jan,11-12

43253 **with transendoscopic ultrasound-guided transmural injection of diagnostic or therapeutic substance(s) (eg, anesthetic, neurolytic agent) or fiducial marker(s) (includes endoscopic ultrasound examination of the esophagus, stomach, and either the duodenum or a surgically altered stomach where the jejunum is examined distal to the anastomosis)**

EXCLUDES   *Transmural fine needle biopsy/aspiration with ultrasound guidance, transendoscopic, esophagus/stomach/duodenum/neighboring structures (43238, 43242)*

Do not report more than one time per operative session
Do not report on same lesion with (43240)
Do not report with (43197-43198, 43235, 43237, 43259, 44360-44379, 76942, 76975)

📖 8.05   ⚕ 8.05   **FUD** 000   ⊙ T G2

AMA: 2015,Jan,16; 2014,Jan,11; 2013,Dec,3

43254 **with endoscopic mucosal resection**

Do not report with (43197-43198, 43235, 44360-44379)
Do not report with on same lesion (43236, 43239, 43251)

📖 8.25   ⚕ 8.25   **FUD** 000   ⊙ T G2

AMA: 2015,Jan,16; 2014,Jan,11; 2013,Dec,3

43255 **with control of bleeding, any method**

Do not report with (43197-43198, 43235, 44360-44379)
Do not report with on same lesion (43236, 43243-43244)

📖 6.17   ⚕ 12.4   **FUD** 000   ⊙ T A2 ▭

AMA: 2015,Jan,16; 2014,Jan,11; 2013,Dec,3; 2013,Jan,11-12; 2010,Jun,4-5

\# **43266** **with placement of endoscopic stent (includes pre- and post-dilation and guide wire passage, when performed)**

Do not report with (43197-43198, 43235, 43240-43241, 43245, 43248-43249, 44360-44379)

⟰ (74360)

📖 6.92   ⚕ 6.92   **FUD** 000   ⊙ J G2

AMA: 2015,Jan,16; 2014,Jan,11; 2013,Dec,3

43257 **with delivery of thermal energy to the muscle of lower esophageal sphincter and/or gastric cardia, for treatment of gastroesophageal reflux disease**

EXCLUDES   *Esophageal lesion ablation (43229, [43270])*

Do not report with (43197-43198, 43235, 44360-44379)

📖 7.11   ⚕ 7.11   **FUD** 000   ⊙ T A2 ▭

AMA: 2015,Jan,16; 2014,Jan,11; 2013,Dec,3; 2013,Jan,11-12

\# **43270** **with ablation of tumor(s), polyp(s), or other lesion(s) (includes pre- and post-dilation and guide wire passage, when performed)**

Code also esophagoscopic photodynamic therapy, when performed (96570-96571)

Do not report with (43197-43198, 43235, 43248-43249, 44360-44379)

📖 7.13   ⚕ 21.7   **FUD** 000   ⊙ T G2

AMA: 2015,Jan,16; 2014,Jan,11; 2013,Dec,3

43259 **with endoscopic ultrasound examination, including the esophagus, stomach, and either the duodenum or a surgically altered stomach where the jejunum is examined distal to the anastomosis**

Do not report more than one time per operative session
Do not report with (43197-43198, 43235, 43237, 43240, 43242, 43253, 44360-44379, 76975)

📖 6.93   ⚕ 6.93   **FUD** 000   ⊙ T A2 ▭

AMA: 2015,Jan,16; 2014,Jan,11; 2013,Dec,3; 2013,Jan,11-12

● \# **43210** **with esophagogastric fundoplasty, partial or complete, includes duodenoscopy when performed**

📖 0.00   ⚕ 0.00   **FUD** 000

Do not report with (43180, 43191, 43197, 43200, 43235)

● New Code   ▲ Revised Code   ○ Reinstated   M Maternity   A Age Edit   Unlisted   Not Covered   \# Resequenced
⊘ AMA Mod 51 Exempt   51 Optum Mod 51 Exempt   63 Mod 63 Exempt   ⊙ Mod Sedation   + Add-on   ▭ CCI   PQ PQRS   FUD Follow-up Days

© 2015 Optum360, LLC (Blue Text)   CPT © 2015 American Medical Association. All Rights Reserved. (Black Text)   Medicare (Red Text)   167

43260-43278 [43274, 43275, 43276, 43277, 43278]
Endoscopic Procedures: ERCP

INCLUDES Diagnostic endoscopy with surgical endoscopy
Pancreaticobiliary system:
 Biliary tree (right and left hepatic ducts, cystic duct/gallbladder, and common bile ducts)
 Pancreas (major and minor ducts)

EXCLUDES *ERCP via Roux-en-Y anatomy (for instance post-gastric or bariatric bypass or post total gastrectomy) or via gastrostomy (open or laparoscopic) (47999, 48999)*
Optical endomicroscopy of biliary tract and pancreas, report one time per session (0397T)
Percutaneous biliary catheter procedures (47490-47544)

Code also appropriate endoscopy of each anatomic site examined
Code also sphincteroplasty or ductal stricture dilation, when performed prior to the debris/stone removal from the duct ([43277])
Code also the appropriate ERCP procedure when performed on altered postoperative anatomy (i.e. Billroth II gastroenterostomy)
⊠ (74328-74330)

43260 **Endoscopic retrograde cholangiopancreatography (ERCP); diagnostic, including collection of specimen(s) by brushing or washing, when performed (separate procedure)**

Do not report with (43261-43270 [43274, 43275, 43276, 43277, 43278])

⊅ 9.82   **⊗** 9.82   **FUD** 000   ⊙ T A2 ▭ P0

AMA: 2015,Jan,16; 2014,Jan,11; 2013,Dec,3; 2013,Jan,11-12; 2012,Jan,11-12; 2012,Jan,15-42; 2011,Jan,11

43261 **with biopsy, single or multiple**

EXCLUDES *Percutaneous endoluminal biopsy of biliary tree (47543)*
Do not report with (43260)

⊅ 10.2   **⊗** 10.2   **FUD** 000   ⊙ T A2 ▭ P0

AMA: 2015,Jan,16; 2014,Jan,11; 2013,Dec,3; 2013,Jan,11-12; 2012,Jan,15-42; 2011,Jun,13

43262 **with sphincterotomy/papillotomy**

EXCLUDES *Percutaneous balloon dilation biliary duct or ampulla (47542)*
Code also procedure performed with sphincterotomy (43261, 43263-43265, [43275], [43278])
Do not report with (43260, [43277])
Do not report with placement or exchange of stent in same location ([43274], [43276])

⊅ 10.8   **⊗** 10.8   **FUD** 000   ⊙ T A2 ▭ P0

AMA: 2015,Jan,16; 2014,Jan,11; 2013,Dec,3; 2013,Jan,11-12; 2012,Jan,15-42; 2011,Jan,11

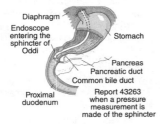

Diaphragm
Endoscope entering the sphincter of Oddi
Stomach
Pancreas
Pancreatic duct
Common bile duct
Proximal duodenum
Report 43263 when a pressure measurement is made of the sphincter

An endoscope is fed through the stomach and into the duodenum. Usually a smaller sub-scope is fed up the sphincter of Oddi and into the ducts that drain the pancreas and the gallbladder (common bile).

43263 **with pressure measurement of sphincter of Oddi**

Do not report more than one time per session
Do not report with (43260)

⊅ 10.8   **⊗** 10.8   **FUD** 000   ⊙ T A2 ▭ P0

AMA: 2015,Jan,16; 2014,Jan,11; 2013,Dec,3; 2013,Jan,11-12

43264 **with removal of calculi/debris from biliary/pancreatic duct(s)**

INCLUDES Incidental dilation due to passage of instrument
EXCLUDES *Percutaneous calculus/debris removal (47544)*
Code also sphincteroplasty when dilation is necessary in order to access the area of debris/stones ([43277])
Do not report if debris or calculi are not found, even if balloon was used
Do not report with (43260, 43265)

⊅ 11.0   **⊗** 11.0   **FUD** 000   ⊙ T A2 ▭ P0

AMA: 2015,Jan,16; 2014,Jan,11; 2013,Dec,3; 2013,Jan,11-12; 2012,Jan,15-42; 2011,Jan,11

43265 **with destruction of calculi, any method (eg, mechanical, electrohydraulic, lithotripsy)**

INCLUDES Incidental dilation due to passage of instrument
 Stone removal when in the same ductal system
EXCLUDES *Percutaneous calculus/debris removal (47544)*
Code also sphincteroplasty when dilation is necessary in order to access the area of debris/stones ([43277])
Do not report if debris or calculi are not found, even if balloon was used
Do not report with (43260, 43264)

⊅ 13.1   **⊗** 13.1   **FUD** 000   ⊙ T A2 ▭ P0

AMA: 2015,Jan,16; 2014,Jan,11; 2013,Dec,3; 2013,Jan,11-12

43266 **Resequenced code. See code following 43255.**

**43274** **with placement of endoscopic stent into biliary or pancreatic duct, including pre- and post-dilation and guide wire passage, when performed, including sphincterotomy, when performed, each stent**

INCLUDES Balloon dilation when in the same duct
 Tube placement for naso-pancreatic or naso-biliary drainage
EXCLUDES *Percutaneous placement biliary stent (47538-47540)*
Code also for each additional stent placement in different ducts or side by side in same duct in same session/day, using modifier 59 with ([43274])
Do not report with the following procedures for stent placement or exchange in the same duct (43262, 43270 [43275, 43276, 43277])

⊅ 14.0   **⊗** 14.0   **FUD** 000   ⊙ J 62

AMA: 2015,Jan,16; 2014,Jan,11; 2013,Dec,3

**43275** **with removal of foreign body(s) or stent(s) from biliary/pancreatic duct(s)**

EXCLUDES *Pancreatic or biliary duct stent removal without ERCP (43247)*
Percutaneous calculus/debris removal (47544)
Do not report more than one time per session
Do not report with (43260, [43274], [43276])

⊅ 11.4   **⊗** 11.4   **FUD** 000   ⊙ T 62

AMA: 2015,Jan,16; 2014,Jan,11; 2013,Dec,3

**43276** **with removal and exchange of stent(s), biliary or pancreatic duct, including pre- and post-dilation and guide wire passage, when performed, including sphincterotomy, when performed, each stent exchanged**

INCLUDES Balloon dilation when in the same duct
 Stent placement or exchange of one stent
Code also each additional stent exchanged in same session/day, using modifier 59 with ([43276])
Do not report for stent insertion or exchange of stent in same duct (43262, [43274])
Do not report with (43260, [43275])

⊅ 14.5   **⊗** 14.5   **FUD** 000   ⊙ J 62

AMA: 2015,Jan,16; 2014,Jan,11; 2013,Dec,3

43270 **Resequenced code. See code following 43257.**

26/TC PC/TC Comp Only   A2-Z3 ASC Pmt   50 Bilateral   ♂ Male Only   ♀ Female Only   ⊅ Facility RVU   ⊗ Non-Facility RVU
AMA: CPT Asst   **CMS:** Pub 100   A-Y OPPSI   80/80 Surg Assist Allowed / w/Doc   ◪ Lab Crosswalk   ⊠ Radiology Crosswalk

with trans-endoscopic balloon dilation of biliary/pancreatic duct(s) or of ampulla (sphincterotomy), including sphincterotomy, when performed, each duct

 # 43277

> *EXCLUDES* *Percutaneous dilation biliary duct/ampulla (47542)*

Code also both right and left hepatic duct (bilateral) balloon dilation, using ([43277]) and append modifier 59 to second procedure

Code also each additional balloon dilation in different ducts or side by side in same duct in same session/day, using modifier 59 with ([43277])

Code also same session sphincterotomy without sphincteroplasty in different duct, using modifier 59 with (43262)

Do not report for same lesion ([43278])

Do not report with (43260, 43262, [43274], [43276])

Do not report with removal of stone/debris when dilation incidental to instrument passage (43264-43265)

⏣ 11.4 ⚘ 11.4 **FUD** 000 ⊙ T 62

AMA: 2015,Jan,16; 2014,Jan,11; 2013,Dec,3

 # 43278 with ablation of tumor(s), polyp(s), or other lesion(s), including pre- and post-dilation and guide wire passage, when performed

> *EXCLUDES* *Ampullectomy (43254)*

Do not report on same lesion with ([43277])

Do not report with (43260)

⏣ 13.1 ⚘ 13.1 **FUD** 000 ⊙ T 62

AMA: 2015,Jan,16; 2014,Jan,11; 2013,Dec,3

+ 43273 Endoscopic cannulation of papilla with direct visualization of pancreatic/common bile duct(s) (List separately in addition to code(s) for primary procedure)

Code first (43260-43270 [43274, 43275, 43276, 43277, 43278])

Do not report more than one time per session

⏣ 3.58 ⚘ 3.58 **FUD** ZZZ ⊙ N M 80

AMA: 2015,Jan,16; 2014,Jan,11; 2013,Dec,3; 2013,Jan,11-12; 2012,Jan,15-42; 2011,Jan,11

43274 Resequenced code. See code following 43265.

43275 Resequenced code. See code following 43265.

43276 Resequenced code. See code following 43265.

43277 Resequenced code. See code before 43273.

43278 Resequenced code. See code before 43273.

43279-43289 Laparoscopic Procedures of Esophagus

> *INCLUDES* Diagnostic laparoscopy with surgical laparoscopy

43279 Laparoscopy, surgical, esophagomyotomy (Heller type), with fundoplasty, when performed

> *EXCLUDES* *Esophagomyotomy, open method (43330-43331)*

Do not report with (43280)

⏣ 37.4 ⚘ 37.4 **FUD** 090 C 80 PQ

AMA: 2015,Jan,16; 2014,Jan,11; 2013,Jan,11-12; 2012,Feb,3-7; 2011,Jun,8-10

43280 Laparoscopy, surgical, esophagogastric fundoplasty (eg, Nissen, Toupet procedures)

> *EXCLUDES* *Esophageal sphincter augmentation (0392T-0393T)*
>
> *Esophagogastric fundoplasty, open method (43327-43328)*
>
> *Esophagogastroduodenoscopy fundoplasty, transoral (43210)*

Do not report with (43279)

⏣ 31.3 ⚘ 31.3 **FUD** 090 T 80 □ PQ

AMA: 2015,Jan,16; 2014,Dec,16; 2014,Dec,16; 2014,Jan,11; 2013,Jan,11-12; 2012,Feb,3-7; 2011,Jun,8-10

43281 Laparoscopy, surgical, repair of paraesophageal hernia, includes fundoplasty, when performed; without implantation of mesh

> *EXCLUDES* *Transabdominal repair of paraesophageal hiatal hernia (43332-43333)*
>
> *Transthoracic repair of diaphragmatic hernia (43334-43335)*

Do not report with (43280, 43450, 43453, 49568)

⏣ 44.7 ⚘ 44.7 **FUD** 090 T 80 PQ

AMA: 2015,Jan,16; 2014,Dec,16; 2014,Dec,16; 2014,Jan,11; 2013,Jan,11-12; 2012,Feb,3-7; 2011,Jun,8-10

43282 with implantation of mesh

> *EXCLUDES* *Transabdominal paraesophageal hernia repair (43332-43333)*
>
> *Transthoracic paraesophageal hernia repair (43334-43335)*

Do not report with (43280, 43450, 43453, 49568)

⏣ 50.3 ⚘ 50.3 **FUD** 090 C 80 PQ

AMA: 2015,Jan,16; 2014,Dec,16; 2014,Dec,16; 2014,Jan,11; 2013,Jan,11-12; 2012,Feb,3-7; 2011,Jun,8-10

+ 43283 Laparoscopy, surgical, esophageal lengthening procedure (eg, Collis gastroplasty or wedge gastroplasty) (List separately in addition to code for primary procedure)

Code first (43280-43282)

⏣ 4.62 ⚘ 4.62 **FUD** ZZZ C 80

AMA: 2015,Jan,16; 2014,Jan,11; 2013,Jan,11-12; 2012,Feb,3-7; 2011,Jun,8-10

43289 Unlisted laparoscopy procedure, esophagus

⏣ 0.00 ⚘ 0.00 **FUD** YYY T 80 50

AMA: 2015,Jan,16; 2014,Dec,16; 2014,Dec,16; 2014,Jan,11; 2013,Jan,11-12

43300-43425 Open Esophageal Repair Procedures

43300 Esophagoplasty (plastic repair or reconstruction), cervical approach; without repair of tracheoesophageal fistula

⏣ 17.8 ⚘ 17.8 **FUD** 090 C 80 □ PQ

AMA: 2014,Jan,11; 2013,Jan,11-12

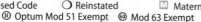

Proximal esophagus

Intestinal esophagus

Diaphragm

Stomach

Thyroid cartilage
Cricoid cartilage
Trachea
Esophagus

43305 with repair of tracheoesophageal fistula

⏣ 31.6 ⚘ 31.6 **FUD** 090 C 80 □ PQ

AMA: 2014,Jan,11; 2013,Jan,11-12

43310 Esophagoplasty (plastic repair or reconstruction), thoracic approach; without repair of tracheoesophageal fistula

⏣ 43.0 ⚘ 43.0 **FUD** 090 C 80 □ PQ

AMA: 2014,Jan,11; 2013,Jan,11-12

43312 with repair of tracheoesophageal fistula

⏣ 46.7 ⚘ 46.7 **FUD** 090 C 80 □ PQ

AMA: 2014,Jan,11; 2013,Jan,11-12

43313 Esophagoplasty for congenital defect (plastic repair or reconstruction), thoracic approach; without repair of congenital tracheoesophageal fistula

⏣ 75.2 ⚘ 75.2 **FUD** 090 63 C 80 □ PQ

AMA: 2014,Jan,11; 2013,Jan,11-12

43314 with repair of congenital tracheoesophageal fistula

⏣ 81.2 ⚘ 81.2 **FUD** 090 63 C 80 □ PQ

AMA: 2014,Jan,11; 2013,Jan,11-12

43320   **Esophagogastrostomy (cardioplasty), with or without vagotomy and pyloroplasty, transabdominal or transthoracic approach**
EXCLUDES   *Laparoscopic approach (43280)*
🏥 40.4   ⚕ 40.4   **FUD** 090   C 80 ▭ PQ
AMA: 2014,Jan,11; 2013,Jan,11-12

43325   **Esophagogastric fundoplasty, with fundic patch (Thal-Nissen procedure)**
EXCLUDES   *Myotomy, cricopharyngeal (43030)*
🏥 38.9   ⚕ 38.9   **FUD** 090   C 80 ▭ PQ
AMA: 2014,Jan,11; 2013,Jan,11-12

43327   **Esophagogastric fundoplasty partial or complete; laparotomy**
🏥 23.6   ⚕ 23.6   **FUD** 090   C 80 PQ
AMA: 2015,Jan,16; 2014,Jan,11; 2013,Jan,11-12; 2012,Feb,3-7; 2011,Jun,8-10

43328   **thoracotomy**
EXCLUDES   *Esophagogastroduodenoscopy fundoplasty, transoral (43210)*
🏥 33.0   ⚕ 33.0   **FUD** 090   C 80 PQ
AMA: 2015,Jan,16; 2014,Jan,11; 2013,Jan,11-12; 2012,Feb,3-7; 2011,Jun,8-10

43330   **Esophagomyotomy (Heller type); abdominal approach**
EXCLUDES   *Esophagomyotomy, laparoscopic method (43279)*
🏥 38.6   ⚕ 38.6   **FUD** 090   C 80 ▭ PQ
AMA: 2015,Jan,16; 2014,Jan,11; 2013,Jan,11-12; 2012,Feb,3-7; 2011,Jun,8-10

43331   **thoracic approach**
EXCLUDES   *Thoracoscopy with esophagomyotomy (32665)*
🏥 39.1   ⚕ 39.1   **FUD** 090   C 80 ▭ PQ
AMA: 2015,Jan,16; 2014,Jan,11; 2013,Jan,11-12; 2012,Feb,3-7; 2011,Jun,8-10

43332   **Repair, paraesophageal hiatal hernia (including fundoplication), via laparotomy, except neonatal; without implantation of mesh or other prosthesis**
EXCLUDES   *Neonatal diaphragmatic hernia repair (39503)*
🏥 33.6   ⚕ 33.6   **FUD** 090   C 80 PQ
AMA: 2015,Jan,16; 2014,Jan,11; 2013,Jan,11-12; 2012,Feb,3-7; 2011,Jun,8-10

43333   **with implantation of mesh or other prosthesis**
EXCLUDES   *Neonatal diaphragmatic hernia repair (39503)*
🏥 36.6   ⚕ 36.6   **FUD** 090   C 80 PQ
AMA: 2015,Jan,16; 2014,Jan,11; 2013,Jan,11-12; 2012,Feb,3-7; 2011,Jun,8-10

43334   **Repair, paraesophageal hiatal hernia (including fundoplication), via thoracotomy, except neonatal; without implantation of mesh or other prosthesis**
EXCLUDES   *Neonatal diaphragmatic hernia repair (39503)*
🏥 36.4   ⚕ 36.4   **FUD** 090   C 80 ▭ PQ
AMA: 2015,Jan,16; 2014,Jan,11; 2013,Jan,11-12; 2012,Feb,3-7; 2011,Jun,8-10

43335   **with implantation of mesh or other prosthesis**
EXCLUDES   *Neonatal diaphragmatic hernia repair (39503)*
🏥 39.2   ⚕ 39.2   **FUD** 090   C 80 PQ
AMA: 2015,Jan,16; 2014,Jan,11; 2013,Jan,11-12; 2012,Feb,3-7; 2011,Jun,8-10

43336   **Repair, paraesophageal hiatal hernia, (including fundoplication), via thoracoabdominal incision, except neonatal; without implantation of mesh or other prosthesis**
EXCLUDES   *Neonatal diaphragmatic hernia repair (39503)*
🏥 44.1   ⚕ 44.1   **FUD** 090   C 80 PQ
AMA: 2015,Jan,16; 2014,Jan,11; 2013,Jan,11-12; 2012,Feb,3-7; 2011,Jun,8-10

43337   **with implantation of mesh or other prosthesis**
EXCLUDES   *Neonatal diaphragmatic hernia repair (39503)*
🏥 47.4   ⚕ 47.4   **FUD** 090   C 80 PQ
AMA: 2015,Jan,16; 2014,Jan,11; 2013,Jan,11-12; 2012,Feb,3-7; 2011,Jun,8-10

+ **43338**   **Esophageal lengthening procedure (eg, Collis gastroplasty or wedge gastroplasty) (List separately in addition to code for primary procedure)**
Code first (43280, 43327-43337)
🏥 3.38   ⚕ 3.38   **FUD** ZZZ   C 80
AMA: 2015,Jan,16; 2014,Jan,11; 2013,Jan,11-12; 2012,Feb,3-7; 2011,Jun,8-10

43340   **Esophagojejunostomy (without total gastrectomy); abdominal approach**
🏥 39.9   ⚕ 39.9   **FUD** 090   C 80 ▭ PQ
AMA: 2014,Jan,11; 2013,Jan,11-12

43341   **thoracic approach**
🏥 42.9   ⚕ 42.9   **FUD** 090   C 80 ▭ PQ
AMA: 2014,Jan,11; 2013,Jan,11-12

43351   **Esophagostomy, fistulization of esophagus, external; thoracic approach**
🏥 40.3   ⚕ 40.3   **FUD** 090   C 80 ▭ PQ
AMA: 2014,Jan,11; 2013,Jan,11-12

43352   **cervical approach**
🏥 31.1   ⚕ 31.1   **FUD** 090   C 80 ▭ PQ
AMA: 2014,Jan,11; 2013,Jan,11-12

43360   **Gastrointestinal reconstruction for previous esophagectomy, for obstructing esophageal lesion or fistula, or for previous esophageal exclusion; with stomach, with or without pyloroplasty**
🏥 69.1   ⚕ 69.1   **FUD** 090   C 80 ▭ PQ
AMA: 2014,Jan,11; 2013,Jan,11-12

43361   **with colon interposition or small intestine reconstruction, including intestine mobilization, preparation, and anastomosis(es)**
🏥 74.5   ⚕ 74.5   **FUD** 090   C 80 ▭ PQ
AMA: 2014,Jan,11; 2013,Jan,11-12

43400   **Ligation, direct, esophageal varices**
🏥 44.1   ⚕ 44.1   **FUD** 090   C 80 ▭ PQ
AMA: 2014,Jan,11; 2013,Jan,11-12

43401   **Transection of esophagus with repair, for esophageal varices**
🏥 45.5   ⚕ 45.5   **FUD** 090   C 80 ▭ PQ
AMA: 2014,Jan,11; 2013,Jan,11-12

43405   **Ligation or stapling at gastroesophageal junction for pre-existing esophageal perforation**
🏥 44.6   ⚕ 44.6   **FUD** 090   C 80 ▭ PQ
AMA: 2014,Jan,11; 2013,Jan,11-12

43410   **Suture of esophageal wound or injury; cervical approach**
🏥 30.5   ⚕ 30.5   **FUD** 090   C 80 ▭ PQ
AMA: 2015,Jan,16; 2014,Jan,11; 2013,Jan,11-12

43415   **transthoracic or transabdominal approach**
🏥 74.6   ⚕ 74.6   **FUD** 090   C 80 ▭ PQ
AMA: 2014,Jan,11; 2013,Jan,11-12

43420   **Closure of esophagostomy or fistula; cervical approach**
EXCLUDES   *Paraesophageal hiatal hernia repair:*
             Transabdominal (43332-43333)
             Transthoracic (43334-43335)
🏥 29.5   ⚕ 29.5   **FUD** 090   T 80 ▭ PQ
AMA: 2014,Jan,11; 2013,Jan,11-12

43425   **transthoracic or transabdominal approach**
EXCLUDES   *Paraesophageal hiatal hernia repair:*
             Transabdominal (43332-43333)
             Transthoracic (43334-43335)
🏥 42.2   ⚕ 42.2   **FUD** 090   C 80 ▭ PQ
AMA: 2014,Jan,11; 2013,Jan,11-12

43450-43453 Esophageal Dilation

43450 Dilation of esophagus, by unguided sound or bougie, single or multiple passes

📷 (74220, 74360)

💰 2.54 ⚕ 6.12 **FUD** 000   T A2 ▢

AMA: 2015,Jan,16; 2014,Jan,11; 2013,Dec,3; 2013,Jan,11-12; 2012,Jan,15-42; 2011,Jan,11

43453 Dilation of esophagus, over guide wire

EXCLUDES *Dilation performed with direct visualization (43195, 43226)*

Endoscopic dilation by dilator or balloon:
Balloon diameter 30 mm or larger (43214, 43233)
Balloon diameter less than 30 mm (43195, 43220, 43249)

📷 (74220, 74360)

💰 2.73 ⚕ 27.9 **FUD** 000   ⊙ T A2 ▢

AMA: 2015,Jan,16; 2014,Jan,11; 2013,Dec,3; 2013,Jan,11-12; 2012,Jan,15-42; 2011,Jan,11

43460-43499 Other/Unlisted Esophageal Procedures

43460 Esophagogastric tamponade, with balloon (Sengstaken type)

EXCLUDES *Removal of foreign body of the esophagus with balloon catheter (43499, 74235)*

📷 (74220)

💰 6.38 ⚕ 6.38 **FUD** 000   C ▢

AMA: 2014,Jan,11; 2013,Jan,11-12

In 43460, laryngoscope guides tube through vocal cords

Gastric aspiration tube
Endotracheal tube
Tube to gastric balloon
Esophagus
Tube to esophageal balloon
Inflated cuff
Esophageal balloon
Diaphragm
Fundus of stomach
Side view schematic (above) of inflated endotracheal cuff generally used to provide air passage and prevent tracheal collapse
Inferior esophageal sphincter
Cutaway view of Sengstaken-type esophagogastric tamponade with balloons inflated
Gastric balloon and aspiration tube

43496 Free jejunum transfer with microvascular anastomosis

INCLUDES Operating microscope (69990)

💰 0.00 ⚕ 0.00 **FUD** 090   C 80 ▢ PQ

AMA: 2015,Jan,16; 2014,Jan,11; 2013,Jan,11-12

43499 Unlisted procedure, esophagus

💰 0.00 ⚕ 0.00 **FUD** YYY   T

AMA: 2015,Jan,16; 2014,Jan,11; 2013,Dec,3; 2013,Mar,13; 2013,Jan,11-12; 2012,Jan,15-42; 2011,Dec,19; 2011,May,9; 2011,Jan,11; 2010,Dec,12

43500-43641 Open Gastric Incisional and Resection Procedures

43500 Gastrotomy; with exploration or foreign body removal

💰 22.6 ⚕ 22.6 **FUD** 090   C 80 ▢ PQ

AMA: 2014,Jan,11; 2013,Jan,11-12

Esophagus
Mucosal and muscle layers
Fundus
Esophagus
Cardiac notch
Rugae (folds lining the stomach)
Pyloric sphincter
Diaphragm
Inner stomach
Duodenum

43501 with suture repair of bleeding ulcer

💰 39.0 ⚕ 39.0 **FUD** 090   C 80 ▢ PQ

AMA: 2014,Jan,11; 2013,Jan,11-12

43502 with suture repair of pre-existing esophagogastric laceration (eg, Mallory-Weiss)

💰 44.1 ⚕ 44.1 **FUD** 090   C 80 ▢ PQ

AMA: 2014,Jan,11; 2013,Jan,11-12

43510 with esophageal dilation and insertion of permanent intraluminal tube (eg, Celestin or Mousseaux-Barbin)

💰 27.3 ⚕ 27.3 **FUD** 090   T 80 ▢ PQ

AMA: 2014,Jan,11; 2013,Jan,11-12

43520 Pyloromyotomy, cutting of pyloric muscle (Fredet-Ramstedt type operation)

💰 19.8 ⚕ 19.8 **FUD** 090   63 C 80 ▢ PQ

AMA: 2014,Jan,11; 2013,Jan,11-12

43605 Biopsy of stomach, by laparotomy

💰 24.1 ⚕ 24.1 **FUD** 090   C 80 ▢ PQ

AMA: 2014,Jan,11; 2013,Jan,11-12

43610 Excision, local; ulcer or benign tumor of stomach

💰 28.4 ⚕ 28.4 **FUD** 090   C 80 ▢ PQ

AMA: 2014,Jan,11; 2013,Jan,11-12

43611 malignant tumor of stomach

💰 35.3 ⚕ 35.3 **FUD** 090   C 80 ▢ PQ

AMA: 2014,Jan,11; 2013,Jan,11-12

43620 Gastrectomy, total; with esophagoenterostomy

💰 57.0 ⚕ 57.0 **FUD** 090   C 80 ▢ PQ

AMA: 2014,Jan,11; 2013,Jan,11-12

43621 with Roux-en-Y reconstruction

💰 65.7 ⚕ 65.7 **FUD** 090   C 80 ▢ PQ

AMA: 2014,Jan,11; 2013,Jan,11-12

43622 with formation of intestinal pouch, any type

💰 67.0 ⚕ 67.0 **FUD** 090   C 80 ▢ PQ

AMA: 2014,Jan,11; 2013,Jan,11-12

43631 Gastrectomy, partial, distal; with gastroduodenostomy

INCLUDES Billroth operation

💰 41.9 ⚕ 41.9 **FUD** 090   C 80 ▢ PQ

AMA: 2014,Jan,11; 2013,Jan,11-12

43632 with gastrojejunostomy

INCLUDES Polya anastomosis

💰 58.8 ⚕ 58.8 **FUD** 090   C 80 ▢ PQ

AMA: 2014,Jan,11; 2013,Jan,11-12

43633 with Roux-en-Y reconstruction

💰 55.6 ⚕ 55.6 **FUD** 090   C 80 ▢ PQ

AMA: 2014,Jan,11; 2013,Jan,11-12

43634 with formation of intestinal pouch

💰 61.6 ⚕ 61.6 **FUD** 090   C 80 ▢ PQ

AMA: 2014,Jan,11; 2013,Jan,11-12

+ **43635** Vagotomy when performed with partial distal gastrectomy (List separately in addition to code[s] for primary procedure)

Code first as appropriate (43631-43634)

💰 3.27 ⚕ 3.27 **FUD** ZZZ   C 80 ▢

AMA: 2014,Jan,11; 2013,Jan,11-12

43640 Vagotomy including pyloroplasty, with or without gastrostomy; truncal or selective

EXCLUDES *Pyloroplasty (43800)*
Vagotomy (64755, 64760)

💰 34.0 ⚕ 34.0 **FUD** 090   C 80 ▢ PQ

AMA: 2014,Jan,11; 2013,Jan,11-12

43641 parietal cell (highly selective)

EXCLUDES *Upper gastrointestinal endoscopy (43235-43259 [43233, 43266, 43270])*

💰 34.8 ⚕ 34.8 **FUD** 090   C 80 ▢ PQ

AMA: 2014,Jan,11; 2013,Jan,11-12

Digestive System

43644 — 43760

43644-43645 Laparoscopic Gastric Bypass with Small Bowel Resection

CMS: 100-3,100.1 Bariatric Surgery for Treatment Co-morbid Conditions Due to Morbid Obesity; 100-4,32,150.1 Bariatric Surgery: Treatment of Co-Morbid Conditions Due to Morbid Obesity; 100-4,32,150.2 HCPCS Procedure Codes for Bariatric Surgery; 100-4,32,150.5 ICD-9 Diagnosis Codes for BMI Greater Than or Equal to 35; 100-4,32,150.6 Bariatric Surgery Claims Guidance

INCLUDES Diagnostic laparoscopy

EXCLUDES *Endoscopy, upper gastrointestinal, (esophagus/stomach/duodenum/jejunum) (43235-43259 [43233, 43266, 43270])*

43644 **Laparoscopy, surgical, gastric restrictive procedure; with gastric bypass and Roux-en-Y gastroenterostomy (roux limb 150 cm or less)**

> **EXCLUDES** *Open method (43846)*
> *Roux limb greater than 150 cm (43645)*
> Do not report with (43846, 49320)
> 🔧 50.1 ⚕ 50.1 **FUD** 090   C 80 🖥 P0
> **AMA:** 2014,Jan,11; 2013,Jan,11-12

43645 **with gastric bypass and small intestine reconstruction to limit absorption**

> Do not report with (43847, 49320)
> 🔧 53.5 ⚕ 53.5 **FUD** 090   C 80 🖥 P0
> **AMA:** 2015,Jan,16; 2014,Jan,11; 2013,Jan,11-12

43647-43659 Other and Unlisted Laparoscopic Gastric Procedures

INCLUDES Diagnostic laparoscopy

EXCLUDES *Endoscopy, upper gastrointestinal, (esophagus/stomach/duodenum/jejunum) (43235-43259 [43233, 43266, 43270])*

43647 **Laparoscopy, surgical; implantation or replacement of gastric neurostimulator electrodes, antrum**

> **EXCLUDES** *Electronic analysis/programming gastric neurostimulator (95980-95982)*
> *Insertion gastric neurostimulator pulse generator (64590)*
> *Laparoscopy with implantation, removal, or revision of gastric neurostimulator electrodes on the lesser curvature of the stomach (43659)*
> *Open method (43881)*
> *Vagus nerve blocking pulse generator and/or neurostimulator electrode array implantation, reprogramming, replacement, revision, or removal at the esophagogastric junction performed laparoscopically (0312T-0317T)*
> 🔧 0.00 ⚕ 0.00 **FUD** YYY   J 80
> **AMA:** 2015,Jan,16; 2014,Jan,11; 2013,Jan,11-12; 2012,Jan,15-42; 2011,Jan,11

43648 **revision or removal of gastric neurostimulator electrodes, antrum**

> **EXCLUDES** *Electronic analysis/programming gastric neurostimulator (95980-95982)*
> *Laparoscopy with implantation, removal, or revision of gastric neurostimulator electrodes on the lesser curvature of the stomach (43659)*
> *Open method (43882)*
> *Revision/removal gastric neurostimulator pulse generator (64595)*
> *Vagus nerve blocking pulse generator and/or neurostimulator electrode array implantation, reprogramming, replacement, revision, or removal at the esophagogastric junction performed laparoscopically (0312T-0317T)*
> 🔧 0.00 ⚕ 0.00 **FUD** YYY   02 80
> **AMA:** 2015,Jan,16; 2014,Jan,11; 2013,Jan,11-12

43651 **Laparoscopy, surgical; transection of vagus nerves, truncal**

> 🔧 18.9 ⚕ 18.9 **FUD** 090   T 80 🖥 P0
> **AMA:** 2015,Jan,16; 2014,Jan,11; 2013,Jan,11-12

43652 **transection of vagus nerves, selective or highly selective**

> 🔧 22.1 ⚕ 22.1 **FUD** 090   T 80 🖥 P0
> **AMA:** 2015,Jan,16; 2014,Jan,11; 2013,Jan,11-12

43653 **gastrostomy, without construction of gastric tube (eg, Stamm procedure) (separate procedure)**

> 🔧 16.5 ⚕ 16.5 **FUD** 090   T A2 80 🖥 P0
> **AMA:** 2015,Jan,16; 2014,Jan,11; 2013,Jan,11-12

43659 **Unlisted laparoscopy procedure, stomach**

> 🔧 0.00 ⚕ 0.00 **FUD** YYY   T 80 50
> **AMA:** 2015,Jan,16; 2014,Jan,11; 2013,Jun,13; 2013,Feb,13; 2013,Jan,11-12; 2012,Jan,15-42; 2011,Dec,19; 2011,Jun,8-10; 2011,Jan,11

43752-43761 Nonsurgical Gastric Tube Procedures

43752 **Naso- or oro-gastric tube placement, requiring physician's skill and fluoroscopic guidance (includes fluoroscopy, image documentation and report)**

> **EXCLUDES** *Percutaneous insertion of gastrostomy tube (43246, 49440)*
> *Placement of enteric tube (44500, 74340)*
> Do not report with (99291-99292, 99468-99469, 99471-99472, 99478-99479)
> 🔧 1.19 ⚕ 1.19 **FUD** 000   03 G2 🖥 P0
> **AMA:** 2015,Jan,16; 2014,May,4; 2014,Jan,11; 2013,Jan,11-12; 2012,Jan,15-42; 2011,Sep,3-4; 2011,Jan,11

43753 **Gastric intubation and aspiration(s) therapeutic, necessitating physician's skill (eg, for gastrointestinal hemorrhage), including lavage if performed**

> 🔧 0.62 ⚕ 0.62 **FUD** 000   01 N1 80
> **AMA:** 2015,Jan,16; 2014,May,4; 2014,Jan,11; 2013,Jan,11-12; 2011,Sep,3-4

43754 **Gastric intubation and aspiration, diagnostic; single specimen (eg, acid analysis)**

> **EXCLUDES** *Naso- or oro-gastric tube placement using fluoroscopic guidance (43752)*
> 🔬 (82930)
> 🔧 1.05 ⚕ 3.73 **FUD** 000   01 N1 80
> **AMA:** 2015,Jan,16; 2014,Jan,11; 2013,Jan,11-12; 2011,Sep,3-4; 2010,Dec,7-10

43755 **collection of multiple fractional specimens with gastric stimulation, single or double lumen tube (gastric secretory study) (eg, histamine, insulin, pentagastrin, calcium, secretin), includes drug administration**

> **EXCLUDES** *Naso- or oro-gastric tube placement using fluoroscopic guidance (43752)*
> Code also drugs or substances administered
> 🔬 (82930)
> 🔧 1.80 ⚕ 3.98 **FUD** 000   S G2 80
> **AMA:** 2015,Jan,16; 2014,Jan,11; 2013,Jan,11-12; 2011,Sep,3-4; 2010,Dec,7-10

43756 **Duodenal intubation and aspiration, diagnostic, includes image guidance; single specimen (eg, bile study for crystals or afferent loop culture)**

> 🔬 89049-89240
> 🔧 1.51 ⚕ 5.89 **FUD** 000   S G2 80
> **AMA:** 2015,Jan,16; 2014,Jan,11; 2013,Jan,11-12; 2011,Sep,3-4; 2010,Dec,7-10

43757 **collection of multiple fractional specimens with pancreatic or gallbladder stimulation, single or double lumen tube, includes drug administration**

> Code also drugs or substances administered
> 🔬 (89049-89240)
> 🔧 2.30 ⚕ 8.42 **FUD** 000   S G2 80
> **AMA:** 2015,Jan,16; 2014,Jan,11; 2013,Jan,11-12; 2011,Sep,3-4; 2010,Dec,7-10

43760 **Change of gastrostomy tube, percutaneous, without imaging or endoscopic guidance**

> **EXCLUDES** *Endoscopic placement of gastrostomy tube (43246)*
> *Gastrostomy tube replacement using fluoroscopy (49450)*
> 🔧 1.38 ⚕ 13.9 **FUD** 000   T A2
> **AMA:** 2015,Jan,16; 2014,Jan,11; 2013,Jan,11-12; 2012,Jan,15-42; 2011,Jan,11; 2010,Sep,9

26/TC PC/TC Comp Only	A2-Z3 ASC Pmt	50 Bilateral	♂ Male Only	♀ Female Only	🔧 Facility RVU	⚕ Non-Facility RVU
AMA: CPT Asst	**CMS:** Pub 100	A-Y OPPSI	80/80 Surg Assist Allowed / w/Doc		🔬 Lab Crosswalk	🖥 Radiology Crosswalk

172   Medicare (Red Text)   CPT © 2015 American Medical Association. All Rights Reserved. (Black Text)   © 2015 Optum360, LLC (Blue Text)

43761   Repositioning of a naso- or oro-gastric feeding tube, through the duodenum for enteric nutrition

EXCLUDES   *Gastrostomy tube converted endoscopically to jejunostomy tube (44373)*

Introduction of long gastrointestinal tube into the duodenum (44500)

Do not report with (44500, 49446)

⊞ (76000)

🔪 2.99   ⚬ 3.36   **FUD** 000   🔲 A2 ▣

AMA: 2015,Jan,16; 2014,Jan,11; 2013,Jan,11-12

43770-43775 Laparoscopic Bariatric Procedures

CMS: 100-3,100.1 Bariatric Surgery for Treatment Co-morbid Conditions Due to Morbid Obesity; 100-4,32,150.1 Bariatric Surgery: Treatment of Co-Morbid Conditions Due to Morbid Obesity; 100-4,32,150.2 HCPCS Procedure Codes for Bariatric Surgery; 100-4,32,150.5 ICD-9 Diagnosis Codes for BMI Greater Than or Equal to 35; 100-4,32,150.6 Bariatric Surgery Claims Guidance

INCLUDES   Diagnostic laparoscopy
Stomach/duodenum/jejunum/ileum
Subsequent band adjustments (change of the gastric band component diameter by injection/aspiration of fluid through the subcutaneous port component) during the postoperative period

43770   Laparoscopy, surgical, gastric restrictive procedure; placement of adjustable gastric restrictive device (eg, gastric band and subcutaneous port components)

Code also modifier 52 for placement of individual component

🔪 32.3   ⚬ 32.3   **FUD** 090   🔲 80 🅿🅾

AMA: 2015,Jan,16; 2014,Jan,11; 2013,Jan,11-12; 2012,Jan,15-42; 2011,Jan,11; 2010,Dec,12

43771   revision of adjustable gastric restrictive device component only

🔪 36.7   ⚬ 36.7   **FUD** 090   🔲 80 🅿🅾

AMA: 2015,Jan,16; 2014,Jan,11; 2013,Jan,11-12

43772   removal of adjustable gastric restrictive device component only

🔪 27.5   ⚬ 27.5   **FUD** 090   🔲 80 🅿🅾

AMA: 2015,Jan,16; 2014,Jan,11; 2013,Jan,11-12

43773   removal and replacement of adjustable gastric restrictive device component only

Do not report with (43772)

🔪 37.0   ⚬ 37.0   **FUD** 090   🔲 80 🅿🅾

AMA: 2015,Jan,16; 2014,Jan,11; 2013,Jan,11-12

43774   removal of adjustable gastric restrictive device and subcutaneous port components

EXCLUDES   *Removal/replacement of subcutaneous port components and gastric band (43659)*

🔪 27.7   ⚬ 27.7   **FUD** 090   🔲 80 🅿🅾

AMA: 2015,Jan,16; 2014,Jan,11; 2013,Jan,11-12; 2012,Jan,15-42; 2011,Jan,11

43775   longitudinal gastrectomy (ie, sleeve gastrectomy)

EXCLUDES   *Open gastric restrictive procedure for morbid obesity, without gastric bypass, other than vertical-banded gastroplasty (43843)*

Vagus nerve blocking pulse generator and/or neurostimulator electrode array implantation, reprogramming, replacement, revision, or removal at the esophagogastric junction performed laparoscopically (0312T-0317T)

🔪 0.00   ⚬ 0.00   **FUD** YYY   🔲 80

AMA: 2014,Jan,11; 2013,Jan,11-12

43800-43840 Open Gastric Incisional/Repair/Resection Procedures

43800   Pyloroplasty

EXCLUDES   *Vagotomy with pyloroplasty (43640)*

🔪 26.8   ⚬ 26.8   **FUD** 090   🔲 80 ▣ 🅿🅾

AMA: 2014,Jan,11; 2013,Jan,11-12

43810   Gastroduodenostomy

🔪 29.5   ⚬ 29.5   **FUD** 090   🔲 80 ▣ 🅿🅾

AMA: 2014,Jan,11; 2013,Jan,11-12

43820   Gastrojejunostomy; without vagotomy

🔪 38.8   ⚬ 38.8   **FUD** 090   🔲 80 ▣ 🅿🅾

AMA: 2014,Jan,11; 2013,Jan,11-12

43825   with vagotomy, any type

🔪 37.9   ⚬ 37.9   **FUD** 090   🔲 80 ▣ 🅿🅾

AMA: 2014,Jan,11; 2013,Jan,11-12

43830   Gastrostomy, open; without construction of gastric tube (eg, Stamm procedure) (separate procedure)

🔪 20.2   ⚬ 20.2   **FUD** 090   🔲 80 ▣ 🅿🅾

AMA: 2015,Jan,16; 2014,Jan,11; 2013,Jan,11-12

43831   neonatal, for feeding   🅐

EXCLUDES   *Change of gastrostomy tube (43760)*

🔪 17.1   ⚬ 17.1   **FUD** 090   ⑥③ 🔲 80 ▣ 🅿🅾

AMA: 2015,Jan,16; 2014,Jan,11; 2013,Jan,11-12

43832   with construction of gastric tube (eg, Janeway procedure)

EXCLUDES   *Endoscopic placement of percutaneous gastrostomy tube (43246)*

🔪 30.1   ⚬ 30.1   **FUD** 090   🔲 80 ▣ 🅿🅾

AMA: 2015,Jan,16; 2014,Jan,11; 2013,Jan,11-12

43840   Gastrorrhaphy, suture of perforated duodenal or gastric ulcer, wound, or injury

🔪 39.3   ⚬ 39.3   **FUD** 090   🔲 80 ▣ 🅿🅾

AMA: 2014,Jan,11; 2013,Jan,11-12

43842-43848 Open Bariatric Procedures for Morbid Obesity

CMS: 100-3,100.1 Bariatric Surgery for Treatment Co-morbid Conditions Due to Morbid Obesity; 100-4,32,150.1 Bariatric Surgery: Treatment of Co-Morbid Conditions Due to Morbid Obesity; 100-4,32,150.2 HCPCS Procedure Codes for Bariatric Surgery; 100-4,32,150.5 ICD-9 Diagnosis Codes for BMI Greater Than or Equal to 35; 100-4,32,150.6 Bariatric Surgery Claims Guidance

43842   Gastric restrictive procedure, without gastric bypass, for morbid obesity; vertical-banded gastroplasty

🔪 33.0   ⚬ 33.0   **FUD** 090   🅴 ▣

AMA: 2015,Jan,16; 2014,Jan,11; 2013,Jan,11-12

43843   other than vertical-banded gastroplasty

EXCLUDES   *Laparoscopic longitudinal gastrectomy (e.g., sleeve gastrectomy) (43775)*

🔪 37.1   ⚬ 37.1   **FUD** 090   🔲 80 ▣ 🅿🅾

AMA: 2015,Jan,16; 2014,Jan,11; 2013,Jan,11-12

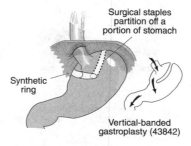

Surgical staples partition off a portion of stomach

Synthetic ring

Vertical-banded gastroplasty (43842)

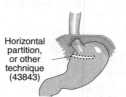

Horizontal partition, or other technique (43843)

The stomach is surgically restricted to treat morbid obesity. A vertical-banded technique is coded 43842 and any other gastroplasty technique that does not employ gastric bypass is coded 43843. These partitioning techniques give the patient a sensation of fullness, thus decreasing daily caloric intake

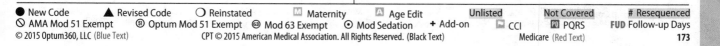

43845   **Gastric restrictive procedure with partial gastrectomy, pylorus-preserving duodenoileostomy and ileoileostomy (50 to 100 cm common channel) to limit absorption (biliopancreatic diversion with duodenal switch)**

Do not report with (43633, 43847, 44130, 49000)

⏚ 56.8   ⚕ 56.8   **FUD** 090   C 80 ▭ P0

AMA: 2015,Jan,16; 2014,Jan,11; 2013,Jan,11-12

43846   **Gastric restrictive procedure, with gastric bypass for morbid obesity; with short limb (150 cm or less) Roux-en-Y gastroenterostomy**

EXCLUDES   *Performed laparoscopically (43644)*
Roux limb more than 150 cm (43847)

⏚ 46.6   ⚕ 46.6   **FUD** 090   C 80 ▭ P0

AMA: 2015,Jan,16; 2014,Jan,11; 2013,Jan,11-12

43847   **with small intestine reconstruction to limit absorption**

EXCLUDES   *Performed laparoscopically (43645)*

⏚ 52.2   ⚕ 52.2   **FUD** 090   C 80 ▭ P0

AMA: 2015,Jan,16; 2014,Jan,11; 2013,Jan,11-12

43848   **Revision, open, of gastric restrictive procedure for morbid obesity, other than adjustable gastric restrictive device (separate procedure)**

EXCLUDES   *Gastric restrictive port procedures (43886-43888)*
Procedures for adjustable gastric restrictive devices (43770-43774)

⏚ 55.7   ⚕ 55.7   **FUD** 090   C 80 ▭ P0

AMA: 2015,Jan,16; 2014,Jan,11; 2013,Jan,11-12

43850-43882 Open Gastric Procedures: Closure/Implantation/Replacement/Revision

43850   **Revision of gastroduodenal anastomosis (gastroduodenostomy) with reconstruction; without vagotomy**

⏚ 47.2   ⚕ 47.2   **FUD** 090   C 80 ▭ P0

AMA: 2014,Jan,11; 2013,Jan,11-12

43855   **with vagotomy**

⏚ 48.9   ⚕ 48.9   **FUD** 090   C 80 ▭ P0

AMA: 2014,Jan,11; 2013,Jan,11-12

43860   **Revision of gastrojejunal anastomosis (gastrojejunostomy) with reconstruction, with or without partial gastrectomy or intestine resection; without vagotomy**

⏚ 47.4   ⚕ 47.4   **FUD** 090   C 80 ▭ P0

AMA: 2014,Jan,11; 2013,Jan,11-12

43865   **with vagotomy**

⏚ 49.5   ⚕ 49.5   **FUD** 090   C 80 ▭ P0

AMA: 2014,Jan,11; 2013,Jan,11-12

43870   **Closure of gastrostomy, surgical**

⏚ 20.6   ⚕ 20.6   **FUD** 090   T A2 80 ▭ P0

AMA: 2014,Jan,11; 2013,Jan,11-12

43880   **Closure of gastrocolic fistula**

⏚ 46.1   ⚕ 46.1   **FUD** 090   C 80 ▭ P0

AMA: 2014,Jan,11; 2013,Jan,11-12

43881   **Implantation or replacement of gastric neurostimulator electrodes, antrum, open**

EXCLUDES   *Electronic analysis and programming (95980-95982)*
Implantation/removal/revision gastric neurostimulator electrodes, lesser curvature or vagal trunk (EGJ):
Laparoscopically (43659)
Open (43999)
Implantation/replacement performed laparoscopically (43647)
Insertion of gastric neurostimulator pulse generator (64590)
Vagus nerve blocking pulse generator and/or neurostimulator electrode array implantation, reprogramming, replacement, revision, or removal at the esophagogastric junction performed laparoscopically (0312T-0317T)

⏚ 0.00   ⚕ 0.00   **FUD** YYY   C 80

AMA: 2015,Jan,16; 2014,Jan,11; 2013,Jan,11-12

43882   **Revision or removal of gastric neurostimulator electrodes, antrum, open**

EXCLUDES   *Electronic analysis and programming (95980-95982)*
Implantation/removal/revision gastric neurostimulator electrodes, lesser curvature or vagal trunk (EGJ):
Laparoscopic (43659)
Open (43999)
Revision/removal gastric neurostimulator electrodes, antrum, performed laparoscopically (43648)
Revision/removal gastric neurostimulator pulse generator (64595)
Vagus nerve blocking pulse generator and/or neurostimulator electrode array implantation, reprogramming, replacement, revision, or removal at the esophagogastric junction performed laparoscopically (0312T-0317T)

⏚ 0.00   ⚕ 0.00   **FUD** YYY   C 80

AMA: 2015,Jan,16; 2014,Jan,11; 2013,Jan,11-12

43886-43999 Bariatric Procedures: Removal/Replacement/Revision Port Components

CMS: 100-4,32,150.1 Bariatric Surgery: Treatment of Co-Morbid Conditions Due to Morbid Obesity; 100-4,32,150.2 HCPCS Procedure Codes for Bariatric Surgery; 100-4,32,150.5 ICD-9 Diagnosis Codes for BMI Greater Than or Equal to 35; 100-4,32,150.6 Bariatric Surgery Claims Guidance

43886   **Gastric restrictive procedure, open; revision of subcutaneous port component only**

⏚ 10.4   ⚕ 10.4   **FUD** 090   T 62 80 P0

AMA: 2015,Jan,16; 2014,Jan,11; 2013,Jan,11-12

43887   **removal of subcutaneous port component only**

EXCLUDES   *Gastric band and subcutaneous port components:*
Removal and replacement performed laparoscopically (43659)
Removal performed laparoscopically (43774)

⏚ 9.43   ⚕ 9.43   **FUD** 090   02 62 80 P0

AMA: 2015,Jan,16; 2014,Jan,11; 2013,Jan,11-12

43888   **removal and replacement of subcutaneous port component only**

EXCLUDES   *Gastric band and subcutaneous port components:*
Removal and replacement performed laparoscopically (43659)
Removal performed laparoscopically (43774)

Do not report with (43774, 43887)

⏚ 13.2   ⚕ 13.2   **FUD** 090   T 62 80 P0

AMA: 2015,Jan,16; 2014,Jan,11; 2013,Jan,11-12

43999   **Unlisted procedure, stomach**

⏚ 0.00   ⚕ 0.00   **FUD** YYY   T 80

AMA: 2015,Jan,16; 2014,Jan,11; 2013,Feb,13; 2013,Jan,11-12; 2012,Jan,15-42; 2011,Jun,13; 2011,Jan,11; 2010,Mar,9-11

44005-44130 Incisional and Resection Procedures of Bowel

44005   **Enterolysis (freeing of intestinal adhesion) (separate procedure)**

EXCLUDES   *Enterolysis performed laparoscopically (44180)*

Do not report with (45136)

⏚ 31.6   ⚕ 31.6   **FUD** 090   C 80 ▭ P0

AMA: 2015,Jan,16; 2014,Jan,11; 2013,Jan,11-12; 2012,Jan,15-42; 2011,Jan,11

44010   **Duodenotomy, for exploration, biopsy(s), or foreign body removal**

⏚ 25.0   ⚕ 25.0   **FUD** 090   C 80 ▭ P0

AMA: 2014,Jan,11; 2013,Jan,11-12

+   **44015**   **Tube or needle catheter jejunostomy for enteral alimentation, intraoperative, any method (List separately in addition to primary procedure)**

Code first the primary procedure

⏚ 4.14   ⚕ 4.14   **FUD** ZZZ   C 80

AMA: 2015,Jan,16; 2014,Jan,11; 2013,Jan,11-12; 2012,Jan,15-42; 2011,Jan,11; 2010,Jul,10

44020   Enterotomy, small intestine, other than duodenum; for exploration, biopsy(s), or foreign body removal
    ⚷ 28.2   ⚖ 28.2   **FUD** 090   C 80 ▢ PQ
    AMA: 2014,Jan,11; 2013,Jan,11-12

44021   for decompression (eg, Baker tube)
    ⚷ 28.2   ⚖ 28.2   **FUD** 090   C 80 ▢ PQ
    AMA: 2014,Jan,11; 2013,Jan,11-12

Anterior abdominal skin   Baker-type tube   Depicted at left is a tube threaded through intestine for decompression
Peritoneum
Bowel lumen   Note that the bowel is sutured to the abdominal wall

44025   Colotomy, for exploration, biopsy(s), or foreign body removal
    INCLUDES   Amussat's operation
    EXCLUDES   *Intestine exteriorization (Mikulicz resection with crushing of spur) (44602-44605)*
    ⚷ 28.5   ⚖ 28.5   **FUD** 090   C 80 ▢ PQ
    AMA: 2014,Jan,11; 2013,Jan,11-12

44050   Reduction of volvulus, intussusception, internal hernia, by laparotomy
    ⚷ 27.0   ⚖ 27.0   **FUD** 090   C 80 ▢ PQ
    AMA: 2014,Jan,11; 2013,Jan,11-12

44055   Correction of malrotation by lysis of duodenal bands and/or reduction of midgut volvulus (eg, Ladd procedure)
    ⚷ 43.0   ⚖ 43.0   **FUD** 090   63 C 80 ▢ PQ
    AMA: 2014,Jan,11; 2013,Jan,11-12

44100   Biopsy of intestine by capsule, tube, peroral (1 or more specimens)
    ⚷ 3.23   ⚖ 3.23   **FUD** 000   T A2 ▢ PQ
    AMA: 2014,Jan,11; 2013,Jan,11-12

44110   Excision of 1 or more lesions of small or large intestine not requiring anastomosis, exteriorization, or fistulization; single enterotomy
    ⚷ 24.6   ⚖ 24.6   **FUD** 090   C 80 ▢ PQ
    AMA: 2014,Jan,11; 2013,Jan,11-12

44111   multiple enterotomies
    ⚷ 28.4   ⚖ 28.4   **FUD** 090   C 80 ▢ PQ
    AMA: 2014,Jan,11; 2013,Jan,11-12

44120   Enterectomy, resection of small intestine; single resection and anastomosis
    Do not report with (45136)
    ⚷ 35.3   ⚖ 35.3   **FUD** 090   C 80 ▢ PQ
    AMA: 2015,Jan,16; 2014,Jan,11; 2013,Jan,11-12

\+ 44121   each additional resection and anastomosis (List separately in addition to code for primary procedure)
    Code first single resection of small intestine (44120)
    ⚷ 7.03   ⚖ 7.03   **FUD** ZZZ   C 80 ▢
    AMA: 2014,Jan,11; 2013,Jan,11-12

44125   with enterostomy
    ⚷ 34.1   ⚖ 34.1   **FUD** 090   C 80 ▢ PQ
    AMA: 2014,Jan,11; 2013,Jan,11-12

44126   Enterectomy, resection of small intestine for congenital atresia, single resection and anastomosis of proximal segment of intestine; without tapering
    ⚷ 71.5   ⚖ 71.5   **FUD** 090   63 C 80 ▢ PQ
    AMA: 2014,Jan,11; 2013,Jan,11-12

44127   with tapering
    ⚷ 82.7   ⚖ 82.7   **FUD** 090   63 C 80 ▢ PQ
    AMA: 2014,Jan,11; 2013,Jan,11-12

\+ 44128   each additional resection and anastomosis (List separately in addition to code for primary procedure)
    Code first single resection of small intestine (44126, 44127)
    ⚷ 7.09   ⚖ 7.09   **FUD** ZZZ   63 C 80 ▢
    AMA: 2014,Jan,11; 2013,Jan,11-12

44130   Enteroenterostomy, anastomosis of intestine, with or without cutaneous enterostomy (separate procedure)
    ⚷ 37.9   ⚖ 37.9   **FUD** 090   C 80 ▢ PQ
    AMA: 2014,Jan,11; 2013,Jan,11-12

44132-44137 Intestine Transplant Procedures

CMS: 100-3,260.5 Intestinal and Multi-Visceral Transplantation; 100-4,3,90.6 Intestinal and Multi-Visceral Transplants

44132   Donor enterectomy (including cold preservation), open; from cadaver donor
    INCLUDES   Graft:
        Cold preservation
        Harvest
    ⚷ 0.00   ⚖ 0.00   **FUD** XXX   C 80 ▢ PQ
    AMA: 2014,Jan,11; 2013,Jan,11-12

44133   partial, from living donor
    INCLUDES   Donor care
        Graft:
        Cold preservation
        Harvest
    EXCLUDES   *Preparation/reconstruction of backbench intestinal graft (44715, 44720-44721)*
    ⚷ 0.00   ⚖ 0.00   **FUD** XXX   C 80 ▢ PQ
    AMA: 2014,Jan,11; 2013,Jan,11-12

44135   Intestinal allotransplantation; from cadaver donor
    INCLUDES   Allograft transplantation
        Recipient care
    ⚷ 0.00   ⚖ 0.00   **FUD** XXX   C 80 ▢ PQ
    AMA: 2014,Jan,11; 2013,Jan,11-12

44136   from living donor
    INCLUDES   Allograft transplantation
        Recipient care
    ⚷ 0.00   ⚖ 0.00   **FUD** XXX   C 80 ▢ PQ
    AMA: 2014,Jan,11; 2013,Jan,11-12

44137   Removal of transplanted intestinal allograft, complete
    EXCLUDES   *Partial removal of transplant allograft (44120-44121, 44140)*
    ⚷ 0.00   ⚖ 0.00   **FUD** XXX   C 80 ▢
    AMA: 2014,Jan,11; 2013,Jan,11-12

44139-44160 Colon Resection Procedures

\+ 44139   Mobilization (take-down) of splenic flexure performed in conjunction with partial colectomy (List separately in addition to primary procedure)
    Code first partial colectomy (44140-44147)
    ⚷ 3.52   ⚖ 3.52   **FUD** ZZZ   C 80 ▢
    AMA: 2014,Jan,11; 2013,Jan,11-12

44140   Colectomy, partial; with anastomosis
    EXCLUDES   *Laparoscopic method (44204)*
    ⚷ 38.8   ⚖ 38.8   **FUD** 090   C 80 ▢ PQ
    AMA: 2015,Jan,16; 2014,Jan,11; 2013,Jan,11-12; 2010,Sep,6-7

44141   with skin level cecostomy or colostomy
    ⚷ 52.8   ⚖ 52.8   **FUD** 090   C 80 ▢ PQ
    AMA: 2015,Jan,16; 2014,Jan,11; 2013,Jan,11-12

44143   with end colostomy and closure of distal segment (Hartmann type procedure)
    EXCLUDES   *Laparoscopic method (44206)*
    ⚷ 48.1   ⚖ 48.1   **FUD** 090   C 80 ▢ PQ
    AMA: 2015,Jan,16; 2014,Jan,11; 2013,Jan,11-12

44144   with resection, with colostomy or ileostomy and creation of mucofistula
    ⚷ 51.2   ⚖ 51.2   **FUD** 090   C 80 ▢ PQ
    AMA: 2015,Jan,16; 2014,Jan,11; 2013,Jan,11-12

Digestive System

44145   **with coloproctostomy (low pelvic anastomosis)**
　　　　EXCLUDES　　*Laparoscopic method (44207)*
　　　　🚗 48.0　　⊰ 48.0　　**FUD** 090　　　　　　　C 80 ▱ P0
　　　　AMA: 2014,Jan,11; 2013,Jan,11-12

44146   **with coloproctostomy (low pelvic anastomosis), with colostomy**
　　　　EXCLUDES　　*Laparoscopic method (44208)*
　　　　🚗 61.4　　⊰ 61.4　　**FUD** 090　　　　　　　C 80 ▱ P0
　　　　AMA: 2015,Jan,16; 2014,Jan,11; 2013,Jan,11-12

44147   **abdominal and transanal approach**
　　　　🚗 56.3　　⊰ 56.3　　**FUD** 090　　　　　　　C 80 ▱ P0
　　　　AMA: 2015,Jan,16; 2014,Jan,11; 2013,Jan,11-12

44150   **Colectomy, total, abdominal, without proctectomy; with ileostomy or ileoproctostomy**
　　　　INCLUDES　　Lane's operation
　　　　EXCLUDES　　*Laparoscopic method (44210)*
　　　　🚗 54.1　　⊰ 54.1　　**FUD** 090　　　　　　　C 80 ▱ P0
　　　　AMA: 2014,Jan,11; 2013,Jan,11-12

44151   **with continent ileostomy**
　　　　🚗 62.3　　⊰ 62.3　　**FUD** 090　　　　　　　C 80 ▱ P0
　　　　AMA: 2014,Jan,11; 2013,Jan,11-12

44155   **Colectomy, total, abdominal, with proctectomy; with ileostomy**
　　　　INCLUDES　　Miles' colectomy
　　　　EXCLUDES　　*Laparoscopic method (44212)*
　　　　🚗 60.2　　⊰ 60.2　　**FUD** 090　　　　　　　C 80 ▱ P0
　　　　AMA: 2014,Jan,11; 2013,Jan,11-12

44156   **with continent ileostomy**
　　　　🚗 67.0　　⊰ 67.0　　**FUD** 090　　　　　　　C 80 ▱ P0
　　　　AMA: 2014,Jan,11; 2013,Jan,11-12

44157   **with ileoanal anastomosis, includes loop ileostomy, and rectal mucosectomy, when performed**
　　　　🚗 63.2　　⊰ 63.2　　**FUD** 090　　　　　　　C 80 P0
　　　　AMA: 2014,Jan,11; 2013,Jan,11-12

44158   **with ileoanal anastomosis, creation of ileal reservoir (S or J), includes loop ileostomy, and rectal mucosectomy, when performed**
　　　　EXCLUDES　　*Laparoscopic method (44211)*
　　　　🚗 61.2　　⊰ 61.2　　**FUD** 090　　　　　　　C 80 P0
　　　　AMA: 2014,Jan,11; 2013,Jan,11-12

44160   **Colectomy, partial, with removal of terminal ileum with ileocolostomy**
　　　　EXCLUDES　　*Laparoscopic method (44205)*
　　　　🚗 35.9　　⊰ 35.9　　**FUD** 090　　　　　　　C 80 ▱ P0
　　　　AMA: 2015,Jan,16; 2014,Jan,11; 2013,Jan,11-12

44180 Laparoscopic Enterolysis

INCLUDES　　Diagnostic laparoscopy
EXCLUDES　　*Laparoscopic salpingolysis/ovariolysis (58660)*

44180   **Laparoscopy, surgical, enterolysis (freeing of intestinal adhesion) (separate procedure)**
　　　　🚗 26.5　　⊰ 26.5　　**FUD** 090　　　　　　　T 80 P0
　　　　AMA: 2015,Jan,16; 2014,Jan,11; 2013,Jan,11-12

44186-44238 Laparoscopic Enterostomy Procedures

INCLUDES　　Diagnostic laparoscopy with surgical laparoscopy

44186   **Laparoscopy, surgical; jejunostomy (eg, for decompression or feeding)**
　　　　🚗 18.8　　⊰ 18.8　　**FUD** 090　　　　　　　T 80 P0
　　　　AMA: 2015,Jan,16; 2014,Jan,11; 2013,Jan,11-12

44187   **ileostomy or jejunostomy, non-tube**
　　　　EXCLUDES　　*Open method (44310)*
　　　　🚗 32.0　　⊰ 32.0　　**FUD** 090　　　　　　　C 80 P0
　　　　AMA: 2015,Jan,16; 2014,Jan,11; 2013,Jan,11-12

44188   **Laparoscopy, surgical, colostomy or skin level cecostomy**
　　　　EXCLUDES　　*Open method (44320)*
　　　　Do not report with (44970)
　　　　🚗 35.4　　⊰ 35.4　　**FUD** 090　　　　　　　C 80 P0
　　　　AMA: 2015,Jan,16; 2014,Jan,11; 2013,Jan,11-12; 2012,Jan,15-42; 2011,Jan,11

44202   **Laparoscopy, surgical; enterectomy, resection of small intestine, single resection and anastomosis**
　　　　EXCLUDES　　*Open method (44120)*
　　　　🚗 40.1　　⊰ 40.1　　**FUD** 090　　　　　　　C 80 ▱ P0
　　　　AMA: 2015,Jan,16; 2014,Jan,11; 2013,Jan,11-12

+ **44203**   **each additional small intestine resection and anastomosis (List separately in addition to code for primary procedure)**
　　　　EXCLUDES　　*Open method (44121)*
　　　　Code first single resection of small intestine (44202)
　　　　🚗 7.09　　⊰ 7.09　　**FUD** ZZZ　　　　　　　C 80 ▱
　　　　AMA: 2015,Jan,16; 2014,Jan,11; 2013,Jan,11-12

44204   **colectomy, partial, with anastomosis**
　　　　EXCLUDES　　*Open method (44140)*
　　　　🚗 44.5　　⊰ 44.5　　**FUD** 090　　　　　　　C 80 ▱ P0
　　　　AMA: 2015,Jan,16; 2014,Jan,11; 2013,Jan,11-12; 2012,Jan,15-42; 2011,Jan,11

44205   **colectomy, partial, with removal of terminal ileum with ileocolostomy**
　　　　EXCLUDES　　*Open method (44160)*
　　　　🚗 38.7　　⊰ 38.7　　**FUD** 090　　　　　　　C 80 ▱ P0
　　　　AMA: 2015,Jan,16; 2014,Jan,11; 2013,Jan,11-12

44206   **colectomy, partial, with end colostomy and closure of distal segment (Hartmann type procedure)**
　　　　EXCLUDES　　*Open method (44143)*
　　　　🚗 50.7　　⊰ 50.7　　**FUD** 090　　　　　　　C 80 ▱ P0
　　　　AMA: 2015,Jan,16; 2014,Jan,11; 2013,Jan,11-12

44207   **colectomy, partial, with anastomosis, with coloproctostomy (low pelvic anastomosis)**
　　　　EXCLUDES　　*Open method (44145)*
　　　　🚗 52.7　　⊰ 52.7　　**FUD** 090　　　　　　　C 80 ▱ P0
　　　　AMA: 2015,Jan,16; 2014,Jan,11; 2013,Jan,11-12

44208   **colectomy, partial, with anastomosis, with coloproctostomy (low pelvic anastomosis) with colostomy**
　　　　EXCLUDES　　*Open method (44146)*
　　　　🚗 57.6　　⊰ 57.6　　**FUD** 090　　　　　　　C 80 ▱ P0
　　　　AMA: 2015,Jan,16; 2014,Jan,11; 2013,Jan,11-12

44210   **colectomy, total, abdominal, without proctectomy, with ileostomy or ileoproctostomy**
　　　　EXCLUDES　　*Open method (44150)*
　　　　🚗 51.5　　⊰ 51.5　　**FUD** 090　　　　　　　C 80 ▱ P0
　　　　AMA: 2015,Jan,16; 2014,Jan,11; 2013,Jan,11-12

44211   **colectomy, total, abdominal, with proctectomy, with ileoanal anastomosis, creation of ileal reservoir (S or J), with loop ileostomy, includes rectal mucosectomy, when performed**
　　　　EXCLUDES　　*Open method (44157, 44158)*
　　　　🚗 62.9　　⊰ 62.9　　**FUD** 090　　　　　　　C 80 ▱ P0
　　　　AMA: 2015,Jan,16; 2014,Jan,11; 2013,Jan,11-12

44212   **colectomy, total, abdominal, with proctectomy, with ileostomy**
　　　　EXCLUDES　　*Open method (44155)*
　　　　🚗 59.4　　⊰ 59.4　　**FUD** 090　　　　　　　C 80 ▱ P0
　　　　AMA: 2015,Jan,16; 2014,Jan,11; 2013,Jan,11-12

44145 — 44212

+ **44213** **Laparoscopy, surgical, mobilization (take-down) of splenic flexure performed in conjunction with partial colectomy (List separately in addition to primary procedure)**

    EXCLUDES   *Open method (44139)*

    Code first partial colectomy (44204-44208)

    🚗 5.48   ✂ 5.48   **FUD** ZZZ   C 80

    AMA: 2015,Jan,16; 2014,Jan,11; 2013,Jan,11-12; 2012,Jan,15-42; 2011,Jan,11

44227 **Laparoscopy, surgical, closure of enterostomy, large or small intestine, with resection and anastomosis**

    EXCLUDES   *Open method (44625-44626)*

    🚗 48.3   ✂ 48.3   **FUD** 090   C 80 P0

    AMA: 2015,Jan,16; 2014,Jan,11; 2013,Jan,11-12

44238 **Unlisted laparoscopy procedure, intestine (except rectum)**

    🚗 0.00   ✂ 0.00   **FUD** YYY   T 80 50

    AMA: 2015,Jan,16; 2014,Jan,11; 2013,Jan,11-12

44300-44346 Open Enterostomy Procedures

44300 **Placement, enterostomy or cecostomy, tube open (eg, for feeding or decompression) (separate procedure)**

    EXCLUDES   *Other gastrointestinal tube(s) placed percutaneously with fluoroscopic imaging guidance (49441-49442)*

    🚗 24.3   ✂ 24.3   **FUD** 090   C 80 P0

    AMA: 2015,Jan,16; 2014,Jan,11; 2013,Jan,11-12; 2012,Jan,15-42; 2011,Jan,11

44310 **Ileostomy or jejunostomy, non-tube**

    EXCLUDES   *Laparoscopic method (44187)*

    Do not report with (44144, 44150-44151, 44155-44156, 45113, 45119, 45136)

    🚗 30.2   ✂ 30.2   **FUD** 090   C 80 P0

    AMA: 2015,Jan,16; 2014,Jan,11; 2013,Jan,11-12; 2012,Jan,15-42; 2011,Jan,11

44312 **Revision of ileostomy; simple (release of superficial scar) (separate procedure)**

    🚗 17.0   ✂ 17.0   **FUD** 090   T A2 80 P0

    AMA: 2014,Jan,11; 2013,Jan,11-12

44314 **complicated (reconstruction in-depth) (separate procedure)**

    🚗 29.0   ✂ 29.0   **FUD** 090   C 80 P0

    AMA: 2014,Jan,11; 2013,Jan,11-12

44316 **Continent ileostomy (Kock procedure) (separate procedure)**

    EXCLUDES   *Fiberoptic evaluation (44385)*

    🚗 40.9   ✂ 40.9   **FUD** 090   C 80 P0

    AMA: 2014,Jan,11; 2013,Jan,11-12

44320 **Colostomy or skin level cecostomy;**

    EXCLUDES   *Laparoscopic method (44188)*

    Do not report with (44141, 44144, 44146, 44605, 45110, 45119, 45126, 45563, 45805, 45825, 50810, 51597, 57307, 58240)

    🚗 34.7   ✂ 34.7   **FUD** 090   C 80 P0

    AMA: 2015,Jan,16; 2014,Jan,11; 2013,Jan,11-12

44322 **with multiple biopsies (eg, for congenital megacolon) (separate procedure)**

    🚗 28.9   ✂ 28.9   **FUD** 090   C 80 P0

    AMA: 2014,Jan,11; 2013,Jan,11-12

44340 **Revision of colostomy; simple (release of superficial scar) (separate procedure)**

    🚗 18.0   ✂ 18.0   **FUD** 090   T A2 P0

    AMA: 2014,Jan,11; 2013,Jan,11-12

44345 **complicated (reconstruction in-depth) (separate procedure)**

    🚗 30.4   ✂ 30.4   **FUD** 090   C 80 P0

    AMA: 2014,Jan,11; 2013,Jan,11-12

44346 **with repair of paracolostomy hernia (separate procedure)**

    🚗 34.2   ✂ 34.2   **FUD** 090   C 80 P0

    AMA: 2015,Jan,16; 2014,Jan,11; 2013,Jan,11-12; 2012,Jan,15-42; 2011,Jan,11

Skin

Herniations that have formed around the site of a colostomy are repaired

The colon is mobilized, trimmed if necessary, and a new stoma is often created

44360-44379 Endoscopy of Small Intestine

INCLUDES   Control of bleeding as result of endoscopic procedure during same operative session

EXCLUDES   *Retrograde exam through anus/colon stoma (44799)*

Do not report with (43235-43259 [43233, 43266, 43270])

44360 **Small intestinal endoscopy, enteroscopy beyond second portion of duodenum, not including ileum; diagnostic, including collection of specimen(s) by brushing or washing, when performed (separate procedure)**

    Do not report with (44376-44379)

    🚗 4.45   ✂ 4.45   **FUD** 000   ⊙ T A2

    AMA: 2015,Jan,16; 2014,Nov,3; 2014,Jan,11; 2013,Dec,3; 2013,Jan,11-12; 2012,Jan,15-42; 2011,Mar,9

44361 **with biopsy, single or multiple**

    Do not report with (44376-44379)

    🚗 4.91   ✂ 4.91   **FUD** 000   ⊙ T A2 P0

    AMA: 2014,Nov,3; 2014,Jan,11; 2013,Dec,3; 2013,Jan,11-12

44363 **with removal of foreign body(s)**

    Do not report with (44376-44379)

    🚗 5.88   ✂ 5.88   **FUD** 000   ⊙ T A2 80

    AMA: 2014,Nov,3; 2014,Jan,11; 2013,Dec,3; 2013,Jan,11-12

44364 **with removal of tumor(s), polyp(s), or other lesion(s) by snare technique**

    Do not report with (44376-44379)

    🚗 6.27   ✂ 6.27   **FUD** 000   ⊙ T A2 80

    AMA: 2014,Nov,3; 2014,Jan,11; 2013,Dec,3; 2013,Jan,11-12

44365 **with removal of tumor(s), polyp(s), or other lesion(s) by hot biopsy forceps or bipolar cautery**

    Do not report with (44376-44379)

    🚗 5.46   ✂ 5.46   **FUD** 000   ⊙ T A2 80

    AMA: 2014,Nov,3; 2014,Jan,11; 2013,Dec,3; 2013,Jan,11-12

44366 **with control of bleeding (eg, injection, bipolar cautery, unipolar cautery, laser, heater probe, stapler, plasma coagulator)**

    Do not report with (44376-44379)

    🚗 7.36   ✂ 7.36   **FUD** 000   ⊙ T A2

    AMA: 2015,Jan,16; 2014,Nov,3; 2014,Jan,11; 2013,Dec,3; 2013,Jan,11-12; 2010,Jun,4-5

44369 **with ablation of tumor(s), polyp(s), or other lesion(s) not amenable to removal by hot biopsy forceps, bipolar cautery or snare technique**

    Do not report with (44376-44379)

    🚗 7.53   ✂ 7.53   **FUD** 000   ⊙ T A2 80

    AMA: 2014,Nov,3; 2014,Jan,11; 2013,Dec,3; 2013,Jan,11-12

44370 **with transendoscopic stent placement (includes predilation)**

    Do not report with (44376-44379)

    🚗 8.14   ✂ 8.14   **FUD** 000   ⊙ J A2 80

    AMA: 2015,Jan,16; 2014,Nov,3; 2014,Jan,11; 2013,Dec,3; 2013,Jan,11-12

Digestive System

44372 — 44391

44372   **with placement of percutaneous jejunostomy tube**
Do not report with (44376-44379)
📋 7.33   ⚗ 7.33   **FUD** 000   ⊙ T A2 ▭
AMA: 2015,Jan,16; 2014,Nov,3; 2014,Jan,11; 2013,Dec,3; 2013,Jan,11-12

44373   **with conversion of percutaneous gastrostomy tube to percutaneous jejunostomy tube**
EXCLUDES   *Jejunostomy, fiberoptic, through stoma (43235)*
Do not report with (44376-44379)
📋 5.88   ⚗ 5.88   **FUD** 000   ⊙ T A2 ▭
AMA: 2015,Jan,16; 2014,Nov,3; 2014,Jan,11; 2013,Dec,3; 2013,Jan,11-12

44376   **Small intestinal endoscopy, enteroscopy beyond second portion of duodenum, including ileum; diagnostic, with or without collection of specimen(s) by brushing or washing (separate procedure)**
Do not report with (44360-44373)
📋 8.62   ⚗ 8.62   **FUD** 000   ⊙ T A2 80 ▭
AMA: 2015,Jan,16; 2014,Nov,3; 2014,Jan,11; 2013,Dec,3; 2013,Jan,11-12; 2011,Mar,9

44377   **with biopsy, single or multiple**
Do not report with (44360-44373)
📋 9.13   ⚗ 9.13   **FUD** 000   ⊙ T A2 80 ▭ P0
AMA: 2015,Jan,16; 2014,Nov,3; 2014,Jan,11; 2013,Dec,3; 2013,Jan,11-12

44378   **with control of bleeding (eg, injection, bipolar cautery, unipolar cautery, laser, heater probe, stapler, plasma coagulator)**
Do not report with (44360-44373)
📋 11.6   ⚗ 11.6   **FUD** 000   ⊙ T A2 80 ▭
AMA: 2015,Jan,16; 2014,Nov,3; 2014,Jan,11; 2013,Dec,3; 2013,Jan,11-12; 2012,Apr,17-18; 2010,Jun,4-5

44379   **with transendoscopic stent placement (includes predilation)**
Do not report with (44360-44373)
📋 12.4   ⚗ 12.4   **FUD** 000   ⊙ J A2 80 ▭
AMA: 2015,Jan,16; 2014,Nov,3; 2014,Jan,11; 2013,Dec,3; 2013,Jan,11-12

44380-44384 [44381] Ileoscopy Via Stoma

INCLUDES   Control of bleeding as result of endoscopic procedure during same operative session
EXCLUDES   *Computed tomographic colonography (74261-74263)*
Code also exam of nonfunctional distal colon/rectum, when performed, with:
   Anoscopy (46600, 46604-46606, 46608-46615)
   Proctosigmoidoscopy (45300-45327)
   Sigmoidoscopy (45330-45347 [45346])

44380   **Ileoscopy, through stoma; diagnostic, including collection of specimen(s) by brushing or washing, when performed (separate procedure)**
Do not report with (44382-44384 [44381])
📋 1.96   ⚗ 1.96   **FUD** 000   ⊙ T A2 ▭
AMA: 2015,Jan,16; 2014,Dec,3; 2014,Nov,3; 2014,Jan,11; 2013,Dec,3; 2013,Jan,11-12

44381   **Resequenced code. See code following 44382.**

44382   **with biopsy, single or multiple**
Do not report with (44380)
📋 2.33   ⚗ 2.33   **FUD** 000   ⊙ T A2 ▭ P0
AMA: 2015,Jan,16; 2014,Dec,3; 2014,Nov,3; 2014,Jan,11; 2013,Dec,3; 2013,Jan,11-12

\# **44381**   **with transendoscopic balloon dilation**
Code also each additional stricture dilated in same session, using modifier 59 with (44381)
Do not report with (44380, 44384)
⚕ (74360)
📋 0.00   ⚗ 0.00   **FUD** 000   ⊙ T G2
AMA: 2015,Jan,16; 2014,Dec,3; 2014,Nov,3

44384   **with placement of endoscopic stent (includes pre- and post-dilation and guide wire passage, when performed)**
Do not report with (44380-44381)
⚕ (74360)
📋 0.00   ⚗ 0.00   **FUD** 000   ⊙ T G2
AMA: 2015,Jan,16; 2014,Dec,3; 2014,Nov,3

44385-44386 Endoscopy of Small Intestinal Pouch

INCLUDES   Control of bleeding as result of the endoscopic procedure during same operative session
EXCLUDES   *Computed tomographic colonography (74261-74263)*

44385   **Endoscopic evaluation of small intestinal pouch (eg, Kock pouch, ileal reservoir [S or J]); diagnostic, including collection of specimen(s) by brushing or washing, when performed (separate procedure)**
Do not report with (44386)
📋 3.10   ⚗ 7.58   **FUD** 000   ⊙ T A2 ▭
AMA: 2015,Jan,16; 2014,Dec,3; 2014,Nov,3; 2014,Jan,11; 2013,Dec,3; 2013,Jan,11-12

44386   **with biopsy, single or multiple**
Do not report with (44385)
📋 3.66   ⚗ 10.1   **FUD** 000   ⊙ T A2 ▭
AMA: 2015,Jan,16; 2014,Dec,3; 2014,Nov,3; 2014,Jan,11; 2013,Dec,3; 2013,Jan,11-12

44388-44408 [44401] Colonoscopy Via Stoma

INCLUDES   Control of bleeding as result of endoscopic procedure during same operative session
EXCLUDES   *Colonoscopy via rectum (45378, 45392-45393 [45390, 45398])*
          Computed tomographic colonography (74261-74263)
Code also exam of nonfunctional distal colon/rectum, when performed, with:
   Anoscopy (46600, 46604-46606, 46608-46615)
   Proctosigmoidoscopy (45300-45327)
   Sigmoidoscopy (45330-45347 [45346])

44388   **Colonoscopy through stoma; diagnostic, including collection of specimen(s) by brushing or washing, when performed (separate procedure)**
Code also modifier 53 when planned total colonoscopy cannot be completed
Do not report with (44389-44408 [44401])
📋 4.80   ⚗ 10.0   **FUD** 000   ⊙ T A2 ▭ P0
AMA: 2015,Jan,16; 2014,Dec,3; 2014,Nov,3; 2014,Jan,11; 2013,Dec,3; 2013,Jan,11-12; 2012,Jan,15-42; 2011,Jan,11

44389   **with biopsy, single or multiple**
Code also modifier 52 when colonoscope fails to reach the junction of the small intestine
Do not report with (44388)
Do not report with on same lesion (44403)
📋 5.30   ⚗ 11.2   **FUD** 000   ⊙ T A2 ▭ P0
AMA: 2015,Jan,16; 2014,Dec,3; 2014,Nov,3; 2014,Jan,11; 2013,Dec,3; 2013,Jan,11-12

44390   **with removal of foreign body(s)**
Code also modifier 52 when colonoscope fails to reach the junction of the small intestine
Do not report with (44388)
⚕ (76000)
📋 6.45   ⚗ 13.2   **FUD** 000   ⊙ T A2 ▭
AMA: 2015,Jan,16; 2014,Dec,3; 2014,Nov,3; 2014,Jan,11; 2013,Dec,3; 2013,Jan,11-12

44391   **with control of bleeding, any method**
Code also modifier 52 when colonoscope fails to reach the junction of the small intestine
Do not report with (44388)
Do not report with on same lesion (44404)
📋 7.20   ⚗ 14.2   **FUD** 000   ⊙ T A2 ▭
AMA: 2015,Jan,16; 2014,Dec,3; 2014,Nov,3; 2014,Jan,11; 2013,Dec,3; 2013,Jan,11-12; 2010,Jun,4-5

44392   **with removal of tumor(s), polyp(s), or other lesion(s) by hot biopsy forceps**

Code also modifier 52 when colonoscope fails to reach the junction of the small intestine

Do not report with (44388)

🖐 6.28   ✂ 12.5   **FUD** 000   ⊙ T A2 🖵 PQ

AMA: 2015,Jan,16; 2014,Dec,3; 2014,Nov,3; 2014,Jan,11; 2013,Dec,3; 2013,Jan,11-12

**44401**   **with ablation of tumor(s), polyp(s), or other lesion(s) (includes pre-and post-dilation and guide wire passage, when performed)**

Code also modifier 52 when colonoscope fails to reach the junction of the small intestine

Do not report with (44388)

Do not report with on same lesion (44405)

🖐 0.00   ✂ 0.00   **FUD** 000   ⊙ T G2

AMA: 2015,Jan,16; 2014,Dec,3; 2014,Nov,3

44394   **with removal of tumor(s), polyp(s), or other lesion(s) by snare technique**

Code also modifier 52 when colonoscope fails to reach the junction of the small intestine

Do not report with (44388)

Do not report with on same lesion (44403)

🖐 7.35   ✂ 14.1   **FUD** 000   ⊙ T A2 🖵 PQ

AMA: 2015,Jan,16; 2014,Dec,3; 2014,Nov,3; 2014,Jan,11; 2013,Dec,3; 2013,Jan,11-12

44401   **Resequenced code. See code following 44392.**

44402   **with endoscopic stent placement (including pre- and post-dilation and guide wire passage, when performed)**

Code also modifier 52 when colonoscope fails to reach the junction of the small intestine

Do not report with (44388, 44405)

📷 (74360)

🖐 0.00   ✂ 0.00   **FUD** 000   ⊙ T G2

AMA: 2015,Jan,16; 2014,Dec,3; 2014,Nov,3

44403   **with endoscopic mucosal resection**

Code also modifier 52 when colonoscope fails to reach the junction of the small intestine

Do not report with (44388)

Do not report with on same lesion (44389, 44394, 44404)

🖐 0.00   ✂ 0.00   **FUD** 000   ⊙ T G2

AMA: 2015,Jan,16; 2014,Dec,3; 2014,Nov,3

44404   **with directed submucosal injection(s), any substance**

Code also modifier 52 when colonoscope fails to reach the junction of the small intestine

Do not report with (44388)

Do not report with on same lesion (44391, 44403)

🖐 0.00   ✂ 0.00   **FUD** 000   ⊙ T G2

AMA: 2015,Jan,16; 2014,Dec,3; 2014,Nov,3

44405   **with transendoscopic balloon dilation**

Code also each additional stricture dilated in same session, using modifier 59 with (44405)

Code also modifier 52 when colonoscope fails to reach the junction of the small intestine

Do not report with (44388, [44401], 44402)

📷 (74360)

🖐 0.00   ✂ 0.00   **FUD** 000   ⊙ T G2

AMA: 2015,Jan,16; 2014,Dec,3; 2014,Nov,3

44406   **with endoscopic ultrasound examination, limited to the sigmoid, descending, transverse, or ascending colon and cecum and adjacent structures**

Code also modifier 52 when colonoscope fails to reach the junction of the small intestine

Do not report more than one time per operative session

Do not report with (44388, 44407, 76975)

🖐 0.00   ✂ 0.00   **FUD** 000   ⊙ T G2

AMA: 2015,Jan,16; 2014,Dec,3; 2014,Nov,3

44407   **with transendoscopic ultrasound guided intramural or transmural fine needle aspiration/biopsy(s), includes endoscopic ultrasound examination limited to the sigmoid, descending, transverse, or ascending colon and cecum and adjacent structures**

Code also modifier 52 when colonoscope fails to reach the junction of the small intestine

Do not report more than one time per operative session

Do not report with (44388, 44406, 76942, 76975)

🖐 0.00   ✂ 0.00   **FUD** 000   ⊙ T G2

AMA: 2015,Jan,16; 2014,Dec,3; 2014,Nov,3

44408   **with decompression (for pathologic distention) (eg, volvulus, megacolon), including placement of decompression tube, when performed**

Do not report more than one time per operative session

Do not report with (44388)

🖐 0.00   ✂ 0.00   **FUD** 000   ⊙ T G2

AMA: 2015,Jan,16; 2014,Dec,3; 2014,Nov,3

44500 Gastrointestinal Intubation

44500   **Introduction of long gastrointestinal tube (eg, Miller-Abbott) (separate procedure)**

EXCLUDES   *Placement of oro- or naso-gastric tube (43752)*

📷 (74340)

🖐 0.71   ✂ 0.71   **FUD** 000   ⊘ ⊙ T G2 80 🖵 PQ

AMA: 2015,Jan,16; 2014,Jan,11; 2013,Dec,3; 2013,Jan,11-12

44602-44680 Open Repair Procedures of Intestines

44602   **Suture of small intestine (enterorrhaphy) for perforated ulcer, diverticulum, wound, injury or rupture; single perforation**

🖐 40.8   ✂ 40.8   **FUD** 090   C 80 🖵 PQ

AMA: 2014,Jan,11; 2013,Dec,3; 2013,Jan,11-12

44603   **multiple perforations**

🖐 46.9   ✂ 46.9   **FUD** 090   C 80 🖵 PQ

AMA: 2014,Jan,11; 2013,Dec,3; 2013,Jan,11-12

44604   **Suture of large intestine (colorrhaphy) for perforated ulcer, diverticulum, wound, injury or rupture (single or multiple perforations); without colostomy**

🖐 30.6   ✂ 30.6   **FUD** 090   C 80 🖵 PQ

AMA: 2014,Jan,11; 2013,Dec,3; 2013,Jan,11-12

44605   **with colostomy**

🖐 37.8   ✂ 37.8   **FUD** 090   C 80 🖵 PQ

AMA: 2014,Jan,11; 2013,Dec,3; 2013,Jan,11-12

44615   **Intestinal stricturoplasty (enterotomy and enterorrhaphy) with or without dilation, for intestinal obstruction**

🖐 31.0   ✂ 31.0   **FUD** 090   C 80 🖵 PQ

AMA: 2014,Jan,11; 2013,Dec,3; 2013,Jan,11-12

44620   **Closure of enterostomy, large or small intestine;**

🖐 25.1   ✂ 25.1   **FUD** 090   C 80 🖵 PQ

AMA: 2014,Jan,11; 2013,Dec,3; 2013,Jan,11-12

44625   **with resection and anastomosis other than colorectal**

EXCLUDES   *Laparoscopic method (44227)*

🖐 29.4   ✂ 29.4   **FUD** 090   C 80 🖵 PQ

AMA: 2014,Jan,11; 2013,Dec,3; 2013,Jan,11-12

44626   **with resection and colorectal anastomosis (eg, closure of Hartmann type procedure)**

EXCLUDES   *Laparoscopic method (44227)*

🖐 46.4   ✂ 46.4   **FUD** 090   C 80 🖵 PQ

AMA: 2014,Jan,11; 2013,Dec,3; 2013,Jan,11-12

44640   **Closure of intestinal cutaneous fistula**

🖐 40.5   ✂ 40.5   **FUD** 090   C 80 🖵 PQ

AMA: 2014,Jan,11; 2013,Dec,3; 2013,Jan,11-12

44650   **Closure of enteroenteric or enterocolic fistula**

🖐 42.0   ✂ 42.0   **FUD** 090   C 80 🖵 PQ

AMA: 2014,Jan,11; 2013,Dec,3; 2013,Jan,11-12

Digestive System

44660   Closure of enterovesical fistula; without intestinal or bladder resection

> EXCLUDES   Closure of fistula:
>   Gastrocolic (43880)
>   Rectovesical (45800, 45805)
>   Renocolic (50525-50526)
>
> 🖐 38.6   ✂ 38.6   **FUD** 090   C 80 🔲 PQ
>
> **AMA:** 2014,Jan,11; 2013,Dec,3; 2013,Jan,11-12

44661   with intestine and/or bladder resection

> EXCLUDES   Closure of fistula:
>   Gastrocolic (43880)
>   Rectovesical (45800, 45805)
>   Renocolic (50525-50526)
>
> 🖐 44.9   ✂ 44.9   **FUD** 090   C 80 🔲 PQ
>
> **AMA:** 2014,Jan,11; 2013,Dec,3; 2013,Jan,11-12

44680   Intestinal plication (separate procedure)

> INCLUDES   Noble intestinal plication
>
> 🖐 30.8   ✂ 30.8   **FUD** 090   C 80 🔲 PQ
>
> **AMA:** 2014,Jan,11; 2013,Dec,3; 2013,Jan,11-12

44700-44705 Other Intestinal Procedures

44700   Exclusion of small intestine from pelvis by mesh or other prosthesis, or native tissue (eg, bladder or omentum)

> EXCLUDES   Therapeutic radiation clinical treatment (77261-77799
>   [77295, 77385, 77386, 77387, 77424, 77425])
>
> 🖐 29.5   ✂ 29.5   **FUD** 090   C 80 🔲 PQ
>
> **AMA:** 2014,Jan,11; 2013,Dec,3; 2013,Jan,11-12

+   **44701**   Intraoperative colonic lavage (List separately in addition to code for primary procedure)

> Code first as appropriate (44140, 44145, 44150, 44604)
> Do not report with (44300, 44950-44960)
>
> 🖐 4.88   ✂ 4.88   **FUD** ZZZ   N N1 80 🔲
>
> **AMA:** 2014,Jan,11; 2013,Dec,3; 2013,Jan,11-12

44705   Preparation of fecal microbiota for instillation, including assessment of donor specimen

> EXCLUDES   Fecal instillation by enema or oro-nasogastric tube
>   (44799)
> Do not report with (74283)
>
> 🖐 0.00   ✂ 0.00   **FUD** XXX   B
>
> **AMA:** 2015,Jan,16; 2014,Jan,11; 2013,Dec,3; 2013,May,12;
> 2013,Jan,11-12

44715-44799 Backbench Transplant Procedures

CMS: 100-4,3,90.6 Intestinal and Multi-Visceral Transplants

44715   Backbench standard preparation of cadaver or living donor intestine allograft prior to transplantation, including mobilization and fashioning of the superior mesenteric artery and vein

> INCLUDES   Mobilization/fashioning of superior mesenteric
>   vein/artery
>
> 🖐 0.00   ✂ 0.00   **FUD** XXX   C 80 🔲
>
> **AMA:** 2014,Jan,11; 2013,Dec,3; 2013,Jan,11-12

44720   Backbench reconstruction of cadaver or living donor intestine allograft prior to transplantation; venous anastomosis, each

> 🖐 7.99   ✂ 7.99   **FUD** XXX   C 80 🔲
>
> **AMA:** 2014,Jan,11; 2013,Dec,3; 2013,Jan,11-12

44721   arterial anastomosis, each

> 🖐 11.1   ✂ 11.1   **FUD** XXX   C 80 🔲
>
> **AMA:** 2015,Jan,16; 2014,Jan,11; 2013,Dec,3; 2013,Jan,11-12

44799   Unlisted procedure, small intestine

> EXCLUDES   Unlisted colon procedure (45399)
>   Unlisted intestinal procedure performed
>   laparoscopically (44238)
>   Unlisted rectal procedure (45499, 45999)
>
> 🖐 0.00   ✂ 0.00   **FUD** XXX   T 🔲
>
> **AMA:** 2015,Jan,16; 2014,Nov,3; 2014,Jan,11; 2013,Dec,3;
> 2013,May,12; 2013,Jan,11-12; 2012,Jan,15-42; 2011,May,9;
> 2011,Mar,9; 2011,Jan,11; 2010,Jul,10; 2010,Mar,9-11

44800-44899 Meckel's Diverticulum and Mesentery Procedures

44800   Excision of Meckel's diverticulum (diverticulectomy) or omphalomesenteric duct

> 🖐 22.1   ✂ 22.1   **FUD** 090   C 80 🔲 PQ
>
> **AMA:** 2014,Jan,11; 2013,Dec,3; 2013,Jan,11-12

44820   Excision of lesion of mesentery (separate procedure)

> EXCLUDES   Resection of intestine (44120-44128, 44140-44160)
>
> 🖐 24.5   ✂ 24.5   **FUD** 090   C 80 🔲 PQ
>
> **AMA:** 2014,Jan,11; 2013,Dec,3; 2013,Jan,11-12

44850   Suture of mesentery (separate procedure)

> EXCLUDES   Internal hernia repair/reduction (44050)
>
> 🖐 21.7   ✂ 21.7   **FUD** 090   C 80 🔲 PQ
>
> **AMA:** 2014,Jan,11; 2013,Dec,3; 2013,Jan,11-12

44899   Unlisted procedure, Meckel's diverticulum and the mesentery

> 🖐 0.00   ✂ 0.00   **FUD** YYY   C 80
>
> **AMA:** 2014,Jan,11; 2013,Dec,3; 2013,Jan,11-12

44900-44979 Open and Endoscopic Appendix Procedures

44900   Incision and drainage of appendiceal abscess, open

> EXCLUDES   Image guided percutaneous catheter drainage (49406)
>
> 🖐 22.4   ✂ 22.4   **FUD** 090   C 80 🔲 PQ
>
> **AMA:** 2014,Jan,11; 2013,Nov,9; 2013,Dec,3; 2013,Jan,11-12

44950   Appendectomy;

> INCLUDES   Battle's operation
> Do not report with other intra-abdominal procedure(s) when
>   appendectomy is incidental
>
> 🖐 18.5   ✂ 18.5   **FUD** 090   T 80 🔲 PQ
>
> **AMA:** 2015,Jan,16; 2014,Jan,11; 2013,Dec,3; 2013,Jan,11-12

Failure to treat appendicitis can lead to peritonitis

Ileum

Ascending colon

Cecum

Free tenia

Appendix and appendicular artery

Mesoappendix

+   **44955**   when done for indicated purpose at time of other major procedure (not as separate procedure) (List separately in addition to code for primary procedure)

> Code first primary procedure
>
> 🖐 2.43   ✂ 2.43   **FUD** ZZZ   N 80 🔲
>
> **AMA:** 2015,Jan,16; 2014,Jan,11; 2013,Dec,3; 2013,Jan,11-12;
> 2012,Jan,13-14

44960   for ruptured appendix with abscess or generalized peritonitis

> INCLUDES   Battle's operation
>
> 🖐 25.2   ✂ 25.2   **FUD** 090   C 80 🔲 PQ
>
> **AMA:** 2015,Jan,16; 2014,Jan,11; 2013,Dec,3; 2013,Jan,11-12

44970   Laparoscopy, surgical, appendectomy

> INCLUDES   Diagnostic laparoscopy
>
> 🖐 17.3   ✂ 17.3   **FUD** 090   T 80 🔲 PQ
>
> **AMA:** 2015,Mar,3; 2015,Jan,16; 2014,Jan,11; 2013,Dec,3;
> 2013,Jan,11-12; 2012,Jan,15-42; 2011,Jan,11

44979   Unlisted laparoscopy procedure, appendix

> 🖐 0.00   ✂ 0.00   **FUD** YYY   T 80 50
>
> **AMA:** 2015,Jan,16; 2014,Jan,11; 2013,Dec,3; 2013,Jan,11-12;
> 2012,Jan,13-14

45000-45190 Open and Transrectal Procedures of Rectum

45000 **Transrectal drainage of pelvic abscess**

EXCLUDES   *Image guided transrectal catheter drainage (49407)*

🔲 12.1   ⚕ 12.1   **FUD** 090   T A2 ▢ P0

AMA: 2014,Jan,11; 2013,Nov,9; 2013,Dec,3; 2013,Jan,11-12

45005 **Incision and drainage of submucosal abscess, rectum**

🔲 4.64   ⚕ 7.77   **FUD** 010   T A2 ▢

AMA: 2014,Jan,11; 2013,Dec,3; Jan,11-12

45020 **Incision and drainage of deep supralevator, pelvirectal, or retrorectal abscess**

EXCLUDES   *Incision and drainage of perianal, ischiorectal, intramural abscess (46050, 46060)*

🔲 16.4   ⚕ 16.4   **FUD** 090   T A2 ▢ P0

AMA: 2014,Jan,11; 2013,Dec,3; 2013,Jan,11-12

45100 **Biopsy of anorectal wall, anal approach (eg, congenital megacolon)**

EXCLUDES   *Biopsy performed endoscopically (45305)*

🔲 8.65   ⚕ 8.65   **FUD** 090   T A2 ▢ P0

AMA: 2014,Jan,11; 2013,Dec,3; 2013,Jan,11-12

45108 **Anorectal myomectomy**

🔲 10.6   ⚕ 10.6   **FUD** 090   T A2 ▢ P0

AMA: 2014,Jan,11; 2013,Dec,3; 2013,Jan,11-12

45110 **Proctectomy; complete, combined abdominoperineal, with colostomy**

EXCLUDES   *Laparoscopic method (45395)*

🔲 53.5   ⚕ 53.5   **FUD** 090   C 80 ▢ P0

AMA: 2014,Jan,11; 2013,Dec,3; 2013,Jan,11-12

45111 **partial resection of rectum, transabdominal approach**

INCLUDES   Luschka proctectomy

🔲 31.4   ⚕ 31.4   **FUD** 090   C 80 ▢ P0

AMA: 2014,Jan,11; 2013,Dec,3; 2013,Jan,11-12

45112 **Proctectomy, combined abdominoperineal, pull-through procedure (eg, colo-anal anastomosis)**

EXCLUDES   *Proctectomy for colo-anal anastomosis with creation of colonic pouch or reservoir (45119)*

🔲 54.5   ⚕ 54.5   **FUD** 090   C 80 ▢ P0

AMA: 2014,Jan,11; 2013,Dec,3; 2013,Jan,11-12

45113 **Proctectomy, partial, with rectal mucosectomy, ileoanal anastomosis, creation of ileal reservoir (S or J), with or without loop ileostomy**

🔲 54.6   ⚕ 54.6   **FUD** 090   C 80 ▢ P0

AMA: 2014,Jan,11; 2013,Dec,3; 2013,Jan,11-12

45114 **Proctectomy, partial, with anastomosis; abdominal and transsacral approach**

🔲 52.6   ⚕ 52.6   **FUD** 090   C 80 ▢ P0

AMA: 2014,Jan,11; 2013,Dec,3; 2013,Jan,11-12

45116 **transsacral approach only (Kraske type)**

🔲 44.8   ⚕ 44.8   **FUD** 090   C 80 ▢ P0

AMA: 2014,Jan,11; 2013,Dec,3; 2013,Jan,11-12

45119 **Proctectomy, combined abdominoperineal pull-through procedure (eg, colo-anal anastomosis), with creation of colonic reservoir (eg, J-pouch), with diverting enterostomy when performed**

EXCLUDES   *Laparoscopic method (45397)*

🔲 56.4   ⚕ 56.4   **FUD** 090   C 80 ▢ P0

AMA: 2015,Jan,16; 2014,Jan,11; 2013,Dec,3; 2013,Jan,11-12

45120 **Proctectomy, complete (for congenital megacolon), abdominal and perineal approach; with pull-through procedure and anastomosis (eg, Swenson, Duhamel, or Soave type operation)**

🔲 46.0   ⚕ 46.0   **FUD** 090   C 80 ▢ P0

AMA: 2014,Jan,11; 2013,Dec,3; 2013,Jan,11-12

45121 **with subtotal or total colectomy, with multiple biopsies**

🔲 47.6   ⚕ 47.6   **FUD** 090   C 80 ▢ P0

AMA: 2014,Jan,11; 2013,Dec,3; 2013,Jan,11-12

45123 **Proctectomy, partial, without anastomosis, perineal approach**

🔲 32.4   ⚕ 32.4   **FUD** 090   C 80 ▢ P0

AMA: 2014,Jan,11; 2013,Dec,3; 2013,Jan,11-12

45126 **Pelvic exenteration for colorectal malignancy, with proctectomy (with or without colostomy), with removal of bladder and ureteral transplantations, and/or hysterectomy, or cervicectomy, with or without removal of tube(s), with or without removal of ovary(s), or any combination thereof**

🔲 78.5   ⚕ 78.5   **FUD** 090   C 80 ▢ P0

AMA: 2014,Jan,11; 2013,Dec,3; 2013,Jan,11-12

45130 **Excision of rectal procidentia, with anastomosis; perineal approach**

INCLUDES   Altemeier procedure

🔲 31.4   ⚕ 31.4   **FUD** 090   C 80 ▢ P0

AMA: 2014,Jan,11; 2013,Dec,3; 2013,Jan,11-12

45135 **abdominal and perineal approach**

INCLUDES   Altemeier procedure

🔲 39.8   ⚕ 39.8   **FUD** 090   C 80 ▢ P0

AMA: 2014,Jan,11; 2013,Dec,3; 2013,Jan,11-12

45136 **Excision of ileoanal reservoir with ileostomy**

Do not report with (44005, 44120, 44310)

🔲 52.1   ⚕ 52.1   **FUD** 090   C 80 ▢ P0

AMA: 2014,Jan,11; 2013,Dec,3; 2013,Jan,11-12

45150 **Division of stricture of rectum**

🔲 10.3   ⚕ 10.3   **FUD** 090   T A2 80 ▢ P0

AMA: 2014,Jan,11; 2013,Dec,3; 2013,Jan,11-12

45160 **Excision of rectal tumor by proctotomy, transsacral or transcoccygeal approach**

🔲 29.6   ⚕ 29.6   **FUD** 090   T A2 80 ▢ P0

AMA: 2014,Jan,11; 2013,Dec,3; 2013,Jan,11-12

45171 **Excision of rectal tumor, transanal approach; not including muscularis propria (ie, partial thickness)**

EXCLUDES   *Transanal destruction of rectal tumor (45190)*
            Transanal endoscopic microsurgical tumor excision (TEMS) (0184T)

🔲 17.3   ⚕ 17.3   **FUD** 090   T G2 80 P0

AMA: 2015,Jan,16; 2014,Jan,11; 2013,Dec,3; 2013,Jan,11-12; 2010,Jun,3

45172 **including muscularis propria (ie, full thickness)**

EXCLUDES   *Transanal destruction of rectal tumor (45190)*
            Transanal endoscopic microsurgical tumor excision (TEMS) (0184T)

🔲 23.4   ⚕ 23.4   **FUD** 090   T G2 80 P0

AMA: 2015,Jan,16; 2014,Jan,11; 2013,Dec,3; 2013,Jan,11-12; 2010,Jun,3

45190 **Destruction of rectal tumor (eg, electrodesiccation, electrosurgery, laser ablation, laser resection, cryosurgery) transanal approach**

EXCLUDES   *Transanal endoscopic microsurgical tumor excision (TEMS) (0184T)*
            Transanal excision of rectal tumor (45171-45172)

🔲 20.0   ⚕ 20.0   **FUD** 090   T A2 ▢ P0

AMA: 2015,Jan,16; 2014,Jan,11; 2013,Dec,3; 2013,Jan,11-12; 2010,Jun,3

45300-45327 Rigid Proctosigmoidoscopy Procedures

INCLUDES   Control of bleeding as result of the endoscopic procedure during same operative session
Exam of:
   Entire rectum
   Portion of sigmoid colon
EXCLUDES   *Computed tomographic colonography (74261-74263)*
Code also examination of colon through stoma:
   Colonoscopy via stoma (44388-44408 [44401])
   Ileoscopy via stoma (44380-44384 [44381])

45300   **Proctosigmoidoscopy, rigid; diagnostic, with or without collection of specimen(s) by brushing or washing (separate procedure)**
         1.56   3.53   **FUD** 000   T P3
         AMA: 2015,Jan,16; 2014,Jan,11; 2013,Dec,3; 2013,Jan,11-12

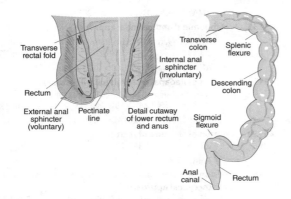

45303   **with dilation (eg, balloon, guide wire, bougie)**
         (74360)
         2.69   27.5   **FUD** 000   ⊙ T P2
         AMA: 2015,Jan,16; 2014,Jan,11; 2013,Dec,3; 2013,Jan,11-12

45305   **with biopsy, single or multiple**
         2.29   5.58   **FUD** 000   ⊙ T A2 P0
         AMA: 2015,Jan,16; 2014,Jan,11; 2013,Dec,3; 2013,Jan,11-12

45307   **with removal of foreign body**
         2.97   6.39   **FUD** 000   ⊙ T A2 80
         AMA: 2015,Jan,16; 2014,Jan,11; 2013,Dec,3; 2013,Jan,11-12

45308   **with removal of single tumor, polyp, or other lesion by hot biopsy forceps or bipolar cautery**
         2.59   6.28   **FUD** 000   ⊙ T A2
         AMA: 2015,Jan,16; 2014,Jan,11; 2013,Dec,3; 2013,Jan,11-12

45309   **with removal of single tumor, polyp, or other lesion by snare technique**
         2.61   6.32   **FUD** 000   ⊙ T A2
         AMA: 2015,Jan,16; 2014,Jan,11; 2013,Dec,3; 2013,Jan,11-12

45315   **with removal of multiple tumors, polyps, or other lesions by hot biopsy forceps, bipolar cautery or snare technique**
         3.25   7.10   **FUD** 000   ⊙ T A2
         AMA: 2015,Jan,16; 2014,Jan,11; 2013,Dec,3; 2013,Jan,11-12

45317   **with control of bleeding (eg, injection, bipolar cautery, unipolar cautery, laser, heater probe, stapler, plasma coagulator)**
         3.40   6.93   **FUD** 000   ⊙ T A2
         AMA: 2015,Jan,16; 2014,Jan,11; 2013,Dec,3; 2013,Jan,11-12

45320   **with ablation of tumor(s), polyp(s), or other lesion(s) not amenable to removal by hot biopsy forceps, bipolar cautery or snare technique (eg, laser)**
         3.21   7.01   **FUD** 000   ⊙ T A2
         AMA: 2015,Jan,16; 2014,Jan,11; 2013,Dec,3; 2013,Jan,11-12

45321   **with decompression of volvulus**
         3.10   3.10   **FUD** 000   ⊙ T A2
         AMA: 2015,Jan,16; 2014,Jan,11; 2013,Dec,3; 2013,Jan,11-12

45327   **with transendoscopic stent placement (includes predilation)**
         3.54   3.54   **FUD** 000   ⊙ J A2
         AMA: 2015,Jan,16; 2014,Jan,11; 2013,Dec,3; 2013,Jan,11-12

45330-45350 [45346] Flexible Sigmoidoscopy Procedures

INCLUDES   Control of bleeding as result of the endoscopic procedure during same operative session
Exam of:
   Entire rectum
   Entire sigmoid colon
   Portion of descending colon (when performed)
EXCLUDES   *Computed tomographic colonography (74261-74263)*
Code also examination of colon through stoma when appropriate:
   Colonoscopy (44388-44408 [44401])
   Ileoscopy (44380-44384 [44381])

45330   **Sigmoidoscopy, flexible; diagnostic, including collection of specimen(s) by brushing or washing, when performed (separate procedure)**
         Do not report with (45331-45349 [45346])
         1.83   3.91   **FUD** 000   T P3
         AMA: 2015,Jan,16; 2014,Dec,3; 2014,Dec,18; 2014,Jan,11; 2013,Dec,3; 2013,Jan,11-12; 2012,Jan,15-42; 2011,Jan,11

45331   **with biopsy, single or multiple**
         Do not report with on same lesion (45349)
         2.16   4.64   **FUD** 000   T A2 P0
         AMA: 2015,Jan,16; 2014,Dec,3; 2014,Dec,18; 2014,Jan,11; 2013,Dec,3; 2013,Jan,11-12; 2012,Jan,15-42; 2011,Jan,11

45332   **with removal of foreign body(s)**
         Do not report with (45330)
         (76000)
         3.18   8.32   **FUD** 000   ⊙ T A2
         AMA: 2015,Jan,16; 2014,Dec,3; 2014,Dec,18; 2014,Jan,11; 2013,Dec,3; 2013,Jan,11-12

45333   **with removal of tumor(s), polyp(s), or other lesion(s) by hot biopsy forceps**
         Do not report with (45330)
         3.17   8.46   **FUD** 000   ⊙ T A2
         AMA: 2015,Jan,16; 2014,Dec,3; 2014,Dec,18; 2014,Jan,11; 2013,Dec,3; 2013,Jan,11-12

45334   **with control of bleeding, any method**
         Do not report with (45330)
         Do not report with on same lesion (45335, 45350)
         4.68   4.68   **FUD** 000   ⊙ T A2
         AMA: 2015,Jan,16; 2014,Dec,3; 2014,Dec,18; 2014,Jan,11; 2013,Dec,3; 2013,Jan,11-12; 2012,Jan,15-42; 2011,Jan,11; 2010,Jun,4-5

45335   **with directed submucosal injection(s), any substance**
         Do not report with (45330)
         Do not report with on same lesion (45334, 45349)
         2.65   7.83   **FUD** 000   ⊙ T A2
         AMA: 2015,Jan,16; 2014,Dec,3; 2014,Dec,18; 2014,Jan,11; 2013,Dec,3; 2013,Jan,11-12; 2012,Jan,15-42; 2011,Jan,11; 2010,Jun,4-5

45337   **with decompression (for pathologic distention) (eg, volvulus, megacolon), including placement of decompression tube, when performed**
         Do not report with (45330)
         Do not report more than one time per operative session
         4.09   4.09   **FUD** 000   ⊙ T A2
         AMA: 2015,Jan,16; 2014,Dec,3; 2014,Dec,18; 2014,Jan,11; 2013,Dec,3; 2013,Jan,11-12

45338   **with removal of tumor(s), polyp(s), or other lesion(s) by snare technique**
         Do not report with (45330)
         Do not report with on same lesion (45349)
         4.04   9.08   **FUD** 000   ⊙ T A2
         AMA: 2015,Jan,16; 2014,Dec,3; 2014,Dec,18; 2014,Jan,11; 2013,Dec,3; 2013,Jan,11-12

Digestive System

**45346** **with ablation of tumor(s), polyp(s), or other lesion(s) (includes pre- and post-dilation and guide wire passage, when performed)**
    Do not report with (45330)
    Do not report with on same lesion (45340)
    ☒ 0.00   ✂ 0.00   **FUD** 000   ⊙ T 62
    AMA: 2015,Jan,16; 2014,Dec,3

45340 **with transendoscopic balloon dilation**
    Code also each additional stricture dilated in same session, using modifier 59 with (45340)
    Do not report with (45330, [45346], 45347)
    ☒ (74360)
    ☒ 3.33   ✂ 13.8   **FUD** 000   ⊙ T A2 ▭
    AMA: 2015,Jan,16; 2014,Dec,3; 2014,Dec,18; 2014,Jan,11; 2013,Dec,3; 2013,Jan,11-12

45341 **with endoscopic ultrasound examination**
    Do not report more than one time per operative session
    Do not report with (45330, 45342, 76872, 76975)
    ☒ 4.46   ✂ 4.46   **FUD** 000   ⊙ T A2 ▭
    AMA: 2015,Jan,16; 2014,Dec,3; 2014,Dec,18; 2014,Jan,11; 2013,Dec,3; 2013,Jan,11-12

45342 **with transendoscopic ultrasound guided intramural or transmural fine needle aspiration/biopsy(s)**
    Do not report with (45330, 45341, 76872, 76942, 76975)
    Do not report more than one time per operative session
    ☒ 6.77   ✂ 6.77   **FUD** 000   ⊙ T A2 ▭
    AMA: 2015,Jan,16; 2014,Dec,3; 2014,Dec,18; 2014,Jan,11; 2013,Dec,3; 2013,Jan,11-12

45346 **Resequenced code. See code following 45338.**

45347 **with placement of endoscopic stent (includes pre- and post-dilation and guide wire passage, when performed)**
    Do not report with (45330, 45340)
    ☒ (74360)
    ☒ 0.00   ✂ 0.00   **FUD** 000   ⊙ T 62
    AMA: 2015,Jan,16; 2014,Dec,3

45349 **with endoscopic mucosal resection**
    Do not report with (45330)
    Do not report with on same lesion (45331, 45335, 45338, 45350)
    ☒ 0.00   ✂ 0.00   **FUD** 000   ⊙ T 62
    AMA: 2015,Jan,16; 2014,Dec,3

45350 **with band ligation(s) (eg, hemorrhoids)**
    EXCLUDES *Bleeding control by band ligation (45334)*
    Do not report more than one time per operative session
    Do not report with (45330, 45349, 46221)
    Do not report with on same lesion (45334)
    ☒ 0.00   ✂ 0.00   **FUD** 000   ⊙ T 62
    AMA: 2015,Jan,16; 2014,Dec,3

45378-45393 [45388, 45390, 45398] Flexible and Rigid Colonoscopy Procedures

  INCLUDES Control of bleeding as result of the endoscopic procedure during same operative session
    Exam of:
      Entire colon (rectum to cecum)
      Terminal ileum (when performed)
  EXCLUDES *Computed tomographic colonography (74261-74263)*
  Code also modifier 53 (physician), or 73, 74 (facility) for an incomplete colonoscopy

45378 **Colonoscopy, flexible; diagnostic, including collection of specimen(s) by brushing or washing, when performed (separate procedure)**

Screening

    EXCLUDES *Decompression for pathological distention (45393)*
    Code also modifier 53 when planned total colonoscopy cannot be completed
    Do not report with (45379-45393 [45388, 45390, 45398])
    ☒ 6.19   ✂ 11.0   **FUD** 000   ⊙ T A2 ▭ P0
    AMA: 2015,Jan,16; 2014,Dec,3; 2014,Nov,3; 2014,Jan,11; 2013,Dec,3; 2013,Jan,11-12; 2012,Jan,15-42; 2011,Apr,12; 2010,Dec,3-6

45379 **with removal of foreign body(s)**
    Code also modifier 52 when colonoscope fails to reach the junction of the small intestine
    Do not report with (45378)
    ☒ (76000)
    ☒ 7.78   ✂ 14.2   **FUD** 000   ⊙ T A2 ▭
    AMA: 2015,Jan,16; 2014,Dec,3; 2014,Jan,11; 2013,Dec,3; 2013,Jan,11-12

45380 **with biopsy, single or multiple**
    Code also modifier 52 when colonoscope fails to reach the junction of the small intestine
    Do not report with (45378)
    Do not report with on same lesion (45390)
    ☒ 7.40   ✂ 13.1   **FUD** 000   ⊙ T A2 ▭ P0
    AMA: 2015,Jan,16; 2014,Dec,3; 2014,Jan,11; 2013,Dec,3; 2013,Jan,11-12; 2012,Jan,15-42; 2011,Jan,11

45381 **with directed submucosal injection(s), any substance** *- Botox / India Ink / Saline*
    Code also modifier 52 when colonoscope fails to reach the junction of the small intestine
    Do not report with (45378)
    Do not report with on same lesion (45382, 45390)
    ☒ 7.01   ✂ 13.2   **FUD** 000   ⊙ T A2 ▭ P0
    AMA: 2015,Jan,16; 2014,Dec,3; 2014,Jan,11; 2013,Dec,3; 2013,Jan,11-12; 2012,Jan,15-42; 2011,Jan,11; 2010,Jun,4-5

45382 **with control of bleeding, any method**
    Code also modifier 52 when colonoscope fails to reach the junction of the small intestine
    Do not report with (45378)
    Do not report with on same lesion (45381, [45398])
    ☒ 9.39   ✂ 17.1   **FUD** 000   ⊙ T A2 ▭
    AMA: 2015,Jan,16; 2014,Dec,3; 2014,Jan,11; 2013,Dec,3; 2013,Jan,11-12; 2010,Jun,4-5

**45388** **with ablation of tumor(s), polyp(s), or other lesion(s) (includes pre- and post-dilation and guide wire passage, when performed)**
    Code also modifier 52 when colonoscope fails to reach the junction of the small intestine
    Do not report (45378, 45386)
    ☒ 0.00   ✂ 0.00   **FUD** 000   ⊙ T 62
    AMA: 2015,Jan,16; 2014,Dec,3

45384 **with removal of tumor(s), polyp(s), or other lesion(s) by hot biopsy forceps**
    Code also modifier 52 when colonoscope fails to reach the junction of the small intestine
    Do not report with (45378)
    ☒ 7.76   ✂ 13.2   **FUD** 000   ⊙ T A2 ▭ P0
    AMA: 2015,Jun,10; 2015,Jan,16; 2014,Dec,3; 2014,Jan,11; 2013,Dec,3; 2013,Jan,11-12; 2012,Jan,15-42; 2011,Apr,12; 2011,Jan,11

45385 **with removal of tumor(s), polyp(s), or other lesion(s) by snare technique**
    Do not report with (45378)
    Do not report with on same lesion (45390)
    ☒ 8.78   ✂ 14.8   **FUD** 000   ⊙ T A2 ▭ P0
    AMA: 2015,Jan,16; 2014,Dec,3; 2014,Jan,11; 2013,Dec,3; 2013,Jan,11-12; 2012,Jan,15-42; 2011,Jan,11; 2010,Jun,4-5

45386 **with transendoscopic balloon dilation**
    Code also each additional stricture dilated in same operative session, using modifier 59 with (45386)
    Do not report with (45378, [45388], 45389)
    ☒ (74360)
    ☒ 7.60   ✂ 18.9   **FUD** 000   ⊙ T A2 ▭
    AMA: 2015,Jan,16; 2014,Dec,3; 2014,Jan,11; 2013,Dec,3; 2013,Jan,11-12

45388 **Resequenced code. See code following 45382.**

45389 **with endoscopic stent placement (includes pre- and post-dilation and guide wire passage, when performed)**
    Do not report with (45378, 45386)
    ☒ (74360)
    ☒ 0.00   ✂ 0.00   **FUD** 000   ⊙ T 62
    AMA: 2015,Jan,16; 2014,Dec,3

Digestive System

45390 — 45805

45390 **Resequenced code. See code following 45392.**

45391 **with endoscopic ultrasound examination limited to the rectum, sigmoid, descending, transverse, or ascending colon and cecum, and adjacent structures**

Do not report more than one time per operative session
Do not report with (45378, 45392, 76872, 76975)
📷 8.43   ⚕ 8.43   **FUD** 000   ⊙ T A2

AMA: 2015,Jan,16; 2014,Dec,3; 2014,Jan,11; 2013,Dec,3; 2013,Jan,11-12

45392 **with transendoscopic ultrasound guided intramural or transmural fine needle aspiration/biopsy(s), includes endoscopic ultrasound examination limited to the rectum, sigmoid, descending, transverse, or ascending colon and cecum, and adjacent structures**

Do not report more than one time per operative session
Do not report with (45378, 45391, 76872, 76942, 76975)
📷 10.7   ⚕ 10.7   **FUD** 000   ⊙ T A2 PQ

AMA: 2015,Jan,16; 2014,Dec,3; 2014,Jan,11; 2013,Dec,3; 2013,Jan,11-12

\# **45390** **with endoscopic mucosal resection**

Do not report when on same lesion with (45380-45381, 45385, [45398])
Do not report with (45378)
📷 0.00   ⚕ 0.00   **FUD** 000   ⊙ T 62

AMA: 2015,Jan,16; 2014,Dec,3

45393 **with decompression (for pathologic distention) (eg, volvulus, megacolon), including placement of decompression tube, when performed**

Do not report more than one time per operative session
Do not report with (45378)
📷 0.00   ⚕ 0.00   **FUD** 000   ⊙ T 62

AMA: 2015,Jan,16; 2014,Dec,3

\# **45398** **with band ligation(s) (eg, hemorrhoids)**

EXCLUDES *Bleeding control by band ligation (45382)*
Code also modifier 52 when colonoscope fails to reach the junction of the small intestine
Do not report more than one time per operative session
Do not report with (45378, 45390, 46221)
Do not report with on same lesion (45382)
📷 0.00   ⚕ 0.00   **FUD** 000   ⊙ T 62

AMA: 2015,Jan,16; 2014,Dec,3

45395-45499 Laparoscopic Procedures of Rectum

INCLUDES Diagnostic laparoscopy

45395 **Laparoscopy, surgical; proctectomy, complete, combined abdominoperineal, with colostomy**

EXCLUDES *Open method (45110)*
📷 57.3   ⚕ 57.3   **FUD** 090   C 80 PQ

AMA: 2015,Jan,16; 2014,Jan,11; 2013,Jan,11-12

45397 **proctectomy, combined abdominoperineal pull-through procedure (eg, colo-anal anastomosis), with creation of colonic reservoir (eg, J-pouch), with diverting enterostomy, when performed**

EXCLUDES *Open method (45119)*
📷 62.4   ⚕ 62.4   **FUD** 090   C 80 PQ

AMA: 2015,Jan,16; 2014,Jan,11; 2013,Jan,11-12; 2012,Jan,15-42; 2011,Jan,11

45398 **Resequenced code. See code following 45393.**

45399 **Resequenced code. See code before 45990.**

45400 **Laparoscopy, surgical; proctopexy (for prolapse)**

EXCLUDES *Open method (45540-45541)*
📷 32.9   ⚕ 32.9   **FUD** 090   C 80 PQ

AMA: 2015,Jan,16; 2014,Jan,11; 2013,Jan,11-12

45402 **proctopexy (for prolapse), with sigmoid resection**

EXCLUDES *Open method (45550)*
📷 44.0   ⚕ 44.0   **FUD** 090   C 80 PQ

AMA: 2015,Jan,16; 2014,Jan,11; 2013,Jan,11-12

45499 **Unlisted laparoscopy procedure, rectum**

EXCLUDES *Unlisted rectal procedure performed via open technique (45999)*
📷 0.00   ⚕ 0.00   **FUD** YYY   T 80

AMA: 2014,Jan,11; 2013,Jan,11-12

45500-45825 Open Repairs of Rectum

45500 **Proctoplasty; for stenosis**

📷 15.1   ⚕ 15.1   **FUD** 090   T A2 80 ▱ PQ

AMA: 2014,Jan,11; 2013,Jan,11-12

45505 **for prolapse of mucous membrane**

📷 17.1   ⚕ 17.1   **FUD** 090   T A2 ▱ PQ

AMA: 2015,Mar,9; 2015,Jan,16; 2014,Jan,11; 2013,Oct,18; 2013,Jan,11-12

45520 **Perirectal injection of sclerosing solution for prolapse**

📷 1.16   ⚕ 4.53   **FUD** 000   T P2 ▱ PQ

AMA: 2015,Jan,16; 2014,Jan,11; 2013,Jan,11-12; 2012,Jan,15-42; 2011,Jan,11

45540 **Proctopexy (eg, for prolapse); abdominal approach**

EXCLUDES *Laparoscopic method (45400)*
📷 30.6   ⚕ 30.6   **FUD** 090   C 80 ▱ PQ

AMA: 2014,Jan,11; 2013,Jan,11-12

45541 **perineal approach**

📷 27.1   ⚕ 27.1   **FUD** 090   T 62 80 ▱ PQ

AMA: 2014,Jan,11; 2013,Jan,11-12

45550 **with sigmoid resection, abdominal approach**

INCLUDES Frickman proctopexy
EXCLUDES *Laparoscopic method (45402)*
📷 42.2   ⚕ 42.2   **FUD** 090   C 80 ▱ PQ

AMA: 2014,Jan,11; 2013,Jan,11-12

45560 **Repair of rectocele (separate procedure)**

EXCLUDES *Posterior colporrhaphy with rectocele repair (57250)*
📷 19.8   ⚕ 19.8   **FUD** 090   T A2 80 ▱ PQ

AMA: 2014,Jan,11; 2013,Jan,11-12

45562 **Exploration, repair, and presacral drainage for rectal injury;**

📷 33.1   ⚕ 33.1   **FUD** 090   C 80 ▱ PQ

AMA: 2014,Jan,11; 2013,Jan,11-12

45563 **with colostomy**

INCLUDES Maydl colostomy
📷 47.7   ⚕ 47.7   **FUD** 090   C 80 ▱ PQ

AMA: 2014,Jan,11; 2013,Jan,11-12

45800 **Closure of rectovesical fistula;**

📷 35.8   ⚕ 35.8   **FUD** 090   C 80 ▱ PQ

AMA: 2014,Jan,11; 2013,Jan,11-12

An anal fistula leading from the rectum to the skin near the anus contains a continual discharge that irritates the skin and causes discomfort or pain

Bladder   Pubic symphysis   Urethra

Rectoperineal fistula

Rectum

45805 **with colostomy**

📷 39.9   ⚕ 39.9   **FUD** 090   C 80 ▱ PQ

AMA: 2014,Jan,11; 2013,Jan,11-12

45820	**Closure of rectourethral fistula;**

EXCLUDES *Closure of fistula, rectovaginal (57300-57308)*
🔧 32.4   ⚕ 32.4   **FUD** 090   C 80 ▭ PQ
AMA: 2014,Jan,11; 2013,Jan,11-12

45825	**with colostomy**

EXCLUDES *Closure of fistula, rectovaginal (57300-57308)*
🔧 41.8   ⚕ 41.8   **FUD** 090   C 80 ▭ PQ
AMA: 2014,Jan,11; 2013,Jan,11-12

45900-45999 [45399] Closed Procedures of Rectum With Anesthesia

45900	**Reduction of procidentia (separate procedure) under anesthesia**

🔧 5.90   ⚕ 5.90   **FUD** 010   T A2 80 ▭
AMA: 2014,Jan,11; 2013,Jan,11-12

45905	**Dilation of anal sphincter (separate procedure) under anesthesia other than local**

🔧 4.89   ⚕ 4.89   **FUD** 010   T A2 ▭
AMA: 2014,Jan,11; 2013,Jan,11-12

45910	**Dilation of rectal stricture (separate procedure) under anesthesia other than local**

🔧 5.62   ⚕ 5.62   **FUD** 010   T A2 ▭
AMA: 2014,Jan,11; 2013,Jan,11-12

45915	**Removal of fecal impaction or foreign body (separate procedure) under anesthesia**

🔧 6.55   ⚕ 9.49   **FUD** 010   T A2 ▭
AMA: 2015,Jan,16; 2014,Jan,11; 2013,Jan,11-12; 2012,Jan,15-42; 2011,Jan,11

#	45399	**Unlisted procedure, colon**

🔧 0.00   ⚕ 0.00   **FUD** XXX   T
AMA: 2015,Jan,16; 2014,Dec,3; 2014,Nov,3

45990	**Anorectal exam, surgical, requiring anesthesia (general, spinal, or epidural), diagnostic**

INCLUDES Diagnostic:
Anoscopy
Proctoscopy, rigid
Exam:
Pelvic (when performed)
Perineal, external
Rectal, digital
Do not report with (45300-45327, 45600, 57410, 99170)
🔧 3.12   ⚕ 3.12   **FUD** 000   T A2 80
AMA: 2015,Jan,16; 2014,Jan,11; 2013,Jan,11-12; 2012,Jan,15-42; 2011,Jan,11

45999	**Unlisted procedure, rectum**

EXCLUDES *Unlisted rectal procedure performed laparoscopically (45499)*
🔧 0.00   ⚕ 0.00   **FUD** YYY   T 80
AMA: 2015,Jan,16; 2014,Jan,11; 2013,Jan,11-12

46020-46083 Surgical Incision of Anus

EXCLUDES *Cryosurgical destruction of hemorrhoid(s) (46999)*
Fistulotomy, subcutaneous (46270)
Hemorrhoidopexy ([46947])
Injection of hemorrhoid(s) (46500)
Thermal energy destruction of internal hemorrhoid(s) (46930)

46020	**Placement of seton**

Do not report with (46060, 46280, 46600, 0249T)
🔧 6.75   ⚕ 7.92   **FUD** 010   T A2 ▭
AMA: 2014,Jan,11; 2013,Jan,11-12

46030	**Removal of anal seton, other marker**

🔧 2.61   ⚕ 3.99   **FUD** 010   T A2 80 ▭
AMA: 2014,Jan,11; 2013,Jan,11-12

46040	**Incision and drainage of ischiorectal and/or perirectal abscess (separate procedure)**

🔧 11.9   ⚕ 15.3   **FUD** 090   T A2 ▭
AMA: 2014,Jan,11; 2013,Jan,11-12

46045	**Incision and drainage of intramural, intramuscular, or submucosal abscess, transanal, under anesthesia**

🔧 12.5   ⚕ 12.5   **FUD** 090   T A2 ▭
AMA: 2014,Jan,11; 2013,Jan,11-12

46050	**Incision and drainage, perianal abscess, superficial**

EXCLUDES *Incision and drainage abscess:*
Ischiorectal/intramural (46060)
Supralevator/pelvirectal/retrorectal (45020)
🔧 2.81   ⚕ 5.76   **FUD** 010   T A2 ▭
AMA: 2014,Jan,11; 2013,Jan,11-12

46060	**Incision and drainage of ischiorectal or intramural abscess, with fistulectomy or fistulotomy, submuscular, with or without placement of seton**

EXCLUDES *Incision and drainage abscess:*
Supralevator/pelvirectal/retrorectal (45020)
Do not report with (46020)
🔧 13.7   ⚕ 13.7   **FUD** 090   T A2 ▭
AMA: 2014,Jan,11; 2013,Jan,11-12

46070	**Incision, anal septum (infant)**	A

EXCLUDES *Anoplasty (46700-46705)*
🔧 6.33   ⚕ 6.33   **FUD** 090   63 T 62 80 ▭
AMA: 2014,Jan,11; 2013,Jan,11-12

46080	**Sphincterotomy, anal, division of sphincter (separate procedure)**

🔧 4.59   ⚕ 7.08   **FUD** 010   T A2 ▭
AMA: 2014,Jan,11; 2013,Jan,11-12

46083	**Incision of thrombosed hemorrhoid, external**

🔧 3.06   ⚕ 5.02   **FUD** 010   T P2 ▭
AMA: 2015,Jan,16; 2014,Jan,11; 2013,Jan,11-12; 2012,Jan,15-42; 2011,Jan,11

46200-46262 [46220, 46320, 46945, 46946] Anal Resection and Hemorrhoidectomies

EXCLUDES *Cryosurgical destruction of hemorrhoid(s) (46999)*
Hemorrhoidopexy ([46947])
Injection of hemorrhoid(s) (46500)
Thermal energy destruction of internal hemorrhoid(s) (46930)

46200	**Fissurectomy, including sphincterotomy, when performed**

🔧 9.37   ⚕ 12.7   **FUD** 090   T A2 ▭
AMA: 2014,Jan,11; 2013,Jan,11-12

46220	*Resequenced code. See code before 46230.*

46221	**Hemorrhoidectomy, internal, by rubber band ligation(s)**

EXCLUDES *Ligation of hemorrhoidal vascular bundles including ultrasound guidance (0249T)*
Do not report with (45350, [45398])
🔧 5.53   ⚕ 7.73   **FUD** 010   T P3 ▭
AMA: 2015,Apr,10; 2015,Jan,16; 2014,Dec,3; 2014,Jan,11; 2013,Jan,11-12

#	46945	**Hemorrhoidectomy, internal, by ligation other than rubber band; single hemorrhoid column/group**

EXCLUDES *Other hemorrhoid procedures:*
Destruction (46930)
Excision (46250-46262)
Injection sclerosing solution (46500)
Do not report with (0249T)
🔧 6.49   ⚕ 8.84   **FUD** 090   T P3 ▭
AMA: 2015,Apr,10; 2014,Jan,11; 2013,Jan,11-12

#	46946	**2 or more hemorrhoid columns/groups**

Do not report with (0249T)
🔧 6.52   ⚕ 9.03   **FUD** 090   T A2 ▭
AMA: 2015,Apr,10; 2014,Jan,11; 2013,Jan,11-12

#	46220	**Excision of single external papilla or tag, anus**

🔧 3.43   ⚕ 5.90   **FUD** 010   T A2 ▭
AMA: 2014,Jan,11; 2013,Jan,11-12

46230	**Excision of multiple external papillae or tags, anus**

🔧 4.99   ⚕ 7.81   **FUD** 010   T A2 ▭
AMA: 2014,Jan,11; 2013,Jan,11-12

● New Code   ▲ Revised Code   ○ Reinstated   M Maternity   A Age Edit   Unlisted   Not Covered   # Resequenced
Ⓢ AMA Mod 51 Exempt   ⑨ Optum Mod 51 Exempt   63 Mod 63 Exempt   ⊙ Mod Sedation   + Add-on   ▭ CCI   PQ PQRS   FUD Follow-up Days

Digestive System

46320 — 46608

| # | 46320 | **Excision of thrombosed hemorrhoid, external** |

🔲 3.20 ✂ 5.25 **FUD** 010 ☐ T P3 ☐

AMA: 2014,Jan,11; 2013,Jan,11-12

46250 **Hemorrhoidectomy, external, 2 or more columns/groups**

EXCLUDES *Hemorrhoidectomy, external, single column/group (46999)*

Do not report with (0249T)

🔲 9.06 ✂ 13.2 **FUD** 090 ☐ T A2 ☐

AMA: 2014,Jan,11; 2013,Jan,11-12

46255 **Hemorrhoidectomy, internal and external, single column/group;**

Do not report with (0249T)

🔲 10.1 ✂ 14.5 **FUD** 090 ☐ T A2 ☐

AMA: 2015,Jan,16; 2014,Oct,14; 2014,Jan,11; 2013,Jan,11-12

46257 **with fissurectomy**

Do not report with (0249T)

🔲 12.1 ✂ 12.1 **FUD** 090 ☐ T A2 ☐

AMA: 2014,Jan,11; 2013,Jan,11-12

46258 **with fistulectomy, including fissurectomy, when performed**

Do not report with (0249T)

🔲 13.4 ✂ 13.4 **FUD** 090 ☐ T A2 80 ☐

AMA: 2014,Jan,11; 2013,Jan,11-12

46260 **Hemorrhoidectomy, internal and external, 2 or more columns/groups;**

INCLUDES Whitehead hemorrhoidectomy

Do not report with (0249T)

🔲 13.7 ✂ 13.7 **FUD** 090 ☐ T A2 ☐

AMA: 2014,Jan,11; 2013,Jan,11-12

46261 **with fissurectomy**

Do not report with (0249T)

🔲 15.0 ✂ 15.0 **FUD** 090 ☐ T A2 ☐

AMA: 2014,Jan,11; 2013,Jan,11-12

46262 **with fistulectomy, including fissurectomy, when performed**

Do not report with (0249T)

🔲 15.9 ✂ 15.9 **FUD** 090 ☐ T A2 ☐

AMA: 2015,Jan,16; 2014,Jan,11; 2013,Jan,11-12

46270-46320 Resection of Anal Fistula

46270 **Surgical treatment of anal fistula (fistulectomy/fistulotomy); subcutaneous**

🔲 11.2 ✂ 14.5 **FUD** 090 ☐ T A2 ☐

AMA: 2014,Jan,11; 2013,Jan,11-12

46275 **intersphincteric**

🔲 11.9 ✂ 15.4 **FUD** 090 ☐ T A2 ☐

AMA: 2014,Jan,11; 2013,Jan,11-12

46280 **transsphincteric, suprasphincteric, extrasphincteric or multiple, including placement of seton, when performed**

Do not report with (46020)

🔲 13.5 ✂ 13.5 **FUD** 090 ☐ T A2 ☐

AMA: 2014,Jan,11; 2013,Jan,11-12

46285 **second stage**

🔲 11.8 ✂ 15.3 **FUD** 090 ☐ T A2 ☐

AMA: 2014,Jan,11; 2013,Jan,11-12

46288 **Closure of anal fistula with rectal advancement flap**

🔲 15.8 ✂ 15.8 **FUD** 090 ☐ T A2 ☐

AMA: 2014,Jan,11; 2013,Jan,11-12

46320 **Resequenced code. See code following 46230.**

46500 Other Hemorrhoid Procedures

EXCLUDES *Anoscopic injection of bulking agent, submucosal, for fecal incontinence (0377T)*

46500 **Injection of sclerosing solution, hemorrhoids**

🔲 3.73 ✂ 6.85 **FUD** 010 ☐ T P3 ☐

AMA: 2015,Jan,16; 2014,Jan,11; 2013,Jan,11-12

Rectum

Valve cusps become
incompetent in the
varicose vein causing
blood to pool

Anal
sphincter

Internal
hemorrhoid

External
hemorrhoid

Thrombus
(blood clot)

46505 Chemodenervation Anal Sphincter

EXCLUDES *Chemodenervation of:*
Extremity muscles (64642-64645)
Muscles/facial nerve (64612)
Neck muscles (64616)
Other peripheral nerve/branch (64640)
Pudendal nerve (64630)
Trunk muscles (64646-64647)

Code also drug(s)/substance(s) given

46505 **Chemodenervation of internal anal sphincter**

🔲 6.86 ✂ 8.15 **FUD** 010 ☐ T G2 50

AMA: 2015,Jan,16; 2014,Jan,11; 2013,Jan,11-12

46600-46615 Anoscopic Procedures

INCLUDES Diagnostic endoscopy with surgical endoscopy

EXCLUDES *Delivery of thermal energy via anoscope to the muscle of the anal canal (0288T)*
Injection of bulking agent, submucosal, for fecal incontinence (0377T)

46600 **Anoscopy; diagnostic, including collection of specimen(s) by brushing or washing, when performed (separate procedure)**

EXCLUDES *High-resolution anoscopy (HRA), diagnostic (46601)*

Do not report during same session with (46020-46942 [46220, 46320, 46945, 46946, 46947], 0184T, 0249T, 0377T)

🔲 1.17 ✂ 2.52 **FUD** 000 ☐ Q1 N1

AMA: 2015,Jan,16; 2014,Jan,11; 2013,Jan,11-12; 2012,Jan,15-42; 2011,Aug,9-10; 2010,Jun,3

46601 **diagnostic, with high-resolution magnification (HRA) (eg, colposcope, operating microscope) and chemical agent enhancement, including collection of specimen(s) by brushing or washing, when performed**

🔲 0.00 ✂ 0.00 **FUD** 000 ☐ Q1 N1

INCLUDES Operating microscope (69990)

46604 **with dilation (eg, balloon, guide wire, bougie)**

🔲 1.92 ✂ 17.8 **FUD** 000 ☐ T P2 ☐

AMA: 2015,Jan,16; 2014,Jan,11; 2013,Jan,11-12

46606 **with biopsy, single or multiple**

EXCLUDES *High resolution anoscopy (HRA) with biopsy (46607)*

🔲 2.20 ✂ 6.43 **FUD** 000 ☐ T P3 ☐ P0

AMA: 2015,Jan,16; 2014,Jan,11; 2013,Jan,11-12

46607 **with high-resolution magnification (HRA) (eg, colposcope, operating microscope) and chemical agent enhancement, with biopsy, single or multiple**

🔲 0.00 ✂ 0.00 **FUD** 000 ☐ T G2

INCLUDES Operating microscope (69990)

46608 **with removal of foreign body**

🔲 2.44 ✂ 6.79 **FUD** 000 ☐ T A2 ☐

AMA: 2015,Jan,16; 2014,Jan,11; 2013,Jan,11-12

46610   with removal of single tumor, polyp, or other lesion by hot biopsy forceps or bipolar cautery
    2.36 6.46 **FUD** 000   T A2 ▯
    AMA: 2015,Jan,16; 2014,Jan,11; 2013,Jan,11-12

46611   with removal of single tumor, polyp, or other lesion by snare technique
    2.36 4.99 **FUD** 000   T A2 ▯
    AMA: 2015,Jan,16; 2014,Jan,11; 2013,Jan,11-12

46612   with removal of multiple tumors, polyps, or other lesions by hot biopsy forceps, bipolar cautery or snare technique
    2.76 7.85 **FUD** 000   T A2 ▯
    AMA: 2015,Jan,16; 2014,Jan,11; 2013,Jan,11-12

46614   with control of bleeding (eg, injection, bipolar cautery, unipolar cautery, laser, heater probe, stapler, plasma coagulator)
    1.87 3.68 **FUD** 000   T P3 ▯
    AMA: 2015,Jan,16; 2014,Jan,11; 2013,Jan,11-12

46615   with ablation of tumor(s), polyp(s), or other lesion(s) not amenable to removal by hot biopsy forceps, bipolar cautery or snare technique
    2.69 4.13 **FUD** 000   T A2 ▯
    AMA: 2015,Jan,16; 2014,Jan,11; 2013,Jan,11-12

46700-46762 [46947] Anal Repairs and Stapled Hemorrhoidopexy

46700   Anoplasty, plastic operation for stricture; adult
    18.8 18.8 **FUD** 090   T A2 ▯
    AMA: 2014,Jan,11; 2013,Jan,11-12

46705   infant   A
    EXCLUDES Anal septum incision (46070)
    13.9 13.9 **FUD** 090   63 C 80 ▯
    AMA: 2014,Jan,11; 2013,Jan,11-12

46706   Repair of anal fistula with fibrin glue
    5.07 5.07 **FUD** 010   T A2 ▯
    AMA: 2014,Jan,11; 2013,Jan,11-12

46707   Repair of anorectal fistula with plug (eg, porcine small intestine submucosa [SIS])
    13.6 13.6 **FUD** 090   T 62 80
    AMA: 2015,Jan,16; 2014,Jan,11; 2013,Oct,15; 2013,Jan,11-12; 2012,Jan,6-10

46710   Repair of ileoanal pouch fistula/sinus (eg, perineal or vaginal), pouch advancement; transperineal approach
    30.2 30.2 **FUD** 090   C 80
    AMA: 2015,Jan,16; 2014,Jan,11; 2013,Jan,11-12

46712   combined transperineal and transabdominal approach
    57.8 57.8 **FUD** 090   C 80
    AMA: 2015,Jan,16; 2014,Jan,11; 2013,Jan,11-12

46715   Repair of low imperforate anus; with anoperineal fistula (cut-back procedure)
    15.6 15.6 **FUD** 090   63 C 80 ▯ P0
    AMA: 2014,Jan,11; 2013,Jan,11-12

46716   with transposition of anoperineal or anovestibular fistula
    30.7 30.7 **FUD** 090   63 C 80 ▯ P0
    AMA: 2014,Jan,11; 2013,Jan,11-12

46730   Repair of high imperforate anus without fistula; perineal or sacroperineal approach
    56.7 56.7 **FUD** 090   63 C 80 ▯ P0
    AMA: 2014,Jan,11; 2013,Jan,11-12

46735   combined transabdominal and sacroperineal approaches
    58.4 58.4 **FUD** 090   63 C 80 ▯ P0
    AMA: 2014,Jan,11; 2013,Jan,11-12

46740   Repair of high imperforate anus with rectourethral or rectovaginal fistula; perineal or sacroperineal approach
    62.0 62.0 **FUD** 090   63 C 80 ▯ P0
    AMA: 2014,Jan,11; 2013,Jan,11-12

46742   combined transabdominal and sacroperineal approaches
    64.2 64.2 **FUD** 090   63 C 80 ▯ P0
    AMA: 2014,Jan,11; 2013,Jan,11-12

46744   Repair of cloacal anomaly by anorectovaginoplasty and urethroplasty, sacroperineal approach   ♀
    101. 101. **FUD** 090   63 C 80 ▯ P0
    AMA: 2014,Jan,11; 2013,Jan,11-12

46746   Repair of cloacal anomaly by anorectovaginoplasty and urethroplasty, combined abdominal and sacroperineal approach;   ♀
    100. 100. **FUD** 090   C 80 ▯ P0
    AMA: 2014,Jan,11; 2013,Jan,11-12

46748   with vaginal lengthening by intestinal graft or pedicle flaps   ♀
    109. 109. **FUD** 090   C 80 ▯ P0
    AMA: 2014,Jan,11; 2013,Jan,11-12

46750   Sphincteroplasty, anal, for incontinence or prolapse; adult
    21.7 21.7 **FUD** 090   T A2 80 ▯ P0
    AMA: 2014,Jan,11; 2013,Jan,11-12

46751   child   A
    16.5 16.5 **FUD** 090   C 80 ▯ P0
    AMA: 2014,Jan,11; 2013,Jan,11-12

46753   Graft (Thiersch operation) for rectal incontinence and/or prolapse
    16.6 16.6 **FUD** 090   T A2 ▯ P0
    AMA: 2014,Jan,11; 2013,Jan,11-12

46754   Removal of Thiersch wire or suture, anal canal
    6.55 8.48 **FUD** 010   T A2 80 ▯ P0
    AMA: 2014,Jan,11; 2013,Jan,11-12

46760   Sphincteroplasty, anal, for incontinence, adult; muscle transplant
    31.5 31.5 **FUD** 090   T A2 80 ▯ P0
    AMA: 2014,Jan,11; 2013,Jan,11-12

46761   levator muscle imbrication (Park posterior anal repair)
    26.6 26.6 **FUD** 090   T A2 80 ▯ P0
    AMA: 2014,Jan,11; 2013,Jan,11-12

46762   implantation artificial sphincter
    EXCLUDES Anoscopic injection of bulking agent, submucosal, for fecal incontinence (0377T)
    26.6 26.6 **FUD** 090   T A2 80 ▯ P0
    AMA: 2014,Jan,11; 2013,Jan,11-12

\# **46947** **Hemorrhoidopexy (eg, for prolapsing internal hemorrhoids) by stapling**
    10.9 10.9 **FUD** 090   T A2 ▯
    AMA: 2015,Jan,16; 2014,Jan,11; 2013,Jan,11-12; 2012,Jan,15-42; 2011,Jan,11

46900-46999 Destruction Procedures: Anus

46900   Destruction of lesion(s), anus (eg, condyloma, papilloma, molluscum contagiosum, herpetic vesicle), simple; chemical
    3.97 6.95 **FUD** 010   T P2 ▯
    AMA: 2014,Jan,11; 2013,Jan,11-12

46910   electrodesiccation
    3.85 7.31 **FUD** 010   T P3 ▯
    AMA: 2014,Jan,11; 2013,Jan,11-12

46916   cryosurgery
    4.11 6.52 **FUD** 010   T P2 ▯
    AMA: 2014,Jan,11; 2013,Jan,11-12

46917   laser surgery
    3.82 12.8 **FUD** 010   T A2 ▯
    AMA: 2014,Jan,11; 2013,Jan,11-12

Digestive System *(side tab)*

46922 — 47140 *(side tab)*

46922   **surgical excision**
     3.91   7.63   **FUD** 010   T A2
     AMA: 2014,Jan,11; 2013,Jan,11-12

46924   **Destruction of lesion(s), anus (eg, condyloma, papilloma, molluscum contagiosum, herpetic vesicle), extensive (eg, laser surgery, electrosurgery, cryosurgery, chemosurgery)**
     5.32   15.3   **FUD** 010   T A2
     AMA: 2014,Jan,11; 2013,Jan,11-12

46930   **Destruction of internal hemorrhoid(s) by thermal energy (eg, infrared coagulation, cautery, radiofrequency)**
     EXCLUDES   *Other hemorrhoid procedures:*
         Cryosurgery destruction (46999)
         Excision ([46320], 46250-46262)
         Hemorrhoidopexy ([46947])
         Incision (46083)
         Injection sclerosing solution (46500)
         Ligation (46221, [46945, 46946])
     4.27   5.91   **FUD** 090   T P3 80
     AMA: 2015,Apr,10; 2014,Jan,11; 2013,Jan,11-12

46940   **Curettage or cautery of anal fissure, including dilation of anal sphincter (separate procedure); initial**
     4.23   6.57   **FUD** 090   T P3
     AMA: 2014,Jan,11; 2013,Jan,11-12

46942   **subsequent**
     3.81   6.22   **FUD** 010   T P3 80
     AMA: 2014,Jan,11; 2013,Jan,11-12

46945   **Resequenced code. See code following 46221.**

46946   **Resequenced code. See code following 46221.**

46947   **Resequenced code. See code following 46762.**

46999   **Unlisted procedure, anus**
     0.00   0.00   **FUD** YYY   T 80
     AMA: 2015,Apr,10; 2015,Jan,16; 2014,Jan,11; 2013,Jan,11-12

47000-47001 Needle Biopsy of Liver

EXCLUDES   *Fine needle aspiration (10021, 10022)*

47000   **Biopsy of liver, needle; percutaneous**
     (76942, 77002, 77012, 77021)
     (88172-88173)
     3.00   10.3   **FUD** 000   ⊙ T A2 PQ
     AMA: 2015,Jan,16; 2014,Jan,11; 2013,Jan,11-12; 2012,Jan,15-42; 2011,Jan,11

Neck of cystic duct / Cystic artery / Infundibulum / Fundus / Cystic duct / Portal vein / Hepatic artery / Common bile duct / Gallbladder

47001   **when done for indicated purpose at time of other major procedure (List separately in addition to code for primary procedure)**
     Code first primary procedure
     (76942, 77002)
     (88172-88173)
     3.02   3.02   **FUD** ZZZ   N N1 PQ
     AMA: 2015,Jan,16; 2014,Jan,11; 2013,Jan,11-12; 2012,Jan,15-42; 2011,Jan,11

47010-47130 Open Incisional and Resection Procedures of Liver

47010   **Hepatotomy, for open drainage of abscess or cyst, 1 or 2 stages**
     EXCLUDES   *Image guided percutaneous catheter drainage (49505)*
     34.8   34.8   **FUD** 090   C 80 PQ
     AMA: 2014,Jan,11; 2013,Nov,9; 2013,Jan,11-12

47015   **Laparotomy, with aspiration and/or injection of hepatic parasitic (eg, amoebic or echinococcal) cyst(s) or abscess(es)**
     33.6   33.6   **FUD** 090   C 80
     AMA: 2014,Jan,11; 2013,Jan,11-12

Inferior vena cava / Hepatic veins / Diaphragm / Caudate lobe / Gallbladder / Portal vein / Common bile duct / Medial segment / Lateral segment / Right lobe / Left lobe

47100   **Biopsy of liver, wedge**
     24.4   24.4   **FUD** 090   C 80 PQ
     AMA: 2014,Jan,11; 2013,Jan,11-12

47120   **Hepatectomy, resection of liver; partial lobectomy**
     67.4   67.4   **FUD** 090   C 80 PQ
     AMA: 2015,Jan,16; 2014,Sep,13; 2014,Jan,11; 2013,Jan,11-12; 2012,Jan,15-42; 2011,Jan,11

47122   **trisegmentectomy**
     99.3   99.3   **FUD** 090   C 80 PQ
     AMA: 2014,Jan,11; 2013,Jan,11-12

47125   **total left lobectomy**
     88.9   88.9   **FUD** 090   C 80 PQ
     AMA: 2014,Jan,11; 2013,Jan,11-12

47130   **total right lobectomy**
     95.5   95.5   **FUD** 090   C 80 PQ
     AMA: 2014,Jan,11; 2013,Jan,11-12

47133-47147 Liver Transplant Procedures

CMS: 100-3,260.1 Adult Liver Transplantation; 100-3,260.2 Pediatric Liver Transplantation; 100-4,3,90.4 Liver Transplants; 100-4,3,90.4.1 Standard Liver Acquisition Charge; 100-4,3,90.4.2 Billing for Liver Transplant and Acquisition Services; 100-4,3,90.6 Intestinal and Multi-Visceral Transplants

47133   **Donor hepatectomy (including cold preservation), from cadaver donor**
     INCLUDES   Graft:
         Cold preservation
         Harvest
     0.00   0.00   **FUD** XXX   C
     AMA: 2014,Jan,11; 2013,Jan,11-12

47135   **Liver allotransplantation, orthotopic, partial or whole, from cadaver or living donor, any age**
     INCLUDES   Partial/whole recipient hepatectomy
         Partial/whole transplant of allograft
         Recipient care
     141.   141.   **FUD** 090   C 80 PQ
     AMA: 2015,Jan,16; 2014,Jan,11; 2013,Jan,11-12; 2012,Jan,15-42

47136   ~~heterotopic, partial or whole, from cadaver or living donor, any age~~
     To report, see ~47399

47140   **Donor hepatectomy (including cold preservation), from living donor; left lateral segment only (segments II and III)**
     INCLUDES   Donor care
         Graft:
         Cold preservation
         Harvest
     92.8   92.8   **FUD** 090   C 80 PQ
     AMA: 2015,Jan,16; 2014,Jan,11; 2013,Jan,11-12; 2012,Jan,15-42

26/TC PC/TC Comp Only   A2-Z3 ASC Pmt   50 Bilateral   ♂ Male Only   ♀ Female Only   Facility RVU   Non-Facility RVU
AMA: CPT Asst   **CMS:** Pub 100   A-Y OPPSI   80/80 Surg Assist Allowed / w/Doc   Lab Crosswalk   Radiology Crosswalk

188   Medicare (Red Text)   CPT © 2015 American Medical Association. All Rights Reserved. (Black Text)   © 2015 Optum360, LLC (Blue Text)

47141 total left lobectomy (segments II, III and IV)

INCLUDES Donor care
Graft:
Cold preservation
Harvest
🔧 123. ⚕ 123. **FUD** 090 C 80 ▢ PQ
AMA: 2014,Jan,11; 2013,Jan,11-12

47142 total right lobectomy (segments V, VI, VII and VIII)

INCLUDES Donor care
Graft:
Cold preservation
Harvest
🔧 136. ⚕ 136. **FUD** 090 C 80 ▢ PQ
AMA: 2014,Jan,11; 2013,Jan,11-12

47143 Backbench standard preparation of cadaver donor whole liver graft prior to allotransplantation, including cholecystectomy, if necessary, and dissection and removal of surrounding soft tissues to prepare the vena cava, portal vein, hepatic artery, and common bile duct for implantation; without trisegment or lobe split

Do not report with (47120-47125, 47600, 47610)
🔧 0.00 ⚕ 0.00 **FUD** XXX C 80 ▢
AMA: 2015,Jan,16; 2014,Jan,11; 2013,Jan,11-12

47144 with trisegment split of whole liver graft into 2 partial liver grafts (ie, left lateral segment [segments II and III] and right trisegment [segments I and IV through VIII])

Do not report with (47120-47125, 47600, 47610)
🔧 0.00 ⚕ 0.00 **FUD** 090 C 80 ▢
AMA: 2014,Jan,11; 2013,Jan,11-12

47145 with lobe split of whole liver graft into 2 partial liver grafts (ie, left lobe [segments II, III, and IV] and right lobe [segments I and V through VIII])

Do not report with (47120-47125, 47600, 47610)
🔧 0.00 ⚕ 0.00 **FUD** XXX C 80 ▢
AMA: 2014,Jan,11; 2013,Jan,11-12

47146 Backbench reconstruction of cadaver or living donor liver graft prior to allotransplantation; venous anastomosis, each

Do not report with (47120-47125, 47600, 47610)
🔧 9.59 ⚕ 9.59 **FUD** XXX C 80 ▢
AMA: 2014,Jan,11; 2013,Jan,11-12

47147 arterial anastomosis, each

Do not report with (47120-47125, 47600, 47610)
🔧 11.1 ⚕ 11.1 **FUD** XXX C 80 ▢
AMA: 2014,Jan,11; 2013,Jan,11-12

47300-47362 Open Repair of Liver

47300 Marsupialization of cyst or abscess of liver
🔧 32.8 ⚕ 32.8 **FUD** 090 C 80 ▢ PQ
AMA: 2014,Jan,11; 2013,Jan,11-12

47350 Management of liver hemorrhage; simple suture of liver wound or injury
🔧 39.6 ⚕ 39.6 **FUD** 090 C 80 ▢ PQ
AMA: 2014,Jan,11; 2013,Jan,11-12

47360 complex suture of liver wound or injury, with or without hepatic artery ligation
🔧 54.1 ⚕ 54.1 **FUD** 090 C 80 ▢ PQ
AMA: 2014,Jan,11; 2013,Jan,11-12

47361 exploration of hepatic wound, extensive debridement, coagulation and/or suture, with or without packing of liver
🔧 87.7 ⚕ 87.7 **FUD** 090 C 80 ▢ PQ
AMA: 2014,Jan,11; 2013,Jan,11-12

47362 re-exploration of hepatic wound for removal of packing
🔧 41.9 ⚕ 41.9 **FUD** 090 C 80 ▢ PQ
AMA: 2014,Jan,11; 2013,Jan,11-12

47370-47379 Laparoscopic Ablation Liver Tumors

INCLUDES Diagnostic laparoscopy

47370 Laparoscopy, surgical, ablation of 1 or more liver tumor(s); radiofrequency
🔧 (76940)
🔧 36.0 ⚕ 36.0 **FUD** 090 T 80 ▢ PQ
AMA: 2015,Jan,16; 2014,Jan,11; 2013,Jan,11-12

47371 cryosurgical
🔧 (76940)
🔧 36.3 ⚕ 36.3 **FUD** 090 T 80 ▢ PQ
AMA: 2014,Jan,11; 2013,Jan,11-12

47379 Unlisted laparoscopic procedure, liver
🔧 0.00 ⚕ 0.00 **FUD** YYY T 80
AMA: 2015,Jan,16; 2014,Dec,18; 2014,Jan,11; 2013,Jan,11-12; 2012,Jan,15-42; 2011,Jan,11

47380-47399 Open/Percutaneous Ablation Liver Tumors

47380 Ablation, open, of 1 or more liver tumor(s); radiofrequency
🔧 (76940)
🔧 41.6 ⚕ 41.6 **FUD** 090 C 80 ▢ PQ
AMA: 2015,Jan,16; 2014,Jan,11; 2013,Jan,11-12

47381 cryosurgical
🔧 (76940)
🔧 38.9 ⚕ 38.9 **FUD** 090 C 80 ▢ PQ
AMA: 2014,Jan,11; 2013,Jan,11-12

47382 Ablation, 1 or more liver tumor(s), percutaneous, radiofrequency
🔧 (76940, 77013, 77022)
🔧 22.4 ⚕ 142. **FUD** 010 ⊙ T 62 ▢ PQ
AMA: 2015,Jan,16; 2014,Jan,11; 2013,Jan,11-12

47383 Ablation, 1 or more liver tumor(s), percutaneous, cryoablation
🔧 (76940, 77013, 77022)
🔧 13.8 ⚕ 215. **FUD** 010 ⊙ T 62
AMA: 2015,Jan,16; 2014,Dec,18

47399 Unlisted procedure, liver
🔧 0.00 ⚕ 0.00 **FUD** YYY T
AMA: 2015,Jan,16; 2014,Dec,18; 2014,Jan,11; 2013,Jan,11-12

47400-47490 Biliary Tract Procedures

47400 Hepaticotomy or hepaticostomy with exploration, drainage, or removal of calculus
🔧 62.4 ⚕ 62.4 **FUD** 090 C 80 ▢ PQ
AMA: 2014,Jan,11; 2013,Jan,11-12

47420 Choledochotomy or choledochostomy with exploration, drainage, or removal of calculus, with or without cholecystotomy; without transduodenal sphincterotomy or sphincteroplasty
🔧 38.8 ⚕ 38.8 **FUD** 090 C 80 ▢ PQ
AMA: 2014,Jan,11; 2013,Jan,11-12

47425 with transduodenal sphincterotomy or sphincteroplasty
🔧 39.5 ⚕ 39.5 **FUD** 090 C 80 ▢ PQ
AMA: 2014,Jan,11; 2013,Jan,11-12

47460 Transduodenal sphincterotomy or sphincteroplasty, with or without transduodenal extraction of calculus (separate procedure)
🔧 36.7 ⚕ 36.7 **FUD** 090 C 80 ▢ PQ
AMA: 2014,Jan,11; 2013,Jan,11-12

47480 Cholecystotomy or cholecystostomy, open, with exploration, drainage, or removal of calculus (separate procedure)

> EXCLUDES *Percutaneous cholecystostomy (47490)*
>
> 🔲 25.3   🔲 25.3   **FUD** 090   C 80 🔲 P0
>
> **AMA:** 2015,Jan,16; 2014,Jan,11; 2013,Jan,11-12; 2012,Jan,15-42; 2011,Apr,12

R. hepatic duct
Gallbladder
L. hepatic duct
Common hepatic duct
Drainage tube
Cystic duct
Common bile duct (choledochus)
Calculi (stones) are removed if present

47490 Cholecystostomy, percutaneous, complete procedure, including imaging guidance, catheter placement, cholecystogram when performed, and radiological supervision and interpretation

> EXCLUDES *Open cholecystostomy (47480)*
>
> Do not report with (47531-47532, 75989, 76942, 77002, 77012, 77021)
>
> 🔲 9.62   🔲 9.62   **FUD** 010   T 🔲
>
> **AMA:** 2015,Jan,16; 2014,Jan,11; 2013,Nov,9; 2013,Jan,11-12; 2012,Jan,15-42; 2011,Apr,12

47500-47532 Injection/Insertion Procedures of Biliary Tract

47500 ~~Injection procedure for percutaneous transhepatic cholangiography~~

> To report, see ~47531-47541

47505 ~~Injection procedure for cholangiography through an existing catheter (eg, percutaneous transhepatic or T-tube)~~

> To report, see ~47531-47541

47510 ~~Introduction of percutaneous transhepatic catheter for biliary drainage~~

> To report, see ~47531-47541

47511 ~~Introduction of percutaneous transhepatic stent for internal and external biliary drainage~~

> To report, see ~47531-47541

47525 ~~Change of percutaneous biliary drainage catheter~~

> To report, see ~47531-47541

47530 ~~Revision and/or reinsertion of transhepatic tube~~

> To report, see ~47531-47541

47531 Injection procedure for cholangiography, percutaneous, complete diagnostic procedure including imaging guidance (eg, ultrasound and/or fluoroscopy) and all associated radiological supervision and interpretation; existing access

> INCLUDES Contrast material injection
> Radiologic supervision and interpretation
>
> EXCLUDES *Intraoperative cholangiography (74300-74301)*
>
> Do not report with when performed via same access (47490, 47533-47541)
>
> 🔲 0.00   🔲 0.00   **FUD** 000   ☉

47532 new access (eg, percutaneous transhepatic cholangiogram)

> INCLUDES Contrast material injection
> Radiologic supervision and interpretation
>
> EXCLUDES *Intraoperative cholangiography (74300-74301)*
>
> Do not report with when performed via same access (47490, 47533-47541)
>
> 🔲 0.00   🔲 0.00   **FUD** 000   ☉

47533-47544 Percutaneous Procedures of the Biliary Tract

47533 Placement of biliary drainage catheter, percutaneous, including diagnostic cholangiography when performed, imaging guidance (eg, ultrasound and/or fluoroscopy), and all associated radiological supervision and interpretation; external

> EXCLUDES *Conversion to internal-external drainage catheter (47535)*
> *Percutaneous placment stent in bile duct (47538)*
> *Replacement existing interal drainage catheter (47536)*
>
> 🔲 0.00   🔲 0.00   **FUD** 000   ☉

47534 internal-external

> EXCLUDES *Conversion to external only drainage catheter (47536)*
> *Percutaneous placement stent in bile duct (47538)*
>
> 🔲 0.00   🔲 0.00   **FUD** 000   ☉

47535 Conversion of external biliary drainage catheter to internal-external biliary drainage catheter, percutaneous, including diagnostic cholangiography when performed, imaging guidance (eg, fluoroscopy), and all associated radiological supervision and interpretation

> 🔲 0.00   🔲 0.00   **FUD** 000   ☉

47536 Exchange of biliary drainage catheter (eg, external, internal-external, or conversion of internal-external to external only), percutaneous, including diagnostic cholangiography when performed, imaging guidance (eg, fluoroscopy), and all associated radiological supervision and interpretation

> 🔲 0.00   🔲 0.00   **FUD** 000   ☉
>
> INCLUDES Exchange of one drainage catheter
> Code also exchange of additional catheters in same session with modifier 59 (47536)
> Do not report with (47538)

47537 Removal of biliary drainage catheter, percutaneous, requiring fluoroscopic guidance (eg, with concurrent indwelling biliary stents), including diagnostic cholangiography when performed, imaging guidance (eg, fluoroscopy), and all associated radiological supervision and interpretation

> EXCLUDES *Removal without use of fluoroscopic guidance; report with appropriate E&M service code*
> Do not report with for the same percutaneous access site (47538)
>
> 🔲 0.00   🔲 0.00   **FUD** 000   ☉

47538 Placement of stent(s) into a bile duct, percutaneous, including diagnostic cholangiography, imaging guidance (eg, fluoroscopy and/or ultrasound), balloon dilation, catheter exchange(s) and catheter removal(s) when performed, and all associated radiological supervision and interpretation, each stent; existing access

> Do not report for the same access site (47536-47537)
> Do not report if drainage catheter is inserted following stent placement (47536)
> Do not report more than one time per session for serial stents or stents that overlap
> Do not report with treatment of same lesion in same session ([43277], 47542, 47555-47556)
>
> 🔲 0.00   🔲 0.00   **FUD** 000   ☉

47539 new access, without placement of separate biliary drainage catheter

> Do not report more than one time per session for serial stents or stents that overlap
> Do not report with treatment of same lesion in same session ([43277], 47542, 47555-47556)
>
> 🔲 0.00   🔲 0.00   **FUD** 000   ☉

47540 new access, with placement of separate biliary drainage catheter (eg, external or internal-external)

> Do not report for the same percutaneous access site (47533-47534)
> Do not report more than one time per session for serial stents or stent that overlap
> Do not report with treatment of same lesion in same session ([43277], 47542, 47555-47556)
>
> 🔲 0.00   🔲 0.00   **FUD** 000   ☉

● **47541** **Placement of access through the biliary tree and into small bowel to assist with an endoscopic biliary procedure (eg, rendezvous procedure), percutaneous, including diagnostic cholangiography when performed, imaging guidance (eg, ultrasound and/or fluoroscopy), and all associated radiological supervision and interpretation, new access**

🔖 0.00 ⚕ 0.00 **FUD** 000 ⊙

> **EXCLUDES** *Access through biliary tree into small bowel for endoscopic biliary procedure (47535-47537)*
> Do not report when previous catheter access exists
> Do not report with (47531-47540)

● + **47542** **Balloon dilation of biliary duct(s) or of ampulla (sphincteroplasty), percutaneous, including imaging guidance (eg, fluoroscopy), and all associated radiological supervision and interpretation, each duct (List separately in addition to code for primary procedure)**

🔖 0.00 ⚕ 0.00 **FUD** 000 ⊙

> **EXCLUDES** *Endoscopic balloon dilation ([43277], 47555-47556)*
> Code also one additional dilation when more than one dilation performed in same session, using modifier 59 with (47542)
> Code first (47531-47537, 47541)
> Do not report when balloon used to remove calculi, debris, sludge without dilation (47544)
> Do not report with (43262, [43277], 47538-47540, 47555-47556)

● + **47543** **Endoluminal biopsy(ies) of biliary tree, percutaneous, any method(s) (eg, brush, forceps, and/or needle), including imaging guidance (eg, fluoroscopy), and all associated radiological supervision and interpretation, single or multiple (List separately in addition to code for primary procedure)**

🔖 0.00 ⚕ 0.00 **FUD** 000 ⊙

> **EXCLUDES** *Endoscopic biopsy (46261, 47553)*
> *Endoscopic brushings (43260, 47552)*
> Code first (47531-47540)
> Do not report more than one time per session

● + **47544** **Removal of calculi/debris from biliary duct(s) and/or gallbladder, percutaneous, including destruction of calculi by any method (eg, mechanical, electrohydraulic, lithotripsy) when performed, imaging guidance (eg, fluoroscopy), and all associated radiological supervision and interpretation (List separately in addition to code for primary procedure)**

🔖 0.00 ⚕ 0.00 **FUD** 000 ⊙

> **EXCLUDES** *Endoscopic calculi removal/destruction (43264-43265, 47554)*
> Code first (47531-47540)
> Do not report for incidental debris/sludge removal (47531-47543)
> Do not report if no calculi/debris found despite device deployment
> Do not report with (43264, 47554)

47550-47556 Endoscopic Procedures of the Biliary Tract

INCLUDES Diagnostic endoscopy with surgical endoscopy
EXCLUDES *Endoscopic retrograde cholangiopancreatography (ERCP) (43260-43265, [43274], [43275], [43276], [43277], [43278], 74328-74330, 74363)*

+ **47550** **Biliary endoscopy, intraoperative (choledochoscopy) (List separately in addition to code for primary procedure)**
> Code first primary procedure
> 🔖 4.81 ⚕ 4.81 **FUD** ZZZ C 80
> **AMA:** 2014,Jan,11; 2013,Jan,11-12

47552 **Biliary endoscopy, percutaneous via T-tube or other tract; diagnostic, with collection of specimen(s) by brushing and/or washing, when performed (separate procedure)**
> 🔖 9.13 ⚕ 9.13 **FUD** 000 T A2 ▭
> **AMA:** 2015,Jan,16; 2014,Jan,11; 2013,Jan,11-12; 2012,Jan,15-42; 2011,Jan,11

47553 **with biopsy, single or multiple**
> 🔖 9.06 ⚕ 9.06 **FUD** 000 T A2 ▭ P0
> **AMA:** 2015,Jan,16; 2014,Jan,11; 2013,Jan,11-12; 2012,Jan,15-42; 2011,Jan,11

47554 **with removal of calculus/calculi**
> 🔖 13.9 ⚕ 13.9 **FUD** 000 T A2 ▭
> **AMA:** 2015,Jan,16; 2014,Jan,11; 2013,Jan,11-12; 2012,Jan,15-42; 2011,Jan,11

47555 **with dilation of biliary duct stricture(s) without stent**
> 🔖 10.7 ⚕ 10.7 **FUD** 000 T A2 ▭
> **AMA:** 2015,Jan,16; 2014,Jan,11; 2013,Jan,11-12; 2012,Jan,15-42; 2011,Jan,11

47556 **with dilation of biliary duct stricture(s) with stent**
> ☒ (74363)
> 🔖 12.2 ⚕ 12.2 **FUD** 000 T A2 ▭
> **AMA:** 2015,Jan,16; 2014,Jan,11; 2013,Jan,11-12; 2012,Jan,15-42; 2011,Jan,11

47560-47579 Laparoscopic Gallbladder Procedures

CMS: 100-3,100.13 Laparoscopic Cholecystectomy
INCLUDES Diagnostic laparoscopy

47560 ~~Laparoscopy, surgical; with guided transhepatic cholangiography, without biopsy~~
> To report, see ~47579

47561 ~~with guided transhepatic cholangiography with biopsy~~
> To report, see ~47579

47562 **Laparoscopy, surgical; cholecystectomy**
> 🔖 19.0 ⚕ 19.0 **FUD** 090 T 62 80 ▭ P0
> **AMA:** 2015,Jan,16; 2014,Jan,11; 2013,Jan,11-12; 2012,Jan,15-42; 2011,Jan,11

47563 **cholecystectomy with cholangiography**
> **EXCLUDES** *Percutaneous cholangiography (47531-47532)*
> Code also intraoperative radiology supervision and interpretation (74300-74301)
> 🔖 20.6 ⚕ 20.6 **FUD** 090 T 62 80 ▭ P0
> **AMA:** 2015,Jan,16; 2014,Jan,11; 2013,Jan,11-12; 2012,Jan,15-42; 2011,Jan,11

47564 **cholecystectomy with exploration of common duct**
> 🔖 32.1 ⚕ 32.1 **FUD** 090 T 62 80 ▭ P0
> **AMA:** 2015,Jan,16; 2014,Jan,11; 2013,Jan,11-12; 2012,Jan,15-42; 2011,Jan,11

47570 **cholecystoenterostomy**
> 🔖 22.4 ⚕ 22.4 **FUD** 090 C 80 ▭ P0
> **AMA:** 2015,Jan,16; 2014,Jan,11; 2013,Jan,11-12

47579 **Unlisted laparoscopy procedure, biliary tract**
> 🔖 0.00 ⚕ 0.00 **FUD** YYY T 80 50
> **AMA:** 2015,Jan,16; 2014,Jan,11; 2013,Jan,11-12

47600-47620 Open Gallbladder Procedures

47600 **Cholecystectomy;**
> **EXCLUDES** *Laparoscopic method (47562-47564)*
> 🔖 30.8 ⚕ 30.8 **FUD** 090 C 80 ▭ P0
> **AMA:** 2015,Jan,16; 2014,Jan,11; 2013,Jan,11-12

Liver, Gallbladder, Duodenum, Stomach, Stone in neck of cystic duct, Cystic artery, Infundibulum, Cystic duct, Fundus, Portal vein, Common bile duct, Gallstones

Digestive System

47605   **with cholangiography**

> EXCLUDES   *Laparoscopic method (47563-47564)*

> 🔧 32.4   ⚕ 32.4   **FUD** 090   C 80 📖 PQ

> **AMA:** 2015,Jan,16; 2014,Jan,11; 2013,Jan,11-12; 2012,Jan,15-42; 2011,Jan,11

47610   **Cholecystectomy with exploration of common duct;**

> EXCLUDES   *Laparoscopic method (47564)*

> Code also biliary endoscopy when performed in conjunction with cholecystectomy with exploration of common duct (47550)

> 🔧 36.3   ⚕ 36.3   **FUD** 090   C 80 📖 PQ

> **AMA:** 2015,Jan,16; 2014,Jan,11; 2013,Jan,11-12; 2012,Jan,15-42; 2011,Jan,11

47612   **with choledochoenterostomy**

> 🔧 36.7   ⚕ 36.7   **FUD** 090   C 80 📖 PQ

> **AMA:** 2014,Jan,11; 2013,Jan,11-12

47620   **with transduodenal sphincterotomy or sphincteroplasty, with or without cholangiography**

> 🔧 39.9   ⚕ 39.9   **FUD** 090   C 80 📖 PQ

> **AMA:** 2014,Jan,11; 2013,Jan,11-12

47630-47999 Open Resection and Repair of Biliary Tract

47630   ~~Biliary duct stone extraction, percutaneous via T-tube tract, basket, or snare (eg, Burhenne technique)~~

> To report, see ~47544

47700   **Exploration for congenital atresia of bile ducts, without repair, with or without liver biopsy, with or without cholangiography**

> 🔧 30.4   ⚕ 30.4   **FUD** 090   63 C 80 📖 PQ

> **AMA:** 2014,Jan,11; 2013,Jan,11-12

47701   **Portoenterostomy (eg, Kasai procedure)**

> 🔧 50.2   ⚕ 50.2   **FUD** 090   63 C 80 📖 PQ

> **AMA:** 2014,Jan,11; 2013,Jan,11-12

47711   **Excision of bile duct tumor, with or without primary repair of bile duct; extrahepatic**

> EXCLUDES   *Anastomosis (47760-47800)*

> 🔧 44.9   ⚕ 44.9   **FUD** 090   C 80 📖 PQ

> **AMA:** 2014,Jan,11; 2013,Jan,11-12

47712   **intrahepatic**

> EXCLUDES   *Anastomosis (47760-47800)*

> 🔧 57.9   ⚕ 57.9   **FUD** 090   C 80 📖 PQ

> **AMA:** 2014,Jan,11; 2013,Jan,11-12

47715   **Excision of choledochal cyst**

> 🔧 38.5   ⚕ 38.5   **FUD** 090   C 80 📖 PQ

> **AMA:** 2015,Jan,16; 2014,Jan,11; 2013,Jan,11-12; 2012,Jan,15-42; 2011,Jan,11

47720   **Cholecystoenterostomy; direct**

> EXCLUDES   *Laparoscopic method (47570)*

> 🔧 33.4   ⚕ 33.4   **FUD** 090   C 80 📖 PQ

> **AMA:** 2015,Jan,16; 2014,Jan,11; 2013,Jan,11-12

47721   **with gastroenterostomy**

> 🔧 39.2   ⚕ 39.2   **FUD** 090   C 80 📖 PQ

> **AMA:** 2014,Jan,11; 2013,Jan,11-12

47740   **Roux-en-Y**

> 🔧 38.0   ⚕ 38.0   **FUD** 090   C 80 📖 PQ

> **AMA:** 2014,Jan,11; 2013,Jan,11-12

47741   **Roux-en-Y with gastroenterostomy**

> 🔧 42.7   ⚕ 42.7   **FUD** 090   C 80 📖 PQ

> **AMA:** 2014,Jan,11; 2013,Jan,11-12

47760   **Anastomosis, of extrahepatic biliary ducts and gastrointestinal tract**

> 🔧 65.3   ⚕ 65.3   **FUD** 090   C 80 📖 PQ

> **AMA:** 2014,Jan,11; 2013,Jan,11-12

47765   **Anastomosis, of intrahepatic ducts and gastrointestinal tract**

> INCLUDES   *Longmire anastomosis*

> 🔧 88.1   ⚕ 88.1   **FUD** 090   C 80 📖 PQ

> **AMA:** 2014,Jan,11; 2013,Jan,11-12

47780   **Anastomosis, Roux-en-Y, of extrahepatic biliary ducts and gastrointestinal tract**

> 🔧 71.5   ⚕ 71.5   **FUD** 090   C 80 📖 PQ

> **AMA:** 2014,Jan,11; 2013,Jan,11-12

47785   **Anastomosis, Roux-en-Y, of intrahepatic biliary ducts and gastrointestinal tract**

> 🔧 94.0   ⚕ 94.0   **FUD** 090   C 80 📖 PQ

> **AMA:** 2014,Jan,11; 2013,Jan,11-12

47800   **Reconstruction, plastic, of extrahepatic biliary ducts with end-to-end anastomosis**

> 🔧 45.7   ⚕ 45.7   **FUD** 090   C 80 📖 PQ

> **AMA:** 2014,Jan,11; 2013,Jan,11-12

47801   **Placement of choledochal stent**

> 🔧 29.0   ⚕ 29.0   **FUD** 090   C 80 📖 PQ

> **AMA:** 2015,Jan,16; 2014,Jan,11; 2013,Jan,11-12; 2012,Jan,15-42; 2010,Dec,12

47802   **U-tube hepaticoenterostomy**

> 🔧 44.2   ⚕ 44.2   **FUD** 090   C 80 📖 PQ

> **AMA:** 2014,Jan,11; 2013,Jan,11-12

47900   **Suture of extrahepatic biliary duct for pre-existing injury (separate procedure)**

> 🔧 39.7   ⚕ 39.7   **FUD** 090   C 80 📖 PQ

> **AMA:** 2014,Jan,11; 2013,Jan,11-12

47999   **Unlisted procedure, biliary tract**

> 🔧 0.00   ⚕ 0.00   **FUD** YYY   T

> **AMA:** 2015,Jan,16; 2014,Jan,11; 2013,Jan,11-12; 2012,Jan,15-42; 2011,May,9

48000-48548 Open Procedures of the Pancreas

> EXCLUDES   *Peroral pancreatic procedures performed endoscopically (43260-43265, 43270 [43274, 43275, 43276, 43277, 43278])*

48000   **Placement of drains, peripancreatic, for acute pancreatitis;**

> 🔧 54.4   ⚕ 54.4   **FUD** 090   C 80 📖 PQ

> **AMA:** 2014,Jan,11; 2013,Jan,11-12

Pancreas

48001   **with cholecystostomy, gastrostomy, and jejunostomy**

> 🔧 66.9   ⚕ 66.9   **FUD** 090   C 80 📖 PQ

> **AMA:** 2014,Jan,11; 2013,Jan,11-12

48020 **Removal of pancreatic calculus**
🚑 34.0 ✂ 34.0 **FUD** 090 Ⓒ 80 🖥 PQ
AMA: 2014,Jan,11; 2013,Jan,11-12

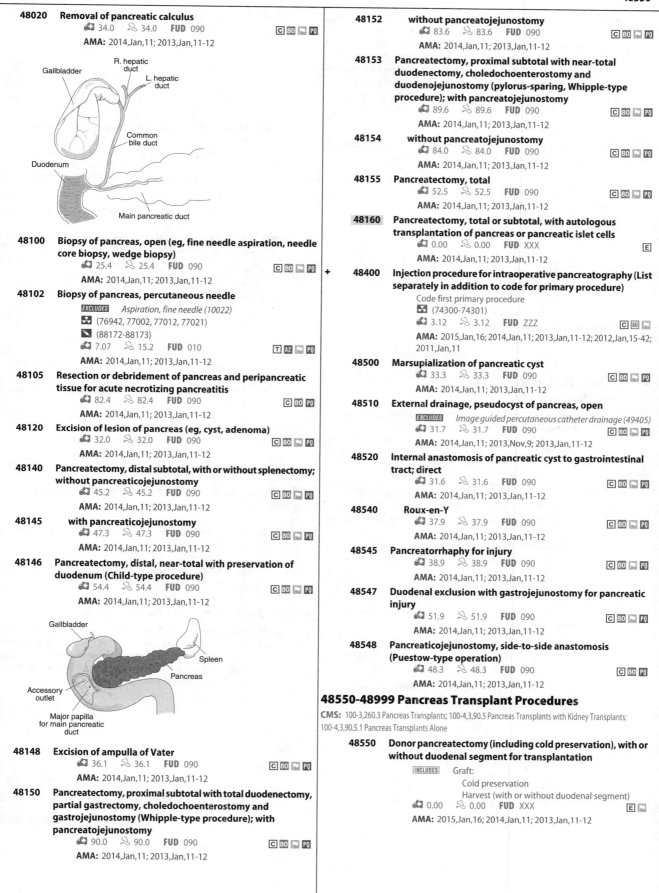

Labels: Gallbladder; R. hepatic duct; L. hepatic duct; Common bile duct; Duodenum; Main pancreatic duct

48100 **Biopsy of pancreas, open (eg, fine needle aspiration, needle core biopsy, wedge biopsy)**
🚑 25.4 ✂ 25.4 **FUD** 090 Ⓒ 80 🖥 PQ
AMA: 2014,Jan,11; 2013,Jan,11-12

48102 **Biopsy of pancreas, percutaneous needle**
EXCLUDES Aspiration, fine needle (10022)
🔀 (76942, 77002, 77012, 77021)
🔳 (88172-88173)
🚑 7.07 ✂ 15.2 **FUD** 010 Ⓣ A2 🖥 PQ
AMA: 2014,Jan,11; 2013,Jan,11-12

48105 **Resection or debridement of pancreas and peripancreatic tissue for acute necrotizing pancreatitis**
🚑 82.4 ✂ 82.4 **FUD** 090 Ⓒ 80 PQ
AMA: 2014,Jan,11; 2013,Jan,11-12

48120 **Excision of lesion of pancreas (eg, cyst, adenoma)**
🚑 32.0 ✂ 32.0 **FUD** 090 Ⓒ 80 🖥 PQ
AMA: 2014,Jan,11; 2013,Jan,11-12

48140 **Pancreatectomy, distal subtotal, with or without splenectomy; without pancreaticojejunostomy**
🚑 45.2 ✂ 45.2 **FUD** 090 Ⓒ 80 🖥 PQ
AMA: 2014,Jan,11; 2013,Jan,11-12

48145 **with pancreaticojejunostomy**
🚑 47.3 ✂ 47.3 **FUD** 090 Ⓒ 80 🖥 PQ
AMA: 2014,Jan,11; 2013,Jan,11-12

48146 **Pancreatectomy, distal, near-total with preservation of duodenum (Child-type procedure)**
🚑 54.4 ✂ 54.4 **FUD** 090 Ⓒ 80 🖥 PQ
AMA: 2014,Jan,11; 2013,Jan,11-12

Labels: Gallbladder; Spleen; Pancreas; Accessory outlet; Major papilla for main pancreatic duct

48148 **Excision of ampulla of Vater**
🚑 36.1 ✂ 36.1 **FUD** 090 Ⓒ 80 🖥 PQ
AMA: 2014,Jan,11; 2013,Jan,11-12

48150 **Pancreatectomy, proximal subtotal with total duodenectomy, partial gastrectomy, choledochoenterostomy and gastrojejunostomy (Whipple-type procedure); with pancreatojejunostomy**
🚑 90.0 ✂ 90.0 **FUD** 090 Ⓒ 80 🖥 PQ
AMA: 2014,Jan,11; 2013,Jan,11-12

48152 **without pancreatojejunostomy**
🚑 83.6 ✂ 83.6 **FUD** 090 Ⓒ 80 🖥 PQ
AMA: 2014,Jan,11; 2013,Jan,11-12

48153 **Pancreatectomy, proximal subtotal with near-total duodenectomy, choledochoenterostomy and duodenojejunostomy (pylorus-sparing, Whipple-type procedure); with pancreatojejunostomy**
🚑 89.6 ✂ 89.6 **FUD** 090 Ⓒ 80 🖥 PQ
AMA: 2014,Jan,11; 2013,Jan,11-12

48154 **without pancreatojejunostomy**
🚑 84.0 ✂ 84.0 **FUD** 090 Ⓒ 80 🖥 PQ
AMA: 2014,Jan,11; 2013,Jan,11-12

48155 **Pancreatectomy, total**
🚑 52.5 ✂ 52.5 **FUD** 090 Ⓒ 80 🖥 PQ
AMA: 2014,Jan,11; 2013,Jan,11-12

48160 **Pancreatectomy, total or subtotal, with autologous transplantation of pancreas or pancreatic islet cells**
🚑 0.00 ✂ 0.00 **FUD** XXX Ⓔ
AMA: 2014,Jan,11; 2013,Jan,11-12

+ **48400** **Injection procedure for intraoperative pancreatography (List separately in addition to code for primary procedure)**
Code first primary procedure
🔀 (74300-74301)
🚑 3.12 ✂ 3.12 **FUD** ZZZ Ⓒ 80 🖥
AMA: 2015,Jan,16; 2014,Jan,11; 2013,Jan,11-12; 2012,Jan,15-42; 2011,Jan,11

48500 **Marsupialization of pancreatic cyst**
🚑 33.3 ✂ 33.3 **FUD** 090 Ⓒ 80 🖥 PQ
AMA: 2014,Jan,11; 2013,Jan,11-12

48510 **External drainage, pseudocyst of pancreas, open**
EXCLUDES Image guided percutaneous catheter drainage (49405)
🚑 31.7 ✂ 31.7 **FUD** 090 Ⓒ 80 🖥 PQ
AMA: 2014,Jan,11; 2013,Nov,9; 2013,Jan,11-12

48520 **Internal anastomosis of pancreatic cyst to gastrointestinal tract; direct**
🚑 31.6 ✂ 31.6 **FUD** 090 Ⓒ 80 🖥 PQ
AMA: 2014,Jan,11; 2013,Jan,11-12

48540 **Roux-en-Y**
🚑 37.9 ✂ 37.9 **FUD** 090 Ⓒ 80 🖥 PQ
AMA: 2014,Jan,11; 2013,Jan,11-12

48545 **Pancreatorrhaphy for injury**
🚑 38.9 ✂ 38.9 **FUD** 090 Ⓒ 80 🖥 PQ
AMA: 2014,Jan,11; 2013,Jan,11-12

48547 **Duodenal exclusion with gastrojejunostomy for pancreatic injury**
🚑 51.9 ✂ 51.9 **FUD** 090 Ⓒ 80 🖥 PQ
AMA: 2014,Jan,11; 2013,Jan,11-12

48548 **Pancreaticojejunostomy, side-to-side anastomosis (Puestow-type operation)**
🚑 48.3 ✂ 48.3 **FUD** 090 Ⓒ 80 PQ
AMA: 2014,Jan,11; 2013,Jan,11-12

48550-48999 Pancreas Transplant Procedures

CMS: 100-3,260.3 Pancreas Transplants; 100-4,3,90.5 Pancreas Transplants with Kidney Transplants; 100-4,3,90.5.1 Pancreas Transplants Alone

48550 **Donor pancreatectomy (including cold preservation), with or without duodenal segment for transplantation**
INCLUDES Graft:
Cold preservation
Harvest (with or without duodenal segment)
🚑 0.00 ✂ 0.00 **FUD** XXX Ⓔ 🖥
AMA: 2015,Jan,16; 2014,Jan,11; 2013,Jan,11-12

48551 Backbench standard preparation of cadaver donor pancreas allograft prior to transplantation, including dissection of allograft from surrounding soft tissues, splenectomy, duodenotomy, ligation of bile duct, ligation of mesenteric vessels, and Y-graft arterial anastomoses from iliac artery to superior mesenteric artery and to splenic artery

Do not report with (35531, 35563, 35685, 38100-38102, 44010, 44820, 44850, 47460, 47550-47556, 48100-48120, 48545)

⏣ 0.00　⚚ 0.00　**FUD** XXX　　　　　　C 80 ▣

AMA: 2014,Jan,11; 2013,Jan,11-12

48552 Backbench reconstruction of cadaver donor pancreas allograft prior to transplantation, venous anastomosis, each

Do not report with (35531, 35563, 35685, 38100-38102, 44010, 44820, 44850, 47460, 47550-47556, 48100-48120, 48545)

⏣ 6.87　⚚ 6.87　**FUD** XXX　　　　　　C 80 ▣

AMA: 2014,Jan,11; 2013,Jan,11-12

48554 Transplantation of pancreatic allograft

INCLUDES　Allograft transplant
　　　　　Recipient care

⏣ 73.9　⚚ 73.9　**FUD** 090　　　　C 80 ▣ PQ

AMA: 2014,Jan,11; 2013,Jan,11-12

48556 Removal of transplanted pancreatic allograft

⏣ 36.8　⚚ 36.8　**FUD** 090　　　　C 80 ▣ PQ

AMA: 2014,Jan,11; 2013,Jan,11-12

48999 Unlisted procedure, pancreas

⏣ 0.00　⚚ 0.00　**FUD** YYY　　　　　T 80

AMA: 2015,Jan,16; 2014,Jan,11; 2013,Feb,13; 2013,Jan,11-12; 2012,Jan,15-42; 2011,May,9; 2011,Jan,11

49000-49084 Exploratory and Drainage Procedures: Abdomen/Peritoneum

49000 Exploratory laparotomy, exploratory celiotomy with or without biopsy(s) (separate procedure)

EXCLUDES　Exploration of penetrating wound without laparotomy (20102)
　　　　　Percutaneous iamge-guided drainage of peritoneal abscess/peritonitis via catheter (49406)
　　　　　Transrectal/transvaginal image-guided drainage of peritoneal abscess via catheter (49407)

⏣ 22.2　⚚ 22.2　**FUD** 090　　　　C 80 ▣ PQ

AMA: 2015,Jan,16; 2014,Jan,11; 2013,Jan,11-12; 2012,Oct,3-8; 2012,Sep,11-13; 2012,Jan,15-42; 2011,Jan,11

49002 Reopening of recent laparotomy

EXCLUDES　Hepatic wound re-exploration for packing removal (47362)

⏣ 30.2　⚚ 30.2　**FUD** 090　　　　C 80 ▣ PQ

AMA: 2015,Jan,16; 2014,Jan,11; 2013,Jan,11-12

49010 Exploration, retroperitoneal area with or without biopsy(s) (separate procedure)

EXCLUDES　Exploration of penetrating wound without laparotomy (20102)

⏣ 26.9　⚚ 26.9　**FUD** 090　　　　C 80 ▣ PQ

AMA: 2014,Jan,11; 2013,Jan,11-12

49020 Drainage of peritoneal abscess or localized peritonitis, exclusive of appendiceal abscess, open

EXCLUDES　Appendiceal abscess (44900)
　　　　　Image guided percutaneous catheter drainage of abscess/peritonitis via catheter (49406)
　　　　　Image-guided transrectal/transvaginal drainage of peritoneal abscess via catheter (49407)

⏣ 46.0　⚚ 46.0　**FUD** 090　　　　C 80 ▣ PQ

AMA: 2014,Jan,11; 2013,Nov,9; 2013,Jan,11-12

49040 Drainage of subdiaphragmatic or subphrenic abscess, open

EXCLUDES　Image-guided percutaneous drainage of subdiaphragmatic/subphrenic abscess via catheter (49406)

⏣ 28.9　⚚ 28.9　**FUD** 090　　　　C 80 ▣ PQ

AMA: 2014,Jan,11; 2013,Nov,9; 2013,Jan,11-12

49060 Drainage of retroperitoneal abscess, open

EXCLUDES　Drainage performed laparoscopically (49323)
　　　　　Image-guided percutaneous drainage of retroperitoneal abscess via catheter (49406)
　　　　　Transrectal/transvaginal image-guided drainage of retroperitoneal abscess via catheter (49407)

⏣ 31.7　⚚ 31.7　**FUD** 090　　　　C ▣ PQ

AMA: 2015,Jan,16; 2014,Jan,11; 2013,Nov,9; 2013,Jan,11-12; 2012,Jan,15-42; 2011,Jan,11

49062 Drainage of extraperitoneal lymphocele to peritoneal cavity, open

EXCLUDES　Drainage of lymphocele to peritoneal cavity, laparoscopic (49323)
　　　　　Image-guided percutaneous drainage of retroperitoneal lymphocele via catheter (49406)

⏣ 21.4　⚚ 21.4　**FUD** 090　　　　C 80 ▣

AMA: 2015,Jan,16; 2014,Jan,11; 2013,Jan,11-12; 2012,Jan,15-42; 2011,Jan,11

49082 Abdominal paracentesis (diagnostic or therapeutic); without imaging guidance

⏣ 2.17　⚚ 5.51　**FUD** 000　　　　T 62

AMA: 2015,Jan,16; 2014,Jan,11; 2013,Nov,9; 2013,Jan,11-12; 2012,Dec,9-10

49083 with imaging guidance

EXCLUDES　Image-guided percutaneous drainage of retroperitoneal abscess via catheter (49406)

Do not report with (76942, 77002, 77012, 77021)

⏣ 3.16　⚚ 8.34　**FUD** 000　　　　T 62

AMA: 2015,Jan,16; 2014,Mar,13; 2014,Jan,11; 2013,Nov,9; 2013,Jan,11-12; 2012,Dec,9-10

49084 Peritoneal lavage, including imaging guidance, when performed

EXCLUDES　Image-guided percutaneous drainage of retroperitoneal abscess via catheter (49406)

Do not report with (76942, 77002, 77012, 77021)

⏣ 3.16　⚚ 3.16　**FUD** 000　　　　T 62

AMA: 2015,Jan,16; 2014,Jan,11; 2013,Nov,9; 2013,Jan,11-12; 2012,Dec,9-10

49180 Biopsy of Mass: Abdomen/Retroperitoneum

EXCLUDES　Aspiration, fine needle (10021, 10022)
　　　　　Lysis of intestinal adhesions (44005)

49180 Biopsy, abdominal or retroperitoneal mass, percutaneous needle

✦ (76942, 77002, 77012, 77021)

✦ (88172-88173)

⏣ 2.50　⚚ 4.68　**FUD** 000　　　　T A2 ▣ PQ

AMA: 2015,Jan,16; 2014,Jan,11; 2013,Jan,11-12

49185 Sclerotherapy of a Fluid Collection

● **49185** Sclerotherapy of a fluid collection (eg, lymphocele, cyst, or seroma), percutaneous, including contrast injection(s), sclerosant injection(s), diagnostic study, imaging guidance (eg, ultrasound, fluoroscopy) and radiological supervision and interpretation when performed

INCLUDES　Mulitple lesions treated via same access

EXCLUDES　Sclerotherapy of lymphatic/vascular malformation (37241)
　　　　　Sclerosis of veins/endoveinous ablation of incompetent veins of extremity (36468, 36470-36471, 36475-36476, 36478-36479)
　　　　　Pleurodesis (32560)

Code also access or drainage via needle or catheter (10030, 10160, 49405-49407, 50390)

Code also existing catheter exchange pre- or post-sclerosant injection (49423, 75984)

Code also modifier 59 for treatment of multiple lesions in same session via separate access

Do not report with (49424, 76080)

⏣ 0.00　⚚ 0.00　**FUD** 000

49203-49205 Open Destruction or Excision: Abdominal Tumors

> *EXCLUDES* Cryoablation of renal tumor (50250, 50593)
> Lysis of intestinal adhesions (44005)
> Primary, recurrent ovarian, uterine, or tubal resection (58957-58958)

Code also colectomy (44140)
Code also nephrectomy (50220, 50240)
Code also small bowel resection (44120)
Code also vena caval resection with reconstruction (37799)
Do not report with (38770, 38780, 49000, 49010, 49215, 50010, 50205, 50225, 50236, 50250, 50290, 58900-58960)

49203 **Excision or destruction, open, intra-abdominal tumors, cysts or endometriomas, 1 or more peritoneal, mesenteric, or retroperitoneal primary or secondary tumors; largest tumor 5 cm diameter or less**
  34.6   34.6   **FUD** 090   C 80 PQ
  AMA: 2015,Jan,16; 2014,Jan,11; 2013,Jan,11-12; 2010,Dec,12

49204 **largest tumor 5.1-10.0 cm diameter**
  44.3   44.3   **FUD** 090   C 80 PQ
  AMA: 2015,Jan,16; 2014,Jan,11; 2013,Jan,11-12; 2010,Dec,12

49205 **largest tumor greater than 10.0 cm diameter**
  50.8   50.8   **FUD** 090   C 80 PQ
  AMA: 2015,Jan,16; 2014,Jan,11; 2013,Jan,11-12; 2010,Dec,12

49215 Resection Presacral/Sacrococcygeal Tumor

49215 **Excision of presacral or sacrococcygeal tumor**
  63.6   63.6   **FUD** 090   63 C 80 ☐ PQ
  AMA: 2014,Jan,11; 2013,Jan,11-12

49220-49255 Other Open Abdominal Procedures

> *EXCLUDES* Lysis of intestinal adhesions (44005)

49220 **Staging laparotomy for Hodgkins disease or lymphoma (includes splenectomy, needle or open biopsies of both liver lobes, possibly also removal of abdominal nodes, abdominal node and/or bone marrow biopsies, ovarian repositioning)**
  28.1   28.1   **FUD** 090   C 80 ☐ PQ
  AMA: 2014,Jan,11; 2013,Jan,11-12

49250 **Umbilectomy, omphalectomy, excision of umbilicus (separate procedure)**
  16.8   16.8   **FUD** 090   T A2 ☐ PQ
  AMA: 2014,Jan,11; 2013,Jan,11-12

49255 **Omentectomy, epiploectomy, resection of omentum (separate procedure)**
  22.8   22.8   **FUD** 090   C 80 ☐ PQ
  AMA: 2015,Jan,16; 2014,Jan,11; 2013,Jan,11-12

49320-49329 Laparoscopic Procedures of the Abdomen/Peritoneum/Omentum

> *INCLUDES* Diagnostic laparoscopy
> *EXCLUDES* Fulguration/excision of lesions of ovary/pelvic viscera/peritoneal surface, performed laparoscopically (58662)

49320 **Laparoscopy, abdomen, peritoneum, and omentum, diagnostic, with or without collection of specimen(s) by brushing or washing (separate procedure)**
  9.38   9.38   **FUD** 010   T A2 80 ☐ PQ
  AMA: 2015,Jan,16; 2014,Jan,11; 2013,Jan,11-12; 2012,Jan,15-42; 2011,Jan,11; 2010,Jun,6-7

49321 **Laparoscopy, surgical; with biopsy (single or multiple)**
  9.94   9.94   **FUD** 010   T A2 80 ☐ PQ
  AMA: 2015,Jan,16; 2014,Jan,11; 2013,Jan,11-12

49322 **with aspiration of cavity or cyst (eg, ovarian cyst) (single or multiple)**
  10.6   10.6   **FUD** 010   T A2 80 ☐ PQ
  AMA: 2015,Jan,16; 2014,Jan,11; 2013,Jan,11-12

49323 **with drainage of lymphocele to peritoneal cavity**
> *EXCLUDES* Open drainage of lymphocele to peritoneal cavity (49062)
  18.4   18.4   **FUD** 090   T 80 ☐ PQ
  AMA: 2015,Jan,16; 2014,Jan,11; 2013,Jan,11-12; 2012,Jan,15-42; 2011,Jan,11

49324 **with insertion of tunneled intraperitoneal catheter**
> *EXCLUDES* Open approach (49421)
Code also insertion of subcutaneous extension to intraperitoneal cannula with remote chest exit site, when appropriate (49435)
  11.2   11.2   **FUD** 010   T 62 80
  AMA: 2014,Jan,11; 2013,Jan,11-12

49325 **with revision of previously placed intraperitoneal cannula or catheter, with removal of intraluminal obstructive material if performed**
  12.0   12.0   **FUD** 010   T 62 80
  AMA: 2014,Jan,11; 2013,Jan,11-12

+ **49326** **with omentopexy (omental tacking procedure) (List separately in addition to code for primary procedure)**
Code first laparoscopy with permanent intraperitoneal cannula or catheter insertion or revision of previously placed catheter/cannula (49324, 49325)
  5.50   5.50   **FUD** ZZZ   N N1 80
  AMA: 2014,Jan,11; 2013,Jan,11-12

+ **49327** **with placement of interstitial device(s) for radiation therapy guidance (eg, fiducial markers, dosimeter), intra-abdominal, intrapelvic, and/or retroperitoneum, including imaging guidance, if performed, single or multiple (List separately in addition to code for primary procedure)**
> *EXCLUDES* Open approach (49412)
> Percutaneous approach (49411)
Code first laparoscopic abdominal, pelvic or retroperitoneal procedures
  3.79   3.79   **FUD** ZZZ   N N1 80
  AMA: 2014,Jan,11; 2013,Jan,11-12

49329 **Unlisted laparoscopy procedure, abdomen, peritoneum and omentum**
  0.00   0.00   **FUD** YYY   T 80 50
  AMA: 2015,Jan,16; 2014,Jan,11; 2013,Oct,18; 2013,Jan,11-12; 2012,Jan,15-42; 2011,Dec,14-18; 2011,Jan,11

49400-49436 Peritoneal and Visceral Procedures: Drainage/Insertion/Modifications/Removal

49400 **Injection of air or contrast into peritoneal cavity (separate procedure)**
  ☒ (74190)
  2.75   3.92   **FUD** 000   N N1 ☐
  AMA: 2015,Jan,16; 2014,Jan,11; 2013,Jan,11-12; 2012,Jan,15-42; 2011,Jan,11; 2010,Dec,12

49402 **Removal of peritoneal foreign body from peritoneal cavity**
> *EXCLUDES* Enterolysis (44005)
> Percutaneous or open drainage or lavage (49020, 49040, 49082-49084, 49406)
> Percutaneous tunneled intraperitoneal catheter insertion without subcutaneous port (49418)
  24.7   24.7   **FUD** 090   T A2
  AMA: 2014,Jan,11; 2013,Jan,11-12

49405 **Image-guided fluid collection drainage by catheter (eg, abscess, hematoma, seroma, lymphocele, cyst); visceral (eg, kidney, liver, spleen, lung/mediastinum), percutaneous**
> *EXCLUDES* Open drainage (32200, 47010, 48510, 50020)
> Percutaneous cholecystostomy (47490)
> Percutaneous pleural drainage (32556-32557)
> Pneumonostomy (32200)
> Thoracentesis (32554-32555)
Code also each individual collection drained per separate catheter
Do not report with (75989, 76942, 77002-77003, 77012, 77021)
  6.19   24.8   **FUD** 000   ⊙ T
  AMA: 2015,Jan,16; 2014,May,9; 2014,Jan,11; 2013,Nov,9

49406   **peritoneal or retroperitoneal, percutaneous**

> **EXCLUDES**   *Diagnostic or therapeutic percutaneous abdominal paracentesis (49082-49083)*
> *Open peritoneal/retroperitoneal drainage (44900, 49020-49062, 49040-49084, 50020, 58805, 58822)*
> *Open transrectal drainage pelvic abscess (45000)*
> *Percutaneous tunneled intraperitoneal catheter insertion without subcutaneous port (49418)*
> *Transrectal/transvaginal image-guided pertoneal/retroperitoneal drainage via catheter (49407)*
>
> Code also each individual collection drained per separate catheter
> Do not report with (75989, 76942, 77002-77003, 77012, 77021)

   6.20   24.9   **FUD** 000   ⊙ T

AMA: 2015,Jan,16; 2014,May,9; 2014,Jan,11; 2013,Nov,9

49407   **peritoneal or retroperitoneal, transvaginal or transrectal**

> **EXCLUDES**   *Image guided percutaneous catheter drainage of soft tissue (ie, abdominal wall, neck, extremity) (10030)*
> *Open transrectal/transvaginal drainage (45000, 58800, 58820)*
> *Percutaneous pleural drainage (32556-32557)*
> *Peritoneal drainage or lavage, open or percutaneous (49020, 49040, 49082)*
> *Thoracentesis (32554-32555)*
>
> Code also each individual collection drained per separate catheter
> Do not report with (75989, 76942, 77002-77003, 77012, 77021)

   6.58   20.8   **FUD** 000   ⊙ T G2

AMA: 2015,Jan,16; 2014,May,9; 2014,Jan,11; 2013,Nov,9

49411   **Placement of interstitial device(s) for radiation therapy guidance (eg, fiducial markers, dosimeter), percutaneous, intra-abdominal, intra-pelvic (except prostate), and/or retroperitoneum, single or multiple**

> **EXCLUDES**   *Placement (percutaneous) of interstitial device(s) for intrathoracic radiation therapy guidance (32553)*
> Code also supply of device
> **⊞** (76942, 77002, 77012, 77021)

   5.74   15.6   **FUD** 000   ⊙ S P3 80

AMA: 2015,Jan,16; 2014,Jan,11; 2013,Jan,11-12; 2010,Jan,6; 2010,Jan,7-8

+ 49412   **Placement of interstitial device(s) for radiation therapy guidance (eg, fiducial markers, dosimeter), open, intra-abdominal, intrapelvic, and/or retroperitoneum, including image guidance, if performed, single or multiple (List separately in addition to code for primary procedure)**

> **EXCLUDES**   *Laparoscopic approach (49327)*
> *Percutaneous approach (49411)*
> Code first open abdominal, pelvic or retroperitoneal procedure(s)

   2.39   2.39   **FUD** ZZZ   C 80

AMA: 2014,Jan,11; 2013,Jan,11-12

49418   **Insertion of tunneled intraperitoneal catheter (eg, dialysis, intraperitoneal chemotherapy instillation, management of ascites), complete procedure, including imaging guidance, catheter placement, contrast injection when performed, and radiological supervision and interpretation, percutaneous**

   6.36   40.7   **FUD** 000   ⊙ T G2 80

AMA: 2014,Jan,11; 2013,Nov,9; 2013,Jan,11-12

49419   **Insertion of tunneled intraperitoneal catheter, with subcutaneous port (ie, totally implantable)**

> **EXCLUDES**   *Removal of catheter/cannula (49422)*

   12.8   12.8   **FUD** 090   T A2

AMA: 2014,Jan,11; 2013,Jan,11-12

49421   **Insertion of tunneled intraperitoneal catheter for dialysis, open**

> **EXCLUDES**   *Laparoscopic approach (49324)*
> Code also insertion of subcutaneous extension to intraperitoneal cannula with remote chest exit site, when appropriate (49435)

   6.69   6.69   **FUD** 000   T G2

AMA: 2015,Jan,16; 2014,Jan,11; 2013,Jan,11-12; 2012,Jan,15-42; 2011,Jan,11

49422   **Removal of tunneled intraperitoneal catheter**

> **EXCLUDES**   *Removal temporary catheter or cannula (Use appropriate E&M code)*

   10.9   10.9   **FUD** 010   02 A2

AMA: 2014,Jan,11; 2013,Jan,11-12

49423   **Exchange of previously placed abscess or cyst drainage catheter under radiological guidance (separate procedure)**

> **⊞** (75984)

   2.11   15.6   **FUD** 000   T G2 80

AMA: 2015,Jan,16; 2014,Jan,11; 2013,Jan,11-12

49424   **Contrast injection for assessment of abscess or cyst via previously placed drainage catheter or tube (separate procedure)**

> **⊞** (76080)

   1.11   4.16   **FUD** 000   N N1 80

AMA: 2015,Jan,16; 2014,Jan,11; 2013,Jan,11-12; 2012,Jan,15-42; 2011,Jan,11

49425   **Insertion of peritoneal-venous shunt**

   21.0   21.0   **FUD** 090   C 80

AMA: 2014,Jan,11; 2013,Jan,11-12

49426   **Revision of peritoneal-venous shunt**

> **EXCLUDES**   *Shunt patency test (78291)*

   17.6   17.6   **FUD** 090   T A2

AMA: 2014,Jan,11; 2013,Jan,11-12

49427   **Injection procedure (eg, contrast media) for evaluation of previously placed peritoneal-venous shunt**

> **⊞** (75809, 78291)

   1.31   1.31   **FUD** 000   N N1 80

AMA: 2014,Jan,11; 2013,Jan,11-12

49428   **Ligation of peritoneal-venous shunt**

   15.4   15.4   **FUD** 010   C

AMA: 2014,Jan,11; 2013,Jan,11-12

49429   **Removal of peritoneal-venous shunt**

   13.2   13.2   **FUD** 010   02 G2

AMA: 2014,Jan,11; 2013,Jan,11-12

+ 49435   **Insertion of subcutaneous extension to intraperitoneal cannula or catheter with remote chest exit site (List separately in addition to code for primary procedure)**

> Code first permanent insertion of intraperitoneal catheter/cannula (49324, 49421)

   3.47   3.47   **FUD** ZZZ   N N1 80

AMA: 2014,Jan,11; 2013,Jan,11-12

49436   **Delayed creation of exit site from embedded subcutaneous segment of intraperitoneal cannula or catheter**

   5.40   5.40   **FUD** 010   T G2 80

AMA: 2014,Jan,11; 2013,Jan,11-12

49440-49442 Insertion of Percutaneous Gastrointestinal Tube

Do not report with (43752)

49440   **Insertion of gastrostomy tube, percutaneous, under fluoroscopic guidance including contrast injection(s), image documentation and report**

> **INCLUDES**   Needle placement with fluoroscopic guidance (77002)
> Code also gastrostomy to gastro-jejunostomy tube conversion with initial gastrostomy tube insertion, when performed (49446)

   6.48   29.6   **FUD** 010   ⊙ T G2 80 PQ

AMA: 2015,Jan,16; 2014,Dec,18; 2014,Sep,5; 2014,Jan,11; 2013,Jan,11-12; 2012,Jan,15-42; 2011,Jan,11; 2010,Sep,9

26/TC PC/TC Comp Only	A2-Z3 ASC Pmt	50 Bilateral	♂ Male Only	♀ Female Only	🖪 Facility RVU	🖎 Non-Facility RVU
AMA: CPT Asst	**CMS:** Pub 100	A-Y OPPSI	80/80 Surg Assist Allowed / w/Doc		🖪 Lab Crosswalk	🖪 Radiology Crosswalk

196   Medicare (Red Text)   CPT © 2015 American Medical Association. All Rights Reserved. (Black Text)   © 2015 Optum360, LLC (Blue Text)

49441 Insertion of duodenostomy or jejunostomy tube, percutaneous, under fluoroscopic guidance including contrast injection(s), image documentation and report

> *EXCLUDES* *Gastrostomy tube to gastrojejunostomy tube conversion (49446)*

🛏 7.47 ⚕ 33.1 **FUD** 010 ⊙ T 63 80 PQ

AMA: 2015,Jan,16; 2014,Dec,18; 2014,Sep,5; 2014,Jan,11; 2013,Jan,11-12; 2012,Jan,15-42; 2011,Jan,11

49442 Insertion of cecostomy or other colonic tube, percutaneous, under fluoroscopic guidance including contrast injection(s), image documentation and report

🛏 6.47 ⚕ 27.5 **FUD** 010 ⊙ T 63 80 PQ

AMA: 2015,Jan,16; 2014,Dec,18; 2014,Sep,5; 2014,Jan,11; 2013,Jan,11-12; 2012,Jan,15-42; 2011,Jan,11

49446 Percutaneous Conversion: Gastrostomy to Gastro-jejunostomy Tube

> *EXCLUDES* *Code also initial gastrostomy tube insertion (49440) when conversion is performed at the same time*

49446 Conversion of gastrostomy tube to gastro-jejunostomy tube, percutaneous, under fluoroscopic guidance including contrast injection(s), image documentation and report

🛏 4.75 ⚕ 28.4 **FUD** 000 ⊙ T 63 80 PQ

AMA: 2015,Jan,16; 2014,Sep,5; 2014,Jan,11; 2013,Jan,11-12; 2012,Jan,15-42; 2011,Jan,11

49450-49452 Replacement Gastrointestinal Tube

> *EXCLUDES* *Placement of new tube whether gastrostomy, jejunostomy, duodenostomy, gastro-jejunostomy, or cecostomy at different percutaneous site (49440-49442)*

49450 Replacement of gastrostomy or cecostomy (or other colonic) tube, percutaneous, under fluoroscopic guidance including contrast injection(s), image documentation and report

> *EXCLUDES* *Change of gastrostomy tube, percutaneous, without imaging or endoscopic guidance (43760)*

🛏 1.96 ⚕ 18.9 **FUD** 000 T 63 80 PQ

AMA: 2015,Jan,16; 2014,Sep,5; 2014,Jan,11; 2013,Dec,16; 2013,Jan,11-12; 2012,Jan,15-42; 2011,Jan,11; 2010,Sep,9

49451 Replacement of duodenostomy or jejunostomy tube, percutaneous, under fluoroscopic guidance including contrast injection(s), image documentation and report

🛏 2.65 ⚕ 20.6 **FUD** 000 T 63 80 PQ

AMA: 2015,Jan,16; 2014,Dec,18; 2014,Sep,5; 2014,Jan,11; 2013,Jan,11-12; 2012,Jan,15-42; 2011,Jan,11; 2010,Jul,10

49452 Replacement of gastro-jejunostomy tube, percutaneous, under fluoroscopic guidance including contrast injection(s), image documentation and report

🛏 4.10 ⚕ 25.6 **FUD** 000 T 63 80 PQ

AMA: 2015,Jan,16; 2014,Sep,5; 2014,Jan,11; 2013,Jan,11-12; 2012,Jan,15-42; 2011,Jan,11; 2010,Mar,9-11

49460-49465 Removal of Obstruction/Injection for Contrast Through Gastrointestinal Tube

49460 Mechanical removal of obstructive material from gastrostomy, duodenostomy, jejunostomy, gastro-jejunostomy, or cecostomy (or other colonic) tube, any method, under fluoroscopic guidance including contrast injection(s), if performed, image documentation and report

Do not report with (49450-49452, 49465)

🛏 1.40 ⚕ 20.8 **FUD** 000 T 63 80 PQ

AMA: 2015,Jan,16; 2014,Sep,5; 2014,Jan,11; 2013,Jan,11-12

49465 Contrast injection(s) for radiological evaluation of existing gastrostomy, duodenostomy, jejunostomy, gastro-jejunostomy, or cecostomy (or other colonic) tube, from a percutaneous approach including image documentation and report

Do not report with (49450-49460)

🛏 0.90 ⚕ 4.62 **FUD** 000 S 63 80 PQ

AMA: 2015,Jan,16; 2014,Sep,5; 2014,Jan,11; 2013,Jan,11-12

49491-49492 Inguinal Hernia Repair on Premature Infant

> *INCLUDES* Hernia repairs done on preterm infants younger than or equal to 50 weeks postconception age but younger than 6 months of age since birth
> Initial repair: no previous repair required
> Mesh or other prosthesis
> *EXCLUDES* *Abdominal wall debridement (11042, 11043)*
> *Intra-abdominal hernia repair/reduction (44050)*
> Code also repair or excision of testicle(s), intestine, ovaries if performed (44120, 54520, 58940)

49491 Repair, initial inguinal hernia, preterm infant (younger than 37 weeks gestation at birth), performed from birth up to 50 weeks postconception age, with or without hydrocelectomy; reducible [A]

🛏 21.5 ⚕ 21.5 **FUD** 090 63 T 80 50

AMA: 2015,Jan,16; 2014,Jan,11; 2013,Jan,11-12; 2012,Jan,15-42; 2011,Jan,11

49492 incarcerated or strangulated [A]

🛏 24.7 ⚕ 24.7 **FUD** 090 63 T 80 50

AMA: 2015,Jan,16; 2014,Jan,11; 2013,Jan,11-12

49495-49557 Hernia Repair: Femoral/Inguinal /Lumbar

> *INCLUDES* Initial repair: no previous repair required
> Mesh or other prosthesis
> Recurrent repair: required previous repair(s)
> *EXCLUDES* *Abdominal wall debridement (11042, 11043)*
> *Intra-abdominal hernia repair/reduction (44050)*
> Code also repair or excision of testicle(s), intestine, ovaries if performed (44120, 54520, 58940)

49495 Repair, initial inguinal hernia, full term infant younger than age 6 months, or preterm infant older than 50 weeks postconception age and younger than age 6 months at the time of surgery, with or without hydrocelectomy; reducible [A]

> *INCLUDES* Hernia repairs done on preterm infants older than 50 weeks postconception age and younger than 6 months

🛏 10.7 ⚕ 10.7 **FUD** 090 63 T A2 80 50

AMA: 2015,Jan,16; 2014,Jan,11; 2013,Jan,11-12; 2012,Jan,15-42; 2011,Jan,11

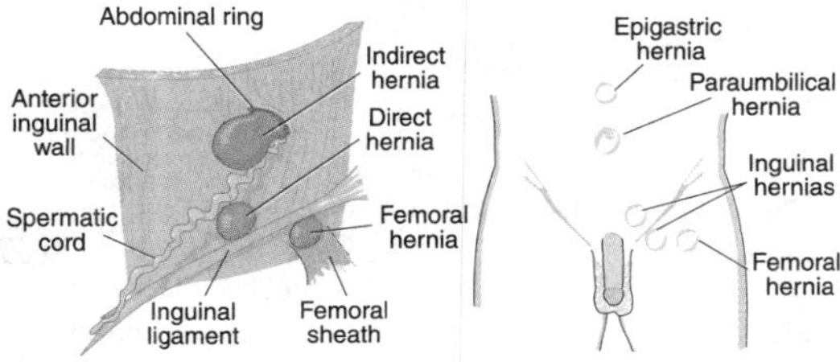

A hernia is a protrusion, usually through an abdominal wall containment

49496 incarcerated or strangulated [A]

> *INCLUDES* Hernia repairs done on preterm infants older than 50 weeks postconception age and younger than 6 months

🛏 15.7 ⚕ 15.7 **FUD** 090 63 T A2 80 50

AMA: 2015,Jan,16; 2014,Jan,11; 2013,Jan,11-12; 2012,Jan,15-42; 2011,Jan,11

49500 Repair initial inguinal hernia, age 6 months to younger than 5 years, with or without hydrocelectomy; reducible [A]

> *INCLUDES* Repairs performed on patients 6 months to younger than 5 years old

🛏 11.8 ⚕ 11.8 **FUD** 090 T A2 80 50

AMA: 2015,Jan,16; 2014,Nov,14; 2014,Jan,11; 2013,Jan,11-12; 2012,Jan,15-42; 2011,Jan,11

49501 incarcerated or strangulated [A]

> *INCLUDES* Repairs performed on patients 6 months to younger than 5 years old

🛏 17.5 ⚕ 17.5 **FUD** 090 T A2 80 50

AMA: 2015,Jan,16; 2014,Jan,11; 2013,Jan,11-12; 2012,Jan,15-42; 2011,Jan,11

● New Code ▲ Revised Code ○ Reinstated Ⓜ Maternity Ⓐ Age Edit Unlisted # Resequenced
⊘ AMA Mod 51 Exempt ⑤ Optum Mod 51 Exempt ⑥ Mod 63 Exempt ⊙ Mod Sedation + Add-on CCI PQ PQRS FUD Follow-up Days
Not Covered

© 2015 Optum360, LLC (Blue Text) CPT © 2015 American Medical Association. All Rights Reserved. (Black Text) Medicare (Red Text) **197**

Digestive System

49505 — 49590

49505   **Repair initial inguinal hernia, age 5 years or older; reducible**   A

     INCLUDES   MacEwen hernia repair
     Code also when performed:
       Excision of hydrocele (55040)
       Excision of spermatocele (54840)
       Simple orchiectomy (54520)
     15.0   15.0   **FUD** 090   T A2 80 50
     AMA: 2015,Jan,16; 2014,Jan,11; 2013,Jan,11-12; 2012,Jan,15-42; 2011,Jan,11

49507   **incarcerated or strangulated**   A

     Code also when performed:
       Excision of hydrocele (55040)
       Excision of spermatocele (54840)
       Simple orchiectomy (54520)
     16.8   16.8   **FUD** 090   T A2 80 50
     AMA: 2015,Jan,16; 2014,Jan,11; 2013,Jan,11-12; 2012,Jan,15-42; 2011,Jan,11

49520   **Repair recurrent inguinal hernia, any age; reducible**
     18.2   18.2   **FUD** 090   T A2 80 50
     AMA: 2015,Jan,16; 2014,Jan,11; 2013,Jan,11-12; 2012,Jan,15-42; 2011,Jan,11

49521   **incarcerated or strangulated**
     20.6   20.6   **FUD** 090   T A2 80 50
     AMA: 2015,Jan,16; 2014,Jan,11; 2013,Jan,11-12; 2012,Jan,15-42; 2011,Jan,11

49525   **Repair inguinal hernia, sliding, any age**
     EXCLUDES   Inguinal hernia repair, incarcerated/strangulated (49496, 49501, 49507, 49521)
     16.5   16.5   **FUD** 090   T A2 80 50
     AMA: 2015,Jan,16; 2014,Jan,11; 2013,Jan,11-12; 2012,Jan,15-42; 2011,Jan,11

Sliding inguinal hernia
Anterior inguinal wall
Spermatic cord
Inguinal ligament
Femoral sheath
Peritoneal lining is forced through a defect in the inguinal wall
A peritoneal sac is created
Because the bowel is attached to the peritoneum, it is pulled through the abdominal defect as well

49540   **Repair lumbar hernia**
     19.4   19.4   **FUD** 090   T A2 80 50
     AMA: 2015,Jan,16; 2014,Jan,11; 2013,Jan,11-12

49550   **Repair initial femoral hernia, any age; reducible**
     16.6   16.6   **FUD** 090   T A2 80 50
     AMA: 2015,Jan,16; 2014,Jan,11; 2013,Jan,11-12

49553   **incarcerated or strangulated**
     18.2   18.2   **FUD** 090   T A2 80 50
     AMA: 2015,Jan,16; 2014,Jan,11; 2013,Jan,11-12

49555   **Repair recurrent femoral hernia; reducible**
     17.2   17.2   **FUD** 090   T A2 80 50
     AMA: 2015,Jan,16; 2014,Jan,11; 2013,Jan,11-12

49557   **incarcerated or strangulated**
     20.8   20.8   **FUD** 090   T A2 80 50
     AMA: 2015,Jan,16; 2014,Jan,11; 2013,Jan,11-12

49560-49568 Hernia Repair: Incisional/Ventral

INCLUDES   Initial repair: no previous repair required
          Recurrent repair: required previous repair(s)
EXCLUDES   Abdominal wall debridement (11042, 11043)
          Intra-abdominal hernia repair/reduction (44050)
Code also repair or excision of testicle(s), intestine, ovaries if performed (44120, 54520, 58940)

49560   **Repair initial incisional or ventral hernia; reducible**
     Code also implantation of mesh or other prosthesis if performed (49568)
     21.2   21.2   **FUD** 090   T A2 80 50 P0
     AMA: 2015,Jan,16; 2014,Jan,11; 2013,Oct,15; 2013,Jan,11-12; 2012,Jan,6-10

49561   **incarcerated or strangulated**
     Code also implantation of mesh or other prosthesis if performed (49568)
     26.8   26.8   **FUD** 090   T A2 80 50 P0
     AMA: 2015,Jan,16; 2014,Jan,11; 2013,Oct,15; 2013,Jan,11-12; 2012,Jan,6-10

49565   **Repair recurrent incisional or ventral hernia; reducible**
     Code also implantation of mesh or other prosthesis if performed (49568)
     22.1   22.1   **FUD** 090   T A2 80 50 P0
     AMA: 2015,Jan,16; 2014,Jan,11; 2013,Oct,15; 2013,Jan,11-12; 2012,Jan,6-10

49566   **incarcerated or strangulated**
     Code also implantation of mesh or other prosthesis if performed (49568)
     27.1   27.1   **FUD** 090   T A2 80 50 P0
     AMA: 2015,Jan,16; 2014,Jan,11; 2013,Oct,15; 2013,Jan,11-12; 2012,Jan,6-10

+ 49568   **Implantation of mesh or other prosthesis for open incisional or ventral hernia repair or mesh for closure of debridement for necrotizing soft tissue infection (List separately in addition to code for the incisional or ventral hernia repair)**
     Code first (11004-11006, 49560-49566)
     7.76   7.76   **FUD** ZZZ   N N1 80 P0
     AMA: 2015,Jan,16; 2014,Jan,11; 2013,Oct,15; 2013,Jan,11-12; 2012,Jan,6-10; 2012,Jan,15-42; 2011,Jan,11

49570-49590 Hernia Repair: Epigastric/Lateral Ventral/Umbilical

INCLUDES   Mesh or other prosthesis
EXCLUDES   Abdominal wall debridement (11042, 11043)
          Intra-abdominal hernia repair/reduction (44050)
Code also repair or excision of testicle(s), intestine, ovaries if performed (44120, 54520, 58940)

49570   **Repair epigastric hernia (eg, preperitoneal fat); reducible (separate procedure)**
     11.9   11.9   **FUD** 090   T A2 80 50 P0
     AMA: 2015,Jan,16; 2014,Jan,11; 2013,Jan,11-12

49572   **incarcerated or strangulated**
     14.8   14.8   **FUD** 090   T A2 80 50
     AMA: 2015,Jan,16; 2014,Jan,11; 2013,Jan,11-12

49580   **Repair umbilical hernia, younger than age 5 years; reducible**   A
     9.58   9.58   **FUD** 090   T A2 80
     AMA: 2015,Jan,16; 2014,Jan,11; 2013,Jan,11-12

49582   **incarcerated or strangulated**   A
     13.9   13.9   **FUD** 090   T A2 80
     AMA: 2015,Jan,16; 2014,Jan,11; 2013,Jan,11-12

49585   **Repair umbilical hernia, age 5 years or older; reducible**   A
     INCLUDES   Mayo hernia repair
     12.8   12.8   **FUD** 090   T A2 80
     AMA: 2015,Jan,16; 2014,Jan,11; 2013,Jan,11-12

49587   **incarcerated or strangulated**   A
     13.7   13.7   **FUD** 090   T A2 80
     AMA: 2015,Jan,16; 2014,Jan,11; 2013,Jan,11-12

49590   **Repair spigelian hernia**
     16.5   16.5   **FUD** 090   T A2 80 50
     AMA: 2015,Jan,16; 2014,Jan,11; 2013,Jan,11-12

49600-49611 Repair Birth Defect Abdominal Wall: Omphalocele/Gastroschisis

INCLUDES Mesh or other prosthesis

EXCLUDES *Abdominal wall debridement (11042, 11043)*
Intra-abdominal hernia repair/reduction (44050)
Repair of:
Diaphragmatic or hiatal hernia (39503, 43332-43337)
Omentum (49999)

49600 **Repair of small omphalocele, with primary closure**
🚑 20.0 ⚕ 20.0 **FUD** 090 ⑥③ T A2 80 ▭

AMA: 2015,Jan,16; 2014,Jan,11; 2013,Jan,11-12

49605 **Repair of large omphalocele or gastroschisis; with or without prosthesis**
🚑 143. ⚕ 143. **FUD** 090 ⑥③ C 80 ▭

AMA: 2015,Jan,16; 2014,Jan,11; 2013,Jan,11-12

49606 **with removal of prosthesis, final reduction and closure, in operating room**
🚑 32.8 ⚕ 32.8 **FUD** 090 ⑥③ C 80 ▭

AMA: 2015,Jan,16; 2014,Jan,11; 2013,Jan,11-12

49610 **Repair of omphalocele (Gross type operation); first stage**
🚑 19.8 ⚕ 19.8 **FUD** 090 ⑥③ C 80 ▭

AMA: 2015,Jan,16; 2014,Jan,11; 2013,Jan,11-12

49611 **second stage**
🚑 15.5 ⚕ 15.5 **FUD** 090 ⑥③ C 80 ▭

AMA: 2015,Jan,16; 2014,Jan,11; 2013,Jan,11-12; 2012,Jan,15-42; 2011,Jan,11

49650-49659 Laparoscopic Hernia Repair

INCLUDES Diagnostic laparoscopy

49650 **Laparoscopy, surgical; repair initial inguinal hernia**
🚑 12.3 ⚕ 12.3 **FUD** 090 T A2 80 50 ▭

AMA: 2015,Jan,16; 2014,Jul,5; 2014,Jan,11; 2013,Jan,11-12

49651 **repair recurrent inguinal hernia**
🚑 16.0 ⚕ 16.0 **FUD** 090 T A2 80 50 ▭

AMA: 2015,Jan,16; 2014,Jan,11; 2013,Jan,11-12

49652 **Laparoscopy, surgical, repair, ventral, umbilical, spigelian or epigastric hernia (includes mesh insertion, when performed); reducible**
Do not report with (44180, 49568)
🚑 21.4 ⚕ 21.4 **FUD** 090 T 62 80 50

AMA: 2014,Jan,11; 2013,Jan,11-12

49653 **incarcerated or strangulated**
Do not report with (44180, 49568)
🚑 26.8 ⚕ 26.8 **FUD** 090 T 62 80 50

AMA: 2014,Jan,11; 2013,Jan,11-12

49654 **Laparoscopy, surgical, repair, incisional hernia (includes mesh insertion, when performed); reducible**
Do not report with (44180, 49568)
🚑 24.4 ⚕ 24.4 **FUD** 090 T 62 80 50

AMA: 2014,Jan,11; 2013,Jan,11-12

49655 **incarcerated or strangulated**
Do not report with (44180, 49568)
🚑 29.8 ⚕ 29.8 **FUD** 090 T 62 80 50

AMA: 2014,Jan,11; 2013,Jan,11-12

49656 **Laparoscopy, surgical, repair, recurrent incisional hernia (includes mesh insertion, when performed); reducible**
Do not report with (44180, 49568)
🚑 26.5 ⚕ 26.5 **FUD** 090 T 62 80 50

AMA: 2014,Jan,11; 2013,Jan,11-12

49657 **incarcerated or strangulated**
Do not report with (44180, 49568)
🚑 38.1 ⚕ 38.1 **FUD** 090 T 62 80 50

AMA: 2014,Jan,11; 2013,Jan,11-12

49659 **Unlisted laparoscopy procedure, hernioplasty, herniorrhaphy, herniotomy**
🚑 0.00 ⚕ 0.00 **FUD** YYY T 80 50

AMA: 2015,Jan,16; 2014,Dec,16; 2014,Dec,16; 2014,Jul,5; 2014,Jan,11; 2013,Jan,11-12; 2012,Jan,15-42; 2011,Jan,11

49900 Surgical Repair Abdominal Wall

EXCLUDES *Abdominal wall debridement (11042, 11043)*
Suture of ruptured diaphragm (39540-39541)

49900 **Suture, secondary, of abdominal wall for evisceration or dehiscence**
🚑 23.5 ⚕ 23.5 **FUD** 090 C 80 ▭

AMA: 2015,Jan,16; 2014,Jan,11; 2013,Jan,11-12; 2010,Sep,6-7

49904-49999 Harvesting of Omental Flap

49904 **Omental flap, extra-abdominal (eg, for reconstruction of sternal and chest wall defects)**

INCLUDES Harvest and transfer

EXCLUDES *Omental flap harvest by second surgeon: both surgeons code 49904 with modifier 62*
🚑 41.1 ⚕ 41.1 **FUD** 090 C ▭

AMA: 2014,Jan,11; 2013,Jan,11-12

+ 49905 **Omental flap, intra-abdominal (List separately in addition to code for primary procedure)**
Code first primary procedure
Do not report with (44700)
🚑 10.2 ⚕ 10.2 **FUD** ZZZ C 80 ▭

AMA: 2015,Jan,16; 2014,Jan,11; 2013,Jan,11-12; 2012,Jan,15-42; 2011,Jan,11

49906 **Free omental flap with microvascular anastomosis**

INCLUDES Operating microscope (69990)
🚑 0.00 ⚕ 0.00 **FUD** 090 C ▭

AMA: 2015,Jan,16; 2014,Jan,11; 2013,Jan,11-12

49999 **Unlisted procedure, abdomen, peritoneum and omentum**
🚑 0.00 ⚕ 0.00 **FUD** YYY T

AMA: 2015,Jan,16; 2014,Jan,9; 2014,Jan,11; 2013,Jan,11-12; 2012,Jan,15-42; 2011,Jun,13; 2011,Jan,11; 2010,Dec,12; 2010,Apr,10

50010-50045 Kidney Procedures for Exploration or Drainage

EXCLUDES Retroperitoneal
Abscess drainage (49060)
Exploration (49010)
Tumor/cyst excision (49203-49205)

50010 **Renal exploration, not necessitating other specific procedures**
EXCLUDES Laparoscopic ablation of mass lesions of kidney (50542)
🔧 21.4   ✂ 21.4   **FUD** 090   C 80 50 ▭
AMA: 2014,Jan,11

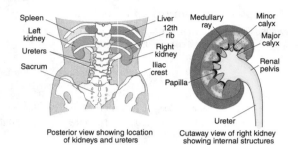

Spleen
Left kidney
Ureters
Sacrum
Liver
12th rib
Right kidney
Iliac crest
Medullary ray
Minor calyx
Major calyx
Renal pelvis
Papilla
Ureter

Posterior view showing location of kidneys and ureters

Cutaway view of right kidney showing internal structures

50020 **Drainage of perirenal or renal abscess, open**
EXCLUDES Image-guided percutaneous of perirenal or renal abscess (49405)
🔧 29.0   ✂ 29.0   **FUD** 090   T ▭ P0
AMA: 2015,Jan,16; 2014,May,9; 2014,Jan,11; 2013,Nov,9

50040 **Nephrostomy, nephrotomy with drainage**
🔧 26.6   ✂ 26.6   **FUD** 090   C 50 ▭
AMA: 2015,Jan,16; 2014,Jan,11

50045 **Nephrotomy, with exploration**
EXCLUDES Renal endoscopy through nephrotomy (50570-50580)
🔧 26.7   ✂ 26.7   **FUD** 090   C 80 50 ▭
AMA: 2015,Jan,16; 2014,Jan,11

50060-50081 Treatment of Kidney Stones

CMS: 100-3,230.1 NCD for Treatment of Kidney Stones
EXCLUDES Retroperitoneal:
Abscess drainage (49060)
Exploration (49010)
Tumor/cyst excision (49203-49205)

50060 **Nephrolithotomy; removal of calculus**
🔧 32.7   ✂ 32.7   **FUD** 090   C 80 50 ▭
AMA: 2015,Jan,16; 2014,Jan,11

50065 **secondary surgical operation for calculus**
🔧 34.7   ✂ 34.7   **FUD** 090   C 80 50 ▭
AMA: 2015,Jan,16; 2014,Jan,11

50070 **complicated by congenital kidney abnormality**
🔧 34.0   ✂ 34.0   **FUD** 090   C 80 50 ▭
AMA: 2015,Jan,16; 2014,Jan,11

50075 **removal of large staghorn calculus filling renal pelvis and calyces (including anatrophic pyelolithotomy)**
🔧 41.8   ✂ 41.8   **FUD** 090   C 80 50 ▭
AMA: 2015,Jan,16; 2014,Jan,11

50080 **Percutaneous nephrostolithotomy or pyelostolithotomy, with or without dilation, endoscopy, lithotripsy, stenting, or basket extraction; up to 2 cm**
EXCLUDES Nephrostomy without nephrostolithotomy (50040, 50395, 52334)
📷 (76000, 76001)
🔧 24.9   ✂ 24.9   **FUD** 090   T 62 50 ▭
AMA: 2015,Jan,16; 2014,Jan,11; 2012,Jan,15-42; 2011,Jan,11

50081 **over 2 cm**
EXCLUDES Nephrostomy without nephrostolithotomy (50040, 50395, 52334)
📷 (76000, 76001)
🔧 36.6   ✂ 36.6   **FUD** 090   62 80 50 ▭
AMA: 2015,Jan,16; 2014,Jan,11; 2012,Jan,15-42; 2011,Jan,11

50100 Repair of Anomalous Vessels of the Kidney

EXCLUDES Retroperitoneal:
Abscess drainage (49060)
Exploration (49010)
Tumor/cyst excision (49203-49205)

50100 **Transection or repositioning of aberrant renal vessels (separate procedure)**
🔧 31.1   ✂ 31.1   **FUD** 090   C 80 50 ▭
AMA: 2015,Jan,16; 2014,Jan,11

50120-50135 Procedures of Renal Pelvis

EXCLUDES Retroperitoneal:
Abscess drainage (49060)
Exploration (49010)
Tumor/cyst excision (49203-49205)

50120 **Pyelotomy; with exploration**
INCLUDES Gol-Vernet pyelotomy
EXCLUDES Renal endoscopy through pyelotomy (50570-50580)
🔧 27.2   ✂ 27.2   **FUD** 090   C 80 50 ▭
AMA: 2015,Jan,16; 2014,Jan,11

50125 **with drainage, pyelostomy**
🔧 28.2   ✂ 28.2   **FUD** 090   C 80 50 ▭
AMA: 2015,Jan,16; 2014,Jan,11

50130 **with removal of calculus (pyelolithotomy, pelviolithotomy, including coagulum pyelolithotomy)**
🔧 29.6   ✂ 29.6   **FUD** 090   C 80 50 ▭
AMA: 2015,Jan,16; 2014,Jan,11

50135 **complicated (eg, secondary operation, congenital kidney abnormality)**
🔧 32.2   ✂ 32.2   **FUD** 090   C 80 50 ▭
AMA: 2015,Jan,16; 2014,Jan,11

50200-50205 Biopsy of Kidney

EXCLUDES Laparoscopic renal mass lesion ablation (50542)
Retroperitoneal tumor/cyst excision (49203-49205)

50200 **Renal biopsy; percutaneous, by trocar or needle**
EXCLUDES Fine needle aspiration (10022)
📷 (76942, 77002, 77012, 77021)
🔬 (88172-88173)
🔧 4.15   ✂ 17.4   **FUD** 000   ⊙ T A2 50 ▭ P0
AMA: 2015,Jan,16; 2014,Jan,11; 2010,Jan,7-8

50205 **by surgical exposure of kidney**
🔧 21.7   ✂ 21.7   **FUD** 090   C 80 50 ▭ P0
AMA: 2015,Jan,16; 2014,Jan,11

50220-50240 Nephrectomy Procedures

EXCLUDES Laparoscopic renal mass lesion ablation (50542)
Retroperitoneal tumor/cyst excision (49203-49205)

50220 **Nephrectomy, including partial ureterectomy, any open approach including rib resection;**
🔧 30.0   ✂ 30.0   **FUD** 090   C 80 50 ▭ P0
AMA: 2015,Jan,16; 2014,Jan,11

50225 **complicated because of previous surgery on same kidney**
🔧 34.4   ✂ 34.4   **FUD** 090   C 80 50 ▭ P0
AMA: 2015,Jan,16; 2014,Jan,11

50230 **radical, with regional lymphadenectomy and/or vena caval thrombectomy**
EXCLUDES Vena caval resection with reconstruction (37799)
🔧 36.8   ✂ 36.8   **FUD** 090   C 80 50 ▭ P0
AMA: 2015,Jan,16; 2014,Jan,11

50234 **Nephrectomy with total ureterectomy and bladder cuff; through same incision**

🔧 37.3 ✂ 37.3 **FUD** 090 C 80 50 ▣ PQ

AMA: 2015,Jan,16; 2014,Jan,11

50236 **through separate incision**

🔧 42.1 ✂ 42.1 **FUD** 090 C 80 50 ▣ PQ

AMA: 2015,Jan,16; 2014,Jan,11

50240 **Nephrectomy, partial**

EXCLUDES *Laparoscopic partial nephrectomy (50543)*

🔧 37.9 ✂ 37.9 **FUD** 090 C 80 50 ▣ PQ

AMA: 2015,Jan,16; 2014,Jan,11

50250-50290 Open Removal Kidney Lesions

EXCLUDES *Open destruction or excision intra-abdominal tumors (49203-49205)*

50250 **Ablation, open, 1 or more renal mass lesion(s), cryosurgical, including intraoperative ultrasound guidance and monitoring, if performed**

EXCLUDES *Laparoscopic renal mass lesion ablation (50542)*
Percutaneous renal tumor ablation (50592-50593)

🔧 34.9 ✂ 34.9 **FUD** 090 C 80

AMA: 2015,Jan,16; 2014,Jan,11; 2012,Jan,15-42; 2011,Jan,11

50280 **Excision or unroofing of cyst(s) of kidney**

EXCLUDES *Renal cyst laparoscopic ablation (50541)*

🔧 27.4 ✂ 27.4 **FUD** 090 C 80 50 ▣

AMA: 2015,Jan,16; 2014,Jan,11

50290 **Excision of perinephric cyst**

🔧 25.7 ✂ 25.7 **FUD** 090 C 80 ▣

AMA: 2015,Jan,16; 2014,Jan,11

50300-50380 Kidney Transplant Procedures

CMS: 100-4,3,90.1 Kidney Transplant - General; 100-4,3,90.1.1 Standard Kidney Acquisition Charge; 100-4,3,90.1.2 Billing for Kidney Transplant and Acquisition Services; 100-4,3,90.5 Pancreas Transplants with Kidney Transplants

EXCLUDES *Dialysis procedures (90935-90999)*
Donor nephrectomy performed laparoscopically (50547)
Lymphocele drainage to peritoneal cavity performed laparoscopically (49323)

50300 **Donor nephrectomy (including cold preservation); from cadaver donor, unilateral or bilateral**

INCLUDES Graft:
Cold preservation
Harvesting

🔧 0.00 ✂ 0.00 **FUD** XXX C ▣

AMA: 2015,Jan,16; 2014,Jan,11

50320 **open, from living donor**

INCLUDES Donor care
Graft:
Cold preservation
Harvesting

EXCLUDES *Donor nephrectomy performed laparoscopically (50547)*

🔧 43.4 ✂ 43.4 **FUD** 090 C 80 50 ▣ PQ

AMA: 2015,Jan,16; 2014,Jan,11

50323 **Backbench standard preparation of cadaver donor renal allograft prior to transplantation, including dissection and removal of perinephric fat, diaphragmatic and retroperitoneal attachments, excision of adrenal gland, and preparation of ureter(s), renal vein(s), and renal artery(s), ligating branches, as necessary**

Do not report with (60540, 60545)

🔧 0.00 ✂ 0.00 **FUD** XXX C 80 ▣

AMA: 2015,Jan,16; 2014,Jan,11

50325 **Backbench standard preparation of living donor renal allograft (open or laparoscopic) prior to transplantation, including dissection and removal of perinephric fat and preparation of ureter(s), renal vein(s), and renal artery(s), ligating branches, as necessary**

🔧 0.00 ✂ 0.00 **FUD** XXX C 80 ▣

AMA: 2014,Jan,11

50327 **Backbench reconstruction of cadaver or living donor renal allograft prior to transplantation; venous anastomosis, each**

🔧 6.29 ✂ 6.29 **FUD** XXX C 80 ▣

AMA: 2014,Jan,11

50328 **arterial anastomosis, each**

🔧 5.51 ✂ 5.51 **FUD** XXX C 80 ▣

AMA: 2014,Jan,11

50329 **ureteral anastomosis, each**

🔧 5.31 ✂ 5.31 **FUD** XXX C 80 ▣

AMA: 2014,Jan,11

50340 **Recipient nephrectomy (separate procedure)**

🔧 27.3 ✂ 27.3 **FUD** 090 C 80 50 ▣ PQ

AMA: 2014,Jan,11

50360 **Renal allotransplantation, implantation of graft; without recipient nephrectomy**

INCLUDES Allograft transplantation
Recipient care
Code also backbench work (50323, 50325, 50327-50329)
Code also donor nephrectomy (cadaver or living donor) (50300, 50320, 50547)

🔧 69.9 ✂ 69.9 **FUD** 090 C 80 PQ

AMA: 2014,Jan,11

50365 **with recipient nephrectomy**

INCLUDES Allograft transplantation
Recipient care

🔧 81.9 ✂ 81.9 **FUD** 090 C 80 50 ▣ PQ

AMA: 2015,Jan,16; 2014,Jan,11

50370 **Removal of transplanted renal allograft**

🔧 34.6 ✂ 34.6 **FUD** 090 C 80 ▣ PQ

AMA: 2014,Jan,11

50380 **Renal autotransplantation, reimplantation of kidney**

INCLUDES Reimplantation of autograft

EXCLUDES *Secondary backbench procedures:*
Nephrolithotomy (50060-50075)
Partial nephrectomy (50240, 50543)

🔧 57.8 ✂ 57.8 **FUD** 090 C 80 ▣ PQ

AMA: 2015,Jan,16; 2014,Jan,11

50382-50386 Removal With/Without Replacement Internal Ureteral Stent

INCLUDES Radiological supervision and interpretation

50382 **Removal (via snare/capture) and replacement of internally dwelling ureteral stent via percutaneous approach, including radiological supervision and interpretation**

EXCLUDES *Removal and replacement of an internally dwelling ureteral stent using a transurethral approach (50385)*

Do not report with (50395)

🔧 7.90 ✂ 33.7 **FUD** 000 ⊙ T 62 50 PQ

AMA: 2015,Jan,16; 2014,Jan,11

50384 **Removal (via snare/capture) of internally dwelling ureteral stent via percutaneous approach, including radiological supervision and interpretation**

EXCLUDES *Removal of an internally dwelling ureteral stent using a transurethral approach (50386)*

Do not report with (50395)

🔧 7.15 ✂ 26.8 **FUD** 000 ⊙ 02 62 50 PQ

AMA: 2015,Jan,16; 2014,Jan,11

50385 **Removal (via snare/capture) and replacement of internally dwelling ureteral stent via transurethral approach, without use of cystoscopy, including radiological supervision and interpretation**

🔧 6.75 ✂ 32.4 **FUD** 000 ⊙ T 62 80 50 PQ

AMA: 2015,Jan,16; 2014,Jan,11

50386 Removal (via snare/capture) of internally dwelling ureteral stent via transurethral approach, without use of cystoscopy, including radiological supervision and interpretation
  5.10   21.1   **FUD** 000   ⊙ 02 P2 80 50 P0
  AMA: 2015,Jan,16; 2014,Jan,11

50387 Remove/Replace Accessible Ureteral Stent

EXCLUDES   *Removal and replacement of ureteral stent through ureterostomy tube or ileal conduit (50688)*
  Removal without replacement of externally accessible ureteral stent without fluoroscopic guidance, report with appropriate E&M code

▲ **50387** Removal and replacement of externally accessible nephroureteral catheter (eg, external/internal stent) requiring fluoroscopic guidance, including radiological supervision and interpretation
  2.84   15.4   **FUD** 000   ⊙ T 02 80 50 P0
  AMA: 2015,Jan,16; 2014,Jan,11; 2012,Mar,9-10

50389-50398 [50430, 50431, 50432, 50433, 50434, 50435] Percutaneous and Injection Procedures With/Without Indwelling Tube/Catheter Access

50389 Removal of nephrostomy tube, requiring fluoroscopic guidance (eg, with concurrent indwelling ureteral stent)
  EXCLUDES   *Nephrostomy tube removal without fluoroscopic guidance, report with appropriate E&M code*
  1.58   8.44   **FUD** 000   02 62 50 P0
  AMA: 2015,Jan,16; 2014,Jan,11

50390 Aspiration and/or injection of renal cyst or pelvis by needle, percutaneous
  EXCLUDES   *Antegrade nephrostogram/pyelogram ([50430, 50431])*
  ⚕ (74425, 74470, 76942, 77002, 77012, 77021)
  2.81   2.81   **FUD** 000   T A2 50
  AMA: 2015,Jan,16; 2014,Jan,11

50391 Instillation(s) of therapeutic agent into renal pelvis and/or ureter through established nephrostomy, pyelostomy or ureterostomy tube (eg, anticarcinogenic or antifungal agent)
  Code also therapeutic agent
  2.85   3.50   **FUD** 000   T P3 50
  AMA: 2015,Jan,16; 2014,Jan,11

~~**50392** Introduction of intracatheter or catheter into renal pelvis for drainage and/or injection, percutaneous~~
  To report, see ~[50432]

~~**50393** Introduction of ureteral catheter or stent into ureter through renal pelvis for drainage and/or injection, percutaneous~~
  To report, see ~50693-50695

~~**50394** Injection procedure for pyelography (as nephrostogram, pyelostogram, antegrade pyeloureterograms) through nephrostomy or pyelostomy tube, or indwelling ureteral catheter~~
  To report, see ~[50430, 50431]

50395 Introduction of guide into renal pelvis and/or ureter with dilation to establish nephrostomy tract, percutaneous
  EXCLUDES   *Percutaneous nephrostolithotomy (50080, 50081)*
  Renal endoscopy (50551-50561)
  Retrograde percutaneous nephrostomy (52334)
  Do not report with (50382, 50384, [50432, 50433])
  ⚕ (74485)
  5.19   5.19   **FUD** 000   T A2 50
  AMA: 2015,Jan,16; 2014,Jan,11; 2012,Jan,15-42; 2011,Jan,11

50396 Manometric studies through nephrostomy or pyelostomy tube, or indwelling ureteral catheter
  ⚕ (74425)
  3.44   3.44   **FUD** 000   T A2 80 50
  AMA: 2015,Jan,16; 2014,Jan,11

● # **50430** Injection procedure for antegrade nephrostogram and/or ureterogram, complete diagnostic procedure including imaging guidance (eg, ultrasound and fluoroscopy) and all associated radiological supervision and interpretation; new access
  0.00   0.00   **FUD** 000   ⊙
  INCLUDES   Renal pelvis and associated ureter as a single element
  Do not report with for same renal collecting system/ureter ([50432, 50433, 50434, 50435], 50693-50695, 74425)

● # **50431** existing access
  0.00   0.00   **FUD** 000
  INCLUDES   Renal pelvis and associated ureter as a single element
  Do not report with for same renal collecting system/ureter ([50432, 50433, 50434, 50435], 50693-50695, 74425)

● # **50432** Placement of nephrostomy catheter, percutaneous, including diagnostic nephrostogram and/or ureterogram when performed, imaging guidance (eg, ultrasound and/or fluoroscopy) and all associated radiological supervision and interpretation
  0.00   0.00   **FUD** 000   ⊙
  INCLUDES   Renal pelvis and associated ureter as a single element
  Do not report with for dilation of nephrostomy tube tract (50395)
  Do not report with for same renal collecting system/ureter ([50430, 50431], [50433], 50694-50695, 74425)

● # **50433** Placement of nephroureteral catheter, percutaneous, including diagnostic nephrostogram and/or ureterogram when performed, imaging guidance (eg, ultrasound and/or fluoroscopy) and all associated radiological supervision and interpretation, new access
  0.00   0.00   **FUD** 000   ⊙
  INCLUDES   Renal pelvis and associated ureter as a single element
  EXCLUDES   *Nephroureteral catheter removal/replacement (50387)*
  Do not report with for dilation of nephroureteral catheter tract (50395)
  Do not report with for same renal collecting system/ureter ([50430, 50431, 50432], 50693-50695, 74425)

● # **50434** Convert nephrostomy catheter to nephroureteral catheter, percutaneous, including diagnostic nephrostogram and/or ureterogram when performed, imaging guidance (eg, ultrasound and/or fluoroscopy) and all associated radiological supervision and interpretation, via pre-existing nephrostomy tract
  0.00   0.00   **FUD** 000   ⊙
  INCLUDES   Renal pelvis and associated ureter as a single element
  Do not report with for same renal collecting system/ureter ([50430, 50431], [50435], 50684, 50693, 74425)

● # **50435** Exchange nephrostomy catheter, percutaneous, including diagnostic nephrostogram and/or ureterogram when performed, imaging guidance (eg, ultrasound and/or fluoroscopy) and all associated radiological supervision and interpretation
  0.00   0.00   **FUD** 000
  INCLUDES   Renal pelvis and associated ureter as a single element
  EXCLUDES   *Removal nephrostomy catheter that requires fluoroscopic guidance (50389)*
  Do not report with for same renal collecting system/ureter ([50430, 50431], [50434], 50693, 74425)

~~**50398** Change of nephrostomy or pyelostomy tube~~
  To report, see ~[50435]

50400-50540 Open Surgical Procedures of Kidney

50400 Pyeloplasty (Foley Y-pyeloplasty), plastic operation on renal pelvis, with or without plastic operation on ureter, nephropexy, nephrostomy, pyelostomy, or ureteral splinting; simple
  EXCLUDES   *Laparoscopic pyeloplasty (50544)*
  33.1   33.1   **FUD** 090   C 80 50
  AMA: 2015,Jan,16; 2014,Jan,11

Urinary System

50386 — 50400

50405 complicated (congenital kidney abnormality, secondary pyeloplasty, solitary kidney, calycoplasty)

EXCLUDES *Laparoscopic pyeloplasty (50544)*

⚕ 40.1   ✂ 40.1   **FUD** 090   C 80 50 ▭

AMA: 2015,Jan,16; 2014,Jan,11

50430 Resequenced code. See code following 50396.

50431 Resequenced code. See code following 50396.

50432 Resequenced code. See code following 50396.

50433 Resequenced code. See code following 50396.

50434 Resequenced code. See code following 50396.

50435 Resequenced code. See code following 50396.

50500 Nephrorrhaphy, suture of kidney wound or injury

⚕ 33.1   ✂ 33.1   **FUD** 090   C 80 ▭

AMA: 2014,Jan,11

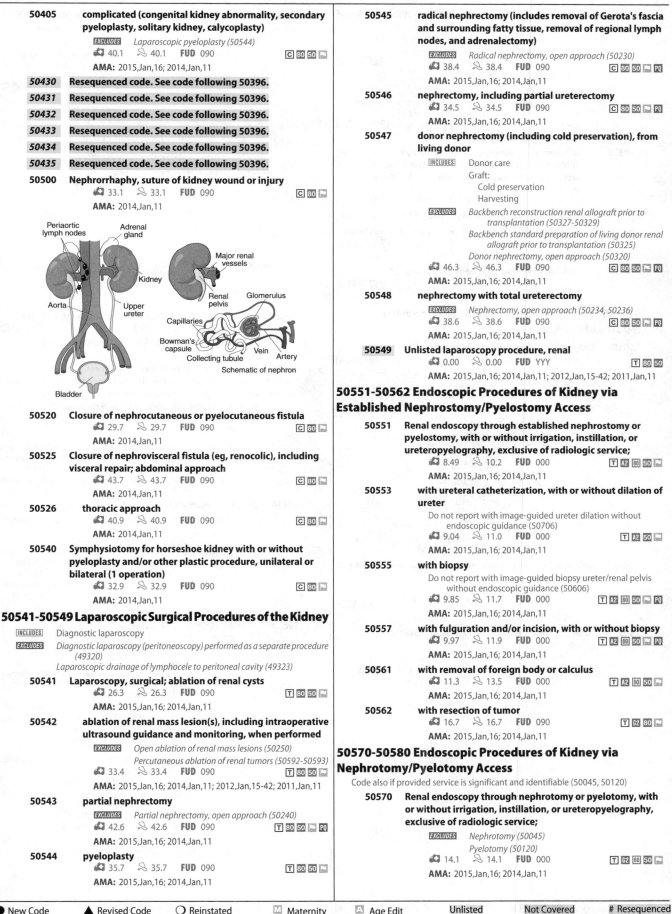

Periaortic lymph nodes
Adrenal gland
Major renal vessels
Kidney
Aorta
Upper ureter
Renal pelvis
Glomerulus
Capillaries
Bowman's capsule
Collecting tubule
Vein
Artery
Schematic of nephron
Bladder

50520 Closure of nephrocutaneous or pyelocutaneous fistula

⚕ 29.7   ✂ 29.7   **FUD** 090   C 80 ▭

AMA: 2014,Jan,11

50525 Closure of nephrovisceral fistula (eg, renocolic), including visceral repair; abdominal approach

⚕ 43.7   ✂ 43.7   **FUD** 090   C 80 ▭

AMA: 2014,Jan,11

50526 thoracic approach

⚕ 40.9   ✂ 40.9   **FUD** 090   C 80 ▭

AMA: 2014,Jan,11

50540 Symphysiotomy for horseshoe kidney with or without pyeloplasty and/or other plastic procedure, unilateral or bilateral (1 operation)

⚕ 32.9   ✂ 32.9   **FUD** 090   C 80 ▭

AMA: 2014,Jan,11

50541-50549 Laparoscopic Surgical Procedures of the Kidney

INCLUDES Diagnostic laparoscopy

EXCLUDES *Diagnostic laparoscopy (peritoneoscopy) performed as a separate procedure (49320)*
Laparoscopic drainage of lymphocele to peritoneal cavity (49323)

50541 Laparoscopy, surgical; ablation of renal cysts

⚕ 26.3   ✂ 26.3   **FUD** 090   T 80 50 ▭

AMA: 2015,Jan,16; 2014,Jan,11

50542 ablation of renal mass lesion(s), including intraoperative ultrasound guidance and monitoring, when performed

EXCLUDES *Open ablation of renal mass lesions (50250)*
Percutaneous ablation of renal tumors (50592-50593)

⚕ 33.4   ✂ 33.4   **FUD** 090   T 80 50 ▭

AMA: 2015,Jan,16; 2014,Jan,11; 2012,Jan,15-42; 2011,Jan,11

50543 partial nephrectomy

EXCLUDES *Partial nephrectomy, open approach (50240)*

⚕ 42.6   ✂ 42.6   **FUD** 090   T 80 50 ▭ PQ

AMA: 2015,Jan,16; 2014,Jan,11

50544 pyeloplasty

⚕ 35.7   ✂ 35.7   **FUD** 090   T 80 50 ▭

AMA: 2015,Jan,16; 2014,Jan,11

50545 radical nephrectomy (includes removal of Gerota's fascia and surrounding fatty tissue, removal of regional lymph nodes, and adrenalectomy)

EXCLUDES *Radical nephrectomy, open approach (50230)*

⚕ 38.4   ✂ 38.4   **FUD** 090   C 80 50 ▭ PQ

AMA: 2015,Jan,16; 2014,Jan,11

50546 nephrectomy, including partial ureterectomy

⚕ 34.5   ✂ 34.5   **FUD** 090   C 80 50 ▭ PQ

AMA: 2015,Jan,16; 2014,Jan,11

50547 donor nephrectomy (including cold preservation), from living donor

INCLUDES Donor care
Graft:
Cold preservation
Harvesting

EXCLUDES *Backbench reconstruction renal allograft prior to transplantation (50327-50329)*
Backbench standard preparation of living donor renal allograft prior to transplantation (50325)
Donor nephrectomy, open approach (50320)

⚕ 46.3   ✂ 46.3   **FUD** 090   C 80 50 ▭ PQ

AMA: 2015,Jan,16; 2014,Jan,11

50548 nephrectomy with total ureterectomy

EXCLUDES *Nephrectomy, open approach (50234, 50236)*

⚕ 38.6   ✂ 38.6   **FUD** 090   C 80 50 ▭ PQ

AMA: 2015,Jan,16; 2014,Jan,11

50549 Unlisted laparoscopy procedure, renal

⚕ 0.00   ✂ 0.00   **FUD** YYY   T 80 50

AMA: 2015,Jan,16; 2014,Jan,11; 2012,Jan,15-42; 2011,Jan,11

50551-50562 Endoscopic Procedures of Kidney via Established Nephrostomy/Pyelostomy Access

50551 Renal endoscopy through established nephrostomy or pyelostomy, with or without irrigation, instillation, or ureteropyelography, exclusive of radiologic service;

⚕ 8.49   ✂ 10.2   **FUD** 000   T A2 80 50 ▭

AMA: 2015,Jan,16; 2014,Jan,11

50553 with ureteral catheterization, with or without dilation of ureter

Do not report with image-guided ureter dilation without endoscopic guidance (50706)

⚕ 9.04   ✂ 11.0   **FUD** 000   T A2 50 ▭

AMA: 2015,Jan,16; 2014,Jan,11

50555 with biopsy

Do not report with image-guided biopsy ureter/renal pelvis without endoscopic guidance (50606)

⚕ 9.85   ✂ 11.7   **FUD** 000   T A2 80 50 ▭ PQ

AMA: 2015,Jan,16; 2014,Jan,11

50557 with fulguration and/or incision, with or without biopsy

⚕ 9.97   ✂ 11.9   **FUD** 000   T A2 80 50 ▭ PQ

AMA: 2015,Jan,16; 2014,Jan,11

50561 with removal of foreign body or calculus

⚕ 11.3   ✂ 13.5   **FUD** 000   T A2 80 50 ▭

AMA: 2015,Jan,16; 2014,Jan,11

50562 with resection of tumor

⚕ 16.7   ✂ 16.7   **FUD** 090   T 63 80 ▭

AMA: 2015,Jan,16; 2014,Jan,11

50570-50580 Endoscopic Procedures of Kidney via Nephrotomy/Pyelotomy Access

Code also if provided service is significant and identifiable (50045, 50120)

50570 Renal endoscopy through nephrotomy or pyelotomy, with or without irrigation, instillation, or ureteropyelography, exclusive of radiologic service;

EXCLUDES *Nephrotomy (50045)*
Pyelotomy (50120)

⚕ 14.1   ✂ 14.1   **FUD** 000   T 63 80 50 ▭

AMA: 2015,Jan,16; 2014,Jan,11

50572   **with ureteral catheterization, with or without dilation of ureter**

Do not report with image-guided ureter dilation without endoscopic guidance (50706)

🔷 15.3   ⚬ 15.3   **FUD** 000   T G2 80 50 ⬜

AMA: 2015,Jan,16; 2014,Jan,11

50574   **with biopsy**

Do not report with image-guide ureter/renal pelvis biopsy without endoscopic guidance (50606)

🔷 16.2   ⚬ 16.2   **FUD** 000   T G2 80 50 ⬜ P0

AMA: 2015,Jan,16; 2014,Jan,11

50575   **with endopyelotomy (includes cystoscopy, ureteroscopy, dilation of ureter and ureteral pelvic junction, incision of ureteral pelvic junction and insertion of endopyelotomy stent)**

🔷 20.5   ⚬ 20.5   **FUD** 000   T G2 50 ⬜ P0

AMA: 2015,Jan,16; 2014,Jan,11; 2012,Jan,15-42; 2011,Jan,11

50576   **with fulguration and/or incision, with or without biopsy**

🔷 16.2   ⚬ 16.2   **FUD** 000   T G2 80 50 ⬜ P0

AMA: 2015,Jan,16; 2014,Jan,11

50580   **with removal of foreign body or calculus**

🔷 17.4   ⚬ 17.4   **FUD** 000   T G2 80 50 ⬜

AMA: 2015,Jan,16; 2014,Jan,11

50590-50593 Noninvasive and Minimally Invasive Procedures of the Kidney

50590   **Lithotripsy, extracorporeal shock wave**

🔷 16.2   ⚬ 20.5   **FUD** 090   T G2 50 ⬜ P0

AMA: 2015,Jan,16; 2014,Jan,11; 2012,Jan,15-42; 2011,Jan,11

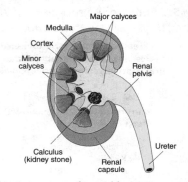

Major calyces
Medulla
Cortex
Minor calyces
Renal pelvis
Calculus (kidney stone)
Ureter
Renal capsule

50592   **Ablation, 1 or more renal tumor(s), percutaneous, unilateral, radiofrequency**

🔲 (76940, 77013, 77022)

🔷 10.5   ⚬ 89.3   **FUD** 010   ⊙ T G2 50

AMA: 2014,Jan,11

50593   **Ablation, renal tumor(s), unilateral, percutaneous, cryotherapy**

🔲 (76940, 77013, 77022)

🔷 13.9   ⚬ 131.   **FUD** 010   ⊙ T G2 80 50

AMA: 2014,Jan,11

50600-50940 Open and Injection Procedures of Ureter

50600   **Ureterotomy with exploration or drainage (separate procedure)**

Code also ureteral endoscopy through ureterotomy when procedures constitute a significant identifiable service (50970-50980)

🔷 26.9   ⚬ 26.9   **FUD** 090   C 80 50 ⬜

AMA: 2014,Jan,11

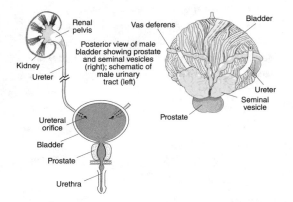

Renal pelvis
Vas deferens
Bladder
Kidney
Ureter
Posterior view of male bladder showing prostate and seminal vesicles (right); schematic of male urinary tract (left)
Ureteral orifice
Bladder
Prostate
Urethra
Ureter
Seminal vesicle
Prostate

50605   **Ureterotomy for insertion of indwelling stent, all types**

🔷 28.3   ⚬ 28.3   **FUD** 090   C 80 50 ⬜

AMA: 2015,Jan,16; 2014,Jan,11; 2012,Apr,17-18; 2012,Jan,15-42; 2011,Jan,11

● + **50606**   **Endoluminal biopsy of ureter and/or renal pelvis, non-endoscopic, including imaging guidance (eg, ultrasound and/or fluoroscopy) and all associated radiological supervision and interpretation (List separately in addition to code for primary procedure)**

🔷 0.00   ⚬ 0.00   **FUD** 000   ⊙

INCLUDES   Renal pelvis and associated ureter as a single element

Code first (50382-50389, [50430, 50431, 50432, 50433, 50434, 50435], 50684, 50688, 50690, 50693-50695, 51610)

Do not report for same renal collecting system/associated ureter with (50555, 50574, 50955, 50974, 52007, 74425)

50610   **Ureterolithotomy; upper one-third of ureter**

EXCLUDES   *Cystotomy with calculus basket extraction of ureteral calculus (51065)*
           Transvesical ureterolithotomy (51060)
           Ureteral calculus manipulation/extraction performed endoscopically (50080-50081, 50561, 50961, 50980, 52320-52330, 52352-52353, [52356])
           Ureterolithotomy performed laparoscopically (50945)

🔷 27.1   ⚬ 27.1   **FUD** 090   C 80 50 ⬜

AMA: 2015,Jan,16; 2014,Jan,11

50620   **middle one-third of ureter**

EXCLUDES   *Cystotomy with calculus basket extraction of ureteral calculus (51065)*
           Transvesical ureterolithotomy (51060)
           Ureteral calculus manipulation/extraction performed endoscopically (50080-50081, 50561, 50961, 50980, 52320-52330, 52352-52353, [52356])
           Ureterolithotomy performed laparoscopically (50945)

🔷 25.9   ⚬ 25.9   **FUD** 090   C 80 50 ⬜

AMA: 2015,Jan,16; 2014,Jan,11

50630   **lower one-third of ureter**

EXCLUDES   *Cystotomy with calculus basket extraction of ureteral calculus (51065)*
           Transvesical ureterolithotomy (51060)
           Ureteral calculus manipulation/extraction performed endoscopically (50080-50081, 50561, 50961, 50980, 52320-52330, 52352-52353, [52356])
           Ureterolithotomy performed laparoscopically (50945)

🔷 25.6   ⚬ 25.6   **FUD** 090   C 80 50 ⬜

AMA: 2015,Jan,16; 2014,May,3; 2014,Jan,11

50572 — 50630

50650 **Ureterectomy, with bladder cuff (separate procedure)**
EXCLUDES *Ureterocele (51535, 52300)*
🔲 29.7   ⚖ 29.7   **FUD** 090   C 80 50 🔲
AMA: 2014,Jan,11

50660 **Ureterectomy, total, ectopic ureter, combination abdominal, vaginal and/or perineal approach**
EXCLUDES *Ureterocele (51535, 52300)*
🔲 32.8   ⚖ 32.8   **FUD** 090   C 80 🔲
AMA: 2014,Jan,11

50684 **Injection procedure for ureterography or ureteropyelography through ureterostomy or indwelling ureteral catheter**
Do not report with ([50433, 50434], 50693-50695)
🔲 (74425)
🔲 1.44   ⚖ 3.01   **FUD** 000   N N1 50 🔲
AMA: 2014,Jan,11

50686 **Manometric studies through ureterostomy or indwelling ureteral catheter**
🔲 2.71   ⚖ 4.50   **FUD** 000   T P2 80 🔲
AMA: 2014,Jan,11

50688 **Change of ureterostomy tube or externally accessible ureteral stent via ileal conduit**
🔲 (75984)
🔲 2.30   ⚖ 2.30   **FUD** 010   T A2 🔲
AMA: 2014,Jan,11

50690 **Injection procedure for visualization of ileal conduit and/or ureteropyelography, exclusive of radiologic service**
🔲 (74425)
🔲 2.04   ⚖ 2.81   **FUD** 000   N N1 🔲
AMA: 2014,Jan,11

● **50693** **Placement of ureteral stent, percutaneous, including diagnostic nephrostogram and/or ureterogram when performed, imaging guidance (eg, ultrasound and/or fluoroscopy), and all associated radiological supervision and interpretation; pre-existing nephrostomy tract**
🔲 0.00   ⚖ 0.00   **FUD** 000   ⊙
INCLUDES Renal pelvis and associated ureter as a single element
Do not report with for the same renal collecting system/ureter ([50430, 50431, 50432, 50433, 50434, 50435], 50684, 74425)

● **50694** **new access, without separate nephrostomy catheter**
🔲 0.00   ⚖ 0.00   **FUD** 000   ⊙
INCLUDES Renal pelvis and associated ureter as a single element
Do not report with for the same renal collecting system/ureter ([50430, 50431, 50432, 50433, 50434, 50435], 50684, 74425)

● **50695** **new access, with separate nephrostomy catheter**
🔲 0.00   ⚖ 0.00   **FUD** 000   ⊙
INCLUDES Placement of separate ureteral stent and nephrostomy catheter into a ureter/associated renal pelvis through a new access
Renal pelvis and associated ureter as a single element
Do not report with for the same renal collecting system/ureter ([50430, 50431, 50432, 50433, 50434, 50435], 50684, 74425)

50700 **Ureteroplasty, plastic operation on ureter (eg, stricture)**
🔲 26.5   ⚖ 26.5   **FUD** 090   C 80 50 🔲
AMA: 2014,Jan,11

● + **50705** **Ureteral embolization or occlusion, including imaging guidance (eg, ultrasound and/or fluoroscopy) and all associated radiological supervision and interpretation (List separately in addition to code for primary procedure)**
🔲 0.00   ⚖ 0.00   **FUD** 000   ⊙
INCLUDES Renal pelvis and associated ureter as a single element
EXCLUDES *Percutaneous nephrostomy/nephroureteral catheter/ureteral catheter placement (50385, 50387, [50432, 50433, 50434, 50435], 50693-50695)*
Code also when performed:
  additional catheter insertions
  diagnostic pyelography/ureterography
  other interventions
Code first (50382-50389, [50430, 50431, 50432, 50433, 50434, 50435], 50684, 50688, 50690, 50693-50695, 51610)

● + **50706** **Balloon dilation, ureteral stricture, including imaging guidance (eg, ultrasound and/or fluoroscopy) and all associated radiological supervision and interpretation (List separately in addition to code for primary procedure)**
🔲 0.00   ⚖ 0.00   **FUD** 000   ⊙
INCLUDES Renal pelvis and associated ureter as a single element
EXCLUDES *Percutaneous nephrostomy/nephroureteral catheter/ureteral catheter placement (50385, 50387, [50432, 50433, 50434, 50435], 50693-50695)*
Code also when performed:
  additional catheter insertions
  diagnostic pyelography/ureterography
  other interventions
Code first (50382-50389, [50430, 50431, 50432, 50433, 50434, 50435], 50684, 50688, 50690, 50693-50695, 51610)
Do not report with (50553, 50572, 50953, 50972, 52341, 52344-52345, 74485)

50715 **Ureterolysis, with or without repositioning of ureter for retroperitoneal fibrosis**
🔲 35.1   ⚖ 35.1   **FUD** 090   C 80 50 🔲 PQ
AMA: 2014,Jan,11

50722 **Ureterolysis for ovarian vein syndrome**   ♀
🔲 29.6   ⚖ 29.6   **FUD** 090   C 80 🔲 PQ
AMA: 2014,Jan,11

50725 **Ureterolysis for retrocaval ureter, with reanastomosis of upper urinary tract or vena cava**
🔲 31.9   ⚖ 31.9   **FUD** 090   C 80 🔲 PQ
AMA: 2014,Jan,11

50727 **Revision of urinary-cutaneous anastomosis (any type urostomy);**
🔲 14.5   ⚖ 14.5   **FUD** 090   T G2 80 🔲 PQ
AMA: 2014,Jan,11

50728 **with repair of fascial defect and hernia**
🔲 20.0   ⚖ 20.0   **FUD** 090   C 80 🔲 PQ
AMA: 2014,Jan,11

50740 **Ureteropyelostomy, anastomosis of ureter and renal pelvis**
🔲 35.3   ⚖ 35.3   **FUD** 090   C 80 50 🔲
AMA: 2015,Jan,16; 2014,Jan,11

50750 **Ureterocalycostomy, anastomosis of ureter to renal calyx**
🔲 33.1   ⚖ 33.1   **FUD** 090   C 80 50 🔲
AMA: 2015,Jan,16; 2014,Jan,11

50760 **Ureteroureterostomy**
🔲 32.4   ⚖ 32.4   **FUD** 090   C 80 50 🔲
AMA: 2015,Jan,16; 2014,Jan,11

50770 **Transureteroureterostomy, anastomosis of ureter to contralateral ureter**
🔲 33.1   ⚖ 33.1   **FUD** 090   C 80 🔲 PQ
AMA: 2014,Jan,11

50780 **Ureteroneocystostomy; anastomosis of single ureter to bladder**
> INCLUDES Minor procedures to prevent vesicoureteral reflux
> EXCLUDES *Cystourethroplasty with ureteroneocystostomy (51820)*
> 🚑 31.8 ⚚ 31.8 **FUD** 090 C 80 50 ▢ P0
> **AMA:** 2015,Jan,16; 2014,Jan,11

50782 **anastomosis of duplicated ureter to bladder**
> INCLUDES Minor procedures to prevent vesicoureteral reflux
> 🚑 32.1 ⚚ 32.1 **FUD** 090 C 80 50 ▢ P0
> **AMA:** 2015,Jan,16; 2014,Jan,11

50783 **with extensive ureteral tailoring**
> INCLUDES Minor procedures to prevent vesicoureteral reflux
> 🚑 32.3 ⚚ 32.3 **FUD** 090 C 80 50 ▢ P0
> **AMA:** 2015,Jan,16; 2014,Jan,11

50785 **with vesico-psoas hitch or bladder flap**
> INCLUDES Minor procedures to prevent vesicoureteral reflux
> 🚑 34.8 ⚚ 34.8 **FUD** 090 C 80 50 ▢ P0
> **AMA:** 2015,Jan,16; 2014,Jan,11

50800 **Ureteroenterostomy, direct anastomosis of ureter to intestine**
> EXCLUDES *Cystectomy with ureterosigmoidostomy/ureteroileal conduit (51580-51595)*
> 🚑 26.6 ⚚ 26.6 **FUD** 090 C 80 50 ▢ P0
> **AMA:** 2015,Jan,16; 2014,Jan,11

50810 **Ureterosigmoidostomy, with creation of sigmoid bladder and establishment of abdominal or perineal colostomy, including intestine anastomosis**
> EXCLUDES *Cystectomy with ureterosigmoidostomy/ureteroileal conduit (51580-51595)*
> 🚑 40.4 ⚚ 40.4 **FUD** 090 C 80 ▢ P0
> **AMA:** 2015,Jan,16; 2014,Jan,11

50815 **Ureterocolon conduit, including intestine anastomosis**
> EXCLUDES *Cystectomy with ureterosigmoidostomy/ureteroileal conduit (51580-51595)*
> 🚑 35.0 ⚚ 35.0 **FUD** 090 C 80 50 ▢ P0
> **AMA:** 2015,Jan,16; 2014,Jan,11

50820 **Ureteroileal conduit (ileal bladder), including intestine anastomosis (Bricker operation)**
> EXCLUDES *Cystectomy with ureterosigmoidostomy/ureteroileal conduit (51580-51595)*
> 🚑 37.8 ⚚ 37.8 **FUD** 090 C 80 50 ▢ P0
> **AMA:** 2015,Jan,16; 2014,Jan,11

50825 **Continent diversion, including intestine anastomosis using any segment of small and/or large intestine (Kock pouch or Camey enterocystoplasty)**
> 🚑 47.5 ⚚ 47.5 **FUD** 090 C 80 ▢
> **AMA:** 2015,Jan,16; 2014,Jan,11

50830 **Urinary undiversion (eg, taking down of ureteroileal conduit, ureterosigmoidostomy or ureteroenterostomy with ureteroureterostomy or ureteroneocystostomy)**
> 🚑 51.7 ⚚ 51.7 **FUD** 090 C 80 ▢
> **AMA:** 2015,Jan,16; 2014,Jan,11

50840 **Replacement of all or part of ureter by intestine segment, including intestine anastomosis**
> 🚑 35.2 ⚚ 35.2 **FUD** 090 C 80 50 ▢
> **AMA:** 2015,Jan,16; 2014,Jan,11

50845 **Cutaneous appendico-vesicostomy**
> INCLUDES Mitrofanoff operation
> 🚑 35.8 ⚚ 35.8 **FUD** 090 C 80 ▢
> **AMA:** 2014,Jan,11

50860 **Ureterostomy, transplantation of ureter to skin**
> 🚑 27.1 ⚚ 27.1 **FUD** 090 C 80 50 ▢
> **AMA:** 2014,Jan,11

50900 **Ureterorrhaphy, suture of ureter (separate procedure)**
> 🚑 24.3 ⚚ 24.3 **FUD** 090 C 80 50 ▢
> **AMA:** 2014,Jan,11

50920 **Closure of ureterocutaneous fistula**
> 🚑 25.2 ⚚ 25.2 **FUD** 090 C 80 ▢
> **AMA:** 2014,Jan,11

50930 **Closure of ureterovisceral fistula (including visceral repair)**
> 🚑 31.6 ⚚ 31.6 **FUD** 090 C 80 ▢
> **AMA:** 2014,Jan,11

50940 **Deligation of ureter**
> EXCLUDES *Ureteroplasty/ureterolysis (50700-50860)*
> 🚑 25.4 ⚚ 25.4 **FUD** 090 C 80 50 ▢
> **AMA:** 2014,Jan,11

50945-50949 Laparoscopic Procedures of Ureter
> INCLUDES Diagnostic laparoscopy
> EXCLUDES *Diagnostic laparoscopy (peritoneoscopy) performed as a separate procedure (49320)*
> *Ureteroneocystostomy, open approach (50780-50785)*

50945 **Laparoscopy, surgical; ureterolithotomy**
> 🚑 27.9 ⚚ 27.9 **FUD** 090 T 80 50 ▢
> **AMA:** 2015,Jan,16; 2014,Jan,11; 2012,Jan,15-42; 2011,Jan,11

50947 **ureteroneocystostomy with cystoscopy and ureteral stent placement**
> 🚑 39.8 ⚚ 39.8 **FUD** 090 T A2 80 50 ▢ P0
> **AMA:** 2015,Jan,16; 2014,Jan,11

50948 **ureteroneocystostomy without cystoscopy and ureteral stent placement**
> 🚑 36.6 ⚚ 36.6 **FUD** 090 T A2 80 50 ▢ P0
> **AMA:** 2015,Jan,16; 2014,Jan,11

50949 **Unlisted laparoscopy procedure, ureter**
> 🚑 0.00 ⚚ 0.00 **FUD** YYY T 80 50
> **AMA:** 2015,Jan,16; 2014,Jan,11

50951-50961 Endoscopic Procedures of Ureter via Established Ureterostomy Access

50951 **Ureteral endoscopy through established ureterostomy, with or without irrigation, instillation, or ureteropyelography, exclusive of radiologic service;**
> 🚑 8.85 ⚚ 10.7 **FUD** 000 T A2 80 50 ▢
> **AMA:** 2015,Jan,16; 2014,Jan,11; 2012,Jan,15-42; 2011,Jan,11

50953 **with ureteral catheterization, with or without dilation of ureter**
> Do not report with image-guided ureter dilation without endoscopic guidance (50706)
> 🚑 9.42 ⚚ 11.3 **FUD** 000 T A2 80 50 ▢
> **AMA:** 2015,Jan,16; 2014,Jan,11

50955 **with biopsy**
> Do not report with image-guided biopsy of ureter and/or renal pelvis without endoscopic guidance (50606)
> 🚑 10.1 ⚚ 12.1 **FUD** 000 T A2 80 50 ▢ P0
> **AMA:** 2015,Jan,16; 2014,Jan,11

50957 **with fulguration and/or incision, with or without biopsy**
> 🚑 10.2 ⚚ 12.2 **FUD** 000 T A2 80 50 ▢ P0
> **AMA:** 2015,Jan,16; 2014,Jan,11

50961 **with removal of foreign body or calculus**
> 🚑 9.16 ⚚ 11.0 **FUD** 000 T A2 80 50 ▢
> **AMA:** 2015,Jan,16; 2014,Jan,11; 2012,Jan,15-42; 2011,Jan,11

50970-50980 Endoscopic Procedures of Ureter via Ureterotomy
> EXCLUDES *Ureterotomy (50600)*

50970 **Ureteral endoscopy through ureterotomy, with or without irrigation, instillation, or ureteropyelography, exclusive of radiologic service;**
> 🚑 10.6 ⚚ 10.6 **FUD** 000 T A2 80 50 ▢
> **AMA:** 2015,Jan,16; 2014,Jan,11

50972 with ureteral catheterization, with or without dilation of ureter

> Do not report with image-guided ureter dilation without endoscopic guidance (50706)

🔧 10.3 ⚕ 10.3 **FUD** 000   T A2 80 50 ▣

AMA: 2015,Jan,16; 2014,Jan,11

50974 with biopsy

> Do not report with image-guided biopsy of ureter and/or renal pelvis without endoscopic guidance (50606)

🔧 13.6 ⚕ 13.6 **FUD** 000   T A2 80 50 ▣ P0

AMA: 2015,Jan,16; 2014,Jan,11

50976 with fulguration and/or incision, with or without biopsy

🔧 13.4 ⚕ 13.4 **FUD** 000   T A2 80 50 ▣ P0

AMA: 2015,Jan,16; 2014,Jan,11

50980 with removal of foreign body or calculus

🔧 10.2 ⚕ 10.2 **FUD** 000   T A2 80 50 ▣

AMA: 2015,Jan,16; 2014,Jan,11

51020-51080 Open Incisional Procedures of Bladder

51020 Cystotomy or cystostomy; with fulguration and/or insertion of radioactive material

🔧 13.4 ⚕ 13.4 **FUD** 090   T A2 80 ▣

AMA: 2014,Jan,11

51030 with cryosurgical destruction of intravesical lesion

🔧 13.4 ⚕ 13.4 **FUD** 090   T A2 80 ▣

AMA: 2014,Jan,11

51040 Cystostomy, cystotomy with drainage

🔧 8.27 ⚕ 8.27 **FUD** 090   T A2 80 ▣

AMA: 2014,Jan,11

51045 Cystotomy, with insertion of ureteral catheter or stent (separate procedure)

🔧 14.0 ⚕ 14.0 **FUD** 090   T A2 80 ▣

AMA: 2014,Jan,11

51050 Cystolithotomy, cystotomy with removal of calculus, without vesical neck resection

🔧 13.5 ⚕ 13.5 **FUD** 090   T A2 80 ▣

AMA: 2014,Jan,11

51060 Transvesical ureterolithotomy

🔧 16.6 ⚕ 16.6 **FUD** 090   T 80 ▣

AMA: 2014,Jan,11

51065 Cystotomy, with calculus basket extraction and/or ultrasonic or electrohydraulic fragmentation of ureteral calculus

🔧 16.5 ⚕ 16.5 **FUD** 090   T A2 80 ▣

AMA: 2014,Jan,11

51080 Drainage of perivesical or prevesical space abscess

> EXCLUDES Image-guided percutaneous catheter drainage (49406)

🔧 11.6 ⚕ 11.6 **FUD** 090   T A2 80 ▣

AMA: 2014,Jan,11

51100-51102 Bladder Aspiration Procedures

51100 Aspiration of bladder; by needle

📷 (76942, 77002, 77012)

🔧 1.13 ⚕ 1.77 **FUD** 000   T P3

AMA: 2015,Jan,16; 2014,Jan,11

Diaphragm
Umbilicus
Access is from above the pubic bone
Pubic bone
Hip and pubic bone
Ovary
Uterus
Rectouterine pouch
Bladder
Cervix
Rectum
Pubic bone
Urethral orifice
Labia majora
Anus
Vaginal canal

51101 by trocar or intracatheter

📷 (76942, 77002, 77012)

🔧 1.50 ⚕ 3.55 **FUD** 000   T P2

51102 with insertion of suprapubic catheter

📷 (76942, 77002, 77012)

🔧 4.18 ⚕ 6.46 **FUD** 000   T A2

AMA: 2015,Jan,16; 2014,Jan,11

51500-51597 Open Excisional Procedures of Bladder

51500 Excision of urachal cyst or sinus, with or without umbilical hernia repair

🔧 18.2 ⚕ 18.2 **FUD** 090   T A2 80 ▣

AMA: 2014,Jan,11

51520 Cystotomy; for simple excision of vesical neck (separate procedure)

🔧 17.0 ⚕ 17.0 **FUD** 090   T A2 80 ▣

AMA: 2014,Jan,11

51525 for excision of bladder diverticulum, single or multiple (separate procedure)

> EXCLUDES Transurethral resection (52305)

🔧 24.6 ⚕ 24.6 **FUD** 090   C 80 ▣

AMA: 2014,Jan,11

51530 for excision of bladder tumor

> EXCLUDES Transurethral resection (52234-52240, 52305)

🔧 22.4 ⚕ 22.4 **FUD** 090   C 80 ▣

AMA: 2014,Jan,11

51535 Cystotomy for excision, incision, or repair of ureterocele

> EXCLUDES Transurethral excision (52300)

🔧 22.3 ⚕ 22.3 **FUD** 090   T 62 80 50 ▣

AMA: 2014,Jan,11

51550 Cystectomy, partial; simple

🔧 27.6 ⚕ 27.6 **FUD** 090   C 80 ▣ P0

AMA: 2014,Jan,11

51555 complicated (eg, postradiation, previous surgery, difficult location)

🔧 36.4 ⚕ 36.4 **FUD** 090   C 80 ▣ P0

AMA: 2014,Jan,11

51565 Cystectomy, partial, with reimplantation of ureter(s) into bladder (ureteroneocystostomy)

🔧 37.3 ⚕ 37.3 **FUD** 090   C 80 ▣ P0

AMA: 2014,Jan,11

51570 Cystectomy, complete; (separate procedure)

🔧 42.4 ⚕ 42.4 **FUD** 090   C 80 ▣ P0

AMA: 2014,Jan,11

51575 with bilateral pelvic lymphadenectomy, including external iliac, hypogastric, and obturator nodes

🔧 52.3 ⚕ 52.3 **FUD** 090   C 80 ▣ P0

AMA: 2014,Jan,11

51580 Cystectomy, complete, with ureterosigmoidostomy or ureterocutaneous transplantations;

🔧 54.4 ⚕ 54.4 **FUD** 090   C 80 ▣ P0

AMA: 2014,Jan,11

51585 with bilateral pelvic lymphadenectomy, including external iliac, hypogastric, and obturator nodes

🔧 60.6 ⚕ 60.6 **FUD** 090   C 80 ▣ P0

AMA: 2014,Jan,11

51590 Cystectomy, complete, with ureteroileal conduit or sigmoid bladder, including intestine anastomosis;

🔧 55.5 ⚕ 55.5 **FUD** 090   C 80 ▣ P0

AMA: 2014,Jan,11

51595 with bilateral pelvic lymphadenectomy, including external iliac, hypogastric, and obturator nodes

🔧 62.8 ⚕ 62.8 **FUD** 090   C 80 ▣ P0

AMA: 2014,Jan,11

51596 Cystectomy, complete, with continent diversion, any open technique, using any segment of small and/or large intestine to construct neobladder
📷 67.4 ⚓ 67.4 **FUD** 090 [C] [80] [▣] [P0]
AMA: 2014,Jan,11

51597 Pelvic exenteration, complete, for vesical, prostatic or urethral malignancy, with removal of bladder and ureteral transplantations, with or without hysterectomy and/or abdominoperineal resection of rectum and colon and colostomy, or any combination thereof
EXCLUDES Pelvic exenteration for gynecologic malignancy (58240)
📷 65.9 ⚓ 65.9 **FUD** 090 [C] [80] [▣] [P0]
AMA: 2014,Jan,11

51600-51720 Injection/Insertion/Instillation Procedures of Bladder

51600 Injection procedure for cystography or voiding urethrocystography
📷 (74430, 74455)
📷 1.29 ⚓ 5.20 **FUD** 000 [N] [N1] [▣]
AMA: 2014,Jan,11

51605 Injection procedure and placement of chain for contrast and/or chain urethrocystography
📷 (74430)
📷 1.09 ⚓ 1.09 **FUD** 000 [N] [N1] [▣]
AMA: 2014,Jan,11

51610 Injection procedure for retrograde urethrocystography
📷 (74450)
📷 1.86 ⚓ 3.04 **FUD** 000 [N] [N1] [▣]
AMA: 2014,Jan,11

51700 Bladder irrigation, simple, lavage and/or instillation
📷 1.29 ⚓ 2.36 **FUD** 000 [T] [P3] [▣]
AMA: 2014,Jan,11

51701 Insertion of non-indwelling bladder catheter (eg, straight catheterization for residual urine)
EXCLUDES Catheterization for specimen collection (P9612)
Do not report with insertion of catheter as an inclusive component of another procedure
📷 0.79 ⚓ 1.54 **FUD** 000 [01] [N1] [▣]
AMA: 2015,Jan,16; 2014,Jan,11; 2012,Jan,15-42; 2011,Jan,11

51702 Insertion of temporary indwelling bladder catheter; simple (eg, Foley)
Do not report with (0071T-0072T)
Do not report with insertion of catheter as an inclusive component of another procedure
📷 0.86 ⚓ 1.98 **FUD** 000 [01] [N1] [▣]
AMA: 2015,Jan,16; 2014,May,3; 2014,Jan,11; 2012,Jan,15-42; 2011,Jan,11

51703 complicated (eg, altered anatomy, fractured catheter/balloon)   *← enlarged prostate*
📷 2.34 ⚓ 3.68 **FUD** 000 [T] [P2] [▣]
AMA: 2015,Jan,16; 2014,Jan,11

51705 Change of cystostomy tube; simple
📷 1.49 ⚓ 2.58 **FUD** 000 [T] [P3] [▣]
AMA: 2015,Jan,16; 2014,Jan,11; 2012,Jan,15-42; 2011,Jan,11

51710 complicated
📷 (75984)
📷 2.30 ⚓ 3.65 **FUD** 000 [T] [A2] [▣]
AMA: 2015,Jan,16; 2014,Jan,11

51715 Endoscopic injection of implant material into the submucosal tissues of the urethra and/or bladder neck
EXCLUDES Injection of bulking agent (submucosal) for fecal incontinence, via anoscope (0377T)
📷 5.77 ⚓ 8.27 **FUD** 000 [T] [A2] [80] [▣]
AMA: 2014,Jan,11

51720 Bladder instillation of anticarcinogenic agent (including retention time)
Code also bacillus Calmette-Guerin vaccine (BCG) (90586)
📷 2.30 ⚓ 3.10 **FUD** 000 [T] [P3] [80] [P0]
AMA: 2015,Jan,16; 2014,Jan,11; 2012,Jan,15-42; 2011,Jan,11

51725-51798 [51797] Uroflowmetric Evaluations

INCLUDES Equipment
Fees for services of technician
Medications
Supplies
Code also modifier 26 if physician/other qualified health care professional provides only interpretation of results and/or operates the equipment

51725 Simple cystometrogram (CMG) (eg, spinal manometer)
📷 5.31 ⚓ 5.31 **FUD** 000 [T] [P3] [80] [▣]
AMA: 2015,Jan,16; 2014,Jan,11; 2010,Jan,7-8

51726 Complex cystometrogram (ie, calibrated electronic equipment);
📷 7.43 ⚓ 7.43 **FUD** 000 [T] [A2] [▣]
AMA: 2015,Jan,16; 2014,Jan,11; 2010,Jan,7-8; 2010,Jan,3-5

51727 with urethral pressure profile studies (ie, urethral closure pressure profile), any technique
📷 8.80 ⚓ 8.80 **FUD** 000 [T] [P2] [80] [▣]
AMA: 2015,Jan,16; 2014,Jan,11; 2010,Jan,7-8; 2010,Jan,3-5

51728 with voiding pressure studies (ie, bladder voiding pressure), any technique
📷 8.87 ⚓ 8.87 **FUD** 000 [T] [P2] [80] [▣]
AMA: 2015,Jan,16; 2014,Jan,11; 2010,Jan,7-8; 2010,Jan,3-5

51729 with voiding pressure studies (ie, bladder voiding pressure) and urethral pressure profile studies (ie, urethral closure pressure profile), any technique
📷 9.61 ⚓ 9.61 **FUD** 000 [T] [P2] [80] [▣]
AMA: 2015,Jan,16; 2014,Jan,11; 2010,Jan,7-8; 2010,Jan,3-5

+ # **51797** Voiding pressure studies, intra-abdominal (ie, rectal, gastric, intraperitoneal) (List separately in addition to code for primary procedure)
Code first (51728-51729)
📷 3.16 ⚓ 3.16 **FUD** ZZZ [N] [N1] [80] [▣]
AMA: 2015,Jan,16; 2014,Jan,11; 2012,Jan,15-42; 2011,Jan,11; 2010,Jan,7-8

51736 Simple uroflowmetry (UFR) (eg, stop-watch flow rate, mechanical uroflowmeter)
📷 0.44 ⚓ 0.44 **FUD** XXX [01] [N1] [80] [▣]
AMA: 2015,Jan,16; 2014,Jan,11; 2010,Jan,7-8

51741 Complex uroflowmetry (eg, calibrated electronic equipment)
📷 0.45 ⚓ 0.45 **FUD** XXX [T] [P3] [▣]
AMA: 2015,Jan,16; 2014,Sep,13; 2014,Jan,11; 2010,Jan,7-8

51784 Electromyography studies (EMG) of anal or urethral sphincter, other than needle, any technique
Do not report with (51792)
📷 5.44 ⚓ 5.44 **FUD** 000 [T] [P2] [▣]
AMA: 2015,Jan,16; 2014,Sep,13; 2014,Feb,11; 2014,Jan,11; 2010,Jan,7-8

51785 Needle electromyography studies (EMG) of anal or urethral sphincter, any technique
📷 7.14 ⚓ 7.14 **FUD** 000 [T] [A2] [80] [▣]
AMA: 2015,Jan,16; 2014,Jan,11; 2012,Jan,15-42; 2011,Jan,11; 2010,Jan,7-8

51792 Stimulus evoked response (eg, measurement of bulbocavernosus reflex latency time)
Do not report with (51784)
📷 5.96 ⚓ 5.96 **FUD** 000 [T] [P2] [80] [▣]
AMA: 2015,Jan,16; 2014,Feb,11; 2014,Jan,11; 2010,Jan,7-8

51797 Resequenced code, See code following 51729.

51798 Measurement of post-voiding residual urine and/or bladder capacity by ultrasound, non-imaging
📷 0.53 ⚓ 0.53 **FUD** XXX [01] [N1] [80] [TC]
AMA: 2015,Jan,16; 2014,Jan,11; 2010,Jan,7-8

---

[26]/[TC] PC/TC Comp Only   [A2]-[Z3] ASC Pmt   [50] Bilateral   ♂ Male Only   ♀ Female Only   📷 Facility RVU   ⚓ Non-Facility RVU
AMA: CPT Asst   **CMS:** Pub 100   [A]-[Y] OPPSI   [80]/[80] Surg Assist Allowed / w/Doc   [▣] Lab Crosswalk   [📷] Radiology Crosswalk

Medicare (Red Text)   CPT © 2015 American Medical Association. All Rights Reserved. (Black Text)   © 2015 Optum360, LLC (Blue Text)

51800-51980 Open Repairs Urinary System

51800 **Cystoplasty or cystourethroplasty, plastic operation on bladder and/or vesical neck (anterior Y-plasty, vesical fundus resection), any procedure, with or without wedge resection of posterior vesical neck**
🔧 29.9 ✂ 29.9 **FUD** 090
C 80 ▣ PQ
AMA: 2014,Jan,11

51820 **Cystourethroplasty with unilateral or bilateral ureteroneocystostomy**
🔧 35.0 ✂ 35.0 **FUD** 090
C 80 ▣ PQ
AMA: 2014,Jan,11

51840 **Anterior vesicourethropexy, or urethropexy (eg, Marshall-Marchetti-Krantz, Burch); simple**
EXCLUDES   Pereyra type urethropexy (57289)
🔧 18.8 ✂ 18.8 **FUD** 090
C 80 ▣
AMA: 2015,Jan,16; 2014,Jan,11; 2012,Aug,13-14; 2012,Jan,15-42; 2011,Jan,11; 2010,Jun,6-7

51841 **complicated (eg, secondary repair)**
EXCLUDES   Pereyra type urethropexy (57289)
🔧 22.2 ✂ 22.2 **FUD** 090
C 80 ▣
AMA: 2015,Jan,16; 2014,Jan,11; 2012,Aug,13-14; 2010,Jun,6-7

51845 **Abdomino-vaginal vesical neck suspension, with or without endoscopic control (eg, Stamey, Raz, modified Pereyra)** ♀
🔧 16.8 ✂ 16.8 **FUD** 090
J 80 ▣
AMA: 2015,Jan,16; 2014,Jan,11

51860 **Cystorrhaphy, suture of bladder wound, injury or rupture; simple**
🔧 21.4 ✂ 21.4 **FUD** 090
T 80 ▣
AMA: 2014,Jan,11

51865 **complicated**
🔧 25.7 ✂ 25.7 **FUD** 090
C 80 ▣
AMA: 2014,Jan,11

51880 **Closure of cystostomy (separate procedure)**
🔧 13.4 ✂ 13.4 **FUD** 090
T A2 80 ▣
AMA: 2014,Jan,11

51900 **Closure of vesicovaginal fistula, abdominal approach** ♀
EXCLUDES   Vesicovaginal fistula closure, vaginal approach (57320-57330)
🔧 23.9 ✂ 23.9 **FUD** 090
C 80 ▣ PQ
AMA: 2014,Jan,11

51920 **Closure of vesicouterine fistula;** ♀
EXCLUDES   Enterovesical fistula closure (44660-44661)
          Rectovesical fistula closure (45800-45805)
🔧 21.8 ✂ 21.8 **FUD** 090
C 80 ▣ PQ
AMA: 2014,Jan,11

51925 **with hysterectomy** ♀
EXCLUDES   Enterovesical fistula closure (44660-44661)
          Rectovesical fistula closure (45800-45805)
🔧 32.3 ✂ 32.3 **FUD** 090
C 80 ▣ PQ
AMA: 2014,Jan,11

51940 **Closure, exstrophy of bladder**
EXCLUDES   Epispadias reconstruction with exstrophy of bladder (54390)
🔧 47.1 ✂ 47.1 **FUD** 090
C 80 ▣
AMA: 2014,Jan,11

51960 **Enterocystoplasty, including intestinal anastomosis**
🔧 39.8 ✂ 39.8 **FUD** 090
C 80 ▣ PQ
AMA: 2014,Jan,11

51980 **Cutaneous vesicostomy**
🔧 20.4 ✂ 20.4 **FUD** 090
C 80 ▣
AMA: 2014,Jan,11

51990-51999 Laparoscopic Procedures of Urinary System

CMS: 100-3,230.10 Incontinence Control Devices
INCLUDES   Diagnostic laparoscopy
EXCLUDES   Diagnostic laparoscopy (peritoneoscopy) performed as a separate procedure (49320)

51990 **Laparoscopy, surgical; urethral suspension for stress incontinence**
🔧 21.5 ✂ 21.5 **FUD** 090
T 80 ▣
AMA: 2015,Jan,16; 2014,Jan,11; 2012,Aug,13-14; 2012,Mar,9-10; 2010,Jun,6-7

51992 **sling operation for stress incontinence (eg, fascia or synthetic)**
EXCLUDES   Removal/revision of sling for stress incontinence (57287)
          Sling operation for stress incontinence, open approach (57288)
🔧 24.1 ✂ 24.1 **FUD** 090
T A2 80 ▣
AMA: 2015,Jan,16; 2014,Jan,11; 2012,Aug,13-14; 2012,Mar,9-10

51999 **Unlisted laparoscopy procedure, bladder**
🔧 0.00 ✂ 0.00 **FUD** YYY
T 80
AMA: 2014,Jan,11

52000-52318 Endoscopic Procedures via Urethra: Bladder and Urethra

INCLUDES   Diagnostic and therapeutic endoscopy of bowel segments utilized as replacements for native bladder

52000 **Cystourethroscopy (separate procedure)**
Do not report with (52001, 52320, 52325, 52327, 52330, 52332, 52334, 52341-52343, [52356])
🔧 3.63 ✂ 5.80 **FUD** 000
T A2 ▣
AMA: 2015,Jan,16; 2014,May,3; 2014,Jan,11; 2013,Mar,13; 2012,Jan,15-42; 2011,Jan,11

52001 **Cystourethroscopy with irrigation and evacuation of multiple obstructing clots**
Do not report with (52000)
🔧 8.28 ✂ 10.5 **FUD** 000
T A2 ▣
AMA: 2014,Jan,11

52005 **Cystourethroscopy, with ureteral catheterization, with or without irrigation, instillation, or ureteropyelography, exclusive of radiologic service;**
INCLUDES   Howard test
🔧 3.83 ✂ 7.51 **FUD** 000
T A2 ▣
AMA: 2015,Jan,16; 2014,Jan,11; 2012,Jan,15-42; 2011,Jan,11; 2010,Dec,12

52007 **with brush biopsy of ureter and/or renal pelvis**
EXCLUDES   Image-guided ureter/renal pelvis biopsy without endoscopic guidance (50606)
🔧 4.77 ✂ 12.5 **FUD** 000
T A2 50 ▣ PQ
AMA: 2015,Jan,16; 2014,Jan,11

52010 **Cystourethroscopy, with ejaculatory duct catheterization, with or without irrigation, instillation, or duct radiography, exclusive of radiologic service** ♂
📷 (74440)
🔧 4.76 ✂ 10.3 **FUD** 000
T A2 ▣
AMA: 2015,Jan,16; 2014,Jan,11

52204 **Cystourethroscopy, with biopsy(s)**
🔧 4.09 ✂ 10.4 **FUD** 000
T A2 ▣ PQ
AMA: 2015,Jan,16; 2014,Jan,11; 2012,Jan,15-42; 2011,Jan,11

52214 **Cystourethroscopy, with fulguration (including cryosurgery or laser surgery) of trigone, bladder neck, prostatic fossa, urethra, or periurethral glands**
Code also modifier 78 when performed by same physician:
During postoperative period (52601, 52630)
During the postoperative period of a related surgical procedure
For postoperative bleeding
🔧 5.06 ✂ 18.6 **FUD** 000
T A2 ▣
AMA: 2015,Jan,16; 2014,Jan,11

52224 Cystourethroscopy, with fulguration (including cryosurgery or laser surgery) or treatment of MINOR (less than 0.5 cm) lesion(s) with or without biopsy
🔲 5.88 ⚕ 19.4 **FUD** 000 Ⓣ A2 ▭ P0
AMA: 2015,Jan,16; 2014,Jan,11; 2012,Jan,15-42; 2011,Jan,11

52234 Cystourethroscopy, with fulguration (including cryosurgery or laser surgery) and/or resection of; SMALL bladder tumor(s) (0.5 up to 2.0 cm)
EXCLUDES *Bladder tumor excision through cystotomy (51530)*
🔲 7.08 ⚕ 7.08 **FUD** 000 Ⓣ A2 ▭
AMA: 2015,Jan,16; 2014,Jan,11; 2012,Jan,15-42; 2011,Jan,11

52235 MEDIUM bladder tumor(s) (2.0 to 5.0 cm)
EXCLUDES *Bladder tumor excision through cystotomy (51530)*
🔲 8.31 ⚕ 8.31 **FUD** 000 Ⓣ A2 ▭
AMA: 2015,Jan,16; 2014,Jan,11

52240 LARGE bladder tumor(s)
EXCLUDES *Bladder tumor excision through cystotomy (51530)*
🔲 11.2 ⚕ 11.2 **FUD** 000 Ⓣ A2 ▭
AMA: 2015,Jan,16; 2014,Jan,11

52250 Cystourethroscopy with insertion of radioactive substance, with or without biopsy or fulguration
🔲 6.90 ⚕ 6.90 **FUD** 000 Ⓣ A2 ▭ P0
AMA: 2015,Jan,16; 2014,Jan,11

52260 Cystourethroscopy, with dilation of bladder for interstitial cystitis; general or conduction (spinal) anesthesia
🔲 6.07 ⚕ 6.07 **FUD** 000 Ⓣ A2 ▭
AMA: 2015,Jan,16; 2014,Jan,11; 2012,Jan,15-42; 2011,Jan,11

52265 local anesthesia
🔲 4.68 ⚕ 10.3 **FUD** 000 Ⓣ P3 ▭
AMA: 2015,Jan,16; 2014,Jan,11

52270 Cystourethroscopy, with internal urethrotomy; female ♀
🔲 5.23 ⚕ 10.0 **FUD** 000 Ⓣ A2 ▭
AMA: 2015,Jan,16; 2014,Jan,11

52275 male ♂
🔲 7.16 ⚕ 13.5 **FUD** 000 Ⓣ A2 ▭
AMA: 2015,Jan,16; 2014,Jan,11

52276 Cystourethroscopy with direct vision internal urethrotomy
🔲 7.62 ⚕ 7.62 **FUD** 000 Ⓣ A2 ▭
AMA: 2015,Jan,16; 2014,Jan,11; 2012,Jan,15-42; 2011,Jan,11; 2010,Jan,7-8

52277 Cystourethroscopy, with resection of external sphincter (sphincterotomy)
🔲 9.32 ⚕ 9.32 **FUD** 000 Ⓣ A2 80 ▭
AMA: 2015,Jan,16; 2014,Jan,11

52281 Cystourethroscopy, with calibration and/or dilation of urethral stricture or stenosis, with or without meatotomy, with or without injection procedure for cystography, male or female
🔲 4.38 ⚕ 7.70 **FUD** 000 Ⓣ A2 ▭
AMA: 2015,Jan,16; 2014,Jan,11; 2012,Jan,15-42; 2011,Jan,11

52282 Cystourethroscopy, with insertion of permanent urethral stent
EXCLUDES *Placement of temporary prostatic urethral stent (53855)*
🔲 9.71 ⚕ 9.71 **FUD** 000 Ⓣ A2 ▭
AMA: 2015,Jun,5; 2015,Jan,16; 2014,Jan,11; 2010,Jan,7-8

52283 Cystourethroscopy, with steroid injection into stricture
🔲 5.79 ⚕ 7.84 **FUD** 000 Ⓣ A2 ▭
AMA: 2015,Mar,9; 2015,Jan,16; 2014,Jan,11

52285 Cystourethroscopy for treatment of the female urethral syndrome with any or all of the following: urethral meatotomy, urethral dilation, internal urethrotomy, lysis of urethrovaginal septal fibrosis, lateral incisions of the bladder neck, and fulguration of polyp(s) of urethra, bladder neck, and/or trigone ♀
🔲 5.64 ⚕ 7.92 **FUD** 000 Ⓣ A2 ▭
AMA: 2015,Jan,16; 2014,Jan,11

52287 Cystourethroscopy, with injection(s) for chemodenervation of the bladder
Code also supply of chemodenervation agent
🔲 4.87 ⚕ 8.81 **FUD** 000 Ⓣ G2
AMA: 2014,Jan,11

52290 Cystourethroscopy; with ureteral meatotomy, unilateral or bilateral
🔲 7.03 ⚕ 7.03 **FUD** 000 Ⓣ A2 ▭
AMA: 2015,Jan,16; 2014,Jan,11

52300 with resection or fulguration of orthotopic ureterocele(s), unilateral or bilateral
🔲 8.08 ⚕ 8.08 **FUD** 000 Ⓣ A2 80 ▭
AMA: 2015,Jan,16; 2014,Jan,11

52301 with resection or fulguration of ectopic ureterocele(s), unilateral or bilateral
🔲 8.37 ⚕ 8.37 **FUD** 000 Ⓣ A2 80 ▭
AMA: 2015,Jan,16; 2014,Jan,11

52305 with incision or resection of orifice of bladder diverticulum, single or multiple
🔲 8.02 ⚕ 8.02 **FUD** 000 Ⓣ A2 ▭
AMA: 2015,Jan,16; 2014,Jan,11

Diverticulum of bladder
Bladder
Pubic bone
Rectum
Urethra

52310 Cystourethroscopy, with removal of foreign body, calculus, or ureteral stent from urethra or bladder (separate procedure); simple
Code also modifier 58 for removal of a self-retaining, indwelling ureteral stent
🔲 4.36 ⚕ 6.89 **FUD** 000 Ⓣ A2 ▭
AMA: 2015,Jun,5; 2015,Jan,16; 2014,Jan,11

52315 complicated
Code also modifier 58 for removal of a self-retaining, indwelling ureteral stent
🔲 7.91 ⚕ 11.7 **FUD** 000 Ⓣ A2 ▭
AMA: 2015,Jan,16; 2014,Jan,11

52317 Litholapaxy: crushing or fragmentation of calculus by any means in bladder and removal of fragments; simple or small (less than 2.5 cm)
🔲 10.0 ⚕ 22.7 **FUD** 000 Ⓣ A2 ▭
AMA: 2015,Jan,16; 2014,Jan,11; 2012,Feb,11

52318 complicated or large (over 2.5 cm)
🔲 13.6 ⚕ 13.6 **FUD** 000 Ⓣ A2 ▭
AMA: 2015,Jan,16; 2014,Jan,11; 2012,Feb,11

52320-52356 [52356] Endoscopic Procedures via Urethra: Renal Pelvis and Ureter

INCLUDES Diagnostic cystourethroscopy when performed with therapeutic cystourethroscopy
Insertion/removal of temporary ureteral catheter
EXCLUDES *Diagnostic cystourethroscopy only (52000)*
Self-retaining/indwelling ureteral stent removal by cystourethroscope, with modifier 58 if appropriate (52310, 52315)
Code also the insertion of an indwelling stent performed in addition to other procedures within this section (52332)
Do not report with (52005)

26/TC PC/TC Comp Only	A2-Z3 ASC Pmt	50 Bilateral	♂ Male Only	♀ Female Only	🔲 Facility RVU	⚕ Non-Facility RVU
AMA: CPT Asst	**CMS:** Pub 100	A-Y OPPSI	80/80 Surg Assist Allowed / w/Doc		🔳 Lab Crosswalk	🔳 Radiology Crosswalk

210 Medicare (Red Text) CPT © 2015 American Medical Association. All Rights Reserved. (Black Text) © 2015 Optum360, LLC (Blue Text)

52320 Cystourethroscopy (including ureteral catheterization); with removal of ureteral calculus
Do not report with (52000)
📇 7.10   ⚕ 7.10   **FUD** 000
T A2 50 ▭
AMA: 2015,Jan,16; 2014,Jan,11; 2012,Jan,15-42; 2011,Jan,11

52325 with fragmentation of ureteral calculus (eg, ultrasonic or electro-hydraulic technique)
Do not report with (52000)
📇 9.24   ⚕ 9.24   **FUD** 000
T A2 50 ▭
AMA: 2015,Jan,16; 2014,Jan,11; 2012,Jan,15-42; 2011,Jan,11

52327 with subureteric injection of implant material
Do not report with (52000)
📇 7.55   ⚕ 7.55   **FUD** 000
T A2 50 ▭
AMA: 2015,Jan,16; 2014,Jan,11

52330 with manipulation, without removal of ureteral calculus
Do not report with (52000)
📇 7.59   ⚕ 13.9   **FUD** 000
T A2 50 ▭
AMA: 2015,Jan,16; 2014,May,3; 2014,Jan,11; 2012,Jan,15-42; 2011,Jan,11

52332 Cystourethroscopy, with insertion of indwelling ureteral stent (eg, Gibbons or double-J type)
Do not report when performed on the same side with (52000, 52353, [52356])
📇 4.48   ⚕ 13.7   **FUD** 000
T A2 50 ▭
AMA: 2015,Jan,16; 2014,May,3; 2014,Jan,11; 2012,Jan,15-42; 2011,Jan,11

52334 Cystourethroscopy with insertion of ureteral guide wire through kidney to establish a percutaneous nephrostomy, retrograde
EXCLUDES *Cystourethroscopy with incision/fulguration/resection of congenital posterior urethral valves/obstructive hypertrophic mucosal folds (52400)*
Cystourethroscopy with pyeloscopy and/or ureteroscopy (52351-52353 [52356])
Nephrostomy tract establishment only (50395)
Percutaneous nephrostolithotomy (50080, 50081)
Do not report with (52000, 52351)
📇 7.37   ⚕ 7.37   **FUD** 000
T A2 50 ▭
AMA: 2015,Jan,16; 2014,May,3; 2014,Jan,11

52341 Cystourethroscopy; with treatment of ureteral stricture (eg, balloon dilation, laser, electrocautery, and incision)
Do not report with (50706, 52000, 52351)
📇 8.17   ⚕ 8.17   **FUD** 000
T A2 50 ▭
AMA: 2015,Jan,16; 2014,Jan,11

52342 with treatment of ureteropelvic junction stricture (eg, balloon dilation, laser, electrocautery, and incision)
EXCLUDES *Balloon dilation with imaging guidance (50706)*
Do not report with (52000, 52351)
📇 8.91   ⚕ 8.91   **FUD** 000
T A2 50 ▭
AMA: 2015,Jan,16; 2014,Jan,11; 2012,Jan,15-42; 2011,Jan,11

52343 with treatment of intra-renal stricture (eg, balloon dilation, laser, electrocautery, and incision)
EXCLUDES *Balloon dilation with imaging guidance (50706)*
Do not report with (52000, 52351)
📇 9.92   ⚕ 9.92   **FUD** 000
T A2 50 ▭
AMA: 2015,Jan,16; 2014,May,3; 2014,Jan,11

52344 Cystourethroscopy with ureteroscopy; with treatment of ureteral stricture (eg, balloon dilation, laser, electrocautery, and incision)
EXCLUDES *Cystourethroscopy with transurethral resection or incision of ejaculatory ducts (52402)*
Do not report with (50706, 52351)
📇 10.6   ⚕ 10.6   **FUD** 000
T A2 50 ▭
AMA: 2015,Jan,16; 2014,Jan,11

52345 with treatment of ureteropelvic junction stricture (eg, balloon dilation, laser, electrocautery, and incision)
EXCLUDES *Cystourethroscopy with transurethral resection or incision of ejaculatory ducts (52402)*
Do not report with (50706, 52351)
📇 11.3   ⚕ 11.3   **FUD** 000
T A2 80 50 ▭
AMA: 2015,Jan,16; 2014,Jan,11

52346 with treatment of intra-renal stricture (eg, balloon dilation, laser, electrocautery, and incision)
EXCLUDES *Balloon dilation with imaging guidance (50706)*
Cystourethroscopy with transurethral resection or incision of ejaculatory ducts (52402)
Do not report with (52351)
📇 12.8   ⚕ 12.8   **FUD** 000
T A2 80 50 ▭
AMA: 2015,Jan,16; 2014,May,3; 2014,Jan,11

52351 Cystourethroscopy, with ureteroscopy and/or pyeloscopy; diagnostic
Do not report with (52341-52346, 52352-52353 [52356])
💠 (74485)
📇 8.72   ⚕ 8.72   **FUD** 000
T A2
AMA: 2015,Jan,16; 2014,May,3; 2014,Jan,11

52352 with removal or manipulation of calculus (ureteral catheterization is included)
Do not report with (52351)
📇 10.2   ⚕ 10.2   **FUD** 000
T A2 50 ▭
AMA: 2015,Jan,16; 2014,Jan,11; 2012,Jan,15-42; 2011,Jan,11; 2010,Jan,12-15

52353 with lithotripsy (ureteral catheterization is included)
Do not report when performed on the same side with (52332, [52356])
Do not report with (52351)
📇 11.2   ⚕ 11.2   **FUD** 000
T A2 50 ▭
AMA: 2015,Jan,16; 2014,May,3; 2014,Jan,11; 2012,Jan,15-42; 2011,Jan,11

52356 with lithotripsy including insertion of indwelling ureteral stent (eg, Gibbons or double-J type)
Do not report when performed on the same side with (52332, 52353)
Do not report with (52000, 52351)
📇 11.9   ⚕ 11.9   **FUD** 000
T 62 50
AMA: 2015,Jan,16; 2014,May,3; 2014,Jan,11

52354 with biopsy and/or fulguration of ureteral or renal pelvic lesion
EXCLUDES *Image guided biopsy without endoscopic guidance (50606)*
Do not report with (52351)
📇 12.0   ⚕ 12.0   **FUD** 000
T A2 50 ▭ PQ
AMA: 2015,Jan,16; 2014,May,3; 2014,Jan,11

52355 with resection of ureteral or renal pelvic tumor
Do not report with (52351)
📇 13.4   ⚕ 13.4   **FUD** 000
T A2 50 ▭
AMA: 2015,Jan,16; 2014,May,3; 2014,Jan,11

52356 Resequenced code. See code following 52353.

52400-52700 Endoscopic Procedures via Urethra: Prostate and Vesical Neck

52400 Cystourethroscopy with incision, fulguration, or resection of congenital posterior urethral valves, or congenital obstructive hypertrophic mucosal folds
📇 13.7   ⚕ 13.7   **FUD** 090
T A2
AMA: 2015,Jan,16; 2014,Jan,11

52402 Cystourethroscopy with transurethral resection or incision of ejaculatory ducts   ♂
📇 7.68   ⚕ 7.68   **FUD** 000
T A2
AMA: 2014,Jan,11

52441 Cystourethroscopy, with insertion of permanent adjustable transprostatic implant; single implant
📇 6.54   ⚕ 34.9   **FUD** 000
B
AMA: 2015,Jun,5

Urinary System

52442 — 53220

+ 52442   each additional permanent adjustable transprostatic implant (List separately in addition to code for primary procedure)

> EXCLUDES   Permanent urethral stent insertion (52282)
> Removal of stent, calculus or foreign body (implant) (52310)
> Temporary prostatic urethral stent insertion (53855)

Code first (52441)

 1.75   26.6   **FUD** ZZZ   B

AMA: 2015,Jun,5

52450   Transurethral incision of prostate   ♂

 13.4   13.4   **FUD** 090   T A2 P0

AMA: 2015,Jun,5; 2015,Jan,16; 2014,Jan,11; 2012,Jan,15-42; 2011,Jan,11

52500   Transurethral resection of bladder neck (separate procedure)

 13.9   13.9   **FUD** 090   T A2

AMA: 2015,Jan,16; 2014,Jan,11; 2012,Jan,15-42; 2011,Jan,11

52601   Transurethral electrosurgical resection of prostate, including control of postoperative bleeding, complete (vasectomy, meatotomy, cystourethroscopy, urethral calibration and/or dilation, and internal urethrotomy are included)   ♂

> INCLUDES   Stage 1 of partial transurethral resection of prostate
> EXCLUDES   Excision of prostate (55801-55845)
> Transurethral fulguration of prostate (52214)

Code also modifier 58 for stage 2 partial transurethral resection of prostate

 24.2   24.2   **FUD** 090   T A2 P0

AMA: 2015,Jun,5; 2015,Jan,16; 2014,Jan,11; 2012,Jan,15-42; 2011,Oct,10

52630   Transurethral resection; residual or regrowth of obstructive prostate tissue including control of postoperative bleeding, complete (vasectomy, meatotomy, cystourethroscopy, urethral calibration and/or dilation, and internal urethrotomy are included)   ♂

> EXCLUDES   Excision of prostate (55801-55845)

Code also modifier 78 when performed by same physician within the postoperative period of a related procedure

 11.4   11.4   **FUD** 090   T A2 P0

AMA: 2015,Jan,16; 2014,Jan,11

52640   of postoperative bladder neck contracture

> EXCLUDES   Excision of prostate (55801-55845)

 9.01   9.01   **FUD** 090   T A2

AMA: 2015,Jan,16; 2014,Jan,11

52647   Laser coagulation of prostate, including control of postoperative bleeding, complete (vasectomy, meatotomy, cystourethroscopy, urethral calibration and/or dilation, and internal urethrotomy are included if performed)   ♂

 18.5   50.2   **FUD** 090   T A2 P0

AMA: 2015,Jan,16; 2014,Jan,11; 2012,Jan,15-42; 2011,Jan,11

52648   Laser vaporization of prostate, including control of postoperative bleeding, complete (vasectomy, meatotomy, cystourethroscopy, urethral calibration and/or dilation, internal urethrotomy and transurethral resection of prostate are included if performed)   ♂

 19.7   51.7   **FUD** 090   T A2 P0

AMA: 2015,Jun,5; 2015,Jan,16; 2014,Jan,11; 2012,Jan,15-42; 2011,Jan,11

52649   Laser enucleation of the prostate with morcellation, including control of postoperative bleeding, complete (vasectomy, meatotomy, cystourethroscopy, urethral calibration and/or dilation, internal urethrotomy and transurethral resection of prostate are included if performed)   ♂

Do not report with (52000, 52276, 52281, 52601, 52647-52648, 53020, 55250)

 23.6   23.6   **FUD** 090   T 62 80 P0

AMA: 2015,Jun,5; 2014,Jan,11

52700   Transurethral drainage of prostatic abscess   ♂

> EXCLUDES   Litholapaxy (52317, 52318)

 12.6   12.6   **FUD** 090   T A2 80

AMA: 2015,Jan,16; 2014,Jan,11

Bladder   Prostate   Urethra

53000-53520 Open Surgical Procedures of Urethra

> EXCLUDES   Endoscopic procedures; cystoscopy, urethroscopy, cystourethroscopy (52000-52700 [52356])
> Urethrocystography injection procedure (51600-51610)

53000   Urethrotomy or urethrostomy, external (separate procedure); pendulous urethra

 4.26   4.26   **FUD** 010   T A2

AMA: 2014,Jan,11

53010   perineal urethra, external

 8.43   8.43   **FUD** 090   T A2

AMA: 2014,Jan,11

53020   Meatotomy, cutting of meatus (separate procedure); except infant

 2.78   2.78   **FUD** 000   T A2

AMA: 2014,Jan,11

53025   infant   A

 1.96   1.96   **FUD** 000   63 T R2 80

AMA: 2014,Jan,11

53040   Drainage of deep periurethral abscess

> EXCLUDES   Incision and drainage of subcutaneous abscess (10060-10061)

 11.2   11.2   **FUD** 090   T A2 80

AMA: 2014,Jan,11

53060   Drainage of Skene's gland abscess or cyst

 4.74   5.26   **FUD** 010   T P3

AMA: 2014,Jan,11

53080   Drainage of perineal urinary extravasation; uncomplicated (separate procedure)

 12.2   12.2   **FUD** 090   T A2

AMA: 2014,Jan,11

53085   complicated

 18.6   18.6   **FUD** 090   T 62 80

AMA: 2014,Jan,11

53200   Biopsy of urethra

 4.10   4.48   **FUD** 000   T A2 P0

AMA: 2014,Jan,11

53210   Urethrectomy, total, including cystostomy; female   ♀

 22.1   22.1   **FUD** 090   T A2 80

AMA: 2014,Jan,11

53215   male   ♂

 26.6   26.6   **FUD** 090   T A2 80

AMA: 2014,Jan,11

53220   Excision or fulguration of carcinoma of urethra

 13.0   13.0   **FUD** 090   T A2 80

AMA: 2014,Jan,11

26/TC PC/TC Comp Only   A2-Z3 ASC Pmt   50 Bilateral   ♂ Male Only   ♀ Female Only   Facility RVU   Non-Facility RVU
AMA: CPT Asst   **CMS:** Pub 100   A-Y OPPSI   80/80 Surg Assist Allowed / w/Doc   Lab Crosswalk   Radiology Crosswalk
Medicare (Red Text)   CPT © 2015 American Medical Association. All Rights Reserved. (Black Text)   © 2015 Optum360, LLC (Blue Text)

53230 Excision of urethral diverticulum (separate procedure); female ♀

⚕ 17.3 ⚖ 17.3 **FUD** 090 T A2 80 ▢

AMA: 2014,Jan,11

53235 male ♂

⚕ 18.1 ⚖ 18.1 **FUD** 090 T A2 80 ▢

AMA: 2014,Jan,11

53240 Marsupialization of urethral diverticulum, male or female

⚕ 12.1 ⚖ 12.1 **FUD** 090 T A2 ▢

AMA: 2014,Jan,11

53250 Excision of bulbourethral gland (Cowper's gland)

⚕ 11.3 ⚖ 11.3 **FUD** 090 T A2 ▢

AMA: 2014,Jan,11

53260 Excision or fulguration; urethral polyp(s), distal urethra

EXCLUDES *Endoscopic method (52214, 52224)*

⚕ 5.16 ⚖ 5.74 **FUD** 010 T A2 ▢

AMA: 2014,Jan,11

53265 urethral caruncle

EXCLUDES *Endoscopic method (52214, 52224)*

⚕ 5.34 ⚖ 6.22 **FUD** 010 T A2 ▢

AMA: 2014,Jan,11

53270 Skene's glands

EXCLUDES *Endoscopic method (52214, 52224)*

⚕ 5.27 ⚖ 5.87 **FUD** 010 T A2 ▢

AMA: 2014,Jan,11

53275 urethral prolapse

EXCLUDES *Endoscopic method (52214, 52224)*

⚕ 7.54 ⚖ 7.54 **FUD** 010 T A2 ▢

AMA: 2014,Jan,11

53400 Urethroplasty; first stage, for fistula, diverticulum, or stricture (eg, Johannsen type)

EXCLUDES *Hypospadias repair (54300-54352)*

⚕ 22.9 ⚖ 22.9 **FUD** 090 T A2 80 ▢

AMA: 2014,Jan,11

53405 second stage (formation of urethra), including urinary diversion

EXCLUDES *Hypospadias repair (54300-54352)*

⚕ 25.0 ⚖ 25.0 **FUD** 090 T A2 80 ▢

AMA: 2014,Jan,11

53410 Urethroplasty, 1-stage reconstruction of male anterior urethra ♂

EXCLUDES *Hypospadias repair (54300-54352)*

⚕ 28.1 ⚖ 28.1 **FUD** 090 T A2 80 ▢

AMA: 2014,Jan,11

53415 Urethroplasty, transpubic or perineal, 1-stage, for reconstruction or repair of prostatic or membranous urethra ♂

⚕ 32.4 ⚖ 32.4 **FUD** 090 C 80 ▢

AMA: 2014,Jan,11

53420 Urethroplasty, 2-stage reconstruction or repair of prostatic or membranous urethra; first stage ♂

⚕ 24.1 ⚖ 24.1 **FUD** 090 T A2 ▢

AMA: 2014,Jan,11

53425 second stage ♂

⚕ 26.8 ⚖ 26.8 **FUD** 090 T A2 80 ▢

AMA: 2014,Jan,11

53430 Urethroplasty, reconstruction of female urethra ♀

⚕ 27.6 ⚖ 27.6 **FUD** 090 T A2 80 ▢

AMA: 2014,Jan,11

53431 Urethroplasty with tubularization of posterior urethra and/or lower bladder for incontinence (eg, Tenago, Leadbetter procedure)

⚕ 33.1 ⚖ 33.1 **FUD** 090 T A2 80 ▢

AMA: 2014,Jan,11

53440 Sling operation for correction of male urinary incontinence (eg, fascia or synthetic) ♂

⚕ 21.6 ⚖ 21.6 **FUD** 090 J J8 80 ▢

AMA: 2014,Jan,11

53442 Removal or revision of sling for male urinary incontinence (eg, fascia or synthetic) ♂

⚕ 22.4 ⚖ 22.4 **FUD** 090 T A2 80 ▢

AMA: 2014,Jan,11

53444 Insertion of tandem cuff (dual cuff)

⚕ 22.7 ⚖ 22.7 **FUD** 090 J J8 80 ▢

AMA: 2014,Jan,11

53445 Insertion of inflatable urethral/bladder neck sphincter, including placement of pump, reservoir, and cuff

⚕ 21.6 ⚖ 21.6 **FUD** 090 J J8 80 ▢

AMA: 2014,Jan,11

53446 Removal of inflatable urethral/bladder neck sphincter, including pump, reservoir, and cuff

⚕ 18.4 ⚖ 18.4 **FUD** 090 02 A2 80 ▢

AMA: 2014,Jan,11

53447 Removal and replacement of inflatable urethral/bladder neck sphincter including pump, reservoir, and cuff at the same operative session

⚕ 23.1 ⚖ 23.1 **FUD** 090 J J8 80 ▢

AMA: 2014,Jan,11

53448 Removal and replacement of inflatable urethral/bladder neck sphincter including pump, reservoir, and cuff through an infected field at the same operative session including irrigation and debridement of infected tissue

Do not report with (11042, 11043)

⚕ 36.7 ⚖ 36.7 **FUD** 090 C 80 ▢

AMA: 2014,Jan,11

53449 Repair of inflatable urethral/bladder neck sphincter, including pump, reservoir, and cuff

⚕ 17.5 ⚖ 17.5 **FUD** 090 T A2 80 ▢

AMA: 2014,Jan,11

53450 Urethromeatoplasty, with mucosal advancement

EXCLUDES *Meatotomy (53020, 53025)*

⚕ 11.7 ⚖ 11.7 **FUD** 090 T A2 ▢

AMA: 2015,Jan,16; 2014,Jan,11; 2012,Oct,14; 2012,Sep,16

53460 Urethromeatoplasty, with partial excision of distal urethral segment (Richardson type procedure)

⚕ 13.1 ⚖ 13.1 **FUD** 090 T A2 80 ▢

AMA: 2014,Jan,11

53500 Urethrolysis, transvaginal, secondary, open, including cystourethroscopy (eg, postsurgical obstruction, scarring)

EXCLUDES *Retropubic approach (53899)*

Do not report with (52000)

⚕ 21.4 ⚖ 21.4 **FUD** 090 T 80 ▢

AMA: 2015,Jan,16; 2014,Jan,11

53502 Urethrorrhaphy, suture of urethral wound or injury, female ♀

⚕ 13.9 ⚖ 13.9 **FUD** 090 T A2 ▢

AMA: 2014,Jan,11

53505 Urethrorrhaphy, suture of urethral wound or injury; penile ♂

⚕ 13.9 ⚖ 13.9 **FUD** 090 T A2 80 ▢

AMA: 2014,Jan,11

53510 perineal ♂

⚕ 18.0 ⚖ 18.0 **FUD** 090 T A2 80 ▢

AMA: 2014,Jan,11

53515 prostatomembranous ♂

⚕ 22.8 ⚖ 22.8 **FUD** 090 T A2 80 ▢

AMA: 2014,Jan,11

● New Code ▲ Revised Code ○ Reinstated M Maternity A Age Edit Unlisted Not Covered # Resequenced
⊘ AMA Mod 51 Exempt ⑤ Optum Mod 51 Exempt ⑥③ Mod 63 Exempt ⊙ Mod Sedation + Add-on ▢ CCI P0 PQRS FUD Follow-up Days

Urinary System

53520   **Closure of urethrostomy or urethrocutaneous fistula, male (separate procedure)** ♂

> EXCLUDES   *Closure of fistula:*
> *Urethrorectal (45820, 45825)*
> *Urethrovaginal (57310)*

   🖥 15.9   ⚕ 15.9   **FUD** 090   T A2 ▭

   AMA: 2014,Jan,11

53600-53665 Urethral Dilation

> EXCLUDES   *Endoscopic procedures; cystoscopy, urethroscopy, cystourethroscopy*
> *(52000-52700 [52356])*
> *Urethral catheterization (51701-51703)*
> *Urethrocystography injection procedure (51600-51610)*
> ▨ *(74485)*

53600   **Dilation of urethral stricture by passage of sound or urethral dilator, male; initial** ♂

   🖥 1.84   ⚕ 2.37   **FUD** 000   T P3 ▭

   AMA: 2014,Jan,11

53601   **subsequent** ♂

   🖥 1.54   ⚕ 2.30   **FUD** 000   T P3 ▭

   AMA: 2014,Jan,11

53605   **Dilation of urethral stricture or vesical neck by passage of sound or urethral dilator, male, general or conduction (spinal) anesthesia** ♂

> EXCLUDES   *Procedure performed under local anesthesia*
> *(53600-53601, 53620-53621)*

   🖥 1.86   ⚕ 1.86   **FUD** 000   T A2 ▭

   AMA: 2014,Jan,11

53620   **Dilation of urethral stricture by passage of filiform and follower, male; initial** ♂

   🖥 2.51   ⚕ 3.30   **FUD** 000   T P3 ▭

   AMA: 2014,Jan,11

53621   **subsequent** ♂

   🖥 2.07   ⚕ 3.11   **FUD** 000   T P3 ▭

   AMA: 2014,Jan,11

53660   **Dilation of female urethra including suppository and/or instillation; initial** ♀

   🖥 1.19   ⚕ 1.99   **FUD** 000   T P3 ▭

   AMA: 2014,Jan,11

53661   **subsequent** ♀

   🖥 1.15   ⚕ 1.95   **FUD** 000   T P3 ▭

   AMA: 2014,Jan,11

53665   **Dilation of female urethra, general or conduction (spinal) anesthesia** ♀

> EXCLUDES   *Procedure performed under local anesthesia*
> *(53660-53661)*

   🖥 1.12   ⚕ 1.12   **FUD** 000   T A2 ▭

   AMA: 2014,Jan,11

53850-53899 Transurethral Procedures

> EXCLUDES   *Endoscopic procedures; cystoscopy, urethroscopy, cystourethroscopy*
> *(52000-52700 [52356])*

53850   **Transurethral destruction of prostate tissue; by microwave thermotherapy** ♂

   ▨ (81020)

   🖥 17.4   ⚕ 58.4   **FUD** 090   T P2 ▭

   AMA: 2015,Jun,5; 2015,Jan,16; 2014,Jan,11; 2010,Jan,7-8

53852   **by radiofrequency thermotherapy** ♂

   ▨ (81020)

   🖥 17.8   ⚕ 53.8   **FUD** 090   T P3 ▭

   AMA: 2015,Jun,5; 2015,Jan,16; 2014,Jan,11

53855   **Insertion of a temporary prostatic urethral stent, including urethral measurement** ♂

> EXCLUDES   *Permanent urethral stent insertion (52282)*

   🖥 2.37   ⚕ 21.8   **FUD** 000   T P2 80

   AMA: 2015,Jun,5; 2015,Jan,16; 2014,Jan,11; 2010,Jan,7-8

53860   **Transurethral radiofrequency micro-remodeling of the female bladder neck and proximal urethra for stress urinary incontinence** ♀

   🖥 6.47   ⚕ 44.1   **FUD** 090   T P2 80

   AMA: 2014,Jan,11

53899   **Unlisted procedure, urinary system**

   🖥 0.00   ⚕ 0.00   **FUD** YYY   T 80

   AMA: 2015,Jun,5; 2015,Mar,9; 2015,Jan,16; 2014,Jan,11; 2012,Jan,15-42; 2011,Jan,11; 2010,May,9

Kidney, Ureter, Bladder, Prostate, Urethra, Testis, Pubic bone, Corpus cavernosus, Corpus spongiosum, Glans penis, Foreskin (prepuce), Urethra, Septa and lobules of testes, Bladder, Rectum, Prostate

54000-54015 Procedures of Penis: Incisional

EXCLUDES *Debridement of abdominal perineal gangrene (11004-11006)*

54000 Slitting of prepuce, dorsal or lateral (separate procedure); newborn ♂ Ⓐ
🚗 3.10 ⚖ 4.21 **FUD** 010 ⑥③ T A2 80 ▭
AMA: 2014,Jan,11

Prostate
Dorsal surface
Ventral surface
Reservoir
An implanted, inflatable penile prosthesis (left); schematic of the main features of the penis (far left)
Corpus spongiosum
Corpus cavernosum
Pump in scrotum
Prepuce
Glans
External urethral orifice

54001 except newborn ♂
🚗 3.98 ⚖ 5.25 **FUD** 010 T A2 ▭
AMA: 2014,Jan,11

54015 Incision and drainage of penis, deep ♂
EXCLUDES *Abscess, skin/subcutaneous (10060-10160)*
🚗 8.78 ⚖ 8.78 **FUD** 010 T A2 80 ▭
AMA: 2014,Jan,11

54050-54065 Destruction of Penis Lesions: Multiple Methods

EXCLUDES *Excision/destruction other lesions (11420-11426, 11620-11626, 17000-17250, 17270-17276)*

54050 Destruction of lesion(s), penis (eg, condyloma, papilloma, molluscum contagiosum, herpetic vesicle), simple; chemical ♂
🚗 3.02 ⚖ 3.76 **FUD** 010 T P2 ▭
AMA: 2014,Jan,11

54055 electrodesiccation ♂
🚗 2.66 ⚖ 3.38 **FUD** 010 T P3 ▭
AMA: 2014,Jan,11

54056 cryosurgery ♂
🚗 3.17 ⚖ 4.03 **FUD** 010 01 N1 ▭
AMA: 2014,Jan,11

54057 laser surgery ♂
🚗 2.71 ⚖ 3.84 **FUD** 010 T A2 ▭
AMA: 2014,Jan,11

54060 surgical excision ♂
🚗 3.73 ⚖ 5.09 **FUD** 010 T A2 ▭
AMA: 2014,Jan,11

54065 Destruction of lesion(s), penis (eg, condyloma, papilloma, molluscum contagiosum, herpetic vesicle), extensive (eg, laser surgery, electrosurgery, cryosurgery, chemosurgery) ♂
🚗 4.95 ⚖ 6.20 **FUD** 010 T A2 ▭
AMA: 2014,Jan,11

54100-54115 Procedures of Penis: Excisional

54100 Biopsy of penis; (separate procedure) ♂
🚗 3.61 ⚖ 5.63 **FUD** 000 T A2 ▭ P0
AMA: 2015,Jan,16; 2014,Jan,11

54105 deep structures ♂
🚗 6.12 ⚖ 7.52 **FUD** 010 T A2 ▭ P0
AMA: 2014,Jan,11

54110 Excision of penile plaque (Peyronie disease); ♂
🚗 17.8 ⚖ 17.8 **FUD** 090 T A2 80 ▭
AMA: 2014,Jan,11

54111 with graft to 5 cm in length ♂
🚗 22.9 ⚖ 22.9 **FUD** 090 T A2 80 ▭
AMA: 2015,Jan,16; 2014,Jan,11; 2012,Jan,15-42; 2011,Jan,11

54112 with graft greater than 5 cm in length ♂
🚗 26.9 ⚖ 26.9 **FUD** 090 T A2 80 ▭
AMA: 2014,Jan,11

54115 Removal foreign body from deep penile tissue (eg, plastic implant) ♂
🚗 12.1 ⚖ 12.9 **FUD** 090 T A2 80 ▭
AMA: 2014,Jan,11

54120-54135 Amputation of Penis

EXCLUDES *Lymphadenectomy (separate procedure) (38760-38770)*

54120 Amputation of penis; partial ♂
🚗 18.1 ⚖ 18.1 **FUD** 090 T A2 80 ▭
AMA: 2014,Jan,11

54125 complete ♂
🚗 23.3 ⚖ 23.3 **FUD** 090 C 80 ▭
AMA: 2014,Jan,11

54130 Amputation of penis, radical; with bilateral inguinofemoral lymphadenectomy ♂
🚗 34.2 ⚖ 34.2 **FUD** 090 C 80 ▭
AMA: 2014,Jan,11

54135 in continuity with bilateral pelvic lymphadenectomy, including external iliac, hypogastric and obturator nodes ♂
🚗 43.4 ⚖ 43.4 **FUD** 090 C 80 ▭
AMA: 2014,Jan,11

54150-54164 Circumcision Procedures

54150 Circumcision, using clamp or other device with regional dorsal penile or ring block ♂
Code also modifier 52 when performed without dorsal penile or ring block
🚗 2.81 ⚖ 4.39 **FUD** 000 ⑥③ T A2 80 ▭
AMA: 2015,Jan,16; 2014,Jan,11; 2012,Jan,15-42; 2011,Jan,11

54160 Circumcision, surgical excision other than clamp, device, or dorsal slit; neonate (28 days of age or less) Ⓐ ♂
🚗 4.14 ⚖ 6.24 **FUD** 010 ⑥③ T A2 ▭
AMA: 2015,Jan,16; 2014,Jan,11; 2012,Jan,15-42; 2011,Jan,11

54161 older than 28 days of age Ⓐ ♂
🚗 5.64 ⚖ 5.64 **FUD** 010 T A2 ▭
AMA: 2015,Jan,16; 2014,Jan,11; 2012,Jan,15-42; 2011,Jan,11

54162 Lysis or excision of penile post-circumcision adhesions ♂
🚗 5.71 ⚖ 7.29 **FUD** 010 T A2 ▭
AMA: 2014,Jan,11

54163 Repair incomplete circumcision ♂
🚗 6.26 ⚖ 6.26 **FUD** 010 T A2 ▭
AMA: 2014,Jan,11

54164 Frenulotomy of penis ♂
Do not report with (54150-54163)
🚗 5.54 ⚖ 5.54 **FUD** 010 T A2 ▭
AMA: 2014,Jan,11

54200-54250 Evaluation and Treatment of Erectile Abnormalities

54200 Injection procedure for Peyronie disease; ♂
🚗 2.40 ⚖ 3.04 **FUD** 010 T P3 ▭
AMA: 2014,Jan,11

54205 with surgical exposure of plaque ♂
🚗 15.2 ⚖ 15.2 **FUD** 090 T A2 80 ▭
AMA: 2014,Jan,11

54220 Irrigation of corpora cavernosa for priapism ♂
🔲 3.87   ⚕ 5.82   **FUD** 000   [T] [A2] 🔲
AMA: 2014,Jan,11

54230 Injection procedure for corpora cavernosography ♂
🔀 (74445)
🔲 2.30   ⚕ 2.76   **FUD** 000   [N] [N1] 🔲
AMA: 2014,Jan,11

54231 Dynamic cavernosometry, including intracavernosal injection of vasoactive drugs (eg, papaverine, phentolamine) ♂
🔲 3.35   ⚕ 4.00   **FUD** 000   [T] [P3] 🔲
AMA: 2014,Jan,11

54235 Injection of corpora cavernosa with pharmacologic agent(s) (eg, papaverine, phentolamine) ♂
🔲 2.12   ⚕ 2.58   **FUD** 000   [T] [P3] 🔲
AMA: 2015,Jan,16; 2014,Jan,11; 2012,Jan,15-42; 2011,Jan,11

54240 Penile plethysmography ♂
🔲 2.83   ⚕ 2.83   **FUD** 000   [T] [P3] [80] 🔲
AMA: 2014,Jan,11

54250 Nocturnal penile tumescence and/or rigidity test ♂
🔲 3.46   ⚕ 3.46   **FUD** 000   [T] [P3] [80] 🔲
AMA: 2014,Jan,11

54300-54390 Hypospadias Repair and Related Procedures

[EXCLUDES] Other urethroplasties (53400-53430)
Revascularization of penis (37788)

54300 Plastic operation of penis for straightening of chordee (eg, hypospadias), with or without mobilization of urethra ♂
🔲 18.4   ⚕ 18.4   **FUD** 090   [T] [A2] [80] 🔲
AMA: 2015,Jan,16; 2014,Dec,16; 2014,Dec,16; 2014,Jan,11

External urethral orifice
Glans penis
This type of defect often occurs along the raphe of the penis
Penile hypospadias
Raphe
Scrotum
Chordee is characterized by a twisted downward appearance

54304 Plastic operation on penis for correction of chordee or for first stage hypospadias repair with or without transplantation of prepuce and/or skin flaps ♂
🔲 21.5   ⚕ 21.5   **FUD** 090   [T] [A2] [80] 🔲
AMA: 2014,Jan,11

54308 Urethroplasty for second stage hypospadias repair (including urinary diversion); less than 3 cm ♂
🔲 20.5   ⚕ 20.5   **FUD** 090   [T] [A2] [80] 🔲
AMA: 2014,Jan,11

54312 greater than 3 cm ♂
🔲 23.4   ⚕ 23.4   **FUD** 090   [T] [A2] [80] 🔲
AMA: 2014,Jan,11

54316 Urethroplasty for second stage hypospadias repair (including urinary diversion) with free skin graft obtained from site other than genitalia ♂
🔲 28.6   ⚕ 28.6   **FUD** 090   [T] [A2] [80] 🔲
AMA: 2014,Jan,11

54318 Urethroplasty for third stage hypospadias repair to release penis from scrotum (eg, third stage Cecil repair) ♂
🔲 20.6   ⚕ 20.6   **FUD** 090   [T] [A2] [80] 🔲
AMA: 2014,Jan,11

54322 1-stage distal hypospadias repair (with or without chordee or circumcision); with simple meatal advancement (eg, Magpi, V-flap) ♂
🔲 22.4   ⚕ 22.4   **FUD** 090   [T] [A2] [80] 🔲
AMA: 2014,Jan,11

54324 with urethroplasty by local skin flaps (eg, flip-flap, prepucial flap) ♂
[INCLUDES] Browne's operation
🔲 27.8   ⚕ 27.8   **FUD** 090   [T] [A2] [80] 🔲
AMA: 2014,Jan,11

54326 with urethroplasty by local skin flaps and mobilization of urethra ♂
🔲 27.1   ⚕ 27.1   **FUD** 090   [T] [A2] [80] 🔲
AMA: 2014,Jan,11

54328 with extensive dissection to correct chordee and urethroplasty with local skin flaps, skin graft patch, and/or island flap ♂
[EXCLUDES] Urethroplasty/straightening of chordee (54308)
🔲 26.9   ⚕ 26.9   **FUD** 090   [T] [A2] [80] 🔲
AMA: 2015,Jan,16; 2014,Jan,11; 2012,Jan,15-42; 2011,Jan,11

54332 1-stage proximal penile or penoscrotal hypospadias repair requiring extensive dissection to correct chordee and urethroplasty by use of skin graft tube and/or island flap ♂
🔲 29.1   ⚕ 29.1   **FUD** 090   [T] [80] 🔲
AMA: 2015,Jan,16; 2014,Jan,11; 2012,Jan,15-42; 2011,Jan,11

54336 1-stage perineal hypospadias repair requiring extensive dissection to correct chordee and urethroplasty by use of skin graft tube and/or island flap ♂
🔲 34.1   ⚕ 34.1   **FUD** 090   [T] [80] 🔲
AMA: 2015,Jan,16; 2014,Jan,11; 2012,Jan,15-42; 2011,Jan,11

54340 Repair of hypospadias complications (ie, fistula, stricture, diverticula); by closure, incision, or excision, simple ♂
🔲 16.3   ⚕ 16.3   **FUD** 090   [T] [A2] [80] 🔲
AMA: 2014,Jan,11

54344 requiring mobilization of skin flaps and urethroplasty with flap or patch graft ♂
🔲 27.2   ⚕ 27.2   **FUD** 090   [T] [A2] [80] 🔲
AMA: 2014,Jan,11

54348 requiring extensive dissection and urethroplasty with flap, patch or tubed graft (includes urinary diversion) ♂
🔲 29.3   ⚕ 29.3   **FUD** 090   [T] [A2] [80] 🔲
AMA: 2014,Jan,11

54352 Repair of hypospadias cripple requiring extensive dissection and excision of previously constructed structures including re-release of chordee and reconstruction of urethra and penis by use of local skin as grafts and island flaps and skin brought in as flaps or grafts ♂
🔲 40.6   ⚕ 40.6   **FUD** 090   [T] [A2] [80] 🔲
AMA: 2014,Jan,11

54360 Plastic operation on penis to correct angulation ♂
🔲 20.6   ⚕ 20.6   **FUD** 090   [T] [A2] [80] 🔲
AMA: 2014,Jan,11

54380 Plastic operation on penis for epispadias distal to external sphincter; ♂
[INCLUDES] Lowsley's operation
🔲 22.9   ⚕ 22.9   **FUD** 090   [T] [A2] [80] 🔲
AMA: 2014,Jan,11

54385 with incontinence ♂
🔲 29.8   ⚕ 29.8   **FUD** 090   [T] [A2] [80] 🔲
AMA: 2014,Jan,11

| 54390 | with exstrophy of bladder | ♂ |

    35.9   35.9 **FUD** 090   C 80

AMA: 2014,Jan,11

54400-54417 Procedures to Treat Impotence

CMS: 100-3,230.4 Diagnosis and Treatment of Impotence

EXCLUDES *Other urethroplasties (53400-53430)*
Revascularization of penis (37788)

| 54400 | Insertion of penile prosthesis; non-inflatable (semi-rigid) | ♂ |

    EXCLUDES *Replacement/removal penile prosthesis (54415, 54416)*
    15.1   15.1 **FUD** 090   J J8

AMA: 2014,Jan,11

| 54401 | inflatable (self-contained) | ♂ |

    EXCLUDES *Replacement/removal penile prosthesis (54415, 54416)*
    18.7   18.7 **FUD** 090   J J8 PQ

AMA: 2014,Jan,11

| 54405 | Insertion of multi-component, inflatable penile prosthesis, including placement of pump, cylinders, and reservoir | ♂ |

    Code also modifier 52 for reduced services
    23.1   23.1 **FUD** 090   J J8 80 PQ

AMA: 2014,Jan,11

| 54406 | Removal of all components of a multi-component, inflatable penile prosthesis without replacement of prosthesis | ♂ |

    Code also modifier 52 for reduced services
    20.9   20.9 **FUD** 090   02 A2 80 PQ

AMA: 2014,Jan,11

| 54408 | Repair of component(s) of a multi-component, inflatable penile prosthesis | ♂ |

    22.6   22.6 **FUD** 090   T A2 80 PQ

AMA: 2014,Jan,11

| 54410 | Removal and replacement of all component(s) of a multi-component, inflatable penile prosthesis at the same operative session | ♂ |

    24.6   24.6 **FUD** 090   J J8 80 PQ

AMA: 2014,Jan,11

| 54411 | Removal and replacement of all components of a multi-component inflatable penile prosthesis through an infected field at the same operative session, including irrigation and debridement of infected tissue | ♂ |

    Code also modifier 52 for reduced services
    Do not report with (11042, 11043)
    29.4   29.4 **FUD** 090   C 80

AMA: 2014,Jan,11

| 54415 | Removal of non-inflatable (semi-rigid) or inflatable (self-contained) penile prosthesis, without replacement of prosthesis | ♂ |

    15.1   15.1 **FUD** 090   02 A2 80 PQ

AMA: 2014,Jan,11

| 54416 | Removal and replacement of non-inflatable (semi-rigid) or inflatable (self-contained) penile prosthesis at the same operative session | ♂ |

    20.3   20.3 **FUD** 090   J J8 80 PQ

AMA: 2014,Jan,11

| 54417 | Removal and replacement of non-inflatable (semi-rigid) or inflatable (self-contained) penile prosthesis through an infected field at the same operative session, including irrigation and debridement of infected tissue | ♂ |

    Do not report with (11042, 11043)
    25.7   25.7 **FUD** 090   C 80

AMA: 2014,Jan,11

54420-54450 Other Procedures of the Penis

EXCLUDES *Other urethroplasties (53400-53430)*
Revascularization of penis (37788)

| 54420 | Corpora cavernosa-saphenous vein shunt (priapism operation), unilateral or bilateral | ♂ |

    20.2   20.2 **FUD** 090   T A2 80

AMA: 2014,Jan,11

| 54430 | Corpora cavernosa-corpus spongiosum shunt (priapism operation), unilateral or bilateral | ♂ |

    18.3   18.3 **FUD** 090   C 80

AMA: 2014,Jan,11

| 54435 | Corpora cavernosa-glans penis fistulization (eg, biopsy needle, Winter procedure, rongeur, or punch) for priapism | ♂ |

    11.9   11.9 **FUD** 090   T A2

AMA: 2014,Jan,11

● | 54437 | Repair of traumatic corporeal tear(s) |

    EXCLUDES *Urethral repair (53410, 53415)*

● | 54438 | Replantation, penis, complete amputation including urethral repair |

    EXCLUDES *Replantation/repair of corporeal tear in incomplete amputation penis (54437)*
    Replantation/urethral repair in incomplete amputation penis (53410-53415)

| 54440 | Plastic operation of penis for injury | ♂ |

    0.00   0.00 **FUD** 090   T A2 80

AMA: 2014,Jan,11

| 54450 | Foreskin manipulation including lysis of preputial adhesions and stretching | ♂ |

    1.65   1.99 **FUD** 000   T A2

AMA: 2014,Jan,11

54500-54560 Testicular Procedures: Incisional

EXCLUDES *Debridement of abdominal perineal gangrene (11004-11006)*

| 54500 | Biopsy of testis, needle (separate procedure) | ♂ |

    EXCLUDES *Fine needle aspiration (10021, 10022)*
    (88172-88173)
    2.15   2.15 **FUD** 000   T A2 80 50 PQ

AMA: 2014,Jan,11

| 54505 | Biopsy of testis, incisional (separate procedure) | ♂ |

    Code also when combined with epididymogram, seminal vesiculogram or vasogram (55300)
    6.01   6.01 **FUD** 010   T A2 80 50 PQ

AMA: 2015,Jan,16; 2014,Jan,11

| 54512 | Excision of extraparenchymal lesion of testis | ♂ |

    15.5   15.5 **FUD** 090   T A2 50

AMA: 2015,Jan,16; 2014,Jan,11; 2012,Jan,15-42; 2011,Jan,11

| 54520 | Orchiectomy, simple (including subcapsular), with or without testicular prosthesis, scrotal or inguinal approach | ♂ |

    INCLUDES Huggins' orchiectomy
    EXCLUDES *Lymphadenectomy, radical retroperitoneal (38780)*
    Code also hernia repair if performed (49505, 49507)
    9.36   9.36 **FUD** 090   T A2 50

AMA: 2015,Jan,16; 2014,Jan,11

| 54522 | Orchiectomy, partial | ♂ |

    EXCLUDES *Lymphadenectomy, radical retroperitoneal (38780)*
    16.9   16.9 **FUD** 090   T A2 80 50

AMA: 2015,Jan,16; 2014,Jan,11

| 54530 | Orchiectomy, radical, for tumor; inguinal approach | ♂ |

    EXCLUDES *Lymphadenectomy, radical retroperitoneal (38780)*
    14.4   14.4 **FUD** 090   T A2 80 50

AMA: 2015,Jan,16; 2014,Jan,11

| 54535 | with abdominal exploration | ♂ |

    EXCLUDES *Lymphadenectomy, radical retroperitoneal (38780)*
    21.3   21.3 **FUD** 090   T 80 50

AMA: 2015,Jan,16; 2014,Jan,11

54550

Exploration for undescended testis (inguinal or scrotal area) ♂

🚑 14.1   ✂ 14.1   **FUD** 090   T A2 80 50 ▢

AMA: 2015,Jan,16; 2014,Jan,11

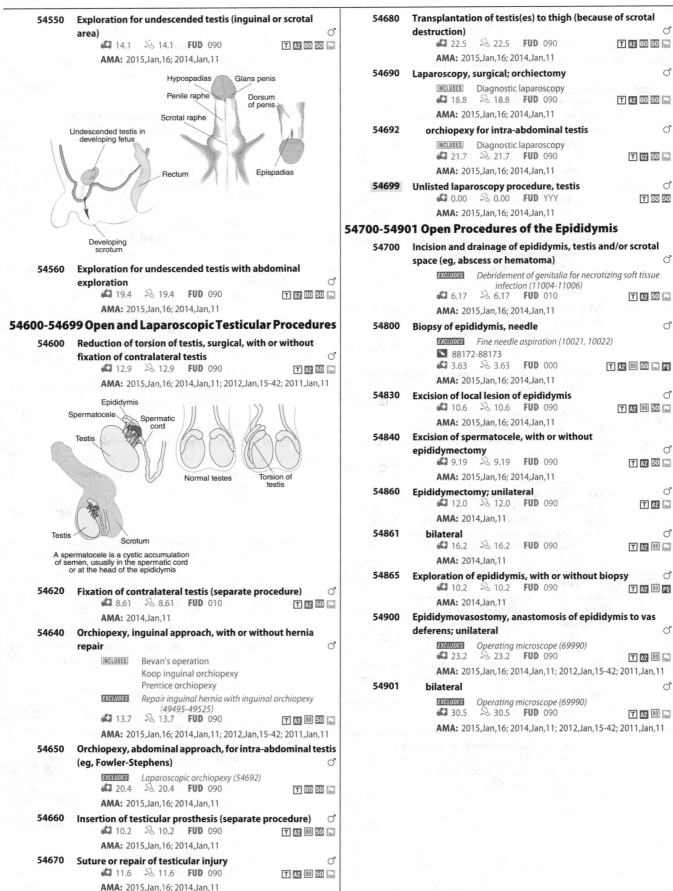

Undescended testis in developing fetus

Hypospadias — Glans penis
Penile raphe — Dorsum of penis
Scrotal raphe
Rectum — Epispadias
Developing scrotum

54560

Exploration for undescended testis with abdominal exploration ♂

🚑 19.4   ✂ 19.4   **FUD** 090   T G2 80 50 ▢

AMA: 2015,Jan,16; 2014,Jan,11

54600-54699 Open and Laparoscopic Testicular Procedures

54600

Reduction of torsion of testis, surgical, with or without fixation of contralateral testis ♂

🚑 12.9   ✂ 12.9   **FUD** 090   T A2 50 ▢

AMA: 2015,Jan,16; 2014,Jan,11; 2012,Jan,15-42; 2011,Jan,11

Epididymis
Spermatocele
Spermatic cord
Testis
Normal testes
Torsion of testis
Testis
Scrotum

A spermatocele is a cystic accumulation of semen, usually in the spermatic cord or at the head of the epididymis

54620

Fixation of contralateral testis (separate procedure) ♂

🚑 8.61   ✂ 8.61   **FUD** 010   T A2 50 ▢

AMA: 2014,Jan,11

54640

Orchiopexy, inguinal approach, with or without hernia repair ♂

INCLUDES   Bevan's operation
Koop inguinal orchiopexy
Prentice orchiopexy

EXCLUDES   *Repair inguinal hernia with inguinal orchiopexy (49495-49525)*

🚑 13.7   ✂ 13.7   **FUD** 090   T A2 80 50 ▢

AMA: 2015,Jan,16; 2014,Jan,11; 2012,Jan,15-42; 2011,Jan,11

54650

Orchiopexy, abdominal approach, for intra-abdominal testis (eg, Fowler-Stephens) ♂

EXCLUDES   *Laparoscopic orchiopexy (54692)*

🚑 20.4   ✂ 20.4   **FUD** 090   T 80 50 ▢

AMA: 2015,Jan,16; 2014,Jan,11

54660

Insertion of testicular prosthesis (separate procedure) ♂

🚑 10.2   ✂ 10.2   **FUD** 090   T A2 80 50 ▢

AMA: 2015,Jan,16; 2014,Jan,11

54670

Suture or repair of testicular injury ♂

🚑 11.6   ✂ 11.6   **FUD** 090   T A2 80 50 ▢

AMA: 2015,Jan,16; 2014,Jan,11

54680

Transplantation of testis(es) to thigh (because of scrotal destruction) ♂

🚑 22.5   ✂ 22.5   **FUD** 090   T A2 80 50 ▢

AMA: 2015,Jan,16; 2014,Jan,11

54690

Laparoscopy, surgical; orchiectomy ♂

INCLUDES   Diagnostic laparoscopy

🚑 18.8   ✂ 18.8   **FUD** 090   T A2 80 50 ▢

AMA: 2015,Jan,16; 2014,Jan,11

54692

orchiopexy for intra-abdominal testis ♂

INCLUDES   Diagnostic laparoscopy

🚑 21.7   ✂ 21.7   **FUD** 090   T G2 50 ▢

AMA: 2015,Jan,16; 2014,Jan,11

54699

Unlisted laparoscopy procedure, testis ♂

🚑 0.00   ✂ 0.00   **FUD** YYY   T 80 50

AMA: 2015,Jan,16; 2014,Jan,11

54700-54901 Open Procedures of the Epididymis

54700

Incision and drainage of epididymis, testis and/or scrotal space (eg, abscess or hematoma) ♂

EXCLUDES   *Debridement of genitalia for necrotizing soft tissue infection (11004-11006)*

🚑 6.17   ✂ 6.17   **FUD** 010   T A2 50 ▢

AMA: 2015,Jan,16; 2014,Jan,11

54800

Biopsy of epididymis, needle ♂

EXCLUDES   *Fine needle aspiration (10021, 10022)*

📠 88172-88173

🚑 3.63   ✂ 3.63   **FUD** 000   T A2 80 50 ▢ PQ

AMA: 2015,Jan,16; 2014,Jan,11

54830

Excision of local lesion of epididymis ♂

🚑 10.6   ✂ 10.6   **FUD** 090   T A2 80 50 ▢

AMA: 2015,Jan,16; 2014,Jan,11

54840

Excision of spermatocele, with or without epididymectomy ♂

🚑 9.19   ✂ 9.19   **FUD** 090   T A2 50 ▢

AMA: 2015,Jan,16; 2014,Jan,11

54860

Epididymectomy; unilateral ♂

🚑 12.0   ✂ 12.0   **FUD** 090   T A2

AMA: 2014,Jan,11

54861

bilateral ♂

🚑 16.2   ✂ 16.2   **FUD** 090   T A2 80

AMA: 2014,Jan,11

54865

Exploration of epididymis, with or without biopsy ♂

🚑 10.2   ✂ 10.2   **FUD** 090   T A2 80 PQ

AMA: 2014,Jan,11

54900

Epididymovasostomy, anastomosis of epididymis to vas deferens; unilateral ♂

EXCLUDES   *Operating microscope (69990)*

🚑 23.2   ✂ 23.2   **FUD** 090   T A2 80 ▢

AMA: 2015,Jan,16; 2014,Jan,11; 2012,Jan,15-42; 2011,Jan,11

54901

bilateral ♂

EXCLUDES   *Operating microscope (69990)*

🚑 30.5   ✂ 30.5   **FUD** 090   T A2 80 ▢

AMA: 2015,Jan,16; 2014,Jan,11; 2012,Jan,15-42; 2011,Jan,11

55000-55180 Procedures of the Tunica Vaginalis and Scrotum

55000 **Puncture aspiration of hydrocele, tunica vaginalis, with or without injection of medication** ♂
    2.45   3.34   **FUD** 000   T P3 50
    AMA: 2014,Jan,11

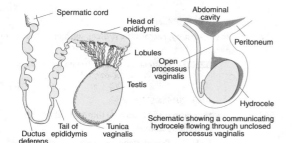

Spermatic cord
Head of epididymis
Abdominal cavity
Peritoneum
Lobules
Open processus vaginalis
Testis
Hydrocele
Ductus deferens
Tail of epididymis
Tunica vaginalis

Schematic showing a communicating hydrocele flowing through unclosed processus vaginalis

55040 **Excision of hydrocele; unilateral** ♂
    EXCLUDES   *Repair of hernia with hydrocelectomy (49495-49501)*
    9.70   9.70   **FUD** 090   T A2
    AMA: 2015,Jan,16; 2014,Jan,11

55041 **bilateral** ♂
    EXCLUDES   *Repair of hernia with hydrocelectomy (49495-49501)*
    14.6   14.6   **FUD** 090   T A2
    AMA: 2014,Jan,11

55060 **Repair of tunica vaginalis hydrocele (Bottle type)** ♂
    10.9   10.9   **FUD** 090   T A2 80 50
    AMA: 2015,Jan,16; 2014,Nov,14; 2014,Jan,11

55100 **Drainage of scrotal wall abscess** ♂
    EXCLUDES   *Debridement of genitalia for necrotizing soft tissue infection (11004-11006)*
    Incision and drainage of scrotal space (54700)
    4.78   6.13   **FUD** 010   T A2
    AMA: 2014,Jan,11

55110 **Scrotal exploration** ♂
    11.1   11.1   **FUD** 090   T A2
    AMA: 2014,Jan,11

55120 **Removal of foreign body in scrotum** ♂
    10.2   10.2   **FUD** 090   T A2 80
    AMA: 2014,Jan,11

55150 **Resection of scrotum** ♂
    EXCLUDES   *Lesion excision of skin of scrotum (11420-11426, 11620-11626)*
    14.1   14.1   **FUD** 090   T A2 80
    AMA: 2014,Jan,11

55175 **Scrotoplasty; simple** ♂
    10.3   10.3   **FUD** 090   T A2 80
    AMA: 2015,Jan,16; 2014,Dec,16; 2014,Dec,16; 2014,Jan,11

55180 **complicated** ♂
    19.7   19.7   **FUD** 090   T A2 80
    AMA: 2014,Jan,11

55200-55680 Procedures of Other Male Genital Ducts and Glands

55200 **Vasotomy, cannulization with or without incision of vas, unilateral or bilateral (separate procedure)** ♂
    7.99   12.3   **FUD** 090   T A2 80
    AMA: 2014,Jan,11

55250 **Vasectomy, unilateral or bilateral (separate procedure), including postoperative semen examination(s)** ♂
    6.51   10.8   **FUD** 090   T A2
    AMA: 2015,Jan,16; 2014,Jan,11; 2012,Jan,15-42; 2011,Jan,11

55300 **Vasotomy for vasograms, seminal vesiculograms, or epididymograms, unilateral or bilateral** ♂
    Code also biopsy of testis and modifier 51 when combined (54505)
    (74440)
    5.38   5.38   **FUD** 000   N N1 80
    AMA: 2014,Jan,11

55400 **Vasovasostomy, vasovasorrhaphy** ♂
    EXCLUDES   *Operating microscope (69990)*
    14.2   14.2   **FUD** 090   T A2 80 50
    AMA: 2015,Jan,16; 2014,Jan,11; 2012,Jan,15-42; 2011,Jan,11

55450 **Ligation (percutaneous) of vas deferens, unilateral or bilateral (separate procedure)** ♂
    7.39   10.1   **FUD** 010   T P3 80
    AMA: 2014,Jan,11

55500 **Excision of hydrocele of spermatic cord, unilateral (separate procedure)** ♂
    11.3   11.3   **FUD** 090   T A2 80 50
    AMA: 2015,Jan,16; 2014,Jan,11

55520 **Excision of lesion of spermatic cord (separate procedure)** ♂
    13.0   13.0   **FUD** 090   T A2 80 50
    AMA: 2015,Jan,16; 2014,Jan,11; 2012,Jan,15-42; 2011,Jan,11

55530 **Excision of varicocele or ligation of spermatic veins for varicocele; (separate procedure)** ♂
    10.1   10.1   **FUD** 090   T A2 50
    AMA: 2015,Jan,16; 2014,Jan,11

55535 **abdominal approach** ♂
    12.3   12.3   **FUD** 090   T A2 80 50
    AMA: 2015,Jan,16; 2014,Jan,11

55540 **with hernia repair** ♂
    15.9   15.9   **FUD** 090   T A2 50
    AMA: 2015,Jan,16; 2014,Jan,11

55550 **Laparoscopy, surgical, with ligation of spermatic veins for varicocele** ♂
    INCLUDES   Diagnostic laparoscopy
    12.2   12.2   **FUD** 090   T A2 80 50
    AMA: 2015,Jan,16; 2014,Jan,11

55559 **Unlisted laparoscopy procedure, spermatic cord** ♂
    0.00   0.00   **FUD** YYY   T 80 50
    AMA: 2015,Jan,16; 2014,Jan,11

55600 **Vesiculotomy;** ♂
    12.0   12.0   **FUD** 090   T R2 80 50
    AMA: 2014,Jan,11

55605 **complicated** ♂
    15.1   15.1   **FUD** 090   C 80 50
    AMA: 2014,Jan,11

55650 **Vesiculectomy, any approach** ♂
    20.5   20.5   **FUD** 090   C 80 50
    AMA: 2014,Jan,11

55680 **Excision of Mullerian duct cyst** ♂
    EXCLUDES   *Injection procedure (52010, 55300)*
    10.0   10.0   **FUD** 090   T A2 80 50
    AMA: 2014,Jan,11

55700-55725 Procedures of Prostate: Incisional

55700 Biopsy, prostate; needle or punch, single or multiple, any approach ♂

 EXCLUDES Fine needle aspiration (10021, 10022)
 Needle biopsy of prostate, saturation sampling for prostate mapping (55706)

 (76942)

 (88172-88173)

 4.01 6.18 **FUD** 000 T A2 ▭ P0

 AMA: 2015,Jan,16; 2014,Jan,11; 2010,Nov,5

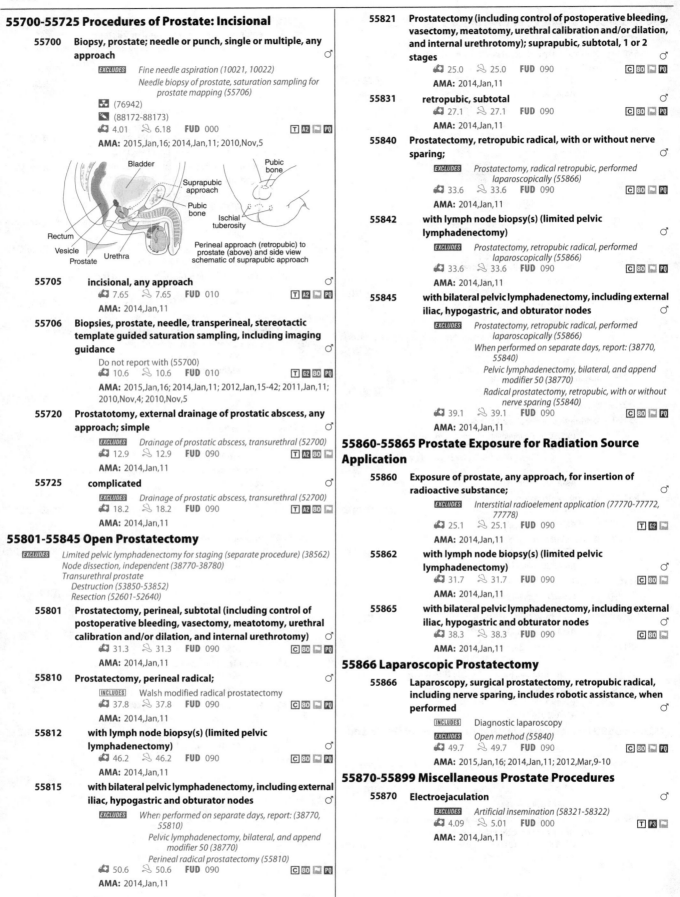

Bladder
Pubic bone
Suprapubic approach
Pubic bone
Ischial tuberosity
Rectum
Vesicle
Prostate
Urethra

Perineal approach (retropubic) to prostate (above) and side view schematic of suprapubic approach

55705 incisional, any approach ♂

 7.65 7.65 **FUD** 010 T A2 ▭ P0

 AMA: 2014,Jan,11

55706 Biopsies, prostate, needle, transperineal, stereotactic template guided saturation sampling, including imaging guidance ♂

 Do not report with (55700)

 10.6 10.6 **FUD** 010 T G2 80 P0

 AMA: 2015,Jan,16; 2014,Jan,11; 2012,Jan,15-42; 2011,Jan,11; 2010,Nov,4; 2010,Nov,5

55720 Prostatotomy, external drainage of prostatic abscess, any approach; simple ♂

 EXCLUDES Drainage of prostatic abscess, transurethral (52700)

 12.9 12.9 **FUD** 090 T A2 80 ▭

 AMA: 2014,Jan,11

55725 complicated ♂

 EXCLUDES Drainage of prostatic abscess, transurethral (52700)

 18.2 18.2 **FUD** 090 T A2 80 ▭

 AMA: 2014,Jan,11

55801-55845 Open Prostatectomy

 EXCLUDES Limited pelvic lymphadenectomy for staging (separate procedure) (38562)
 Node dissection, independent (38770-38780)
 Transurethral prostate
 Destruction (53850-53852)
 Resection (52601-52640)

55801 Prostatectomy, perineal, subtotal (including control of postoperative bleeding, vasectomy, meatotomy, urethral calibration and/or dilation, and internal urethrotomy) ♂

 31.3 31.3 **FUD** 090 C 80 ▭ P0

 AMA: 2014,Jan,11

55810 Prostatectomy, perineal radical; ♂

 INCLUDES Walsh modified radical prostatectomy

 37.8 37.8 **FUD** 090 C 80 ▭ P0

 AMA: 2014,Jan,11

55812 with lymph node biopsy(s) (limited pelvic lymphadenectomy) ♂

 46.2 46.2 **FUD** 090 C 80 ▭ P0

 AMA: 2014,Jan,11

55815 with bilateral pelvic lymphadenectomy, including external iliac, hypogastric and obturator nodes ♂

 EXCLUDES When performed on separate days, report: (38770, 55810)
 Pelvic lymphadenectomy, bilateral, and append modifier 50 (38770)
 Perineal radical prostatectomy (55810)

 50.6 50.6 **FUD** 090 C 80 ▭ P0

 AMA: 2014,Jan,11

55821 Prostatectomy (including control of postoperative bleeding, vasectomy, meatotomy, urethral calibration and/or dilation, and internal urethrotomy); suprapubic, subtotal, 1 or 2 stages ♂

 25.0 25.0 **FUD** 090 C 80 ▭ P0

 AMA: 2014,Jan,11

55831 retropubic, subtotal ♂

 27.1 27.1 **FUD** 090 C 80 ▭ P0

 AMA: 2014,Jan,11

55840 Prostatectomy, retropubic radical, with or without nerve sparing; ♂

 EXCLUDES Prostatectomy, radical retropubic, performed laparoscopically (55866)

 33.6 33.6 **FUD** 090 C 80 ▭ P0

 AMA: 2014,Jan,11

55842 with lymph node biopsy(s) (limited pelvic lymphadenectomy) ♂

 EXCLUDES Prostatectomy, retropubic radical, performed laparoscopically (55866)

 33.6 33.6 **FUD** 090 C 80 ▭ P0

 AMA: 2014,Jan,11

55845 with bilateral pelvic lymphadenectomy, including external iliac, hypogastric, and obturator nodes ♂

 EXCLUDES Prostatectomy, retropubic radical, performed laparoscopically (55866)
 When performed on separate days, report: (38770, 55840)
 Pelvic lymphadenectomy, bilateral, and append modifier 50 (38770)
 Radical prostatectomy, retropubic, with or without nerve sparing (55840)

 39.1 39.1 **FUD** 090 C 80 ▭ P0

 AMA: 2014,Jan,11

55860-55865 Prostate Exposure for Radiation Source Application

55860 Exposure of prostate, any approach, for insertion of radioactive substance; ♂

 EXCLUDES Interstitial radioelement application (77770-77772, 77778)

 25.1 25.1 **FUD** 090 T G2 ▭

 AMA: 2014,Jan,11

55862 with lymph node biopsy(s) (limited pelvic lymphadenectomy) ♂

 31.7 31.7 **FUD** 090 C 80 ▭

 AMA: 2014,Jan,11

55865 with bilateral pelvic lymphadenectomy, including external iliac, hypogastric and obturator nodes ♂

 38.3 38.3 **FUD** 090 C 80 ▭

 AMA: 2014,Jan,11

55866 Laparoscopic Prostatectomy

55866 Laparoscopy, surgical prostatectomy, retropubic radical, including nerve sparing, includes robotic assistance, when performed ♂

 INCLUDES Diagnostic laparoscopy

 EXCLUDES Open method (55840)

 49.7 49.7 **FUD** 090 C 80 ▭ P0

 AMA: 2015,Jan,16; 2014,Jan,11; 2012,Mar,9-10

55870-55899 Miscellaneous Prostate Procedures

55870 Electroejaculation ♂

 EXCLUDES Artificial insemination (58321-58322)

 4.09 5.01 **FUD** 000 T P3 ▭

 AMA: 2014,Jan,11

55873 **Cryosurgical ablation of the prostate (includes ultrasonic guidance and monitoring)** ♂
  🔲 22.0 ✂ 200. **FUD** 090   J J8 ▭ P0
  AMA: 2015,Jan,16; 2014,Jan,11; 2010,Jan,7-8

55875 **Transperineal placement of needles or catheters into prostate for interstitial radioelement application, with or without cystoscopy** ♂
  Code also interstitial radioelement application (77770-77772, 77778)
  ⟲ (76965)
  🔲 21.8 ✂ 21.8 **FUD** 090   Q3 A2 80 P0
  AMA: 2015,Jan,16; 2014,Jan,11

55876 **Placement of interstitial device(s) for radiation therapy guidance (eg, fiducial markers, dosimeter), prostate (via needle, any approach), single or multiple** ♂
  Code also supply of device
  ⟲ (76942, 77002, 77012, 77021)
  🔲 2.89 ✂ 3.85 **FUD** 000   S P3 P0
  AMA: 2015,Jan,16; 2014,Jan,11; 2012,Jan,15-42; 2011,Jan,11; 2010,Jan,7-8; 2010,Jan,12-15

55899 **Unlisted procedure, male genital system** ♂
  🔲 0.00 ✂ 0.00 **FUD** YYY   T 80
  AMA: 2015,Jun,5; 2015,Jan,16; 2014,Jan,11

55920 Insertion Brachytherapy Catheters/Needles Pelvis/Genitalia, Male/Female

55920 **Placement of needles or catheters into pelvic organs and/or genitalia (except prostate) for subsequent interstitial radioelement application**
  EXCLUDES   Insertion of Heyman capsules for purposes of brachytherapy (58346)
  Insertion of vaginal ovoids and/or uterine tandems for purposes of brachytherapy (57155)
  Placement of catheters or needles, prostate (55875)
  🔲 12.7 ✂ 12.7 **FUD** 000   T G2 80
  AMA: 2015,Jan,16; 2014,Jan,11

55970-55980 Transsexual Surgery

CMS: 100-2,16,10 Exclusions from Coverage; 100-2,16,180 Services Related to Noncovered Procedures

55970 **Intersex surgery; male to female** ♂
  🔲 0.00 ✂ 0.00 **FUD** YYY   T
  AMA: 2014,Jan,11

55980 **female to male** ♀
  🔲 0.00 ✂ 0.00 **FUD** YYY   T
  AMA: 2014,Jan,11

56405-56420 Incision and Drainage of Abscess

EXCLUDES   Incision and drainage Skene's gland cyst/abscess (53060)
  Incision and drainage subcutaneous abscess/cyst/furuncle (10040, 10060, 10061)

56405 **Incision and drainage of vulva or perineal abscess** ♀
  🔲 3.10 ✂ 3.12 **FUD** 010   T P3 ▭
  AMA: 2014,Jan,11

56420 **Incision and drainage of Bartholin's gland abscess** ♀
  🔲 2.60 ✂ 3.46 **FUD** 010   T P3 ▭
  AMA: 2014,Jan,11

56440-56442 Other Female Genital Incisional Procedures

EXCLUDES   Incision and drainage subcutaneous abscess/cyst/furuncle (10040, 10060, 10061)

56440 **Marsupialization of Bartholin's gland cyst** ♀
  🔲 5.19 ✂ 5.19 **FUD** 010   T A2
  AMA: 2014,Jan,11

56441 **Lysis of labial adhesions** ♀
  🔲 3.98 ✂ 4.13 **FUD** 010   T A2 80 ▭
  AMA: 2014,Jan,11

56442 **Hymenotomy, simple incision** ♀
  🔲 1.35 ✂ 1.35 **FUD** 000   T A2 80
  AMA: 2014,Jan,11

56501-56515 Destruction of Vulvar Lesions, Any Method

EXCLUDES   Excision/fulguration/destruction
  Skene's glands (53270)
  Urethral caruncle (53265)

56501 **Destruction of lesion(s), vulva; simple (eg, laser surgery, electrosurgery, cryosurgery, chemosurgery)** ♀
  🔲 3.27 ✂ 3.72 **FUD** 010   T P3 ▭
  AMA: 2014,Jan,11

56515 **extensive (eg, laser surgery, electrosurgery, cryosurgery, chemosurgery)** ♀
  🔲 5.75 ✂ 6.45 **FUD** 010   T A2 ▭
  AMA: 2014,Jan,11

56605-56606 Vulvar and Perineal Biopsies

EXCLUDES   Excision local lesion (11420-11426, 11620-11626)

56605 **Biopsy of vulva or perineum (separate procedure); 1 lesion** ♀
  🔲 1.73 ✂ 2.34 **FUD** 000   T P3 ▭ P0
  AMA: 2015,Jan,16; 2014,Jan,11

+ 56606 **each separate additional lesion (List separately in addition to code for primary procedure)** ♀
  Code first (56605)
  🔲 0.84 ✂ 1.07 **FUD** ZZZ   N N1 ▭
  AMA: 2014,Jan,11

56620-56640 Vulvectomy Procedures

INCLUDES   Removal of:
  Greater than 80% of the vulvar area - complete procedure
  Less than 80% of the vulvar area - partial procedure
  Skin and deep subcutaneous tissue - radical procedure
  Skin and superficial subcutaneous tissues - simple procedure
EXCLUDES   Skin graft (15004-15005, 15120-15121, 15240-15241)

56620 **Vulvectomy simple; partial** ♀
  🔲 14.8 ✂ 14.8 **FUD** 090   T A2 80 ▭
  AMA: 2015,Jan,16; 2014,Jan,11; 2013,Dec,14

56625 **complete** ♀
  🔲 18.0 ✂ 18.0 **FUD** 090   T A2 80 ▭
  AMA: 2014,Jan,11

56630 **Vulvectomy, radical, partial;** ♀
  🔲 26.6 ✂ 26.6 **FUD** 090   C 80 ▭ P0
  AMA: 2014,Jan,11

56631 with unilateral inguinofemoral lymphadenectomy ♀
- INCLUDES Bassett's operation
- 🔧 33.8 ✂ 33.8 **FUD** 090
- C 80 ▦ P0
- AMA: 2014,Jan,11

56632 with bilateral inguinofemoral lymphadenectomy ♀
- INCLUDES Bassett's operation
- 🔧 39.6 ✂ 39.6 **FUD** 090
- C 80 ▦ P0
- AMA: 2014,Jan,11

56633 Vulvectomy, radical, complete; ♀
- INCLUDES Bassett's operation
- 🔧 34.8 ✂ 34.8 **FUD** 090
- C 80 ▦ P0
- AMA: 2014,Jan,11

56634 with unilateral inguinofemoral lymphadenectomy ♀
- INCLUDES Bassett's operation
- 🔧 37.5 ✂ 37.5 **FUD** 090
- C 80 ▦ P0
- AMA: 2014,Jan,11

56637 with bilateral inguinofemoral lymphadenectomy ♀
- INCLUDES Bassett's operation
- 🔧 43.5 ✂ 43.5 **FUD** 090
- C 80 ▦ P0
- AMA: 2014,Jan,11

56640 Vulvectomy, radical, complete, with inguinofemoral, iliac, and pelvic lymphadenectomy ♀
- INCLUDES Bassett's operation
- EXCLUDES Lymphadenectomy (38760-38780)
- 🔧 43.9 ✂ 43.9 **FUD** 090
- C 80 50 ▦ P0
- AMA: 2014,Jan,11

56700-56740 Other Excisional Procedures: External Female Genitalia

56700 Partial hymenectomy or revision of hymenal ring ♀
- 🔧 5.31 ✂ 5.31 **FUD** 010
- T A2 80 ▦
- AMA: 2014,Jan,11

56740 Excision of Bartholin's gland or cyst ♀
- EXCLUDES Excision/fulguration/marsupialization:
  - Skene's glands (53270)
  - Urethral carcinoma (53220)
  - Urethral caruncle (53265)
  - Urethral diverticulum (53230, 53240)
- 🔧 8.58 ✂ 8.58 **FUD** 010
- T A2 50 ▦
- AMA: 2014,Jan,11

Urethra

Vagina

Bartholin's gland cyst

Anus

56800-56810 Repair/Reconstruction External Female Genitalia

EXCLUDES Repair of urethra for mucosal prolapse (53275)

56800 Plastic repair of introitus ♀
- INCLUDES Emmet's operation
- 🔧 6.87 ✂ 6.87 **FUD** 010
- T A2 80 ▦
- AMA: 2014,Jan,11

56805 Clitoroplasty for intersex state ♀
- 🔧 32.4 ✂ 32.4 **FUD** 090
- T G2 80 ▦
- AMA: 2014,Jan,11

56810 Perineoplasty, repair of perineum, nonobstetrical (separate procedure) ♀
- INCLUDES Emmet's operation
- EXCLUDES Genitalia wound repair (12001-12007, 12041-12047, 13131-13133)
  - Introitus plastic repair (56800)
  - Sphincteroplasty, anal (46750-46751)
  - Vaginal/perineum recent injury repair, nonobstetrical (57210)
  - Vulva/perineum episiorrhaphy/episioperineorrhaphy for recent injury, nonobstetrical (57210)
- 🔧 7.40 ✂ 7.40 **FUD** 010
- T A2 80 ▦
- AMA: 2014,Jan,11

56820-56821 Vulvar Colposcopy with/without Biopsy

EXCLUDES Colposcopic procedures and/or examinations:
- Cervix (57452-57461)
- Vagina (57420-57421)

56820 Colposcopy of the vulva; ♀
- 🔧 2.48 ✂ 3.19 **FUD** 000
- T P3 ▦
- AMA: 2015,Jan,16; 2014,Jan,11

56821 with biopsy(s) ♀
- 🔧 3.31 ✂ 4.21 **FUD** 000
- T P3 ▦ P0
- AMA: 2015,Jan,16; 2014,Jan,11

57000-57023 Incisional Procedures: Vagina

57000 Colpotomy; with exploration ♀
- 🔧 5.25 ✂ 5.25 **FUD** 010
- T A2 80 ▦
- AMA: 2015,Jan,16; 2014,Jan,11

57010 with drainage of pelvic abscess ♀
- INCLUDES Laroyenne operation
- 🔧 12.3 ✂ 12.3 **FUD** 090
- T A2 80 ▦
- AMA: 2014,Jan,11

57020 Colpocentesis (separate procedure) ♀
- 🔧 2.30 ✂ 2.63 **FUD** 000
- T A2 80 ▦
- AMA: 2014,Jan,11

57022 Incision and drainage of vaginal hematoma; obstetrical/postpartum ♀
- 🔧 4.78 ✂ 4.78 **FUD** 010
- T R2 80 ▦
- AMA: 2014,Jan,11

57023 non-obstetrical (eg, post-trauma, spontaneous bleeding) ♀
- 🔧 8.84 ✂ 8.84 **FUD** 010
- T A2 80 ▦
- AMA: 2014,Jan,11

57061-57065 Destruction of Vaginal Lesions, Any Method

CMS: 100-3,140.5 Laser Procedures

57061 Destruction of vaginal lesion(s); simple (eg, laser surgery, electrosurgery, cryosurgery, chemosurgery) ♀
- 🔧 2.81 ✂ 3.24 **FUD** 010
- T P3 ▦
- AMA: 2015,Jan,16; 2014,Jan,11; 2012,Jan,15-42; 2011,Jan,11

57065 extensive (eg, laser surgery, electrosurgery, cryosurgery, chemosurgery) ♀
- 🔧 5.00 ✂ 5.58 **FUD** 010
- T A2 ▦
- AMA: 2015,Jan,16; 2014,Jan,11; 2012,Jan,15-42; 2011,Jan,11

57100-57135 Excisional Procedures: Vagina

57100 Biopsy of vaginal mucosa; simple (separate procedure) ♀
- 🔧 1.92 ✂ 2.54 **FUD** 000
- T P3 ▦ P0
- AMA: 2014,Jan,11

| 57105 | extensive, requiring suture (including cysts) ♀ |

🔪 3.61 ⚕ 3.88 **FUD** 010 T A2 ▢ PQ

AMA: 2014,Jan,11

57106 Vaginectomy, partial removal of vaginal wall; ♀

🔪 14.1 ⚕ 14.1 **FUD** 090 T 80 ▢

AMA: 2015,Jan,16; 2014,Jan,11

57107 with removal of paravaginal tissue (radical vaginectomy) ♀

🔪 41.7 ⚕ 41.7 **FUD** 090 T 80 ▢

AMA: 2015,Jan,16; 2014,Jan,11

57109 with removal of paravaginal tissue (radical vaginectomy) with bilateral total pelvic lymphadenectomy and para-aortic lymph node sampling (biopsy) ♀

🔪 50.3 ⚕ 50.3 **FUD** 090 T 80 ▢

AMA: 2015,Jan,16; 2014,Jan,11

57110 Vaginectomy, complete removal of vaginal wall; ♀

🔪 25.4 ⚕ 25.4 **FUD** 090 C 80 ▢

AMA: 2015,Jan,16; 2014,Jan,11

57111 with removal of paravaginal tissue (radical vaginectomy) ♀

🔪 45.5 ⚕ 45.5 **FUD** 090 C 80 ▢

AMA: 2015,Jan,16; 2014,Jan,11

57112 with removal of paravaginal tissue (radical vaginectomy) with bilateral total pelvic lymphadenectomy and para-aortic lymph node sampling (biopsy) ♀

🔪 53.8 ⚕ 53.8 **FUD** 090 C 80 ▢

AMA: 2015,Jan,16; 2014,Jan,11

57120 Colpocleisis (Le Fort type) ♀

🔪 14.4 ⚕ 14.4 **FUD** 090 J 80 ▢

AMA: 2014,Jan,11

57130 Excision of vaginal septum ♀

🔪 4.53 ⚕ 5.03 **FUD** 010 T A2 80 ▢

AMA: 2014,Jan,11

57135 Excision of vaginal cyst or tumor ♀

🔪 4.93 ⚕ 5.45 **FUD** 010 T A2 ▢

AMA: 2014,Jan,11

57150-57180 Irrigation/Insertion/Introduction Vaginal Medication or Supply

57150 Irrigation of vagina and/or application of medicament for treatment of bacterial, parasitic, or fungoid disease ♀

🔪 0.82 ⚕ 1.28 **FUD** 000 T P3 ▢

AMA: 2014,Jan,11

57155 Insertion of uterine tandem and/or vaginal ovoids for clinical brachytherapy ♀

EXCLUDES *Insertion of radioelement sources or ribbons (77761-77763, 77770-77772)*
The placement of needles or catheters into the pelvic organs and/or genitalia (except for the prostate) for interstitial radioelement application (55920)

🔪 8.26 ⚕ 12.1 **FUD** 000 ☉ T A2 ▢

AMA: 2015,Jan,16; 2014,Jan,11

57156 Insertion of a vaginal radiation afterloading apparatus for clinical brachytherapy ♀

🔪 4.16 ⚕ 5.58 **FUD** 000 T G2 80

AMA: 2014,Jan,11

57160 Fitting and insertion of pessary or other intravaginal support device ♀

🔪 1.35 ⚕ 2.17 **FUD** 000 T P3 ▢

AMA: 2015,Jan,16; 2014,Jan,11; 2012,Jan,15-42; 2011,Jan,11; 2010,May,9

57170 Diaphragm or cervical cap fitting with instructions ♀

🔪 1.38 ⚕ 1.72 **FUD** 000 T P3 80 ▢

AMA: 2014,Jan,11

57180 Introduction of any hemostatic agent or pack for spontaneous or traumatic nonobstetrical vaginal hemorrhage (separate procedure) ♀

🔪 3.02 ⚕ 4.00 **FUD** 010 T A2

AMA: 2015,Jan,16; 2014,Jan,11

57200-57335 Vaginal Repair and Reconstruction

EXCLUDES *Marshall-Marchetti-Kranz type urethral suspension, abdominal approach (51840-51841)*
Urethral suspension performed laparoscopically (51990)

57200 Colporrhaphy, suture of injury of vagina (nonobstetrical) ♀

🔪 8.61 ⚕ 8.61 **FUD** 090 T A2 80 ▢

AMA: 2014,Jan,11

57210 Colpoperineorrhaphy, suture of injury of vagina and/or perineum (nonobstetrical) ♀

🔪 10.4 ⚕ 10.4 **FUD** 090 T A2 80 ▢

AMA: 2014,Jan,11

57220 Plastic operation on urethral sphincter, vaginal approach (eg, Kelly urethral plication) ♀

🔪 9.06 ⚕ 9.06 **FUD** 090 J A2 80 ▢

AMA: 2014,Jan,11

57230 Plastic repair of urethrocele ♀

🔪 11.2 ⚕ 11.2 **FUD** 090 T A2 80 ▢

AMA: 2014,Jan,11

57240 Anterior colporrhaphy, repair of cystocele with or without repair of urethrocele ♀

🔪 19.1 ⚕ 19.1 **FUD** 090 J A2 80 ▢

AMA: 2015,Jan,16; 2014,Jan,11; 2010,Jun,6-7

57250 Posterior colporrhaphy, repair of rectocele with or without perineorrhaphy ♀

EXCLUDES *Rectocele repair (separate procedure) without posterior colporrhaphy (45560)*

🔪 19.2 ⚕ 19.2 **FUD** 090 J A2 80 ▢

AMA: 2015,Jan,16; 2014,Jan,11; 2012,Jan,15-42; 2011,May,9

57260 Combined anteroposterior colporrhaphy; ♀

🔪 23.7 ⚕ 23.7 **FUD** 090 J A2 80 ▢

AMA: 2015,Jan,16; 2014,Jan,11; 2010,Jun,6-7

57265 with enterocele repair ♀

🔪 25.9 ⚕ 25.9 **FUD** 090 J A2 80 ▢

AMA: 2015,Jan,16; 2014,Jan,11; 2010,Jun,6-7

+ **57267** Insertion of mesh or other prosthesis for repair of pelvic floor defect, each site (anterior, posterior compartment), vaginal approach (List separately in addition to code for primary procedure) ♀

Code first (45560, 57240-57265, 57285)

🔪 7.31 ⚕ 7.31 **FUD** ZZZ N N1 80

AMA: 2015,Jan,16; 2014,Jan,11; 2013,Oct,15; 2012,Jan,6-10; 2012,Jan,15-42; 2011,May,9; 2011,Jan,11

57268 Repair of enterocele, vaginal approach (separate procedure) ♀

🔪 13.7 ⚕ 13.7 **FUD** 090 T A2 80 ▢

AMA: 2015,Jan,16; 2014,Jan,11

57270 Repair of enterocele, abdominal approach (separate procedure) ♀

🔪 22.6 ⚕ 22.6 **FUD** 090 C 80 ▢

AMA: 2015,Jan,16; 2014,Jan,11

57280 Colpopexy, abdominal approach ♀

🔪 27.1 ⚕ 27.1 **FUD** 090 C 80 ▢

AMA: 2015,Jan,16; 2014,Jan,11

57282 Colpopexy, vaginal; extra-peritoneal approach (sacrospinous, iliococcygeus) ♀

🔪 14.2 ⚕ 14.2 **FUD** 090 J 80 ▢

AMA: 2015,Jan,16; 2014,Jan,11

57283 intra-peritoneal approach (uterosacral, levator myorrhaphy) ♀
Do not report with (57556, 58263, 58270, 58280, 58292, 58294)
🚑 19.6 ⚕ 19.6 **FUD** 090 J 80 💻
AMA: 2015,Jan,16; 2014,Jan,11; 2012,Jan,15-42; 2011,May,9

57284 Paravaginal defect repair (including repair of cystocele, if performed); open abdominal approach ♀
Do not report with (51840-51841, 51990, 57240, 57260-57265, 58152, 58267)
🚑 23.2 ⚕ 23.2 **FUD** 090 J 80 💻
AMA: 2015,Jan,16; 2014,Jan,11; 2012,Jan,15-42; 2011,Jan,11; 2010,Jun,6-7

57285 vaginal approach ♀
Do not report with (51990, 57240, 57260-57265, 58267)
🚑 19.1 ⚕ 19.1 **FUD** 090 J 80
AMA: 2015,Jan,16; 2014,Jan,11; 2010,Jun,6-7

57287 Removal or revision of sling for stress incontinence (eg, fascia or synthetic) ♀
🚑 19.3 ⚕ 19.3 **FUD** 090 02 G2 80
AMA: 2015,Jan,16; 2014,Jan,11; 2012,Jan,15-42; 2011,Jan,11

57288 Sling operation for stress incontinence (eg, fascia or synthetic) ♀
INCLUDES Millin-Read operation
EXCLUDES Sling operation for stress incontinence performed laparoscopically (51992)
🚑 20.3 ⚕ 20.3 **FUD** 090 J A2 80 💻
AMA: 2015,Jan,16; 2014,Jan,11; 2012,Jan,15-42; 2011,Jan,11

57289 Pereyra procedure, including anterior colporrhaphy ♀
🚑 20.9 ⚕ 20.9 **FUD** 090 J A2 80 💻
AMA: 2015,Jan,16; 2014,Jan,11

57291 Construction of artificial vagina; without graft ♀
INCLUDES McIndoe vaginal construction
🚑 15.0 ⚕ 15.0 **FUD** 090 T A2 80 💻
AMA: 2014,Jan,11

57292 with graft ♀
🚑 23.1 ⚕ 23.1 **FUD** 090 J 80
AMA: 2014,Jan,11

57295 Revision (including removal) of prosthetic vaginal graft; vaginal approach ♀
EXCLUDES Laparoscopic approach (57426)
🚑 13.5 ⚕ 13.5 **FUD** 090 T G2 80
AMA: 2014,Jan,11

57296 open abdominal approach ♀
EXCLUDES Laparoscopic approach (57426)
🚑 26.5 ⚕ 26.5 **FUD** 090 C 80
AMA: 2014,Jan,11

57300 Closure of rectovaginal fistula; vaginal or transanal approach ♀
🚑 16.2 ⚕ 16.2 **FUD** 090 T A2 80 💻
AMA: 2014,Jan,11

57305 abdominal approach ♀
🚑 26.8 ⚕ 26.8 **FUD** 090 C 80
AMA: 2014,Jan,11

57307 abdominal approach, with concomitant colostomy ♀
🚑 30.9 ⚕ 30.9 **FUD** 090 C 80
AMA: 2014,Jan,11

57308 transperineal approach, with perineal body reconstruction, with or without levator plication ♀
🚑 18.1 ⚕ 18.1 **FUD** 090 C 80 💻
AMA: 2014,Jan,11

57310 Closure of urethrovaginal fistula; ♀
🚑 13.1 ⚕ 13.1 **FUD** 090 J 80 💻
AMA: 2014,Jan,11

57311 with bulbocavernosus transplant ♀
🚑 15.0 ⚕ 15.0 **FUD** 090 C 80 💻
AMA: 2014,Jan,11

57320 Closure of vesicovaginal fistula; vaginal approach ♀
EXCLUDES Cystostomy, concomitant (51020-51040, 51101-51102)
🚑 15.1 ⚕ 15.1 **FUD** 090 J G2 80 💻
AMA: 2014,Jan,11

57330 transvesical and vaginal approach ♀
EXCLUDES Vesicovaginal fistula closure, abdominal approach (51900)
🚑 21.2 ⚕ 21.2 **FUD** 090 J 80 💻
AMA: 2014,Jan,11

57335 Vaginoplasty for intersex state ♀
🚑 31.8 ⚕ 31.8 **FUD** 090 T 80 💻
AMA: 2014,Jan,11

57400-57415 Treatment of Vaginal Disorders Under Anesthesia

57400 Dilation of vagina under anesthesia (other than local) ♀
🚑 3.79 ⚕ 3.79 **FUD** 000 T A2 80 💻
AMA: 2014,Jan,11

57410 Pelvic examination under anesthesia (other than local) ♀
🚑 3.09 ⚕ 3.09 **FUD** 000 T A2
AMA: 2015,Jan,16; 2014,Jan,11

57415 Removal of impacted vaginal foreign body (separate procedure) under anesthesia (other than local) ♀
EXCLUDES Removal of impacted vaginal foreign body without anesthesia, report with appropriate E&M code
🚑 4.56 ⚕ 4.56 **FUD** 010 T A2 80 💻
AMA: 2014,Jan,11

57420-57426 Endoscopic Vaginal Procedures

57420 Colposcopy of the entire vagina, with cervix if present; ♀
EXCLUDES Colposcopic procedures and/or examinations:
Cervix (57452-57461)
Vulva (56820-56821)
Code also endometrial sampling (biopsy) performed at the same time as colposcopy (58110)
Code also modifier 51 for colposcopic procedures of different sites, as appropriate
🚑 2.65 ⚕ 3.37 **FUD** 000 T P3
AMA: 2015,Jan,16; 2014,Jan,11

57421 with biopsy(s) of vagina/cervix ♀
EXCLUDES Colposcopic procedures and/or examinations:
Cervix (57452-57461)
Vulva (56820-56821)
Code also endometrial sampling (biopsy) performed at the same time as colposcopy (58110)
Code also modifier 51 for colposcopic procedures of multiple sites, as appropriate
🚑 3.56 ⚕ 4.49 **FUD** 000 T P3 💻 P0
AMA: 2015,Jan,16; 2014,Jan,11; 2012,Jan,15-42; 2011,Jan,11

57423 Paravaginal defect repair (including repair of cystocele, if performed), laparoscopic approach ♀
Do not report with (49320, 51840-51841, 51990, 57240, 57260, 58152, 58267)
🚑 26.0 ⚕ 26.0 **FUD** 090 T 80
AMA: 2015,Jan,16; 2014,Jan,11; 2010,Jun,6-7

57425 Laparoscopy, surgical, colpopexy (suspension of vaginal apex) ♀
🚑 27.5 ⚕ 27.5 **FUD** 090 T 80 💻
AMA: 2014,Jan,11

57426 Revision (including removal) of prosthetic vaginal graft, laparoscopic approach ♀
EXCLUDES Open abdominal approach (57296)
Vaginal approach (57295)
🚑 24.0 ⚕ 24.0 **FUD** 090 J G2 80 💻
AMA: 2014,Jan,11

57452-57461 Endoscopic Cervical Procedures

EXCLUDES   Colposcopic procedures and/or examinations:
          Vagina (57420-57421)
          Vulva (56820-56821)
Code also endometrial sampling (biopsy) performed at the same time as colposcopy (58110)

57452   Colposcopy of the cervix including upper/adjacent vagina;   ♀
Do not report with (57454-57461)
🚗 2.64   ✂ 3.10   **FUD** 000   T P3 ⬜
AMA: 2015,Jan,16; 2014,Jan,11

57454   with biopsy(s) of the cervix and endocervical curettage   ♀
🚗 3.89   ✂ 4.35   **FUD** 000   T P3 ⬜ P0
AMA: 2015,Jan,16; 2014,Jan,11; 2012,Jan,15-42; 2011,Aug,9-10

57455   with biopsy(s) of the cervix   ♀
🚗 3.17   ✂ 4.07   **FUD** 000   T P3 ⬜ P0
AMA: 2015,Jan,16; 2014,Jan,11

57456   with endocervical curettage   ♀
Do not report with (57461)
🚗 2.95   ✂ 3.83   **FUD** 000   T P3 ⬜
AMA: 2015,Jan,16; 2014,Jan,11; 2012,Jan,15-42; 2011,Jan,11

57460   with loop electrode biopsy(s) of the cervix   ♀
🚗 4.64   ✂ 8.00   **FUD** 000   T P3 ⬜ P0
AMA: 2015,Jan,16; 2014,Jan,11; 2012,Jan,15-42; 2011,Jan,11

57461   with loop electrode conization of the cervix   ♀
Do not report with (57456)
🚗 5.37   ✂ 9.06   **FUD** 000   T P3 ⬜
AMA: 2015,Jan,16; 2014,Jan,11; 2012,Jan,15-42; 2011,Jan,11

57500-57556 Cervical Procedures: Multiple Techniques

EXCLUDES   Radical surgical procedures (58200-58240)

57500   Biopsy of cervix, single or multiple, or local excision of lesion, with or without fulguration (separate procedure)   ♀
🚗 2.17   ✂ 3.63   **FUD** 000   T P3 ⬜ P0
AMA: 2014,Jan,11

57505   Endocervical curettage (not done as part of a dilation and curettage)   ♀
🚗 2.62   ✂ 2.89   **FUD** 010   T P3 ⬜
AMA: 2015,Jan,16; 2014,Jan,11; 2012,Jan,15-42; 2011,Jan,11

57510   Cautery of cervix; electro or thermal   ♀
🚗 3.29   ✂ 3.72   **FUD** 010   T P3 ⬜
AMA: 2014,Jan,11

57511   cryocautery, initial or repeat   ♀
🚗 3.77   ✂ 4.13   **FUD** 010   T P3 ⬜
AMA: 2014,Jan,11

57513   laser ablation   ♀
🚗 3.83   ✂ 4.13   **FUD** 010   T A2 ⬜
AMA: 2014,Jan,11

57520   Conization of cervix, with or without fulguration, with or without dilation and curettage, with or without repair; cold knife or laser   ♀
EXCLUDES   Dilation and curettage, diagnostic/therapeutic, nonobstetrical (58120)
🚗 7.84   ✂ 8.71   **FUD** 090   T A2 ⬜ P0
AMA: 2015,Jan,16; 2014,Jan,11

57522   loop electrode excision   ♀
🚗 6.94   ✂ 7.47   **FUD** 090   T A2 ⬜
AMA: 2015,Jan,16; 2014,Jan,11; 2012,Jan,15-42; 2011,Jan,11

57530   Trachelectomy (cervicectomy), amputation of cervix (separate procedure)   ♀
🚗 9.92   ✂ 9.92   **FUD** 090   T A2 80 ⬜
AMA: 2014,Jan,11

57531   Radical trachelectomy, with bilateral total pelvic lymphadenectomy and para-aortic lymph node sampling biopsy, with or without removal of tube(s), with or without removal of ovary(s)   ♀
🚗 53.1   ✂ 53.1   **FUD** 090   C 80 ⬜
AMA: 2014,Jan,11

57540   Excision of cervical stump, abdominal approach;   ♀
🚗 22.8   ✂ 22.8   **FUD** 090   C 80 ⬜
AMA: 2014,Jan,11

57545   with pelvic floor repair   ♀
🚗 23.3   ✂ 23.3   **FUD** 090   C 80 ⬜
AMA: 2014,Jan,11

57550   Excision of cervical stump, vaginal approach;   ♀
🚗 11.5   ✂ 11.5   **FUD** 090   T A2 80 ⬜
AMA: 2014,Jan,11

57555   with anterior and/or posterior repair   ♀
🚗 17.0   ✂ 17.0   **FUD** 090   J 80 ⬜
AMA: 2014,Jan,11

57556   with repair of enterocele   ♀
EXCLUDES   Insertion of hemostatic agent/pack for spontaneous/traumatic nonobstetrical vaginal hemorrhage (57180)
          Intrauterine device insertion (58300)
🚗 16.1   ✂ 16.1   **FUD** 090   J A2 80 ⬜
AMA: 2014,Jan,11

57558-57800 Cervical Procedures: Dilation, Suturing, or Instrumentation

57558   Dilation and curettage of cervical stump   ♀
EXCLUDES   Radical surgical procedures (58200-58240)
🚗 3.23   ✂ 3.55   **FUD** 010   T A2
AMA: 2014,Jan,11

57700   Cerclage of uterine cervix, nonobstetrical   ♀
INCLUDES   McDonald cerclage
          Shirodker operation
🚗 8.80   ✂ 8.80   **FUD** 090   T A2 80 ⬜
AMA: 2014,Jan,11

57720   Trachelorrhaphy, plastic repair of uterine cervix, vaginal approach   ♀
INCLUDES   Emmet operation
🚗 8.70   ✂ 8.70   **FUD** 090   T A2 80 ⬜
AMA: 2014,Jan,11

57800   Dilation of cervical canal, instrumental (separate procedure)   ♀
🚗 1.40   ✂ 1.73   **FUD** 000   T P3 ⬜
AMA: 2014,Jan,11

58100-58120 Procedures Involving the Endometrium

58100   Endometrial sampling (biopsy) with or without endocervical sampling (biopsy), without cervical dilation, any method (separate procedure)   ♀
EXCLUDES   Endocervical curettage only (57505)
          Endometrial sampling (biopsy) performed in conjunction with colposcopy (58110)
🚗 2.49   ✂ 3.09   **FUD** 000   T P3 ⬜ P0
AMA: 2014,Jan,11

+ **58110**   Endometrial sampling (biopsy) performed in conjunction with colposcopy (List separately in addition to code for primary procedure)   ♀
Code first colposcopy (57420-57421, 57452-57461)
🚗 1.18   ✂ 1.37   **FUD** ZZZ   N N1 80
AMA: 2015,Jan,16; 2014,Jan,11

Genital System

58120   58120 — 58294

58120   **Dilation and curettage, diagnostic and/or therapeutic (nonobstetrical)** ♀

> **EXCLUDES**   *Postpartum hemorrhage (59160)*

🚗 6.25   ☙ 7.34   **FUD** 010   T A2

AMA: 2015,Jan,16; 2014,Jan,11; 2012,Jan,15-42; 2011,Jan,11

58140-58146 Myomectomy Procedures

58140   **Myomectomy, excision of fibroid tumor(s) of uterus, 1 to 4 intramural myoma(s) with total weight of 250 g or less and/or removal of surface myomas; abdominal approach** ♀

🚗 26.2   ☙ 26.2   **FUD** 090   C 80

AMA: 2015,Jan,16; 2014,Jan,11; 2012,Jan,15-42; 2011,Jan,11

58145   **vaginal approach** ♀

🚗 15.5   ☙ 15.5   **FUD** 090   T A2 80

AMA: 2014,Jan,11

58146   **Myomectomy, excision of fibroid tumor(s) of uterus, 5 or more intramural myomas and/or intramural myomas with total weight greater than 250 g, abdominal approach** ♀

Do not report with (58140-58145, 58150-58240)

🚗 32.7   ☙ 32.7   **FUD** 090   C 80

AMA: 2015,Jan,16; 2014,Jan,11; 2012,Jan,15-42; 2011,Jan,11

58150-58294 Abdominal and Vaginal Hysterectomies

CMS: 100-3,230.3 Sterilization

> **EXCLUDES**   *Destruction/excision of endometriomas, open method (49203-49205, 58957-58958)*
> *Paracentesis (49082-49084)*
> *Pelvic laparotomy (49000)*
> *Secondary closure disruption or evisceration of abdominal wall (49900)*

58150   **Total abdominal hysterectomy (corpus and cervix), with or without removal of tube(s), with or without removal of ovary(s);** ♀

🚗 28.9   ☙ 28.9   **FUD** 090   C 80 P0

AMA: 2015,Jan,16; 2014,Jan,11; 2012,Jan,15-42; 2011,Jan,11

58152   **with colpo-urethrocystopexy (eg, Marshall-Marchetti-Krantz, Burch)** ♀

> **EXCLUDES**   *Urethrocystopexy without hysterectomy (51840-51841)*

🚗 35.6   ☙ 35.6   **FUD** 090   C 80 P0

AMA: 2015,Jan,16; 2014,Jan,11; 2010,Jun,6-7

58180   **Supracervical abdominal hysterectomy (subtotal hysterectomy), with or without removal of tube(s), with or without removal of ovary(s)** ♀

🚗 27.4   ☙ 27.4   **FUD** 090   C 80 P0

AMA: 2014,Jan,11

58200   **Total abdominal hysterectomy, including partial vaginectomy, with para-aortic and pelvic lymph node sampling, with or without removal of tube(s), with or without removal of ovary(s)** ♀

🚗 39.2   ☙ 39.2   **FUD** 090   C 80 P0

AMA: 2014,Jan,11

58210   **Radical abdominal hysterectomy, with bilateral total pelvic lymphadenectomy and para-aortic lymph node sampling (biopsy), with or without removal of tube(s), with or without removal of ovary(s)** ♀

> **INCLUDES**   Wertheim hysterectomy
> **EXCLUDES**   *Chemotherapy (96401-96549)*
> *Hysterectomy, radical, with transposition of ovary(s) (58825)*

🚗 52.8   ☙ 52.8   **FUD** 090   C 80 P0

AMA: 2015,Jan,16; 2014,Jan,11; 2012,May,14-15

58240   **Pelvic exenteration for gynecologic malignancy, with total abdominal hysterectomy or cervicectomy, with or without removal of tube(s), with or without removal of ovary(s), with removal of bladder and ureteral transplantations, and/or abdominoperineal resection of rectum and colon and colostomy, or any combination thereof** ♀

> **EXCLUDES**   *Chemotherapy (96401-96549)*
> *Pelvic exenteration for male genital malignancy or lower urinary tract (51597)*

🚗 83.6   ☙ 83.6   **FUD** 090   C 80 P0

AMA: 2014,Jan,11

58260   **Vaginal hysterectomy, for uterus 250 g or less;** ♀

🚗 23.4   ☙ 23.4   **FUD** 090   J 80 P0

AMA: 2015,Jan,16; 2014,Jan,11; 2011,May,9

58262   **with removal of tube(s), and/or ovary(s)** ♀

🚗 26.2   ☙ 26.2   **FUD** 090   J 80 P0

AMA: 2014,Jan,11

58263   **with removal of tube(s), and/or ovary(s), with repair of enterocele** ♀

🚗 28.1   ☙ 28.1   **FUD** 090   J 80 P0

AMA: 2014,Jan,11

58267   **with colpo-urethrocystopexy (Marshall-Marchetti-Krantz type, Pereyra type) with or without endoscopic control** ♀

🚗 30.0   ☙ 30.0   **FUD** 090   C 80 P0

AMA: 2015,Jan,16; 2014,Jan,11; 2010,Jun,6-7

58270   **with repair of enterocele** ♀

> **EXCLUDES**   *Vaginal hysterectomy with repair of enterocele and removal of tubes and/or ovaries (58263)*

🚗 25.0   ☙ 25.0   **FUD** 090   J 80 P0

AMA: 2014,Jan,11

58275   **Vaginal hysterectomy, with total or partial vaginectomy;** ♀

🚗 28.0   ☙ 28.0   **FUD** 090   C 80 P0

AMA: 2014,Jan,11

58280   **with repair of enterocele** ♀

🚗 29.8   ☙ 29.8   **FUD** 090   C 80 P0

AMA: 2014,Jan,11

58285   **Vaginal hysterectomy, radical (Schauta type operation)** ♀

🚗 41.1   ☙ 41.1   **FUD** 090   C 80 P0

AMA: 2015,Jan,16; 2014,Jan,11

58290   **Vaginal hysterectomy, for uterus greater than 250 g;** ♀

🚗 32.6   ☙ 32.6   **FUD** 090   J 80 P0

AMA: 2014,Jan,11

58291   **with removal of tube(s) and/or ovary(s)** ♀

🚗 35.3   ☙ 35.3   **FUD** 090   J 80 P0

AMA: 2014,Jan,11

58292   **with removal of tube(s) and/or ovary(s), with repair of enterocele** ♀

🚗 37.2   ☙ 37.2   **FUD** 090   J 80 P0

AMA: 2014,Jan,11

58293   **with colpo-urethrocystopexy (Marshall-Marchetti-Krantz type, Pereyra type) with or without endoscopic control** ♀

🚗 38.7   ☙ 38.7   **FUD** 090   C 80 P0

AMA: 2014,Jan,11

58294   **with repair of enterocele** ♀

🚗 34.5   ☙ 34.5   **FUD** 090   J 80 P0

AMA: 2014,Jan,11

26/TC PC/TC Comp Only	A2-Z4 ASC Pmt	50 Bilateral	♂ Male Only	♀ Female Only	🚗 Facility RVU	☙ Non-Facility RVU
AMA: CPT Asst	CMS: Pub 100	A-Y OPPSI	80/80 Surg Assist Allowed / w/Doc		🔬 Lab Crosswalk	☢ Radiology Crosswalk

226   Medicare (Red Text)   CPT © 2015 American Medical Association. All Rights Reserved. (Black Text)   © 2015 Optum360, LLC (Blue Text)

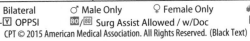
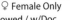
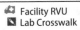

58300-58323 Contraception and Reproduction Procedures

58300   Insertion of intrauterine device (IUD)   ♀

> **EXCLUDES**   *Insertion non-biodegradeable contraceptive drug delivery implant (11981)*
> *Removal of implantable contraceptive capsules (11976, 11982)*
>
> 🔧 1.46   ⚖ 1.98   **FUD** XXX   E
>
> **AMA:** 2015,Jan,16; 2014,Jan,11; 2012,Jan,15-42; 2011,Jan,11

58301   Removal of intrauterine device (IUD)   ♀

> **EXCLUDES**   *Insertion and/or removal of implantable contraceptive capsules (11976, 11981)*
>
> 🔧 1.93   ⚖ 2.69   **FUD** 000   02 P3 80
>
> **AMA:** 2015,Jan,16; 2014,Jan,11; 2012,Jan,15-42; 2011,Jan,11

58321   Artificial insemination; intra-cervical   ♀

> 🔧 1.39   ⚖ 2.16   **FUD** 000   T P3 80
>
> **AMA:** 2014,Jan,11

58322   intra-uterine   ♀

> 🔧 1.67   ⚖ 2.43   **FUD** 000   T P3 80
>
> **AMA:** 2014,Jan,11

58323   Sperm washing for artificial insemination   ♀

> 🔧 0.35   ⚖ 0.44   **FUD** 000   T P3 80
>
> **AMA:** 2014,Jan,11

58340-58350 Fallopian Tube Patency and Brachytherapy Procedures

58340   Catheterization and introduction of saline or contrast material for saline infusion sonohysterography (SIS) or hysterosalpingography   ♀

HSG (handwritten)

> 📷 (74740, 76831)
>
> 🔧 1.66   ⚖ 3.36   **FUD** 000   N N1
>
> **AMA:** 2015,Jan,16; 2014,Jan,11; 2012,Jan,15-42; 2011,Jan,11

(handwritten margin note:) se 76831 for ...ologic supervision ...interp.

58345   Transcervical introduction of fallopian tube catheter for diagnosis and/or re-establishing patency (any method), with or without hysterosalpingography   ♀

> 📷 (74742)
>
> 🔧 7.92   ⚖ 7.92   **FUD** 010   T R2 80 50
>
> **AMA:** 2015,Jan,16; 2014,Jan,11; 2012,Jan,15-42; 2011,Jan,11

58346   Insertion of Heyman capsules for clinical brachytherapy   ♀

> **EXCLUDES**   *Insertion of radioelement sources or ribbons (77761-77763, 77770-77772)*
> *The placement of needles or catheters into the pelvic organs and/or genitalia (except for the prostate) for interstitial radioelement application (55920)*
>
> 🔧 12.5   ⚖ 12.5   **FUD** 090   T A2
>
> **AMA:** 2015,Jan,16; 2014,Jan,11

58350   Chromotubation of oviduct, including materials   ♀

> 🔧 2.24   ⚖ 2.74   **FUD** 010   J A2 50
>
> **AMA:** 2015,Jan,16; 2014,Jan,11; 2012,Jan,15-42; 2011,Jan,11

Mild pressure drives solution into tubes
Uterus
Ovary
Cervix
Delivery apparatus
Saline or medicated solution is injected into uterus

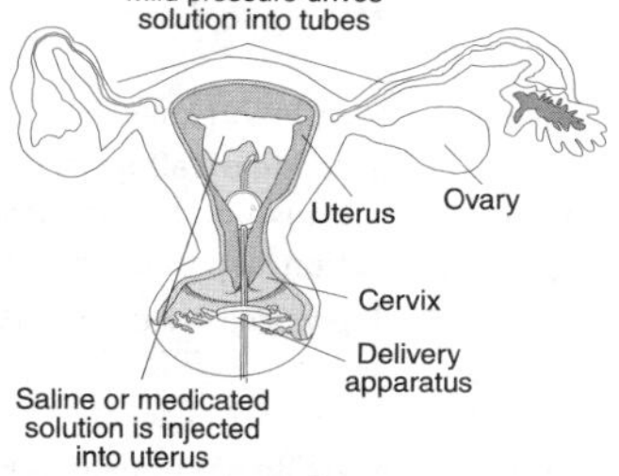

58353-58356 Ablation of Endometrium

> **EXCLUDES**   *Destruction/excision of endometriomas, open method (49203-49205)*

58353   Endometrial ablation, thermal, without hysteroscopic guidance   ♀

> **EXCLUDES**   *Endometrial ablation performed hysteroscopically (58563)*
>
> 🔧 6.23   ⚖ 28.3   **FUD** 010   J A2
>
> **AMA:** 2015,Jan,16; 2014,Jan,11; 2012,Jan,15-42; 2011,Jan,11

58356   Endometrial cryoablation with ultrasonic guidance, including endometrial curettage, when performed   ♀

> Do not report with (58100, 58120, 58340, 76700, 76856)
>
> 🔧 9.83   ⚖ 52.9   **FUD** 010   J P3 80
>
> **AMA:** 2014,Jan,11

58400-58540 Uterine Repairs: Vaginal and Abdominal

58400   Uterine suspension, with or without shortening of round ligaments, with or without shortening of sacrouterine ligaments; (separate procedure)   ♀

> **INCLUDES**   Alexander's operation
> Baldy-Webster operation
> Manchester colporrhaphy
>
> **EXCLUDES**   *Anastomosis of tubes to uterus (58752)*
>
> 🔧 12.4   ⚖ 12.4   **FUD** 090   C 80
>
> **AMA:** 2014,Jan,11

58410   with presacral sympathectomy   ♀

> **INCLUDES**   Alexander's operation
>
> **EXCLUDES**   *Anastomosis of tubes to uterus (58752)*
>
> 🔧 22.8   ⚖ 22.8   **FUD** 090   C 80
>
> **AMA:** 2015,Jan,16; 2014,Jan,11; 2012,Jan,15-42; 2011,Jan,11

58520   Hysterorrhaphy, repair of ruptured uterus (nonobstetrical)   ♀

> 🔧 22.7   ⚖ 22.7   **FUD** 090   C 80
>
> **AMA:** 2014,Jan,11

58540   Hysteroplasty, repair of uterine anomaly (Strassman type)   ♀

> **INCLUDES**   Strassman type
>
> **EXCLUDES**   *Vesicouterine fistula closure (51920)*
>
> 🔧 25.7   ⚖ 25.7   **FUD** 090   C 80
>
> **AMA:** 2014,Jan,11

58541-58554 Laparoscopic Procedures of the Uterus

CMS: 100-3,230.3 Sterilization

> **INCLUDES**   Diagnostic laparoscopy
>
> **EXCLUDES**   *Hysteroscopy (58555-58565)*

58541   Laparoscopy, surgical, supracervical hysterectomy, for uterus 250 g or less;   ♀

> Do not report with (49320, 57000, 57180, 57410, 58140-58146, 58545-58546, 58561, 58661, 58670-58671)
>
> 🔧 20.3   ⚖ 20.3   **FUD** 090   T R2 80
>
> **AMA:** 2015,Jan,16; 2014,Jan,11

58542   with removal of tube(s) and/or ovary(s)   ♀

> Do not report with (49320, 57000, 57180, 57410, 58140-58146, 58545-58546, 58561, 58661, 58670-58671)
>
> 🔧 23.2   ⚖ 23.2   **FUD** 090   T R2 80
>
> **AMA:** 2015,Jan,16; 2014,Jan,11

58543   Laparoscopy, surgical, supracervical hysterectomy, for uterus greater than 250 g;   ♀

> Do not report with (49320, 57000, 57180, 57410, 58140-58146, 58545-58546, 58561, 58661, 58670-58671)
>
> 🔧 23.5   ⚖ 23.5   **FUD** 090   T 80
>
> **AMA:** 2015,Jan,16; 2014,Jan,11

58544   with removal of tube(s) and/or ovary(s)   ♀

> Do not report with (49320, 57000, 57180, 57410, 58140-58146, 58545-58546, 58561, 58661, 58670-58671)
>
> 🔧 25.7   ⚖ 25.7   **FUD** 090   T 80
>
> **AMA:** 2015,Jan,16; 2014,Jan,11

58545   Laparoscopy, surgical, myomectomy, excision; 1 to 4 intramural myomas with total weight of 250 g or less and/or removal of surface myomas   ♀

> 🔧 25.8   ⚖ 25.8   **FUD** 090   T A2 80
>
> **AMA:** 2014,Jan,11

58546   5 or more intramural myomas and/or intramural myomas with total weight greater than 250 g   ♀

> 🔧 31.9   ⚖ 31.9   **FUD** 090   T A2 80
>
> **AMA:** 2015,Jan,16; 2014,Jan,11; 2012,Jan,15-42; 2011,Jan,11

58548 Laparoscopy, surgical, with radical hysterectomy, with bilateral total pelvic lymphadenectomy and para-aortic lymph node sampling (biopsy), with removal of tube(s) and ovary(s), if performed ♀

Do not report with (38570-38572, 58210, 58285, 58550-58554)

📋 54.5 ✂ 54.5 **FUD** 090 [C] [80]

AMA: 2015,Jan,16; 2014,Jan,11

58550 Laparoscopy, surgical, with vaginal hysterectomy, for uterus 250 g or less; ♀

Do not report with (49320, 57000, 57180, 57410, 58140-58146, 58545-58546, 58561, 58661, 58670-58671)

📋 25.0 ✂ 25.0 **FUD** 090 [T] [A2] [80]

AMA: 2015,Jan,16; 2014,Jan,11

58552 with removal of tube(s) and/or ovary(s) ♀

Do not report with (49320, 57000, 57180, 57410, 58140-58146, 58545-58546, 58561, 58661, 58670-58671)

📋 28.1 ✂ 28.1 **FUD** 090 [T] [62] [80]

AMA: 2015,Jan,16; 2014,Jan,11

58553 Laparoscopy, surgical, with vaginal hysterectomy, for uterus greater than 250 g; ♀

Do not report with (49320, 57000, 57180, 57410, 58140-58146, 58545-58546, 58561, 58661, 58670-58671)

📋 32.2 ✂ 32.2 **FUD** 090 [T] [80]

AMA: 2014,Jan,11

58554 with removal of tube(s) and/or ovary(s) ♀

Do not report with (49320, 57000, 57180, 57410, 58140-58146, 58545-58546, 58561, 58661, 58670-58671)

📋 37.7 ✂ 37.7 **FUD** 090 [T] [80]

AMA: 2014,Jan,11

58555-58565 Hysteroscopy

INCLUDES Diagnostic hysteroscopy
EXCLUDES Laparoscopy (58541-58554, 58570-58578)

58555 Hysteroscopy, diagnostic (separate procedure) ♀

📋 5.41 ✂ 8.59 **FUD** 000 [T] [A2] [80]

AMA: 2015,Jan,16; 2014,Jan,11

Some common sites of endometriosis, in descending order of frequency:
(1) ovary,
(2) cul de sac,
(3) uterosacral ligaments,
(4) broad ligaments,
(5) fallopian tube,
(6) uterovesical fold,
(7) round ligament,
(8) vermiform appendix,
(9) vagina,
(10) rectovaginal septum

58558 Hysteroscopy, surgical; with sampling (biopsy) of endometrium and/or polypectomy, with or without D & C ♀

📋 7.60 ✂ 11.2 **FUD** 000 [T] [A2] [P0]

AMA: 2015,Jan,16; 2014,Jan,11; 2012,Jan,15-42; 2011,Jan,11

58559 with lysis of intrauterine adhesions (any method) ♀

📋 9.71 ✂ 9.71 **FUD** 000 [J] [A2]

AMA: 2015,Jan,16; 2014,Jan,11

58560 with division or resection of intrauterine septum (any method) ♀

📋 10.9 ✂ 10.9 **FUD** 000 [J] [A2] [80]

AMA: 2015,Jan,16; 2014,Jan,11

58561 with removal of leiomyomata *Myosure* ♀

📋 15.5 ✂ 15.5 **FUD** 000 [J] [A2] [80]

AMA: 2015,Jan,16; 2014,Jan,11 → *Fibroid*

58562 with removal of impacted foreign body ♀

📋 8.27 ✂ 11.6 **FUD** 000 [T] [A2]

AMA: 2015,Jan,16; 2014,Jan,11; 2012,Jan,15-42; 2011,Jan,11

58563 with endometrial ablation (eg, endometrial resection, electrosurgical ablation, thermoablation) *Novasure* ♀

📋 9.73 ✂ 46.8 **FUD** 000 [J] [A2] [80]

AMA: 2015,Jan,13; 2015,Jan,16; 2014,Jan,11; 2012,Feb,11; 2012,Jan,15-42; 2011,Jan,11

58565 with bilateral fallopian tube cannulation to induce occlusion by placement of permanent implants ♀

Code also modifier 52 when a unilateral procedure is performed
Do not report with (57800, 58555)

📋 12.2 ✂ 52.6 **FUD** 090 [J] [A2]

AMA: 2015,Jan,16; 2014,Jan,11; 2012,Feb,11; 2012,Jan,15-42; 2011,Jan,9-10

58570-58579 Other Uterine Endoscopy

INCLUDES Diagnostic laparoscopy
EXCLUDES Hysteroscopy (58555-58565)

58570 Laparoscopy, surgical, with total hysterectomy, for uterus 250 g or less; ♀

Do not report with (49320, 57000, 57180, 57410, 58140-58146, 58150, 58545-58546, 58561, 58661, 58670-58671)

📋 22.1 ✂ 22.1 **FUD** 090 [T] [62] [80]

AMA: 2014,Jan,11

58571 with removal of tube(s) and/or ovary(s) ♀

Do not report with (49320, 57100, 57180, 57410, 58140-58146, 58150, 58545-58546, 58561, 58661, 58670-58671)

📋 25.6 ✂ 25.6 **FUD** 090 [T] [62] [80]

AMA: 2015,Jan,16; 2014,Jan,11; 2012,Aug,13-14; 2012,May,14-15

58572 Laparoscopy, surgical, with total hysterectomy, for uterus greater than 250 g; ♀

Do not report with (49320, 57000, 57180, 57410, 58140-58146, 58150, 58545-58546, 58561, 58661, 58670-58671)

📋 28.9 ✂ 28.9 **FUD** 090 [T] [80]

AMA: 2014,Jan,11

58573 with removal of tube(s) and/or ovary(s) ♀

Do not report with (49320, 57000, 57180, 57410, 58140-58146, 58150, 58545-58546, 58561, 58661, 58670-58671)

📋 34.6 ✂ 34.6 **FUD** 090 [T] [80]

AMA: 2015,Jan,16; 2014,Jan,11; 2012,Aug,13-14; 2012,May,14-15

58578 Unlisted laparoscopy procedure, uterus ♀

📋 0.00 ✂ 0.00 **FUD** YYY [T] [80] [50]

AMA: 2015,Jan,16; 2014,Jan,11; 2012,Jan,15-42; 2011,Jan,11

58579 Unlisted hysteroscopy procedure, uterus ♀

📋 0.00 ✂ 0.00 **FUD** YYY [T] [80] [50]

AMA: 2015,Jan,16; 2014,Jan,11

58600-58615 Sterilization by Tubal Interruption

CMS: 100-3,230.3 Sterilization

EXCLUDES Destruction/excision of endometriomas, open method (49203-49205, 58957-58958)

58600 Ligation or transection of fallopian tube(s), abdominal or vaginal approach, unilateral or bilateral ♀

INCLUDES Madlener operation

📋 10.3 ✂ 10.3 **FUD** 090 [T] [62] [80]

AMA: 2015,Jan,16; 2014,Jan,11

58605 Ligation or transection of fallopian tube(s), abdominal or vaginal approach, postpartum, unilateral or bilateral, during same hospitalization (separate procedure) ♀

EXCLUDES Laparoscopic methods (58670-58671)

📋 9.35 ✂ 9.35 **FUD** 090 [C] [80]

AMA: 2015,Jan,16; 2014,Jan,11

+ 58611 Ligation or transection of fallopian tube(s) when done at the time of cesarean delivery or intra-abdominal surgery (not a separate procedure) (List separately in addition to code for primary procedure) ♀

Code first primary procedure

📋 2.20 ✂ 2.20 **FUD** ZZZ [C] [80]

AMA: 2014,Jan,11

58615 **Occlusion of fallopian tube(s) by device (eg, band, clip, Falope ring) vaginal or suprapubic approach** ♀

EXCLUDES Laparoscopic method (58671)
Lysis of adnexal adhesions (58740)
🚑 6.92 ⚕ 6.92 **FUD** 010 [T] [G2] [80] [▯]
AMA: 2015,Jan,16; 2014,Jan,11

58660-58679 Endoscopic Procedures Fallopian Tubes and/or Ovaries

CMS: 100-3,230.3 Sterilization

INCLUDES Diagnostic laparoscopy
EXCLUDES Laparoscopy with biopsy of fallopian tube or ovary (49321)
Laparoscopy with ovarian cyst aspiration (49322)

58660 **Laparoscopy, surgical; with lysis of adhesions (salpingolysis, ovariolysis) (separate procedure)**
🚑 19.1 ⚕ 19.1 **FUD** 090 [T] [A2] [80] [▯]
AMA: 2015,Jan,16; 2014,Jan,11; 2012,Jan,15-42; 2011,Dec,14-18; 2011,Jan,11

58661 **with removal of adnexal structures (partial or total oophorectomy and/or salpingectomy)** ♀
🚑 18.5 ⚕ 18.5 **FUD** 010 [T] [A2] [80] [50] [▯]
AMA: 2015,Jan,16; 2014,Jan,11; 2012,Jan,15-42; 2011,Jan,11; 2010,May,9

58662 **with fulguration or excision of lesions of the ovary, pelvic viscera, or peritoneal surface by any method** ♀
🚑 20.2 ⚕ 20.2 **FUD** 090 [T] [A2] [80] [▯]
AMA: 2015,Jan,16; 2014,Jan,11

58670 **with fulguration of oviducts (with or without transection)** ♀
🚑 10.3 ⚕ 10.3 **FUD** 090 [T] [A2]
AMA: 2015,Jan,16; 2014,Jan,11

58671 **with occlusion of oviducts by device (eg, band, clip, or Falope ring)** ♀
🚑 10.3 ⚕ 10.3 **FUD** 090 [T] [A2] [▯]
AMA: 2015,Jan,16; 2014,Jan,11

58672 **with fimbrioplasty** ♀
🚑 20.8 ⚕ 20.8 **FUD** 090 [T] [A2] [80] [50] [▯]
AMA: 2015,Jan,16; 2014,Jan,11

58673 **with salpingostomy (salpingoneostomy)** ♀
🚑 22.6 ⚕ 22.6 **FUD** 090 [T] [A2] [80] [50] [▯]
AMA: 2015,Jan,16; 2014,Jan,11; 2012,Jan,15-42; 2011,Jan,11

58679 **Unlisted laparoscopy procedure, oviduct, ovary** ♀
🚑 0.00 ⚕ 0.00 **FUD** YYY [T] [80] [50]
AMA: 2015,Jan,16; 2014,Jan,11

58700-58770 Open Procedures Fallopian Tubes, with/without Ovaries

EXCLUDES Destruction/excision of endometriomas, open method (49203-49205, 58957-58958)

58700 **Salpingectomy, complete or partial, unilateral or bilateral (separate procedure)** ♀
🚑 22.3 ⚕ 22.3 **FUD** 090 [C] [80] [▯]
AMA: 2014,Jan,11

58720 **Salpingo-oophorectomy, complete or partial, unilateral or bilateral (separate procedure)** ♀
🚑 21.0 ⚕ 21.0 **FUD** 090 [C] [80] [▯]
AMA: 2015,Jan,16; 2014,Jan,11; 2012,Jan,15-42; 2011,Jan,11

58740 **Lysis of adhesions (salpingolysis, ovariolysis)** ♀
EXCLUDES Excision/fulguration of lesions performed laparoscopically (58662)
Laparoscopic method (58660)
🚑 25.2 ⚕ 25.2 **FUD** 090 [C] [80] [▯]
AMA: 2015,Jan,16; 2014,Jan,11

58750 **Tubotubal anastomosis** ♀
🚑 25.9 ⚕ 25.9 **FUD** 090 [C] [80] [50]
AMA: 2014,Jan,11

Occluded section of tube is excised

Ovary

Tube ends are sutured

58752 **Tubouterine implantation** ♀
🚑 24.7 ⚕ 24.7 **FUD** 090 [C] [80] [50]
AMA: 2014,Jan,11

58760 **Fimbrioplasty** ♀
EXCLUDES Laparoscopic method (58672)
🚑 22.9 ⚕ 22.9 **FUD** 090 [C] [80] [50]
AMA: 2015,Jan,16; 2014,Jan,11

58770 **Salpingostomy (salpingoneostomy)** ♀
EXCLUDES Laparoscopic method (58673)
🚑 24.1 ⚕ 24.1 **FUD** 090 [T] [80] [50]
AMA: 2015,Jan,16; 2014,Jan,11

58800-58925 Open Procedures: Ovary

CMS: 100-3,230.3 Sterilization

EXCLUDES Destruction/excision of endometriomas, open method (49203-49205, 58957-58958)

58800 **Drainage of ovarian cyst(s), unilateral or bilateral (separate procedure); vaginal approach** ♀
🚑 8.46 ⚕ 9.01 **FUD** 090 [T] [A2]
AMA: 2014,Jan,11; 2013,Nov,9

58805 **abdominal approach** ♀
🚑 11.4 ⚕ 11.4 **FUD** 090 [T] [G2] [80] [▯]
AMA: 2014,Jan,11; 2013,Nov,9

58820 **Drainage of ovarian abscess; vaginal approach, open** ♀
🚑 8.84 ⚕ 8.84 **FUD** 090 [T] [A2] [80] [50] [▯]
AMA: 2014,Jan,11; 2013,Nov,9

58822 **abdominal approach** ♀
🚑 19.8 ⚕ 19.8 **FUD** 090 [C] [80] [50] [▯]
AMA: 2014,Jan,11; 2013,Nov,9

58825 **Transposition, ovary(s)** ♀
🚑 21.7 ⚕ 21.7 **FUD** 090 [C] [80]
AMA: 2014,Jan,11

58900 **Biopsy of ovary, unilateral or bilateral (separate procedure)** ♀
EXCLUDES Laparoscopy with biopsy of fallopian tube or ovary (49321)
🚑 11.7 ⚕ 11.7 **FUD** 090 [T] [A2] [80] [▯] [PQ]
AMA: 2015,Jan,16; 2014,Jan,11

58920 **Wedge resection or bisection of ovary, unilateral or bilateral** ♀
🚑 20.2 ⚕ 20.2 **FUD** 090 [J] [80] [▯]
AMA: 2014,Jan,11

58925 **Ovarian cystectomy, unilateral or bilateral** ♀
🚑 21.3 ⚕ 21.3 **FUD** 090 [J] [80] [▯]
AMA: 2014,Jan,11

Genital System

58940 — 59025

58940-58960 Removal Ovary(s) with/without Multiple Procedures for Malignancy

CMS: 100-3,230.3 Sterilization

EXCLUDES   Chemotherapy (96401-96549)
Destruction/excision of tumors, cysts, or endometriomas, open method (49203-49205)

58940   Oophorectomy, partial or total, unilateral or bilateral;   ♀

EXCLUDES   Oophorectomy with tumor debulking for ovarian malignancy (58952)

🔲 15.0   ⚖ 15.0   **FUD** 090   C 80 ▣

AMA: 2015,Jan,16; 2014,Jan,11

58943   for ovarian, tubal or primary peritoneal malignancy, with para-aortic and pelvic lymph node biopsies, peritoneal washings, peritoneal biopsies, diaphragmatic assessments, with or without salpingectomy(s), with or without omentectomy   ♀

🔲 33.6   ⚖ 33.6   **FUD** 090   C 80 ▣

AMA: 2014,Jan,11; 2011,Jan,11; 2010,Dec,12

58950   Resection (initial) of ovarian, tubal or primary peritoneal malignancy with bilateral salpingo-oophorectomy and omentectomy;   ♀

EXCLUDES   Resection/tumor debulking of recurrent ovarian/tubal/primary peritoneal/uterine malignancy (58957-58958)

🔲 32.4   ⚖ 32.4   **FUD** 090   C 80 ▣

AMA: 2014,Jan,11; 2011,Jan,11; 2010,Dec,12

58951   with total abdominal hysterectomy, pelvic and limited para-aortic lymphadenectomy   ♀

EXCLUDES   Resection/tumor debulking of recurrent ovarian/tubal/primary peritoneal/uterine malignancy (58957-58958)

🔲 41.6   ⚖ 41.6   **FUD** 090   C 80 ▣ PQ

AMA: 2015,Jan,16; 2014,Jan,11; 2012,Jan,15-42; 2011,Jan,11; 2010,Dec,12

58952   with radical dissection for debulking (ie, radical excision or destruction, intra-abdominal or retroperitoneal tumors)   ♀

EXCLUDES   Resection/tumor debulking of recurrent ovarian/tubal/primary peritoneal/uterine malignancy (58957-58958)

🔲 47.1   ⚖ 47.1   **FUD** 090   C 80 ▣

AMA: 2015,Jan,16; 2014,Jan,11; 2012,Jan,15-42; 2011,Jan,11; 2010,Dec,12

58953   Bilateral salpingo-oophorectomy with omentectomy, total abdominal hysterectomy and radical dissection for debulking;   ♀

🔲 58.3   ⚖ 58.3   **FUD** 090   C 80 ▣ PQ

AMA: 2015,Jan,16; 2014,May,10; 2014,Jan,11; 2011,Jan,11; 2010,Dec,12

58954   with pelvic lymphadenectomy and limited para-aortic lymphadenectomy   ♀

🔲 63.2   ⚖ 63.2   **FUD** 090   C 80 ▣ PQ

AMA: 2015,Jan,16; 2014,Jan,11; 2011,Jan,11; 2010,Dec,12

58956   Bilateral salpingo-oophorectomy with total omentectomy, total abdominal hysterectomy for malignancy   ♀

Do not report with (49255, 58150, 58180, 58262-58263, 58550, 58661, 58700, 58720, 58900, 58925, 58940, 58957-58958)

🔲 39.6   ⚖ 39.6   **FUD** 090   C 80 ▣ PQ

AMA: 2015,Jan,16; 2014,May,10; 2014,Jan,11

58957   Resection (tumor debulking) of recurrent ovarian, tubal, primary peritoneal, uterine malignancy (intra-abdominal, retroperitoneal tumors), with omentectomy, if performed;   ♀

Do not report with (38770, 38780, 44005, 49000, 49203-49215, 49255, 58900-58960)

🔲 45.6   ⚖ 45.6   **FUD** 090   C 80

AMA: 2014,Jan,11

58958   with pelvic lymphadenectomy and limited para-aortic lymphadenectomy   ♀

Do not report with (38770, 38780, 44005, 49000, 49203-49215, 49255, 58900-58960)

🔲 50.0   ⚖ 50.0   **FUD** 090   C 80

AMA: 2014,Jan,11

58960   Laparotomy, for staging or restaging of ovarian, tubal, or primary peritoneal malignancy (second look), with or without omentectomy, peritoneal washing, biopsy of abdominal and pelvic peritoneum, diaphragmatic assessment with pelvic and limited para-aortic lymphadenectomy   ♀

Do not report with (58957-58958)

🔲 28.0   ⚖ 28.0   **FUD** 090   C 80 ▣

AMA: 2014,Jan,11

58970-58999 Procedural Components: In Vitro Fertilization

58970   Follicle puncture for oocyte retrieval, any method   M ♀

🔯 (76948)

🔲 5.72   ⚖ 6.32   **FUD** 000   T A2 80 ▣

AMA: 2014,Jan,11

58974   Embryo transfer, intrauterine   M ♀

🔲 0.00   ⚖ 0.00   **FUD** 000   T A2 80 ▣

AMA: 2014,Jan,11

58976   Gamete, zygote, or embryo intrafallopian transfer, any method   M ♀

EXCLUDES   Adnexal procedures performed laparoscopically (58660-58673)

🔲 5.97   ⚖ 6.94   **FUD** 000   T A2 80 ▣

AMA: 2015,Jan,16; 2014,Jan,11

58999   Unlisted procedure, female genital system (nonobstetrical)   ♀

🔲 0.00   ⚖ 0.00   **FUD** YYY   T

AMA: 2015,Jan,16; 2014,Jan,11; 2012,Jan,15-42; 2011,Jan,11; 2010,Dec,12

59000-59001 Aspiration of Amniotic Fluid

EXCLUDES   Intrauterine fetal transfusion (36460)
Unlisted fetal invasive procedure (59897)

59000   Amniocentesis; diagnostic   M ♀

🔯 (76946)

🔲 2.35   ⚖ 3.61   **FUD** 000   T P3 ▣

AMA: 2015,Jan,16; 2014,Jan,11

59001   therapeutic amniotic fluid reduction (includes ultrasound guidance)   M ♀

🔲 5.24   ⚖ 5.24   **FUD** 000   T R2

AMA: 2015,Jan,16; 2014,Jan,11

59012-59076 Fetal Testing and Treatment

EXCLUDES   Intrauterine fetal transfusion (36460)
Unlisted fetal invasive procedures (59897)

59012   Cordocentesis (intrauterine), any method   M ♀

🔯 (76941)

🔲 5.91   ⚖ 5.91   **FUD** 000   T R2 80 ▣

AMA: 2014,Jan,11

59015   Chorionic villus sampling, any method   M ♀

🔯 (76945)

🔲 3.85   ⚖ 4.50   **FUD** 000   T P3 80 ▣ PQ

AMA: 2015,Jan,16; 2014,Jan,11

59020   Fetal contraction stress test   M ♀

🔲 2.04   ⚖ 2.04   **FUD** 000   T P3 80 ▣

AMA: 2015,Jan,16; 2014,Jan,11

59025   Fetal non-stress test   M ♀

🔲 1.38   ⚖ 1.38   **FUD** 000   T P3 80 ▣

AMA: 2015,Jan,16; 2014,Jan,11; 2012,Jan,15-42; 2011,Jan,11

26/TC PC/TC Comp Only   A2-Z3 ASC Pmt   50 Bilateral   ♂ Male Only   ♀ Female Only   🔲 Facility RVU   ⚖ Non-Facility RVU
AMA: CPT Asst   **CMS:** Pub 100   A-Y OPPSI   80/80 Surg Assist Allowed / w/Doc   ▣ Lab Crosswalk   🔯 Radiology Crosswalk

230   Medicare (Red Text)   CPT © 2015 American Medical Association. All Rights Reserved. (Black Text)   © 2015 Optum360, LLC (Blue Text)

59030 **Fetal scalp blood sampling** Ⓜ ♀

Code also modifier 76 or 77, as appropriate, for repeat fetal scalp blood sampling

🔧 2.89 ⚖ 2.89 **FUD** 000

Ⓣ 80 ▯

AMA: 2014,Jan,11

59050 **Fetal monitoring during labor by consulting physician (ie, non-attending physician) with written report; supervision and interpretation** Ⓜ ♀

🔧 1.48 ⚖ 1.48 **FUD** XXX

Ⓜ 80 ▯

AMA: 2014,Jan,11

59051 **interpretation only** Ⓜ ♀

🔧 1.22 ⚖ 1.22 **FUD** XXX

Ⓑ 80 ▯

AMA: 2014,Jan,11

59070 **Transabdominal amnioinfusion, including ultrasound guidance** Ⓜ ♀

🔧 9.04 ⚖ 11.8 **FUD** 000

Ⓣ 62 80 ▯

AMA: 2015,Jan,16; 2014,Jan,11; 2012,Jan,15-42; 2011,Jan,11

59072 **Fetal umbilical cord occlusion, including ultrasound guidance** Ⓜ ♀

🔧 13.4 ⚖ 13.4 **FUD** 000

Ⓣ 62 ▯

AMA: 2015,Jan,16; 2014,Jan,11; 2012,Jan,15-42; 2011,Jan,11

59074 **Fetal fluid drainage (eg, vesicocentesis, thoracocentesis, paracentesis), including ultrasound guidance** Ⓜ ♀

🔧 9.05 ⚖ 11.3 **FUD** 000

Ⓣ 62 80 ▯

AMA: 2015,Jan,16; 2014,Jan,11; 2012,Jan,15-42; 2011,Jan,11

59076 **Fetal shunt placement, including ultrasound guidance** Ⓜ ♀

🔧 13.4 ⚖ 13.4 **FUD** 000

Ⓣ 62 80 ▯

AMA: 2015,Jan,16; 2014,Jan,11; 2012,Jan,15-42; 2011,Jan,11

59100-59151 Tubal Pregnancy/Hysterotomy Procedures

CMS: 100-3,230.3 Sterilization

59100 **Hysterotomy, abdominal (eg, for hydatidiform mole, abortion)** Ⓜ ♀

Code also ligation of fallopian tubes when performed at the same time as hysterotomy (58611)

🔧 24.1 ⚖ 24.1 **FUD** 090

Ⓣ A2 80 ▯

AMA: 2014,Jan,11

59120 **Surgical treatment of ectopic pregnancy; tubal or ovarian, requiring salpingectomy and/or oophorectomy, abdominal or vaginal approach** Ⓜ ♀

🔧 23.0 ⚖ 23.0 **FUD** 090

Ⓒ 80 ▯

AMA: 2014,Jan,11

59121 **tubal or ovarian, without salpingectomy and/or oophorectomy** Ⓜ ♀

🔧 23.0 ⚖ 23.0 **FUD** 090

Ⓒ 80 ▯

AMA: 2014,Jan,11

59130 **abdominal pregnancy** Ⓜ ♀

🔧 24.1 ⚖ 24.1 **FUD** 090

Ⓒ 80 ▯

AMA: 2014,Jan,11

59135 **interstitial, uterine pregnancy requiring total hysterectomy** Ⓜ ♀

🔧 23.8 ⚖ 23.8 **FUD** 090

Ⓒ 80 ▯

AMA: 2014,Jan,11

59136 **interstitial, uterine pregnancy with partial resection of uterus** Ⓜ ♀

🔧 25.4 ⚖ 25.4 **FUD** 090

Ⓒ 80 ▯

AMA: 2014,Jan,11

59140 **cervical, with evacuation** Ⓜ ♀

🔧 11.6 ⚖ 11.6 **FUD** 090

Ⓒ 80 ▯

AMA: 2014,Jan,11

59150 **Laparoscopic treatment of ectopic pregnancy; without salpingectomy and/or oophorectomy** Ⓜ ♀

🔧 22.3 ⚖ 22.3 **FUD** 090

Ⓣ 62 80 ▯

AMA: 2015,Jan,16; 2014,Jan,11

59151 **with salpingectomy and/or oophorectomy** Ⓜ ♀

🔧 21.6 ⚖ 21.6 **FUD** 090

Ⓣ 62 80 ▯

AMA: 2014,Jan,11

59160-59200 Procedures of Uterus Prior To/After Delivery

59160 **Curettage, postpartum** Ⓜ ♀

🔧 5.03 ⚖ 5.88 **FUD** 010

Ⓣ A2 80 ▯

AMA: 2015,Jan,16; 2014,Jan,11; 2012,Jan,15-42; 2011,Jan,11

59200 **Insertion of cervical dilator (eg, laminaria, prostaglandin) (separate procedure)** Ⓜ ♀

EXCLUDES Fetal transfusion, intrauterine (36460)

Hypertonic solution/prostaglandin introduction for labor initiation (59850-59857)

🔧 1.31 ⚖ 2.07 **FUD** 000

Ⓣ P3 ▯

AMA: 2015,Jan,16; 2014,Jan,11

59300-59350 Postpartum Vaginal/Cervical/Uterine Repairs

EXCLUDES Nonpregnancy-related cerclage (57700)

59300 **Episiotomy or vaginal repair, by other than attending** Ⓜ ♀

🔧 4.33 ⚖ 5.58 **FUD** 000

Ⓣ P3 80 ▯

AMA: 2014,Jan,11

59320 **Cerclage of cervix, during pregnancy; vaginal** Ⓜ ♀

🔧 4.44 ⚖ 4.44 **FUD** 000

Ⓣ A2 80 ▯

AMA: 2015,Jan,16; 2014,Jan,11; 2012,Jan,15-42; 2011,Jan,11

59325 **abdominal** Ⓜ ♀

🔧 7.06 ⚖ 7.06 **FUD** 000

Ⓒ 80 ▯

AMA: 2015,Jan,16; 2014,Jan,11; 2012,Jan,15-42; 2011,Jan,11

59350 **Hysterorrhaphy of ruptured uterus** Ⓜ ♀

🔧 8.20 ⚖ 8.20 **FUD** 000

Ⓒ 80 ▯

AMA: 2014,Jan,11

59400-59410 Vaginal Delivery: Comprehensive and Component Services

CMS: 100-2,15,180 Nurse-Midwife (CNM) Services; 100-2,15,20.1 Physician Expense for Surgery, Childbirth, and Treatment for Infertility

INCLUDES Care provided for an uncomplicated pregnancy including delivery as well as antepartum and postpartum care:

Admission history

Admission to hospital

Artificial rupture of membranes

Management of uncomplicated labor

Physical exam

Vaginal delivery with or without episiotomy or forceps

EXCLUDES Medical complications of pregnancy, labor, and delivery:

Cardiac problems

Diabetes

Hyperemesis

Hypertension

Neurological problems

Premature rupture of membranes

Pre-term labor

Toxemia

Trauma

Newborn circumcision (54150, 54160)

Services incidental to or unrelated to the pregnancy

Genital System

59400   **Routine obstetric care including antepartum care, vaginal delivery (with or without episiotomy, and/or forceps) and postpartum care**   Ⓜ ♀

INCLUDES   Fetal heart tones
Hospital/office visits following cesarean section or vaginal delivery
Initial/subsequent history
Physical exams
Recording of weight/blood pressures
Routine chemical urinalysis
Routine prenatal visits:
     Each month up to 28 weeks gestation
     Every other week from 29 to 36 weeks gestation
     Weekly from 36 weeks until delivery

🖐 60.6   ✂ 60.6   **FUD** MMM   Ⓑ ▭

AMA: 2015,Jan,16; 2014,Jan,11; 2012,Jan,15-42; 2011,Jan,11

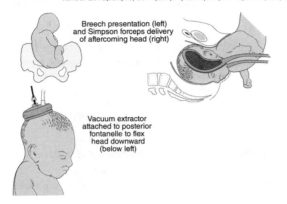

Breech presentation (left) and Simpson forceps delivery of aftercoming head (right)

Vacuum extractor attached to posterior fontanelle to flex head downward (below left)

59409   **Vaginal delivery only (with or without episiotomy and/or forceps);**   Ⓜ ♀

EXCLUDES   Inpatient management after delivery/discharge services (99217-99239 [99224, 99225, 99226])

🖐 23.7   ✂ 23.7   **FUD** MMM   Ⓣ 80 ▭

AMA: 2015,Jan,16; 2014,Jan,11; 2012,Jan,15-42; 2011,Jan,11

59410   **including postpartum care**   Ⓜ ♀

INCLUDES   Hospital/office visits following cesarean section or vaginal delivery

🖐 30.3   ✂ 30.3   **FUD** MMM   Ⓑ ▭

AMA: 2014,Jan,11

59412-59414 Other Maternity Services

CMS: 100-2,15,180 Nurse-Midwife (CNM) Services; 100-2,15,20.1 Physician Expense for Surgery, Childbirth, and Treatment for Infertility

59412   **External cephalic version, with or without tocolysis**   Ⓜ ♀

Code also delivery code(s)

🖐 3.02   ✂ 3.02   **FUD** MMM   Ⓣ 62 80 ▭

AMA: 2014,Jan,11

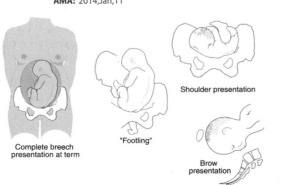

Complete breech presentation at term

Shoulder presentation

"Footling"

Brow presentation

59414   **Delivery of placenta (separate procedure)**   Ⓜ ♀

🖐 2.67   ✂ 2.67   **FUD** MMM   Ⓣ 62 80 ▭

AMA: 2015,Jan,16; 2014,Jan,11; 2012,Jan,15-42; 2011,Jan,11

59425-59430 Prenatal and Postpartum Visits

CMS: 100-2,15,180 Nurse-Midwife (CNM) Services; 100-2,15,20.1 Physician Expense for Surgery, Childbirth, and Treatment for Infertility

INCLUDES   Physician/other qualified health care professional providing all or a portion of antepartum/postpartum care, but no delivery due to:
     Referral to another physician for delivery
     Termination of pregnancy by abortion

EXCLUDES   *Antepartum care, 1-3 visits, report with appropriate evaluation and management service code*
Medical complications of pregnancy, labor, and delivery:
     Cardiac problems
     Diabetes
     Hyperemesis
     Hypertension
     Neurological problems
     Premature rupture of membranes
     Pre-term labor
     Toxemia
     Trauma
Newborn circumcision (54150, 54160)
Services incidental to or unrelated to the pregnancy

59425   **Antepartum care only; 4-6 visits**   Ⓜ ♀

INCLUDES   Fetal heart tones
Initial/subsequent history
Physical exams
Recording of weight/blood pressures
Routine chemical urinalysis
Routine prenatal visits:
     Each month up to 28 weeks gestation
     Every other week from 29 to 36 weeks gestation
     Weekly from 36 weeks until delivery

🖐 10.4   ✂ 13.1   **FUD** MMM   Ⓑ 80 ▭

AMA: 2015,Jan,16; 2014,Jan,11; 2012,Jan,15-42; 2011,Jan,11

59426   **7 or more visits**   Ⓜ ♀

INCLUDES   Biweekly visits to 36 weeks gestation
Fetal heart tones
Initial/subsequent history
Monthly visits up to 28 weeks gestation
Physical exams
Recording of weight/blood pressures
Routine chemical urinalysis
Weekly visits until delivery

🖐 18.3   ✂ 23.5   **FUD** MMM   Ⓑ 80 ▭

AMA: 2015,Jan,16; 2014,Jan,11; 2012,Jan,15-42; 2011,Jan,11

59430   **Postpartum care only (separate procedure)**   Ⓜ ♀

INCLUDES   Office/other outpatient visits following cesarean section or vaginal delivery

🖐 4.07   ✂ 5.35   **FUD** MMM   Ⓑ ▭

AMA: 2015,Jan,16; 2014,Jan,11; 2012,Jan,15-42; 2011,Jan,11

59510-59525 Cesarean Section Delivery: Comprehensive and Components of Care

CMS: 100-2,15,20.1 Physician Expense for Surgery, Childbirth, and Treatment for Infertility

INCLUDES Classic cesarean section
Low cervical cesarean section

EXCLUDES Infant standby attendance (99360)
Medical complications of pregnancy, labor, and delivery:
    Cardiac problems
    Diabetes
    Hyperemesis
    Hypertension
    Neurological problems
    Premature rupture of membranes
    Pre-term labor
    Toxemia
    Trauma
Newborn circumcision (54150, 54160)
Services incidental to or unrelated to the pregnancy
Vaginal delivery after prior cesarean section (59610-59614)

59510   **Routine obstetric care including antepartum care, cesarean delivery, and postpartum care**   M ♀

    INCLUDES   Admission history
         Admission to hospital
         Cesarean delivery
         Fetal heart tones
         Hospital/office visits following cesarean section
         Initial/subsequent history
         Management of uncomplicated labor
         Physical exam
         Recording of weight/blood pressures
         Routine chemical urinalysis
         Routine prenatal visits:
            Each month up to 28 weeks gestation
            Every other week 29 to 36 weeks gestation
            Weekly from 36 weeks until delivery

    EXCLUDES Medical problems complicating labor and delivery

    🔲 66.9   ⚕ 66.9   **FUD** MMM   B 🖳

    AMA: 2015,Jan,16; 2014,Jan,11; 2013,Mar,13; 2012,Jan,15-42; 2011,Jan,11

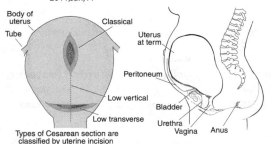

Body of uterus
Tube
Classical
Uterus at term
Peritoneum
Low vertical
Bladder
Urethra
Vagina
Anus
Low transverse

Types of Cesarean section are classified by uterine incision

59514   **Cesarean delivery only;**   M ♀

    INCLUDES   Admission history
         Admission to hospital
         Cesarean delivery
         Management of uncomplicated labor
         Physical exam

    EXCLUDES Inpatient management after delivery/discharge services (99217-99239 [99224, 99225, 99226])
         Medical problems complicating labor and delivery

    🔲 26.6   ⚕ 26.6   **FUD** MMM   C 80 🖳

    AMA: 2015,Jan,16; 2014,Jan,11; 2013,Mar,13; 2012,Jan,15-42; 2011,Jan,11

59515   **including postpartum care**   M ♀

    INCLUDES   Admission history
         Admission to hospital
         Cesarean delivery
         Hospital/office visits following cesarean section or vaginal delivery
         Management of uncomplicated labor
         Physical exam

    EXCLUDES Medical problems complicating labor and delivery

    🔲 36.6   ⚕ 36.6   **FUD** MMM   B 🖳

    AMA: 2015,Jan,16; 2014,Jan,11; 2013,Mar,13

+ **59525**   **Subtotal or total hysterectomy after cesarean delivery (List separately in addition to code for primary procedure)**   M ♀

    Code first cesarean delivery (59510, 59514, 59515, 59618, 59620, 59622)

    🔲 14.1   ⚕ 14.1   **FUD** ZZZ   C 80 🖳

    AMA: 2014,Jan,11

59610-59614 Vaginal Delivery After Prior Cesarean Section: Comprehensive and Components of Care

CMS: 100-2,15,180 Nurse-Midwife (CNM) Services; 100-2,15,20.1 Physician Expense for Surgery, Childbirth, and Treatment for Infertility

INCLUDES Admission history
Admission to hospital
Management of uncomplicated labor
Patients with previous cesarean delivery who present with the expectation of a vaginal delivery
Physical exam
Successful vaginal delivery after previous cesarean delivery (VBAC)
Vaginal delivery with or without episiotomy or forceps

EXCLUDES Elective cesarean delivery (59510, 59514, 59515)
Medical complications of pregnancy, labor, and delivery:
    Cardiac problems
    Diabetes
    Hyperemesis
    Hypertension
    Neurological problems
    Premature rupture of membranes
    Pre-term labor
    Toxemia
    Trauma
Newborn circumcision (54150, 54160)
Services incidental to or unrelated to the pregnancy

59610   **Routine obstetric care including antepartum care, vaginal delivery (with or without episiotomy, and/or forceps) and postpartum care, after previous cesarean delivery**   M ♀

    INCLUDES   Fetal heart tones
         Hospital/office visits following cesarean section or vaginal delivery
         Initial/subsequent history
         Physical exams
         Recording of weight/blood pressures
         Routine chemical urinalysis
         Routine prenatal visits:
            Each month up to 28 weeks gestation
            Every other week 29 to 36 weeks gestation
            Weekly from 36 weeks until delivery

    🔲 63.5   ⚕ 63.5   **FUD** MMM   B 80 🖳

    AMA: 2015,Jan,16; 2014,Jan,11

59612   **Vaginal delivery only, after previous cesarean delivery (with or without episiotomy and/or forceps);**   M ♀

    EXCLUDES Inpatient management after delivery/discharge services (99217-99239 [99224, 99225, 99226])

    🔲 26.6   ⚕ 26.6   **FUD** MMM   T 80 🖳

    AMA: 2015,Jan,16; 2014,Jan,11

59614   **including postpartum care**   M ♀

    INCLUDES   Hospital/office visits following cesarean section or vaginal delivery

    🔲 33.1   ⚕ 33.1   **FUD** MMM   B 80 🖳

    AMA: 2015,Jan,16; 2014,Jan,11

● New Code   ▲ Revised Code   ○ Reinstated   M Maternity   A Age Edit   Unlisted   Not Covered   # Resequenced
⊘ AMA Mod 51 Exempt   51 Optum Mod 51 Exempt   63 Mod 63 Exempt   ⊙ Mod Sedation   + Add-on   CCI   P0 PQRS   FUD Follow-up Days

© 2015 Optum360, LLC (Blue Text)   CPT © 2015 American Medical Association. All Rights Reserved. (Black Text)   Medicare (Red Text)   **233**

59618-59622 Cesarean Section After Attempted Vaginal Birth/Prior C-Section

CMS: 100-2,15,20.1 Physician Expense for Surgery, Childbirth, and Treatment for Infertility

INCLUDES Admission history
Admission to hospital
Cesarean delivery
Cesarean delivery following an unsuccessful vaginal delivery attempt after previous cesarean delivery
Management of uncomplicated labor
Patients with previous cesarean delivery who present with the expectation of a vaginal delivery
Physical exam

EXCLUDES *Elective cesarean delivery (59510, 59514, 59515)*
Medical complications of pregnancy, labor, and delivery:
  Cardiac problems
  Diabetes
  Hyperemesis
  Hypertension
  Neurological problems
  Premature rupture of membranes
  Pre-term labor
  Toxemia
  Trauma
Newborn circumcision (54150, 54160)
Services incidental to or unrelated to the pregnancy

59618   **Routine obstetric care including antepartum care, cesarean delivery, and postpartum care, following attempted vaginal delivery after previous cesarean delivery**   M ♀

INCLUDES Fetal heart tones
Hospital/office visits following cesarean section or vaginal delivery
Initial/subsequent history
Physical exams
Recording of weight/blood pressures
Routine chemical urinalysis
Routine prenatal visits:
  Each month up to 28 weeks gestation
  Every two weeks 29 to 36 weeks gestation
  Weekly from 36 weeks until delivery

🔧 67.9   ✂ 67.9   **FUD** MMM   B 80 🖥

AMA: 2015,Jan,16; 2014,Jan,11

59620   **Cesarean delivery only, following attempted vaginal delivery after previous cesarean delivery;**   M ♀

EXCLUDES *Inpatient management after delivery/discharge services (99217-99239 [99224, 99225, 99226])*

🔧 27.6   ✂ 27.6   **FUD** MMM   C 80

AMA: 2015,Jan,16; 2014,Jan,11

59622   **including postpartum care**   M ♀

INCLUDES Hospital/office visits following cesarean section or vaginal delivery

🔧 37.6   ✂ 37.6   **FUD** MMM   B 80 🖥

AMA: 2015,Jan,16; 2014,Jan,11

59812-59830 Treatment of Miscarriage

CMS: 100-2,15,20.1 Physician Expense for Surgery, Childbirth, and Treatment for Infertility

EXCLUDES *Medical treatment of spontaneous complete abortion, any trimester (99201-99233 [99224, 99225, 99226])*

59812   **Treatment of incomplete abortion, any trimester, completed surgically**   M ♀

INCLUDES Surgical treatment of spontaneous abortion

🔧 8.56   ✂ 9.17   **FUD** 090   T A2 🖥

AMA: 2015,Jan,16; 2014,Jan,11

59820   **Treatment of missed abortion, completed surgically; first trimester**   M ♀

🔧 10.2   ✂ 10.9   **FUD** 090   T A2 🖥

AMA: 2015,Jan,16; 2014,Jan,11

59821   **second trimester**   M ♀

🔧 10.3   ✂ 11.0   **FUD** 090   T A2 80 🖥

AMA: 2015,Jan,16; 2014,Jan,11

59830   **Treatment of septic abortion, completed surgically**   M ♀

🔧 12.6   ✂ 12.6   **FUD** 090   C 80 🖥

AMA: 2015,Jan,16; 2014,Jan,11

59840-59866 Elective Abortions

CMS: 100-2,1,90 Termination of Pregnancy; 100-2,15,20.1 Physician Expense for Surgery, Childbirth, and Treatment for Infertility; 100-3,140.1 Abortion; 100-4,3,100.1 Billing for Abortion Services

59840   **Induced abortion, by dilation and curettage**   M ♀

🔧 6.03   ✂ 6.28   **FUD** 010   T A2 80 🖥

AMA: 2015,Jan,16; 2014,Jan,11; 2012,Jan,15-42; 2011,Jan,11

59841   **Induced abortion, by dilation and evacuation**   M ♀

🔧 10.4   ✂ 11.0   **FUD** 010   T A2 80 🖥

AMA: 2015,Jan,16; 2014,Jan,11

59850   **Induced abortion, by 1 or more intra-amniotic injections (amniocentesis-injections), including hospital admission and visits, delivery of fetus and secundines;**   M ♀

EXCLUDES *Cervical dilator insertion (59200)*

🔧 9.97   ✂ 9.97   **FUD** 090   C 80 🖥

AMA: 2015,Jan,16; 2014,Jan,11

59851   **with dilation and curettage and/or evacuation**   M ♀

EXCLUDES *Cervical dilator insertion (59200)*

🔧 11.5   ✂ 11.5   **FUD** 090   C 80 🖥

AMA: 2015,Jan,16; 2014,Jan,11

59852   **with hysterotomy (failed intra-amniotic injection)**   M ♀

EXCLUDES *Cervical dilator insertion (59200)*

🔧 14.4   ✂ 14.4   **FUD** 090   C 80 🖥

AMA: 2015,Jan,16; 2014,Jan,11

59855   **Induced abortion, by 1 or more vaginal suppositories (eg, prostaglandin) with or without cervical dilation (eg, laminaria), including hospital admission and visits, delivery of fetus and secundines;**   M ♀

🔧 12.0   ✂ 12.0   **FUD** 090   C 80 🖥

AMA: 2014,Jan,11

59856   **with dilation and curettage and/or evacuation**   M ♀

🔧 14.1   ✂ 14.1   **FUD** 090   C 80 🖥

AMA: 2014,Jan,11

59857   **with hysterotomy (failed medical evacuation)**   M ♀

🔧 14.8   ✂ 14.8   **FUD** 090   C 80 🖥

AMA: 2014,Jan,11

59866   **Multifetal pregnancy reduction(s) (MPR)**   M ♀

🔧 6.22   ✂ 6.22   **FUD** 000   T 62 80 🖥

AMA: 2014,Jan,11

59870-59899 Miscellaneous Obstetrical Procedures

CMS: 100-2,15,20.1 Physician Expense for Surgery, Childbirth, and Treatment for Infertility

59870   **Uterine evacuation and curettage for hydatidiform mole**   M ♀

🔧 13.6   ✂ 13.6   **FUD** 090   T A2 80 🖥

AMA: 2015,Jan,16; 2014,Jan,11; 2012,Jan,15-42; 2011,Jan,11

59871   **Removal of cerclage suture under anesthesia (other than local)**   M ♀

🔧 3.88   ✂ 3.88   **FUD** 000   Q2 A2 80 🖥

AMA: 2015,Jan,16; 2014,Jan,11

59897   **Unlisted fetal invasive procedure, including ultrasound guidance, when performed**   ♀

🔧 0.00   ✂ 0.00   **FUD** YYY   T 🖥

AMA: 2014,Jan,11

59898   **Unlisted laparoscopy procedure, maternity care and delivery**   M ♀

🔧 0.00   ✂ 0.00   **FUD** YYY   T 80 50

AMA: 2015,Jan,16; 2014,Jan,11

59899   **Unlisted procedure, maternity care and delivery**   M ♀

🔧 0.00   ✂ 0.00   **FUD** YYY   T 80

AMA: 2015,Jan,16; 2014,Jan,11; 2013,Oct,3; 2012,Jan,15-42; 2011,Jan,11

60000 I&D of Infected Thyroglossal Cyst

60000 Incision and drainage of thyroglossal duct cyst, infected
🔧 4.12 ⚕ 4.56 **FUD** 010 T A2 80 ▣
AMA: 2014,Jan,11

60100 Core Needle Biopsy: Thyroid

EXCLUDES Fine needle aspiration (10021-10022)

60100 Biopsy thyroid, percutaneous core needle
▣ (76942, 77002, 77012, 77021)
◧ (88172-88173)
🔧 2.30 ⚕ 3.24 **FUD** 000 T P3 ▣
AMA: 2015,Jan,16; 2014,Jan,11; 2012,Jan,15-42; 2011,Jan,11

60200 Surgical Removal Thyroid Cyst or Mass; Division of Isthmus

60200 Excision of cyst or adenoma of thyroid, or transection of isthmus
🔧 19.0 ⚕ 19.0 **FUD** 090 T A2 80 ▣ PQ
AMA: 2015,Jan,16; 2014,Jan,11; 2012,Dec,3-5; 2011,Aug,9-10

60210-60225 Subtotal Thyroidectomy

60210 Partial thyroid lobectomy, unilateral; with or without isthmusectomy
🔧 20.3 ⚕ 20.3 **FUD** 090 T 62 80 ▣ PQ
AMA: 2015,Jan,16; 2014,Jan,11; 2012,Dec,3-5; 2012,Jan,15-42; 2011,Aug,9-10

60212 with contralateral subtotal lobectomy, including isthmusectomy
🔧 29.1 ⚕ 29.1 **FUD** 090 T 62 80 ▣ PQ
AMA: 2015,Jan,16; 2014,Jan,11; 2012,Dec,3-5

60220 Total thyroid lobectomy, unilateral; with or without isthmusectomy
🔧 20.3 ⚕ 20.3 **FUD** 090 T 62 80 ▣ PQ
AMA: 2015,Jan,16; 2014,Jan,11; 2012,Dec,3-5; 2012,Jan,15-42; 2011,Aug,9-10; 2011,Jan,11; 2010,Dec,12

60225 with contralateral subtotal lobectomy, including isthmusectomy
🔧 26.9 ⚕ 26.9 **FUD** 090 T 62 80 ▣ PQ
AMA: 2015,Jan,16; 2014,Jan,11; 2012,Dec,3-5

60240-60271 Complete Thyroidectomy Procedures

60240 Thyroidectomy, total or complete
EXCLUDES Subtotal or partial thyroidectomy (60271)
🔧 26.5 ⚕ 26.5 **FUD** 090 T 62 80 ▣ PQ
AMA: 2015,Jan,16; 2014,Jan,11; 2012,Dec,3-5

60252 Thyroidectomy, total or subtotal for malignancy; with limited neck dissection
🔧 38.1 ⚕ 38.1 **FUD** 090 T 80 ▣ PQ
AMA: 2015,Jan,16; 2014,Jan,11; 2012,Dec,3-5; 2012,Jan,15-42; 2011,Jan,11

60254 with radical neck dissection
🔧 48.4 ⚕ 48.4 **FUD** 090 C 80 ▣ PQ
AMA: 2015,Jan,16; 2014,Jan,11; 2012,Dec,3-5; 2012,Jan,15-42; 2011,Jan,11

60260 Thyroidectomy, removal of all remaining thyroid tissue following previous removal of a portion of thyroid
🔧 31.5 ⚕ 31.5 **FUD** 090 T 80 50 ▣ PQ
AMA: 2015,Jan,16; 2014,Jan,11; 2012,Dec,3-5; 2012,Jan,15-42; 2011,Jan,11; 2010,Dec,12

60270 Thyroidectomy, including substernal thyroid; sternal split or transthoracic approach
🔧 39.5 ⚕ 39.5 **FUD** 090 C 80 ▣ PQ
AMA: 2015,Jan,16; 2014,Jan,11; 2012,Dec,3-5

60271 cervical approach
🔧 30.5 ⚕ 30.5 **FUD** 090 T 80 ▣ PQ
AMA: 2015,Jan,16; 2014,Jan,11; 2012,Dec,3-5

60280-60300 Treatment of Cyst/Sinus of Thyroid

60280 Excision of thyroglossal duct cyst or sinus;
EXCLUDES Thyroid ultrasound (76536)
🔧 12.7 ⚕ 12.7 **FUD** 090 T A2 80 ▣ PQ
AMA: 2014,Jan,11

60281 recurrent
EXCLUDES Thyroid ultrasound (76536)
🔧 16.9 ⚕ 16.9 **FUD** 090 T A2 80 ▣ PQ
AMA: 2014,Jan,11

60300 Aspiration and/or injection, thyroid cyst
EXCLUDES Fine needle aspiration (10021-10022)
▣ (76942, 77012)
🔧 1.45 ⚕ 3.39 **FUD** 000 T P3
AMA: 2014,Jan,11

60500-60512 Parathyroid Procedures

60500 Parathyroidectomy or exploration of parathyroid(s);
🔧 27.8 ⚕ 27.8 **FUD** 090 T 62 80 ▣ PQ
AMA: 2015,Jan,16; 2014,Jan,11; 2012,Dec,3-5

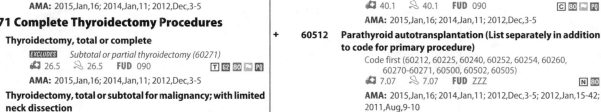

Posterior view of pharynx, thyroid glands, and parathyroid glands

60502 re-exploration
🔧 37.1 ⚕ 37.1 **FUD** 090 T 80 ▣ PQ
AMA: 2015,Jan,16; 2014,Jan,11; 2012,Dec,3-5

60505 with mediastinal exploration, sternal split or transthoracic approach
🔧 40.1 ⚕ 40.1 **FUD** 090 C 80 ▣ PQ
AMA: 2015,Jan,16; 2014,Jan,11; 2012,Dec,3-5

+ **60512** Parathyroid autotransplantation (List separately in addition to code for primary procedure)
Code first (60212, 60225, 60240, 60252, 60254, 60260, 60270-60271, 60500, 60502, 60505)
🔧 7.07 ⚕ 7.07 **FUD** ZZZ N 80
AMA: 2015,Jan,16; 2014,Jan,11; 2012,Dec,3-5; 2012,Jan,15-42; 2011,Aug,9-10

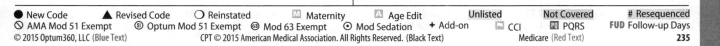

60520-60522 Thymus Procedures

> **EXCLUDES** Surgical thoracoscopy (video-assisted thoracic surgery (VATS) thymectomy (32673)

60520 **Thymectomy, partial or total; transcervical approach (separate procedure)**
 📣 30.2   ✂ 30.2   **FUD** 090   T 80 ▭ P0
 AMA: 2014,Jan,11; 2012,Oct,9-11; 2012,Sep,3-8

60521 **sternal split or transthoracic approach, without radical mediastinal dissection (separate procedure)**
 📣 32.6   ✂ 32.6   **FUD** 090   C 80 ▭ P0
 AMA: 2015,Jan,16; 2014,Jan,11; 2012,Oct,9-11; 2012,Sep,3-8; 2012,Jan,15-42; 2011,Jan,11

60522 **sternal split or transthoracic approach, with radical mediastinal dissection (separate procedure)**
 📣 39.5   ✂ 39.5   **FUD** 090   C 80 ▭ P0
 AMA: 2014,Jan,11; 2012,Oct,9-11; 2012,Sep,3-8

60540-60545 Adrenal Gland Procedures

> **EXCLUDES** Laparoscopic approach (60650)
> Removal of remote or disseminated pheochromocytoma (49203-49205)

Do not report with (50323)

60540 **Adrenalectomy, partial or complete, or exploration of adrenal gland with or without biopsy, transabdominal, lumbar or dorsal (separate procedure);**
 📣 30.5   ✂ 30.5   **FUD** 090   C 80 50 ▭ P0
 AMA: 2014,Jan,11

60545 **with excision of adjacent retroperitoneal tumor**
 📣 35.1   ✂ 35.1   **FUD** 090   C 80 50 ▭ P0
 AMA: 2014,Jan,11

60600-60605 Carotid Body Procedures

60600 **Excision of carotid body tumor; without excision of carotid artery**
 📣 40.6   ✂ 40.6   **FUD** 090   C 80 ▭ P0
 AMA: 2014,Jan,11

60605 **with excision of carotid artery**
 📣 57.9   ✂ 57.9   **FUD** 090   C 80 ▭ P0
 AMA: 2014,Jan,11

60650-60699 Laparoscopic and Unlisted Procedures

> **INCLUDES** Diagnostic laparoscopy

60650 **Laparoscopy, surgical, with adrenalectomy, partial or complete, or exploration of adrenal gland with or without biopsy, transabdominal, lumbar or dorsal**
> **EXCLUDES** Peritoneoscopy performed as separate procedure (49320)

 📣 34.3   ✂ 34.3   **FUD** 090   C 80 50 ▭ P0
 AMA: 2015,Jan,16; 2014,Jan,11

60659 **Unlisted laparoscopy procedure, endocrine system**
 📣 0.00   ✂ 0.00   **FUD** YYY   T 80 50
 AMA: 2015,Jan,16; 2014,Jan,11

60699 **Unlisted procedure, endocrine system**
 📣 0.00   ✂ 0.00   **FUD** YYY   T 80
 AMA: 2015,Jan,16; 2014,Jan,11; 2012,Jan,15-42; 2011,Jan,11

61000-61253 Transcranial Access via Puncture, Burr Hole, Twist Hole, or Trephine

EXCLUDES Injection for:
Cerebral angiography (36100-36218)

61000 Subdural tap through fontanelle, or suture, infant, unilateral or bilateral; initial ⒜

EXCLUDES Injection for:
Pneumoencephalography (61055)
Ventriculography (61026, 61120)

🔲 3.15   ⚕ 3.15   **FUD** 000   T R2 ▢

AMA: 2014,Jan,11

Overhead view of newborn skull

An initial tap through to the subdural level is performed on an infant via a fontanelle or suture, either unilateral or bilateral.

61001 subsequent taps ⒜

🔲 2.35   ⚕ 2.35   **FUD** 000   T R2 ▢

AMA: 2014,Jan,11

61020 Ventricular puncture through previous burr hole, fontanelle, suture, or implanted ventricular catheter/reservoir; without injection

🔲 3.07   ⚕ 3.07   **FUD** 000   T A2 ▢

AMA: 2014,Jan,11

61026 with injection of medication or other substance for diagnosis or treatment

INCLUDES Injection for ventriculography

🔲 2.99   ⚕ 2.99   **FUD** 000   T A2 ▢

AMA: 2014,Jan,11

61050 Cisternal or lateral cervical (C1-C2) puncture; without injection (separate procedure)

🔲 2.47   ⚕ 2.47   **FUD** 000   T A2 80 ▢

AMA: 2014,Jan,11

61055 with injection of medication or other substance for diagnosis or treatment

INCLUDES Injection for pneumoencephalography

EXCLUDES Radiology procedures except when furnished by a different provider
Do not report with (62302-62305)

🔲 3.52   ⚕ 3.52   **FUD** 000   T A2 ▢

AMA: 2014,Sep,3; 2014,Jan,11

61070 Puncture of shunt tubing or reservoir for aspiration or injection procedure

🔁 (75809)

🔲 1.67   ⚕ 1.67   **FUD** 000   T A2 ▢

AMA: 2015,Jan,16; 2014,Jan,11; 2012,Jan,15-42; 2011,Jan,11

61105 Twist drill hole for subdural or ventricular puncture

🔲 13.7   ⚕ 13.7   **FUD** 090   C 80 ▢

AMA: 2014,Jan,11

61107 Twist drill hole(s) for subdural, intracerebral, or ventricular puncture; for implanting ventricular catheter, pressure recording device, or other intracerebral monitoring device

Code also intracranial neuroendoscopic ventricular catheter insertion or reinsertion, when performed (62160)

🔲 9.35   ⚕ 9.35   **FUD** 000   ⊘ C ▢

AMA: 2014,Jan,11

61108 for evacuation and/or drainage of subdural hematoma

🔲 26.9   ⚕ 26.9   **FUD** 090   C ▢

AMA: 2014,Jan,11

61120 Burr hole(s) for ventricular puncture (including injection of gas, contrast media, dye, or radioactive material)

INCLUDES Includes: Injection for ventriculography

🔲 22.1   ⚕ 22.1   **FUD** 090   C 80 ▢

AMA: 2014,Jan,11

61140 Burr hole(s) or trephine; with biopsy of brain or intracranial lesion

🔲 37.2   ⚕ 37.2   **FUD** 090   C 80 ▢ PQ

AMA: 2014,Jan,11

61150 with drainage of brain abscess or cyst

🔲 40.2   ⚕ 40.2   **FUD** 090   C ▢

AMA: 2014,Jan,11

61151 with subsequent tapping (aspiration) of intracranial abscess or cyst

🔲 29.5   ⚕ 29.5   **FUD** 090   C ▢

AMA: 2014,Jan,11

61154 Burr hole(s) with evacuation and/or drainage of hematoma, extradural or subdural

🔲 37.5   ⚕ 37.5   **FUD** 090   C 80 50 ▢ PQ

AMA: 2014,Jan,11

61156 Burr hole(s); with aspiration of hematoma or cyst, intracerebral

🔲 37.0   ⚕ 37.0   **FUD** 090   C 80 ▢

AMA: 2014,Jan,11

61210 for implanting ventricular catheter, reservoir, EEG electrode(s), pressure recording device, or other cerebral monitoring device (separate procedure)

Code also intracranial neuroendoscopic ventricular catheter insertion or reinsertion, when performed (62160)

🔲 11.0   ⚕ 11.0   **FUD** 000   C ▢

AMA: 2015,Jan,16; 2014,Jan,11; 2012,Jan,15-42; 2011,Jan,11

61215 Insertion of subcutaneous reservoir, pump or continuous infusion system for connection to ventricular catheter

EXCLUDES Chemotherapy (96450)
Refilling and maintenance of implantable infusion pump (95990)

🔲 14.8   ⚕ 14.8   **FUD** 090   T A2 ▢

AMA: 2015,Jan,16; 2014,Jan,11

61250 Burr hole(s) or trephine, supratentorial, exploratory, not followed by other surgery

EXCLUDES Burr hole or trephine followed by craniotomy at same operative session (61304-61321)

🔲 25.7   ⚕ 25.7   **FUD** 090   C 80 50 ▢

AMA: 2014,Jan,11

61253 Burr hole(s) or trephine, infratentorial, unilateral or bilateral

EXCLUDES Burr hole or trephine followed by craniotomy at same operative session (61304-61321)

🔲 27.4   ⚕ 27.4   **FUD** 090   C 80 ▢

AMA: 2015,Jan,16; 2014,Jan,11; 2012,Jan,15-42; 2011,Jan,11

● New Code   ▲ Revised Code   ○ Reinstated   M Maternity   A Age Edit   Unlisted   # Resequenced
⊘ AMA Mod 51 Exempt   ⑨ Optum Mod 51 Exempt   ⑥③ Mod 63 Exempt   ☉ Mod Sedation   + Add-on   ▢ CCI   PQ PQRS   Not Covered   **FUD** Follow-up Days

© 2015 Optum360, LLC (Blue Text)   CPT © 2015 American Medical Association. All Rights Reserved. (Black Text)   Medicare (Red Text)   **237**

61304-61323 Craniectomy/Craniotomy: By Indication/Specific Area of Brain

EXCLUDES *Injection for:*
Cerebral angiography (36100-36218)
Pneumoencephalography (61055)
Ventriculography (61026, 61120)

61304 Craniectomy or craniotomy, exploratory; supratentorial
Do not report with another craniectomy/craniotomy procedure when performed at the same anatomical site and same surgical encounter
🔧 48.4 ⚕ 48.4 **FUD** 090 C 80 ▱
AMA: 2014,Jan,11

61305 infratentorial (posterior fossa)
Do not report with another craniectomy/craniotomy procedure when performed at the same anatomical site and same surgical encounter
🔧 59.7 ⚕ 59.7 **FUD** 090 C 80 ▱
AMA: 2014,Jan,11

61312 Craniectomy or craniotomy for evacuation of hematoma, supratentorial; extradural or subdural
🔧 61.5 ⚕ 61.5 **FUD** 090 C 80 ▱ P0
AMA: 2015,Jan,16; 2014,Jan,11

61313 intracerebral
🔧 58.6 ⚕ 58.6 **FUD** 090 C 80 ▱ P0
AMA: 2014,Jan,11

61314 Craniectomy or craniotomy for evacuation of hematoma, infratentorial; extradural or subdural
🔧 53.9 ⚕ 53.9 **FUD** 090 C 80 ▱
AMA: 2014,Jan,11

61315 intracerebellar
🔧 61.2 ⚕ 61.2 **FUD** 090 C 80 ▱ P0
AMA: 2014,Jan,11

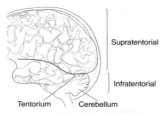

Supratentorial

Infratentorial

Tentorium   Cerebellum

The tentorium is a dural septum that separates the cerebellum from the occipital lobes

+ 61316 Incision and subcutaneous placement of cranial bone graft (List separately in addition to code for primary procedure)
Code first (61304, 61312-61313, 61322-61323, 61340, 61570-61571, 61680-61705)
🔧 2.62 ⚕ 2.62 **FUD** ZZZ C ▱
AMA: 2014,Jan,11

61320 Craniectomy or craniotomy, drainage of intracranial abscess; supratentorial
🔧 56.0 ⚕ 56.0 **FUD** 090 C 80 ▱
AMA: 2014,Jan,11

61321 infratentorial
🔧 63.3 ⚕ 63.3 **FUD** 090 C 80 ▱
AMA: 2014,Jan,11

61322 Craniectomy or craniotomy, decompressive, with or without duraplasty, for treatment of intracranial hypertension, without evacuation of associated intraparenchymal hematoma; without lobectomy
EXCLUDES *Subtemporal decompression (61340)*
Do not report with (61313)
🔧 70.3 ⚕ 70.3 **FUD** 090 C 80 ▱
AMA: 2014,Jan,11

61323 with lobectomy
EXCLUDES *Subtemporal decompression (61340)*
Do not report with (61313)
🔧 71.0 ⚕ 71.0 **FUD** 090 C ▱
AMA: 2014,Jan,11

61330-61530 Craniectomy/Craniotomy/Decompression Brain By Surgical Approach/Specific Area of Brain

EXCLUDES *Injection for:*
Cerebral angiography (36100-36218)
Pneumoencephalography (61055)
Ventriculography (61026, 61120)

61330 Decompression of orbit only, transcranial approach
INCLUDES Naffziger operation
🔧 44.3 ⚕ 44.3 **FUD** 090 T G2 80 50 ▱
AMA: 2014,Jan,11

61332 Exploration of orbit (transcranial approach); with biopsy
🔧 51.3 ⚕ 51.3 **FUD** 090 C 80 50 ▱
AMA: 2014,Jan,11

61333 with removal of lesion
🔧 52.4 ⚕ 52.4 **FUD** 090 C 80 50 ▱
AMA: 2014,Jan,11

61340 Subtemporal cranial decompression (pseudotumor cerebri, slit ventricle syndrome)
EXCLUDES *Decompression craniotomy or craniectomy for intracranial hypertension, without hematoma removal (61322-61323)*
🔧 42.9 ⚕ 42.9 **FUD** 090 C 80 50 ▱
AMA: 2014,Jan,11

61343 Craniectomy, suboccipital with cervical laminectomy for decompression of medulla and spinal cord, with or without dural graft (eg, Arnold-Chiari malformation)
🔧 64.9 ⚕ 64.9 **FUD** 090 C 80 ▱
AMA: 2014,Jan,11

61345 Other cranial decompression, posterior fossa
EXCLUDES *Kroenlein procedure (67445)*
Orbital decompression using a lateral wall approach (67445)
🔧 60.6 ⚕ 60.6 **FUD** 090 C 80 ▱
AMA: 2014,Jan,11

61450 Craniectomy, subtemporal, for section, compression, or decompression of sensory root of gasserian ganglion
INCLUDES Frazier-Spiller procedure
Hartley-Krause
Krause decompression
Taarnhoj procedure
🔧 57.2 ⚕ 57.2 **FUD** 090 C 80 ▱
AMA: 2014,Jan,11

61458 Craniectomy, suboccipital; for exploration or decompression of cranial nerves
INCLUDES Jannetta decompression
🔧 59.4 ⚕ 59.4 **FUD** 090 C 80 ▱
AMA: 2014,Jan,11

61460 **for section of 1 or more cranial nerves**
    62.6   62.6 **FUD** 090   C 80
    AMA: 2014,Jan,11

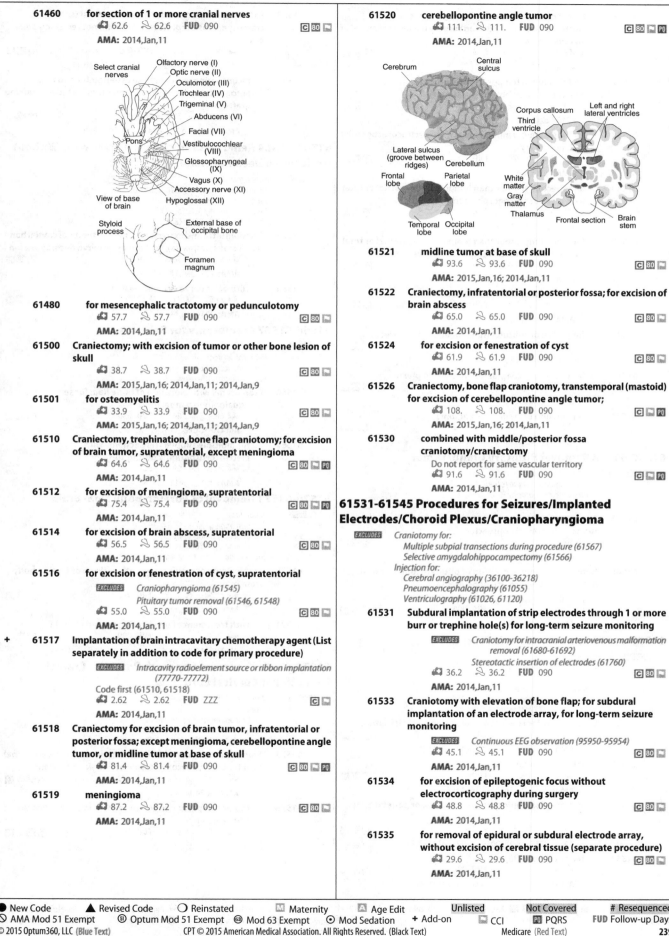

61480 **for mesencephalic tractotomy or pedunculotomy**
    57.7   57.7 **FUD** 090   C 80
    AMA: 2014,Jan,11

61500 **Craniectomy; with excision of tumor or other bone lesion of skull**
    38.7   38.7 **FUD** 090   C 80
    AMA: 2015,Jan,16; 2014,Jan,11; 2014,Jan,9

61501 **for osteomyelitis**
    33.9   33.9 **FUD** 090   C 80
    AMA: 2015,Jan,16; 2014,Jan,11; 2014,Jan,9

61510 **Craniectomy, trephination, bone flap craniotomy; for excision of brain tumor, supratentorial, except meningioma**
    64.6   64.6 **FUD** 090   C 80 PQ
    AMA: 2014,Jan,11

61512 **for excision of meningioma, supratentorial**
    75.4   75.4 **FUD** 090   C 80 PQ
    AMA: 2014,Jan,11

61514 **for excision of brain abscess, supratentorial**
    56.5   56.5 **FUD** 090   C 80
    AMA: 2014,Jan,11

61516 **for excision or fenestration of cyst, supratentorial**
    EXCLUDES *Craniopharyngioma (61545)*
    Pituitary tumor removal (61546, 61548)
    55.0   55.0 **FUD** 090   C 80
    AMA: 2014,Jan,11

+ **61517** **Implantation of brain intracavitary chemotherapy agent (List separately in addition to code for primary procedure)**
    EXCLUDES *Intracavity radioelement source or ribbon implantation (77770-77772)*
    Code first (61510, 61518)
    2.62   2.62 **FUD** ZZZ   C
    AMA: 2014,Jan,11

61518 **Craniectomy for excision of brain tumor, infratentorial or posterior fossa; except meningioma, cerebellopontine angle tumor, or midline tumor at base of skull**
    81.4   81.4 **FUD** 090   C 80 PQ
    AMA: 2014,Jan,11

61519 **meningioma**
    87.2   87.2 **FUD** 090   C 80
    AMA: 2014,Jan,11

61520 **cerebellopontine angle tumor**
    111.   111. **FUD** 090   C 80 PQ
    AMA: 2014,Jan,11

61521 **midline tumor at base of skull**
    93.6   93.6 **FUD** 090   C 80
    AMA: 2015,Jan,16; 2014,Jan,11

61522 **Craniectomy, infratentorial or posterior fossa; for excision of brain abscess**
    65.0   65.0 **FUD** 090   C 80
    AMA: 2014,Jan,11

61524 **for excision or fenestration of cyst**
    61.9   61.9 **FUD** 090   C 80
    AMA: 2014,Jan,11

61526 **Craniectomy, bone flap craniotomy, transtemporal (mastoid) for excision of cerebellopontine angle tumor;**
    108.   108. **FUD** 090   C PQ
    AMA: 2015,Jan,16; 2014,Jan,11

61530 **combined with middle/posterior fossa craniotomy/craniectomy**
    Do not report for same vascular territory
    91.6   91.6 **FUD** 090   C PQ
    AMA: 2014,Jan,11

61531-61545 Procedures for Seizures/Implanted Electrodes/Choroid Plexus/Craniopharyngioma

    EXCLUDES *Craniotomy for:*
    Multiple subpial transections during procedure (61567)
    Selective amygdalohippocampectomy (61566)
    Injection for:
    Cerebral angiography (36100-36218)
    Pneumoencephalography (61055)
    Ventriculography (61026, 61120)

61531 **Subdural implantation of strip electrodes through 1 or more burr or trephine hole(s) for long-term seizure monitoring**
    EXCLUDES *Craniotomy for intracranial arteriovenous malformation removal (61680-61692)*
    Stereotactic insertion of electrodes (61760)
    36.2   36.2 **FUD** 090   C 80
    AMA: 2014,Jan,11

61533 **Craniotomy with elevation of bone flap; for subdural implantation of an electrode array, for long-term seizure monitoring**
    EXCLUDES *Continuous EEG observation (95950-95954)*
    45.1   45.1 **FUD** 090   C 80
    AMA: 2014,Jan,11

61534 **for excision of epileptogenic focus without electrocorticography during surgery**
    48.8   48.8 **FUD** 090   C 80
    AMA: 2014,Jan,11

61535 **for removal of epidural or subdural electrode array, without excision of cerebral tissue (separate procedure)**
    29.6   29.6 **FUD** 090   C 80
    AMA: 2014,Jan,11

61536   for excision of cerebral epileptogenic focus, with electrocorticography during surgery (includes removal of electrode array)
🔷 76.7   ⚖ 76.7   **FUD** 090   © 80 ▭
AMA: 2014,Jan,11

61537   for lobectomy, temporal lobe, without electrocorticography during surgery
🔷 72.7   ⚖ 72.7   **FUD** 090   © 80 ▭
AMA: 2014,Jan,11

61538   for lobectomy, temporal lobe, with electrocorticography during surgery
🔷 79.5   ⚖ 79.5   **FUD** 090   © 80 ▭
AMA: 2014,Jan,11

61539   for lobectomy, other than temporal lobe, partial or total, with electrocorticography during surgery
🔷 70.2   ⚖ 70.2   **FUD** 090   © 80 ▭
AMA: 2014,Jan,11

61540   for lobectomy, other than temporal lobe, partial or total, without electrocorticography during surgery
🔷 64.9   ⚖ 64.9   **FUD** 090   © 80 ▭
AMA: 2014,Jan,11

61541   for transection of corpus callosum
🔷 63.9   ⚖ 63.9   **FUD** 090   © 80 ▭
AMA: 2014,Jan,11

61543   for partial or subtotal (functional) hemispherectomy
🔷 64.6   ⚖ 64.6   **FUD** 090   © 80 ▭
AMA: 2014,Jan,11

61544   for excision or coagulation of choroid plexus
🔷 56.5   ⚖ 56.5   **FUD** 090   © 80 ▭
AMA: 2014,Jan,11

61545   for excision of craniopharyngioma
🔷 94.7   ⚖ 94.7   **FUD** 090   © 80 ▭
AMA: 2014,Jan,11

61546-61548 Removal Pituitary Gland/Tumor

EXCLUDES   Injection for:
Cerebral angiography (36100-36218)
Pneumoencephalography (61055)
Ventriculography (61026, 61120)

61546   Craniotomy for hypophysectomy or excision of pituitary tumor, intracranial approach
🔷 68.6   ⚖ 68.6   **FUD** 090   © 80 ▭
AMA: 2014,Jan,11

61548   Hypophysectomy or excision of pituitary tumor, transnasal or transseptal approach, nonstereotactic
INCLUDES   Operating microscope (69990)
🔷 46.2   ⚖ 46.2   **FUD** 090   © 80 ▭ P0
AMA: 2014,Jan,11

61550-61559 Craniosynostosis Procedures

EXCLUDES   Injection for:
Cerebral angiography (36100-36218)
Pneumoencephalography (61055)
Ventriculography (61026, 61120)
Orbital hypertelorism reconstruction (21260-21263)
Reconstruction (21172-21180)

61550   Craniectomy for craniosynostosis; single cranial suture
🔷 28.1   ⚖ 28.1   **FUD** 090   © 80 ▭
AMA: 2015,Jan,16; 2014,Jan,11; 2012,Feb,11

61552   multiple cranial sutures
🔷 32.1   ⚖ 32.1   **FUD** 090   © 80 ▭
AMA: 2015,Jan,16; 2014,Jan,11; 2012,Feb,11

61556   Craniotomy for craniosynostosis; frontal or parietal bone flap
🔷 50.6   ⚖ 50.6   **FUD** 090   © 80 ▭
AMA: 2015,Jan,16; 2014,Jan,11; 2012,Feb,11

61557   bifrontal bone flap
🔷 49.9   ⚖ 49.9   **FUD** 090   © 80 ▭
AMA: 2015,Jan,16; 2014,Jan,11; 2012,Feb,11

61558   Extensive craniectomy for multiple cranial suture craniosynostosis (eg, cloverleaf skull); not requiring bone grafts
🔷 49.4   ⚖ 49.4   **FUD** 090   © 80 ▭
AMA: 2015,Jan,16; 2014,Jan,11; 2012,Feb,11

61559   recontouring with multiple osteotomies and bone autografts (eg, barrel-stave procedure) (includes obtaining grafts)
🔷 71.0   ⚖ 71.0   **FUD** 090   © 80 ▭
AMA: 2015,Jan,16; 2014,Jan,11; 2012,Feb,11

61563-61564 Removal Cranial Bone Tumor With/Without Optic Nerve Decompression

EXCLUDES   Injection for:
Cerebral angiography (36100-36218)
Pneumoencephalography (61055)
Ventriculography (61026, 61120)
Reconstruction (21181-21183)

61563   Excision, intra and extracranial, benign tumor of cranial bone (eg, fibrous dysplasia); without optic nerve decompression
🔷 58.8   ⚖ 58.8   **FUD** 090   © 80 ▭
AMA: 2014,Jan,11

61564   with optic nerve decompression
🔷 71.5   ⚖ 71.5   **FUD** 090   © 80 50 ▭
AMA: 2014,Jan,11

61566-61567 Craniotomy for Seizures

EXCLUDES   Injection for:
Cerebral angiography (36100-36218)
Pneumoencephalography (61055)
Ventriculography (61026, 61120)

61566   Craniotomy with elevation of bone flap; for selective amygdalohippocampectomy
🔷 66.9   ⚖ 66.9   **FUD** 090   © 80 ▭
AMA: 2014,Jan,11

61567   for multiple subpial transections, with electrocorticography during surgery
🔷 69.8   ⚖ 69.8   **FUD** 090   © 80 ▭
AMA: 2014,Jan,11

61570-61571 Removal of Foreign Body from Brain

EXCLUDES   Injection for:
Cerebral angiography (36100-36218)
Pneumoencephalography (61055)
Ventriculography (61026, 61120)
Sequestrectomy for osteomyelitis (61501)

61570   Craniectomy or craniotomy; with excision of foreign body from brain
🔷 55.5   ⚖ 55.5   **FUD** 090   © 80 ▭
AMA: 2014,Jan,11

61571   with treatment of penetrating wound of brain
🔷 59.1   ⚖ 59.1   **FUD** 090   © 80 ▭
AMA: 2014,Jan,11

61575-61576 Transoral Approach Posterior Cranial Fossa/Upper Cervical Cord

EXCLUDES   Arthrodesis (22548)
Injection for:
Cerebral angiography (36100-36218)
Pneumoencephalography (61055)
Ventriculography (61026, 61120)

61575   Transoral approach to skull base, brain stem or upper spinal cord for biopsy, decompression or excision of lesion;
🔷 74.5   ⚖ 74.5   **FUD** 090   © 80 ▭ P0
AMA: 2014,Jan,11

61576   requiring splitting of tongue and/or mandible (including tracheostomy)
🔷 98.8   ⚖ 98.8   **FUD** 090   © 80 ▭ P0
AMA: 2014,Jan,11

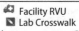

61580-61598 Surgical Approach: Cranial Fossae

EXCLUDES Definitive surgery (61600-61616)
Dural repair and/or reconstruction (61618-61619)
Injection for:
　Cerebral angiography (36100-36218)
　Pneumoencephalography (61055)
　Ventriculography (61026, 61120)
Primary closure (15732, 15756-15758)

61580 Craniofacial approach to anterior cranial fossa; extradural, including lateral rhinotomy, ethmoidectomy, sphenoidectomy, without maxillectomy or orbital exenteration
　72.6 　72.6 **FUD** 090 　　　　C 50 □
AMA: 2015,Jan,16; 2014,Jan,11

61581 extradural, including lateral rhinotomy, orbital exenteration, ethmoidectomy, sphenoidectomy and/or maxillectomy
　76.2 　76.2 **FUD** 090 　　　　C 50 □
AMA: 2015,Jan,16; 2014,Jan,11

61582 extradural, including unilateral or bifrontal craniotomy, elevation of frontal lobe(s), osteotomy of base of anterior cranial fossa
　88.7 　88.7 **FUD** 090 　　　　C 80 □
AMA: 2015,Jan,16; 2014,Jan,11

61583 intradural, including unilateral or bifrontal craniotomy, elevation or resection of frontal lobe, osteotomy of base of anterior cranial fossa
　85.2 　85.2 **FUD** 090 　　　　C 80 □
AMA: 2015,Jan,16; 2014,Jan,11

61584 Orbitocranial approach to anterior cranial fossa, extradural, including supraorbital ridge osteotomy and elevation of frontal and/or temporal lobe(s); without orbital exenteration
　84.1 　84.1 **FUD** 090 　　　C 80 50 □
AMA: 2015,Jan,16; 2014,Jan,11

61585 with orbital exenteration
　95.2 　95.2 **FUD** 090 　　　C 80 50 □
AMA: 2015,Jan,16; 2014,Jan,11

61586 Bicoronal, transzygomatic and/or LeFort I osteotomy approach to anterior cranial fossa with or without internal fixation, without bone graft
　71.1 　71.1 **FUD** 090 　　　　C 80 □
AMA: 2014,Jan,11

61590 Infratemporal pre-auricular approach to middle cranial fossa (parapharyngeal space, infratemporal and midline skull base, nasopharynx), with or without disarticulation of the mandible, including parotidectomy, craniotomy, decompression and/or mobilization of the facial nerve and/or petrous carotid artery
　88.1 　88.1 **FUD** 090 　　　C 80 50 □
AMA: 2015,Jan,16; 2014,Jan,11

61591 Infratemporal post-auricular approach to middle cranial fossa (internal auditory meatus, petrous apex, tentorium, cavernous sinus, parasellar area, infratemporal fossa) including mastoidectomy, resection of sigmoid sinus, with or without decompression and/or mobilization of contents of auditory canal or petrous carotid artery
　90.5 　90.5 **FUD** 090 　　C 80 50 □ P0
AMA: 2015,Jan,16; 2014,Jan,11

61592 Orbitocranial zygomatic approach to middle cranial fossa (cavernous sinus and carotid artery, clivus, basilar artery or petrous apex) including osteotomy of zygoma, craniotomy, extra- or intradural elevation of temporal lobe
　93.8 　93.8 **FUD** 090 　　　C 80 50 □
AMA: 2015,Jan,16; 2014,Jan,11

61595 Transtemporal approach to posterior cranial fossa, jugular foramen or midline skull base, including mastoidectomy, decompression of sigmoid sinus and/or facial nerve, with or without mobilization
　68.7 　68.7 **FUD** 090 　　　C 50 □ P0
AMA: 2015,Jan,16; 2014,Jan,11

61596 Transcochlear approach to posterior cranial fossa, jugular foramen or midline skull base, including labyrinthectomy, decompression, with or without mobilization of facial nerve and/or petrous carotid artery
　70.7 　70.7 **FUD** 090 　　C 80 50 □ P0
AMA: 2015,Jan,16; 2014,Jan,11

61597 Transcondylar (far lateral) approach to posterior cranial fossa, jugular foramen or midline skull base, including occipital condylectomy, mastoidectomy, resection of C1-C3 vertebral body(s), decompression of vertebral artery, with or without mobilization
　85.4 　85.4 **FUD** 090 　　　C 80 50 □
AMA: 2015,Jan,16; 2014,Jan,11

61598 Transpetrosal approach to posterior cranial fossa, clivus or foramen magnum, including ligation of superior petrosal sinus and/or sigmoid sinus
　84.0 　84.0 **FUD** 090 　　　C 80 □ P0
AMA: 2015,Jan,16; 2014,Jan,11

61600-61616 Definitive Procedures: Cranial Fossae

EXCLUDES Dural repair and/or reconstruction (61618-61619)
Injection for:
　Cerebral angiography (36100-36218)
　Pneumoencephalography (61055)
　Ventriculography (61026, 61120)
Primary closure (15732, 15756-15758)
Surgical approach (61580-61598)

61600 Resection or excision of neoplastic, vascular or infectious lesion of base of anterior cranial fossa; extradural
　61.8 　61.8 **FUD** 090 　　　　C 80 □
AMA: 2015,Jan,16; 2014,Jan,11

61601 intradural, including dural repair, with or without graft
　70.8 　70.8 **FUD** 090 　　　　C 80 □
AMA: 2015,Jan,16; 2014,Jan,11

61605 Resection or excision of neoplastic, vascular or infectious lesion of infratemporal fossa, parapharyngeal space, petrous apex; extradural
　62.9 　62.9 **FUD** 090 　　　　C 80 □
AMA: 2015,Jan,16; 2014,Jan,11

61606 intradural, including dural repair, with or without graft
　89.9 　89.9 **FUD** 090 　　　C 80 □ P0
AMA: 2015,Jan,16; 2014,Jan,11

61607 Resection or excision of neoplastic, vascular or infectious lesion of parasellar area, cavernous sinus, clivus or midline skull base; extradural
　78.1 　78.1 **FUD** 090 　　　　C 80 □
AMA: 2015,Jan,16; 2014,Jan,11

61608 intradural, including dural repair, with or without graft
　96.2 　96.2 **FUD** 090 　　　　C 80 □
AMA: 2015,Jan,16; 2014,Jan,11

+ 61610 Transection or ligation, carotid artery in cavernous sinus, with repair by anastomosis or graft (List separately in addition to code for primary procedure)
Code first (61605-61608)
　55.5 　55.5 **FUD** ZZZ 　　　　C 80 □
AMA: 2015,Jan,16; 2014,Jan,11

+ 61611 Transection or ligation, carotid artery in petrous canal; without repair (List separately in addition to code for primary procedure)
Code first (61605-61608)
　10.7 　10.7 **FUD** ZZZ 　　　　C 80 □
AMA: 2015,Jan,16; 2014,Jan,11

+ 61612 with repair by anastomosis or graft (List separately in addition to code for primary procedure)

Code first (61605-61608)
📋 40.3 ✂ 40.3 **FUD** ZZZ [C] [80] 🖥

AMA: 2015,Jan,16; 2014,Jan,11

61613 Obliteration of carotid aneurysm, arteriovenous malformation, or carotid-cavernous fistula by dissection within cavernous sinus
📋 97.5 ✂ 97.5 **FUD** 090 [C] [80] [50] 🖥

AMA: 2015,Jan,16; 2014,Jan,11

61615 Resection or excision of neoplastic, vascular or infectious lesion of base of posterior cranial fossa, jugular foramen, foramen magnum, or C1-C3 vertebral bodies; extradural
📋 79.7 ✂ 79.7 **FUD** 090 [C] [80] 🖥

AMA: 2015,Jan,16; 2014,Jan,11

61616 intradural, including dural repair, with or without graft
📋 97.6 ✂ 97.6 **FUD** 090 [C] [80] 🖥 [P0]

AMA: 2015,Jan,16; 2014,Jan,11

61618-61619 Reconstruction Post-Surgical Cranial Fossae Defects

EXCLUDES *Definitive surgery (61600-61616)*
Injection for:
  Cerebral angiography (36100-36218)
  Pneumoencephalography (61055)
  Ventriculography (61026, 61120)
Primary closure (15732, 15756-15758)
Surgical approach (61580-61598)

61618 Secondary repair of dura for cerebrospinal fluid leak, anterior, middle or posterior cranial fossa following surgery of the skull base; by free tissue graft (eg, pericranium, fascia, tensor fascia lata, adipose tissue, homologous or synthetic grafts)
📋 38.0 ✂ 38.0 **FUD** 090 [C] [80] 🖥 [P0]

AMA: 2015,Jan,16; 2014,Jan,11; 2012,Jan,15-42; 2011,Jan,11

61619 by local or regionalized vascularized pedicle flap or myocutaneous flap (including galea, temporalis, frontalis or occipitalis muscle)
📋 42.1 ✂ 42.1 **FUD** 090 [C] [80] 🖥 [P0]

AMA: 2015,Jan,16; 2014,Jan,11; 2012,Jan,15-42; 2011,Jan,11

61623-61651 Neurovascular Interventional Procedures

61623 Endovascular temporary balloon arterial occlusion, head or neck (extracranial/intracranial) including selective catheterization of vessel to be occluded, positioning and inflation of occlusion balloon, concomitant neurological monitoring, and radiologic supervision and interpretation of all angiography required for balloon occlusion and to exclude vascular injury post occlusion

EXCLUDES *Diagnostic angiography of target artery just before temporary occlusion; report only radiological supervision and interpretation*
Selective catheterization and angiography of artery besides the target artery; report catheterization and radiological supervision and interpretation codes as appropriate
📋 16.4 ✂ 16.4 **FUD** 000 [J] 🖥 [P0]

AMA: 2015,Jan,16; 2014,Jan,11

Pericallosal artery
Right anterior cerebral artery
Basilar artery
Superior cerebellar artery
Posterior cerebral artery
Left vertebral artery

61624 Transcatheter permanent occlusion or embolization (eg, for tumor destruction, to achieve hemostasis, to occlude a vascular malformation), percutaneous, any method; central nervous system (intracranial, spinal cord)

EXCLUDES *Non-central nervous system transcatheter occlusion or embolization other than head or neck (37241-37244)*
🔀 (75894)
📋 33.3 ✂ 33.3 **FUD** 000 [C] 🖥

AMA: 2015,Jan,16; 2014,Jan,11; 2013,Nov,6; 2012,Jan,15-42; 2011,Jan,11

61626 non-central nervous system, head or neck (extracranial, brachiocephalic branch)

EXCLUDES *Non-central nervous system transcatheter occlusion or embolization other than head or neck (37241-37244)*
🔀 (75894)
📋 25.0 ✂ 25.0 **FUD** 000 [J] 🖥

AMA: 2015,Jan,16; 2014,Jan,11; 2013,Nov,6

61630 Balloon angioplasty, intracranial (eg, atherosclerotic stenosis), percutaneous

INCLUDES Diagnostic arteriogram if stent or angioplasty is necessary
Radiology services for arteriography of target vascular family
Selective catheterization of the target vascular family

EXCLUDES *Diagnostic arteriogram if stent or angioplasty is not necessary (use applicable code for selective catheterization and radiology services)*
Do not report for procedure performed in the same vascular territory as (61645)
📋 38.5 ✂ 38.5 **FUD** XXX [C] [80]

AMA: 2015,Jan,16; 2014,Jan,11

61635 Transcatheter placement of intravascular stent(s), intracranial (eg, atherosclerotic stenosis), including balloon angioplasty, if performed

INCLUDES Diagnostic arteriogram if stent or angioplasty is necessary
Radiology services for arteriography of target vascular family
Selective catheterization of the target vascular family

EXCLUDES *Diagnostic arteriogram if stent or angioplasty is not necessary (use applicable code for selective catheterization and radiology services)*
Do not report for procedure performed in the same vascular territory as (61545)
📋 40.6 ✂ 40.6 **FUD** XXX [C] [80]

AMA: 2015,Jan,16; 2014,Mar,8; 2014,Jan,11

61640 Balloon dilatation of intracranial vasospasm, percutaneous; initial vessel

INCLUDES Angiography after dilation of vessel
Fluoroscopic guidance
Injection of contrast material
Roadmapping
Selective catheterization of target vessel
Vessel analysis
Do not report for procedure performed in the same vascular territory as (61650-61651)
📋 17.8 ✂ 17.8 **FUD** 000 [E]

AMA: 2015,Jan,16; 2014,May,10; 2014,Jan,11

+ 61641 each additional vessel in same vascular family (List separately in addition to code for primary procedure)

INCLUDES Angiography after dilation of vessel
Fluoroscopic guidance
Injection of contrast material
Roadmapping
Selective catheterization of target vessel
Vessel analysis
Code first (61640)
📋 6.29 ✂ 6.29 **FUD** ZZZ [E]

AMA: 2015,Jan,16; 2014,May,10; 2014,Jan,11

+ 61642 each additional vessel in different vascular family (List separately in addition to code for primary procedure)

INCLUDES Angiography after dilation of vessel
Fluoroscopic guidance
Injection of contrast material
Roadmapping
Selective catheterization of target vessel
Vessel analysis

Code first (61640)

Do not report with procedure performed in the same vascular territory as (61650-61651)

🚑 12.5 ✂ 12.5 **FUD** ZZZ ▣E

AMA: 2015,Jan,16; 2014,May,10; 2014,Jan,11

● 61645 Percutaneous arterial transluminal mechanical thrombectomy and/or infusion for thrombolysis, intracranial, any method, including diagnostic angiography, fluoroscopic guidance, catheter placement, and intraprocedural pharmacological thrombolytic injection(s)

INCLUDES Interventions performed in an intracranial artery including:
Angiography with radiologic supervision and interpretation (diagnostic and subsequent)
Closure of arteriotomy by any method
Fluoroscopy
Patient monitoring
Procedures performed in vascular territories:
Left carotid
Right carotid
Vertebro-basilar

EXCLUDES Venous thrombectomy or thrombolysis (37187-37188, [37212], [37214])

Do not report with for the same vascular target area (36221-36228, 37184, 37186, 61630, 61635, 61650-61651)

🚑 0.00 ✂ 0.00 **FUD** 000

● 61650 Endovascular intracranial prolonged administration of pharmacologic agent(s) other than for thrombolysis, arterial, including catheter placement, diagnostic angiography, and imaging guidance; initial vascular territory

INCLUDES Interventions performed in an intracranial artery, including:
Angiography with radiologic supervision and interpretation (diagnostic and subsequent)
Closure of arteriotomy by any method
Fluoroscopy
Patient monitoring
Procedures performed in vascular territories:
Left carotid
Right carotid
Vertebro-basilar
Prolonged (at least 10 minutes) arterial administration of non-thrombolytic agents

EXCLUDES Venous thrombectomy or thrombolysis

Do not report in same vascular territory as (36221-36228, 37184, 37186, 61640-61642, 61645, 96420-96425)

Do not report for treatment of an iatrogenic condition

🚑 0.00 ✂ 0.00 **FUD** 000

● **+** 61651 each additional vascular territory (List separately in addition to code for primary procedure)

🚑 0.00 ✂ 0.00 **FUD** 000

INCLUDES Interventions performed in an intracranial artery including:
Angiography with radiologic supervision and interpretation (diagnostic and subsequent)
Closure of arteriotomy by any method
Fluoroscopy
Patient monitoring
Procedures performed in vascular territories:
Left carotid
Right carotid
Vertebro-basilar
Prolonged (at least 10 minutes) arterial administration of non-thrombolytic agents

EXCLUDES Venous thrombectomy or thrombolysis

Code first (61650)

Do not report for treatment of an iatrogenic condition

Do not report in same vascular territory as (36221-36226, 37184, 37186, 61640-61642, 61645, 96420-96425)

61680-61692 Surgical Treatment of Arteriovenous Malformation of the Brain

INCLUDES Craniotomy

61680 Surgery of intracranial arteriovenous malformation; supratentorial, simple

🚑 66.5 ✂ 66.5 **FUD** 090 C 80 ▣

AMA: 2014,Jan,11

61682 supratentorial, complex

🚑 123. ✂ 123. **FUD** 090 C 80 ▣

AMA: 2015,Jan,16; 2014,Jan,11; 2013,Jun,13

61684 infratentorial, simple

🚑 84.6 ✂ 84.6 **FUD** 090 C 80 ▣

AMA: 2014,Jan,11

61686 infratentorial, complex

🚑 134. ✂ 134. **FUD** 090 C 80 ▣

AMA: 2015,Jan,16; 2014,Jan,11; 2013,Jun,13

61690 dural, simple

🚑 65.0 ✂ 65.0 **FUD** 090 C 80 ▣

AMA: 2014,Jan,11

61692 dural, complex

🚑 109. ✂ 109. **FUD** 090 C 80 ▣

AMA: 2015,Jan,16; 2014,Jan,11; 2013,Jun,13

61697-61703 Surgical Treatment Brain Aneurysm

INCLUDES Craniotomy

61697 Surgery of complex intracranial aneurysm, intracranial approach; carotid circulation

INCLUDES Aneurysms bigger than 15 mm
Calcification of the aneurysm neck
Inclusion of normal vessels in aneurysm neck
Surgery needing temporary vessel occlusion, trapping, or cardiopulmonary bypass to treat aneurysm

🚑 125. ✂ 125. **FUD** 090 C 80 ▣ PQ

AMA: 2014,Jan,11

61698 vertebrobasilar circulation

INCLUDES Aneurysm bigger than 15 mm
Calcification of aneurysm neck
Inclusion of normal vessels into aneurysm neck
Surgery needing temporary vessel occlusion, trapping, or cardiopulmonary bypass to treat aneurysm

🚑 138. ✂ 138. **FUD** 090 C 80 ▣

AMA: 2014,Jan,11

61700 Surgery of simple intracranial aneurysm, intracranial approach; carotid circulation

🚑 101. ✂ 101. **FUD** 090 C 80 ▣ PQ

AMA: 2015,Jan,16; 2014,Jan,11; 2012,Jan,15-42; 2011,Jan,11

61702 vertebrobasilar circulation

  ⏢ 120. ✂ 120. **FUD** 090   C 80 ▢

AMA: 2014,Jan,11

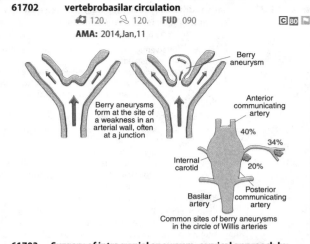

Berry aneurysm

Berry aneurysms form at the site of a weakness in an arterial wall, often at a junction

Anterior communicating artery

40%

34%

Internal carotid

20%

Basilar artery

Posterior communicating artery

Common sites of berry aneurysms in the circle of Willis arteries

61703 Surgery of intracranial aneurysm, cervical approach by application of occluding clamp to cervical carotid artery (Selverstone-Crutchfield type)

  EXCLUDES *Cervical approach for direct ligation of carotid artery (37600-37606)*

  ⏢ 40.3 ✂ 40.3 **FUD** 090   C 80 ▢

AMA: 2014,Jan,11

61705-61710 Other Procedures for Aneurysm, Arteriovenous Malformation, and Carotid-Cavernous Fistula

INCLUDES Craniotomy

61705 Surgery of aneurysm, vascular malformation or carotid-cavernous fistula; by intracranial and cervical occlusion of carotid artery

  ⏢ 77.5 ✂ 77.5 **FUD** 090   C 80 ▢

AMA: 2014,Jan,11

61708 by intracranial electrothrombosis

  EXCLUDES *Ligation or gradual occlusion of internal or common carotid artery (37605-37606)*

  ⏢ 75.7 ✂ 75.7 **FUD** 090   C 80 ▢

AMA: 2014,Jan,11

61710 by intra-arterial embolization, injection procedure, or balloon catheter

  ⏢ 64.0 ✂ 64.0 **FUD** 090   C 80 ▢

AMA: 2015,Jan,16; 2014,Jan,11; 2013,Nov,6

61711 Extracranial-Intracranial Bypass

CMS: 100-2,16,10 Exclusions from Coverage; 100-3,20.2 Extracranial-intracranial (EC-IC) Arterial Bypass Surgery

INCLUDES Craniotomy

EXCLUDES *Carotid or vertebral thromboendarterectomy (35301)*

Code also operating microscope when appropriate (69990)

61711 Anastomosis, arterial, extracranial-intracranial (eg, middle cerebral/cortical) arteries

  ⏢ 76.8 ✂ 76.8 **FUD** 090   C 80 ▢

AMA: 2014,Jan,11

61720-61791 Stereotactic Procedures of the Brain

61720 Creation of lesion by stereotactic method, including burr hole(s) and localizing and recording techniques, single or multiple stages; globus pallidus or thalamus

  ⏢ 37.7 ✂ 37.7 **FUD** 090   T ▢

AMA: 2015,Jan,16; 2014,Jul,8; 2014,Jan,11; 2011,Jul,12-13

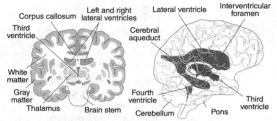

Corpus callosum
Left and right lateral ventricles
Lateral ventricle
Interventricular foramen
Third ventricle
Cerebral aqueduct
White matter
Gray matter
Thalamus
Brain stem
Cerebellum
Fourth ventricle
Pons
Third ventricle

Frontal secion of the brain (left) and lateral view schematic showing the ventricular system in blue (right)

61735 subcortical structure(s) other than globus pallidus or thalamus

  ⏢ 47.2 ✂ 47.2 **FUD** 090   C ▢

AMA: 2014,Jul,8; 2014,Jan,11; 2011,Jul,12-13

61750 Stereotactic biopsy, aspiration, or excision, including burr hole(s), for intracranial lesion;

  ⏢ 41.5 ✂ 41.5 **FUD** 090   C ▢ P0

AMA: 2015,Jan,16; 2014,Jul,8; 2014,Jan,11; 2011,Jul,12-13

61751 with computed tomography and/or magnetic resonance guidance

  ▦ (70450, 70460, 70470, 70551-70553)

  ⏢ 40.8 ✂ 40.8 **FUD** 090   C ▢ P0

AMA: 2015,Jan,16; 2014,Jul,8; 2014,Jan,11; 2012,Jan,15-42; 2011,Jul,12-13; 2011,Jan,11

61760 Stereotactic implantation of depth electrodes into the cerebrum for long-term seizure monitoring

  ⏢ 47.0 ✂ 47.0 **FUD** 090   C ▢

AMA: 2014,Jul,8; 2014,Jan,11; 2011,Jul,12-13

61770 Stereotactic localization, including burr hole(s), with insertion of catheter(s) or probe(s) for placement of radiation source

  ⏢ 48.3 ✂ 48.3 **FUD** 090   T 82 ▢

AMA: 2015,Jan,16; 2014,Jul,8; 2014,Jan,11; 2011,Jul,12-13

+ **61781** Stereotactic computer-assisted (navigational) procedure; cranial, intradural (List separately in addition to code for primary procedure)

  Code first primary procedure

  Do not report for same surgical session by same individual (61782)

  Do not report with (61720-61791, 61796-61799, 61863-61868, 62201, 77371-77373, 77432)

  ⏢ 7.01 ✂ 7.01 **FUD** ZZZ   N N1 80

AMA: 2015,Jan,16; 2014,Sep,13; 2014,Jul,8; 2014,Jan,11; 2011,Jul,12-13; 2010,Oct,3-4

+ **61782** cranial, extradural (List separately in addition to code for primary procedure)

  Code first primary procedure

  Do not report for same surgical session by same individual (61781)

  Do not report with (61796-61799)

  ⏢ 5.10 ✂ 5.10 **FUD** ZZZ   N N1 80

AMA: 2015,Jan,16; 2014,Jul,8; 2014,Jan,11; 2011,Jul,12-13; 2010,Oct,3-4

+ **61783** spinal (List separately in addition to code for primary procedure)

  Code first primary procedure

  Do not report with (61796-61799, 63620-63621)

  ⏢ 6.91 ✂ 6.91 **FUD** ZZZ   N N1 80

AMA: 2015,Jan,16; 2014,Jul,8; 2014,Jan,11; 2011,Jul,12-13; 2010,Oct,3-4

61790 **Creation of lesion by stereotactic method, percutaneous, by neurolytic agent (eg, alcohol, thermal, electrical, radiofrequency); gasserian ganglion**

🔧 25.9 ⚕ 25.9 **FUD** 090 T A2 50 📷

AMA: 2014,Jul,8; 2014,Jan,11; 2011,Jul,12-13

61791 **trigeminal medullary tract**

🔧 33.3 ⚕ 33.3 **FUD** 090 T A2 80 50 📷

AMA: 2015,Jan,16; 2014,Jul,8; 2014,Jan,11; 2011,Jul,12-13

61796-61800 Stereotactic Radiosurgery (SRS): Brain

INCLUDES Planning, dosimetry, targeting, positioning or blocking performed by the neurosurgeon

EXCLUDES *Intensity modulated beam delivery plan and treatment (77301, 77385-77386)*
Stereotactic body radiation therapy (77373, 77435)
Treatment planning, physics and dosimetry, and treatment delivery performed by the radiation oncologist

Do not report radiation treatment management and radiosurgery by the same provider (77427-77435)

Do not report with (20660)

61796 **Stereotactic radiosurgery (particle beam, gamma ray, or linear accelerator); 1 simple cranial lesion**

INCLUDES Lesions < 3.5 cm

EXCLUDES *Treatment of complex lesions: (61798-61799)*
Arteriovenous malformations (AVM)
Brainstem lesions
Cavernous sinus/parasellar/petroclival tumors, glomus tumors, pituitary tumors, and tumors of pineal region
Lesions located <= 5 mm from the optic nerve, chasm, or tract
Schwannomas

Code also stereotactic headframe application, when performed (61800)

Do not report more than one time per treatment course

Do not report with (61781-61783, 61798)

🔧 30.0 ⚕ 30.0 **FUD** 090 B 80

AMA: 2015,Jun,6; 2015,Jan,16; 2014,Jul,8; 2014,Jan,11; 2012,Apr,11-13; 2011,Jul,12-13

+ **61797** **each additional cranial lesion, simple (List separately in addition to code for primary procedure)**

INCLUDES Lesions < 3.5 cm

EXCLUDES *Treatment of complex lesions: (61798-61799)*
Arteriovenous malformations (AVM)
Brainstem lesion
Cavernous sinus/parasellar/petroclival tumors, glomus tumors, pituitary tumor, tumors of pineal region
Lesions located <= 5 mm from the optic nerve, chasm, or tract
Schwannomas

Code first (61796, 61798)

Do not report more than four times in total per treatment course when used alone or in combination with (61799)

Do not report more than one time per lesion per treatment course

Do not report with (61781-61783)

🔧 6.60 ⚕ 6.60 **FUD** ZZZ B 80

AMA: 2015,Jun,6; 2015,Jan,16; 2014,Jul,8; 2014,Jan,11; 2012,Apr,11-13; 2011,Jul,12-13

61798 **1 complex cranial lesion**

INCLUDES All therapeutic lesion creation procedures
Treatment of complex lesions:
Arteriovenous malformations (AVM)
Brainstem lesions
Cavernous sinus, parasellar, petroclival, glomus, pineal region, and pituitary tumors
Lesions located <= 5 mm from the optic nerve, chasm, or tract
Lesions >= 3.5 cm
Schwannomas
Treatment of multiple lesions as long as one is complex

Code also stereotactic headframe application, when performed (61800)

Do not report more than one time per treatment course

Do not report with (61781-61783, 61796)

🔧 41.0 ⚕ 41.0 **FUD** 090 B 80

AMA: 2015,Jun,6; 2015,Jan,16; 2014,Jul,8; 2014,Jan,11; 2012,Apr,11-13; 2011,Jul,12-13

+ **61799** **each additional cranial lesion, complex (List separately in addition to code for primary procedure)**

INCLUDES All therapeutic lesion creation procedures
Treatment of complex lesions:
Arteriovenous malformations (AVM)
Brainstem lesions
Cavernous sinus, parasellar, petroclival, glomus, pineal region, and pituitary tumors
Lesions located <= 5 mm from the optic nerve, chasm, or tract
Lesions >= 3.5 cm
Schwannomas

Code first (61798)

Do not report more than four times in total per treatment course when used alone or in combination with (61799)

Do not report more than once per lesion per treatment course

Do not report with (61781-61783)

🔧 9.09 ⚕ 9.09 **FUD** ZZZ B 80

AMA: 2015,Jun,6; 2015,Jan,16; 2014,Jul,8; 2014,Jan,11; 2012,Apr,11-13; 2011,Jul,12-13

+ **61800** **Application of stereotactic headframe for stereotactic radiosurgery (List separately in addition to code for primary procedure)**

Code first (61796, 61798)

🔧 4.60 ⚕ 4.60 **FUD** ZZZ B 80

AMA: 2015,Jun,6; 2015,Jan,16; 2014,Jan,11; 2012,Apr,11-13

61850-61888 Intracranial Neurostimulation

INCLUDES Microelectrode recording by operating surgeon

EXCLUDES *Electronic analysis and reprogramming of neurostimulator pulse generator (95970-95975)*
Neurophysiological mapping by another physician/qualified health care professional (95961-95962)

61850 **Twist drill or burr hole(s) for implantation of neurostimulator electrodes, cortical**

🔧 29.1 ⚕ 29.1 **FUD** 090 C 80 📷

AMA: 2015,Jan,16; 2014,Jan,11

61860 **Craniectomy or craniotomy for implantation of neurostimulator electrodes, cerebral, cortical**

🔧 46.5 ⚕ 46.5 **FUD** 090 C 80 📷

AMA: 2015,Jan,16; 2014,Jan,11

61863 **Twist drill, burr hole, craniotomy, or craniectomy with stereotactic implantation of neurostimulator electrode array in subcortical site (eg, thalamus, globus pallidus, subthalamic nucleus, periventricular, periaqueductal gray), without use of intraoperative microelectrode recording; first array**

🔧 44.5 ⚕ 44.5 **FUD** 090 C 80 50 📷

AMA: 2015,Jan,16; 2014,Jul,8; 2014,Jan,11; 2012,Jan,15-42; 2011,Jul,12-13; 2011,Jan,11; 2010,Oct,9

+ 61864 **each additional array (List separately in addition to primary procedure)**
Code first (61863)
🏥 8.52   ⚕ 8.52   **FUD** ZZZ   C 80 ▣
AMA: 2014,Jul,8; 2014,Jan,11; 2011,Jul,12-13

61867 **Twist drill, burr hole, craniotomy, or craniectomy with stereotactic implantation of neurostimulator electrode array in subcortical site (eg, thalamus, globus pallidus, subthalamic nucleus, periventricular, periaqueductal gray), with use of intraoperative microelectrode recording; first array**
🏥 67.5   ⚕ 67.5   **FUD** 090   C 80 50 ▣ PQ
AMA: 2014,Jul,8; 2014,Jan,11; 2011,Jul,12-13

+ 61868 **each additional array (List separately in addition to primary procedure)**
Code first (61867)
🏥 14.8   ⚕ 14.8   **FUD** ZZZ   C 80 ▣
AMA: 2015,Jan,16; 2014,Jul,8; 2014,Jan,11; 2011,Jul,12-13

61870 **Craniectomy for implantation of neurostimulator electrodes, cerebellar, cortical**
🏥 35.1   ⚕ 35.1   **FUD** 090   C 80 ▣
AMA: 2014,Jan,11

61880 **Revision or removal of intracranial neurostimulator electrodes**
🏥 16.7   ⚕ 16.7   **FUD** 090   02 62 80 50 ▣
AMA: 2014,Jan,11

61885 **Insertion or replacement of cranial neurostimulator pulse generator or receiver, direct or inductive coupling; with connection to a single electrode array**
EXCLUDES *Percutaneous procedure to place cranial nerve neurostimulator electrode(s) (64553)*
Revision or replacement cranial neurostimulator electrode array (64569)
🏥 15.1   ⚕ 15.1   **FUD** 090   J J8 80 50 ▣
AMA: 2015,Jan,16; 2014,Jan,11; 2012,Jan,15-42; 2011,Sep,9-10; 2011,Sep,8; 2011,Feb,4-5; 2010,Dec,12

61886 **with connection to 2 or more electrode arrays**
EXCLUDES *Percutaneous procedure to place cranial nerve neurostimulator electrode(s) (64553)*
Revision or replacement cranial neurostimulator electrode array (64569)
🏥 24.8   ⚕ 24.8   **FUD** 090   J J8 80 ▣
AMA: 2015,Jan,16; 2014,Jan,11; 2012,Jan,15-42; 2011,Sep,9-10; 2011,Sep,8; 2011,Feb,4-5

61888 **Revision or removal of cranial neurostimulator pulse generator or receiver**
Do not report with (61885-61886)
🏥 11.6   ⚕ 11.6   **FUD** 010   J J8 50 ▣
AMA: 2015,Jan,16; 2014,Jan,11; 2012,Jan,15-42; 2011,Sep,8; 2011,Sep,9-10; 2011,Feb,4-5

62000-62148 Repair of Skull and/or Cerebrospinal Fluid Leaks

62000 **Elevation of depressed skull fracture; simple, extradural**
🏥 30.5   ⚕ 30.5   **FUD** 090   T ▣
AMA: 2014,Jan,11

62005 **compound or comminuted, extradural**
🏥 37.7   ⚕ 37.7   **FUD** 090   C 80 ▣
AMA: 2014,Jan,11

62010 **with repair of dura and/or debridement of brain**
🏥 45.5   ⚕ 45.5   **FUD** 090   C 80 ▣
AMA: 2014,Jan,11

62100 **Craniotomy for repair of dural/cerebrospinal fluid leak, including surgery for rhinorrhea/otorrhea**
EXCLUDES *Repair of spinal fluid leak (63707, 63709)*
🏥 47.2   ⚕ 47.2   **FUD** 090   C 80 ▣
AMA: 2014,Jan,11

62115 **Reduction of craniomegalic skull (eg, treated hydrocephalus); not requiring bone grafts or cranioplasty**
🏥 39.8   ⚕ 39.8   **FUD** 090   C 80 ▣
AMA: 2014,Jan,11

62117 **requiring craniotomy and reconstruction with or without bone graft (includes obtaining grafts)**
🏥 58.3   ⚕ 58.3   **FUD** 090   C 80 ▣
AMA: 2014,Jan,11

62120 **Repair of encephalocele, skull vault, including cranioplasty**
🏥 48.0   ⚕ 48.0   **FUD** 090   C 80 ▣
AMA: 2014,Jan,11

62121 **Craniotomy for repair of encephalocele, skull base**
🏥 47.0   ⚕ 47.0   **FUD** 090   C 80 ▣
AMA: 2014,Jan,11

62140 **Cranioplasty for skull defect; up to 5 cm diameter**
🏥 30.4   ⚕ 30.4   **FUD** 090   C 80 ▣
AMA: 2015,Jan,16; 2014,Jan,11; 2014,Jan,9

62141 **larger than 5 cm diameter**
🏥 33.7   ⚕ 33.7   **FUD** 090   C 80 ▣
AMA: 2015,Jan,16; 2014,Jan,11; 2014,Jan,9

62142 **Removal of bone flap or prosthetic plate of skull**
🏥 26.0   ⚕ 26.0   **FUD** 090   C 80 ▣
AMA: 2015,Jan,16; 2014,Jan,11; 2014,Jan,9

62143 **Replacement of bone flap or prosthetic plate of skull**
🏥 30.8   ⚕ 30.8   **FUD** 090   C 80 ▣
AMA: 2015,Jan,16; 2014,Jan,11; 2014,Jan,9

62145 **Cranioplasty for skull defect with reparative brain surgery**
🏥 41.7   ⚕ 41.7   **FUD** 090   C 80 ▣
AMA: 2015,Jan,16; 2014,Jan,11; 2014,Jan,9

62146 **Cranioplasty with autograft (includes obtaining bone grafts); up to 5 cm diameter**
🏥 36.4   ⚕ 36.4   **FUD** 090   C 80 ▣
AMA: 2015,Jan,16; 2014,Jan,11; 2014,Jan,9

62147 **larger than 5 cm diameter**
🏥 43.3   ⚕ 43.3   **FUD** 090   C 80 ▣
AMA: 2015,Jan,16; 2014,Jan,11; 2014,Jan,9

+ 62148 **Incision and retrieval of subcutaneous cranial bone graft for cranioplasty (List separately in addition to code for primary procedure)**
Code first (62140-62147)
🏥 3.79   ⚕ 3.79   **FUD** ZZZ   C ▣
AMA: 2014,Jan,11

62160-62165 Neuroendoscopic Brain Procedures

INCLUDES Diagnostic endoscopy

+ 62160 **Neuroendoscopy, intracranial, for placement or replacement of ventricular catheter and attachment to shunt system or external drainage (List separately in addition to code for primary procedure)**
Code first (61107, 61210, 62220-62230, 62258)
🏥 5.69   ⚕ 5.69   **FUD** ZZZ   N III ▣
AMA: 2015,Jan,16; 2014,Jan,11; 2012,Dec,12; 2012,Jan,15-42; 2011,Jan,11

62161 **Neuroendoscopy, intracranial; with dissection of adhesions, fenestration of septum pellucidum or intraventricular cysts (including placement, replacement, or removal of ventricular catheter)**
🏥 45.1   ⚕ 45.1   **FUD** 090   C 80 ▣
AMA: 2014,Jan,11

62162 **with fenestration or excision of colloid cyst, including placement of external ventricular catheter for drainage**
🏥 56.1   ⚕ 56.1   **FUD** 090   C 80 ▣
AMA: 2014,Jan,11

62163 **with retrieval of foreign body**
🏥 36.3   ⚕ 36.3   **FUD** 090   C 80 ▣
AMA: 2014,Jan,11

62164	with excision of brain tumor, including placement of external ventricular catheter for drainage
	62.0 62.0 **FUD** 090 C 80 ▢
	AMA: 2014,Jan,11

62165	with excision of pituitary tumor, transnasal or trans-sphenoidal approach
	45.3 45.3 **FUD** 090 C 80 ▢
	AMA: 2014,Jan,11

62180-62258 Cerebrospinal Fluid Diversion Procedures

62180	Ventriculocisternostomy (Torkildsen type operation)
	47.5 47.5 **FUD** 090 C 80 ▢
	AMA: 2014,Jan,11

62190	Creation of shunt; subarachnoid/subdural-atrial, -jugular, -auricular
	16.9 16.9 **FUD** 090 C ▢
	AMA: 2014,Jan,11

Origin of shunt is subarachnoid/subdural

Shunt to pleura, peritoneum, or other site (62192)

Shunt to jugular, atria, or auricle (62190)

62192	subarachnoid/subdural-peritoneal, -pleural, other terminus
	28.8 28.8 **FUD** 090 C 80 ▢
	AMA: 2014,Jan,11

62194	Replacement or irrigation, subarachnoid/subdural catheter
	14.3 14.3 **FUD** 010 T A2 80 ▢
	AMA: 2015,Jan,16; 2014,Jan,11; 2011,Dec,6-7

62200	Ventriculocisternostomy, third ventricle;
	INCLUDES Dandy ventriculocisternostomy
	40.9 40.9 **FUD** 090 C 80 ▢
	AMA: 2014,Jan,11

62201	stereotactic, neuroendoscopic method
	EXCLUDES Intracranial neuroendoscopic surgery (62161-62165)
	35.6 35.6 **FUD** 090 C ▢
	AMA: 2015,Jan,16; 2014,Jul,8; 2014,Jan,11; 2012,Jan,15-42; 2011,Jul,12-13; 2011,Jan,11

62220	Creation of shunt; ventriculo-atrial, -jugular, -auricular
	Code also intracranial neuroendoscopic ventricular catheter insertion, when performed (62160)
	30.2 30.2 **FUD** 090 C 80 ▢
	AMA: 2014,Jan,11

62223	ventriculo-peritoneal, -pleural, other terminus
	Code also intracranial neuroendoscopic ventricular catheter insertion, when performed (62160)
	30.9 30.9 **FUD** 090 C 80 ▢ P0
	AMA: 2014,Jan,11

62225	Replacement or irrigation, ventricular catheter
	Code also intracranial neuroendoscopic ventricular catheter insertion, when performed (62160)
	15.4 15.4 **FUD** 090 T A2 ▢
	AMA: 2015,Jan,16; 2014,Jan,11; 2012,Jan,15-42; 2011,Dec,6-7

62230	Replacement or revision of cerebrospinal fluid shunt, obstructed valve, or distal catheter in shunt system
	Code also intracranial neuroendoscopic ventricular catheter insertion, when performed (62160)
	24.8 24.8 **FUD** 090 T A2 80 ▢ P0
	AMA: 2015,Jan,16; 2014,Jan,11; 2012,Dec,12; 2012,Jan,15-42; 2011,Dec,6-7

62252	Reprogramming of programmable cerebrospinal shunt
	2.46 2.46 **FUD** XXX S P3 80 ▢
	AMA: 2014,Jan,11

62256	Removal of complete cerebrospinal fluid shunt system; without replacement
	EXCLUDES Reprogramming cerebrospinal fluid (CSF) shunt (62252)
	17.7 17.7 **FUD** 090 C 80 ▢
	AMA: 2014,Jan,11

62258	with replacement by similar or other shunt at same operation
	EXCLUDES Reprogramming of a cerebrospinal fluid (CSF) shunt (62252)
	Code also intracranial neuroendoscopic ventricular catheter insertion, when performed (62160)
	33.1 33.1 **FUD** 090 C 80 ▢
	AMA: 2015,Jan,16; 2014,Jan,11; 2012,Jan,15-42; 2011,Dec,6-7

62263-62264 Lysis of Epidural Lesions with Injection of Solution/Mechanical Methods

INCLUDES Contrast injection during fluoroscopic guidance/localization
Percutaneous mechanical lysis
Code also fluoroscopic guidance and localization unless a formal contrast study is performed (77003)

62263	Percutaneous lysis of epidural adhesions using solution injection (eg, hypertonic saline, enzyme) or mechanical means (eg, catheter) including radiologic localization (includes contrast when administered), multiple adhesiolysis sessions; 2 or more days
	INCLUDES All adhesiolysis treatments, injections, and infusions during course of treatment
	Percutaneous epidural catheter insertion and removal for neurolytic agent injections during a series of treatment sessions
	Do not report more than one time for the complete series spanning two or more treatment days
	9.59 18.0 **FUD** 010 T A2 ▢ P0
	AMA: 2015,Jan,16; 2014,Jan,11; 2012,Jun,12-13; 2012,Jan,15-42; 2011,Jan,11; 2011,Jan,8; 2010,Nov,1; 2010,Nov,3

62264	1 day
	INCLUDES Multiple treatment sessions performed on the same day
	Do not report with (62263)
	6.84 11.9 **FUD** 010 T A2 ▢ P0
	AMA: 2015,Jan,16; 2014,Jan,11; 2012,Jun,12-13; 2012,Jan,15-42; 2011,Jan,11; 2011,Jan,8; 2010,Nov,1; 2010,Nov,3

62267-62269 Percutaneous Procedures of Spinal Cord

62267 **Percutaneous aspiration within the nucleus pulposus, intervertebral disc, or paravertebral tissue for diagnostic purposes**

> **INCLUDES** Contrast injection during fluoroscopic guidance/localization
>
> Code also fluoroscopic guidance and localization unless a formal contrast study is performed (77003)
>
> Do not report with (10022, 20225, 62287, 62290-62291)
>
> ☒ (77003)

🔲 4.65   ⚬ 7.14   **FUD** 000   T 🔲 🔲

AMA: 2015,Jan,16; 2014,Jan,11; 2012,Jul,3-6; 2011,Jan,8; 2010,Nov,1; 2010,Nov,3

62268 **Percutaneous aspiration, spinal cord cyst or syrinx**

> ☒ (76942, 77002, 77012)

🔲 7.60   ⚬ 7.60   **FUD** 000   T 🔲 🔲

AMA: 2014,Jan,11

62269 **Biopsy of spinal cord, percutaneous needle**

> **EXCLUDES** Fine needle aspiration (10021-10022)
>
> ☒ (76942, 77002, 77012)
>
> ☒ (88172-88173)

🔲 7.80   ⚬ 7.80   **FUD** 000   T 🔲 🔲 🔲 🔲

AMA: 2014,Jan,11

62270-62272 Spinal Puncture, Subarachnoid Space, Diagnostic/Therapeutic

> **INCLUDES** Contrast injection during fluoroscopic guidance/localization
>
> Code also fluoroscopic guidance and localization unless a formal contrast study is performed (77003)

62270 **Spinal puncture, lumbar, diagnostic**

🔲 2.27   ⚬ 4.56   **FUD** 000   T 🔲 🔲

AMA: 2015,Jan,16; 2014,Sep,3; 2014,Jan,11; 2012,Mar,4-7; 2011,Jan,8; 2010,Nov,1; 2010,Nov,3

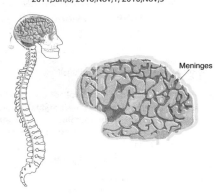

Meninges

62272 **Spinal puncture, therapeutic, for drainage of cerebrospinal fluid (by needle or catheter)**

🔲 2.44   ⚬ 5.75   **FUD** 000   T 🔲 🔲

AMA: 2015,Jan,16; 2014,Jan,11; 2013,Dec,14; 2011,Jan,8; 2010,Nov,1; 2010,Nov,3

62273 Epidural Blood Patch

CMS: 100-3,10.5 NCD for Autogenous Epidural Blood Graft (10.5)

> **INCLUDES** Contrast injection during fluoroscopic guidance/localization
>
> **EXCLUDES** Injection of diagnostic or therapeutic material (62310-62311, 62318-62319)
>
> Code also fluoroscopic guidance and localization unless a formal contrast study is performed (77003)

62273 **Injection, epidural, of blood or clot patch**

🔲 3.28   ⚬ 4.94   **FUD** 000   T 🔲 🔲

AMA: 2015,Jan,16; 2014,Jan,11; 2011,Jan,8; 2010,Nov,1; 2010,Nov,3

62280-62282 Neurolysis

> **INCLUDES** Contrast injection during fluoroscopic guidance/localization
>
> **EXCLUDES** Injection of diagnostic or therapeutic material only (62310-62311, 62318-62319)
>
> Code also fluoroscopic guidance and localization unless a formal contrast study is performed (77003)

62280 **Injection/infusion of neurolytic substance (eg, alcohol, phenol, iced saline solutions), with or without other therapeutic substance; subarachnoid**

🔲 4.56   ⚬ 8.54   **FUD** 010   T 🔲 🔲 🔲

AMA: 2015,Jan,16; 2014,Jan,11; 2012,Jun,12-13; 2011,Jan,8; 2010,Nov,1; 2010,Nov,3; 2010,Jan,9-11

62281 **epidural, cervical or thoracic**

🔲 4.42   ⚬ 6.66   **FUD** 010   T 🔲 🔲 🔲

AMA: 2015,Jan,16; 2014,Jan,11; 2012,Jun,12-13; 2011,Jan,8; 2010,Nov,1; 2010,Nov,3; 2010,May,9; 2010,Jan,12-15; 2010,Jan,9-11

62282 **epidural, lumbar, sacral (caudal)**

🔲 4.22   ⚬ 8.39   **FUD** 010   T 🔲 🔲 🔲

AMA: 2015,Jan,16; 2014,Jan,11; 2012,Jun,12-13; 2012,Jan,15-42; 2011,Jan,11; 2011,Jan,8; 2010,Nov,1; 2010,Nov,3; 2010,Jan,9-11

62284-62294 Injection/Aspiration of Spine, Diagnostic/Therapeutic

62284 **Injection procedure for myelography and/or computed tomography, lumbar**

> **EXCLUDES** Injection at C1-C2 (61055)
>
> Do not report with (62302-62305, 72240, 72255, 72265, 72270)

🔲 2.50   ⚬ 5.21   **FUD** 000   N 🔲 🔲

AMA: 2015,Jan,16; 2014,Sep,3; 2014,Jan,11; 2012,Jan,15-42; 2011,Jan,11

62287 **Decompression procedure, percutaneous, of nucleus pulposus of intervertebral disc, any method utilizing needle based technique to remove disc material under fluoroscopic imaging or other form of indirect visualization, with the use of an endoscope, with discography and/or epidural injection(s) at the treated level(s), when performed, single or multiple levels, lumbar**

> **INCLUDES** Endoscopic approach
>
> **EXCLUDES** Percutaneous decompression of nucleus pulposus of an intervertebral disc, non-needle based technique (0274T-0275T)
>
> Do not report with (62267, 62290, 62311, 72295, 77003, 77012)

🔲 16.5   ⚬ 16.5   **FUD** 090   T 🔲

AMA: 2015,Mar,9; 2015,Jan,16; 2014,Apr,10; 2014,Jan,11; 2012,Oct,14; 2012,Jul,3-6; 2012,Jan,15-42; 2011,Jan,11; 2010,Oct,9

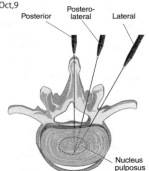

Posterior   Postero-lateral   Lateral

Nucleus pulposus

62290 **Injection procedure for discography, each level; lumbar**

> ☒ (72295)

🔲 4.97   ⚬ 9.52   **FUD** 000   N 🔲 🔲

AMA: 2015,Jan,16; 2014,Jan,11; 2012,Jul,3-6; 2012,Jan,15-42; 2011,Mar,7; 2011,Jan,11

62291 **cervical or thoracic**

> ☒ (72285)

🔲 4.96   ⚬ 9.61   **FUD** 000   N 🔲 🔲

AMA: 2015,Jan,16; 2014,Jan,11; 2011,Mar,7

| 26 /TC PC/TC Comp Only | A2-Z3 ASC Pmt | 50 Bilateral | ♂ Male Only | ♀ Female Only | 🔲 Facility RVU | ⚬ Non-Facility RVU |
| **AMA:** CPT Asst | **CMS:** Pub 100 | A-Y OPPSI | 80 /80 Surg Assist Allowed / w/Doc | | 🔲 Lab Crosswalk | ☒ Radiology Crosswalk |

248   Medicare (Red Text)   CPT © 2015 American Medical Association. All Rights Reserved. (Black Text)   © 2015 Optum360, LLC (Blue Text)

62292 Injection procedure for chemonucleolysis, including discography, intervertebral disc, single or multiple levels, lumbar

    16.7   16.7   **FUD** 090   T R2 80

AMA: 2015,Jan,16; 2014,Jan,11; 2012,Jan,15-42; 2011,Jan,11

62294 Injection procedure, arterial, for occlusion of arteriovenous malformation, spinal

    22.8   22.8   **FUD** 090   T A2

AMA: 2014,Jan,11

62302-62305 Myelography

EXCLUDES   C1-C2 injection (61055)
Lumbar myelogram furnished by other providers (62284, 72240, 72255, 72265, 72270)

62302 Myelography via lumbar injection, including radiological supervision and interpretation; cervical

    3.61   6.95   **FUD** 000   Q2 N1

Do not report with (62303-62305)

62303 thoracic

    3.66   7.22   **FUD** 000   Q2 N1

Do not report with (62302, 62304-62305)

62304 lumbosacral

    3.55   6.86   **FUD** 000   Q2 N1

Do not report with (62302-62303, 62305)

62305 2 or more regions (eg, lumbar/thoracic, cervical/thoracic, lumbar/cervical, lumbar/thoracic/cervical)

    3.72   7.49   **FUD** 000   Q2 N1

Do not report with (62302-62305)

62310-62319 Injection/Infusion Diagnostic/Therapeutic Material

INCLUDES   Contrast injection during fluoroscopic guidance/localization
EXCLUDES   Daily management of continuous epidural or subarachnoid drug administration (01996)
Epidurography (72275)
Transforaminal epidural injection (64479-64484)
Code also fluoroscopic guidance and localization unless a formal contrast study is performed (77003)
Do not report more than once, even when catheter tip or substance injected moves into another spinal region

62310 Injection(s), of diagnostic or therapeutic substance(s) (including anesthetic, antispasmodic, opioid, steroid, other solution), not including neurolytic substances, including needle or catheter placement, includes contrast for localization when performed, epidural or subarachnoid; cervical or thoracic

INCLUDES   Placement and use of a catheter to administer epidural or subarachnoid injection(s), even if more than one injection on a single calendar day
Placement of catheter into the epidural space and then removing the catheter after injecting substance(s) at one or more levels
Do not report with (62318)

    3.13   6.83   **FUD** 000   T A2

AMA: 2015,Jan,16; 2014,Jan,11; 2012,Jul,3-6; 2012,Jan,15-42; 2011,Feb,4-5; 2011,Jan,11; 2011,Jan,8; 2010,Nov,1; 2010,Nov,3; 2010,May,9; 2010,Jan,12-15

62311 lumbar or sacral (caudal)

INCLUDES   Placement and use of a catheter to administer epidural or subarachnoid injection(s), even if more than one injection on a single calendar day
Placement of catheter into the epidural space and then removing the catheter after injecting substance(s) at one or more levels
Do not report with (62319)

    2.58   6.29   **FUD** 000   T A2

AMA: 2015,Jan,16; 2014,Jan,11; 2012,Jul,3-6; 2012,Jan,15-42; 2011,Feb,4-5; 2011,Jan,11; 2011,Jan,8; 2010,Nov,1; 2010,Nov,3

62318 Injection(s), including indwelling catheter placement, continuous infusion or intermittent bolus, of diagnostic or therapeutic substance(s) (including anesthetic, antispasmodic, opioid, steroid, other solution), not including neurolytic substances, includes contrast for localization when performed, epidural or subarachnoid; cervical or thoracic

INCLUDES   Placement of catheter into the epidural space with delivery of substances for more than one calendar day, either continuously or by intermittent bolus
Do not report with (62310)

    2.86   6.52   **FUD** 000   T A2

AMA: 2015,Jan,16; 2014,Jan,11; 2012,Oct,14; 2012,Jul,3-6; 2012,Jan,15-42; 2011,Jan,11; 2011,Jan,8; 2010,Nov,1; 2010,Nov,3

62319 lumbar or sacral (caudal)

INCLUDES   Placement of catheter into the epidural space with delivery of substances for more than one calendar day, either continuously or by intermittent bolus
Do not report with (62311)

    2.76   4.77   **FUD** 000   T A2

AMA: 2015,Jan,16; 2014,Jan,11; 2012,Jul,3-6; 2012,Jan,15-42; 2011,Jan,11; 2011,Jan,8; 2010,Nov,1; 2010,Nov,3

62350-62370 Procedures Related to Epidural and Intrathecal Catheters

EXCLUDES   Infusion pump refilling and maintenance without reprogramming (95990-95991)
Percutaneous insertion of intrathecal or epidural catheter (62270-62273, 62280-62284, 62310-62319)

62350 Implantation, revision or repositioning of tunneled intrathecal or epidural catheter, for long-term medication administration via an external pump or implantable reservoir/infusion pump; without laminectomy

    11.6   11.6   **FUD** 010   T A2

AMA: 2015,Jan,16; 2014,Jan,11

62351 with laminectomy

    25.1   25.1   **FUD** 090   T 80

AMA: 2015,Jan,16; 2014,Jan,11

62355 Removal of previously implanted intrathecal or epidural catheter

    7.83   7.83   **FUD** 010   Q2 A2 80

AMA: 2014,Jan,11

62360 Implantation or replacement of device for intrathecal or epidural drug infusion; subcutaneous reservoir

    8.82   8.82   **FUD** 010   T A2 80

AMA: 2014,Jan,11

62361 nonprogrammable pump

    12.6   12.6   **FUD** 010   J J8 80

AMA: 2014,Jan,11

62362 programmable pump, including preparation of pump, with or without programming

    11.2   11.2   **FUD** 010   J J8 80

AMA: 2015,Jan,16; 2014,Jan,11; 2012,Jan,15-42; 2011,Jan,11

62365 Removal of subcutaneous reservoir or pump, previously implanted for intrathecal or epidural infusion

    8.65   8.65   **FUD** 010   Q2 A2 80

AMA: 2014,Jan,11

62367 Electronic analysis of programmable, implanted pump for intrathecal or epidural drug infusion (includes evaluation of reservoir status, alarm status, drug prescription status); without reprogramming or refill

    0.72   1.16   **FUD** XXX   S P3

AMA: 2015,Jan,16; 2014,Jan,11; 2012,Aug,10-12; 2012,Jul,3-6

62368 with reprogramming

    1.01   1.61   **FUD** XXX   S P3

AMA: 2015,Jan,16; 2014,Jan,11; 2012,Aug,10-12; 2012,Jul,3-6; 2012,Jan,15-42; 2011,Jan,11

62369   **with reprogramming and refill**
🔧 1.02   ✂ 3.43   **FUD** XXX   S P3
AMA: 2015,Jan,16; 2014,Jan,11; 2012,Aug,10-12; 2012,Jul,3-6

62370   **with reprogramming and refill (requiring skill of a physician or other qualified health care professional)**
🔧 1.35   ✂ 3.62   **FUD** XXX   S P3
AMA: 2015,Jan,16; 2014,Jan,11; 2012,Aug,10-12; 2012,Jul,3-6

63001-63048 Posterior Midline Approach: Laminectomy/Laminotomy/Decompression

INCLUDES   Endoscopic assistance through open and direct visualization
EXCLUDES   Arthrodesis (22590-22614)
           Percutaneous laminotomy/hemilaminectomy with imaging guidance and/or endoscope only (0274T, 0275T)

63001   **Laminectomy with exploration and/or decompression of spinal cord and/or cauda equina, without facetectomy, foraminotomy or discectomy (eg, spinal stenosis), 1 or 2 vertebral segments; cervical**
🔧 36.5   ✂ 36.5   **FUD** 090   T G2 80 ▣
AMA: 2015,Jan,16; 2014,Jan,11; 2013,Jul,3-5; 2012,Jul,3-6; 2012,Jan,15-42; 2011,Jul,12-13; 2011,Jan,11

63003   **thoracic**
🔧 36.3   ✂ 36.3   **FUD** 090   T G2 80 ▣
AMA: 2015,Jan,16; 2014,Jan,11; 2013,Jul,3-5; 2012,Jul,3-6; 2012,Jan,15-42; 2011,Jul,12-13; 2011,Jan,11

63005   **lumbar, except for spondylolisthesis**
🔧 34.6   ✂ 34.6   **FUD** 090   T G2 80 ▣
AMA: 2015,Jan,16; 2014,Jan,11; 2013,Dec,16; 2013,Jul,3-5; 2012,Jul,3-6; 2012,Jan,15-42; 2011,Jul,12-13; 2011,Jan,11

63011   **sacral**
🔧 32.1   ✂ 32.1   **FUD** 090   T 80 ▣
AMA: 2015,Jan,16; 2014,Jan,11; 2013,Jul,3-5; 2012,Jan,15-42; 2011,Jul,12-13; 2011,Jan,11

63012   **Laminectomy with removal of abnormal facets and/or pars inter-articularis with decompression of cauda equina and nerve roots for spondylolisthesis, lumbar (Gill type procedure)**
🔧 34.8   ✂ 34.8   **FUD** 090   T 80 ▣
AMA: 2015,Jan,16; 2014,Jan,11; 2013,Jul,3-5; 2012,Jan,15-42; 2011,Jul,12-13; 2011,Jan,11

63015   **Laminectomy with exploration and/or decompression of spinal cord and/or cauda equina, without facetectomy, foraminotomy or discectomy (eg, spinal stenosis), more than 2 vertebral segments; cervical**
🔧 43.6   ✂ 43.6   **FUD** 090   T 80 ▣ P0
AMA: 2015,Jan,16; 2014,Jan,11; 2013,Jul,3-5; 2012,Jan,15-42; 2011,Jul,12-13; 2011,Jan,11

63016   **thoracic**
🔧 44.6   ✂ 44.6   **FUD** 090   T 80 ▣
AMA: 2015,Jan,16; 2014,Jan,11; 2013,Jul,3-5; 2012,Jan,15-42; 2011,Jul,12-13; 2011,Jan,11

63017   **lumbar**
🔧 36.8   ✂ 36.8   **FUD** 090   T 80 ▣
AMA: 2015,Jan,16; 2014,Jan,11; 2013,Jul,3-5; 2012,Jan,15-42; 2011,Jul,12-13; 2011,Jan,11

Nerve root problems in C₅ through C₇ cause paralysis of the upper limb

Atlas (C₁)
Axis (C₂)
C₁ to C₄
C₅ to C₇
The specialized atlas allows for rotary motion, which turns the head

63020   **Laminotomy (hemilaminectomy), with decompression of nerve root(s), including partial facetectomy, foraminotomy and/or excision of herniated intervertebral disc; 1 interspace, cervical**
🔧 34.1   ✂ 34.1   **FUD** 090   T G2 80 50 ▣ PQ
AMA: 2015,Jan,16; 2014,Jan,11; 2013,Jul,3-5; 2012,Dec,12; 2012,Jul,3-6; 2012,Jan,15-42; 2011,Jul,12-13; 2011,Jan,11

63030   **1 interspace, lumbar**
🔧 28.2   ✂ 28.2   **FUD** 090   T G2 80 50 ▣ PQ
AMA: 2015,Jan,16; 2014,Jan,11; 2013,Dec,16; 2013,Jul,3-5; 2012,Dec,12; 2012,Jul,3-6; 2012,Jan,15-42; 2011,Jul,12-13; 2011,Mar,7; 2011,Jan,11; 2010,Nov,4

+ **63035**   **each additional interspace, cervical or lumbar (List separately in addition to code for primary procedure)**
Code first (63020-63030)
🔧 5.64   ✂ 5.64   **FUD** ZZZ   N 80 50 ▣
AMA: 2015,Jan,16; 2014,Jan,11; 2012,Jul,3-6; 2012,Jan,15-42; 2011,Jul,12-13; 2011,Jan,11

63040   **Laminotomy (hemilaminectomy), with decompression of nerve root(s), including partial facetectomy, foraminotomy and/or excision of herniated intervertebral disc, reexploration, single interspace; cervical**
🔧 40.8   ✂ 40.8   **FUD** 090   T 80 50 ▣
AMA: 2015,Jan,16; 2014,Jan,11; 2013,Jul,3-5; 2012,Jan,15-42; 2011,Jul,12-13; 2011,Jan,11

63042   **lumbar**
🔧 37.8   ✂ 37.8   **FUD** 090   T G2 80 50 ▣ PQ
AMA: 2015,Jan,16; 2014,Jan,11; 2013,Jul,3-5; 2012,Jan,15-42; 2011,Jul,12-13; 2011,Jan,11

+ **63043**   **each additional cervical interspace (List separately in addition to code for primary procedure)**
Code first (63040)
🔧 0.00   ✂ 0.00   **FUD** ZZZ   N 80 50 ▣
AMA: 2015,Jan,16; 2014,Jan,11; 2012,Jan,15-42; 2011,Jul,12-13; 2011,Jan,11

+ **63044**   **each additional lumbar interspace (List separately in addition to code for primary procedure)**
Code first (63042)
🔧 0.00   ✂ 0.00   **FUD** ZZZ   N NI 80 50 ▣
AMA: 2015,Jan,16; 2014,Jan,11; 2012,Jan,15-42; 2011,Jul,12-13; 2011,Jan,11

63045   **Laminectomy, facetectomy and foraminotomy (unilateral or bilateral with decompression of spinal cord, cauda equina and/or nerve root[s], [eg, spinal or lateral recess stenosis]), single vertebral segment; cervical**
🔧 37.4   ✂ 37.4   **FUD** 090   T G2 80 ▣ PQ
AMA: 2015,Jan,16; 2014,Jan,11; 2013,Jul,3-5; 2012,Dec,12; 2012,Jan,15-42; 2011,Jul,12-13; 2011,Jan,11

63046   **thoracic**
🔧 35.3   ✂ 35.3   **FUD** 090   T 80 ▣
AMA: 2015,Jan,16; 2014,Jan,11; 2013,Jul,3-5; 2012,Dec,12; 2012,Jan,15-42; 2011,Jul,12-13; 2011,Jan,11

63047   **lumbar**
🔧 32.2   ✂ 32.2   **FUD** 090   T G2 80 ▣ PQ
AMA: 2015,Jan,16; 2014,Dec,16; 2014,Dec,16; 2014,Jan,11; 2013,Dec,16; 2013,Jul,3-5; 2012,Dec,12; 2012,Jan,15-42; 2011,Jul,12-13; 2011,Jan,11; 2010,Nov,4

+ **63048**   **each additional segment, cervical, thoracic, or lumbar (List separately in addition to code for primary procedure)**
Code first (63045-63047)
🔧 6.24   ✂ 6.24   **FUD** ZZZ   N 80 ▣
AMA: 2015,Jan,16; 2014,Jan,11; 2012,Dec,12; 2012,Jan,15-42; 2011,Jul,12-13; 2011,Jan,11

63050-63051 Cervical Laminoplasty: Posterior Midline Approach

Do not report with procedure performed on the same vertebral segment(s) (22600, 22614, 22840-22842, 63001, 63015, 63045, 63048, 63295)

63050 **Laminoplasty, cervical, with decompression of the spinal cord, 2 or more vertebral segments;**
🔧 43.4 ⚖ 43.4 **FUD** 090   C 80 🖵
AMA: 2015,Jan,16; 2014,Jan,11; 2013,Jul,3-5; 2011,Jul,12-13

63051 **with reconstruction of the posterior bony elements (including the application of bridging bone graft and non-segmental fixation devices [eg, wire, suture, mini-plates], when performed)**
🔧 50.1 ⚖ 50.1 **FUD** 090   C 80 🖵
AMA: 2015,Jan,16; 2014,Jan,11; 2013,Jul,3-5; 2011,Jul,12-13

63055-63066 Spinal Cord/Nerve Root Decompression: Costovertebral or Transpedicular Approach

63055 **Transpedicular approach with decompression of spinal cord, equina and/or nerve root(s) (eg, herniated intervertebral disc), single segment; thoracic**
🔧 47.9 ⚖ 47.9 **FUD** 090   T 80 🖵
AMA: 2015,Jan,16; 2014,Jan,11; 2013,Jul,3-5

63056 **lumbar (including transfacet, or lateral extraforaminal approach) (eg, far lateral herniated intervertebral disc)**
🔧 43.4 ⚖ 43.4 **FUD** 090   T 62 80 🖵 PQ
AMA: 2015,Jan,16; 2014,Jan,9; 2014,Jan,11; 2013,Jul,3-5; 2012,Jul,3-6; 2012,Jan,15-42

+ **63057** **each additional segment, thoracic or lumbar (List separately in addition to code for primary procedure)**
Code first (63055-63056)
🔧 9.41 ⚖ 9.41 **FUD** ZZZ   N 80 🖵
AMA: 2015,Jan,16; 2014,Jan,11

63064 **Costovertebral approach with decompression of spinal cord or nerve root(s) (eg, herniated intervertebral disc), thoracic; single segment**
EXCLUDES Laminectomy with intraspinal thoracic lesion removal (63266, 63271, 63276, 63281, 63286)
🔧 51.9 ⚖ 51.9 **FUD** 090   T 80 🖵
AMA: 2015,Jan,16; 2014,Jan,11; 2013,Jul,3-5

+ **63066** **each additional segment (List separately in addition to code for primary procedure)**
EXCLUDES Laminectomy with intraspinal thoracic lesion removal (63266, 63271, 63276, 63281, 63286)
Code first (63064)
🔧 6.17 ⚖ 6.17 **FUD** ZZZ   N 80 🖵
AMA: 2014,Jan,11

63075-63078 Discectomy: Anterior or Anterolateral Approach

INCLUDES Operating microscope (69990)

63075 **Discectomy, anterior, with decompression of spinal cord and/or nerve root(s), including osteophytectomy; cervical, single interspace**
EXCLUDES Anterior cervical discectomy and anterior interbody fusion at same level during same operative session (22551)
Do not report with anterior interbody arthrodesis (even by another provider) (22554)
🔧 39.6 ⚖ 39.6 **FUD** 090   T 80 🖵 PQ
AMA: 2015,Apr,7; 2015,Jan,16; 2014,Jan,11; 2013,Jul,3-5; 2012,Jan,15-42; 2011,Jan,11

+ **63076** **cervical, each additional interspace (List separately in addition to code for primary procedure)**
EXCLUDES Anterior cervical discectomy and anterior interbody fusion at same level during same operative session (22552)
Code first (63075)
Do not report with anterior interbody arthrodesis (even by another provider) (22554)
🔧 7.27 ⚖ 7.27 **FUD** ZZZ   N 80 🖵
AMA: 2015,Jan,16; 2014,Jan,11; 2012,Jan,15-42; 2011,Jan,11

63077 **thoracic, single interspace**
🔧 43.9 ⚖ 43.9 **FUD** 090   C 80 🖵
AMA: 2015,Jan,16; 2014,Jan,11; 2013,Jul,3-5; 2012,Jan,15-42; 2011,Jan,11

+ **63078** **thoracic, each additional interspace (List separately in addition to code for primary procedure)**
Code first (63077)
🔧 5.56 ⚖ 5.56 **FUD** ZZZ   C 80 🖵
AMA: 2015,Jan,16; 2014,Jan,11; 2012,Jan,15-42; 2011,Jan,11

63081-63091 Vertebral Corpectomy, All Levels, Anterior Approach

INCLUDES Disc removal at the level below and/or above vertebral segment
EXCLUDES Arthrodesis (22548-22812)
Code also reconstruction (20930-20938, 22548-22812, 22840-22855)

63081 **Vertebral corpectomy (vertebral body resection), partial or complete, anterior approach with decompression of spinal cord and/or nerve root(s); cervical, single segment**
EXCLUDES Transoral approach (61575-61576)
🔧 51.4 ⚖ 51.4 **FUD** 090   C 80 🖵 PQ
AMA: 2015,Jun,10; 2015,Jan,16; 2014,Jan,11; 2013,Jul,3-5

+ **63082** **cervical, each additional segment (List separately in addition to code for primary procedure)**
EXCLUDES Transoral approach (61575-61576)
Code first (63081)
🔧 7.85 ⚖ 7.85 **FUD** ZZZ   C 80 🖵
AMA: 2015,Jan,16; 2014,Jan,11

63085 **Vertebral corpectomy (vertebral body resection), partial or complete, transthoracic approach with decompression of spinal cord and/or nerve root(s); thoracic, single segment**
🔧 56.0 ⚖ 56.0 **FUD** 090   C 80 🖵
AMA: 2015,Jan,16; 2014,Jan,11; 2013,Jul,3-5

+ **63086** **thoracic, each additional segment (List separately in addition to code for primary procedure)**
Code first (63085)
🔧 5.61 ⚖ 5.61 **FUD** ZZZ   C 80 🖵
AMA: 2015,Jan,16; 2014,Jan,11

63087 **Vertebral corpectomy (vertebral body resection), partial or complete, combined thoracolumbar approach with decompression of spinal cord, cauda equina or nerve root(s), lower thoracic or lumbar; single segment**
🔧 70.5 ⚖ 70.5 **FUD** 090   C 80 🖵
AMA: 2015,Jan,16; 2014,Jan,11; 2013,Jul,3-5

+ **63088** **each additional segment (List separately in addition to code for primary procedure)**
Code first (63087)
🔧 7.71 ⚖ 7.71 **FUD** ZZZ   C 80 🖵
AMA: 2015,Jan,16; 2014,Jan,11

63090 **Vertebral corpectomy (vertebral body resection), partial or complete, transperitoneal or retroperitoneal approach with decompression of spinal cord, cauda equina or nerve root(s), lower thoracic, lumbar, or sacral; single segment**
🔧 56.8 ⚖ 56.8 **FUD** 090   C 80 🖵
AMA: 2015,Jan,16; 2014,Jan,11; 2013,Jul,3-5

+ **63091** **each additional segment (List separately in addition to code for primary procedure)**
Code first (63090)
🔧 5.18 ⚖ 5.18 **FUD** ZZZ   C 80 🖵
AMA: 2015,Jan,16; 2014,Jan,11

63101-63103 Corpectomy: Lateral Extracavitary Approach

63101 **Vertebral corpectomy (vertebral body resection), partial or complete, lateral extracavitary approach with decompression of spinal cord and/or nerve root(s) (eg, for tumor or retropulsed bone fragments); thoracic, single segment**
🔧 68.2 ⚖ 68.2 **FUD** 090   C 80 🖵
AMA: 2015,Jan,16; 2014,Jan,11; 2013,Jul,3-5

Nervous System (vertical, left margin)

63102 — 63278 (vertical, left margin)

63102	**lumbar, single segment**	
	66.6 66.6 **FUD** 090	C 80
	AMA: 2015,Jan,16; 2014,Jan,11; 2013,Jul,3-5	
+ 63103	**thoracic or lumbar, each additional segment (List separately in addition to code for primary procedure)**	
	Code first (63101-63102)	
	8.67 8.67 **FUD** ZZZ	C 80
	AMA: 2014,Jan,11	

63170-63295 Laminectomies

63170	**Laminectomy with myelotomy (eg, Bischof or DREZ type), cervical, thoracic, or thoracolumbar**	
	47.3 47.3 **FUD** 090	C 80
	AMA: 2015,Jan,16; 2014,Jan,11; 2013,Jul,3-5	
63172	**Laminectomy with drainage of intramedullary cyst/syrinx; to subarachnoid space**	
	42.1 42.1 **FUD** 090	C 80
	AMA: 2015,Jan,16; 2014,Jan,11; 2013,Jul,3-5	
63173	**to peritoneal or pleural space**	
	51.3 51.3 **FUD** 090	C 80
	AMA: 2015,Jan,16; 2014,Jan,11; 2013,Jul,3-5	
63180	**Laminectomy and section of dentate ligaments, with or without dural graft, cervical; 1 or 2 segments**	
	44.1 44.1 **FUD** 090	C 80
	AMA: 2015,Jan,16; 2014,Jan,11; 2013,Jul,3-5	
63182	**more than 2 segments**	
	48.4 48.4 **FUD** 090	C 80
	AMA: 2015,Jan,16; 2014,Jan,11; 2013,Jul,3-5	
63185	**Laminectomy with rhizotomy; 1 or 2 segments**	
	INCLUDES Dana rhizotomy	
	Stoffel rhizotomy	
	33.3 33.3 **FUD** 090	C 80
	AMA: 2015,Jan,16; 2014,Jan,11; 2013,Jul,3-5	
63190	**more than 2 segments**	
	36.7 36.7 **FUD** 090	C 80
	AMA: 2015,Jan,16; 2014,Jan,11; 2013,Jul,3-5	
63191	**Laminectomy with section of spinal accessory nerve**	
	EXCLUDES Division of sternocleidomastoid muscle for torticollis (21720)	
	40.9 40.9 **FUD** 090	C 80 50
	AMA: 2015,Jan,16; 2014,Jan,11; 2013,Jul,3-5	
63194	**Laminectomy with cordotomy, with section of 1 spinothalamic tract, 1 stage; cervical**	
	47.4 47.4 **FUD** 090	C 80
	AMA: 2015,Jan,16; 2014,Jan,11; 2013,Jul,3-5	
63195	**thoracic**	
	33.6 33.6 **FUD** 090	C 80
	AMA: 2015,Jan,16; 2014,Jan,11; 2013,Jul,3-5	
63196	**Laminectomy with cordotomy, with section of both spinothalamic tracts, 1 stage; cervical**	
	39.1 39.1 **FUD** 090	C 80
	AMA: 2015,Jan,16; 2014,Jan,11; 2013,Jul,3-5	
63197	**thoracic**	
	50.8 50.8 **FUD** 090	C 80
	AMA: 2015,Jan,16; 2014,Jan,11; 2013,Jul,3-5	
63198	**Laminectomy with cordotomy with section of both spinothalamic tracts, 2 stages within 14 days; cervical**	
	INCLUDES Keen laminectomy	
	46.0 46.0 **FUD** 090	C 80
	AMA: 2015,Jan,16; 2014,Jan,11; 2013,Jul,3-5	
63199	**thoracic**	
	48.3 48.3 **FUD** 090	C 80
	AMA: 2015,Jan,16; 2014,Jan,11; 2013,Jul,3-5	
63200	**Laminectomy, with release of tethered spinal cord, lumbar**	
	45.2 45.2 **FUD** 090	C 80
	AMA: 2015,Jan,16; 2014,Jan,11; 2013,Jul,3-5	

63250	**Laminectomy for excision or occlusion of arteriovenous malformation of spinal cord; cervical**	
	88.4 88.4 **FUD** 090	C 80
	AMA: 2015,Jan,16; 2014,Jan,11; 2013,Jul,3-5	

Cervical C₁ to C₇ / Thoracic T₁ to T₁₂ / Lumbar L₁ to L₅ / Sacrum / Nerve roots / Pia mater / Arachnoid / Dura mater (reflected) / White matter / Gray matter / Schematic of spinal cord layers

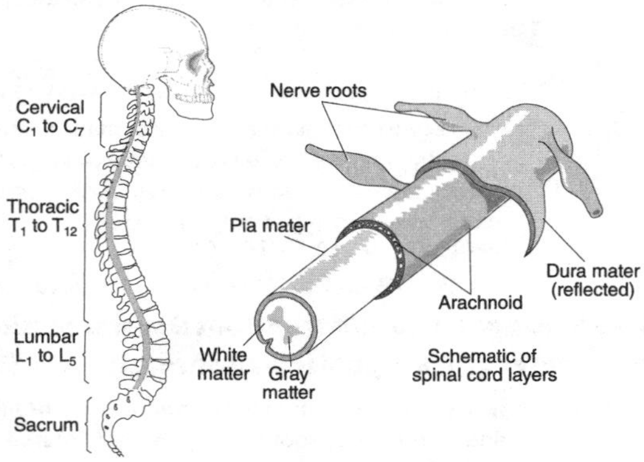

63251	**thoracic**	
	90.3 90.3 **FUD** 090	C 80
	AMA: 2015,Jan,16; 2014,Jan,11; 2013,Jul,3-5	
63252	**thoracolumbar**	
	90.3 90.3 **FUD** 090	C 80
	AMA: 2015,Jan,16; 2014,Jan,11; 2013,Jul,3-5	
63265	**Laminectomy for excision or evacuation of intraspinal lesion other than neoplasm, extradural; cervical**	
	49.1 49.1 **FUD** 090	C 80
	AMA: 2015,Jan,16; 2014,Jan,11; 2013,Jul,3-5	
63266	**thoracic**	
	50.6 50.6 **FUD** 090	C 80
	AMA: 2014,Jan,11; 2013,Jul,3-5	
63267	**lumbar**	
	40.2 40.2 **FUD** 090	C 80 PQ
	AMA: 2015,Jan,16; 2014,Jan,11; 2013,Jul,3-5	
63268	**sacral**	
	42.7 42.7 **FUD** 090	C 80
	AMA: 2015,Jan,16; 2014,Jan,11; 2013,Jul,3-5	
63270	**Laminectomy for excision of intraspinal lesion other than neoplasm, intradural; cervical**	
	61.7 61.7 **FUD** 090	C 80
	AMA: 2015,Jan,16; 2014,Jan,11; 2013,Jul,3-5	
63271	**thoracic**	
	61.3 61.3 **FUD** 090	C 80
	AMA: 2015,Jan,16; 2014,Jan,11; 2013,Jul,3-5	
63272	**lumbar**	
	55.6 55.6 **FUD** 090	C 80
	AMA: 2015,Jan,16; 2014,Jan,11; 2013,Jul,3-5	
63273	**sacral**	
	55.4 55.4 **FUD** 090	C 80
	AMA: 2015,Jan,16; 2014,Jan,11; 2013,Jul,3-5	
63275	**Laminectomy for biopsy/excision of intraspinal neoplasm; extradural, cervical**	
	53.2 53.2 **FUD** 090	C 80 PQ
	AMA: 2015,Jan,16; 2014,Jan,11; 2013,Jul,3-5	
63276	**extradural, thoracic**	
	52.7 52.7 **FUD** 090	C 80 PQ
	AMA: 2015,Jan,16; 2014,Jan,11; 2013,Jul,3-5	
63277	**extradural, lumbar**	
	45.6 45.6 **FUD** 090	C 80 PQ
	AMA: 2015,Jan,16; 2014,Jan,11; 2013,Jul,3-5	
63278	**extradural, sacral**	
	47.2 47.2 **FUD** 090	C 80 PQ
	AMA: 2015,Jan,16; 2014,Jan,11; 2013,Jul,3-5	

26/TC PC/TC Comp Only	A2-Z3 ASC Pmt	50 Bilateral	♂ Male Only	♀ Female Only	Facility RVU	Non-Facility RVU
AMA: CPT Asst	CMS: Pub 100	A-Y OPPSI	80/80 Surg Assist Allowed / w/Doc		Lab Crosswalk	Radiology Crosswalk

252   Medicare (Red Text)   CPT © 2015 American Medical Association. All Rights Reserved. (Black Text)   © 2015 Optum360, LLC (Blue Text)

63280 intradural, extramedullary, cervical
62.7   62.7   **FUD** 090   C 80 ▢ PQ
AMA: 2015,Jan,16; 2014,Jan,11; 2013,Jul,3-5

63281 intradural, extramedullary, thoracic
61.8   61.8   **FUD** 090   C 80 ▢ PQ
AMA: 2015,Jan,16; 2014,Jan,11; 2013,Jul,3-5

63282 intradural, extramedullary, lumbar
58.1   58.1   **FUD** 090   C 80 ▢ PQ
AMA: 2015,Jan,16; 2014,Jan,11; 2013,Jul,3-5

63283 intradural, sacral
56.4   56.4   **FUD** 090   C 80 ▢ PQ
AMA: 2015,Jan,16; 2014,Jan,11; 2013,Jul,3-5

63285 intradural, intramedullary, cervical
77.8   77.8   **FUD** 090   C 80 ▢ PQ
AMA: 2015,Jan,16; 2014,Jan,11; 2013,Jul,3-5

63286 intradural, intramedullary, thoracic
77.0   77.0   **FUD** 090   C 80 ▢ PQ
AMA: 2015,Jan,16; 2014,Jan,11; 2013,Jul,3-5

63287 intradural, intramedullary, thoracolumbar
81.7   81.7   **FUD** 090   C 80 ▢ PQ
AMA: 2015,Jan,16; 2014,Jan,11; 2013,Jul,3-5

63290 combined extradural-intradural lesion, any level
EXCLUDES Drainage intermedullary cyst or syrinx (63172-63173)
83.1   83.1   **FUD** 090   C 80 ▢ PQ
AMA: 2015,Jan,16; 2014,Jan,11; 2013,Jul,3-5

+ **63295** Osteoplastic reconstruction of dorsal spinal elements, following primary intraspinal procedure (List separately in addition to code for primary procedure)
Code first (63172-63173, 63185, 63190, 63200-63290)
Do not report with procedure performed at the same vertebral segment(s) (22590-22614, 22840-22844, 63050-63051)
9.98   9.98   **FUD** ZZZ   C 80
AMA: 2014,Jan,11

63300-63308 Vertebral Corpectomy for Intraspinal Lesion: Anterior/Anterolateral Approach

EXCLUDES Arthrodesis (22548-22585)
Spinal reconstruction (20930-20938)

63300 Vertebral corpectomy (vertebral body resection), partial or complete, for excision of intraspinal lesion, single segment; extradural, cervical
54.1   54.1   **FUD** 090   C 80 ▢
AMA: 2015,Jan,16; 2014,Jan,11; 2013,Jul,3-5

63301 extradural, thoracic by transthoracic approach
64.0   64.0   **FUD** 090   C 80 ▢
AMA: 2015,Jan,16; 2014,Jan,11; 2013,Jul,3-5

63302 extradural, thoracic by thoracolumbar approach
64.8   64.8   **FUD** 090   C 80 ▢
AMA: 2015,Jan,16; 2014,Jan,11; 2013,Jul,3-5

63303 extradural, lumbar or sacral by transperitoneal or retroperitoneal approach
68.8   68.8   **FUD** 090   C 80 ▢
AMA: 2015,Jan,16; 2014,Jan,11; 2013,Jul,3-5

63304 intradural, cervical
69.9   69.9   **FUD** 090   C 80 ▢
AMA: 2015,Jan,16; 2014,Jan,11; 2013,Jul,3-5

63305 intradural, thoracic by transthoracic approach
74.4   74.4   **FUD** 090   C 80 ▢
AMA: 2015,Jan,16; 2014,Jan,11; 2013,Jul,3-5

63306 intradural, thoracic by thoracolumbar approach
58.0   58.0   **FUD** 090   C 80 ▢
AMA: 2015,Jan,16; 2014,Jan,11; 2013,Jul,3-5

63307 intradural, lumbar or sacral by transperitoneal or retroperitoneal approach
63.8   63.8   **FUD** 090   C 80 ▢
AMA: 2015,Jan,16; 2014,Jan,11; 2013,Jul,3-5

+ **63308** each additional segment (List separately in addition to codes for single segment)
Code first (63300-63307)
9.57   9.57   **FUD** ZZZ   C 80 ▢
AMA: 2014,Jan,11

63600-63615 Stereotactic Procedures of the Spinal Cord

63600 Creation of lesion of spinal cord by stereotactic method, percutaneous, any modality (including stimulation and/or recording)
26.2   26.2   **FUD** 090   T A2 80 ▢
AMA: 2014,Jan,11

63610 Stereotactic stimulation of spinal cord, percutaneous, separate procedure not followed by other surgery
11.2   11.2   **FUD** 000   T A2 80 ▢ PQ
AMA: 2014,Jan,11

63615 Stereotactic biopsy, aspiration, or excision of lesion, spinal cord
31.0   31.0   **FUD** 090   T R2 ▢ PQ
AMA: 2014,Jan,11

63620-63621 Stereotactic Radiosurgery (SRS): Spine

INCLUDES Computer assisted planning
Planning dosimetry, targeting, positioning, or blocking by neurosurgeon
EXCLUDES Arteriovenous malformations (see Radiation Oncology Section)
Intensity modulated beam delivery plan and treatment (77301, 77385-77386)
Stereotactic body radiation therapy (77373, 77435)
Treatment planning, physics, dosimetry, treatment delivery and management provided by the radiation oncologist (77261-77790 [77295, 77385, 77386, 77387, 77424, 77425])
Do not report stereotactic radiosurgery services with radiation treatment management by the same provider (77427-77432)
Do not report with (61781-61783)

63620 Stereotactic radiosurgery (particle beam, gamma ray, or linear accelerator); 1 spinal lesion
Do not report more than one time per treatment course
32.9   32.9   **FUD** 090   B 80
AMA: 2015,Jun,6; 2015,Jan,16; 2014,Jan,11; 2011,Jul,12-13; 2010,Oct,3-4

+ **63621** each additional spinal lesion (List separately in addition to code for primary procedure)
Code first (63620)
Do not report more than one time per lesion
Do not report more than two times per entire treatment course
7.54   7.54   **FUD** ZZZ   B 80
AMA: 2015,Jun,6; 2015,Jan,16; 2014,Jan,11; 2011,Jul,12-13; 2010,Oct,3-4

63650-63688 Spinal Neurostimulation

INCLUDES Complex and simple neurostimulators
EXCLUDES Analysis and programming of neurostimulator pulse generator (95970-95975)

63650 Percutaneous implantation of neurostimulator electrode array, epidural
INCLUDES The following are components of a neurostimulator system:
Collection of contacts of which four or more provide the electrical stimulation in the epidural space
Contacts on a catheter-type lead (array)
Extension
External controller
Implanted neurostimulator
11.8   37.7   **FUD** 010   J J8 ▢
AMA: 2015,Jan,16; 2014,Jan,11; 2013,Oct,18; 2012,Jan,15-42; 2011,Apr,10-11; 2011,Apr,9; 2011,Jan,11; 2010,Dec,12; 2010,Aug,8&15; 2010,Jan,9-11

63655 **Laminectomy for implantation of neurostimulator electrodes, plate/paddle, epidural**

    INCLUDES   The following are components of a neurostimulator system:

        Collection of contacts of which four or more provide the electrical stimulation in the epidural space

        Contacts on a plate or paddle-shaped surface for systems placed by open exposure

        Extension

        External controller

        Implanted neurostimulator

    🔧 24.1   ✂ 24.1   **FUD** 090   J J8 80 ▱

    AMA: 2015,Jan,16; 2014,Jan,11; 2012,Jan,15-42; 2011,Apr,10-11; 2011,Apr,9; 2010,Aug,8&15; 2010,Dec,12; 2010,Jan,9-11

63661 **Removal of spinal neurostimulator electrode percutaneous array(s), including fluoroscopy, when performed**

    INCLUDES   The following are components of a neurostimulator system:

        Collection of contacts of which four or more provide the electrical stimulation in the epidural space

        Contacts on a catheter-type lead (array)

        Extension

        External controller

        Implanted neurostimulator

    Do not report when removing or replacing a temporary array placed percutaneously for an external generator

    🔧 9.28   ✂ 16.5   **FUD** 010   02 02 80

    AMA: 2015,Jan,16; 2014,Jan,11; 2011,Apr,10-11; 2011,Apr,9; 2011,Jan,8; 2010,Nov,1; 2010,Aug,8&15; 2010,Jan,9-11

63662 **Removal of spinal neurostimulator electrode plate/paddle(s) placed via laminotomy or laminectomy, including fluoroscopy, when performed**

    INCLUDES   The following are components of a neurostimulator system:

        Collection of contacts of which four or more provide the electrical stimulation in the epidural space

        Contacts on a plate or paddle-shaped surface for systems placed by open exposure

        Extension

        External controller

        Implanted neurostimulator

    🔧 24.5   ✂ 24.5   **FUD** 090   02 02 80

    AMA: 2015,Jan,16; 2014,Jan,11; 2011,Apr,10-11; 2011,Apr,9; 2011,Jan,8; 2010,Nov,1; 2010,Aug,8&15; 2010,Jan,9-11

63663 **Revision including replacement, when performed, of spinal neurostimulator electrode percutaneous array(s), including fluoroscopy, when performed**

    INCLUDES   The following are components of a neurostimulator system:

        Collection of contacts of which four or more provide the electrical stimulation in the epidural space

        Contacts on a catheter-type lead (array)

        Extension

        External controller

        Implanted neurostimulator

    Do not report at same level with (63661-63662)

    Do not report when removing or replacing a temporary array placed percutaneously for an external generator

    🔧 13.0   ✂ 22.4   **FUD** 010   J J8 80

    AMA: 2015,Jan,16; 2014,Jan,11; 2011,Apr,10-11; 2011,Apr,9; 2011,Jan,8; 2010,Nov,1; 2010,Aug,8&15; 2010,Jan,9-11

63664 **Revision including replacement, when performed, of spinal neurostimulator electrode plate/paddle(s) placed via laminotomy or laminectomy, including fluoroscopy, when performed**

    INCLUDES   The following are components of a neurostimulator system:

        Collection of contacts of which four or more provide the electrical stimulation in the epidural space

        Contacts on a plate or paddle-shaped surface for systems placed by open exposure

        Extension

        External controller

        Implanted neurostimulator

    Do not report at same level with (63661-63662)

    🔧 25.0   ✂ 25.0   **FUD** 090   J J8 80

    AMA: 2015,Jan,16; 2014,Jan,11; 2011,Apr,10-11; 2011,Apr,9; 2011,Jan,8; 2010,Nov,1; 2010,Aug,8&15; 2010,Jan,9-11

63685 **Insertion or replacement of spinal neurostimulator pulse generator or receiver, direct or inductive coupling**

    Do not report with for the same pulse generator or receiver (63688)

    🔧 10.6   ✂ 10.6   **FUD** 010   J J8 80 ▱

    AMA: 2015,Jan,16; 2014,Jan,11; 2012,Jan,15-42; 2011,Apr,10-11; 2011,Jan,11; 2010,Dec,12; 2010,Jan,9-11

63688 **Revision or removal of implanted spinal neurostimulator pulse generator or receiver**

    Do not report with for the same pulse generator or receiver (63685)

    🔧 10.7   ✂ 10.7   **FUD** 010   02 A2 ▱

    AMA: 2015,Jan,16; 2014,Jan,11; 2011,Apr,10-11; 2010,Jan,9-11

63700-63706 Repair Congenital Neural Tube Defects

    EXCLUDES   *Complex skin repair (see appropriate integumentary closure code)*

63700 **Repair of meningocele; less than 5 cm diameter**

    🔧 33.8   ✂ 33.8   **FUD** 090   63 C 80 ▱

    AMA: 2014,Jan,11

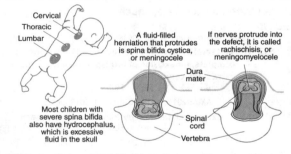

Cervical / Thoracic / Lumbar

A fluid-filled herniation that protrudes is spina bifida cystica, or meningocele

If nerves protrude into the defect, it is called rachischisis, or meningomyelocele

Dura mater

Most children with severe spina bifida also have hydrocephalus, which is excessive fluid in the skull

Spinal cord

Vertebra

63702 **larger than 5 cm diameter**

    🔧 41.4   ✂ 41.4   **FUD** 090   63 C 80 ▱

    AMA: 2014,Jan,11

63704 **Repair of myelomeningocele; less than 5 cm diameter**

    🔧 43.1   ✂ 43.1   **FUD** 090   63 C 80 ▱

    AMA: 2014,Jan,11

63706 **larger than 5 cm diameter**

    🔧 48.9   ✂ 48.9   **FUD** 090   63 C 80 ▱

    AMA: 2014,Jan,11

63707-63710 Repair Dural Cerebrospinal Fluid Leak

63707 **Repair of dural/cerebrospinal fluid leak, not requiring laminectomy**

    🔧 26.8   ✂ 26.8   **FUD** 090   C 80 ▱

    AMA: 2014,Jan,11

63709 **Repair of dural/cerebrospinal fluid leak or pseudomeningocele, with laminectomy**

    🔧 32.1   ✂ 32.1   **FUD** 090   C 80 ▱

    AMA: 2014,Jan,11

63710 Dural graft, spinal

> EXCLUDES Laminectomy and section of dentate ligament (63180, 63182)

🔧 31.5 ✂ 31.5 **FUD** 090 C 80 📋

AMA: 2014,Jan,11

63740-63746 Cerebrospinal Fluid (CSF) Shunt: Lumbar

> EXCLUDES Placement of subarachnoid catheter with reservoir and/or pump:
> Not requiring laminectomy (62350, 62360-62362)
> With laminectomy (62351, 62360-62362)

63740 Creation of shunt, lumbar, subarachnoid-peritoneal, -pleural, or other; including laminectomy

🔧 28.2 ✂ 28.2 **FUD** 090 C 80 📋

AMA: 2014,Jan,11

63741 percutaneous, not requiring laminectomy

🔧 19.9 ✂ 19.9 **FUD** 090 T 80 📋

AMA: 2014,Jan,11

63744 Replacement, irrigation or revision of lumbosubarachnoid shunt

🔧 19.9 ✂ 19.9 **FUD** 090 T A2 80 📋

AMA: 2014,Jan,11

63746 Removal of entire lumbosubarachnoid shunt system without replacement

🔧 17.7 ✂ 17.7 **FUD** 090 02 A2 80 📋

AMA: 2014,Jan,11

64400-64463 Nerve Blocks

> EXCLUDES Epidural or subarachnoid injection (62310-62319)
> Nerve destruction (62280-62282, 64600-64681 [64633, 64634, 64635, 64636])

64400 Injection, anesthetic agent; trigeminal nerve, any division or branch *Dental*

🔧 2.04 ✂ 3.63 **FUD** 000 P3 50 📋

AMA: 2015,Jan,16; 2014,Jan,11; 2013,Jan,13-14; 2012,Jan,15-42; 2011,Feb,4-5; 2011,Jan,11; 2010,Jan,9-11

64402 facial nerve

🔧 2.25 ✂ 3.71 **FUD** 000 01 M1 50 📋

AMA: 2015,Jan,16; 2014,Jan,11; 2013,Jan,13-14; 2012,Jan,15-42; 2011,Feb,4-5; 2011,Jan,11; 2010,Jan,9-11

64405 greater occipital nerve

🔧 1.82 ✂ 2.88 **FUD** 000 T P3 50 📋

AMA: 2015,Jan,16; 2014,Jan,11; 2013,Jan,13-14; 2012,Jan,15-42; 2011,Feb,4-5; 2011,Jan,11; 2010,Jan,9-11

64408 vagus nerve

🔧 2.47 ✂ 3.32 **FUD** 000 T P3 80 50 📋

AMA: 2015,Jan,16; 2014,Jan,11; 2013,Jan,13-14; 2012,Jan,15-42; 2011,Feb,4-5; 2011,Jan,11; 2010,Jan,9-11

64410 phrenic nerve

🔧 1.97 ✂ 3.42 **FUD** 000 T A2 80 50 📋

AMA: 2015,Jan,16; 2014,Jan,11; 2013,Jan,13-14; 2012,Jan,15-42; 2011,Feb,4-5; 2011,Jan,11; 2010,Jan,9-11

64412 spinal accessory nerve

To report, see ~64999

64413 cervical plexus

🔧 2.37 ✂ 3.68 **FUD** 000 T P3 50 📋

AMA: 2015,Jan,16; 2014,Jan,11; 2013,Jan,13-14; 2012,Jan,15-42; 2011,Feb,4-5; 2011,Jan,11; 2010,Jan,9-11

64415 brachial plexus, single

🔧 1.86 ✂ 3.34 **FUD** 000 T A2 50 📋

AMA: 2015,Jan,16; 2014,Jan,11; 2013,Jan,13-14; 2012,Jan,15-42; 2011,Feb,4-5; 2011,Jan,11; 2010,Jan,9-11

64416 brachial plexus, continuous infusion by catheter (including catheter placement)

Do not report with (01996)

🔧 2.27 ✂ 2.27 **FUD** 000 T G2 50 📋

AMA: 2015,Jan,16; 2014,Jan,11; 2013,Jan,13-14; 2012,Jan,15-42; 2011,Feb,4-5; 2011,Jan,11; 2010,Jan,9-11

64417 axillary nerve

🔧 2.02 ✂ 3.67 **FUD** 000 T A2 50 📋

AMA: 2015,Jan,16; 2014,Jan,11; 2013,Jan,13-14; 2012,Jan,15-42; 2011,Feb,4-5; 2011,Jan,11; 2010,Jan,9-11

64418 suprascapular nerve

🔧 2.21 ✂ 4.17 **FUD** 000 T P3 50 📋

AMA: 2015,Jan,16; 2014,Jan,11; 2013,Jan,13-14; 2012,Jan,15-42; 2011,Feb,4-5; 2011,Jan,11; 2010,Jan,9-11

64420 intercostal nerve, single

🔧 1.95 ✂ 3.20 **FUD** 000 T A2 📋

AMA: 2015,Jun,3; 2015,Jan,16; 2014,Jan,11; 2013,Jan,13-14; 2012,Jan,15-42; 2011,Feb,4-5; 2011,Jan,11; 2010,Aug,12; 2010,Nov,8; 2010,Aug,12; 2010,Jan,9-11

64421 intercostal nerves, multiple, regional block

🔧 2.63 ✂ 4.26 **FUD** 000 T A2 50 📋

AMA: 2015,Jun,3; 2015,Jan,16; 2014,Jan,11; 2013,Jan,13-14; 2012,Jan,15-42; 2011,Feb,4-5; 2011,Jan,11; 2010,Nov,8; 2010,Aug,12; 2010,Jan,9-11

64425 ilioinguinal, iliohypogastric nerves

🔧 2.67 ✂ 3.74 **FUD** 000 T P3 50 📋

AMA: 2015,Jun,3; 2015,Jan,16; 2014,Jan,11; 2013,Jan,13-14; 2012,Jan,15-42; 2011,Feb,4-5; 2011,Jan,11; 2010,Jan,9-11

64430 pudendal nerve

🔧 2.39 ✂ 3.98 **FUD** 000 T A2 50 📋

AMA: 2015,Jan,16; 2014,Jan,11; 2013,Jan,13-14; 2012,Jan,15-42; 2011,Feb,4-5; 2011,Jan,11; 2010,Jan,9-11

64435 paracervical (uterine) nerve ♀

🔧 2.40 ✂ 3.85 **FUD** 000 T P3 50 📋

AMA: 2015,Jan,16; 2014,Jan,11; 2013,Jan,13-14; 2012,Feb,11; 2012,Jan,15-42; 2011,Feb,4-5; 2011,Jan,11; 2010,Jan,9-11

64445 sciatic nerve, single

🔧 2.07 ✂ 3.84 **FUD** 000 T P3 50 📋

AMA: 2015,Jan,16; 2014,Jan,11; 2013,Jan,13-14; 2012,Apr,19; 2011,Dec,8-9; 2011,Feb,4-5; 2010,Jan,9-11

64446 sciatic nerve, continuous infusion by catheter (including catheter placement)

Do not report with (01996)

🔧 2.28 ✂ 2.28 **FUD** 000 T G2 50 📋

AMA: 2015,Jan,16; 2014,Jan,11; 2013,Jan,13-14; 2011,Feb,4-5; 2010,Jan,9-11

64447 femoral nerve, single

Do not report with (01996)

🔧 1.89 ✂ 3.39 **FUD** 000 T P3 50 📋

AMA: 2015,Jan,16; 2014,Dec,16; 2014,Dec,16; 2014,Nov,14; 2014,Jan,11; 2013,Jan,13-14; 2011,Feb,4-5; 2010,Jan,9-11

64448 femoral nerve, continuous infusion by catheter (including catheter placement)

Do not report with (01996)

🔧 2.03 ✂ 2.03 **FUD** 000 T G2 50 📋

AMA: 2015,Jan,16; 2014,Dec,16; 2014,Dec,16; 2014,Nov,14; 2014,Jan,11; 2013,Jan,13-14; 2011,Feb,4-5; 2010,Jan,9-11

64449 lumbar plexus, posterior approach, continuous infusion by catheter (including catheter placement)

Do not report with (01996)

🔧 2.40 ✂ 2.40 **FUD** 000 T G2 50 📋

AMA: 2015,Jan,16; 2014,Jan,11; 2013,Jan,13-14; 2011,Feb,4-5; 2010,Jan,9-11

64450 other peripheral nerve or branch

> EXCLUDES Morton's neuroma (64455, 64632)

🔧 1.31 ✂ 2.28 **FUD** 000 T P3 50 📋

AMA: 2015,Jun,3; 2015,Jan,16; 2014,Jan,11; 2013,Jan,13-14; 2012,Jan,15-42; 2011,Feb,4-5; 2011,Jan,11; 2010,Jan,9-11

64455 Injection(s), anesthetic agent and/or steroid, plantar common digital nerve(s) (eg, Morton's neuroma)

Do not report with (64632)

🔧 0.99 ✂ 1.35 **FUD** 000 T P3 80 50 📋

AMA: 2015,Jan,16; 2014,Jan,11; 2013,Nov,14; 2013,Jan,13-14; 2012,Sep,14-15; 2012,Sep,14-15; 2011,Feb,4-5; 2010,Jan,9-11

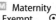
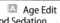
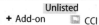
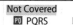

64461   Resequenced code. See code following 64484.

64462   Resequenced code. See code following 64484.

64463   Resequenced code. See code following 64484.

64479-64484 Transforaminal Injection

INCLUDES   Imaging guidance (fluoroscopy or CT) and contrast injection

EXCLUDES   *Epidural or subarachnoid injection (62310-62319)*
Nerve destruction (62280-62282, 64600-64681 [64633, 64634, 64635, 64636])

64479   **Injection(s), anesthetic agent and/or steroid, transforaminal epidural, with imaging guidance (fluoroscopy or CT); cervical or thoracic, single level**

EXCLUDES   *Transforaminal epidural injection using ultrasonic guidance (0228T)*

⚙ 3.82   ⚗ 6.70   **FUD** 000   T A2 50 🔲

AMA: 2015,Jan,16; 2014,Jan,11; 2012,Jul,3-6; 2012,Jan,15-42; 2011,Jul,16-17; 2011,Feb,4-5; 2011,Jan,8; 2010,Nov,1; 2010,Jan,9-11

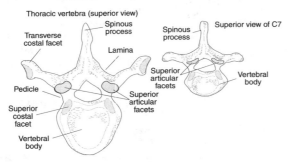

+   64480   **cervical or thoracic, each additional level (List separately in addition to code for primary procedure)**

EXCLUDES   *Transforaminal epidural injection at T12-L1 level (64479)*
Transforaminal epidural injection using ultrasonic guidance (0229T)

Code first (64479)
⚙ 1.82   ⚗ 3.21   **FUD** ZZZ   N N1 50 🔲

AMA: 2015,Jan,16; 2014,Jan,11; 2012,Jul,3-6; 2012,Jan,15-42; 2011,Jul,16-17; 2011,Feb,4-5; 2011,Jan,11; 2011,Jan,8; 2010,Nov,1; 2010,Jan,9-11

64483   **lumbar or sacral, single level**

EXCLUDES   *Transforaminal epidural injection using ultrasonic guidance (0230T)*

⚙ 3.25   ⚗ 6.22   **FUD** 000   T A2 50 🔲

AMA: 2015,Jan,16; 2014,Jan,11; 2012,Jul,3-6; 2012,May,14-15; 2011,Jul,16-17; 2011,Feb,4-5; 2011,Jan,8; 2010,Nov,1; 2010,Jan,9-11

+   64484   **lumbar or sacral, each additional level (List separately in addition to code for primary procedure)**

EXCLUDES   *Transforaminal epidural injection using ultrasonic guidance (0231T)*

Code first (64483)
⚙ 1.49   ⚗ 2.48   **FUD** ZZZ   N N1 50 🔲

AMA: 2015,Jan,16; 2014,Jan,11; 2012,Jul,3-6; 2012,Jan,15-42; 2011,Jul,16-17; 2011,Feb,4-5; 2011,Jan,11; 2010,Jan,9-11

[64461, 64462, 64463] Paravertebral Blocks

Do not report with (62310, 62318, 64420-64421, 64479-64480, 64490-64492, 76942, 77002-77003)

● # **64461**   **Paravertebral block (PVB) (paraspinous block), thoracic; single injection site (includes imaging guidance, when performed)**

⚙ 0.00   ⚗ 0.00   **FUD** 000

● + # **64462**   **second and any additional injection site(s) (includes imaging guidance, when performed) (List separately in addition to code for primary procedure)**

⚙ 0.00   ⚗ 0.00   **FUD** 000

Code first (64461)
Do not report more than one time per day

● # **64463**   **continuous infusion by catheter (includes imaging guidance, when performed)**

⚙ 0.00   ⚗ 0.00   **FUD** 000

64486-64489 Transversus Abdominis Plane (TAP) Block

64486   **Transversus abdominis plane (TAP) block (abdominal plane block, rectus sheath block) unilateral; by injection(s) (includes imaging guidance, when performed)**

⚙ 1.81   ⚗ 3.53   **FUD** 000   N N1 50

AMA: 2015,Jun,3

64487   **by continuous infusion(s) (includes imaging guidance, when performed)**

⚙ 2.08   ⚗ 4.31   **FUD** 000   N N1 50

AMA: 2015,Jun,3

64488   **Transversus abdominis plane (TAP) block (abdominal plane block, rectus sheath block) bilateral; by injections (includes imaging guidance, when performed)**

⚙ 2.27   ⚗ 4.34   **FUD** 000   N N1

AMA: 2015,Jun,3

64489   **by continuous infusions (includes imaging guidance, when performed)**

⚙ 2.55   ⚗ 6.03   **FUD** 000   N N1

AMA: 2015,Jun,3

64490-64495 Paraspinal Nerve Injections

INCLUDES   Image guidance (CT or fluoroscopy) and any contrast injection

EXCLUDES   *Injection without imaging (20552-20553)*
Ultrasonic guidance (0213T-0218T)

64490   **Injection(s), diagnostic or therapeutic agent, paravertebral facet (zygapophyseal) joint (or nerves innervating that joint) with image guidance (fluoroscopy or CT), cervical or thoracic; single level**

INCLUDES   Injection of T12-L1 joint and nerves that innervate that joint

⚙ 3.08   ⚗ 5.41   **FUD** 000   T G2 80 50

AMA: 2015,Jan,16; 2014,Jan,11; 2012,Oct,14; 2012,Jun,10-11; 2012,Jan,15-42; 2011,Feb,4-5; 2011,Jan,8; 2011,Jan,11; 2010,Nov,1; 2010,Aug,12; 2010,Dec,12; 2010,Aug,12; 2010,Jan,9-11

+   64491   **second level (List separately in addition to code for primary procedure)**

Code first (64490)
⚙ 1.74   ⚗ 2.68   **FUD** ZZZ   N N1 80 50

AMA: 2015,Jan,16; 2014,Jan,11; 2012,Oct,14; 2012,Jun,10-11; 2012,Jan,15-42; 2011,Feb,4-5; 2011,Jan,8; 2011,Jan,11; 2010,Nov,1; 2010,Aug,12; 2010,Aug,12; 2010,Jan,9-11

+   64492   **third and any additional level(s) (List separately in addition to code for primary procedure)**

Code also when appropriate (64491)
Code first (64490)
Do not report more than one time per day
⚙ 1.76   ⚗ 2.69   **FUD** ZZZ   N N1 80 50

AMA: 2015,Jan,16; 2014,Jan,11; 2012,Oct,14; 2012,Jun,10-11; 2012,Jan,15-42; 2011,Feb,4-5; 2011,Jan,8; 2010,Nov,1; 2010,Aug,12; 2010,Aug,12; 2010,Jan,9-11

64493   **Injection(s), diagnostic or therapeutic agent, paravertebral facet (zygapophyseal) joint (or nerves innervating that joint) with image guidance (fluoroscopy or CT), lumbar or sacral; single level**

⚙ 2.63   ⚗ 4.90   **FUD** 000   T G2 80 50

AMA: 2015,Jan,16; 2014,Jan,11; 2012,Oct,14; 2012,Jun,10-11; 2012,Jan,15-42; 2011,Feb,4-5; 2011,Feb,8-9; 2011,Jan,8; 2010,Nov,1; 2010,Aug,12; 2010,Aug,12; 2010,Jan,9-11

+   64494   **second level (List separately in addition to code for primary procedure)**

Code first (64493)
⚙ 1.50   ⚗ 2.47   **FUD** ZZZ   N N1 80 50

AMA: 2015,Jan,16; 2014,Jan,11; 2012,Oct,14; 2012,Jun,10-11; 2011,Feb,4-5; 2011,Jan,8; 2010,Nov,1; 2010,Aug,12; 2010,Aug,12; 2010,Jan,9-11

+ **64495** **third and any additional level(s) (List separately in addition to code for primary procedure)**
Code also when appropriate (64494)
Code first (64493)
Do not report more than one time per day
🚑 1.52   ⚕ 2.48   **FUD** ZZZ   N N1 80 50

AMA: 2015,Jan,16; 2014,Jan,11; 2012,Oct,14; 2012,Jun,10-11; 2011,Feb,4-5; 2011,Jan,8; 2010,Nov,1; 2010,Aug,12; 2010,Aug,12; 2010,Jan,9-11

64505-64530 Sympathetic Nerve Blocks

64505 **Injection, anesthetic agent; sphenopalatine ganglion**
🚑 2.49   ⚕ 2.98   **FUD** 000   T P3 50 ▢

AMA: 2015,Jan,16; 2014,Jul,8; 2014,Jan,11; 2013,Jan,13-14; 2012,Jan,15-42; 2011,Feb,4-5; 2011,Jan,11

64508 **carotid sinus (separate procedure)**
🚑 2.11   ⚕ 1.80   **FUD** 000   T P3 80 50 ▢

AMA: 2015,Jan,16; 2014,Jan,11; 2013,Jan,13-14; 2011,Feb,4-5

64510 **stellate ganglion (cervical sympathetic)**
🚑 2.12   ⚕ 3.62   **FUD** 000   T A2 50 ▢

AMA: 2015,Jan,16; 2014,Jan,11; 2013,Jan,13-14; 2011,Feb,4-5

64517 **superior hypogastric plexus**
🚑 3.52   ⚕ 5.14   **FUD** 000   T A2 ▢

AMA: 2015,Jan,16; 2014,Jan,11; 2013,Jan,13-14; 2012,Jan,15-42; 2011,Feb,4-5; 2011,Jan,11

64520 **lumbar or thoracic (paravertebral sympathetic)**
🚑 2.33   ⚕ 5.28   **FUD** 000   T A2 50 ▢

AMA: 2015,Jan,16; 2014,Jan,11; 2013,Jan,13-14; 2012,Jan,15-42; 2011,Feb,4-5; 2011,Jan,11; 2010,Dec,12

64530 **celiac plexus, with or without radiologic monitoring**
EXCLUDES Transmural anesthetic injection with transendoscopic ultrasound-guidance (43253)
🚑 2.66   ⚕ 5.42   **FUD** 000   T A2 ▢

AMA: 2015,Jan,16; 2014,Jan,11; 2013,Jan,13-14; 2012,Jan,15-42; 2011,Feb,4-5; 2011,Jan,11

64550 Transcutaneous Electrical Nerve Stimulation

CMS: 100-3,10.2 Transcutaneous Electrical Nerve Stimulation (TENS) for Acute Postoperative Pain
EXCLUDES Analysis and programming neurostimulator pulse generator (95970-95975)
Implantation of electrode array(s), either trial or permanent, with pulse generator for peripheral subcutaneous field stimulation (0282T-0284T)

64550 **Application of surface (transcutaneous) neurostimulator**
🚑 0.25   ⚕ 0.45   **FUD** 000   A ▢

AMA: 2015,Jan,16; 2014,Jan,11; 2012,Jan,15-42; 2011,Feb,4-5; 2011,Jan,11

64553-64570 Electrical Nerve Stimulation: Insertion/Replacement/Removal/Revision

INCLUDES Simple and complex neurostimulators
EXCLUDES Analysis and programming of neurostimulator pulse generator (95970-95975)
Implantation of electrode array(s), either trial or permanent, with pulse generator for peripheral subcutaneous field stimulation (0282T-0284T)

64553 **Percutaneous implantation of neurostimulator electrode array; cranial nerve**
EXCLUDES Open procedure (61885-61886)
🚑 4.60   ⚕ 6.09   **FUD** 010   J J8 80 ▢

AMA: 2015,Jan,16; 2014,Jan,11; 2011,Feb,4-5; 2010,Jan,9-11

64555 **peripheral nerve (excludes sacral nerve)**
Do not report with (64566)
🚑 4.43   ⚕ 6.03   **FUD** 010   J J8 ▢

AMA: 2015,Jan,13; 2015,Jan,16; 2014,Jan,11; 2012,Jan,15-42; 2011,Feb,4-5; 2010,Jan,9-11

64561 **sacral nerve (transforaminal placement) including image guidance, if performed**
🚑 8.70   ⚕ 23.2   **FUD** 010   J J8 50 ▢

AMA: 2015,Jan,16; 2014,Sep,5; 2014,Jan,11; 2012,Dec,12; 2011,Feb,4-5; 2010,Jan,9-11

64565 **neuromuscular**
🚑 3.81   ⚕ 5.40   **FUD** 010   J J8

AMA: 2015,Jan,16; 2014,Jan,11; 2012,Jan,15-42; 2011,Feb,4-5; 2011,Jan,11; 2010,Jan,9-11

64566 **Posterior tibial neurostimulation, percutaneous needle electrode, single treatment, includes programming**
Do not report with (64555, 95970-95972)
🚑 0.87   ⚕ 3.44   **FUD** 000   T P3 80

AMA: 2015,Jan,16; 2014,Jan,11; 2011,Sep,8; 2011,Feb,4-5

64568 **Incision for implantation of cranial nerve (eg, vagus nerve) neurostimulator electrode array and pulse generator**
Do not report with (61885-61886, 64570)
🚑 19.3   ⚕ 19.3   **FUD** 090   J J8 80 50

AMA: 2015,Jan,16; 2014,Jan,11; 2012,Jan,15-42; 2011,Sep,9-10; 2011,Sep,11-12; 2011,Sep,8; 2011,Feb,4-5

64569 **Revision or replacement of cranial nerve (eg, vagus nerve) neurostimulator electrode array, including connection to existing pulse generator**
EXCLUDES Replacement of pulse generator (61885)
Do not report with (61888, 64570)
🚑 22.9   ⚕ 22.9   **FUD** 090   J J8 80 50

AMA: 2015,Jan,16; 2014,Jan,11; 2011,Sep,8; 2011,Sep,9-10; 2011,Feb,4-5

64570 **Removal of cranial nerve (eg, vagus nerve) neurostimulator electrode array and pulse generator**
EXCLUDES Laparoscopic revision, replacement, removal, or implantation of vagus nerve blocking neurostimulator pulse generator and/or electrode array at the esophagogastric junction (0312T-0317T)
Do not report with (61888)
🚑 19.5   ⚕ 19.5   **FUD** 090   Q2 G2 80 50

AMA: 2015,Jan,16; 2014,Jan,11; 2011,Sep,8; 2011,Sep,9-10; 2011,Feb,4-5

64575-64595 Implantation/Revision/Removal Neurostimulators: Incisional

INCLUDES Simple and complex neurostimulators
EXCLUDES Analysis and programming neurostimulator pulse generator (95970-95975)
Implantation of electrode array(s), either trial or permanent, with pulse generator for peripheral subcutaneous field stimulation (0282T-0284T)

64575 **Incision for implantation of neurostimulator electrode array; peripheral nerve (excludes sacral nerve)**
🚑 9.20   ⚕ 9.20   **FUD** 090   J J8 ▢

AMA: 2014,Jan,11; 2011,Feb,4-5

64580 **neuromuscular**
🚑 8.67   ⚕ 8.67   **FUD** 090   J J8 80 ▢

AMA: 2014,Jan,11; 2011,Feb,4-5

64581 **sacral nerve (transforaminal placement)**
🚑 19.0   ⚕ 19.0   **FUD** 090   J J8 ▢

AMA: 2015,Jan,16; 2014,Sep,5; 2014,Jan,11; 2012,Dec,12; 2011,Feb,4-5

64585 **Revision or removal of peripheral neurostimulator electrode array**
🚑 4.13   ⚕ 6.98   **FUD** 010   Q2 A2 ▢

AMA: 2014,Jan,11; 2011,Feb,4-5

64590 **Insertion or replacement of peripheral or gastric neurostimulator pulse generator or receiver, direct or inductive coupling**
Do not report with (64595)
🚑 4.63   ⚕ 7.54   **FUD** 010   J J8 ▢

AMA: 2015,Jan,13; 2015,Jan,16; 2014,Jan,11; 2012,Dec,12; 2012,Jan,15-42; 2011,Sep,9-10; 2011,Feb,4-5

64595 **Revision or removal of peripheral or gastric neurostimulator pulse generator or receiver**
Do not report with (64590)
🚑 3.64   ⚕ 6.99   **FUD** 010   Q2 A2 ▢

AMA: 2015,Jan,16; 2014,Jan,11; 2012,Jan,15-42; 2011,Feb,4-5; 2011,Jan,11

Nervous System

64600-64610 Chemical Denervation Trigeminal Nerve

INCLUDES Injection of therapeutic medication

EXCLUDES *The following chemodenervation procedures:*
Anal sphincter (46505)
Bladder (52287)
Muscle electrical stimulation or EMG with needle guidance (95873, 95874)
Strabismus that involves the extraocular muscles (67345)
Treatments that do not destroy the target nerve (64999)

Code also chemodenervation agent

64600 **Destruction by neurolytic agent, trigeminal nerve; supraorbital, infraorbital, mental, or inferior alveolar branch**

🖩 6.31   ✂ 10.9   **FUD** 010   T A2 🖵

AMA: 2015,Jan,16; 2014,Jan,11; 2012,Sep,14-15; 2012,Sep,14-15; 2011,Feb,4-5; 2010,Jan,9-11

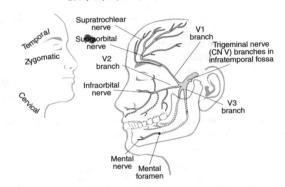

Supratrochlear nerve
Supraorbital nerve
Temporal
Zygomatic
V2 branch
Cervical
Infraorbital nerve
V1 branch
Trigeminal nerve (CN V) branches in infratemporal fossa
V3 branch
Mental nerve
Mental foramen

64605 **second and third division branches at foramen ovale**

🖩 10.2   ✂ 16.7   **FUD** 010   T A2 80 50 🖵

AMA: 2015,Jan,16; 2014,Jan,11; 2012,Sep,14-15; 2012,Sep,14-15; 2011,Feb,4-5; 2010,Jan,9-11

64610 **second and third division branches at foramen ovale under radiologic monitoring**

🖩 14.1   ✂ 20.8   **FUD** 010   T A2 50 🖵 P0

AMA: 2015,Jan,16; 2014,Jan,11; 2012,Sep,14-15; 2012,Sep,14-15; 2011,Feb,4-5; 2010,Jan,9-11

64611-64617 Chemical Denervation Procedures Head and Neck

INCLUDES Injection of therapeutic medication

EXCLUDES *Electromyography or muscle electric stimulation guidance (95873-95874)*
Nerve destruction of:
Anal sphincter (46505)
Bladder (52287)
Extraocular muscles to treat strabismus (67345)
Treatments that do not destroy the target nerve (64999)

64611 **Chemodenervation of parotid and submandibular salivary glands, bilateral**

Code also modifier 52 for injection of fewer than four salivary glands

🖩 2.94   ✂ 3.35   **FUD** 010   T P3 80

AMA: 2015,Jan,16; 2014,Jan,11; 2012,Sep,14-15; 2012,Sep,14-15; 2011,Feb,4-5

64612 **Chemodenervation of muscle(s); muscle(s) innervated by facial nerve, unilateral (eg, for blepharospasm, hemifacial spasm)**

🖩 3.36   ✂ 3.74   **FUD** 010   T P3 50 🖵

AMA: 2015,Jan,16; 2014,May,5; 2014,Jan,6; 2014,Jan,11; 2013,Dec,10; 2013,Apr,5-6; 2012,Sep,14-15; 2012,Sep,14-15; 2012,Jan,15-42; 2011,Dec,19; 2011,Feb,4-5; 2011,Jan,11; 2010,Jan,9-11; 2010,Jan,12-15

64615 **muscle(s) innervated by facial, trigeminal, cervical spinal and accessory nerves, bilateral (eg, for chronic migraine)**

Code also any guidance performed but report only once (95873-95874)

Do not report more than one time per session

Do not report with (64612, 64616-64617, 64642-64647)

🖩 3.65   ✂ 4.21   **FUD** 010   T P3

AMA: 2015,Jan,16; 2014,Jan,11; 2014,Jan,6; 2013,Apr,5-6

64616 **neck muscle(s), excluding muscles of the larynx, unilateral (eg, for cervical dystonia, spasmodic torticollis)**

Code also guidance by muscle electrical stimulation or needle electromyography, but report only once (95873-95874)

🖩 3.12   ✂ 3.57   **FUD** 010   T P3 50

AMA: 2015,Jan,16; 2014,May,5; 2014,Jan,11; 2014,Jan,6

64617 **larynx, unilateral, percutaneous (eg, for spasmodic dysphonia), includes guidance by needle electromyography, when performed**

EXCLUDES *Chemodenervation of larynx via direct laryngoscopy (31570-31571)*
Diagnostic needle electromyography of larynx (95865)

Do not report with (95873-95874)

🖩 3.31   ✂ 5.42   **FUD** 010   T P3 50

AMA: 2015,Jan,16; 2014,Jan,11; 2014,Jan,6

64620-64640 [64633, 64634, 64635, 64636] Chemical Denervation Intercostal, Facet Joint, Plantar, and Pudendal Nerve(s)

INCLUDES Injection of therapeutic medication

64620 **Destruction by neurolytic agent, intercostal nerve**

🖩 4.96   ✂ 5.87   **FUD** 010   T A2 🖵 P0

AMA: 2015,Jan,16; 2014,Jan,6; 2014,Jan,11; 2012,Sep,14-15; 2012,Sep,14-15; 2011,Feb,4-5

\# **64633** **Destruction by neurolytic agent, paravertebral facet joint nerve(s), with imaging guidance (fluoroscopy or CT); cervical or thoracic, single facet joint**

INCLUDES Imaging guidance (fluoroscopy or CT) and contrast injection
Paravertebral facet destruction of T12-L1 joint or nerve(s) that innervate that joint

EXCLUDES *Denervation performed using chemical, low grade thermal, or pulsed radiofrequency methods (64999)*
Destruction of paravertebral facet joint nerve(s) without imaging guidance (64999)

Code first ([64633])

Do not report with (77003, 77012)

🖩 6.53   ✂ 11.8   **FUD** 010   T 62 50

AMA: 2015,Feb,9; 2015,Jan,16; 2014,Jan,11; 2013,Apr,10-11; 2012,Sep,14-15; 2012,Sep,14-15; 2012,Jul,3-6; 2012,Jun,10-11

+ \# **64634** **cervical or thoracic, each additional facet joint (List separately in addition to code for primary procedure)**

INCLUDES Imaging guidance (fluoroscopy or CT) and contrast injection

EXCLUDES *Denervation performed using chemical, low grade thermal, or pulsed radiofrequency methods (64999)*
Destruction of paravertebral facet joint nerve(s) without imaging guidance (64999)

Code first ([64633])

Do not report with (77003, 77012)

🖩 1.96   ✂ 5.29   **FUD** ZZZ   N N1 50

AMA: 2015,Feb,9; 2015,Jan,16; 2014,Jan,11; 2013,Apr,10-11; 2012,Sep,14-15; 2012,Sep,14-15; 2012,Jul,3-6; 2012,Jun,10-11

lumbar or sacral, single facet joint | 64635

INCLUDES Imaging guidance (fluoroscopy or CT) and contrast injection

EXCLUDES Denervation performed using chemical, low grade thermal, or pulsed radiofrequency methods (64999)

Destruction of individual nerves, sacroiliac joint, by neurolytic agent (61640)

Destruction of paravertebral facet joint nerve(s) without imaging guidance (64999)

Do not report with (77003, 77012)

🚑 6.45   ⚕ 11.7   **FUD** 010   T G2 50

AMA: 2015,Feb,9; 2015,Jan,16; 2014,Jan,11; 2013,Apr,10-11; 2012,Sep,14-15; 2012,Sep,14-15; 2012,Jul,3-6; 2012,Jun,10-11

+ # 64636   **lumbar or sacral, each additional facet joint (List separately in addition to code for primary procedure)**

INCLUDES Imaging guidance (fluoroscopy or CT) with contrast injection

EXCLUDES Denervation performed using chemical, low grade thermal, or pulsed radiofrequency methods (64999)

Destruction of individual nerves, sacroiliac joint, by neurolytic agent (61640)

Destruction of paravertebral facet joint nerve(s) without imaging guidance (64999)

Code first ([64635])

Do not report with (77003, 77012)

🚑 1.73   ⚕ 4.84   **FUD** ZZZ   N N1 50

AMA: 2015,Feb,9; 2015,Jan,16; 2014,Jan,11; 2013,Apr,10-11; 2012,Sep,14-15; 2012,Sep,14-15; 2012,Jul,3-6; 2012,Jun,10-11

64630   **Destruction by neurolytic agent; pudendal nerve**

🚑 5.56   ⚕ 6.66   **FUD** 010   T A2 80 ▱

AMA: 2015,Jan,16; 2014,Jan,11; 2012,Sep,14-15; 2012,Sep,14-15; 2011,Feb,4-5; 2010,Jan,9-11

64632   **plantar common digital nerve**

Do not report with (64455)

🚑 1.98   ⚕ 2.44   **FUD** 010   T P3 80 50

AMA: 2015,Jul,10; 2015,Jan,16; 2014,Jan,11; 2013,Nov,14; 2013,Jan,13-14; 2012,Sep,14-15; 2012,Sep,14-15; 2011,Feb,4-5; 2010,Jan,9-11

64633	**Resequenced code. See code following 64620.**
64634	**Resequenced code. See code following 64620.**
64635	**Resequenced code. See code following 64620.**
64636	**Resequenced code. See code before 64630.**

64640   **other peripheral nerve or branch**

INCLUDES Neurolytic destruction of nerves of sacroiliac joint

🚑 2.67   ⚕ 3.79   **FUD** 010   T P3 50 ▱

AMA: 2015,Jan,16; 2014,Jan,11; 2012,Sep,14-15; 2012,Sep,14-15; 2012,Jun,15-16; 2012,Jan,15-42; 2011,Feb,4-5; 2011,Jan,11; 2010,Jan,9-11

64642-64645 Chemical Denervation Extremity Muscles

INCLUDES Trunk muscles include erector spine, obliques, paraspinal and rectus abdominus. The rest of the muscles are considered neck, head or extremity muscles.

EXCLUDES Chemodenervation with needle-guided electromyography or with guidance provided by muscle electrical stimulation (95873-95874)

Code also other extremities when appropriate, up to a total of 4 units per patient (if all extremities are injected) (64642-64645)

Do not report more than once per extremity

Do not report with modifier 50

64642   **Chemodenervation of one extremity; 1-4 muscle(s)**

Do not report more than one base code per session (64642, 64646)

🚑 3.13   ⚕ 4.04   **FUD** 000   T P3

AMA: 2015,Jan,16; 2014,Oct,14; 2014,Jan,11; 2014,Jan,6

+ 64643   **each additional extremity, 1-4 muscle(s) (List separately in addition to code for primary procedure)**

Code first (64642, 64644)

🚑 2.13   ⚕ 2.68   **FUD** ZZZ   N N1

AMA: 2015,Jan,16; 2014,Oct,14; 2014,Jan,11; 2014,Jan,6

64644   **Chemodenervation of one extremity; 5 or more muscles**

🚑 3.44   ⚕ 4.65   **FUD** 000   T P3

AMA: 2015,Jan,16; 2014,Oct,14; 2014,Jan,11; 2014,Jan,6

+ 64645   **each additional extremity, 5 or more muscles (List separately in addition to code for primary procedure)**

Code first (64644)

🚑 2.41   ⚕ 3.26   **FUD** ZZZ   N N1

AMA: 2015,Jan,16; 2014,Oct,14; 2014,Jan,11; 2014,Jan,6

64646-64647 Chemical Denervation Trunk Muscles

Do not report more than one time per session

Do not report with modifier 50

64646   **Chemodenervation of trunk muscle(s); 1-5 muscle(s)**

Do not report more than one base code per session (64642, 64646)

🚑 3.41   ⚕ 4.39   **FUD** 000   T P3

AMA: 2015,Jan,16; 2014,Jan,11; 2014,Jan,6

64647   **6 or more muscles**

🚑 3.94   ⚕ 5.07   **FUD** 000   T P3

AMA: 2015,Jan,16; 2014,Jan,11; 2014,Jan,6

64650-64653 Chemical Denervation Eccrine Glands

INCLUDES Injection of therapeutic medication

EXCLUDES Chemodenervation of extremities (64999)

Code also drugs or other substances used

64650   **Chemodenervation of eccrine glands; both axillae**

🚑 1.20   ⚕ 2.22   **FUD** 000   T P3 80

AMA: 2015,Jan,16; 2014,Jan,11; 2012,Sep,14-15; 2012,Sep,14-15; 2011,Feb,4-5; 2010,Jan,9-11

64653   **other area(s) (eg, scalp, face, neck), per day**

EXCLUDES Bladder chemodenervation (52287)

Hands or feet (64999)

🚑 1.55   ⚕ 2.71   **FUD** 000   T P3 80

AMA: 2015,Jan,16; 2014,Jan,11; 2012,Sep,14-15; 2012,Sep,14-15; 2011,Feb,4-5; 2010,Jan,9-11

64680-64681 Neurolysis: Celiac Plexus, Superior Hypogastric Plexus

INCLUDES Injection of therapeutic medication

Only for lesions that abut the dura matter or that affect the spinal neural tissue

Planning, dosimetry, targeting, positioning, or blocking performed by the surgeon

Radiation treatment management by the same physician (77427-77432)

64680   **Destruction by neurolytic agent, with or without radiologic monitoring; celiac plexus**

EXCLUDES Transmural neurolytic agent injection with transendoscopic ultrasound guidance (43253)

🚑 4.85   ⚕ 8.93   **FUD** 010   T A2 ▱

AMA: 2015,Jan,16; 2014,Jan,11; 2012,Sep,14-15; 2012,Sep,14-15; 2012,Jan,15-42; 2011,Feb,4-5; 2011,Jan,11; 2010,Jan,9-11

64681   **superior hypogastric plexus**

🚑 6.63   ⚕ 11.5   **FUD** 010   T A2 ▱

AMA: 2015,Jan,16; 2014,Jan,11; 2012,Sep,14-15; 2012,Sep,14-15; 2012,Jan,15-42; 2011,Feb,4-5; 2011,Jan,11; 2010,Jan,9-11

64702-64727 Decompression and/or Transposition of Nerve

INCLUDES External neurolysis and/or transposition to repair or restore a nerve

Neuroplasty with nerve wrapping

Surgical decompression/freeing of nerve from scar tissue

EXCLUDES Facial nerve decompression (69720)

Neuroplasty with operating microscope (64727)

Percutaneous neurolysis (62263-62264, 62280-62282)

64702   **Neuroplasty; digital, 1 or both, same digit**

🚑 14.3   ⚕ 14.3   **FUD** 090   T A2 ▱

AMA: 2015,Jan,16; 2014,Jan,11; 2012,Jan,15-42; 2011,Jan,11; 2010,Jan,3-5

64704   **nerve of hand or foot**

🚑 9.07   ⚕ 9.07   **FUD** 090   T A2 80 ▱

AMA: 2015,Jan,16; 2014,Jan,11; 2012,Jan,15-42; 2011,Jan,11; 2010,Jan,3-5

64708 **Neuroplasty, major peripheral nerve, arm or leg, open; other than specified**
🔧 14.3 ⚕ 14.3 **FUD** 090 ⊤ G2 80 ▣
AMA: 2015,Jan,16; 2014,Jan,11; 2012,Jun,12-13; 2012,Jan,15-42; 2011,Jan,11; 2010,Jan,3-5

64712 **sciatic nerve**
🔧 16.4 ⚕ 16.4 **FUD** 090 ⊤ G2 80 50 ▣
AMA: 2015,Jan,16; 2014,Jan,11; 2012,Jun,12-13; 2012,Jan,15-42; 2011,Jan,11; 2010,Jan,3-5

64713 **brachial plexus**
🔧 20.7 ⚕ 20.7 **FUD** 090 ⊤ G2 80 50 ▣
AMA: 2015,Jan,16; 2014,Jan,11; 2013,May,12; 2012,Jun,12-13; 2012,Jan,15-42; 2011,Jan,11; 2010,Jan,3-5

64714 **lumbar plexus**
🔧 18.6 ⚕ 18.6 **FUD** 090 G2 80 50 ▣
AMA: 2015,Jan,16; 2014,Jan,11; 2013,Dec,16; 2012,Jun,12-13; 2012,Jan,15-42; 2011,Jan,11; 2010,Jan,3-5

64716 **Neuroplasty and/or transposition; cranial nerve (specify)**
🔧 15.3 ⚕ 15.3 **FUD** 090 ⊤ A2 80 ▣
AMA: 2015,Jan,16; 2014,Jan,11; 2012,Jan,15-42; 2011,Jan,11; 2010,Jan,3-5

64718 **ulnar nerve at elbow**
🔧 17.0 ⚕ 17.0 **FUD** 090 ⊤ A2 80 50 ▣
AMA: 2015,Jan,16; 2014,Jan,11; 2012,Jan,15-42; 2011,Jan,11; 2010,Jan,3-5

64719 **ulnar nerve at wrist**
🔧 11.4 ⚕ 11.4 **FUD** 090 ⊤ A2 50 ▣
AMA: 2015,Jan,16; 2014,Jan,11; 2012,Jan,15-42; 2011,Jan,11; 2010,Jan,3-5

64721 **median nerve at carpal tunnel**
EXCLUDES Arthroscopic procedure (29848)
🔧 12.2 ⚕ 12.3 **FUD** 090 ⊤ A2 50 ▣
AMA: 2015,Jul,10; 2015,Jan,16; 2014,Jan,11; 2013,Dec,14; 2012,Oct,14; 2012,Sep,16; 2012,Jun,15-16; 2012,Jan,15-42; 2011,Jan,11; 2010,Jan,3-5

64722 **Decompression; unspecified nerve(s) (specify)**
🔧 10.6 ⚕ 10.6 **FUD** 090 ⊤ A2 80 ▣
AMA: 2015,Jan,16; 2014,Jan,11; 2012,Jan,15-42; 2011,Jan,11; 2010,Jan,3-5

64726 **plantar digital nerve**
🔧 7.91 ⚕ 7.91 **FUD** 090 ⊤ A2 ▣
AMA: 2015,Jan,16; 2014,Jan,11; 2012,Jan,15-42; 2011,Jan,11; 2010,Jan,3-5

+ 64727 **Internal neurolysis, requiring use of operating microscope (List separately in addition to code for neuroplasty) (Neuroplasty includes external neurolysis)**
INCLUDES Operating microscope (69990)
Code first neuroplasty (64702-64721)
🔧 5.35 ⚕ 5.35 **FUD** ZZZ N N1 ▣
AMA: 2015,Jan,16; 2014,Jan,11; 2012,Jun,12-13; 2012,Jan,15-42; 2011,Jan,11; 2010,Jan,3-5

64732-64772 Surgical Avulsion/Transection of Nerve

EXCLUDES Stereotactic lesion of gasserian ganglion (61790)

64732 **Transection or avulsion of; supraorbital nerve**
🔧 10.9 ⚕ 10.9 **FUD** 090 ⊤ A2 80 50 ▣
AMA: 2015,Jan,16; 2014,Jan,11

64734 **infraorbital nerve**
🔧 14.6 ⚕ 14.6 **FUD** 090 ⊤ A2 80 50 ▣
AMA: 2014,Jan,11

64736 **mental nerve**
🔧 11.4 ⚕ 11.4 **FUD** 090 ⊤ A2 80 50 ▣
AMA: 2014,Jan,11

64738 **inferior alveolar nerve by osteotomy**
🔧 13.2 ⚕ 13.2 **FUD** 090 ⊤ A2 80 50 ▣
AMA: 2014,Jan,11

64740 **lingual nerve**
🔧 13.1 ⚕ 13.1 **FUD** 090 ⊤ A2 80 50 ▣
AMA: 2014,Jan,11

64742 **facial nerve, differential or complete**
🔧 13.1 ⚕ 13.1 **FUD** 090 ⊤ A2 80 50 ▣
AMA: 2014,Jan,11

64744 **greater occipital nerve**
🔧 14.5 ⚕ 14.5 **FUD** 090 ⊤ A2 80 50 ▣
AMA: 2014,Jan,11

64746 **phrenic nerve**
EXCLUDES Section of recurrent unilateral laryngeal nerve (31595)
🔧 12.5 ⚕ 12.5 **FUD** 090 ⊤ A2 80 50 ▣ PQ
AMA: 2014,Jan,11

64755 **vagus nerves limited to proximal stomach (selective proximal vagotomy, proximal gastric vagotomy, parietal cell vagotomy, supra- or highly selective vagotomy)**
EXCLUDES Laparoscopic procedure (43652)
🔧 26.5 ⚕ 26.5 **FUD** 090 C 80 ▣
AMA: 2015,Jan,16; 2014,Jan,11

64760 **vagus nerve (vagotomy), abdominal**
EXCLUDES Laparoscopic procedure (43651)
🔧 14.8 ⚕ 14.8 **FUD** 090 C 80 ▣
AMA: 2015,Jan,16; 2014,Jan,11

64763 **Transection or avulsion of obturator nerve, extrapelvic, with or without adductor tenotomy**
🔧 14.6 ⚕ 14.6 **FUD** 090 ⊤ G2 80 50 ▣
AMA: 2014,Jan,11

64766 **Transection or avulsion of obturator nerve, intrapelvic, with or without adductor tenotomy**
🔧 16.3 ⚕ 16.3 **FUD** 090 ⊤ G2 80 50 ▣
AMA: 2014,Jan,11

64771 **Transection or avulsion of other cranial nerve, extradural**
🔧 17.1 ⚕ 17.1 **FUD** 090 ⊤ A2 80 ▣
AMA: 2014,Jan,11

64772 **Transection or avulsion of other spinal nerve, extradural**
EXCLUDES Removal of tender scar and soft tissue including neuroma if necessary (11400-11446, 13100-13153)
🔧 16.4 ⚕ 16.4 **FUD** 090 ⊤ A2 80 ▣
AMA: 2015,Apr,10; 2014,Jan,11

64774-64823 Excisional Nerve Procedures

EXCLUDES Morton neuroma excision (28080)

64774 **Excision of neuroma; cutaneous nerve, surgically identifiable**
🔧 11.9 ⚕ 11.9 **FUD** 090 ⊤ A2 ▣
AMA: 2014,Jan,11

64776 **digital nerve, 1 or both, same digit**
🔧 11.1 ⚕ 11.1 **FUD** 090 ⊤ A2 80 ▣
AMA: 2014,Jan,11

+ 64778 **digital nerve, each additional digit (List separately in addition to code for primary procedure)**
Code first (64776)
🔧 4.10 ⚕ 4.10 **FUD** ZZZ N N1 ▣
AMA: 2014,Jan,11

64782 **hand or foot, except digital nerve**
🔧 12.9 ⚕ 12.9 **FUD** 090 ⊤ A2 ▣
AMA: 2014,Jan,11

+ 64783 **hand or foot, each additional nerve, except same digit (List separately in addition to code for primary procedure)**
Code first (64782)
🔧 6.35 ⚕ 6.35 **FUD** ZZZ N N1 ▣
AMA: 2014,Jan,11

64784 **major peripheral nerve, except sciatic**
🔧 20.9 ⚕ 20.9 **FUD** 090 ⊤ A2 80 ▣
AMA: 2014,Jan,11

| 26 /TC PC/TC Comp Only | A2-Z3 ASC Pmt | 50 Bilateral | ♂ Male Only | ♀ Female Only | 🔧 Facility RVU | ⚕ Non-Facility RVU |
| AMA: CPT Asst | CMS: Pub 100 | A-Y OPPSI | 80 /80 Surg Assist Allowed / w/Doc | | ▣ Lab Crosswalk | Radiology Crosswalk |

260   Medicare (Red Text)   CPT © 2015 American Medical Association. All Rights Reserved. (Black Text)   © 2015 Optum360, LLC (Blue Text)

64786	sciatic nerve

⚙ 31.2 ⅀ 31.2 **FUD** 090 [T] [A2] [80] [50] [▣]
AMA: 2014,Jan,11

+ 64787 Implantation of nerve end into bone or muscle (List separately in addition to neuroma excision)
Code also, when appropriate (64774-64786)
⚙ 7.08 ⅀ 7.08 **FUD** ZZZ [N] [N1] [80] [▣]
AMA: 2014,Jan,11

64788 Excision of neurofibroma or neurolemmoma; cutaneous nerve
⚙ 11.7 ⅀ 11.7 **FUD** 090 [T] [A2]
AMA: 2014,Jan,11

64790 major peripheral nerve
⚙ 24.3 ⅀ 24.3 **FUD** 090 [T] [A2] [80] [▣]
AMA: 2014,Jan,11

64792 extensive (including malignant type)
⚙ 31.1 ⅀ 31.1 **FUD** 090 [T] [A2] [80] [▣]
AMA: 2014,Jan,11

64795 Biopsy of nerve
⚙ 5.57 ⅀ 5.57 **FUD** 000 [T] [A2] [▣] [PQ]
AMA: 2014,Jan,11

64802 Sympathectomy, cervical
⚙ 19.1 ⅀ 19.1 **FUD** 090 [T] [A2] [80] [50] [▣]
AMA: 2014,Jan,11

64804 Sympathectomy, cervicothoracic
⚙ 27.1 ⅀ 27.1 **FUD** 090 [T] [80] [50] [▣]
AMA: 2014,Jan,11

64809 Sympathectomy, thoracolumbar
[INCLUDES] Leriche sympathectomy
⚙ 32.2 ⅀ 32.2 **FUD** 090 [C] [80] [50] [▣]
AMA: 2014,Jan,11

64818 Sympathectomy, lumbar
⚙ 15.9 ⅀ 15.9 **FUD** 090 [C] [80] [50] [▣]
AMA: 2014,Jan,11

64820 Sympathectomy; digital arteries, each digit
[INCLUDES] Operating microscope (69990)
⚙ 20.9 ⅀ 20.9 **FUD** 090 [T] [G2] [▣]
AMA: 2015,Jan,16; 2014,Jan,11; 2012,Jan,15-42; 2011,Jan,11

64821 radial artery
[INCLUDES] Operating microscope (69990)
⚙ 19.7 ⅀ 19.7 **FUD** 090 [T] [A2] [50] [▣]
AMA: 2014,Jan,11

64822 ulnar artery
[INCLUDES] Operating microscope (69990)
⚙ 19.7 ⅀ 19.7 **FUD** 090 [T] [G2] [50] [▣]
AMA: 2014,Jan,11

64823 superficial palmar arch
[INCLUDES] Operating microscope (69990)
⚙ 22.7 ⅀ 22.7 **FUD** 090 [T] [G2] [50] [▣]
AMA: 2014,Jan,11

64831-64907 Nerve Repair: Suture and Nerve Grafts

64831 Suture of digital nerve, hand or foot; 1 nerve
⚙ 19.6 ⅀ 19.6 **FUD** 090 [T] [A2] [50] [▣]
AMA: 2015,Jan,16; 2014,Sep,13; 2014,Jan,11

+ 64832 each additional digital nerve (List separately in addition to code for primary procedure)
Code first (64831)
⚙ 9.76 ⅀ 9.76 **FUD** ZZZ [N] [N1] [80] [▣]
AMA: 2015,Jan,16; 2014,Jan,11

64834 Suture of 1 nerve; hand or foot, common sensory nerve
⚙ 21.2 ⅀ 21.2 **FUD** 090 [T] [A2] [80] [50] [▣]
AMA: 2014,Jan,11

64835 median motor thenar
⚙ 23.5 ⅀ 23.5 **FUD** 090 [T] [A2] [80] [50] [▣]
AMA: 2014,Jan,11

64836 ulnar motor
⚙ 23.5 ⅀ 23.5 **FUD** 090 [T] [A2] [80] [50] [▣]
AMA: 2014,Jan,11

+ 64837 Suture of each additional nerve, hand or foot (List separately in addition to code for primary procedure)
Code first (64834-64836)
⚙ 10.9 ⅀ 10.9 **FUD** ZZZ [N] [N1] [80] [▣]
AMA: 2014,Jan,11

64840 Suture of posterior tibial nerve
⚙ 27.8 ⅀ 27.8 **FUD** 090 [T] [A2] [80] [50] [▣]
AMA: 2014,Jan,11

64856 Suture of major peripheral nerve, arm or leg, except sciatic; including transposition
⚙ 29.2 ⅀ 29.2 **FUD** 090 [T] [A2]
AMA: 2014,Jan,11

64857 without transposition
⚙ 30.2 ⅀ 30.2 **FUD** 090 [T] [A2] [80] [▣]
AMA: 2014,Jan,11

64858 Suture of sciatic nerve
⚙ 34.1 ⅀ 34.1 **FUD** 090 [T] [A2] [80] [50] [▣]
AMA: 2014,Jan,11

+ 64859 Suture of each additional major peripheral nerve (List separately in addition to code for primary procedure)
Code first (64856-64857)
⚙ 7.31 ⅀ 7.31 **FUD** ZZZ [N] [N1] [80] [▣]
AMA: 2014,Jan,11

64861 Suture of; brachial plexus
⚙ 36.5 ⅀ 36.5 **FUD** 090 [T] [A2] [80] [50] [▣]
AMA: 2014,Jan,11

64862 lumbar plexus
⚙ 33.1 ⅀ 33.1 **FUD** 090 [T] [A2] [80] [50] [▣]
AMA: 2014,Jan,11

64864 Suture of facial nerve; extracranial
⚙ 25.1 ⅀ 25.1 **FUD** 090 [T] [A2] [80] [▣]
AMA: 2014,Jan,11

64865 infratemporal, with or without grafting
⚙ 31.9 ⅀ 31.9 **FUD** 090 [T] [A2] [80] [▣]
AMA: 2014,Jan,11

64866 Anastomosis; facial-spinal accessory
⚙ 33.1 ⅀ 33.1 **FUD** 090 [C] [80] [▣]
AMA: 2014,Jan,11

64868 facial-hypoglossal
[INCLUDES] Korte-Ballance anastomosis
⚙ 29.2 ⅀ 29.2 **FUD** 090 [C] [80] [▣]
AMA: 2014,Jan,11

+ 64872 Suture of nerve; requiring secondary or delayed suture (List separately in addition to code for primary neurorrhaphy)
Code also when appropriate (64831-64865)
⚙ 3.43 ⅀ 3.43 **FUD** ZZZ [N] [N1] [80] [▣]
AMA: 2014,Jan,11

+ 64874 requiring extensive mobilization, or transposition of nerve (List separately in addition to code for nerve suture)
Code first (64831-64865)
⚙ 4.77 ⅀ 4.77 **FUD** ZZZ [N] [N1] [80] [▣]
AMA: 2014,Jan,11

+ 64876 requiring shortening of bone of extremity (List separately in addition to code for nerve suture)
Code also when appropriate (64831-64865)
⚙ 4.89 ⅀ 4.89 **FUD** ZZZ [N] [N1] [80] [▣]
AMA: 2014,Jan,11

64885 Nerve graft (includes obtaining graft), head or neck; up to 4 cm in length
⚙ 32.2 ⅀ 32.2 **FUD** 090 [T] [A2] [80] [▣]
AMA: 2015,Jan,16; 2014,Jan,11; 2012,Jan,15-42; 2011,Jan,11

Nervous System

64886 — 64999

64886	**more than 4 cm length**
	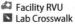 37.4 ✂ 37.4 **FUD** 090 T A2 80 ▭
	AMA: 2015,Jan,16; 2014,Jan,11; 2012,Jan,15-42; 2011,Jan,11

64890	**Nerve graft (includes obtaining graft), single strand, hand or foot; up to 4 cm length**
	31.5 ✂ 31.5 **FUD** 090 T A2 80 ▭
	AMA: 2015,Aug,8; 2015,Apr,10; 2014,Jan,11

64891	**more than 4 cm length**
	33.5 ✂ 33.5 **FUD** 090 T A2 80 ▭
	AMA: 2014,Jan,11

64892	**Nerve graft (includes obtaining graft), single strand, arm or leg; up to 4 cm length**
	30.4 ✂ 30.4 **FUD** 090 T A2 80 ▭
	AMA: 2014,Jan,11

64893	**more than 4 cm length**
	32.7 ✂ 32.7 **FUD** 090 T A2 80 ▭
	AMA: 2014,Jan,11

64895	**Nerve graft (includes obtaining graft), multiple strands (cable), hand or foot; up to 4 cm length**
	38.9 ✂ 38.9 **FUD** 090 T A2 80 ▭
	AMA: 2015,Jan,16; 2014,Jan,11

64896	**more than 4 cm length**
	46.9 ✂ 46.9 **FUD** 090 T A2 80 ▭
	AMA: 2015,Jan,16; 2014,Jan,11

64897	**Nerve graft (includes obtaining graft), multiple strands (cable), arm or leg; up to 4 cm length**
	36.5 ✂ 36.5 **FUD** 090 T A2 80 ▭
	AMA: 2015,Jan,16; 2014,Jan,11

64898	**more than 4 cm length**
	39.6 ✂ 39.6 **FUD** 090 T A2 80 ▭
	AMA: 2015,Jan,16; 2014,Jan,11

+ 64901	**Nerve graft, each additional nerve; single strand (List separately in addition to code for primary procedure)**
	Code first (64885-64893)
	16.2 ✂ 16.2 **FUD** ZZZ N N1 80 ▭
	AMA: 2015,Jan,16; 2014,Jan,11

+ 64902	**multiple strands (cable) (List separately in addition to code for primary procedure)**
	Code first (64885-64886, 64895-64898)
	18.7 ✂ 18.7 **FUD** ZZZ N N1 80 ▭
	AMA: 2015,Jan,16; 2014,Jan,11

64905	**Nerve pedicle transfer; first stage**
	29.5 ✂ 29.5 **FUD** 090 T A2 80 ▭
	AMA: 2014,Jan,11

64907	**second stage**
	42.6 ✂ 42.6 **FUD** 090 T A2 80 ▭
	AMA: 2014,Jan,11

64910-64999 Nerve Repair: Synthetic and Vein Grafts

64910	**Nerve repair; with synthetic conduit or vein allograft (eg, nerve tube), each nerve**
	INCLUDES Operating microscope (69990)
	23.7 ✂ 23.7 **FUD** 090 T 02 80
	AMA: 2015,Aug,8; 2015,Apr,10; 2015,Jan,16; 2014,Jan,11

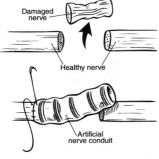

Damaged nerve

Healthy nerve

Artificial nerve conduit

A synthetic "bridge" is affixed to each end of a
severed nerve with sutures
This procedure is performed using an operating
microscope

64911	**with autogenous vein graft (includes harvest of vein graft), each nerve**
	INCLUDES Operating microscope (69990)
	29.2 ✂ 29.2 **FUD** 090 T 80
	AMA: 2015,Jan,16; 2014,Jan,11

64999	**Unlisted procedure, nervous system**
	0.00 ✂ 0.00 **FUD** YYY T 80
	AMA: 2015,Aug,8; 2015,Jul,10; 2015,Apr,10; 2015,Feb,9; 2015,Jan,16; 2014,Jul,8; 2014,Feb,11; 2014,Jan,11; 2014,Jan,9; 2014,Jan,8; 2013,Nov,14; 2013,Dec,14; 2013,Jun,13; 2013,Apr,10-11; 2013,Apr,5-6; 2012,Dec,12; 2012,Sep,14-15; 2012,Oct,14; 2012,Sep,14-15; 2012,Sep,16; 2012,May,14-15; 2012,Feb,11; 2012,Jan,13-14; 2012,Jan,15-42; 2011,Sep,11-12; 2011,Jul,16-17; 2011,Jul,12-13; 2011,Apr,12; 2011,Jan,11; 2010,Nov,4; 2010,Sep,9; 2010,Jun,8

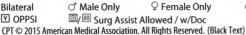

65091-65093 Surgical Removal of Eyeball Contents

INCLUDES Operating microscope (69990)

65091 Evisceration of ocular contents; without implant

    17.9   17.9   **FUD** 090   T A2 80 50

    AMA: 2014,Jan,11

Conjunctiva
Sclera
Muscles are severed at their attachment to the eyeball

Evisceration involves removal of the contents of the eyeball: the vitreous; retina; choroid; lens; iris; and ciliary muscle. Only the scleral shell remains. A temporary or permanent implant is usually inserted

Enucleation involves severing the extraorbital muscles and optic nerve with removal of the eyeball. An implant is usually inserted and, if permanent, may involve attachment to the severed extraorbital muscles

65093 with implant

    17.7   17.7   **FUD** 090   T A2 50

    AMA: 2014,Jan,11

65101-65105 Surgical Removal of Eyeball

INCLUDES Operating microscope (69990)

EXCLUDES Conjunctivoplasty following enucleation (68320-68328)

65101 Enucleation of eye; without implant

    20.8   20.8   **FUD** 090   T A2 50

    AMA: 2014,Jan,11

65103 with implant, muscles not attached to implant

    21.7   21.7   **FUD** 090   T A2 50

    AMA: 2014,Jan,11

65105 with implant, muscles attached to implant

    23.9   23.9   **FUD** 090   T A2 80 50

    AMA: 2014,Jan,11

65110-65114 Surgical Removal of Orbital Contents

INCLUDES Operating microscope (69990)

EXCLUDES Free full thickness graft (15260-15261)
Repair more extensive than skin (67930-67975)
Skin graft (15120-15121)

65110 Exenteration of orbit (does not include skin graft), removal of orbital contents; only

    34.4   34.4   **FUD** 090   T A2 80 50

    AMA: 2014,Jan,11

65112 with therapeutic removal of bone

    40.0   40.0   **FUD** 090   T A2 80 50

    AMA: 2014,Jan,11

65114 with muscle or myocutaneous flap

    41.9   41.9   **FUD** 090   T A2 80 50

    AMA: 2014,Jan,11

65125-65175 Implant Procedures: Insertion, Removal, and Revision

INCLUDES Operating microscope (69990)

EXCLUDES Orbital implant insertion outside muscle cone (67550)
Orbital implant removal or revision outside muscle cone (67560)

65125 Modification of ocular implant with placement or replacement of pegs (eg, drilling receptacle for prosthesis appendage) (separate procedure)

    8.26   12.8   **FUD** 090   T G2 50

    AMA: 2014,Jan,11

65130 Insertion of ocular implant secondary; after evisceration, in scleral shell

    20.6   20.6   **FUD** 090   T A2 50

    AMA: 2014,Jan,11

65135 after enucleation, muscles not attached to implant

    20.9   20.9   **FUD** 090   T A2 50

    AMA: 2014,Jan,11

65140 after enucleation, muscles attached to implant

    22.7   22.7   **FUD** 090   T A2 50

    AMA: 2014,Jan,11

65150 Reinsertion of ocular implant; with or without conjunctival graft

    16.2   16.2   **FUD** 090   T A2 80 50

    AMA: 2014,Jan,11

65155 with use of foreign material for reinforcement and/or attachment of muscles to implant

    23.8   23.8   **FUD** 090   T A2 50

    AMA: 2014,Jan,11

65175 Removal of ocular implant

    18.5   18.5   **FUD** 090   T A2 50

    AMA: 2014,Jan,11

65205-65265 Foreign Body Removal By Area of Eye

INCLUDES Operating microscope (69990)

EXCLUDES Removal:
Anterior segment implant (65920)
Ocular implant (65175)
Orbital implant outside muscle cone (67560)
Posterior segment implant (67120)
Removal of foreign body:
Eyelid (67938)
Lacrimal system (68530)
Orbit:
Lateral approach (67430)
Frontal approach (67413)

65205 Removal of foreign body, external eye; conjunctival superficial

    (70030, 76529)

    1.25   1.58   **FUD** 000   01 N1 50

    AMA: 2015,Jan,16; 2014,Jan,11; 2013,Oct,18; 2012,Jan,15-42; 2011,Jan,11

65210 conjunctival embedded (includes concretions), subconjunctival, or scleral nonperforating

    (70030, 76529)

    1.51   1.94   **FUD** 000   01 N1 50

    AMA: 2014,Jan,11

65220 corneal, without slit lamp

    EXCLUDES Repair of corneal wound with foreign body (65275)

    (70030, 76529)

    1.19   1.63   **FUD** 000   01 N1 50

    AMA: 2015,Jan,16; 2014,Jan,11; 2012,Jan,15-42; 2011,Jan,11

65222 corneal, with slit lamp

    EXCLUDES Repair of corneal wound with foreign body (65275)

    (70030, 76529)

    1.48   1.89   **FUD** 000   01 N1 50

    AMA: 2015,Jan,16; 2014,Jan,11; 2012,Jan,15-42; 2011,Jan,11

65235 Removal of foreign body, intraocular; from anterior chamber of eye or lens

    (70030, 76529)

    20.1   20.1   **FUD** 090   T A2 80 50

    AMA: 2015,Jan,16; 2014,Jan,11

65260 from posterior segment, magnetic extraction, anterior or posterior route

    (70030, 76529)

    27.0   27.0   **FUD** 090   S A2 80 50

    AMA: 2014,Jan,11

65265 from posterior segment, nonmagnetic extraction

    (70030, 76529)

    30.5   30.5   **FUD** 090   T A2 80 50

    AMA: 2014,Jan,11

● New Code   ▲ Revised Code   ○ Reinstated   M Maternity   ◣ Age Edit Edit   Unlisted   Not Covered   # Resequenced
Ⓝ AMA Mod 51 Exempt   ⑪ Optum Mod 51 Exempt   ⓢ Mod 63 Exempt   ⊙ Mod Sedation   + Add-on   CCI   P0 PQRS   **FUD** Follow-up Days

© 2015 Optum360, LLC (Blue Text)   CPT © 2015 American Medical Association. All Rights Reserved. (Black Text)   Medicare (Red Text)   **263**

65270-65290 Laceration Repair External Eye

INCLUDES Conjunctival flap
Operating microscope (69990)
Restoration of anterior chamber with air or saline injection

EXCLUDES Repair:
Ciliary body or iris (66680)
Eyelid laceration (12011-12018, 12051-12057, 13151-13160, 67930, 67935)
Lacrimal system injury (68700)
Surgical wound (66250)
Treatment of orbit fracture (21385-21408)

65270 **Repair of laceration; conjunctiva, with or without nonperforating laceration sclera, direct closure**
🚗 3.99 ⚕ 7.53 **FUD** 010 T A2 80 50 🖳
AMA: 2015,Jan,16; 2014,Jan,11; 2012,Aug,9

65272 **conjunctiva, by mobilization and rearrangement, without hospitalization**
🚗 9.92 ⚕ 14.1 **FUD** 090 T A2 50 🖳
AMA: 2014,Jan,11

65273 **conjunctiva, by mobilization and rearrangement, with hospitalization**
🚗 10.7 ⚕ 10.7 **FUD** 090 C 50 🖳
AMA: 2014,Jan,11

65275 **cornea, nonperforating, with or without removal foreign body**
🚗 13.0 ⚕ 16.3 **FUD** 090 T A2 80 50 🖳
AMA: 2014,Jan,11

65280 **cornea and/or sclera, perforating, not involving uveal tissue**
Do not report for surgical wound repair
🚗 19.0 ⚕ 19.0 **FUD** 090 T A2 80 50 🖳
AMA: 2015,Jan,16; 2014,Jan,11; 2012,Aug,9

65285 **cornea and/or sclera, perforating, with reposition or resection of uveal tissue**
Do not report for surgical wound repair
🚗 31.3 ⚕ 31.3 **FUD** 090 T A2 50 🖳
AMA: 2015,Jan,16; 2014,Jan,11; 2012,Aug,9

65286 **application of tissue glue, wounds of cornea and/or sclera**
🚗 14.0 ⚕ 19.8 **FUD** 090 T P2 50 🖳
AMA: 2015,Jan,16; 2014,Jan,11

65290 **Repair of wound, extraocular muscle, tendon and/or Tenon's capsule**
🚗 13.8 ⚕ 13.8 **FUD** 090 T A2 50 🖳
AMA: 2014,Jan,11

65400-65600 Removal Corneal Lesions

INCLUDES Operating microscope (69990)

65400 **Excision of lesion, cornea (keratectomy, lamellar, partial), except pterygium**
🚗 17.0 ⚕ 19.1 **FUD** 090 T A2 50 🖳
AMA: 2015,Jan,16; 2014,Jan,11

65410 **Biopsy of cornea**
🚗 2.96 ⚕ 4.04 **FUD** 000 T A2 80 50 🖳 P0
AMA: 2015,Jan,16; 2014,Jan,11

65420 **Excision or transposition of pterygium; without graft**
🚗 10.6 ⚕ 14.5 **FUD** 090 T A2 50 🖳
AMA: 2015,Jan,16; 2014,Jan,11; 2012,Jan,15-42; 2011,Jan,11

Conjunctiva

Cornea

The conjunctiva is subject to numerous acute and chronic irritations and disorders

Pterygium

Lens

Posterior chamber

Iris

Anterior chamber

65426 **with graft**
🚗 13.5 ⚕ 18.4 **FUD** 090 T A2 50 🖳
AMA: 2015,Jan,16; 2014,Jan,11

65430 **Scraping of cornea, diagnostic, for smear and/or culture**
🚗 2.93 ⚕ 3.24 **FUD** 000 Q1 N1 50 🖳
AMA: 2014,Jan,11

65435 **Removal of corneal epithelium; with or without chemocauterization (abrasion, curettage)**
Do not report with (0402T)
🚗 1.96 ⚕ 2.24 **FUD** 000 T P3 50 🖳
AMA: 2015,Jan,16; 2014,Jan,11; 2012,Jan,15-42; 2011,Jan,11

65436 **with application of chelating agent (eg, EDTA)**
🚗 10.5 ⚕ 10.9 **FUD** 090 T P3 50 🖳
AMA: 2014,Jan,11

65450 **Destruction of lesion of cornea by cryotherapy, photocoagulation or thermocauterization**
🚗 9.09 ⚕ 9.19 **FUD** 090 T G2 50 🖳
AMA: 2014,Jan,11

65600 **Multiple punctures of anterior cornea (eg, for corneal erosion, tattoo)**
🚗 9.73 ⚕ 11.1 **FUD** 090 T P3 50 🖳
AMA: 2014,Jan,11

65710-65757 Corneal Transplants

CMS: 100-3,80.7 Refractive Keratoplasty
INCLUDES Operating microscope (69990)
EXCLUDES Processing, preserving, and transporting corneal tissue (V2785)
Do not report with (92025)

65710 **Keratoplasty (corneal transplant); anterior lamellar**
INCLUDES Use and preparation of fresh or preserved graft
EXCLUDES Refractive keratoplasty surgery (65760-65767)
🚗 31.2 ⚕ 31.2 **FUD** 090 T A2 80 50 🖳
AMA: 2015,Jan,16; 2014,Jan,11; 2012,Aug,9

65730 **penetrating (except in aphakia or pseudophakia)**
INCLUDES Use and preparation of fresh or preserved graft
EXCLUDES Refractive keratoplasty surgery (65760-65767)
🚗 34.7 ⚕ 34.7 **FUD** 090 T A2 80 50 🖳
AMA: 2015,Jan,16; 2014,Jan,11; 2012,Aug,9; 2012,Jan,15-42; 2011,Jan,11

65750 **penetrating (in aphakia)**
INCLUDES Use and preparation of fresh or preserved graft
EXCLUDES Refractive keratoplasty surgery (65760-65767)
🚗 34.8 ⚕ 34.8 **FUD** 090 T A2 80 50 🖳
AMA: 2015,Jan,16; 2014,Jan,11; 2012,Aug,9; 2011,Jan,11

65755 **penetrating (in pseudophakia)**
INCLUDES Use and preparation of fresh or preserved graft
EXCLUDES Refractive keratoplasty surgery (65760-65767)
🚗 34.7 ⚕ 34.7 **FUD** 090 T A2 80 50 🖳
AMA: 2015,Jan,16; 2014,Jan,11; 2012,Aug,9

65756 **endothelial**
EXCLUDES Refractive keratoplasty surgery (65760-65767)
Code also donor material
Code also if appropriate (65757)
🚗 33.5 ⚕ 33.5 **FUD** 090 T G2 80 50
AMA: 2015,Jan,16; 2014,Jan,11; 2012,Jan,15-42; 2011,Jan,11

+ 65757 **Backbench preparation of corneal endothelial allograft prior to transplantation (List separately in addition to code for primary procedure)**
Code first (65756)
🚗 0.00 ⚕ 0.00 **FUD** ZZZ N N1 80
AMA: 2015,Jan,16; 2014,Aug,14; 2014,Jan,11; 2012,Jan,15-42; 2011,Jan,11

| 26 TC PC/TC Component Only | A2-Z3 ASC Payment | 50 Bilateral | ♂ Male Only | ♀ Female Only | 🚗 Facility RVU | ⚕ Non-Facility RVU |
| **AMA:** CPT Assistant References | **CMS:** Pub 100 | A-Y OPPSI | 80 /80 Surg Assist Allowed / w/Doc | | 🖳 Lab crosswalk | Radiology crosswalk |

264 Medicare (Red Text) CPT © 2015 American Medical Association. All Rights Reserved. (Black Text) © 2015 Optum360, LLC (Blue Text)

65760-65785 Corneal Refractive Procedures

CMS: 100-3,80.7 Refractive Keratoplasty

INCLUDES Operating microscope (69990)
EXCLUDES *Unlisted corneal procedures (66999)*

65760 **Keratomileusis**
Do not report with (92025)
🔲 0.00   ⚖ 0.00   **FUD** XXX   E
AMA: 2014,Jan,11

65765 **Keratophakia**
Do not report with (92025)
🔲 0.00   ⚖ 0.00   **FUD** XXX   E
AMA: 2014,Jan,11

65767 **Epikeratoplasty**
Do not report with (92025)
🔲 0.00   ⚖ 0.00   **FUD** XXX   E
AMA: 2014,Jan,11

65770 **Keratoprosthesis**
Do not report with (92025)
🔲 39.7   ⚖ 39.7   **FUD** 090   J J8 80 50 ▭
AMA: 2014,Jan,11

65771 **Radial keratotomy**
Do not report with (92025)
🔲 0.00   ⚖ 0.00   **FUD** XXX   E
AMA: 2014,Jan,11

65772 **Corneal relaxing incision for correction of surgically induced astigmatism**
🔲 11.4   ⚖ 12.7   **FUD** 090   T A2 50 ▭
AMA: 2014,Jan,11

65775 **Corneal wedge resection for correction of surgically induced astigmatism**
EXCLUDES *Fitting of contact lens to treat disease (92071-92072)*
🔲 15.6   ⚖ 15.6   **FUD** 090   T A2 50 ▭
AMA: 2015,Jan,16; 2014,Jan,11; 2012,Aug,9

65778 **Placement of amniotic membrane on the ocular surface; without sutures**
EXCLUDES *Use of tissue glue to place amniotic membrane (66999)*
Do not report with (65430, 65435, 65780)
🔲 1.99   ⚖ 38.9   **FUD** 010   Q2 N1 80 50
AMA: 2015,Jan,16; 2014,May,5; 2014,Jan,11

65779 **single layer, sutured**
EXCLUDES *Use of tissue glue to place amniotic membrane (66999)*
Do not report with (65430, 65435, 65780)
🔲 8.02   ⚖ 34.5   **FUD** 010   Q2 N1 80 50
AMA: 2015,Jan,16; 2014,May,5; 2014,Jan,11

65780 **Ocular surface reconstruction; amniotic membrane transplantation, multiple layers**
🔲 25.1   ⚖ 25.1   **FUD** 090   T A2 50 ▭
AMA: 2015,Jan,16; 2014,May,5; 2014,Jan,11; 2012,Jan,15-42; 2011,Jan,11

65781 **limbal stem cell allograft (eg, cadaveric or living donor)**
🔲 37.7   ⚖ 37.7   **FUD** 090   T A2 80 50 ▭
AMA: 2015,Jan,16; 2014,Jan,11

65782 **limbal conjunctival autograft (includes obtaining graft)**
EXCLUDES *Conjunctival allograft harvest from a living donor (68371)*
🔲 32.5   ⚖ 32.5   **FUD** 090   T A2 50 ▭
AMA: 2015,Jan,16; 2014,Jan,11; 2012,Jan,15-42; 2011,Jan,11

● **65785** **Implantation of intrastromal corneal ring segments**
🔲 0.00   ⚖ 0.00   **FUD** 000

65800-66030 Anterior Segment Procedures

INCLUDES Operating microscope (69990)
EXCLUDES *Unlisted procedures of anterior segment (66999)*

65800 **Paracentesis of anterior chamber of eye (separate procedure); with removal of aqueous**
Do not report with (0308T)
🔲 2.60   ⚖ 3.37   **FUD** 000   S A2 50 ▭
AMA: 2015,Jan,16; 2014,Jan,11; 2013,Mar,6-7; 2012,Nov,10

65810 **with removal of vitreous and/or discission of anterior hyaloid membrane, with or without air injection**
Do not report with (0308T)
🔲 13.1   ⚖ 13.1   **FUD** 090   T A2 50 ▭
AMA: 2015,Jan,16; 2014,Jan,11; 2012,Nov,10

65815 **with removal of blood, with or without irrigation and/or air injection**
EXCLUDES *Injection only (66020-66030)*
Removal of blood clot only (65930)
Do not report with (0308T)
🔲 13.5   ⚖ 18.0   **FUD** 090   T A2 50 ▭
AMA: 2015,Jan,16; 2014,Jan,11; 2012,Nov,10

65820 **Goniotomy**
INCLUDES Barkan's operation
Code also ophthalmic endoscope if used (69990)
🔲 21.1   ⚖ 21.1   **FUD** 090   63 T A2 80 50 ▭
AMA: 2015,Jan,16; 2014,Jan,11

65850 **Trabeculotomy ab externo**
🔲 23.7   ⚖ 23.7   **FUD** 090   T A2 50 ▭
AMA: 2014,Jan,11

▲ **65855** **Trabeculoplasty by laser surgery**
EXCLUDES *Trabeculectomy ab externo (66170)*
Code also modifier 22 Increased procedural services, or 52 Reduced services, as appropriate, for re-treatment after several months for advancing disease
Do not report with (65860-65880)
🔲 8.41   ⚖ 9.55   **FUD** 010   T P3 50 ▭
AMA: 2015,Jan,16; 2014,Jan,11; 2012,Jan,15-42; 2011,Jan,11

65860 **Severing adhesions of anterior segment, laser technique (separate procedure)**
🔲 7.17   ⚖ 8.73   **FUD** 090   T P3 80 50 ▭
AMA: 2014,Jan,11

65865 **Severing adhesions of anterior segment of eye, incisional technique (with or without injection of air or liquid) (separate procedure); goniosynechiae**
EXCLUDES *Laser trabeculectomy (65855)*
🔲 13.3   ⚖ 13.3   **FUD** 090   T A2 50 ▭
AMA: 2014,Jan,11

65870 **anterior synechiae, except goniosynechiae**
🔲 16.7   ⚖ 16.7   **FUD** 090   T A2 50 ▭
AMA: 2014,Jan,11

65875 **posterior synechiae**
Code also ophthalmic endoscope if used (66990)
🔲 17.8   ⚖ 17.8   **FUD** 090   T A2 50 ▭
AMA: 2015,Jan,16; 2014,Jan,11

65880 **corneovitreal adhesions**
EXCLUDES *Laser procedure (66821)*
🔲 18.7   ⚖ 18.7   **FUD** 090   T A2 50 ▭
AMA: 2014,Jan,11

65900 **Removal of epithelial downgrowth, anterior chamber of eye**
🔲 27.2   ⚖ 27.2   **FUD** 090   T A2 80 50 ▭
AMA: 2014,Jan,11

65920 **Removal of implanted material, anterior segment of eye**
Code also ophthalmic endoscope if used (66990)
🔲 22.2   ⚖ 22.2   **FUD** 090   T A2 50 ▭
AMA: 2015,Jan,16; 2014,Jan,11

65930 **Removal of blood clot, anterior segment of eye**
🔲 18.0   ⚖ 18.0   **FUD** 090   T A2 50 ▭
AMA: 2014,Jan,11

66020 **Injection, anterior chamber of eye (separate procedure); air or liquid**
Do not report with (0308T)
🔲 3.72   ⚖ 5.25   **FUD** 010   T A2 50 ▭
AMA: 2015,Jan,16; 2014,Jan,11; 2012,Nov,10

66030   medication
Do not report with (0308T)
📷 3.14   ✂ 4.68   **FUD** 010
AMA: 2014,Jan,11; 2012,Nov,10   T A2 50 ▫

66130 Excision Scleral Lesion

INCLUDES Operating microscope (69990)
EXCLUDES *Intraocular foreign body removal (65235)*
          Surgery on posterior sclera (67250, 67255)

66130   **Excision of lesion, sclera**
📷 16.1   ✂ 19.6   **FUD** 090   T A2 80 50 ▫
AMA: 2014,Jan,11

66150-66185 Procedures for Glaucoma

INCLUDES Operating microscope (69990)
EXCLUDES *Intraocular foreign body removal (65235)*
          Surgery on posterior sclera (67250, 67255)

66150   **Fistulization of sclera for glaucoma; trephination with iridectomy**
📷 24.6   ✂ 24.6   **FUD** 090   T A2 50 ▫
AMA: 2014,Jan,11

66155   **thermocauterization with iridectomy**
📷 24.7   ✂ 24.7   **FUD** 090   T A2 50 ▫
AMA: 2014,Jan,11

66160   **sclerectomy with punch or scissors, with iridectomy**
INCLUDES Knapp's operation
📷 27.9   ✂ 27.9   **FUD** 090   T A2 50 ▫
AMA: 2014,Jan,11

66170   **trabeculectomy ab externo in absence of previous surgery**
EXCLUDES *Repair of surgical wound (66250)*
          Trabeculectomy ab externo (65850)
📷 33.9   ✂ 33.9   **FUD** 090   T A2 80 50 ▫
AMA: 2015,Jan,16; 2014,Jan,11; 2012,Dec,12

66172   **trabeculectomy ab externo with scarring from previous ocular surgery or trauma (includes injection of antifibrotic agents)**
📷 42.8   ✂ 42.8   **FUD** 090   T A2 80 50 ▫
AMA: 2015,Jan,16; 2014,Jan,11; 2012,Dec,12

66174   **Transluminal dilation of aqueous outflow canal; without retention of device or stent**
📷 26.8   ✂ 26.8   **FUD** 090   T A2 80 50
AMA: 2014,Jan,11

66175   **with retention of device or stent**
📷 28.0   ✂ 28.0   **FUD** 090   T A2 80 50
AMA: 2014,Jan,11

66179   **Aqueous shunt to extraocular equatorial plate reservoir, external approach; without graft**
📷 30.4   ✂ 30.4   **FUD** 090   T 62 80 50
AMA: 2015,Jan,10

66180   **with graft**
Do not report with (67255)
📷 32.1   ✂ 32.1   **FUD** 090   T A2 80 50 ▫
AMA: 2015,Jan,10; 2015,Jan,16; 2014,Jan,11; 2012,Jun,15-16

66183   **Insertion of anterior segment aqueous drainage device, without extraocular reservoir, external approach**
📷 29.1   ✂ 29.1   **FUD** 090   T 62 80 50
AMA: 2015,Jan,16; 2014,May,5; 2014,Jan,11

66184   **Revision of aqueous shunt to extraocular equatorial plate reservoir; without graft**
📷 22.1   ✂ 22.1   **FUD** 090   T 62 80 50
AMA: 2015,Jan,10

66185   **with graft**
EXCLUDES *Implanted shunt removal (67120)*
Do not report with (67255)
📷 23.8   ✂ 23.8   **FUD** 090   T A2 80 50 ▫
AMA: 2015,Jan,10; 2014,Jan,11

66220-66225 Staphyloma Repair

INCLUDES Operating microscope (69990)
EXCLUDES *Scleral procedures with retinal procedures (67101-67228)*
          Scleral reinforcement (67250, 67255)

66220   **Repair of scleral staphyloma; without graft**
📷 21.0   ✂ 21.0   **FUD** 090   T A2 80 50 ▫
AMA: 2014,Jan,11

66225   **with graft**
📷 26.3   ✂ 26.3   **FUD** 090   T A2 50 ▫
AMA: 2014,Jan,11

66250 Anterior Segment Operative Wound Revision or Repair

INCLUDES Operating microscope (69990)
EXCLUDES *Unlisted procedures of anterior sclera (66999)*

66250   **Revision or repair of operative wound of anterior segment, any type, early or late, major or minor procedure**
📷 15.7   ✂ 21.1   **FUD** 090   T A2 50 ▫
AMA: 2015,Jan,16; 2014,Jan,11; 2012,Jan,15-42; 2011,Jan,11; 2010,Dec,12

66500-66505 Iridotomy With/Without Transfixion

INCLUDES Operating microscope (69990)
EXCLUDES *Photocoagulation iridotomy (66761)*

66500   **Iridotomy by stab incision (separate procedure); except transfixion**
📷 10.0   ✂ 10.0   **FUD** 090   S A2 50 ▫
AMA: 2014,Jan,11

66505   **with transfixion as for iris bombe**
📷 10.9   ✂ 10.9   **FUD** 090   T A2 50 ▫
AMA: 2014,Jan,11

66600-66635 Iridectomy Procedures

INCLUDES Operating microscope (69990)
EXCLUDES *Photocoagulation coreoplasty (66762)*
Do not report with (0308T)

66600   **Iridectomy, with corneoscleral or corneal section; for removal of lesion**
📷 23.5   ✂ 23.5   **FUD** 090   T A2 50 ▫
AMA: 2014,Jan,11

66605   **with cyclectomy**
📷 29.8   ✂ 29.8   **FUD** 090   T A2 50 ▫
AMA: 2014,Jan,11

66625   **peripheral for glaucoma (separate procedure)**
📷 12.1   ✂ 12.1   **FUD** 090   T A2 50 ▫
AMA: 2014,Jan,11

66630   **sector for glaucoma (separate procedure)**
📷 16.1   ✂ 16.1   **FUD** 090   T A2 50 ▫
AMA: 2014,Jan,11

66635   **optical (separate procedure)**
📷 16.2   ✂ 16.2   **FUD** 090   T A2 50 ▫
AMA: 2014,Jan,11

66680-66770 Other Procedures of the Uveal Tract

INCLUDES Operating microscope (69990)
EXCLUDES *Unlisted procedures of ciliary body or iris (66999)*

66680   **Repair of iris, ciliary body (as for iridodialysis)**
EXCLUDES *Resection or repositioning of uveal tissue for perforating laceration of cornea and/or sclera (65285)*
📷 14.6   ✂ 14.6   **FUD** 090   T A2 50 ▫
AMA: 2014,Jan,11

66682   **Suture of iris, ciliary body (separate procedure) with retrieval of suture through small incision (eg, McCannel suture)**
📷 18.0   ✂ 18.0   **FUD** 090   T A2 50 ▫
AMA: 2014,Jan,11

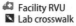

66700 **Ciliary body destruction; diathermy**

INCLUDES Heine's operation

🔧 11.1   ⚖ 12.7   **FUD** 090   T A2 80 50 ▭

AMA: 2014,Jan,11

66710 **cyclophotocoagulation, transscleral**

🔧 11.1   ⚖ 12.4   **FUD** 090   T A2 50 ▭

AMA: 2015,Jan,16; 2014,Jan,11; 2012,Jan,15-42; 2011,Jan,11

66711 **cyclophotocoagulation, endoscopic**

🔧 18.1   ⚖ 18.1   **FUD** 090   T A2 50 ▭

AMA: 2015,Jan,16; 2014,Jan,11; 2012,Jan,15-42; 2011,Jan,11

66720 **cryotherapy**

🔧 11.9   ⚖ 13.4   **FUD** 090   ⊙ T A2 50 ▭

AMA: 2014,Jan,11

66740 **cyclodialysis**

🔧 11.1   ⚖ 12.3   **FUD** 090   T A2 50 ▭

AMA: 2014,Jan,11

66761 **Iridotomy/iridectomy by laser surgery (eg, for glaucoma) (per session)**

Do not report with (0308T)

🔧 6.67   ⚖ 8.36   **FUD** 010   T P3 50 ▭

AMA: 2015,Jan,16; 2014,Jan,11

66762 **Iridoplasty by photocoagulation (1 or more sessions) (eg, for improvement of vision, for widening of anterior chamber angle)**

🔧 12.0   ⚖ 13.4   **FUD** 090   T P2 50 ▭

AMA: 2015,Jan,16; 2014,Jan,11

66770 **Destruction of cyst or lesion iris or ciliary body (nonexcisional procedure)**

EXCLUDES Excision:
Epithelial downgrowth (65900)
Iris, ciliary body lesion (66600-66605)

🔧 13.6   ⚖ 14.9   **FUD** 090   T P2 50 ▭

AMA: 2014,Jan,11

66820-66825 Post-Cataract Surgery Procedures

INCLUDES Operating microscope (69990)

66820 **Discission of secondary membranous cataract (opacified posterior lens capsule and/or anterior hyaloid); stab incision technique (Ziegler or Wheeler knife)**

🔧 11.1   ⚖ 11.1   **FUD** 090   S G2 50 ▭

AMA: 2014,Jan,11

Cataract — Iris — Lens — Artificial lens — Cornea — Opaque lens capsule — Iris

An after-cataract is a cataract that develops in a lens tissue that remains after most of the lens has already been removed

66821 **laser surgery (eg, YAG laser) (1 or more stages)**

🔧 8.80   ⚖ 9.32   **FUD** 090   T A2 50 ▭

AMA: 2014,Jan,11

66825 **Repositioning of intraocular lens prosthesis, requiring an incision (separate procedure)**

Do not report with (0308T)

🔧 21.4   ⚖ 21.4   **FUD** 090   T A2 80 50 ▭

AMA: 2014,Jan,11

66830-66940 Cataract Extraction; Without Insertion Intraocular Lens

CMS: 100-3,80.10 Phacoemulsification Procedure--Cataract Extraction

INCLUDES Anterior and/or posterior capsulotomy
Enzymatic zonulysis
Iridectomy/iridotomy
Lateral canthotomy
Medications
Operating microscope (69990)
Subconjunctival injection
Subtenon injection
Use of viscoelastic material

EXCLUDES Removal of intralenticular foreign body without lens excision (65235)
Repair of surgical laceration (66250)

66830 **Removal of secondary membranous cataract (opacified posterior lens capsule and/or anterior hyaloid) with corneo-scleral section, with or without iridectomy (iridocapsulotomy, iridocapsulectomy)**

INCLUDES Graefe's operation

🔧 20.1   ⚖ 20.1   **FUD** 090   T A2 50 ▭

AMA: 2014,Jan,11

Cataract — Iris — Lens — Coloboma

A congenital keyhole pupil is also called a coloboma of the iris

66840 **Removal of lens material; aspiration technique, 1 or more stages**

INCLUDES Fukala's operation

🔧 19.7   ⚖ 19.7   **FUD** 090   T A2 50 ▭ P0

AMA: 2015,Jan,16; 2014,Jan,11; 2012,Jan,15-42; 2011,Jan,11

66850 **phacofragmentation technique (mechanical or ultrasonic) (eg, phacoemulsification), with aspiration**

🔧 22.4   ⚖ 22.4   **FUD** 090   T A2 50 ▭ P0

AMA: 2015,Jan,16; 2014,Jan,11; 2012,Jan,15-42; 2011,Jan,11

66852 **pars plana approach, with or without vitrectomy**

🔧 23.8   ⚖ 23.8   **FUD** 090   T A2 80 50 ▭ P0

AMA: 2015,Jan,16; 2014,Jan,11; 2012,Jan,15-42; 2011,Jan,11

66920 **intracapsular**

🔧 21.3   ⚖ 21.3   **FUD** 090   T A2 80 50 ▭ P0

AMA: 2015,Jan,16; 2014,Jan,11; 2012,Jan,15-42; 2011,Jan,11

66930 **intracapsular, for dislocated lens**

🔧 24.2   ⚖ 24.2   **FUD** 090   T A2 80 50 ▭ P0

AMA: 2015,Jan,16; 2014,Jan,11; 2012,Jan,15-42; 2011,Jan,11

66940 **extracapsular (other than 66840, 66850, 66852)**

🔧 22.1   ⚖ 22.1   **FUD** 090   T A2 80 50 ▭ P0

AMA: 2015,Jan,16; 2014,Jan,11; 2012,Jan,15-42; 2011,Jan,11

Eye and Ocular Adnexa

66982 — 67036

66982-66984 Cataract Extraction: With Insertion Intraocular Lens

CMS: 100-3,80.10 Phacoemulsification Procedure--Cataract Extraction; 100-4,32,120.2 PC-IOL and A-C IOL Billing

INCLUDES   Anterior or posterior capsulotomy
Enzymatic zonulysis
Iridectomy/iridotomy
Lateral canthotomy
Medications
Operating microscope (69990)
Subconjunctival injection
Subtenon injection
Use of viscoelastic material

EXCLUDES   *Implanted material removal from the anterior segment (65920)*
Ocular telescope prosthesis insertion with lens removal (0308T)
Secondary fixation (66682)
Supply of intraocular lens

Do not report with (0308T)

66982   **Extracapsular cataract removal with insertion of intraocular lens prosthesis (1-stage procedure), manual or mechanical technique (eg, irrigation and aspiration or phacoemulsification), complex, requiring devices or techniques not generally used in routine cataract surgery (eg, iris expansion device, suture support for intraocular lens, or primary posterior capsulorrhexis) or performed on patients in the amblyogenic developmental stage**

    (76519)
    ⚕ 22.4   ✂ 22.4   **FUD** 090   T A2 50 🔲 P0

AMA: 2015,Jan,16; 2014,Jan,11; 2013,Mar,6-7; 2012,Jan,15-42; 2011,Jan,11

66983   **Intracapsular cataract extraction with insertion of intraocular lens prosthesis (1 stage procedure)**

    (76519)
    ⚕ 20.7   ✂ 20.7   **FUD** 090   T A2 50 🔲 P0

AMA: 2015,Jan,16; 2014,Jan,11; 2013,Mar,6-7; 2012,Jan,15-42; 2011,Jan,11

66984   **Extracapsular cataract removal with insertion of intraocular lens prosthesis (1 stage procedure), manual or mechanical technique (eg, irrigation and aspiration or phacoemulsification)**

EXCLUDES   *Complex extracapsular cataract removal (66982)*
    (76519)
    ⚕ 18.1   ✂ 18.1   **FUD** 090   T A2 50 🔲 P0

AMA: 2015,Jan,16; 2014,Jan,11; 2013,Mar,6-7; 2012,Jan,15-42; 2011,Jan,11

66985-66986 Secondary Insertion or Replacement of Intraocular Lens

CMS: 100-3,80.10 Phacoemulsification Procedure--Cataract Extraction; 100-3,80.12 Intraocular Lenses (IOLs); 100-4,32,120.2 PC-IOL and A-C IOL Billing

INCLUDES   Operating microscope (69990)

EXCLUDES   *Implanted material removal from the anterior segment (65920)*
Secondary fixation (66682)
Supply of intraocular lens

Code also ophthalmic endoscope if used (66990)
Do not report with (0308T)

66985   **Insertion of intraocular lens prosthesis (secondary implant), not associated with concurrent cataract removal**

EXCLUDES   *Insertion of lens at the time of cataract procedure (66982-66984)*
    (76519)
    ⚕ 21.7   ✂ 21.7   **FUD** 090   T A2 50 🔲

AMA: 2015,Jan,16; 2014,Jan,11; 2013,Mar,6-7; 2012,Jan,15-42; 2011,Dec,14-18; 2011,Jan,11

66986   **Exchange of intraocular lens**

    (76519)
    ⚕ 25.6   ✂ 25.6   **FUD** 090   T A2 50 🔲

AMA: 2015,Jan,16; 2014,Jan,11

66990-66999 Ophthalmic Endoscopy

INCLUDES   Operating microscope (69990)

+   **66990**   **Use of ophthalmic endoscope (List separately in addition to code for primary procedure)**

Code first (65820, 65875, 65920, 66985-66986, 67036, 67039-67043, 67113)
    ⚕ 2.57   ✂ 2.57   **FUD** ZZZ   N N1

AMA: 2015,Jan,16; 2014,Jan,11; 2012,Jan,15-42; 2011,Jan,11

66999   **Unlisted procedure, anterior segment of eye**

    ⚕ 0.00   ✂ 0.00   **FUD** YYY   T 80 50

AMA: 2015,Jan,16; 2014,Jan,11

67005-67015 Vitrectomy: Partial and Subtotal

INCLUDES   Operating microscope (69990)

67005   **Removal of vitreous, anterior approach (open sky technique or limbal incision); partial removal**

EXCLUDES   *Anterior chamber vitrectomy by paracentesis (65810)*
Severing of corneovitreal adhesions (65880)
    ⚕ 13.3   ✂ 13.3   **FUD** 090   T A2 50 🔲

AMA: 2015,Jan,16; 2014,Jan,11

67010   **subtotal removal with mechanical vitrectomy**

EXCLUDES   *Anterior chamber vitrectomy by paracentesis (65810)*
Severing of corneovitreal adhesions (65880)
    ⚕ 15.3   ✂ 15.3   **FUD** 090   T A2 50 🔲

AMA: 2015,Jan,16; 2014,Jan,11

67015   **Aspiration or release of vitreous, subretinal or choroidal fluid, pars plana approach (posterior sclerotomy)**

    ⚕ 16.4   ✂ 16.4   **FUD** 090   T A2 50 🔲

AMA: 2014,Jan,11

67025-67028 Intravitreal Injection/Implantation

INCLUDES   Operating microscope (69990)

67025   **Injection of vitreous substitute, pars plana or limbal approach (fluid-gas exchange), with or without aspiration (separate procedure)**

    ⚕ 17.9   ✂ 20.5   **FUD** 090   T A2 50 🔲

AMA: 2014,Jan,11

67027   **Implantation of intravitreal drug delivery system (eg, ganciclovir implant), includes concomitant removal of vitreous**

EXCLUDES   *Removal of drug delivery system (67121)*
    ⚕ 24.0   ✂ 24.0   **FUD** 090   T A2 80 50 🔲

AMA: 2015,Jan,16; 2014,Jan,11; 2012,Jan,15-42; 2011,Jan,11

67028   **Intravitreal injection of a pharmacologic agent (separate procedure)**

    ⚕ 2.83   ✂ 2.88   **FUD** 000   S P3 50 🔲

AMA: 2015,Jan,16; 2014,Jan,11; 2012,Oct,14

67030-67031 Incision of Vitreous Strands/Membranes

INCLUDES   Operating microscope (69990)

67030   **Discission of vitreous strands (without removal), pars plana approach**

    ⚕ 15.0   ✂ 15.0   **FUD** 090   T A2 50 🔲

AMA: 2014,Jan,11

67031   **Severing of vitreous strands, vitreous face adhesions, sheets, membranes or opacities, laser surgery (1 or more stages)**

    ⚕ 10.0   ✂ 10.9   **FUD** 090   T A2 50 🔲

AMA: 2014,Jan,11

67036-67043 Pars Plana Mechanical Vitrectomy

INCLUDES   Operating microscope (69990)

EXCLUDES   *Foreign body removal (65260, 65265)*
Lens removal (66850)
Unlisted vitreal procedures (67299)
Vitrectomy in retinal detachment (67108, 67113)

Code also ophthalmic endoscope if used (66990)

67036   **Vitrectomy, mechanical, pars plana approach;**

Code also placement of intraocular radiation source applicator (0190T)
    ⚕ 25.4   ✂ 25.4   **FUD** 090   T A2 80 50 🔲 P0

AMA: 2015,Jan,16; 2014,Jan,11

67039   with focal endolaser photocoagulation
🔪 27.3   ✂ 27.3   **FUD** 090   T A2 80 50 ▣ PQ
AMA: 2015,Jan,16; 2014,Jan,11; 2012,Jan,15-42; 2011,Jan,11

67040   with endolaser panretinal photocoagulation
🔪 29.5   ✂ 29.5   **FUD** 090   T A2 80 50 ▣ PQ
AMA: 2015,Jan,16; 2014,Jan,11; 2012,Jan,15-42; 2011,Jan,11

67041   with removal of preretinal cellular membrane (eg, macular pucker)
🔪 32.6   ✂ 32.6   **FUD** 090   T G2 80 50 PQ
AMA: 2015,Jan,16; 2014,Jan,11

67042   with removal of internal limiting membrane of retina (eg, for repair of macular hole, diabetic macular edema), includes, if performed, intraocular tamponade (ie, air, gas or silicone oil)
🔪 32.6   ✂ 32.6   **FUD** 090   T G2 80 50 PQ
AMA: 2015,Jan,16; 2014,Jan,11

67043   with removal of subretinal membrane (eg, choroidal neovascularization), includes, if performed, intraocular tamponade (ie, air, gas or silicone oil) and laser photocoagulation
🔪 34.4   ✂ 34.4   **FUD** 090   T G2 80 50 PQ
AMA: 2015,Jan,16; 2014,Jan,11

67101-67115 Detached Retina Repair

INCLUDES   Operating microscope (69990)
Primary technique when cryotherapy and/or diathermy and/or photocoagulation are used in combination

▲ **67101**   Repair of retinal detachment, 1 or more sessions; cryotherapy or diathermy, including drainage of subretinal fluid, when performed
🔪 19.0   ✂ 22.1   **FUD** 090   T P3 50 ▣
AMA: 2015,Jan,16; 2014,Jan,11

Vitreous
Optic nerve
Optic disc
Choroid
Sclera
Retina
Pars plana

Posterior chamber

▲ **67105**   photocoagulation, including drainage of subretinal fluid, when performed
🔪 18.2   ✂ 20.3   **FUD** 090   T P2 50 ▣
AMA: 2015,Jan,16; 2014,Jan,11

▲ **67107**   Repair of retinal detachment; scleral buckling (such as lamellar scleral dissection, imbrication or encircling procedure), including, when performed, implant, cryotherapy, photocoagulation, and drainage of subretinal fluid
INCLUDES   Gonin's operation
🔪 34.3   ✂ 34.3   **FUD** 090   T A2 80 50 ▣
AMA: 2014,Jan,11

▲ **67108**   with vitrectomy, any method, including, when performed, air or gas tamponade, focal endolaser photocoagulation, cryotherapy, drainage of subretinal fluid, scleral buckling, and/or removal of lens by same technique
🔪 45.3   ✂ 45.3   **FUD** 090   T A2 80 50 ▣
AMA: 2015,Jan,16; 2014,Jan,11; 2012,Mar,9-10; 2012,Jan,15-42; 2011,Jan,11

67110   by injection of air or other gas (eg, pneumatic retinopexy)
🔪 21.9   ✂ 24.5   **FUD** 090   T P3 50 ▣
AMA: 2014,Jan,11

~~67112~~   ~~by scleral buckling or vitrectomy, on patient having previous ipsilateral retinal detachment repair(s) using scleral buckling or vitrectomy techniques~~
To report, see ~67107-67113

▲ **67113**   Repair of complex retinal detachment (eg, proliferative vitreoretinopathy, stage C-1 or greater, diabetic traction retinal detachment, retinopathy of prematurity, retinal tear of greater than 90 degrees), with vitrectomy and membrane peeling, including, when performed, air, gas, or silicone oil tamponade, cryotherapy, endolaser photocoagulation, drainage of subretinal fluid, scleral buckling, and/or removal of lens
EXCLUDES   *Vitrectomy for other than retinal detachment, pars plana approach (67036-67043)*
Code also ophthalmic endoscope if used (66990)
🔪 49.3   ✂ 49.3   **FUD** 090   T G2 80 50
AMA: 2015,Jan,16; 2014,Jan,11

67115   Release of encircling material (posterior segment)
🔪 14.1   ✂ 14.1   **FUD** 090   T A2 50 ▣
AMA: 2014,Jan,11

67120-67121 Removal of Previously Implanted Prosthetic Device

INCLUDES   Operating microscope (69990)
EXCLUDES   *Foreign body removal (65260, 65265)*
Removal of implanted material anterior segment (65920)

67120   Removal of implanted material, posterior segment; extraocular
🔪 15.7   ✂ 18.5   **FUD** 090   T A2 50 ▣
AMA: 2014,Jan,11

67121   intraocular
🔪 25.6   ✂ 25.6   **FUD** 090   T A2 80 50 ▣
AMA: 2014,Jan,11

67141-67145 Retinal Detachment: Preventative Procedures

INCLUDES   Operating microscope (69990)
Treatment at one or more sessions that may occur at different encounters
Do not report more than one time during a defined period of treatment

67141   Prophylaxis of retinal detachment (eg, retinal break, lattice degeneration) without drainage, 1 or more sessions; cryotherapy, diathermy
🔪 13.8   ✂ 14.8   **FUD** 090   T A2 50 ▣
AMA: 2015,Jan,16; 2014,Jan,11

67145   photocoagulation (laser or xenon arc)
🔪 14.0   ✂ 14.9   **FUD** 090   T P2 50 ▣
AMA: 2015,Jan,16; 2014,Jan,11

67208-67218 Destruction of Retinal Lesions

INCLUDES   Operating microscope (69990)
Treatment at one or more sessions that may occur at different encounters
EXCLUDES   *Unlisted retinal procedures (67299)*
Do not report more than one time during a defined period of treatment

67208   Destruction of localized lesion of retina (eg, macular edema, tumors), 1 or more sessions; cryotherapy, diathermy
🔪 16.3   ✂ 16.9   **FUD** 090   T P2 50 ▣
AMA: 2015,Jan,16; 2014,Jan,11

67210   photocoagulation
🔪 14.1   ✂ 14.6   **FUD** 090   T P2 50 ▣
AMA: 2015,Jan,16; 2014,Jan,11; 2012,Jan,3-5

67218   radiation by implantation of source (includes removal of source)
🔪 39.1   ✂ 39.1   **FUD** 090   T A2 50 ▣
AMA: 2015,Jan,16; 2014,Jan,11

67220-67225 Destruction of Choroidal Lesions

INCLUDES   Operating microscope (69990)

67220   **Destruction of localized lesion of choroid (eg, choroidal neovascularization); photocoagulation (eg, laser), 1 or more sessions**

INCLUDES   Treatment at one or more sessions that may occur at different encounters

Do not report more than one time during a defined period of treatment

⊞ 14.1   ⊗ 15.1   **FUD** 090   T P2 50 ▭

AMA: 2015,Jan,16; 2014,Jan,11; 2012,Jan,3-5; 2012,Jan,15-42; 2011,Jan,11

67221   **photodynamic therapy (includes intravenous infusion)**

⊞ 6.07   ⊗ 8.11   **FUD** 000   T P3 ▭

AMA: 2015,Jan,16; 2014,Jan,11; 2012,Jan,15-42; 2011,Jan,11

+   **67225**   **photodynamic therapy, second eye, at single session (List separately in addition to code for primary eye treatment)**

Code first (67221)

⊞ 0.79   ⊗ 0.84   **FUD** ZZZ   N N1 ▭

AMA: 2015,Jan,16; 2014,Jan,11; 2012,Jan,15-42; 2011,Jan,11

67227-67229 Destruction Retinopathy

INCLUDES   Operating microscope (69990)
EXCLUDES   Unlisted retinal procedures (67299)

▲   **67227**   **Destruction of extensive or progressive retinopathy (eg, diabetic retinopathy), cryotherapy, diathermy**

⊞ 16.1   ⊗ 17.2   **FUD** 090   T A2 50 ▭

AMA: 2015,Jan,16; 2014,Jan,11; 2012,Jan,15-42; 2011,Jan,11

▲   **67228**   **Treatment of extensive or progressive retinopathy (eg, diabetic retinopathy), photocoagulation**

⊞ 26.7   ⊗ 28.2   **FUD** 090   T P2 50 ▭

AMA: 2015,Jan,16; 2014,Jan,11

67229   **Treatment of extensive or progressive retinopathy, 1 or more sessions, preterm infant (less than 37 weeks gestation at birth), performed from birth up to 1 year of age (eg, retinopathy of prematurity), photocoagulation or cryotherapy**

Do not report more than one time during a defined period of treatment

⊞ 32.9   ⊗ 32.9   **FUD** 090   T R2 50

AMA: 2015,Jan,16; 2014,Jan,11

67250-67255 Reinforcement of Posterior Sclera

INCLUDES   Operating microscope (69990)
EXCLUDES   Removal of lesion of sclera (66130)
             Repair scleral staphyloma (66220, 66225)

67250   **Scleral reinforcement (separate procedure); without graft**

⊞ 22.0   ⊗ 22.0   **FUD** 090   T A2 50 ▭

AMA: 2014,Jan,11

67255   **with graft**

Do not report with (66180, 66185)

⊞ 19.3   ⊗ 19.3   **FUD** 090   T A2 80 50 ▭

AMA: 2015,Jan,16; 2015,Jan,10; 2014,Jan,11; 2012,Jun,15-16

67299 Unlisted Posterior Segment Procedure

CMS: 100-4,4,180.3 Unlisted Service or Procedure
INCLUDES   Operating microscope (69990)

67299   **Unlisted procedure, posterior segment**

⊞ 0.00   ⊗ 0.00   **FUD** YYY   T 80 50 ▭

AMA: 2015,Jan,16; 2014,Jan,11; 2012,Jan,15-42; 2011,Jan,11

67311-67334 Strabismus Procedures on Extraocular Muscles

INCLUDES   Operating microscope (69990)
Code also adjustable sutures (67335)

67311   **Strabismus surgery, recession or resection procedure; 1 horizontal muscle**

⊞ 16.9   ⊗ 16.9   **FUD** 090   T A2 50 ▭

AMA: 2015,Jan,16; 2014,Jan,11; 2012,Jan,15-42; 2011,Jan,11

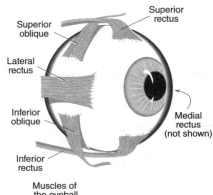

Superior oblique
Superior rectus
Lateral rectus
Inferior oblique
Inferior rectus
Medial rectus (not shown)

Muscles of the eyeball (right eye shown)

67312   **2 horizontal muscles**

⊞ 20.1   ⊗ 20.1   **FUD** 090   T A2 50 ▭

AMA: 2015,Jan,16; 2014,Jan,11; 2012,Jan,15-42; 2011,Jan,11

67314   **1 vertical muscle (excluding superior oblique)**

⊞ 19.0   ⊗ 19.0   **FUD** 090   T A2 50 ▭

AMA: 2015,Jan,16; 2014,Jan,11

67316   **2 or more vertical muscles (excluding superior oblique)**

⊞ 22.6   ⊗ 22.6   **FUD** 090   T A2 80 50 ▭

AMA: 2015,Jan,16; 2014,Jan,11

67318   **Strabismus surgery, any procedure, superior oblique muscle**

⊞ 19.9   ⊗ 19.9   **FUD** 090   T A2 50 ▭

AMA: 2015,Jan,16; 2014,Jan,11

+   **67320**   **Transposition procedure (eg, for paretic extraocular muscle), any extraocular muscle (specify) (List separately in addition to code for primary procedure)**

Code first (67311-67318)

⊞ 9.14   ⊗ 9.14   **FUD** ZZZ   N N1 ▭

AMA: 2015,Jan,16; 2014,Jan,11

+   **67331**   **Strabismus surgery on patient with previous eye surgery or injury that did not involve the extraocular muscles (List separately in addition to code for primary procedure)**

Code first (67311-67318)

⊞ 8.67   ⊗ 8.67   **FUD** ZZZ   N N1 50 ▭

AMA: 2015,Jan,16; 2014,Jan,11

+   **67332**   **Strabismus surgery on patient with scarring of extraocular muscles (eg, prior ocular injury, strabismus or retinal detachment surgery) or restrictive myopathy (eg, dysthyroid ophthalmopathy) (List separately in addition to code for primary procedure)**

Code first (67311-67318)

⊞ 9.41   ⊗ 9.41   **FUD** ZZZ   N N1 50 ▭

AMA: 2015,Jan,16; 2014,Jan,11

+   **67334**   **Strabismus surgery by posterior fixation suture technique, with or without muscle recession (List separately in addition to code for primary procedure)**

Code first (67311-67318)

⊞ 8.55   ⊗ 8.55   **FUD** ZZZ   N N1 50 ▭

AMA: 2015,Jan,16; 2014,Jan,11

67335-67399 Other Procedures of Extraocular Muscles

INCLUDES   Operating microscope (69990)

+   **67335**   **Placement of adjustable suture(s) during strabismus surgery, including postoperative adjustment(s) of suture(s) (List separately in addition to code for specific strabismus surgery)**

Code first (67311-67334)

⊞ 4.23   ⊗ 4.23   **FUD** ZZZ   N N1 50 ▭

AMA: 2015,Jan,16; 2014,Jan,11

Eye and Ocular Adnexa

67220 — 67335

+ 67340 Strabismus surgery involving exploration and/or repair of detached extraocular muscle(s) (List separately in addition to code for primary procedure)

INCLUDES Hummelsheim operation
Code first (67311-67334)
🔧 10.1 ⚕ 10.1 **FUD** ZZZ

[N] [N1] [80] ▢

AMA: 2015,Jan,16; 2014,Jan,11

67343 Release of extensive scar tissue without detaching extraocular muscle (separate procedure)

Code also if these procedures are performed on other than the affected muscle (67311-67340)
🔧 18.4 ⚕ 18.4 **FUD** 090

[T] [A2] [50] ▢

AMA: 2015,Jan,16; 2014,Jan,11

67345 Chemodenervation of extraocular muscle

EXCLUDES Nerve destruction for blepharospasm and other neurological disorders (64612, 64616)
🔧 6.21 ⚕ 6.88 **FUD** 010

[T] [P3] [50] ▢

AMA: 2015,Jan,16; 2014,May,5; 2014,Jan,11; 2013,Dec,10; 2012,Jan,15-42; 2011,Jan,11; 2010,Jan,12-15

67346 Biopsy of extraocular muscle

EXCLUDES Repair laceration extraocular muscle, tendon, or Tenon's capsule (65290)
🔧 5.51 ⚕ 5.51 **FUD** 000

[T] [A2] [80] [50] ▢ [P0]

AMA: 2014,Jan,11

67399 Unlisted procedure, extraocular muscle

🔧 0.00 ⚕ 0.00 **FUD** YYY

[T] [80] [50]

AMA: 2014,Jan,11

67400-67415 Frontal Orbitotomy

INCLUDES Operating microscope (69990)

67400 Orbitotomy without bone flap (frontal or transconjunctival approach); for exploration, with or without biopsy
🔧 26.2 ⚕ 26.2 **FUD** 090

[T] [A2] [50] ▢ [P0]

AMA: 2014,Jan,11

67405 with drainage only
🔧 22.4 ⚕ 22.4 **FUD** 090

[T] [A2] [50] ▢

AMA: 2015,Jan,16; 2014,Jan,11; 2012,Jan,15-42; 2011,Jan,11

67412 with removal of lesion
🔧 24.0 ⚕ 24.0 **FUD** 090

[T] [A2] [50] ▢

AMA: 2014,Jan,11

67413 with removal of foreign body
🔧 24.1 ⚕ 24.1 **FUD** 090

[T] [A2] [80] [50] ▢

AMA: 2014,Jan,11

67414 with removal of bone for decompression
🔧 37.4 ⚕ 37.4 **FUD** 090

[T] [G2] [80] [50] ▢

AMA: 2015,Jan,16; 2014,Jan,11; 2012,Jan,15-42; 2011,Jan,11

67415 Fine needle aspiration of orbital contents

EXCLUDES Decompression optic nerve (67570)
Exenteration, enucleation, and repair (65101-65175)
🔧 2.97 ⚕ 2.97 **FUD** 000

[T] [A2] [80] [50] ▢ [P0]

AMA: 2014,Jan,11

67420-67450 Lateral Orbitotomy

INCLUDES Operating microscope (69990)
EXCLUDES Orbital implant (67550, 67560)
Surgical removal of all or some of the orbital contents or repair after removal (65091-65175)
Transcranial approach orbitotomy (61330-61333)

67420 Orbitotomy with bone flap or window, lateral approach (eg, Kroenlein); with removal of lesion
🔧 45.7 ⚕ 45.7 **FUD** 090

[T] [A2] [80] [50] ▢

AMA: 2014,Jan,11

67430 with removal of foreign body
🔧 35.2 ⚕ 35.2 **FUD** 090

[T] [A2] [80] [50] ▢

AMA: 2014,Jan,11

67440 with drainage
🔧 34.0 ⚕ 34.0 **FUD** 090

[T] [A2] [80] [50] ▢

AMA: 2014,Jan,11

67445 with removal of bone for decompression

EXCLUDES Decompression optic nerve sheath (67570)
🔧 39.6 ⚕ 39.6 **FUD** 090

[T] [A2] [80] [50] ▢

AMA: 2014,Jan,11

67450 for exploration, with or without biopsy
🔧 35.4 ⚕ 35.4 **FUD** 090

[T] [A2] [80] [50] ▢ [P0]

AMA: 2014,Jan,11

67500-67515 Eye Injections

INCLUDES Operating microscope (69990)

67500 Retrobulbar injection; medication (separate procedure, does not include supply of medication)
🔧 2.05 ⚕ 2.22 **FUD** 000

[T] [G2] [50] ▢

AMA: 2015,Jan,16; 2014,Jan,11; 2012,Nov,10

67505 alcohol
🔧 2.31 ⚕ 2.52 **FUD** 000

[T] [P3] [50] ▢

AMA: 2014,Jan,11

67515 Injection of medication or other substance into Tenon's capsule

EXCLUDES Subconjunctival injection (68200)
🔧 2.53 ⚕ 2.74 **FUD** 000

[T] [P3] [50] ▢

AMA: 2015,Jan,16; 2014,Jan,11; 2012,Nov,10

67550-67560 Orbital Implant

INCLUDES Operating microscope (69990)
EXCLUDES Fracture repair malar area, orbit (21355-21408)
Ocular implant inside muscle cone (65093-65105, 65130-65175)

67550 Orbital implant (implant outside muscle cone); insertion
🔧 27.2 ⚕ 27.2 **FUD** 090

[T] [A2] [50] ▢

AMA: 2014,Jan,11

67560 removal or revision
🔧 27.9 ⚕ 27.9 **FUD** 090

[T] [A2] [80] [50] ▢

AMA: 2014,Jan,11

67570-67599 Other and Unlisted Orbital Procedures

INCLUDES Operating microscope (69990)

67570 Optic nerve decompression (eg, incision or fenestration of optic nerve sheath)
🔧 32.6 ⚕ 32.6 **FUD** 090

[T] [A2] [80] [50] ▢

AMA: 2014,Jan,11

67599 Unlisted procedure, orbit
🔧 0.00 ⚕ 0.00 **FUD** YYY

[T] [80] [50]

AMA: 2014,Jan,11

67700-67715 [67810] Incisional Procedures of Eyelids

INCLUDES Operating microscope (69990)

67700 Blepharotomy, drainage of abscess, eyelid
🔧 3.29 ⚕ 7.54 **FUD** 010

[T] [P2] [50] ▢

AMA: 2015,Jan,16; 2014,Jan,11; 2013,Mar,6-7

67710 Severing of tarsorrhaphy
🔧 2.75 ⚕ 6.28 **FUD** 010

[T] [P3] [50] ▢

AMA: 2015,Jan,16; 2014,Jan,11; 2013,Mar,6-7

67715 Canthotomy (separate procedure)

EXCLUDES Canthoplasty (67950)
Symblepharon division (68340)
🔧 3.07 ⚕ 6.70 **FUD** 010

[T] [A2] [50] ▢

AMA: 2015,Jan,16; 2014,Jan,11; 2013,Mar,6-7

 # 67810 Incisional biopsy of eyelid skin including lid margin

EXCLUDES Biopsy of eyelid skin (11100-11101, 11310-11313)
🔧 2.04 ⚕ 4.84 **FUD** 000

[T] [P3] [50] ▢ [P0]

AMA: 2015,Jan,16; 2014,Jan,11; 2013,Mar,6-7; 2013,Feb,16-17; 2012,Jan,15-42; 2011,Jan,11

Eye and Ocular Adnexa

67800 — 67914

67800-67808 Excision of Chalazion (Meibomian Cyst)

INCLUDES Lesion removal requiring more than skin:
　　Lid margin
　　Palpebral conjunctiva
　　Tarsus
　　Operating microscope (69990)

EXCLUDES *Blepharoplasty, graft, or reconstructive procedures (67930-67975)*
Excision skin lesion of eyelid (11310-11313, 11440-11446, 11640-11646, 17000-17004)

67800 **Excision of chalazion; single**
🔧 2.93 　✂ 3.59 　**FUD** 010 　　　　　T P3 ▢
AMA: 2015,Jan,16; 2014,Jan,11; 2013,Mar,6-7; 2012,Jan,15-42; 2011,Jan,11

67801 **multiple, same lid**
🔧 3.79 　✂ 4.58 　**FUD** 010 　　　　　T P3 ▢
AMA: 2014,Jan,11; 2013,Mar,6-7

67805 **multiple, different lids**
🔧 4.68 　✂ 5.69 　**FUD** 010 　　　　　T P3 ▢
AMA: 2015,Jan,16; 2014,Jan,11; 2013,Mar,6-7; 2012,Jan,15-42; 2011,Jan,11

67808 **under general anesthesia and/or requiring hospitalization, single or multiple**
🔧 10.4 　✂ 10.4 　**FUD** 090 　　　　　T A2 ▢
AMA: 2014,Jan,11; 2013,Mar,6-7

67810-67850 Other Eyelid Procedures

INCLUDES Operating microscope (69990)

67810 **Resequenced code. See code following 67715.**

67820 **Correction of trichiasis; epilation, by forceps only**
🔧 1.51 　✂ 1.41 　**FUD** 000 　　　　　01 N1 50 ▢
AMA: 2015,Jan,16; 2014,Jan,11; 2012,Jan,15-42; 2011,Jan,11

67825 **epilation by other than forceps (eg, by electrosurgery, cryotherapy, laser surgery)**
🔧 3.45 　✂ 3.64 　**FUD** 010 　　　　　T P3 50 ▢
AMA: 2015,Jan,16; 2014,Jan,11; 2012,Jan,15-42; 2011,Jan,11

67830 **incision of lid margin**
🔧 3.92 　✂ 7.50 　**FUD** 010 　　　　　T A2 50 ▢
AMA: 2014,Jan,11

67835 **incision of lid margin, with free mucous membrane graft**
🔧 12.4 　✂ 12.4 　**FUD** 090 　　　　　T A2 80 50 ▢
AMA: 2014,Jan,11

67840 **Excision of lesion of eyelid (except chalazion) without closure or with simple direct closure**
EXCLUDES *Eyelid resection and reconstruction (67961, 67966)*
🔧 4.49 　✂ 7.75 　**FUD** 010 　　　　　T P3 50 ▢
AMA: 2014,Jan,11

67850 **Destruction of lesion of lid margin (up to 1 cm)**
EXCLUDES *Mohs micro procedures (17311-17315)*
Topical chemotherapy (99201-99215)
🔧 3.86 　✂ 6.04 　**FUD** 010 　　　　　T P3 50 ▢
AMA: 2014,Jan,11

67875-67882 Suturing of the Eyelids

INCLUDES Operating microscope (69990)
EXCLUDES *Canthoplasty (67950)*
Canthotomy (67715)
Severing of tarsorrhaphy (67710)

67875 **Temporary closure of eyelids by suture (eg, Frost suture)**
🔧 2.76 　✂ 4.82 　**FUD** 000 　　　　　T G2 50 ▢
AMA: 2014,Jan,11

67880 **Construction of intermarginal adhesions, median tarsorrhaphy, or canthorrhaphy;**
🔧 10.4 　✂ 12.9 　**FUD** 090 　　　　　T A2 50 ▢
AMA: 2014,Jan,11

67882 **with transposition of tarsal plate**
🔧 13.3 　✂ 15.9 　**FUD** 090 　　　　　T A2 50 ▢
AMA: 2014,Jan,11

67900-67912 Repair of Ptosis/Retraction Eyelids, Eyebrows

INCLUDES Operating microscope (69990)

67900 **Repair of brow ptosis (supraciliary, mid-forehead or coronal approach)**
EXCLUDES *Forehead rhytidectomy (15824)*
🔧 14.4 　✂ 18.0 　**FUD** 090 　　　　　T A2 50 ▢
AMA: 2015,Jan,16; 2014,Jan,11; 2012,Jan,15-42; 2011,Jan,11

Labels: Superior fornix of conjunctiva; Orbital part of superior eyelid; Sulcus of eyelid; Tarsal part of superior eyelid; Lacrimal puncta; Pupil; Iris; Opening of tarsal gland; Cornea; Lens; Iris; Lower eyelid; Inferior fornix of conjunctiva

67901 **Repair of blepharoptosis; frontalis muscle technique with suture or other material (eg, banked fascia)**
🔧 16.3 　✂ 21.3 　**FUD** 090 　　　　　T A2 50 ▢
AMA: 2015,Jan,16; 2014,Jan,11

67902 **frontalis muscle technique with autologous fascial sling (includes obtaining fascia)**
🔧 20.4 　✂ 20.4 　**FUD** 090 　　　　　T A2 50 ▢
AMA: 2015,Jan,16; 2014,Jan,11

67903 **(tarso) levator resection or advancement, internal approach**
🔧 13.6 　✂ 16.7 　**FUD** 090 　　　　　T A2 50 ▢
AMA: 2015,Jan,16; 2014,Jan,11

67904 **(tarso) levator resection or advancement, external approach**
INCLUDES Everbusch's operation
🔧 16.9 　✂ 20.6 　**FUD** 090 　　　　　T A2 50 ▢
AMA: 2015,Jan,16; 2014,Jan,11; 2011,Aug,8

67906 **superior rectus technique with fascial sling (includes obtaining fascia)**
🔧 14.3 　✂ 14.3 　**FUD** 090 　　　　　T A2 50 ▢
AMA: 2015,Jan,16; 2014,Jan,11

67908 **conjunctivo-tarso-Muller's muscle-levator resection (eg, Fasanella-Servat type)**
🔧 11.9 　✂ 13.9 　**FUD** 090 　　　　　T A2 50 ▢
AMA: 2015,Jan,16; 2014,Jan,11

67909 **Reduction of overcorrection of ptosis**
🔧 12.4 　✂ 15.1 　**FUD** 090 　　　　　T A2 50 ▢
AMA: 2015,Jan,16; 2014,Jan,11

67911 **Correction of lid retraction**
EXCLUDES *Graft harvest (20920, 20922, 20926)*
Mucous membrane graft repair of trichiasis (67835)
🔧 15.9 　✂ 15.9 　**FUD** 090 　　　　　T A2 50 ▢
AMA: 2015,Jan,16; 2014,Jan,11

67912 **Correction of lagophthalmos, with implantation of upper eyelid lid load (eg, gold weight)**
🔧 13.9 　✂ 24.8 　**FUD** 090 　　　　　T A2 50 ▢
AMA: 2015,Jan,16; 2014,Jan,11; 2012,Jan,15-42; 2011,Jan,11

67914-67924 Repair Ectropion/Entropion

INCLUDES Operating microscope (69990)
EXCLUDES *Cicatricial ectropion or entropion with scar excision or graft (67961-67966)*

67914 **Repair of ectropion; suture**
🔧 9.27 　✂ 13.2 　**FUD** 090 　　　　　T A2 50 ▢
AMA: 2015,Jan,16; 2014,Jan,11

67915 thermocauterization
🚑 5.59 ✂ 8.23 **FUD** 090 T P3 50 ▭
AMA: 2015,Jan,16; 2014,Jan,11

67916 excision tarsal wedge
🚑 12.2 ✂ 16.7 **FUD** 090 T A2 50 ▭
AMA: 2015,Jan,16; 2014,Jan,11; 2012,Jan,15-42; 2011,Jan,11

67917 extensive (eg, tarsal strip operations)
EXCLUDES Repair of everted punctum (68705)
🚑 12.9 ✂ 17.0 **FUD** 090 T A2 50 ▭
AMA: 2015,Jan,16; 2014,Jan,11; 2012,Jan,15-42; 2011,Jan,11

67921 Repair of entropion; suture
🚑 8.77 ✂ 12.9 **FUD** 090 T A2 50 ▭
AMA: 2015,Jan,16; 2014,Jan,11

67922 thermocauterization
🚑 5.57 ✂ 8.15 **FUD** 090 T P3 50 ▭
AMA: 2015,Jan,16; 2014,Jan,11

67923 excision tarsal wedge
🚑 12.1 ✂ 16.6 **FUD** 090 T A2 50 ▭
AMA: 2015,Jan,16; 2014,Jan,11

67924 extensive (eg, tarsal strip or capsulopalpebral fascia repairs operation)
🚑 12.9 ✂ 17.7 **FUD** 090 T A2 50 ▭
AMA: 2015,Jan,16; 2014,Jan,11

67930-67935 Repair Eyelid Wound

INCLUDES Operating microscope (69990)
Repairs involving more than skin:
    Lid margin
    Palpebral conjunctiva
    Tarsus
EXCLUDES Blepharoplasty for entropion or ectropion (67916-67917, 67923-67924)
Correction of lid retraction and blepharoptosis (67901-67911)
Free graft (15120-15121, 15260-15261)
Graft preparation (15004)
Plastic repair of lacrimal canaliculi (68700)
Removal of eyelid lesion (67800 [67810], 67840-67850)
Repair involving skin of eyelid (12011-12018, 12051-12057, 13151-13153)
Repair of blepharochalasis (15820-15823)
Skin adjacent tissue transfer (14060-14061)
Tarsorrhaphy, canthorrhaphy (67880, 67882)

67930 Suture of recent wound, eyelid, involving lid margin, tarsus, and/or palpebral conjunctiva direct closure; partial thickness
🚑 6.83 ✂ 10.2 **FUD** 010 T P3 50 ▭
AMA: 2014,Jan,11

67935 full thickness
🚑 12.5 ✂ 16.7 **FUD** 090 T A2 50 ▭
AMA: 2014,Jan,11

67938-67999 Eyelid Reconstruction/Repair/Removal Deep Foreign Body

INCLUDES Operating microscope (69990)
EXCLUDES Blepharoplasty for entropion or ectropion (67916-67917, 67923-67924)
Correction of lid retraction and blepharoptosis (67901-67911)
Free graft (15120-15121, 15260-15261)
Graft preparation (15004)
Plastic repair of lacrimal canaliculi (68700)
Removal of eyelid lesion (67800-67808, 67840-67850)
Repair involving skin of eyelid (12011-12018, 12051-12057, 13151-13153)
Repair of blepharochalasis (15820-15823)
Skin adjacent tissue transfer (14060-14061)
Tarsorrhaphy, canthorrhaphy (67880, 67882)

67938 Removal of embedded foreign body, eyelid
🚑 3.25 ✂ 6.78 **FUD** 010 T P2 50 ▭
AMA: 2015,Jan,16; 2014,May,5; 2014,Jan,11

67950 Canthoplasty (reconstruction of canthus)
🚑 13.1 ✂ 16.1 **FUD** 090 T A2 50 ▭
AMA: 2014,Jan,11

67961 Excision and repair of eyelid, involving lid margin, tarsus, conjunctiva, canthus, or full thickness, may include preparation for skin graft or pedicle flap with adjacent tissue transfer or rearrangement; up to one-fourth of lid margin
EXCLUDES Canthoplasty (67950)
Delay flap (15630)
Flap attachment (15650)
Free skin grafts (15120-15121, 15260-15261)
Tubed pedicle flap preparation (15576)
🚑 12.8 ✂ 16.2 **FUD** 090 T A2 80 50 ▭
AMA: 2015,Jan,16; 2014,Jan,11

67966 over one-fourth of lid margin
EXCLUDES Canthoplasty (67950)
Delay flap (15630)
Flap attachment (15650)
Free skin grafts (15120-15121, 15260-15261)
Tubed pedicle flap preparation (15576)
🚑 18.6 ✂ 21.7 **FUD** 090 T A2 50 ▭
AMA: 2015,Jan,16; 2014,Jan,11; 2012,Nov,13-14

67971 Reconstruction of eyelid, full thickness by transfer of tarsoconjunctival flap from opposing eyelid; up to two-thirds of eyelid, 1 stage or first stage
INCLUDES Dupuy-Dutemp reconstruction
Landboldt's operation
🚑 20.4 ✂ 20.4 **FUD** 090 T A2 50 ▭
AMA: 2014,Jan,11

67973 total eyelid, lower, 1 stage or first stage
INCLUDES Landboldt's operation
🚑 26.3 ✂ 26.3 **FUD** 090 T A2 80 50 ▭
AMA: 2014,Jan,11

67974 total eyelid, upper, 1 stage or first stage
INCLUDES Landboldt's operation
🚑 26.2 ✂ 26.2 **FUD** 090 T A2 80 50 ▭
AMA: 2014,Jan,11

67975 second stage
INCLUDES Landboldt's operation
🚑 19.4 ✂ 19.4 **FUD** 090 T A2 50 ▭
AMA: 2014,Jan,11

67999 Unlisted procedure, eyelids
🚑 0.00 ✂ 0.00 **FUD** YYY T 80 50
AMA: 2015,Jan,16; 2014,Jan,11; 2012,Jan,15-42; 2011,Jan,11

68020-68200 Conjunctival Biopsy/Injection/Treatment of Lesions

INCLUDES Operating microscope (69990)
EXCLUDES Foreign body removal (65205-65265)

68020 Incision of conjunctiva, drainage of cyst
🚑 3.13 ✂ 3.38 **FUD** 010 T P3 50 ▭
AMA: 2014,Jan,11

68040 Expression of conjunctival follicles (eg, for trachoma)
EXCLUDES Automated evacuation meibomian glands with heat/pressure (0207T)
🚑 1.44 ✂ 1.76 **FUD** 000 T P3 50 ▭
AMA: 2015,Jan,16; 2014,May,5; 2014,Jan,11

68100 Biopsy of conjunctiva
🚑 2.76 ✂ 4.78 **FUD** 000 T P3 50 ▭ PQ
AMA: 2014,Jan,11

68110 Excision of lesion, conjunctiva; up to 1 cm
🚑 4.23 ✂ 6.35 **FUD** 010 T P3 50 ▭
AMA: 2014,Jan,11

68115 over 1 cm
🚑 5.21 ✂ 8.76 **FUD** 010 T A2 50 ▭
AMA: 2014,Jan,11

68130 with adjacent sclera
🚑 11.6 ✂ 15.1 **FUD** 090 T A2 50 ▭
AMA: 2014,Jan,11

68135 **Destruction of lesion, conjunctiva**
　🗗 4.29　　⅃ 4.43　　**FUD** 010　　T P3 50 ▭
AMA: 2014,Jan,11

68200 **Subconjunctival injection**
　EXCLUDES　Retrobulbar or Tenon's capsule injection (67500-67515)
　🗗 0.98　　⅃ 1.16　　**FUD** 000　　Q1 N1 50 ▭
AMA: 2015,Jan,16; 2014,Jan,11; 2012,Nov,10; 2012,Jan,15-42; 2011,Jan,11

68320-68340 Conjunctivoplasty Procedures
　INCLUDES　Operating microscope (69990)
　EXCLUDES　Conjunctival foreign body removal (65205, 65210)
　　Laceration repair (65270-65273)

68320 **Conjunctivoplasty; with conjunctival graft or extensive rearrangement**
　🗗 15.2　　⅃ 20.4　　**FUD** 090　　T A2 50 ▭
AMA: 2015,Jan,16; 2014,Jan,11; 2012,Jan,15-42; 2011,Jan,11

68325 **with buccal mucous membrane graft (includes obtaining graft)**
　🗗 18.6　　⅃ 18.6　　**FUD** 090　　T A2 50 ▭
AMA: 2014,Jan,11

68326 **Conjunctivoplasty, reconstruction cul-de-sac; with conjunctival graft or extensive rearrangement**
　🗗 18.2　　⅃ 18.2　　**FUD** 090　　T A2 50 ▭
AMA: 2014,Jan,11

68328 **with buccal mucous membrane graft (includes obtaining graft)**
　🗗 20.0　　⅃ 20.0　　**FUD** 090　　T A2 80 50 ▭
AMA: 2014,Jan,11

68330 **Repair of symblepharon; conjunctivoplasty, without graft**
　🗗 13.0　　⅃ 17.0　　**FUD** 090　　T A2 80 50 ▭
AMA: 2014,Jan,11

68335 **with free graft conjunctiva or buccal mucous membrane (includes obtaining graft)**
　🗗 18.3　　⅃ 18.3　　**FUD** 090　　T A2 50 ▭
AMA: 2014,Jan,11

68340 **division of symblepharon, with or without insertion of conformer or contact lens**
　🗗 11.2　　⅃ 15.3　　**FUD** 090　　T A2 80 50 ▭
AMA: 2014,Jan,11

68360-68399 Conjunctival Flaps and Unlisted Procedures
　INCLUDES　Operating microscope (69990)

68360 **Conjunctival flap; bridge or partial (separate procedure)**
　EXCLUDES　Conjunctival flap for injury (65280, 65285)
　　Conjunctival foreign body removal (65205, 65210)
　　Surgical wound repair (66250)
　🗗 11.6　　⅃ 14.9　　**FUD** 090　　T A2 50 ▭
AMA: 2014,Jan,11

68362 **total (such as Gunderson thin flap or purse string flap)**
　EXCLUDES　Conjunctival flap for injury (65280, 65285)
　　Conjunctival foreign body removal (65205, 65210)
　　Surgical wound repair (66250)
　🗗 18.5　　⅃ 18.5　　**FUD** 090　　T A2 50 ▭
AMA: 2015,Jan,16; 2014,Jan,11

68371 **Harvesting conjunctival allograft, living donor**
　🗗 11.6　　⅃ 11.6　　**FUD** 010　　T A2 50 ▭
AMA: 2015,Jan,16; 2014,Jan,11

68399 **Unlisted procedure, conjunctiva**
　🗗 0.00　　⅃ 0.00　　**FUD** YYY　　T 80 50
AMA: 2015,Jan,16; 2014,Jan,11

68400-68899 Nasolacrimal System Procedures
　INCLUDES　Operating microscope (69990)

68400 **Incision, drainage of lacrimal gland**
　🗗 3.75　　⅃ 8.01　　**FUD** 010　　T P3 50 ▭
AMA: 2014,Jan,11

Left eye — diagram of lacrimal system: Superior and inferior lobes of lacrimal gland; Lacrimal ducts; Lacrimal canaliculi; Nasolacrimal sac; Medial angle; Lacrimal caruncle; Superior, inferior lacrimal puncta

68420 **Incision, drainage of lacrimal sac (dacryocystotomy or dacryocystostomy)**
　🗗 4.78　　⅃ 9.04　　**FUD** 010　　T P3 50 ▭
AMA: 2014,Jan,11

68440 **Snip incision of lacrimal punctum**
　🗗 2.80　　⅃ 2.88　　**FUD** 010　　T P3 50 ▭
AMA: 2014,Jan,11

68500 **Excision of lacrimal gland (dacryoadenectomy), except for tumor; total**
　🗗 27.5　　⅃ 27.5　　**FUD** 090　　T A2 50 ▭
AMA: 2014,Jan,11

68505 **partial**
　🗗 27.4　　⅃ 27.4　　**FUD** 090　　T A2 50 ▭
AMA: 2014,Jan,11

68510 **Biopsy of lacrimal gland**
　🗗 8.29　　⅃ 12.5　　**FUD** 000　　T A2 80 50 ▭ P0
AMA: 2014,Jan,11

68520 **Excision of lacrimal sac (dacryocystectomy)**
　🗗 19.4　　⅃ 19.4　　**FUD** 090　　T A2 80 50 ▭
AMA: 2014,Jan,11

68525 **Biopsy of lacrimal sac**
　🗗 7.49　　⅃ 7.49　　**FUD** 000　　T A2 50 ▭ P0
AMA: 2014,Jan,11

68530 **Removal of foreign body or dacryolith, lacrimal passages**
　INCLUDES　Meller's excision
　🗗 7.29　　⅃ 12.0　　**FUD** 010　　T P2 50 ▭
AMA: 2014,Jan,11

68540 **Excision of lacrimal gland tumor; frontal approach**
　🗗 26.2　　⅃ 26.2　　**FUD** 090　　T A2 50 ▭
AMA: 2014,Jan,11

68550 **involving osteotomy**
　🗗 30.4　　⅃ 30.4　　**FUD** 090　　T A2 50 ▭
AMA: 2014,Jan,11

68700 **Plastic repair of canaliculi**
　🗗 17.0　　⅃ 17.0　　**FUD** 090　　T A2 50 ▭
AMA: 2014,Jan,11

68705 **Correction of everted punctum, cautery**
　🗗 4.72　　⅃ 6.66　　**FUD** 010　　T P3 50 ▭
AMA: 2015,Jan,16; 2014,Jan,11

68720 **Dacryocystorhinostomy (fistulization of lacrimal sac to nasal cavity)**
　🗗 21.3　　⅃ 21.3　　**FUD** 090　　T A2 80 50 ▭
AMA: 2015,Jan,16; 2014,Jan,11; 2012,Jan,15-42; 2011,Jan,11

68745 **Conjunctivorhinostomy (fistulization of conjunctiva to nasal cavity); without tube**
　🗗 21.4　　⅃ 21.4　　**FUD** 090　　T A2 80 50 ▭
AMA: 2014,Jan,11

68750 **with insertion of tube or stent**
　🗗 22.2　　⅃ 22.2　　**FUD** 090　　T A2 80 50 ▭
AMA: 2015,Jan,16; 2014,Jan,11; 2012,Jan,15-42; 2011,Jan,11

26/TC PC/TC Component Only　　A2-Z3 ASC Payment　　50 Bilateral　　♂ Male Only　　♀ Female Only　　🗗 Facility RVU　　⅃ Non-Facility RVU
AMA: CPT Assistant References　　CMS: Pub 100　　A-Y OPPSI　　80/80 Surg Assist Allowed / w/Doc　　▪ Lab crosswalk　　▣ Radiology crosswalk

274　　Medicare (Red Text)　　CPT © 2015 American Medical Association. All Rights Reserved. (Black Text)　　© 2015 Optum360, LLC (Blue Text)

68760	**Closure of the lacrimal punctum; by thermocauterization, ligation, or laser surgery**
	4.14 5.66 **FUD** 010 T P3 50
	AMA: 2014,Jan,11

68761	**by plug, each**
	EXCLUDES *Drug-eluting lacrimal implant (0356T)*
	3.37 4.17 **FUD** 010 T P3 80 50
	AMA: 2015,Jan,16; 2014,Jan,11; 2012,Jan,15-42; 2011,Jan,11

68770	**Closure of lacrimal fistula (separate procedure)**
	17.8 17.8 **FUD** 090 T A2 80 50
	AMA: 2014,Jan,11

68801	**Dilation of lacrimal punctum, with or without irrigation**
	3.04 3.51 **FUD** 010 01 N1 50
	AMA: 2014,Jan,11

68810	**Probing of nasolacrimal duct, with or without irrigation;**
	EXCLUDES *Ophthalmological exam under anesthesia (92018)*
	5.31 6.81 **FUD** 010 T A2 50
	AMA: 2015,Jan,16; 2014,Jan,11

68811	**requiring general anesthesia**
	EXCLUDES *Ophthalmological exam under anesthesia (92018)*
	5.83 5.83 **FUD** 010 T A2 50
	AMA: 2015,Jan,16; 2014,Jan,11; 2012,Jan,15-42; 2011,Jan,11

68815	**with insertion of tube or stent**
	EXCLUDES *Ophthalmological exam under anesthesia (92018)*
	7.28 12.6 **FUD** 010 T A2 50
	AMA: 2015,Jan,16; 2014,Jan,11; 2012,Jan,15-42; 2011,Jan,11; 2010,Nov,8

68816	**with transluminal balloon catheter dilation**
	Do not report with (68810-68811, 68815)
	7.08 20.9 **FUD** 010 T 62 50
	AMA: 2015,Jan,16; 2014,Jan,11

68840	**Probing of lacrimal canaliculi, with or without irrigation**
	3.31 3.61 **FUD** 010 T P3 50
	AMA: 2014,Jan,11

68850	**Injection of contrast medium for dacryocystography**
	(70170, 78660)
	1.59 1.73 **FUD** 000 N N1 50
	AMA: 2015,Jan,16; 2014,Jan,11; 2012,Jan,15-42; 2011,Jan,11

68899	**Unlisted procedure, lacrimal system**
	0.00 0.00 **FUD** YYY T 80 50
	AMA: 2014,Jan,11

69000-69020 Treatment External Abscess/Hematoma

69000	**Drainage external ear, abscess or hematoma; simple**
	3.41 5.32 **FUD** 010 T P2 50
	AMA: 2015,Jan,16; 2014,Jan,11; 2012,Jan,15-42; 2011,Jan,11

External acoustic meatus
Tympanic membrane (ear drum)
Coronal cutaway schematic of left ear and meatus
Lobule
Helix
Scaphoid fossa
Antihelix
Opening to external acoustic meatus
Tragus
Antitragus
Concha
Lobule

69005	**complicated**
	4.53 6.13 **FUD** 010 T P3 50
	AMA: 2014,Jan,11

69020	**Drainage external auditory canal, abscess**
	4.09 6.63 **FUD** 010 T P2 50
	AMA: 2015,Jan,16; 2014,Jan,11; 2012,Jan,15-42; 2011,Jan,11

69090 Cosmetic Ear Piercing

CMS: 100-2,16,10 Exclusions from Coverage; 100-2,16,120 Cosmetic Procedures

69090	**Ear piercing**
	0.00 0.00 **FUD** XXX E
	AMA: 2014,Jan,11

69100-69222 External Ear/Auditory Canal Procedures

EXCLUDES *Reconstruction of ear (see integumentary section codes)*

69100	**Biopsy external ear**
	1.40 2.85 **FUD** 000 T P3 PQ
	AMA: 2014,Jan,11

69105	**Biopsy external auditory canal**
	1.83 4.01 **FUD** 000 T P3 50 PQ
	AMA: 2014,Jan,11

69110	**Excision external ear; partial, simple repair**
	9.28 13.0 **FUD** 090 T A2 50
	AMA: 2014,Jan,11

69120	**complete amputation**
	11.5 11.5 **FUD** 090 T A2
	AMA: 2014,Jan,11

69140	**Excision exostosis(es), external auditory canal**
	25.2 25.2 **FUD** 090 T A2 80 50
	AMA: 2014,Jan,11

69145	**Excision soft tissue lesion, external auditory canal**
	7.16 11.3 **FUD** 090 T A2 50
	AMA: 2014,Jan,11

69150	**Radical excision external auditory canal lesion; without neck dissection**
	EXCLUDES *Skin graft (15004-15261)*
	Temporal bone resection (69535)
	30.1 30.1 **FUD** 090 T A2
	AMA: 2014,Jan,11

69155	**with neck dissection**
	EXCLUDES *Skin graft (15004-15261)*
	Temporal bone resection (69535)
	47.9 47.9 **FUD** 090 C 80
	AMA: 2014,Jan,11

69200	**Removal foreign body from external auditory canal; without general anesthesia**
	1.66 3.50 **FUD** 000 01 N1 50
	AMA: 2014,Jan,11

69205	**with general anesthesia**
	2.92 2.92 **FUD** 010 T A2 50
	AMA: 2015,Jan,16; 2014,Jan,11; 2013,Apr,10-11

● 69209	**Removal impacted cerumen using irrigation/lavage, unilateral**
	EXCLUDES *Removal impacted cerumen using instrumentation (69210)*
	Removal of nonimpacted cerumen (see appropriate E&M code(s)) (99201-99233 [99224, 99225, 99226], 99241-99255, 99281-99285, 99304-99318, 99324-99337, 99341-99350)
	Do not report for same ear as (69210)

Bilat–50

69210	**Removal impacted cerumen requiring instrumentation, unilateral**
	EXCLUDES *Removal of impacted cerumen using irrigation or lavage (69209)*
	Removal of nonimpacted cerumen (see appropriate E&M code(s)) (99201-99233 [99224, 99225, 99226], 99241-99255, 99281-99285, 99304-99318, 99324-99337, 99341-99350)
	Do not report with for same ear (69209)
	0.94 1.40 **FUD** 000 01 N1
	AMA: 2015,Jan,16; 2014,Nov,14; 2014,Jan,11; 2013,Oct,14; 2012,Jan,15-42; 2011,Jan,11

69220	**Debridement, mastoidectomy cavity, simple (eg, routine cleaning)**
	1.78 3.91 **FUD** 000 01 N1 50
	AMA: 2014,Jan,11

69222   **Debridement, mastoidectomy cavity, complex (eg, with anesthesia or more than routine cleaning)**
         ⚕ 3.94   ⚗ 6.27   **FUD** 010   T P3 50 ▣
         AMA: 2014,Jan,11

69300 Plastic Surgery for Prominent Ears

CMS: 100-2,16,120 Cosmetic Procedures; 100-2,16,180 Services Related to Noncovered Procedures
EXCLUDES   Suture of laceration of external ear (12011-14302)

69300   **Otoplasty, protruding ear, with or without size reduction**
         ⚕ 13.6   ⚗ 20.9   **FUD** YYY   ⊙ T A2 80 50 ▣
         AMA: 2014,Jan,11

69310-69399 Reconstruction Auditory Canal: Postaural Approach

EXCLUDES   Suture of laceration of external ear (12011-14302)

69310   **Reconstruction of external auditory canal (meatoplasty) (eg, for stenosis due to injury, infection) (separate procedure)**
         ⚕ 31.3   ⚗ 31.3   **FUD** 090   T A2 50 ▣
         AMA: 2015,Jan,16; 2014,Jul,8; 2014,Jan,11; 2014,Jan,9

69320   **Reconstruction external auditory canal for congenital atresia, single stage**
         EXCLUDES   Other reconstruction surgery with graft (13151-15760, 21230-21235)
                    Tympanoplasty (69631, 69641)
         ⚕ 43.9   ⚗ 43.9   **FUD** 090   T A2 80 50 ▣
         AMA: 2014,Jan,11

69399   **Unlisted procedure, external ear**
         EXCLUDES   Otoscopy under general anesthesia (92502)
         ⚕ 0.00   ⚗ 0.00   **FUD** YYY   T 80
         AMA: 2014,Jan,11

69420-69450 Ear Drum Procedures

69420   **Myringotomy including aspiration and/or eustachian tube inflation**
         ⚕ 3.48   ⚗ 5.47   **FUD** 010   T P3 50 ▣
         AMA: 2015,Jan,16; 2014,Jan,11; 2011,May,8

69421   **Myringotomy including aspiration and/or eustachian tube inflation requiring general anesthesia**
         ⚕ 4.30   ⚗ 4.30   **FUD** 010   T A2 50 ▣
         AMA: 2015,Jan,16; 2014,Jan,11; 2011,May,8

69424   **Ventilating tube removal requiring general anesthesia**
         Do not report with (69205, 69210, 69420-69421, 69433-69676, 69710-69745, 69801-69930)
         ⚕ 1.78   ⚗ 3.65   **FUD** 000   02 P3 50 ▣
         AMA: 2015,Jan,16; 2014,Jan,11; 2012,Jan,15-42; 2011,Jan,11; 2010,Nov,8; 2010,Jun,8

69433   **Tympanostomy (requiring insertion of ventilating tube), local or topical anesthesia**
         ⚕ 3.81   ⚗ 5.78   **FUD** 010   T P3 50 ▣
         AMA: 2015,Jan,16; 2014,Jan,11; 2011,May,8

69436   **Tympanostomy (requiring insertion of ventilating tube), general anesthesia**
         ⚕ 4.63   ⚗ 4.63   **FUD** 010   T A2 50 ▣
         AMA: 2015,Jan,16; 2014,Jan,11; 2012,May,14-15; 2011,May,8

69440   **Middle ear exploration through postauricular or ear canal incision**
         EXCLUDES   Atticotomy (69601-69605)
         ⚕ 19.8   ⚗ 19.8   **FUD** 090   T A2 50 ▣
         AMA: 2014,Jan,11

69450   **Tympanolysis, transcanal**
         ⚕ 15.6   ⚗ 15.6   **FUD** 090   T A2 80 50 ▣
         AMA: 2014,Jan,11

69501-69530 Transmastoid Excision

EXCLUDES   Mastoidectomy cavity debridement (69220, 69222)
           Skin graft (15004-15770)

69501   **Transmastoid antrotomy (simple mastoidectomy)**
         ⚕ 21.0   ⚗ 21.0   **FUD** 090   T A2 50 ▣
         AMA: 2015,Jan,16; 2014,Jan,11

69502   **Mastoidectomy; complete**
         ⚕ 28.0   ⚗ 28.0   **FUD** 090   T A2 80 50 ▣
         AMA: 2015,Jan,16; 2014,Jan,11

69505   **modified radical**
         ⚕ 34.6   ⚗ 34.6   **FUD** 090   T A2 80 50 ▣
         AMA: 2015,Jan,16; 2014,Jan,11

69511   **radical**
         ⚕ 35.4   ⚗ 35.4   **FUD** 090   T A2 80 50 ▣
         AMA: 2015,Jan,16; 2014,Jan,11

69530   **Petrous apicectomy including radical mastoidectomy**
         ⚕ 47.5   ⚗ 47.5   **FUD** 090   T A2 80 50 ▣
         AMA: 2014,Jan,11

69535-69554 Polyp and Glomus Tumor Removal

69535   **Resection temporal bone, external approach**
         EXCLUDES   Middle fossa approach (69950-69970)
         ⚕ 77.2   ⚗ 77.2   **FUD** 090   C 50 ▣
         AMA: 2014,Jan,11

69540   **Excision aural polyp**
         ⚕ 3.65   ⚗ 5.95   **FUD** 010   T P3 50 ▣
         AMA: 2014,Jan,11

69550   **Excision aural glomus tumor; transcanal**
         ⚕ 29.9   ⚗ 29.9   **FUD** 090   T A2 80 50 ▣
         AMA: 2014,Jan,11

69552   **transmastoid**
         ⚕ 45.2   ⚗ 45.2   **FUD** 090   T A2 80 50 ▣
         AMA: 2014,Jan,11

69554   **extended (extratemporal)**
         ⚕ 72.6   ⚗ 72.6   **FUD** 090   C 80 50 ▣
         AMA: 2014,Jan,11

69601-69605 Revised Mastoidectomy

EXCLUDES   Skin graft (15120-15121, 15260-15261)

69601   **Revision mastoidectomy; resulting in complete mastoidectomy**
         ⚕ 30.1   ⚗ 30.1   **FUD** 090   T A2 80 50 ▣
         AMA: 2015,Jan,16; 2014,Jan,11

Squamous part of temporal bone · Internal acoustic canal · Petrous part of temporal bone · Petrous apex · Mastoid · Mastoid process · Petrous part of temporal bone · Cutaway of mastoid process · Oval window · Plane of view above · Mastoid air cells · Facial nerve canal

69602   **resulting in modified radical mastoidectomy**
         ⚕ 31.3   ⚗ 31.3   **FUD** 090   T A2 80 50 ▣
         AMA: 2015,Jan,16; 2014,Jan,11

69603   **resulting in radical mastoidectomy**
         ⚕ 36.2   ⚗ 36.2   **FUD** 090   T A2 80 50 ▣
         AMA: 2015,Jan,16; 2014,Jan,11

69604   **resulting in tympanoplasty**
         EXCLUDES   Secondary tympanoplasty following mastoidectomy (69631-69632)
         ⚕ 32.0   ⚗ 32.0   **FUD** 090   T A2 50 ▣
         AMA: 2015,Jan,16; 2014,Jan,11

69605   **with apicectomy**
         ⚕ 44.9   ⚗ 44.9   **FUD** 090   T A2 80 50 ▣
         AMA: 2014,Jan,11

69610-69646 Eardrum Repair with/without Other Procedures

69610 Tympanic membrane repair, with or without site preparation of perforation for closure, with or without patch

🔧 8.39   ⚕ 11.0   **FUD** 010   T P3 50 ▢

AMA: 2015,May,10; 2015,Apr,10; 2015,Jan,16; 2014,Jan,11; 2012,Jan,15-42; 2011,Jan,11

69620 Myringoplasty (surgery confined to drumhead and donor area)

🔧 14.0   ⚕ 19.8   **FUD** 090   T A2 50 ▢

AMA: 2015,May,10; 2015,Apr,10; 2015,Jan,16; 2014,Jan,11; 2012,Jan,15-42; 2011,Jan,11

69631 Tympanoplasty without mastoidectomy (including canalplasty, atticotomy and/or middle ear surgery), initial or revision; without ossicular chain reconstruction

🔧 25.4   ⚕ 25.4   **FUD** 090   T A2 50 ▢

AMA: 2015,Jan,16; 2014,Jan,11; 2012,Dec,11; 2012,Jan,15-42; 2011,Jan,11

69632 with ossicular chain reconstruction (eg, postfenestration)

🔧 31.0   ⚕ 31.0   **FUD** 090   T A2 50 ▢

AMA: 2015,Jan,16; 2014,Jan,11

69633 with ossicular chain reconstruction and synthetic prosthesis (eg, partial ossicular replacement prosthesis [PORP], total ossicular replacement prosthesis [TORP])

🔧 30.0   ⚕ 30.0   **FUD** 090   T A2 50 ▢

AMA: 2015,Jan,16; 2014,Jan,11

69635 Tympanoplasty with antrotomy or mastoidotomy (including canalplasty, atticotomy, middle ear surgery, and/or tympanic membrane repair); without ossicular chain reconstruction

🔧 35.4   ⚕ 35.4   **FUD** 090   T A2 50 ▢

AMA: 2015,Jan,16; 2014,Jan,11

69636 with ossicular chain reconstruction

🔧 39.7   ⚕ 39.7   **FUD** 090   T A2 80 50 ▢

AMA: 2015,Jan,16; 2014,Jan,11

69637 with ossicular chain reconstruction and synthetic prosthesis (eg, partial ossicular replacement prosthesis [PORP], total ossicular replacement prosthesis [TORP])

🔧 40.4   ⚕ 40.4   **FUD** 090   T A2 80 50 ▢

AMA: 2015,Jan,16; 2014,Jan,11

69641 Tympanoplasty with mastoidectomy (including canalplasty, middle ear surgery, tympanic membrane repair); without ossicular chain reconstruction

🔧 29.9   ⚕ 29.9   **FUD** 090   T A2 50 ▢

AMA: 2015,Jan,16; 2014,Jan,11

69642 with ossicular chain reconstruction

🔧 38.5   ⚕ 38.5   **FUD** 090   T A2 50 ▢

AMA: 2015,Jan,16; 2014,Jan,11

69643 with intact or reconstructed wall, without ossicular chain reconstruction

🔧 35.2   ⚕ 35.2   **FUD** 090   T A2 50 ▢

AMA: 2015,Jan,16; 2014,Jan,11

69644 with intact or reconstructed canal wall, with ossicular chain reconstruction

🔧 42.6   ⚕ 42.6   **FUD** 090   T A2 50 ▢

AMA: 2015,Jan,16; 2014,Jan,11

69645 radical or complete, without ossicular chain reconstruction

🔧 41.9   ⚕ 41.9   **FUD** 090   T A2 50 ▢

AMA: 2015,Jan,16; 2014,Jan,11

69646 radical or complete, with ossicular chain reconstruction

🔧 44.4   ⚕ 44.4   **FUD** 090   T A2 80 50 ▢

AMA: 2015,Jan,16; 2014,Jan,11

69650-69662 Stapes Procedures

69650 Stapes mobilization

🔧 23.1   ⚕ 23.1   **FUD** 090   T A2 50 ▢

AMA: 2014,Jan,11

69660 Stapedectomy or stapedotomy with reestablishment of ossicular continuity, with or without use of foreign material;

🔧 26.7   ⚕ 26.7   **FUD** 090   T A2 50 ▢

AMA: 2014,Jan,11

69661 with footplate drill out

🔧 34.7   ⚕ 34.7   **FUD** 090   T A2 80 50 ▢

AMA: 2014,Jan,11

69662 Revision of stapedectomy or stapedotomy

🔧 33.4   ⚕ 33.4   **FUD** 090   T A2 50 ▢

AMA: 2014,Jan,11

69666-69700 Other Inner Ear Procedures

69666 Repair oval window fistula

🔧 23.3   ⚕ 23.3   **FUD** 090   T A2 80 50 ▢

AMA: 2014,Jan,11

69667 Repair round window fistula

🔧 23.3   ⚕ 23.3   **FUD** 090   T A2 80 50 ▢

AMA: 2014,Jan,11

69670 Mastoid obliteration (separate procedure)

🔧 27.1   ⚕ 27.1   **FUD** 090   T A2 80 50 ▢

AMA: 2014,Jan,11

69676 Tympanic neurectomy

🔧 23.9   ⚕ 23.9   **FUD** 090   T A2 50 ▢

AMA: 2014,Jan,11

69700 Closure postauricular fistula, mastoid (separate procedure)

🔧 19.7   ⚕ 19.7   **FUD** 090   T A2 50 ▢

AMA: 2014,Jan,11

69710-69718 Procedures Related to Hearing Aids/Auditory Implants

CMS: 100-2,16,100 Hearing Devices

69710 Implantation or replacement of electromagnetic bone conduction hearing device in temporal bone

INCLUDES   Removal of existing device when performing replacement procedure

🔧 0.00   ⚕ 0.00   **FUD** XXX   E

AMA: 2014,Jan,11

69711 Removal or repair of electromagnetic bone conduction hearing device in temporal bone

🔧 24.8   ⚕ 24.8   **FUD** 090   02 A2 80 50 ▢

AMA: 2014,Jan,11

69714 Implantation, osseointegrated implant, temporal bone, with percutaneous attachment to external speech processor/cochlear stimulator; without mastoidectomy

🔧 31.0   ⚕ 31.0   **FUD** 090   J J8 50 ▢

AMA: 2015,Jan,16; 2014,Jan,11; 2013,Oct,18

69715 with mastoidectomy

🔧 38.3   ⚕ 38.3   **FUD** 090   J J8 50 ▢

AMA: 2014,Jan,11

69717 Replacement (including removal of existing device), osseointegrated implant, temporal bone, with percutaneous attachment to external speech processor/cochlear stimulator; without mastoidectomy

  🔧 32.5   ⚕ 32.5   **FUD** 090   T G2 50 ▭

  AMA: 2014,Jan,11

69718 with mastoidectomy

  🔧 38.6   ⚕ 38.6   **FUD** 090   J J8 50 ▭

  AMA: 2014,Jan,11

69720-69799 Procedures of the Facial Nerve

EXCLUDES Extracranial suture of facial nerve (64864)

69720 Decompression facial nerve, intratemporal; lateral to geniculate ganglion

  🔧 34.5   ⚕ 34.5   **FUD** 090   T A2 80 50 ▭ P0

  AMA: 2014,Jan,11

69725 including medial to geniculate ganglion

  🔧 54.2   ⚕ 54.2   **FUD** 090   T 80 50 ▭

  AMA: 2014,Jan,11

69740 Suture facial nerve, intratemporal, with or without graft or decompression; lateral to geniculate ganglion

  🔧 33.6   ⚕ 33.6   **FUD** 090   T A2 80 50 ▭

  AMA: 2014,Jan,11

69745 including medial to geniculate ganglion

  🔧 35.7   ⚕ 35.7   **FUD** 090   T A2 80 50 ▭

  AMA: 2014,Jan,11

69799 Unlisted procedure, middle ear

  🔧 0.00   ⚕ 0.00   **FUD** YYY   T 80 50

  AMA: 2015,Jan,16; 2014,Jan,11

69801-69915 Procedures of the Labyrinth

69801 Labyrinthotomy, with perfusion of vestibuloactive drug(s), transcanal

  Do not report more than one time per day

  Do not report when performed on the same ear (69420-69421, 69433, 69436)

  🔧 3.64   ⚕ 5.61   **FUD** 000   T P3 80 50 ▭

  AMA: 2015,Jan,16; 2014,Jan,11; 2012,Jan,15-42; 2011,May,8; 2011,May,7; 2011,Jan,11

Anterior semicircular canal / Lateral semicircular canal / Window / Posterior semicircular canal / Cochlea

Side view schematic of semicircular canals (left). Sound (below) as registered in the cochlea
- Low tone
- Mid range
- High tones

Petrous apex / Internal acoustic canal / Mastoid

69805 Endolymphatic sac operation; without shunt

  🔧 30.3   ⚕ 30.3   **FUD** 090   T A2 80 50 ▭

  AMA: 2014,Jan,11

69806 with shunt

  🔧 27.2   ⚕ 27.2   **FUD** 090   T A2 50 ▭

  AMA: 2014,Jan,11

69820 Fenestration semicircular canal

  INCLUDES Lempert's fenestration

  🔧 24.6   ⚕ 24.6   **FUD** 090   T A2 80 50 ▭

  AMA: 2014,Jan,11

69840 Revision fenestration operation

  🔧 26.2   ⚕ 26.2   **FUD** 090   T A2 80 50 ▭

  AMA: 2014,Jan,11

69905 Labyrinthectomy; transcanal

  🔧 26.4   ⚕ 26.4   **FUD** 090   T A2 50 ▭

  AMA: 2014,Jan,11

69910 with mastoidectomy

  🔧 29.3   ⚕ 29.3   **FUD** 090   T A2 80 50 ▭

  AMA: 2014,Jan,11

69915 Vestibular nerve section, translabyrinthine approach

  EXCLUDES Transcranial approach (69950)

  🔧 44.3   ⚕ 44.3   **FUD** 090   T A2 80 50 ▭

  AMA: 2014,Jan,11

69930-69949 Cochlear Implantation

CMS: 100-2,16,100 Hearing Devices

69930 Cochlear device implantation, with or without mastoidectomy

  🔧 35.3   ⚕ 35.3   **FUD** 090   J J8 80 50 ▭ P0

  AMA: 2014,Jan,11

69949 Unlisted procedure, inner ear

  🔧 0.00   ⚕ 0.00   **FUD** YYY   T 80 50

  AMA: 2014,Jan,11

69950-69979 Inner Ear Procedures via Craniotomy

EXCLUDES External approach (69535)

69950 Vestibular nerve section, transcranial approach

  🔧 51.4   ⚕ 51.4   **FUD** 090   C 80 50 ▭

  AMA: 2014,Jan,11

69955 Total facial nerve decompression and/or repair (may include graft)

  🔧 57.0   ⚕ 57.0   **FUD** 090   T 80 50 ▭ P0

  AMA: 2014,Jan,11

69960 Decompression internal auditory canal

  🔧 55.5   ⚕ 55.5   **FUD** 090   T 80 50 ▭ P0

  AMA: 2014,Jan,11

69970 Removal of tumor, temporal bone

  🔧 61.8   ⚕ 61.8   **FUD** 090   T 80 50 ▭ P0

  AMA: 2014,Jan,11

69979 Unlisted procedure, temporal bone, middle fossa approach

  🔧 0.00   ⚕ 0.00   **FUD** YYY   T 80 50

  AMA: 2015,Jan,16; 2014,Sep,13; 2014,Jan,11

69990 Operating Microscope

EXCLUDES Magnifying loupes

Do not report with (15756-15758, 15842, 19364, 19368, 20955-20962, 20969-20973, 22551-22552, 22856-22861 [22858], 26551-26554, 26556, 31526, 31531, 31536, 31541, 31545-31546, 31561, 31571, 43116, 43180, 43496, 46601, 46607, 49906, 61548, 63075-63078, 64727, 64820-64823, 65091-68850 [67810], 0184T, 0308T, 0402T)

+ 69990 Microsurgical techniques, requiring use of operating microscope (List separately in addition to code for primary procedure)

  Code first primary procedure

  🔧 6.51   ⚕ 6.51   **FUD** ZZZ   N N1 80

  AMA: 2015,Jan,16; 2014,Sep,13; 2014,Apr,10; 2014,Jan,8; 2014,Jan,11; 2013,Oct,14; 2012,Dec,12; 2012,Jun,12-13; 2012,Mar,9-10; 2012,Jan,15-42; 2011,Jan,11

70010-70015 Radiography: Neurodiagnostic

70010 **Myelography, posterior fossa, radiological supervision and interpretation**
🔲 2.05 ⚕ 2.05 **FUD** XXX [Q2] [N1] [80] [⬚] [PQ]
AMA: 2015,Jan,16; 2014,Jan,11; 2012,Feb,9-10

70015 **Cisternography, positive contrast, radiological supervision and interpretation**
🔲 4.34 ⚕ 4.34 **FUD** XXX [Q2] [N1] [80] [⬚] [PQ]
AMA: 2014,Jan,11; 2012,Feb,9-10

70030-70390 Radiography: Head, Neck, Orofacial Structures

[INCLUDES] Minimum number of views or more views when needed to adequately complete the study
Radiographs that have to be repeated during the encounter due to substandard quality; only one unit of service is reported

[EXCLUDES] *Obtaining more films after review of initial films, based on the discretion of the radiologist, an order for the test, and a change in the patient's condition*

70030 **Radiologic examination, eye, for detection of foreign body**
🔲 0.77 ⚕ 0.77 **FUD** XXX [Q1] [N1] [80]
AMA: 2014,Jan,11; 2012,Feb,9-10

70100 **Radiologic examination, mandible; partial, less than 4 views**
🔲 0.92 ⚕ 0.92 **FUD** XXX [Q1] [N1] [80]
AMA: 2014,Jan,11; 2012,Feb,9-10

70110 **complete, minimum of 4 views**
🔲 1.06 ⚕ 1.06 **FUD** XXX [Q1] [N1] [80] [⬚]
AMA: 2014,Jan,11; 2012,Feb,9-10

70120 **Radiologic examination, mastoids; less than 3 views per side**
🔲 0.95 ⚕ 0.95 **FUD** XXX [Q1] [N1] [80]
AMA: 2014,Jan,11; 2012,Feb,9-10

70130 **complete, minimum of 3 views per side**
🔲 1.53 ⚕ 1.53 **FUD** XXX [Q1] [N1] [80] [⬚]
AMA: 2014,Jan,11; 2012,Feb,9-10

70134 **Radiologic examination, internal auditory meati, complete**
🔲 1.44 ⚕ 1.44 **FUD** XXX [Q1] [N1] [80]
AMA: 2014,Jan,11; 2012,Feb,9-10

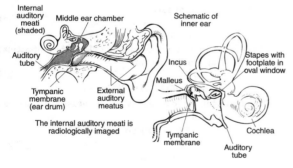

The internal auditory meati is radiologically imaged

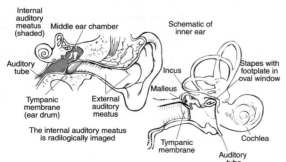

The internal auditory meatus is radiologically imaged

70140 **Radiologic examination, facial bones; less than 3 views**
🔲 0.83 ⚕ 0.83 **FUD** XXX [Q1] [N1] [80]
AMA: 2014,Jan,11; 2012,Feb,9-10

An x-ray of the facial bones is performed

70150 **complete, minimum of 3 views**
🔲 1.16 ⚕ 1.16 **FUD** XXX [Q1] [N1] [80] [⬚]
AMA: 2014,Jan,11; 2012,Feb,9-10

70160 **Radiologic examination, nasal bones, complete, minimum of 3 views**
🔲 0.91 ⚕ 0.91 **FUD** XXX [Q1] [N1] [80]
AMA: 2014,Jan,11; 2012,Feb,9-10

70170 **Dacryocystography, nasolacrimal duct, radiological supervision and interpretation**
[EXCLUDES] *Injection of contrast (68850)*
🔲 0.00 ⚕ 0.00 **FUD** XXX [Q2] [N1] [80] [⬚] [PQ]
AMA: 2014,Jan,11; 2012,Feb,9-10

70190 **Radiologic examination; optic foramina**
🔲 0.98 ⚕ 0.98 **FUD** XXX [Q1] [N1] [80]
AMA: 2014,Jan,11; 2012,Feb,9-10

70200 **orbits, complete, minimum of 4 views**
🔲 1.18 ⚕ 1.18 **FUD** XXX [Q1] [N1] [80]
AMA: 2014,Jan,11; 2012,Feb,9-10

An x-ray of the orbits is performed

70210 **Radiologic examination, sinuses, paranasal, less than 3 views**
🔲 0.83 ⚕ 0.83 **FUD** XXX [Q1] [N1] [80]
AMA: 2014,Jan,11; 2012,Feb,9-10

70220 **Radiologic examination, sinuses, paranasal, complete, minimum of 3 views**
🔲 1.04 ⚕ 1.04 **FUD** XXX [Q1] [N1] [80] [⬚]
AMA: 2014,Jan,11; 2012,Feb,9-10

70240 **Radiologic examination, sella turcica**
🔲 0.84 ⚕ 0.84 **FUD** XXX [Q1] [N1] [80]
AMA: 2014,Jan,11; 2012,Feb,9-10

70250 **Radiologic examination, skull; less than 4 views**
🔲 1.00 ⚕ 1.00 **FUD** XXX [Q1] [N1] [80]
AMA: 2014,Jan,11; 2012,Feb,9-10

70260 **complete, minimum of 4 views**
🔲 1.26 ⚕ 1.26 **FUD** XXX [Q1] [N1] [80] [⬚]
AMA: 2014,Jan,11; 2012,Feb,9-10

70300 Radiologic examination, teeth; single view

🔷 0.42 ⚖ 0.42 **FUD** XXX `Q1` `N1` `80`

AMA: 2014,Jan,11; 2012,Feb,9-10

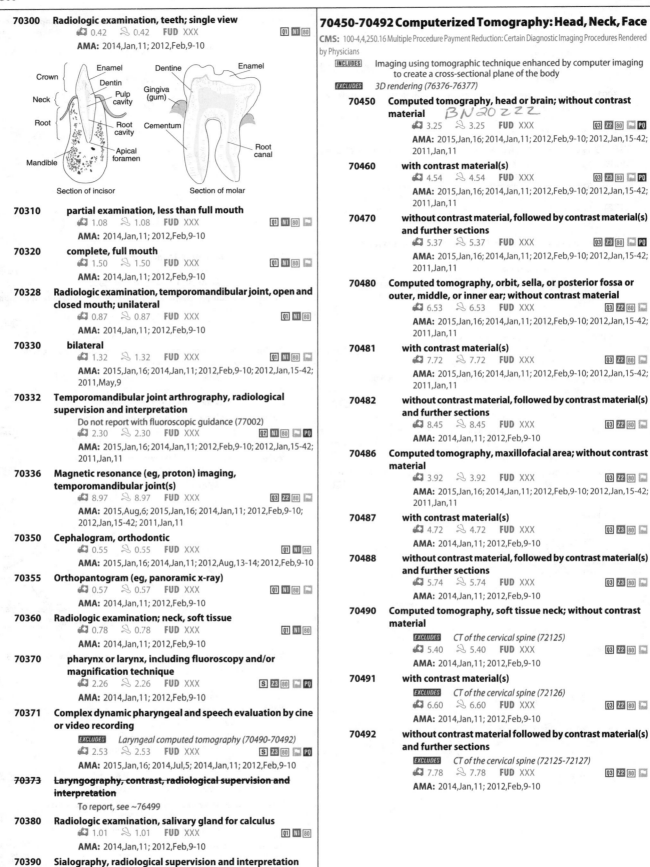

Crown
Enamel
Dentin
Neck
Pulp cavity
Root
Root cavity
Mandible
Apical foramen

Dentine
Enamel
Gingiva (gum)
Cementum
Root canal

Section of incisor
Section of molar

70310 partial examination, less than full mouth

🔷 1.08 ⚖ 1.08 **FUD** XXX `Q1` `N1` `80` 🖵

AMA: 2014,Jan,11; 2012,Feb,9-10

70320 complete, full mouth

🔷 1.50 ⚖ 1.50 **FUD** XXX `Q1` `N1` `80` 🖵

AMA: 2014,Jan,11; 2012,Feb,9-10

70328 Radiologic examination, temporomandibular joint, open and closed mouth; unilateral

🔷 0.87 ⚖ 0.87 **FUD** XXX `Q1` `N1` `80`

AMA: 2014,Jan,11; 2012,Feb,9-10

70330 bilateral

🔷 1.32 ⚖ 1.32 **FUD** XXX `Q1` `N1` `80` 🖵

AMA: 2015,Jan,16; 2014,Jan,11; 2012,Feb,9-10; 2012,Jan,15-42; 2011,May,9

70332 Temporomandibular joint arthrography, radiological supervision and interpretation

Do not report with fluoroscopic guidance (77002)

🔷 2.30 ⚖ 2.30 **FUD** XXX `Q2` `N1` `80` 🖵 `P0`

AMA: 2015,Jan,16; 2014,Jan,11; 2012,Feb,9-10; 2012,Jan,15-42; 2011,Jan,11

70336 Magnetic resonance (eg, proton) imaging, temporomandibular joint(s)

🔷 8.97 ⚖ 8.97 **FUD** XXX `Q3` `Z2` `80` 🖵

AMA: 2015,Aug,6; 2015,Jan,16; 2014,Jan,11; 2012,Feb,9-10; 2012,Jan,15-42; 2011,Jan,11

70350 Cephalogram, orthodontic

🔷 0.55 ⚖ 0.55 **FUD** XXX `Q1` `N1` `80`

AMA: 2015,Jan,16; 2014,Jan,11; 2012,Aug,13-14; 2012,Feb,9-10

70355 Orthopantogram (eg, panoramic x-ray)

🔷 0.57 ⚖ 0.57 **FUD** XXX `Q1` `N1` `80` 🖵

AMA: 2014,Jan,11; 2012,Feb,9-10

70360 Radiologic examination; neck, soft tissue

🔷 0.78 ⚖ 0.78 **FUD** XXX `Q1` `N1` `80`

AMA: 2014,Jan,11; 2012,Feb,9-10

70370 pharynx or larynx, including fluoroscopy and/or magnification technique

🔷 2.26 ⚖ 2.26 **FUD** XXX `S` `Z3` `80` 🖵 `P0`

AMA: 2014,Jan,11; 2012,Feb,9-10

70371 Complex dynamic pharyngeal and speech evaluation by cine or video recording

EXCLUDES *Laryngeal computed tomography (70490-70492)*

🔷 2.53 ⚖ 2.53 **FUD** XXX `S` `Z3` `80` 🖵 `P0`

AMA: 2015,Jan,16; 2014,Jul,5; 2014,Jan,11; 2012,Feb,9-10

70373 ~~Laryngography, contrast, radiological supervision and interpretation~~

To report, see ~76499

70380 Radiologic examination, salivary gland for calculus

🔷 1.01 ⚖ 1.01 **FUD** XXX `Q1` `N1` `80`

AMA: 2014,Jan,11; 2012,Feb,9-10

70390 Sialography, radiological supervision and interpretation

🔷 2.63 ⚖ 2.63 **FUD** XXX `Q2` `N1` `80` 🖵 `P0`

AMA: 2014,Jan,11; 2012,Feb,9-10

70450-70492 Computerized Tomography: Head, Neck, Face

CMS: 100-4,4,250.16 Multiple Procedure Payment Reduction: Certain Diagnostic Imaging Procedures Rendered by Physicians

INCLUDES Imaging using tomographic technique enhanced by computer imaging to create a cross-sectional plane of the body

EXCLUDES *3D rendering (76376-76377)*

70450 Computed tomography, head or brain; without contrast material *BN20ZZZ*

🔷 3.25 ⚖ 3.25 **FUD** XXX `Q3` `Z2` `80` 🖵 `P0`

AMA: 2015,Jan,16; 2014,Jan,11; 2012,Feb,9-10; 2012,Jan,15-42; 2011,Jan,11

70460 with contrast material(s)

🔷 4.54 ⚖ 4.54 **FUD** XXX `Q3` `Z3` `80` 🖵 `P0`

AMA: 2015,Jan,16; 2014,Jan,11; 2012,Feb,9-10; 2012,Jan,15-42; 2011,Jan,11

70470 without contrast material, followed by contrast material(s) and further sections

🔷 5.37 ⚖ 5.37 **FUD** XXX `Q3` `Z3` `80` 🖵 `P0`

AMA: 2015,Jan,16; 2014,Jan,11; 2012,Feb,9-10; 2012,Jan,15-42; 2011,Jan,11

70480 Computed tomography, orbit, sella, or posterior fossa or outer, middle, or inner ear; without contrast material

🔷 6.53 ⚖ 6.53 **FUD** XXX `Q3` `Z2` `80` 🖵

AMA: 2015,Jan,16; 2014,Jan,11; 2012,Feb,9-10; 2012,Jan,15-42; 2011,Jan,11

70481 with contrast material(s)

🔷 7.72 ⚖ 7.72 **FUD** XXX `Q3` `Z2` `80` 🖵

AMA: 2015,Jan,16; 2014,Jan,11; 2012,Feb,9-10; 2012,Jan,15-42; 2011,Jan,11

70482 without contrast material, followed by contrast material(s) and further sections

🔷 8.45 ⚖ 8.45 **FUD** XXX `Q3` `Z2` `80` 🖵

AMA: 2014,Jan,11; 2012,Feb,9-10

70486 Computed tomography, maxillofacial area; without contrast material

🔷 3.92 ⚖ 3.92 **FUD** XXX `Q3` `Z2` `80` 🖵

AMA: 2015,Jan,16; 2014,Jan,11; 2012,Feb,9-10; 2012,Jan,15-42; 2011,Jan,11

70487 with contrast material(s)

🔷 4.72 ⚖ 4.72 **FUD** XXX `Q3` `Z3` `80` 🖵

AMA: 2014,Jan,11; 2012,Feb,9-10

70488 without contrast material, followed by contrast material(s) and further sections

🔷 5.74 ⚖ 5.74 **FUD** XXX `Q3` `Z3` `80` 🖵

AMA: 2014,Jan,11; 2012,Feb,9-10

70490 Computed tomography, soft tissue neck; without contrast material

EXCLUDES *CT of the cervical spine (72125)*

🔷 5.40 ⚖ 5.40 **FUD** XXX `Q3` `Z2` `80` 🖵

AMA: 2014,Jan,11; 2012,Feb,9-10

70491 with contrast material(s)

EXCLUDES *CT of the cervical spine (72126)*

🔷 6.60 ⚖ 6.60 **FUD** XXX `Q3` `Z2` `80` 🖵

AMA: 2014,Jan,11; 2012,Feb,9-10

70492 without contrast material followed by contrast material(s) and further sections

EXCLUDES *CT of the cervical spine (72125-72127)*

🔷 7.78 ⚖ 7.78 **FUD** XXX `Q3` `Z2` `80` 🖵

AMA: 2014,Jan,11; 2012,Feb,9-10

`26`/`TC` PC/TC Comp Only	`A2`-`Z3` ASC Pmt	`50` Bilateral	♂ Male Only	♀ Female Only	🔷 Facility RVU	⚖ Non-Facility RVU
AMA: CPT Asst	**CMS:** Pub 100	`A`-`Y` OPPSI	`80`/`80` Surg Assist Allowed / w/Doc		🖵 Lab Crosswalk	🔀 Radiology Crosswalk

Medicare (Red Text)   CPT © 2015 American Medical Association. All Rights Reserved. (Black Text)   © 2015 Optum360, LLC (Blue Text)

70496-70498 Computerized Tomographic Angiography: Head and Neck

CMS: 100-4,4,250.16 Multiple Procedure Payment Reduction: Certain Diagnostic Imaging Procedures Rendered by Physicians

INCLUDES Multiple rapid thin section CT scans to create cross-sectional images of bones, organs and tissues

70496 **Computed tomographic angiography, head, with contrast material(s), including noncontrast images, if performed, and image postprocessing** *B32RYZZ*
  ⚷ 8.28   ⚖ 8.28   **FUD** XXX   Q3 Z2 80 ▭
  AMA: 2015,Jan,16; 2014,Jan,11; 2012,Feb,9-10

70498 **Computed tomographic angiography, neck, with contrast material(s), including noncontrast images, if performed, and image postprocessing** *B320YZZ*
  ⚷ 8.23   ⚖ 8.23   **FUD** XXX   Q3 Z2 80 ▭ PQ
  AMA: 2015,Jan,16; 2014,Jan,11; 2012,Feb,9-10

70540-70543 Magnetic Resonance Imaging: Face, Neck, Orbits

CMS: 100-4,13,40 Magnetic Resonance Imaging (MRI); 100-4,4,250.16 Multiple Procedure Payment Reduction: Certain Diagnostic Imaging Procedures Rendered by Physicians

INCLUDES Application of an external magnetic field that forces alignment of hydrogen atom nuclei in soft tissues which converts to sets of tomographic images that can be displayed as three-dimensional images
EXCLUDES Magnetic resonance angiography head/neck (70544-70549)
Do not report more than one time per session

70540 **Magnetic resonance (eg, proton) imaging, orbit, face, and/or neck; without contrast material(s)**
  ⚷ 10.0   ⚖ 10.0   **FUD** XXX   Q3 Z2 80 ▭
  AMA: 2015,Jan,16; 2014,Jan,11; 2012,Feb,9-10; 2012,Jan,15-42; 2010,Sep,9

70542 **with contrast material(s)**
  ⚷ 11.2   ⚖ 11.2   **FUD** XXX   Q3 Z2 80 ▭
  AMA: 2015,Jan,16; 2014,Jan,11; 2012,Feb,9-10; 2012,Jan,15-42; 2010,Sep,9

70543 **without contrast material(s), followed by contrast material(s) and further sequences**
  ⚷ 13.7   ⚖ 13.7   **FUD** XXX   Q3 Z2 80 ▭
  AMA: 2015,Jan,16; 2014,Jan,11; 2012,Feb,9-10; 2012,Jan,15-42; 2010,Sep,9

70544-70549 Magnetic Resonance Angiography: Head and Neck

CMS: 100-4,13,40.1.1 Magnetic Resonance Angiography; 100-4,13,40.1.2 HCPCS Coding Requirements; 100-4,4,250.16 Multiple Procedure Payment Reduction: Certain Diagnostic Imaging Procedures Rendered by Physicians

INCLUDES Use of magnetic fields and radio waves to produce detailed cross-sectional images of internal body structures

70544 **Magnetic resonance angiography, head; without contrast material(s)**
  ⚷ 11.0   ⚖ 11.0   **FUD** XXX   Q3 Z2 80 ▭
  AMA: 2015,Jan,16; 2014,Jan,11; 2012,Feb,9-10

70545 **with contrast material(s)**
  ⚷ 10.8   ⚖ 10.8   **FUD** XXX   Q3 Z2 80 ▭
  AMA: 2015,Jan,16; 2014,Jan,11; 2012,Feb,9-10

70546 **without contrast material(s), followed by contrast material(s) and further sequences**
  ⚷ 16.8   ⚖ 16.8   **FUD** XXX   Q3 Z2 80 ▭
  AMA: 2015,Jan,16; 2014,Jan,11; 2012,Feb,9-10

70547 **Magnetic resonance angiography, neck; without contrast material(s)**
  ⚷ 11.0   ⚖ 11.0   **FUD** XXX   Q3 Z2 80 ▭ PQ
  AMA: 2015,Jan,16; 2014,Jan,11; 2012,Feb,9-10

70548 **with contrast material(s)**
  ⚷ 11.5   ⚖ 11.5   **FUD** XXX   Q3 Z2 80 ▭ PQ
  AMA: 2015,Jan,16; 2014,Jan,11; 2012,Feb,9-10

70549 **without contrast material(s), followed by contrast material(s) and further sequences**
  ⚷ 16.8   ⚖ 16.8   **FUD** XXX   Q3 Z2 80 ▭ PQ
  AMA: 2015,Jan,16; 2014,Jan,11; 2012,Feb,9-10

70551-70553 Magnetic Resonance Imaging: Brain and Brain Stem

CMS: 100-4,13,40 Magnetic Resonance Imaging (MRI); 100-4,4,250.16 Multiple Procedure Payment Reduction: Certain Diagnostic Imaging Procedures Rendered by Physicians

INCLUDES Application of an external magnetic field that forces alignment of hydrogen atom nuclei in soft tissues which converts to sets of tomographic images that can be displayed as three-dimensional images
EXCLUDES Magnetic spectroscopy (76390)

70551 **Magnetic resonance (eg, proton) imaging, brain (including brain stem); without contrast material**
  ⚷ 6.44   ⚖ 6.44   **FUD** XXX   Q3 Z3 80 ▭ PQ
  AMA: 2015,Jan,16; 2014,Jan,11; 2012,Feb,9-10; 2012,Jan,15-42; 2011,Jan,11

70552 **with contrast material(s)**
  ⚷ 8.97   ⚖ 8.97   **FUD** XXX   Q3 Z3 80 ▭ PQ
  AMA: 2015,Jan,16; 2014,Jan,11; 2012,Feb,9-10; 2012,Jan,15-42; 2011,Jan,11

70553 **without contrast material, followed by contrast material(s) and further sequences**
  ⚷ 10.5   ⚖ 10.5   **FUD** XXX   Q3 Z3 80 ▭ PQ
  AMA: 2015,Jan,16; 2014,Jan,11; 2012,Feb,9-10; 2012,Jan,15-42; 2011,Jan,11

70554-70555 Magnetic Resonance Imaging: Brain Mapping

INCLUDES Neuroimaging technique using MRI to identify and map signals related to brain activity
Do not report with the following codes unless a separate diagnostic MRI is performed (70551-70553)

70554 **Magnetic resonance imaging, brain, functional MRI; including test selection and administration of repetitive body part movement and/or visual stimulation, not requiring physician or psychologist administration**
  EXCLUDES Testing performed by a physician or psychologist (70555)
  Do not report with functional brain mapping (96020)
  ⚷ 12.6   ⚖ 12.6   **FUD** XXX   Q3 Z2 80
  AMA: 2015,Jan,16; 2014,Jan,11; 2012,Feb,9-10; 2012,Jan,15-42; 2011,Jan,11

70555 **requiring physician or psychologist administration of entire neurofunctional testing**
  EXCLUDES Testing performed by a technologist, nonphysician, or nonpsychologist (70554)
  Code also (96020)
  ⚷ 0.00   ⚖ 0.00   **FUD** XXX   S Z2 80
  AMA: 2015,Jan,16; 2014,Jan,11; 2012,Feb,9-10

70557-70559 Magnetic Resonance Imaging: Intraoperative

EXCLUDES Intracranial lesion stereotaxic biopsy with magnetic resonance guidance (61751)
Do not report more than one time per surgical encounter
Do not report unless a separate report is generated
Do not report with (61751, 77021-77022)

70557 **Magnetic resonance (eg, proton) imaging, brain (including brain stem and skull base), during open intracranial procedure (eg, to assess for residual tumor or residual vascular malformation); without contrast material**
  ⚷ 0.00   ⚖ 0.00   **FUD** XXX   S Z2 80 ▭
  AMA: 2014,Jan,11; 2012,Feb,9-10

70558 **with contrast material(s)**
  ⚷ 0.00   ⚖ 0.00   **FUD** XXX   S Z2 80 ▭
  AMA: 2014,Jan,11; 2012,Feb,9-10

70559 **without contrast material(s), followed by contrast material(s) and further sequences**
  ⚷ 0.00   ⚖ 0.00   **FUD** XXX   S Z2 80 ▭
  AMA: 2014,Jan,11; 2012,Feb,9-10

Radiology

71010-71130 Radiography: Thorax

> *EXCLUDES* *Needle placement guidance (76942, 77002)*

71010 **Radiologic examination, chest; single view, frontal**
> *EXCLUDES* *Concurrent computer-aided detection (0174T)*
> Do not report with (99291-99292)
> Do not report with remotely performed CAD (0175T)
> 🔴 0.63 ⚕ 0.63 **FUD** XXX `03` `Z3` `80` ▭
> **AMA:** 2015,Jan,16; 2014,May,4; 2014,Jan,11; 2013,Sep,17; 2012,Feb,9-10; 2012,Jan,15-42; 2011,Jan,11

71015 **stereo, frontal**
> Do not report with (99291-99292)
> 🔴 0.77 ⚕ 0.77 **FUD** XXX `03` `Z3` `80` ▭
> **AMA:** 2015,Jan,16; 2014,May,4; 2014,Jan,11; 2012,Feb,9-10

71020 **Radiologic examination, chest, 2 views, frontal and lateral;**
> *EXCLUDES* *Concurrent computer-aided detection (0174T)*
> Do not report with (99291-99292)
> Do not report with remotely performed CAD (0175T)
> 🔴 0.78 ⚕ 0.78 **FUD** XXX `03` `Z3` `80` ▭
> **AMA:** 2015,Jan,16; 2014,Jun,14; 2014,May,4; 2014,Jan,11; 2013,Sep,17; 2012,Feb,9-10; 2012,Jan,15-42; 2011,Jan,11; 2010,Sep,6-7

71021 **with apical lordotic procedure**
> *EXCLUDES* *Concurrent computer-aided detection (0174T)*
> Do not report with remotely performed CAD (0175T)
> 🔴 0.95 ⚕ 0.95 **FUD** XXX `01` `N1` `80` ▭
> **AMA:** 2014,Jan,11; 2012,Feb,9-10

71022 **with oblique projections**
> *EXCLUDES* *Concurrent computer-aided detection (0174T)*
> Do not report with remotely performed CAD (0175T)
> 🔴 1.17 ⚕ 1.17 **FUD** XXX `01` `N1` `80` ▭
> **AMA:** 2015,Jan,16; 2014,Jan,11; 2012,Feb,9-10

71023 **with fluoroscopy**
> 🔴 1.78 ⚕ 1.78 **FUD** XXX `01` `N1` `80` ▭ `PQ`
> **AMA:** 2015,Jan,16; 2014,Sep,5; 2014,Jan,11; 2013,Sep,17; 2013,Mar,10-11; 2013,Feb,3-6; 2012,Feb,9-10; 2012,Jan,15-42; 2011,Jul,3-11; 2011,Jan,11

71030 **Radiologic examination, chest, complete, minimum of 4 views;**
> *EXCLUDES* *Concurrent computer-aided detection (0174T)*
> Do not report with remotely performed CAD (0175T)
> 🔴 1.16 ⚕ 1.16 **FUD** XXX `01` `N1` `80` ▭
> **AMA:** 2015,Jan,16; 2014,Jan,11; 2012,Feb,9-10; 2011,Jan,11

71034 **with fluoroscopy**
> *EXCLUDES* *Separate fluoroscopy of chest (76000)*
> 🔴 2.36 ⚕ 2.36 **FUD** XXX `S` `Z3` `80` ▭ `PQ`
> **AMA:** 2015,Jan,16; 2014,Sep,5; 2014,Jan,11; 2013,Sep,17; 2013,Mar,10-11; 2013,Feb,3-6; 2012,Feb,9-10; 2012,Jan,15-42; 2011,Jul,3-11; 2011,Jan,11

71035 **Radiologic examination, chest, special views (eg, lateral decubitus, Bucky studies)**
> 🔴 0.91 ⚕ 0.91 **FUD** XXX `01` `N1` `80`
> **AMA:** 2015,Jan,16; 2014,Jan,11; 2013,Sep,17; 2012,Feb,9-10; 2012,Jan,15-42; 2011,Jan,11

71100 **Radiologic examination, ribs, unilateral; 2 views**
> 🔴 0.85 ⚕ 0.85 **FUD** XXX `01` `N1` `80` ▭
> **AMA:** 2014,Jan,11; 2012,Feb,9-10

Hyoid bone
Laryngeal cartilage — Cricoid cartilage
Clavicle — Trachea
Manubrium of sternum
Sternum
Rib cage — Xiphoid process
Costal cartilages

71101 **including posteroanterior chest, minimum of 3 views**
> 🔴 1.01 ⚕ 1.01 **FUD** XXX `01` `N1` `80` ▭
> **AMA:** 2014,Jan,11; 2012,Feb,9-10

71110 **Radiologic examination, ribs, bilateral; 3 views**
> 🔴 1.04 ⚕ 1.04 **FUD** XXX `01` `N1` `80` ▭
> **AMA:** 2014,Jan,11; 2012,Feb,9-10

71111 **including posteroanterior chest, minimum of 4 views**
> 🔴 1.32 ⚕ 1.32 **FUD** XXX `01` `N1` `80` ▭
> **AMA:** 2014,Jan,11; 2012,Feb,9-10

71120 **Radiologic examination; sternum, minimum of 2 views**
> 🔴 0.82 ⚕ 0.82 **FUD** XXX `01` `N1` `80`
> **AMA:** 2014,Jan,11; 2012,Feb,9-10

71130 **sternoclavicular joint or joints, minimum of 3 views**
> 🔴 1.01 ⚕ 1.01 **FUD** XXX `01` `N1` `80`
> **AMA:** 2014,Jan,11; 2012,Feb,9-10

71250-71270 Computerized Tomography: Thorax

CMS: 100-4,4,250.16 Multiple Procedure Payment Reduction: Certain Diagnostic Imaging Procedures Rendered by Physicians

> *INCLUDES* Imaging using tomographic technique enhanced by computer imaging to create a cross-sectional plane of the body
> *EXCLUDES* *3D rendering (76376-76377)*
> *CT of the heart (75571-75574)*

71250 **Computed tomography, thorax; without contrast material**
> 🔴 5.04 ⚕ 5.04 **FUD** XXX `03` `Z2` `80` ▭
> **AMA:** 2015,Jan,16; 2014,Jan,11; 2012,Feb,9-10; 2012,Jan,15-42; 2011,Aug,9-10; 2011,Jan,11

71260 **with contrast material(s)**
> 🔴 6.42 ⚕ 6.42 **FUD** XXX `03` `Z2` `80` ▭
> **AMA:** 2015,Jan,16; 2014,Jan,11; 2012,Feb,9-10; 2012,Jan,15-42; 2011,Jan,11

71270 **without contrast material, followed by contrast material(s) and further sections**
> 🔴 7.70 ⚕ 7.70 **FUD** XXX `03` `Z2` `80` ▭
> **AMA:** 2015,Jan,16; 2014,Jan,11; 2012,Feb,9-10; 2012,Jan,15-42; 2011,Jan,11

71275 Computerized Tomographic Angiography: Thorax

CMS: 100-4,4,250.16 Multiple Procedure Payment Reduction: Certain Diagnostic Imaging Procedures Rendered by Physicians

> *INCLUDES* Multiple rapid thin section CT scans to create cross-sectional images of bones, organs and tissues
> *EXCLUDES* *CT angiography of coronary arteries that includes calcification score and/or cardiac morphology (75574)*

71275 **Computed tomographic angiography, chest (noncoronary), with contrast material(s), including noncontrast images, if performed, and image postprocessing**
> 🔴 8.41 ⚕ 8.41 **FUD** XXX `03` `Z2` `80` ▭
> **AMA:** 2015,Jan,16; 2014,Jan,11; 2012,Feb,9-10; 2011,Aug,9-10; 2011,Jan,11

71550-71552 Magnetic Resonance Imaging: Thorax

CMS: 100-4,13,40 Magnetic Resonance Imaging (MRI); 100-4,4,250.16 Multiple Procedure Payment Reduction: Certain Diagnostic Imaging Procedures Rendered by Physicians

> *INCLUDES* Application of an external magnetic field that forces alignment of hydrogen atom nuclei in soft tissues which converts to sets of tomographic images that can be displayed as three-dimensional images
> *EXCLUDES* *MRI of the breast (77058-77059)*

71550 **Magnetic resonance (eg, proton) imaging, chest (eg, for evaluation of hilar and mediastinal lymphadenopathy); without contrast material(s)**
> 🔴 11.6 ⚕ 11.6 **FUD** XXX `03` `Z2` `80` ▭
> **AMA:** 2015,Jan,16; 2014,Jan,11; 2012,Feb,9-10; 2012,Jan,15-42; 2011,Jan,11; 2010,Sep,9; 2010,Apr,10

71551 **with contrast material(s)**
> 🔴 12.8 ⚕ 12.8 **FUD** XXX `03` `Z2` `80` ▭
> **AMA:** 2015,Jan,16; 2014,Jan,11; 2012,Feb,9-10; 2012,Jan,15-42; 2011,Jan,11; 2010,Sep,9; 2010,Apr,10

71010 — 71551

PC/TC Comp Only	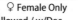 ASC Pmt	🚺 Bilateral ♂ Male Only ♀ Female Only 🔴 Facility RVU ⚕ Non-Facility RVU
AMA: CPT Asst	**CMS:** Pub 100	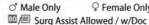 OPPSI 80/80 Surg Assist Allowed / w/Doc ▣ Lab Crosswalk ➕ Radiology Crosswalk

282 Medicare (Red Text) CPT © 2015 American Medical Association. All Rights Reserved. (Black Text) © 2015 Optum360, LLC (Blue Text)

71552 without contrast material(s), followed by contrast material(s) and further sequences
🚑 16.2 🔪 16.2 **FUD** XXX 〔03〕〔Z2〕〔80〕⊡
AMA: 2015,Jan,16; 2014,Jan,11; 2012,Feb,9-10; 2012,Jan,15-42; 2011,Jan,11; 2010,Sep,9; 2010,Apr,10

71555 Magnetic Resonance Angiography: Thorax

CMS: 100-4,13,40.1.1 Magnetic Resonance Angiography; 100-4,13,40.1.2 HCPCS Coding Requirements; 100-4,4,250.16 Multiple Procedure Payment Reduction: Certain Diagnostic Imaging Procedures Rendered by Physicians

71555 Magnetic resonance angiography, chest (excluding myocardium), with or without contrast material(s)
🚑 11.1 🔪 11.1 **FUD** XXX 〔B〕〔80〕⊡
AMA: 2015,Jan,16; 2014,Jan,11; 2012,Feb,9-10

72010-72120 Radiography: Spine

INCLUDES Minimum number of views or more views when needed to adequately complete the study
Radiographs that have to be repeated during the encounter due to substandard quality; only one unit of service is reported

EXCLUDES Obtaining more films after review of initial films, based on the discretion of the radiologist, an order for the test, and a change in the patient's condition

~~**72010** Radiologic examination, spine, entire, survey study, anteroposterior and lateral~~
To report, see ~72082

72020 Radiologic examination, spine, single view, specify level
EXCLUDES Single view of entire thoracic and lumbar spine (72081)
🚑 0.61 🔪 0.61 **FUD** XXX 〔01〕〔N1〕〔80〕
AMA: 2015,Jan,16; 2014,Jan,11; 2013,Jul,10; 2012,Feb,9-10

72040 Radiologic examination, spine, cervical; 2 or 3 views
🚑 0.93 🔪 0.93 **FUD** XXX 〔01〕〔N1〕〔80〕
AMA: 2015,Jan,16; 2014,Jan,11; 2013,Jul,10; 2012,Feb,9-10

Detail of top two vertebrae — C-1—C-4
Odontoid process — C-5—C-7
Atlas
Axis — T-1—T-12
Spinous process

An x-ray of the cervical spine is performed

72050 4 or 5 views
🚑 1.25 🔪 1.25 **FUD** XXX 〔01〕〔N1〕〔80〕⊡
AMA: 2014,Jan,11; 2012,Feb,9-10

72052 6 or more views
🚑 1.57 🔪 1.57 **FUD** XXX 〔01〕〔N1〕〔80〕⊡
AMA: 2014,Jan,11; 2012,Feb,9-10

~~**72069** Radiologic examination, spine, thoracolumbar, standing (scoliosis)~~
To report, see ~72081-72084

72070 Radiologic examination, spine; thoracic, 2 views
🚑 0.88 🔪 0.88 **FUD** XXX 〔01〕〔N1〕〔80〕⊡
AMA: 2015,Jan,16; 2014,Jan,11; 2012,Feb,9-10

72072 thoracic, 3 views
🚑 0.96 🔪 0.96 **FUD** XXX 〔01〕〔N1〕〔80〕⊡
AMA: 2015,Jan,16; 2014,Jan,11; 2012,Feb,9-10

72074 thoracic, minimum of 4 views
🚑 1.09 🔪 1.09 **FUD** XXX 〔01〕〔N1〕〔80〕⊡
AMA: 2015,Jan,16; 2014,Jan,11; 2012,Feb,9-10

▲ **72080** thoracolumbar junction, minimum of 2 views
EXCLUDES Single view of thoracolumbar junction (72020)
🚑 0.94 🔪 0.94 **FUD** XXX 〔01〕〔N1〕〔80〕⊡
AMA: 2015,Jan,16; 2014,Jan,11; 2012,Feb,9-10

● **72081** Radiologic examination, spine, entire thoracic and lumbar, including skull, cervical and sacral spine if performed (eg, scoliosis evaluation); one view

● **72082** 2 or 3 views

● **72083** 4 or 5 views

● **72084** minimum of 6 views

~~**72090** scoliosis study, including supine and erect studies~~
To report, see ~72081-72084

72100 Radiologic examination, spine, lumbosacral; 2 or 3 views
🚑 0.98 🔪 0.98 **FUD** XXX 〔01〕〔N1〕〔80〕⊡
AMA: 2015,Jan,16; 2014,Jan,11; 2012,Feb,9-10

Superior articular process   Tranverse process
L-1—L-5
Spinal cord
Lateral view of lumbar vertebrae
Disc
Spinous process
Sacrum
Body of vertebra

72110 minimum of 4 views
🚑 1.37 🔪 1.37 **FUD** XXX 〔01〕〔N1〕〔80〕⊡
AMA: 2015,Jan,16; 2014,Jan,11; 2012,Feb,9-10

72114 complete, including bending views, minimum of 6 views
🚑 1.75 🔪 1.75 **FUD** XXX 〔01〕〔N1〕〔80〕⊡
AMA: 2014,Jan,11; 2012,Feb,9-10

72120 bending views only, 2 or 3 views
🚑 1.13 🔪 1.13 **FUD** XXX 〔01〕〔N1〕〔80〕⊡
AMA: 2014,Jan,11; 2012,Feb,9-10

72125-72133 Computerized Tomography: Spine

CMS: 100-4,4,250.16 Multiple Procedure Payment Reduction: Certain Diagnostic Imaging Procedures Rendered by Physicians

INCLUDES Imaging using tomographic technique enhanced by computer imaging to create a cross-sectional plane of the body
EXCLUDES 3D rendering (76376-76377)
Code also intrathecal injection procedure when performed (61055, 62284)

72125 Computed tomography, cervical spine; without contrast material
🚑 5.16 🔪 5.16 **FUD** XXX 〔03〕〔Z2〕〔80〕⊡
AMA: 2014,Jan,11; 2012,Feb,9-10

72126 with contrast material
🚑 6.42 🔪 6.42 **FUD** XXX 〔03〕〔Z2〕〔80〕⊡
AMA: 2015,Jan,16; 2014,Jan,11; 2012,Feb,9-10

72127 without contrast material, followed by contrast material(s) and further sections
🚑 7.57 🔪 7.57 **FUD** XXX 〔03〕〔Z2〕〔80〕⊡
AMA: 2014,Jan,11; 2012,Feb,9-10

72128 Computed tomography, thoracic spine; without contrast material
🚑 5.04 🔪 5.04 **FUD** XXX 〔03〕〔Z2〕〔80〕⊡
AMA: 2014,Jan,11; 2012,Feb,9-10

72129 with contrast material
🚑 6.42 🔪 6.42 **FUD** XXX 〔03〕〔Z2〕〔80〕⊡
AMA: 2015,Jan,16; 2014,Jan,11; 2012,Feb,9-10

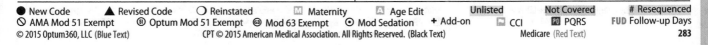

72130   **without contrast material, followed by contrast material(s) and further sections**
    🚗 7.58   ✂ 7.58   **FUD** XXX   03 Z2 80 ▭
    AMA: 2014,Jan,11; 2012,Feb,9-10

72131   **Computed tomography, lumbar spine; without contrast material**
    🚗 5.01   ✂ 5.01   **FUD** XXX   03 Z2 80 ▭
    AMA: 2014,Jan,11; 2012,Feb,9-10

72132   **with contrast material**
    🚗 6.40   ✂ 6.40   **FUD** XXX   03 Z2 80 ▭
    AMA: 2015,Jan,16; 2014,Jan,11; 2012,Feb,9-10

72133   **without contrast material, followed by contrast material(s) and further sections**
    🚗 7.58   ✂ 7.58   **FUD** XXX   03 Z2 80 ▭
    AMA: 2014,Jan,11; 2012,Feb,9-10

72141-72158 Magnetic Resonance Imaging: Spine

CMS: 100-4,13,40 Magnetic Resonance Imaging (MRI); 100-4,4,250.16 Multiple Procedure Payment Reduction: Certain Diagnostic Imaging Procedures Rendered by Physicians

INCLUDES   Application of an external magnetic field that forces alignment of hydrogen atom nuclei in soft tissues which converts to sets of tomographic images that can be displayed as three-dimensional images
Code also intrathecal injection procedure when performed (61055, 62284)

72141   **Magnetic resonance (eg, proton) imaging, spinal canal and contents, cervical; without contrast material**
    🚗 6.25   ✂ 6.25   **FUD** XXX   03 Z3 80 ▭
    AMA: 2015,Jan,16; 2014,Jun,14; 2014,Jan,11; 2012,Feb,9-10; 2010,Apr,10

72142   **with contrast material(s)**
    EXCLUDES   *MRI of cervical spinal canal performed without contrast followed by repeating the study with contrast (72156)*
    🚗 9.07   ✂ 9.07   **FUD** XXX   03 Z3 80 ▭
    AMA: 2015,Jan,16; 2014,Jan,11; 2012,Feb,9-10; 2010,Apr,10

72146   **Magnetic resonance (eg, proton) imaging, spinal canal and contents, thoracic; without contrast material**
    🚗 6.25   ✂ 6.25   **FUD** XXX   03 Z3 80 ▭
    AMA: 2015,Jan,16; 2014,Jun,14; 2014,Jan,11; 2012,Feb,9-10; 2010,Apr,10

72147   **with contrast material(s)**
    EXCLUDES   *MRI of thoracic spinal canal performed without contrast followed by repeating the study with contrast (72157)*
    🚗 9.01   ✂ 9.01   **FUD** XXX   03 Z3 80 ▭
    AMA: 2015,Jan,16; 2014,Jan,11; 2012,Feb,9-10; 2012,Jan,15-42; 2011,Jan,11; 2010,Apr,10

72148   **Magnetic resonance (eg, proton) imaging, spinal canal and contents, lumbar; without contrast material**
    🚗 6.22   ✂ 6.22   **FUD** XXX   03 Z3 80 ▭
    AMA: 2015,Jan,16; 2014,Jun,14; 2014,Jan,11; 2012,Feb,9-10; 2012,Jan,15-42; 2011,Jan,11

72149   **with contrast material(s)**
    EXCLUDES   *MRI of lumbar spinal canal performed without contrast followed by repeating the study with contrast (72158)*
    🚗 8.96   ✂ 8.96   **FUD** XXX   03 Z3 80 ▭
    AMA: 2014,Jan,11; 2012,Feb,9-10

72156   **Magnetic resonance (eg, proton) imaging, spinal canal and contents, without contrast material, followed by contrast material(s) and further sequences; cervical**
    🚗 10.6   ✂ 10.6   **FUD** XXX   03 Z3 80 ▭
    AMA: 2014,Jan,11; 2012,Feb,9-10

72157   **thoracic**
    🚗 10.6   ✂ 10.6   **FUD** XXX   03 Z2 80 ▭
    AMA: 2014,Jan,11; 2012,Feb,9-10

72158   **lumbar**
    🚗 10.6   ✂ 10.6   **FUD** XXX   03 Z3 80 ▭
    AMA: 2014,Jan,11; 2012,Feb,9-10

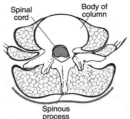

Spinal cord   Body of column

Spinous process

Superior view of thoracic spine and surrounding paraspinal muscles

72159 Magnetic Resonance Angiography: Spine

CMS: 100-4,13,40.1.1 Magnetic Resonance Angiography; 100-4,13,40.1.2 HCPCS Coding Requirements; 100-4,4,250.16 Multiple Procedure Payment Reduction: Certain Diagnostic Imaging Procedures Rendered by Physicians

72159   **Magnetic resonance angiography, spinal canal and contents, with or without contrast material(s)**
    🚗 11.7   ✂ 11.7   **FUD** XXX   B 80
    AMA: 2015,Jan,16; 2014,Jan,11; 2012,Feb,9-10

72170-72190 Radiography: Pelvis

INCLUDES   Minimum number of views or more views when needed to adequately complete the study
    Radiographs that have to be repeated during the encounter due to substandard quality; only one unit of service is reported
EXCLUDES   *Combined CT or CT angiography of abdomen and pelvis (74174, 74176-74178)*
    Obtaining more films after review of initial films, based on the discretion of the radiologist, an order for the test, and a change in the patient's condition
    Pelvimetry (74710)
Do not report with a second interpretation by the requesting physician (included in E&M service)

72170   **Radiologic examination, pelvis; 1 or 2 views**
    🚗 0.77   ✂ 0.77   **FUD** XXX   Q1 N1 80
    AMA: 2015,Jan,16; 2014,Jan,11; 2012,Feb,9-10; 2012,Jan,15-42; 2011,Jan,11

72190   **complete, minimum of 3 views**
    🚗 1.07   ✂ 1.07   **FUD** XXX   Q1 N1 80 ▭
    AMA: 2014,Jan,11; 2012,Feb,9-10

72191 Computerized Tomographic Angiography: Pelvis

CMS: 100-4,4,250.16 Multiple Procedure Payment Reduction: Certain Diagnostic Imaging Procedures Rendered by Physicians

INCLUDES   Multiple rapid thin section CT scans to create cross-sectional images of bones, organs and tissues
Do not report with (73706, 74174-74175, 75635)

72191   **Computed tomographic angiography, pelvis, with contrast material(s), including noncontrast images, if performed, and image postprocessing**
    🚗 8.53   ✂ 8.53   **FUD** XXX   03 Z2 80 ▭
    AMA: 2015,Jan,16; 2014,Jan,11; 2012,Feb,9-10

72192-72194 Computerized Tomography: Pelvis

CMS: 100-4,4,250.16 Multiple Procedure Payment Reduction: Certain Diagnostic Imaging Procedures Rendered by Physicians

EXCLUDES   *3D rendering (76376-76377)*
    Combined CT of abdomen and pelvis (74176-74178)
    CT colonography, diagnostic (74261-74262)
    CT colonography, screening (74263)
Do not report with (74261-74263)

72192   **Computed tomography, pelvis; without contrast material**
    🚗 4.10   ✂ 4.10   **FUD** XXX   03 Z2 80 ▭
    AMA: 2015,Jan,16; 2014,Jan,11; 2012,Oct,12; 2012,Feb,9-10; 2012,Jan,15-42; 2011,Jan,11; 2010,Apr,9

72193   with contrast material(s)
🚑 6.32   ⚕ 6.32   **FUD** XXX   [03] [Z2] [80] ▭
AMA: 2015,Jan,16; 2014,Jan,11; 2012,Oct,12; 2012,Feb,9-10; 2010,Apr,9

72194   without contrast material, followed by contrast material(s) and further sections
🚑 7.29   ⚕ 7.29   **FUD** XXX   [03] [Z2] [80] ▭
AMA: 2015,Jan,16; 2014,Jan,11; 2012,Oct,12; 2012,Feb,9-10; 2012,Jan,15-42; 2011,Jan,11; 2010,Apr,9

72195-72197 Magnetic Resonance Imaging: Pelvis

CMS: 100-4,13,40 Magnetic Resonance Imaging (MRI); 100-4,4,250.16 Multiple Procedure Payment Reduction: Certain Diagnostic Imaging Procedures Rendered by Physicians

INCLUDES   Application of an external magnetic field that forces alignment of hydrogen atom nuclei in soft tissues which converts to sets of tomographic images that can be displayed as three-dimensional images

EXCLUDES   *Magnetic resonance imaging of fetus(es) (74712-74713)*
Do not report with (74712-74713)

72195   Magnetic resonance (eg, proton) imaging, pelvis; without contrast material(s)
🚑 10.5   ⚕ 10.5   **FUD** XXX   [03] [Z2] [80] ▭
AMA: 2015,Jan,16; 2014,Jun,14; 2014,Jan,11; 2012,Feb,9-10; 2012,Jan,15-42; 2011,Jan,11

72196   with contrast material(s)
🚑 11.5   ⚕ 11.5   **FUD** XXX   [03] [Z2] [80] ▭
AMA: 2015,Jan,16; 2014,Jan,11; 2012,Feb,9-10; 2012,Jan,15-42; 2011,Jan,11

72197   without contrast material(s), followed by contrast material(s) and further sequences
🚑 14.1   ⚕ 14.1   **FUD** XXX   [03] [Z2] [80] ▭
AMA: 2015,Jan,16; 2014,Jan,11; 2012,Feb,9-10

72198 Magnetic Resonance Angiography: Pelvis

CMS: 100-4,13,40.1.1 Magnetic Resonance Angiography; 100-4,13,40.1.2 HCPCS Coding Requirements; 100-4,4,250.16 Multiple Procedure Payment Reduction: Certain Diagnostic Imaging Procedures Rendered by Physicians

INCLUDES   Use of magnetic fields and radio waves to produce detailed cross-sectional images of internal body structures

72198   Magnetic resonance angiography, pelvis, with or without contrast material(s)
🚑 11.2   ⚕ 11.2   **FUD** XXX   [B] [80] ▭
AMA: 2015,Jan,16; 2014,Jan,11; 2012,Feb,9-10

72200-72220 Radiography: Pelvisacral

INCLUDES   Minimum number of views or more views when needed to adequately complete the study
Radiographs that have to be repeated during the encounter due to substandard quality; only one unit of service is reported

EXCLUDES   *Obtaining more films after review of initial films, based on the discretion of the radiologist, an order for the test, and a change in the patient's condition*
Do not report with second interpretation by the requesting physician (included in E&M service)

72200   Radiologic examination, sacroiliac joints; less than 3 views
🚑 0.79   ⚕ 0.79   **FUD** XXX   [01] [N1] [80]
AMA: 2014,Jan,11; 2012,Feb,9-10

72202   3 or more views
🚑 0.92   ⚕ 0.92   **FUD** XXX   [01] [N1] [80] ▭
AMA: 2014,Jan,11; 2012,Feb,9-10

72220   Radiologic examination, sacrum and coccyx, minimum of 2 views
🚑 0.78   ⚕ 0.78   **FUD** XXX   [01] [N1] [80]
AMA: 2014,Jan,11; 2012,Feb,9-10

72240-72270 Myelography with Contrast: Spinal Cord

CMS: 100-4,13,30.1.3.1 Payment for Low Osmolar Contrast Material

INCLUDES   Fluoroscopic guidance for subarachnoid puncture for diagnostic radiographic myelography (77003)
Code also injection for myelogram at C1-C2 when appropriate (61055)
Do not report with (62284, 62302-62305)

72240   Myelography, cervical, radiological supervision and interpretation
🚑 2.76   ⚕ 2.76   **FUD** XXX   [02] [N1] [80] ▭ [PQ]
AMA: 2015,Jan,16; 2014,Sep,3; 2014,Jan,11; 2012,Feb,9-10

72255   Myelography, thoracic, radiological supervision and interpretation
🚑 2.74   ⚕ 2.74   **FUD** XXX   [02] [N1] [80] ▭ [PQ]
AMA: 2015,Jan,16; 2014,Sep,3; 2014,Jan,11; 2012,Feb,9-10

72265   Myelography, lumbosacral, radiological supervision and interpretation
🚑 2.58   ⚕ 2.58   **FUD** XXX   [02] [N1] [80] ▭ [PQ]
AMA: 2015,Jan,16; 2014,Sep,3; 2014,Jan,11; 2012,Feb,9-10

72270   Myelography, 2 or more regions (eg, lumbar/thoracic, cervical/thoracic, lumbar/cervical, lumbar/thoracic/cervical), radiological supervision and interpretation
🚑 3.57   ⚕ 3.57   **FUD** XXX   [02] [N1] [80] ▭ [PQ]
AMA: 2015,Jan,16; 2014,Sep,3; 2014,Jan,11; 2012,Feb,9-10

72275 Radiography: Epidural Space

INCLUDES   Epidurogram, documentation of images, formal written report
Fluoroscopic guidance (77003)
Code also injection procedure as appropriate (62280-62282, 62310-62319, 64479-64484)
Do not report with (22586, 0195T-0196T, 0309T)

72275   Epidurography, radiological supervision and interpretation
🚑 3.24   ⚕ 3.24   **FUD** XXX   [N] [N1] ▭ [PQ]
AMA: 2015,Jan,16; 2014,Jan,11; 2012,Jul,3-6; 2012,Jun,12-13; 2012,Feb,9-10; 2012,Jan,15-42; 2011,Jan,11; 2010,May,9; 2010,Jan,12-15

72285 Radiography: Intervertebral Disc (Cervical/Thoracic)

CMS: 100-4,13,30.1.3.1 Payment for Low Osmolar Contrast Material
Code also discography injection procedure (62291)

72285   Discography, cervical or thoracic, radiological supervision and interpretation
🚑 3.21   ⚕ 3.21   **FUD** XXX   [02] [N1] [80] ▭ [PQ]
AMA: 2015,Jan,16; 2014,Jan,11; 2012,Feb,9-10; 2011,Mar,7

72295 Radiography: Intervertebral Disc (Lumbar)

CMS: 100-4,13,30.1.3.1 Payment for Low Osmolar Contrast Material
Code also discography injection procedure (62290)

72295   Discography, lumbar, radiological supervision and interpretation
🚑 2.75   ⚕ 2.75   **FUD** XXX   [02] [N1] [80] ▭ [PQ]
AMA: 2015,Jan,16; 2014,Jan,11; 2012,Jul,3-6; 2012,Feb,9-10; 2012,Jan,15-42; 2011,Mar,7; 2011,Jan,11

73000-73085 Radiography: Shoulder and Upper Arm

INCLUDES   Minimum number of views or more views when needed to adequately complete the study
Radiographs that have to be repeated during the encounter due to substandard quality; only one unit of service is reported

EXCLUDES   *Obtaining more films after review of initial films, based on the discretion of the radiologist, an order for the test, and a change in the patient's condition*
Stress views of upper body joint(s), when performed (77071)
Do not report with a second interpretation by the requesting physician (included in E&M service)

73000   Radiologic examination; clavicle, complete
🚑 0.78   ⚕ 0.78   **FUD** XXX   [01] [N1] [80]
AMA: 2014,Jan,11; 2012,Feb,9-10

● New Code   ▲ Revised Code   ○ Reinstated   Ⓜ Maternity   🅰 Age Edit   Unlisted   Not Covered   # Resequenced
⊘ AMA Mod 51 Exempt   ⑤ Optum Mod 51 Exempt   ⑥³ Mod 63 Exempt   ⊙ Mod Sedation   + Add-on   ▭ CCI   [PQ] PQRS   **FUD** Follow-up Days

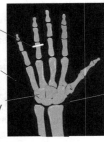
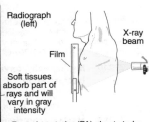

Gold wedding band absorbs all x-rays (white)

Radiograph (left)

X-ray beam

Film

Air allows all rays to reach film (black)

Calcium in bone absorbs most of rays and is nearly white

Soft tissues absorb part of rays and will vary in gray intensity

Posterioranterior (PA) chest study; lateral views also common

73010   **scapula, complete**
             0.84   0.84   **FUD** XXX   Q1 N1 80
             AMA: 2014,Jan,11; 2012,Feb,9-10

73020   **Radiologic examination, shoulder; 1 view**
             0.65   0.65   **FUD** XXX   Q1 N1 80
             AMA: 2014,Jan,11; 2012,Feb,9-10

73030   **complete, minimum of 2 views**
             0.81   0.81   **FUD** XXX   Q1 N1 80
             AMA: 2014,Jan,11; 2012,Feb,9-10

73040   **Radiologic examination, shoulder, arthrography, radiological supervision and interpretation**
             Code also arthrography injection procedure (23350)
             Do not report with (77002)
             2.82   2.82   **FUD** XXX   Q2 N1 80 P0
             AMA: 2015,Jan,16; 2014,Jan,11; 2012,Feb,9-10; 2012,Jan,15-42; 2011,Jan,11

73050   **Radiologic examination; acromioclavicular joints, bilateral, with or without weighted distraction**
             1.00   1.00   **FUD** XXX   Q1 N1 80
             AMA: 2014,Jan,11; 2012,Feb,9-10

73060   **humerus, minimum of 2 views**
             0.75   0.75   **FUD** XXX   Q1 N1 80
             AMA: 2014,Jan,11; 2012,Feb,9-10

73070   **Radiologic examination, elbow; 2 views**
             0.77   0.77   **FUD** XXX   Q1 N1 80
             AMA: 2015,Jan,16; 2014,Jan,11; 2012,Feb,9-10

73080   **complete, minimum of 3 views**
             0.88   0.88   **FUD** XXX   Q1 N1 80
             AMA: 2014,Jan,11; 2012,Feb,9-10

73085   **Radiologic examination, elbow, arthrography, radiological supervision and interpretation**
             Do not report with (77002)
             Code also arthrography injection procedure (24220)
             2.76   2.76   **FUD** XXX   Q2 N1 80 P0
             AMA: 2015,Jan,16; 2014,Jan,11; 2012,Feb,9-10

73090-73140 Radiography: Forearm and Hand

INCLUDES   Minimum number of views or more views when needed to adequately complete the study
           Radiographs that have to be repeated during the encounter due to substandard quality; only one unit of service is reported

EXCLUDES   *Obtaining more films after review of initial films, based on the discretion of the radiologist, an order for the test, and a change in the patient's condition*
           Stress views of upper body joint(s), when performed (77071)
           Do not report with a second interpretation by the requesting physician (included in E&M service)

73090   **Radiologic examination; forearm, 2 views**
             0.72   0.72   **FUD** XXX   Q1 N1 80
             AMA: 2015,Jan,16; 2014,Jan,11; 2012,Feb,9-10

73092   **upper extremity, infant, minimum of 2 views**   A
             0.76   0.76   **FUD** XXX   Q1 N1 80
             AMA: 2014,Jan,11; 2012,Feb,9-10

73100   **Radiologic examination, wrist; 2 views**
             0.82   0.82   **FUD** XXX   Q1 N1 80
             AMA: 2015,Jan,16; 2014,Jan,11; 2012,Feb,9-10

73110   **complete, minimum of 3 views**
             0.99   0.99   **FUD** XXX   Q1 N1 80
             AMA: 2015,Jan,16; 2014,Jan,11; 2012,Feb,9-10; 2012,Jan,15-42; 2011,Jan,11

73115   **Radiologic examination, wrist, arthrography, radiological supervision and interpretation**
             Code also arthrography injection procedure (25246)
             Do not report with (77002)
             3.00   3.00   **FUD** XXX   Q2 N1 80 P0
             AMA: 2015,Jan,16; 2014,Jan,11; 2012,Feb,9-10

73120   **Radiologic examination, hand; 2 views**
             0.73   0.73   **FUD** XXX   Q1 N1 80
             AMA: 2014,Jan,11; 2012,Feb,9-10

73130   **minimum of 3 views**
             0.85   0.85   **FUD** XXX   Q1 N1 80
             AMA: 2014,Jan,11; 2012,Feb,9-10

73140   **Radiologic examination, finger(s), minimum of 2 views**
             0.87   0.87   **FUD** XXX   Q1 N1 80
             AMA: 2015,Jan,16; 2014,Jan,11; 2012,Feb,9-10

73200-73202 Computerized Tomography: Shoulder, Arm, Hand

CMS: 100-4,4,250.16 Multiple Procedure Payment Reduction: Certain Diagnostic Imaging Procedures Rendered by Physicians

INCLUDES   Imaging using tomographic technique enhanced by computer imaging to create a cross-sectional plane of the body
           Intravascular, intrathecal, or intra-articular contrast materials when noted in code descriptor

EXCLUDES   *3D rendering (76376-76377)*

73200   **Computed tomography, upper extremity; without contrast material**
             5.01   5.01   **FUD** XXX   Q3 Z2 80
             AMA: 2015,Jan,16; 2014,Jan,11; 2012,Feb,9-10; 2012,Jan,15-42; 2011,Jul,16-17; 2011,Feb,8-9

73201   **with contrast material(s)**
             6.23   6.23   **FUD** XXX   Q3 Z2 80
             AMA: 2015,Aug,6; 2015,Jan,16; 2014,Jan,11; 2012,Feb,9-10; 2012,Jan,15-42; 2011,Jul,16-17

73202   **without contrast material, followed by contrast material(s) and further sections**
             7.78   7.78   **FUD** XXX   Q3 Z2 80
             AMA: 2014,Jan,11; 2012,Feb,9-10; 2011,Jul,16-17

73206 Computerized Tomographic Angiography: Shoulder, Arm, and Hand

CMS: 100-4,4,250.16 Multiple Procedure Payment Reduction: Certain Diagnostic Imaging Procedures Rendered by Physicians

INCLUDES   Intravascular, intrathecal, or intra-articular contrast materials when noted in code descriptor
           Multiple rapid thin section CT scans to create cross-sectional images of bones, organs and tissues

73206   **Computed tomographic angiography, upper extremity, with contrast material(s), including noncontrast images, if performed, and image postprocessing**
             9.15   9.15   **FUD** XXX   Q3 Z2 80
             AMA: 2015,Jan,16; 2014,Jan,11; 2012,Feb,9-10

73218-73223 Magnetic Resonance Imaging: Shoulder, Arm, Hand

CMS: 100-4,13,40 Magnetic Resonance Imaging (MRI); 100-4,4,250.16 Multiple Procedure Payment Reduction: Certain Diagnostic Imaging Procedures Rendered by Physicians

INCLUDES   Application of an external magnetic field that forces alignment of hydrogen atom nuclei in soft tissues which converts to sets of tomographic images that can be displayed as three-dimensional images
           Intravascular, intrathecal, or intra-articular contrast materials when noted in code descriptor

73218 Magnetic resonance (eg, proton) imaging, upper extremity, other than joint; without contrast material(s)

    📷 10.2   ⚕ 10.2   **FUD** XXX   Q3 Z2 80 ▣

    AMA: 2015,Jan,16; 2014,Jan,11; 2012,Feb,9-10; 2012,Jan,15-42; 2011,Feb,8-9; 2010,Sep,9

73219   with contrast material(s)

    📷 11.3   ⚕ 11.3   **FUD** XXX   Q3 Z2 80 ▣

    AMA: 2015,Jan,16; 2014,Jan,11; 2012,Feb,9-10; 2012,Jan,15-42; 2010,Sep,9

73220   without contrast material(s), followed by contrast material(s) and further sequences

    📷 14.0   ⚕ 14.0   **FUD** XXX   Q3 Z2 80 ▣

    AMA: 2015,Jan,16; 2014,Jan,11; 2012,Feb,9-10; 2010,Sep,9

73221 Magnetic resonance (eg, proton) imaging, any joint of upper extremity; without contrast material(s)

    📷 6.60   ⚕ 6.60   **FUD** XXX   Q3 Z2 80 ▣

    AMA: 2015,Jan,16; 2014,Jan,11; 2012,Feb,9-10; 2012,Jan,15-42; 2011,Feb,8-9; 2010,Sep,9

73222   with contrast material(s)

    📷 10.6   ⚕ 10.6   **FUD** XXX   Q3 Z2 80 ▣

    AMA: 2015,Aug,6; 2015,Jan,16; 2014,Jan,11; 2012,Feb,9-10; 2010,Sep,9

73223   without contrast material(s), followed by contrast material(s) and further sequences

    📷 13.1   ⚕ 13.1   **FUD** XXX   Q3 Z2 80 ▣

    AMA: 2015,Jan,16; 2014,Jan,11; 2012,Feb,9-10; 2010,Sep,9

73225 Magnetic Resonance Angiography: Shoulder, Arm, Hand

CMS: 100-4,13,40.1.1 Magnetic Resonance Angiography; 100-4,4,250.16 Multiple Procedure Payment Reduction: Certain Diagnostic Imaging Procedures Rendered by Physicians

INCLUDES   Intravascular, intrathecal, or intra-articular contrast materials when noted in code descriptor
Use of magnetic fields and radio waves to produce detailed cross-sectional images of internal body structures

73225 Magnetic resonance angiography, upper extremity, with or without contrast material(s)

    📷 11.3   ⚕ 11.3   **FUD** XXX   B 80

    AMA: 2015,Jan,16; 2014,Jan,11; 2012,Feb,9-10

73500-73552 Radiography: Pelvic Region and Thigh

EXCLUDES   Stress views of lower body joint(s), when performed (77071)

~~**73500** Radiologic examination, hip, unilateral; 1 view~~
    To report, see ~73501

● **73501** Radiologic examination, hip, unilateral, with pelvis when performed; 1 view

● **73502**   2-3 views

● **73503**   minimum of 4 views

~~**73510** complete, minimum of 2 views~~
    To report, see ~73502-73503

~~**73520** Radiologic examination, hips, bilateral, minimum of 2 views of each hip, including anteroposterior view of pelvis~~
    To report, see ~73521-73523

● **73521** Radiologic examination, hips, bilateral, with pelvis when performed; 2 views

● **73522**   3-4 views

● **73523**   minimum of 5 views

73525 Radiologic examination, hip, arthrography, radiological supervision and interpretation
    Do not report with (77002)

    📷 2.85   ⚕ 2.85   **FUD** XXX   Q2 N1 80 ▣ PQ

    AMA: 2015,Jan,16; 2014,Jan,11; 2012,Jun,14; 2012,Feb,9-10

~~**73530** Radiologic examination, hip, during operative procedure~~
    To report, see ~73501-73503

~~**73540** Radiologic examination, pelvis and hips, infant or child, minimum of 2 views~~
    To report, see ~73501-73503

~~**73550** Radiologic examination, femur, 2 views~~
    To report, see ~73551-73552

● **73551** Radiologic examination, femur; 1 view

● **73552**   minimum 2 views

73560-73660 Radiography: Lower Leg, Ankle, and Foot

EXCLUDES   Stress views of lower body joint(s), when performed (77071)

73560 Radiologic examination, knee; 1 or 2 views

    📷 0.82   ⚕ 0.82   **FUD** XXX   01 N1 80 ▣

    AMA: 2015,May,10; 2015,Feb,10; 2014,Jan,11; 2012,Feb,9-10

73562   3 views

    📷 0.96   ⚕ 0.96   **FUD** XXX   01 N1 80 ▣

    AMA: 2014,Jan,11; 2012,Feb,9-10

73564   complete, 4 or more views

    📷 1.12   ⚕ 1.12   **FUD** XXX   01 N1 80 ▣

    AMA: 2015,May,10; 2015,Feb,10; 2015,Jan,16; 2014,Jan,11; 2012,Feb,9-10; 2012,Jan,15-42; 2011,Jan,11

73565   both knees, standing, anteroposterior

    📷 0.92   ⚕ 0.92   **FUD** XXX   01 N1 80 ▣

    AMA: 2015,May,10; 2015,Feb,10; 2014,Jan,11; 2012,Feb,9-10

73580 Radiologic examination, knee, arthrography, radiological supervision and interpretation
    Do not report with (77002)

    📷 3.22   ⚕ 3.22   **FUD** XXX   02 N1 80 ▣ PQ

    AMA: 2015,Aug,6; 2015,Jan,16; 2014,Jan,11; 2012,Feb,9-10

73590 Radiologic examination; tibia and fibula, 2 views

    📷 0.74   ⚕ 0.74   **FUD** XXX   01 N1 80 ▣

    AMA: 2015,Jan,16; 2014,Jan,11; 2012,Feb,9-10

73592   lower extremity, infant, minimum of 2 views   ▲

    📷 0.76   ⚕ 0.76   **FUD** XXX   01 N1 80 ▣

    AMA: 2014,Jan,11; 2012,Feb,9-10

73600 Radiologic examination, ankle; 2 views

    📷 0.76   ⚕ 0.76   **FUD** XXX   01 N1 80 ▣

    AMA: 2015,Jan,16; 2014,Jan,11; 2012,Feb,9-10

73610   complete, minimum of 3 views

    📷 0.88   ⚕ 0.88   **FUD** XXX   01 N1 80 ▣

    AMA: 2015,Jan,16; 2014,Jan,11; 2012,Feb,9-10

73615 Radiologic examination, ankle, arthrography, radiological supervision and interpretation
    Do not report with (77002)

    📷 2.77   ⚕ 2.77   **FUD** XXX   02 N1 80 ▣ PQ

    AMA: 2015,Jan,16; 2014,Jan,11; 2012,Feb,9-10

73620 Radiologic examination, foot; 2 views

    📷 0.72   ⚕ 0.72   **FUD** XXX   01 N1 80 ▣

    AMA: 2015,Jan,16; 2014,Jan,11; 2012,Feb,9-10

73630   complete, minimum of 3 views

    📷 0.81   ⚕ 0.81   **FUD** XXX   01 N1 80 ▣

    AMA: 2014,Jan,11; 2012,Feb,9-10

73650 Radiologic examination; calcaneus, minimum of 2 views

    📷 0.75   ⚕ 0.75   **FUD** XXX   01 N1 80

    AMA: 2014,Jan,11; 2012,Feb,9-10

73660   toe(s), minimum of 2 views

    📷 0.78   ⚕ 0.78   **FUD** XXX   01 N1 80

    AMA: 2014,Jan,11; 2012,Feb,9-10

73700-73702 Computerized Tomography: Leg, Ankle, and Foot

CMS: 100-4,4,250.16 Multiple Procedure Payment Reduction: Certain Diagnostic Imaging Procedures Rendered by Physicians

EXCLUDES   3D rendering (76376-76377)

73700 Computed tomography, lower extremity; without contrast material

    📷 5.01   ⚕ 5.01   **FUD** XXX   Q3 Z2 80 ▣

    AMA: 2015,Jan,16; 2014,Jan,11; 2012,Feb,9-10; 2012,Jan,15-42; 2011,Jul,16-17

Radiology

73701   **with contrast material(s)**
    📷 6.32   ✂ 6.32   **FUD** XXX   03 Z2 80 ▢
    AMA: 2015,Jan,16; 2014,Jan,11; 2012,Feb,9-10; 2011,Jul,16-17

73702   **without contrast material, followed by contrast material(s) and further sections**
    📷 7.65   ✂ 7.65   **FUD** XXX   03 Z2 80 ▢
    AMA: 2015,Jan,16; 2014,Jan,11; 2012,Feb,9-10; 2011,Jul,16-17

73706 Computerized Tomographic Angiography: Leg, Ankle, and Foot

CMS: 100-4,4,250.16 Multiple Procedure Payment Reduction: Certain Diagnostic Imaging Procedures Rendered by Physicians

EXCLUDES   CT angiography for aorto-iliofemoral runoff (75635)

73706   **Computed tomographic angiography, lower extremity, with contrast material(s), including noncontrast images, if performed, and image postprocessing**
    📷 9.84   ✂ 9.84   **FUD** XXX   03 Z2 80 ▢
    AMA: 2015,Jan,16; 2014,Jan,11; 2012,Feb,9-10; 2012,Jan,15-42; 2011,Apr,12; 2011,Jan,11

73718-73723 Magnetic Resonance Imaging: Leg, Ankle, and Foot

CMS: 100-4,13,40 Magnetic Resonance Imaging (MRI); 100-4,4,250.16 Multiple Procedure Payment Reduction: Certain Diagnostic Imaging Procedures Rendered by Physicians

73718   **Magnetic resonance (eg, proton) imaging, lower extremity other than joint; without contrast material(s)**
    📷 10.2   ✂ 10.2   **FUD** XXX   03 Z2 80 ▢
    AMA: 2015,Jan,16; 2014,Jan,11; 2012,Feb,9-10

73719   **with contrast material(s)**
    📷 11.3   ✂ 11.3   **FUD** XXX   03 Z2 80 ▢
    AMA: 2015,Jan,16; 2014,Jan,11; 2012,Feb,9-10

73720   **without contrast material(s), followed by contrast material(s) and further sequences**
    📷 14.0   ✂ 14.0   **FUD** XXX   03 Z2 80 ▢
    AMA: 2015,Jan,16; 2014,Jan,11; 2012,Feb,9-10

73721   **Magnetic resonance (eg, proton) imaging, any joint of lower extremity; without contrast material**
    📷 6.59   ✂ 6.59   **FUD** XXX   03 Z2 80 ▢
    AMA: 2015,Jan,16; 2014,Jan,11; 2012,Feb,9-10; 2012,Jan,15-42; 2011,Jan,11

73722   **with contrast material(s)**
    📷 10.7   ✂ 10.7   **FUD** XXX   03 Z2 80 ▢
    AMA: 2015,Aug,6; 2015,Jan,16; 2014,Jan,11; 2012,Feb,9-10

73723   **without contrast material(s), followed by contrast material(s) and further sequences**
    📷 13.2   ✂ 13.2   **FUD** XXX   03 Z2 80 ▢
    AMA: 2015,Jan,16; 2014,Jan,11; 2012,Feb,9-10

73725 Magnetic Resonance Angiography: Leg, Ankle, and Foot

CMS: 100-4,13,40.1.2 HCPCS Coding Requirements; 100-4,4,250.16 Multiple Procedure Payment Reduction: Certain Diagnostic Imaging Procedures Rendered by Physicians

73725   **Magnetic resonance angiography, lower extremity, with or without contrast material(s)**
    📷 11.3   ✂ 11.3   **FUD** XXX   B 80 ▢
    AMA: 2015,Jan,16; 2014,Jan,11; 2012,Feb,9-10

74000-74022 Radiography: Abdomen--General

74000   **Radiologic examination, abdomen; single anteroposterior view**
    📷 0.66   ✂ 0.66   **FUD** XXX   01 N1 80
    AMA: 2014,Jan,11; 2012,Feb,9-10

74010   **anteroposterior and additional oblique and cone views**
    📷 0.98   ✂ 0.98   **FUD** XXX   01 N1 80 ▢
    AMA: 2015,Jan,16; 2014,Jun,14; 2014,Jan,11; 2012,Feb,9-10

74020   **complete, including decubitus and/or erect views**
    📷 1.04   ✂ 1.04   **FUD** XXX   01 N1 80 ▢
    AMA: 2014,Jan,11; 2012,Feb,9-10

74022   **complete acute abdomen series, including supine, erect, and/or decubitus views, single view chest**
    📷 1.23   ✂ 1.23   **FUD** XXX   01 N1 80 ▢
    AMA: 2014,Jan,11; 2012,Feb,9-10

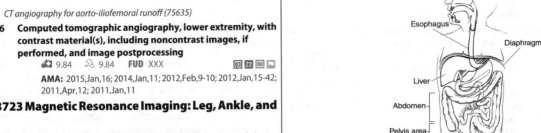

Esophagus — Diaphragm — Liver — Abdomen — Pelvis area

74150-74170 Computerized Tomography: Abdomen–General

CMS: 100-4,4,250.16 Multiple Procedure Payment Reduction: Certain Diagnostic Imaging Procedures Rendered by Physicians

EXCLUDES   3D rendering (76376-76377)
          Combined CT of abdomen and pelvis (74176-74178)
          CT colonography, diagnostic (74261-74262)
          CT colonography, screening (74263)
Do not report with CT colonography (74261-74263)

74150   **Computed tomography, abdomen; without contrast material**
    📷 4.20   ✂ 4.20   **FUD** XXX   03 Z2 80 ▢
    AMA: 2015,Jan,16; 2014,Jan,11; 2012,Oct,12; 2012,Feb,9-10; 2012,Jan,15-42; 2011,Jan,11; 2010,Apr,9

74160   **with contrast material(s)**
    📷 6.46   ✂ 6.46   **FUD** XXX   03 Z2 80 ▢
    AMA: 2015,Jan,16; 2014,Jan,11; 2012,Oct,12; 2012,Feb,9-10; 2010,Apr,9

74170   **without contrast material, followed by contrast material(s) and further sections**
    📷 7.35   ✂ 7.35   **FUD** XXX   03 Z2 80 ▢
    AMA: 2015,Jan,16; 2014,Jan,11; 2012,Oct,12; 2012,Feb,9-10; 2010,Apr,9

74174-74175 Computerized Tomographic Angiography: Abdomen and Pelvis

CMS: 100-4,4,250.16 Multiple Procedure Payment Reduction: Certain Diagnostic Imaging Procedures Rendered by Physicians

EXCLUDES   CT angiography for aorto-iliofemoral runoff (75635)

74174   **Computed tomographic angiography, abdomen and pelvis, with contrast material(s), including noncontrast images, if performed, and image postprocessing**
    Do not report with (72191, 73706, 74175, 75635, 76376-76377)
    📷 10.9   ✂ 10.9   **FUD** XXX   S Z2 80
    AMA: 2014,Jan,11; 2012,Feb,9-10

74175   **Computed tomographic angiography, abdomen, with contrast material(s), including noncontrast images, if performed, and image postprocessing**
    EXCLUDES   Combined CT angiography study of abdomen and pelvis (74174)
    Do not report with (72191, 73706, 75635)
    📷 8.60   ✂ 8.60   **FUD** XXX   03 Z2 80 ▢
    AMA: 2015,Jan,16; 2014,Jan,11; 2012,Feb,9-10; 2012,Jan,15-42; 2011,Apr,12

| 26/TC PC/TC Comp Only | A2-Z3 ASC Pmt | 50 Bilateral | ♂ Male Only | ♀ Female Only | 📷 Facility RVU | ✂ Non-Facility RVU |
| **AMA:** CPT Asst | **CMS:** Pub 100 | A-Y OPPSI | 80/180 Surg Assist Allowed / w/Doc | | ▣ Lab Crosswalk | ▣ Radiology Crosswalk |

288   Medicare (Red Text)   CPT © 2015 American Medical Association. All Rights Reserved. (Black Text)   © 2015 Optum360, LLC (Blue Text)

74176-74178 Computerized Tomography: Abdomen and Pelvis

CMS: 100-4,4,250.16 Multiple Procedure Payment Reduction: Certain Diagnostic Imaging Procedures Rendered by Physicians

Do not report more than one time for each combined examination of the abdomen and pelvis

Do not report with (72192-72194, 74150-74170)

74176 Computed tomography, abdomen and pelvis; without contrast material

🚑 5.62 ⚖ 5.62 **FUD** XXX

[Q3] [Z3]

AMA: 2015,Jan,16; 2014,Jan,11; 2012,Feb,9-10

74177 with contrast material(s)

🚑 8.74 ⚖ 8.74 **FUD** XXX

[Q3] [Z2]

AMA: 2015,Jan,16; 2014,Jan,11; 2012,Feb,9-10

74178 without contrast material in one or both body regions, followed by contrast material(s) and further sections in one or both body regions

🚑 9.89 ⚖ 9.89 **FUD** XXX

[Q3] [Z2]

AMA: 2015,Jan,16; 2014,Jan,11; 2012,Feb,9-10

74181-74183 Magnetic Resonance Imaging: Abdomen–General

CMS: 100-4,13,40 Magnetic Resonance Imaging (MRI); 100-4,4,250.16 Multiple Procedure Payment Reduction: Certain Diagnostic Imaging Procedures Rendered by Physicians

74181 Magnetic resonance (eg, proton) imaging, abdomen; without contrast material(s)

🚑 9.32 ⚖ 9.32 **FUD** XXX

[Q3] [Z2] [80] ▭

AMA: 2015,Jan,16; 2014,Jan,11; 2012,Feb,9-10; 2012,Jan,15-42; 2011,Jan,11

74182 with contrast material(s)

🚑 12.7 ⚖ 12.7 **FUD** XXX

[Q3] [Z2] [80] ▭

AMA: 2015,Jan,16; 2014,Jan,11; 2012,Feb,9-10; 2012,Jan,15-42; 2011,Jan,11

74183 without contrast material(s), followed by with contrast material(s) and further sequences

🚑 14.2 ⚖ 14.2 **FUD** XXX

[Q3] [Z2] [80] ▭

AMA: 2015,Jan,16; 2014,Jan,11; 2012,Feb,9-10

74185 Magnetic Resonance Angiography: Abdomen–General

CMS: 100-4,13,40.1.1 Magnetic Resonance Angiography; 100-4,13,40.1.2 HCPCS Coding Requirements; 100-4,4,250.16 Multiple Procedure Payment Reduction: Certain Diagnostic Imaging Procedures Rendered by Physicians

74185 Magnetic resonance angiography, abdomen, with or without contrast material(s)

🚑 11.3 ⚖ 11.3 **FUD** XXX

[B] [80] ▭

AMA: 2015,Jan,16; 2014,Jan,11; 2012,Feb,9-10

74190 Peritoneography

74190 Peritoneogram (eg, after injection of air or contrast), radiological supervision and interpretation

EXCLUDES Computed tomography, pelvis or abdomen (72192, 74150)

Code also injection procedure (49400)

🚑 0.00 ⚖ 0.00 **FUD** XXX

[02] [N1] [80] ▭ [PQ]

AMA: 2015,Jan,16; 2014,Jan,11; 2012,Feb,9-10; 2012,Jan,15-42; 2011,Jan,11; 2010,Dec,12

74210-74235 Radiography: Throat and Esophagus

EXCLUDES Percutaneous placement of gastrostomy tube, endoscopic (43246)
Percutaneous placement of gastrostomy tube, fluoroscopic guidance (49440)

74210 Radiologic examination; pharynx and/or cervical esophagus

🚑 2.17 ⚖ 2.17 **FUD** XXX

[S] [Z2] [80] [PQ]

AMA: 2014,Jan,11; 2012,Feb,9-10

74220 esophagus

🚑 2.48 ⚖ 2.48 **FUD** XXX

[S] [Z2] [80] ▭ [PQ]

AMA: 2014,Jan,11; 2012,Feb,9-10

74230 Swallowing function, with cineradiography/videoradiography

🚑 3.60 ⚖ 3.60 **FUD** XXX

[S] [Z2] [80] ▭ [PQ]

AMA: 2015,Jan,16; 2014,Jul,5; 2014,Jan,11; 2012,Feb,9-10

74235 Removal of foreign body(s), esophageal, with use of balloon catheter, radiological supervision and interpretation

Code also procedure (43499)

🚑 0.00 ⚖ 0.00 **FUD** XXX

[N] [N1] [80] ▭ [PQ]

AMA: 2014,Jan,11; 2012,Feb,9-10

74240-74283 Radiography: Intestines

EXCLUDES Percutaneous placement of gastrostomy tube, endoscopic (43246)
Percutaneous placement of gastrostomy tube, fluoroscopic guidance (49440)

▲ **74240** Radiologic examination, gastrointestinal tract, upper; with or without delayed images, without KUB

🚑 3.19 ⚖ 3.19 **FUD** XXX

[S] [Z3] [80] ▭ [PQ]

AMA: 2014,Jan,11; 2012,Feb,9-10

▲ **74241** with or without delayed images, with KUB

🚑 3.29 ⚖ 3.29 **FUD** XXX

[S] [Z3] [80] ▭ [PQ]

AMA: 2014,Jan,11; 2012,Feb,9-10

▲ **74245** with small intestine, includes multiple serial images

🚑 4.80 ⚖ 4.80 **FUD** XXX

[S] [Z2] [80] ▭ [PQ]

AMA: 2014,Jan,11; 2012,Feb,9-10

▲ **74246** Radiological examination, gastrointestinal tract, upper, air contrast, with specific high density barium, effervescent agent, with or without glucagon; with or without delayed images, without KUB

INCLUDES Moynihan test

🚑 3.59 ⚖ 3.59 **FUD** XXX

[S] [Z2] [80] ▭ [PQ]

AMA: 2014,Jan,11; 2012,Feb,9-10

▲ **74247** with or without delayed images, with KUB

🚑 3.95 ⚖ 3.95 **FUD** XXX

[S] [Z2] [80] ▭ [PQ]

AMA: 2014,Jan,11; 2012,Feb,9-10

74249 with small intestine follow-through

🚑 5.14 ⚖ 5.14 **FUD** XXX

[S] [Z2] [80] ▭ [PQ]

AMA: 2014,Jan,11; 2012,Feb,9-10

▲ **74250** Radiologic examination, small intestine, includes multiple serial images;

🚑 2.92 ⚖ 2.92 **FUD** XXX

[S] [Z2] [80] ▭ [PQ]

AMA: 2014,Jan,11; 2012,Feb,9-10

▲ **74251** via enteroclysis tube

🚑 11.7 ⚖ 11.7 **FUD** XXX

[S] [Z2] [80] ▭ [PQ]

AMA: 2014,Jan,11; 2012,Feb,9-10

74260 Duodenography, hypotonic

🚑 9.80 ⚖ 9.80 **FUD** XXX

[S] [Z2] [80] ▭ [PQ]

AMA: 2014,Jan,11; 2012,Feb,9-10

74261 Computed tomographic (CT) colonography, diagnostic, including image postprocessing; without contrast material

Do not report with (72192-72194, 74150-74170, 74263, 76376-76377)

🚑 13.6 ⚖ 13.6 **FUD** XXX

[Q3] [Z2] [80]

AMA: 2015,Jan,16; 2014,Jan,11; 2012,Feb,9-10; 2010,Apr,6-8; 2010,Apr,9

74262 with contrast material(s) including non-contrast images, if performed

Do not report with (72192-72194, 74150-74170, 74263, 76376-76377)

🚑 15.2 ⚖ 15.2 **FUD** XXX

[Q3] [Z2] [80]

AMA: 2015,Jan,16; 2014,Jan,11; 2012,Feb,9-10; 2010,Apr,6-8; 2010,Apr,9

74263 Computed tomographic (CT) colonography, screening, including image postprocessing

Do not report with (72192-72194, 74150-74170, 74261-74262, 76376-76377)

🚑 21.1 ⚖ 21.1 **FUD** XXX

[E]

AMA: 2015,Jan,16; 2014,Jan,11; 2012,Feb,9-10; 2010,Apr,6-8; 2010,Apr,9

Radiology

74270 — 74450

74270 Radiologic examination, colon; contrast (eg, barium) enema, with or without KUB
📷 4.20 ⚕ 4.20 **FUD** XXX [S][Z2][80][💻][PQ]
AMA: 2015,Jan,16; 2014,Jan,11; 2012,Feb,9-10; 2012,Jan,15-42; 2011,Jan,11

74280 air contrast with specific high density barium, with or without glucagon
📷 5.95 ⚕ 5.95 **FUD** XXX [S][Z2][80][💻][PQ]
AMA: 2014,Jan,11; 2012,Feb,9-10

74283 Therapeutic enema, contrast or air, for reduction of intussusception or other intraluminal obstruction (eg, meconium ileus)
📷 5.82 ⚕ 5.82 **FUD** XXX [S][Z2][80][PQ]
AMA: 2014,Jan,11; 2012,Feb,9-10

74290-74330 Radiography: Biliary Tract

74290 Cholecystography, oral contrast
📷 1.96 ⚕ 1.96 **FUD** XXX [S][Z2][80][PQ]
AMA: 2014,Jan,11; 2012,Feb,9-10

74300 Cholangiography and/or pancreatography; intraoperative, radiological supervision and interpretation
📷 0.00 ⚕ 0.00 **FUD** XXX [N][N1][80][💻][PQ]
AMA: 2015,Jan,16; 2014,Jan,11; 2012,Feb,9-10; 2012,Jan,15-42; 2011,Jan,11

+ 74301 additional set intraoperative, radiological supervision and interpretation (List separately in addition to code for primary procedure)
Code first (74300)
📷 0.00 ⚕ 0.00 **FUD** ZZZ [N][N1][80][💻]
AMA: 2014,Jan,11; 2012,Feb,9-10

74305 ~~through existing catheter, radiological supervision and interpretation~~
To report, see ~47531

74320 ~~Cholangiography, percutaneous, transhepatic, radiological supervision and interpretation~~
To report, see ~47532

74327 ~~Postoperative biliary duct calculus removal, percutaneous via T-tube tract, basket, or snare (eg, Burhenne technique), radiological supervision and interpretation~~
To report, see ~47544

74328 Endoscopic catheterization of the biliary ductal system, radiological supervision and interpretation
Code also ERCP (43260-43270 [43274, 43275, 43276, 43277, 43278])
📷 0.00 ⚕ 0.00 **FUD** XXX [N][N1][80][💻][PQ]
AMA: 2015,Jan,16; 2014,Jan,11; 2012,Feb,9-10; 2012,Jan,15-42; 2011,Jan,11

74329 Endoscopic catheterization of the pancreatic ductal system, radiological supervision and interpretation
Code also ERCP (43260-43270 [43274, 43275, 43276, 43277, 43278])
📷 0.00 ⚕ 0.00 **FUD** XXX [N][N1][80][💻][PQ]
AMA: 2014,Jan,11; 2012,Feb,9-10

74330 Combined endoscopic catheterization of the biliary and pancreatic ductal systems, radiological supervision and interpretation
Code also ERCP (43260-43270 [43274, 43275, 43276, 43277, 43278])
📷 0.00 ⚕ 0.00 **FUD** XXX [N][N1][80][💻][PQ]
AMA: 2014,Jan,11; 2012,Feb,9-10

74340-74363 Radiography: Bilidigestive Intubation

EXCLUDES *Percutaneous insertion of gastrostomy tube, endoscopic (43246)*
Percutaneous placement of gastrotomy tube, fluoroscopic guidance (49440)

▲ 74340 Introduction of long gastrointestinal tube (eg, Miller-Abbott), including multiple fluoroscopies and images, radiological supervision and interpretation
Code also placement of tube (44500)
📷 0.00 ⚕ 0.00 **FUD** XXX [N][N1][80][💻][PQ]
AMA: 2014,Jan,11; 2012,Feb,9-10

74355 Percutaneous placement of enteroclysis tube, radiological supervision and interpretation
INCLUDES Fluoroscopic guidance (77002)
📷 0.00 ⚕ 0.00 **FUD** XXX [N][N1][80][💻][PQ]
AMA: 2015,Jan,16; 2014,Jan,11; 2012,Feb,9-10; 2011,Jan,8; 2010,Nov,1; 2010,Nov,3

74360 Intraluminal dilation of strictures and/or obstructions (eg, esophagus), radiological supervision and interpretation
Do not report with (43213-43214, 43233)
📷 0.00 ⚕ 0.00 **FUD** XXX [N][N1][80][💻][PQ]
AMA: 2015,Jan,16; 2014,Jan,11; 2012,Feb,9-10

74363 Percutaneous transhepatic dilation of biliary duct stricture with or without placement of stent, radiological supervision and interpretation
EXCLUDES Surgical procedure (47555-47556)
📷 0.00 ⚕ 0.00 **FUD** XXX [N][N1][80][💻][PQ]
AMA: 2014,Jan,11; 2012,Feb,9-10

74400-74775 Radiography: Urogenital

74400 Urography (pyelography), intravenous, with or without KUB, with or without tomography
📷 3.06 ⚕ 3.06 **FUD** XXX [S][Z2][80][💻]
AMA: 2014,Jan,11; 2012,Feb,9-10

74410 Urography, infusion, drip technique and/or bolus technique;
📷 2.98 ⚕ 2.98 **FUD** XXX [S][Z2][80][💻]
AMA: 2014,Jan,11; 2012,Feb,9-10

74415 with nephrotomography
📷 3.82 ⚕ 3.82 **FUD** XXX [S][Z2][80][💻]
AMA: 2014,Jan,11; 2012,Feb,9-10

74420 Urography, retrograde, with or without KUB
📷 0.00 ⚕ 0.00 **FUD** XXX [S][Z2][80][💻]
AMA: 2015,Jan,16; 2014,Jan,11; 2012,Feb,9-10; 2012,Jan,15-42; 2011,Jan,11; 2010,Dec,12

74425 Urography, antegrade (pyelostogram, nephrostogram, loopogram), radiological supervision and interpretation
Do not report with ([50430, 50431, 50432, 50433, 50434, 50435], 50693-50695)
📷 0.00 ⚕ 0.00 **FUD** XXX [02][N1][80][💻][PQ]
AMA: 2015,Jan,16; 2014,Jan,11; 2012,Feb,9-10

74430 Cystography, minimum of 3 views, radiological supervision and interpretation
📷 1.04 ⚕ 1.04 **FUD** XXX [02][N1][80][💻][PQ]
AMA: 2014,Jan,11; 2012,Feb,9-10

74440 Vasography, vesiculography, or epididymography, radiological supervision and interpretation ♂
📷 2.23 ⚕ 2.23 **FUD** XXX [02][N1][80][💻][PQ]
AMA: 2014,Jan,11; 2012,Feb,9-10

74445 Corpora cavernosography, radiological supervision and interpretation ♂
INCLUDES Needle placement with fluoroscopic guidance (77002)
📷 0.00 ⚕ 0.00 **FUD** XXX [02][N1][80][💻][PQ]
AMA: 2015,Jan,16; 2014,Jan,11; 2012,Feb,9-10; 2011,Jan,8; 2010,Nov,1; 2010,Nov,3

74450 Urethrocystography, retrograde, radiological supervision and interpretation
📷 0.00 ⚕ 0.00 **FUD** XXX [02][N1][80][💻][PQ]
AMA: 2014,Jan,11; 2012,Feb,9-10

Radiology

74455 **Urethrocystography, voiding, radiological supervision and interpretation**
    2.28   2.28   **FUD** XXX   02 N1 80 PQ
    AMA: 2014,Jan,11; 2012,Feb,9-10

74470 **Radiologic examination, renal cyst study, translumbar, contrast visualization, radiological supervision and interpretation**
    INCLUDES   Needle placement with fluoroscopic guidance (77002)
    0.00   0.00   **FUD** XXX   02 N1 80 PQ
    AMA: 2015,Jan,16; 2014,Jan,11; 2012,Feb,9-10; 2011,Jan,8; 2010,Nov,1; 2010,Nov,3

74475 ~~Introduction of intracatheter or catheter into renal pelvis for drainage and/or injection, percutaneous, radiological supervision and interpretation~~
    To report, see ~[50432, 50433, 50434, 50435], 50606, 50693-50695

74480 ~~Introduction of ureteral catheter or stent into ureter through renal pelvis for drainage and/or injection, percutaneous, radiological supervision and interpretation~~
    To report, see ~[50432, 50433, 50434, 50435], 50606, 50693-50695

74485 **Dilation of nephrostomy, ureters, or urethra, radiological supervision and interpretation**
    EXCLUDES   Change of pyelostomy/nephrostomy tube ([50435])
             Ureter dilation without radiologic guidance (52341, 52344)
    2.57   2.57   **FUD** XXX   02 N1 80 PQ
    AMA: 2015,Jan,16; 2014,Jan,11; 2012,Feb,9-10; 2012,Jan,15-42; 2011,Jan,11

74710 **Pelvimetry, with or without placental localization** ♀
    EXCLUDES   Imaging procedures on abdomen and pelvis (72170-72190, 74000-74170)
    1.12   1.12   **FUD** XXX   01 N1 80
    AMA: 2014,Jan,11; 2012,Feb,9-10

● **74712** **Magnetic resonance (eg, proton) imaging, fetal, including placental and maternal pelvic imaging when performed; single or first gestation**
    EXCLUDES   Imaging of maternal pelvis or placenta without fetal imaging (72195-72197)
    Do not report with (72195-72197)

● + **74713** **each additional gestation (List separately in addition to code for primary procedure)**
    0.00   0.00   **FUD** 000
    EXCLUDES   Imaging of maternal pelvis or placent without fetal imaging (72195-72197)
    Code first (74712)
    Do not report with (72195-72197)

74740 **Hysterosalpingography, radiological supervision and interpretation** ♀
    EXCLUDES   Imaging procedures on abdomen and pelvis (72170-72190, 74000-74170)
    Code also injection of saline/contrast (58340)
    2.11   2.11   **FUD** XXX   02 N1 80 PQ
    AMA: 2015,Jan,16; 2014,Jan,11; 2012,Feb,9-10; 2012,Jan,15-42; 2011,Jan,11

Tube   Contrast

Ovary

Delivery apparatus

Uterus

Cervix

Vaginal canal

Hysterosalpingography (imaging of the uterus and tubes) is performed. Report for radiological supervision and interpretation

74742 **Transcervical catheterization of fallopian tube, radiological supervision and interpretation** ♀
    EXCLUDES   Imaging procedures on abdomen and pelvis (72170-72190, 74000-74170)
    Code also (58345)
    0.00   0.00   **FUD** XXX   N N1 80 PQ
    AMA: 2015,Jan,16; 2014,Jan,11; 2012,Feb,9-10

74775 **Perineogram (eg, vaginogram, for sex determination or extent of anomalies)** M ♀
    EXCLUDES   Imaging procedures on abdomen and pelvis (72170-72190, 74000-74170)
    0.00   0.00   **FUD** XXX   S Z2 80
    AMA: 2014,Jan,11; 2012,Feb,9-10

75557-75565 Magnetic Resonance Imaging: Heart Structure and Physiology

CMS: 100-4,13,40 Magnetic Resonance Imaging (MRI)
INCLUDES   Physiologic evaluation of cardiac function
EXCLUDES   Cardiac catheterization procedures (93451-93572)
Code also separate vascular injection (36000-36299)
Do not report more than one code in this group per session
Do not report with (76376-76377)

75557 **Cardiac magnetic resonance imaging for morphology and function without contrast material;**
    8.92   8.92   **FUD** XXX   03 Z2 80
    AMA: 2015,Jan,16; 2014,Jan,11; 2012,Feb,9-10; 2010,Jul,7-8

75559 **with stress imaging**
    INCLUDES   Pharmacologic wall motion stress evaluation without contrast
    Code also stress testing when performed (93015-93018)
    12.1   12.1   **FUD** XXX   03 Z2 80
    AMA: 2015,Jan,16; 2014,Jan,11; 2012,Feb,9-10; 2010,Jul,7-8

75561 **Cardiac magnetic resonance imaging for morphology and function without contrast material(s), followed by contrast material(s) and further sequences;**
    11.9   11.9   **FUD** XXX   03 Z2 80
    AMA: 2015,Jan,16; 2014,Jan,11; 2012,Feb,9-10; 2010,Jul,7-8

75563 **with stress imaging**
    INCLUDES   Pharmacologic perfusion stress evaluation with contrast
    Code also stress testing when performed (93015-93018)
    14.1   14.1   **FUD** XXX   03 Z3 80
    AMA: 2015,Jan,16; 2014,Jan,11; 2012,Feb,9-10; 2010,Jul,7-8

74455 — 75563

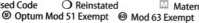
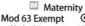

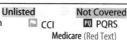

+ **75565** Cardiac magnetic resonance imaging for velocity flow mapping (List separately in addition to code for primary procedure)

Code first (75557, 75559, 75561, 75563)

⚕ 1.55   ⚕ 1.55   **FUD** ZZZ   N N1 80

AMA: 2015,Jan,16; 2014,Jan,11; 2012,Feb,9-10; 2010,Jul,7-8

75571-75574 Computed Tomographic Imaging: Heart

CMS: 100-4,4,250.16 Multiple Procedure Payment Reduction: Certain Diagnostic Imaging Procedures Rendered by Physicians

Do not report more than one code in this group per session
Do not report with (76376-76377)

75571 Computed tomography, heart, without contrast material, with quantitative evaluation of coronary calcium

⚕ 2.82   ⚕ 2.82   **FUD** XXX   Q1 N1 80

AMA: 2015,Jan,16; 2014,Jan,11; 2012,Feb,9-10; 2010,Jul,7-8

75572 Computed tomography, heart, with contrast material, for evaluation of cardiac structure and morphology (including 3D image postprocessing, assessment of cardiac function, and evaluation of venous structures, if performed)

⚕ 7.98   ⚕ 7.98   **FUD** XXX   S Z2 80

AMA: 2015,Jan,16; 2014,Jan,11; 2012,Feb,9-10; 2010,Jul,7-8

75573 Computed tomography, heart, with contrast material, for evaluation of cardiac structure and morphology in the setting of congenital heart disease (including 3D image postprocessing, assessment of LV cardiac function, RV structure and function and evaluation of venous structures, if performed)

⚕ 10.9   ⚕ 10.9   **FUD** XXX   S Z2 80

AMA: 2015,Jan,16; 2014,Jan,11; 2012,Feb,9-10; 2010,Jul,7-8

75574 Computed tomographic angiography, heart, coronary arteries and bypass grafts (when present), with contrast material, including 3D image postprocessing (including evaluation of cardiac structure and morphology, assessment of cardiac function, and evaluation of venous structures, if performed)

⚕ 11.7   ⚕ 11.7   **FUD** XXX   S Z2 80

AMA: 2015,Jan,16; 2014,Jan,11; 2012,Feb,9-10; 2010,Jul,7-8

75600-75791 Radiography: Arterial

INCLUDES Diagnostic angiography specifically included in the interventional code description
The following diagnostic procedures with interventional supervision and interpretation:
Angiography
Contrast injection
Fluoroscopic guidance for intervention
Post-angioplasty/atherectomy/stent angiography
Roadmapping
Vessel measurement

EXCLUDES Catheterization codes for diagnostic angiography of lower extremity when an access site other than the site used for the therapy is required
Diagnostic angiogram during a separate encounter from the interventional procedure
Diagnostic angiography with interventional procedure if:
1. No previous catheter-based angiogram is accessible and a complete diagnostic procedure is performed and the decision to proceed with an interventional procedure is based on the diagnostic service, OR
2. The previous diagnostic angiogram is accessible but the documentation in the medical record specifies that:
   A. the patient's condition has changed
   B. there is insufficient imaging of the patient's anatomy and/or disease, OR
   C. there is a clinical change during the procedure that necessitates a new examination away from the site of the intervention
3. Modifier 59 is appended to the code(s) for the diagnostic radiological supervision and interpretation service to indicate the guidelines were met
Intra-arterial procedures (36100-36248)
Intravenous procedures (36000, 36005-36015)

75600 Aortography, thoracic, without serialography, radiological supervision and interpretation

EXCLUDES Supravalvular aortography (93567)

⚕ 5.62   ⚕ 5.62   **FUD** XXX   Q2 N1 80

AMA: 2014,Jan,11; 2012,Feb,9-10

75605 Aortography, thoracic, by serialography, radiological supervision and interpretation

EXCLUDES Supravalvular aortography (93567)

⚕ 3.92   ⚕ 3.92   **FUD** XXX   Q2 N1 80 PO

AMA: 2015,Jan,16; 2014,Jan,11; 2013,Jan,6-8; 2012,Feb,9-10; 2012,Jan,15-42; 2011,Jan,11

75625 Aortography, abdominal, by serialography, radiological supervision and interpretation

EXCLUDES Supravalvular aortography (93567)

⚕ 3.92   ⚕ 3.92   **FUD** XXX   Q2 N1 80 PO

AMA: 2015,Jan,16; 2014,Jan,11; 2013,Feb,16-17; 2013,Jan,6-8; 2012,Feb,9-10; 2012,Jan,15-42; 2011,Jul,3-11; 2011,Jan,11

75630 Aortography, abdominal plus bilateral iliofemoral lower extremity, catheter, by serialography, radiological supervision and interpretation

EXCLUDES Supravalvular aortography (93567)

⚕ 4.85   ⚕ 4.85   **FUD** XXX   Q2 N1 80 PO

AMA: 2015,Jan,16; 2014,Jan,11; 2012,Feb,9-10; 2012,Jan,15-42; 2011,Jul,3-11; 2011,Jan,11

75635 Computed tomographic angiography, abdominal aorta and bilateral iliofemoral lower extremity runoff, with contrast material(s), including noncontrast images, if performed, and image postprocessing

Do not report with (72191, 73706, 74174-74175, 76376-76377)

⚕ 10.6   ⚕ 10.6   **FUD** XXX   Q2 N1 80

AMA: 2015,Jan,16; 2014,Jan,11; 2012,Feb,9-10; 2012,Jan,15-42; 2011,Apr,12

75658 Angiography, brachial, retrograde, radiological supervision and interpretation

⚕ 4.70   ⚕ 4.70   **FUD** XXX   Q2 N1 80 PO

AMA: 2014,Jan,11; 2012,Feb,9-10

75705 Angiography, spinal, selective, radiological supervision and interpretation

⚕ 6.64   ⚕ 6.64   **FUD** XXX   Q2 N1 80 PO

AMA: 2014,Jan,11; 2012,Feb,9-10

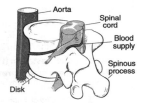

An angiography of a specific area of the spine is performed

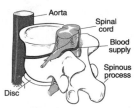

Angiography of a specific area of the spine is performed

75710 Angiography, extremity, unilateral, radiological supervision and interpretation

⚕ 4.53   ⚕ 4.53   **FUD** XXX   Q2 N1 80 PO

AMA: 2015,Jan,16; 2014,Jan,11; 2012,Feb,9-10; 2012,Jan,15-42; 2011,Jan,11

75716 Angiography, extremity, bilateral, radiological supervision and interpretation

⚕ 5.25   ⚕ 5.25   **FUD** XXX   Q2 N1 80 PO

AMA: 2015,Jan,16; 2014,Jan,11; 2012,Feb,9-10; 2012,Jan,15-42; 2011,Jan,11

75726 Angiography, visceral, selective or supraselective (with or without flush aortogram), radiological supervision and interpretation

> EXCLUDES Selective angiography, each additional visceral vessel examined after basic examination (75774)

4.23 4.23 **FUD** XXX [02] [N1] [80] [🖳] [PQ]

AMA: 2014,Jan,11; 2012,Feb,9-10

75731 Angiography, adrenal, unilateral, selective, radiological supervision and interpretation

4.80 4.80 **FUD** XXX [02] [N1] [80] [🖳] [PQ]

AMA: 2014,Jan,11; 2012,Feb,9-10

75733 Angiography, adrenal, bilateral, selective, radiological supervision and interpretation

5.14 5.14 **FUD** XXX [02] [N1] [80] [🖳] [PQ]

AMA: 2014,Jan,11; 2012,Feb,9-10

75736 Angiography, pelvic, selective or supraselective, radiological supervision and interpretation

4.59 4.59 **FUD** XXX [02] [N1] [80] [🖳] [PQ]

AMA: 2014,Jan,11; 2012,Feb,9-10

75741 Angiography, pulmonary, unilateral, selective, radiological supervision and interpretation

4.28 4.28 **FUD** XXX [02] [N1] [80] [🖳] [PQ]

AMA: 2015,Jan,16; 2014,Jan,11; 2013,Jan,6-8; 2012,Feb,9-10; 2012,Mar,9-10

75743 Angiography, pulmonary, bilateral, selective, radiological supervision and interpretation

4.79 4.79 **FUD** XXX [02] [N1] [80] [🖳] [PQ]

AMA: 2015,Jan,16; 2014,Jan,11; 2013,Jan,6-8; 2012,Feb,9-10

75746 Angiography, pulmonary, by nonselective catheter or venous injection, radiological supervision and interpretation

> EXCLUDES Nonselective injection procedure or catheter introduction with cardiac cath (93568)

4.31 4.31 **FUD** XXX [02] [N1] [80] [🖳] [PQ]

AMA: 2014,Jan,11; 2012,Feb,9-10

75756 Angiography, internal mammary, radiological supervision and interpretation

> EXCLUDES Internal mammary angiography with cardiac cath (93455, 93457, 93459, 93461, 93564)

4.78 4.78 **FUD** XXX [02] [N1] [80] [🖳] [PQ]

AMA: 2015,Jan,16; 2014,Jan,11; 2012,Feb,9-10; 2011,Dec,9-12

+ 75774 Angiography, selective, each additional vessel studied after basic examination, radiological supervision and interpretation (List separately in addition to code for primary procedure)

> EXCLUDES Angiography (36147, 75600-75756, 75791)
> Cardiac cath procedures (93452-93462, 93531-93533, 93563-93568)
> Catheterizations (36215-36248)

Code first diagnostic angiography of upper extremities and other vascular beds (except cervicocerebral vessels)

Code first initial vessel

Do not report with intracranial and extracranial cervicocerebral diagnostic angiography (36221-36228)

2.47 2.47 **FUD** ZZZ [N] [N1] [80] [🖳]

AMA: 2015,Jan,16; 2014,Jan,11; 2013,Oct,18; 2013,Jun,12; 2013,May,3-5; 2013,Feb,16-17; 2012,Feb,9-10; 2012,Jan,15-42; 2011,Apr,12; 2011,Jan,11

75791 Angiography, arteriovenous shunt (eg, dialysis patient fistula/graft), complete evaluation of dialysis access, including fluoroscopy, image documentation and report (includes injections of contrast and all necessary imaging from the arterial anastomosis and adjacent artery through entire venous outflow including the inferior or superior vena cava), radiological supervision and interpretation

> INCLUDES Radiological evaluation performed via existing access into the shunt or from an access that is not a direct puncture of the shunt

> EXCLUDES Catheter introduction, when performed (36140, 36215-36217, 36245-36247)
> Radiological evaluation with introduction of needle/catheter, AV dialysis shunt, complete procedure (36147)

Do not report with (36147-36148)

9.00 9.00 **FUD** XXX [02] [N1] [80] [PQ]

AMA: 2015,Jan,16; 2014,Jan,11; 2012,Feb,9-10; 2012,Apr,3-9; 2012,Jan,15-42; 2011,Dec,14-18; 2010,Mar,3

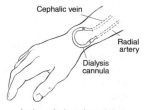

Angiography is performed on an arteriovenous shunt, such as is used in dialysis.

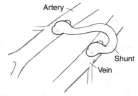

Shunts may be placed for a variety of conditions and are checked radiologically for patency and blood flow

75801-75893 Radiography: Lymphatic and Venous

> INCLUDES Diagnostic venography specifically included in the interventional code description
> The following diagnostic procedures with interventional supervision and interpretation:
> Contrast injection
> Fluoroscopic guidance for intervention
> Post-angioplasty/venography
> Roadmapping
> Venography
> Vessel measurement

> EXCLUDES Diagnostic venogram during a separate encounter from the interventional procedure
> Diagnostic venography with interventional procedure if:
> 1. No previous catheter-based venogram is accessible and a complete diagnostic procedure is performed and the decision to proceed with an interventional procedure is based on the diagnostic service, OR
> 2. The previous diagnostic venogram is accessible but the documentation in the medical record specifies that:
>   A. The patient's condition has changed
>   B. There is insufficient imaging of the patient's anatomy and/or disease, OR
>   C. There is a clinical change during the procedure that necessitates a new examination away from the site of the intervention
> Intravenous procedures (36000-36015, 36400-36510)
> Lymphatic injection procedures (38790)

75801 Lymphangiography, extremity only, unilateral, radiological supervision and interpretation

0.00 0.00 **FUD** XXX [02] [N1] [80] [🖳] [PQ]

AMA: 2014,Jan,11; 2012,Feb,9-10

75803 **Lymphangiography, extremity only, bilateral, radiological supervision and interpretation**
📷 0.00   ✎ 0.00   **FUD** XXX   02 N1 80 ▭ PQ
AMA: 2014,Jan,11; 2012,Feb,9-10

75805 **Lymphangiography, pelvic/abdominal, unilateral, radiological supervision and interpretation**
📷 0.00   ✎ 0.00   **FUD** XXX   02 N1 80 ▭ PQ
AMA: 2014,Jan,11; 2012,Feb,9-10

75807 **Lymphangiography, pelvic/abdominal, bilateral, radiological supervision and interpretation**
📷 0.00   ✎ 0.00   **FUD** XXX   02 N1 80 ▭ PQ
AMA: 2014,Jan,11; 2012,Feb,9-10

75809 **Shuntogram for investigation of previously placed indwelling nonvascular shunt (eg, LeVeen shunt, ventriculoperitoneal shunt, indwelling infusion pump), radiological supervision and interpretation**
INCLUDES   Needle placement with fluoroscopic guidance (77002)
Code also surgical procedure (49427, 61070)
📷 2.78   ✎ 2.78   **FUD** XXX   02 N1 80 ▭ PQ
AMA: 2015,Jan,16; 2014,Jan,11; 2012,Feb,9-10; 2012,Jan,15-42; 2011,Jan,11; 2011,Jan,8; 2010,Nov,1; 2010,Nov,3

75810 **Splenoportography, radiological supervision and interpretation**
INCLUDES   Needle placement with fluoroscopic guidance (77002)
📷 0.00   ✎ 0.00   **FUD** XXX   02 N1 80 ▭ PQ
AMA: 2015,Jan,16; 2014,Jan,11; 2012,Feb,9-10; 2011,Jan,8; 2010,Nov,1; 2010,Nov,3

75820 **Venography, extremity, unilateral, radiological supervision and interpretation**
📷 3.25   ✎ 3.25   **FUD** XXX   02 N1 80 ▭
AMA: 2015,May,3; 2015,Jan,16; 2014,Jan,11; 2012,Feb,9-10; 2012,Jan,15-42; 2011,Jan,11

75822 **Venography, extremity, bilateral, radiological supervision and interpretation**
📷 3.87   ✎ 3.87   **FUD** XXX   02 N1 80 ▭
AMA: 2014,Jan,11; 2012,Feb,9-10

75825 **Venography, caval, inferior, with serialography, radiological supervision and interpretation**
📷 3.86   ✎ 3.86   **FUD** XXX   02 N1 80 ▭ PQ
AMA: 2015,Jan,16; 2014,Jan,11; 2012,Feb,9-10; 2012,Jan,15-42; 2011,Jan,11

75827 **Venography, caval, superior, with serialography, radiological supervision and interpretation**
📷 3.89   ✎ 3.89   **FUD** XXX   02 N1 80 ▭ PQ
AMA: 2015,Jan,16; 2014,Jan,11; 2012,Feb,9-10

75831 **Venography, renal, unilateral, selective, radiological supervision and interpretation**
📷 3.96   ✎ 3.96   **FUD** XXX   02 N1 80 ▭ PQ
AMA: 2014,Jan,11; 2012,Feb,9-10

75833 **Venography, renal, bilateral, selective, radiological supervision and interpretation**
📷 4.75   ✎ 4.75   **FUD** XXX   02 N1 80 ▭ PQ
AMA: 2014,Jan,11; 2012,Feb,9-10

75840 **Venography, adrenal, unilateral, selective, radiological supervision and interpretation**
📷 4.19   ✎ 4.19   **FUD** XXX   02 N1 80 ▭ PQ
AMA: 2014,Jan,11; 2012,Feb,9-10

75842 **Venography, adrenal, bilateral, selective, radiological supervision and interpretation**
📷 5.09   ✎ 5.09   **FUD** XXX   02 N1 80 ▭ PQ
AMA: 2014,Jan,11; 2012,Feb,9-10

75860 **Venography, venous sinus (eg, petrosal and inferior sagittal) or jugular, catheter, radiological supervision and interpretation**
📷 4.06   ✎ 4.06   **FUD** XXX   02 N1 80 ▭ PQ
AMA: 2014,Jan,11; 2012,Feb,9-10

75870 **Venography, superior sagittal sinus, radiological supervision and interpretation**
📷 4.18   ✎ 4.18   **FUD** XXX   02 N1 80 ▭ PQ
AMA: 2014,Jan,11; 2012,Feb,9-10

75872 **Venography, epidural, radiological supervision and interpretation**
📷 4.20   ✎ 4.20   **FUD** XXX   02 N1 80 ▭ PQ
AMA: 2014,Jan,11; 2012,Feb,9-10

75880 **Venography, orbital, radiological supervision and interpretation**
📷 4.10   ✎ 4.10   **FUD** XXX   02 N1 80 ▭ PQ
AMA: 2014,Jan,11; 2012,Feb,9-10

75885 **Percutaneous transhepatic portography with hemodynamic evaluation, radiological supervision and interpretation**
INCLUDES   Needle placement with fluoroscopic guidance (77002)
📷 4.45   ✎ 4.45   **FUD** XXX   02 N1 80 ▭ PQ
AMA: 2015,Jan,16; 2014,Jan,11; 2012,Feb,9-10; 2012,Jan,15-42; 2011,Jan,11; 2011,Jan,8; 2010,Nov,1; 2010,Nov,3

Schematic showing the portal vein

75887 **Percutaneous transhepatic portography without hemodynamic evaluation, radiological supervision and interpretation**
INCLUDES   Needle placement with fluoroscopic guidance (77002)
📷 4.51   ✎ 4.51   **FUD** XXX   02 N1 80 ▭ PQ
AMA: 2015,Jan,16; 2014,Jan,11; 2012,Feb,9-10; 2012,Jan,15-42; 2011,Jan,11; 2011,Jan,8; 2010,Nov,1; 2010,Nov,3

75889 **Hepatic venography, wedged or free, with hemodynamic evaluation, radiological supervision and interpretation**
📷 4.06   ✎ 4.06   **FUD** XXX   02 N1 80 ▭ PQ
AMA: 2014,Jan,11; 2012,Feb,9-10

75891 **Hepatic venography, wedged or free, without hemodynamic evaluation, radiological supervision and interpretation**
📷 4.11   ✎ 4.11   **FUD** XXX   02 N1 80 ▭ PQ
AMA: 2014,Jan,11; 2012,Feb,9-10

75893 **Venous sampling through catheter, with or without angiography (eg, for parathyroid hormone, renin), radiological supervision and interpretation**
Code also surgical procedure (36500)
📷 3.34   ✎ 3.34   **FUD** XXX   02 N1 80 ▭ PQ
AMA: 2014,Jan,11; 2012,Feb,9-10

75894-75946 Transcatheter Procedures

INCLUDES   The following diagnostic procedures with interventional supervision and interpretation:
Angiography/venography
Completion angiography/venography except for those services allowed by (75898)
Contrast injection
Fluoroscopic guidance for intervention
Roadmapping
Vessel measurement

EXCLUDES   *Diagnostic angiography/venography performed at the same session as transcatheter therapy unless it is specifically included in the code descriptor or is excluded in the venography/angiography notes (75600-75893)*

75894 Transcatheter therapy, embolization, any method, radiological supervision and interpretation

Do not report with (35475-35476, 36478-36479, 37241-37244)

⚙ 0.00   ⚕ 0.00   **FUD** XXX   N N1 80 🖥 PQ

AMA: 2015,Jan,16; 2014,Oct,6; 2014,Jan,11; 2013,Nov,6; 2013,Nov,14; 2012,Feb,9-10; 2012,Apr,3-9

75896 ~~Transcatheter therapy, infusion, other than for thrombolysis, radiological supervision and interpretation~~

To report, see ~[37211, 37212, 37213, 37214], 61650-61651

75898 Angiography through existing catheter for follow-up study for transcatheter therapy, embolization or infusion, other than for thrombolysis

EXCLUDES   *Noncoronary thrombolysis infusion ([37211, 37212, 37213, 37214], 61645)*
Non-thrombolyis infusion other than coronary (61650-61651)

Do not report with ([37211, 37212, 37213, 37214], 37241-37244, 61645, 61650-61651)

⚙ 0.00   ⚕ 0.00   **FUD** XXX   Q1 N1 80 🖥 PQ

AMA: 2015,Jan,16; 2014,Oct,6; 2014,Jan,11; 2013,Nov,6; 2013,Nov,14; 2012,Feb,9-10; 2012,Jan,15-42; 2011,Jan,11

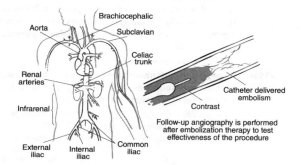

Follow-up angiography is performed after embolization therapy to test effectiveness of the procedure

75901 Mechanical removal of pericatheter obstructive material (eg, fibrin sheath) from central venous device via separate venous access, radiologic supervision and interpretation

EXCLUDES   *Venous catheterization (36010-36012)*

Code also surgical procedure (36595)

⚙ 4.91   ⚕ 4.91   **FUD** XXX   N N1 80 🖥 PQ

AMA: 2015,Jan,16; 2014,Jan,11; 2012,Feb,9-10

75902 Mechanical removal of intraluminal (intracatheter) obstructive material from central venous device through device lumen, radiologic supervision and interpretation

EXCLUDES   *Venous catheterization (36010-36012)*

Code also surgical procedure (36596)

⚙ 2.01   ⚕ 2.01   **FUD** XXX   N N1 80 🖥 PQ

AMA: 2015,Jan,16; 2014,Jan,11; 2012,Feb,9-10

75945 ~~Intravascular ultrasound (non-coronary vessel), radiological supervision and interpretation; initial vessel~~

To report, see ~37252-37253

75946 ~~each additional non-coronary vessel (List separately in addition to code for primary procedure)~~

To report, see ~37252-37253

75952-75959 Endovascular Aneurysm Repair

INCLUDES   The following diagnostic procedures with interventional supervision and interpretation:
Angiography/venography
Completion angiography/venography except for those services allowed by (75898)
Contrast injection
Fluoroscopic guidance for intervention
Roadmapping
Vessel measurement

EXCLUDES   *Diagnostic angiography/venography performed at the same session as transcatheter therapy unless it is specifically included in the code descriptor (75600-75893)*

75952 Endovascular repair of infrarenal abdominal aortic aneurysm or dissection, radiological supervision and interpretation

EXCLUDES   *Endovascular repair of visceral aorta with or without infrarenal abdominal aorta repair, radiologic supervision and interpretation (34841-34848)*
Implantation endovascular grafts (34800-34805)

Do not report with (34841-34848)

⚙ 0.00   ⚕ 0.00   **FUD** XXX   C 80 🖥 PQ

AMA: 2015,Jan,16; 2014,Jan,11; 2013,Dec,8; 2012,Apr,3-9; 2012,Feb,9-10

75953 Placement of proximal or distal extension prosthesis for endovascular repair of infrarenal aortic or iliac artery aneurysm, pseudoaneurysm, or dissection, radiological supervision and interpretation

EXCLUDES   *Placement of endovascular extension prostheses (34825-34826)*

⚙ 0.00   ⚕ 0.00   **FUD** XXX   C 80 🖥 PQ

AMA: 2015,Jan,16; 2014,Jan,11; 2013,Dec,8; 2012,Feb,9-10

75954 Endovascular repair of iliac artery aneurysm, pseudoaneurysm, arteriovenous malformation, or trauma, using ilio-iliac tube endoprosthesis, radiological supervision and interpretation

EXCLUDES   *Endovascular repair of iliac artery aneurysm, arteriovenous malformation, pseudoaneurysm, or trauma with bifurcated endoprosthesis, radiological supervision and interpretation (0255T)*
Placement of endovascular graft (34900)

⚙ 0.00   ⚕ 0.00   **FUD** XXX   C 80 🖥 PQ

AMA: 2015,Jan,16; 2014,Jan,11; 2012,Feb,9-10

75956 Endovascular repair of descending thoracic aorta (eg, aneurysm, pseudoaneurysm, dissection, penetrating ulcer, intramural hematoma, or traumatic disruption); involving coverage of left subclavian artery origin, initial endoprosthesis plus descending thoracic aortic extension(s), if required, to level of celiac artery origin, radiological supervision and interpretation

INCLUDES   All angiography
Fluoroscopy for component delivery

Code also endovascular graft implantation (33880)

⚙ 0.00   ⚕ 0.00   **FUD** XXX   C 80 PQ

AMA: 2015,Jan,16; 2014,Jan,11; 2012,Feb,9-10

75957 not involving coverage of left subclavian artery origin, initial endoprosthesis plus descending thoracic aortic extension(s), if required, to level of celiac artery origin, radiological supervision and interpretation

INCLUDES   All angiography
Fluoroscopy for component delivery

Code also endovascular graft implantation (33881)

⚙ 0.00   ⚕ 0.00   **FUD** XXX   C 80 PQ

AMA: 2015,Jan,16; 2014,Jan,11; 2012,Feb,9-10

75958 Placement of proximal extension prosthesis for endovascular repair of descending thoracic aorta (eg, aneurysm, pseudoaneurysm, dissection, penetrating ulcer, intramural hematoma, or traumatic disruption), radiological supervision and interpretation

Code also placement of each additional proximal extension(s) (75958)
Code also proximal endovascular extension implantation (33883-33884)

⚙ 0.00   ⚕ 0.00   **FUD** XXX   C 80 PQ

AMA: 2015,Jan,16; 2014,Jan,11; 2012,Feb,9-10

75959   **Placement of distal extension prosthesis(s) (delayed) after endovascular repair of descending thoracic aorta, as needed, to level of celiac origin, radiological supervision and interpretation**

> INCLUDES   Corresponding services for placement of distal thoracic endovascular extension(s) placed during procedure following the principal procedure
> Code also placement of distal endovascular extension (33886)
> Do not report more than one time no matter how many modules are deployed
> Do not report with endovascular repair (75956-75957)
> 📷 0.00   ⚕ 0.00   **FUD** XXX   C 80 PQ
> **AMA:** 2015,Jan,16; 2014,Jan,11; 2012,Feb,9-10

75962-75978 Percutaneous Transluminal Angioplasty

> INCLUDES   The following diagnostic procedures with interventional supervision and interpretation:
> Angiography/venography
> Completion angiography/venography except for those services allowed by (75898)
> Contrast injection
> Fluoroscopic guidance for intervention
> Roadmapping
> Vessel measurement
> EXCLUDES   *Diagnostic angiography/venography performed at the same session as transcatheter therapy unless it is specifically included in the code descriptor (75600-75893)*
> *Radiological supervision and interpretation for transluminal balloon angioplasty in:*
> *Femoral/popliteal arteries (37224-37227)*
> *Iliac artery (37220-37223)*
> *Tibial/peroneal artery (37228-37235)*

75962   **Transluminal balloon angioplasty, peripheral artery other than renal, or other visceral artery, iliac or lower extremity, radiological supervision and interpretation**

> Code also surgical procedure (35458, 35475)
> Do not report with (37217)
> 📷 3.89   ⚕ 3.89   **FUD** XXX   N N1 80 PQ
> **AMA:** 2015,Jan,16; 2014,Mar,8; 2014,Jan,11; 2012,Apr,3-9; 2012,Feb,9-10; 2012,Jan,15-42; 2011,Jul,3-11; 2011,Jan,11

+   **75964**   **Transluminal balloon angioplasty, each additional peripheral artery other than renal or other visceral artery, iliac or lower extremity, radiological supervision and interpretation (List separately in addition to code for primary procedure)**

> Code first primary procedure (75962)
> 📷 2.42   ⚕ 2.42   **FUD** ZZZ   N N1 80
> **AMA:** 2015,Jan,16; 2014,Jan,11; 2012,Apr,3-9; 2012,Feb,9-10; 2012,Jan,15-42; 2011,Jul,3-11; 2011,Jan,11

75966   **Transluminal balloon angioplasty, renal or other visceral artery, radiological supervision and interpretation**

> 📷 4.82   ⚕ 4.82   **FUD** XXX   N N1 80 PQ
> **AMA:** 2014,Jan,11; 2012,Feb,9-10

+   **75968**   **Transluminal balloon angioplasty, each additional visceral artery, radiological supervision and interpretation (List separately in addition to code for primary procedure)**

> EXCLUDES   *Percutaneous transluminal coronary angioplasty (92920-92944)*
> Code first primary procedure (75966)
> 📷 2.49   ⚕ 2.49   **FUD** ZZZ   N N1 80
> **AMA:** 2014,Jan,11; 2012,Feb,9-10

75970   **Transcatheter biopsy, radiological supervision and interpretation**

> EXCLUDES   *Injection procedure only for transcatheter therapy or biopsy (36100-36299)*
> *Percutaneous needle biopsy*
> *Pancreas (48102)*
> *Retroperitoneal lymph node/mass (49180)*
> *Transcatheter renal/ureteral biopsy (52007)*
> 📷 0.00   ⚕ 0.00   **FUD** XXX   N N1 80 PQ
> **AMA:** 2014,Jan,11; 2012,Feb,9-10

75978   **Transluminal balloon angioplasty, venous (eg, subclavian stenosis), radiological supervision and interpretation**

> 📷 3.85   ⚕ 3.85   **FUD** XXX   02 N1 80 PQ
> **AMA:** 2015,Jan,16; 2014,Jan,11; 2012,Apr,3-9; 2012,Feb,9-10; 2012,Jan,15-42; 2011,Dec,14-18

75980-75989 Percutaneous Drainage

> INCLUDES   The following diagnostic procedures with interventional supervision and interpretation:
> Angiography/venography
> Completion angiography/venography except for those services allowed by (75898)
> Contrast injection
> Fluoroscopic guidance for intervention
> Roadmapping
> Vessel measurement
> EXCLUDES   *Diagnostic angiography/venography performed at the same session as transcatheter therapy unless it is specifically included in the code descriptor (75600-75893)*

75980   ~~Percutaneous transhepatic biliary drainage with contrast monitoring, radiological supervision and interpretation~~

> To report, see ~47533-47537

75982   ~~Percutaneous placement of drainage catheter for combined internal and external biliary drainage or of a drainage stent for internal biliary drainage in patients with an inoperable mechanical biliary obstruction, radiological supervision and interpretation~~

> To report, see ~47533-47540

75984   **Change of percutaneous tube or drainage catheter with contrast monitoring (eg, genitourinary system, abscess), radiological supervision and interpretation**

> EXCLUDES   *Change only of nephrostomy/pyelostomy tube ([50435])*
> *Cholecystostomy, percutaneous (47490)*
> *Introduction procedure only for percutaneous biliary drainage (47531-47544)*
> *Nephrostolithotomy/pyelostolithotomy, percutaneous (50080-50081)*
> *Percutaneous replacement of gastrointestinal tube using fluoroscopic guidance (49450-49452)*
> *Removal and/or replacement of internal ureteral stent using transurethral approach (50385-50386)*
> 📷 2.99   ⚕ 2.99   **FUD** XXX   N N1 80 PQ
> **AMA:** 2014,Jan,11; 2012,Feb,9-10

75989   **Radiological guidance (ie, fluoroscopy, ultrasound, or computed tomography), for percutaneous drainage (eg, abscess, specimen collection), with placement of catheter, radiological supervision and interpretation**

> INCLUDES   Needle placement with fluoroscopic guidance (77002)
> Do not report with (10030, 32554-32557, 47490, 49405-49407)
> 📷 3.41   ⚕ 3.41   **FUD** XXX   N N1 80
> **AMA:** 2015,Jan,16; 2014,May,9; 2014,Jan,11; 2013,Nov,9; 2012,Nov,3-5; 2012,Feb,9-10; 2012,Jan,15-42; 2011,Apr,12; 2011,Jan,8; 2010,Nov,1; 2010,Nov,3

76000-76140 Miscellaneous Techniques

> EXCLUDES   *Arthrography:*
> *Ankle (73615)*
> *Elbow (73085)*
> *Hip (73525)*
> *Knee (73580)*
> *Shoulder (73040)*
> *Wrist (73115)*
> *CT cerebral perfusion test (0042T)*

76000   **Fluoroscopy (separate procedure), up to 1 hour physician or other qualified health care professional time, other than 71023 or 71034 (eg, cardiac fluoroscopy)**

> Do not report with (33957-33959, [33962, 33963, 33964])
> 📷 1.32   ⚕ 1.32   **FUD** XXX   S Z3 80 PQ
> **AMA:** 2015,May,3; 2015,Jan,16; 2014,Dec,3; 2014,Nov,5; 2014,Oct,6; 2014,Sep,5; 2014,Jan,11; 2013,Sep,17; 2013,Mar,10-11; 2013,Feb,3-6; 2012,Feb,9-10; 2012,Jan,15-42; 2011,Jul,3-11; 2011,Jan,11; 2011,Jan,8; 2010,Nov,1; 2010,Dec,12; 2010,Aug,8&15; 2010,Nov,3

76001 Fluoroscopy, physician or other qualified health care professional time more than 1 hour, assisting a nonradiologic physician or other qualified health care professional (eg, nephrostolithotomy, ERCP, bronchoscopy, transbronchial biopsy)

Do not report with (33957-33959, [33962, 33963, 33964])

🔗 0.00   ⚕ 0.00   **FUD** XXX   N N1 80 ▢ P0

AMA: 2015,Jan,16; 2014,Oct,6; 2014,Sep,5; 2014,Jan,11; 2013,Mar,10-11; 2013,Feb,3-6; 2012,Feb,9-10; 2012,Jan,15-42; 2011,Jan,11; 2011,Jan,8; 2010,Nov,1

76010 Radiologic examination from nose to rectum for foreign body, single view, child   A

🔗 0.73   ⚕ 0.73   **FUD** XXX   Q1 N1 80 A

AMA: 2015,Jan,16; 2014,Jan,11; 2012,Feb,9-10; 2012,Jan,15-42; 2011,Jan,11; 2010,Jan,12-15

76080 Radiologic examination, abscess, fistula or sinus tract study, radiological supervision and interpretation

EXCLUDES *Contrast injections, radiology evaluation, and guidance via fluoroscopy of gastrostomy, duodenostomy, jejunostomy, gastro-jejunostomy, or cecostomy tube (49465)*

🔗 1.55   ⚕ 1.55   **FUD** XXX   Q2 N1 80 ▢ P0

AMA: 2015,Jan,16; 2014,Jan,11; 2012,Feb,9-10; 2012,Jan,15-42; 2011,Jan,11

76098 Radiological examination, surgical specimen

Do not report with (19081-19086)

🔗 0.46   ⚕ 0.46   **FUD** XXX   Q2 N1 80

AMA: 2012,Feb,9-10

76100 Radiologic examination, single plane body section (eg, tomography), other than with urography

🔗 2.60   ⚕ 2.60   **FUD** XXX   Q1 N1 80 ▢

AMA: 2012,Feb,9-10

76101 Radiologic examination, complex motion (ie, hypercycloidal) body section (eg, mastoid polytomography), other than with urography; unilateral

EXCLUDES *Nephrotomography (74415)*
Panoramic x-ray (70355)

Do not report more than one time per day

🔗 3.72   ⚕ 3.72   **FUD** XXX   S Z3 80

AMA: 2012,Feb,9-10

76102 bilateral

EXCLUDES *Nephrotomography (74415)*
Panoramic x-ray (70355)

Do not report more than one time per day

🔗 4.89   ⚕ 4.89   **FUD** XXX   S Z3 80 ▢

AMA: 2012,Feb,9-10

76120 Cineradiography/videoradiography, except where specifically included

🔗 2.55   ⚕ 2.55   **FUD** XXX   S Z3 80 ▢ P0

AMA: 2015,Jan,16; 2014,Jan,11; 2012,Feb,9-10; 2011,Apr,13

+ **76125** Cineradiography/videoradiography to complement routine examination (List separately in addition to code for primary procedure)

Code first primary procedure

🔗 0.00   ⚕ 0.00   **FUD** ZZZ   N N1 80 ▢

AMA: 2015,Jan,16; 2014,Jan,11; 2012,Feb,9-10

76140 Consultation on X-ray examination made elsewhere, written report

🔗 0.00   ⚕ 0.00   **FUD** XXX   E

AMA: 2015,Jan,16; 2014,Jan,11; 2012,Feb,9-10; 2012,Jan,15-42; 2011,Jan,11

76376-76377 Three-dimensional Manipulation

INCLUDES Concurrent physician supervision of image postprocessing
3D manipulation of volumetric data set
Rendering of image

EXCLUDES *Arthrography:*
Ankle (73615)
Elbow (73085)
Hip (73525)
Knee (73580)
Shoulder (73040)
Wrist (73115)
Computer-aided detection of MRI data for lesion, breast MRI (0159T)
CT cerebral perfusion test (0042T)

Code also base imaging procedure(s)

76376 3D rendering with interpretation and reporting of computed tomography, magnetic resonance imaging, ultrasound, or other tomographic modality with image postprocessing under concurrent supervision; not requiring image postprocessing on an independent workstation

Do not report with (31627, 34839, 70496, 70498, 70544-70549, 71275, 71555, 72159, 72191, 72198, 73206, 73225, 73706, 73725, 74174-74175, 74185, 74261-74263, 75557, 75559, 75561, 75563, 75565, 75571-75574, 75635, 76377, 77061-77063, 78012-78999, 93355, 0159T)

🔗 0.64   ⚕ 0.64   **FUD** XXX   N N1 80

AMA: 2015,Jan,16; 2014,Jan,11; 2013,Jun,12; 2013,May,3-5; 2012,Feb,9-10; 2012,Jan,15-42; 2011,Jan,11; 2010,Jul,7-8; 2010,Apr,9; 2010,Apr,5; 2010,Jan,6

76377 requiring image postprocessing on an independent workstation

Do not report with (34839, 70496, 70498, 70544-70549, 71275, 71555, 72159, 72191, 72198, 73206, 73225, 73706, 73725, 74174-74175, 74185, 74261-74263, 75557, 75559, 75561, 75563, 75565, 75571-75574, 75635, 76376, 77061-77063, 78012-78999, 93355, 0159T)

🔗 1.80   ⚕ 1.80   **FUD** XXX   N N1 80

AMA: 2015,Jan,16; 2014,Jan,11; 2013,Jun,12; 2013,May,3-5; 2012,Feb,9-10; 2012,Jan,15-42; 2011,Jan,11; 2010,Jul,7-8; 2010,Apr,9; 2010,Apr,5; 2010,Jan,6

76380 Computerized Tomography: Delimited

EXCLUDES *Arthrography:*
Ankle (73615)
Elbow (73085)
Hip (73525)
Knee (73580)
Shoulder (73040)
Wrist (73115)
CT cerebral perfusion test (0042T)

76380 Computed tomography, limited or localized follow-up study

🔗 4.11   ⚕ 4.11   **FUD** XXX   Q1 N1 80

AMA: 2015,Jan,16; 2014,Jan,11; 2012,Feb,9-10

76390 Magnetic Resonance Spectroscopy

CMS: 100-3,220.2.1 Magnetic Resonance Spectroscopy

EXCLUDES *Arthrography:*
Ankle (73615)
Elbow (73085)
Hip (73525)
Knee (73580)
Shoulder (73040)
Wrist (73115)
CT cerebral perfusion test (0042T)

76390 Magnetic resonance spectroscopy

EXCLUDES *MRI*

🔗 12.4   ⚕ 12.4   **FUD** XXX   E

AMA: 2012,Feb,9-10

76496-76499 Unlisted Radiology Procedures

76496 Unlisted fluoroscopic procedure (eg, diagnostic, interventional)

🔗 0.00   ⚕ 0.00   **FUD** XXX   S Z2 80 P0

AMA: 2012,Feb,9-10

76497 Unlisted computed tomography procedure (eg, diagnostic, interventional)

    📷 0.00   🔶 0.00   **FUD** XXX   01 N1 80

    AMA: 2015,Jan,16; 2014,Jan,11; 2012,Feb,9-10; 2012,Jan,15-42; 2011,Jan,11

76498 Unlisted magnetic resonance procedure (eg, diagnostic, interventional)

    📷 0.00   🔶 0.00   **FUD** XXX   S Z2 80

    AMA: 2015,Jan,16; 2014,Jan,11; 2012,Feb,9-10; 2012,Jan,15-42; 2011,Dec,14-18; 2011,Jan,11

76499 Unlisted diagnostic radiographic procedure

    📷 0.00   🔶 0.00   **FUD** XXX   01 N1 80

    AMA: 2015,Jan,16; 2014,Jan,11; 2013,Dec,16; 2012,Feb,9-10; 2012,Jan,15-42; 2011,Dec,14-18; 2011,Jan,11

76506 Ultrasound: Brain

INCLUDES   Required permanent documentation of ultrasound images except when diagnostic purpose is biometric measurement
Written documentation

EXCLUDES   *Noninvasive vascular studies, diagnostic (93880-93990)*
Ultrasound exam that does not include thorough assessment of organ or site, recorded image, and written report

76506 Echoencephalography, real time with image documentation (gray scale) (for determination of ventricular size, delineation of cerebral contents, and detection of fluid masses or other intracranial abnormalities), including A-mode encephalography as secondary component where indicated

    📷 3.35   🔶 3.35   **FUD** XXX   S Z2 80

    AMA: 2015,Jan,16; 2014,Jan,11; 2012,Feb,9-10

76510-76529 Ultrasound: Eyes

INCLUDES   Required permanent documentation of ultrasound images except when diagnostic purpose is biometric measurement
Written documentation

76510 Ophthalmic ultrasound, diagnostic; B-scan and quantitative A-scan performed during the same patient encounter

    📷 4.80   🔶 4.80   **FUD** XXX   01 N1 80

    AMA: 2015,Jan,16; 2014,Jan,11; 2012,Feb,9-10

76511 quantitative A-scan only

    📷 2.90   🔶 2.90   **FUD** XXX   S Z3 80

    AMA: 2015,Jan,16; 2014,Jan,11; 2012,Feb,9-10

76512 B-scan (with or without superimposed non-quantitative A-scan)

    📷 2.62   🔶 2.62   **FUD** XXX   S Z3 80

    AMA: 2015,Jan,16; 2014,Jan,11; 2012,Feb,9-10

76513 anterior segment ultrasound, immersion (water bath) B-scan or high resolution biomicroscopy

    EXCLUDES   *Computerized ophthalmic testing other than by ultrasound (92132-92134)*

    📷 2.71   🔶 2.71   **FUD** XXX   S Z3 80

    AMA: 2015,Jan,16; 2014,Jan,11; 2013,Apr,7; 2012,Feb,9-10; 2012,Jan,15-42; 2011,Jan,11

76514 corneal pachymetry, unilateral or bilateral (determination of corneal thickness)

    INCLUDES   Biometric measurement for which permanent documentation of images is not required
    Do not report with (0402T)

    📷 0.43   🔶 0.43   **FUD** XXX   01 N1 80

    AMA: 2015,Jan,16; 2014,Jan,11; 2012,Feb,9-10; 2012,Jan,15-42; 2011,Jan,11

76516 Ophthalmic biometry by ultrasound echography, A-scan;

    INCLUDES   Biometric measurement for which permanent documentation of images is not required

    📷 2.22   🔶 2.22   **FUD** XXX   01 N1 80

    AMA: 2015,Jan,16; 2014,Jan,11; 2012,Feb,9-10; 2012,Jan,15-42; 2011,Jan,11

76519 with intraocular lens power calculation

    INCLUDES   Biometric measurement for which permanent documentation of images is not required
    Written prescription that satisfies requirement for written report

    EXCLUDES   *Partial coherence interferometry (92136)*

    📷 2.38   🔶 2.38   **FUD** XXX   01 N1 80

    AMA: 2015,Jan,16; 2014,Jan,11; 2012,Feb,9-10; 2012,Jan,15-42; 2011,Jan,11

76529 Ophthalmic ultrasonic foreign body localization

    📷 2.25   🔶 2.25   **FUD** XXX   S Z3 80

    AMA: 2015,Jan,16; 2014,Jan,11; 2012,Feb,9-10

76536-76800 Ultrasound: Neck, Thorax, Abdomen, and Spine

INCLUDES   Required permanent documentation of ultrasound images except when diagnostic purpose is biometric measurement
Written documentation

EXCLUDES   *Focused ultrasound ablation of uterine leiomyomata (0071T-0072T)*
Ultrasound exam that does not include thorough assessment of organ or site, recorded image, and written report

76536 Ultrasound, soft tissues of head and neck (eg, thyroid, parathyroid, parotid), real time with image documentation

    📷 3.28   🔶 3.28   **FUD** XXX   S Z2 80

    AMA: 2015,Jan,16; 2014,Jan,11; 2012,Feb,9-10

76604 Ultrasound, chest (includes mediastinum), real time with image documentation

    📷 2.49   🔶 2.49   **FUD** XXX   03 Z3 80

    AMA: 2015,Jan,16; 2014,Jan,11; 2012,Nov,3-5; 2012,Feb,9-10

76641 Ultrasound, breast, unilateral, real time with image documentation, including axilla when performed; complete

    INCLUDES   Complete examination of all four quadrants, retroareolar region, and axilla when performed
    Do not report more than one time per breast per session

    📷 3.06   🔶 3.06   **FUD** XXX   01 N1 80

    AMA: 2015,Aug,8

76642 limited

    📷 2.52   🔶 2.52   **FUD** XXX   01 N1 80

    INCLUDES   Examination not including all of the elements in complete examination
    Do not report more than one time per breast per session

76700 Ultrasound, abdominal, real time with image documentation; complete

    INCLUDES   Real time scans of:
        Common bile duct
        Gall bladder
        Inferior vena cava
        Kidneys
        Liver
        Pancreas
        Spleen
        Upper abdominal aorta

    📷 3.47   🔶 3.47   **FUD** XXX   03 Z2 80

    AMA: 2015,Jan,16; 2014,Jan,11; 2012,Feb,9-10

76705 limited (eg, single organ, quadrant, follow-up)

    📷 2.59   🔶 2.59   **FUD** XXX   03 Z3 80

    AMA: 2015,Jan,16; 2014,Jan,11; 2012,Dec,9-10; 2012,Mar,9-10; 2012,Feb,9-10; 2012,Jan,15-42; 2011,Jan,11

76770 Ultrasound, retroperitoneal (eg, renal, aorta, nodes), real time with image documentation; complete

    INCLUDES   Complete assessment of kidneys and bladder if history indicates urinary pathology
    Real time scans of:
        Abdominal aorta
        Common iliac artery origins
        Inferior vena cava
        Kidneys

    📷 3.19   🔶 3.19   **FUD** XXX   03 Z2 80

    AMA: 2015,Jan,16; 2014,Jan,11; 2012,Feb,9-10

76775 **limited**

    1.62   1.62   **FUD** XXX   03 Z3 80

AMA: 2015,Jan,16; 2014,Jan,11; 2012,Feb,9-10; 2012,Jan,15-42; 2011,Jan,11

76776 **Ultrasound, transplanted kidney, real time and duplex Doppler with image documentation**

    EXCLUDES   *Transplanted kidney ultrasound without duplex doppler (76775)*

    Do not report with abdominal/pelvic/scrotal contents/retroperitoneal duplex scan (93975, 93976)

    4.42   4.42   **FUD** XXX   03 Z2 80

    AMA: 2015,Jan,16; 2014,Jan,11; 2012,Feb,9-10

76800 **Ultrasound, spinal canal and contents**

    3.89   3.89   **FUD** XXX   Q1 N1 80

    AMA: 2015,Jan,16; 2014,Jan,11; 2012,Feb,9-10; 2012,Jan,15-42; 2011,Jan,11

76801-76802 Ultrasound: Pregnancy Less Than 14 Weeks

INCLUDES   Determination of the number of gestational sacs and fetuses
Gestational sac/fetal measurement appropriate for gestational age (younger than 14 weeks 0 days)
Inspection of the maternal uterus and adnexa
Quality analysis of amniotic fluid volume/gestational sac shape
Visualization of fetal and placental anatomic formation
Written documentation of each component of exam

EXCLUDES   *Focused ultrasound ablation of uterine leiomyomata (0071T-0072T)*
Ultrasound exam that does not include thorough assessment of organ or site, recorded image, and written report

76801 **Ultrasound, pregnant uterus, real time with image documentation, fetal and maternal evaluation, first trimester (< 14 weeks 0 days), transabdominal approach; single or first gestation**   M ♀

    EXCLUDES   *Fetal nuchal translucency measurement, first trimester (76813)*

    3.52   3.52   **FUD** XXX   S Z3 80

    AMA: 2015,Jan,16; 2014,Jan,11; 2012,Feb,9-10; 2012,Jan,15-42; 2011,Jan,11

+ 76802 **each additional gestation (List separately in addition to code for primary procedure)**   M ♀

    EXCLUDES   *Fetal nuchal translucency measurement, first trimester (76814)*

    Code first (76801)

    1.86   1.86   **FUD** ZZZ   N N1 80

    AMA: 2015,Jan,16; 2014,Jan,11; 2012,Feb,9-10; 2012,Jan,15-42; 2011,Jan,11

76805-76810 Ultrasound: Pregnancy of 14 Weeks or More

INCLUDES   Determination of the number of gestational/chorionic sacs and fetuses
Evaluation of:
  Amniotic fluid
  Four chambered heart
  Intracranial, spinal, abdominal anatomy
  Placenta location
  Umbilical cord insertion site
Examination of maternal adnexa if visible
Gestational sac/fetal measurement appropriate for gestational age (older than or equal to 14 weeks 0 days)
Written documentation of each component of exam

EXCLUDES   *Focused ultrasound ablation of uterine leiomyomata (0071T-0072T)*
Ultrasound exam that does not include thorough assessment of organ or site, recorded image, and written report

76805 **Ultrasound, pregnant uterus, real time with image documentation, fetal and maternal evaluation, after first trimester (> or = 14 weeks 0 days), transabdominal approach; single or first gestation**   M ♀

    4.04   4.04   **FUD** XXX   S Z2 80

    AMA: 2015,Jan,16; 2014,Jan,11; 2012,Feb,9-10

+ 76810 **each additional gestation (List separately in addition to code for primary procedure)**   M ♀

    Code first (76805)

    2.69   2.69   **FUD** ZZZ   N N1 80

    AMA: 2015,Jan,16; 2014,Jan,11; 2012,Feb,9-10

76811-76812 Ultrasound: Pregnancy, with Additional Studies of Fetus

INCLUDES   Determination of the number of gestational/chorionic sacs and fetuses
Evaluation of:
  Abdominal organ specific anatomy
  Amniotic fluid
  Chest anatomy
  Face
  Fetal brain/ventricles
  Four chambered heart
  Heart/outflow tracts and chest anatomy
  Intracranial, spinal, abdominal anatomy
  Limbs including number, length, and architecture
  Other fetal anatomy as indicated
  Placenta location
  Umbilical cord insertion site
Examination of maternal adnexa if visible
Gestational sac/fetal measurement appropriate for gestational age (older than or equal to 14 weeks 0 days)
Written documentation of each component of exam, including reason for nonvisualization, when applicable

EXCLUDES   *Focused ultrasound ablation of uterine leiomyomata (0071T-0072T)*
Ultrasound exam that does not include thorough assessment organ or site, recorded image, and written report

76811 **Ultrasound, pregnant uterus, real time with image documentation, fetal and maternal evaluation plus detailed fetal anatomic examination, transabdominal approach; single or first gestation**   M ♀

    5.16   5.16   **FUD** XXX   S Z3 80

    AMA: 2015,Jan,16; 2014,Jan,11; 2012,Feb,9-10

+ 76812 **each additional gestation (List separately in addition to code for primary procedure)**   M ♀

    Code first (76811)

    5.85   5.85   **FUD** ZZZ   N N1 80

    AMA: 2015,Jan,16; 2014,Jan,11; 2012,Feb,9-10

76813-76828 Ultrasound: Other Fetal Evaluations

INCLUDES   Required permanent documentation of ultrasound images except when diagnostic purpose is biometric measurement
Written documentation

EXCLUDES   *Focused ultrasound ablation of uterine leiomyomata (0071T-0072T)*
Ultrasound exam that does not include thorough assessment of organ or site, recorded image, and written report

76813 **Ultrasound, pregnant uterus, real time with image documentation, first trimester fetal nuchal translucency measurement, transabdominal or transvaginal approach; single or first gestation**   M ♀

    3.45   3.45   **FUD** XXX   S Z3 80

    AMA: 2015,Jan,16; 2014,Jan,11; 2012,Feb,9-10

+ 76814 **each additional gestation (List separately in addition to code for primary procedure)**   M ♀

    Code first (76813)

    2.32   2.32   **FUD** XXX   N N1 80

    AMA: 2015,Jan,16; 2014,Jan,11; 2012,Feb,9-10

76815 **Ultrasound, pregnant uterus, real time with image documentation, limited (eg, fetal heart beat, placental location, fetal position and/or qualitative amniotic fluid volume), 1 or more fetuses**   M ♀

    INCLUDES   Exam concentrating on one or more elements
              Reporting only one time per exam, instead of per element

    EXCLUDES   *Fetal nuchal translucency measurement, first trimester (76813-76814)*

    2.40   2.40   **FUD** XXX   S Z3 80

    AMA: 2015,Jan,16; 2014,Jan,11; 2012,Feb,9-10; 2012,Jan,15-42; 2011,Jan,11; 2010,May,9

Radiology

76816 — 76872

76816 Ultrasound, pregnant uterus, real time with image documentation, follow-up (eg, re-evaluation of fetal size by measuring standard growth parameters and amniotic fluid volume, re-evaluation of organ system(s) suspected or confirmed to be abnormal on a previous scan), transabdominal approach, per fetus   M ♀

    INCLUDES Re-evaluation of fetal size, interval growth, or aberrancies noted on a prior ultrasound

    Code also modifier 59 for examination of each additional fetus in a multiple pregnancy

    ⚕ 3.26   ✂ 3.26   **FUD** XXX   01 N1 80 ▱

    AMA: 2015,Jan,16; 2014,Jan,11; 2012,Feb,9-10; 2012,Jan,15-42; 2011,Jan,11; 2010,May,9

76817 Ultrasound, pregnant uterus, real time with image documentation, transvaginal   M ♀

    EXCLUDES Transvaginal ultrasound, non-obstetrical (76830)

    Code also transabdominal obstetrical ultrasound, if performed

    ⚕ 2.76   ✂ 2.76   **FUD** XXX   S Z3 80 ▱

    AMA: 2015,Jan,16; 2014,Jan,11; 2012,Feb,9-10; 2012,Jan,15-42

76818 Fetal biophysical profile; with non-stress testing   M ♀

    Code also modifier 59 for each additional fetus

    ⚕ 3.45   ✂ 3.45   **FUD** XXX   S Z3 80 ▱

    AMA: 2015,Jan,16; 2014,Jan,11; 2012,Feb,9-10; 2012,Jan,15-42; 2011,Jan,11

76819 without non-stress testing   M ♀

    EXCLUDES Amniotic fluid index without non-stress test (76815)

    Code also modifier 59 for each additional fetus

    ⚕ 2.52   ✂ 2.52   **FUD** XXX   S Z3 80 ▱

    AMA: 2015,Jan,16; 2014,Jan,11; 2012,Feb,9-10; 2012,Jan,15-42; 2011,Jan,11

76820 Doppler velocimetry, fetal; umbilical artery   M

    ⚕ 1.34   ✂ 1.34   **FUD** XXX   01 N1 80

    AMA: 2015,Jan,16; 2014,Jan,11; 2012,Feb,9-10

76821 middle cerebral artery   M

    ⚕ 2.63   ✂ 2.63   **FUD** XXX   01 N1 80

    AMA: 2015,Jan,16; 2014,Jan,11; 2012,Feb,9-10

76825 Echocardiography, fetal, cardiovascular system, real time with image documentation (2D), with or without M-mode recording;   M ♀

    ⚕ 7.85   ✂ 7.85   **FUD** XXX   S Z3 80 ▱

    AMA: 2015,Jan,16; 2014,Jan,11; 2012,Feb,9-10; 2010,Jan,8-10

76826 follow-up or repeat study   M ♀

    ⚕ 4.65   ✂ 4.65   **FUD** XXX   S Z3 80 ▱

    AMA: 2012,Feb,9-10; 2010,Jan,8-10

76827 Doppler echocardiography, fetal, pulsed wave and/or continuous wave with spectral display; complete   M ♀

    ⚕ 2.16   ✂ 2.16   **FUD** XXX   01 N1 80 ▱

    AMA: 2015,Jan,16; 2014,Jan,11; 2012,Feb,9-10; 2010,Jan,8-10

76828 follow-up or repeat study   M ♀

    EXCLUDES Color mapping (93325)

    ⚕ 1.52   ✂ 1.52   **FUD** XXX   01 N1 80 ▱

    AMA: 2015,Jan,16; 2014,Jan,11; 2012,Feb,9-10; 2010,Jan,8-10

76830-76873 Ultrasound: Male and Female Genitalia

INCLUDES Required permanent documentation of ultrasound images except when diagnostic purpose is biometric measurement
Written documentation

EXCLUDES Focused ultrasound ablation of uterine leiomyomata (0071T-0072T)
Ultrasound exam that does not include thorough assessment of organ or site, recorded image, and written report

76830 Ultrasound, transvaginal   ♀

    EXCLUDES Transvaginal ultrasound, obstetric (76817)

    Code also transabdominal non-obstetrical ultrasound, if performed

    ⚕ 3.46   ✂ 3.46   **FUD** XXX   S Z3 80 ▱

    AMA: 2015,Jan,16; 2014,Jan,11; 2012,Feb,9-10; 2012,Jan,15-42; 2011,Jan,11

Nonpregnant uterus

Ovary

Pubic bone

Bladder

Rectum

Ultrasonic lead in vaginal canal

Ultrasound is performed in real time with image documentation by a transvaginal approach

76831 Saline infusion sonohysterography (SIS), including color flow Doppler, when performed   ♀

    Code also saline introduction for saline infusion sonohysterography (58340)

    ⚕ 3.36   ✂ 3.36   **FUD** XXX   03 Z3 80 ▱

    AMA: 2015,Jan,16; 2014,Jan,11; 2012,Feb,9-10; 2012,Jan,15-42; 2011,Jan,11

76856 Ultrasound, pelvic (nonobstetric), real time with image documentation; complete

    INCLUDES Total examination of the female pelvic anatomy which includes:
        Bladder measurement
        Description and measurement of the uterus and adnexa
        Description of any pelvic pathology
        Measurement of the endometrium
    Total examination of the male pelvis which includes:
        Bladder measurement
        Description of any pelvic pathology
        Evaluation of prostate and seminal vesicles

    ⚕ 3.10   ✂ 3.10   **FUD** XXX   03 Z2 80 ▱

    AMA: 2015,Jan,16; 2014,Jan,11; 2012,Feb,9-10; 2012,Jan,15-42; 2011,Jan,11

76857 limited or follow-up (eg, for follicles)

    INCLUDES Focused evaluation limited to:
        Evaluation of one or more elements listed in 76856 and/or
        Reevaluation of one or more pelvic aberrancies noted on a prior ultrasound
        Urinary bladder alone

    EXCLUDES Bladder volume or post-voided residual measurement without imaging the bladder (51798)
        Urinary bladder and kidneys (76770)

    ⚕ 1.33   ✂ 1.33   **FUD** XXX   03 Z3 80 ▱

    AMA: 2015,Jan,16; 2014,Jan,11; 2012,Feb,9-10; 2012,Jan,15-42; 2011,Jan,11

76870 Ultrasound, scrotum and contents   ♂

    ⚕ 1.88   ✂ 1.88   **FUD** XXX   03 Z3 80 ▱

    AMA: 2012,Feb,9-10

76872 Ultrasound, transrectal;

    Do not report with (45341-45342, 45391-45392, 0249T)

    ⚕ 2.64   ✂ 2.64   **FUD** XXX   S Z3 80 ▱

    AMA: 2015,Jan,16; 2014,Jan,11; 2012,Feb,9-10

26/TC PC/TC Comp Only   A2-Z4 ASC Pmt   50 Bilateral   ♂ Male Only   ♀ Female Only   ⚕ Facility RVU   ✂ Non-Facility RVU
AMA: CPT Asst   **CMS:** Pub 100   A-Y OPPSI   80/80 Surg Assist Allowed / w/Doc   Lab Crosswalk   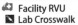 Radiology Crosswalk

300   Medicare (Red Text)   CPT © 2015 American Medical Association. All Rights Reserved. (Black Text)   © 2015 Optum360, LLC (Blue Text)

76873 prostate volume study for brachytherapy treatment planning (separate procedure) ♂

⌗ 4.69 ☒ 4.69 **FUD** XXX [S][Z3]

AMA: 2015,Jan,16; 2014,Jan,11; 2012,Feb,9-10

76881-76886 Ultrasound: Extremities

EXCLUDES *Doppler studies of the extremities (93925-93926, 93930-93931, 93970-93971)*

76881 Ultrasound, extremity, nonvascular, real-time with image documentation; complete

INCLUDES Real time scans of a specific joint including assessment of:
Joint
Muscles
Other soft tissue
Tendons

⌗ 3.29 ☒ 3.29 **FUD** XXX [S][Z2]

AMA: 2012,Feb,9-10

76882 limited, anatomic specific

INCLUDES Limited examination of a certain anatomical structure (e.g. muscle or tendon) or for evaluation of a soft-tissue mass

⌗ 1.02 ☒ 1.02 **FUD** XXX [Q1][N1]

AMA: 2012,Feb,9-10

76885 Ultrasound, infant hips, real time with imaging documentation; dynamic (requiring physician or other qualified health care professional manipulation) [A]

⌗ 4.08 ☒ 4.08 **FUD** XXX [Q1][N1][80][□]

AMA: 2012,Feb,9-10

76886 limited, static (not requiring physician or other qualified health care professional manipulation) [A]

⌗ 3.01 ☒ 3.01 **FUD** XXX [Q1][N1][80][□]

AMA: 2012,Feb,9-10

76930-76970 Imaging Guidance: Ultrasound

INCLUDES Required permanent documentation of ultrasound images except when diagnostic purpose is biometric measurement
Written documentation

EXCLUDES *Focused ultrasound ablation of uterine leiomyomata (0071T-0072T)*
Ultrasound exam that does not include thorough assessment of organ or site, recorded image, and written report

76930 Ultrasonic guidance for pericardiocentesis, imaging supervision and interpretation

⌗ 0.00 ☒ 0.00 **FUD** XXX [N][N1][80][□]

AMA: 2012,Feb,9-10

76932 Ultrasonic guidance for endomyocardial biopsy, imaging supervision and interpretation

⌗ 0.00 ☒ 0.00 **FUD** YYY [N][N1][80][□]

AMA: 2012,Feb,9-10

76936 Ultrasound guided compression repair of arterial pseudoaneurysm or arteriovenous fistulae (includes diagnostic ultrasound evaluation, compression of lesion and imaging)

⌗ 7.74 ☒ 7.74 **FUD** XXX [S][Z3][80][□]

AMA: 2012,Feb,9-10

+ 76937 Ultrasound guidance for vascular access requiring ultrasound evaluation of potential access sites, documentation of selected vessel patency, concurrent realtime ultrasound visualization of vascular needle entry, with permanent recording and reporting (List separately in addition to code for primary procedure)

EXCLUDES *Extremity venous non-invasive vascular diagnostic study performed separately from venous access guidance (93965, 93970-93971)*

Code first primary procedure
Do not report with (37191-37193, 37760-37761, 76942)

⌗ 0.91 ☒ 0.91 **FUD** ZZZ [N][N1][80][□]

AMA: 2015,Jul,10; 2015,Jan,16; 2014,Oct,6; 2014,Jan,11; 2013,Sep,17; 2013,Jun,12; 2013,May,3-5; 2013,Feb,3-6; 2012,Feb,9-10; 2012,Apr,3-9; 2011,Jan,8; 2010,Nov,1; 2010,Nov,3; 2010,Jul,6

76940 Ultrasound guidance for, and monitoring of, parenchymal tissue ablation

EXCLUDES *Ablation (32998, 47370-47383, 50592-50593)*
Do not report with (20982-20983, 50250, 50542, 76942, 76998, 0340T)

⌗ 0.00 ☒ 0.00 **FUD** YYY [N][N1][80][□]

AMA: 2015,Jul,8; 2015,Jan,16; 2014,Jan,11; 2012,Feb,9-10

76941 Ultrasonic guidance for intrauterine fetal transfusion or cordocentesis, imaging supervision and interpretation [M] ♀

Code also surgical procedure (36460, 59012)

⌗ 0.00 ☒ 0.00 **FUD** XXX [N][N1][80][□]

AMA: 2012,Feb,9-10

76942 Ultrasonic guidance for needle placement (eg, biopsy, aspiration, injection, localization device), imaging supervision and interpretation

EXCLUDES *Platelet rich plasma injection(s) (0232T)*
Do not report with (10030, 19083, 19285, 20604, 20606, 20611, 27096, 32554-32557, 37760-37761, 43232, 43237, 43242, 45341-45342, 64479-64484, 64490-64495, 76975, 0213T-0218T, 0228T, 0231T-0232T, 0249T, 0301T)

⌗ 1.70 ☒ 1.70 **FUD** XXX [N][N1][80][□]

AMA: 2015,Aug,8; 2015,Feb,6; 2015,Jan,16; 2014,Oct,6; 2014,Jan,11; 2013,Nov,9; 2013,Dec,3; 2012,Dec,9-10; 2012,Nov,3-5; 2012,Feb,9-10; 2012,Jan,15-42; 2011,Apr,12; 2011,Mar,9; 2011,Feb,4-5; 2011,Jan,11; 2010,Jul,6; 2010,Mar,9-11; 2010,Jan,6

76945 Ultrasonic guidance for chorionic villus sampling, imaging supervision and interpretation [M] ♀

Code also surgical procedure (59015)

⌗ 0.00 ☒ 0.00 **FUD** XXX [N][N1][80][□]

AMA: 2012,Feb,9-10

76946 Ultrasonic guidance for amniocentesis, imaging supervision and interpretation [M] ♀

⌗ 0.93 ☒ 0.93 **FUD** XXX [N][N1][80][□]

AMA: 2012,Feb,9-10

76948 Ultrasonic guidance for aspiration of ova, imaging supervision and interpretation [M] ♀

⌗ 0.93 ☒ 0.93 **FUD** XXX [N][N1][80][□]

AMA: 2012,Feb,9-10

76965 Ultrasonic guidance for interstitial radioelement application

⌗ 2.54 ☒ 2.54 **FUD** XXX [N][N1][80][□]

AMA: 2012,Feb,9-10

76970 Ultrasound study follow-up (specify)

⌗ 2.63 ☒ 2.63 **FUD** XXX [Q1][N1][80][□]

AMA: 2012,Feb,9-10

76975 Endoscopic Ultrasound

CMS: 100-4,12,30.1 Upper Gastrointestinal Endoscopy Including Endoscopic Ultrasound (EUS)

INCLUDES Required permanent documentation of ultrasound images except when diagnostic purpose is biometric measurement
Written documentation

EXCLUDES *Focused ultrasound ablation of uterine leiomyomata (0071T-0072T)*
Ultrasound exam that does not include thorough assessment of organ or site, recorded image, and written report

76975 Gastrointestinal endoscopic ultrasound, supervision and interpretation

Do not report with (43231-43232, 43237-43238, 43240, 43242, 43259, 44406-44407, 45341-45342, 45391-45392, 76942)

⌗ 0.00 ☒ 0.00 **FUD** XXX [Q2][N1][80][□]

AMA: 2015,Jan,16; 2014,Jan,11; 2013,Dec,3; 2012,Feb,9-10

76977 Bone Density Measurements: Ultrasound

CMS: 100-2,15,80.5.5 Frequency Standards; 100-4,13,30.1.3.1 Payment for Low Osmolar Contrast Material

INCLUDES   Required permanent documentation of ultrasound images except when diagnostic purpose is biometric measurement
Written documentation

EXCLUDES   *Ultrasound exam that does not include thorough assessment of organ or site, recorded image, and written report*

76977   **Ultrasound bone density measurement and interpretation, peripheral site(s), any method**

    0.20   0.20   **FUD** XXX   [S] [Z3] [80] ▢

    AMA: 2012,Feb,9-10

76998-76999 Imaging Guidance During Surgery: Ultrasound

INCLUDES   Required permanent documentation of ultrasound images except when diagnostic purpose is biometric measurement
Written documentation

EXCLUDES   *Focused ultrasound ablation of uterine leiomyomata (0071T-0072T)*
Ultrasound exam that does not include thorough assessment of organ or site, recorded image, and written report

76998   **Ultrasonic guidance, intraoperative**

    EXCLUDES   *Radiofrequency tissue ablation, open/laparoscopic, ultrasonic guidance (76940)*
    Do not report with (36475, 36479, 37760-37761, 47370-47382, 0249T, 0301T)

    0.00   0.00   **FUD** XXX   [N] [N1] [80]

    AMA: 2015,Aug,8; 2015,Jan,16; 2014,Oct,6; 2014,Jan,11; 2014,Jan,5; 2013,Jan,6-8; 2012,Feb,9-10; 2010,Jul,6

76999   **Unlisted ultrasound procedure (eg, diagnostic, interventional)**

    0.00   0.00   **FUD** XXX   [01] [N1] [80]

    AMA: 2015,Jan,16; 2014,Jan,11; 2012,Feb,9-10

77001-77022 Imaging Guidance Techniques

+ **77001**   **Fluoroscopic guidance for central venous access device placement, replacement (catheter only or complete), or removal (includes fluoroscopic guidance for vascular access and catheter manipulation, any necessary contrast injections through access site or catheter with related venography radiologic supervision and interpretation, and radiographic documentation of final catheter position) (List separately in addition to code for primary procedure)**

    EXCLUDES   *Formal extremity venography performed separately from venous access and interpreted separately (36005, 75820, 75822, 75825, 75827)*
    Code first primary procedure
    Do not report with (33957-33959, [33962, 33963, 33964], 77002)
    Do not report with procedure codes that include fluoroscopic guidance in the code descriptor

    1.97   1.97   **FUD** ZZZ   [N] [N1] [PQ]

    AMA: 2015,Jan,16; 2014,Jan,11; 2012,Feb,9-10; 2012,Jan,15-42; 2011,Jan,8; 2011,Jan,11; 2010,Nov,1; 2010,Nov,3

77002   **Fluoroscopic guidance for needle placement (eg, biopsy, aspiration, injection, localization device)**

    EXCLUDES   *Platelet rich plasma injection(s) (0232T)*
    Code also surgical procedure
    Do not report with (10030, 19081-19086, 19281-19288, 20982-20983, 32554-32557, 70332, 73040, 73085, 73115, 73525, 73580, 73615, 0232T)
    Do not report with arthrography procedure(s)
    Do not report with codes that include 77002 in the radiological supervision and interpretation (49440, 74355, 74445, 74470, 75809-75810, 75885, 75887, 75989)

    2.59   2.59   **FUD** XXX   [N] [N1] [PQ]

    AMA: 2015,Aug,6; 2015,Jul,8; 2015,Feb,6; 2015,Feb,10; 2015,Jan,16; 2014,Jan,11; 2013,Nov,9; 2012,Dec,9-10; 2012,Nov,3-5; 2012,Jun,14; 2012,Feb,11; 2012,Apr,19; 2012,Feb,9-10; 2012,Jan,15-42; 2011,Apr,12; 2011,Jan,8; 2011,Jan,11; 2010,Nov,1; 2010,Nov,3; 2010,Jan,6

77003   **Fluoroscopic guidance and localization of needle or catheter tip for spine or paraspinous diagnostic or therapeutic injection procedures (epidural or subarachnoid)**

    EXCLUDES   *Destruction of paravertebral facet joint nerve by neurolysis ([64633, 64634, 64635, 64636])*
Injection and needle/catheter placement, epidural/subarachnoid (62270-62282, 62310-62319)
Injection, paravertebral facet joint (64490-64495)
Sacroiliac joint arthrography (27096)
Subarachnoid guidance puncture for myelography (72240-72270)
Transforaminal epidural needle placement/injection (64479-64484)
    Do not report with (10030, 22586, 27096, 64479-64484, 64490-64495, [64633, 64634, 64635, 64636], 0195T-0196T, 0309T)
    Do not report with procedure codes that include fluoroscopic guidance in the code descriptor

    2.40   2.40   **FUD** XXX   [N] [N1] [PQ]

    AMA: 2015,Jan,16; 2014,Jan,11; 2013,Nov,9; 2013,Dec,14; 2012,Sep,14-15; 2012,Sep,14-15; 2012,Jul,3-6; 2012,Jun,12-13; 2012,Feb,9-10; 2011,Jul,16-17; 2011,Mar,7; 2011,Feb,4-5; 2011,Jan,8; 2011,Jan,11; 2010,Nov,1; 2010,Aug,8&15; 2010,Dec,12; 2010,Nov,3; 2010,May,9; 2010,Jan,12-15; 2010,Jan,9-11

77011   **Computed tomography guidance for stereotactic localization**

    Do not report with (22586, 0195T-0196T, 0309T)

    6.17   6.17   **FUD** XXX   [N] [N1]

    AMA: 2015,Jan,16; 2014,Jan,11; 2012,Feb,9-10

77012   **Computed tomography guidance for needle placement (eg, biopsy, aspiration, injection, localization device), radiological supervision and interpretation**

    EXCLUDES   *Platelet rich plasma injection(s) (0232T)*
    Do not report with (10030, 22586, 27096, 32554-32557, 64479-64484, 64490-64495, [64633, 64634, 64635, 64636], 0195T-0196T, 0232T, 0309T)

    3.50   3.50   **FUD** XXX   [N] [N1]

    AMA: 2015,Feb,6; 2015,Jan,16; 2014,Jan,11; 2013,Nov,9; 2012,Dec,9-10; 2012,Nov,3-5; 2012,Sep,14-15; 2012,Sep,14-15; 2012,Jul,3-6; 2012,Feb,9-10; 2012,Jan,15-42; 2011,Apr,12; 2010,Jan,6

77013   **Computed tomography guidance for, and monitoring of, parenchymal tissue ablation**

    EXCLUDES   *Percutaneous radiofrequency ablation (32998, 47382-47383, 50592-50593)*
    Do not report with (20982-20983, 0340T)

    0.00   0.00   **FUD** XXX   [N] [N1] [80]

    AMA: 2015,Jul,8; 2015,Jan,16; 2014,Jan,11; 2012,Feb,9-10

77014   **Computed tomography guidance for placement of radiation therapy fields**

    Code also placement of interstitial device(s) for radiation therapy guidance (31627, 32553, 49411, 55876)

    3.28   3.28   **FUD** XXX   [N] [N1]

    AMA: 2015,Apr,10; 2015,Jan,16; 2014,Jan,11; 2012,Feb,9-10

77021   **Magnetic resonance guidance for needle placement (eg, for biopsy, needle aspiration, injection, or placement of localization device) radiological supervision and interpretation**

    EXCLUDES   *Platelet rich plasma injection(s) (0232T)*
Surgical procedure
    Do not report with (10030, 19085, 19287, 32554-32557, 0232T)

    11.5   11.5   **FUD** XXX   [N] [N1]

    AMA: 2015,Feb,6; 2015,Jan,16; 2014,Jan,11; 2013,Nov,9; 2012,Dec,9-10; 2012,Nov,3-5; 2012,Feb,9-10; 2011,Apr,12; 2010,Jan,6

[26]/[TC] PC/TC Comp Only   [A2]-[Z3] ASC Pmt   [50] Bilateral   ♂ Male Only   ♀ Female Only   Facility RVU   Non-Facility RVU
AMA: CPT Asst   **CMS:** Pub 100   [A]-[Y] OPPSI   [80]/[80] Surg Assist Allowed / w/Doc   Lab Crosswalk   Radiology Crosswalk

302   Medicare (Red Text)   CPT © 2015 American Medical Association. All Rights Reserved. (Black Text)   © 2015 Optum360, LLC (Blue Text)

77022 Magnetic resonance guidance for, and monitoring of, parenchymal tissue ablation

> EXCLUDES Ablation:
>> Percutaneous radiofrequency (32998, 47382-47383, 50592-50593)
>> Uterine leiomyomata by focused ablation (0071T, 0072T)
>
> Do not report with (20982-20983, 0071T-0072T, 0340T)
>
> 📖 0.00 ⚖ 0.00 **FUD** XXX [N] [N1] [80]
>
> **AMA:** 2015,Jul,8; 2015,Jan,16; 2014,Oct,6; 2014,Jan,11; 2012,Feb,9-10

77051-77063 Radiography: Breast

+ **77051** Computer-aided detection (computer algorithm analysis of digital image data for lesion detection) with further review for interpretation, with or without digitization of film radiographic images; diagnostic mammography (List separately in addition to code for primary procedure)

> Code first mammography (77055, 77056)
>
> 📖 0.25 ⚖ 0.25 **FUD** ZZZ [A]
>
> **AMA:** 2015,Jan,16; 2014,Jun,14; 2014,Jan,11; 2012,Feb,9-10

+ **77052** screening mammography (List separately in addition to code for primary procedure)

> Code first screening mammography (77057)
>
> 📖 0.25 ⚖ 0.25 **FUD** ZZZ [A]
>
> **AMA:** 2015,Jan,16; 2014,Jun,14; 2014,Jan,11; 2012,Feb,9-10

77053 Mammary ductogram or galactogram, single duct, radiological supervision and interpretation

> Code also injection procedure (19030)
>
> 📖 1.63 ⚖ 1.63 **FUD** XXX [Q2] [N1]
>
> **AMA:** 2015,Jan,16; 2014,Jan,11; 2012,Feb,9-10

77054 Mammary ductogram or galactogram, multiple ducts, radiological supervision and interpretation

> 📖 2.14 ⚖ 2.14 **FUD** XXX [Q2] [N1]
>
> **AMA:** 2015,Jan,16; 2014,Jan,11; 2012,Feb,9-10

77055 Mammography; unilateral

> Do not report with (77063)
>
> Code also computer-aided detection applied to diagnostic mammogram, if performed (77051)
>
> 📖 2.52 ⚖ 2.52 **FUD** XXX [A]
>
> **AMA:** 2015,Jan,16; 2014,Jun,14; 2014,Jan,11; 2012,Feb,9-10

77056 bilateral

> Code also computer-aided detection applied to diagnostic mammogram, if performed (77051)
>
> Do not report with (77063)
>
> 📖 3.24 ⚖ 3.24 **FUD** XXX [A]
>
> **AMA:** 2015,Jan,16; 2014,Jun,14; 2014,Jan,11; 2012,Feb,9-10

▲ **77057** Screening mammography, bilateral (2-view study of each breast) ♀

> Code also computer-aided detection applied to screening mammogram, if performed (77052)
>
> EXCLUDES Breast electrical impedance scan (76499)
>
> Do not report with (77061-77062)
>
> 📖 2.31 ⚖ 2.31 **FUD** XXX [A] [P0]
>
> **AMA:** 2015,Jan,16; 2014,Jun,14; 2014,Jan,11; 2012,Feb,9-10

77058 Magnetic resonance imaging, breast, without and/or with contrast material(s); unilateral

> 📖 15.1 ⚖ 15.1 **FUD** XXX [B]
>
> **AMA:** 2015,Jan,16; 2014,Jan,11; 2012,Feb,9-10

77059 bilateral

> 📖 15.0 ⚖ 15.0 **FUD** XXX [B]
>
> **AMA:** 2015,Jan,16; 2014,Jan,11; 2012,Feb,9-10

77061 Digital breast tomosynthesis; unilateral

> 📖 0.00 ⚖ 0.00 **FUD** XXX [E]
>
> Do not report with (76376-76377, 77057)

77062 bilateral

> 📖 0.00 ⚖ 0.00 **FUD** XXX [E]
>
> Do not report with (76376-76377, 77057)

+ **77063** Screening digital breast tomosynthesis, bilateral (List separately in addition to code for primary procedure)

> 📖 1.57 ⚖ 1.57 **FUD** XXX [A]
>
> Code first (77057)
>
> Do not report with (76376-76377, 77055-77056)

77071-77086 [77085, 77086] Additional Evaluations of Bones and Joints

77071 Manual application of stress performed by physician or other qualified health care professional for joint radiography, including contralateral joint if indicated

> Code also interpretation of stressed images according to anatomical site and number of views
>
> 📖 1.36 ⚖ 1.36 **FUD** XXX [01] [N1] [80] [26]
>
> **AMA:** 2015,Jan,16; 2014,Jan,11; 2012,Feb,9-10

77072 Bone age studies

> 📖 0.65 ⚖ 0.65 **FUD** XXX [01] [N1] [80]
>
> **AMA:** 2015,Jan,16; 2014,Jan,11; 2012,Feb,9-10

77073 Bone length studies (orthoroentgenogram, scanogram)

> 📖 1.02 ⚖ 1.02 **FUD** XXX [01] [N1] [80]
>
> **AMA:** 2015,Jan,16; 2014,Jan,11; 2012,Feb,9-10

77074 Radiologic examination, osseous survey; limited (eg, for metastases)

> 📖 1.79 ⚖ 1.79 **FUD** XXX [01] [N1] [80]
>
> **AMA:** 2015,Jan,16; 2014,Jan,11; 2012,Feb,9-10

77075 complete (axial and appendicular skeleton)

> 📖 2.44 ⚖ 2.44 **FUD** XXX [S] [Z3] [80]
>
> **AMA:** 2015,Jan,16; 2014,Jan,11; 2012,Feb,9-10

77076 Radiologic examination, osseous survey, infant

> 📖 2.67 ⚖ 2.67 **FUD** XXX [01] [N1] [80]
>
> **AMA:** 2015,Jan,16; 2014,Jan,11; 2012,Feb,9-10

77077 Joint survey, single view, 2 or more joints (specify)

> 📖 1.06 ⚖ 1.06 **FUD** XXX [01] [N1] [80]
>
> **AMA:** 2015,Jan,16; 2014,Jan,11; 2012,Feb,9-10

77078 Computed tomography, bone mineral density study, 1 or more sites, axial skeleton (eg, hips, pelvis, spine)

> 📖 3.19 ⚖ 3.19 **FUD** XXX [S] [Z2] [80]
>
> **AMA:** 2015,Jan,16; 2014,Jan,11; 2012,Feb,9-10

77080 Dual-energy X-ray absorptiometry (DXA), bone density study, 1 or more sites; axial skeleton (eg, hips, pelvis, spine)

> Do not report with ([77085], [77086])
>
> 📖 1.16 ⚖ 1.16 **FUD** XXX [S] [Z3] [80]
>
> **AMA:** 2015,Jan,16; 2014,Jan,11; 2012,Feb,9-10

77081 appendicular skeleton (peripheral) (eg, radius, wrist, heel)

> 📖 0.79 ⚖ 0.79 **FUD** XXX [S] [Z3] [80]
>
> **AMA:** 2015,Jan,16; 2014,Jan,11; 2012,Feb,9-10

\# **77085** axial skeleton (eg, hips, pelvis, spine), including vertebral fracture assessment

> 📖 1.58 ⚖ 1.58 **FUD** XXX [01] [N1] [80]
>
> Do not report with (77080, [77086])

\# **77086** Vertebral fracture assessment via dual-energy X-ray absorptiometry (DXA)

> 📖 1.00 ⚖ 1.00 **FUD** XXX [01] [N1] [80]
>
> Do not report with (77080, [77085])

77084 Magnetic resonance (eg, proton) imaging, bone marrow blood supply

> 📖 10.9 ⚖ 10.9 **FUD** XXX [S] [Z2] [80]
>
> **AMA:** 2015,Jan,16; 2014,Jan,11; 2012,Feb,9-10

77085 **Resequenced code. See code following 77081.**

77086 **Resequenced code. See code before 77084.**

Radiology

77261 — 77332

77261-77263 Therapeutic Radiology: Treatment Planning

INCLUDES Determination of:
Appropriate treatment devices
Number and size of treatment ports
Treatment method
Treatment time/dosage
Treatment volume
Interpretation of special testing
Tumor localization
Do not report with (77401, 0394T-0395T)

77261   Therapeutic radiology treatment planning; simple

INCLUDES Planning for single treatment area included in a single port or simple parallel opposed ports with simple or no blocking

🔾 2.13   ⅍ 2.13   **FUD** XXX   B 80 2G 🖵 P0

AMA: 2015,Jan,16; 2014,Jan,11; 2012,Feb,9-10; 2010,Oct,3-4

77262   intermediate

INCLUDES Planning for three or more converging ports, two separate treatment sites, multiple blocks, or special time dose constraints

🔾 3.17   ⅍ 3.17   **FUD** XXX   B 80 2G 🖵 P0

AMA: 2015,Jan,16; 2014,Jan,11; 2012,Feb,9-10; 2010,Oct,3-4

77263   complex

INCLUDES Planning for very complex blocking, custom shielding blocks, tangential ports, special wedges or compensators, three or more separate treatment areas, rotational or special beam considerations, combination of treatment modalities

🔾 4.64   ⅍ 4.64   **FUD** XXX   B 80 2G 🖵 P0

AMA: 2015,Jan,16; 2014,Jan,11; 2012,Feb,9-10; 2010,Oct,3-4

77280-77299 Radiation Therapy Simulation

CMS: 100-4,4,200.3.2 Additional Billing Instructions for IMRT Planning and Delivery

77280   Therapeutic radiology simulation-aided field setting; simple

INCLUDES Simulation of a single treatment site

🔾 7.59   ⅍ 7.59   **FUD** XXX   S Z2 80 🖵

AMA: 2015,Apr,10; 2015,Jan,16; 2014,Jan,11; 2013,Nov,11; 2012,Feb,9-10; 2012,Jan,15-42; 2011,Jan,11; 2010,Oct,3-4

77285   intermediate

INCLUDES Two different treatment sites

🔾 11.9   ⅍ 11.9   **FUD** XXX   S Z2 80 🖵

AMA: 2015,Apr,10; 2015,Jan,16; 2014,Jan,11; 2013,Nov,11; 2012,Feb,9-10; 2010,Oct,3-4

77290   complex

INCLUDES Brachytherapy
Complex blocking
Contrast material
Custom shielding blocks
Hyperthermia probe verification
Rotation, arc or particle therapy
Simulation to >= 3 treatment sites

🔾 14.2   ⅍ 14.2   **FUD** XXX   S Z2 80 🖵

AMA: 2015,Apr,10; 2015,Jan,16; 2014,Jan,11; 2013,Nov,11; 2012,Feb,9-10; 2012,Jan,15-42; 2011,Jan,11; 2010,Oct,3-4

+ ### 77293   Respiratory motion management simulation (List separately in addition to code for primary procedure)

Code first (77295, 77301)

🔾 12.9   ⅍ 12.9   **FUD** ZZZ   N 80

AMA: 2013,Nov,11

77295   Resequenced code. See code before 77300.

77299   Unlisted procedure, therapeutic radiology clinical treatment planning

🔾 0.00   ⅍ 0.00   **FUD** XXX   S Z2 80

AMA: 2015,Jan,16; 2014,Jan,11; 2013,Nov,11; 2012,Feb,9-10; 2012,Jan,15-42; 2011,Jan,11; 2010,Oct,3-4

77300-77370 [77295] Radiation Physics Services

CMS: 100-4,13,70.5 Radiation Physics Services

\# ### 77295   3-dimensional radiotherapy plan, including dose-volume histogram

🔾 13.6   ⅍ 13.6   **FUD** XXX   S Z3 80 🖵 P0

AMA: 2015,Jun,6; 2015,Jan,16; 2014,Jan,11; 2013,Nov,11; 2012,Feb,9-10; 2010,Oct,3-4

77300   Basic radiation dosimetry calculation, central axis depth dose calculation, TDF, NSD, gap calculation, off axis factor, tissue inhomogeneity factors, calculation of non-ionizing radiation surface and depth dose, as required during course of treatment, only when prescribed by the treating physician

Do not report with (77306-77307, 77316-77318, 77321, 77767-77772, 0394T-0395T)

🔾 1.77   ⅍ 1.77   **FUD** XXX   S Z3 80 🖵

AMA: 2015,Jan,16; 2014,Jan,11; 2013,Nov,11; 2012,Feb,9-10; 2012,Jan,15-42; 2011,Jan,11; 2010,Oct,3-4

77301   Intensity modulated radiotherapy plan, including dose-volume histograms for target and critical structure partial tolerance specifications

🔾 54.2   ⅍ 54.2   **FUD** XXX   S Z2 80 🖵

AMA: 2015,Jan,16; 2014,Jan,11; 2013,Nov,11; 2012,Feb,9-10; 2012,Jan,15-42; 2011,Jan,11; 2010,Oct,3-4

77306   Teletherapy isodose plan; simple (1 or 2 unmodified ports directed to a single area of interest), includes basic dosimetry calculation(s)

🔾 4.07   ⅍ 4.07   **FUD** XXX   S Z2 80

Do not report more than one time for treatment to a specific area
Do not report with (77300, 77401, 0394T-0395T)

77307   complex (multiple treatment areas, tangential ports, the use of wedges, blocking, rotational beam, or special beam considerations), includes basic dosimetry calculation(s)

🔾 7.97   ⅍ 7.97   **FUD** XXX   S Z2 80

Do not report more than one time for treatment to a specific area
Do not report with (77300, 77401, 0394T-0395T)

77316   Brachytherapy isodose plan; simple (calculation[s] made from 1 to 4 sources, or remote afterloading brachytherapy, 1 channel), includes basic dosimetry calculation(s)

🔾 5.22   ⅍ 5.22   **FUD** XXX   S Z2 80

Do not report with (77300, 77401, 0394T-0395T)

77317   intermediate (calculation[s] made from 5 to 10 sources, or remote afterloading brachytherapy, 2-12 channels), includes basic dosimetry calculation(s)

🔾 6.83   ⅍ 6.83   **FUD** XXX   S Z3 80

Do not report with (77300, 77401, 0394T-0395T)

77318   complex (calculation[s] made from over 10 sources, or remote afterloading brachytherapy, over 12 channels), includes basic dosimetry calculation(s)

🔾 9.87   ⅍ 9.87   **FUD** XXX   S Z2 80

Do not report with (77300, 77401, 0394T-0395T)

77321   Special teletherapy port plan, particles, hemibody, total body

🔾 2.58   ⅍ 2.58   **FUD** XXX   S Z3 80 🖵

AMA: 2015,Jan,16; 2014,Jan,11; 2013,Nov,11; 2012,Feb,9-10; 2010,Oct,3-4

77331   Special dosimetry (eg, TLD, microdosimetry) (specify), only when prescribed by the treating physician

🔾 1.79   ⅍ 1.79   **FUD** XXX   S Z3 80 🖵

AMA: 2015,Jun,6; 2015,Jan,16; 2014,Jan,11; 2013,Nov,11; 2012,Feb,9-10; 2010,Oct,3-4

77332   Treatment devices, design and construction; simple (simple block, simple bolus)

Do not report with (77401, 0394T-0395T)

🔾 2.31   ⅍ 2.31   **FUD** XXX   S Z3 80 🖵

AMA: 2015,Jan,16; 2014,Jan,11; 2013,Nov,11; 2012,Feb,9-10; 2012,Jan,15-42; 2010,Oct,3-4

77333 intermediate (multiple blocks, stents, bite blocks, special bolus)

Do not report with (77401, 0394T-0395T)

🚗 1.48 ⚕ 1.48 **FUD** XXX

[S] [Z3] [80] [⬜]

AMA: 2015,Jan,16; 2014,Jan,11; 2013,Nov,11; 2012,Feb,9-10; 2010,Oct,3-4

77334 complex (irregular blocks, special shields, compensators, wedges, molds or casts)

Do not report with (77401, 0394T-0395T)

🚗 4.26 ⚕ 4.26 **FUD** XXX

[S] [Z3] [80] [⬜]

AMA: 2015,Jan,16; 2014,Jan,11; 2013,Nov,11; 2012,Feb,9-10; 2012,Jan,15-42; 2010,Dec,12; 2010,Oct,3-4

77336 Continuing medical physics consultation, including assessment of treatment parameters, quality assurance of dose delivery, and review of patient treatment documentation in support of the radiation oncologist, reported per week of therapy

Do not report with (77401, 0394T-0395T)

🚗 2.15 ⚕ 2.15 **FUD** XXX

[S] [Z2] [80] [TC] [⬜]

AMA: 2015,Jan,16; 2014,Jan,11; 2013,Nov,11; 2012,Feb,9-10; 2010,Oct,3-4

77338 Multi-leaf collimator (MLC) device(s) for intensity modulated radiation therapy (IMRT), design and construction per IMRT plan

EXCLUDES *Immobilization in IMRT treatment (77332-77334)*

Do not report with (77385)

Do not report more than one time per IMRT plan

🚗 14.1 ⚕ 14.1 **FUD** XXX

[S] [Z2] [80]

AMA: 2015,Jan,16; 2014,Jan,11; 2013,Nov,11; 2012,Feb,9-10; 2012,Jan,15-42; 2011,Jan,11; 2010,Dec,12; 2010,Oct,3-4

77370 Special medical radiation physics consultation

🚗 3.27 ⚕ 3.27

[S] [Z2] [80] [TC] [⬜]

AMA: 2015,Jun,6; 2015,Jan,16; 2014,Jan,11; 2013,Nov,11; 2012,Feb,9-10; 2012,Jan,15-42; 2011,Jan,11; 2010,Oct,3-4

77371-77399 Stereotactic Radiosurgery (SRS) Planning and Delivery

CMS: 100-4,13,70.5 Radiation Physics Services

77371 Radiation treatment delivery, stereotactic radiosurgery (SRS), complete course of treatment of cranial lesion(s) consisting of 1 session; multi-source Cobalt 60 based

🚗 0.00 ⚕ 0.00 **FUD** XXX

[⊙] [J] [Z2] [80] [TC]

AMA: 2015,Jan,16; 2014,Jul,8; 2014,Jan,11; 2012,Feb,9-10; 2011,Jul,12-13; 2010,Oct,3-4

77372 linear accelerator based

EXCLUDES *Radiation treatment supervision (77432)*

🚗 29.7 ⚕ 29.7 **FUD** XXX

[J] [Z3] [80] [TC]

AMA: 2015,Jan,16; 2014,Jul,8; 2014,Jan,11; 2012,Feb,9-10; 2011,Jul,12-13; 2010,Oct,3-4

77373 Stereotactic body radiation therapy, treatment delivery, per fraction to 1 or more lesions, including image guidance, entire course not to exceed 5 fractions

EXCLUDES *Single fraction cranial lesion(s) (77371-77372)*

Do not report with (77385-77386, 77401-77402, 77407, 77412)

🚗 37.7 ⚕ 37.7 **FUD** XXX

[S] [Z2] [80] [TC]

AMA: 2015,Jun,6; 2015,Jan,16; 2014,Jul,8; 2014,Jan,11; 2012,Feb,9-10; 2011,Jul,12-13; 2010,Oct,3-4

77385 Resequenced code. See code following 77417.

77386 Resequenced code. See code following 77417.

77387 Resequenced code. See code following 77417.

77399 Unlisted procedure, medical radiation physics, dosimetry and treatment devices, and special services

🚗 0.00 ⚕ 0.00 **FUD** XXX

[S] [Z2] [80]

AMA: 2015,Jan,16; 2014,Jan,11; 2012,Feb,9-10; 2010,Oct,3-4

77401-77417 [77385, 77386, 77387, 77424, 77425] Radiation Treatment

INCLUDES Technical component and assorted energy levels

EXCLUDES *Intra-fraction localization and target tracking (77387)*

77401 Radiation treatment delivery, superficial and/or ortho voltage, per day

Code also E&M codes when performed alone, as appropriate

Do not report with (77261-77263, 77306-77307, 77316-77318, 77332-77334, 77336, 77373, 77427, 77431-77432, 77435, 77469-77470, 77499)

🚗 0.58 ⚕ 0.58 **FUD** XXX

[S] [Z3] [80] [TC] [⬜]

AMA: 2015,Jan,16; 2014,Jan,11; 2012,Feb,9-10; 2010,Oct,3-4

77402 Radiation treatment delivery,=>1 MeV; simple

Do not report with (77373)

🚗 0.00 ⚕ 0.00 **FUD** XXX

[S] [Z2] [80] [TC] [⬜]

AMA: 2015,Jan,16; 2014,Jan,11; 2012,Feb,9-10; 2010,Oct,3-4

77407 intermediate

Do not report with (77373)

🚗 0.00 ⚕ 0.00 **FUD** XXX

[S] [Z2] [80] [TC] [⬜]

AMA: 2015,Jan,16; 2014,Jan,11; 2012,Feb,9-10; 2010,Oct,3-4

77412 complex

Do not report with (77373)

🚗 0.00 ⚕ 0.00 **FUD** XXX

[S] [Z2] [80] [TC] [⬜]

AMA: 2015,Jan,16; 2014,Jan,11; 2012,Feb,9-10; 2010,Oct,3-4

▲ **77417** Therapeutic radiology port image(s)

EXCLUDES *Intensity modulated treatment planning (77301)*

🚗 0.30 ⚕ 0.30 **FUD** XXX

[N] [N1] [80] [TC] [⬜]

AMA: 2015,Jan,16; 2014,Jan,11; 2012,Feb,9-10; 2012,Jan,15-42; 2011,Jan,11; 2010,Oct,3-4

\# **77385** Intensity modulated radiation treatment delivery (IMRT), includes guidance and tracking, when performed; simple

🚗 0.00 ⚕ 0.00 **FUD** XXX

[S] [Z2] [80] [TC]

Code also modifier 26 for professional component tracking and guidance with (77387)

Do not report with (77371-77373)

\# **77386** complex

🚗 0.00 ⚕ 0.00 **FUD** XXX

[S] [Z2] [80] [TC]

Code also modifier 26 for professional component tracking and guidance with (77387)

Do not report with (77371-77373)

\# **77387** Guidance for localization of target volume for delivery of radiation treatment delivery, includes intrafraction tracking, when performed

🚗 0.00 ⚕ 0.00 **FUD** XXX

[N] [N1] [80]

Do not report technical component with (77371-77373, 77385-77386)

\# **77424** Intraoperative radiation treatment delivery, x-ray, single treatment session

🚗 0.00 ⚕ 0.00 **FUD** XXX

[J] [Z2]

AMA: 2012,Feb,9-10

\# **77425** Intraoperative radiation treatment delivery, electrons, single treatment session

🚗 0.00 ⚕ 0.00 **FUD** XXX

[J] [Z2]

AMA: 2015,Jan,16; 2014,Jan,11; 2012,Feb,9-10

77422-77425 Neutron Therapy

77422 High energy neutron radiation treatment delivery; single treatment area using a single port or parallel-opposed ports with no blocks or simple blocking

🚗 0.94 ⚕ 0.94 **FUD** XXX

[S] [Z3] [80] [TC]

AMA: 2015,Jan,16; 2014,Jan,11; 2012,Feb,9-10; 2010,Oct,3-4

77423 1 or more isocenter(s) with coplanar or non-coplanar geometry with blocking and/or wedge, and/or compensator(s)

🚗 1.83 ⚕ 1.83 **FUD** XXX

[S] [Z3] [80] [TC]

AMA: 2015,Jan,16; 2014,Jan,11; 2012,Feb,9-10; 2010,Oct,3-4

77424 Resequenced code. See code before 77422.

77425 Resequenced code. See code before 77422.

Radiology

7742 — 77610

77427-77499 Radiation Therapy Management

INCLUDES Assessment of patient for medical evaluation and management (at least one per treatment management service) that includes:
Coordination of care/treatment
Evaluation of patient's response to treatment
Review of:
Dose delivery
Dosimetry
Lab tests
Patient treatment set-up
Port film
Treatment parameters
X-rays
Units of five fractions or treatment sessions regardless of time. Two or more fractions performed on the same day can be counted separately provided there is a distinct break in service between sessions and the fractions are of the character usually furnished on different days.
Do not report with (77401, 0394T-0395T)

77427 **Radiation treatment management, 5 treatments**

INCLUDES 3 or 4 fractions beyond a multiple of five at the end of a treatment period
Do not report separately when one or two more fractions are provided beyond a multiple of five at the end of a course of treatment

⚕ 5.22   ⚕ 5.22   **FUD** XXX   Ⓑ 26 🔲 P0

AMA: 2015,Jun,6; 2015,Jan,16; 2014,Jan,11; 2012,Feb,9-10; 2010,Oct,3-4

77431 **Radiation therapy management with complete course of therapy consisting of 1 or 2 fractions only**

Do not report when used to fill in the last week of a protracted therapy course

⚕ 2.86   ⚕ 2.86   **FUD** XXX   Ⓑ 80 26 🔲 P0

AMA: 2015,Jun,6; 2015,Jan,16; 2014,Jan,11; 2012,Feb,9-10; 2010,Oct,3-4

77432 **Stereotactic radiation treatment management of cranial lesion(s) (complete course of treatment consisting of 1 session)**

INCLUDES Guidance for localization of target volume for radiation delivery (professional component)
EXCLUDES Stereotactic body radiation therapy treatment (77435)
Code also technical component of guidance for localization of target volume by appending modifier TC to (77387)
Do not report with stereotactic radiosurgery by same physician (61796-61800)

⚕ 11.7   ⚕ 11.7   **FUD** XXX   Ⓑ 80 26 🔲 P0

AMA: 2015,Jun,6; 2015,Jan,16; 2014,Jul,8; 2014,Jan,11; 2012,Feb,9-10; 2012,Jan,15-42; 2011,Jul,12-13; 2011,Jan,11; 2010,Oct,3-4; 2010,Oct,9

77435 **Stereotactic body radiation therapy, treatment management, per treatment course, to 1 or more lesions, including image guidance, entire course not to exceed 5 fractions**

INCLUDES Guidance for localization of target volume for radiation delivery (professional component)
Code also technical component of guidance for localization of target volume by appending modifier TC to (77387)
Do not report with (77427-77432)
Do not report with stereotactic radiosurgery by same physician (32701, 61796-61800, 63620-63621)

⚕ 17.6   ⚕ 17.6   **FUD** XXX   Ⓝ N1 80 26 P0

AMA: 2015,Jun,6; 2015,Jan,16; 2014,Jan,11; 2012,Feb,9-10; 2012,Jan,15-42; 2010,Oct,3-4; 2010,Oct,9

77469 **Intraoperative radiation treatment management**

EXCLUDES Medical evaluation and management provided outside of the intraoperative treatment management

⚕ 9.01   ⚕ 9.01   **FUD** XXX   Ⓑ 80

AMA: 2015,Jun,6; 2012,Feb,9-10

77470 **Special treatment procedure (eg, total body irradiation, hemibody radiation, per oral or endocavitary irradiation)**

EXCLUDES Daily or weekly patient management
Intraoperative radiation treatment delivery and management ([77424, 77425], 77469)
Do not report more than one time per course of therapy

⚕ 4.36   ⚕ 4.36   **FUD** XXX   Ⓢ Z3 80 🔲 P0

AMA: 2015,Jun,6; 2015,Jan,16; 2014,Jan,11; 2012,Feb,9-10; 2010,Oct,3-4

77499 **Unlisted procedure, therapeutic radiology treatment management**

⚕ 0.00   ⚕ 0.00   **FUD** XXX   Ⓑ 80

AMA: 2015,Jun,6; 2015,Jan,16; 2014,Jan,11; 2012,Feb,9-10; 2010,Oct,3-4

77520-77525 Proton Therapy

EXCLUDES High dose rate electronic brachytherapy, per fraction (0394T-0395T)

77520 **Proton treatment delivery; simple, without compensation**

INCLUDES Single treatment site using:
Single nontangential/oblique port

⚕ 0.00   ⚕ 0.00   **FUD** XXX   Ⓢ Z2 80 TC

AMA: 2015,Jan,16; 2014,Jan,11; 2012,Feb,9-10; 2010,Oct,3-4

77522 **simple, with compensation**

INCLUDES Single treatment site using:
Custom block with compensation
Single nontangential/oblique port

⚕ 0.00   ⚕ 0.00   **FUD** XXX   Ⓢ Z2 80 TC 🔲

AMA: 2012,Feb,9-10; 2010,Oct,3-4

77523 **intermediate**

INCLUDES One or more treatment sites using:
One or more tangential/oblique ports with custom blocks and compensators OR
Two or more ports with custom blocks and compensators

⚕ 0.00   ⚕ 0.00   **FUD** XXX   Ⓢ Z2 80 TC 🔲

AMA: 2015,Jan,16; 2014,Jan,11; 2012,Feb,9-10; 2010,Oct,3-4

77525 **complex**

INCLUDES One or more treatment sites using:
Two or more ports with matching or patching fields and custom blocks and compensators

⚕ 0.00   ⚕ 0.00   **FUD** XXX   Ⓢ Z2 80 TC 🔲

AMA: 2012,Feb,9-10; 2010,Oct,3-4

77600-77620 Hyperthermia Treatment

CMS: 100-3,110.1 Hyperthermia for Treatment of Cancer

INCLUDES Interstitial insertion of temperature sensors
Management during the course of therapy
Normal follow-up care for three months after completion
Physics planning
Use of heat generating devices
EXCLUDES Initial evaluation and management service
Radiation therapy treatment (77371-77373, 77401-77412, 77422-77423)

77600 **Hyperthermia, externally generated; superficial (ie, heating to a depth of 4 cm or less)**

⚕ 11.3   ⚕ 11.3   **FUD** XXX   ⊙ Ⓢ Z2 80 🔲

AMA: 2015,Jan,16; 2014,Jan,11; 2013,Dec,16; 2012,Feb,9-10; 2010,Oct,3-4

77605 **deep (ie, heating to depths greater than 4 cm)**

EXCLUDES Microwave thermotherapy of the breast (0301T)

⚕ 21.3   ⚕ 21.3   **FUD** XXX   ⊙ Ⓢ Z2 80 🔲

AMA: 2015,Jan,16; 2014,Jan,11; 2013,Dec,16; 2012,Feb,9-10; 2010,Oct,3-4

77610 **Hyperthermia generated by interstitial probe(s); 5 or fewer interstitial applicators**

⚕ 28.8   ⚕ 28.8   **FUD** XXX   ⊙ Ⓢ Z2 80 🔲

AMA: 2015,Jan,16; 2014,Jan,11; 2013,Dec,16; 2012,Feb,9-10; 2010,Oct,3-4

77615 more than 5 interstitial applicators
28.3   28.3   **FUD** XXX   ⊙ S Z2 80 ▯
AMA: 2015,Jan,16; 2014,Jan,11; 2013,Dec,16; 2012,Feb,9-10; 2010,Oct,3-4

77620 Hyperthermia generated by intracavitary probe(s)
13.0   13.0   **FUD** XXX   S Z2 80 ▯
AMA: 2015,Jan,16; 2014,Jan,11; 2013,Dec,16; 2012,Feb,9-10; 2010,Oct,3-4

77750-77799 Brachytherapy

CMS: 100-4,13,70.4 Clinical Brachytherapy; 100-4,4,61.4.4 Billing for Brachytherapy Source Supervision, Handling and Loading Costs

INCLUDES Hospital admission and daily visits
EXCLUDES Placement of:
Heyman capsules (58346)
Ovoids and tandems (57155)

77750 Infusion or instillation of radioelement solution (includes 3-month follow-up care)
EXCLUDES Monoclonal antibody infusion (79403)
Nonantibody radiopharmaceutical therapy infusion without follow-up care (79101)
10.3   10.3   **FUD** 090   S Z2 80 ▯
AMA: 2015,Jan,16; 2014,Jan,11; 2012,Feb,9-10; 2010,Oct,3-4

77761 Intracavitary radiation source application; simple
INCLUDES One to four sources/ribbons
Do not report with (0394T-0395T)
10.8   10.8   **FUD** 090   S Z3 80 ▯
AMA: 2015,Jan,16; 2014,Jan,11; 2012,Feb,9-10; 2012,Jan,15-42; 2011,Jan,11; 2010,Oct,3-4

77762 intermediate
INCLUDES Five to ten sources/ribbons
Do not report with (0394T-0395T)
15.3   15.3   **FUD** 090   S Z2 80 ▯
AMA: 2015,Jan,16; 2014,Jan,11; 2012,Feb,9-10; 2010,Oct,3-4

77763 complex
INCLUDES More than ten sources/ribbons
Do not report with (0394T-0395T)
20.4   20.4   **FUD** 090   S Z2 80 ▯
AMA: 2015,Jan,16; 2014,Jan,11; 2012,Feb,9-10; 2010,Oct,3-4

● **77767** Remote afterloading high dose rate radionuclide skin surface brachytherapy, includes basic dosimetry, when performed; lesion diameter up to 2.0 cm or 1 channel
EXCLUDES Superficial non-brachytherapy superficial treatment delivery (77401)
Do not report with (77300, 0394T-0395T)

● **77768** lesion diameter over 2.0 cm and 2 or more channels, or multiple lesions
EXCLUDES Superficial non-brachytherapy superficial treatment delivery (77401)
Do not report with (77300, 0394T-0395T)

● **77770** Remote afterloading high dose rate radionuclide interstitial or intracavitary brachytherapy, includes basic dosimetry, when performed; 1 channel
EXCLUDES Superficial non-brachytherapy superficial treatment delivery (77401)
Do not report with (77300, 0394T-0395T)

● **77771** 2-12 channels
EXCLUDES Superficial non-brachytherapy superficial treatment delivery (77401)
Do not report with (77300, 0394T-0395T)

● **77772** over 12 channels
EXCLUDES Superficial non-brachytherapy superficial treatment delivery (77401)
Do not report with (77300, 0394T-0395T)

77776 Interstitial radiation source application; simple
To report, see ~77799

77777 intermediate
To report, see ~77799

▲ **77778** Interstitial radiation source application, complex, includes supervision, handling, loading of radiation source, when performed
INCLUDES More than ten sources/ribbons
Do not report with (77790, 0394T-0395T)
24.4   24.4   **FUD** 090   Q3 Z3 80 ▯ PQ
AMA: 2015,Jan,16; 2014,Jan,11; 2012,Feb,9-10; 2010,Oct,3-4

77785 Remote afterloading high dose rate radionuclide brachytherapy; 1 channel
To report, see ~77770-77772

77786 2-12 channels
To report, see ~77770-77772

77787 over 12 channels
To report, see ~77770-77772

▲ **77789** Surface application of low dose rate radionuclide source
Do not report with (77401, 77767-77768, 0394T-0395T)
3.33   3.33   **FUD** 000   S Z3 80 ▯
AMA: 2015,Jan,16; 2014,Jan,11; 2012,Feb,9-10; 2010,Oct,3-4

77790 Supervision, handling, loading of radiation source
Do not report with (77778)
2.71   2.71   **FUD** XXX   N N1 80 ▯
AMA: 2015,Jan,16; 2014,Jan,11; 2012,Feb,9-10; 2010,Oct,3-4

77799 Unlisted procedure, clinical brachytherapy
0.00   0.00   **FUD** XXX   S Z2 80
AMA: 2015,Jan,16; 2014,Jan,11; 2012,Feb,9-10

78012-78099 Nuclear Radiology: Thyroid, Parathyroid, Adrenal

EXCLUDES Diagnostic services (see appropriate sections)
Follow-up care (see appropriate section)
Radioimmunoassays (82009-84999 [82652])
Code also radiopharmaceutical(s) and/or drug(s) supplied

78012 Thyroid uptake, single or multiple quantitative measurement(s) (including stimulation, suppression, or discharge, when performed)
2.31   2.31   **FUD** XXX   S Z2 80
AMA: 2015,Jan,16; 2013,Jun,9-11

78013 Thyroid imaging (including vascular flow, when performed);
5.51   5.51   **FUD** XXX   S Z2 80
AMA: 2015,Jan,16; 2013,Jun,9-11

78014 with single or multiple uptake(s) quantitative measurement(s) (including stimulation, suppression, or discharge, when performed)
6.99   6.99   **FUD** XXX   S Z2 80
AMA: 2015,Jan,16; 2013,Jun,9-11

78015 Thyroid carcinoma metastases imaging; limited area (eg, neck and chest only)
6.39   6.39   **FUD** XXX   S Z2 80 ▯
AMA: 2015,Jan,16; 2014,Jan,11; 2012,Feb,9-10

78016 with additional studies (eg, urinary recovery)
8.21   8.21   **FUD** XXX   S Z2 80 ▯
AMA: 2015,Jan,16; 2014,Jan,11; 2012,Feb,9-10

78018 whole body
9.04   9.04   **FUD** XXX   S Z2 80 ▯
AMA: 2015,Jan,16; 2014,Jan,11; 2012,Feb,9-10

+ **78020** Thyroid carcinoma metastases uptake (List separately in addition to code for primary procedure)
Code first (78018)
2.42   2.42   **FUD** ZZZ   N N1 80 ▯
AMA: 2015,Jan,16; 2014,Jan,11; 2012,Feb,9-10; 2012,Jan,15-42; 2011,Jan,11

78070 Parathyroid planar imaging (including subtraction, when performed);
8.72   8.72   **FUD** XXX   S Z2 80 ▯
AMA: 2015,Jan,16; 2014,Jan,11; 2012,Feb,9-10

● New Code   ▲ Revised Code   ○ Reinstated   M Maternity   A Age Edit   Unlisted   Not Covered   # Resequenced
⊘ AMA Mod 51 Exempt   ⑤ Optum Mod 51 Exempt   ⑥ Mod 63 Exempt   ⊙ Mod Sedation   + Add-on   ▯ CCI   PQ PQRS   FUD Follow-up Days

Radiology

78071   with tomographic (SPECT)
    📷 10.3   ⚖ 10.3   **FUD** XXX   S Z2 80

78072   with tomographic (SPECT), and concurrently acquired computed tomography (CT) for anatomical localization
    📷 11.8   ⚖ 11.8   **FUD** XXX   S Z2 80

78075   Adrenal imaging, cortex and/or medulla
    📷 13.1   ⚖ 13.1   **FUD** XXX   S Z2 80 💻
    AMA: 2015,Jan,16; 2014,Jan,11; 2012,Feb,9-10

78099   Unlisted endocrine procedure, diagnostic nuclear medicine
    📷 0.00   ⚖ 0.00   **FUD** XXX   S Z2 80
    AMA: 2015,Jan,16; 2014,Jan,11; 2012,Feb,9-10

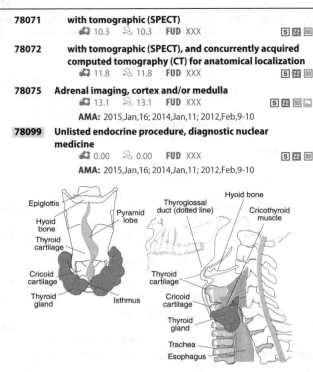

Epiglottis, Hyoid bone, Pyramid lobe, Thyroid cartilage, Cricoid cartilage, Thyroid gland, Isthmus — Thyroglossal duct (dotted line), Hyoid bone, Cricothyroid muscle, Thyroid cartilage, Cricoid cartilage, Thyroid gland, Trachea, Esophagus

78102-78199 Nuclear Radiology: Blood Forming Organs

EXCLUDES   *Diagnostic services (see appropriate sections)*
Follow-up care (see appropriate section)
Radioimmunoassays (82009-84999 [82652])
Code also radiopharmaceutical(s) and/or drug(s) supplied

78102   Bone marrow imaging; limited area
    📷 4.92   ⚖ 4.92   **FUD** XXX   S Z2 80 💻
    AMA: 2015,Jan,16; 2014,Jan,11; 2012,Feb,9-10

78103   multiple areas
    📷 6.40   ⚖ 6.40   **FUD** XXX   S Z2 80 💻
    AMA: 2012,Feb,9-10

78104   whole body
    📷 7.10   ⚖ 7.10   **FUD** XXX   S Z2 80 💻
    AMA: 2012,Feb,9-10

78110   Plasma volume, radiopharmaceutical volume-dilution technique (separate procedure); single sampling
    📷 2.98   ⚖ 2.98   **FUD** XXX   S Z2 80 💻
    AMA: 2012,Feb,9-10

78111   multiple samplings
    📷 2.79   ⚖ 2.79   **FUD** XXX   S Z2 80 💻
    AMA: 2012,Feb,9-10

78120   Red cell volume determination (separate procedure); single sampling
    📷 2.72   ⚖ 2.72   **FUD** XXX   S Z2 80 💻
    AMA: 2012,Feb,9-10

78121   multiple samplings
    📷 3.05   ⚖ 3.05   **FUD** XXX   S Z2 80 💻
    AMA: 2012,Feb,9-10

78122   Whole blood volume determination, including separate measurement of plasma volume and red cell volume (radiopharmaceutical volume-dilution technique)
    📷 2.78   ⚖ 2.78   **FUD** XXX   S Z2 80 💻
    AMA: 2012,Feb,9-10

78130   Red cell survival study;
    📷 4.56   ⚖ 4.56   **FUD** XXX   S Z2 80 💻
    AMA: 2012,Feb,9-10

78135   differential organ/tissue kinetics (eg, splenic and/or hepatic sequestration)
    📷 10.1   ⚖ 10.1   **FUD** XXX   S Z2 80 💻
    AMA: 2012,Feb,9-10

78140   Labeled red cell sequestration, differential organ/tissue (eg, splenic and/or hepatic)
    📷 3.93   ⚖ 3.93   **FUD** XXX   S Z2 80 💻
    AMA: 2012,Feb,9-10

78185   Spleen imaging only, with or without vascular flow
    EXCLUDES   *Liver imaging (78215-78216)*
    📷 6.15   ⚖ 6.15   **FUD** XXX   S Z2 80 💻
    AMA: 2012,Feb,9-10

78190   Kinetics, study of platelet survival, with or without differential organ/tissue localization
    📷 11.4   ⚖ 11.4   **FUD** XXX   S Z2 80 💻
    AMA: 2012,Feb,9-10

78191   Platelet survival study
    📷 4.83   ⚖ 4.83   **FUD** XXX   S Z2 80 💻
    AMA: 2012,Feb,9-10

78195   Lymphatics and lymph nodes imaging
    EXCLUDES   *Sentinel node identification without scintigraphy (38792)*
        Sentinel node removal (38500-38542)
    📷 10.3   ⚖ 10.3   **FUD** XXX   S Z2 80 💻
    AMA: 2015,Jan,16; 2014,Jan,11; 2012,Feb,9-10

78199   Unlisted hematopoietic, reticuloendothelial and lymphatic procedure, diagnostic nuclear medicine
    📷 0.00   ⚖ 0.00   **FUD** XXX   S Z2 80
    AMA: 2015,Jan,16; 2014,Jan,11; 2012,Feb,9-10

78201-78299 Nuclear Radiology: Digestive System

EXCLUDES   *Diagnostic services (see appropriate sections)*
Follow-up care (see appropriate section)
Radioimmunoassays (82009-84999 [82652])
Code also radiopharmaceutical(s) and/or drug(s) supplied

78201   Liver imaging; static only
    EXCLUDES   *Spleen imaging only (78185)*
    📷 5.46   ⚖ 5.46   **FUD** XXX   S Z2 80 💻
    AMA: 2015,Jan,16; 2014,Jan,11; 2012,Feb,9-10

78202   with vascular flow
    EXCLUDES   *Spleen imaging only (78185)*
    📷 5.82   ⚖ 5.82   **FUD** XXX   S Z2 80 💻
    AMA: 2012,Feb,9-10

78205   Liver imaging (SPECT);
    📷 6.10   ⚖ 6.10   **FUD** XXX   S Z2 80 💻
    AMA: 2012,Feb,9-10

78206   with vascular flow
    📷 9.97   ⚖ 9.97   **FUD** XXX   S Z2 80 💻
    AMA: 2012,Feb,9-10

78215   Liver and spleen imaging; static only
    📷 5.63   ⚖ 5.63   **FUD** XXX   S Z2 80 💻
    AMA: 2012,Feb,9-10

78216   with vascular flow
    📷 3.64   ⚖ 3.64   **FUD** XXX   S Z2 80 💻
    AMA: 2012,Feb,9-10

78226   Hepatobiliary system imaging, including gallbladder when present;
    📷 9.62   ⚖ 9.62   **FUD** XXX   S Z2 80
    AMA: 2012,Feb,9-10

78227   with pharmacologic intervention, including quantitative measurement(s) when performed
    📷 13.0   ⚖ 13.0   **FUD** XXX   S Z2 80
    AMA: 2012,Feb,9-10

78230   Salivary gland imaging;
    📷 5.01   ⚖ 5.01   **FUD** XXX   S Z2 80 💻
    AMA: 2012,Feb,9-10

78231	**with serial images**

    3.75   3.75 **FUD** XXX   S Z2 80

AMA: 2012,Feb,9-10

78232 Salivary gland function study

    2.86   2.86 **FUD** XXX   S Z2 80

AMA: 2012,Feb,9-10

78258 Esophageal motility

    6.38   6.38 **FUD** XXX   S Z2 80

AMA: 2012,Feb,9-10

78261 Gastric mucosa imaging

    7.34   7.34 **FUD** XXX   S Z2 80

AMA: 2012,Feb,9-10

78262 Gastroesophageal reflux study

    7.07   7.07 **FUD** XXX   S Z2 80

AMA: 2012,Feb,9-10

▲ **78264 Gastric emptying imaging study (eg, solid, liquid, or both);**

Do not report more than one time per study

    8.40   8.40 **FUD** XXX   S Z2 80

AMA: 2012,Feb,9-10

● **78265 with small bowel transit**

Do not report more than one time per study

● **78266 with small bowel and colon transit, multiple days**

Do not report more than one time per study

78267 Urea breath test, C-14 (isotopic); acquisition for analysis

EXCLUDES *Breath hydrogen/methane test (91065)*

    0.00   0.00 **FUD** XXX   A

AMA: 2015,Jan,16; 2014,Jan,11; 2012,Feb,9-10

78268 analysis

EXCLUDES *Breath hydrogen/methane test (91065)*

    0.00   0.00 **FUD** XXX   A

AMA: 2015,Jan,16; 2014,Jan,11; 2012,Feb,9-10

78270 Vitamin B-12 absorption study (eg, Schilling test); without intrinsic factor

    2.94   2.94 **FUD** XXX   S Z2 80

AMA: 2012,Feb,9-10

78271 with intrinsic factor

    2.62   2.62 **FUD** XXX   S Z2 80

AMA: 2012,Feb,9-10

78272 Vitamin B-12 absorption studies combined, with and without intrinsic factor

    2.81   2.81 **FUD** XXX   S Z2 80

AMA: 2012,Feb,9-10

78278 Acute gastrointestinal blood loss imaging

    10.1   10.1 **FUD** XXX   S Z2 80

AMA: 2012,Feb,9-10

78282 Gastrointestinal protein loss

    0.00   0.00 **FUD** XXX   S Z2 80

AMA: 2012,Feb,9-10

78290 Intestine imaging (eg, ectopic gastric mucosa, Meckel's localization, volvulus)

    9.66   9.66 **FUD** XXX   S Z2 80

AMA: 2012,Feb,9-10

78291 Peritoneal-venous shunt patency test (eg, for LeVeen, Denver shunt)

Code also (49427)

    7.22   7.22 **FUD** XXX   S Z2 80

AMA: 2012,Feb,9-10

78299 Unlisted gastrointestinal procedure, diagnostic nuclear medicine

    0.00   0.00 **FUD** XXX   S Z2 80

AMA: 2015,Jan,16; 2014,Jan,11; 2012,Feb,9-10

78300-78399 Nuclear Radiology: Bones and Joints

EXCLUDES *Diagnostic services (see appropriate sections)*
Follow-up care (see appropriate section)
Radioimmunoassays (82009-84999 [82652])

Code also radiopharmaceutical(s) and/or drug(s) supplied

78300 Bone and/or joint imaging; limited area

    5.23   5.23 **FUD** XXX   S Z2 80 PQ

AMA: 2015,Jan,16; 2014,Jan,11; 2012,Feb,9-10; 2012,Jan,15-42; 2011,Jan,11

78305 multiple areas

    6.69   6.69 **FUD** XXX   S Z2 80 PQ

AMA: 2015,Jan,16; 2014,Jan,11; 2012,Feb,9-10

78306 whole body

    7.31   7.31 **FUD** XXX   S Z2 80 PQ

AMA: 2015,Jan,16; 2014,Jan,11; 2012,Feb,9-10; 2012,Jan,15-42; 2011,Jan,11

78315 3 phase study

    10.0   10.0 **FUD** XXX   S Z2 80 PQ

AMA: 2015,Jan,16; 2014,Jan,11; 2012,Feb,9-10; 2012,Jan,15-42; 2011,Jan,11

78320 tomographic (SPECT)

    6.61   6.61 **FUD** XXX   S Z2 80 PQ

AMA: 2015,Jan,16; 2014,Jan,11; 2012,Feb,9-10; 2012,Jan,15-42; 2011,Jan,11

78350 Bone density (bone mineral content) study, 1 or more sites; single photon absorptiometry

    0.93   0.93 **FUD** XXX   E

AMA: 2012,Feb,9-10

78351 dual photon absorptiometry, 1 or more sites

    0.43   0.43 **FUD** XXX   E

AMA: 2012,Feb,9-10

78399 Unlisted musculoskeletal procedure, diagnostic nuclear medicine

    0.00   0.00 **FUD** XXX   S Z2 80

AMA: 2015,Jan,16; 2014,Jan,11; 2012,Feb,9-10

78414-78499 Nuclear Radiology: Heart and Vascular

EXCLUDES *Diagnostic services (see appropriate sections)*
Follow-up care (see appropriate section)
Radioimmunoassays (82009-84999 [82652])

Code also radiopharmaceutical(s) and/or drug(s) supplied

78414 Determination of central c-v hemodynamics (non-imaging) (eg, ejection fraction with probe technique) with or without pharmacologic intervention or exercise, single or multiple determinations

    0.00   0.00 **FUD** XXX   S Z2 80

AMA: 2015,Jan,16; 2014,Jan,11; 2012,Feb,9-10; 2010,May,5-6

78428 Cardiac shunt detection

    5.24   5.24 **FUD** XXX   S Z2 80

AMA: 2015,Jan,16; 2014,Jan,11; 2012,Feb,9-10; 2010,May,5-6

78445 Non-cardiac vascular flow imaging (ie, angiography, venography)

    5.21   5.21 **FUD** XXX   S Z2 80

AMA: 2015,Jan,16; 2014,Jan,11; 2012,Feb,9-10; 2010,May,5-6

78451 Myocardial perfusion imaging, tomographic (SPECT) (including attenuation correction, qualitative or quantitative wall motion, ejection fraction by first pass or gated technique, additional quantification, when performed); single study, at rest or stress (exercise or pharmacologic)

Code also stress testing when performed (93015-93018)

    9.90   9.90 **FUD** XXX   S Z2 80

AMA: 2015,Jan,16; 2014,Jan,11; 2012,Feb,9-10; 2012,Jan,15-42; 2011,Feb,8-9; 2010,May,5-6; 2010,Jan,3-5

 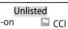 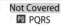

78452 — Radiology
78452 — 78597 (side tab)

78452 multiple studies, at rest and/or stress (exercise or pharmacologic) and/or redistribution and/or rest reinjection
Code also stress testing when performed (93015-93018)
13.7   13.7   **FUD** XXX   S Z2 80
AMA: 2015,Jan,16; 2014,Jan,11; 2012,Feb,9-10; 2012,Jan,15-42; 2011,Feb,8-9; 2010,May,5-6; 2010,Jan,3-5

78453 Myocardial perfusion imaging, planar (including qualitative or quantitative wall motion, ejection fraction by first pass or gated technique, additional quantification, when performed); single study, at rest or stress (exercise or pharmacologic)
Code also stress testing when performed (93015-93018)
8.83   8.83   **FUD** XXX   S Z2 80
AMA: 2015,Jan,16; 2014,Jan,11; 2012,Feb,9-10; 2010,May,5-6; 2010,Jan,3-5

78454 multiple studies, at rest and/or stress (exercise or pharmacologic) and/or redistribution and/or rest reinjection
Code also stress testing when performed (93015-93018)
12.6   12.6   **FUD** XXX   S Z2 80
AMA: 2015,Jan,16; 2014,Jan,11; 2012,Feb,9-10; 2010,May,5-6; 2010,Jan,3-5

78456 Acute venous thrombosis imaging, peptide
9.30   9.30   **FUD** XXX   S Z2
AMA: 2015,Jan,16; 2014,Jan,11; 2012,Feb,9-10; 2010,May,5-6

78457 Venous thrombosis imaging, venogram; unilateral
5.08   5.08   **FUD** XXX   S Z2 80
AMA: 2015,Jan,16; 2014,Jan,11; 2012,Feb,9-10; 2010,May,5-6

78458 bilateral
5.95   5.95   **FUD** XXX   S Z2 80
AMA: 2015,Jan,16; 2014,Jan,11; 2012,Feb,9-10; 2010,May,5-6

78459 Myocardial imaging, positron emission tomography (PET), metabolic evaluation
EXCLUDES Myocardial perfusion studies (78491-78492)
0.00   0.00   **FUD** XXX   S Z2 80
AMA: 2015,Jan,16; 2014,Jan,11; 2012,Feb,9-10; 2010,May,5-6

78466 Myocardial imaging, infarct avid, planar; qualitative or quantitative
5.65   5.65   **FUD** XXX   S Z2 80
AMA: 2012,Feb,9-10; 2010,May,5-6

78468 with ejection fraction by first pass technique
5.60   5.60   **FUD** XXX   S Z2 80
AMA: 2015,Jan,16; 2014,Jan,11; 2012,Feb,9-10; 2010,May,5-6

78469 tomographic SPECT with or without quantification
EXCLUDES Myocardial sympathetic innervation imaging (0331T-0332T)
6.60   6.60   **FUD** XXX   S Z2 80
AMA: 2015,Jan,16; 2014,Jan,11; 2012,Feb,9-10; 2010,May,5-6

78472 Cardiac blood pool imaging, gated equilibrium; planar, single study at rest or stress (exercise and/or pharmacologic), wall motion study plus ejection fraction, with or without additional quantitative processing
EXCLUDES Right ventricular ejection fraction by first pass technique (78496)
Code also stress testing when performed (93015-93018)
Do not report with (78451-78454, 78481, 78483, 78494)
6.67   6.67   **FUD** XXX   S Z2 80
AMA: 2015,Jan,16; 2014,Jan,11; 2012,Feb,9-10; 2010,May,5-6

78473 multiple studies, wall motion study plus ejection fraction, at rest and stress (exercise and/or pharmacologic), with or without additional quantification
Code also stress testing when performed (93015-93018)
Do not report with (78451-78454, 78481, 78483, 78494)
8.37   8.37   **FUD** XXX   S Z2 80
AMA: 2015,Jan,16; 2014,Jan,11; 2012,Feb,9-10; 2010,May,5-6

78481 Cardiac blood pool imaging (planar), first pass technique; single study, at rest or with stress (exercise and/or pharmacologic), wall motion study plus ejection fraction, with or without quantification
Code also stress testing when performed (93015-93018)
Do not report with (78451-78454)
5.06   5.06   **FUD** XXX   S Z2 80
AMA: 2015,Jan,16; 2014,Jan,11; 2012,Feb,9-10; 2010,May,5-6

78483 multiple studies, at rest and with stress (exercise and/or pharmacologic), wall motion study plus ejection fraction, with or without quantification
EXCLUDES Blood flow studies of the brain (78610)
Code also stress testing when performed (93015-93018)
Do not report with (78451-78454)
6.89   6.89   **FUD** XXX   S Z2 80
AMA: 2015,Jan,16; 2014,Jan,11; 2012,Feb,9-10; 2010,May,5-6

78491 Myocardial imaging, positron emission tomography (PET), perfusion; single study at rest or stress
Code also stress testing when performed (93015-93018)
0.00   0.00   **FUD** XXX   S Z2 80
AMA: 2015,Jan,16; 2014,Jan,11; 2012,Feb,9-10; 2010,May,5-6

78492 multiple studies at rest and/or stress
Code also stress testing when performed (93015-93018)
0.00   0.00   **FUD** XXX   S Z2 80
AMA: 2015,Jan,16; 2014,Jan,11; 2012,Feb,9-10; 2010,May,5-6

78494 Cardiac blood pool imaging, gated equilibrium, SPECT, at rest, wall motion study plus ejection fraction, with or without quantitative processing
6.49   6.49   **FUD** XXX   S Z2 80
AMA: 2015,Jan,16; 2014,Jan,11; 2012,Feb,9-10; 2010,May,5-6

+ **78496** Cardiac blood pool imaging, gated equilibrium, single study, at rest, with right ventricular ejection fraction by first pass technique (List separately in addition to code for primary procedure)
Code first (78472)
1.28   1.28   **FUD** ZZZ   N N1 80
AMA: 2015,Jan,16; 2014,Jan,11; 2012,Feb,9-10; 2012,Jan,15-42; 2011,Jan,11; 2010,May,5-6

78499 Unlisted cardiovascular procedure, diagnostic nuclear medicine
0.00   0.00   **FUD** XXX   S Z2 80
AMA: 2015,Jan,16; 2014,Jan,11; 2012,Feb,9-10; 2010,May,5-6

78579-78599 Nuclear Radiology: Lungs

EXCLUDES Diagnostic services (see appropriate sections)
Follow-up care (see appropriate sections)
Radioimmunoassays (82009-84999 [82652])
Code also radiopharmaceutical(s) and/or drug(s) supplied

78579 Pulmonary ventilation imaging (eg, aerosol or gas)
Do not report more than one time per imaging session
5.35   5.35   **FUD** XXX   S Z2 80
AMA: 2012,Feb,9-10

78580 Pulmonary perfusion imaging (eg, particulate)
Do not report more than one time per imaging session
Do not report with (78451-78454)
6.92   6.92   **FUD** XXX   S Z2 80
AMA: 2015,Jan,16; 2014,Jan,11; 2012,Feb,9-10; 2010,May,5-6

78582 Pulmonary ventilation (eg, aerosol or gas) and perfusion imaging
Do not report more than one time per imaging session
Do not report with (78451-78454)
9.72   9.72   **FUD** XXX   S Z2 80
AMA: 2012,Feb,9-10

78597 Quantitative differential pulmonary perfusion, including imaging when performed
Do not report more than one time per imaging session
Do not report with (78451-78454)
5.86   5.86   **FUD** XXX   S Z2 80
AMA: 2012,Feb,9-10

78598 Quantitative differential pulmonary perfusion and ventilation (eg, aerosol or gas), including imaging when performed

> Do not report more than one time per imaging session
> Do not report with (78451-78454)
> 🏷 8.89 ⚖ 8.89 **FUD** XXX [S] [Z2] [80]
>
> **AMA:** 2012,Feb,9-10

78599 Unlisted respiratory procedure, diagnostic nuclear medicine

> 🏷 0.00 ⚖ 0.00 **FUD** XXX [S] [Z2] [80]
>
> **AMA:** 2015,Jan,16; 2014,Jan,11; 2012,Feb,9-10

78600-78650 Nuclear Radiology: Brain/Cerebrospinal Fluid

EXCLUDES *Diagnostic services (see appropriate sections)*
Follow-up care (see appropriate sections)
Radioimmunoassays (82009-84999 [82652])
Code also radiopharmaceutical(s) and/or drug(s) supplied

78600 Brain imaging, less than 4 static views;

> 🏷 5.34 ⚖ 5.34 **FUD** XXX [S] [Z2] [80] 🖳
>
> **AMA:** 2015,Jan,16; 2014,Jan,11; 2012,Feb,9-10

Diagram of tomography principal (left)

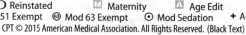

X-ray beam
Plane of study
Focal point
Detection plate

Schematic of frontal coronal CT section of skull

78601 with vascular flow

> 🏷 6.23 ⚖ 6.23 **FUD** XXX [S] [Z2] [80] 🖳
>
> **AMA:** 2012,Feb,9-10

78605 Brain imaging, minimum 4 static views;

> 🏷 5.76 ⚖ 5.76 **FUD** XXX [S] [Z2] [80] 🖳
>
> **AMA:** 2012,Feb,9-10

78606 with vascular flow

> 🏷 9.66 ⚖ 9.66 **FUD** XXX [S] [Z2] [80] 🖳
>
> **AMA:** 2012,Feb,9-10

78607 Brain imaging, tomographic (SPECT)

> 🏷 10.2 ⚖ 10.2 **FUD** XXX [S] [Z2] [80] 🖳
>
> **AMA:** 2012,Feb,9-10

78608 Brain imaging, positron emission tomography (PET); metabolic evaluation

> 🏷 0.00 ⚖ 0.00 **FUD** XXX [S] [Z2] [80] 🖳
>
> **AMA:** 2012,Feb,9-10

78609 perfusion evaluation

> 🏷 2.17 ⚖ 2.17 **FUD** XXX [E] 🖳
>
> **AMA:** 2012,Feb,9-10

78610 Brain imaging, vascular flow only

> 🏷 5.05 ⚖ 5.05 **FUD** XXX [S] [Z2] [80] 🖳
>
> **AMA:** 2012,Feb,9-10

78630 Cerebrospinal fluid flow, imaging (not including introduction of material); cisternography

> Code also injection procedure (61000-61070, 62270-62319)
> 🏷 9.86 ⚖ 9.86 **FUD** XXX [S] [Z2] [80] 🖳
>
> **AMA:** 2012,Feb,9-10

78635 ventriculography

> Code also injection procedure (61000-61070, 62270-62294)
> 🏷 9.89 ⚖ 9.89 **FUD** XXX [S] [Z2] [80] 🖳
>
> **AMA:** 2012,Feb,9-10

78645 shunt evaluation

> Code also injection procedure (61000-61070, 62270-62294)
> 🏷 9.40 ⚖ 9.40 **FUD** XXX [S] [Z2] [80] 🖳
>
> **AMA:** 2012,Feb,9-10

78647 tomographic (SPECT)

> 🏷 10.1 ⚖ 10.1 **FUD** XXX [S] [Z2] [80] 🖳
>
> **AMA:** 2012,Feb,9-10

78650 Cerebrospinal fluid leakage detection and localization

> Code also injection procedure (61000-61070, 62270-62294)
> 🏷 9.70 ⚖ 9.70 **FUD** XXX [S] [Z2] [80] 🖳
>
> **AMA:** 2012,Feb,9-10

78660-78699 Nuclear Radiology: Lacrimal Duct System

Code also radiopharmaceutical(s) and/or drug(s) supplied

78660 Radiopharmaceutical dacryocystography

> 🏷 5.11 ⚖ 5.11 **FUD** XXX [S] [Z2] [80] 🖳
>
> **AMA:** 2012,Feb,9-10

78699 Unlisted nervous system procedure, diagnostic nuclear medicine

> 🏷 0.00 ⚖ 0.00 **FUD** XXX [S] [Z2] [80]
>
> **AMA:** 2015,Jan,16; 2014,Jan,11; 2012,Feb,9-10

78700-78725 Nuclear Radiology: Renal Anatomy and Function

EXCLUDES *Diagnostic services (see appropriate sections)*
Follow-up care (see appropriate section)
Radioimmunoassays (82009-84999 [82652])
Renal endoscopy with insertion of radioactive substances (77778)
Code also radiopharmaceutical(s) and/or drug(s) supplied

78700 Kidney imaging morphology;

> 🏷 4.97 ⚖ 4.97 **FUD** XXX [S] [Z2] [80] 🖳
>
> **AMA:** 2015,Jan,16; 2014,Jan,11; 2012,Feb,9-10

78701 with vascular flow

> 🏷 6.10 ⚖ 6.10 **FUD** XXX [S] [Z2] [80] 🖳
>
> **AMA:** 2012,Feb,9-10

78707 with vascular flow and function, single study without pharmacological intervention

> 🏷 6.73 ⚖ 6.73 **FUD** XXX [S] [Z2] [80] 🖳
>
> **AMA:** 2015,Jan,16; 2014,Jan,11; 2012,Feb,9-10

78708 with vascular flow and function, single study, with pharmacological intervention (eg, angiotensin converting enzyme inhibitor and/or diuretic)

> 🏷 5.03 ⚖ 5.03 **FUD** XXX [S] [Z2] [80] 🖳
>
> **AMA:** 2015,Jan,16; 2014,Jan,11; 2012,Feb,9-10

78709 with vascular flow and function, multiple studies, with and without pharmacological intervention (eg, angiotensin converting enzyme inhibitor and/or diuretic)

> 🏷 10.4 ⚖ 10.4 **FUD** XXX [S] [Z2] [80] 🖳
>
> **AMA:** 2015,Jan,16; 2014,Jan,11; 2012,Feb,9-10

78710 tomographic (SPECT)

> 🏷 5.73 ⚖ 5.73 **FUD** XXX [S] [Z2] [80] 🖳
>
> **AMA:** 2015,Jan,16; 2014,Jan,11; 2012,Feb,9-10

78725 Kidney function study, non-imaging radioisotopic study

> 🏷 3.13 ⚖ 3.13 **FUD** XXX [S] [Z2] [80] 🖳
>
> **AMA:** 2012,Feb,9-10

78730-78799 Nuclear Radiology: Urogenital

EXCLUDES *Diagnostic services (see appropriate sections)*
Follow-up care (see appropriate section)
Radioimmunoassays (82009-84999 [82652])
Code also radiopharmaceutical(s) and/or drug(s) supplied

+ 78730 Urinary bladder residual study (List separately in addition to code for primary procedure)

> EXCLUDES *Measurement of postvoid residual urine and/or bladder capacity using ultrasound (51798)*
> *Ultrasound imaging of the bladder only with measurement of postvoid residual urine (76857)*
> Code first (78740)
> 🏷 2.22 ⚖ 2.22 **FUD** ZZZ [N] [N1] [80] 🖳
>
> **AMA:** 2015,Jan,16; 2014,Jan,11; 2012,Feb,9-10

78740 Ureteral reflux study (radiopharmaceutical voiding cystogram)

> EXCLUDES *Catheterization (51701-51703)*
> Code also urinary bladder residual study (78730)
> 🏷 6.34 ⚖ 6.34 **FUD** XXX [S] [Z2] [80] 🖳
>
> **AMA:** 2012,Feb,9-10

● New Code ▲ Revised Code ○ Reinstated Ⓜ Maternity 🅐 Age Edit Unlisted Not Covered # Resequenced
◌ AMA Mod 51 Exempt ⑨ Optum Mod 51 Exempt ⑥ Mod 63 Exempt ⊙ Mod Sedation + Add-on 🖳 CCI ⑳ PQRS **FUD** Follow-up Days

© 2015 Optum360, LLC (Blue Text) CPT © 2015 American Medical Association. All Rights Reserved. (Black Text) Medicare (Red Text) **311**

Radiology

78761 — 79200

78761 Testicular imaging with vascular flow ♂
   6.11   6.11 **FUD** XXX   S Z2 80
AMA: 2015,Jan,16; 2014,Jan,11; 2012,Feb,9-10

78799 Unlisted genitourinary procedure, diagnostic nuclear medicine
   0.00   0.00 **FUD** XXX   S Z2 80
AMA: 2015,Jan,16; 2014,Jan,11; 2012,Feb,9-10

78800-78804 Nuclear Radiology: Tumor Localization
Code also radiopharmaceutical(s) and/or drug(s) supplied

78800 Radiopharmaceutical localization of tumor or distribution of radiopharmaceutical agent(s); limited area
  INCLUDES Ocular radiophosphorus tumor identification
  EXCLUDES Specific organ (see appropriate site)
   5.52   5.52 **FUD** XXX   S Z2 80
AMA: 2015,Jan,16; 2014,Jan,11; 2012,Feb,9-10; 2012,Jan,15-42; 2011,Dec,14-18

78801 multiple areas
   7.55   7.55 **FUD** XXX   S Z2 80
AMA: 2015,Jan,16; 2014,Jan,11; 2012,Feb,9-10; 2012,Jan,15-42; 2011,Dec,14-18

78802 whole body, single day imaging
   9.42   9.42 **FUD** XXX   S Z2 80
AMA: 2012,Feb,9-10

78803 tomographic (SPECT)
   9.89   9.89 **FUD** XXX   S Z2 80
AMA: 2012,Feb,9-10

78804 whole body, requiring 2 or more days imaging
   16.5   16.5 **FUD** XXX   S Z2 80
AMA: 2012,Feb,9-10

78805-78807 Nuclear Radiology: Inflammation and Infection
  EXCLUDES Imaging bone infectious or inflammatory disease with bone imaging radiopharmaceutical (78300, 78305-78306)
Code also radiopharmaceutical(s) and/or drug(s) supplied

78805 Radiopharmaceutical localization of inflammatory process; limited area
   5.27   5.27 **FUD** XXX   S Z2 80
AMA: 2015,Jan,16; 2014,Jan,11; 2012,Feb,9-10

78806 whole body
   9.68   9.68 **FUD** XXX   S Z2 80
AMA: 2015,Jan,16; 2014,Jan,11; 2012,Feb,9-10

78807 tomographic (SPECT)
   9.90   9.90 **FUD** XXX   S Z2 80
AMA: 2012,Feb,9-10

78808 Intravenous Injection for Radiopharmaceutical Localization
Code also radiopharmaceutical(s) and/or drug(s) supplied

78808 Injection procedure for radiopharmaceutical localization by non-imaging probe study, intravenous (eg, parathyroid adenoma)
  EXCLUDES Identification of sentinel node (38792)
   1.27   1.27 **FUD** XXX   Q1 N1 80
AMA: 2012,Feb,9-10

78811-78999 Nuclear Radiology: Diagnosis, Staging, Restaging or Monitoring Cancer
CMS: 100-3,220.6.17 Positron Emission Tomography (FDG) for Oncologic Conditions; 100-3,220.6.19 NaF-18 PET to Identify Bone Metastasis of Cancer; 100-3,220.6.9 FDG PET for Refractory Seizures; 100-4,13,60 Positron Emission Tomography (PET) Scans - General Information; 100-4,13,60.13 Billing for PET Scans for Specific Indications of Cervical Cancer; 100-4,13,60.15 Billing for CMS-Approved Clinical Trials for PET Scans; 100-4,13,60.16 Billing and Coverage for PET Scans After April 3, 2009; 100-4,13,60.17 Billing and Coverage Changes for PET Scans for Cervical Cancer; 100-4,13,60.18 Billing and Coverage for PET (NaF-18) Scans to Identify Bone Metastasis; 100-4,13,60.2 Use of Gamma Cameras, Full and Partial Ring PET Scanners; 100-4,13,60.3 PET Scan Qualifying Conditions; 100-4,13,60.3.1 Appropriate Codes for PET Scans; 100-4,13,60.3.2 Tracer Codes Required for PET Scans

  EXCLUDES CT scan performed for other than attenuation correction and anatomical localization (report with the appropriate site-specific CT code and modifier 59)
    Ocular radiophosphorus tumor identification (78800)
    PET brain scan (78608-78609)
    PET myocardial imaging (78459, 78491-78492)
Code also radiopharmaceutical(s) and/or drug(s) supplied
Do not report with procedure performed more than one time per session

78811 Positron emission tomography (PET) imaging; limited area (eg, chest, head/neck)
   0.00   0.00 **FUD** XXX   S Z2 80
AMA: 2015,Jan,16; 2014,Jan,11; 2012,Feb,9-10

78812 skull base to mid-thigh
   0.00   0.00 **FUD** XXX   S Z2 80
AMA: 2015,Jan,16; 2014,Jan,11; 2013,Feb,16-17; 2012,Feb,9-10

78813 whole body
   0.00   0.00 **FUD** XXX   S Z2 80
AMA: 2015,Jan,16; 2014,Jan,11; 2013,Feb,16-17; 2012,Feb,9-10

78814 Positron emission tomography (PET) with concurrently acquired computed tomography (CT) for attenuation correction and anatomical localization imaging; limited area (eg, chest, head/neck)
   0.00   0.00 **FUD** XXX   S Z2 80
AMA: 2015,Jan,16; 2014,Jan,11; 2013,Feb,16-17; 2012,Feb,9-10; 2012,Jan,15-42; 2011,Jan,11

78815 skull base to mid-thigh
   0.00   0.00 **FUD** XXX   S Z2 80
AMA: 2015,Jan,16; 2014,Jan,11; 2013,Feb,16-17; 2012,Feb,9-10; 2012,Jan,15-42; 2011,Jan,11

78816 whole body
   0.00   0.00 **FUD** XXX   S Z2 80
AMA: 2015,Jan,16; 2014,Jan,11; 2013,Feb,16-17; 2012,Feb,9-10; 2012,Jan,15-42; 2011,Jan,11

78999 Unlisted miscellaneous procedure, diagnostic nuclear medicine
   0.00   0.00 **FUD** XXX   S Z2 80
AMA: 2015,Jan,16; 2014,Jan,11; 2012,Feb,9-10

79005-79999 Systemic Radiopharmaceutical Therapy
  EXCLUDES Imaging guidance
    Injection into artery, body cavity, or joint (see appropriate injection codes)
    Radiological supervision and interpretation

79005 Radiopharmaceutical therapy, by oral administration
  EXCLUDES Monoclonal antibody treatment (79403)
   3.86   3.86 **FUD** XXX   S Z3 80
AMA: 2015,Jan,16; 2014,Jan,11; 2012,Feb,9-10

79101 Radiopharmaceutical therapy, by intravenous administration
  EXCLUDES Administration of nonantibody radioelement solution including follow-up care (77750)
    Radiolabeled monoclonal antibody IV infusion (79403)
  Do not report with (36400, 36410, 79403, 96360, 96374-96375, 96409)
   4.03   4.03 **FUD** XXX   S Z3 80
AMA: 2015,Jan,16; 2014,Jan,11; 2012,Feb,9-10

79200 Radiopharmaceutical therapy, by intracavitary administration
   3.84   3.84 **FUD** XXX   S Z3 80
AMA: 2015,Jan,16; 2014,Jan,11; 2012,Feb,9-10

| 26/TC PC/TC Comp Only | A2-Z1 ASC Pmt | 50 Bilateral | ♂ Male Only | ♀ Female Only | Facility RVU | Non-Facility RVU |
| AMA: CPT Asst | CMS: Pub 100 | A-Y OPPSI | 80/80 Surg Assist Allowed / w/Doc | | Lab Crosswalk | Radiology Crosswalk |

312   Medicare (Red Text)   CPT © 2015 American Medical Association. All Rights Reserved. (Black Text)   © 2015 Optum360, LLC (Blue Text)

79300	**Radiopharmaceutical therapy, by interstitial radioactive colloid administration** 0.00 0.00 **FUD** XXX S Z2 80 **AMA:** 2015,Jan,16; 2014,Jan,11; 2012,Feb,9-10
79403	**Radiopharmaceutical therapy, radiolabeled monoclonal antibody by intravenous infusion** *EXCLUDES* *Pretreatment imaging (78802, 78804)* Do not report with (79101) 5.38 5.38 **FUD** XXX S Z3 80 **AMA:** 2015,Jan,16; 2014,Jan,11; 2012,Feb,9-10
79440	**Radiopharmaceutical therapy, by intra-articular administration** 3.64 3.64 **FUD** XXX S Z3 80 **AMA:** 2015,Jan,16; 2014,Jan,11; 2012,Feb,9-10
79445	**Radiopharmaceutical therapy, by intra-arterial particulate administration** *EXCLUDES* *Procedural and radiological supervision and interpretation for angiographic and interventional procedures before intra-arterial radiopharmaceutical therapy* Do not report with (96373, 96420) 0.00 0.00 **FUD** XXX S Z2 80 **AMA:** 2015,Jan,16; 2014,Jan,11; 2013,Nov,6; 2012,Feb,9-10
79999	**Radiopharmaceutical therapy, unlisted procedure** 0.00 0.00 **FUD** XXX S Z2 80 **AMA:** 2015,Jan,16; 2014,Jan,11; 2012,Feb,9-10

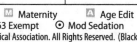
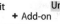
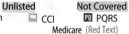

Pathology and Laboratory

80047 — 80081

80047-80081 [80081] Multi-test Laboratory Panels

EXCLUDES   Test codes:
For testing performed at a frequency greater than the number specified by panel definition
Not specified by panel definition
Do not report two or more panel codes comprising the same tests; report the panel with the highest number of tests to meet the definition of the code, and report the remaining tests individually

80047   Basic metabolic panel (Calcium, ionized)

INCLUDES   Calcium, ionized (82330)
Carbon dioxide (bicarbonate) (82374)
Chloride (82435)
Creatinine (82565)
Glucose (82947)
Potassium (84132)
Sodium (84295)
Urea nitrogen (BUN) (84520)

🚑 0.00   ⚕ 0.00   **FUD** XXX   ☒ Ⓝ

AMA: 2015,Jan,16; 2014,Jan,11; 2013,Apr,10-11

80048   Basic metabolic panel (Calcium, total)

INCLUDES   Calcium, total (82310)
Carbon dioxide (bicarbonate) (82374)
Chloride (82435)
Creatinine (82565)
Glucose (82947)
Potassium (84132)
Sodium (84295)
Urea nitrogen (BUN) (84520)

🚑 0.00   ⚕ 0.00   **FUD** XXX   ☒ Ⓝ ⬚

AMA: 2015,Jan,16; 2014,Jan,11

80050   General health panel

INCLUDES   Complete blood count (CBC), automated, with:
Manual differential WBC count
Blood smear with manual differential AND complete (CBC), automated (85007, 85027)
Manual differential WBC count, buffy coat AND complete (CBC), automated (85009, 85027)
OR
Automated differential WBC count
Automated differential WBC count AND complete (CBC), automated/automated differential WBC count (85004, 85025)
Automated differential WBC count AND complete (CBC), automated (85004, 85027)
Comprehensive metabolic profile (80053)
Thyroid stimulating hormone (84443)

🚑 0.00   ⚕ 0.00   **FUD** XXX   Ⓔ

AMA: 2015,Jan,16; 2014,Jan,11; 2012,Jan,15-42; 2011,Jan,11

80051   Electrolyte panel

INCLUDES   Carbon dioxide (bicarbonate) (82374)
Chloride (82435)
Potassium (84132)
Sodium (84295)

🚑 0.00   ⚕ 0.00   **FUD** XXX   ☒ Ⓝ ⬚

AMA: 2015,Jan,16; 2014,Jan,11; 2012,Jan,15-42; 2011,Jan,11

80053   Comprehensive metabolic panel

INCLUDES   Albumin (82040)
Bilirubin, total (82247)
Calcium, total (82310)
Carbon dioxide (bicarbonate) (82374)
Chloride (82435)
Creatinine (82565)
Glucose (82947)
Phosphatase, alkaline (84075)
Potassium (84132)
Protein, total (84155)
Sodium (84295)
Transferase, alanine amino (ALT) (SGPT) (84460)
Transferase, aspartate amino (AST) (SGOT) (84450)
Urea nitrogen (BUN) (84520)

🚑 0.00   ⚕ 0.00   **FUD** XXX   ☒ Ⓝ ⬚

AMA: 2015,Jan,16; 2014,Jan,11; 2013,Apr,10-11; 2012,Jan,15-42; 2011,Jan,11; 2010,Apr,10

80055   Obstetric panel   Ⓜ ♀

INCLUDES   Complete blood count (CBC), automated, with:
Manual differential WBC count
Blood smear with manual differential AND complete (CBC), automated (85007, 85027)
Manual differential WBC count, buffy coat AND complete (CBC), automated (85009, 85027)
OR
Automated differential WBC count
Automated differential WBC count AND complete (CBC), automated/automated differential WBC count (85004, 85025)
Automated differential WBC count AND complete (CBC), automated (85004, 85027)
Blood typing, ABO and Rh (86900-86901)
Hepatitis B surface antigen (HBsAg) (87340)
RBC antibody screen, each serum technique (86850)
Rubella antibody (86762)
Syphilis test, non-treponemal antibody qualitative (86592)
Do not report panel code 80055 when syphilis screening is provided using a treponemal antibody approach (86780) report individual codes for tests performed in the OB panel instead (80055, 86780)

🚑 0.00   ⚕ 0.00   **FUD** XXX   Ⓔ

AMA: 2015,Jan,16; 2014,Jan,11; 2012,Jan,15-42; 2011,Jan,11

● # 80081   Obstetric panel (includes HIV testing)

🚑 0.00   ⚕ 0.00   **FUD** 000

INCLUDES   Complete blood count (CBC), automated, with:
Manual differential WBC count
Blood smear with manual differential AND complete (CBC), automated (85007, 85027)
Manual differential WBC count, buffy count AND complete (CBC), automated (85009, 85027)
OR
Automated differential WBC count
Automated differential WBC count AND complete (CBC), automated/automated differential WBC count (85004, 85025)
Automated differential WBC count AND complete (CBC), automated (85004, 85027)
Blood typing, ABO and Rh (86900-86901)
Hepatitis B surface antigen (HBsAg) (87340)
HIV-1 antigens, with HIV-1 and HIV-2 antibodies, single result (87389)
RBC antibody screen, each serum technique (86850)
Rubella antibody (86762)
Syphilis test, non-treponemal antibody qualitative (86592)
Do not report panel code 80055 when syphilis screening is provided using a treponemal antibody approach (86780); report individual codes for tests performed in the OB panel instead

80061 Lipid panel

INCLUDES
Cholesterol, serum, total (82465)
Lipoprotein, direct measurement, high density cholesterol (HDL cholesterol) (83718)
Triglycerides (84478)

🔁 0.00 ⚕ 0.00 **FUD** XXX   Ⓧ Ⓝ ▱

AMA: 2015,Jan,16; 2014,Jan,11; 2012,Jan,15-42; 2011,Jan,11

80069 Renal function panel

INCLUDES
Albumin (82040)
Calcium, total (82310)
Carbon dioxide (bicarbonate) (82374)
Chloride (82435)
Creatinine (82565)
Glucose (82947)
Phosphorus inorganic (phosphate) (84100)
Potassium (84132)
Sodium (84295)
Urea nitrogen (BUN) (84520)

🔁 0.00 ⚕ 0.00 **FUD** XXX   Ⓧ Ⓝ ▱

AMA: 2015,Jan,16; 2014,Jan,11; 2012,Jan,15-42; 2011,Jan,11

80074 Acute hepatitis panel

INCLUDES
Hepatitis A antibody (HAAb) IgM (86709)
Hepatitis B core antibody (HBcAb), IgM (86705)
Hepatitis B surface antigen (HBsAg) (87340)
Hepatitis C antibody (86803)

🔁 0.00 ⚕ 0.00 **FUD** XXX   Ⓝ ▱

AMA: 2015,Jan,16; 2014,Jan,11; 2012,Jan,15-42; 2011,Jan,11

80076 Hepatic function panel

INCLUDES
Albumin (82040)
Bilirubin, direct (82248)
Bilirubin, total (82247)
Phosphatase, alkaline (84075)
Protein, total (84155)
Transferase, alanine amino (ALT) (SGPT) (84460)
Transferase, aspartate amino (AST) (SGOT) (84450)

🔁 0.00 ⚕ 0.00 **FUD** XXX   Ⓝ ▱

AMA: 2015,Jan,16; 2014,Jan,11; 2012,Jan,15-42; 2011,Jan,11

80081 *Resequenced code. See code following 80055.*

[80300, 80301, 80302, 80303, 80304] Nonspecific Drug Screening

INCLUDES
Analytic procedure to identify drugs and drug metabolites in biological specimens based on an antibody-antigen reaction that establishes if a drug metabolite is present

List A drugs
Amphetamines
Alcohol
Barbiturates
Benzodiazepines
Buprenorphine
Cocaine metabolite
Heroin metabolite
Methadone and methadone metabolite
Methamphetamine
Methaqualone
Methylenedioxymethamphetamine (MDMA)
Opiates
Oxycodone
Phencyclidine
Propoxyphene (not available in U.S. after 11/19/2010)
Marijuana (THC metabolites)
Tricyclic antidepressants

List B drugs
Acetaminophen
Carisoprodol/meprobamate
Ethyl glucuronide
Fentanyl
Ketamine
Meperidine (Demerol)
Methylphenidate
Nicotine and metabolite (Cotinine)
Salicylate
Synthetic cannabinoids (K2, spice)
Tarpentadol
Tramadol
Zolpidem
Other drugs that are not elsewhere classified

\# **80300 Drug screen, any number of drug classes from Drug Class List A; any number of non-TLC devices or procedures, (eg, immunoassay) capable of being read by direct optical observation, including instrumented-assisted when performed (eg, dipsticks, cups, cards, cartridges), per date of service**

🔁 0.00 ⚕ 0.00 **FUD** XXX   Ⓑ

Do not report more than one time per day

\# **80301 single drug class method, by instrumented test systems (eg, discrete multichannel chemistry analyzers utilizing immunoassay or enzyme assay), per date of service**

🔁 0.00 ⚕ 0.00 **FUD** XXX   Ⓑ

\# **80302 Drug screen, presumptive, single drug class from Drug Class List B, by immunoassay (eg, ELISA) or non-TLC chromatography without mass spectrometry (eg, GC, HPLC), each procedure**

🔁 0.00 ⚕ 0.00 **FUD** XXX   Ⓑ

\# **80303 Drug screen, any number of drug classes, presumptive, single or multiple drug class method; thin layer chromatography procedure(s) (TLC) (eg, acid, neutral, alkaloid plate), per date of service**

🔁 0.00 ⚕ 0.00 **FUD** XXX   Ⓑ

\# **80304 not otherwise specified presumptive procedure (eg, TOF, MALDI, LDTD, DESI, DART), each procedure**

🔁 0.00 ⚕ 0.00 **FUD** XXX   Ⓑ

AMA: 2015,Jun,10

[80320, 80321, 80322, 80323, 80324, 80325, 80326, 80327, 80328, 80329, 80330, 80331, 80332, 80333, 80334, 80335, 80336, 80337, 80338, 80339, 80340, 80341, 80342, 80343, 80344, 80345, 80346, 80347, 80348, 80349, 80350, 80351, 80352, 80353, 80354, 80355, 80356, 80357, 80358, 80359, 80360, 80361, 80362, 80363, 80364, 80365, 80366, 80367, 80368, 80369, 80370, 80371, 80372, 80373, 80374, 80375, 80376, 80377, 83992] **Confirmatory Drug Testing**

INCLUDES   Antihistamine drug tests ([80375, 80376, 80377])
Detection of specific drugs using methods other than immunoassay or enzymatic technique
Do not report metabolites separate from the code for the drug except when a distinct code is available

\# **80320** **Alcohols**
🚑 0.00   ⚖ 0.00   **FUD** XXX   B
AMA: 2015,Apr,3

\# **80321** **Alcohol biomarkers; 1 or 2**
🚑 0.00   ⚖ 0.00   **FUD** XXX   B
AMA: 2015,Apr,3

\# **80322** **3 or more**
🚑 0.00   ⚖ 0.00   **FUD** XXX   B
AMA: 2015,Apr,3

\# **80323** **Alkaloids, not otherwise specified**
🚑 0.00   ⚖ 0.00   **FUD** XXX   B
AMA: 2015,Apr,3

\# **80324** **Amphetamines; 1 or 2**
🚑 0.00   ⚖ 0.00   **FUD** XXX   B
AMA: 2015,Apr,3

\# **80325** **3 or 4**
🚑 0.00   ⚖ 0.00   **FUD** XXX   B
AMA: 2015,Apr,3

\# **80326** **5 or more**
🚑 0.00   ⚖ 0.00   **FUD** XXX   B
AMA: 2015,Apr,3

\# **80327** **Anabolic steroids; 1 or 2**
🚑 0.00   ⚖ 0.00   **FUD** XXX   B
AMA: 2015,Apr,3

\# **80328** **3 or more**
🚑 0.00   ⚖ 0.00   **FUD** XXX   B
AMA: 2015,Apr,3

\# **80329** **Analgesics, non-opioid; 1 or 2**
🚑 0.00   ⚖ 0.00   **FUD** XXX   B
AMA: 2015,Apr,3

\# **80330** **3-5**
🚑 0.00   ⚖ 0.00   **FUD** XXX   B
AMA: 2015,Apr,3

\# **80331** **6 or more**
🚑 0.00   ⚖ 0.00   **FUD** XXX   B
AMA: 2015,Apr,3

\# **80332** **Antidepressants, serotonergic class; 1 or 2**
🚑 0.00   ⚖ 0.00   **FUD** XXX   B
AMA: 2015,Apr,3

\# **80333** **3-5**
🚑 0.00   ⚖ 0.00   **FUD** XXX   B
AMA: 2015,Apr,3

\# **80334** **6 or more**
🚑 0.00   ⚖ 0.00   **FUD** XXX   B
AMA: 2015,Apr,3

\# **80335** **Antidepressants, tricyclic and other cyclicals; 1 or 2**
🚑 0.00   ⚖ 0.00   **FUD** XXX   B
AMA: 2015,Apr,3

\# **80336** **3-5**
🚑 0.00   ⚖ 0.00   **FUD** XXX   B
AMA: 2015,Apr,3

\# **80337** **6 or more**
🚑 0.00   ⚖ 0.00   **FUD** XXX   B
AMA: 2015,Apr,3

\# **80338** **Antidepressants, not otherwise specified**
🚑 0.00   ⚖ 0.00   **FUD** XXX   B
AMA: 2015,Apr,3

\# **80339** **Antiepileptics, not otherwise specified; 1-3**
🚑 0.00   ⚖ 0.00   **FUD** XXX   B
AMA: 2015,Apr,3

\# **80340** **4-6**
🚑 0.00   ⚖ 0.00   **FUD** XXX   B
AMA: 2015,Apr,3

\# **80341** **7 or more**
🚑 0.00   ⚖ 0.00   **FUD** XXX   B
AMA: 2015,Apr,3

\# **80342** **Antipsychotics, not otherwise specified; 1-3**
🚑 0.00   ⚖ 0.00   **FUD** XXX   B
AMA: 2015,Apr,3

\# **80343** **4-6**
🚑 0.00   ⚖ 0.00   **FUD** XXX   B
AMA: 2015,Apr,3

\# **80344** **7 or more**
🚑 0.00   ⚖ 0.00   **FUD** XXX   B
AMA: 2015,Apr,3

\# **80345** **Barbiturates**
🚑 0.00   ⚖ 0.00   **FUD** XXX   B
AMA: 2015,Apr,3

\# **80346** **Benzodiazepines; 1-12**
🚑 0.00   ⚖ 0.00   **FUD** XXX   B
AMA: 2015,Apr,3

\# **80347** **13 or more**
🚑 0.00   ⚖ 0.00   **FUD** XXX   B
AMA: 2015,Apr,3

\# **80348** **Buprenorphine**
🚑 0.00   ⚖ 0.00   **FUD** XXX   B
AMA: 2015,Apr,3

\# **80349** **Cannabinoids, natural**
🚑 0.00   ⚖ 0.00   **FUD** XXX   B
AMA: 2015,Apr,3

\# **80350** **Cannabinoids, synthetic; 1-3**
🚑 0.00   ⚖ 0.00   **FUD** XXX   B
AMA: 2015,Apr,3

\# **80351** **4-6**
🚑 0.00   ⚖ 0.00   **FUD** XXX   B
AMA: 2015,Apr,3

\# **80352** **7 or more**
🚑 0.00   ⚖ 0.00   **FUD** XXX   B
AMA: 2015,Apr,3

\# **80353** **Cocaine**
🚑 0.00   ⚖ 0.00   **FUD** XXX   B
AMA: 2015,Apr,3

\# **80354** **Fentanyl**
🚑 0.00   ⚖ 0.00   **FUD** XXX   B
AMA: 2015,Apr,3

\# **80355** **Gabapentin, non-blood**
🚑 0.00   ⚖ 0.00   **FUD** XXX   B
AMA: 2015,Apr,3

\# **80356** **Heroin metabolite**
🚑 0.00   ⚖ 0.00   **FUD** XXX   B
AMA: 2015,Apr,3

Pathology and Laboratory

\# **80357** **Ketamine and norketamine**
📋 0.00 🔪 0.00 **FUD** XXX [B]
AMA: 2015,Apr,3

\# **80358** **Methadone**
📋 0.00 🔪 0.00 **FUD** XXX [B]
AMA: 2015,Apr,3

\# **80359** **Methylenedioxyamphetamines (MDA, MDEA, MDMA)**
📋 0.00 🔪 0.00 **FUD** XXX [B]
AMA: 2015,Apr,3

\# **80360** **Methylphenidate**
📋 0.00 🔪 0.00 **FUD** XXX [B]
AMA: 2015,Apr,3

\# **80361** **Opiates, 1 or more**
📋 0.00 🔪 0.00 **FUD** XXX [B]
AMA: 2015,Apr,3

\# **80362** **Opioids and opiate analogs; 1 or 2**
📋 0.00 🔪 0.00 **FUD** XXX [B]
AMA: 2015,Apr,3

\# **80363** **3 or 4**
📋 0.00 🔪 0.00 **FUD** XXX [B]
AMA: 2015,Apr,3

\# **80364** **5 or more**
📋 0.00 🔪 0.00 **FUD** XXX [B]
AMA: 2015,Apr,3

\# **80365** **Oxycodone**
📋 0.00 🔪 0.00 **FUD** XXX [B]
AMA: 2015,Apr,3

\# **83992** **Phencyclidine (PCP)**
📋 0.00 🔪 0.00 **FUD** XXX [N]
AMA: 2015,Jun,10; 2015,Apr,3; 2010,Dec,7-10

\# **80366** **Pregabalin**
📋 0.00 🔪 0.00 **FUD** XXX [B]
AMA: 2015,Apr,3

\# **80367** **Propoxyphene**
📋 0.00 🔪 0.00 **FUD** XXX [B]
AMA: 2015,Apr,3

\# **80368** **Sedative hypnotics (non-benzodiazepines)**
📋 0.00 🔪 0.00 **FUD** XXX [B]
AMA: 2015,Apr,3

\# **80369** **Skeletal muscle relaxants; 1 or 2**
📋 0.00 🔪 0.00 **FUD** XXX [B]
AMA: 2015,Apr,3

\# **80370** **3 or more**
📋 0.00 🔪 0.00 **FUD** XXX [B]
AMA: 2015,Apr,3

\# **80371** **Stimulants, synthetic**
📋 0.00 🔪 0.00 **FUD** XXX [B]
AMA: 2015,Apr,3

\# **80372** **Tapentadol**
📋 0.00 🔪 0.00 **FUD** XXX [B]
AMA: 2015,Apr,3

\# **80373** **Tramadol**
📋 0.00 🔪 0.00 **FUD** XXX [B]
AMA: 2015,Apr,3

\# **80374** **Stereoisomer (enantiomer) analysis, single drug class**
Code also index drug analysis if appropriate
📋 0.00 🔪 0.00 **FUD** XXX [B]
AMA: 2015,Apr,3

\# **80375** **Drug(s) or substance(s), definitive, qualitative or quantitative, not otherwise specified; 1-3**
📋 0.00 🔪 0.00 **FUD** XXX [B]
AMA: 2015,Apr,3

\# **80376** **4-6**
📋 0.00 🔪 0.00 **FUD** XXX [B]
AMA: 2015,Apr,3

\# **80377** **7 or more**
📋 0.00 🔪 0.00 **FUD** XXX [B]
AMA: 2015,Apr,3

80150-80377 [80164, 80165, 80171] Therapeutic Drug Levels

INCLUDES Testing of drug and metabolite(s) in primary code
Tests on specimens from blood and blood components, and spinal fluid

80150 **Amikacin**
📋 0.00 🔪 0.00 **FUD** XXX [N]
AMA: 2015,Apr,3; 2015,Jan,16; 2014,Jan,11; 2012,Jan,15-42; 2011,Mar,9; 2010,Dec,7-10

80155 **Caffeine**
📋 0.00 🔪 0.00 **FUD** XXX [A]
AMA: 2015,Apr,3; 2014,Jan,11

80156 **Carbamazepine; total**
📋 0.00 🔪 0.00 **FUD** XXX [N]
AMA: 2015,Apr,3; 2015,Jan,16; 2014,Jan,11; 2011,Mar,9; 2010,Dec,7-10

80157 **free**
📋 0.00 🔪 0.00 **FUD** XXX [N]
AMA: 2015,Apr,3; 2015,Jan,16; 2014,Jan,11; 2011,Mar,9; 2010,Dec,7-10

80158 **Cyclosporine**
📋 0.00 🔪 0.00 **FUD** XXX [N]
AMA: 2015,Apr,3; 2015,Jan,16; 2014,Jan,11; 2011,Mar,9; 2010,Dec,7-10

80159 **Clozapine**
📋 0.00 🔪 0.00 **FUD** XXX [A]
AMA: 2015,Apr,3; 2014,Jan,11

80162 **Digoxin; total**
📋 0.00 🔪 0.00 **FUD** XXX [N]
AMA: 2015,Apr,3; 2015,Jan,16; 2014,Jan,11; 2011,Mar,9; 2010,Dec,7-10

80163 **free**
📋 0.00 🔪 0.00 **FUD** XXX [N]
AMA: 2015,Apr,3

80164 **Resequenced code. See code following 80201.**

80165 **Resequenced code. See code following 80201.**

80168 **Ethosuximide**
📋 0.00 🔪 0.00 **FUD** XXX [N]
AMA: 2015,Apr,3; 2015,Jan,16; 2014,Jan,11; 2011,Mar,9; 2010,Dec,7-10

80169 **Everolimus**
📋 0.00 🔪 0.00 **FUD** XXX [A]
AMA: 2015,Apr,3; 2014,Jan,11

\# **80171** **Gabapentin, whole blood, serum, or plasma**
📋 0.00 🔪 0.00 **FUD** XXX [A]
AMA: 2015,Apr,3; 2014,Jan,11

80170 **Gentamicin**
📋 0.00 🔪 0.00 **FUD** XXX [N]
AMA: 2015,Apr,3; 2015,Jan,16; 2014,Jan,11; 2011,Mar,9; 2010,Dec,7-10

80171 **Resequenced code. See code following 80169.**

80173 **Haloperidol**
📋 0.00 🔪 0.00 **FUD** XXX [N]
AMA: 2015,Apr,3; 2015,Jan,16; 2014,Jan,11; 2011,Mar,9; 2010,Dec,7-10

80175 **Lamotrigine**
📋 0.00 🔪 0.00 **FUD** XXX [A]
AMA: 2015,Apr,3; 2014,Jan,11

80176 **Lidocaine**
  0.00   0.00   **FUD** XXX   N
  AMA: 2015,Apr,3; 2015,Jan,16; 2014,Jan,11; 2011,Mar,9; 2010,Dec,7-10

80177 **Levetiracetam**
  0.00   0.00   **FUD** XXX   A
  AMA: 2015,Apr,3; 2014,Jan,11

80178 **Lithium**
  0.00   0.00   **FUD** XXX   ☒ N
  AMA: 2015,Apr,3; 2015,Jan,16; 2014,Jan,11; 2011,Mar,9; 2010,Dec,7-10

80180 **Mycophenolate (mycophenolic acid)**
  0.00   0.00   **FUD** XXX   A
  AMA: 2015,Apr,3; 2014,Jan,11

80183 **Oxcarbazepine**
  0.00   0.00   **FUD** XXX   A
  AMA: 2015,Apr,3; 2014,Jan,11

80184 **Phenobarbital**
  0.00   0.00   **FUD** XXX   N
  AMA: 2015,Apr,3; 2015,Jan,16; 2014,Jan,11; 2011,Mar,9; 2010,Dec,7-10

80185 **Phenytoin; total**
  0.00   0.00   **FUD** XXX   N
  AMA: 2015,Apr,3; 2015,Jan,16; 2014,Jan,11; 2011,Mar,9; 2010,Dec,7-10

80186   **free**
  0.00   0.00   **FUD** XXX   N
  AMA: 2015,Apr,3; 2015,Jan,16; 2014,Jan,11; 2011,Mar,9; 2010,Dec,7-10

80188 **Primidone**
  0.00   0.00   **FUD** XXX   N
  AMA: 2015,Apr,3; 2015,Jan,16; 2014,Jan,11; 2011,Mar,9; 2010,Dec,7-10

80190 **Procainamide;**
  0.00   0.00   **FUD** XXX   N
  AMA: 2015,Apr,3; 2015,Jan,16; 2014,Jan,11; 2011,Mar,9; 2010,Dec,7-10

80192   **with metabolites (eg, n-acetyl procainamide)**
  0.00   0.00   **FUD** XXX   N ▭
  AMA: 2015,Apr,3; 2015,Jan,16; 2014,Jan,11; 2011,Mar,9; 2010,Dec,7-10

80194 **Quinidine**
  0.00   0.00   **FUD** XXX   N
  AMA: 2015,Apr,3; 2015,Jan,16; 2014,Jan,11; 2011,Mar,9; 2010,Dec,7-10

80195 **Sirolimus**
  0.00   0.00   **FUD** XXX   N
  AMA: 2015,Apr,3; 2015,Jan,16; 2014,Jan,11; 2011,Mar,9; 2010,Dec,7-10

80197 **Tacrolimus**
  0.00   0.00   **FUD** XXX   N
  AMA: 2015,Apr,3; 2015,Jan,16; 2014,Jan,11; 2011,Mar,9; 2010,Dec,7-10

80198 **Theophylline**
  0.00   0.00   **FUD** XXX   N
  AMA: 2015,Apr,3; 2015,Jan,16; 2014,Jan,11; 2011,Mar,9; 2010,Dec,7-10

80199 **Tiagabine**
  0.00   0.00   **FUD** XXX   A
  AMA: 2015,Apr,3; 2014,Jan,11

80200 **Tobramycin**
  0.00   0.00   **FUD** XXX   N
  AMA: 2015,Apr,3; 2015,Jan,16; 2014,Jan,11; 2011,Mar,9; 2010,Dec,7-10

80201 **Topiramate**
  0.00   0.00   **FUD** XXX   N
  AMA: 2015,Apr,3; 2015,Jan,16; 2014,Jan,11; 2011,Mar,9; 2010,Dec,7-10

\# **80164** **Valproic acid (dipropylacetic acid); total**
  0.00   0.00   **FUD** XXX   N
  AMA: 2015,Apr,3; 2015,Jan,16; 2014,Jan,11; 2011,Mar,9; 2010,Dec,7-10

\# **80165**   **free**
  0.00   0.00   **FUD** XXX   N
  AMA: 2015,Apr,3

80202 **Vancomycin**
  0.00   0.00   **FUD** XXX   N
  AMA: 2015,Apr,3; 2015,Jan,16; 2014,Jan,11; 2012,Jan,15-42; 2011,Mar,9; 2010,Dec,7-10

80203 **Zonisamide**
  0.00   0.00   **FUD** XXX   A
  AMA: 2015,Apr,3; 2014,Jan,11

80299 **Quantitation of therapeutic drug, not elsewhere specified**
  0.00   0.00   **FUD** XXX   N
  AMA: 2015,Apr,3; 2015,Jan,16; 2014,Jan,11; 2012,Jan,15-42; 2011,Mar,9; 2011,Jan,11; 2010,Dec,7-10

80300 Resequenced code. See code before 80150.
80301 Resequenced code. See code before 80150.
80302 Resequenced code. See code before 80150.
80303 Resequenced code. See code before 80150.
80304 Resequenced code. See code before 80150.
80320 Resequenced code. See code before 80150.
80321 Resequenced code. See code before 80150.
80322 Resequenced code. See code before 80150.
80323 Resequenced code. See code before 80150.
80324 Resequenced code. See code before 80150.
80325 Resequenced code. See code before 80150.
80326 Resequenced code. See code before 80150.
80327 Resequenced code. See code before 80150.
80328 Resequenced code. See code before 80150.
80329 Resequenced code. See code before 80150.
80330 Resequenced code. See code before 80150.
80331 Resequenced code. See code before 80150.
80332 Resequenced code. See code before 80150.
80333 Resequenced code. See code before 80150.
80334 Resequenced code. See code before 80150.
80335 Resequenced code. See code before 80150.
80336 Resequenced code. See code before 80150.
80337 Resequenced code. See code before 80150.
80338 Resequenced code. See code before 80150.
80339 Resequenced code. See code before 80150.
80340 Resequenced code. See code before 80150.
80341 Resequenced code. See code before 80150.
80342 Resequenced code. See code before 80150.
80343 Resequenced code. See code before 80150.
80344 Resequenced code. See code before 80150.
80345 Resequenced code. See code before 80150.
80346 Resequenced code. See code before 80150.
80347 Resequenced code. See code before 80150.
80348 Resequenced code. See code before 80150.
80349 Resequenced code. See code before 80150.
80350 Resequenced code. See code before 80150.

80351	Resequenced code. See code before 80150.
80352	Resequenced code. See code before 80150.
80353	Resequenced code. See code before 80150.
80354	Resequenced code. See code before 80150.
80355	Resequenced code. See code before 80150.
80356	Resequenced code. See code before 80150.
80357	Resequenced code. See code before 80150.
80358	Resequenced code. See code before 80150.
80359	Resequenced code. See code before 80150.
80360	Resequenced code. See code before 80150.
80361	Resequenced code. See code before 80150.
80362	Resequenced code. See code before 80150.
80363	Resequenced code. See code before 80150.
80364	Resequenced code. See code before 80150.
80365	Resequenced code. See code following 80364.
80366	Resequenced code. See code following 83992.
80367	Resequenced code. See code following 80366.
80368	Resequenced code. See code following 80367.
80369	Resequenced code. See code following 80368.
80370	Resequenced code. See code following 80369.
80371	Resequenced code. See code following 80370.
80372	Resequenced code. See code following 80371.
80373	Resequenced code. See code following 80372.
80374	Resequenced code. See code following 80373.
80375	Resequenced code. See code following 80374.
80376	Resequenced code. See code following 80375.
80377	Resequenced code. See code following 80376.

80400-80439 Stimulation and Suppression Test Panels

EXCLUDES *Administration of evocative or suppressive material (96365-96368, 96372, 96374-96376, C8957)*
Evocative or suppression test substances, as applicable
Physician monitoring and attendance during the test (see Evaluation and Management codes)

80400 **ACTH stimulation panel; for adrenal insufficiency**
INCLUDES Cortisol x 2 (82533)
0.00   0.00   **FUD** XXX   N ▢
AMA: 2015,Jan,16; 2014,Jan,11

80402 **for 21 hydroxylase deficiency**
INCLUDES 17 hydroxyprogesterone X 2 (83498)
Cortisol x 2 (82533)
0.00   0.00   **FUD** XXX   N ▢
AMA: 2014,Jan,11

80406 **for 3 beta-hydroxydehydrogenase deficiency**
INCLUDES 17 hydroxypregnenolone x 2 (84143)
Cortisol x 2 (82533)
0.00   0.00   **FUD** XXX   N ▢
AMA: 2014,Jan,11

80408 **Aldosterone suppression evaluation panel (eg, saline infusion)**
INCLUDES Aldosterone x 2 (82088)
Renin x 2 (84244)
0.00   0.00   **FUD** XXX   N ▢
AMA: 2014,Jan,11

80410 **Calcitonin stimulation panel (eg, calcium, pentagastrin)**
INCLUDES Calcitonin x 3 (82308)
0.00   0.00   **FUD** XXX   N ▢
AMA: 2014,Jan,11

80412 **Corticotropic releasing hormone (CRH) stimulation panel**
INCLUDES Adrenocorticotropic hormone (ACTH) x 6 (82024)
Cortisol x 6 (82533)
0.00   0.00   **FUD** XXX   N ▢
AMA: 2014,Jan,11

80414 **Chorionic gonadotropin stimulation panel; testosterone response**
INCLUDES Testosterone x 2 on three pooled blood samples (84403)
0.00   0.00   **FUD** XXX   N ▢
AMA: 2014,Jan,11

80415 **estradiol response**
INCLUDES Estradiol x 2 on three pooled blood samples (82670)
0.00   0.00   **FUD** XXX   N ▢
AMA: 2014,Jan,11

80416 **Renal vein renin stimulation panel (eg, captopril)**
INCLUDES Renin x 6 (84244)
0.00   0.00   **FUD** XXX   N ▢
AMA: 2014,Jan,11

80417 **Peripheral vein renin stimulation panel (eg, captopril)**
INCLUDES Renin x 2 (84244)
0.00   0.00   **FUD** XXX   N ▢
AMA: 2014,Jan,11

80418 **Combined rapid anterior pituitary evaluation panel**
INCLUDES Adrenocorticotropic hormone (ACTH) x 4 (82024)
Cortisol x 4 (82533)
Follicle stimulating hormone (FSH) x 4 (83001)
Human growth hormone x 4 (83003)
Luteinizing hormone (LH) x 4 (83002)
Prolactin x 4 (84146)
Thyroid stimulating hormone (TSH) x 4 (84443)
0.00   0.00   **FUD** XXX   N ▢
AMA: 2014,Jan,11

80420 **Dexamethasone suppression panel, 48 hour**
INCLUDES Cortisol x 2 (82533)
Free cortisol, urine x 2 (82530)
Volume measurement for timed collection x 2 (81050)
EXCLUDES *Single dose dexamethasone (82533)*
0.00   0.00   **FUD** XXX   N ▢
AMA: 2014,Jan,11

80422 **Glucagon tolerance panel; for insulinoma**
INCLUDES Glucose x 3 (82947)
Insulin x 3 (83525)
0.00   0.00   **FUD** XXX   N ▢
AMA: 2014,Jan,11

80424 **for pheochromocytoma**
INCLUDES Catecholamines, fractionated x 2 (82384)
0.00   0.00   **FUD** XXX   N ▢
AMA: 2014,Jan,11

80426 **Gonadotropin releasing hormone stimulation panel**
INCLUDES Follicle stimulating hormone (FSH) x 4 (83001)
Luteinizing hormone (LH) x 4 (83002)
0.00   0.00   **FUD** XXX   N ▢
AMA: 2014,Jan,11

80428 **Growth hormone stimulation panel (eg, arginine infusion, l-dopa administration)**
INCLUDES Human growth hormone (HGH) x 4 (83003)
0.00   0.00   **FUD** XXX   N ▢
AMA: 2014,Jan,11

80430 **Growth hormone suppression panel (glucose administration)**
INCLUDES Glucose x 3 (82947)
Human growth hormone (HGH) x 4 (83003)
0.00   0.00   **FUD** XXX   N ▢
AMA: 2014,Jan,11

80432 **Insulin-induced C-peptide suppression panel**
> INCLUDES C-peptide x 5 (84681)
> Glucose x 5 (82947)
> Insulin (83525)
> 🔧 0.00 ⚕ 0.00 **FUD** XXX   N ▱
> **AMA:** 2014,Jan,11

80434 **Insulin tolerance panel; for ACTH insufficiency**
> INCLUDES Cortisol x 5 (82533)
> Glucose x 5 (82947)
> 🔧 0.00 ⚕ 0.00 **FUD** XXX   N ▱
> **AMA:** 2014,Jan,11

80435 **for growth hormone deficiency**
> INCLUDES Glucose x 5 (82947)
> Human growth hormone (HGH) x 5 (83003)
> 🔧 0.00 ⚕ 0.00 **FUD** XXX   N ▱
> **AMA:** 2014,Jan,11

80436 **Metyrapone panel**
> INCLUDES 11 deoxycortisol x 2 (82634)
> Cortisol x 2 (82533)
> 🔧 0.00 ⚕ 0.00 **FUD** XXX   N ▱
> **AMA:** 2014,Jan,11

80438 **Thyrotropin releasing hormone (TRH) stimulation panel; 1 hour**
> INCLUDES Thyroid stimulating hormone (TSH) x 3 (84443)
> 🔧 0.00 ⚕ 0.00 **FUD** XXX   N ▱
> **AMA:** 2014,Jan,11

80439 **2 hour**
> INCLUDES Thyroid stimulating hormone (TSH) x 4 (84443)
> 🔧 0.00 ⚕ 0.00 **FUD** XXX   N ▱
> **AMA:** 2014,Jan,11

80500-80502 Consultation By Clinical Pathologist

> INCLUDES Pharmacokinetic consultations
> Written report by pathologist for tests requiring additional medical judgment and requested by a physician or other qualified health care professional
> Do not report for consultations that include patient examination
> Do not report when a medical interpretive assessment is not provided

80500 **Clinical pathology consultation; limited, without review of patient's history and medical records**
> 🔧 0.56 ⚕ 0.65 **FUD** XXX   01 80 ▱
> **AMA:** 2015,Jan,16; 2014,Jan,11

80502 **comprehensive, for a complex diagnostic problem, with review of patient's history and medical records**
> 🔧 1.96 ⚕ 2.05 **FUD** XXX   01 80 ▱
> **AMA:** 2015,Jan,16; 2014,Jan,11

81000-81099 Urine Tests

81000 **Urinalysis, by dip stick or tablet reagent for bilirubin, glucose, hemoglobin, ketones, leukocytes, nitrite, pH, protein, specific gravity, urobilinogen, any number of these constituents; non-automated, with microscopy**
> 🔧 0.00 ⚕ 0.00 **FUD** XXX   N ▱
> **AMA:** 2015,Jan,16; 2014,Jan,11

81001 **automated, with microscopy**
> 🔧 0.00 ⚕ 0.00 **FUD** XXX   N ▱
> **AMA:** 2014,Jan,11

81002 **non-automated, without microscopy**
> INCLUDES Mosenthal test
> 🔧 0.00 ⚕ 0.00 **FUD** XXX   ✖ N ▱
> **AMA:** 2015,Jan,16; 2014,Jan,11

81003 **automated, without microscopy**
> 🔧 0.00 ⚕ 0.00 **FUD** XXX   ✖ N ▱
> **AMA:** 2015,Jan,16; 2014,Jan,11

81005 **Urinalysis; qualitative or semiquantitative, except immunoassays**
> INCLUDES Benedict test for dextrose
> EXCLUDES *Immunoassay, qualitative or semiquantitative (83518)*
> *Microalbumin (82043-82044)*
> *Nonimmunoassay reagent strip analysis (81000, 81002)*
> 🔧 0.00 ⚕ 0.00 **FUD** XXX   N ▱
> **AMA:** 2015,Jan,16; 2014,Jan,11

81007 **bacteriuria screen, except by culture or dipstick**
> EXCLUDES *Culture (87086-87088)*
> *Dipstick (81000, 81002)*
> 🔧 0.00 ⚕ 0.00 **FUD** XXX   ✖ N ▱
> **AMA:** 2014,Jan,11

81015 **microscopic only**
> EXCLUDES *Sperm evaluation for retrograde ejaculation (89331)*
> 🔧 0.00 ⚕ 0.00 **FUD** XXX   N
> **AMA:** 2014,Jan,11

81020 **2 or 3 glass test**
> INCLUDES Valentine's test
> 🔧 0.00 ⚕ 0.00 **FUD** XXX   N ▱
> **AMA:** 2014,Jan,11

81025 **Urine pregnancy test, by visual color comparison methods**   M ♀
> 🔧 0.00 ⚕ 0.00 **FUD** XXX   ✖ N
> **AMA:** 2015,Jan,16; 2014,Jan,11

81050 **Volume measurement for timed collection, each**
> 🔧 0.00 ⚕ 0.00 **FUD** XXX   N
> **AMA:** 2014,Jan,11

81099 **Unlisted urinalysis procedure**
> 🔧 0.00 ⚕ 0.00 **FUD** XXX   N
> **AMA:** 2015,Jan,16; 2014,Jan,11

81161-81355 [81161, 81162, 81287, 81288] Gene Analysis: Tier 1 Procedures

> INCLUDES All analytical procedures in the evaluation such as:
> Amplification
> Cell lysis
> Detection
> Digestion
> Extraction
> Nucleic acid stabilization
> Code selection based on specific gene being reviewed
> Evaluation of constitutional or somatic gene variations
> Evaluation of the presence of gene variants using the common gene variant name
> Examples of proteins or diseases in the code description that are not all inclusive
> Generally all the listed gene variants in the code description would be tested but lists are not all inclusive
> Gene specific and genomic testing
> Genes described using Human Genome Organization (HUGO) approved names
> Qualitative results unless otherwise stated
> Tier 1 molecular pathology codes (81200-81355 [81161, 81162, 81287, 81288])
>
> EXCLUDES *In situ hybridization analyses (88271-88275, 88365-88368 [88364, 88373, 88374])*
> *Microbial identification (87149-87153, 87470-87801 [87623, 87624, 87625], 87900-87904 [87906, 87910, 87912])*
> *Tier 1 molecular pathology codes (81370-81383)*
> *Tier 2 codes (81400-81408)*
> *Unlisted molecular pathology procedures ([81479])*
> Code also modifier 26 when only interpretation and report are performed
> Code also services required before cell lysis
> Do not report full gene sequencing using separately gene variant assessment codes unless it is specifically stated in the code description
> Do not report other related gene variants not listed in code

81161 **Resequenced code. See code following 81229.**

81162 **Resequenced code. See code following 81211.**

● **81170** *ABL1 (ABL proto-oncogene 1, non-receptor tyrosine kinase) (eg, acquired imatinib tyrosine kinase inhibitor resistance), gene analysis, variants in the kinase domain*

81200   *ASPA (aspartoacylase) (eg, Canavan disease) gene analysis, common variants (eg, E285A, Y231X)*
🔲 0.00   ✂ 0.00   **FUD** XXX   Ⓐ
     AMA: 2015,Jan,16; 2014,Jan,11; 2013,Sep,3-12; 2012,May,3-10

81201   *APC (adenomatous polyposis coli) (eg, familial adenomatosis polyposis [FAP], attenuated FAP) gene analysis; full gene sequence*
🔲 0.00   ✂ 0.00   **FUD** XXX   Ⓐ
     AMA: 2015,Jan,16; 2014,Jan,11; 2013,Sep,3-12

81202   **known familial variants**
🔲 0.00   ✂ 0.00   **FUD** XXX   Ⓐ
     AMA: 2015,Jan,16; 2014,Jan,11; 2013,Sep,3-12

81203   **duplication/deletion variants**
🔲 0.00   ✂ 0.00   **FUD** XXX   Ⓐ
     AMA: 2015,Jan,16; 2014,Jan,11; 2013,Sep,3-12

81205   *BCKDHB (branched-chain keto acid dehydrogenase E1, beta polypeptide) (eg, maple syrup urine disease) gene analysis, common variants (eg, R183P, G278S, E422X)*
🔲 0.00   ✂ 0.00   **FUD** XXX   Ⓐ
     AMA: 2015,Jan,16; 2014,Jan,11; 2013,Sep,3-12; 2012,May,3-10

81206   *BCR/ABL1 (t(9;22)) (eg, chronic myelogenous leukemia) translocation analysis; major breakpoint, qualitative or quantitative*
🔲 0.00   ✂ 0.00   **FUD** XXX   Ⓐ
     AMA: 2015,Jan,16; 2014,Jan,11; 2013,Sep,3-12; 2012,May,3-10

81207   **minor breakpoint, qualitative or quantitative**
🔲 0.00   ✂ 0.00   **FUD** XXX   Ⓐ
     AMA: 2015,Jan,16; 2014,Jan,11; 2013,Sep,3-12; 2012,May,3-10

81208   **other breakpoint, qualitative or quantitative**
🔲 0.00   ✂ 0.00   **FUD** XXX   Ⓐ
     AMA: 2015,Jan,16; 2014,Jan,11; 2013,Sep,3-12; 2012,May,3-10

81209   *BLM (Bloom syndrome, RecQ helicase-like) (eg, Bloom syndrome) gene analysis, 2281del6ins7 variant*
🔲 0.00   ✂ 0.00   **FUD** XXX   Ⓐ
     AMA: 2015,Jan,16; 2014,Jan,11; 2013,Sep,3-12; 2012,May,3-10

▲ 81210   *BRAF (B-Raf proto-oncogene, serine/threonine kinase) (eg, colon cancer, melanoma), gene analysis, V600 variant(s)*
🔲 0.00   ✂ 0.00   **FUD** XXX   Ⓐ
     AMA: 2015,Jan,16; 2014,Jan,11; 2013,Sep,3-12; 2012,May,3-10

81211   *BRCA1, BRCA2 (breast cancer 1 and 2) (eg, hereditary breast and ovarian cancer) gene analysis; full sequence analysis and common duplication/deletion variants in BRCA1 (ie, exon 13 del 3.835kb, exon 13 dup 6kb, exon 14-20 del 26kb, exon 22 del 510bp, exon 8-9 del 7.1kb)*
     Do not report with (81162)
🔲 0.00   ✂ 0.00   **FUD** XXX   Ⓐ
     AMA: 2015,Jan,16; 2014,Jan,11; 2013,Sep,3-12; 2012,May,3-10

● # 81162   **full sequence analysis and full duplication/deletion analysis**
🔲 0.00   ✂ 0.00   **FUD** 000
     Do not report with (81211, 81213-81214, 81216)

81212   **185delAG, 5385insC, 6174delT variants**
🔲 0.00   ✂ 0.00   **FUD** XXX   Ⓐ
     AMA: 2015,Jan,16; 2014,Jan,11; 2013,Sep,3-12; 2012,May,3-10

81213   **uncommon duplication/deletion variants**
     Do not report with (81162)
🔲 0.00   ✂ 0.00   **FUD** XXX   Ⓐ
     AMA: 2015,Jan,16; 2014,Jan,11; 2013,Sep,3-12; 2012,May,3-10

81214   *BRCA1 (breast cancer 1) (eg, hereditary breast and ovarian cancer) gene analysis; full sequence analysis and common duplication/deletion variants (ie, exon 13 del 3.835kb, exon 13 dup 6kb, exon 14-20 del 26kb, exon 22 del 510bp, exon 8-9 del 7.1kb)*
     EXCLUDES   *BRCA1 with BRCA2 full sequence testing (81162, 81211)*
     Do not report with (81162)
🔲 0.00   ✂ 0.00   **FUD** XXX   Ⓐ
     AMA: 2015,Jan,16; 2014,Jan,11; 2013,Sep,3-12; 2012,May,3-10

81215   **known familial variant**
🔲 0.00   ✂ 0.00   **FUD** XXX   Ⓐ
     AMA: 2015,Jan,16; 2014,Jan,11; 2013,Sep,3-12; 2012,May,3-10

81216   *BRCA2 (breast cancer 2) (eg, hereditary breast and ovarian cancer) gene analysis; full sequence analysis*
     EXCLUDES   *BRCA1 with BRCA2 full sequence testing (81162, 81211)*
     Do not report with (81162)
🔲 0.00   ✂ 0.00   **FUD** XXX   Ⓐ
     AMA: 2015,Jan,16; 2014,Jan,11; 2013,Sep,3-12; 2012,May,3-10

81217   **known familial variant**
🔲 0.00   ✂ 0.00   **FUD** XXX   Ⓐ
     AMA: 2015,Jan,16; 2014,Jan,11; 2013,Sep,3-12; 2012,May,3-10

● 81218   *CEBPA (CCAAT/enhancer binding protein [C/EBP], alpha) (eg, acute myeloid leukemia), gene analysis, full gene sequence*

● 81219   *CALR (calreticulin) (eg, myeloproliferative disorders), gene analysis, common variants in exon 9*

81220   *CFTR (cystic fibrosis transmembrane conductance regulator) (eg, cystic fibrosis) gene analysis; common variants (eg, ACMG/ACOG guidelines)*
     Do not report with Intron 8 poly-T analysis performed on a R117H positive patient with (81224)
🔲 0.00   ✂ 0.00   **FUD** XXX   Ⓐ
     AMA: 2015,Jan,16; 2014,Jan,11; 2013,Sep,3-12; 2012,May,3-10

81221   **known familial variants**
🔲 0.00   ✂ 0.00   **FUD** XXX   Ⓐ
     AMA: 2015,Jan,16; 2014,Jan,11; 2013,Sep,3-12; 2012,May,3-10

81222   **duplication/deletion variants**
🔲 0.00   ✂ 0.00   **FUD** XXX   Ⓐ
     AMA: 2015,Jan,16; 2014,Jan,11; 2013,Sep,3-12; 2012,May,3-10

81223   **full gene sequence**
🔲 0.00   ✂ 0.00   **FUD** XXX   Ⓐ
     AMA: 2015,Jan,16; 2014,Jan,11; 2013,Sep,3-12; 2012,May,3-10

81224   **intron 8 poly-T analysis (eg, male infertility)**
🔲 0.00   ✂ 0.00   **FUD** XXX   Ⓐ
     AMA: 2015,Jan,16; 2014,Jan,11; 2013,Sep,3-12; 2012,May,3-10

81225   *CYP2C19 (cytochrome P450, family 2, subfamily C, polypeptide 19) (eg, drug metabolism), gene analysis, common variants (eg, *2, *3, *4, *8, *17)*
🔲 0.00   ✂ 0.00   **FUD** XXX   Ⓐ
     AMA: 2015,Jan,16; 2014,Jan,11; 2013,Sep,3-12; 2012,May,3-10

81226   *CYP2D6 (cytochrome P450, family 2, subfamily D, polypeptide 6) (eg, drug metabolism), gene analysis, common variants (eg, *2, *3, *4, *5, *6, *9, *10, *17, *19, *29, *35, *41, *1XN, *2XN, *4XN)*
🔲 0.00   ✂ 0.00   **FUD** XXX   Ⓐ
     AMA: 2015,Jan,16; 2014,Jan,11; 2013,Sep,3-12; 2012,May,3-10

81227   *CYP2C9 (cytochrome P450, family 2, subfamily C, polypeptide 9) (eg, drug metabolism), gene analysis, common variants (eg, *2, *3, *5, *6)*
🔲 0.00   ✂ 0.00   **FUD** XXX   Ⓐ
     AMA: 2015,Jan,16; 2014,Jan,11; 2013,Sep,3-12; 2012,May,3-10

81228   **Cytogenomic constitutional (genome-wide) microarray analysis; interrogation of genomic regions for copy number variants (eg, bacterial artificial chromosome [BAC] or oligo-based comparative genomic hybridization [CGH] microarray analysis)**
     EXCLUDES   *Cytogenomic constitutional microarray analysis (not genome-wide), report code for targeted analysis or unlisted molecular pathology (81405, [81479])*
     Do not report with (81229, 88271)
     Do not report with analyte-specific procedures when the analytes are included in the microarray analysis
🔲 0.00   ✂ 0.00   **FUD** XXX   Ⓐ
     AMA: 2015,Jan,16; 2014,Jan,11; 2013,Sep,3-12; 2012,May,3-10

81229 interrogation of genomic regions for copy number and single nucleotide polymorphism (SNP) variants for chromosomal abnormalities

> EXCLUDES *Cytogenomic constitutional microarray analysis (not genome-wide), report code for targeted analysis or unlisted molecular pathology (81405, [81479])*
>
> Do not report with (81228, 88271)
>
> Do not report with analyte-specific procedures when the analytes are included in the microarray analysis

  0.00   0.00   **FUD** XXX   [A]

AMA: 2015,Jan,16; 2014,Jan,11; 2013,Sep,3-12; 2012,May,3-10

\# **81161** *DMD (dystrophin) (eg, Duchenne/Becker muscular dystrophy) deletion analysis, and duplication analysis, if performed*

  0.00   0.00   **FUD** XXX   [E]

AMA: 2014,Jan,11

81235 *EGFR (epidermal growth factor receptor) (eg, non-small cell lung cancer) gene analysis, common variants (eg, exon 19 LREA deletion, L858R, T790M, G719A, G719S, L861Q)*

  0.00   0.00   **FUD** XXX   [A]

AMA: 2015,Jan,16; 2014,Jan,11; 2013,Sep,3-12

81240 *F2 (prothrombin, coagulation factor II) (eg, hereditary hypercoagulability) gene analysis, 20210G>A variant*

  0.00   0.00   **FUD** XXX   [A]

AMA: 2015,Jan,16; 2014,Jan,11; 2013,Sep,3-12; 2012,May,3-10

81241 *F5 (coagulation factor V) (eg, hereditary hypercoagulability) gene analysis, Leiden variant*

  0.00   0.00   **FUD** XXX   [A]

AMA: 2015,Jan,16; 2014,Jan,11; 2013,Sep,3-12; 2012,May,3-10

81242 *FANCC (Fanconi anemia, complementation group C) (eg, Fanconi anemia, type C) gene analysis, common variant (eg, IVS4+4A>T)*

  0.00   0.00   **FUD** XXX   [A]

AMA: 2015,Jan,16; 2014,Jan,11; 2013,Sep,3-12; 2012,May,3-10

81243 *FMR1 (fragile X mental retardation 1) (eg, fragile X mental retardation) gene analysis; evaluation to detect abnormal (eg, expanded) alleles*

> INCLUDES Testing for detection and characterization of abnormal alleles using a single assay such as PCR

  0.00   0.00   **FUD** XXX   [A]

AMA: 2015,Jan,16; 2014,Jan,11; 2013,Sep,3-12; 2012,May,3-10

81244 characterization of alleles (eg, expanded size and methylation status)

> EXCLUDES *Testing for detection and characterization of abnormal alleles using a single assay such as PCR (81243)*

  0.00   0.00   **FUD** XXX   [A]

AMA: 2015,Jan,16; 2014,Jan,11; 2013,Sep,3-12; 2012,May,3-10

81245 *FLT3 (fms-related tyrosine kinase 3) (eg, acute myeloid leukemia), gene analysis; internal tandem duplication (ITD) variants (ie, exons 14, 15)*

  0.00   0.00   **FUD** XXX   [A]

AMA: 2015,Jan,16; 2015,Jan,3; 2014,Jan,11; 2013,Sep,3-12; 2012,May,3-10

81246 tyrosine kinase domain (TKD) variants (eg, D835, I836)

  0.00   0.00   **FUD** XXX   [A]

AMA: 2015,Jan,3

81250 *G6PC (glucose-6-phosphatase, catalytic subunit) (eg, Glycogen storage disease, type 1a, von Gierke disease) gene analysis, common variants (eg, R83C, Q347X)*

  0.00   0.00   **FUD** XXX   [A]

AMA: 2015,Jan,16; 2014,Jan,11; 2013,Sep,3-12; 2012,May,3-10

81251 *GBA (glucosidase, beta, acid) (eg, Gaucher disease) gene analysis, common variants (eg, N370S, 84GG, L444P, IVS2+1G>A)*

  0.00   0.00   **FUD** XXX   [A]

AMA: 2015,Jan,16; 2014,Jan,11; 2013,Sep,3-12; 2012,May,3-10

81252 *GJB2 (gap junction protein, beta 2, 26kDa, connexin 26) (eg, nonsyndromic hearing loss) gene analysis; full gene sequence*

  0.00   0.00   **FUD** XXX   [A]

AMA: 2015,Jan,16; 2014,Jan,11; 2013,Sep,3-12

81253 known familial variants

  0.00   0.00   **FUD** XXX   [A]

AMA: 2015,Jan,16; 2014,Jan,11; 2013,Sep,3-12

81254 *GJB6 (gap junction protein, beta 6, 30kDa, connexin 30) (eg, nonsyndromic hearing loss) gene analysis, common variants (eg, 309kb [del(GJB6-D13S1830)] and 232kb [del(GJB6-D13S1854)])*

  0.00   0.00   **FUD** XXX   [A]

AMA: 2015,Jan,16; 2014,Jan,11; 2013,Sep,3-12

81255 *HEXA (hexosaminidase A [alpha polypeptide]) (eg, Tay-Sachs disease) gene analysis, common variants (eg, 1278insTATC, 1421+1G>C, G269S)*

  0.00   0.00   **FUD** XXX   [A]

AMA: 2015,Jan,16; 2014,Jan,11; 2013,Sep,3-12; 2012,May,3-10

81256 *HFE (hemochromatosis) (eg, hereditary hemochromatosis) gene analysis, common variants (eg, C282Y, H63D)*

  0.00   0.00   **FUD** XXX   [A]

AMA: 2015,Jan,16; 2014,Jan,11; 2013,Sep,3-12; 2012,May,3-10

81257 *HBA1/HBA2 (alpha globin 1 and alpha globin 2) (eg, alpha thalassemia, Hb Bart hydrops fetalis syndrome, HbH disease), gene analysis, for common deletions or variant (eg, Southeast Asian, Thai, Filipino, Mediterranean, alpha3.7, alpha4.2, alpha20.5, and Constant Spring)*

  0.00   0.00   **FUD** XXX   [A]

AMA: 2015,Jan,16; 2014,Jan,11; 2013,Sep,3-12; 2012,May,3-10

81260 *IKBKAP (inhibitor of kappa light polypeptide gene enhancer in B-cells, kinase complex-associated protein) (eg, familial dysautonomia) gene analysis, common variants (eg, 2507+6T>C, R696P)*

  0.00   0.00   **FUD** XXX   [A]

AMA: 2015,Jan,16; 2014,Jan,11; 2013,Sep,3-12; 2012,May,3-10

81261 *IGH@ (Immunoglobulin heavy chain locus) (eg, leukemias and lymphomas, B-cell), gene rearrangement analysis to detect abnormal clonal population(s); amplified methodology (eg, polymerase chain reaction)*

  0.00   0.00   **FUD** XXX   [A]

AMA: 2015,Jan,16; 2014,Jan,11; 2013,Sep,3-12; 2012,May,3-10

81262 direct probe methodology (eg, Southern blot)

  0.00   0.00   **FUD** XXX   [A]

AMA: 2015,Jan,16; 2014,Jan,11; 2013,Sep,3-12; 2012,May,3-10

81263 *IGH@ (Immunoglobulin heavy chain locus) (eg, leukemia and lymphoma, B-cell), variable region somatic mutation analysis*

  0.00   0.00   **FUD** XXX   [A]

AMA: 2015,Jan,16; 2014,Jan,11; 2013,Sep,3-12; 2012,May,3-10

81264 *IGK@ (Immunoglobulin kappa light chain locus) (eg, leukemia and lymphoma, B-cell), gene rearrangement analysis, evaluation to detect abnormal clonal population(s)*

> EXCLUDES *Immunoglobulin kappa deleting element (IGKDEL) analysis ([81479])*
> *Immunoglobulin lambda gene (IGL@) rearrangement ([81479])*

  0.00   0.00   **FUD** XXX   [A]

AMA: 2015,Jan,16; 2014,Jan,11; 2013,Sep,3-12; 2012,May,3-10

81265 Comparative analysis using Short Tandem Repeat (STR) markers; patient and comparative specimen (eg, pre-transplant recipient and donor germline testing, post-transplant non-hematopoietic recipient germline [eg, buccal swab or other germline tissue sample] and donor testing, twin zygosity testing, or maternal cell contamination of fetal cells)

Code also the following codes for chimerism testing if comparative short tandem repeat (STR) analysis of recipient (using buccal swab or other germline tissue sample) and donor are performed after hematopoietic stem cell transplantation (81266-81268)

  0.00 0.00 **FUD** XXX [A]

AMA: 2015,Jan,16; 2014,Jan,11; 2013,Sep,3-12; 2012,May,3-10

+ 81266 each additional specimen (eg, additional cord blood donor, additional fetal samples from different cultures, or additional zygosity in multiple birth pregnancies) (List separately in addition to code for primary procedure)

Code also the following codes for chimerism testing if comparative short tandem repeat (STR) analysis of recipient (using buccal swab or other germline tissue sample) and donor are performed after hematopoietic stem cell transplantation (81267-81268)

Code first (81265)

  0.00 0.00 **FUD** XXX [A]

AMA: 2015,Jan,16; 2014,Jan,11; 2013,Sep,3-12; 2012,May,3-10

81267 Chimerism (engraftment) analysis, post transplantation specimen (eg, hematopoietic stem cell), includes comparison to previously performed baseline analyses; without cell selection

Code also the following codes for chimerism testing if comparative short tandem repeat (STR) analysis of recipient (using buccal swab or other germline tissue sample) and donor are performed after hematopoietic stem cell transplantation (81265-81266, 81268)

  0.00 0.00 **FUD** XXX [A]

AMA: 2015,Jan,16; 2014,Jan,11; 2013,Sep,3-12; 2012,May,3-10

81268 with cell selection (eg, CD3, CD33), each cell type

Code also the following codes for chimerism testing if comparative short tandem repeat (STR) analysis of recipient (using buccal swab or other germline tissue sample) and donor are performed after hematopoietic stem cell transplantation (81265-81267)

  0.00 0.00 **FUD** XXX [A]

AMA: 2015,Jan,16; 2014,Jan,11; 2013,Sep,3-12; 2012,May,3-10

81270 *JAK2 (Janus kinase 2)* (eg, myeloproliferative disorder) gene analysis, p.Val617Phe (V617F) variant

  0.00 0.00 **FUD** XXX [A]

AMA: 2015,Jan,16; 2014,Jan,11; 2013,Sep,3-12; 2012,May,3-10

● **81272** *KIT (v-kit Hardy-Zuckerman 4 feline sarcoma viral oncogene homolog)* (eg, gastrointestinal stromal tumor [GIST], acute myeloid leukemia, melanoma), gene analysis, targeted sequence analysis (eg, exons 8, 11, 13, 17, 18)

● **81273** *KIT (v-kit Hardy-Zuckerman 4 feline sarcoma viral oncogene homolog)* (eg, mastocytosis), gene analysis, D816 variant

▲ **81275** *KRAS (Kirsten rat sarcoma viral oncogene homolog)* (eg, carcinoma) gene analysis; variants in exon 2 (eg, codons 12 and 13)

  0.00 0.00 **FUD** XXX [A]

AMA: 2015,Jan,16; 2014,Jan,11; 2013,Sep,3-12; 2012,May,3-10

● **81276** additional variant(s) (eg, codon 61, codon 146)

81280 Long QT syndrome gene analyses (eg, *KCNQ1, KCNH2, SCN5A, KCNE1, KCNE2, KCNJ2, CACNA1C, CAV3, SCN4B, AKAP, SNTA1, and ANK2)*; full sequence analysis

  0.00 0.00 **FUD** XXX [A]

AMA: 2015,Jan,16; 2014,Jan,11; 2013,Sep,3-12; 2012,May,3-10

81281 known familial sequence variant

  0.00 0.00 **FUD** XXX [A]

AMA: 2015,Jan,16; 2014,Jan,11; 2013,Sep,3-12; 2012,May,3-10

81282 duplication/deletion variants

  0.00 0.00 **FUD** XXX [A]

AMA: 2015,Jan,16; 2014,Jan,11; 2013,Sep,3-12; 2012,May,3-10

81287 Resequenced code. See code following 81290.

81288 Resequenced code. See code following 81292.

81290 *MCOLN1 (mucolipin 1)* (eg, Mucolipidosis, type IV) gene analysis, common variants (eg, IVS3-2A>G, del6.4kb)

  0.00 0.00 **FUD** XXX [A]

AMA: 2015,Jan,16; 2014,Jan,11; 2013,Sep,3-12; 2012,May,3-10

81287 *MGMT (O-6-methylguanine-DNA methyltransferase)* (eg, glioblastoma multiforme), methylation analysis

  0.00 0.00 **FUD** XXX [A]

AMA: 2014,Jan,11

81291 *MTHFR (5,10-methylenetetrahydrofolate reductase)* (eg, hereditary hypercoagulability) gene analysis, common variants (eg, 677T, 1298C)

  0.00 0.00 **FUD** XXX [A]

AMA: 2015,Jan,16; 2014,Jan,11; 2013,Sep,3-12; 2012,May,3-10

81292 *MLH1 (mutL homolog 1, colon cancer, nonpolyposis type 2)* (eg, hereditary non-polyposis colorectal cancer, Lynch syndrome) gene analysis; full sequence analysis

  0.00 0.00 **FUD** XXX [A]

AMA: 2015,Jan,16; 2015,Jan,3; 2014,Jan,11; 2013,Sep,3-12; 2012,May,3-10

81288 promoter methylation analysis

  0.00 0.00 **FUD** XXX [A]

AMA: 2015,Jan,3

81293 known familial variants

  0.00 0.00 **FUD** XXX [A]

AMA: 2015,Jan,16; 2014,Jan,11; 2013,Sep,3-12; 2012,May,3-10

81294 duplication/deletion variants

  0.00 0.00 **FUD** XXX [A]

AMA: 2015,Jan,16; 2014,Jan,11; 2013,Sep,3-12; 2012,May,3-10

81295 *MSH2 (mutS homolog 2, colon cancer, nonpolyposis type 1)* (eg, hereditary non-polyposis colorectal cancer, Lynch syndrome) gene analysis; full sequence analysis

  0.00 0.00 **FUD** XXX [A]

AMA: 2015,Jan,16; 2014,Jan,11; 2013,Sep,3-12; 2012,May,3-10

81296 known familial variants

  0.00 0.00 **FUD** XXX [A]

AMA: 2015,Jan,16; 2014,Jan,11; 2013,Sep,3-12; 2012,May,3-10

81297 duplication/deletion variants

  0.00 0.00 **FUD** XXX [A]

AMA: 2015,Jan,16; 2014,Jan,11; 2013,Sep,3-12; 2012,May,3-10

81298 *MSH6 (mutS homolog 6 [E. coli])* (eg, hereditary non-polyposis colorectal cancer, Lynch syndrome) gene analysis; full sequence analysis

  0.00 0.00 **FUD** XXX [A]

AMA: 2015,Jan,16; 2014,Jan,11; 2013,Sep,3-12; 2012,May,3-10

81299 known familial variants

  0.00 0.00 **FUD** XXX [A]

AMA: 2015,Jan,16; 2014,Jan,11; 2013,Sep,3-12; 2012,May,3-10

81300 duplication/deletion variants

  0.00 0.00 **FUD** XXX [A]

AMA: 2015,Jan,16; 2014,Jan,11; 2013,Sep,3-12; 2012,May,3-10

81301 Microsatellite instability analysis (eg, hereditary non-polyposis colorectal cancer, Lynch syndrome) of markers for mismatch repair deficiency (eg, BAT25, BAT26), includes comparison of neoplastic and normal tissue, if performed

  0.00 0.00 **FUD** XXX [A]

AMA: 2015,Jan,16; 2014,Jan,11; 2013,Sep,3-12; 2012,May,3-10

81302 *MECP2 (methyl CpG binding protein 2)* (eg, Rett syndrome) gene analysis; full sequence analysis

  0.00 0.00 **FUD** XXX [A]

AMA: 2015,Jan,16; 2014,Jan,11; 2013,Sep,3-12; 2012,May,3-10

81303	**known familial variant**
	🔲 0.00 🔲 0.00 **FUD** XXX [A]
	AMA: 2015,Jan,16; 2014,Jan,11; 2013,Sep,3-12; 2012,May,3-10

81304	**duplication/deletion variants**
	🔲 0.00 🔲 0.00 **FUD** XXX [A]
	AMA: 2015,Jan,16; 2014,Jan,11; 2013,Sep,3-12; 2012,May,3-10

81310 *NPM1 (nucleophosmin) (eg, acute myeloid leukemia) gene analysis, exon 12 variants*
🔲 0.00   🔲 0.00   **FUD** XXX   [A]
AMA: 2015,Jan,16; 2014,Jan,11; 2013,Sep,3-12; 2012,May,3-10

● 81311 *NRAS (neuroblastoma RAS viral [v-ras] oncogene homolog) (eg, colorectal carcinoma), gene analysis, variants in exon 2 (eg, codons 12 and 13) and exon 3 (eg, codon 61)*

81313 *PCA3/KLK3 (prostate cancer antigen 3 [non-protein coding]/kallikrein-related peptidase 3 [prostate specific antigen]) ratio (eg, prostate cancer)*
🔲 0.00   🔲 0.00   **FUD** XXX   [A]
AMA: 2015,Jan,3

● 81314 *PDGFRA (platelet-derived growth factor receptor, alpha polypeptide) (eg, gastrointestinal stromal tumor [GIST]), gene analysis, targeted sequence analysis (eg, exons 12, 18)*

81315 *PML/RARalpha, (t(15;17)), (promyelocytic leukemia/retinoic acid receptor alpha) (eg, promyelocytic leukemia) translocation analysis; common breakpoints (eg, intron 3 and intron 6), qualitative or quantitative*
INCLUDES   Intron 3 and 6 (and exon 6 if performed) testing
🔲 0.00   🔲 0.00   **FUD** XXX   [A]
AMA: 2015,Jan,16; 2014,Jan,11; 2013,Sep,3-12; 2012,May,3-10

81316	**single breakpoint (eg, intron 3, intron 6 or exon 6), qualitative or quantitative**
	EXCLUDES Intron 3 and 6 (and exon 6 if performed) testing (81315)
	Do not report more than one unit of this code for testing intron 6 and exon 6 without intron 3 (81316)
	🔲 0.00 🔲 0.00 **FUD** XXX [A]
	AMA: 2015,Jan,16; 2014,Jan,11; 2013,Sep,3-12; 2012,May,3-10

81317 *PMS2 (postmeiotic segregation increased 2 [S. cerevisiae]) (eg, hereditary non-polyposis colorectal cancer, Lynch syndrome) gene analysis; full sequence analysis*
🔲 0.00   🔲 0.00   **FUD** XXX   [A]
AMA: 2015,Jan,16; 2014,Jan,11; 2013,Sep,3-12; 2012,May,3-10

81318	**known familial variants**
	🔲 0.00 🔲 0.00 **FUD** XXX [A]
	AMA: 2015,Jan,16; 2014,Jan,11; 2013,Sep,3-12; 2012,May,3-10

81319	**duplication/deletion variants**
	🔲 0.00 🔲 0.00 **FUD** XXX [A]
	AMA: 2015,Jan,16; 2014,Jan,11; 2013,Sep,3-12; 2012,May,3-10

81321 *PTEN (phosphatase and tensin homolog) (eg, Cowden syndrome, PTEN hamartoma tumor syndrome) gene analysis; full sequence analysis*
🔲 0.00   🔲 0.00   **FUD** XXX   [A]
AMA: 2015,Jan,16; 2014,Jan,11; 2013,Sep,3-12

81322	**known familial variant**
	🔲 0.00 🔲 0.00 **FUD** XXX [A]
	AMA: 2015,Jan,16; 2014,Jan,11; 2013,Sep,3-12

81323	**duplication/deletion variant**
	🔲 0.00 🔲 0.00 **FUD** XXX [A]
	AMA: 2015,Jan,16; 2014,Jan,11; 2013,Sep,3-12

81324 *PMP22 (peripheral myelin protein 22) (eg, Charcot-Marie-Tooth, hereditary neuropathy with liability to pressure palsies) gene analysis; duplication/deletion analysis*
🔲 0.00   🔲 0.00   **FUD** XXX   [A]
AMA: 2015,Jan,16; 2014,Jan,11; 2013,Sep,3-12

81325	**full sequence analysis**
	🔲 0.00 🔲 0.00 **FUD** XXX [A]
	AMA: 2015,Jan,16; 2014,Jan,11; 2013,Sep,3-12

81326	**known familial variant**
	🔲 0.00 🔲 0.00 **FUD** XXX [A]
	AMA: 2015,Jan,16; 2014,Jan,11; 2013,Sep,3-12

81330 *SMPD1(sphingomyelin phosphodiesterase 1, acid lysosomal) (eg, Niemann-Pick disease, Type A) gene analysis, common variants (eg, R496L, L302P, fsP330)*
🔲 0.00   🔲 0.00   **FUD** XXX   [A]
AMA: 2015,Jan,16; 2014,Jan,11; 2013,Sep,3-12; 2012,May,3-10

81331 *SNRPN/UBE3A (small nuclear ribonucleoprotein polypeptide N and ubiquitin protein ligase E3A) (eg, Prader-Willi syndrome and/or Angelman syndrome), methylation analysis*
🔲 0.00   🔲 0.00   **FUD** XXX   [A]
AMA: 2015,Jan,16; 2014,Jan,11; 2013,Sep,3-12; 2012,May,3-10

81332 *SERPINA1 (serpin peptidase inhibitor, clade A, alpha-1 antiproteinase, antitrypsin, member 1) (eg, alpha-1-antitrypsin deficiency), gene analysis, common variants (eg, *S and *Z)*
🔲 0.00   🔲 0.00   **FUD** XXX   [A]
AMA: 2015,Jan,16; 2014,Jan,11; 2013,Sep,3-12; 2012,May,3-10

81340 *TRB@ (T cell antigen receptor, beta) (eg, leukemia and lymphoma), gene rearrangement analysis to detect abnormal clonal population(s); using amplification methodology (eg, polymerase chain reaction)*
🔲 0.00   🔲 0.00   **FUD** XXX   [A]
AMA: 2015,Jan,16; 2014,Jan,11; 2013,Sep,3-12; 2012,May,3-10

81341	**using direct probe methodology (eg, Southern blot)**
	🔲 0.00 🔲 0.00 **FUD** XXX [A]
	AMA: 2015,Jan,16; 2014,Jan,11; 2013,Sep,3-12; 2012,May,3-10

81342 *TRG@ (T cell antigen receptor, gamma) (eg, leukemia and lymphoma), gene rearrangement analysis, evaluation to detect abnormal clonal population(s)*
EXCLUDES   T cell antigen alpha [TRA@] gene arrangement testing ([81479])
T cell antigen delta [TRD@] gene arrangement testing (81402)
🔲 0.00   🔲 0.00   **FUD** XXX   [A]
AMA: 2015,Jan,16; 2014,Jan,11; 2013,Sep,3-12; 2012,May,3-10

81350 *UGT1A1 (UDP glucuronosyltransferase 1 family, polypeptide A1) (eg, irinotecan metabolism), gene analysis, common variants (eg, *28, *36, *37)*
🔲 0.00   🔲 0.00   **FUD** XXX   [A]
AMA: 2015,Jan,16; 2014,Jan,11; 2013,Sep,3-12; 2012,May,3-10

▲ 81355 *VKORC1 (vitamin K epoxide reductase complex, subunit 1) (eg, warfarin metabolism), gene analysis, common variant(s) (eg, -1639G>A, c.173+1000C>T)*
🔲 0.00   🔲 0.00   **FUD** XXX   [A]
AMA: 2015,Jan,16; 2014,Jan,11; 2013,Sep,3-12; 2012,May,3-10

81370-81383 Human Leukocyte Antigen (HLA) Testing

INCLUDES Additional testing that must be performed to resolve ambiguous allele combinations for high-resolution typing
All analytical procedures in the evaluation such as:
Amplification
Cell lysis
Detection
Digestion
Extraction
Nucleic acid stabilization
Analysis to identify human leukocyte antigen (HLA) alleles and allele groups connected to specific diseases and individual response to drug therapy in addition to other clinical uses
Code selection based on specific gene being reviewed
Evaluation of the presence of gene variants using the common gene variant name
Examples of proteins or diseases in the code description that are not all inclusive
Generally all the listed gene variants in the code description would be tested but lists are not all inclusive
Genes described using Human Genome Organization (HUGO) approved names
High-resolution typing resolves the common well-defined (CWD) alleles and is usually identified by at least four-digits. There are some instances when high-resolution typing may include some ambiguities for rare alleles, and those may be reported as a string of alleles or an NMDP code
Histocompatibility antigen testing
Intermediate resolution HLA testing is identified by a string of alleles or a National Marrow Donor Program (NMDP) code
Low and intermediate resolution are considered low resolution for code assignment
Low-resolution HLA type reporting is identified by two-digit HLA name
Multiple variant alleles or allele groups that can be identified by typing
One or more HLA genes in specific clinical circumstances
Qualitative results unless otherwise stated
Typing performed to determine the compatibility of recipients and potential donors undergoing solid organ or hematopoietic stem cell pretransplantation testing

EXCLUDES HLA antigen typing by nonmolecular pathology methods (86812-86822)
Microbial identification (87149-87153, 87470-87801 [87623, 87624, 87625], 87900-87904 [87906, 87910, 87912])
Tier 1 molecular pathology codes (81200-81355 [81161, 81162, 81287, 81288])
Tier 2 and unlisted mocular pathology procedures (81400-81408, [81479])
Code also modifier 26 when only interpretation and report are performed
Code also services required before cell lysis
Do not report full gene sequencing separately using gene variant assessment codes unless it is specifically stated in the code description
Do not report other related gene variants not listed in code

81370 **HLA Class I and II typing, low resolution (eg, antigen equivalents); *HLA-A, -B, -C, -DRB1/3/4/5, and -DQB1***
    0.00   0.00   **FUD** XXX   A
    AMA: 2015,Jan,16; 2014,Jan,11; 2013,Sep,3-12; 2012,May,3-10; 2012,Jun,15-16

81371 ***HLA-A, -B, and -DRB1 (eg, verification typing)***
    0.00   0.00   **FUD** XXX   A
    AMA: 2015,Jan,16; 2014,Jan,11; 2013,Sep,3-12; 2012,May,3-10; 2012,Jun,15-16

81372 **HLA Class I typing, low resolution (eg, antigen equivalents); complete *(ie, HLA-A, -B, and -C)***
    EXCLUDES *Class I and II low-resolution HLA typing for HLA-A, -B, -C, -DRB1/3/4/5, and -DQB1 (81370)*
    0.00   0.00   **FUD** XXX   A
    AMA: 2015,Jan,16; 2014,Jan,11; 2013,Sep,3-12; 2012,May,3-10; 2012,Jun,15-16

81373 **one locus *(eg, HLA-A, -B, or -C)*, each**
    EXCLUDES *A complete Class 1 (HLA-A, -B, and -C) low-resolution typing (81372)*
    Reporting the presence or absence of a single antigen equivalent using low-resolution methodology (81374)
    0.00   0.00   **FUD** XXX   A
    AMA: 2015,Jan,16; 2014,Jan,11; 2013,Sep,3-12; 2012,May,3-10; 2012,Jun,15-16

81374 **one antigen equivalent *(eg, B*27)*, each**
    EXCLUDES *Testing for the presence or absence of more than 2 antigen equivalents at a locus, use the following code for each locus test (81373)*
    0.00   0.00   **FUD** XXX   A
    AMA: 2015,Jan,16; 2014,Jan,11; 2013,Sep,3-12; 2012,May,3-10; 2012,Jun,15-16

81375 **HLA Class II typing, low resolution (eg, antigen equivalents); *HLA-DRB1/3/4/5 and -DQB1***
    EXCLUDES *Class I and II low-resolution HLA typing for HLA-A, -B, -C, -DRB 1/3/4/5, and DQB1 (81370)*
    0.00   0.00   **FUD** XXX   A
    AMA: 2015,Jan,16; 2014,Jan,11; 2013,Sep,3-12; 2012,May,3-10; 2012,Jun,15-16

81376 **one locus *(eg, HLA-DRB1, -DRB3/4/5, -DQB1, -DQA1, -DPB1, or -DPA1)*, each**
    INCLUDES Low-resolution typing, HLA-DRB1/3/4/5 reported as a single locus
    EXCLUDES *Low-resolution typing for HLA-DRB1/3/4/5 and -DQB1 (81375)*
    0.00   0.00   **FUD** XXX   A
    AMA: 2015,Jan,16; 2014,Jan,11; 2013,Sep,3-12; 2012,May,3-10; 2012,Jun,15-16

81377 **one antigen equivalent, each**
    EXCLUDES *Testing for presence or absence of more than two antigen equivalents at a locus (81376)*
    0.00   0.00   **FUD** XXX   A
    AMA: 2015,Jan,16; 2014,Jan,11; 2013,Sep,3-12; 2012,May,3-10; 2012,Jun,15-16

81378 **HLA Class I and II typing, high resolution (ie, alleles or allele groups), *HLA-A, -B, -C, and -DRB1***
    0.00   0.00   **FUD** XXX   A
    AMA: 2015,Jan,16; 2014,Jan,11; 2013,Sep,3-12; 2012,May,3-10; 2012,Jun,15-16

81379 **HLA Class I typing, high resolution (ie, alleles or allele groups); complete *(ie, HLA-A, -B, and -C)***
    0.00   0.00   **FUD** XXX   A
    AMA: 2015,Jan,16; 2014,Jan,11; 2013,Sep,3-12; 2012,May,3-10; 2012,Jun,15-16

81380 **one locus *(eg, HLA-A, -B, or -C)*, each**
    EXCLUDES *Complete Class I high-resolution typing for HLA-A, -B, and -C (81379)*
    Testing for presence or absence of a single allele or allele group using high-resolution methodology (81381)
    0.00   0.00   **FUD** XXX   A
    AMA: 2015,Jan,16; 2014,Jan,11; 2013,Sep,3-12; 2012,May,3-10; 2012,Jun,15-16

81381 **one allele or allele group *(eg, B*57:01P)*, each**
    EXCLUDES *Testing for the presence or absence of more than two alleles or allele groups of locus, report the following code for each locus (81380)*
    0.00   0.00   **FUD** XXX   A
    AMA: 2015,Jan,16; 2014,Jan,11; 2013,Sep,3-12; 2012,May,3-10; 2012,Jun,15-16

81382 **HLA Class II typing, high resolution (ie, alleles or allele groups); one locus *(eg, HLA-DRB1, -DRB3/4/5, -DQB1, -DQA1, -DPB1, or -DPA1)*, each**
    INCLUDES Typing of one or all of the DRB3/4/5 genes is regarded as one locus
    EXCLUDES *Testing for just the presence or absence of a single allele or allele group using high-resolution methodology (81383)*
    0.00   0.00   **FUD** XXX   A
    AMA: 2015,Jan,16; 2014,Jan,11; 2013,Sep,3-12; 2012,May,3-10; 2012,Jun,15-16

81383 one allele or allele group (eg, *HLA-DQB1*06:02P*), each

EXCLUDES For testing for the presence or absence of more than two alleles or allele groups at a locus, report the following code for each locus (81382)

💬 0.00 ✂ 0.00 **FUD** XXX Ⓐ

AMA: 2015,Jan,16; 2014,Jan,11; 2013,Sep,3-12; 2012,May,3-10; 2012,Jun,15-16

81400-81408 [81479] Molecular Pathology Tier 2 Procedures

INCLUDES All analytical procedures in the evaluation such as:
Amplification
Cell lysis
Detection
Digestion
Extraction
Nucleic acid stabilization
Code selection based on specific gene being reviewed
Codes that are arranged by level of technical resources and work involved
Evaluation of the presence of a gene variant using the common gene variant name
Examples in parentheses at/near the beginning of the code descriptions that are not all-inclusive
Examples of proteins or diseases in the code description that are not all inclusive
Generally all the listed gene variants in the code description would be tested but lists are not all inclusive
Genes described using the Human Genome Organization (HUGO) approved names
Histocompatibility testing
Qualitative results unless otherwise stated
Specific analytes listed after the code description to use for selecting the appropriate molecular pathology procedure
Targeted genomic testing (81410-81471)
Testing for diseases that are more rare

EXCLUDES Microbial identification (87149-87153, 87470-87801 [87623, 87624, 87625], 87900-87904 [87906, 87910, 87912])
Tier 1 molecular pathology (81200-81383 [81161, 81162, 81287, 81288])
Tier 2 codes (Error)
Unlisted molecular pathology procedures ([81479])
Code also modifier 26 when only interpretation and report are performed
Code also services required before cell lysis
Do not report full gene sequencing using gene variant assessment codes unless it is specifically stated in the code description
Do not report other related gene variants not listed in the code description

81400 Molecular pathology procedure, Level 1(eg, identification of single germline variant [eg, SNP] by techniques such as restriction enzyme digestion or melt curve analysis)

INCLUDES *ACADM (acyl-CoA dehydrogenase, C-4 to C-12 straight chain, MCAD)* (eg, medium chain acyl dehydrogenase deficiency), K304E variant
ACE (angiotensin converting enzyme) (eg, hereditary blood pressure regulation), insertion/deletion variant
AGTR1 (angiotensin II receptor, type 1) (eg, essential hypertension), 1166A>C variant
BCKDHA (branched chain keto acid dehydrogenase E1, alpha polypeptide) (eg, maple syrup urine disease, type 1A), Y438N variant
CCR5 (chemokine C-C motif receptor 5) (eg, HIV resistance), 32-bp deletion mutation/794 825del32 deletion
CLRN1 (clarin 1) (eg, Usher syndrome, type 3), N48K variant
DPYD (dihydropyrimidine dehydrogenase) (eg, 5-fluorouracil/5-FU and capecitabine drug metabolism), IVS14+1G>A variant
F2 (coagulation factor 2) (eg, hereditary hypercoagulability), 1199G>A variant
F5 (coagulation factor V) (eg, hereditary hypercoagulability), HR2 variant
F7 (coagulation factor VII [serum prothrombin conversion accelerator]) (eg, hereditary hypercoagulability), R353Q variant
F13B (coagulation factor XIII, B polypeptide) (eg, hereditary hypercoagulability), V34L variant
FGB (fibrinogen beta chain) (eg, hereditary ischemic heart disease), -455G>A variant

FGFR1 (fibroblast growth factor receptor 1) (eg, Pfeiffer syndrome type 1, craniosynostosis), P252R variant
FGFR3 (fibroblast growth factor receptor 3) (eg, Muenke syndrome), P250R variant
FKTN (fukutin) (eg, Fukuyama congenital muscular dystrophy), retrotransposon insertion variant
GNE (glucosamine [UDP-N-acetyl]-2 -epimerase/N-acetylmannosamine kinase) (eg, inclusion body myopathy 2 [IBM2], Nonaka myopathy), M712T variant
Human platelet antigen 1 genotyping (HPA-1), ITGB3 (integrin, beta 3 [platelet glycoprotein IIIa], antigen CD61 [GPIIIa]) (eg, neonatal alloimmune thrombocytopenia [NAIT], post-transfusion purpura), HPA-1a/b (L33P)
Human platelet antigen 2 genotyping (HPA-2), GP1BA (glycoprotein Ib [platelet], alpha polypeptide [GPIba]) (eg, neonatal alloimmune thrombocytopenia [NAIT], post-transfusion purpura), HPA-2a/b (T145M)
Human platelet antigen 3 genotyping (HPA-3), ITGA2B (integrin, alpha 2b [platelet glycoprotein IIb of IIb/IIIa complex], antigen CD41 [GPIIb]) (eg, neonatal alloimmune thrombocytopenia [NAIT], post-transfusion purpura), HPA-3a/b (I843S)
Human platelet antigen 4 genotyping (HPA-4), ITGB3 (integrin, beta 3 [platelet glycoprotein IIIa], antigen CD61 [GPIIIa]) (eg, neonatal alloimmune thrombocytopenia [NAIT], post-transfusion purpura), HPA-4a/b (R143Q)
Human platelet antigen 5 genotyping (HPA-5), ITGA2 (integrin, alpha 2 [CD49B, alpha 2 subunit of VLA-2 receptor] [GPIa]) (eg, neonatal alloimmune thrombocytopenia [NAIT], post-transfusion purpura), HPA-5a/b (K505E)
Human platelet antigen 6 genotyping (HPA-6w), ITGB3 (integrin, beta 3 [platelet glycoprotein IIIa, antigen CD61] [GPIIIa]) (eg, neonatal alloimmune thrombocytopenia [NAIT], post-transfusion purpura), HPA-6a/b (R489Q)
Human platelet antigen 9 genotyping (HPA-9w), ITGA2B (integrin, alpha 2b [platelet glycoprotein IIb of IIb/IIIa complex, antigen CD41] [GPIIb]) (eg, neonatal alloimmune thrombocytopenia [NAIT], post-transfusion purpura), HPA-9a/b (V837M)
Human platelet antigen 15 genotyping (HPA-15), CD109 (CD109 molecule) (eg, neonatal alloimmune thrombocytopenia [NAIT], post-transfusion purpura), HPA-15a/b(S682Y)
IL28B (interleukin 28B [interferon, lambda 3]) (eg, drug response), rs12979860 variant
IVD (isovaleryl-CoA dehydrogenase) (eg, isovaleric acidemia), A282V variant
LCT (lactase-phlorizin hydrolase) (eg, lactose intolerance), 13910 C>T variant
NEB (nebulin) (eg, nemaline myopathy 2), exon 55 deletion variant
PCDH15 (protocadherin-related 15) (eg, Usher syndrome type 1F), R245X variant
SERPINE1 (serpine peptidase inhibitor clade E, member 1, plasminogen activator inhibitor -1, PAI-1) (eg, thrombophilia), 4G variant
SHOC2 (soc-2 suppressor of clear homolog) (eg, Noonan-like syndrome with loose anagen hair), S2G variant
SLCO1B1 (solute carrier organic anion transporter family, member 1B1) (eg, adverse drug reaction), V174A variant
SMN1 (survival of motor neuron 1, telomeric) (eg, spinal muscular atrophy), exon 7 deletion
SRY (sex determining region Y) (eg, 46,XX testicular disorder of sex development, gonadal dysgenesis), gene analysis
TOR1A (torsin family 1, member A [torsin A]) (eg, early-onset primary dystonia [DYT1]), 907_909delGAG (904_906delGAG) variant

💬 0.00 ✂ 0.00 **FUD** XXX Ⓐ

AMA: 2015,Jan,16; 2015,Jan,3; 2014,Jan,11; 2013,Sep,3-12; 2013,Jul,11-12; 2012,May,3-10

▲ 81401 **Molecular pathology procedure, Level 2 (eg, 2-10 SNPs, 1 methylated variant, or 1 somatic variant [typically using nonsequencing target variant analysis], or detection of a dynamic mutation disorder/triplet repeat)**

INCLUDES

ABCC8 (ATP-binding cassette, sub-family C [CFTR/MRP], member 8) (eg, familial hyperinsulinism), common variants (eg, c.3898-9G>A [c.3992-9G>A], F1388del)

ABL1 (ABL proto oncogene 1, non-receptor tyrosine kinase) (eg, acquired imatinib resistance), T315I variant

ACADM (acyl-CoA dehydrogenase, C-4 to C-12 straight chain, MCAD) (eg, medium chain acyl dehydrogenase deficiency), common variants (eg, K304E, Y42H)

ADRB2 (adrenergic beta-2 receptor surface) (eg, drug metabolism), common variants (eg, G16R, Q27E)

AFF2 (AF4/FMR2 family, member 2 [FMR2]) (eg, fragile X mental retardation 2 [FRAXE]), evaluation to detect abnormal (eg, expanded) alleles

APOB (apolipoprotein B) (eg, familial hypercholesterolemia type B), common variants (eg, R3500Q, R3500W)

APOE (apolipoprotein E) (eg, hyperlipoproteinemia type III, cardiovascular disease, Alzheimer disease), common variants (eg, *2, *3, *4)

AR (androgen receptor) (eg, spinal and bulbar muscular atrophy, Kennedy disease, X chromosome inactivation), characterization of alleles (eg, expanded size or methylation status)

ATN1 (atrophin 1) (eg, dentatorubral-pallidoluysian atrophy), evaluation to detect abnormal (eg, expanded) alleles

ATXN1 (ataxin 1) (eg, spinocerebellar ataxia), evaluation to detect abnormal (eg, expanded) alleles

ATXN2 (ataxin 2) (eg, spinocerebellar ataxia), evaluation to detect abnormal (eg, expanded) alleles

ATXN3 (ataxin 3) (eg, spinocerebellar ataxia, Machado-Joseph disease), evaluation to detect abnormal (eg, expanded) alleles

ATXN7 (ataxin 7) (eg, spinocerebellar ataxia), evaluation to detect abnormal (eg, expanded) alleles

ATXN8OS (ATXN8 opposite strand [non-protein coding]) (eg, spinocerebellar ataxia), evaluation to detect abnormal (eg, expanded) alleles

ATXN10 (ataxin 10) (eg, spinocerebellar ataxia), evaluation to detect abnormal (eg, expanded) alleles

CACNA1A (calcium channel, voltage-dependent, P/Q type, alpha 1A subunit) (eg, spinocerebellar ataxia), evaluation to detect abnormal (eg, expanded) alleles

CBFB/MYH11 (inv(16)) (eg, acute myeloid leukemia), qualitative, and quantitative, if performed

CBS (cystathionine-beta-synthase) (eg, homocystinuria, cystathionine beta-synthase deficiency), common variants (eg, I278T, G307S)

CCND1/IGH (BCL1/IgH, t(11;14)) (eg, mantle cell lymphoma) translocation analysis, major breakpoint, qualitative and quantitative, if performed

CFH/ARMS2 (complement factor H/age-related maculopathy susceptibility 2) (eg, macular degeneration), common variants (eg, Y402H [CFH], A69S [ARMS2])

CNBP (CCHC-type zinc finger, nucleic acid binding protein) (eg, myotonic dystrophy type 2), evaluation to detect abnormal (eg, expanded) alleles

CSTB (cystatin B [stefin B]) (eg, Unverricht-Lundborg disease), evaluation to detect abnormal (eg, expanded) alleles

CYP3A4 (cytochrome P450, family 3, subfamily A, polypeptide 4) (eg, drug metabolism), common variants (eg, *2, *3, *4, *5, *6)

CYP3A5 (cytochrome P450, family 3, subfamily A, polypeptide 5) (eg, drug metabolism), common variants (eg, *2, *3, *4, *5, *6)

DEK/NUP214 (t(6;9)) (eg, acute myeloid leukemia), translocation analysis, qualitative, and quantitative, if performed

DMPK (dystrophia myotonica-protein kinase) (eg, myotonic dystrophy, type 1), evaluation to detect abnormal (eg, expanded) alleles

E2A/PBX1 (t(1;19)) (eg, acute lymphocytic leukemia), translocation analysis, qualitative, and quantitative, if performed

EML4/ALK (inv(2)) (eg, non-small cell lung cancer), translocation or inversion analysis

ETV6/NTRK3 (t(12;15)) (eg, congenital/infantile fibrosarcoma), translocation analysis, qualitative, and quantitative, if performed

ETV6/RUNX1 (t(12;21)) (eg, acute lymphocytic leukemia), translocation analysis, qualitative and quantitative, if performed

EWSR1/ATF1 (t(12;22)) (eg, clear cell sarcoma), translocation analysis, qualitative, and quantitative, if performed

EWSR1/ERG (t(21;22)) (eg, Ewing sarcoma/peripheral neuroectodermal tumor), translocation analysis, qualitative and quantitative, if performed

EWSR1/FLI1 (t(11;22)) (eg, Ewing sarcoma/peripheral neuroectodermal tumor), translocation analysis, qualitative and quantitative, if performed

EWSR1/WT1 (t(11;22)) (eg, desmoplastic small round cell tumor), translocation analysis, qualitative and quantitative, if performed

F11 (coagulation factor XI) (eg, coagulation disorder), common variants (eg, E117X [Type II], F283L [Type III], IVS14del14, and IVS14+1G>A [Type I])

FGFR3 (fibroblast growth factor receptor 3) (eg, achondroplasia, hypochondroplasia), common variants (eg, 1138G>A, 1138G>C, 1620C>A, 1620C>G)

FIP1L1/PDGFRA (del[4q12]) (eg, imatinib-sensitive chronic eosinophilic leukemia), qualitative and quantitative, if performed

FLG (filaggrin) (eg, ichthyosis vulgaris), common variants (eg, R501X, 2282del4, R2447X, S3247X, 3702delG)

FOXO1/PAX3 (t(2;13)) (eg, alveolar rhabdomyosarcoma), translocation analysis, qualitative and quantitative, if performed

FOXO1/PAX7 (t(1;13)) (eg, alveolar rhabdomyosarcoma), translocation analysis, qualitative and quantitative, if performed

FUS/DDIT3 (t(12;16)) (eg, myxoid liposarcoma), translocation analysis, qualitative, and quantitative, if performed

FXN (frataxin) (eg, Friedreich ataxia), evaluation to detect abnormal (expanded) alleles

GALC (galactosylceramidase) (eg, Krabbe disease), common variants (eg, c.857G>A, 30-kb deletion)

GALT (galactose-1-phosphate uridylyltransferase) (eg, galactosemia), common variants (eg, Q188R, S135L, K285N, T138M, L195P, Y209C, IVS2-2A>G, P171S, del5kb, N314D, L218L/N314D)

H19 (imprinted maternally expressed transcript [non-protein coding]) (eg, Beckwith-Wiedemann syndrome), methylation analysis

HBB (hemoglobin, beta) (eg, sickle cell anemia, hemoglobin C, hemoglobin E), common variants (eg, HbS, HbC, HbE)

HTT (huntingtin) (eg, Huntington disease), evaluation to detect abnormal (eg, expanded) alleles

IGH@/BCL2 (t(14;18)) (eg, follicular lymphoma), translocation and analysis; single breakpoint (eg) major breakpoint region [MBR] or minor cluster region [mcr]), qualitative or quantitative(When both MBR and mcr breakpoints are performed, use 81402)

KCNQ1OT1 (KCNQ1 overlapping transcript 1 [non-protein coding]) (e.g, Beckwith-Wiedemann syndrome), methylation analysis

LRRK2 (leucine-rich repeat kinase 2) (eg, Parkinson disease), common variants (eg, R1441G, G2019S, I2020T)

MED12 (mediator complex subunit 12) (eg, FG syndrome type 1, Lujan syndrome), common variants (eg, R961W, N1007S)

MEG3/DLK1 (maternally expressed 3 [non-protein coding]/delta-like 1 homolog [Drosophila]) (eg, intrauterine growth retardation), methylation analysis

MLL/AFF1 (t(4;11)) (eg acute lymphoblastic leukemia), translocation analysis, qualitative and quantitative, if performed

MLL/MLLT3 (t(9;11)) (eg, acute myeloid leukemia) translocation analysis, qualitative and quantitative, if performed

MT-RNR1 (mitochondrially encoded 12S RNA) (eg, nonsyndromic hearing loss), common variants (eg, m.1555>G, m1494C>T)

MUTYH (mutY homolog [E.coli]) (eg, MYH-associated polyposis), common variants (eg, Y165C, G382D)

MT-ATP6 (mitochondrially encoded ATP synthase 6) (eg, neuropathy with ataxia and retinitis pigmentosa [NARP], Leigh syndrome), common variants (eg, m.8993T>G, m.8993T>C)

MT-ND4, MT-ND6 (mitochondrially encoded NADH dehydrogenase 4, mitochondrially encoded NADH dehydrogenase 6) (eg, Leber hereditary optic neuropathy [LHON]), common variants (eg m.11778G>A, m3460G>A, m14484T>C)

MT-ND5 (mitochondrially encoded tRNA leucine 1 [UUA/G], mitochondrially encoded NADH dehydrogenase 5) (eg, mitochondrial encephalopathy with lactic acidosis and stroke-like episodes [MELAS]), common variants (eg, m.3243A>G, m.3271T>C, m.3252A>G, m.13513G>A)

MT-TK (mitochondrially encoded tRNA lysine) (eg, myoclonic epilepsy with ragged-red fibers [MERRF]), common variants (eg, m8344A>G, m.8356T>C)

MT-TL1 (mitochondrially encoded tRNA leucine 1[UUA/G]) (eg, diabetes and hearing loss), common variants (eg, m.3243A>G, m.14709 T>C) MT-TL1

MT-TS1, MT-RNR1 (mitochondrially encoded tRNA serine 1 [UCN], mitochondrially encoded 12S RNA) (eg, nonsyndromic sensorineural deafness [including aminoglycoside-induced nonsyndromic deafness]) common variants (eg, m.7445A>G, m.1555A>G)

NOD2 (nucleotide-binding oligomerization domain containing 2) (eg, Crohn's disease, Blau syndrome), common variants (eg, SNP 8, SNP 12, SNP 13)

NPM/ALK (t(2;5)) (eg, anaplastic large cell lymphoma), translocation analysis

PABPN1 (poly[A] binding protein, nuclear 1) (eg, oculopharyngeal muscular dystrophy), evaluation to detect abnormal (eg, expanded) alleles

PAX8/PPARG (t(2;3) (q13;p25)) (eg, follicular thyroid carcinoma), translocation analysis

PPP2R2B (protein phosphatase 2, regulatory subunit B, beta) (eg, spinocerebellar ataxia), evaluation to detect abnormal (eg, expanded) alleles

PRSS1 (protease, serine, 1 [trypsin 1]) (eg, hereditary pancreatitis), common variants (eg, N29I, A16V, R122H)

PYGM (phosphorylase, glycogen, muscle) (eg, glycogen storage disease type V, McArdle disease), common variants (eg, R50X, G205S)

RUNX1/RUNX1T1 (t(8;21)) (eg, acute myeloid leukemia) translocation analysis, qualitative and quantitative, if performed

SEPT9 (septin 9) (eg, colon cancer), methylation analysis

SMN1/SMN2 (survival of motor neuron 1, telomeric/survival of motor neuron 2, centromeric) (eg, spinal muscular atrophy), dosage analysis (eg, carrier testing)

SMN1/SMN2 duplication/deletion analysis

SS18/SSX1 (t(X;18)) (eg, synovial sarcoma), translocation analysis, qualitative and quantitative, if performed

SS18/SSX2 (t(X;18)) (eg, synovial sarcoma), translocation analysis, qualitative and quantitative, if performed

TBP (TATA box binding protein) (eg, spinocerebellar ataxia), evaluation to detect abnormal (eg, expanded) alleles

*TPMT (thiopurine S-methyltransferase) (eg, drug metabolism), common variants (eg, *2, *3)*

TYMS (thymidylate synthetase) (eg, 5-fluorouracil/5-FU drug metabolism), tandem repeat variant

VWF (von Willebrand factor) (eg, von Willebrand disease type 2N), common variants (eg, T791M, R816W, R854Q)

🔒 0.00   ⚕ 0.00   **FUD** XXX   Ⓐ

AMA: 2015,Jan,16; 2015,Jan,3; 2014,Jan,11; 2013,Sep,3-12; 2013,Jul,11-12; 2012,May,3-10

▲ **81402**   **Molecular pathology procedure, Level 3 (eg, >10 SNPs, 2-10 methylated variants, or 2-10 somatic variants [typically using non-sequencing target variant analysis], immunoglobulin and T-cell receptor gene rearrangements, duplication/deletion variants of 1 exon, loss of heterozygosity [LOH], uniparental disomy [UPD])**

INCLUDES   *Chromosome 1p-/19q- (eg, glial tumors), deletion analysis*

Chromosome 18q- (eg, D18S55, D18S58, D18S61, D18S64, and D18S69) (eg, colon cancer), allelic imbalance assessment (ie, loss of heterozygosity)

COL1A1/PDGFB (t(17;22)) (eg, dermatofibrosarcoma protuberans), translocation analysis, multiple breakpoints, qualitative, and quantitative, if performed

CYP21A2 (cytochrome P450, family 21, subfamily A, polypeptide 2) (eg, congenital adrenal hyperplasia, 21-hydroxylase deficiency), common variants (eg, IVS2-13G, P30L, I172N, exon 6 mutation cluster [I235N, V236E, M238K], V281L, L307FfsX6, Q318X, R356W, P453S, G110VfsX21, 30-kb deletion variant)

ESR1/PGR (receptor 1/progesterone receptor) ratio (eg, breast cancer)

IGH@/BCL2 (t(14;18)) (eg, follicular lymphoma), translocation analysis; major breakpoint region (MBR) and minor cluster region (mcr) breakpoints, qualitative or quantitative

MEFV (Mediterranean fever) (eg, familial Mediterranean fever), common variants (eg, E148Q, P369S, F479L, M680I, I692del, M694V, M694I, K695R, V726A, A744S, R761H)

MPL (myeloproliferative leukemia virus oncogene, thrombopoietin receptor, TPOR) (eg, myeloproliferative disorder), common variants (eg, W515A, W515K, W515L, W515R)

TRD@ (T cell antigen receptor, delta) (eg, leukemia and lymphoma), gene rearrangement analysis, evaluation to detect abnormal clonal population

Uniparental disomy (UPD) (eg, Russell-Silver syndrome, Prader-Willi/Angelman syndrome), short tandem repeat (STR) analysis

🔒 0.00   ⚕ 0.00   **FUD** XXX   Ⓐ

AMA: 2015,Jan,16; 2015,Jan,3; 2014,Jan,11; 2013,Sep,3-12; 2013,Jul,11-12; 2012,May,3-10

26/TC PC/TC Comp Only   ❌ CLIA Waived   ♂ Male Only   ♀ Female Only
AMA: CPT Asst   CMS: Pub 100   Ⓐ-Ⓨ OPPSI   ❎ Radiology Crosswalk

328   Medicare (Red Text)   CPT © 2015 American Medical Association. All Rights Reserved. (Black Text)   © 2015 Optum360, LLC (Blue Text)

▲ 81403 **Molecular pathology procedure, Level 4 (eg, analysis of single exon by DNA sequence analysis, analysis of >10 amplicons using multiplex PCR in 2 or more independent reactions, mutation scanning or duplication/deletion variants of 2-5 exons)**

INCLUDES ANG (angiogenin, ribonuclease, RNase A family, 5) (eg, amyotrophic lateral sclerosis), full gene sequence

ARX (aristaless-related homeobox) (eg, X-linked lissencephaly with ambiguous genitalia, X-linked mental retardation), duplication/deletion analysis

CEL (carboxyl ester lipase [bile salt-stimulated lipase]) (eg, maturity-onset diabetes of the young [MODY]), targeted sequence analysis of exon 11 (eg, c.1785delC, c.1686delT)

CTNNB1 (catenin [cadherin-associated protein], beta 1, 88kDa) (eg, desmoid tumors), targeted sequence analysis (eg, exon 3)

DAZ/SRY (deleted in azoospermia and sex determining region Y) (eg, male infertility), common deletions (eg, AZFa, AZFb, AZFc, AZFd)

DNMT3A (DNA [cytosine-5-]-methyltransferase 3 alpha) (eg, acute myeloid leukemia), targeted sequence analysis (eg, exon 23)

EPCAM (epithelial cell adhesion molecule) (eg, Lynch syndrome), duplication/deletion analysis

F8 (coagulation factor VIII) (eg, hemophilia A), inversion analysis, intron 1 and intron 22A

F12 (coagulation factor XII [Hageman factor]) (eg, angioedema, hereditary, type III; factor XII deficiency), targeted sequence analysis of exon 9

FGFR3 (fibroblast growth factor receptor 3) (eg, isolated craniosynostosis), targeted sequence analysis (eg, exon 7)

Excludes targeted sequence analysis of multiple FGFR3 exons (81404)

GJB1 (gap junction protein, beta 1) (eg, Charcot-Marie-Tooth X-linked), full gene sequence

GNAQ (guanine nucleotide-binding protein G[q] subunit alpha) (eg, uveal melanoma), common variants (eg, R183, Q209)

HBB (hemoglobin, beta, beta-globin) (eg, beta thalassemia), duplication/deletion analysis

Human erythrocyte antigen gene analyses (eg, SLC14A1 [Kidd blood group], BCAM [Lutheran blood group], ICAM4 [Landsteiner-Wiener blood group], SLC4A1 [Diego blood group], AQP1 [Colton blood group], ERMAP [Scianna blood group], RHCE [Rh blood group, CcEe antigens], KEL [Kell blood group], DARC [Duffy blood group], GYPA, GYPB, GYPE [MNS blood group], ART4 [Dombrock blood group]) (eg, sickle-cell disease, thalassemia, hemolytic transfusion reactions, hemolytic disease of the fetus or newborn), common variants

HRAS (v-Ha-ras Harvey rat sarcoma viral oncogene homolog) (eg, Costello syndrome), exon 2 sequence

IDH1 (isocitrate dehydrogenase 1 [NADP+], soluble) (eg, glioma), common exon 4 variants (eg, R132H, R132C)

IDH2 (isocitrate dehydrogenase 2 [NADP+], mitochondrial) (eg, glioma), common exon 4 variants (eg, R140W, R172M)

JAK2 (Janus kinase 2) (eg, myeloproliferative disorder), exon 12 sequence and exon 13 sequence, if performed

KCNC3 (potassium voltage-gated channel, Shaw-related subfamily, member 3) (eg, spinocerebellar ataxia), targeted sequence analysis (eg, exon 2)

KCNJ2 (potassium inwardly-rectifying channel, subfamily J, member 2) (eg, Andersen-Tawil syndrome), full gene sequence

KCNJ11 (potassium inwardly-rectifying channel, subfamily J, member 11) (eg, familial hyperinsulinism), full gene sequence

Killer cell immunoglobulin-like receptor (KIR) gene family (eg, hematopoietic stem cell transplantation), genotyping of KIR family genes

Includes known familial variant, not otherwise specified, for gene listed in Tier 1 or Tier 2, DNA sequence analysis, each variant exon

Excludes specific Tier 1 or Tier 2 code for known common variant

MC4R (melanocortin 4 receptor) (eg, obesity), full gene sequence

MICA (MHC class I polypeptide-related sequence A) (eg, solid organ transplantation), common variants (eg, *001, *002)

MPL (myeloproliferative leukemia virus oncogene, thrombopoietin receptor, TPOR) (eg, myeloproliferative disorder), exon 10 sequence

MT-RNR1 (mitochondrially encoded 12S RNA) (eg, nonsyndromic hearing loss), full gene sequence

MT-TS1 (mitochondrially encoded tRNA serine 1) (eg, nonsyndromic hearing loss), full gene sequence

NDP (Norrie disease [pseudoglioma]) (eg, Norrie disease), duplication/deletion analysis

NHLRC1 (NHL repeat containing 1) (eg, progressive myoclonus epilepsy), full gene sequence

PHOX2B (paired-like homeobox 2b) (eg, congenital central hypoventilation syndrome), duplication/deletion analysis

PLN (phospholamban) (eg, dilated cardiomyopathy, hypertrophic cardiomyopathy), full gene sequence

RHD (Rh blood group, D antigen) (eg, hemolytic disease of the fetus and newborn, Rh maternal/fetal compatibility), deletion analysis (eg, exons 4, 5, and 7, pseudogene)

RHD (Rh blood group, D antigen) (eg, hemolytic disease of the fetus and newborn, Rh maternal/fetal compatibility), deletion analysis (eg, exons 4, 5, and 7, pseudogene), performed on cell-free fetal DNA in maternal blood

(For human erythrocyte gene analysis of RHD, use a separate unit of 81403)

SH2D1A (SH2 domain containing 1A) (eg, X-linked lymphoproliferative syndrome), duplication/deletion analysis

SMN1 (survival of motor neuron 1, telomeric) (eg, spinal muscular atrophy), known familial sequence variant(s)

TWIST1 (twist homolog 1 [Drosophila]) (eg, Saethre-Chotzen syndrome), duplication/deletion analysis

UBA1 (ubiquitin-like modifier activating enzyme 1) (eg, spinal muscular atrophy, X-linked), targeted sequence analysis (eg, exon 15)

VHL (von Hippel-Lindau tumor suppressor) (eg, von Hippel-Lindau familial cancer syndrome), deletion/duplication analysis

VWF (von Willebrand factor) (eg, von Willebrand disease types 2A, 2B, 2M), targeted sequence analysis (eg, exon 28)

📷 0.00 　 ⬡ 0.00 　 **FUD** XXX 　 Ⓐ

AMA: 2015,Jan,16; 2015,Jan,3; 2014,Jan,11; 2013,Sep,3-12; 2013,Jul,11-12; 2012,May,3-10

▲ 81404 **Molecular pathology procedure, Level 5 (eg, analysis of 2-5 exons by DNA sequence analysis, mutation scanning or duplication/deletion variants of 6-10 exons, or characterization of a dynamic mutation disorder/triplet repeat by Southern blot analysis)**

INCLUDES *ACADS (acyl-CoA dehydrogenase, C-2 to C-3 short chain)* (eg, short chain acyl-CoA dehydrogenase deficiency), targeted sequence analysis (eg, exons 5 and 6)

AFF2 (AF4/FMR2 family, member 2 [FMR2]) (eg, fragile X mental retardation 2 [FRAXE]), characterization of alleles (eg, expanded size and methylation status)

AQP2 (aquaporin 2 [collecting duct]) (eg, nephrogenic diabetes insipidus), full gene sequence

ARX (aristaless related homeobox) (eg, X-linked lissencephaly with ambiguous genitalia, X-linked mental retardation), full gene sequence

AVPR2 (arginine vasopressin receptor 2) (eg, nephrogenic diabetes insipidus), full gene sequence

BBS10 (Bardet-Biedl syndrome 10) (eg, Bardet-Biedl syndrome), full gene sequence

BTD (biotinidase) (eg, biotinidase deficiency), full gene sequence

C10orf2 (chromosome 10 open reading frame 2) (eg, mitochondrial DNA depletion syndrome), full gene sequence

CAV3 (caveolin 3) (eg, CAV3-related distal myopathy, limb-girdle muscular dystrophy type 1C), full gene sequence

CD40LG (CD40 ligand) (eg, X-linked hyper IgM syndrome), full gene sequence

CDKN2A (cyclin-dependent kinase inhibitor 2A) (eg, CDKN2A-related cutaneous malignant melanoma, familial atypical mole-malignant melanoma syndrome), full gene sequence

CLRN1 (clarin 1) (eg, Usher syndrome, type 3), full gene sequence

COX6B1 (cytochrome c oxidase subunit VIb polypeptide 1) (eg, mitochondrial respiratory chain complex IV deficiency), full gene sequence

CPT2 (carnitine palmitoyltransferase 2) (eg, carnitine palmitoyltransferase II deficiency), full gene sequence

CRX (cone-rod homeobox) (eg, cone-rod dystrophy 2, Leber congenital amaurosis), full gene sequence

CSTB (cystatin B [stefin B]) (eg, Unverricht-Lundborg disease), full gene sequence

CYP1B1 (cytochrome P450, family 1, subfamily B, polypeptide 1) (eg, primary congenital glaucoma), full gene sequence

DMPK (dystrophia myotonica-protein kinase) (eg, myotonic dystrophy type 1), characterization of abnormal (eg, expanded) alleles

EGR2 (early growth response 2) (eg, Charcot-Marie-Tooth), full gene sequence

EMD (emerin) (eg, Emery-Dreifuss muscular dystrophy), duplication/deletion analysis

EPM2A (epilepsy, progressive myoclonus type 2A, Lafora disease [laforin]) (eg, progressive myoclonus epilepsy), full gene sequence

FGF23 (fibroblast growth factor 23) (eg, hypophosphatemic rickets), full gene sequence

FGFR2 (fibroblast growth factor receptor 2) (eg, craniosynostosis, Apert syndrome, Crouzon syndrome), targeted sequence analysis (eg, exons 8, 10)

FGFR3 (fibroblast growth factor receptor 3) (eg, achondroplasia, hypochondroplasia), targeted sequence analysis (eg, exons 8, 11, 12, 13)

FHL1 (four and a half LIM domains 1) (eg, Emery-Dreifuss muscular dystrophy), full gene sequence

FKRP (Fukutin related protein) (eg, congenital muscular dystrophy type 1C [MDC1C], limb-girdle muscular dystrophy [LGMD] type 2I), full gene sequence

FOXG1 (forkhead box G1) (eg, Rett syndrome), full gene sequence

FSHMD1A (facioscapulohumeral muscular dystrophy 1A) (eg, facioscapulohumeral muscular dystrophy), evaluation to detect abnormal (eg, deleted) alleles

FSHMD1A (facioscapulohumeral muscular dystrophy 1A) (eg, facioscapulohumeral muscular dystrophy), characterization of haplotype(s) (ie, chromosome 4A and 4B haplotypes)

FXN (frataxin) (eg, Friedreich ataxia), full gene sequence

GH1 (growth hormone 1) (eg, growth hormone deficiency), full gene sequence

GP1BB (glycoprotein Ib [platelet], beta polypeptide) (eg, Bernard-Soulier syndrome type B), full gene sequence

HBA1/HBA2 (alpha globin 1 and alpha globin 2) (eg, alpha thalassemia), duplication/deletion analysis

Excludes common deletion variants of alpha globin 1 and 2 genes (81257)

HBB (hemoglobin, beta, beta-globin) (eg, thalassemia), full gene sequence

HNF1B (HNF1 homeobox B) (eg, maturity-onset diabetes of the young [MODY]), duplication/deletion analysis

HRAS (v-Ha-ras Harvey rat sarcoma viral oncogene homolog) (eg, Costello syndrome), full gene sequence

HSD3B2 (hydroxy-delta-5-steroid dehydrogenase, 3 beta- and steroid delta-isomerase 2) (eg, 3-beta-hydroxysteroid dehydrogenase type II deficiency), full gene sequence

HSD11B2 (hydroxysteroid [11-beta] dehydrogenase 2) (eg, mineralocorticoid excess syndrome), full gene sequence

HSPB1 (heat shock 27kDa protein 1) (eg, Charcot-Marie-Tooth disease), full gene sequence

INS (insulin) (eg, diabetes mellitus), full gene sequence

KCNJ1 (potassium inwardly-rectifying channel, subfamily J, member 1) (eg, Bartter syndrome), full gene sequence

KCNJ10 (potassium inwardly-rectifying channel, subfamily J, member 10) (eg, SeSAME syndrome, EAST syndrome, sensorineural hearing loss), full gene sequence

LITAF (lipopolysaccharide-induced TNF factor) (eg, Charcot-Marie-Tooth), full gene sequence

MEFV (Mediterranean fever) (eg, familial Mediterranean fever), full gene sequence

MEN1 (multiple endocrine neoplasia I) (eg, multiple endocrine neoplasia type 1, Wermer syndrome), duplication/deletion analysis

MMACHC (methylmalonic aciduria [cobalamin deficiency] cblC type, with homocystinuria) (eg, methylmalonic acidemia and homocystinuria), full gene sequence

MPV17 (MpV17 mitochondrial inner membrane protein) (eg, mitochondrial DNA depletion syndrome), duplication/deletion analysis

NDP (Norrie disease [pseudoglioma]) (eg, Norrie disease), full gene sequence

NDUFA1 (NADH dehydrogenase [ubiquinone] 1 alpha subcomplex, 1, 7.5kDa) (eg, Leigh syndrome, mitochondrial complex I deficiency), full gene sequence

NDUFAF2 (NADH dehydrogenase [ubiquinone] 1 alpha subcomplex, assembly factor 2) (eg, Leigh syndrome, mitochondrial complex I deficiency), full gene sequence

NDUFS4 (NADH dehydrogenase [ubiquinone] Fe-S protein 4, 18kDa [NADH-coenzyme Q reductase]) (eg, Leigh syndrome, mitochondrial complex I deficiency), full gene sequence

NIPA1 (non-imprinted in Prader-Willi/Angelman syndrome 1) (eg, spastic paraplegia), full gene sequence

NLGN4X (neuroligin 4, X-linked) (eg, autism spectrum disorders), duplication/deletion analysis

NPC2 (Niemann-Pick disease, type C2 [epididymal secretory protein E1]) (eg, Niemann-Pick disease type C2), full gene sequence

NR0B1 (nuclear receptor subfamily 0, group B, member 1) (eg, congenital adrenal hypoplasia), full gene sequence

PDX1 (pancreatic and duodenal homeobox 1) (eg, maturity-onset diabetes of the young [MODY]), full gene sequence

PHOX2B (paired-like homeobox 2b) (eg, congenital central hypoventilation syndrome), full gene sequence

PIK3CA (phosphatidylinositol-4,5-bisphosphate 3-kinase, catalytic subunit alpha) (eg, colorectal cancer), targeted sequence analysis (eg, exons 9 and 20)

PLP1 (proteolipid protein 1) (eg, Pelizaeus-Merzbacher disease, spastic paraplegia), duplication/deletion analysis

PQBP1 (polyglutamine binding protein 1) (eg, Renpenning syndrome), duplication/deletion analysis

PRNP (prion protein) (eg, genetic prion disease), full gene sequence

PROP1 (PROP paired-like homeobox 1) (eg, combined pituitary hormone deficiency), full gene sequence

PRPH2 (peripherin 2 [retinal degeneration, slow]) (eg, retinitis pigmentosa), full gene sequence

PRSS1 (protease, serine, 1 [trypsin 1]) (eg, hereditary pancreatitis), full gene sequence

RAF1 (v-raf-1 murine leukemia viral oncogene homolog 1) (eg, LEOPARD syndrome), targeted sequence analysis (eg, exons 7, 12, 14, 17)

RET (ret proto-oncogene) (eg, multiple endocrine neoplasia, type 2B and familial medullary thyroid carcinoma), common variants (eg, M918T, 2647_2648delinsTT, A883F)

RHO (rhodopsin) (eg, retinitis pigmentosa), full gene sequence

RP1 (retinitis pigmentosa 1) (eg, retinitis pigmentosa), full gene sequence

SCN1B (sodium channel, voltage-gated, type I, beta) (eg, Brugada syndrome), full gene sequence

SCO2 (SCO cytochrome oxidase deficient homolog 2 [SCO1L]) (eg, mitochondrial respiratory chain complex IV deficiency), full gene sequence

SDHC (succinate dehydrogenase complex, subunit C, integral membrane protein, 15kDa) (eg, hereditary paraganglioma-pheochromocytoma syndrome), duplication/deletion analysis

SDHD (succinate dehydrogenase complex, subunit D, integral membrane protein) (eg, hereditary paraganglioma), full gene sequence

SGCG (sarcoglycan, gamma [35kDa dystrophin-associated glycoprotein]) (eg, limb-girdle muscular dystrophy), duplication/deletion analysis

SH2D1A (SH2 domain containing 1A) (eg, X-linked lymphoproliferative syndrome), full gene sequence

SLC16A2 (solute carrier family 16, member 2 [thyroid hormone transporter]) (eg, specific thyroid hormone cell transporter deficiency, Allan-Herndon-Dudley syndrome), duplication/deletion analysis

SLC25A20 (solute carrier family 25 [carnitine/acylcarnitine translocase], member 20) (eg, carnitine-acylcarnitine translocase deficiency), duplication/deletion analysis

SLC25A4 (solute carrier family 25 [mitochondrial carrier; adenine nucleotide translocation], member 4) (eg, progressive external ophthalmoplegia), full gene sequence

SOD1 (superoxide dismutase 1, soluble) (eg, amyotrophic lateral sclerosis), full gene sequence

SPINK1 (serine peptidase inhibitor, Kazal type 1) (eg, hereditary pancreatitis), full gene sequence

STK11 (serine/threonine kinase 11) (eg, Peutz-Jeghers syndrome), duplication/deletion analysis

TACO1 (translational activator of mitochondrial encoded cytochrome c oxidase I) (eg, mitochondrial respiratory chain complex IV deficiency), full gene sequence

THAP1 (THAP domain containing, apoptosis associated protein 1) (eg, torsion dystonia), full gene sequence

TOR1A (torsin family 1, member A [torsin A]) (eg, torsion dystonia), full gene sequence

TP53 (tumor protein 53) (eg, tumor samples), targeted sequence analysis of 2-5 exons

TTPA (tocopherol [alpha] transfer protein) (eg, ataxia), full gene sequence

TTR (transthyretin) (eg, familial transthyretin amyloidosis), full gene sequence

TWIST1 (twist homolog 1 [Drosophila]) (eg, Saethre-Chotzen syndrome), full gene sequence

TYR (tyrosinase [oculocutaneous albinism IA]) (eg, oculocutaneous albinism IA), full gene sequence

USH1G (Usher syndrome 1G [autosomal recessive]) (eg, Usher syndrome, type 1), full gene sequence

VWF (von Willebrand factor) (eg, von Willebrand disease type 1C), targeted sequence analysis (eg, exons 26, 27, 37)

VHL (von Hippel-Lindau tumor suppressor) (eg, von Hippel-Lindau familial cancer syndrome), full gene sequence

ZEB2 (zinc finger E-box binding homeobox 2) (eg, Mowat-Wilson syndrome), duplication/deletion analysis

ZNF41 (zinc finger protein 41) (eg, X-linked mental retardation 89), full gene sequence

🏢 0.00 🩺 0.00 **FUD** XXX [A]

AMA: 2015,Jan,16; 2015,Jan,3; 2014,Jan,11; 2013,Sep,3-12; 2013,Jul,11-12; 2012,May,3-10

▲ **81405** **Molecular pathology procedure, Level 6 (eg, analysis of 6-10 exons by DNA sequence analysis, mutation scanning or duplication/deletion variants of 11-25 exons, regionally targeted cytogenomic array analysis)**

INCLUDES *ABCD1 (ATP-binding cassette, sub-family D [ALD], member 1)* (eg, adrenoleukodystrophy), full gene sequence

ACADS (acyl-CoA dehydrogenase, C-2 to C-3 short chain) (eg, short chain acyl-CoA dehydrogenase deficiency), full gene sequence

ACTA2 (actin, alpha 2, smooth muscle, aorta) (eg, thoracic aortic aneurysms and aortic dissections), full gene sequence

ACTC1 (actin, alpha, cardiac muscle 1) (eg, familial hypertrophic cardiomyopathy), full gene sequence

ANKRD1 (ankyrin repeat domain 1) (eg, dilated cardiomyopathy), full gene sequence

APTX (aprataxin) (eg, ataxia with oculomotor apraxia 1), full gene sequence

AR (androgen receptor) (eg, androgen insensitivity syndrome), full gene sequence

ARSA (arylsulfatase A) (eg, arylsulfatase A deficiency), full gene sequence

BCKDHA (branched chain keto acid dehydrogenase E1, alpha polypeptide) (eg, maple syrup urine disease, type 1A), full gene sequence

BCS1L (BCS1-like [S. cerevisiae]) (eg, Leigh syndrome, mitochondrial complex III deficiency, GRACILE syndrome), full gene sequence

BMPR2 (bone morphogenetic protein receptor, type II [serine/threonine kinase]) (eg, heritable pulmonary arterial hypertension), duplication/deletion analysis

CASQ2 (calsequestrin 2 [cardiac muscle]) (eg, catecholaminergic polymorphic ventricular tachycardia), full gene sequence

CASR (calcium-sensing receptor) (eg, hypocalcemia), full gene sequence

CDKL5 (cyclin-dependent kinase-like 5) (eg, early infantile epileptic encephalopathy), duplication/deletion analysis

CHRNA4 (cholinergic receptor, nicotinic, alpha 4) (eg, nocturnal frontal lobe epilepsy), full gene sequence

CHRNB2 (cholinergic receptor, nicotinic, beta 2 [neuronal]) (eg, nocturnal frontal lobe epilepsy), full gene sequence

COX10 (COX10 homolog, cytochrome c oxidase assembly protein) (eg, mitochondrial respiratory chain complex IV deficiency), full gene sequence

COX15 (COX15 homolog, cytochrome c oxidase assembly protein) (eg, mitochondrial respiratory chain complex IV deficiency), full gene sequence

CYP11B1 (cytochrome P450, family 11, subfamily B, polypeptide 1) (eg, congenital adrenal hyperplasia), full gene sequence

CYP17A1 (cytochrome P450, family 17, subfamily A, polypeptide 1) (eg, congenital adrenal hyperplasia), full gene sequence

CYP21A2 (cytochrome P450, family 21, subfamily A, polypeptide2) (eg, steroid 21-hydroxylase isoform, congenital adrenal hyperplasia), full gene sequence

Cytogenomic constitutional targeted microarray analysis of chromosome 22q13 by interrogation of genomic regions for copy number and single nucleotide polymorphism (SNP) variants for chromosomal abnormalities

Excludes genome-wide cytogenomic constitutional microarray analysis (81228-81229)

Do not report analyte-specific molecular pathology services separately when the analytes are part of the microarray analysis of chromosome 22q13

Do not report with (88271)

DBT (dihydrolipoamide branched chain transacylase E2) (eg, maple syrup urine disease, type 2), duplication/deletion analysis

DCX (doublecortin) (eg, X-linked lissencephaly), full gene sequence

DES (desmin) (eg, myofibrillar myopathy), full gene sequence

DFNB59 (deafness, autosomal recessive 59) (eg, autosomal recessive nonsyndromic hearing impairment), full gene sequence

DGUOK (deoxyguanosine kinase) (eg, hepatocerebral mitochondrial DNA depletion syndrome), full gene sequence

DHCR7 (7-dehydrocholesterol reductase) (eg, Smith-Lemli-Opitz syndrome), full gene sequence

EIF2B2 (eukaryotic translation initiation factor 2B, subunit 2 beta, 39kDa) (eg, leukoencephalopathy with vanishing white matter), full gene sequence

EMD (emerin) (eg, Emery-Dreifuss muscular dystrophy), full gene sequence

ENG (endoglin) (eg, hereditary hemorrhagic telangiectasia, type 1), duplication/deletion analysis

EYA1 (eyes absent homolog 1 [Drosophila]) (eg, branchio-oto-renal [BOR] spectrum disorders), duplication/deletion analysis

F9 (coagulation factor IX) (eg, hemophilia B), full gene sequence

FGFR1 (fibroblast growth factor receptor 1) (eg, Kallmann syndrome 2), full gene sequence

FH (fumarate hydratase) (eg, fumarate hydratase deficiency, hereditary leiomyomatosis with renal cell cancer), full gene sequence

FKTN (fukutin) (eg, limb-girdle muscular dystrophy [LGMD] type 2M or 2L), full gene sequence

FTSJ1 (FtsJ RNA methyltransferase homolog 1 [E. coli]) (eg, X-linked mental retardation 9), duplication/deletion analysis

GABRG2 (gamma-aminobutyric acid [GABA] A receptor, gamma 2) (eg, generalized epilepsy with febrile seizures), full gene sequence

GCH1 (GTP cyclohydrolase 1) (eg, autosomal dominant dopa-responsive dystonia), full gene sequence

GDAP1 (ganglioside-induced differentiation-associated protein 1) (eg, Charcot-Marie-Tooth disease), full gene sequence

GFAP (glial fibrillary acidic protein) (eg, Alexander disease), full gene sequence

GHR (growth hormone receptor) (eg, Laron syndrome), full gene sequence

GHRHR (growth hormone releasing hormone receptor) (eg, growth hormone deficiency), full gene sequence

GLA (galactosidase, alpha) (eg, Fabry disease), full gene sequence

HBA1/HBA2 (alpha globin 1 and alpha globin 2) (eg, thalassemia), full gene sequence

HNF1A (HNF1 homeobox A) (eg, maturity-onset diabetes of the young [MODY]), full gene sequence

HNF1B (HNF1 homeobox B) (eg, maturity-onset diabetes of the young [MODY]), full gene sequence

HTRA1 (HtrA serine peptidase 1) (eg, macular degeneration), full gene sequence

IDS (iduronate 2-sulfatase) (eg, mucopolysaccharidosis, type II), full gene sequence

IL2RG (interleukin 2 receptor, gamma) (eg, X-linked severe combined immunodeficiency), full gene sequence

ISPD (isoprenoid synthase domain containing) (eg, muscle-eye-brain disease, Walker-Warburg syndrome), full gene sequence

KRAS (Kirsten rat sarcoma viral oncogene homolog) (eg, Noonan syndrome), full gene sequence

LAMP2 (lysosomal-associated membrane protein 2) (eg, Danon disease), full gene sequence

LDLR (low density lipoprotein receptor) (eg, familial hypercholesterolemia), duplication/deletion analysis

MEN1 (multiple endocrine neoplasia I) (eg, multiple endocrine neoplasia type 1, Wermer syndrome), full gene sequence

MMAA (methylmalonic aciduria [cobalamine deficiency] type A) (eg, MMAA-related methylmalonic acidemia), full gene sequence

MMAB (methylmalonic aciduria [cobalamine deficiency] type B) (eg, MMAA-related methylmalonic acidemia), full gene sequence

MPI (mannose phosphate isomerase) (eg, congenital disorder of glycosylation 1b), full gene sequence

MPV17 (MpV17 mitochondrial inner membrane protein) (eg, mitochondrial DNA depletion syndrome), full gene sequence

MPZ (myelin protein zero) (eg, Charcot-Marie-Tooth), full gene sequence

MTM1 (myotubularin 1) (eg, X-linked centronuclear myopathy), duplication/deletion analysis

MYL2 (myosin, light chain 2, regulatory, cardiac, slow) (eg, familial hypertrophic cardiomyopathy), full gene sequence

MYL3 (myosin, light chain 3, alkali, ventricular, skeletal, slow) (eg, familial hypertrophic cardiomyopathy), full gene sequence

MYOT (myotilin) (eg, limb-girdle muscular dystrophy), full gene sequence

NDUFS7 (NADH dehydrogenase [ubiquinone] Fe-S protein 7, 20kDa [NADH-coenzyme Q reductase]) (eg, Leigh syndrome, mitochondrial complex I deficiency), full gene sequence

NDUFS8 (NADH dehydrogenase [ubiquinone] Fe-S protein 8, 23kDa [NADH-coenzyme Q reductase]) (eg, Leigh syndrome, mitochondrial complex I deficiency), full gene sequence

NDUFV1 (NADH dehydrogenase [ubiquinone] flavoprotein 1, 51kDa) (eg, Leigh syndrome, mitochondrial complex I deficiency), full gene sequence

NEFL (neurofilament, light polypeptide) (eg, Charcot-Marie-Tooth), full gene sequence

NF2 (neurofibromin 2 [merlin]) (eg, neurofibromatosis, type 2), duplication/deletion analysis

NLGN3 (neuroligin 3) (eg, autism spectrum disorders), full gene sequence

NLGN4X (neuroligin 4, X-linked) (eg, autism spectrum disorders), full gene sequence

NPHP1 (nephronophthisis 1 [juvenile]) (eg, Joubert syndrome), deletion analysis, and duplication analysis, if performed

NPHS2 (nephrosis 2, idiopathic, steroid-resistant [podocin]) (eg, steroid-resistant nephrotic syndrome), full gene sequence

NSD1 (nuclear receptor binding SET domain protein 1) (eg, Sotos syndrome), duplication/deletion analysis

OTC (ornithine carbamoyltransferase) (eg, ornithine transcarbamylase deficiency), full gene sequence

PAFAH1B1 (platelet-activating factor acetylhydrolase 1b, regulatory subunit 1 [45kDa]) (eg, lissencephaly, Miller-Dieker syndrome), duplication/deletion analysis

PARK2 (Parkinson protein 2, E3 ubiquitin protein ligase [parkin]) (eg, Parkinson disease), duplication/deletion analysis

PCCA (propionyl CoA carboxylase, alpha polypeptide) (eg, propionic acidemia, type 1), duplication/deletion analysis

PCDH19 (protocadherin 19) (eg, epileptic encephalopathy), full gene sequence

PDHA1 (pyruvate dehydrogenase [lipoamide] alpha 1) (eg, lactic acidosis), duplication/deletion analysis

PDHB (pyruvate dehydrogenase [lipoamide] beta) (eg, lactic acidosis), full gene sequence

PINK1 (PTEN induced putative kinase 1) (eg, Parkinson disease), full gene sequence

PLP1 (proteolipid protein 1) (eg, Pelizaeus-Merzbacher disease, spastic paraplegia), full gene sequence

POU1F1 (POU class 1 homeobox 1) (eg, combined pituitary hormone deficiency), full gene sequence

PQBP1 (polyglutamine binding protein 1) (eg, Renpenning syndrome), full gene sequence

PRX (periaxin) (eg, Charcot-Marie-Tooth disease), full gene sequence

PSEN1 (presenilin 1) (eg, Alzheimer's disease), full gene sequence

RAB7A (RAB7A, member RAS oncogene family) (eg, Charcot-Marie-Tooth disease), full gene sequence

RAI1 (retinoic acid induced 1) (eg, Smith-Magenis syndrome), full gene sequence

REEP1 (receptor accessory protein 1) (eg, spastic paraplegia), full gene sequence

RET (ret proto-oncogene) (eg, multiple endocrine neoplasia, type 2A and familial medullary thyroid carcinoma), targeted sequence analysis (eg, exons 10, 11, 13-16)

RPS19 (ribosomal protein S19) (eg, Diamond-Blackfan anemia), full gene sequence

RRM2B (ribonucleotide reductase M2 B [TP53 inducible]) (eg, mitochondrial DNA depletion), full gene sequence

SCO1 (SCO cytochrome oxidase deficient homolog 1) (eg, mitochondrial respiratory chain complex IV deficiency), full gene sequence

SDHB (succinate dehydrogenase complex, subunit B, iron sulfur) (eg, hereditary paraganglioma), full gene sequence

SDHC (succinate dehydrogenase complex, subunit C, integral membrane protein, 15kDa) (eg, hereditary paraganglioma-pheochromocytoma syndrome), full gene sequence

SGCA (sarcoglycan, alpha [50kDa dystrophin-associated glycoprotein]) (eg, limb-girdle muscular dystrophy), full gene sequence

SGCB (sarcoglycan, beta [43kDa dystrophin-associated glycoprotein]) (eg, limb-girdle muscular dystrophy), full gene sequence

SGCD (sarcoglycan, delta [35kDa dystrophin-associated glycoprotein]) (eg, limb-girdle muscular dystrophy), full gene sequence

SGCE (sarcoglycan, epsilon) (eg, myoclonic dystonia), duplication/deletion analysis

SGCG (sarcoglycan, gamma [35kDa dystrophin-associated glycoprotein]) (eg, limb-girdle muscular dystrophy), full gene sequence

SHOC2 (soc-2 suppressor of clear homolog) (eg, Noonan-like syndrome with loose anagen hair), full gene sequence

SHOX (short stature homeobox) (eg, Langer mesomelic dysplasia), full gene sequence

SIL1 (SIL1 homolog, endoplasmic reticulum chaperone [S. cerevisiae]) (eg, ataxia), full gene sequence

SLC2A1 (solute carrier family 2 [facilitated glucose transporter], member 1) (eg, glucose transporter type 1 [GLUT 1] deficiency syndrome), full gene sequence

SLC16A2 (solute carrier family 16, member 2 [thyroid hormone transporter]) (eg, specific thyroid hormone cell transporter deficiency, Allan-Herndon-Dudley syndrome), full gene sequence

SLC22A5 (solute carrier family 22 [organic cation/carnitine transporter], member 5) (eg, systemic primary carnitine deficiency), full gene sequence

SLC25A20 (solute carrier family 25 [carnitine/acylcarnitine translocase], member 20) (eg, carnitine-acylcarnitine translocase deficiency), full gene sequence

SMAD4 (SMAD family member 4) (eg, hemorrhagic telangiectasia syndrome, juvenile polyposis), duplication/deletion analysis

SMN1 (survival of motor neuron 1, telomeric) (eg, spinal muscular atrophy), full gene sequence

SPAST (spastin) (eg, spastic paraplegia), duplication/deletion analysis

SPG7 (spastic paraplegia 7 [pure and complicated autosomal recessive]) (eg, spastic paraplegia), duplication/deletion analysis

SPRED1 (sprouty-related, EVH1 domain containing 1) (eg, Legius syndrome), full gene sequence

STAT3 (signal transducer and activator of transcription 3 [acute-phase response factor]) (eg, autosomal dominant hyper-IgE syndrome), targeted sequence analysis (eg, exons 12, 13, 14, 16, 17, 20, 21)

STK11 (serine/threonine kinase 11) (eg, Peutz-Jeghers syndrome), full gene sequence

SURF1 (surfeit 1) (eg, mitochondrial respiratory chain complex IV deficiency), full gene sequence

TARDBP (TAR DNA binding protein) (eg, amyotrophic lateral sclerosis), full gene sequence

TBX5 (T-box 5) (eg, Holt-Oram syndrome), full gene sequence

TCF4 (transcription factor 4) (eg, Pitt-Hopkins syndrome), duplication/deletion analysis

TGFBR1 (transforming growth factor, beta receptor 1) (eg, Marfan syndrome), full gene sequence

TGFBR2 (transforming growth factor, beta receptor 2) (eg, Marfan syndrome), full gene sequence

THRB (thyroid hormone receptor, beta) (eg, thyroid hormone resistance, thyroid hormone beta receptor deficiency), full gene sequence or targeted sequence analysis of >5 exons

TK2 (thymidine kinase 2, mitochondrial) (eg, mitochondrial DNA depletion syndrome), full gene sequence

TNNC1 (troponin C type 1 [slow]) (eg, hypertrophic cardiomyopathy or dilated cardiomyopathy), full gene sequence

TNNI3 (troponin 1, type 3 [cardiac]) (eg, familial hypertrophic cardiomyopathy), full gene sequence

TP53 (tumor protein 53) (eg, Li-Fraumeni syndrome, tumor samples), full gene sequence or targeted sequence analysis of >5 exons

TPM1 (tropomyosin 1 [alpha]) (eg, familial hypertrophic cardiomyopathy), full gene sequence

TSC1 (tuberous sclerosis 1) (eg, tuberous sclerosis), duplication/deletion analysis

TYMP (thymidine phosphorylase) (eg, mitochondrial DNA depletion syndrome), full gene sequence

VWF (von Willebrand factor) (eg, von Willebrand disease type 2N), targeted sequence analysis (eg, exons 18-20, 23-25)

WT1 (Wilms tumor 1) (eg, Denys-Drash syndrome, familial Wilms tumor), full gene sequence

ZEB2 (zinc finger E-box binding homeobox 2) (eg, Mowat-Wilson syndrome), full gene sequence

📷 0.00 ⚖ 0.00 **FUD** XXX ◻A◻

AMA: 2015,Jan,16; 2015,Jan,3; 2014,Jan,11; 2013,Sep,3-12; 2013,Jul,11-12; 2012,May,3-10

▲ 81406 **Molecular pathology procedure, Level 7 (eg, analysis of 11-25 exons by DNA sequence analysis, mutation scanning or duplication/deletion variants of 26-50 exons, cytogenomic array analysis for neoplasia)**

[INCLUDES] *ACADVL (acyl-CoA dehydrogenase, very long chain)* (eg, very long chain acyl-coenzyme A dehydrogenase deficiency), full gene sequence

ACTN4 (actinin, alpha 4) (eg, focal segmental glomerulosclerosis), full gene sequence

AFG3L2 (AFG3 ATPase family gene 3-like 2 [S. cerevisiae]) (eg, spinocerebellar ataxia), full gene sequence

AIRE (autoimmune regulator) (eg, autoimmune polyendocrinopathy syndrome type 1), full gene sequence

ALDH7A1 (aldehyde dehydrogenase 7 family, member A1) (eg, pyridoxine-dependent epilepsy), full gene sequence

ANO5 (anoctamin 5) (eg, limb-girdle muscular dystrophy), full gene sequence

APP (amyloid beta [A4] precursor protein) (eg, Alzheimer's disease), full gene sequence

ASS1 (argininosuccinate synthase 1) (eg, citrullinemia type I), full gene sequence

ATL1 (atlastin GTPase 1) (eg, spastic paraplegia), full gene sequence

ATP1A2 (ATPase, Na+/K+ transporting, alpha 2 polypeptide) (eg, familial hemiplegic migraine), full gene sequence

ATP7B (ATPase, Cu++ transporting, beta polypeptide) (eg, Wilson disease), full gene sequence

BBS1 (Bardet-Biedl syndrome 1) (eg, Bardet-Biedl syndrome), full gene sequence

BBS2 (Bardet-Biedl syndrome 2) (eg, Bardet-Biedl syndrome), full gene sequence

BCKDHB (branched-chain keto acid dehydrogenase E1, beta polypeptide) (eg, maple syrup urine disease, type 1B), full gene sequence

BEST1 (bestrophin 1) (eg, vitelliform macular dystrophy), full gene sequence

BMPR2 (bone morphogenetic protein receptor, type II [serine/threonine kinase]) (eg, heritable pulmonary arterial hypertension), full gene sequence

BRAF (B-Raf proto-oncogene, serine/threonine kinase) (eg, Noonan syndrome), full gene sequence

BSCL2 (Berardinelli-Seip congenital lipodystrophy 2 [seipin]) (eg, Berardinelli-Seip congenital lipodystrophy), full gene sequence

BTK (Bruton agammaglobulinemia tyrosine kinase) (eg, X-linked agammaglobulinemia), full gene sequence

CACNB2 (calcium channel, voltage-dependent, beta 2 subunit) (eg, Brugada syndrome), full gene sequence

CAPN3 (calpain 3) (eg, limb-girdle muscular dystrophy [LGMD] type 2A, calpainopathy), full gene sequence

CBS (cystathionine-beta-synthase) (eg, homocystinuria, cystathionine beta-synthase deficiency), full gene sequence

CDH1 (cadherin 1, type 1, E-cadherin [epithelial]) (eg, hereditary diffuse gastric cancer), full gene sequence

CDKL5 (cyclin-dependent kinase-like 5) (eg, early infantile epileptic encephalopathy), full gene sequence

CLCN1 (chloride channel 1, skeletal muscle) (eg, myotonia congenita), full gene sequence

CLCNKB (chloride channel, voltage-sensitive Kb) (eg, Bartter syndrome 3 and 4b), full gene sequence

CNTNAP2 (contactin-associated protein-like 2) (eg, Pitt-Hopkins-like syndrome 1), full gene sequence

COL6A2 (collagen, type VI, alpha 2) (eg, collagen type VI-related disorders), duplication/deletion analysis

CPT1A (carnitine palmitoyltransferase 1A [liver]) (eg, carnitine palmitoyltransferase 1A [CPT1A] deficiency), full gene sequence

CRB1 (crumbs homolog 1 [Drosophila]) (eg, Leber congenital amaurosis), full gene sequence

CREBBP (CREB binding protein) (eg, Rubinstein-Taybi syndrome), duplication/deletion analysis

Cytogenomic microarray analysis, neoplasia (eg, interrogation of copy number, and loss-of-heterozygosity via single nucleotide polymorphism [SNP]-based comparative genomic hybridization [CGH] microarray analysis)

> Do not report analyte-specific molecular pathology services separately when the analytes are part of the cytogenomic microarray analysis for neoplasia

> Do not report with (88271)

DBT (dihydrolipoamide branched chain transacylase E2) (eg, maple syrup urine disease, type 2), full gene sequence

DLAT (dihydrolipoamide S-acetyltransferase) (eg, pyruvate dehydrogenase E2 deficiency), full gene sequence

DLD (dihydrolipoamide dehydrogenase) (eg, maple syrup urine disease, type III), full gene sequence

DSC2 (desmocollin) (eg, arrhythmogenic right ventricular dysplasia/cardiomyopathy 11), full gene sequence

DSG2 (desmoglein 2) (eg, arrhythmogenic right ventricular dysplasia/cardiomyopathy 10), full gene sequence

DSP (desmoplakin) (eg, arrhythmogenic right ventricular dysplasia/cardiomyopathy 8), full gene sequence

EFHC1 (EF-hand domain [C-terminal] containing 1) (eg, juvenile myoclonic epilepsy), full gene sequence

EIF2B3 (eukaryotic translation initiation factor 2B, subunit 3 gamma, 58kDa) (eg, leukoencephalopathy with vanishing white matter), full gene sequence

EIF2B4 (eukaryotic translation initiation factor 2B, subunit 4 delta, 67kDa) (eg, leukoencephalopathy with vanishing white matter), full gene sequence

EIF2B5 (eukaryotic translation initiation factor 2B, subunit 5 epsilon, 82kDa) (eg, childhood ataxia with central nervous system hypomyelination/vanishing white matter), full gene sequence

ENG (endoglin) (eg, hereditary hemorrhagic telangiectasia, type 1), full gene sequence

EYA1 (eyes absent homolog 1 [Drosophila]) (eg, branchio-oto-renal [BOR] spectrum disorders), full gene sequence

F8 (coagulation factor VIII) (eg, hemophilia A), duplication/deletion analysis

FAH (fumarylacetoacetate hydrolase [fumarylacetoacetase]) (eg, tyrosinemia, type 1), full gene sequence

FASTKD2 (FAST kinase domains 2) (eg, mitochondrial respiratory chain complex IV deficiency), full gene sequence

FIG4 (FIG4 homolog, SAC1 lipid phosphatase domain containing [S. cerevisiae]) (eg, Charcot-Marie-Tooth disease), full gene sequence

FTSJ1 (FtsJ RNA methyltransferase homolog 1 [E. coli]) (eg, X-linked mental retardation 9), full gene sequence

FUS (fused in sarcoma) (eg, amyotrophic lateral sclerosis), full gene sequence

GAA (glucosidase, alpha; acid) (eg, glycogen storage disease type II [Pompe disease]), full gene sequence

GALC (galactosylceramidase) (eg, Krabbe disease), full gene sequence

GALT (galactose-1-phosphate uridylyltransferase) (eg, galactosemia), full gene sequence

GARS (glycyl-tRNA synthetase) (eg, Charcot-Marie-Tooth disease), full gene sequence

GCDH (glutaryl-CoA dehydrogenase) (eg, glutaricacidemia type 1), full gene sequence

GCK (glucokinase [hexokinase 4]) (eg, maturity-onset diabetes of the young [MODY]), full gene sequence

GLUD1 (glutamate dehydrogenase 1) (eg, familial hyperinsulinism), full gene sequence

GNE (glucosamine [UDP-N-acetyl]-2-epimerase/N-acetylmannosamine kinase) (eg, inclusion body myopathy 2 [IBM2], Nonaka myopathy), full gene sequence

GRN (granulin) (eg, frontotemporal dementia), full gene sequence

HADHA (hydroxyacyl-CoA dehydrogenase/3-ketoacyl-CoA thiolase/enoyl-CoA hydratase [trifunctional protein] alpha subunit) (eg, long chain acyl-coenzyme A dehydrogenase deficiency), full gene sequence

HADHB (hydroxyacyl-CoA dehydrogenase/3-ketoacyl-CoA thiolase/enoyl-CoA hydratase [trifunctional protein], beta subunit) (eg, trifunctional protein deficiency), full gene sequence

HEXA (hexosaminidase A, alpha polypeptide) (eg, Tay-Sachs disease), full gene sequence

HLCS (HLCS holocarboxylase synthetase) (eg, holocarboxylase synthetase deficiency), full gene sequence

HNF4A (hepatocyte nuclear factor 4, alpha) (eg, maturity-onset diabetes of the young [MODY]), full gene sequence

IDUA (iduronidase, alpha-L-) (eg, mucopolysaccharidosis type I), full gene sequence

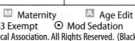

INF2 (inverted formin, FH2 and WH2 domain containing) (eg, focal segmental glomerulosclerosis), full gene sequence

IVD (isovaleryl-CoA dehydrogenase) (eg, isovaleric acidemia), full gene sequence

JAG1 (jagged 1) (eg, Alagille syndrome), duplication/deletion analysis

JUP (junction plakoglobin) (eg, arrhythmogenic right ventricular dysplasia/cardiomyopathy 11), full gene sequence

KAL1 (Kallmann syndrome 1 sequence) (eg, Kallmann syndrome), full gene sequence

KCNH2 (potassium voltage-gated channel, subfamily H [eag-related], member 2) (eg, short QT syndrome, long QT syndrome), full gene sequence

Do not report with (81280)

KCNQ1 (potassium voltage-gated channel, KQT-like subfamily, member 1) (eg, short QT syndrome, long QT syndrome), full gene sequence

Do not report with (81280)

KCNQ2 (potassium voltage-gated channel, KQT-like subfamily, member 2) (eg, epileptic encephalopathy), full gene sequence

LDB3 (LIM domain binding 3) (eg, familial dilated cardiomyopathy, myofibrillar myopathy), full gene sequence

LDLR (low density lipoprotein receptor) (eg, familial hypercholesterolemia), full gene sequence

LEPR (leptin receptor (eg, obesity with hypogonadism), full gene sequence

LHCGR (luteinizing hormone/choriogonadotropin receptor) (eg, precocious male puberty), full gene sequence

LMNA (lamin A/C) (eg, Emery-Dreifuss muscular dystrophy [EDMD1, 2 and 3] limb-girdle muscular dystrophy [LGMD] type 1B, dilated cardiomyopathy [CMD1A], familial partial lipodystrophy [FPLD2]), full gene sequence

LRP5 (low density lipoprotein receptor-related protein 5) (eg, osteopetrosis), full gene sequence

MAP2K1 (mitogen-activated protein kinase 1) (eg, cardiofaciocutaneous syndrome), full gene sequence

MAP2K2 (mitogen-activated protein kinase 2) (eg, cardiofaciocutaneous syndrome), full gene sequence

MAPT (microtubule-associated protein tau) (eg, frontotemporal dementia), full gene sequence

MCCC1 (methylcrotonoyl-CoA carboxylase 1 [alpha]) (eg, 3-methylcrotonyl-CoA carboxylase deficiency), full gene sequence

MCCC2 (methylcrotonoyl-CoA carboxylase 2 [beta]) (eg, 3-methylcrotonyl carboxylase deficiency), full gene sequence

MFN2 (mitofusin 2) (eg, Charcot-Marie-Tooth disease), full gene sequence

MTM1 (myotubularin 1) (eg, X-linked centronuclear myopathy), full gene sequence

MUT (methylmalonyl CoA mutase) (eg, methylmalonic acidemia), full gene sequence

MUTYH (mutY homolog [E. coli]) (eg, MYH-associated polyposis), full gene sequence

NDUFS1 (NADH dehydrogenase [ubiquinone] Fe-S protein 1, 75kDa [NADH-coenzyme Q reductase]) (eg, Leigh syndrome, mitochondrial complex I deficiency), full gene sequence

NF2 (neurofibromin 2 [merlin]) (eg, neurofibromatosis, type 2), full gene sequence

NOTCH3 (notch 3) (eg, cerebral autosomal dominant arteriopathy with subcortical infarcts and leukoencephalopathy [CADASIL]), targeted sequence analysis (eg, exons 1-23)

NPC1 (Niemann-Pick disease, type C1) (eg, Niemann-Pick disease), full gene sequence

NPHP1 (nephronophthisis 1 [juvenile]) (eg, Joubert syndrome), full gene sequence

NSD1 (nuclear receptor binding SET domain protein 1) (eg, Sotos syndrome), full gene sequence

OPA1 (optic atrophy 1) (eg, optic atrophy), duplication/deletion analysis

OPTN (optineurin) (eg, amyotrophic lateral sclerosis), full gene sequence

PAFAH1B1 (platelet-activating factor acetylhydrolase 1b, regulatory subunit 1 [45kDa]) (eg, lissencephaly, Miller-Dieker syndrome), full gene sequence

PAH (phenylalanine hydroxylase) (eg, phenylketonuria), full gene sequence

PALB2 (partner and localizer of BRCA2) (eg, breast and pancreatic cancer), full gene sequence

PARK2 (Parkinson protein 2, E3 ubiquitin protein ligase [parkin]) (eg, Parkinson disease), full gene sequence

PAX2 (paired box 2) (eg, renal coloboma syndrome), full gene sequence

PC (pyruvate carboxylase) (eg, pyruvate carboxylase deficiency), full gene sequence

PCCA (propionyl CoA carboxylase, alpha polypeptide) (eg, propionic acidemia, type 1), full gene sequence

PCCB (propionyl CoA carboxylase, beta polypeptide) (eg, propionic acidemia), full gene sequence

PCDH15 (protocadherin-related 15) (eg, Usher syndrome type 1F), duplication/deletion analysis

PCSK9 (proprotein convertase subtilisin/kexin type 9) (eg familial hypercholesterolemia), full gene sequence

PDHA1 (pyruvate dehydrogenase [lipoamide] alpha 1) (eg, lactic acidosis), full gene sequence

PDHX (pyruvate dehydrogenase complex, component X) (eg, lactic acidosis), full gene sequence

PHEX (phosphate-regulating endopeptidase homolog, X-linked) (eg, hypophosphatemic rickets), full gene sequence

PKD2 (polycystic kidney disease 2 [autosomal dominant]) (eg, polycystic kidney disease), full gene sequence

PKP2 (plakophilin 2) (eg, arrhythmogenic right ventricular dysplasia/cardiomyopathy 9), full gene sequence

PNKD (eg, paroxysmal nonkinesigenic dyskinesia), full gene sequence

POLG (polymerase [DNA directed], gamma) (eg, Alpers-Huttenlocher syndrome, autosomal dominant progressive external ophthalmoplegia), full gene sequence

POMGNT1 (protein O-linked mannose beta1, 2-N acetylglucosaminyltransferase) (eg, muscle-eye-brain disease, Walker-Warburg syndrome), full gene sequence

POMT1 (protein-O-mannosyltransferase 1) (eg, limb-girdle muscular dystrophy [LGMD] type 2K, Walker-Warburg syndrome), full gene sequence

POMT2 (protein-O-mannosyltransferase 2) (eg, limb-girdle muscular dystrophy [LGMD] type 2N, Walker-Warburg syndrome), full gene sequence

PRKAG2 (protein kinase, AMP-activated, gamma 2 non-catalytic subunit) (eg, familial hypertrophic cardiomyopathy with Wolff-Parkinson-White syndrome, lethal congenital glycogen storage disease of heart), full gene sequence

PRKCG (protein kinase C, gamma) (eg, spinocerebellar ataxia), full gene sequence

PSEN2 (presenilin 2[Alzheimer's disease 4]) (eg, Alzheimer's disease), full gene sequence

PTPN11 (protein tyrosine phosphatase, non-receptor type 11) (eg, Noonan syndrome, LEOPARD syndrome), full gene sequence

PYGM (phosphorylase, glycogen, muscle) (eg, glycogen storage disease type V, McArdle disease), full gene sequence

RAF1 (v-raf-1 murine leukemia viral oncogene homolog 1) (eg, LEOPARD syndrome), full gene sequence

RET (ret proto-oncogene) (eg, Hirschsprung disease), full gene sequence

RPE65 (retinal pigment epithelium-specific protein 65kDa) (eg, retinitis pigmentosa, Leber congenital amaurosis), full gene sequence

RYR1 (ryanodine receptor 1, skeletal) (eg, malignant hyperthermia), targeted sequence analysis of exons with functionally-confirmed mutations

SCN4A (sodium channel, voltage-gated, type IV, alpha subunit) (eg, hyperkalemic periodic paralysis), full gene sequence

SCNN1A (sodium channel, nonvoltage-gated 1 alpha) (eg, pseudohypoaldosteronism), full gene sequence

SCNN1B (sodium channel, nonvoltage-gated 1, beta) (eg, Liddle syndrome, pseudohypoaldosteronism), full gene sequence

SCNN1G (sodium channel, nonvoltage-gated 1, gamma) (eg, Liddle syndrome, pseudohypoaldosteronism), full gene sequence

SDHA (succinate dehydrogenase complex, subunit A, flavoprotein [Fp]) (eg, Leigh syndrome, mitochondrial complex II deficiency), full gene sequence

SETX (senataxin) (eg, ataxia), full gene sequence

SGCE (sarcoglycan, epsilon) (eg, myoclonic dystonia), full gene sequence

SH3TC2 (SH3 domain and tetratricopeptide repeats 2) (eg, Charcot-Marie-Tooth disease), full gene sequence

SLC9A6 (solute carrier family 9 [sodium/hydrogen exchanger], member 6) (eg, Christianson syndrome), full gene sequence

SLC26A4 (solute carrier family 26, member 4) (eg, Pendred syndrome), full gene sequence

SLC37A4 (solute carrier family 37 [glucose-6-phosphate transporter], member 4) (eg, glycogen storage disease type Ib), full gene sequence

SMAD4 (SMAD family member 4) (eg, hemorrhagic telangiectasia syndrome, juvenile polyposis), full gene sequence

SOS1 (son of sevenless homolog 1) (eg, Noonan syndrome, gingival fibromatosis), full gene sequence

SPAST (spastin) (eg, spastic paraplegia), full gene sequence

SPG7 (spastic paraplegia 7 [pure and complicated autosomal recessive]) (eg, spastic paraplegia), full gene sequence

STXBP1 (syntaxin-binding protein 1) (eg, epileptic encephalopathy), full gene sequence

TAZ (tafazzin) (eg, methylglutaconic aciduria type 2, Barth syndrome), full gene sequence

TCF4 (transcription factor 4) (eg, Pitt-Hopkins syndrome), full gene sequence

TH (tyrosine hydroxylase) (eg, Segawa syndrome), full gene sequence

TMEM43 (transmembrane protein 43) (eg, arrhythmogenic right ventricular cardiomyopathy), full gene sequence

TNNT2 (troponin T, type 2 [cardiac]) (eg, familial hypertrophic cardiomyopathy), full gene sequence

TRPC6 (transient receptor potential cation channel, subfamily C, member 6) (eg, focal segmental glomerulosclerosis), full gene sequence

TSC1 (tuberous sclerosis 1) (eg, tuberous sclerosis), full gene sequence

TSC2 (tuberous sclerosis 2) (eg, tuberous sclerosis), duplication/deletion analysis

UBE3A (ubiquitin protein ligase E3A) (eg, Angelman syndrome) full gene sequence

UMOD (uromodulin) (eg, glomerulocystic kidney disease with hyperuricemia and isosthenuria), full gene sequence

VWF (von Willebrand factor) (von Willebrand disease type 2A), extended targeted sequence analysis (eg, exons 11-16, 24-26, 51, 52)

WAS (Wiskott-Aldrich syndrome [eczema-thrombocytopenia]) (eg, Wiskott-Aldrich syndrome), full gene sequence

🔲 0.00   ⬚ 0.00   **FUD** XXX   Ⓐ

AMA: 2015,Jan,16; 2015,Jan,3; 2014,Jan,11; 2013,Sep,3-12; 2013,Jul,11-12; 2012,May,3-10

81407 **Molecular pathology procedure, Level 8 (eg, analysis of 26-50 exons by DNA sequence analysis, mutation scanning or duplication/deletion variants of >50 exons, sequence analysis of multiple genes on one platform)**

INCLUDES ABCC8 (ATP-binding cassette, sub-family C [CFTR/MRP], member 8) (eg, familial hyperinsulinism), full gene sequence

AGL (amylo-alpha-1, 6-glucosidase, 4-alpha-glucanotransferase) (eg, glycogen storage disease type III), full gene sequence

AHI1 (Abelson helper integration site 1) (eg, Joubert syndrome), full gene sequence

ASPM (asp [abnormal spindle] homolog, microcephaly associated [Drosophila]) (eg, primary microcephaly), full gene sequence

CACNA1A (calcium channel, voltage-dependent, P/Q type, alpha 1A subunit) (eg, familial hemiplegic migraine), full gene sequence

CHD7 (chromodomain helicase DNA binding protein 7) (eg, CHARGE syndrome), full gene sequence

COL4A4 (collagen, type IV, alpha 4) (eg, Alport syndrome), full gene sequence

COL4A5 (collagen, type IV, alpha 5) (eg, Alport syndrome), duplication/deletion analysis

COL6A1 (collagen, type VI, alpha 1) (eg, collagen type VI-related disorders), full gene sequence

COL6A2 (collagen, type VI, alpha 2) (eg, collagen type VI-related disorders), full gene sequence

COL6A3 (collagen, type VI, alpha 3) (eg, collagen type VI-related disorders), full gene sequence

CREBBP (CREB binding protein) (eg, Rubinstein-Taybi syndrome), full gene sequence

F8 (coagulation factor VIII) (eg, hemophilia A), full gene sequence

JAG1 (jagged 1) (eg, Alagille syndrome), full gene sequence

KDM5C (lysine [K]-specific demethylase 5C) (eg, X-linked mental retardation), full gene sequence

KIAA0196 (KIAA0196) (eg, spastic paraplegia), full gene sequence

L1CAM (L1 cell adhesion molecule) (eg, MASA syndrome, X-linked hydrocephaly), full gene sequence

LAMB2 (laminin, beta 2 [laminin S]) (eg, Pierson syndrome), full gene sequence

MYBPC3 (myosin binding protein C, cardiac) (eg, familial hypertrophic cardiomyopathy), full gene sequence

MYH6 (myosin, heavy chain 6, cardiac muscle, alpha) (eg, familial dilated cardiomyopathy), full gene sequence

MYH7 (myosin, heavy chain 7, cardiac muscle, beta) (eg, familial hypertrophic cardiomyopathy, Liang distal myopathy), full gene sequence

MYO7A (myosin VIIA) (eg, Usher syndrome, type 1), full gene sequence

NOTCH1 (notch 1) (eg, aortic valve disease), full gene sequence

NPHS1 (nephrosis 1, congenital, Finnish type [nephrin]) (eg, congenital Finnish nephrosis), full gene sequence

OPA1 (optic atrophy 1) (eg, optic atrophy), full gene sequence

PCDH15 (protocadherin-related 15) (eg, Usher syndrome, type 1), full gene sequence

PKD1 (polycystic kidney disease 1 [autosomal dominant]) (eg, polycystic kidney disease), full gene sequence

PLCE1 (phospholipase C, epsilon 1) (eg, nephrotic syndrome type 3), full gene sequence

SCN1A (sodium channel, voltage-gated, type 1, alpha subunit) (eg, generalized epilepsy with febrile seizures), full gene sequence

SCN5A (sodium channel, voltage-gated, type V, alpha subunit) (eg, familial dilated cardiomyopathy), full gene sequence

SLC12A1 (solute carrier family 12 [sodium/potassium/chloride transporters], member 1) (eg, Bartter syndrome), full gene sequence

SLC12A3 (solute carrier family 12 [sodium/chloride transporters], member 3) (eg, Gitelman syndrome), full gene sequence

SPG11 (spastic paraplegia 11 [autosomal recessive]) (eg, spastic paraplegia), full gene sequence

SPTBN2 (spectrin, beta, non-erythrocytic 2) (eg, spinocerebellar ataxia), full gene sequence

TMEM67 (transmembrane protein 67) (eg, Joubert syndrome), full gene sequence

TSC2 (tuberous sclerosis 2) (eg, tuberous sclerosis), full gene sequence

USH1C (Usher syndrome 1C [autosomal recessive, severe]) (eg, Usher syndrome, type 1), full gene sequence

VPS13B (vacuolar protein sorting 13 homolog B [yeast]) (eg, Cohen syndrome), duplication/deletion analysis

WDR62 (WD repeat domain 62) (eg, primary autosomal recessive microcephaly), full gene sequence

🔪 0.00   ⚕ 0.00   **FUD** XXX   [A]

AMA: 2015,Jan,16; 2015,Jan,3; 2014,Jan,11; 2013,Sep,3-12; 2013,Jul,11-12; 2012,May,3-10

81408   **Molecular pathology procedure, Level 9 (eg, analysis of >50 exons in a single gene by DNA sequence analysis)**

[INCLUDES]   ABCA4 (ATP-binding cassette, sub-family A [ABC1], member 4) (eg, Stargardt disease, age-related macular degeneration), full gene sequence

ATM (ataxia telangiectasia mutated) (eg, ataxia telangiectasia), full gene sequence

CDH23 (cadherin-related 23) (eg, Usher syndrome, type 1), full gene sequence

CEP290 (centrosomal protein 290kDa) (eg, Joubert syndrome), full gene sequence

COL1A1 (collagen, type I, alpha 1) (eg, osteogenesis imperfecta, type I), full gene sequence

COL1A2 (collagen, type I, alpha 2) (eg, osteogenesis imperfecta, type I), full gene sequence

COL4A1 (collagen, type IV, alpha 1) (eg, brain small-vessel disease with hemorrhage), full gene sequence

COL4A3 (collagen, type IV, alpha 3 [Goodpasture antigen]) (eg, Alport syndrome), full gene sequence

COL4A5 (collagen, type IV, alpha 5) (eg, Alport syndrome), full gene sequence

DMD (dystrophin) (eg, Duchenne/Becker muscular dystrophy), full gene sequence

DYSF (dysferlin, limb girdle muscular dystrophy 2B [autosomal recessive]) (eg, limb-girdle muscular dystrophy), full gene sequence

FBN1 (fibrillin 1) (eg, Marfan syndrome), full gene sequence

ITPR1 (inositol 1,4,5-trisphosphate receptor, type 1) (eg, spinocerebellar ataxia), full gene sequence

LAMA2 (laminin, alpha 2) (eg, congenital muscular dystrophy), full gene sequence

LRRK2 (leucine-rich repeat kinase 2) (eg, Parkinson disease), full gene sequence

MYH11 (myosin, heavy chain 11, smooth muscle) (eg, thoracic aortic aneurysms and aortic dissections), full gene sequence

NEB (nebulin) (eg, nemaline myopathy 2), full gene sequence

NF1 (neurofibromin 1) (eg, neurofibromatosis, type 1), full gene sequence

PKHD1 (polycystic kidney and hepatic disease 1) (eg, autosomal recessive polycystic kidney disease), full gene sequence

RYR1 (ryanodine receptor 1, skeletal) (eg, malignant hyperthermia), full gene sequence

RYR2 (ryanodine receptor 2 [cardiac]) (eg, catecholaminergic polymorphic ventricular tachycardia, arrhythmogenic right ventricular dysplasia), full gene sequence or targeted sequence analysis of > 50 exons

USH2A (Usher syndrome 2A [autosomal recessive, mild]) (eg, Usher syndrome, type 2), full gene sequence

VPS13B (vacuolar protein sorting 13 homolog B [yeast]) (eg, Cohen syndrome), full gene sequence

VWF (von Willebrand factor) (eg, von Willebrand disease types 1 and 3), full gene sequence

🔪 0.00   ⚕ 0.00   **FUD** XXX   [A]

AMA: 2015,Jan,16; 2015,Jan,3; 2014,Jan,11; 2013,Sep,3-12; 2013,Jul,11-12; 2012,May,3-10

81445

#	**81479** **Unlisted molecular pathology procedure**

 0.00 0.00 **FUD** XXX

[A]

AMA: 2015,Jan,16; 2015,Jan,3; 2014,Jan,11; 2013,Sep,3-12; 2013,Jul,11-12

81410-81479 Genomic Sequencing

81410 **Aortic dysfunction or dilation (eg, Marfan syndrome, Loeys Dietz syndrome, Ehler Danlos syndrome type IV, arterial tortuosity syndrome); genomic sequence analysis panel, must include sequencing of at least 9 genes, including** *FBN1, TGFBR1, TGFBR2, COL3A1, MYH11, ACTA2, SLC2A10, SMAD3,* **and** *MYLK*

 0.00 0.00 **FUD** XXX

[A]

AMA: 2015,Jan,3

81411 **duplication/deletion analysis panel, must include analyses for** *TGFBR1, TGFBR2, MYH11, and COL3A1*

 0.00 0.00 **FUD** XXX

[A]

AMA: 2015,Jan,3

● **81412** **Ashkenazi Jewish associated disorders (eg, Bloom syndrome, Canavan disease, cystic fibrosis, familial dysautonomia, Fanconi anemia group C, Gaucher disease, Tay-Sachs disease), genomic sequence analysis panel, must include sequencing of at least 9 genes, including** *ASPA, BLM, CFTR, FANCC, GBA, HEXA, IKBKAP, MCOLN1,* **and** *SMPD1*

81415 **Exome (eg, unexplained constitutional or heritable disorder or syndrome); sequence analysis**

 0.00 0.00 **FUD** XXX

[A]

AMA: 2015,Jan,3

+ **81416** **sequence analysis, each comparator exome (eg, parents, siblings) (List separately in addition to code for primary procedure)**

Code first (81415)

 0.00 0.00 **FUD** XXX

[A]

AMA: 2015,Jan,3

81417 **re-evaluation of previously obtained exome sequence (eg, updated knowledge or unrelated condition/syndrome)**

Do not report for results that are incidental

 0.00 0.00 **FUD** XXX

[A]

AMA: 2015,Jan,3

81420 **Fetal chromosomal aneuploidy (eg, trisomy 21, monosomy X) genomic sequence analysis panel, circulating cell-free fetal DNA in maternal blood, must include analysis of chromosomes 13, 18, and 21**

[M]

 0.00 0.00 **FUD** XXX

[A]

AMA: 2015,Jan,3

81425 **Genome (eg, unexplained constitutional or heritable disorder or syndrome); sequence analysis**

 0.00 0.00 **FUD** XXX

[A]

AMA: 2015,Jan,3

+ **81426** **sequence analysis, each comparator genome (eg, parents, siblings) (List separately in addition to code for primary procedure)**

Code first (81425)

 0.00 0.00 **FUD** XXX

[A]

AMA: 2015,Jan,3

81427 **re-evaluation of previously obtained genome sequence (eg, updated knowledge or unrelated condition/syndrome)**

EXCLUDES *Genome-wide microarray analysis (81228-81229)*

Do not report for results that are incidental

 0.00 0.00 **FUD** XXX

[A]

AMA: 2015,Jan,3

81430 **Hearing loss (eg, nonsyndromic hearing loss, Usher syndrome, Pendred syndrome); genomic sequence analysis panel, must include sequencing of at least 60 genes, including** *CDH23, CLRN1, GJB2, GPR98, MTRNR1, MYO7A, MYO15A, PCDH15, OTOF, SLC26A4, TMC1, TMPRSS3, USH1C, USH1G, USH2A,* **and** *WFS1*

 0.00 0.00 **FUD** XXX

[A]

AMA: 2015,Jan,3; 2012,May,3-10

81431 **duplication/deletion analysis panel, must include copy number analyses for** *STRC* **and** *DFNB1* **deletions in** *GJB2* **and** *GJB6* **genes**

 0.00 0.00 **FUD** XXX

[A]

AMA: 2015,Jan,3

● **81432** **Hereditary breast cancer-related disorders (eg, hereditary breast cancer, hereditary ovarian cancer, hereditary endometrial cancer); genomic sequence analysis panel, must include sequencing of at least 14 genes, including** *ATM, BRCA1, BRCA2, BRIP1, CDH1, MLH1, MSH2, MSH6, NBN, PALB2, PTEN, RAD51C, STK11,* **and** *TP53*

● **81433** **duplication/deletion analysis panel, must include analyses for** *BRCA1, BRCA2, MLH1, MSH2,* **and** *STK11*

● **81434** **Hereditary retinal disorders (eg, retinitis pigmentosa, Leber congenital amaurosis, cone-rod dystrophy), genomic sequence analysis panel, must include sequencing of at least 15 genes, including** *ABCA4, CNGA1, CRB1, EYS, PDE6A, PDE6B, PRPF31, PRPH2, RDH12, RHO, RP1, RP2, RPE65, RPGR,* **and** *USH2A*

▲ **81435** **Hereditary colon cancer disorders (eg Lynch syndrome, PTEN hamartoma syndrome, Cowden syndrome, familial adenomatosis polyposis); carcinoma, malignant genomic sequence analysis panel, must include sequencing of at least 10 genes, including** *APC, BMPR1A, CDH1, MLH1, MSH2, MSH6, MUTYH, PTEN, SMAD4,* **and** *STK11*

[A]

 0.00 0.00 **FUD** XXX

AMA: 2015,Jan,3

▲ **81436** **duplication/deletion analysis panel, must include analysis of at least 5 genes, including** *MLH1, MSH2, EPCAM, SMAD4,* **and** *STK11*

 0.00 0.00 **FUD** XXX

[A]

AMA: 2015,Jan,3

● **81437** **Hereditary neuroendocrine tumor disorders (eg, medullary thyroid carcinoma, parathyroid carcinoma, malignant pheochromocytoma or paraganglioma); genomic sequence analysis panel, must include sequencing of at least 6 genes, including** *MAX, SDHB, SDHC, SDHD, TMEM127,* **and** *VHL*

● **81438** **duplication/deletion analysis panel, must include analyses for** *SDHB, SDHC, SDHD,* **and** *VHL*

81440 **Nuclear encoded mitochondrial genes (eg, neurologic or myopathic phenotypes), genomic sequence panel, must include analysis of at least 100 genes, including** *BCS1L, C10orf2, COQ2, COX10, DGUOK, MPV17, OPA1, PDSS2, POLG, POLG2, RRM2B, SCO1, SCO2, SLC25A4, SUCLA2, SUCLG1, TAZ, TK2,* **and** *TYMP*

 0.00 0.00 **FUD** XXX

[A]

AMA: 2015,Jan,3

● **81442** **Noonan spectrum disorders (eg, Noonan syndrome, cardio-facio-cutaneous syndrome, Costello syndrome, LEOPARD syndrome, Noonan-like syndrome), genomic sequence analysis panel, must include sequencing of at least 12 genes, including** *BRAF, CBL, HRAS, KRAS, MAP2K1, MAP2K2, NRAS, PTPN11, RAF1, RIT1, SHOC2,* **and** *SOS1*

▲ **81445** **Targeted genomic sequence analysis panel, solid organ neoplasm, DNA analysis, and RNA analysis when performed, 5-50 genes (eg,** *ALK, BRAF, CDKN2A, EGFR, ERBB2, KIT, KRAS, NRAS, MET, PDGFRA, PDGFRB, PGR, PIK3CA, PTEN, RET),* **interrogation for sequence variants and copy number variants or rearrangements, if performed**

 0.00 0.00 **FUD** XXX

[A]

AMA: 2015,Jan,3

Pathology and Laboratory

81450 — 81512

▲ **81450** Targeted genomic sequence analysis panel, hematolymphoid neoplasm or disorder, DNA analysis, and RNA analysis when performed, 5-50 genes (eg, *BRAF, CEBPA, DNMT3A, EZH2, FLT3, IDH1, IDH2, JAK2, KRAS, KIT, MLL, NRAS, NPM1, NOTCH1*), interrogation for sequence variants, and copy number variants or rearrangements, or isoform expression or mRNA expression levels, if performed

EXCLUDES *Microarray copy number assessment (81406)*
🖻 0.00   ⚕ 0.00   **FUD** XXX   Ⓐ
AMA: 2015,Jan,3

▲ **81455** Targeted genomic sequence analysis panel, solid organ or hematolymphoid neoplasm, DNA analysis, and RNA analysis when performed, 51 or greater genes (eg, *ALK, BRAF, CDKN2A, CEBPA, DNMT3A, EGFR, ERBB2, EZH2, FLT3, IDH1, IDH2, JAK2, KIT, KRAS, MLL, NPM1, NRAS, MET, NOTCH1, PDGFRA, PDGFRB, PGR, PIK3CA, PTEN, RET*), interrogation for sequence variants and copy number variants or rearrangements, if performed

EXCLUDES *Microarray copy number assessment (81406)*
🖻 0.00   ⚕ 0.00   **FUD** XXX   Ⓐ
AMA: 2015,Jan,3

81460 Whole mitochondrial genome (eg, Leigh syndrome, mitochondrial encephalomyopathy, lactic acidosis, and stroke-like episodes [MELAS], myoclonic epilepsy with ragged-red fibers [MERFF], neuropathy, ataxia, and retinitis pigmentosa [NARP], Leber hereditary optic neuropathy [LHON]), genomic sequence, must include sequence analysis of entire mitochondrial genome with heteroplasmy detection

🖻 0.00   ⚕ 0.00   **FUD** XXX   Ⓐ
AMA: 2015,Jan,3

81465 Whole mitochondrial genome large deletion analysis panel (eg, Kearns-Sayre syndrome, chronic progressive external ophthalmoplegia), including heteroplasmy detection, if performed

🖻 0.00   ⚕ 0.00   **FUD** XXX   Ⓐ
AMA: 2015,Jan,3

81470 X-linked intellectual disability (XLID) (eg, syndromic and non-syndromic XLID); genomic sequence analysis panel, must include sequencing of at least 60 genes, including *ARX, ATRX, CDKL5, FGD1, FMR1, HUWE1, IL1RAPL, KDM5C, L1CAM, MECP2, MED12, MID1, OCRL, RPS6KA3*, and *SLC16A2*

🖻 0.00   ⚕ 0.00   **FUD** XXX   Ⓐ
AMA: 2015,Jan,3

81471 duplication/deletion gene analysis, must include analysis of at least 60 genes, including *ARX, ATRX, CDKL5, FGD1, FMR1, HUWE1, IL1RAPL, KDM5C, L1CAM, MECP2, MED12, MID1, OCRL, RPS6KA3*, and *SLC16A2*

🖻 0.00   ⚕ 0.00   **FUD** XXX   Ⓐ
AMA: 2015,Jan,3

81479 Resequenced code. See code following 81408.

81490-81599 Multianalyte Assays

INCLUDES Procedures using results of multiple assay panels (eg, molecular pathology, fluorescent in situ hybridization, non-nucleic acid-based) and other patient information to perform algorithmic analysis
Required analytical services (eg, amplification, cell lysis, detection, digestion, extraction, hybridization, nucleic acid stabilization) and algorithmic analysis

EXCLUDES *Genomic resequencing tests (81410-81471)*
Multianalyte assays with algorithmic analyses without a Category 1 code
Multianalyte assays with algorithmic analyses without a Category 1 or alphanumeric code (81599)
Code also procedures performed prior to cell lysis (eg, microdissection) (88380-88381)

● **81490** Autoimmune (rheumatoid arthritis), analysis of 12 biomarkers using immunoassays, utilizing serum, prognostic algorithm reported as a disease activity score

Do not report with (86140)

● **81493** Coronary artery disease, mRNA, gene expression profiling by real-time RT-PCR of 23 genes, utilizing whole peripheral blood, algorithm reported as a risk score

81500 Oncology (ovarian), biochemical assays of two proteins (CA-125 and HE4), utilizing serum, with menopausal status, algorithm reported as a risk score   ♀

Do not report with (86304-86305)
🖻 0.00   ⚕ 0.00   **FUD** XXX   Ⓔ
AMA: 2015,Jan,3; 2014,Jan,11

81503 Oncology (ovarian), biochemical assays of five proteins (CA-125, apolipoprotein A1, beta-2 microglobulin, transferrin, and pre-albumin), utilizing serum, algorithm reported as a risk score   ♀

Do not report with (82172, 82232, 83695, 83700, 84134, 84466, 86304)
🖻 0.00   ⚕ 0.00   **FUD** XXX   Ⓔ
AMA: 2015,Jan,3; 2014,Jan,11

81504 Oncology (tissue of origin), microarray gene expression profiling of > 2000 genes, utilizing formalin-fixed paraffin-embedded tissue, algorithm reported as tissue similarity scores

🖻 0.00   ⚕ 0.00   **FUD** XXX   Ⓐ
AMA: 2015,Jan,3; 2014,Jan,11

81506 Endocrinology (type 2 diabetes), biochemical assays of seven analytes (glucose, HbA1c, insulin, hs-CRP, adiponectin, ferritin, interleukin 2-receptor alpha), utilizing serum or plasma, algorithm reporting a risk score

Do not report with (82728, 82947, 83036, 83520, 83525, 84999, 86141)
🖻 0.00   ⚕ 0.00   **FUD** XXX   Ⓔ
AMA: 2015,Jan,3; 2014,Jan,11

81507 Fetal aneuploidy (trisomy 21, 18, and 13) DNA sequence analysis of selected regions using maternal plasma, algorithm reported as a risk score for each trisomy   ♀

🖻 0.00   ⚕ 0.00   **FUD** XXX   Ⓐ
AMA: 2015,Jan,3; 2014,Jan,11

81508 Fetal congenital abnormalities, biochemical assays of two proteins (PAPP-A, hCG [any form]), utilizing maternal serum, algorithm reported as a risk score   ♀

Do not report with (84163, 84702)
🖻 0.00   ⚕ 0.00   **FUD** XXX   Ⓔ
AMA: 2015,Jan,3; 2014,Jan,11

81509 Fetal congenital abnormalities, biochemical assays of three proteins (PAPP-A, hCG [any form], DIA), utilizing maternal serum, algorithm reported as a risk score   ♀

Do not report with (84163, 84702, 86336)
🖻 0.00   ⚕ 0.00   **FUD** XXX   Ⓔ
AMA: 2015,Jan,3; 2014,Jan,11

81510 Fetal congenital abnormalities, biochemical assays of three analytes (AFP, uE3, hCG [any form]), utilizing maternal serum, algorithm reported as a risk score   ♀

Do not report with (82105, 82677, 84702)
🖻 0.00   ⚕ 0.00   **FUD** XXX   Ⓔ
AMA: 2015,Jan,3; 2014,Jan,11

81511 Fetal congenital abnormalities, biochemical assays of four analytes (AFP, uE3, hCG [any form], DIA) utilizing maternal serum, algorithm reported as a risk score (may include additional results from previous biochemical testing)   ♀

Do not report with (82105, 82677, 84702, 86336)
🖻 0.00   ⚕ 0.00   **FUD** XXX   Ⓔ
AMA: 2015,Jan,3; 2014,Jan,11

81512 Fetal congenital abnormalities, biochemical assays of five analytes (AFP, uE3, total hCG, hyperglycosylated hCG, DIA) utilizing maternal serum, algorithm reported as a risk score   ♀

Do not report with (82105, 82677, 84702, 86336)
🖻 0.00   ⚕ 0.00   **FUD** XXX   Ⓔ
AMA: 2015,Jan,3; 2014,Jan,11

81519 Oncology (breast), mRNA, gene expression profiling by real-time RT-PCR of 21 genes, utilizing formalin-fixed paraffin embedded tissue, algorithm reported as recurrence score

    🔧 0.00   ⚕ 0.00   **FUD** XXX   A

    AMA: 2015,Jan,3

● **81525** Oncology (colon), mRNA, gene expression profiling by real-time RT-PCR of 12 genes (7 content and 5 housekeeping), utilizing formalin-fixed paraffin-embedded tissue, algorithm reported as a recurrence score

● **81528** Oncology (colorectal) screening, quantitative real-time target and signal amplification of 10 DNA markers (*KRAS* mutations, promoter methylation of *NDRG4* and *BMP3*) and fecal hemoglobin, utilizing stool, algorithm reported as a positive or negative result

    Do not report with (81275, 82274)

● **81535** Oncology (gynecologic), live tumor cell culture and chemotherapeutic response by DAPI stain and morphology, predictive algorithm reported as a drug response score; first single drug or drug combination

● + **81536** each additional single drug or drug combination (List separately in addition to code for primary procedure)

    🔧 0.00   ⚕ 0.00   **FUD** 000

    Code first (81535)

● **81538** Oncology (lung), mass spectrometric 8-protein signature, including amyloid A, utilizing serum, prognostic and predictive algorithm reported as good versus poor overall survival

● **81540** Oncology (tumor of unknown origin), mRNA, gene expression profiling by real-time RT-PCR of 92 genes (87 content and 5 housekeeping) to classify tumor into main cancer type and subtype, utilizing formalin-fixed paraffin-embedded tissue, algorithm reported as a probability of a predicted main cancer type and subtype

● **81545** Oncology (thyroid), gene expression analysis of 142 genes, utilizing fine needle aspirate, algorithm reported as a categorical result (eg, benign or suspicious)

● **81595** Cardiology (heart transplant), mRNA, gene expression profiling by real-time quantitative PCR of 20 genes (11 content and 9 housekeeping), utilizing subfraction of peripheral blood, algorithm reported as a rejection risk score

81599 Unlisted multianalyte assay with algorithmic analysis

    Do not report with other MAAA codes

    🔧 0.00   ⚕ 0.00   **FUD** XXX   E

    AMA: 2015,Jan,3; 2014,Jan,11

82009-82030 Chemistry: Acetaldehyde—Adenosine

INCLUDES Clinical information not requested by the ordering physician
Mathematically calculated results
Quantitative analysis unless otherwise specified
Specimens from any source unless otherwise specified

EXCLUDES *Calculated results that represent a score or probability that was derived by algorithm*
Drug testing ([80300, 80301, 80302, 80303, 80304], [80324, 80325, 80326, 80327, 80328, 80329, 80330, 80331, 80332, 80333, 80334, 80335, 80336, 80337, 80338, 80339, 80340, 80341, 80342, 80343, 80344, 80345, 80346, 80347, 80348, 80349, 80350, 80351, 80352, 80353, 80354, 80355, 80356, 80357, 80358, 80359, 80360, 80361, 80362, 80363, 80364, 80365, 80366, 80367, 80368, 80369, 80370, 80371, 80372, 80373, 80374, 80375, 80376, 80377, 83992])
Organ or disease panels (80048-80076 [80081])
Therapeutic drug assays (80150-80299 [80164, 80165, 80171])
Do not report analytes from nonrequested laboratory analysis

82009 Ketone body(s) (eg, acetone, acetoacetic acid, beta-hydroxybutyrate); qualitative

    🔧 0.00   ⚕ 0.00   **FUD** XXX   N

    AMA: 2015,Jun,10; 2015,Apr,3; 2015,Jan,16; 2014,Jan,11; 2011,Oct,8; 2010,Dec,7-10

82010 quantitative

    🔧 0.00   ⚕ 0.00   **FUD** XXX   ✗ N

    AMA: 2015,Jun,10; 2015,Apr,3; 2015,Jan,16; 2014,Jan,11; 2011,Oct,8; 2010,Dec,7-10

82013 Acetylcholinesterase

    EXCLUDES *Acid phosphatase (84060-84066)*
        Gastric acid analysis (82930)

    🔧 0.00   ⚕ 0.00   **FUD** XXX   N

    AMA: 2015,Jun,10; 2015,Apr,3; 2014,Jan,11; 2010,Dec,7-10

82016 Acylcarnitines; qualitative, each specimen

    🔧 0.00   ⚕ 0.00   **FUD** XXX   N

    AMA: 2015,Jun,10; 2015,Apr,3; 2014,Jan,11; 2010,Dec,7-10

82017 quantitative, each specimen

    EXCLUDES *Carnitine (82379)*

    🔧 0.00   ⚕ 0.00   **FUD** XXX   N ▢

    AMA: 2015,Jun,10; 2015,Apr,3; 2014,Jan,11; 2010,Dec,7-10

82024 Adrenocorticotropic hormone (ACTH)

    🔧 0.00   ⚕ 0.00   **FUD** XXX   N ▢

    AMA: 2015,Jun,10; 2015,Apr,3; 2014,Jan,11; 2010,Dec,7-10

82030 Adenosine, 5-monophosphate, cyclic (cyclic AMP)

    🔧 0.00   ⚕ 0.00   **FUD** XXX   N

    AMA: 2015,Jun,10; 2015,Apr,3; 2014,Jan,11; 2010,Dec,7-10

82040-82045 Chemistry: Albumin

INCLUDES Clinical information not requested by the ordering physician
Mathematically calculated results
Quantitative analysis unless otherwise specified
Specimens from any other sources unless otherwise specified

EXCLUDES *Calculated results that represent a score or probability that was derived by algorithm*
Drug testing ([80300, 80301, 80302, 80303, 80304], [80324, 80325, 80326, 80327, 80328, 80329, 80330, 80331, 80332, 80333, 80334, 80335, 80336, 80337, 80338, 80339, 80340, 80341, 80342, 80343, 80344, 80345, 80346, 80347, 80348, 80349, 80350, 80351, 80352, 80353, 80354, 80355, 80356, 80357, 80358, 80359, 80360, 80361, 80362, 80363, 80364, 80365, 80366, 80367, 80368, 80369, 80370, 80371, 80372, 80373, 80374, 80375, 80376, 80377, 83992])
Organ or disease panels (80048-80076 [80081])
Therapeutic drug assays (80150-80299 [80164, 80165, 80171])
Do not report analytes from nonrequested laboratory analysis

82040 Albumin; serum, plasma or whole blood

    🔧 0.00   ⚕ 0.00   **FUD** XXX   ✗ N

    AMA: 2015,Jun,10; 2015,Apr,3; 2015,Jan,16; 2014,Jan,11; 2010,Dec,7-10

82042 urine or other source, quantitative, each specimen

    🔧 0.00   ⚕ 0.00   **FUD** XXX   N

    AMA: 2015,Jun,10; 2015,Apr,3; 2014,Jan,11; 2010,Dec,7-10

82043 urine, microalbumin, quantitative

    🔧 0.00   ⚕ 0.00   **FUD** XXX   ✗ N ▢

    AMA: 2015,Jun,10; 2015,Apr,3; 2015,Jan,16; 2014,Jan,11; 2010,Dec,7-10

82044 urine, microalbumin, semiquantitative (eg, reagent strip assay)

    EXCLUDES *Prealbumin (84134)*

    🔧 0.00   ⚕ 0.00   **FUD** XXX   ✗ N

    AMA: 2015,Jun,10; 2015,Apr,3; 2015,Jan,16; 2014,Jan,11; 2012,Jan,15-42; 2011,Jan,11; 2010,Dec,7-10

82045 ischemia modified

    🔧 0.00   ⚕ 0.00   **FUD** XXX   N

    AMA: 2015,Jun,10; 2015,Apr,3; 2010,Dec,7-10

82075-82107 Chemistry: Alcohol—Alpha-fetoprotein (AFP)

INCLUDES Clinical information not requested by the ordering physician
Mathematically calculated results
Quantitative analysis unless otherwise specified
Specimens from any source unless otherwise specified

EXCLUDES *Calculated results that represent a score or probability that was derived by algorithm*
Drug testing ([80300, 80301, 80302, 80303, 80304], [80324, 80325, 80326, 80327, 80328, 80329, 80330, 80331, 80332, 80333, 80334, 80335, 80336, 80337, 80338, 80339, 80340, 80341, 80342, 80343, 80344, 80345, 80346, 80347, 80348, 80349, 80350, 80351, 80352, 80353, 80354, 80355, 80356, 80357, 80358, 80359, 80360, 80361, 80362, 80363, 80364, 80365, 80366, 80367, 80368, 80369, 80370, 80371, 80372, 80373, 80374, 80375, 80376, 80377, 83992])
Organ or disease panels (80048-80076 [80081])
Therapeutic drug assays (80150-80299 [80164, 80165, 80171])
Do not report analytes from nonrequested laboratory analysis

82075 **Alcohol (ethanol), breath**
  0.00   0.00 **FUD** XXX   N
  AMA: 2015,Jun,10; 2015,Apr,3; 2010,Dec,7-10

82085 **Aldolase**
  0.00   0.00 **FUD** XXX   N
  AMA: 2015,Jun,10; 2015,Apr,3; 2010,Dec,7-10

82088 **Aldosterone**
  0.00   0.00 **FUD** XXX   N ⬜
  AMA: 2015,Jun,10; 2015,Apr,3; 2010,Dec,7-10

82103 **Alpha-1-antitrypsin; total**
  0.00   0.00 **FUD** XXX   N
  AMA: 2015,Jun,10; 2015,Apr,3; 2010,Dec,7-10

82104 **phenotype**
  0.00   0.00 **FUD** XXX   N
  AMA: 2015,Jun,10; 2015,Apr,3; 2010,Dec,7-10

82105 **Alpha-fetoprotein (AFP); serum**
  0.00   0.00 **FUD** XXX   N ⬜
  AMA: 2015,Jun,10; 2015,Apr,3; 2010,Dec,7-10

82106 **amniotic fluid**   M
  0.00   0.00 **FUD** XXX   N ⬜
  AMA: 2015,Jun,10; 2015,Apr,3; 2010,Dec,7-10

82107 **AFP-L3 fraction isoform and total AFP (including ratio)**
  0.00   0.00 **FUD** XXX   N
  AMA: 2015,Jun,10; 2015,Apr,3; 2010,Dec,7-10

82108 Chemistry: Aluminum

CMS: 100-02,11,20.2 ESRD Laboratory Services

INCLUDES Clinical information not requested by the ordering physician
Mathematically calculated results
Quantitative analysis unless otherwise specified
Specimens from any source unless otherwise specified

EXCLUDES *Calculated results that represent a score or probability that was derived by algorithm*
Drug testing ([80300, 80301, 80302, 80303, 80304], [80324, 80325, 80326, 80327, 80328, 80329, 80330, 80331, 80332, 80333, 80334, 80335, 80336, 80337, 80338, 80339, 80340, 80341, 80342, 80343, 80344, 80345, 80346, 80347, 80348, 80349, 80350, 80351, 80352, 80353, 80354, 80355, 80356, 80357, 80358, 80359, 80360, 80361, 80362, 80363, 80364, 80365, 80366, 80367, 80368, 80369, 80370, 80371, 80372, 80373, 80374, 80375, 80376, 80377, 83992])
Organ or disease panels (80048-80076 [80081])
Therapeutic drug assays (80150-80299 [80164, 80165, 80171])
Do not report analytes from nonrequested laboratory analysis

82108 **Aluminum**
  0.00   0.00 **FUD** XXX   N
  AMA: 2015,Jun,10; 2015,Apr,3; 2010,Dec,7-10

82120-82261 Chemistry: Amines—Biotinidase

INCLUDES Clinical information not requested by the ordering physician
Mathematically calculated results
Quantitative analysis unless otherwise specified
Specimens from any source unless otherwise specified

EXCLUDES *Calculated results that represent a score or probability that was derived by algorithm*
Drug testing ([80300, 80301, 80302, 80303, 80304], [80324, 80325, 80326, 80327, 80328, 80329, 80330, 80331, 80332, 80333, 80334, 80335, 80336, 80337, 80338, 80339, 80340, 80341, 80342, 80343, 80344, 80345, 80346, 80347, 80348, 80349, 80350, 80351, 80352, 80353, 80354, 80355, 80356, 80357, 80358, 80359, 80360, 80361, 80362, 80363, 80364, 80365, 80366, 80367, 80368, 80369, 80370, 80371, 80372, 80373, 80374, 80375, 80376, 80377, 83992])
Organ or disease panels (80048-80076 [80081])
Therapeutic drug assays (80150-80299 [80164, 80165, 80171])
Do not report analytes from nonrequested laboratory analysis

82120 **Amines, vaginal fluid, qualitative**   ♀
  EXCLUDES *Combined pH and amines test for vaginitis (82120, 83986)*
  0.00   0.00 **FUD** XXX   ❌ N
  AMA: 2015,Jun,10; 2015,Apr,3; 2015,Jan,16; 2014,Jan,11; 2010,Dec,7-10

82127 **Amino acids; single, qualitative, each specimen**
  0.00   0.00 **FUD** XXX   N
  AMA: 2015,Jun,10; 2015,Apr,3; 2010,Dec,7-10

82128 **multiple, qualitative, each specimen**
  0.00   0.00 **FUD** XXX   N ⬜
  AMA: 2015,Jun,10; 2015,Apr,3; 2010,Dec,7-10

82131 **single, quantitative, each specimen**
  INCLUDES Van Slyke method
  0.00   0.00 **FUD** XXX   N ⬜
  AMA: 2015,Jun,10; 2015,Apr,3; 2015,Jan,16; 2014,Jan,11; 2012,Jan,15-42; 2011,Jan,11; 2010,Dec,7-10

82135 **Aminolevulinic acid, delta (ALA)**
  0.00   0.00 **FUD** XXX   N
  AMA: 2015,Jun,10; 2015,Apr,3; 2010,Dec,7-10

82136 **Amino acids, 2 to 5 amino acids, quantitative, each specimen**
  0.00   0.00 **FUD** XXX   N ⬜
  AMA: 2015,Jun,10; 2015,Apr,3; 2010,Dec,7-10

82139 **Amino acids, 6 or more amino acids, quantitative, each specimen**
  0.00   0.00 **FUD** XXX   N ⬜
  AMA: 2015,Jun,10; 2015,Apr,3; 2010,Dec,7-10

82140 **Ammonia**
  0.00   0.00 **FUD** XXX   N
  AMA: 2015,Jun,10; 2015,Apr,3; 2010,Dec,7-10

82143 **Amniotic fluid scan (spectrophotometric)**   M ♀
  EXCLUDES *L/S ratio (83661)*
  0.00   0.00 **FUD** XXX   N
  AMA: 2015,Jun,10; 2015,Apr,3; 2010,Dec,7-10

82150 **Amylase**
  0.00   0.00 **FUD** XXX   ❌ N
  AMA: 2015,Jun,10; 2015,Apr,3; 2010,Dec,7-10

82154 **Androstanediol glucuronide**
  0.00   0.00 **FUD** XXX   N
  AMA: 2015,Jun,10; 2015,Apr,3; 2015,Jan,16; 2014,Jan,11; 2010,Dec,7-10

82157 **Androstenedione**
  0.00   0.00 **FUD** XXX   N
  AMA: 2015,Jun,10; 2015,Apr,3; 2010,Dec,7-10

82160 **Androsterone**
  0.00   0.00 **FUD** XXX   N
  AMA: 2015,Jun,10; 2015,Apr,3; 2010,Dec,7-10

82163 **Angiotensin II**
  0.00   0.00 **FUD** XXX   N
  AMA: 2015,Jun,10; 2015,Apr,3; 2010,Dec,7-10

82164 Angiotensin I - converting enzyme (ACE)
0.00   0.00   **FUD** XXX   N

    AMA: 2015,Jun,10; 2015,Apr,3; 2010,Dec,7-10

82172 Apolipoprotein, each
0.00   0.00   **FUD** XXX   N

    AMA: 2015,Jun,10; 2015,Apr,3; 2010,Dec,7-10

82175 Arsenic
    EXCLUDES   *Heavy metal screening (83015)*
0.00   0.00   **FUD** XXX   N

    AMA: 2015,Jun,10; 2015,Apr,3; 2010,Dec,7-10

82180 Ascorbic acid (Vitamin C), blood
0.00   0.00   **FUD** XXX   N

    AMA: 2015,Jun,10; 2015,Apr,3; 2010,Dec,7-10

82190 Atomic absorption spectroscopy, each analyte
0.00   0.00   **FUD** XXX   N

    AMA: 2015,Jun,10; 2015,Apr,3; 2010,Dec,7-10

82232 Beta-2 microglobulin
0.00   0.00   **FUD** XXX   N

    AMA: 2015,Jun,10; 2015,Apr,3; 2010,Dec,7-10

82239 Bile acids; total
0.00   0.00   **FUD** XXX   N

    AMA: 2015,Jun,10; 2015,Apr,3; 2010,Dec,7-10

82240 cholylglycine
    EXCLUDES   *Bile pigments, urine (81000-81005)*
0.00   0.00   **FUD** XXX   N

    AMA: 2015,Jun,10; 2015,Apr,3; 2010,Dec,7-10

82247 Bilirubin; total
    INCLUDES   Van Den Bergh test
0.00   0.00   **FUD** XXX   X N

    AMA: 2015,Jun,10; 2015,Apr,3; 2015,Jan,16; 2014,Jan,11; 2012,Jan,15-42; 2010,Dec,7-10; 2010,Apr,10

82248 direct
0.00   0.00   **FUD** XXX   N

    AMA: 2015,Jun,10; 2015,Apr,3; 2015,Jan,16; 2014,Jan,11; 2012,Jan,15-42; 2010,Dec,7-10; 2010,Apr,10

82252 feces, qualitative
0.00   0.00   **FUD** XXX   N

    AMA: 2015,Jun,10; 2015,Apr,3; 2010,Dec,7-10

82261 Biotinidase, each specimen
0.00   0.00   **FUD** XXX   N

    AMA: 2015,Jun,10; 2015,Apr,3; 2010,Dec,7-10

82270-82274 Chemistry: Occult Blood

CMS: 100-4,16,70.8 CLIA Waived Tests

INCLUDES   Clinical information not requested by the ordering physician
Mathematically calculated results
Quantitative analysis unless otherwise specified
Specimens from any source unless otherwise specified

EXCLUDES   *Calculated results that represent a score or probability that was derived by algorithm*
Drug testing ([80300, 80301, 80302, 80303, 80304], [80324, 80325, 80326, 80327, 80328, 80329, 80330, 80331, 80332, 80333, 80334, 80335, 80336, 80337, 80338, 80339, 80340, 80341, 80342, 80343, 80344, 80345, 80346, 80347, 80348, 80349, 80350, 80351, 80352, 80353, 80354, 80355, 80356, 80357, 80358, 80359, 80360, 80361, 80362, 80363, 80364, 80365, 80366, 80367, 80368, 80369, 80370, 80371, 80372, 80373, 80374, 80375, 80376, 80377, 83992])
Organ or disease panels (80048-80076 [80081])
Therapeutic drug assays (80150-80299 [80164, 80165, 80171])
Do not report analytes from nonrequested laboratory analysis

82270 Blood, occult, by peroxidase activity (eg, guaiac), qualitative; feces, consecutive collected specimens with single determination, for colorectal neoplasm screening (ie, patient was provided 3 cards or single triple card for consecutive collection)
    INCLUDES   Day test
0.00   0.00   **FUD** XXX   X N

    AMA: 2015,Jun,10; 2015,Apr,3; 2015,Jan,16; 2014,Jan,11; 2012,Jan,15-42; 2011,Jan,11; 2010,Dec,7-10

82271 other sources
0.00   0.00   **FUD** XXX   X N

    AMA: 2015,Jun,10; 2015,Apr,3; 2010,Dec,7-10

82272 Blood, occult, by peroxidase activity (eg, guaiac), qualitative, feces, 1-3 simultaneous determinations, performed for other than colorectal neoplasm screening
0.00   0.00   **FUD** XXX   X N

    AMA: 2015,Jun,10; 2015,Apr,3; 2015,Jan,16; 2014,Jan,11; 2012,Jan,15-42; 2011,Jan,11; 2010,Dec,7-10

82274 Blood, occult, by fecal hemoglobin determination by immunoassay, qualitative, feces, 1-3 simultaneous determinations
0.00   0.00   **FUD** XXX   X N

    AMA: 2015,Jun,10; 2015,Apr,3; 2010,Dec,7-10

82286-82308 [82652] Chemistry: Bradykinin—Calcitonin

INCLUDES   Clinical information not requested by the ordering physician
Mathematically calculated results
Quantitative analysis unless otherwise specified
Specimens from any source unless otherwise specified

EXCLUDES   *Calculated results that represent a score or probability that was derived by algorithm*
Drug testing ([80300, 80301, 80302, 80303, 80304], [80324, 80325, 80326, 80327, 80328, 80329, 80330, 80331, 80332, 80333, 80334, 80335, 80336, 80337, 80338, 80339, 80340, 80341, 80342, 80343, 80344, 80345, 80346, 80347, 80348, 80349, 80350, 80351, 80352, 80353, 80354, 80355, 80356, 80357, 80358, 80359, 80360, 80361, 80362, 80363, 80364, 80365, 80366, 80367, 80368, 80369, 80370, 80371, 80372, 80373, 80374, 80375, 80376, 80377, 83992])
Organ or disease panels (80048-80076 [80081])
Therapeutic drug assays (80150-80299 [80164, 80165, 80171])
Do not report analytes from nonrequested laboratory analysis

82286 Bradykinin
0.00   0.00   **FUD** XXX   N

    AMA: 2015,Jun,10; 2015,Apr,3; 2010,Dec,7-10

82300 Cadmium
0.00   0.00   **FUD** XXX   N

    AMA: 2015,Jun,10; 2015,Apr,3; 2010,Dec,7-10

82306 Vitamin D; 25 hydroxy, includes fraction(s), if performed
0.00   0.00   **FUD** XXX   N

    AMA: 2015,Jun,10; 2015,Apr,3; 2010,Dec,7-10

**82652** 1, 25 dihydroxy, includes fraction(s), if performed
0.00   0.00   **FUD** XXX   N

    AMA: 2015,Jun,10; 2015,Apr,3; 2010,Dec,7-10

82308 Calcitonin
0.00   0.00   **FUD** XXX   N

    AMA: 2015,Jun,10; 2015,Apr,3; 2010,Dec,7-10

82310-82373 Chemistry: Calcium, total; Carbohydrate Deficient Transferrin

INCLUDES   Clinical information not requested by the ordering physician
Mathematically calculated results
Quantitative analysis unless otherwise specified
Specimens from any source unless otherwise specified

EXCLUDES   *Calculated results that represent a score or probability that was derived by algorithm*
Drug testing ([80300, 80301, 80302, 80303, 80304], [80324, 80325, 80326, 80327, 80328, 80329, 80330, 80331, 80332, 80333, 80334, 80335, 80336, 80337, 80338, 80339, 80340, 80341, 80342, 80343, 80344, 80345, 80346, 80347, 80348, 80349, 80350, 80351, 80352, 80353, 80354, 80355, 80356, 80357, 80358, 80359, 80360, 80361, 80362, 80363, 80364, 80365, 80366, 80367, 80368, 80369, 80370, 80371, 80372, 80373, 80374, 80375, 80376, 80377, 83992])
Organ or disease panels (80048-80076 [80081])
Therapeutic drug assays (80150-80299 [80164, 80165, 80171])

82310 Calcium; total
0.00   0.00   **FUD** XXX   X N

    AMA: 2015,Jun,10; 2015,Apr,3; 2015,Jan,16; 2014,Jan,11; 2010,Dec,7-10

82330 ionized
0.00   0.00   **FUD** XXX   X N

    AMA: 2015,Jun,10; 2015,Apr,3; 2015,Jan,16; 2014,Jan,11; 2013,Apr,10-11; 2010,Dec,7-10

82331	**after calcium infusion test**
	🚑 0.00 ⚕ 0.00 **FUD** XXX N 💬
	AMA: 2015,Jun,10; 2015,Apr,3; 2010,Dec,7-10

82340	**urine quantitative, timed specimen**
	🚑 0.00 ⚕ 0.00 **FUD** XXX N
	AMA: 2015,Jun,10; 2015,Apr,3; 2010,Dec,7-10

82355	**Calculus; qualitative analysis**
	🚑 0.00 ⚕ 0.00 **FUD** XXX N 💬
	AMA: 2015,Jun,10; 2015,Apr,3; 2010,Dec,7-10

82360	**quantitative analysis, chemical**
	🚑 0.00 ⚕ 0.00 **FUD** XXX N 💬
	AMA: 2015,Jun,10; 2015,Apr,3; 2010,Dec,7-10

82365	**infrared spectroscopy**
	🚑 0.00 ⚕ 0.00 **FUD** XXX N 💬
	AMA: 2015,Jun,10; 2015,Apr,3; 2010,Dec,7-10

82370	**X-ray diffraction**
	🚑 0.00 ⚕ 0.00 **FUD** XXX N 💬
	AMA: 2015,Jun,10; 2015,Apr,3; 2010,Dec,7-10

82373	**Carbohydrate deficient transferrin**
	🚑 0.00 ⚕ 0.00 **FUD** XXX N
	AMA: 2015,Jun,10; 2015,Apr,3; 2010,Dec,7-10

82374 Chemistry: Carbon Dioxide

CMS: 100-02,11,20.2 ESRD Laboratory Services; 100-2,11,30.2.2 Automated Multi-Channel Chemistry (AMCC) Tests; 100-4,16,40.6.1 Automated Multi-Channel Chemistry Tests for ESRD Beneficiaries; 100-4,16,70.8 CLIA Waived Tests

INCLUDES Clinical information not requested by the ordering physician
Mathematically calculated results
Quantitative analysis unless otherwise specified
Specimens from any source unless otherwise specified

EXCLUDES *Calculated results that represent a score or probability that was derived by algorithm*
Drug testing ([80300, 80301, 80302, 80303, 80304], [80324, 80325, 80326, 80327, 80328, 80329, 80330, 80331, 80332, 80333, 80334, 80335, 80336, 80337, 80338, 80339, 80340, 80341, 80342, 80343, 80344, 80345, 80346, 80347, 80348, 80349, 80350, 80351, 80352, 80353, 80354, 80355, 80356, 80357, 80358, 80359, 80360, 80361, 80362, 80363, 80364, 80365, 80366, 80367, 80368, 80369, 80370, 80371, 80372, 80373, 80374, 80375, 80376, 80377, 83992])
Organ or disease panels (80048-80076 [80081])
Therapeutic drug assays (80150-80299 [80164, 80165, 80171])
Do not report analytes from nonrequested laboratory analysis

82374	**Carbon dioxide (bicarbonate)**
	EXCLUDES *Blood gases (82803)*
	🚑 0.00 ⚕ 0.00 **FUD** XXX ✖ N
	AMA: 2015,Jun,10; 2015,Apr,3; 2015,Jan,16; 2014,Jan,11; 2013,Apr,10-11; 2010,Dec,7-10

82375-82376 Chemistry: Carboxyhemoglobin (Carbon Monoxide)

INCLUDES Clinical information not requested by the ordering physician
Mathematically calculated results
Specimens from any source unless otherwise specified

EXCLUDES *Calculated results that represent a score or probability that was derived by algorithm*
Drug testing ([80300, 80301, 80302, 80303, 80304], [80324, 80325, 80326, 80327, 80328, 80329, 80330, 80331, 80332, 80333, 80334, 80335, 80336, 80337, 80338, 80339, 80340, 80341, 80342, 80343, 80344, 80345, 80346, 80347, 80348, 80349, 80350, 80351, 80352, 80353, 80354, 80355, 80356, 80357, 80358, 80359, 80360, 80361, 80362, 80363, 80364, 80365, 80366, 80367, 80368, 80369, 80370, 80371, 80372, 80373, 80374, 80375, 80376, 80377, 83992])
Organ or disease panels (80048-80076 [80081])
Transcutaneous measurement of carboxyhemoglobin (88740)
Do not report analytes from nonrequested laboratory analysis

82375	**Carboxyhemoglobin; quantitative**
	🚑 0.00 ⚕ 0.00 **FUD** XXX N
	AMA: 2015,Jun,10; 2015,Apr,3; 2015,Jan,16; 2014,Jan,11; 2010,Dec,7-10

82376	**qualitative**
	🚑 0.00 ⚕ 0.00 **FUD** XXX N
	AMA: 2015,Jun,10; 2015,Apr,3; 2010,Dec,7-10

82378 Chemistry: Carcinoembryonic Antigen (CEA)

CMS: 100-3,190.26 Carcinoembryonic Antigen (CEA)

INCLUDES Clinical information not requested by the ordering physician

EXCLUDES *Calculated results that represent a score or probability that was derived by algorithm*
Do not report analytes from nonrequested laboratory analysis

82378	**Carcinoembryonic antigen (CEA)**
	🚑 0.00 ⚕ 0.00 **FUD** XXX N
	AMA: 2015,Jun,10; 2015,Apr,3; 2015,Jan,16; 2014,Jan,11; 2012,Jan,15-42; 2011,Jan,11; 2010,Dec,7-10

82379-82415 Chemistry: Carnitine—Chloramphenicol

INCLUDES Clinical information not requested by the ordering physician
Mathematically calculated results
Quantitative analysis unless otherwise specified
Specimens from any source unless otherwise specified

EXCLUDES *Calculated results that represent a score or probability that was derived by algorithm*
Drug testing ([80300, 80301, 80302, 80303, 80304], [80324, 80325, 80326, 80327, 80328, 80329, 80330, 80331, 80332, 80333, 80334, 80335, 80336, 80337, 80338, 80339, 80340, 80341, 80342, 80343, 80344, 80345, 80346, 80347, 80348, 80349, 80350, 80351, 80352, 80353, 80354, 80355, 80356, 80357, 80358, 80359, 80360, 80361, 80362, 80363, 80364, 80365, 80366, 80367, 80368, 80369, 80370, 80371, 80372, 80373, 80374, 80375, 80376, 80377, 83992])
Organ or disease panels (80048-80076 [80081])
Therapeutic drug assays (80150-80299 [80164, 80165, 80171])
Do not report analytes from nonrequested laboratory analysis

82379	**Carnitine (total and free), quantitative, each specimen**
	EXCLUDES *Acylcarnitine (82016-82017)*
	🚑 0.00 ⚕ 0.00 **FUD** XXX N
	AMA: 2015,Jun,10; 2015,Apr,3; 2010,Dec,7-10

82380	**Carotene**
	🚑 0.00 ⚕ 0.00 **FUD** XXX N
	AMA: 2015,Jun,10; 2015,Apr,3; 2010,Dec,7-10

82382	**Catecholamines; total urine**
	🚑 0.00 ⚕ 0.00 **FUD** XXX N
	AMA: 2015,Jun,10; 2015,Apr,3; 2010,Dec,7-10

82383	**blood**
	🚑 0.00 ⚕ 0.00 **FUD** XXX N
	AMA: 2015,Jun,10; 2015,Apr,3; 2010,Dec,7-10

82384	**fractionated**
	EXCLUDES *Urine metabolites (83835, 84585)*
	🚑 0.00 ⚕ 0.00 **FUD** XXX N 💬
	AMA: 2015,Jun,10; 2015,Apr,3; 2010,Dec,7-10

82387	**Cathepsin-D**
	🚑 0.00 ⚕ 0.00 **FUD** XXX N
	AMA: 2015,Jun,10; 2015,Apr,3; 2010,Dec,7-10

82390	**Ceruloplasmin**
	🚑 0.00 ⚕ 0.00 **FUD** XXX N
	AMA: 2015,Jun,10; 2015,Apr,3; 2010,Dec,7-10

82397	**Chemiluminescent assay**
	🚑 0.00 ⚕ 0.00 **FUD** XXX N
	AMA: 2015,Jun,10; 2015,Apr,3; 2015,Jan,16; 2014,Jan,11; 2010,Dec,7-10

82415	**Chloramphenicol**
	🚑 0.00 ⚕ 0.00 **FUD** XXX N
	AMA: 2015,Jun,10; 2015,Apr,3; 2010,Dec,7-10

82435-82438 Chemistry: Chloride

INCLUDES Clinical information not requested by the ordering physician
Mathematically calculated results
Quantitative analysis unless otherwise specified
Specimens from any source unless otherwise specified

EXCLUDES *Calculated results that represent a score or probability that was derived by algorithm*
Organ or disease panels (80048-80076 [80081])
Therapeutic drug assays (80150-80299 [80164, 80165, 80171])
Do not report analytes from nonrequested laboratory analysis

82435	Chloride; blood

🚑 0.00   ⚕ 0.00   **FUD** XXX   ☒ Ⓝ

AMA: 2015,Jun,10; 2015,Apr,3; 2015,Jan,16; 2014,Jan,11; 2013,Apr,10-11; 2010,Dec,7-10

82436	urine

🚑 0.00   ⚕ 0.00   **FUD** XXX   Ⓝ

AMA: 2015,Jun,10; 2015,Apr,3; 2010,Dec,7-10

82438	other source

EXCLUDES   *Sweat collections by iontophoresis (89230)*

🚑 0.00   ⚕ 0.00   **FUD** XXX   Ⓝ

AMA: 2015,Jun,10; 2015,Apr,3; 2015,Jan,16; 2014,Jan,11; 2010,Dec,7-10

82441 Chemistry: Chlorinated Hydrocarbons

INCLUDES   Clinical information not requested by the ordering physician
Mathematically calculated results
Quantitative analysis unless otherwise specified
Specimens from any source unless otherwise specified

EXCLUDES   *Calculated results that represent a score or probability that was derived by algorithm*

Do not report analytes from nonrequested laboratory analysis

82441	Chlorinated hydrocarbons, screen

🚑 0.00   ⚕ 0.00   **FUD** XXX   Ⓝ

AMA: 2015,Jun,10; 2015,Apr,3; 2010,Dec,7-10

82465 Chemistry: Cholesterol, Total

CMS: 100-3,190.23 Lipid Testing; 100-4,16,40.6.1 Automated Multi-Channel Chemistry Tests for ESRD Beneficiaries; 100-4,16,70.8 CLIA Waived Tests

INCLUDES   Clinical information not requested by the ordering physician
Mathematically calculated results
Quantitative analysis unless otherwise specified

EXCLUDES   *Calculated results that represent a score or probability that was derived by algorithm*
Organ or disease panels (80048-80299 [80081, 80164, 80165, 80171, 80300, 80301, 80302, 80303, 80304, 80320, 80321, 80322, 80323, 80324, 80325, 80326, 80327, 80328, 80329, 80330, 80331, 80332, 80333, 80334, 80335, 80336, 80337, 80338, 80339, 80340, 80341, 80342, 80343, 80344, 80345, 80346, 80347, 80348, 80349, 80350, 80351, 80352, 80353, 80354, 80355, 80356, 80357, 80358, 80359, 80360, 80361, 80362, 80363, 80364, 80365, 80366, 80367, 80368, 80369, 80370, 80371, 80372, 80373, 80374, 80375, 80376, 80377, 83992])

Do not report analytes from nonrequested laboratory analysis

82465	Cholesterol, serum or whole blood, total

EXCLUDES   *High density lipoprotein (HDL) (83718)*
🚑 0.00   ⚕ 0.00   **FUD** XXX   ☒ Ⓝ ▢

AMA: 2015,Jun,10; 2015,Apr,3; 2015,Jan,16; 2014,Jan,11; 2012,Jan,15-42; 2011,Jan,11; 2010,Dec,7-10

82480-82492 Chemistry: Cholinesterase—Chromatography

INCLUDES   Clinical information not requested by the ordering physician
Mathematically calculated results
Quantitative analysis unless otherwise specified
Specimens from any source unless otherwise specified

EXCLUDES   *Calculated results that represent a score or probability that was derived by algorithm*
Drug testing ([80300, 80301, 80302, 80303, 80304], [80324, 80325, 80326, 80327, 80328, 80329, 80330, 80331, 80332, 80333, 80334, 80335, 80336, 80337, 80338, 80339, 80340, 80341, 80342, 80343, 80344, 80345, 80346, 80347, 80348, 80349, 80350, 80351, 80352, 80353, 80354, 80355, 80356, 80357, 80358, 80359, 80360, 80361, 80362, 80363, 80364, 80365, 80366, 80367, 80368, 80369, 80370, 80371, 80372, 80373, 80374, 80375, 80376, 80377, 83992])
Organ or disease panels (80048-80076 [80081])
Therapeutic drug assays (80048-80299 [80081, 80164, 80165, 80171, 80300, 80301, 80302, 80303, 80304, 80320, 80321, 80322, 80323, 80324, 80325, 80326, 80327, 80328, 80329, 80330, 80331, 80332, 80333, 80334, 80335, 80336, 80337, 80338, 80339, 80340, 80341, 80342, 80343, 80344, 80345, 80346, 80347, 80348, 80349, 80350, 80351, 80352, 80353, 80354, 80355, 80356, 80357, 80358, 80359, 80360, 80361, 80362, 80363, 80364, 80365, 80366, 80367, 80368, 80369, 80370, 80371, 80372, 80373, 80374, 80375, 80376, 80377, 83992])

Do not report analytes from nonrequested laboratory analysis

82480	Cholinesterase; serum

🚑 0.00   ⚕ 0.00   **FUD** XXX   Ⓝ

AMA: 2015,Jun,10; 2015,Apr,3; 2010,Dec,7-10

82482	RBC

🚑 0.00   ⚕ 0.00   **FUD** XXX   Ⓝ

AMA: 2015,Jun,10; 2015,Apr,3; 2010,Dec,7-10

82485	Chondroitin B sulfate, quantitative

🚑 0.00   ⚕ 0.00   **FUD** XXX   Ⓝ

AMA: 2015,Jun,10; 2015,Apr,3; 2010,Dec,7-10

82486	~~Chromatography, qualitative; column (eg, gas liquid or HPLC), analyte not elsewhere specified~~

To report, see specific analyte or ~82542

82487	~~paper, 1-dimensional, analyte not elsewhere specified~~

To report, see specific analyte or ~84999

82488	~~paper, 2-dimensional, analyte not elsewhere specified~~

To report, see specific analyte or ~84999

82489	~~thin layer, analyte not elsewhere specified~~

To report, see specific analyte or ~84999

82491	~~Chromatography, quantitative, column (eg, gas liquid or HPLC); single analyte not elsewhere specified, single stationary and mobile phase~~

To report, see specific analyte or ~82542

82492	~~multiple analytes, single stationary and mobile phase~~

To report, see specific analytes or ~82542

82495-82507 Chemistry: Chromium—Citrate

INCLUDES   Clinical information not requested by the ordering physician
Mathematically calculated results
Quantitative analysis unless otherwise specified
Specimens from any source unless otherwise specified

EXCLUDES   *Calculated results that represent a score or probability that was derived by algorithm*
Drug testing ([80300, 80301, 80302, 80303, 80304], [80324, 80325, 80326, 80327, 80328, 80329, 80330, 80331, 80332, 80333, 80334, 80335, 80336, 80337, 80338, 80339, 80340, 80341, 80342, 80343, 80344, 80345, 80346, 80347, 80348, 80349, 80350, 80351, 80352, 80353, 80354, 80355, 80356, 80357, 80358, 80359, 80360, 80361, 80362, 80363, 80364, 80365, 80366, 80367, 80368, 80369, 80370, 80371, 80372, 80373, 80374, 80375, 80376, 80377, 83992])
Organ or disease panels (80048-80076 [80081])
Therapeutic drug assays (80150-80299 [80164, 80165, 80171])

Do not report analytes from nonrequested laboratory analysis

82495	Chromium

🚑 0.00   ⚕ 0.00   **FUD** XXX   Ⓝ

AMA: 2015,Jun,10; 2015,Apr,3; 2010,Dec,7-10

82507	Citrate

🚑 0.00   ⚕ 0.00   **FUD** XXX   Ⓝ

AMA: 2015,Jun,10; 2015,Apr,3; 2010,Dec,7-10

82523 Chemistry: Collagen Crosslinks, Any Method

CMS: 100-3,190.19 NCD for Collagen Crosslinks, Any Method; 100-4,16,70.8 CLIA Waived Tests

INCLUDES   Clinical information not requested by the ordering physician
Mathematically calculated results
Quantitative analysis unless otherwise specified
Specimens from any source unless otherwise specified

EXCLUDES   *Calculated results that represent a score or probability that was derived by algorithm*
Organ or disease panels (80048-80076 [80081])
Therapeutic drug assays (80150-80299 [80164, 80165, 80171])

Do not report analytes from nonrequested laboratory analysis

82523	Collagen cross links, any method

🚑 0.00   ⚕ 0.00   **FUD** XXX   ☒ Ⓝ

AMA: 2015,Jun,10; 2015,Apr,3; 2010,Dec,7-10

82525-82946 Chemistry: Copper—Glucagon Tolerance Test

INCLUDES Clinical information not requested by the ordering physician
Mathematically calculated results
Quantitative analysis unless otherwise specified
Specimens from any source unless otherwise specified

EXCLUDES *Calculated results that represent a score or probability that was derived by algorithm*
Drug testing ([80300, 80301, 80302, 80303, 80304], [80324, 80325, 80326, 80327, 80328, 80329, 80330, 80331, 80332, 80333, 80334, 80335, 80336, 80337, 80338, 80339, 80340, 80341, 80342, 80343, 80344, 80345, 80346, 80347, 80348, 80349, 80350, 80351, 80352, 80353, 80354, 80355, 80356, 80357, 80358, 80359, 80360, 80361, 80362, 80363, 80364, 80365, 80366, 80367, 80368, 80369, 80370, 80371, 80372, 80373, 80374, 80375, 80376, 80377, 83992])
Organ or disease panels (80048-80076 [80081])
Therapeutic drug assays (80150-80299 [80164, 80165, 80171])
Do not report analytes from nonrequested laboratory analysis

82525   Copper
0.00   0.00   **FUD** XXX   N
AMA: 2015,Jun,10; 2015,Apr,3; 2010,Dec,7-10

82528   Corticosterone
INCLUDES Porter-Silber test
0.00   0.00   **FUD** XXX   N
AMA: 2015,Jun,10; 2015,Apr,3; 2010,Dec,7-10

82530   Cortisol; free
0.00   0.00   **FUD** XXX   N ▢
AMA: 2015,Jun,10; 2015,Apr,3; 2015,Jan,16; 2014,Jan,11; 2010,Dec,7-10

82533   total
0.00   0.00   **FUD** XXX   N ▢
AMA: 2015,Jun,10; 2015,Apr,3; 2015,Jan,16; 2014,Jan,11; 2010,Dec,7-10

82540   Creatine
0.00   0.00   **FUD** XXX   N
AMA: 2015,Jun,10; 2015,Apr,3; 2010,Dec,7-10

~~82541~~   ~~Column chromatography/mass spectrometry (eg, GC/MS, or HPLC/MS), non-drug analyte not elsewhere specified; qualitative, single stationary and mobile phase~~
To report, see specific analyte or ~82542

▲ **82542   Column chromatography, includes mass spectrometry, if performed (eg, HPLC, LC, LC/MS, LC/MS-MS, GC, GC/MS-MS, GC/MS, HPLC/MS), non-drug analyte(s) not elsewhere specified, qualitative or quantitative, each specimen**
Do not report more than one time per specimen
0.00   0.00   **FUD** XXX   N
AMA: 2015,Jun,10; 2015,Apr,3; 2010,Dec,7-10

~~82543~~   ~~stable isotope dilution, single analyte, quantitative, single stationary and mobile phase~~
To report, see specific analyte or ~82542

~~82544~~   ~~stable isotope dilution, multiple analytes, quantitative, single stationary and mobile phase~~
To report, see specific analytes or ~82542

82550   Creatine kinase (CK), (CPK); total
0.00   0.00   **FUD** XXX   ☒ N ▢
AMA: 2015,Jun,10; 2015,Apr,3; 2015,Jan,16; 2014,Jan,11; 2010,Dec,7-10

82552   isoenzymes
0.00   0.00   **FUD** XXX   N ▢
AMA: 2015,Jun,10; 2015,Apr,3; 2015,Jan,16; 2014,Jan,11; 2010,Dec,7-10

82553   MB fraction only
0.00   0.00   **FUD** XXX   N ▢
AMA: 2015,Jun,10; 2015,Apr,3; 2015,Jan,16; 2014,Jan,11; 2010,Dec,7-10

82554   isoforms
0.00   0.00   **FUD** XXX   N ▢
AMA: 2015,Jun,10; 2015,Apr,3; 2015,Jan,16; 2014,Jan,11; 2010,Dec,7-10

82565   Creatinine; blood
0.00   0.00   **FUD** XXX   ☒ N
AMA: 2015,Jun,10; 2015,Apr,3; 2015,Jan,16; 2014,Jan,11; 2013,Apr,10-11; 2010,Dec,7-10

82570   other source
0.00   0.00   **FUD** XXX   ☒ N
AMA: 2015,Jun,10; 2015,Apr,3; 2010,Dec,7-10

82575   clearance
INCLUDES Holten test
0.00   0.00   **FUD** XXX   N ▢
AMA: 2015,Jun,10; 2015,Apr,3; 2010,Dec,7-10

82585   Cryofibrinogen
0.00   0.00   **FUD** XXX   N
AMA: 2015,Jun,10; 2015,Apr,3; 2010,Dec,7-10

82595   Cryoglobulin, qualitative or semi-quantitative (eg, cryocrit)
EXCLUDES *Quantitative, cryoglobulin (82784-82785)*
0.00   0.00   **FUD** XXX   N
AMA: 2015,Jun,10; 2015,Apr,3; 2010,Dec,7-10

82600   Cyanide
0.00   0.00   **FUD** XXX   N
AMA: 2015,Jun,10; 2015,Apr,3; 2010,Dec,7-10

82607   Cyanocobalamin (Vitamin B-12);
0.00   0.00   **FUD** XXX   N ▢
AMA: 2015,Jun,10; 2015,Apr,3; 2010,Dec,7-10

82608   unsaturated binding capacity
0.00   0.00   **FUD** XXX   N
AMA: 2015,Jun,10; 2015,Apr,3; 2010,Dec,7-10

82610   Cystatin C
0.00   0.00   **FUD** XXX   N
AMA: 2015,Jun,10; 2015,Apr,3; 2015,Jan,16; 2014,Jan,11; 2012,Jan,15-42; 2011,Jan,11; 2010,Dec,7-10

82615   Cystine and homocystine, urine, qualitative
0.00   0.00   **FUD** XXX   N
AMA: 2015,Jun,10; 2015,Apr,3; 2010,Dec,7-10

82626   Dehydroepiandrosterone (DHEA)
Do not report with ([80327, 80328])
0.00   0.00   **FUD** XXX   N
AMA: 2015,Jun,10; 2015,Apr,3; 2015,Jan,16; 2014,Jan,11; 2010,Dec,7-10

82627   Dehydroepiandrosterone-sulfate (DHEA-S)
0.00   0.00   **FUD** XXX   N
AMA: 2015,Jun,10; 2015,Apr,3; 2015,Jan,16; 2014,Jan,11; 2010,Dec,7-10

82633   Desoxycorticosterone, 11-
0.00   0.00   **FUD** XXX   N
AMA: 2015,Jun,10; 2015,Apr,3; 2010,Dec,7-10

82634   Deoxycortisol, 11-
0.00   0.00   **FUD** XXX   N ▢
AMA: 2015,Jun,10; 2015,Apr,3; 2010,Dec,7-10

82638   Dibucaine number
0.00   0.00   **FUD** XXX   N
AMA: 2015,Jun,10; 2015,Apr,3; 2010,Dec,7-10

82652   Resequenced code, See code following 82306.

82656   Elastase, pancreatic (EL-1), fecal, qualitative or semi-quantitative
0.00   0.00   **FUD** XXX   N
AMA: 2015,Jun,10; 2015,Apr,3; 2015,Jan,16; 2014,Jan,11; 2012,Jan,15-42; 2011,Jan,11; 2010,Dec,7-10

82657   Enzyme activity in blood cells, cultured cells, or tissue, not elsewhere specified; nonradioactive substrate, each specimen
0.00   0.00   **FUD** XXX   N
AMA: 2015,Jun,10; 2015,Apr,3; 2010,Dec,7-10

82658	radioactive substrate, each specimen

⚕ 0.00 ⚗ 0.00 **FUD** XXX N

AMA: 2015,Jun,10; 2015,Apr,3; 2010,Dec,7-10

82664	**Electrophoretic technique, not elsewhere specified**

⚕ 0.00 ⚗ 0.00 **FUD** XXX N

AMA: 2015,Jun,10; 2015,Apr,3; 2010,Dec,7-10

82668	**Erythropoietin**

⚕ 0.00 ⚗ 0.00 **FUD** XXX N

AMA: 2015,Jun,10; 2015,Apr,3; 2010,Dec,7-10

82670	**Estradiol**

⚕ 0.00 ⚗ 0.00 **FUD** XXX N ▫

AMA: 2015,Jun,10; 2015,Apr,3; 2010,Dec,7-10

82671	**Estrogens; fractionated**

EXCLUDES *Estrogen receptor assay (84233)*

⚕ 0.00 ⚗ 0.00 **FUD** XXX N

AMA: 2015,Jun,10; 2015,Apr,3; 2010,Dec,7-10

82672	total

EXCLUDES *Estrogen receptor assay (84233)*

⚕ 0.00 ⚗ 0.00 **FUD** XXX N

AMA: 2015,Jun,10; 2015,Apr,3; 2010,Dec,7-10

82677	**Estriol**

⚕ 0.00 ⚗ 0.00 **FUD** XXX N

AMA: 2015,Jun,10; 2015,Apr,3; 2010,Dec,7-10

82679	**Estrone**

⚕ 0.00 ⚗ 0.00 **FUD** XXX ✕ N

AMA: 2015,Jun,10; 2015,Apr,3; 2010,Dec,7-10

82693	**Ethylene glycol**

⚕ 0.00 ⚗ 0.00 **FUD** XXX N

AMA: 2015,Jun,10; 2015,Apr,3; 2010,Dec,7-10

82696	**Etiocholanolone**

EXCLUDES *Fractionation of ketosteroids (83593)*

⚕ 0.00 ⚗ 0.00 **FUD** XXX N

AMA: 2015,Jun,10; 2015,Apr,3; 2010,Dec,7-10

82705	**Fat or lipids, feces; qualitative**

⚕ 0.00 ⚗ 0.00 **FUD** XXX N

AMA: 2015,Jun,10; 2015,Apr,3; 2010,Dec,7-10

82710	quantitative

⚕ 0.00 ⚗ 0.00 **FUD** XXX N

AMA: 2015,Jun,10; 2015,Apr,3; 2010,Dec,7-10

82715	**Fat differential, feces, quantitative**

⚕ 0.00 ⚗ 0.00 **FUD** XXX N

AMA: 2015,Jun,10; 2015,Apr,3; 2010,Dec,7-10

82725	**Fatty acids, nonesterified**

⚕ 0.00 ⚗ 0.00 **FUD** XXX N

AMA: 2015,Jun,10; 2015,Apr,3; 2010,Dec,7-10

82726	**Very long chain fatty acids**

EXCLUDES *Long-chain (C20-22) omega-3 fatty acids in red blood cell (RBC) membranes (0111T)*

⚕ 0.00 ⚗ 0.00 **FUD** XXX N

AMA: 2015,Jun,10; 2015,Apr,3; 2010,Dec,7-10

82728	**Ferritin**

⚕ 0.00 ⚗ 0.00 **FUD** XXX N

AMA: 2015,Jun,10; 2015,Apr,3; 2010,Dec,7-10

82731	**Fetal fibronectin, cervicovaginal secretions, semi-quantitative**

M ♀

⚕ 0.00 ⚗ 0.00 **FUD** XXX N

AMA: 2015,Jun,10; 2015,Apr,3; 2010,Dec,7-10

82735	**Fluoride**

⚕ 0.00 ⚗ 0.00 **FUD** XXX N

AMA: 2015,Jun,10; 2015,Apr,3; 2010,Dec,7-10

82746	**Folic acid; serum**

⚕ 0.00 ⚗ 0.00 **FUD** XXX N

AMA: 2015,Jun,10; 2015,Apr,3; 2010,Dec,7-10

82747	**RBC**

⚕ 0.00 ⚗ 0.00 **FUD** XXX N

AMA: 2015,Jun,10; 2015,Apr,3; 2010,Dec,7-10

82757	**Fructose, semen**

EXCLUDES *Fructosamine (82985)*
Fructose, TLC screen (84375)

⚕ 0.00 ⚗ 0.00 **FUD** XXX N

AMA: 2015,Jun,10; 2015,Apr,3; 2010,Dec,7-10

82759	**Galactokinase, RBC**

⚕ 0.00 ⚗ 0.00 **FUD** XXX N

AMA: 2015,Jun,10; 2015,Apr,3; 2010,Dec,7-10

82760	**Galactose**

⚕ 0.00 ⚗ 0.00 **FUD** XXX N

AMA: 2015,Jun,10; 2015,Apr,3; 2010,Dec,7-10

82775	**Galactose-1-phosphate uridyl transferase; quantitative**

⚕ 0.00 ⚗ 0.00 **FUD** XXX N

AMA: 2015,Jun,10; 2015,Apr,3; 2010,Dec,7-10

82776	screen

⚕ 0.00 ⚗ 0.00 **FUD** XXX N

AMA: 2015,Jun,10; 2015,Apr,3; 2010,Dec,7-10

82777	**Galectin-3**

⚕ 0.00 ⚗ 0.00 **FUD** XXX N

AMA: 2015,Jun,10; 2015,Apr,3

82784	**Gammaglobulin (immunoglobulin); IgA, IgD, IgG, IgM, each**

INCLUDES Farr test

⚕ 0.00 ⚗ 0.00 **FUD** XXX N ▫

AMA: 2015,Jun,10; 2015,Apr,3; 2015,Jan,16; 2014,Jan,11; 2012,Jan,15-42; 2011,Jan,11; 2010,Dec,7-10

82785	IgE

INCLUDES Farr test

EXCLUDES *Allergen specific, IgE (86003, 86005)*

⚕ 0.00 ⚗ 0.00 **FUD** XXX N ▫

AMA: 2015,Jun,10; 2015,Apr,3; 2015,Jan,16; 2014,Jan,11; 2010,Dec,7-10

82787	immunoglobulin subclasses (eg, IgG1, 2, 3, or 4), each

EXCLUDES *Gamma-glutamyltransferase (GGT) (82977)*

⚕ 0.00 ⚗ 0.00 **FUD** XXX N ▫

AMA: 2015,Jun,10; 2015,Apr,3; 2010,Dec,7-10

82800	**Gases, blood, pH only**

⚕ 0.00 ⚗ 0.00 **FUD** XXX N ▫

AMA: 2015,Jun,10; 2015,Apr,3; 2010,Dec,7-10

82803	**Gases, blood, any combination of pH, pCO2, pO2, CO2, HCO3 (including calculated O2 saturation);**

INCLUDES Two or more of the listed analytes

⚕ 0.00 ⚗ 0.00 **FUD** XXX N ▫

AMA: 2015,Jun,10; 2015,Apr,3; 2010,Dec,7-10

82805	with O2 saturation, by direct measurement, except pulse oximetry

⚕ 0.00 ⚗ 0.00 **FUD** XXX N ▫

AMA: 2015,Jun,10; 2015,Apr,3; 2010,Dec,7-10

82810	**Gases, blood, O2 saturation only, by direct measurement, except pulse oximetry**

EXCLUDES *Pulse oximetry (94760)*

⚕ 0.00 ⚗ 0.00 **FUD** XXX N ▫

AMA: 2015,Jun,10; 2015,Apr,3; 2010,Dec,7-10

82820	**Hemoglobin-oxygen affinity (pO2 for 50% hemoglobin saturation with oxygen)**

⚕ 0.00 ⚗ 0.00 **FUD** XXX N ▫

AMA: 2015,Jun,10; 2015,Apr,3; 2010,Dec,7-10

82930	**Gastric acid analysis, includes pH if performed, each specimen**

⚕ 0.00 ⚗ 0.00 **FUD** XXX N

AMA: 2015,Jun,10; 2015,Apr,3; 2015,Jan,16; 2014,Jan,11; 2011,Sep,3-4; 2010,Dec,7-10

● New Code ▲ Revised Code ○ Reinstated M Maternity A Age Edit Unlisted Not Covered # Resequenced
⊘ AMA Mod 51 Exempt ⑤⑪ Optum Mod 51 Exempt ⑥⑬ Mod 63 Exempt ⊙ Mod Sedation + Add-on ▫ CCI PQRS **FUD** Follow-up Days

Pathology and Laboratory

82938 — 83012

82938 **Gastrin after secretin stimulation**
🔲 0.00   🔲 0.00   **FUD** XXX   N
AMA: 2015,Jun,10; 2015,Apr,3; 2010,Dec,7-10

82941 **Gastrin**
EXCLUDES   *Qualitative column chromotography report specific analyte or (82542)*
🔲 0.00   🔲 0.00   **FUD** XXX   N
AMA: 2015,Jun,10; 2015,Apr,3; 2010,Dec,7-10

82943 **Glucagon**
🔲 0.00   🔲 0.00   **FUD** XXX   N
AMA: 2015,Jun,10; 2015,Apr,3; 2010,Dec,7-10

82945 **Glucose, body fluid, other than blood**
🔲 0.00   🔲 0.00   **FUD** XXX   N ▱
AMA: 2015,Jun,10; 2015,Apr,3; 2010,Dec,7-10

82946 **Glucagon tolerance test**
🔲 0.00   🔲 0.00   **FUD** XXX   N
AMA: 2015,Jun,10; 2015,Apr,3; 2010,Dec,7-10

82947-82962 Chemistry: Glucose Testing

CMS: 100-3,190.20 Blood Glucose Testing

INCLUDES   Clinical information not requested by the ordering physician
Mathematically calculated results
Quantitative analysis unless otherwise specified
Specimens from any source unless otherwise specified
EXCLUDES   *Calculated results that represent a score or probability that was derived by algorithm*
Organ or disease panels (80048-80076 [80081])
Therapeutic drug assays (80150-80299 [80164, 80165, 80171])
Code also glucose administration injection (96374)
Do not report analytes from nonrequested laboratory analysis

82947 **Glucose; quantitative, blood (except reagent strip)**
🔲 0.00   🔲 0.00   **FUD** XXX   X N ▱
AMA: 2015,Jun,10; 2015,Apr,3; 2015,Jan,16; 2014,Jan,11; 2013,Apr,10-11; 2010,Dec,7-10

82948 **blood, reagent strip**
🔲 0.00   🔲 0.00   **FUD** XXX   N ▱
AMA: 2015,Jun,10; 2015,Apr,3; 2015,Jan,16; 2014,Jan,11; 2012,Jan,15-42; 2011,Oct,8; 2011,Jan,11; 2010,Dec,7-10; 2010,Nov,8

82950 **post glucose dose (includes glucose)**
🔲 0.00   🔲 0.00   **FUD** XXX   X N ▱
AMA: 2015,Jun,10; 2015,Apr,3; 2015,Jan,16; 2014,Jan,11; 2012,Jan,15-42; 2011,Jan,11; 2010,Dec,7-10

82951 **tolerance test (GTT), 3 specimens (includes glucose)**
🔲 0.00   🔲 0.00   **FUD** XXX   X N ▱
AMA: 2015,Jun,10; 2015,Apr,3; 2015,Jan,16; 2014,Jan,11; 2012,Jan,15-42; 2011,Jan,11; 2010,Dec,7-10

+ **82952** **tolerance test, each additional beyond 3 specimens (List separately in addition to code for primary procedure)**
Code first (82951)
🔲 0.00   🔲 0.00   **FUD** XXX   X N ▱
AMA: 2015,Jun,10; 2015,Apr,3; 2015,Jan,16; 2014,Jan,11; 2012,Jan,15-42; 2011,Jan,11; 2010,Dec,7-10

82955 **Glucose-6-phosphate dehydrogenase (G6PD); quantitative**
🔲 0.00   🔲 0.00   **FUD** XXX   N
AMA: 2015,Jun,10; 2015,Apr,3; 2010,Dec,7-10

82960 **screen**
🔲 0.00   🔲 0.00   **FUD** XXX   N
AMA: 2015,Jun,10; 2015,Apr,3; 2010,Dec,7-10

82962 **Glucose, blood by glucose monitoring device(s) cleared by the FDA specifically for home use**
🔲 0.00   🔲 0.00   **FUD** XXX   X N ▱
AMA: 2015,Jun,10; 2015,Apr,3; 2015,Jan,16; 2014,Jan,11; 2012,Jan,15-42; 2011,Oct,8; 2011,Jan,11; 2010,Dec,7-10; 2010,Nov,8

82963-83690 Chemistry: Glucosidase—Lipase

INCLUDES   Clinical information not requested by the ordering physician
Mathematically calculated results
Quantitative analysis unless otherwise specified
Specimens from any source unless otherwise specified
EXCLUDES   *Calculated results that represent a score or probability that was derived by algorithm*
Drug testing ([80300, 80301, 80302, 80303, 80304], [80324, 80325, 80326, 80327, 80328, 80329, 80330, 80331, 80332, 80333, 80334, 80335, 80336, 80337, 80338, 80339, 80340, 80341, 80342, 80343, 80344, 80345, 80346, 80347, 80348, 80349, 80350, 80351, 80352, 80353, 80354, 80355, 80356, 80357, 80358, 80359, 80360, 80361, 80362, 80363, 80364, 80365, 80366, 80367, 80368, 80369, 80370, 80371, 80372, 80373, 80374, 80375, 80376, 80377, 83992])
Organ or disease panels (80048-80076 [80081])
Therapeutic drug assays (80150-80299 [80164, 80165, 80171])
Do not report analytes from nonrequested laboratory analysis

82963 **Glucosidase, beta**
🔲 0.00   🔲 0.00   **FUD** XXX   N
AMA: 2015,Jun,10; 2015,Apr,3; 2010,Dec,7-10

82965 **Glutamate dehydrogenase**
🔲 0.00   🔲 0.00   **FUD** XXX   N
AMA: 2015,Jun,10; 2015,Apr,3; 2010,Dec,7-10

82977 **Glutamyltransferase, gamma (GGT)**
🔲 0.00   🔲 0.00   **FUD** XXX   X N
AMA: 2015,Jun,10; 2015,Apr,3; 2015,Jan,16; 2014,Jan,11; 2010,Dec,7-10

82978 **Glutathione**
🔲 0.00   🔲 0.00   **FUD** XXX   N
AMA: 2015,Jun,10; 2015,Apr,3; 2010,Dec,7-10

82979 **Glutathione reductase, RBC**
🔲 0.00   🔲 0.00   **FUD** XXX   N
AMA: 2015,Jun,10; 2015,Apr,3; 2010,Dec,7-10

82985 **Glycated protein**
EXCLUDES   *Gonadotropin chorionic (hCG) (84702-84703)*
🔲 0.00   🔲 0.00   **FUD** XXX   X N ▱
AMA: 2015,Jun,10; 2015,Apr,3; 2015,Jan,16; 2014,Jan,11; 2010,Dec,7-10

83001 **Gonadotropin; follicle stimulating hormone (FSH)**
🔲 0.00   🔲 0.00   **FUD** XXX   X N ▱
AMA: 2015,Jun,10; 2015,Apr,3; 2010,Dec,7-10

83002 **luteinizing hormone (LH)**
EXCLUDES   *Luteinizing releasing factor (LRH) (83727)*
🔲 0.00   🔲 0.00   **FUD** XXX   X N ▱
AMA: 2015,Jun,10; 2015,Apr,3; 2010,Dec,7-10

83003 **Growth hormone, human (HGH) (somatotropin)**
EXCLUDES   *Antibody to human growth hormone (86277)*
🔲 0.00   🔲 0.00   **FUD** XXX   N ▱
AMA: 2015,Jun,10; 2015,Apr,3; 2010,Dec,7-10

83006 **Growth stimulation expressed gene 2 (ST2, Interleukin 1 receptor like-1)**
🔲 0.00   🔲 0.00   **FUD** XXX   N
AMA: 2015,Jun,10; 2015,Apr,3

83009 **Helicobacter pylori, blood test analysis for urease activity, non-radioactive isotope (eg, C-13)**
EXCLUDES   *H. pylori, breath test analysis for urease activity (83013-83014)*
🔲 0.00   🔲 0.00   **FUD** XXX   N
AMA: 2015,Jun,10; 2015,Apr,3; 2010,Dec,7-10

83010 **Haptoglobin; quantitative**
🔲 0.00   🔲 0.00   **FUD** XXX   N
AMA: 2015,Jun,10; 2015,Apr,3; 2010,Dec,7-10

83012 **phenotypes**
🔲 0.00   🔲 0.00   **FUD** XXX   N
AMA: 2015,Jun,10; 2015,Apr,3; 2010,Dec,7-10

83013 **Helicobacter pylori; breath test analysis for urease activity, non-radioactive isotope (eg, C-13)**
🚑 0.00   ⊘ 0.00   **FUD** XXX   N ▭
AMA: 2015,Jun,10; 2015,Apr,3; 2015,Jan,16; 2014,Jan,11; 2010,Dec,7-10

83014 **drug administration**
EXCLUDES   *H. pylori:*
Blood test analysis for urease activity (83009)
Enzyme immunoassay (87339)
Liquid scintillation counter (78267-78268)
Stool (87338)
🚑 0.00   ⊘ 0.00   **FUD** XXX   N ▭
AMA: 2015,Jun,10; 2015,Apr,3; 2015,Jan,16; 2014,Jan,11; 2010,Dec,7-10

83015 **Heavy metal (eg, arsenic, barium, beryllium, bismuth, antimony, mercury); screen**
INCLUDES   Reinsch test
🚑 0.00   ⊘ 0.00   **FUD** XXX   N
AMA: 2015,Jun,10; 2015,Apr,3; 2010,Dec,7-10

83018 **quantitative, each**
🚑 0.00   ⊘ 0.00   **FUD** XXX   N
AMA: 2015,Jun,10; 2015,Apr,3; 2010,Dec,7-10

83020 **Hemoglobin fractionation and quantitation; electrophoresis (eg, A2, S, C, and/or F)**
🚑 0.00   ⊘ 0.00   **FUD** XXX   N ▭
AMA: 2015,Jun,10; 2015,Apr,3; 2010,Dec,7-10

83021 **chromatography (eg, A2, S, C, and/or F)**
EXCLUDES   *Analysis of glycosylated (A1c) hemoglobin by chromatography or electrophoresis without an identified hemoglobin variant (83036)*
🚑 0.00   ⊘ 0.00   **FUD** XXX   N ▭
AMA: 2015,Jun,10; 2015,Apr,3; 2015,Jan,16; 2014,Jan,11; 2010,Dec,7-10

83026 **Hemoglobin; by copper sulfate method, non-automated**
🚑 0.00   ⊘ 0.00   **FUD** XXX   ☒ N
AMA: 2015,Jun,10; 2015,Apr,3; 2010,Dec,7-10

83030 **F (fetal), chemical**
🚑 0.00   ⊘ 0.00   **FUD** XXX   N ▭
AMA: 2015,Jun,10; 2015,Apr,3; 2010,Dec,7-10

83033 **F (fetal), qualitative**
🚑 0.00   ⊘ 0.00   **FUD** XXX   N ▭
AMA: 2015,Jun,10; 2015,Apr,3; 2010,Dec,7-10

83036 **glycosylated (A1C)**
EXCLUDES   *Analysis of glycosylated (A1c) hemoglobin by chromatography or electrophoresis without an identified hemoglobin variant (83021)*
Detection of hemoglobin, fecal, by immunoassay (82274)
🚑 0.00   ⊘ 0.00   **FUD** XXX   ☒ N
AMA: 2015,Jun,10; 2015,Apr,3; 2015,Jan,16; 2014,Jan,11; 2010,Dec,7-10

83037 **glycosylated (A1C) by device cleared by FDA for home use**
🚑 0.00   ⊘ 0.00   **FUD** XXX   ☒ N
AMA: 2015,Jun,10; 2015,Apr,3; 2015,Jan,16; 2014,Jan,11; 2012,Jan,15-42; 2011,Jan,11; 2010,Dec,7-10

83045 **methemoglobin, qualitative**
🚑 0.00   ⊘ 0.00   **FUD** XXX   N
AMA: 2015,Jun,10; 2015,Apr,3; 2010,Dec,7-10

83050 **methemoglobin, quantitative**
EXCLUDES   *Transcutaneous methemoglobin test (88741)*
🚑 0.00   ⊘ 0.00   **FUD** XXX   N
AMA: 2015,Jun,10; 2015,Apr,3; 2015,Jan,16; 2014,Jan,11; 2010,Dec,7-10

83051 **plasma**
🚑 0.00   ⊘ 0.00   **FUD** XXX   N
AMA: 2015,Jun,10; 2015,Apr,3; 2010,Dec,7-10

83060 **sulfhemoglobin, quantitative**
🚑 0.00   ⊘ 0.00   **FUD** XXX   N
AMA: 2015,Jun,10; 2015,Apr,3; 2010,Dec,7-10

83065 **thermolabile**
🚑 0.00   ⊘ 0.00   **FUD** XXX   N
AMA: 2015,Jun,10; 2015,Apr,3; 2010,Dec,7-10

83068 **unstable, screen**
🚑 0.00   ⊘ 0.00   **FUD** XXX   N ▭
AMA: 2015,Jun,10; 2015,Apr,3; 2010,Dec,7-10

83069 **urine**
🚑 0.00   ⊘ 0.00   **FUD** XXX   N
AMA: 2015,Jun,10; 2015,Apr,3; 2010,Dec,7-10

83070 **Hemosiderin, qualitative**
EXCLUDES   *Qualitative column chromatography report specific analyte or (82542)*
🚑 0.00   ⊘ 0.00   **FUD** XXX   N
AMA: 2015,Jun,10; 2015,Apr,3; 2010,Dec,7-10

83080 **b-Hexosaminidase, each assay**
🚑 0.00   ⊘ 0.00   **FUD** XXX   N
AMA: 2015,Jun,10; 2015,Apr,3; 2010,Dec,7-10

83088 **Histamine**
🚑 0.00   ⊘ 0.00   **FUD** XXX   N
AMA: 2015,Jun,10; 2015,Apr,3; 2010,Dec,7-10

83090 **Homocysteine**
🚑 0.00   ⊘ 0.00   **FUD** XXX   N ▭
AMA: 2015,Jun,10; 2015,Apr,3; 2015,Jan,16; 2014,Jan,11; 2012,Jan,15-42; 2011,Jan,11; 2010,Dec,7-10

83150 **Homovanillic acid (HVA)**
🚑 0.00   ⊘ 0.00   **FUD** XXX   N
AMA: 2015,Jun,10; 2015,Apr,3; 2010,Dec,7-10

83491 **Hydroxycorticosteroids, 17- (17-OHCS)**
EXCLUDES   *Cortisol (82530, 82533)*
Deoxycortisol (82634)
🚑 0.00   ⊘ 0.00   **FUD** XXX   N
AMA: 2015,Jun,10; 2015,Apr,3; 2010,Dec,7-10

83497 **Hydroxyindolacetic acid, 5-(HIAA)**
EXCLUDES   *Urine qualitative test (81005)*
🚑 0.00   ⊘ 0.00   **FUD** XXX   N
AMA: 2015,Jun,10; 2015,Apr,3; 2010,Dec,7-10

83498 **Hydroxyprogesterone, 17-d**
🚑 0.00   ⊘ 0.00   **FUD** XXX   N ▭
AMA: 2015,Jun,10; 2015,Apr,3; 2010,Dec,7-10

83499 **Hydroxyprogesterone, 20-**
🚑 0.00   ⊘ 0.00   **FUD** XXX   N
AMA: 2015,Jun,10; 2015,Apr,3; 2010,Dec,7-10

83500 **Hydroxyproline; free**
🚑 0.00   ⊘ 0.00   **FUD** XXX   N
AMA: 2015,Jun,10; 2015,Apr,3; 2010,Dec,7-10

83505 **total**
🚑 0.00   ⊘ 0.00   **FUD** XXX   N
AMA: 2015,Jun,10; 2015,Apr,3; 2010,Dec,7-10

83516 **Immunoassay for analyte other than infectious agent antibody or infectious agent antigen; qualitative or semiquantitative, multiple step method**
🚑 0.00   ⊘ 0.00   **FUD** XXX   ☒ N ▭
AMA: 2015,Jun,10; 2015,Apr,3; 2010,Dec,7-10

83518 **qualitative or semiquantitative, single step method (eg, reagent strip)**
🚑 0.00   ⊘ 0.00   **FUD** XXX   N
AMA: 2015,Jun,10; 2015,Apr,3; 2010,Dec,7-10

83519 **quantitative, by radioimmunoassay (eg, RIA)**
🚑 0.00   ⊘ 0.00   **FUD** XXX   N ▭
AMA: 2015,Jun,10; 2015,Apr,3; 2015,Jan,16; 2014,Jan,11; 2010,Dec,7-10

83520	**quantitative, not otherwise specified**

🔲 0.00   🖎 0.00   **FUD** XXX   N ▢

AMA: 2015,Jun,10; 2015,Apr,3; 2010,Dec,7-10

83525	**Insulin; total**

EXCLUDES   *Proinsulin (84206)*

🔲 0.00   🖎 0.00   **FUD** XXX   N ▢

AMA: 2015,Jun,10; 2015,Apr,3; 2010,Dec,7-10

83527	**free**

🔲 0.00   🖎 0.00   **FUD** XXX   N

AMA: 2015,Jun,10; 2015,Apr,3; 2015,Jan,16; 2014,Jan,11;
2010,Dec,7-10

83528	**Intrinsic factor**

EXCLUDES   *Intrinsic factor antibodies (86340)*

🔲 0.00   🖎 0.00   **FUD** XXX   N

AMA: 2015,Jun,10; 2015,Apr,3; 2010,Dec,7-10

83540	**Iron**

🔲 0.00   🖎 0.00   **FUD** XXX   N

AMA: 2015,Jun,10; 2015,Apr,3; 2015,Jan,16; 2014,Jan,11;
2010,Dec,7-10

83550	**Iron binding capacity**

🔲 0.00   🖎 0.00   **FUD** XXX   N

AMA: 2015,Jun,10; 2015,Apr,3; 2010,Dec,7-10

83570	**Isocitric dehydrogenase (IDH)**

🔲 0.00   🖎 0.00   **FUD** XXX   N

AMA: 2015,Jun,10; 2015,Apr,3; 2010,Dec,7-10

83582	**Ketogenic steroids, fractionation**

🔲 0.00   🖎 0.00   **FUD** XXX   N

AMA: 2015,Jun,10; 2015,Apr,3; 2010,Dec,7-10

83586	**Ketosteroids, 17- (17-KS); total**

🔲 0.00   🖎 0.00   **FUD** XXX   N

AMA: 2015,Jun,10; 2015,Apr,3; 2010,Dec,7-10

83593	**fractionation**

🔲 0.00   🖎 0.00   **FUD** XXX   N

AMA: 2015,Jun,10; 2015,Apr,3; 2010,Dec,7-10

83605	**Lactate (lactic acid)**

🔲 0.00   🖎 0.00   **FUD** XXX   ✖ N

AMA: 2015,Jun,10; 2015,Apr,3; 2010,Dec,7-10

83615	**Lactate dehydrogenase (LD), (LDH);**

🔲 0.00   🖎 0.00   **FUD** XXX   N

AMA: 2015,Jun,10; 2015,Apr,3; 2015,Jan,16; 2014,Jan,11;
2010,Dec,7-10

83625	**isoenzymes, separation and quantitation**

🔲 0.00   🖎 0.00   **FUD** XXX   N ▢

AMA: 2015,Jun,10; 2015,Apr,3; 2015,Jan,16; 2014,Jan,11;
2010,Dec,7-10

83630	**Lactoferrin, fecal; qualitative**

🔲 0.00   🖎 0.00   **FUD** XXX   N

AMA: 2015,Jun,10; 2015,Apr,3; 2015,Jan,16; 2014,Jan,11;
2010,Dec,7-10

83631	**quantitative**

🔲 0.00   🖎 0.00   **FUD** XXX   N

AMA: 2015,Jun,10; 2015,Apr,3; 2015,Jan,16; 2014,Jan,11;
2012,Jan,15-42; 2011,Jan,11; 2010,Dec,7-10

83632	**Lactogen, human placental (HPL) human chorionic somatomammotropin**

🔲 0.00   🖎 0.00   **FUD** XXX   N

AMA: 2015,Jun,10; 2015,Apr,3; 2010,Dec,7-10

83633	**Lactose, urine, qualitative**

🔲 0.00   🖎 0.00   **FUD** XXX   N

AMA: 2015,Jun,10; 2015,Apr,3; 2010,Dec,7-10

83655	**Lead**

🔲 0.00   🖎 0.00   **FUD** XXX   ✖ N

AMA: 2015,Jun,10; 2015,Apr,3; 2010,Dec,7-10

83661	**Fetal lung maturity assessment; lecithin sphingomyelin (L/S) ratio**

🔲 0.00   🖎 0.00   **FUD** XXX   N ▢

AMA: 2015,Jun,10; 2015,Apr,3; 2015,Jan,16; 2014,Jan,11;
2010,Dec,7-10

83662	**foam stability test**

🔲 0.00   🖎 0.00   **FUD** XXX   N ▢

AMA: 2015,Jun,10; 2015,Apr,3; 2010,Dec,7-10

83663	**fluorescence polarization**

🔲 0.00   🖎 0.00   **FUD** XXX   N ▢

AMA: 2015,Jun,10; 2015,Apr,3; 2010,Dec,7-10

83664	**lamellar body density**

EXCLUDES   *Phosphatidylglycerol (84081)*

🔲 0.00   🖎 0.00   **FUD** XXX   N ▢

AMA: 2015,Jun,10; 2015,Apr,3; 2010,Dec,7-10

83670	**Leucine aminopeptidase (LAP)**

🔲 0.00   🖎 0.00   **FUD** XXX   N

AMA: 2015,Jun,10; 2015,Apr,3; 2010,Dec,7-10

83690	**Lipase**

🔲 0.00   🖎 0.00   **FUD** XXX   N

AMA: 2015,Jun,10; 2015,Apr,3; 2010,Dec,7-10

83695-83727 Chemistry: Lipoprotein—Luteinizing Releasing Factor

INCLUDES   Clinical information not requested by the ordering physician
Mathematically calculated results
Quantitative analysis unless otherwise specified
Specimens from any source unless otherwise specified

EXCLUDES   *Calculated results that represent a score or probability that was derived by algorithm*
Organ or disease panels (80048-80076 [80081])
Therapeutic drug assays (80150-80299 [80164, 80165, 80171])
Do not report analytes from nonrequested laboratory analysis

83695	**Lipoprotein (a)**

🔲 0.00   🖎 0.00   **FUD** XXX   N

AMA: 2015,Jun,10; 2015,Apr,3; 2015,Jan,16; 2014,Jan,11;
2010,Dec,7-10

83698	**Lipoprotein-associated phospholipase A2 (Lp-PLA2)**

🔲 0.00   🖎 0.00   **FUD** XXX   N

AMA: 2015,Jun,10; 2015,Apr,3; 2010,Dec,7-10

83700	**Lipoprotein, blood; electrophoretic separation and quantitation**

🔲 0.00   🖎 0.00   **FUD** XXX   N

AMA: 2015,Jun,10; 2015,Apr,3; 2015,Jan,16; 2014,Jan,11;
2010,Dec,7-10

83701	**high resolution fractionation and quantitation of lipoproteins including lipoprotein subclasses when performed (eg, electrophoresis, ultracentrifugation)**

🔲 0.00   🖎 0.00   **FUD** XXX   N

AMA: 2015,Jun,10; 2015,Apr,3; 2015,Jan,16; 2014,Jan,11;
2010,Dec,7-10

83704	**quantitation of lipoprotein particle numbers and lipoprotein particle subclasses (eg, by nuclear magnetic resonance spectroscopy)**

🔲 0.00   🖎 0.00   **FUD** XXX   N

AMA: 2015,Jun,10; 2015,Apr,3; 2015,Jan,16; 2014,Jan,11;
2010,Dec,7-10

83718	**Lipoprotein, direct measurement; high density cholesterol (HDL cholesterol)**

🔲 0.00   🖎 0.00   **FUD** XXX   ✖ N ▢

AMA: 2015,Jun,10; 2015,Apr,3; 2015,Jan,16; 2014,Jan,11;
2013,Feb,3-6; 2012,Jan,15-42; 2011,Jan,11; 2010,Dec,7-10

83719	**VLDL cholesterol**

🔲 0.00   🖎 0.00   **FUD** XXX   N ▢

AMA: 2015,Jun,10; 2015,Apr,3; 2015,Jan,16; 2014,Jan,11;
2013,Feb,3-6; 2012,Jan,15-42; 2011,Jan,11; 2010,Dec,7-10

83721	**LDL cholesterol**
	EXCLUDES *Fractionation by high resolution electrophoresis or ultracentrifugation (83701)*
	Lipoprotein particle numbers and subclasses analysis by nuclear magnetic resonance spectroscopy (83704)

0.00   0.00   **FUD** XXX   ☒ N ▯

AMA: 2015,Jun,10; 2015,Apr,3; 2015,Jan,16; 2014,Jan,11; 2013,Feb,3-6; 2012,Jan,15-42; 2011,Jan,11; 2010,Dec,7-10

| 83727 | **Luteinizing releasing factor (LRH)** |

0.00   0.00   **FUD** XXX   N

AMA: 2015,Jun,10; 2015,Apr,3; 2010,Dec,7-10

83735-83885 Chemistry: Magnesium—Nickel

INCLUDES Clinical information not requested by the ordering physician
Mathematically calculated results
Quantitative analysis unless otherwise specified
Specimens from any source unless otherwise specified

EXCLUDES *Calculated results that represent a score or probability that was derived by algorithm*
Organ or disease panels (80048-80076 [80081])
Therapeutic drug assays (80150-80299 [80164, 80165, 80171])
Do not report analytes from nonrequested laboratory analysis

| 83735 | **Magnesium** |

0.00   0.00   **FUD** XXX   N

AMA: 2015,Jun,10; 2015,Apr,3; 2010,Dec,7-10

| 83775 | **Malate dehydrogenase** |

0.00   0.00   **FUD** XXX   N

AMA: 2015,Jun,10; 2015,Apr,3; 2010,Dec,7-10

| 83785 | **Manganese** |

0.00   0.00   **FUD** XXX   N

AMA: 2015,Jun,10; 2015,Apr,3; 2010,Dec,7-10

| 83788 | ~~Mass spectrometry and tandem mass spectrometry (MS, MS/MS), analyte not elsewhere specified; qualitative, each specimen~~ |

To report, see specific analyte or ~83789

▲ | 83789 | **Mass spectrometry and tandem mass spectrometry (eg, MS, MS/MS, MALDI, MS-TOF, QTOF), non-drug analyte(s) not elsewhere specified, qualitative or quantitative, each specimen** |

Do not report more than one time per specimen

0.00   0.00   **FUD** XXX   N ▯

AMA: 2015,Jun,10; 2015,Apr,3; 2010,Dec,7-10

| 83825 | **Mercury, quantitative** |
| | EXCLUDES *Mercury screen (83015)* |

0.00   0.00   **FUD** XXX   N

AMA: 2015,Jun,10; 2015,Apr,3; 2010,Dec,7-10

| 83835 | **Metanephrines** |
| | EXCLUDES *Catecholamines (82382-82384)* |

0.00   0.00   **FUD** XXX   N

AMA: 2015,Jun,10; 2015,Apr,3; 2010,Dec,7-10

| 83857 | **Methemalbumin** |

0.00   0.00   **FUD** XXX   N

AMA: 2015,Jun,10; 2015,Apr,3; 2010,Dec,7-10

| 83861 | **Microfluidic analysis utilizing an integrated collection and analysis device, tear osmolarity** |

Code also when performed on both eyes 83861 X 2

0.00   0.00   **FUD** XXX   ☒ N

AMA: 2015,Jun,10; 2015,Apr,3; 2010,Dec,7-10; 2010,Dec,11

| 83864 | **Mucopolysaccharides, acid, quantitative** |

0.00   0.00   **FUD** XXX   N

AMA: 2015,Jun,10; 2015,Apr,3; 2010,Dec,7-10

| 83872 | **Mucin, synovial fluid (Ropes test)** |

0.00   0.00   **FUD** XXX   N

AMA: 2015,Jun,10; 2015,Apr,3; 2010,Dec,7-10

| 83873 | **Myelin basic protein, cerebrospinal fluid** |
| | EXCLUDES *Oligoclonal bands (83916)* |

0.00   0.00   **FUD** XXX   N

AMA: 2015,Jun,10; 2015,Apr,3; 2010,Dec,7-10

| 83874 | **Myoglobin** |

0.00   0.00   **FUD** XXX   N

AMA: 2015,Jun,10; 2015,Apr,3; 2015,Jan,16; 2014,Jan,11; 2010,Dec,7-10

| 83876 | **Myeloperoxidase (MPO)** |

0.00   0.00   **FUD** XXX   N

AMA: 2015,Jun,10; 2015,Apr,3; 2010,Dec,7-10

| 83880 | **Natriuretic peptide** |

0.00   0.00   **FUD** XXX   ☒ N

AMA: 2015,Jun,10; 2015,Apr,3; 2015,Jan,16; 2014,Jan,11; 2010,Dec,7-10

| 83883 | **Nephelometry, each analyte not elsewhere specified** |

0.00   0.00   **FUD** XXX   N

AMA: 2015,Jun,10; 2015,Apr,3; 2010,Dec,7-10

| 83885 | **Nickel** |

0.00   0.00   **FUD** XXX   N

AMA: 2015,Jun,10; 2015,Apr,3; 2010,Dec,7-10

83915-84066 Chemistry: Nucleotidase 5'- —Phosphatase (Acid)

INCLUDES Clinical information not requested by the ordering physician
Mathematically calculated results
Quantitative analysis unless otherwise specified
Specimens from any source unless otherwise specified

EXCLUDES *Calculated results that represent a score or probability that was derived by algorithm*
Drug testing ([80300, 80301, 80302, 80303, 80304], [80324, 80325, 80326, 80327, 80328, 80329, 80330, 80331, 80332, 80333, 80334, 80335, 80336, 80337, 80338, 80339, 80340, 80341, 80342, 80343, 80344, 80345, 80346, 80347, 80348, 80349, 80350, 80351, 80352, 80353, 80354, 80355, 80356, 80357, 80358, 80359, 80360, 80361, 80362, 80363, 80364, 80365, 80366, 80367, 80368, 80369, 80370, 80371, 80372, 80373, 80374, 80375, 80376, 80377, 83992])
Organ or disease panels (80048-80299 [80081, 80164, 80165, 80171, 80300, 80301, 80302, 80303, 80304, 80320, 80321, 80322, 80323, 80324, 80325, 80326, 80327, 80328, 80329, 80330, 80331, 80332, 80333, 80334, 80335, 80336, 80337, 80338, 80339, 80340, 80341, 80342, 80343, 80344, 80345, 80346, 80347, 80348, 80349, 80350, 80351, 80352, 80353, 80354, 80355, 80356, 80357, 80358, 80359, 80360, 80361, 80362, 80363, 80364, 80365, 80366, 80367, 80368, 80369, 80370, 80371, 80372, 80373, 80374, 80375, 80376, 80377, 83992])
Therapeutic drug assays (80150-80299 [80164, 80165, 80171])
Do not report analytes from nonrequested laboratory analysis

| 83915 | **Nucleotidase 5'-** |

0.00   0.00   **FUD** XXX   N

AMA: 2015,Jun,10; 2015,Apr,3; 2010,Dec,7-10

| 83916 | **Oligoclonal immune (oligoclonal bands)** |

0.00   0.00   **FUD** XXX   N ▯

AMA: 2015,Jun,10; 2015,Apr,3; 2010,Dec,7-10

| 83918 | **Organic acids; total, quantitative, each specimen** |

0.00   0.00   **FUD** XXX   N ▯

AMA: 2015,Jun,10; 2015,Apr,3; 2015,Jan,16; 2014,Jan,11; 2012,Jan,15-42; 2011,Jan,11; 2010,Dec,7-10

| 83919 | **qualitative, each specimen** |

0.00   0.00   **FUD** XXX   N

AMA: 2015,Jun,10; 2015,Apr,3; 2010,Dec,7-10

| 83921 | **Organic acid, single, quantitative** |

0.00   0.00   **FUD** XXX   N ▯

AMA: 2015,Jun,10; 2015,Apr,3; 2010,Dec,7-10

| 83930 | **Osmolality; blood** |
| | EXCLUDES *Tear osmolarity (83861)* |

0.00   0.00   **FUD** XXX   N

AMA: 2015,Jun,10; 2015,Apr,3; 2010,Dec,7-10

| 83935 | **urine** |
| | EXCLUDES *Tear osmolarity (83861)* |

0.00   0.00   **FUD** XXX   N

AMA: 2015,Jun,10; 2015,Apr,3; 2010,Dec,7-10

| 83937 | **Osteocalcin (bone g1a protein)** |

0.00   0.00   **FUD** XXX   N

AMA: 2015,Jun,10; 2015,Apr,3; 2015,Jan,16; 2014,Jan,11; 2010,Dec,7-10

83945   **Oxalate**
     🚑 0.00   ⚗ 0.00   **FUD** XXX   N
     AMA: 2015,Jun,10; 2015,Apr,3; 2010,Dec,7-10

83950   **Oncoprotein; HER-2/neu**
     EXCLUDES   *Tissue (88342, 88365)*
     🚑 0.00   ⚗ 0.00   **FUD** XXX   N ▫
     AMA: 2015,Jun,10; 2015,Apr,3; 2010,Dec,7-10

83951   **des-gamma-carboxy-prothrombin (DCP)**
     🚑 0.00   ⚗ 0.00   **FUD** XXX   N
     AMA: 2015,Jun,10; 2015,Apr,3; 2010,Dec,7-10

83970   **Parathormone (parathyroid hormone)**
     🚑 0.00   ⚗ 0.00   **FUD** XXX   N
     AMA: 2015,Jun,10; 2015,Apr,3; 2010,Dec,7-10

83986   **pH; body fluid, not otherwise specified**
     EXCLUDES   *Blood pH (82800, 82803)*
     🚑 0.00   ⚗ 0.00   **FUD** XXX   ✕ N
     AMA: 2015,Jun,10; 2015,Apr,3; 2015,Jan,16; 2013,Sep,13-14; 2010,Dec,7-10

83987   **exhaled breath condensate**
     🚑 0.00   ⚗ 0.00   **FUD** XXX   N
     AMA: 2015,Jun,10; 2015,Apr,3; 2010,Dec,7-10

83992   **Resequenced code. See code following 80365.**

83993   **Calprotectin, fecal**
     🚑 0.00   ⚗ 0.00   **FUD** XXX   N
     AMA: 2015,Jun,10; 2015,Apr,3; 2015,Jan,16; 2014,Jan,11; 2010,Dec,7-10

84030   **Phenylalanine (PKU), blood**
     INCLUDES   Guthrie test
     EXCLUDES   *Phenylalanine-tyrosine ratio (84030, 84510)*
     🚑 0.00   ⚗ 0.00   **FUD** XXX   N
     AMA: 2015,Jun,10; 2015,Apr,3; 2010,Dec,7-10

84035   **Phenylketones, qualitative**
     🚑 0.00   ⚗ 0.00   **FUD** XXX   N
     AMA: 2015,Jun,10; 2015,Apr,3; 2010,Dec,7-10

84060   **Phosphatase, acid; total**
     🚑 0.00   ⚗ 0.00   **FUD** XXX   N
     AMA: 2015,Jun,10; 2015,Apr,3; 2010,Dec,7-10

84061   **forensic examination**
     🚑 0.00   ⚗ 0.00   **FUD** XXX   N
     AMA: 2015,Jun,10; 2015,Apr,3; 2010,Dec,7-10

84066   **prostatic**
     🚑 0.00   ⚗ 0.00   **FUD** XXX   N
     AMA: 2015,Jun,10; 2015,Apr,3; 2010,Dec,7-10

84075-84080 Chemistry: Phosphatase (Alkaline)

CMS: 100-3,160.17 Payment for L-Dopa /Associated Inpatient Hospital Services

INCLUDES   Clinical information not requested by the ordering physician
               Mathematically calculated results
               Quantitative analysis unless otherwise specified
               Specimens from any source unless otherwise specified
EXCLUDES   *Calculated results that represent a score or probability that was derived by algorithm*
               Organ or disease panels (80048-80076 [80081])
Do not report analytes from nonrequested laboratory analysis

84075   **Phosphatase, alkaline;**
     🚑 0.00   ⚗ 0.00   **FUD** XXX   ✕ N
     AMA: 2015,Jun,10; 2015,Apr,3; 2015,Jan,16; 2014,Jan,11; 2010,Dec,7-10

84078   **heat stable (total not included)**
     🚑 0.00   ⚗ 0.00   **FUD** XXX   N
     AMA: 2015,Jun,10; 2015,Apr,3; 2010,Dec,7-10

84080   **isoenzymes**
     🚑 0.00   ⚗ 0.00   **FUD** XXX   N ▫
     AMA: 2015,Jun,10; 2015,Apr,3; 2010,Dec,7-10

84081-84150 Chemistry: Phosphatidylglycerol—Prostaglandin

INCLUDES   Clinical information not requested by the ordering physician
               Mathematically calculated results
               Quantitative analysis unless otherwise specified
               Specimens from any source unless otherwise specified
EXCLUDES   *Calculated results that represent a score or probability that was derived by algorithm*
               Organ or disease panels (80048-80076 [80081])
               Therapeutic drug assays (80150-80299 [80164, 80165, 80171])
Do not report analytes from nonrequested laboratory analysis

84081   **Phosphatidylglycerol**
     🚑 0.00   ⚗ 0.00   **FUD** XXX   N
     AMA: 2015,Jun,10; 2015,Apr,3; 2010,Dec,7-10

84085   **Phosphogluconate, 6-, dehydrogenase, RBC**
     🚑 0.00   ⚗ 0.00   **FUD** XXX   N
     AMA: 2015,Jun,10; 2015,Apr,3; 2010,Dec,7-10

84087   **Phosphohexose isomerase**
     🚑 0.00   ⚗ 0.00   **FUD** XXX   N
     AMA: 2015,Jun,10; 2015,Apr,3; 2010,Dec,7-10

84100   **Phosphorus inorganic (phosphate);**
     🚑 0.00   ⚗ 0.00   **FUD** XXX   N
     AMA: 2015,Jun,10; 2015,Apr,3; 2015,Jan,16; 2014,Jan,11; 2010,Dec,7-10

84105   **urine**
     🚑 0.00   ⚗ 0.00   **FUD** XXX   N
     AMA: 2015,Jun,10; 2015,Apr,3; 2010,Dec,7-10

84106   **Porphobilinogen, urine; qualitative**
     🚑 0.00   ⚗ 0.00   **FUD** XXX   N
     AMA: 2015,Jun,10; 2015,Apr,3; 2010,Dec,7-10

84110   **quantitative**
     🚑 0.00   ⚗ 0.00   **FUD** XXX   N
     AMA: 2015,Jun,10; 2015,Apr,3; 2010,Dec,7-10

84112   **Evaluation of cervicovaginal fluid for specific amniotic fluid protein(s) (eg, placental alpha microglobulin-1 [PAMG-1], placental protein 12 [PP12], alpha-fetoprotein), qualitative, each specimen**   ♀
     🚑 0.00   ⚗ 0.00   **FUD** XXX   N
     AMA: 2015,Jun,10; 2015,Apr,3; 2010,Dec,7-10

84119   **Porphyrins, urine; qualitative**
     🚑 0.00   ⚗ 0.00   **FUD** XXX   N
     AMA: 2015,Jun,10; 2015,Apr,3; 2010,Dec,7-10

84120   **quantitation and fractionation**
     🚑 0.00   ⚗ 0.00   **FUD** XXX   N
     AMA: 2015,Jun,10; 2015,Apr,3; 2010,Dec,7-10

84126   **Porphyrins, feces, quantitative**
     🚑 0.00   ⚗ 0.00   **FUD** XXX   N
     AMA: 2015,Jun,10; 2015,Apr,3; 2010,Dec,7-10

84132   **Potassium; serum, plasma or whole blood**
     🚑 0.00   ⚗ 0.00   **FUD** XXX   ✕ N
     AMA: 2015,Jun,10; 2015,Apr,3; 2015,Jan,16; 2014,Jan,11; 2013,Apr,10-11; 2010,Dec,7-10

84133   **urine**
     🚑 0.00   ⚗ 0.00   **FUD** XXX   N
     AMA: 2015,Jun,10; 2015,Apr,3; 2010,Dec,7-10

84134   **Prealbumin**
     EXCLUDES   *Microalbumin (82043-82044)*
     🚑 0.00   ⚗ 0.00   **FUD** XXX   N
     AMA: 2015,Jun,10; 2015,Apr,3; 2010,Dec,7-10

84135   **Pregnanediol**   ♀
     🚑 0.00   ⚗ 0.00   **FUD** XXX   N
     AMA: 2015,Jun,10; 2015,Apr,3; 2010,Dec,7-10

84138   **Pregnanetriol**   ♀
     🚑 0.00   ⚗ 0.00   **FUD** XXX   N
     AMA: 2015,Jun,10; 2015,Apr,3; 2010,Dec,7-10

84140 **Pregnenolone**

🔧 0.00   ⚗ 0.00   **FUD** XXX   Ⓝ

AMA: 2015,Jun,10; 2015,Apr,3; 2015,Jan,16; 2014,Jan,11; 2010,Dec,7-10

84143 **17-hydroxypregnenolone**

🔧 0.00   ⚗ 0.00   **FUD** XXX   Ⓝ

AMA: 2015,Jun,10; 2015,Apr,3; 2015,Jan,16; 2014,Jan,11; 2010,Dec,7-10

84144 **Progesterone**

EXCLUDES   *Progesterone receptor assay (84234)*

🔧 0.00   ⚗ 0.00   **FUD** XXX   Ⓝ

AMA: 2015,Jun,10; 2015,Apr,3; 2010,Dec,7-10

84145 **Procalcitonin (PCT)**

🔧 0.00   ⚗ 0.00   **FUD** XXX   Ⓝ

AMA: 2015,Jun,10; 2015,Apr,3; 2010,Dec,7-10

84146 **Prolactin**

🔧 0.00   ⚗ 0.00   **FUD** XXX   Ⓝ ▱

AMA: 2015,Jun,10; 2015,Apr,3; 2010,Dec,7-10

84150 **Prostaglandin, each**

🔧 0.00   ⚗ 0.00   **FUD** XXX   Ⓝ

AMA: 2015,Jun,10; 2015,Apr,3; 2010,Dec,7-10

84152-84154 Chemistry: Prostate Specific Antigen

CMS: 100-3,190.31 Prostate Specific Antigen (PSA); 100-3,210.1 Prostate Cancer Screening Tests

INCLUDES   Clinical information not requested by the ordering physician
Mathematically calculated results
Quantitative analysis unless otherwise specified
EXCLUDES   *Calculated results that represent a score or probability that was derived by algorithm*
Do not report analytes from nonrequested laboratory analysis

84152 **Prostate specific antigen (PSA); complexed (direct measurement)**   ♂

🔧 0.00   ⚗ 0.00   **FUD** XXX   Ⓝ

AMA: 2015,Jun,10; 2015,Apr,3; 2010,Dec,7-10

84153 **total**   ♂

🔧 0.00   ⚗ 0.00   **FUD** XXX   Ⓝ

AMA: 2015,Jun,10; 2015,Apr,3; 2015,Jan,16; 2014,Jan,11; 2012,Jan,15-42; 2011,Jan,11; 2010,Dec,7-10

84154 **free**   ♂

🔧 0.00   ⚗ 0.00   **FUD** XXX   Ⓝ

AMA: 2015,Jun,10; 2015,Apr,3; 2015,Jan,16; 2014,Jan,11; 2012,Jan,15-42; 2011,Jan,11; 2010,Dec,7-10

84155-84157 Chemistry: Protein, Total (Not by Refractometry)

INCLUDES   Clinical information not requested by the ordering physician
Mathematically calculated results
EXCLUDES   *Calculated results that represent a score or probability that was derived by algorithm*
Organ or disease panels (80048-80076 [80081])
Do not report analytes from nonrequested laboratory analysis

84155 **Protein, total, except by refractometry; serum, plasma or whole blood**

🔧 0.00   ⚗ 0.00   **FUD** XXX   ☒ Ⓝ ▱

AMA: 2015,Jun,10; 2015,Apr,3; 2015,Jan,16; 2014,Jan,11; 2010,Dec,7-10

84156 **urine**

🔧 0.00   ⚗ 0.00   **FUD** XXX   Ⓝ

AMA: 2015,Jun,10; 2015,Apr,3; 2010,Dec,7-10

84157 **other source (eg, synovial fluid, cerebrospinal fluid)**

🔧 0.00   ⚗ 0.00   **FUD** XXX   Ⓝ

AMA: 2015,Jun,10; 2015,Apr,3; 2010,Dec,7-10

84160-84432 Chemistry: Protein, Total (Refractometry)—Thyroglobulin

INCLUDES   Clinical information not requested by the ordering physician
Mathematically calculated results
Quantitative analysis unless otherwise specified
Specimens from any source unless otherwise specified
EXCLUDES   *Calculated results that represent a score or probability that was derived by algorithm*
Drug testing ([80300, 80301, 80302, 80303, 80304], [80324, 80325, 80326, 80327, 80328, 80329, 80330, 80331, 80332, 80333, 80334, 80335, 80336, 80337, 80338, 80339, 80340, 80341, 80342, 80343, 80344, 80345, 80346, 80347, 80348, 80349, 80350, 80351, 80352, 80353, 80354, 80355, 80356, 80357, 80358, 80359, 80360, 80361, 80362, 80363, 80364, 80365, 80366, 80367, 80368, 80369, 80370, 80371, 80372, 80373, 80374, 80375, 80376, 80377, 83992])
Organ or disease panels (80048-80076 [80081])
Therapeutic drug assays (80150-80299 [80164, 80165, 80171])
Do not report analytes from nonrequested laboratory analysis

84160 **Protein, total, by refractometry, any source**

EXCLUDES   *Dipstick urine protein (81000-81003)*

🔧 0.00   ⚗ 0.00   **FUD** XXX   Ⓝ ▱

AMA: 2015,Jun,10; 2015,Apr,3; 2010,Dec,7-10

84163 **Pregnancy-associated plasma protein-A (PAPP-A)**   ♀

🔧 0.00   ⚗ 0.00   **FUD** XXX   Ⓝ

AMA: 2015,Jun,10; 2015,Apr,3; 2010,Dec,7-10

84165 **Protein; electrophoretic fractionation and quantitation, serum**

🔧 0.00   ⚗ 0.00   **FUD** XXX   Ⓝ ▱

AMA: 2015,Jun,10; 2015,Apr,3; 2010,Dec,7-10

84166 **electrophoretic fractionation and quantitation, other fluids with concentration (eg, urine, CSF)**

🔧 0.00   ⚗ 0.00   **FUD** XXX   Ⓝ ▱

AMA: 2015,Jun,10; 2015,Apr,3; 2010,Dec,7-10

84181 **Western Blot, with interpretation and report, blood or other body fluid**

🔧 0.00   ⚗ 0.00   **FUD** XXX   Ⓝ ▱

AMA: 2015,Jun,10; 2015,Apr,3; 2010,Dec,7-10

84182 **Western Blot, with interpretation and report, blood or other body fluid, immunological probe for band identification, each**

EXCLUDES   *Western Blot tissue testing (88371)*

🔧 0.00   ⚗ 0.00   **FUD** XXX   Ⓝ ▱

AMA: 2015,Jun,10; 2015,Apr,3; 2010,Dec,7-10

84202 **Protoporphyrin, RBC; quantitative**

🔧 0.00   ⚗ 0.00   **FUD** XXX   Ⓝ

AMA: 2015,Jun,10; 2015,Apr,3; 2010,Dec,7-10

84203 **screen**

🔧 0.00   ⚗ 0.00   **FUD** XXX   Ⓝ

AMA: 2015,Jun,10; 2015,Apr,3; 2010,Dec,7-10

84206 **Proinsulin**

🔧 0.00   ⚗ 0.00   **FUD** XXX   Ⓝ

AMA: 2015,Jun,10; 2015,Apr,3; 2010,Dec,7-10

84207 **Pyridoxal phosphate (Vitamin B-6)**

🔧 0.00   ⚗ 0.00   **FUD** XXX   Ⓝ ▱

AMA: 2015,Jun,10; 2015,Apr,3; 2010,Dec,7-10

84210 **Pyruvate**

🔧 0.00   ⚗ 0.00   **FUD** XXX   Ⓝ

AMA: 2015,Jun,10; 2015,Apr,3; 2010,Dec,7-10

84220 **Pyruvate kinase**

🔧 0.00   ⚗ 0.00   **FUD** XXX   Ⓝ

AMA: 2015,Jun,10; 2015,Apr,3; 2010,Dec,7-10

84228 **Quinine**

🔧 0.00   ⚗ 0.00   **FUD** XXX   Ⓝ

AMA: 2015,Jun,10; 2015,Apr,3; 2010,Dec,7-10

84233 **Receptor assay; estrogen**

🔧 0.00   ⚗ 0.00   **FUD** XXX   Ⓝ ▱

AMA: 2015,Jun,10; 2015,Apr,3; 2010,Dec,7-10

84234 **progesterone**
🚑 0.00 ⚕ 0.00 **FUD** XXX   N ▢
AMA: 2015,Jun,10; 2015,Apr,3; 2010,Dec,7-10

84235 **endocrine, other than estrogen or progesterone (specify hormone)**
🚑 0.00 ⚕ 0.00 **FUD** XXX   N ▢
AMA: 2015,Jun,10; 2015,Apr,3; 2010,Dec,7-10

84238 **non-endocrine (specify receptor)**
🚑 0.00 ⚕ 0.00 **FUD** XXX   N ▢
AMA: 2015,Jun,10; 2015,Apr,3; 2015,Jan,16; 2014,Jan,11; 2012,Jan,15-42; 2011,Jan,11; 2010,Dec,7-10

84244 **Renin**
🚑 0.00 ⚕ 0.00 **FUD** XXX   N ▢
AMA: 2015,Jun,10; 2015,Apr,3; 2010,Dec,7-10

84252 **Riboflavin (Vitamin B-2)**
🚑 0.00 ⚕ 0.00 **FUD** XXX   N ▢
AMA: 2015,Jun,10; 2015,Apr,3; 2010,Dec,7-10

84255 **Selenium**
🚑 0.00 ⚕ 0.00 **FUD** XXX   N
AMA: 2015,Jun,10; 2015,Apr,3; 2010,Dec,7-10

84260 **Serotonin**
EXCLUDES   *Urine metabolites (HIAA) (83497)*
🚑 0.00 ⚕ 0.00 **FUD** XXX   N
AMA: 2015,Jun,10; 2015,Apr,3; 2010,Dec,7-10

84270 **Sex hormone binding globulin (SHBG)**
🚑 0.00 ⚕ 0.00 **FUD** XXX   N
AMA: 2015,Jun,10; 2015,Apr,3; 2015,Jan,16; 2014,Jan,11; 2010,Dec,7-10

84275 **Sialic acid**
🚑 0.00 ⚕ 0.00 **FUD** XXX   N
AMA: 2015,Jun,10; 2015,Apr,3; 2010,Dec,7-10

84285 **Silica**
🚑 0.00 ⚕ 0.00 **FUD** XXX   N
AMA: 2015,Jun,10; 2015,Apr,3; 2010,Dec,7-10

84295 **Sodium; serum, plasma or whole blood**
🚑 0.00 ⚕ 0.00 **FUD** XXX   ☒ N
AMA: 2015,Jun,10; 2015,Apr,3; 2015,Jan,16; 2014,Jan,11; 2013,Apr,10-11; 2010,Dec,7-10

84300 **urine**
🚑 0.00 ⚕ 0.00 **FUD** XXX   N
AMA: 2015,Jun,10; 2015,Apr,3; 2010,Dec,7-10

84302 **other source**
🚑 0.00 ⚕ 0.00 **FUD** XXX   N
AMA: 2015,Jun,10; 2015,Apr,3; 2015,Jan,16; 2014,Jan,11; 2010,Dec,7-10

84305 **Somatomedin**
🚑 0.00 ⚕ 0.00 **FUD** XXX   N
AMA: 2015,Jun,10; 2015,Apr,3; 2015,Jan,16; 2014,Jan,11; 2010,Dec,7-10

84307 **Somatostatin**
🚑 0.00 ⚕ 0.00 **FUD** XXX   N
AMA: 2015,Jun,10; 2015,Apr,3; 2015,Jan,16; 2014,Jan,11; 2010,Dec,7-10

84311 **Spectrophotometry, analyte not elsewhere specified**
🚑 0.00 ⚕ 0.00 **FUD** XXX   N
AMA: 2015,Jun,10; 2015,Apr,3; 2010,Dec,7-10

84315 **Specific gravity (except urine)**
EXCLUDES   *Urine specific gravity (81000-81003)*
🚑 0.00 ⚕ 0.00 **FUD** XXX   N
AMA: 2015,Jun,10; 2015,Apr,3; 2010,Dec,7-10

84375 **Sugars, chromatographic, TLC or paper chromatography**
🚑 0.00 ⚕ 0.00 **FUD** XXX   N
AMA: 2015,Jun,10; 2015,Apr,3; 2010,Dec,7-10

84376 **Sugars (mono-, di-, and oligosaccharides); single qualitative, each specimen**
🚑 0.00 ⚕ 0.00 **FUD** XXX   N
AMA: 2015,Jun,10; 2015,Apr,3; 2015,Jan,16; 2014,Jan,11; 2010,Dec,7-10

84377 **multiple qualitative, each specimen**
🚑 0.00 ⚕ 0.00 **FUD** XXX   N ▢
AMA: 2015,Jun,10; 2015,Apr,3; 2015,Jan,16; 2014,Jan,11; 2010,Dec,7-10

84378 **single quantitative, each specimen**
🚑 0.00 ⚕ 0.00 **FUD** XXX   N ▢
AMA: 2015,Jun,10; 2015,Apr,3; 2010,Dec,7-10

84379 **multiple quantitative, each specimen**
🚑 0.00 ⚕ 0.00 **FUD** XXX   N ▢
AMA: 2015,Jun,10; 2015,Apr,3; 2015,Jan,16; 2014,Jan,11; 2010,Dec,7-10

84392 **Sulfate, urine**
🚑 0.00 ⚕ 0.00 **FUD** XXX   N
AMA: 2015,Jun,10; 2015,Apr,3; 2010,Dec,7-10

84402 **Testosterone; free**
Do not report with ([80327, 80328])
🚑 0.00 ⚕ 0.00 **FUD** XXX   N
AMA: 2015,Jun,10; 2015,Apr,3; 2010,Dec,7-10

84403 **total**
Do not report with ([80327, 80328])
🚑 0.00 ⚕ 0.00 **FUD** XXX   N ▢
AMA: 2015,Jun,10; 2015,Apr,3; 2010,Dec,7-10

84425 **Thiamine (Vitamin B-1)**
🚑 0.00 ⚕ 0.00 **FUD** XXX   N ▢
AMA: 2015,Jun,10; 2015,Apr,3; 2010,Dec,7-10

84430 **Thiocyanate**
🚑 0.00 ⚕ 0.00 **FUD** XXX   N
AMA: 2015,Jun,10; 2015,Apr,3; 2010,Dec,7-10

84431 **Thromboxane metabolite(s), including thromboxane if performed, urine**
Code also for determination of concurrent urine creatinine (82570)
🚑 0.00 ⚕ 0.00 **FUD** XXX   N
AMA: 2015,Jun,10; 2015,Apr,3; 2010,Dec,7-10

84432 **Thyroglobulin**
EXCLUDES   *Thyroglobulin antibody (86800)*
🚑 0.00 ⚕ 0.00 **FUD** XXX   N
AMA: 2015,Jun,10; 2015,Apr,3; 2015,Jan,16; 2014,Jan,11; 2010,Dec,7-10

84436-84445 Chemistry: Thyroid Tests

CMS: 100-3,190.22 Thyroid Testing

INCLUDES   Clinical information not requested by the ordering physician
Mathematically calculated results
Quantitative analysis unless otherwise specified
Specimens from any source unless otherwise specified

EXCLUDES   *Calculated results that represent a score or probability that was derived by algorithm*
Organ or disease panels (80048-80076 [80081])
Therapeutic drug assays (80150-80299 [80164, 80165, 80171])
Do not report analytes from nonrequested laboratory analysis

84436 **Thyroxine; total**
🚑 0.00 ⚕ 0.00 **FUD** XXX   N ▢
AMA: 2015,Jun,10; 2015,Apr,3; 2015,Jan,16; 2014,Jan,11; 2010,Dec,7-10

84437 **requiring elution (eg, neonatal)**
🚑 0.00 ⚕ 0.00 **FUD** XXX   N
AMA: 2015,Jun,10; 2015,Apr,3; 2010,Dec,7-10

84439 **free**
🚑 0.00 ⚕ 0.00 **FUD** XXX   N ▢
AMA: 2015,Jun,10; 2015,Apr,3; 2010,Dec,7-10

84442 **Thyroxine binding globulin (TBG)**
🚑 0.00 ⚕ 0.00 **FUD** XXX   N
AMA: 2015,Jun,10; 2015,Apr,3; 2010,Dec,7-10

84443 Thyroid stimulating hormone (TSH)
⚏ 0.00   ⚒ 0.00   **FUD** XXX   ☒ N
AMA: 2015,Jun,10; 2015,Apr,3; 2010,Dec,7-10

84445 Thyroid stimulating immune globulins (TSI)
⚏ 0.00   ⚒ 0.00   **FUD** XXX   N ▭
AMA: 2015,Jun,10; 2015,Apr,3; 2015,Jan,16; 2014,Jan,11; 2010,Dec,7-10

84446-84449 Chemistry: Tocopherol Alpha—Transcortin

INCLUDES Clinical information not requested by the ordering physician
Mathematically calculated results
Quantitative analysis unless otherwise specified
Specimens from any source unless otherwise specified
EXCLUDES *Calculated results that represent a score or probability that was derived by algorithm*
Organ or disease panels (80048-80076 [80081])
Therapeutic drug assays (80150-80299 [80164, 80165, 80171])
Do not report analytes from nonrequested laboratory analysis

84446 Tocopherol alpha (Vitamin E)
⚏ 0.00   ⚒ 0.00   **FUD** XXX   N ▭
AMA: 2015,Jun,10; 2015,Apr,3; 2010,Dec,7-10

84449 Transcortin (cortisol binding globulin)
⚏ 0.00   ⚒ 0.00   **FUD** XXX   N
AMA: 2015,Jun,10; 2015,Apr,3; 2015,Jan,16; 2014,Jan,11; 2010,Dec,7-10

84450-84460 Chemistry: Transferase

CMS: 100-2,11,30.2.2 Automated Multi-Channel Chemistry (AMCC) Tests; 100-3,160.17 Payment for L-Dopa /Associated Inpatient Hospital Services; 100-4,16,40.6.1 Automated Multi-Channel Chemistry Tests for ESRD Beneficiaries; 100-4,16,70.8 CLIA Waived Tests
INCLUDES Clinical information not requested by the ordering physician
Mathematically calculated results
Quantitative analysis unless otherwise specified
EXCLUDES *Calculated results that represent a score or probability that was derived by algorithm*
Do not report analytes from nonrequested laboratory analysis

84450 Transferase; aspartate amino (AST) (SGOT)
⚏ 0.00   ⚒ 0.00   **FUD** XXX   ☒ N
AMA: 2015,Jun,10; 2015,Apr,3; 2015,Jan,16; 2014,Jan,11; 2010,Dec,7-10

84460 alanine amino (ALT) (SGPT)
⚏ 0.00   ⚒ 0.00   **FUD** XXX   ☒ N
AMA: 2015,Jun,10; 2015,Apr,3; 2015,Jan,16; 2014,Jan,11; 2010,Dec,7-10

84466 Chemistry: Transferrin

CMS: 100-02,11,20.2 ESRD Laboratory Services; 100-3,190.18 Serum Iron Studies
INCLUDES Clinical information not requested by the ordering physician
Mathematically calculated results
Quantitative analysis unless otherwise specified
EXCLUDES *Calculated results that represent a score or probability that was derived by algorithm*
Do not report analytes from nonrequested laboratory analysis

84466 Transferrin
EXCLUDES *Iron binding capacity (83550)*
⚏ 0.00   ⚒ 0.00   **FUD** XXX   N ▭
AMA: 2015,Jun,10; 2015,Apr,3; 2015,Jan,16; 2014,Jan,11; 2010,Dec,7-10

84478 Chemistry: Triglycerides

CMS: 100-2,11,30.2.2 Automated Multi-Channel Chemistry (AMCC) Tests; 100-3,190.23 Lipid Testing; 100-4,16,70.8 CLIA Waived Tests
INCLUDES Clinical information not requested by the ordering physician
Mathematically calculated results
EXCLUDES *Calculated results that represent a score or probability that was derived by algorithm*
Organ or disease panels (80048-80076 [80081])
Do not report analytes from nonrequested laboratory analysis

84478 Triglycerides
⚏ 0.00   ⚒ 0.00   **FUD** XXX   ☒ N ▭
AMA: 2015,Jun,10; 2015,Apr,3; 2015,Jan,16; 2014,Jan,11; 2012,Jan,15-42; 2011,Jan,11; 2010,Dec,7-10

84479-84482 Chemistry: Thyroid Hormone—Triiodothyronine

CMS: 100-3,190.22 Thyroid Testing
INCLUDES Clinical information not requested by the ordering physician
Mathematically calculated results
Quantitative analysis unless otherwise specified
Specimens from any source unless otherwise specified
EXCLUDES *Calculated results that represent a score or probability that was derived by algorithm*
Organ or disease panels (80048-80076 [80081])
Do not report analytes from nonrequested laboratory analysis

84479 Thyroid hormone (T3 or T4) uptake or thyroid hormone binding ratio (THBR)
⚏ 0.00   ⚒ 0.00   **FUD** XXX   N ▭
AMA: 2015,Jun,10; 2015,Apr,3; 2015,Jan,16; 2014,Jan,11; 2010,Dec,7-10

84480 Triiodothyronine T3; total (TT-3)
⚏ 0.00   ⚒ 0.00   **FUD** XXX   N ▭
AMA: 2015,Jun,10; 2015,Apr,3; 2010,Dec,7-10

84481 free
⚏ 0.00   ⚒ 0.00   **FUD** XXX   N ▭
AMA: 2015,Jun,10; 2015,Apr,3; 2010,Dec,7-10

84482 reverse
⚏ 0.00   ⚒ 0.00   **FUD** XXX   N ▭
AMA: 2015,Jun,10; 2015,Apr,3; 2015,Jan,16; 2014,Jan,11; 2010,Dec,7-10

84484-84512 Chemistry: Troponin (Quantitative)—Troponin (Qualitative)

INCLUDES Clinical information not requested by the ordering physician
Mathematically calculated results
Specimens from any source unless otherwise specified
EXCLUDES *Calculated results that represent a score or probability that was derived by algorithm*
Organ or disease panels
Do not report analytes from nonrequested laboratory analysis

84484 Troponin, quantitative
EXCLUDES *Qualitative troponin assay (84512)*
⚏ 0.00   ⚒ 0.00   **FUD** XXX   N
AMA: 2015,Jun,10; 2015,Apr,3; 2015,Jan,16; 2014,Jan,11; 2010,Dec,7-10

84485 Trypsin; duodenal fluid
⚏ 0.00   ⚒ 0.00   **FUD** XXX   N
AMA: 2015,Jun,10; 2015,Apr,3; 2010,Dec,7-10

84488 feces, qualitative
⚏ 0.00   ⚒ 0.00   **FUD** XXX   N
AMA: 2015,Jun,10; 2015,Apr,3; 2010,Dec,7-10

84490 feces, quantitative, 24-hour collection
⚏ 0.00   ⚒ 0.00   **FUD** XXX   N
AMA: 2015,Jun,10; 2015,Apr,3; 2010,Dec,7-10

84510 Tyrosine
EXCLUDES *Urate crystal identification (89060)*
⚏ 0.00   ⚒ 0.00   **FUD** XXX   N
AMA: 2015,Jun,10; 2015,Apr,3; 2010,Dec,7-10

84512 Troponin, qualitative
EXCLUDES *Quantitative troponin assay (84484)*
⚏ 0.00   ⚒ 0.00   **FUD** XXX   N
AMA: 2015,Jun,10; 2015,Apr,3; 2015,Jan,16; 2014,Jan,11; 2010,Dec,7-10

84520-84525 Chemistry: Urea Nitrogen (Blood)

CMS: 100-3,160.17 Payment for L-Dopa /Associated Inpatient Hospital Services
INCLUDES Clinical information not requested by the ordering physician
Mathematically calculated results
EXCLUDES *Calculated results that represent a score or probability that was derived by algorithm*
Organ or disease panels (80048-80076 [80081])
Do not report analytes from nonrequested laboratory analysis

84520 Urea nitrogen; quantitative
⚏ 0.00   ⚒ 0.00   **FUD** XXX   ☒ N
AMA: 2015,Jun,10; 2015,Apr,3; 2015,Jan,16; 2014,Jan,11; 2013,Apr,10-11; 2010,Dec,7-10

84525   **semiquantitative (eg, reagent strip test)**
          INCLUDES   Patterson's test
          🚗 0.00   ⚗ 0.00   **FUD** XXX   N
          AMA: 2015,Jun,10; 2015,Apr,3; 2015,Jan,16; 2014,Jan,11;
          2010,Dec,7-10

84540-84630 Chemistry: Urea Nitrogen (Urine)—Zinc

INCLUDES   Clinical information not requested by the ordering physician
          Mathematically calculated results
          Quantitative analysis unless otherwise specified
          Specimens from any source unless otherwise specified
EXCLUDES   *Calculated results that represent a score or probability that was derived by*
          algorithm
          Organ or disease panels (80048-80076 [80081])
          Therapeutic drug assays (80150-80299 [80164, 80165, 80171])
Do not report analytes from nonrequested laboratory analysis

84540   **Urea nitrogen, urine**
          🚗 0.00   ⚗ 0.00   **FUD** XXX   N
          AMA: 2015,Jun,10; 2015,Apr,3; 2010,Dec,7-10

84545   **Urea nitrogen, clearance**
          🚗 0.00   ⚗ 0.00   **FUD** XXX   N
          AMA: 2015,Jun,10; 2015,Apr,3; 2010,Dec,7-10

84550   **Uric acid; blood**
          🚗 0.00   ⚗ 0.00   **FUD** XXX   ☒ N
          AMA: 2015,Jun,10; 2015,Apr,3; 2015,Jan,16; 2014,Jan,11;
          2010,Dec,7-10

84560   **other source**
          🚗 0.00   ⚗ 0.00   **FUD** XXX   N
          AMA: 2015,Jun,10; 2015,Apr,3; 2010,Dec,7-10

84577   **Urobilinogen, feces, quantitative**
          🚗 0.00   ⚗ 0.00   **FUD** XXX   N
          AMA: 2015,Jun,10; 2015,Apr,3; 2010,Dec,7-10

84578   **Urobilinogen, urine; qualitative**
          🚗 0.00   ⚗ 0.00   **FUD** XXX   N
          AMA: 2015,Jun,10; 2015,Apr,3; 2010,Dec,7-10

84580   **quantitative, timed specimen**
          🚗 0.00   ⚗ 0.00   **FUD** XXX   N ▭
          AMA: 2015,Jun,10; 2015,Apr,3; 2010,Dec,7-10

84583   **semiquantitative**
          🚗 0.00   ⚗ 0.00   **FUD** XXX   N
          AMA: 2015,Jun,10; 2015,Apr,3; 2010,Dec,7-10

84585   **Vanillylmandelic acid (VMA), urine**
          🚗 0.00   ⚗ 0.00   **FUD** XXX   N
          AMA: 2015,Jun,10; 2015,Apr,3; 2010,Dec,7-10

84586   **Vasoactive intestinal peptide (VIP)**
          🚗 0.00   ⚗ 0.00   **FUD** XXX   N
          AMA: 2015,Jun,10; 2015,Apr,3; 2015,Jan,16; 2014,Jan,11;
          2010,Dec,7-10

84588   **Vasopressin (antidiuretic hormone, ADH)**
          🚗 0.00   ⚗ 0.00   **FUD** XXX   N
          AMA: 2015,Jun,10; 2015,Apr,3; 2010,Dec,7-10

84590   **Vitamin A**
          🚗 0.00   ⚗ 0.00   **FUD** XXX   N ▭
          AMA: 2015,Jun,10; 2015,Apr,3; 2010,Dec,7-10

84591   **Vitamin, not otherwise specified**
          🚗 0.00   ⚗ 0.00   **FUD** XXX   N
          AMA: 2015,Jun,10; 2015,Apr,3; 2010,Dec,7-10

84597   **Vitamin K**
          🚗 0.00   ⚗ 0.00   **FUD** XXX   N ▭
          AMA: 2015,Jun,10; 2015,Apr,3; 2010,Dec,7-10

84600   **Volatiles (eg, acetic anhydride, diethylether)**
          EXCLUDES   *Carbon tetrachloride, dichloroethane, dichloromethane*
                    (82441)
                    Isopropyl alcohol and methanol ([80320])
          🚗 0.00   ⚗ 0.00   **FUD** XXX   N
          AMA: 2015,Jun,10; 2015,Apr,3; 2010,Dec,7-10

84620   **Xylose absorption test, blood and/or urine**
          EXCLUDES   *Administration (99070)*
          🚗 0.00   ⚗ 0.00   **FUD** XXX   N ▭
          AMA: 2015,Jun,10; 2015,Apr,3; 2010,Dec,7-10

84630   **Zinc**
          🚗 0.00   ⚗ 0.00   **FUD** XXX   N
          AMA: 2015,Jun,10; 2015,Apr,3; 2010,Dec,7-10

84681-84999 Other and Unlisted Chemistry Tests

INCLUDES   Clinical information not requested by the ordering physician
          Mathematically calculated results
          Quantitative analysis unless otherwise specified
          Specimens from any source unless otherwise specified
EXCLUDES   *Calculated results that represent a score or probability that was derived by*
          algorithm
          Confirmatory testing of a not otherwise specified drug ([80375, 80376,
          80377], 80299)
          Organ or disease panels (80048-80076 [80081])
Do not report analytes from nonrequested laboratory analysis

84681   **C-peptide**
          🚗 0.00   ⚗ 0.00   **FUD** XXX   N ▭
          AMA: 2015,Jun,10; 2015,Apr,3; 2010,Dec,7-10

84702   **Gonadotropin, chorionic (hCG); quantitative**
          🚗 0.00   ⚗ 0.00   **FUD** XXX   N ▭
          AMA: 2015,Jun,10; 2015,Apr,3; 2010,Dec,7-10

84703   **qualitative**
          EXCLUDES   *Urine pregnancy test by visual color comparison (81025)*
          🚗 0.00   ⚗ 0.00   **FUD** XXX   ☒ N
          AMA: 2015,Jun,10; 2015,Apr,3; 2010,Dec,7-10

84704   **free beta chain**
          🚗 0.00   ⚗ 0.00   **FUD** XXX   N
          AMA: 2015,Jun,10; 2015,Apr,3; 2015,Jan,16; 2014,Jan,11;
          2012,Jan,15-42; 2011,Jan,11; 2010,Dec,7-10

84830   **Ovulation tests, by visual color comparison methods for**
          human luteinizing hormone   ♀
          🚗 0.00   ⚗ 0.00   **FUD** XXX   ☒ N
          AMA: 2015,Jun,10; 2015,Apr,3; 2010,Dec,7-10

84999   **Unlisted chemistry procedure**
          🚗 0.00   ⚗ 0.00   **FUD** XXX   N
          AMA: 2015,Apr,3; 2015,Jan,16; 2014,Jan,11; 2012,Jan,15-42;
          2011,Jan,11; 2010,Dec,7-10

85002 Bleeding Time Test

EXCLUDES   *Agglutinins (86000, 86156-86157)*
          Antiplasmin (85410)
          Antithrombin III (85300-85301)
          Blood banking procedures (86850-86999)

85002   **Bleeding time**
          🚗 0.00   ⚗ 0.00   **FUD** XXX   N
          AMA: 2015,Jan,16; 2014,Jan,11

85004-85049 Blood Counts

CMS: 100-3,190.15 Blood Counts
EXCLUDES   *Agglutinins (86000, 86156-86157)*
          Antiplasmin (85410)
          Antithrombin III (85300-85301)
          Blood banking procedures (86850-86999)

85004   **Blood count; automated differential WBC count**
          🚗 0.00   ⚗ 0.00   **FUD** XXX   N ▭
          AMA: 2015,Jan,16; 2014,Jan,11; 2012,Jan,15-42; 2011,Jan,11

85007   **blood smear, microscopic examination with manual**
          differential WBC count
          🚗 0.00   ⚗ 0.00   **FUD** XXX   N ▭
          AMA: 2015,Jan,16; 2014,Jan,11; 2012,Jan,15-42; 2011,Jan,11

85008 blood smear, microscopic examination without manual differential WBC count

EXCLUDES Cell count other fluids (eg, CSF) (89050-89051)

⚕ 0.00   ⚖ 0.00   **FUD** XXX   N ▢

AMA: 2015,Jan,16; 2014,Jan,11; 2012,Jan,15-42; 2011,Jan,11

85009 manual differential WBC count, buffy coat

EXCLUDES Eosinophils, nasal smear (89190)

⚕ 0.00   ⚖ 0.00   **FUD** XXX   N ▢

AMA: 2015,Jan,16; 2014,Jan,11; 2012,Jan,15-42; 2011,Jan,11

85013 spun microhematocrit

⚕ 0.00   ⚖ 0.00   **FUD** XXX   X N

AMA: 2005,Aug,7-8; 2005,Jul,11-12

85014 hematocrit (Hct)

⚕ 0.00   ⚖ 0.00   **FUD** XXX   X N ▢

AMA: 2015,Jan,16; 2014,Jan,11

85018 hemoglobin (Hgb)

EXCLUDES Immunoassay, hemoglobin, fecal (82274)
Other hemoglobin determination (83020-83069)
Transcutaneous hemoglobin measurement (88738)

⚕ 0.00   ⚖ 0.00   **FUD** XXX   X N ▢

AMA: 2015,Jan,16; 2014,Jan,11; 2010,Oct,6

85025 complete (CBC), automated (Hgb, Hct, RBC, WBC and platelet count) and automated differential WBC count

⚕ 0.00   ⚖ 0.00   **FUD** XXX   N ▢

AMA: 2015,Jan,16; 2014,Jan,11; 2012,Jan,15-42; 2011,Jul,16-17; 2011,Jan,11

85027 complete (CBC), automated (Hgb, Hct, RBC, WBC and platelet count)

⚕ 0.00   ⚖ 0.00   **FUD** XXX   N ▢

AMA: 2015,Jan,16; 2014,Jan,11

85032 manual cell count (erythrocyte, leukocyte, or platelet) each

⚕ 0.00   ⚖ 0.00   **FUD** XXX   N ▢

AMA: 2015,Jan,16; 2014,Jan,11; 2012,Jan,15-42; 2011,Jan,11

85041 red blood cell (RBC), automated

Do not report with (85025, 85027)

⚕ 0.00   ⚖ 0.00   **FUD** XXX   N ▢

AMA: 2015,Jan,16; 2014,Jan,11

85044 reticulocyte, manual

⚕ 0.00   ⚖ 0.00   **FUD** XXX   N

AMA: 2015,Jan,16; 2014,Jan,11

85045 reticulocyte, automated

⚕ 0.00   ⚖ 0.00   **FUD** XXX   N ▢

AMA: 2015,Jan,16; 2014,Jan,11

85046 reticulocytes, automated, including 1 or more cellular parameters (eg, reticulocyte hemoglobin content [CHr], immature reticulocyte fraction [IRF], reticulocyte volume [MRV], RNA content), direct measurement

⚕ 0.00   ⚖ 0.00   **FUD** XXX   N ▢

AMA: 2005,Aug,7-8; 2005,Jul,11-12

85048 leukocyte (WBC), automated

⚕ 0.00   ⚖ 0.00   **FUD** XXX   N ▢

AMA: 2015,Jan,16; 2014,Jan,11

85049 platelet, automated

⚕ 0.00   ⚖ 0.00   **FUD** XXX   N ▢

AMA: 2005,Aug,7-8; 2005,Jul,11-12

85055-85705 Coagulopathy Testing

EXCLUDES Agglutinins (86000, 86156-86157)
Antiplasmin (85410)
Antithrombin III (85300-85301)
Blood banking procedures (86850-86999)

85055 Reticulated platelet assay

⚕ 0.00   ⚖ 0.00   **FUD** XXX   N

AMA: 2005,Aug,7-8; 2005,Jul,11-12

85060 Blood smear, peripheral, interpretation by physician with written report

⚕ 0.70   ⚖ 0.70   **FUD** XXX   B 80

AMA: 2005,Aug,7-8; 2005,Jul,11-12

85097 Bone marrow, smear interpretation

EXCLUDES Bone biopsy (20220, 20225, 20240, 20245, 20250-20251)
Special stains (88312-88313)

⚕ 1.39   ⚖ 2.50   **FUD** XXX   S 80

AMA: 2015,Jan,16; 2014,Jan,11; 2012,Jan,15-42; 2011,Jan,11

85130 Chromogenic substrate assay

⚕ 0.00   ⚖ 0.00   **FUD** XXX   N ▢

AMA: 2005,Aug,7-8; 2005,Jul,11-12

85170 Clot retraction

⚕ 0.00   ⚖ 0.00   **FUD** XXX   N ▢

AMA: 2005,Aug,7-8; 2005,Jul,11-12

85175 Clot lysis time, whole blood dilution

⚕ 0.00   ⚖ 0.00   **FUD** XXX   N ▢

AMA: 2005,Aug,7-8; 2005,Jul,11-12

85210 Clotting; factor II, prothrombin, specific

EXCLUDES Prothrombin time (85610-85611)
Russell viper venom time (85612-85613)

⚕ 0.00   ⚖ 0.00   **FUD** XXX   N ▢

AMA: 2005,Aug,7-8; 2005,Jul,11-12

85220 factor V (AcG or proaccelerin), labile factor

⚕ 0.00   ⚖ 0.00   **FUD** XXX   N ▢

AMA: 2005,Aug,7-8; 2005,Jul,11-12

85230 factor VII (proconvertin, stable factor)

⚕ 0.00   ⚖ 0.00   **FUD** XXX   N ▢

AMA: 2005,Aug,7-8; 2005,Jul,11-12

85240 factor VIII (AHG), 1-stage

⚕ 0.00   ⚖ 0.00   **FUD** XXX   N ▢

AMA: 2005,Aug,7-8; 2005,Jul,11-12

85244 factor VIII related antigen

⚕ 0.00   ⚖ 0.00   **FUD** XXX   N ▢

AMA: 2005,Aug,7-8; 2005,Jul,11-12

85245 factor VIII, VW factor, ristocetin cofactor

⚕ 0.00   ⚖ 0.00   **FUD** XXX   N ▢

AMA: 2005,Aug,7-8; 2005,Jul,11-12

85246 factor VIII, VW factor antigen

⚕ 0.00   ⚖ 0.00   **FUD** XXX   N ▢

AMA: 2005,Aug,7-8; 2005,Jul,11-12

85247 factor VIII, von Willebrand factor, multimetric analysis

⚕ 0.00   ⚖ 0.00   **FUD** XXX   N ▢

AMA: 2005,Aug,7-8; 2005,Jul,11-12

85250 factor IX (PTC or Christmas)

⚕ 0.00   ⚖ 0.00   **FUD** XXX   N ▢

AMA: 2005,Aug,7-8; 2005,Jul,11-12

85260 factor X (Stuart-Prower)

⚕ 0.00   ⚖ 0.00   **FUD** XXX   N ▢

AMA: 2005,Aug,7-8; 2005,Jul,11-12

85270 factor XI (PTA)

⚕ 0.00   ⚖ 0.00   **FUD** XXX   N ▢

AMA: 2005,Aug,7-8; 2005,Jul,11-12

85280 factor XII (Hageman)

⚕ 0.00   ⚖ 0.00   **FUD** XXX   N ▢

AMA: 2005,Aug,7-8; 2005,Jul,11-12

85290 factor XIII (fibrin stabilizing)

⚕ 0.00   ⚖ 0.00   **FUD** XXX   N ▢

AMA: 2005,Aug,7-8; 2005,Jul,11-12

85291 factor XIII (fibrin stabilizing), screen solubility

⚕ 0.00   ⚖ 0.00   **FUD** XXX   N ▢

AMA: 2005,Aug,7-8; 2005,Jul,11-12

85292 prekallikrein assay (Fletcher factor assay)

⚕ 0.00   ⚖ 0.00   **FUD** XXX   N ▢

AMA: 2005,Aug,7-8; 2005,Jul,11-12

● New Code   ▲ Revised Code   ○ Reinstated   M Maternity   A Age Edit   Unlisted   Not Covered   # Resequenced
⊘ AMA Mod 51 Exempt   51 Optum Mod 51 Exempt   63 Mod 63 Exempt   ⊙ Mod Sedation   + Add-on   ▢ CCI   PQ PQRS   FUD Follow-up Days

Pathology and Laboratory

85293 — 85525

85293 **high molecular weight kininogen assay (Fitzgerald factor assay)**
0.00 0.00 FUD XXX N ▢
AMA: 2005,Aug,7-8; 2005,Jul,11-12

85300 **Clotting inhibitors or anticoagulants; antithrombin III, activity**
0.00 0.00 FUD XXX N ▢
AMA: 2005,Aug,7-8; 2005,Jul,11-12

85301 **antithrombin III, antigen assay**
0.00 0.00 FUD XXX N ▢
AMA: 2005,Aug,7-8; 2005,Jul,11-12

85302 **protein C, antigen**
0.00 0.00 FUD XXX N ▢
AMA: 2005,Aug,7-8; 2005,Jul,11-12

85303 **protein C, activity**
0.00 0.00 FUD XXX N ▢
AMA: 2005,Aug,7-8; 2005,Jul,11-12

85305 **protein S, total**
0.00 0.00 FUD XXX N ▢
AMA: 2005,Jul,11-12; 2005,Aug,7-8

85306 **protein S, free**
0.00 0.00 FUD XXX N ▢
AMA: 2005,Aug,7-8; 2005,Jul,11-12

85307 **Activated Protein C (APC) resistance assay**
0.00 0.00 FUD XXX N ▢
AMA: 2005,Aug,7-8; 2005,Jul,11-12

85335 **Factor inhibitor test**
0.00 0.00 FUD XXX N ▢
AMA: 2005,Aug,7-8; 2005,Jul,11-12

85337 **Thrombomodulin**
EXCLUDES *Mixing studies for inhibitors (85732)*
0.00 0.00 FUD XXX N ▢
AMA: 2005,Aug,7-8; 2005,Jul,11-12

85345 **Coagulation time; Lee and White**
0.00 0.00 FUD XXX N ▢
AMA: 2005,Aug,7-8; 2005,Jul,11-12

85347 **activated**
0.00 0.00 FUD XXX N ▢
AMA: 2005,Aug,7-8; 2005,Jul,11-12

85348 **other methods**
0.00 0.00 FUD XXX N ▢
AMA: 2005,Aug,7-8; 2005,Jul,11-12

85360 **Euglobulin lysis**
0.00 0.00 FUD XXX N ▢
AMA: 2005,Aug,7-8; 2005,Jul,11-12

85362 **Fibrin(ogen) degradation (split) products (FDP) (FSP); agglutination slide, semiquantitative**
EXCLUDES *Immunoelectrophoresis (86320)*
0.00 0.00 FUD XXX N ▢
AMA: 2005,Aug,7-8; 2005,Jul,11-12

85366 **paracoagulation**
0.00 0.00 FUD XXX N ▢
AMA: 2005,Aug,7-8; 2005,Jul,11-12

85370 **quantitative**
0.00 0.00 FUD XXX N ▢
AMA: 2005,Aug,7-8; 2005,Jul,11-12

85378 **Fibrin degradation products, D-dimer; qualitative or semiquantitative**
0.00 0.00 FUD XXX N ▢
AMA: 2015,Jan,16; 2014,Jan,11

85379 **quantitative**
INCLUDES Ultrasensitive and standard sensitivity quantitative D-dimer
0.00 0.00 FUD XXX N ▢
AMA: 2005,Aug,7-8; 2005,Jul,11-12

85380 **ultrasensitive (eg, for evaluation for venous thromboembolism), qualitative or semiquantitative**
0.00 0.00 FUD XXX N ▢
AMA: 2015,Jan,16; 2014,Jan,11

85384 **Fibrinogen; activity**
0.00 0.00 FUD XXX N ▢
AMA: 2005,Jul,11-12; 2005,Aug,7-8

85385 **antigen**
0.00 0.00 FUD XXX N ▢
AMA: 2005,Jul,11-12; 2005,Aug,7-8

85390 **Fibrinolysins or coagulopathy screen, interpretation and report**
0.00 0.00 FUD XXX N ▢
AMA: 2005,Jul,11-12; 2005,Aug,7-8

85396 **Coagulation/fibrinolysis assay, whole blood (eg, viscoelastic clot assessment), including use of any pharmacologic additive(s), as indicated, including interpretation and written report, per day**
0.58 0.58 FUD XXX N 80
AMA: 2005,Aug,7-8; 2005,Jul,11-12

85397 **Coagulation and fibrinolysis, functional activity, not otherwise specified (eg, ADAMTS-13), each analyte**
0.00 0.00 FUD XXX N

85400 **Fibrinolytic factors and inhibitors; plasmin**
0.00 0.00 FUD XXX N ▢
AMA: 2005,Aug,7-8; 2005,Jul,11-12

85410 **alpha-2 antiplasmin**
0.00 0.00 FUD XXX N ▢
AMA: 2005,Aug,7-8; 2005,Jul,11-12

85415 **plasminogen activator**
0.00 0.00 FUD XXX N ▢
AMA: 2005,Aug,7-8; 2005,Jul,11-12

85420 **plasminogen, except antigenic assay**
0.00 0.00 FUD XXX N ▢
AMA: 2005,Aug,7-8; 2005,Jul,11-12

85421 **plasminogen, antigenic assay**
0.00 0.00 FUD XXX N ▢
AMA: 2005,Aug,7-8; 2005,Jul,11-12

85441 **Heinz bodies; direct**
0.00 0.00 FUD XXX N ▢
AMA: 2005,Aug,7-8; 2005,Jul,11-12

85445 **induced, acetyl phenylhydrazine**
0.00 0.00 FUD XXX N ▢
AMA: 2005,Aug,7-8; 2005,Jul,11-12

85460 **Hemoglobin or RBCs, fetal, for fetomaternal hemorrhage; differential lysis (Kleihauer-Betke)** M ♀
EXCLUDES *Hemoglobin F (83030, 83033)*
Hemolysins (86940-86941)
0.00 0.00 FUD XXX N ▢
AMA: 2015,Jan,16; 2014,Jan,11

85461 **rosette** M ♀
0.00 0.00 FUD XXX N ▢
AMA: 2005,Jul,11-12; 2005,Aug,7-8

85475 **Hemolysin, acid**
INCLUDES Ham test
EXCLUDES *Hemolysins and agglutinins (86940-86941)*
0.00 0.00 FUD XXX N ▢
AMA: 2005,Aug,7-8; 2005,Jul,11-12

85520 **Heparin assay**
0.00 0.00 FUD XXX N ▢
AMA: 2005,Aug,7-8; 2005,Jul,11-12

85525 **Heparin neutralization**
0.00 0.00 FUD XXX N ▢
AMA: 2005,Aug,7-8; 2005,Jul,11-12

85530   **Heparin-protamine tolerance test**
   🔲 0.00   ✂ 0.00   **FUD** XXX   N ⬚
   AMA: 2005,Aug,7-8; 2005,Jul,11-12

85536   **Iron stain, peripheral blood**
   EXCLUDES   Iron stains on bone marrow or other tissues with physician evaluation (88313)
   🔲 0.00   ✂ 0.00   **FUD** XXX   N ⬚
   AMA: 2005,Aug,7-8; 2005,Jul,11-12

85540   **Leukocyte alkaline phosphatase with count**
   🔲 0.00   ✂ 0.00   **FUD** XXX   N ⬚
   AMA: 2005,Aug,7-8; 2005,Jul,11-12

85547   **Mechanical fragility, RBC**
   🔲 0.00   ✂ 0.00   **FUD** XXX   N ⬚
   AMA: 2005,Aug,7-8; 2005,Jul,11-12

85549   **Muramidase**
   🔲 0.00   ✂ 0.00   **FUD** XXX   N ⬚
   AMA: 2005,Aug,7-8; 2005,Jul,11-12

85555   **Osmotic fragility, RBC; unincubated**
   🔲 0.00   ✂ 0.00   **FUD** XXX   N ⬚
   AMA: 2005,Aug,7-8; 2005,Jul,11-12

85557   **incubated**
   🔲 0.00   ✂ 0.00   **FUD** XXX   N ⬚
   AMA: 2005,Aug,7-8; 2005,Jul,11-12

85576   **Platelet, aggregation (in vitro), each agent**
   EXCLUDES   Thromboxane metabolite(s), including thromboxane, when performed, in urine (84431)
   🔲 0.00   ✂ 0.00   **FUD** XXX   ✖ N ⬚
   AMA: 2015,Jan,16; 2014,Jan,11; 2012,Jan,15-42; 2011,Jan,11

85597   **Phospholipid neutralization; platelet**
   🔲 0.00   ✂ 0.00   **FUD** XXX   N ⬚
   AMA: 2015,Jan,16; 2014,Jan,11; 2011,Apr,9; 2010,Dec,7-10

85598   **hexagonal phospholipid**
   🔲 0.00   ✂ 0.00   **FUD** XXX   N
   AMA: 2015,Jan,16; 2014,Jan,11; 2011,Apr,3-8; 2011,Apr,9; 2010,Dec,7-10

85610   **Prothrombin time;**
   🔲 0.00   ✂ 0.00   **FUD** XXX   ✖ N ⬚
   AMA: 2005,Aug,7-8; 2005,Jul,11-12

85611   **substitution, plasma fractions, each**
   🔲 0.00   ✂ 0.00   **FUD** XXX   N ⬚
   AMA: 2005,Aug,7-8; 2005,Jul,11-12

85612   **Russell viper venom time (includes venom); undiluted**
   🔲 0.00   ✂ 0.00   **FUD** XXX   N ⬚
   AMA: 2005,Aug,7-8; 2005,Jul,11-12

85613   **diluted**
   🔲 0.00   ✂ 0.00   **FUD** XXX   N ⬚
   AMA: 2005,Aug,7-8; 2005,Jul,11-12

85635   **Reptilase test**
   🔲 0.00   ✂ 0.00   **FUD** XXX   N ⬚
   AMA: 2005,Aug,7-8; 2005,Jul,11-12

85651   **Sedimentation rate, erythrocyte; non-automated**
   🔲 0.00   ✂ 0.00   **FUD** XXX   ✖ N
   AMA: 2005,Aug,7-8; 2005,Jul,11-12

85652   **automated**
   INCLUDES   Westergren test
   🔲 0.00   ✂ 0.00   **FUD** XXX   N ⬚
   AMA: 2005,Aug,7-8; 2005,Jul,11-12

85660   **Sickling of RBC, reduction**
   EXCLUDES   Hemoglobin electrophoresis (83020)
   🔲 0.00   ✂ 0.00   **FUD** XXX   N ⬚
   AMA: 2005,Aug,7-8; 2005,Jul,11-12

85670   **Thrombin time; plasma**
   🔲 0.00   ✂ 0.00   **FUD** XXX   N ⬚
   AMA: 2005,Jul,11-12; 2005,Aug,7-8

85675   **titer**
   🔲 0.00   ✂ 0.00   **FUD** XXX   N ⬚
   AMA: 2005,Jul,11-12; 2005,Aug,7-8

85705   **Thromboplastin inhibition, tissue**
   EXCLUDES   Individual clotting factors (85245-85247)
   🔲 0.00   ✂ 0.00   **FUD** XXX   N ⬚
   AMA: 2005,Aug,7-8; 2005,Jul,11-12

85730-85732 Partial Thromboplastin Time (PTT)

EXCLUDES   Agglutinins (86000, 86156-86157)
   Antiplasmin (85410)
   Antithrombin III (85300-85301)
   Blood banking procedures (86850-86999)

85730   **Thromboplastin time, partial (PTT); plasma or whole blood**
   INCLUDES   Hicks-Pitney test
   🔲 0.00   ✂ 0.00   **FUD** XXX   N ⬚
   AMA: 2005,Aug,7-8; 2005,Jul,11-12

85732   **substitution, plasma fractions, each**
   🔲 0.00   ✂ 0.00   **FUD** XXX   N ⬚
   AMA: 2015,Jan,16; 2014,Jan,11; 2011,Apr,9

85810-85999 Blood Viscosity and Unlisted Hematology Procedures

85810   **Viscosity**
   🔲 0.00   ✂ 0.00   **FUD** XXX   N
   AMA: 2015,Jan,16; 2014,Jan,11; 2012,Jan,15-42; 2011,Jan,11

85999   **Unlisted hematology and coagulation procedure**
   🔲 0.00   ✂ 0.00   **FUD** XXX   N
   AMA: 2015,Jan,16; 2014,Jan,11

86000-86063 Antibody Testing

86000   **Agglutinins, febrile (eg, Brucella, Francisella, Murine typhus, Q fever, Rocky Mountain spotted fever, scrub typhus), each antigen**
   EXCLUDES   Infectious agent antibodies (86602-86804)
   🔲 0.00   ✂ 0.00   **FUD** XXX   N
   AMA: 2015,Jan,16; 2014,Jan,11

86001   **Allergen specific IgG quantitative or semiquantitative, each allergen**
   🔲 0.00   ✂ 0.00   **FUD** XXX   N ⬚
   AMA: 2005,Aug,7-8; 2005,Jul,11-12

86003   **Allergen specific IgE; quantitative or semiquantitative, each allergen**
   EXCLUDES   Total quantitative IgE (82785)
   🔲 0.00   ✂ 0.00   **FUD** XXX   N ⬚
   AMA: 2015,Jan,16; 2014,Jan,11

86005   **qualitative, multiallergen screen (dipstick, paddle, or disk)**
   EXCLUDES   Total qualitative IgE (83518)
   🔲 0.00   ✂ 0.00   **FUD** XXX   N
   AMA: 2015,Jan,16; 2014,Jan,11

86021   **Antibody identification; leukocyte antibodies**
   🔲 0.00   ✂ 0.00   **FUD** XXX   N ⬚
   AMA: 2005,Jul,11-12; 2005,Aug,7-8

86022   **platelet antibodies**
   🔲 0.00   ✂ 0.00   **FUD** XXX   N ⬚
   AMA: 2005,Jul,11-12; 2005,Aug,7-8

86023   **platelet associated immunoglobulin assay**
   🔲 0.00   ✂ 0.00   **FUD** XXX   N ⬚
   AMA: 2005,Jul,11-12; 2005,Aug,7-8

86038   **Antinuclear antibodies (ANA);**
   🔲 0.00   ✂ 0.00   **FUD** XXX   N ⬚
   AMA: 2005,Aug,7-8; 2005,Jul,11-12

86039   **titer**
   🔲 0.00   ✂ 0.00   **FUD** XXX   N ⬚
   AMA: 2005,Aug,7-8; 2005,Jul,11-12

86060	**Antistreptolysin 0; titer**

0.00   0.00   **FUD** XXX   N

AMA: 2005,Jul,11-12; 2005,Aug,7-8

86063	**screen**

0.00   0.00   **FUD** XXX   N

AMA: 2005,Jul,11-12; 2005,Aug,7-8

86077-86079 Blood Bank Services

86077	**Blood bank physician services; difficult cross match and/or evaluation of irregular antibody(s), interpretation and written report**

1.47   1.58   **FUD** XXX   01 80

AMA: 2005,Aug,7-8; 2005,Jul,11-12

86078	**investigation of transfusion reaction including suspicion of transmissible disease, interpretation and written report**

1.46   1.57   **FUD** XXX   01 80

AMA: 2005,Aug,7-8; 2005,Jul,11-12

86079	**authorization for deviation from standard blood banking procedures (eg, use of outdated blood, transfusion of Rh incompatible units), with written report**

1.44   1.54   **FUD** XXX   01 80

AMA: 2005,Aug,7-8; 2005,Jul,11-12

86140-86344 [86152, 86153] Diagnostic Immunology Testing

86140	**C-reactive protein;**

0.00   0.00   **FUD** XXX   N

AMA: 2005,Aug,7-8; 2005,Jul,11-12

86141	**high sensitivity (hsCRP)**

0.00   0.00   **FUD** XXX   N

AMA: 2005,Aug,7-8; 2005,Jul,11-12

86146	**Beta 2 Glycoprotein I antibody, each**

0.00   0.00   **FUD** XXX   N

AMA: 2005,Aug,7-8; 2005,Jul,11-12

86147	**Cardiolipin (phospholipid) antibody, each Ig class**

0.00   0.00   **FUD** XXX   N

AMA: 2005,Aug,7-8; 2005,Jul,11-12

# 86152	**Cell enumeration using immunologic selection and identification in fluid specimen (eg, circulating tumor cells in blood);**

0.00   0.00   **FUD** XXX   N

EXCLUDES   Flow cytometric immunophenotyping (88184-88189)
Flow cytometric quantitation (86355-86357, 86359-86361, 86367)
Code also physician interpretation/report when performed ([86153])

# 86153	**physician interpretation and report, when required**

0.00   0.00   **FUD** 000   B

EXCLUDES   Flow cytometric immunophenotyping (88184-88189)
Flow cytometric quantitation (86355-86357, 86359-86361, 86367)
Code first cell enumeration, when performed ([86152])

86148	**Anti-phosphatidylserine (phospholipid) antibody**

EXCLUDES   Antiprothrombin (phospholipid cofactor) antibody (86849)

0.00   0.00   **FUD** XXX   N

AMA: 2015,Jan,16; 2014,Jan,11

86152	**Resequenced code. See code following 86147.**
86153	**Resequenced code. See code before 86148.**

86155	**Chemotaxis assay, specify method**

0.00   0.00   **FUD** XXX   N

AMA: 2005,Aug,7-8; 2005,Jul,11-12

86156	**Cold agglutinin; screen**

0.00   0.00   **FUD** XXX   N

AMA: 2005,Aug,7-8; 2005,Jul,11-12

86157	**titer**

0.00   0.00   **FUD** XXX   N

AMA: 2005,Aug,7-8; 2005,Jul,11-12

86160	**Complement; antigen, each component**

0.00   0.00   **FUD** XXX   N

AMA: 2005,Aug,7-8; 2005,Jul,11-12

86161	**functional activity, each component**

0.00   0.00   **FUD** XXX   N

AMA: 2005,Aug,7-8; 2005,Jul,11-12

86162	**total hemolytic (CH50)**

0.00   0.00   **FUD** XXX   N

AMA: 2005,Aug,7-8; 2005,Jul,11-12

86171	**Complement fixation tests, each antigen**

0.00   0.00   **FUD** XXX   N

AMA: 2005,Aug,7-8; 2005,Jul,11-12

86185	**Counterimmunoelectrophoresis, each antigen**

0.00   0.00   **FUD** XXX   N

AMA: 2005,Aug,7-8; 2005,Jul,11-12

86200	**Cyclic citrullinated peptide (CCP), antibody**

0.00   0.00   **FUD** XXX   N

AMA: 2015,Jan,16; 2014,Jan,11

86215	**Deoxyribonuclease, antibody**

0.00   0.00   **FUD** XXX   N

AMA: 2005,Aug,7-8; 2005,Jul,11-12

86225	**Deoxyribonucleic acid (DNA) antibody; native or double stranded**

EXCLUDES   HIV antibody tests (86701-86703)

0.00   0.00   **FUD** XXX   N

AMA: 2005,Aug,7-8; 2005,Jul,11-12

86226	**single stranded**

EXCLUDES   Anti D.S, DNA, IFA, eg, using C. Lucilae (86255-86256)

0.00   0.00   **FUD** XXX   N

AMA: 2005,Aug,7-8; 2005,Jul,11-12

86235	**Extractable nuclear antigen, antibody to, any method (eg, nRNP, SS-A, SS-B, Sm, RNP, Sc170, J01), each antibody**

0.00   0.00   **FUD** XXX   N

AMA: 2005,Aug,7-8; 2005,Jul,11-12

86243	**Fc receptor**

0.00   0.00   **FUD** XXX   N

AMA: 2005,Aug,7-8; 2005,Jul,11-12

86255	**Fluorescent noninfectious agent antibody; screen, each antibody**

0.00   0.00   **FUD** XXX   N

AMA: 2005,Aug,9-10; 2005,Aug,7-8

86256	**titer, each antibody**

EXCLUDES   Fluorescent technique for antigen identification in tissue (88346, [88350])
FTA (86780)
Gel (agar) diffusion tests (86331)
Indirect fluorescence (88346, [88350])

0.00   0.00   **FUD** XXX   N

AMA: 2005,Aug,9-10; 2005,Aug,7-8

86277	**Growth hormone, human (HGH), antibody**

0.00   0.00   **FUD** XXX   N

AMA: 2005,Aug,7-8; 2005,Jul,11-12

86280	**Hemagglutination inhibition test (HAI)**

EXCLUDES   Antibodies to infectious agents (86602-86804)
Rubella (86762)

0.00   0.00   **FUD** XXX   N

AMA: 2005,Aug,7-8; 2005,Jul,11-12

86294	**Immunoassay for tumor antigen, qualitative or semiquantitative (eg, bladder tumor antigen)**

EXCLUDES   Qualitative NMP22 protein (86386)

0.00   0.00   **FUD** XXX   ✖ N

AMA: 2005,Aug,7-8; 2005,Jul,11-12

86300 Immunoassay for tumor antigen, quantitative; CA 15-3 (27.29)
    ⚙ 0.00   ⚖ 0.00   **FUD** XXX   N ▣
    AMA: 2005,Aug,7-8; 2005,Jul,11-12

86301 CA 19-9
    ⚙ 0.00   ⚖ 0.00   **FUD** XXX   N ▣
    AMA: 2005,Aug,7-8; 2005,Jul,11-12

86304 CA 125
    EXCLUDES _Measurement of serum HER-2/neu oncoprotein (83950)_
    ⚙ 0.00   ⚖ 0.00   **FUD** XXX   N ▣
    AMA: 2005,Aug,7-8; 2005,Jul,11-12

86305 Human epididymis protein 4 (HE4)
    ⚙ 0.00   ⚖ 0.00   **FUD** XXX   N

86308 Heterophile antibodies; screening
    EXCLUDES _Antibodies to infectious agents (86602-86804)_
    ⚙ 0.00   ⚖ 0.00   **FUD** XXX   ✕ N
    AMA: 2005,Jul,11-12; 2005,Aug,7-8

86309 titer
    EXCLUDES _Antibodies to infectious agents (86602-86804)_
    ⚙ 0.00   ⚖ 0.00   **FUD** XXX   N
    AMA: 2005,Jul,11-12; 2005,Aug,7-8

86310 titers after absorption with beef cells and guinea pig kidney
    EXCLUDES _Antibodies to infectious agents (86602-86804)_
    ⚙ 0.00   ⚖ 0.00   **FUD** XXX   N
    AMA: 2005,Jul,11-12; 2005,Aug,7-8

86316 Immunoassay for tumor antigen, other antigen, quantitative (eg, CA 50, 72-4, 549), each
    ⚙ 0.00   ⚖ 0.00   **FUD** XXX   N ▣
    AMA: 2015,Jan,16; 2014,Jan,11; 2012,Jan,15-42; 2011,Jan,11

86317 Immunoassay for infectious agent antibody, quantitative, not otherwise specified
    EXCLUDES _Immunoassay techniques for antigens (83516, 83518-83520, 87301-87450, 87810-87899)_
    Particle agglutination test (86403)
    ⚙ 0.00   ⚖ 0.00   **FUD** XXX   N ▣
    AMA: 2005,Jul,11-12; 2005,Aug,7-8

86318 Immunoassay for infectious agent antibody, qualitative or semiquantitative, single step method (eg, reagent strip)
    ⚙ 0.00   ⚖ 0.00   **FUD** XXX   ✕ N
    AMA: 2015,Jan,16; 2014,Jan,11; 2012,Jan,15-42; 2011,Jan,11

86320 Immunoelectrophoresis; serum
    ⚙ 0.00   ⚖ 0.00   **FUD** XXX   N ▣
    AMA: 2005,Jul,11-12; 2005,Aug,7-8

86325 other fluids (eg, urine, cerebrospinal fluid) with concentration
    ⚙ 0.00   ⚖ 0.00   **FUD** XXX   N ▣
    AMA: 2005,Jul,11-12; 2005,Aug,7-8

86327 crossed (2-dimensional assay)
    ⚙ 0.00   ⚖ 0.00   **FUD** XXX   N ▣
    AMA: 2005,Jul,11-12; 2005,Aug,7-8

86329 Immunodiffusion; not elsewhere specified
    ⚙ 0.00   ⚖ 0.00   **FUD** XXX   N ▣
    AMA: 2015,Jan,16; 2014,Jan,11; 2012,Jan,15-42; 2011,Jan,11

86331 gel diffusion, qualitative (Ouchterlony), each antigen or antibody
    ⚙ 0.00   ⚖ 0.00   **FUD** XXX   N ▣
    AMA: 2005,Aug,7-8; 2005,Jul,11-12

86332 Immune complex assay
    ⚙ 0.00   ⚖ 0.00   **FUD** XXX   N
    AMA: 2005,Aug,7-8; 2005,Jul,11-12

86334 Immunofixation electrophoresis; serum
    ⚙ 0.00   ⚖ 0.00   **FUD** XXX   N ▣
    AMA: 2005,Jul,11-12; 2005,Aug,7-8

86335 other fluids with concentration (eg, urine, CSF)
    ⚙ 0.00   ⚖ 0.00   **FUD** XXX   N ▣
    AMA: 2005,Aug,7-8; 2005,Jul,11-12

86336 Inhibin A
    ⚙ 0.00   ⚖ 0.00   **FUD** XXX   N
    AMA: 2005,Aug,7-8; 2005,Jul,11-12

86337 Insulin antibodies
    ⚙ 0.00   ⚖ 0.00   **FUD** XXX   N
    AMA: 2005,Aug,7-8; 2005,Jul,11-12

86340 Intrinsic factor antibodies
    ⚙ 0.00   ⚖ 0.00   **FUD** XXX   N
    AMA: 2005,Jul,11-12; 2005,Aug,7-8

86341 Islet cell antibody
    ⚙ 0.00   ⚖ 0.00   **FUD** XXX   N
    AMA: 2015,Jan,16; 2014,Jan,11

86343 Leukocyte histamine release test (LHR)
    ⚙ 0.00   ⚖ 0.00   **FUD** XXX   N
    AMA: 2005,Aug,7-8; 2005,Jul,11-12

86344 Leukocyte phagocytosis
    ⚙ 0.00   ⚖ 0.00   **FUD** XXX   N ▣
    AMA: 2005,Aug,7-8; 2005,Jul,11-12

86352 Assay Cellular Function

86352 Cellular function assay involving stimulation (eg, mitogen or antigen) and detection of biomarker (eg, ATP)
    ⚙ 0.00   ⚖ 0.00   **FUD** XXX   N

86353 Lymphocyte Mitogen Response Assay

CMS: 100-3,190.8 Lymphocyte Mitogen Response Assays

86353 Lymphocyte transformation, mitogen (phytomitogen) or antigen induced blastogenesis
    EXCLUDES _Cellular function assay involving stimulation and detection of biomarker (86352)_
    ⚙ 0.00   ⚖ 0.00   **FUD** XXX   N ▣
    AMA: 2005,Aug,7-8; 2005,Jul,11-12

86355-86593 Additional Diagnostic Immunology Testing

86355 B cells, total count
    Do not report with flow cytometry interpretation (88187-88189)
    ⚙ 0.00   ⚖ 0.00   **FUD** XXX   N
    AMA: 2015,Jan,16; 2014,Jan,11

86356 Mononuclear cell antigen, quantitative (eg, flow cytometry), not otherwise specified, each antigen
    Do not report with flow cytometry interpretation (88187-88189)
    ⚙ 0.00   ⚖ 0.00   **FUD** XXX   N
    AMA: 2015,Jan,16; 2014,Jan,11

86357 Natural killer (NK) cells, total count
    Do not report with flow cytometry interpretation (88187-88189)
    ⚙ 0.00   ⚖ 0.00   **FUD** XXX   N
    AMA: 2015,Jan,16; 2014,Jan,11

86359 T cells; total count
    Do not report with flow cytometry interpretation (88187-88189)
    ⚙ 0.00   ⚖ 0.00   **FUD** XXX   N ▣
    AMA: 2015,Jan,16; 2014,Jan,11

86360 absolute CD4 and CD8 count, including ratio
    Do not report with flow cytometry interpretation (88187-88189)
    ⚙ 0.00   ⚖ 0.00   **FUD** XXX   N ▣
    AMA: 2015,Jan,16; 2014,Jan,11

86361 absolute CD4 count
    Do not report with flow cytometry interpretation (88187-88189)
    ⚙ 0.00   ⚖ 0.00   **FUD** XXX   N ▣
    AMA: 2015,Jan,16; 2014,Jan,11

86367 Stem cells (ie, CD34), total count
    Do not report with flow cytometry interpretation (88187-88189)
    ⚙ 0.00   ⚖ 0.00   **FUD** XXX   N
    AMA: 2015,Jan,16; 2014,Jan,11; 2013,Oct,3

86376 **Microsomal antibodies (eg, thyroid or liver-kidney), each**
🔲 0.00 ⚗ 0.00 **FUD** XXX   Ⓝ ▢
AMA: 2005,Jul,11-12; 2005,Aug,7-8

86378 **Migration inhibitory factor test (MIF)**
🔲 0.00 ⚗ 0.00 **FUD** XXX   Ⓝ ▢
AMA: 2005,Aug,7-8; 2005,Jul,11-12

86382 **Neutralization test, viral**
🔲 0.00 ⚗ 0.00 **FUD** XXX   Ⓝ ▢
AMA: 2005,Aug,7-8; 2005,Jul,11-12

86384 **Nitroblue tetrazolium dye test (NTD)**
🔲 0.00 ⚗ 0.00 **FUD** XXX   Ⓝ ▢
AMA: 2005,Aug,7-8; 2005,Jul,11-12

86386 **Nuclear Matrix Protein 22 (NMP22), qualitative**
🔲 0.00 ⚗ 0.00 **FUD** XXX   ☒ Ⓝ

86403 **Particle agglutination; screen, each antibody**
🔲 0.00 ⚗ 0.00 **FUD** XXX   Ⓝ
AMA: 2005,Jul,11-12; 2005,Aug,7-8

86406 **titer, each antibody**
🔲 0.00 ⚗ 0.00 **FUD** XXX   Ⓝ
AMA: 2005,Jul,11-12; 2005,Aug,7-8

86430 **Rheumatoid factor; qualitative**
🔲 0.00 ⚗ 0.00 **FUD** XXX   Ⓝ
AMA: 2005,Aug,7-8; 2005,Jul,11-12

86431 **quantitative**
🔲 0.00 ⚗ 0.00 **FUD** XXX   Ⓝ
AMA: 2005,Aug,7-8; 2005,Jul,11-12

86480 **Tuberculosis test, cell mediated immunity antigen response measurement; gamma interferon**
🔲 0.00 ⚗ 0.00 **FUD** XXX   Ⓝ
AMA: 2015,Jan,16; 2014,Jan,11; 2010,Dec,7-10

86481 **enumeration of gamma interferon-producing T-cells in cell suspension**
🔲 0.00 ⚗ 0.00 **FUD** XXX   Ⓝ
AMA: 2010,Dec,7-10

86485 **Skin test; candida**
🔲 0.00 ⚗ 0.00 **FUD** XXX   Q1 80 TC
AMA: 2005,Jul,11-12; 2005,Aug,7-8

86486 **unlisted antigen, each**
🔲 0.14 ⚗ 0.14 **FUD** XXX   Q1 80 TC
AMA: 2008,Apr,5-7

86490 **coccidioidomycosis**
🔲 0.19 ⚗ 0.19 **FUD** XXX   Q1 80 TC
AMA: 2005,Aug,7-8; 2005,Jul,11-12

86510 **histoplasmosis**
🔲 0.17 ⚗ 0.17 **FUD** XXX   Q1 80 TC
AMA: 2005,Aug,7-8; 2005,Jul,11-12

86580 **tuberculosis, intradermal**
ᴵᴺᶜᴸᵁᴰᴱˢ Heaf test
Intradermal Mantoux test
ᴱˣᶜᴸᵁᴰᴱˢ Skin test for allergy (95012-95199)
Tuberculosis test, cell mediated immunity measurement of gamma interferon antigen response (86480)
🔲 0.22 ⚗ 0.22 **FUD** XXX   Q1 80 TC ▢
AMA: 2005,Aug,7-8; 2005,Jul,11-12

86590 **Streptokinase, antibody**
ᴱˣᶜᴸᵁᴰᴱˢ Antibodies to infectious agents (86602-86804)
🔲 0.00 ⚗ 0.00 **FUD** XXX   Ⓝ
AMA: 2005,Jul,11-12; 2005,Aug,7-8

86592 **Syphilis test, non-treponemal antibody; qualitative (eg, VDRL, RPR, ART)**
ᴵᴺᶜᴸᵁᴰᴱˢ Wasserman test
ᴱˣᶜᴸᵁᴰᴱˢ Antibodies to infectious agents (86602-86804)
🔲 0.00 ⚗ 0.00 **FUD** XXX   Ⓐ
AMA: 2005,Jul,11-12; 2005,Aug,7-8

86593 **quantitative**
ᴱˣᶜᴸᵁᴰᴱˢ Antibodies to infectious agents (86602-86804)
🔲 0.00 ⚗ 0.00 **FUD** XXX   Ⓐ
AMA: 2005,Jul,11-12; 2005,Aug,7-8

86602-86698 Testing for Antibodies to Infectious Agents: Actinomyces—Histoplasma

ᴵᴺᶜᴸᵁᴰᴱˢ Qualitative or semiquantitative immunoassays performed by multiple-step methods for the detection of antibodies to infectious agents
ᴱˣᶜᴸᵁᴰᴱˢ Detection of:
Antibodies other than those to infectious agents, see specific antibody or method
Infectious agent/antigen (87260-87899 [87623, 87624, 87625, 87806])
Immunoassays by single-step method (86318)

86602 **Antibody; actinomyces**
🔲 0.00 ⚗ 0.00 **FUD** XXX   Ⓝ
AMA: 2015,Jan,16; 2014,Jan,11

86603 **adenovirus**
🔲 0.00 ⚗ 0.00 **FUD** XXX   Ⓝ
AMA: 2005,Jul,11-12; 2005,Aug,7-8

86606 **Aspergillus**
🔲 0.00 ⚗ 0.00 **FUD** XXX   Ⓝ
AMA: 2005,Jul,11-12; 2005,Aug,7-8

86609 **bacterium, not elsewhere specified**
🔲 0.00 ⚗ 0.00 **FUD** XXX   Ⓝ
AMA: 2005,Jul,11-12; 2005,Aug,7-8

86611 **Bartonella**
🔲 0.00 ⚗ 0.00 **FUD** XXX   Ⓝ
AMA: 2005,Jul,11-12; 2005,Aug,7-8

86612 **Blastomyces**
🔲 0.00 ⚗ 0.00 **FUD** XXX   Ⓝ
AMA: 2005,Jul,11-12; 2005,Aug,7-8

86615 **Bordetella**
🔲 0.00 ⚗ 0.00 **FUD** XXX   Ⓝ
AMA: 2005,Jul,11-12; 2005,Aug,7-8

86617 **Borrelia burgdorferi (Lyme disease) confirmatory test (eg, Western Blot or immunoblot)**
🔲 0.00 ⚗ 0.00 **FUD** XXX   Ⓝ
AMA: 2005,Jul,11-12; 2005,Aug,7-8

86618 **Borrelia burgdorferi (Lyme disease)**
🔲 0.00 ⚗ 0.00 **FUD** XXX   ☒ Ⓝ
AMA: 2005,Jul,11-12; 2005,Aug,7-8

86619 **Borrelia (relapsing fever)**
🔲 0.00 ⚗ 0.00 **FUD** XXX   Ⓝ
AMA: 2005,Jul,11-12; 2005,Aug,7-8

86622 **Brucella**
🔲 0.00 ⚗ 0.00 **FUD** XXX   Ⓝ
AMA: 2005,Jul,11-12; 2005,Aug,7-8

86625 **Campylobacter**
🔲 0.00 ⚗ 0.00 **FUD** XXX   Ⓝ
AMA: 2005,Jul,11-12; 2005,Aug,7-8

86628 **Candida**
ᴱˣᶜᴸᵁᴰᴱˢ Candida skin test (86485)
🔲 0.00 ⚗ 0.00 **FUD** XXX   Ⓝ
AMA: 2005,Jul,11-12; 2005,Aug,7-8

86631 **Chlamydia**
🔲 0.00 ⚗ 0.00 **FUD** XXX   Ⓐ
AMA: 2005,Jul,11-12; 2005,Aug,7-8

86632 **Chlamydia, IgM**
ᴱˣᶜᴸᵁᴰᴱˢ Chlamydia antigen (87270, 87320)
Fluorescent antibody technique (86255-86256)
🔲 0.00 ⚗ 0.00 **FUD** XXX   Ⓐ
AMA: 2005,Jul,11-12; 2005,Aug,7-8

86635 **Coccidioides**
🔲 0.00 ⚗ 0.00 **FUD** XXX   Ⓝ
AMA: 2005,Jul,11-12; 2005,Aug,7-8

86638 **Coxiella burnetii (Q fever)**
🔧 0.00 ⚕ 0.00 **FUD** XXX
AMA: 2005,Jul,11-12; 2005,Aug,7-8

86641 **Cryptococcus**
🔧 0.00 ⚕ 0.00 **FUD** XXX
AMA: 2005,Jul,11-12; 2005,Aug,7-8

86644 **cytomegalovirus (CMV)**
🔧 0.00 ⚕ 0.00 **FUD** XXX
AMA: 2005,Jul,11-12; 2005,Aug,7-8

86645 **cytomegalovirus (CMV), IgM**
🔧 0.00 ⚕ 0.00 **FUD** XXX
AMA: 2015,Jan,16; 2014,Jan,11

86648 **Diphtheria**
🔧 0.00 ⚕ 0.00 **FUD** XXX
AMA: 2005,Jul,11-12; 2005,Aug,7-8

86651 **encephalitis, California (La Crosse)**
🔧 0.00 ⚕ 0.00 **FUD** XXX
AMA: 2005,Jul,11-12; 2005,Aug,7-8

86652 **encephalitis, Eastern equine**
🔧 0.00 ⚕ 0.00 **FUD** XXX
AMA: 2005,Jul,11-12; 2005,Aug,7-8

86653 **encephalitis, St. Louis**
🔧 0.00 ⚕ 0.00 **FUD** XXX
AMA: 2005,Jul,11-12; 2005,Aug,7-8

86654 **encephalitis, Western equine**
🔧 0.00 ⚕ 0.00 **FUD** XXX
AMA: 2005,Jul,11-12; 2005,Aug,7-8

86658 **enterovirus (eg, coxsackie, echo, polio)**
EXCLUDES Antibodies to:
Trichinella (86784)
Trypanosoma—see code for specific methodology
Tuberculosis (86580)
Viral—see code for specific methodology
🔧 0.00 ⚕ 0.00 **FUD** XXX
AMA: 2005,Jul,11-12; 2005,Aug,7-8

86663 **Epstein-Barr (EB) virus, early antigen (EA)**
🔧 0.00 ⚕ 0.00 **FUD** XXX
AMA: 2005,Jul,11-12; 2005,Aug,7-8

86664 **Epstein-Barr (EB) virus, nuclear antigen (EBNA)**
🔧 0.00 ⚕ 0.00 **FUD** XXX
AMA: 2005,Jul,11-12; 2005,Aug,7-8

86665 **Epstein-Barr (EB) virus, viral capsid (VCA)**
🔧 0.00 ⚕ 0.00 **FUD** XXX
AMA: 2005,Jul,11-12; 2005,Aug,7-8

86666 **Ehrlichia**
🔧 0.00 ⚕ 0.00 **FUD** XXX
AMA: 2005,Jul,11-12; 2005,Aug,7-8

86668 **Francisella tularensis**
🔧 0.00 ⚕ 0.00 **FUD** XXX
AMA: 2005,Jul,11-12; 2005,Aug,7-8

86671 **fungus, not elsewhere specified**
🔧 0.00 ⚕ 0.00 **FUD** XXX
AMA: 2005,Jul,11-12; 2005,Aug,7-8

86674 **Giardia lamblia**
🔧 0.00 ⚕ 0.00 **FUD** XXX
AMA: 2005,Jul,11-12; 2005,Aug,7-8

86677 **Helicobacter pylori**
🔧 0.00 ⚕ 0.00 **FUD** XXX
AMA: 2015,Jan,16; 2014,Jan,11

86682 **helminth, not elsewhere specified**
🔧 0.00 ⚕ 0.00 **FUD** XXX
AMA: 2005,Jul,11-12; 2005,Aug,7-8

86684 **Haemophilus influenza**
🔧 0.00 ⚕ 0.00 **FUD** XXX
AMA: 2005,Jul,11-12; 2005,Aug,7-8

86687 **HTLV-I**
🔧 0.00 ⚕ 0.00 **FUD** XXX
AMA: 2005,Jul,11-12; 2005,Aug,7-8

86688 **HTLV-II**
🔧 0.00 ⚕ 0.00 **FUD** XXX
AMA: 2005,Jul,11-12; 2005,Aug,7-8

86689 **HTLV or HIV antibody, confirmatory test (eg, Western Blot)**
🔧 0.00 ⚕ 0.00 **FUD** XXX
AMA: 2015,Jan,16; 2014,Jan,11

86692 **hepatitis, delta agent**
EXCLUDES Hepatitis delta agent, antigen (87380)
🔧 0.00 ⚕ 0.00 **FUD** XXX
AMA: 2005,Jul,11-12; 2005,Aug,7-8

86694 **herpes simplex, non-specific type test**
🔧 0.00 ⚕ 0.00 **FUD** XXX
AMA: 2005,Jul,11-12; 2005,Aug,7-8

86695 **herpes simplex, type 1**
🔧 0.00 ⚕ 0.00 **FUD** XXX
AMA: 2015,Jan,16; 2014,Jan,11

86696 **herpes simplex, type 2**
🔧 0.00 ⚕ 0.00 **FUD** XXX
AMA: 2005,Jul,11-12; 2005,Aug,7-8

86698 **histoplasma**
🔧 0.00 ⚕ 0.00 **FUD** XXX
AMA: 2005,Jul,11-12; 2005,Aug,7-8

86701-86703 Testing for HIV Antibodies

CMS: 100-3,190.14 Human Immunodeficiency Virus Testing (Diagnosis); 100-3,190.9 Serologic Testing for Acquired Immunodeficiency Syndrome (AIDS)

INCLUDES Qualitative or semiquantitative immunoassays performed by multiple-step methods for the detection of antibodies to infectious agents

EXCLUDES Confirmatory test for HIV antibody (86689)
Detection of:
Antibodies other than those to infectious agents, see specific antibody or method
Infectious agent/antigen (87260-87899 [87623, 87624, 87625, 87806])
HIV-1 antigen (87390)
HIV-1 antigen(s) with HIV 1 and 2 antibodies, single result (87389)
HIV-2 antigen (87391)
Immunoassays by single-step method (86318)

Code also modifier 92 for test performed using a kit or transportable instrument comprising all or part of a single-use, disposable analytical chamber

86701 **Antibody; HIV-1**
🔧 0.00 ⚕ 0.00 **FUD** XXX ☒
AMA: 2015,Jan,16; 2014,Jan,11

86702 **HIV-2**
🔧 0.00 ⚕ 0.00 **FUD** XXX
AMA: 2015,Jan,16; 2014,Jan,11

86703 **HIV-1 and HIV-2, single result**
🔧 0.00 ⚕ 0.00 **FUD** XXX
AMA: 2015,Jan,16; 2014,Jan,11

86704-86804 Testing for Infectious Disease Antibodies: Hepatitis—Yersinia

INCLUDES Qualitative or semiquantitative immunoassays performed by multiple-step methods for the detection of antibodies to infectious agents

EXCLUDES Detection of:
Antibodies other than those to infectious agents, see specific antibody or method
Infectious agent/antigen (87260-87899 [87623, 87624, 87625, 87806])
Immunoassays by single-step method (86318)

86704 **Hepatitis B core antibody (HBcAb); total**
🔧 0.00 ⚕ 0.00 **FUD** XXX
AMA: 2015,Jan,16; 2014,Jan,11

86705 **IgM antibody**
🔧 0.00 ⚕ 0.00 **FUD** XXX
AMA: 2015,Jan,16; 2014,Jan,11

	86706	**Hepatitis B surface antibody (HBsAb)**				N
		0.00 0.00 **FUD** XXX				
		AMA: 2005,Jul,11-12; 2005,Aug,7-8				

86707 **Hepatitis Be antibody (HBeAb)**
0.00   0.00   **FUD** XXX   N
AMA: 2005,Jul,11-12; 2005,Aug,7-8

▲ 86708 **Hepatitis A antibody (HAAb)**
0.00   0.00   **FUD** XXX   N
AMA: 2015,Jan,16; 2014,Jan,11; 2012,Jan,15-42; 2011,Jan,11

▲ 86709 **Hepatitis A antibody (HAAb), IgM antibody**
0.00   0.00   **FUD** XXX   N
AMA: 2015,Jan,16; 2014,Jan,11; 2012,Jan,15-42; 2011,Jan,11

86710 **Antibody; influenza virus**
0.00   0.00   **FUD** XXX   N
AMA: 2015,Jan,16; 2014,Jan,11

86711 **JC (John Cunningham) virus**
0.00   0.00   **FUD** XXX   N

86713 **Legionella**
0.00   0.00   **FUD** XXX   N
AMA: 2005,Jul,11-12; 2005,Aug,7-8

86717 **Leishmania**
0.00   0.00   **FUD** XXX   N
AMA: 2005,Jul,11-12; 2005,Aug,7-8

86720 **Leptospira**
0.00   0.00   **FUD** XXX   N
AMA: 2005,Jul,11-12; 2005,Aug,7-8

86723 **Listeria monocytogenes**
0.00   0.00   **FUD** XXX   N
AMA: 2005,Jul,11-12; 2005,Aug,7-8

86727 **lymphocytic choriomeningitis**
0.00   0.00   **FUD** XXX   N
AMA: 2005,Jul,11-12; 2005,Aug,7-8

86729 **lymphogranuloma venereum**
0.00   0.00   **FUD** XXX   N
AMA: 2005,Jul,11-12; 2005,Aug,7-8

86732 **mucormycosis**
0.00   0.00   **FUD** XXX   N
AMA: 2005,Jul,11-12; 2005,Aug,7-8

86735 **mumps**
0.00   0.00   **FUD** XXX   N
AMA: 2015,Jan,16; 2014,Jan,11; 2012,Jan,15-42; 2011,Jan,11

86738 **mycoplasma**
0.00   0.00   **FUD** XXX   N
AMA: 2005,Jul,11-12; 2005,Aug,7-8

86741 **Neisseria meningitidis**
0.00   0.00   **FUD** XXX   N
AMA: 2005,Jul,11-12; 2005,Aug,7-8

86744 **Nocardia**
0.00   0.00   **FUD** XXX   N
AMA: 2005,Jul,11-12; 2005,Aug,7-8

86747 **parvovirus**
0.00   0.00   **FUD** XXX   N
AMA: 2005,Jul,11-12; 2005,Aug,7-8

86750 **Plasmodium (malaria)**
0.00   0.00   **FUD** XXX   N
AMA: 2005,Jul,11-12; 2005,Aug,7-8

86753 **protozoa, not elsewhere specified**
0.00   0.00   **FUD** XXX   N
AMA: 2005,Jul,11-12; 2005,Aug,7-8

86756 **respiratory syncytial virus**
0.00   0.00   **FUD** XXX   N
AMA: 2005,Jul,11-12; 2005,Aug,7-8

86757 **Rickettsia**
0.00   0.00   **FUD** XXX   N
AMA: 2005,Jul,11-12; 2005,Aug,7-8

86759 **rotavirus**
0.00   0.00   **FUD** XXX   N
AMA: 2005,Jul,11-12; 2005,Aug,7-8

86762 **rubella**
0.00   0.00   **FUD** XXX   N
AMA: 2005,Jul,11-12; 2005,Aug,7-8

86765 **rubeola**
0.00   0.00   **FUD** XXX   N
AMA: 2005,Jul,11-12; 2005,Aug,7-8

86768 **Salmonella**
0.00   0.00   **FUD** XXX   N
AMA: 2005,Jul,11-12; 2005,Aug,7-8

86771 **Shigella**
0.00   0.00   **FUD** XXX   N
AMA: 2005,Jul,11-12; 2005,Aug,7-8

86774 **tetanus**
0.00   0.00   **FUD** XXX   N
AMA: 2005,Jul,11-12; 2005,Aug,7-8

86777 **Toxoplasma**
0.00   0.00   **FUD** XXX   N
AMA: 2005,Jul,11-12; 2005,Aug,7-8

86778 **Toxoplasma, IgM**
0.00   0.00   **FUD** XXX   N
AMA: 2005,Jul,11-12; 2005,Aug,7-8

86780 **Treponema pallidum** *Syphilis*
0.00   0.00   **FUD** XXX   ☒ A
EXCLUDES   *Nontreponemal antibody analysis syphilis testing (86592-86593)*

86784 **Trichinella**
0.00   0.00   **FUD** XXX   N
AMA: 2005,Jul,11-12; 2005,Aug,7-8

86787 **varicella-zoster**
0.00   0.00   **FUD** XXX   N
AMA: 2005,Jul,11-12; 2005,Aug,7-8

86788 **West Nile virus, IgM**
0.00   0.00   **FUD** XXX   N

86789 **West Nile virus**
0.00   0.00   **FUD** XXX   N

86790 **virus, not elsewhere specified**
0.00   0.00   **FUD** XXX   N
AMA: 2005,Jul,11-12; 2005,Aug,7-8

86793 **Yersinia**
0.00   0.00   **FUD** XXX   N
AMA: 2005,Jul,11-12; 2005,Aug,7-8

86800 **Thyroglobulin antibody**
EXCLUDES   *Thyroglobulin (84432)*
0.00   0.00   **FUD** XXX   N
AMA: 2005,Jul,11-12; 2005,Aug,7-8

86803 **Hepatitis C antibody;**
0.00   0.00   **FUD** XXX   ☒ N
AMA: 2005,Jul,11-12; 2005,Aug,7-8

86804 **confirmatory test (eg, immunoblot)**
0.00   0.00   **FUD** XXX   N
AMA: 2015,Jan,16; 2014,Jan,11

86805-86808 Pre-Transplant Antibody Cross Matching

86805 **Lymphocytotoxicity assay, visual crossmatch; with titration**
0.00   0.00   **FUD** XXX   N ▭
AMA: 2015,Jan,16; 2014,Jan,11

86806 **without titration**
0.00   0.00   **FUD** XXX   N
AMA: 2005,Aug,7-8; 2005,Jul,11-12

| 26 /TC | PC/TC Comp Only | ☒ CLIA Waived | ♂ Male Only | ♀ Female Only |
| AMA: | CPT Asst | CMS: Pub 100 | A-Y OPPSI | ☒ Radiology Crosswalk |

364   Medicare (Red Text)   CPT © 2015 American Medical Association. All Rights Reserved. (Black Text)   © 2015 Optum360, LLC (Blue Text)

86807	Serum screening for cytotoxic percent reactive antibody (PRA); standard method

    0.00   0.00   **FUD** XXX   N

    AMA: 2015,Jan,16; 2014,Jan,11; 2012,Jan,15-42; 2011,Jan,11

86808	quick method

    0.00   0.00   **FUD** XXX   N

    AMA: 2015,Jan,16; 2014,Jan,11; 2012,Jan,15-42; 2011,Jan,11

86812-86826 Histocompatibility Testing

CMS: 100-3,110.8.1 Stem Cell Transplantation; 100-3,190.1 Histocompatibility Testing; 100-4,3,90.3 Stem Cell Transplantation; 100-4,3,90.3.1 Allogeneic Stem Cell Transplantation; 100-4,3,90.3.3 Billing for Allogeneic Stem Cell Transplants; 100-4,32,90 Billing for Stem Cell Transplantation

    EXCLUDES *HLA typing by molecular pathology techniques (81370-81383)*

86812	HLA typing; A, B, or C (eg, A10, B7, B27), single antigen

    0.00   0.00   **FUD** XXX   N

    AMA: 2015,Jan,16; 2014,Jan,11; 2012,May,3-10; 2012,Jan,15-42; 2011,Jan,11

86813	A, B, or C, multiple antigens

    0.00   0.00   **FUD** XXX   N CCI

    AMA: 2015,Jan,16; 2014,Jan,11; 2012,May,3-10; 2012,Jan,15-42; 2011,Jan,11

86816	DR/DQ, single antigen

    0.00   0.00   **FUD** XXX   N

    AMA: 2015,Jan,16; 2014,Jan,11; 2012,May,3-10; 2012,Jan,15-42; 2011,Jan,11

86817	DR/DQ, multiple antigens

    0.00   0.00   **FUD** XXX   N CCI

    AMA: 2015,Jan,16; 2014,Jan,11; 2012,May,3-10; 2012,Jan,15-42; 2011,Jan,11

86821	lymphocyte culture, mixed (MLC)

    0.00   0.00   **FUD** XXX   N

    AMA: 2015,Jan,16; 2014,Jan,11; 2012,Jan,15-42; 2011,Jan,11

86822	lymphocyte culture, primed (PLC)

    0.00   0.00   **FUD** XXX   N

    AMA: 2015,Jan,16; 2014,Jan,11; 2012,Jan,15-42; 2011,Jan,11

86825	Human leukocyte antigen (HLA) crossmatch, non-cytotoxic (eg, using flow cytometry); first serum sample or dilution

    0.00   0.00   **FUD** XXX   N

    INCLUDES Autologous HLA crossmatch

    EXCLUDES *Lymphocytotoxicity visual crossmatch (86805-86806)*

    Do not report with (86355, 86359, 88184-88189)

+	86826	each additional serum sample or sample dilution (List separately in addition to primary procedure)

    0.00   0.00   **FUD** XXX   N

    INCLUDES Autologous HLA crossmatch

    EXCLUDES *Lymphocytotoxicity visual crossmatch (86805-86806)*

    Code first (86825)

    Do not report with (86355, 86359, 88184-88189)

86828-86849 HLA Antibodies

86828	Antibody to human leukocyte antigens (HLA), solid phase assays (eg, microspheres or beads, ELISA, flow cytometry); qualitative assessment of the presence or absence of antibody(ies) to HLA Class I and Class II HLA antigens

    0.00   0.00   **FUD** XXX   N

    Code also solid phase testing of untreated and treated specimens of either class of HLA after treatment (86828-86833)

86829	qualitative assessment of the presence or absence of antibody(ies) to HLA Class I or Class II HLA antigens

    0.00   0.00   **FUD** XXX   N

    Code also solid phase testing of untreated and treated specimens of either class of HLA after treatment (86828-86833)

86830	antibody identification by qualitative panel using complete HLA phenotypes, HLA Class I

    0.00   0.00   **FUD** XXX   N

    Code also solid phase testing of untreated and treated specimens of either class of HLA after treatment (86828-86833)

86831	antibody identification by qualitative panel using complete HLA phenotypes, HLA Class II

    0.00   0.00   **FUD** XXX   N

    Code also solid phase testing of untreated and treated specimens of either class of HLA after treatment (86828-86833)

86832	high definition qualitative panel for identification of antibody specificities (eg, individual antigen per bead methodology), HLA Class I

    0.00   0.00   **FUD** XXX   N

    Code also solid phase testing of untreated and treated specimens of either class of HLA after treatment (86828-86833)

86833	high definition qualitative panel for identification of antibody specificities (eg, individual antigen per bead methodology), HLA Class II

    0.00   0.00   **FUD** XXX   N

    Code also solid phase testing of untreated and treated specimens of either class of HLA after treatment (86828-86833)

86834	semi-quantitative panel (eg, titer), HLA Class I

    0.00   0.00   **FUD** XXX   N

86835	semi-quantitative panel (eg, titer), HLA Class II

    0.00   0.00   **FUD** XXX   N

86849	Unlisted immunology procedure

    0.00   0.00   **FUD** XXX   N

    AMA: 2015,Jan,16; 2014,Jan,11; 2012,Jan,15-42; 2011,Jan,11

86850-86999 Transfusion Services

    EXCLUDES *Apheresis (36511-36512)*

    Therapeutic phlebotomy (99195)

86850	Antibody screen, RBC, each serum technique

    0.00   0.00   **FUD** XXX   01

    AMA: 2015,Jan,16; 2014,Jan,11

86860	Antibody elution (RBC), each elution

    0.00   0.00   **FUD** XXX   S

    AMA: 2005,Jul,11-12; 2005,Aug,7-8

86870	Antibody identification, RBC antibodies, each panel for each serum technique

    0.00   0.00   **FUD** XXX   01

    AMA: 2015,Jan,16; 2014,Jan,11; 2012,Jan,15-42; 2011,Jan,11

86880	Antihuman globulin test (Coombs test); direct, each antiserum

    0.00   0.00   **FUD** XXX   S

    AMA: 2005,Aug,7-8; 2005,Jul,11-12

86885	indirect, qualitative, each reagent red cell

    0.00   0.00   **FUD** XXX   S

    AMA: 2015,Jan,16; 2014,Jan,11

86886	indirect, each antibody titer

    EXCLUDES *Indirect antihuman globulin (Coombs) test for RBC antibody identification using reagent red cell panels (86870)*

    Indirect antihuman globulin (Coombs) test for RBC antibody screening (86850)

    0.00   0.00   **FUD** XXX   01

    AMA: 2015,Jan,16; 2014,Jan,11

86890	Autologous blood or component, collection processing and storage; predeposited

    0.00   0.00   **FUD** XXX   S CCI

    AMA: 2015,Jan,16; 2014,Jan,11

86891	intra- or postoperative salvage

    0.00   0.00   **FUD** XXX   S CCI

    AMA: 2005,Aug,7-8; 2005,Jul,11-12

86900	Blood typing, serologic; ABO

    0.00   0.00   **FUD** XXX   01

    AMA: 2005,Jul,11-12; 2005,Aug,7-8

86901	Rh (D)

    0.00   0.00   **FUD** XXX   01

    AMA: 2015,Jan,16; 2014,Jan,11

86902   **antigen testing of donor blood using reagent serum, each antigen test**
Code also one time for each antigen for each unit when multiple units of blood are tested for the same antigen
🚑 0.00   ⚕ 0.00   **FUD** XXX   [01]
AMA: 2010,Dec,7-10

86904   **antigen screening for compatible unit using patient serum, per unit screened**
🚑 0.00   ⚕ 0.00   **FUD** XXX   [01]
AMA: 2005,Aug,7-8; 2005,Jul,11-12

86905   **RBC antigens, other than ABO or Rh (D), each**
🚑 0.00   ⚕ 0.00   **FUD** XXX   [01]
AMA: 2005,Jul,11-12; 2005,Aug,7-8

86906   **Rh phenotyping, complete**
EXCLUDES   *Use of molecular pathology procedures for human erythrocyte antigen typing (81403)*
🚑 0.00   ⚕ 0.00   **FUD** XXX   [01]
AMA: 2005,Jul,11-12; 2005,Aug,7-8

86910   **Blood typing, for paternity testing, per individual; ABO, Rh and MN**
🚑 0.00   ⚕ 0.00   **FUD** XXX   [E]
AMA: 2005,Jul,11-12; 2005,Aug,7-8

86911   **each additional antigen system**
🚑 0.00   ⚕ 0.00   **FUD** XXX   [E]
AMA: 2005,Jul,11-12; 2005,Aug,7-8

86920   **Compatibility test each unit; immediate spin technique**
🚑 0.00   ⚕ 0.00   **FUD** XXX   [S]
AMA: 2015,Jan,16; 2014,Jan,11

86921   **incubation technique**
🚑 0.00   ⚕ 0.00   **FUD** XXX   [01]
AMA: 2015,Jan,16; 2014,Jan,11

86922   **antiglobulin technique**
🚑 0.00   ⚕ 0.00   **FUD** XXX   [S]
AMA: 2015,Jan,16; 2014,Jan,11

86923   **electronic**
Do not report with (86920-86922)
🚑 0.00   ⚕ 0.00   **FUD** XXX   [S]
AMA: 2015,Jan,16; 2014,Jan,11

86927   **Fresh frozen plasma, thawing, each unit**
🚑 0.00   ⚕ 0.00   **FUD** XXX   [S]
AMA: 2005,Aug,7-8; 2005,Jul,11-12

86930   **Frozen blood, each unit; freezing (includes preparation)**
🚑 0.00   ⚕ 0.00   **FUD** XXX   [01]
AMA: 2015,Jan,16; 2014,Jan,11

86931   **thawing**
🚑 0.00   ⚕ 0.00   **FUD** XXX   [S] 🔲
AMA: 2015,Jan,16; 2014,Jan,11

86932   **freezing (includes preparation) and thawing**
🚑 0.00   ⚕ 0.00   **FUD** XXX   [01] 🔲
AMA: 2015,Jan,16; 2014,Jan,11

86940   **Hemolysins and agglutinins; auto, screen, each**
🚑 0.00   ⚕ 0.00   **FUD** XXX   [N]
AMA: 2005,Aug,7-8; 2005,Jul,11-12

86941   **incubated**
🚑 0.00   ⚕ 0.00   **FUD** XXX   [N]
AMA: 2005,Jul,11-12; 2005,Aug,7-8

86945   **Irradiation of blood product, each unit**
🚑 0.00   ⚕ 0.00   **FUD** XXX   [01]
AMA: 2015,Jan,16; 2014,Jan,11; 2012,Jan,15-42; 2011,Jan,11

86950   **Leukocyte transfusion**
EXCLUDES   *Infusion allogeneic lymphocytes (38242)*
Leukapheresis (36511)
🚑 0.00   ⚕ 0.00   **FUD** XXX   [01] 🔲
AMA: 2015,Jan,16; 2013,Oct,3

86960   **Volume reduction of blood or blood product (eg, red blood cells or platelets), each unit**
🚑 0.00   ⚕ 0.00   **FUD** XXX   [S]
AMA: 2015,Jan,16; 2014,Jan,11

86965   **Pooling of platelets or other blood products**
EXCLUDES   *Injection of platelet rich plasma (0232T)*
🚑 0.00   ⚕ 0.00   **FUD** XXX   [S]
AMA: 2015,Jan,16; 2014,Jan,11; 2010,Dec,7-10

86970   **Pretreatment of RBCs for use in RBC antibody detection, identification, and/or compatibility testing; incubation with chemical agents or drugs, each**
🚑 0.00   ⚕ 0.00   **FUD** XXX   [01]
AMA: 2005,Jul,11-12; 2005,Aug,7-8

86971   **incubation with enzymes, each**
🚑 0.00   ⚕ 0.00   **FUD** XXX   [S]
AMA: 2005,Jul,11-12; 2005,Aug,7-8

86972   **by density gradient separation**
🚑 0.00   ⚕ 0.00   **FUD** XXX   [S]
AMA: 2005,Jul,11-12; 2005,Aug,7-8

86975   **Pretreatment of serum for use in RBC antibody identification; incubation with drugs, each**
🚑 0.00   ⚕ 0.00   **FUD** XXX   [S]
AMA: 2005,Jul,11-12; 2005,Aug,7-8

86976   **by dilution**
🚑 0.00   ⚕ 0.00   **FUD** XXX   [01]
AMA: 2005,Jul,11-12; 2005,Aug,7-8

86977   **incubation with inhibitors, each**
🚑 0.00   ⚕ 0.00   **FUD** XXX   [01]
AMA: 2005,Jul,11-12; 2005,Aug,7-8

86978   **by differential red cell absorption using patient RBCs or RBCs of known phenotype, each absorption**
🚑 0.00   ⚕ 0.00   **FUD** XXX   [01]
AMA: 2005,Jul,11-12; 2005,Aug,7-8

86985   **Splitting of blood or blood products, each unit**
🚑 0.00   ⚕ 0.00   **FUD** XXX   [S]
AMA: 2015,Jan,16; 2014,Jan,11; 2012,May,11-12

86999   **Unlisted transfusion medicine procedure**
🚑 0.00   ⚕ 0.00   **FUD** XXX   [01]
AMA: 2015,Jan,16; 2014,Jan,11; 2012,May,11-12; 2012,Jan,15-42; 2011,Jan,11

87003-87118 Identification of Microorganisms

INCLUDES   Bacteriology, mycology, parasitology, and virology
EXCLUDES   *Additional tests using molecular probes, chromatography, nucleic acid resequencing, or immunologic techniques (87140-87158)*
Code also modifier 59 for multiple specimens or sites
Code also modifier 91 for repeat procedures performed on the same day

87003   **Animal inoculation, small animal, with observation and dissection**
🚑 0.00   ⚕ 0.00   **FUD** XXX   [N] 🔲
AMA: 2005,Aug,7-8; 2005,Jul,11-12

87015   **Concentration (any type), for infectious agents**
Do not report with (87177)
🚑 0.00   ⚕ 0.00   **FUD** XXX   [N]
AMA: 2005,Aug,7-8; 2005,Jul,11-12

87040   **Culture, bacterial; blood, aerobic, with isolation and presumptive identification of isolates (includes anaerobic culture, if appropriate)**
🚑 0.00   ⚕ 0.00   **FUD** XXX   [N] 🔲
AMA: 2015,Jan,16; 2014,Jan,11; 2012,Jan,15-42; 2011,Jan,11; 2010,Dec,12

87045   **stool, aerobic, with isolation and preliminary examination (eg, KIA, LIA), Salmonella and Shigella species**
🚑 0.00   ⚕ 0.00   **FUD** XXX   [N] 🔲
AMA: 2005,Aug,7-8; 2005,Jul,11-12

87046	stool, aerobic, additional pathogens, isolation and presumptive identification of isolates, each plate

🖐 0.00 ⚕ 0.00 **FUD** XXX N ▢

AMA: 2015,Jan,16; 2014,Jan,11

87070 any other source except urine, blood or stool, aerobic, with isolation and presumptive identification of isolates

EXCLUDES *Urine (87088)*

🖐 0.00 ⚕ 0.00 **FUD** XXX N

AMA: 2015,Jan,16; 2014,Jan,11; 2012,Jan,15-42; 2011,Jan,11

87071 quantitative, aerobic with isolation and presumptive identification of isolates, any source except urine, blood or stool

EXCLUDES *Urine (87088)*

🖐 0.00 ⚕ 0.00 **FUD** XXX N ▢

AMA: 2015,Jan,16; 2014,Jan,11

87073 quantitative, anaerobic with isolation and presumptive identification of isolates, any source except urine, blood or stool

EXCLUDES *Definitive identification of isolates (87076, 87077)*
Typing of isolates (87140-87158)

🖐 0.00 ⚕ 0.00 **FUD** XXX N ▢

AMA: 2015,Jan,16; 2014,Jan,11

87075 any source, except blood, anaerobic with isolation and presumptive identification of isolates

🖐 0.00 ⚕ 0.00 **FUD** XXX N

AMA: 2005,Aug,7-8; 2005,Jul,11-12

87076 anaerobic isolate, additional methods required for definitive identification, each isolate

🖐 0.00 ⚕ 0.00 **FUD** XXX N

AMA: 2015,Jan,16; 2014,Jan,11

87077 aerobic isolate, additional methods required for definitive identification, each isolate

🖐 0.00 ⚕ 0.00 **FUD** XXX X N

AMA: 2015,Jan,16; 2014,Jan,11; 2012,Jan,15-42

87081 Culture, presumptive, pathogenic organisms, screening only;

🖐 0.00 ⚕ 0.00 **FUD** XXX N ▢

AMA: 2015,Jan,16; 2014,Jan,11

87084 with colony estimation from density chart

🖐 0.00 ⚕ 0.00 **FUD** XXX N ▢

AMA: 2005,Aug,7-8; 2005,Jul,11-12

87086 Culture, bacterial; quantitative colony count, urine

🖐 0.00 ⚕ 0.00 **FUD** XXX N ▢

AMA: 2015,Jan,16; 2014,Jan,11; 2012,Jan,15-42

87088 with isolation and presumptive identification of each isolate, urine

🖐 0.00 ⚕ 0.00 **FUD** XXX N ▢

AMA: 2015,Jan,16; 2014,Jan,11; 2012,Jan,15-42

87101 Culture, fungi (mold or yeast) isolation, with presumptive identification of isolates; skin, hair, or nail

🖐 0.00 ⚕ 0.00 **FUD** XXX N

AMA: 2015,Jan,16; 2014,Jan,11; 2012,Jan,15-42; 2011,Jan,11

87102 other source (except blood)

🖐 0.00 ⚕ 0.00 **FUD** XXX N

AMA: 2005,Aug,7-8; 2005,Jul,11-12

87103 blood

🖐 0.00 ⚕ 0.00 **FUD** XXX N

AMA: 2005,Aug,7-8; 2005,Jul,11-12

87106 Culture, fungi, definitive identification, each organism; yeast

Code also (87101-87103)

🖐 0.00 ⚕ 0.00 **FUD** XXX N ▢

AMA: 2005,Aug,7-8; 2005,Jul,11-12

87107 mold

🖐 0.00 ⚕ 0.00 **FUD** XXX N

AMA: 2005,Aug,7-8; 2005,Jul,11-12

87109 Culture, mycoplasma, any source

🖐 0.00 ⚕ 0.00 **FUD** XXX N

AMA: 2005,Aug,7-8; 2005,Jul,11-12

87110 Culture, chlamydia, any source

EXCLUDES *Immunofluorescence staining of shell vials (87140)*

🖐 0.00 ⚕ 0.00 **FUD** XXX A

AMA: 2005,Aug,7-8; 2005,Jul,11-12

87116 Culture, tubercle or other acid-fast bacilli (eg, TB, AFB, mycobacteria) any source, with isolation and presumptive identification of isolates

EXCLUDES *Concentration (87015)*

🖐 0.00 ⚕ 0.00 **FUD** XXX N

AMA: 2005,Aug,7-8; 2005,Jul,11-12

87118 Culture, mycobacterial, definitive identification, each isolate

🖐 0.00 ⚕ 0.00 **FUD** XXX N

AMA: 2005,Aug,7-8; 2005,Jul,11-12

87140-87158 Additional Culture Typing Techniques

INCLUDES Bacteriology, mycology, parasitology, and virology
Code also definitive identification
Code also modifier 59 for multiple specimens or sites
Code also modifier 91 for repeat procedures performed on the same day
Do not report molecular procedure codes as a substitute for codes in this range
(81200-81408 [81161, 81162, 81287, 81288])

87140 Culture, typing; immunofluorescent method, each antiserum

🖐 0.00 ⚕ 0.00 **FUD** XXX N ▢

AMA: 2015,Jan,16; 2014,Jan,11

87143 gas liquid chromatography (GLC) or high pressure liquid chromatography (HPLC) method

🖐 0.00 ⚕ 0.00 **FUD** XXX N ▢

AMA: 2005,Aug,7-8; 2005,Jul,11-12

87147 immunologic method, other than immunofluoresence (eg, agglutination grouping), per antiserum

🖐 0.00 ⚕ 0.00 **FUD** XXX N ▢

AMA: 2015,Jan,16; 2014,Jan,11; 2012,Jan,15-42; 2011,Jan,11

87149 identification by nucleic acid (DNA or RNA) probe, direct probe technique, per culture or isolate, each organism probed

Do not report with (81200-81408 [81161, 81162, 81287, 81288])

🖐 0.00 ⚕ 0.00 **FUD** XXX N ▢

AMA: 2015,Jan,16; 2014,Jan,11; 2013,Sep,3-12; 2012,May,3-10

87150 identification by nucleic acid (DNA or RNA) probe, amplified probe technique, per culture or isolate, each organism probed

Do not report with (81200-81408 [81161, 81162, 81287, 81288])

🖐 0.00 ⚕ 0.00 **FUD** XXX N

AMA: 2015,Jan,16; 2014,Jan,11; 2013,Sep,3-12; 2012,May,3-10

87152 identification by pulse field gel typing

Do not report with (81200-81408 [81161, 81162, 81287, 81288])

🖐 0.00 ⚕ 0.00 **FUD** XXX N ▢

AMA: 2015,Jan,16; 2014,Jan,11; 2013,Sep,3-12; 2012,May,3-10

87153 identification by nucleic acid sequencing method, each isolate (eg, sequencing of the 16S rRNA gene)

🖐 0.00 ⚕ 0.00 **FUD** XXX N

AMA: 2015,Jan,16; 2013,Sep,3-12; 2012,May,3-10

87158 other methods

🖐 0.00 ⚕ 0.00 **FUD** XXX N ▢

AMA: 2015,Jan,16; 2014,Jan,11

87164-87255 Identification of Organism from Primary Source and Sensitivity Studies

INCLUDES Bacteriology, mycology, parasitology, and virology
EXCLUDES *Additional tests using molecular probes, chromatography, or immunologic techniques (87140-87158)*
Code also modifier 59 for multiple specimens or sites
Code also modifier 91 for repeat procedures performed on the same day

87164 Dark field examination, any source (eg, penile, vaginal, oral, skin); includes specimen collection
🖫 0.00 ⚖ 0.00 **FUD** XXX ⬚N⬚⬜
AMA: 2005,Jul,11-12; 2005,Aug,7-8

87166 without collection
🖫 0.00 ⚖ 0.00 **FUD** XXX ⬚N⬚⬜
AMA: 2005,Aug,7-8; 2005,Jul,11-12

87168 Macroscopic examination; arthropod
🖫 0.00 ⚖ 0.00 **FUD** XXX ⬚N⬚⬜
AMA: 2005,Aug,7-8; 2005,Jul,11-12

87169 parasite
🖫 0.00 ⚖ 0.00 **FUD** XXX ⬚N⬚⬜
AMA: 2005,Aug,7-8; 2005,Jul,11-12

87172 Pinworm exam (eg, cellophane tape prep)
🖫 0.00 ⚖ 0.00 **FUD** XXX ⬚N⬚⬜
AMA: 2005,Aug,7-8; 2005,Jul,11-12

87176 Homogenization, tissue, for culture
🖫 0.00 ⚖ 0.00 **FUD** XXX ⬚N⬚
AMA: 2005,Aug,7-8; 2005,Jul,11-12

87177 Ova and parasites, direct smears, concentration and identification
EXCLUDES *Coccidia or microsporidia exam (87207)*
Complex special stain (trichrome, iron hematoxylin) (87209)
Direct smears from primary source (87207)
Nucleic acid probes in cytologic material (88365)
Do not report with (87015)
🖫 0.00 ⚖ 0.00 **FUD** XXX ⬚N⬚⬜
AMA: 2015,Jan,16; 2014,Jan,11; 2012,Jan,15-42; 2011,Jan,11

87181 Susceptibility studies, antimicrobial agent; agar dilution method, per agent (eg, antibiotic gradient strip)
🖫 0.00 ⚖ 0.00 **FUD** XXX ⬚N⬚⬜
AMA: 2015,Jan,16; 2014,Jan,11

87184 disk method, per plate (12 or fewer agents)
🖫 0.00 ⚖ 0.00 **FUD** XXX ⬚N⬚⬜
AMA: 2015,Jan,16; 2014,Jan,11

87185 enzyme detection (eg, beta lactamase), per enzyme
🖫 0.00 ⚖ 0.00 **FUD** XXX ⬚N⬚⬜
AMA: 2015,Jan,16; 2014,Jan,11

+ **87186** microdilution or agar dilution (minimum inhibitory concentration [MIC] or breakpoint), each multi-antimicrobial, per plate
🖫 0.00 ⚖ 0.00 **FUD** XXX ⬚N⬚⬜
AMA: 2015,Jan,16; 2014,Jan,11

87187 microdilution or agar dilution, minimum lethal concentration (MLC), each plate (List separately in addition to code for primary procedure)
Code first (87186, 87188)
🖫 0.00 ⚖ 0.00 **FUD** XXX ⬚N⬚
AMA: 2015,Jan,16; 2014,Jan,11

87188 macrobroth dilution method, each agent
🖫 0.00 ⚖ 0.00 **FUD** XXX ⬚N⬚⬜
AMA: 2015,Jan,16; 2014,Jan,11

87190 mycobacteria, proportion method, each agent
EXCLUDES *Other mycobacterial susceptibility studies (87181, 87184, 87186, 87188)*
🖫 0.00 ⚖ 0.00 **FUD** XXX ⬚N⬚
AMA: 2005,Aug,7-8; 2005,Jul,11-12

87197 Serum bactericidal titer (Schlicter test)
🖫 0.00 ⚖ 0.00 **FUD** XXX ⬚N⬚
AMA: 2005,Aug,7-8; 2005,Jul,11-12

87205 Smear, primary source with interpretation; Gram or Giemsa stain for bacteria, fungi, or cell types
🖫 0.00 ⚖ 0.00 **FUD** XXX ⬚N⬚⬜
AMA: 2015,Jan,16; 2014,Jan,11; 2012,Jan,15-42; 2011,Jan,11

87206 fluorescent and/or acid fast stain for bacteria, fungi, parasites, viruses or cell types
🖫 0.00 ⚖ 0.00 **FUD** XXX ⬚N⬚⬜
AMA: 2005,Aug,7-8; 2005,Jul,11-12

87207 special stain for inclusion bodies or parasites (eg, malaria, coccidia, microsporidia, trypanosomes, herpes viruses)
EXCLUDES *Direct smears with concentration and identification (87177)*
Fat, meat, fibers, nasal eosinophils, and starch (see miscellaneous section)
Thick smear preparation (87015)
🖫 0.00 ⚖ 0.00 **FUD** XXX ⬚N⬚⬜
AMA: 2015,Jan,16; 2014,Jan,11

87209 complex special stain (eg, trichrome, iron hemotoxylin) for ova and parasites
🖫 0.00 ⚖ 0.00 **FUD** XXX ⬚N⬚
AMA: 2015,Jan,16; 2014,Jan,11

87210 wet mount for infectious agents (eg, saline, India ink, KOH preps)
EXCLUDES *KOH evaluation of skin, hair, or nails (87220)*
🖫 0.00 ⚖ 0.00 **FUD** XXX ⬛⬚N⬚⬜
AMA: 2005,Aug,7-8; 2005,Jul,11-12

87220 Tissue examination by KOH slide of samples from skin, hair, or nails for fungi or ectoparasite ova or mites (eg, scabies)
🖫 0.00 ⚖ 0.00 **FUD** XXX ⬚N⬚⬜
AMA: 2005,Aug,7-8; 2005,Jul,11-12

87230 Toxin or antitoxin assay, tissue culture (eg, Clostridium difficile toxin)
🖫 0.00 ⚖ 0.00 **FUD** XXX ⬚N⬚
AMA: 2005,Aug,7-8; 2005,Jul,11-12

87250 Virus isolation; inoculation of embryonated eggs, or small animal, includes observation and dissection
🖫 0.00 ⚖ 0.00 **FUD** XXX ⬚N⬚
AMA: 2005,Aug,7-8; 2005,Jul,11-12

87252 tissue culture inoculation, observation, and presumptive identification by cytopathic effect
🖫 0.00 ⚖ 0.00 **FUD** XXX ⬚N⬚
AMA: 2005,Aug,7-8; 2005,Jul,11-12

87253 tissue culture, additional studies or definitive identification (eg, hemabsorption, neutralization, immunofluoresence stain), each isolate
EXCLUDES *Electron microscopy (88348)*
Inclusion bodies in:
Fluids (88106)
Smears (87207-87210)
Tissue sections (88304-88309)
🖫 0.00 ⚖ 0.00 **FUD** XXX ⬚N⬚⬜
AMA: 2005,Aug,7-8; 2005,Jul,11-12

87254 centrifuge enhanced (shell vial) technique, includes identification with immunofluorescence stain, each virus
Code also (87252)
🖫 0.00 ⚖ 0.00 **FUD** XXX ⬚N⬚⬜
AMA: 2015,Jan,16; 2014,Jan,11

87255 including identification by non-immunologic method, other than by cytopathic effect (eg, virus specific enzymatic activity)
🖫 0.00 ⚖ 0.00 **FUD** XXX ⬚N⬚⬜
AMA: 2015,Jan,16; 2014,Jan,11

87260-87300 Fluorescence Microscopy by Organism

INCLUDES Primary source only
EXCLUDES Comparable tests on culture material (87140-87158)
Identification of antibodies (86602-86804)
Nonspecific agent detection (87299, 87449-87450, 87797-87799, 87899)
Code also modifier 59 for different species or strains reported by the same code

87260 Infectious agent antigen detection by immunofluorescent technique; adenovirus
📋 0.00   ⚖ 0.00   **FUD** XXX   N ▭
AMA: 2005,Jul,11-12; 2005,Aug,7-8

87265 Bordetella pertussis/parapertussis
📋 0.00   ⚖ 0.00   **FUD** XXX   N ▭
AMA: 2005,Jul,11-12; 2005,Aug,7-8

87267 Enterovirus, direct fluorescent antibody (DFA)
📋 0.00   ⚖ 0.00   **FUD** XXX   N ▭
AMA: 2015,Jan,16; 2014,Jan,11

87269 giardia
📋 0.00   ⚖ 0.00   **FUD** XXX   N ▭
AMA: 2005,Jul,11-12; 2005,Aug,7-8

87270 Chlamydia trachomatis
📋 0.00   ⚖ 0.00   **FUD** XXX   A ▭
AMA: 2005,Jul,11-12; 2005,Aug,7-8

87271 Cytomegalovirus, direct fluorescent antibody (DFA)
📋 0.00   ⚖ 0.00   **FUD** XXX   N ▭
AMA: 2015,Jan,16; 2014,Jan,11

87272 cryptosporidium
📋 0.00   ⚖ 0.00   **FUD** XXX   N ▭
AMA: 2005,Jul,11-12; 2005,Aug,7-8

87273 Herpes simplex virus type 2
📋 0.00   ⚖ 0.00   **FUD** XXX   N ▭
AMA: 2005,Jul,11-12; 2005,Aug,7-8

87274 Herpes simplex virus type 1
📋 0.00   ⚖ 0.00   **FUD** XXX   N ▭
AMA: 2005,Jul,11-12; 2005,Aug,7-8

87275 influenza B virus
📋 0.00   ⚖ 0.00   **FUD** XXX   N ▭
AMA: 2015,Jan,16; 2014,Jan,11

87276 influenza A virus
📋 0.00   ⚖ 0.00   **FUD** XXX   N ▭
AMA: 2015,Jan,16; 2014,Jan,11

87277 Legionella micdadei
📋 0.00   ⚖ 0.00   **FUD** XXX   N ▭
AMA: 2005,Jul,11-12; 2005,Aug,7-8

87278 Legionella pneumophila
📋 0.00   ⚖ 0.00   **FUD** XXX   N ▭
AMA: 2005,Jul,11-12; 2005,Aug,7-8

87279 Parainfluenza virus, each type
📋 0.00   ⚖ 0.00   **FUD** XXX   N ▭
AMA: 2005,Jul,11-12; 2005,Aug,7-8

87280 respiratory syncytial virus
📋 0.00   ⚖ 0.00   **FUD** XXX   N ▭
AMA: 2005,Jul,11-12; 2005,Aug,7-8

87281 Pneumocystis carinii
📋 0.00   ⚖ 0.00   **FUD** XXX   N ▭
AMA: 2005,Jul,11-12; 2005,Aug,7-8

87283 Rubeola
📋 0.00   ⚖ 0.00   **FUD** XXX   N ▭
AMA: 2005,Jul,11-12; 2005,Aug,7-8

87285 Treponema pallidum
📋 0.00   ⚖ 0.00   **FUD** XXX   N ▭
AMA: 2005,Jul,11-12; 2005,Aug,7-8

87290 Varicella zoster virus
📋 0.00   ⚖ 0.00   **FUD** XXX   N ▭
AMA: 2005,Jul,11-12; 2005,Aug,7-8

87299 not otherwise specified, each organism
📋 0.00   ⚖ 0.00   **FUD** XXX   N ▭
AMA: 2015,Jan,16; 2014,Jan,11

87300 Infectious agent antigen detection by immunofluorescent technique, polyvalent for multiple organisms, each polyvalent antiserum
EXCLUDES Physician evaluation of infectious disease agents by immunofluorescence (88346)
📋 0.00   ⚖ 0.00   **FUD** XXX   N ▭
AMA: 2005,Jul,11-12; 2005,Aug,7-8

87301-87451 Enzyme Immunoassay Technique by Organism

INCLUDES Primary source only
EXCLUDES Comparable tests on culture material (87140-87158)
Identification of antibodies (86602-86804)
Nonspecific agent detection (87449-87450, 87797-87799, 87899)
Code also modifier 59 for different species or strains reported by the same code

▲ **87301** Infectious agent antigen detection by immunoassay technique, (eg, enzyme immunoassay [EIA], enzyme-linked immunosorbent assay [ELISA], immunochemiluminometric assay [IMCA]) qualitative or semiquantitative, multiple-step method; adenovirus enteric types 40/41
📋 0.00   ⚖ 0.00   **FUD** XXX   N
AMA: 2015,Jan,16; 2014,Jan,11

▲ **87305** Aspergillus
📋 0.00   ⚖ 0.00   **FUD** XXX   N

▲ **87320** Chlamydia trachomatis
📋 0.00   ⚖ 0.00   **FUD** XXX   A ▭
AMA: 2005,Jul,11-12; 2005,Aug,7-8

▲ **87324** Clostridium difficile toxin(s)
📋 0.00   ⚖ 0.00   **FUD** XXX   N ▭
AMA: 2005,Jul,11-12; 2005,Aug,7-8

▲ **87327** Cryptococcus neoformans
EXCLUDES Cryptococcus latex agglutination (86403)
📋 0.00   ⚖ 0.00   **FUD** XXX   N
AMA: 2005,Jul,11-12; 2005,Aug,7-8

▲ **87328** cryptosporidium
📋 0.00   ⚖ 0.00   **FUD** XXX   N ▭
AMA: 2005,Jul,11-12; 2005,Aug,7-8

▲ **87329** giardia
📋 0.00   ⚖ 0.00   **FUD** XXX   N ▭
AMA: 2005,Jul,11-12; 2005,Aug,7-8

▲ **87332** cytomegalovirus
📋 0.00   ⚖ 0.00   **FUD** XXX   N ▭
AMA: 2005,Jul,11-12; 2005,Aug,7-8

▲ **87335** Escherichia coli 0157
EXCLUDES Giardia antigen (87329)
📋 0.00   ⚖ 0.00   **FUD** XXX   N
AMA: 2005,Jul,11-12; 2005,Aug,7-8

▲ **87336** Entamoeba histolytica dispar group
📋 0.00   ⚖ 0.00   **FUD** XXX   N
AMA: 2005,Jul,11-12; 2005,Aug,7-8

▲ **87337** Entamoeba histolytica group
📋 0.00   ⚖ 0.00   **FUD** XXX   N
AMA: 2005,Jul,11-12; 2005,Aug,7-8

▲ **87338** Helicobacter pylori, stool
📋 0.00   ⚖ 0.00   **FUD** XXX   N ▭
AMA: 2015,Jan,16; 2014,Jan,11

▲ **87339** Helicobacter pylori
EXCLUDES H. pylori:
Breath and blood by mass spectrometry (83013-83014)
Liquid scintillation counter (78267-78268)
Stool (87338)
📋 0.00   ⚖ 0.00   **FUD** XXX   N ▭
AMA: 2005,Jul,11-12; 2005,Aug,7-8

▲ **87340** hepatitis B surface antigen (HBsAg)
📋 0.00   ⚖ 0.00   **FUD** XXX   N ▭
AMA: 2015,Jan,16; 2014,Jan,11

▲ **87341** **hepatitis B surface antigen (HBsAg) neutralization**
🔲 0.00 ⚕ 0.00 **FUD** XXX [A]
AMA: 2005,Jul,11-12; 2005,Aug,7-8

▲ **87350** **hepatitis Be antigen (HBeAg)**
🔲 0.00 ⚕ 0.00 **FUD** XXX [N] 🖳
AMA: 2005,Jul,11-12; 2005,Aug,7-8

▲ **87380** **hepatitis, delta agent**
🔲 0.00 ⚕ 0.00 **FUD** XXX [N]
AMA: 2005,Jul,11-12; 2005,Aug,7-8

▲ **87385** **Histoplasma capsulatum**
🔲 0.00 ⚕ 0.00 **FUD** XXX [N]
AMA: 2005,Jul,11-12; 2005,Aug,7-8

▲ **87389** **HIV-1 antigen(s), with HIV-1 and HIV-2 antibodies, single result**
🔲 0.00 ⚕ 0.00 **FUD** XXX [N]
Code also modifier 92 for test performed using a kit or transportable instrument that is all or in part consists of a single-use, disposable analytical chamber

▲ **87390** **HIV-1**
🔲 0.00 ⚕ 0.00 **FUD** XXX [N] 🖳
AMA: 2005,Jul,11-12; 2005,Aug,7-8

▲ **87391** **HIV-2**
🔲 0.00 ⚕ 0.00 **FUD** XXX [N]
AMA: 2005,Jul,11-12; 2005,Aug,7-8

▲ **87400** **Influenza, A or B, each**
🔲 0.00 ⚕ 0.00 **FUD** XXX [N] 🖳
AMA: 2015,Jan,16; 2014,Jan,11; 2012,Jan,15-42; 2011,Jan,11

▲ **87420** **respiratory syncytial virus**
🔲 0.00 ⚕ 0.00 **FUD** XXX [N]
AMA: 2005,Jul,11-12; 2005,Aug,7-8

▲ **87425** **rotavirus**
🔲 0.00 ⚕ 0.00 **FUD** XXX [N] 🖳
AMA: 2005,Jul,11-12; 2005,Aug,7-8

▲ **87427** **Shiga-like toxin**
🔲 0.00 ⚕ 0.00 **FUD** XXX [N]
AMA: 2005,Jul,11-12; 2005,Aug,7-8

▲ **87430** **Streptococcus, group A**
🔲 0.00 ⚕ 0.00 **FUD** XXX [N] 🖳
AMA: 2015,Jan,16; 2012,Jan,15-42; 2011,Jan,11

▲ **87449** **Infectious agent antigen detection by immunoassay technique, (eg, enzyme immunoassay [EIA], enzyme-linked immunosorbent assay [ELISA], immunochemiluminometric assay [IMCA]), qualitative or semiquantitative; multiple-step method, not otherwise specified, each organism**
🔲 0.00 ⚕ 0.00 **FUD** XXX ☒ [N] 🖳
AMA: 2015,Jan,16; 2014,Jan,11; 2012,Jan,15-42; 2011,Jan,11

▲ **87450** **single step method, not otherwise specified, each organism**
🔲 0.00 ⚕ 0.00 **FUD** XXX [N]
AMA: 2005,Jul,11-12; 2005,Aug,7-8

▲ **87451** **multiple step method, polyvalent for multiple organisms, each polyvalent antiserum**
🔲 0.00 ⚕ 0.00 **FUD** XXX [N]
AMA: 2005,Jul,11-12; 2005,Aug,7-8

87470-87801 [87623, 87624, 87625] Detection Infectious Agent by Probe Techniques

INCLUDES Primary source only
EXCLUDES *Comparable tests on culture material (87140-87158)*
Identification of antibodies (86602-86804)
Nonspecific agent detection (87299, 87449-87450, 87797-87799, 87899)
Code also modifier 59 for different species or strains reported by the same code
Do not report molecular procedure codes as substitute or with codes in this range (81161-81408 [81161, 81162, 81287, 81288])

87470 **Infectious agent detection by nucleic acid (DNA or RNA); Bartonella henselae and Bartonella quintana, direct probe technique**
🔲 0.00 ⚕ 0.00 **FUD** XXX [N] 🖳
AMA: 2015,Jan,16; 2013,Sep,3-12; 2012,May,3-10

87471 **Bartonella henselae and Bartonella quintana, amplified probe technique**
🔲 0.00 ⚕ 0.00 **FUD** XXX [N] 🖳
AMA: 2015,Jan,16; 2013,Sep,3-12; 2012,May,3-10

87472 **Bartonella henselae and Bartonella quintana, quantification**
🔲 0.00 ⚕ 0.00 **FUD** XXX [N] 🖳
AMA: 2015,Jan,16; 2013,Sep,3-12; 2012,May,3-10

87475 **Borrelia burgdorferi, direct probe technique**
🔲 0.00 ⚕ 0.00 **FUD** XXX [N] 🖳
AMA: 2015,Jan,16; 2013,Sep,3-12; 2012,May,3-10

87476 **Borrelia burgdorferi, amplified probe technique**
🔲 0.00 ⚕ 0.00 **FUD** XXX [N] 🖳
AMA: 2015,Jan,16; 2013,Sep,3-12; 2012,May,3-10

87477 **Borrelia burgdorferi, quantification**
🔲 0.00 ⚕ 0.00 **FUD** XXX [N] 🖳
AMA: 2015,Jan,16; 2013,Sep,3-12; 2012,May,3-10

87480 **Candida species, direct probe technique**
🔲 0.00 ⚕ 0.00 **FUD** XXX [N] 🖳
AMA: 2015,Jan,16; 2013,Sep,3-12; 2012,May,3-10

87481 **Candida species, amplified probe technique**
🔲 0.00 ⚕ 0.00 **FUD** XXX [N] 🖳
AMA: 2015,Jan,16; 2013,Sep,3-12; 2012,May,3-10

87482 **Candida species, quantification**
🔲 0.00 ⚕ 0.00 **FUD** XXX [N] 🖳
AMA: 2015,Jan,16; 2013,Sep,3-12; 2012,May,3-10

87485 **Chlamydia pneumoniae, direct probe technique**
🔲 0.00 ⚕ 0.00 **FUD** XXX [N] 🖳
AMA: 2015,Jan,16; 2013,Sep,3-12; 2012,May,3-10

87486 **Chlamydia pneumoniae, amplified probe technique**
🔲 0.00 ⚕ 0.00 **FUD** XXX [N] 🖳
AMA: 2015,Jan,16; 2013,Sep,3-12; 2012,May,3-10

87487 **Chlamydia pneumoniae, quantification**
🔲 0.00 ⚕ 0.00 **FUD** XXX [N] 🖳
AMA: 2015,Jan,16; 2013,Sep,3-12; 2012,May,3-10

87490 **Chlamydia trachomatis, direct probe technique**
🔲 0.00 ⚕ 0.00 **FUD** XXX [A] 🖳
AMA: 2015,Jan,16; 2013,Sep,3-12; 2012,May,3-10

87491 **Chlamydia trachomatis, amplified probe technique**
🔲 0.00 ⚕ 0.00 **FUD** XXX [A] 🖳
AMA: 2015,Jan,16; 2013,Sep,3-12; 2013,Jun,13; 2012,May,3-10

87492 **Chlamydia trachomatis, quantification**
🔲 0.00 ⚕ 0.00 **FUD** XXX [N] 🖳
AMA: 2015,Jan,16; 2013,Sep,3-12; 2012,May,3-10

87493 **Clostridium difficile, toxin gene(s), amplified probe technique**
🔲 0.00 ⚕ 0.00 **FUD** XXX [N]
AMA: 2015,Jan,16; 2014,Jan,11; 2013,Sep,3-12; 2012,May,3-10; 2010,Sep,8

87495 **cytomegalovirus, direct probe technique**
🔲 0.00 ⚕ 0.00 **FUD** XXX [N] 🖳
AMA: 2015,Jan,16; 2013,Sep,3-12; 2012,May,3-10

87496 **cytomegalovirus, amplified probe technique**
🔲 0.00 ⚕ 0.00 **FUD** XXX [N] 🖳
AMA: 2015,Jan,16; 2013,Sep,3-12; 2012,May,3-10

87497 **cytomegalovirus, quantification**
🔲 0.00 ⚕ 0.00 **FUD** XXX [N] 🖳
AMA: 2015,Jan,16; 2013,Sep,3-12; 2012,May,3-10

87498	**enterovirus, amplified probe technique, includes reverse transcription when performed**
	🖰 0.00 ✂ 0.00 **FUD** XXX [N]
	AMA: 2015,Jan,16; 2013,Sep,3-12; 2012,May,3-10

87500	**vancomycin resistance (eg, enterococcus species van A, van B), amplified probe technique**
	🖰 0.00 ✂ 0.00 **FUD** XXX [N]
	AMA: 2015,Jan,16; 2014,Jan,11; 2013,Sep,3-12; 2012,May,3-10

87501	**influenza virus, includes reverse transcription, when performed, and amplified probe technique, each type or subtype**
	🖰 0.00 ✂ 0.00 **FUD** XXX [N]
	AMA: 2015,Jan,16; 2013,Sep,3-12; 2012,May,3-10; 2010,Dec,7-10

▲ | 87502 | **influenza virus, for multiple types or sub-types, includes multiplex reverse transcription, when performed, and multiplex amplified probe technique, first 2 types or sub-types** |
| | 🖰 0.00   ✂ 0.00   **FUD** XXX   [X][N] |
| | AMA: 2015,Jan,16; 2013,Sep,3-12; 2012,May,3-10; 2010,Dec,7-10 |

▲ + | 87503 | **influenza virus, for multiple types or sub-types, includes multiplex reverse transcription, when performed, and multiplex amplified probe technique, each additional influenza virus type or sub-type beyond 2 (List separately in addition to code for primary procedure)** |
	Code first (87502)
	🖰 0.00 ✂ 0.00 **FUD** XXX [N]
	AMA: 2015,Jan,16; 2013,Sep,3-12; 2012,May,3-10; 2010,Dec,7-10

| 87505 | **gastrointestinal pathogen (eg, Clostridium difficile, E. coli, Salmonella, Shigella, norovirus, Giardia), includes multiplex reverse transcription, when performed, and multiplex amplified probe technique, multiple types or subtypes, 3-5 targets** |
| | 🖰 0.00   ✂ 0.00   **FUD** XXX   [N] |

| 87506 | **gastrointestinal pathogen (eg, Clostridium difficile, E. coli, Salmonella, Shigella, norovirus, Giardia), includes multiplex reverse transcription, when performed, and multiplex amplified probe technique, multiple types or subtypes, 6-11 targets** |
| | 🖰 0.00   ✂ 0.00   **FUD** XXX   [N] |

| 87507 | **gastrointestinal pathogen (eg, Clostridium difficile, E. coli, Salmonella, Shigella, norovirus, Giardia), includes multiplex reverse transcription, when performed, and multiplex amplified probe technique, multiple types or subtypes, 12-25 targets** |
| | 🖰 0.00   ✂ 0.00   **FUD** XXX   [N] |

87510	**Gardnerella vaginalis, direct probe technique**
	🖰 0.00 ✂ 0.00 **FUD** XXX [N][CCI]
	AMA: 2015,Jan,16; 2013,Sep,3-12; 2012,May,3-10

87511	**Gardnerella vaginalis, amplified probe technique**
	🖰 0.00 ✂ 0.00 **FUD** XXX [N][CCI]
	AMA: 2015,Jan,16; 2013,Sep,3-12; 2012,May,3-10

87512	**Gardnerella vaginalis, quantification**
	🖰 0.00 ✂ 0.00 **FUD** XXX [N][CCI]
	AMA: 2015,Jan,16; 2013,Sep,3-12; 2012,May,3-10

87515	**hepatitis B virus, direct probe technique**
	🖰 0.00 ✂ 0.00 **FUD** XXX [N][CCI]
	AMA: 2015,Jan,16; 2013,Sep,3-12; 2012,May,3-10

87516	**hepatitis B virus, amplified probe technique**
	🖰 0.00 ✂ 0.00 **FUD** XXX [N][CCI]
	AMA: 2015,Jan,16; 2013,Sep,3-12; 2012,May,3-10

87517	**hepatitis B virus, quantification**
	🖰 0.00 ✂ 0.00 **FUD** XXX [N][CCI]
	AMA: 2015,Jan,16; 2013,Sep,3-12; 2012,May,3-10

87520	**hepatitis C, direct probe technique**
	🖰 0.00 ✂ 0.00 **FUD** XXX [N][CCI]
	AMA: 2015,Jan,16; 2013,Sep,3-12; 2012,May,3-10

87521	**hepatitis C, amplified probe technique, includes reverse transcription when performed**
	🖰 0.00 ✂ 0.00 **FUD** XXX [N][CCI]
	AMA: 2015,Jan,16; 2013,Sep,3-12; 2012,May,3-10

87522	**hepatitis C, quantification, includes reverse transcription when performed**
	🖰 0.00 ✂ 0.00 **FUD** XXX [N][CCI]
	AMA: 2015,Jan,16; 2013,Sep,3-12; 2012,May,3-10

87525	**hepatitis G, direct probe technique**
	🖰 0.00 ✂ 0.00 **FUD** XXX [N][CCI]
	AMA: 2015,Jan,16; 2013,Sep,3-12; 2012,May,3-10

87526	**hepatitis G, amplified probe technique**
	🖰 0.00 ✂ 0.00 **FUD** XXX [N][CCI]
	AMA: 2015,Jan,16; 2013,Sep,3-12; 2012,May,3-10

87527	**hepatitis G, quantification**
	🖰 0.00 ✂ 0.00 **FUD** XXX [N][CCI]
	AMA: 2015,Jan,16; 2013,Sep,3-12; 2012,May,3-10

87528	**Herpes simplex virus, direct probe technique**
	🖰 0.00 ✂ 0.00 **FUD** XXX [N][CCI]
	AMA: 2015,Jan,16; 2013,Sep,3-12; 2012,May,3-10

87529	**Herpes simplex virus, amplified probe technique**
	🖰 0.00 ✂ 0.00 **FUD** XXX [N][CCI]
	AMA: 2015,Jan,16; 2013,Sep,3-12; 2012,May,3-10

87530	**Herpes simplex virus, quantification**
	🖰 0.00 ✂ 0.00 **FUD** XXX [N][CCI]
	AMA: 2015,Jan,16; 2013,Sep,3-12; 2012,May,3-10

87531	**Herpes virus-6, direct probe technique**
	🖰 0.00 ✂ 0.00 **FUD** XXX [N][CCI]
	AMA: 2015,Jan,16; 2013,Sep,3-12; 2012,May,3-10

87532	**Herpes virus-6, amplified probe technique**
	🖰 0.00 ✂ 0.00 **FUD** XXX [N][CCI]
	AMA: 2015,Jan,16; 2013,Sep,3-12; 2012,May,3-10

87533	**Herpes virus-6, quantification**
	🖰 0.00 ✂ 0.00 **FUD** XXX [N][CCI]
	AMA: 2015,Jan,16; 2013,Sep,3-12; 2012,May,3-10

87534	**HIV-1, direct probe technique**
	🖰 0.00 ✂ 0.00 **FUD** XXX [N][CCI]
	AMA: 2015,Jan,16; 2013,Sep,3-12; 2012,May,3-10

87535	**HIV-1, amplified probe technique, includes reverse transcription when performed**
	🖰 0.00 ✂ 0.00 **FUD** XXX [N][CCI]
	AMA: 2015,Jan,16; 2014,Jan,11; 2013,Sep,3-12; 2012,May,3-10

87536	**HIV-1, quantification, includes reverse transcription when performed**
	🖰 0.00 ✂ 0.00 **FUD** XXX [N][CCI]
	AMA: 2015,Jan,16; 2014,Jan,11; 2013,Sep,3-12; 2012,May,3-10; 2012,Jan,15-42; 2010,Oct,9; 2010,Apr,10

87537	**HIV-2, direct probe technique**
	🖰 0.00 ✂ 0.00 **FUD** XXX [N][CCI]
	AMA: 2015,Jan,16; 2013,Sep,3-12; 2012,May,3-10

87538	**HIV-2, amplified probe technique, includes reverse transcription when performed**
	🖰 0.00 ✂ 0.00 **FUD** XXX [N][CCI]
	AMA: 2015,Jan,16; 2013,Sep,3-12; 2012,May,3-10

87539	**HIV-2, quantification, includes reverse transcription when performed**
	🖰 0.00 ✂ 0.00 **FUD** XXX [N][CCI]
	AMA: 2015,Jan,16; 2013,Sep,3-12; 2012,May,3-10

\# | 87623 | **Human Papillomavirus (HPV), low-risk types (eg, 6, 11, 42, 43, 44)** |
| | 🖰 0.00   ✂ 0.00   **FUD** XXX   [N] |

\# | 87624 | **Human Papillomavirus (HPV), high-risk types (eg, 16, 18, 31, 33, 35, 39, 45, 51, 52, 56, 58, 59, 68)** |
| | 🖰 0.00   ✂ 0.00   **FUD** XXX   [N] |
| | INCLUDES   Low- and high-risk types in one assay |

#	**87625**	**Human Papillomavirus (HPV), types 16 and 18 only, includes type 45, if performed**

🔬 0.00   🔬 0.00   **FUD** XXX   N

AMA: 2015,Jun,10

87540   **Legionella pneumophila, direct probe technique**
🔬 0.00   🔬 0.00   **FUD** XXX   N 🖥

AMA: 2015,Jan,16; 2013,Sep,3-12; 2012,May,3-10

87541   **Legionella pneumophila, amplified probe technique**
🔬 0.00   🔬 0.00   **FUD** XXX   N 🖥

AMA: 2015,Jan,16; 2013,Sep,3-12; 2012,May,3-10

87542   **Legionella pneumophila, quantification**
🔬 0.00   🔬 0.00   **FUD** XXX   N 🖥

AMA: 2015,Jan,16; 2013,Sep,3-12; 2012,May,3-10

87550   **Mycobacteria species, direct probe technique**
🔬 0.00   🔬 0.00   **FUD** XXX   N 🖥

AMA: 2015,Jan,16; 2013,Sep,3-12; 2012,May,3-10

87551   **Mycobacteria species, amplified probe technique**
🔬 0.00   🔬 0.00   **FUD** XXX   N 🖥

AMA: 2015,Jan,16; 2013,Sep,3-12; 2012,May,3-10

87552   **Mycobacteria species, quantification**
🔬 0.00   🔬 0.00   **FUD** XXX   N 🖥

AMA: 2015,Jan,16; 2013,Sep,3-12; 2012,May,3-10

87555   **Mycobacteria tuberculosis, direct probe technique**
🔬 0.00   🔬 0.00   **FUD** XXX   N 🖥

AMA: 2015,Jan,16; 2013,Sep,3-12; 2012,May,3-10

87556   **Mycobacteria tuberculosis, amplified probe technique**
🔬 0.00   🔬 0.00   **FUD** XXX   N 🖥

AMA: 2015,Jan,16; 2013,Sep,3-12; 2012,May,3-10

87557   **Mycobacteria tuberculosis, quantification**
🔬 0.00   🔬 0.00   **FUD** XXX   N 🖥

AMA: 2015,Jan,16; 2013,Sep,3-12; 2012,May,3-10

87560   **Mycobacteria avium-intracellulare, direct probe technique**
🔬 0.00   🔬 0.00   **FUD** XXX   N 🖥

AMA: 2015,Jan,16; 2013,Sep,3-12; 2012,May,3-10

87561   **Mycobacteria avium-intracellulare, amplified probe technique**
🔬 0.00   🔬 0.00   **FUD** XXX   N 🖥

AMA: 2015,Jan,16; 2013,Sep,3-12; 2012,May,3-10

87562   **Mycobacteria avium-intracellulare, quantification**
🔬 0.00   🔬 0.00   **FUD** XXX   N 🖥

AMA: 2015,Jan,16; 2013,Sep,3-12; 2012,May,3-10

87580   **Mycoplasma pneumoniae, direct probe technique**
🔬 0.00   🔬 0.00   **FUD** XXX   N 🖥

AMA: 2015,Jan,16; 2013,Sep,3-12; 2012,May,3-10

87581   **Mycoplasma pneumoniae, amplified probe technique**
🔬 0.00   🔬 0.00   **FUD** XXX   N 🖥

AMA: 2015,Jan,16; 2013,Sep,3-12; 2012,May,3-10

87582   **Mycoplasma pneumoniae, quantification**
🔬 0.00   🔬 0.00   **FUD** XXX   N 🖥

AMA: 2015,Jan,16; 2013,Sep,3-12; 2012,May,3-10

87590   **Neisseria gonorrhoeae, direct probe technique**
🔬 0.00   🔬 0.00   **FUD** XXX   A 🖥

AMA: 2015,Jan,16; 2013,Sep,3-12; 2012,May,3-10

87591   **Neisseria gonorrhoeae, amplified probe technique**
🔬 0.00   🔬 0.00   **FUD** XXX   A 🖥

AMA: 2015,Jan,16; 2013,Sep,3-12; 2013,Jun,13; 2012,May,3-10

87592   **Neisseria gonorrhoeae, quantification**
🔬 0.00   🔬 0.00   **FUD** XXX   N 🖥

AMA: 2015,Jan,16; 2013,Sep,3-12; 2012,May,3-10

87623   **Resequenced code. See code following 87539.**

87624   **Resequenced code. See code following 87539.**

87625   **Resequenced code. See code before 87540.**

87631   **respiratory virus (eg, adenovirus, influenza virus, coronavirus, metapneumovirus, parainfluenza virus, respiratory syncytial virus, rhinovirus), includes multiplex reverse transcription, when performed, and multiplex amplified probe technique, multiple types or subtypes, 3-5 targets**

INCLUDES   Detection of multiple respiratory viruses with one test

EXCLUDES   Assays for typing or subtyping influenza viruses only (87501-87503)
Single test for detection of multiple infectious organisms (87800-87801)

🔬 0.00   🔬 0.00   **FUD** XXX   N

AMA: 2015,Jan,16; 2013,Sep,3-12

87632   **respiratory virus (eg, adenovirus, influenza virus, coronavirus, metapneumovirus, parainfluenza virus, respiratory syncytial virus, rhinovirus), includes multiplex reverse transcription, when performed, and multiplex amplified probe technique, multiple types or subtypes, 6-11 targets**

INCLUDES   Detection of multiple respiratory viruses with one test

EXCLUDES   Assays for typing or subtyping influenza viruses only (87501-87503)
Single test to detect multiple infectious organisms (87800-87801)

🔬 0.00   🔬 0.00   **FUD** XXX   N

AMA: 2015,Jan,16; 2013,Sep,3-12

87633   **respiratory virus (eg, adenovirus, influenza virus, coronavirus, metapneumovirus, parainfluenza virus, respiratory syncytial virus, rhinovirus), includes multiplex reverse transcription, when performed, and multiplex amplified probe technique, multiple types or subtypes, 12-25 targets**

INCLUDES   Detection of multiple respiratory viruses with one test

EXCLUDES   Assays for typing or subtyping influenza viruses only (87501-87503)
Single test to detect multiple infectious organisms (87800-87801)

🔬 0.00   🔬 0.00   **FUD** XXX   N

AMA: 2015,Jan,16; 2013,Sep,3-12

87640   **Staphylococcus aureus, amplified probe technique**
🔬 0.00   🔬 0.00   **FUD** XXX   N

AMA: 2015,Jan,16; 2014,Jan,11; 2013,Sep,3-12; 2012,May,3-10

87641   **Staphylococcus aureus, methicillin resistant, amplified probe technique**

EXCLUDES   Assays that detect methicillin resistance and identify Staphylococcus aureus using a single nucleic acid sequence (87641)

🔬 0.00   🔬 0.00   **FUD** XXX   N

AMA: 2015,Jan,16; 2014,Jan,11; 2013,Sep,3-12; 2012,May,3-10

87650   **Streptococcus, group A, direct probe technique**
🔬 0.00   🔬 0.00   **FUD** XXX   N 🖥

AMA: 2015,Jan,16; 2013,Sep,3-12; 2012,May,3-10

87651   **Streptococcus, group A, amplified probe technique**
🔬 0.00   🔬 0.00   **FUD** XXX   ✖ N 🖥

AMA: 2015,Jan,16; 2013,Sep,3-12; 2012,May,3-10

87652   **Streptococcus, group A, quantification**
🔬 0.00   🔬 0.00   **FUD** XXX   N 🖥

AMA: 2015,Jan,16; 2013,Sep,3-12; 2012,May,3-10

87653   **Streptococcus, group B, amplified probe technique**
🔬 0.00   🔬 0.00   **FUD** XXX   N

AMA: 2015,Jan,16; 2014,Jan,11; 2013,Sep,3-12; 2012,May,3-10

87660   **Trichomonas vaginalis, direct probe technique**
🔬 0.00   🔬 0.00   **FUD** XXX   N 🖥

AMA: 2015,Jan,16; 2013,Sep,3-12; 2012,May,3-10

87661   **Trichomonas vaginalis, amplified probe technique**
🔬 0.00   🔬 0.00   **FUD** XXX   A

87797 Infectious agent detection by nucleic acid (DNA or RNA), not otherwise specified; direct probe technique, each organism

📖 0.00 ✎ 0.00 **FUD** XXX Ⓝ ▯

AMA: 2015,Jan,16; 2014,Jan,11; 2013,Sep,3-12; 2012,May,3-10

87798 amplified probe technique, each organism

📖 0.00 ✎ 0.00 **FUD** XXX Ⓝ ▯

AMA: 2015,Jan,16; 2014,Jan,11; 2013,Sep,3-12; 2012,May,3-10

87799 quantification, each organism

📖 0.00 ✎ 0.00 **FUD** XXX Ⓝ ▯

AMA: 2015,Jan,16; 2013,Sep,3-12; 2012,May,3-10

87800 Infectious agent detection by nucleic acid (DNA or RNA), multiple organisms; direct probe(s) technique

INCLUDES   Single test to detect multiple infectious organisms

EXCLUDES   *Detection of specific infectious agents not otherwise specified (87797-87799)*
Each specific organism nucleic acid detection from a primary source (87470-87660 [87623, 87624, 87625])

📖 0.00 ✎ 0.00 **FUD** XXX Ⓐ ▯

AMA: 2015,Jan,16; 2013,Sep,3-12; 2012,May,3-10

87801 amplified probe(s) technique

INCLUDES   Single test to detect multiple infectious organisms

EXCLUDES   *Detection of multiple respiratory viruses with one test (87631-87633)*
Detection of specific infectious agents not otherwise specified (87797-87799)
Each specific organism nucleic acid detection from a primary source (87470-87660 [87623, 87624, 87625])

📖 0.00 ✎ 0.00 **FUD** XXX Ⓝ ▯

AMA: 2015,Jan,16; 2014,Jan,11; 2013,Sep,3-12; 2013,Jun,13; 2012,May,3-10

87802-87899 [87806] Detection Infectious Agent by Immunoassay with Direct Optical Observation

87802 Infectious agent antigen detection by immunoassay with direct optical observation; Streptococcus, group B

📖 0.00 ✎ 0.00 **FUD** XXX Ⓝ ▯

AMA: 2005,Aug,7-8; 2005,Jul,11-12

87803 Clostridium difficile toxin A

📖 0.00 ✎ 0.00 **FUD** XXX Ⓝ ▯

AMA: 2005,Aug,7-8; 2005,Jul,11-12

\# **87806** HIV-1 antigen(s), with HIV-1 and HIV-2 antibodies

📖 0.00 ✎ 0.00 **FUD** XXX ☒ Ⓝ

87804 Influenza

📖 0.00 ✎ 0.00 **FUD** XXX ☒ Ⓝ ▯

AMA: 2015,Jan,16; 2014,Jan,11; 2012,Jan,15-42; 2011,Jan,11

87806 Resequenced code. See code following 87803.

87807 respiratory syncytial virus

📖 0.00 ✎ 0.00 **FUD** XXX ☒ Ⓝ ▯

AMA: 2005,Jul,11-12; 2005,Aug,7-8

87808 Trichomonas vaginalis

📖 0.00 ✎ 0.00 **FUD** XXX ☒ Ⓝ

87809 adenovirus

📖 0.00 ✎ 0.00 **FUD** XXX ☒ Ⓝ

AMA: 2015,Jan,16; 2014,Jan,11

87810 Chlamydia trachomatis

📖 0.00 ✎ 0.00 **FUD** XXX Ⓐ ▯

AMA: 2015,Jan,16; 2014,Jan,11

87850 Neisseria gonorrhoeae

📖 0.00 ✎ 0.00 **FUD** XXX Ⓐ ▯

AMA: 2015,Jan,16; 2014,Jan,11

87880 Streptococcus, group A

📖 0.00 ✎ 0.00 **FUD** XXX ☒ Ⓝ ▯

AMA: 2015,Jan,16; 2014,Jan,11; 2012,Jan,15-42; 2011,Jan,11

87899 not otherwise specified

📖 0.00 ✎ 0.00 **FUD** XXX ☒ Ⓝ ▯

AMA: 2015,Jan,16; 2014,Jan,11; 2012,Jan,15-42; 2011,Jan,11

87900-87999 [87906, 87910, 87912] Drug Sensitivity Genotype/Phenotype

87900 Infectious agent drug susceptibility phenotype prediction using regularly updated genotypic bioinformatics

📖 0.00 ✎ 0.00 **FUD** XXX Ⓝ

AMA: 2015,Jan,16; 2014,Jan,11; 2013,Sep,3-12; 2012,May,3-10

\# **87910** Infectious agent genotype analysis by nucleic acid (DNA or RNA); cytomegalovirus

📖 0.00 ✎ 0.00 **FUD** XXX Ⓝ

AMA: 2015,Jan,16

87901 HIV-1, reverse transcriptase and protease regions

EXCLUDES   *Infectious agent drug susceptibility phenotype prediction for HIV-1 (87900)*

📖 0.00 ✎ 0.00 **FUD** XXX Ⓝ ▯

AMA: 2015,Jan,16; 2014,Jan,11; 2013,Sep,3-12; 2012,May,3-10; 2010,Dec,7-10

\# **87906** HIV-1, other region (eg, integrase, fusion)

📖 0.00 ✎ 0.00 **FUD** XXX Ⓝ

AMA: 2015,Jan,16; 2010,Dec,7-10

\# **87912** Hepatitis B virus

📖 0.00 ✎ 0.00 **FUD** XXX Ⓝ

AMA: 2015,Jan,16

87902 Hepatitis C virus

📖 0.00 ✎ 0.00 **FUD** XXX Ⓝ ▯

AMA: 2015,Jan,16; 2014,Jan,11; 2013,Sep,3-12; 2012,May,3-10

87903 Infectious agent phenotype analysis by nucleic acid (DNA or RNA) with drug resistance tissue culture analysis, HIV 1; first through 10 drugs tested

📖 0.00 ✎ 0.00 **FUD** XXX Ⓝ ▯

AMA: 2015,Jan,16; 2014,Jan,11; 2013,Sep,3-12; 2012,May,3-10

\+ **87904** each additional drug tested (List separately in addition to code for primary procedure)

Code first (87903)

📖 0.00 ✎ 0.00 **FUD** XXX Ⓝ ▯

AMA: 2015,Jan,16; 2014,Jan,11; 2013,Sep,3-12; 2012,May,3-10; 2012,Jan,15-42; 2011,Jan,11

87905 Infectious agent enzymatic activity other than virus (eg, sialidase activity in vaginal fluid)

📖 0.00 ✎ 0.00 **FUD** XXX ☒ Ⓝ

EXCLUDES   *Isolation of a virus identified by a nonimmunologic method, and by noncytopathic effect (87255)*

87906 Resequenced code. See code following 87901.

87910 Resequenced code. See code following 87900.

87912 Resequenced code. See code before 87902.

87999 Unlisted microbiology procedure

📖 0.00 ✎ 0.00 **FUD** XXX Ⓝ

AMA: 2015,Jan,16; 2014,Jan,11

88000-88099 Autopsy Services

CMS: 100-2,15,80.1 Payment for Clinical Laboratory Services

INCLUDES   Services for physicians only

88000 Necropsy (autopsy), gross examination only; without CNS

📖 0.00 ✎ 0.00 **FUD** XXX Ⓔ

AMA: 2015,Jan,16; 2014,Jan,11

88005 with brain

📖 0.00 ✎ 0.00 **FUD** XXX Ⓔ

AMA: 2005,Jul,11-12; 2005,Aug,7-8

88007 with brain and spinal cord

📖 0.00 ✎ 0.00 **FUD** XXX Ⓔ

AMA: 2005,Jul,11-12; 2005,Aug,7-8

88012 infant with brain 🄰
🖪 0.00 ⚕ 0.00 **FUD** XXX 🄴
AMA: 2005,Jul,11-12; 2005,Aug,7-8

88014 stillborn or newborn with brain 🄰
🖪 0.00 ⚕ 0.00 **FUD** XXX 🄴
AMA: 2005,Jul,11-12; 2005,Aug,7-8

88016 macerated stillborn 🄰
🖪 0.00 ⚕ 0.00 **FUD** XXX 🄴
AMA: 2005,Jul,11-12; 2005,Aug,7-8

88020 Necropsy (autopsy), gross and microscopic; without CNS
🖪 0.00 ⚕ 0.00 **FUD** XXX 🄴
AMA: 2005,Jul,11-12; 2005,Aug,7-8

88025 with brain
🖪 0.00 ⚕ 0.00 **FUD** XXX 🄴
AMA: 2005,Jul,11-12; 2005,Aug,7-8

88027 with brain and spinal cord
🖪 0.00 ⚕ 0.00 **FUD** XXX 🄴
AMA: 2005,Jul,11-12; 2005,Aug,7-8

88028 infant with brain 🄰
🖪 0.00 ⚕ 0.00 **FUD** XXX 🄴
AMA: 2005,Jul,11-12; 2005,Aug,7-8

88029 stillborn or newborn with brain 🄰
🖪 0.00 ⚕ 0.00 **FUD** XXX 🄴
AMA: 2005,Jul,11-12; 2005,Aug,7-8

88036 Necropsy (autopsy), limited, gross and/or microscopic; regional
🖪 0.00 ⚕ 0.00 **FUD** XXX 🄴
AMA: 2005,Jul,11-12; 2005,Aug,7-8

88037 single organ
🖪 0.00 ⚕ 0.00 **FUD** XXX 🄴
AMA: 2005,Jul,11-12; 2005,Aug,7-8

88040 Necropsy (autopsy); forensic examination
🖪 0.00 ⚕ 0.00 **FUD** XXX 🄴
AMA: 2005,Jul,11-12; 2005,Aug,7-8

88045 coroner's call
🖪 0.00 ⚕ 0.00 **FUD** XXX 🄴
AMA: 2005,Jul,11-12; 2005,Aug,7-8

88099 Unlisted necropsy (autopsy) procedure
🖪 0.00 ⚕ 0.00 **FUD** XXX 🄴
AMA: 2015,Jan,16; 2014,Jan,11

88104-88140 Cytopathology: Other Than Cervical/Vaginal

88104 Cytopathology, fluids, washings or brushings, except cervical or vaginal; smears with interpretation
🖪 2.10 ⚕ 2.10 **FUD** XXX 🄾🄾 🄾
AMA: 2015,Jan,16; 2014,Jan,11; 2012,Jan,15-42; 2011,Jan,11

88106 simple filter method with interpretation
EXCLUDES Selective cellular enhancement (nongynecological) including filter transfer techniques (88112)
Do not report with (88104)
🖪 2.46 ⚕ 2.46 **FUD** XXX 🄾🄾
AMA: 2015,Jan,16; 2014,Jan,11

88108 Cytopathology, concentration technique, smears and interpretation (eg, Saccomanno technique)
EXCLUDES Cervical or vaginal smears (88150-88155)
Gastric intubation with lavage (43754-43755)
🖪 (74340)
🖪 2.37 ⚕ 2.37 **FUD** XXX 🄾🄾 🄾
AMA: 2015,Jan,16; 2014,Jan,11

88112 Cytopathology, selective cellular enhancement technique with interpretation (eg, liquid based slide preparation method), except cervical or vaginal
Do not report with (88108)
🖪 1.81 ⚕ 1.81 **FUD** XXX 🄾🄾 🄾
AMA: 2005,Aug,7-8; 2005,Jul,11-12

88120 Cytopathology, in situ hybridization (eg, FISH), urinary tract specimen with morphometric analysis, 3-5 molecular probes, each specimen; manual
EXCLUDES More than five probes (88399)
Morphometric in situ hybridization on specimens other than urinary tract (88367-88368 [88373, 88374])
🖪 17.4 ⚕ 17.4 **FUD** XXX 🄾🄾 🄾
AMA: 2010,Dec,7-10

88121 using computer-assisted technology
EXCLUDES More than five probes (88399)
Morphometric in situ hybridization on specimens other than urinary tract (88367-88368 [88373, 88374])
🖪 15.5 ⚕ 15.5 **FUD** XXX 🄾🄾 🄾
AMA: 2010,Dec,7-10

88125 Cytopathology, forensic (eg, sperm)
🖪 0.74 ⚕ 0.74 **FUD** XXX 🄾🄾 🄾
AMA: 2005,Aug,7-8; 2005,Jul,11-12

88130 Sex chromatin identification; Barr bodies
🖪 0.00 ⚕ 0.00 **FUD** XXX 🄽
AMA: 2005,Aug,7-8; 2005,Jul,11-12

88140 peripheral blood smear, polymorphonuclear drumsticks
EXCLUDES Guard stain (88313)
🖪 0.00 ⚕ 0.00 **FUD** XXX 🄽
AMA: 2015,Jan,16; 2014,Jan,11

88141-88155 Pap Smears

CMS: 100-3,210.2 Screening Pap Smears/Pelvic Examinations for Early Cancer Detection

88141 Cytopathology, cervical or vaginal (any reporting system), requiring interpretation by physician ♀
Code also (88142-88154, 88164-88167, 88174-88175)
🖪 0.91 ⚕ 0.91 **FUD** XXX 🄽 🄾🄾 🄾
AMA: 2015,Jan,16; 2014,Jan,11; 2012,Jan,15-42; 2011,Dec,14-18; 2011,May,9; 2011,Jan,11

88142 Cytopathology, cervical or vaginal (any reporting system), collected in preservative fluid, automated thin layer preparation; manual screening under physician supervision ♀
INCLUDES Bethesda or non-Bethesda method
🖪 0.00 ⚕ 0.00 **FUD** XXX 🄽🄾
AMA: 2015,Jan,16; 2014,Jan,11

88143 with manual screening and rescreening under physician supervision ♀
INCLUDES Bethesda or non-Bethesda method
EXCLUDES Automated screening of automated thin layer preparation (88174-88175)
🖪 0.00 ⚕ 0.00 **FUD** XXX 🄽🄾
AMA: 2015,Jan,16; 2014,Jan,11; 2012,Jan,15-42; 2011,Jan,11

88147 Cytopathology smears, cervical or vaginal; screening by automated system under physician supervision ♀
🖪 0.00 ⚕ 0.00 **FUD** XXX 🄽🄾
AMA: 2015,Jan,16; 2014,Jan,11; 2012,Jan,15-42; 2011,Jan,11

88148 screening by automated system with manual rescreening under physician supervision ♀
🖪 0.00 ⚕ 0.00 **FUD** XXX 🄽🄾
AMA: 2015,Jan,16; 2014,Jan,11

88150 Cytopathology, slides, cervical or vaginal; manual screening under physician supervision ♀
EXCLUDES Bethesda method Pap smears (88164-88167)
🖪 0.00 ⚕ 0.00 **FUD** XXX 🄽🄾
AMA: 2015,Jan,16; 2014,Jan,11

88152 with manual screening and computer-assisted rescreening under physician supervision ♀
EXCLUDES Bethesda method Pap smears (88164-88167)
🖪 0.00 ⚕ 0.00 **FUD** XXX 🄽🄾
AMA: 2015,Jan,16; 2014,Jan,11

88153   with manual screening and rescreening under physician supervision ♀

EXCLUDES   Bethesda method Pap smears (88164-88167)

🚑 0.00   ⚖ 0.00   **FUD** XXX   N 💻

AMA: 2015,Jan,16; 2014,Jan,11; 2012,Jan,15-42; 2011,Jan,11

88154   with manual screening and computer-assisted rescreening using cell selection and review under physician supervision ♀

EXCLUDES   Bethesda method Pap smears (88164-88167)

🚑 0.00   ⚖ 0.00   **FUD** XXX   N 💻

AMA: 2015,Jan,16; 2014,Jan,11

+   88155   Cytopathology, slides, cervical or vaginal, definitive hormonal evaluation (eg, maturation index, karyopyknotic index, estrogenic index) (List separately in addition to code[s] for other technical and interpretation services) ♀

Code first (88142-88154, 88164-88167, 88174-88175)

🚑 0.00   ⚖ 0.00   **FUD** XXX   N 💻

AMA: 2015,Jan,16; 2014,Jan,11; 2012,Jan,15-42; 2011,May,9

88160-88162 Cytopathology Smears (Other Than Pap)

88160   Cytopathology, smears, any other source; screening and interpretation

🚑 1.88   ⚖ 1.88   **FUD** XXX   01 80 💻

AMA: 2006,Dec,10-12; 2005,Jul,11-12

88161   preparation, screening and interpretation

🚑 1.70   ⚖ 1.70   **FUD** XXX   01 80 💻

AMA: 2015,Jan,16; 2014,Jan,11

88162   extended study involving over 5 slides and/or multiple stains

EXCLUDES   Aerosol collection of sputum (89220)
Special stains (88312-88314)

🚑 2.80   ⚖ 2.80   **FUD** XXX   01 80 💻

AMA: 2005,Aug,7-8; 2005,Jul,11-12

88164-88167 Pap Smears: Bethesda System

CMS: 100-3,210.2 Screening Pap Smears/Pelvic Examinations for Early Cancer Detection

EXCLUDES   Non-Bethesda method (88150-88154)

88164   Cytopathology, slides, cervical or vaginal (the Bethesda System); manual screening under physician supervision ♀

🚑 0.00   ⚖ 0.00   **FUD** XXX   N 💻

AMA: 2015,Jan,16; 2014,Jan,11

88165   with manual screening and rescreening under physician supervision ♀

🚑 0.00   ⚖ 0.00   **FUD** XXX   N 💻

AMA: 2015,Jan,16; 2014,Jan,11; 2012,Jan,15-42; 2011,Jan,11

88166   with manual screening and computer-assisted rescreening under physician supervision ♀

🚑 0.00   ⚖ 0.00   **FUD** XXX   N 💻

AMA: 2015,Jan,16; 2014,Jan,11

88167   with manual screening and computer-assisted rescreening using cell selection and review under physician supervision ♀

EXCLUDES   Fine needle aspiration (10021-10022)

🚑 0.00   ⚖ 0.00   **FUD** XXX   N 💻

AMA: 2015,Jan,16; 2014,Jan,11

88172-88173 [88177] Cytopathology of Needle Biopsy

EXCLUDES   Fine needle aspiration (10021-10022)

88172   Cytopathology, evaluation of fine needle aspirate; immediate cytohistologic study to determine adequacy for diagnosis, first evaluation episode, each site

INCLUDES   The submission of a complete set of cytologic material for evaluation regardless of the number of needle passes performed or slides prepared from each site

Do not report with same specimen (88333-88334)

🚑 1.59   ⚖ 1.59   **FUD** XXX   01 80 💻

AMA: 2015,Jan,16; 2014,Jan,11; 2012,Jan,15-42; 2011,Jan,11; 2010,Dec,7-10

88173   interpretation and report

INCLUDES   The interpretation and report from each anatomical site no matter how many passes or evaluation episodes are performed during the aspiration

EXCLUDES   Fine needle aspiration (10021-10022)

Do not report with same specimen (88333-88334)

🚑 4.24   ⚖ 4.24   **FUD** XXX   01 80 💻

AMA: 2015,Jan,16; 2014,Jan,11; 2012,Jan,15-42; 2011,Jan,11; 2010,Dec,7-10

+ #   88177   immediate cytohistologic study to determine adequacy for diagnosis, each separate additional evaluation episode, same site (List separately in addition to code for primary procedure)

Code also each additional immediate repeat evaluation episode(s) required from the same site (e.g., previous sample is inadequate)

Code first (88172)

🚑 0.86   ⚖ 0.86   **FUD** ZZZ   N 80

AMA: 2010,Dec,7-10

88174-88177 Pap Smears: Automated Screening

88174   Cytopathology, cervical or vaginal (any reporting system), collected in preservative fluid, automated thin layer preparation; screening by automated system, under physician supervision ♀

INCLUDES   Bethesda or non-Bethesda method

🚑 0.00   ⚖ 0.00   **FUD** XXX   N 💻

AMA: 2015,Jan,16; 2014,Jan,11

88175   with screening by automated system and manual rescreening or review, under physician supervision ♀

INCLUDES   Bethesda or non-Bethesda method

EXCLUDES   Manual screening (88142-88143)

🚑 0.00   ⚖ 0.00   **FUD** XXX   N 💻

AMA: 2015,Jan,16; 2014,Jan,11; 2012,Jan,15-42; 2011,May,9

88177   Resequenced code, See code following 88173.

88182-88199 Cytopathology Using the Fluorescence-Activated Cell Sorter

88182   Flow cytometry, cell cycle or DNA analysis

EXCLUDES   DNA ploidy analysis by morphometric technique (88358)

🚑 3.04   ⚖ 3.04   **FUD** XXX   S 80 💻

AMA: 2015,Jan,16; 2013,Oct,3

88184   Flow cytometry, cell surface, cytoplasmic, or nuclear marker, technical component only; first marker

🚑 2.63   ⚖ 2.63   **FUD** XXX   01 80 TC

AMA: 2015,Jan,16; 2014,Jan,11; 2013,Oct,3

+   88185   each additional marker (List separately in addition to code for first marker)

Code first (88184)

🚑 1.60   ⚖ 1.60   **FUD** ZZZ   N 80 TC

AMA: 2015,Jan,16; 2014,Jan,11; 2013,Oct,3; 2012,Jan,15-42; 2011,Jan,11

● New Code   ▲ Revised Code   ○ Reinstated   M Maternity   A Age Edit   Unlisted   Not Covered   # Resequenced
⊘ AMA Mod 51 Exempt   ⑤¹ Optum Mod 51 Exempt   ⑥³ Mod 63 Exempt   ⊙ Mod Sedation   + Add-on   CCI   PQ PQRS   FUD Follow-up Days

© 2015 Optum360, LLC (Blue Text)   CPT © 2015 American Medical Association. All Rights Reserved. (Black Text)   Medicare (Red Text)   **375**

Pathology and Laboratory

88187 — 88285

88187 **Flow cytometry, interpretation; 2 to 8 markers**

EXCLUDES *Antibody assessment by flow cytometry (83516-83520, 86000-86849 [86152, 86153])*
Cell enumeration by immunologic selection and identification ([86152, 86153])
Interpretation (86355-86357, 86359-86361, 86367)

🖈 2.02   ⚖ 2.02   **FUD** XXX   B 80 26 💬

AMA: 2015,Jan,16; 2014,Jan,11; 2013,Oct,3; 2012,Jan,15-42; 2011,Jan,11

88188 **9 to 15 markers**

EXCLUDES *Antibody assessment by flow cytometry (83516-83520, 86000-86849 [86152, 86153])*
Cell enumeration by immunologic selection and identification ([86152, 86153])
Interpretation (86355-86357, 86359-86361, 86367)

🖈 2.57   ⚖ 2.57   **FUD** XXX   B 80 26 💬

AMA: 2015,Jan,16; 2014,Jan,11; 2013,Oct,3; 2012,Jan,15-42; 2011,Jan,11

88189 **16 or more markers**

EXCLUDES *Antibody assessment by flow cytometry (83516-83520, 86000-86849 [86152, 86153])*
Cell enumeration using immunologic selection and identification in fluid sample ([86152, 86153])
Interpretation (86355-86357, 86359-86361, 86367)

🖈 3.17   ⚖ 3.17   **FUD** XXX   B 80 26 💬

AMA: 2015,Jan,16; 2014,Jan,11; 2013,Oct,3; 2012,Jan,15-42; 2011,Jan,11

88199 **Unlisted cytopathology procedure**

EXCLUDES *Electron microscopy (88348)*

🖈 0.00   ⚖ 0.00   **FUD** XXX   01 80

AMA: 2015,Jan,16; 2014,Jan,11

88230-88299 Cytogenic Studies

CMS: 100-3,190.3 Cytogenic Studies

EXCLUDES *Acetylcholinesterase (82013)*
Alpha-fetoprotein (amniotic fluid or serum) (82105-82106)
Microdissection (88380)
Molecular pathology codes (81200-81383 [81161, 81162, 81287, 81288], 81400-81408, [81479], 81410-81471, 81500-81512, 81599)

88230 **Tissue culture for non-neoplastic disorders; lymphocyte**

🖈 0.00   ⚖ 0.00   **FUD** XXX   N

AMA: 2015,Jan,16; 2014,Jan,11

88233 **skin or other solid tissue biopsy**

🖈 0.00   ⚖ 0.00   **FUD** XXX   N

AMA: 2015,Jan,16; 2014,Jan,11

88235 **amniotic fluid or chorionic villus cells**   M

🖈 0.00   ⚖ 0.00   **FUD** XXX   N

AMA: 2015,Jan,16; 2014,Jan,11

88237 **Tissue culture for neoplastic disorders; bone marrow, blood cells**

🖈 0.00   ⚖ 0.00   **FUD** XXX   N

AMA: 2015,Jan,16; 2014,Jan,11

88239 **solid tumor**

🖈 0.00   ⚖ 0.00   **FUD** XXX   N

AMA: 2015,Jan,16; 2014,Jan,11

88240 **Cryopreservation, freezing and storage of cells, each cell line**

EXCLUDES *Therapeutic cryopreservation and storage (38207)*

🖈 0.00   ⚖ 0.00   **FUD** XXX   N 💬

AMA: 2015,Jan,16; 2014,Jan,11; 2013,Oct,3

88241 **Thawing and expansion of frozen cells, each aliquot**

EXCLUDES *Therapeutic thawing of prior harvest (38208)*

🖈 0.00   ⚖ 0.00   **FUD** XXX   N 💬

AMA: 2015,Jan,16; 2014,Jan,11; 2013,Oct,3

88245 **Chromosome analysis for breakage syndromes; baseline Sister Chromatid Exchange (SCE), 20-25 cells**

🖈 0.00   ⚖ 0.00   **FUD** XXX   N 💬

AMA: 2015,Jan,16; 2014,Jan,11

88248 **baseline breakage, score 50-100 cells, count 20 cells, 2 karyotypes (eg, for ataxia telangiectasia, Fanconi anemia, fragile X)**

🖈 0.00   ⚖ 0.00   **FUD** XXX   N 💬

AMA: 2015,Jan,16; 2014,Jan,11

88249 **score 100 cells, clastogen stress (eg, diepoxybutane, mitomycin C, ionizing radiation, UV radiation)**

🖈 0.00   ⚖ 0.00   **FUD** XXX   N 💬

AMA: 2015,Jan,16; 2014,Jan,11

88261 **Chromosome analysis; count 5 cells, 1 karyotype, with banding**

🖈 0.00   ⚖ 0.00   **FUD** XXX   N 💬

AMA: 2015,Jan,16; 2014,Jan,11

88262 **count 15-20 cells, 2 karyotypes, with banding**

🖈 0.00   ⚖ 0.00   **FUD** XXX   N 💬

AMA: 2015,Jan,16; 2014,Jan,11; 2012,Jan,15-42; 2011,May,9

88263 **count 45 cells for mosaicism, 2 karyotypes, with banding**

🖈 0.00   ⚖ 0.00   **FUD** XXX   N 💬

AMA: 2015,Jan,16; 2014,Jan,11

88264 **analyze 20-25 cells**

🖈 0.00   ⚖ 0.00   **FUD** XXX   N 💬

AMA: 2015,Jan,16; 2014,Jan,11

88267 **Chromosome analysis, amniotic fluid or chorionic villus, count 15 cells, 1 karyotype, with banding**   M ♀

🖈 0.00   ⚖ 0.00   **FUD** XXX   N 💬

AMA: 2015,Jan,16; 2014,Jan,11

88269 **Chromosome analysis, in situ for amniotic fluid cells, count cells from 6-12 colonies, 1 karyotype, with banding**   M ♀

🖈 0.00   ⚖ 0.00   **FUD** XXX   N 💬

AMA: 2015,Jan,16; 2014,Jan,11

88271 **Molecular cytogenetics; DNA probe, each (eg, FISH)**

EXCLUDES *Cytogenomic microarray analysis (81228-81229, 81405-81406, [81479])*

🖈 0.00   ⚖ 0.00   **FUD** XXX   N 💬

AMA: 2015,Jan,16; 2014,Jan,11; 2013,Sep,3-12; 2012,May,3-10; 2012,Jan,15-42; 2011,Jan,11

88272 **chromosomal in situ hybridization, analyze 3-5 cells (eg, for derivatives and markers)**

🖈 0.00   ⚖ 0.00   **FUD** XXX   N 💬

AMA: 2015,Jan,16; 2014,Jan,11; 2013,Sep,3-12; 2012,May,3-10; 2012,Jan,15-42; 2011,Jan,11

88273 **chromosomal in situ hybridization, analyze 10-30 cells (eg, for microdeletions)**

🖈 0.00   ⚖ 0.00   **FUD** XXX   N 💬

AMA: 2015,Jan,16; 2014,Jan,11; 2013,Sep,3-12; 2012,May,3-10; 2012,Jan,15-42; 2011,Jan,11

88274 **interphase in situ hybridization, analyze 25-99 cells**

🖈 0.00   ⚖ 0.00   **FUD** XXX   N 💬

AMA: 2015,Jan,16; 2014,Jan,11; 2013,Sep,3-12; 2012,May,3-10; 2012,Jan,15-42; 2011,Jan,11

88275 **interphase in situ hybridization, analyze 100-300 cells**

🖈 0.00   ⚖ 0.00   **FUD** XXX   N 💬

AMA: 2015,Jan,16; 2014,Jan,11; 2013,Sep,3-12; 2012,May,3-10; 2012,Jan,15-42; 2011,Jan,11

88280 **Chromosome analysis; additional karyotypes, each study**

🖈 0.00   ⚖ 0.00   **FUD** XXX   N 💬

AMA: 2015,Jan,16; 2014,Jan,11

88283 **additional specialized banding technique (eg, NOR, C-banding)**

🖈 0.00   ⚖ 0.00   **FUD** XXX   N 💬

AMA: 2015,Jan,16; 2014,Jan,11

88285 **additional cells counted, each study**

🖈 0.00   ⚖ 0.00   **FUD** XXX   N 💬

AMA: 2015,Jan,16; 2014,Jan,11; 2012,Jan,15-42; 2011,May,9; 2011,Jan,11

88289   **additional high resolution study**
     🚗 0.00   ⚕ 0.00   **FUD** XXX   N ▢
     AMA: 2015,Jan,16; 2014,Jan,11

88291   **Cytogenetics and molecular cytogenetics, interpretation and report**
     🚗 0.89   ⚕ 0.89   **FUD** XXX   M 80 26 ▢
     AMA: 2015,Jan,16; 2014,Jan,11

88299   **Unlisted cytogenetic study**
     🚗 0.00   ⚕ 0.00   **FUD** XXX   01 80
     AMA: 2015,Jan,16; 2014,Jan,11

88300 Evaluation of Surgical Specimen: Gross Anatomy

CMS: 100-2,15,80.1 Payment for Clinical Laboratory Services

INCLUDES   Attainment, examination, and reporting
       Unit of service is the specimen
EXCLUDES   *Additional procedures (88311-88365 [88341, 88350], 88399)*
       Microscopic exam (88302-88309)

88300   **Level I - Surgical pathology, gross examination only**
     🚗 0.43   ⚕ 0.43   **FUD** XXX   01 80
     AMA: 2015,Jan,16; 2014,Jan,11; 2012,Jan,15-42; 2011,Dec,14-18; 2011,Jan,11

88302-88309 Evaluation of Surgical Specimens: Gross and Microscopic Anatomy

CMS: 100-2,15,80.1 Payment for Clinical Laboratory Services

INCLUDES   Attainment, examination, and reporting
       Unit of service is the specimen
EXCLUDES   *Additional procedures (88311-88365 [88341, 88350], 88399)*
Do not report with Mohs surgery (17311-17315)

88302   **Level II - Surgical pathology, gross and microscopic examination**

       INCLUDES   Confirming identification and absence of disease:
          Appendix, incidental
          Fallopian tube, sterilization
          Fingers or toes traumatic amputation
          Foreskin, newborn
          Hernia sac, any site
          Hydrocele sac
          Nerve
          Skin, plastic repair
          Sympathetic ganglion
          Testis, castration
          Vaginal mucosa, incidental
          Vas deferens, sterilization
     🚗 0.90   ⚕ 0.90   **FUD** XXX   01 80
     AMA: 2015,Jan,16; 2014,Feb,10; 2014,Jan,11; 2012,Jan,15-42; 2011,Dec,14-18; 2011,Jan,11

88304   **Level III - Surgical pathology, gross and microscopic examination**

       INCLUDES   Abortion, induced
          Abscess
          Anal tag
          Aneurysm-atrial/ventricular
          Appendix, other than incidental
          Artery, atheromatous plaque
          Bartholin's gland cyst
          Bone fragment(s), other than pathologic fracture
          Bursa/ synovial cyst
          Carpal tunnel tissue
          Cartilage, shavings
          Cholesteatoma
          Colon, colostomy stoma
          Conjunctiva-biopsy/pterygium
          Cornea
          Diverticulum-esophagus/small intestine
          Dupuytren's contracture tissue
          Femoral head, other than fracture
          Fissure/fistula
          Foreskin, other than newborn
          Gallbladder
          Ganglion cyst
          Hematoma
          Hemorrhoids
          Hydatid of Morgagni
          Intervertebral disc
          Joint, loose body
          Meniscus
          Mucocele, salivary
          Neuroma-Morton's/traumatic
          Pilonidal cyst/sinus
          Polyps, inflammatory-nasal/sinusoidal
          Skin-cyst/tag/debridement
          Soft tissue, debridement
          Soft tissue, lipoma
          Spermatocele
          Tendon/tendon sheath
          Testicular appendage
          Thrombus or embolus
          Tonsil and/or adenoids
          Varicocele
          Vas deferens, other than sterilization
          Vein, varicosity
     🚗 1.28   ⚕ 1.28   **FUD** XXX   01 80 ▢
     AMA: 2015,Jan,16; 2014,Feb,10; 2014,Jan,11; 2012,Jan,15-42; 2011,Dec,14-18; 2011,Jan,11

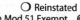
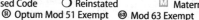

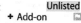
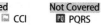
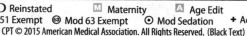

88305 Level IV - Surgical pathology, gross and microscopic examination

INCLUDES
Abortion, spontaneous/missed
Artery, biopsy
Bone exostosis
Bone marrow, biopsy
Brain/meninges, other than for tumor resection
Breast biopsy without microscopic assessment of surgical margin
Breast reduction mammoplasty
Bronchus, biopsy
Cell block, any source
Cervix, biopsy
Colon, biopsy
Duodenum, biopsy
Endocervix, curettings/biopsy
Endometrium, curettings/biopsy
Esophagus, biopsy
Extremity, amputation, traumatic
Fallopian tube, biopsy
Fallopian tube, ectopic pregnancy
Femoral head, fracture
Finger/toes, amputation, nontraumatic
Gingiva/oral mucosa, biopsy
Heart valve
Joint resection
Kidney biopsy
Larynx biopsy
Leiomyoma(s), uterine myomectomy-without uterus
Lip, biopsy/wedge resection
Lung, transbronchial biopsy
Lymph node, biopsy
Muscle, biopsy
Nasal mucosa, biopsy
Nasopharynx/oropharynx, biopsy
Nerve biopsy
Odontogenic/dental cyst
Omentum, biopsy
Ovary, biopsy/wedge resection
Ovary with or without tube, nonneoplastic
Parathyroid gland
Peritoneum, biopsy
Pituitary tumor
Placenta, other than third trimester
Pleura/pericardium-biopsy/tissue
Polyp:
   Cervical/endometrial
   Colorectal
   Stomach/small intestine
Prostate:
   Needle biopsy
   TUR
Salivary gland, biopsy
Sinus, paranasal biopsy
Skin, other than cyst/tag/debridement/plastic repair
Small intestine, biopsy
Soft tissue, other than tumor/mas/lipoma/debridement
Spleen
Stomach biopsy
Synovium
Testis, other than tumor/biopsy, castration
Thyroglossal duct/brachial cleft cyst
Tongue, biopsy
Tonsil, biopsy
Trachea biopsy
Ureter, biopsy
Urethra, biopsy
Urinary bladder, biopsy
Uterus, with or without tubes and ovaries, for prolapse
Vagina biopsy
Vulva/labial biopsy

🖼 2.04　🔬 2.04　**FUD** XXX　　　01 80 ▢ P0

AMA: 2015,Jan,16; 2014,Feb,10; 2014,Jan,11; 2012,Jan,15-42; 2011,Dec,14-18; 2011,Jan,11

88307 Level V - Surgical pathology, gross and microscopic examination

INCLUDES
Adrenal resection
Bone, biopsy/curettings
Bone fragment(s), pathologic fractures
Brain, biopsy
Brain meninges, tumor resection
Breast, excision of lesion, requiring microscopic evaluation of surgical margins
Breast, mastectomy-partial/simple
Cervix, conization
Colon, segmental resection, other than for tumor
Extremity, amputation, nontraumatic
Eye, enucleation
Kidney, partial/total nephrectomy
Larynx, partial/total resection
Liver
   Biopsy, needle/wedge
   Partial resection
Lung, wedge biopsy
Lymph nodes, regional resection
Mediastinum, mass
Myocardium, biopsy
Odontogenic tumor
Ovary with or without tube, neoplastic
Pancreas, biopsy
Placenta, third trimester
Prostate, except radical resection
Salivary gland
Sentinel lymph node
Small intestine, resection, other than for tumor
Soft tissue mass (except lipoma)-biopsy/simple excision
Stomach-subtotal/total resection, other than for tumor
Testis, biopsy
Thymus, tumor
Thyroid, total/lobe
Ureter, resection
Urinary bladder, TUR
Uterus, with or without tubes and ovaries, other than neoplastic/prolapse

🖼 8.56　🔬 8.56　**FUD** XXX　　　01 80 ▢ P0

AMA: 2015,Jan,16; 2014,Feb,10; 2014,Jan,11; 2012,Jan,15-42; 2011,Dec,14-18; 2011,Jan,11

88309 **Level VI - Surgical pathology, gross and microscopic examination**

> INCLUDES Bone resection
> Breast, mastectomy-with regional lymph nodes
> Colon:
>   Segmental resection for tumor
>   Total resection
> Esophagus, partial/total resection
> Extremity, disarticulation
> Fetus, with dissection
> Larynx, partial/total resection-with regional lymph nodes
> Lung-total/lobe/segment resection
> Pancreas, total/subtotal resection
> Prostate, radical resection
> Small intestine, resection for tumor
> Soft tissue tumor, extensive resection
> Stomach, subtotal/total resection for tumor
> Testis, tumor
> Tongue/tonsil, resection for tumor
> Urinary bladder, partial/total resection
> Uterus, with or without tubes and ovaries, neoplastic
> Vulva, total/subtotal resection

> EXCLUDES *Evaluation of fine needle aspirate (88172-88173)*
> *Fine needle aspiration (10021-10022)*

🔲 12.9　　⚖ 12.9　　**FUD** XXX　　　　Ⓢ 80 🔲 P0

AMA: 2015,Jan,16; 2014,Feb,10; 2014,Jan,11; 2012,Jan,15-42; 2011,Dec,14-18; 2011,Jan,11

88311-88399 [88341, 88350, 88364, 88373, 88374, 88377]
Additional Surgical Pathology Services

CMS: 100-2,15,80.1 Payment for Clinical Laboratory Services

+ **88311** **Decalcification procedure (List separately in addition to code for surgical pathology examination)**
> Code first surgical pathology exam (88302-88309)
> 🔲 0.59　　⚖ 0.59　　**FUD** XXX　　　　Ⓝ 80

AMA: 2015,Jan,16; 2014,Jan,11; 2012,Jan,15-42; 2011,Dec,14-18; 2011,Jan,11

88312 **Special stain including interpretation and report; Group I for microorganisms (eg, acid fast, methenamine silver)**
> INCLUDES Reporting one unit for each special stain performed on a surgical pathology block, cytologic sample, or hematologic smear
> 🔲 2.73　　⚖ 2.73　　**FUD** XXX　　　　Ⓠ1 80

AMA: 2015,Jan,16; 2014,Jan,11; 2012,Jan,15-42; 2011,Dec,14-18; 2011,Jan,11

88313 **Group II, all other (eg, iron, trichrome), except stain for microorganisms, stains for enzyme constituents, or immunocytochemistry and immunohistochemistry**
> INCLUDES Reporting one unit for each special stain performed on a surgical pathology block, cytologic sample, or hematologic smear
> EXCLUDES *Immunocytochemistry and immunohistochemistry (88342)*
> 🔲 1.90　　⚖ 1.90　　**FUD** XXX　　　　Ⓠ1 80 🔲

AMA: 2015,Jan,16; 2014,Jan,11; 2012,Jan,15-42; 2011,Dec,14-18; 2011,Jan,11

+ **88314** **histochemical stain on frozen tissue block (List separately in addition to code for primary procedure)**
> INCLUDES Reporting one unit for each special stain on each frozen surgical pathology block
> EXCLUDES *Special stain performed on frozen tissue section specimen to identify enzyme constituents (88319)*
> Code also modifier 59 for nonroutine histochemical stain on frozen section during Mohs surgery
> Code first (17311-17315, 88302-88309, 88331-88332)
> Do not report with routine frozen section stain during Mohs surgery (17311-17315)
> 🔲 2.09　　⚖ 2.09　　**FUD** XXX　　　　Ⓝ 80

AMA: 2015,Jan,16; 2014,Jan,11; 2011,Dec,14-18

88319 **Group III, for enzyme constituents**
> INCLUDES Reporting one unit for each special stain on each frozen surgical pathology block
> EXCLUDES *Detection of enzyme constituents by immunohistochemical or immunocytochemical methodology (88342)*
> 🔲 2.48　　⚖ 2.48　　**FUD** XXX　　　　Ⓢ 80

AMA: 2015,Jan,16; 2014,Jan,11; 2011,Dec,14-18

88321 **Consultation and report on referred slides prepared elsewhere**
> 🔲 2.42　　⚖ 2.70　　**FUD** XXX　　　　Ⓠ1 80 🔲

AMA: 2015,Jan,16; 2014,Jan,11; 2013,Jun,13; 2012,Jan,15-42; 2011,Dec,14-18; 2011,Jan,11; 2010,Jan,11-12

88323 **Consultation and report on referred material requiring preparation of slides**
> 🔲 4.26　　⚖ 4.26　　**FUD** XXX　　　　Ⓠ1 80 🔲

AMA: 2015,Jan,16; 2014,Jan,11; 2013,Jun,13; 2012,Jan,15-42; 2011,Dec,14-18; 2011,Jan,11

88325 **Consultation, comprehensive, with review of records and specimens, with report on referred material**
> 🔲 3.82　　⚖ 6.03　　**FUD** XXX　　　　Ⓠ1 80 🔲

AMA: 2015,Jan,16; 2014,Jan,11; 2013,Jun,13; 2012,Jan,15-42; 2011,Dec,14-18; 2011,Jan,11

88329 **Pathology consultation during surgery;**
> 🔲 1.03　　⚖ 1.65　　**FUD** XXX　　　　Ⓠ1 80 🔲

AMA: 2015,Jan,16; 2014,Feb,10; 2014,Jan,11; 2012,Jan,15-42; 2011,Dec,14-18; 2011,Jan,11; 2010,Oct,5

88331 **first tissue block, with frozen section(s), single specimen**
> Code also cytologic evaluation performed at same time (88334)
> 🔲 2.89　　⚖ 2.89　　**FUD** XXX　　　　Ⓠ1 80 🔲

AMA: 2015,Jan,16; 2014,Feb,10; 2014,Jan,11; 2011,Dec,14-18; 2010,Dec,7-10; 2010,Oct,5

+ **88332** **each additional tissue block with frozen section(s) (List separately in addition to code for primary procedure)**
> Code first (88331)
> 🔲 1.27　　⚖ 1.27　　**FUD** XXX　　　　Ⓝ 80 🔲

AMA: 2015,Jan,16; 2014,Feb,10; 2014,Jan,11; 2011,Dec,14-18; 2010,Dec,7-10; 2010,Oct,5

88333 **cytologic examination (eg, touch prep, squash prep), initial site**
> EXCLUDES *Intraprocedural cytologic evaluation of fine needle aspirate (88172)*
> *Nonintraoperative cytologic examination (88160-88162)*
> 🔲 3.05　　⚖ 3.05　　**FUD** XXX　　　　Ⓢ 80

AMA: 2015,Jan,16; 2014,Feb,10; 2014,Jan,11; 2012,Jan,15-42; 2011,Dec,14-18; 2011,Jan,11; 2010,Dec,7-10; 2010,Oct,5

+ **88334** **cytologic examination (eg, touch prep, squash prep), each additional site (List separately in addition to code for primary procedure)**
> EXCLUDES *Intraprocedural cytologic evaluation of fine needle aspirate (88172)*
> *Nonintraoperative cytologic examination (88160-88162)*
> *Percutaneous needle biopsy requiring intraprocedural cytologic examination (88333)*
> Code first (88331, 88333)
> 🔲 1.87　　⚖ 1.87　　**FUD** XXX　　　　Ⓝ 80

AMA: 2015,Jan,16; 2014,Feb,10; 2014,Jan,11; 2011,Dec,14-18; 2010,Dec,7-10; 2010,Oct,5

88341 **Resequenced code. See code following 88342.**

88342 **Immunohistochemistry or immunocytochemistry, per specimen; initial single antibody stain procedure**
> Do not report more than one time for each specific antibody
> Do not report testing on the same antibody as (88360-88361)
> 🔲 2.53　　⚖ 2.53　　**FUD** XXX　　　　Ⓠ1 80 🔲

AMA: 2015,Jun,10; 2015,Jan,16; 2014,Jun,14; 2014,Jan,11; 2012,Jan,15-42; 2011,Dec,14-18; 2011,Jan,11; 2010,Oct,9

+ # 88341 each additional single antibody stain procedure (List separately in addition to code for primary procedure)
Code first (88342)
Do not report more than one time for each specific antibody
Do not report testing on the same antibody as (88360-88361)
🚗 1.89 ✂ 1.89 **FUD** ZZZ [N] [80]
AMA: 2015,Jun,10

88344 each multiplex antibody stain procedure
INCLUDES Staining with multiple antibodies on the same slide
Do not report more than one time for each specific antibody
Do not report testing on the same antibody as (88360-88361)
🚗 3.27 ✂ 3.27 **FUD** XXX [01] [80]
AMA: 2015,Jun,10

▲ **88346 Immunofluorescence, per specimen; initial single antibody stain procedure**
EXCLUDES Fluorescent in situ hybridization studies (88364-88369 [88364, 88373, 88374, 88377])
Multiple immunofluorescence analysis (88399)
🚗 3.09 ✂ 3.09 **FUD** XXX [01] [80]
AMA: 2015,Jan,16; 2014,Jan,11; 2011,Dec,14-18

● + # **88350 each additional single antibody stain procedure (List separately in addition to code for primary procedure)**
🚗 0.00 ✂ 0.00 **FUD** 000
EXCLUDES Fluorescent in situ hybridization studies (88364-88369 [88364, 88373, 88374, 88377])
Multiple immunofluorescence analysis (88399)
Code first (88346)

88347 indirect method
To report, see ~88346, [88350]

88348 Electron microscopy, diagnostic
🚗 9.70 ✂ 9.70 **FUD** XXX [S] [80]
AMA: 2011,Dec,14-18

88350 Resequenced code. See code following 88346.

88355 Morphometric analysis; skeletal muscle
🚗 4.89 ✂ 4.89 **FUD** XXX [01] [80]
AMA: 2015,Jan,16; 2014,Jan,11; 2011,Dec,14-18

88356 nerve
🚗 5.75 ✂ 5.75 **FUD** XXX [01] [80]
AMA: 2015,Jan,16; 2014,Jun,14; 2014,Jan,11; 2011,Dec,14-18

88358 tumor (eg, DNA ploidy)
Do not report with 88313 unless each procedure is for a different special stain
🚗 2.36 ✂ 2.36 **FUD** XXX [S] [80]
AMA: 2015,Jan,16; 2014,Jan,11; 2012,Jan,15-42; 2011,Dec,14-18; 2011,Jan,11

88360 Morphometric analysis, tumor immunohistochemistry (eg, Her-2/neu, estrogen receptor/progesterone receptor), quantitative or semiquantitative, per specimen, each single antibody stain procedure; manual
EXCLUDES Morphometric analysis using in situ hybridization techniques (88367-88368 [88373, 88374])
Do not report additional stain procedures unless each test is for different antibody (88341, 88342, 88344)
🚗 3.80 ✂ 3.80 **FUD** XXX [01] [80] [PQ]
AMA: 2015,Jun,10; 2015,Jan,16; 2014,Jun,14; 2014,Jan,11; 2011,Dec,14-18

88361 using computer-assisted technology
EXCLUDES Morphometric analysis using in situ hybridization techniques (88367-88368 [88373, 88374])
Do not report additional stain procedures unless each test is for different antibody (88341, 88342, 88344)
🚗 4.74 ✂ 4.74 **FUD** XXX [01] [80] [PQ]
AMA: 2015,Jun,10; 2015,Jan,16; 2014,Jun,14; 2014,Jan,11; 2011,Dec,14-18

88362 Nerve teasing preparations
🚗 8.28 ✂ 8.28 **FUD** XXX [S] [80]
AMA: 2015,Jan,16; 2014,Jan,11; 2011,Dec,14-18

88363 Examination and selection of retrieved archival (ie, previously diagnosed) tissue(s) for molecular analysis (eg, KRAS mutational analysis)
INCLUDES Archival retrieval only
🚗 0.55 ✂ 0.64 **FUD** XXX [01] [80]
AMA: 2015,Jan,16; 2014,Jan,11; 2011,Dec,14-18; 2010,Dec,7-10

88364 Resequenced code. See code following 88365.

88365 In situ hybridization (eg, FISH), per specimen; initial single probe stain procedure
Do not report for the same probe with (88367, [88374], 88368, [88377])
🚗 4.38 ✂ 4.38 **FUD** XXX [01] [80]
AMA: 2015,Jan,16; 2014,Jan,11; 2013,Sep,3-12; 2012,May,3-10; 2012,Jan,15-42; 2011,Dec,14-18; 2011,Jan,11

+ # **88364 each additional single probe stain procedure (List separately in addition to code for primary procedure)**
🚗 2.72 ✂ 2.72 **FUD** ZZZ [N] [80]
Code first (88365)

88366 each multiplex probe stain procedure
🚗 6.53 ✂ 6.53 **FUD** XXX [01] [80]
Do not report for the same probe with (88367, [88374], 88368, [88377])

88367 Morphometric analysis, in situ hybridization (quantitative or semi-quantitative), using computer-assisted technology, per specimen; initial single probe stain procedure
EXCLUDES Morphometric in situ hybridization evaluation of urinary tract cytologic specimens (88120-88121)
Do not report for same probe with (88365, 88366, 88368, [88377])
🚗 3.00 ✂ 3.00 **FUD** XXX [01] [80]
AMA: 2015,Jan,16; 2014,Jan,11; 2013,Sep,3-12; 2012,May,3-10; 2012,Jan,15-42; 2011,Dec,14-18; 2011,Jan,11; 2010,Dec,7-10

+ # **88373 each additional single probe stain procedure (List separately in addition to code for primary procedure)**
🚗 1.69 ✂ 1.69 **FUD** ZZZ [N] [80]
Code first (88367)

88374 each multiplex probe stain procedure
🚗 5.72 ✂ 5.72 **FUD** XXX [01] [80]
Do not report for same probe with (88365, 88366, 88368, [88377])

88368 Morphometric analysis, in situ hybridization (quantitative or semi-quantitative), manual, per specimen; initial single probe stain procedure
EXCLUDES Morphometric in situ hybridization evaluation of urinary tract cytologic specimens (88120-88121)
Do not report for same probe with (88365, 88366-88367, [88374])
🚗 3.04 ✂ 3.04 **FUD** XXX [01] [80]
AMA: 2015,Jan,16; 2014,Jan,11; 2013,Sep,3-12; 2012,May,3-10; 2012,Jan,15-42; 2011,Dec,14-18; 2011,Jan,11; 2010,Dec,7-10

+ **88369 each additional single probe stain procedure (List separately in addition to code for primary procedure)**
🚗 2.06 ✂ 2.06 **FUD** ZZZ [N] [80]
Code first (88368)

88377 each multiplex probe stain procedure
🚗 5.98 ✂ 5.98 **FUD** XXX [01] [80]
Do not report for same probe with (88365, 88366-88367, [88374])

88371 Protein analysis of tissue by Western Blot, with interpretation and report;
  0.00   0.00   **FUD** XXX   N
  AMA: 2015,Jan,16; 2014,Jan,11; 2011,Dec,14-18

88372 immunological probe for band identification, each
  0.00   0.00   **FUD** XXX   N
  AMA: 2015,Jan,16; 2014,Jan,11; 2011,Dec,14-18

88373 Resequenced code. See code following 88367.

88374 Resequenced code. See code following 88367.

88375 Optical endomicroscopic image(s), interpretation and report, real-time or referred, each endoscopic session
  Do not report with (43206, 43252, 0397T)
  1.34   1.34   **FUD** XXX   Q1 80 26
  AMA: 2015,Jan,16; 2013,Aug,5

88377 Resequenced code. See code following 88369.

88380 Microdissection (ie, sample preparation of microscopically identified target); laser capture
  Do not report with (88381)
  3.71   3.71   **FUD** XXX   N 80
  AMA: 2015,Jan,16; 2014,Jan,11; 2013,Sep,3-12; 2012,May,3-10; 2011,Dec,14-18

88381 manual
  Do not report with (88380)
  3.48   3.48   **FUD** XXX   N 80
  AMA: 2015,Jan,16; 2014,Jan,11; 2013,Sep,3-12; 2012,May,14-15; 2012,May,3-10; 2011,Dec,14-18

88387 Macroscopic examination, dissection, and preparation of tissue for non-microscopic analytical studies (eg, nucleic acid-based molecular studies); each tissue preparation (eg, a single lymph node)
  Do not report for tissue preparation for microbiologic cultures or flow cytometric studies
  Do not report with (88329-88334, 88388)
  1.20   1.20   **FUD** XXX   N 80
  AMA: 2015,Jan,16; 2014,Jan,11; 2012,Jan,15-42; 2011,Dec,14-18; 2011,Jan,11; 2010,Oct,5; 2010,Oct,3-4

+ **88388** in conjunction with a touch imprint, intraoperative consultation, or frozen section, each tissue preparation (eg, a single lymph node) (List separately in addition to code for primary procedure)
  Code first (88329-88334)
  Do not report for tissue preparation for microbiologic cultures or flow cytometric studies
  0.96   0.96   **FUD** XXX   N 80
  AMA: 2015,Jan,16; 2014,Jan,11; 2012,Jan,15-42; 2011,Dec,14-18; 2011,Jan,11; 2010,Oct,5; 2010,Oct,3-4

88399 Unlisted surgical pathology procedure
  0.00   0.00   **FUD** XXX   Q1 80
  AMA: 2015,Jan,16; 2014,Jun,14; 2014,Jan,11; 2012,Jan,15-42; 2011,Jan,11; 2010,Dec,7-10

88720-88749 Transcutaneous Procedures

EXCLUDES Transcutaneous oxyhemoglobin measurement in a leg using near infrared spectroscopy (0286T)
Wavelength fluorescent spectroscopy of advanced glycation end products (skin) (88749)

88720 Bilirubin, total, transcutaneous
  EXCLUDES Transdermal oxygen saturation testing (94760-94762)
  0.00   0.00   **FUD** XXX   N
  AMA: 2015,Jan,16; 2014,Jan,11; 2010,Dec,7-10

88738 Hemoglobin (Hgb), quantitative, transcutaneous
  EXCLUDES In vitro hemoglobin measurement (85018)
  0.00   0.00   **FUD** XXX   N
  AMA: 2015,Jan,16; 2014,Jan,11; 2010,Oct,6

88740 Hemoglobin, quantitative, transcutaneous, per day; carboxyhemoglobin
  EXCLUDES In vitro carboxyhemoglobin measurement (82375)
  0.00   0.00   **FUD** XXX   N
  AMA: 2015,Jan,16; 2014,Jan,11; 2010,Oct,6

88741 methemoglobin
  EXCLUDES In vitro quantitative methemoglobin measurement (83050)
  0.00   0.00   **FUD** XXX   N
  AMA: 2015,Jan,16; 2014,Jan,11; 2010,Oct,6

88749 Unlisted in vivo (eg, transcutaneous) laboratory service
  INCLUDES All in vivo measurements not specifically listed
  0.00   0.00   **FUD** XXX   N
  AMA: 2010,Dec,7-10

89049-89240 Other Pathology Services

89049 Caffeine halothane contracture test (CHCT) for malignant hyperthermia susceptibility, including interpretation and report
  1.76   6.76   **FUD** XXX   Q1 80
  AMA: 2015,Jan,16; 2014,Jan,11; 2012,Jan,15-42; 2011,Sep,3-4; 2011,Jan,11

89050 Cell count, miscellaneous body fluids (eg, cerebrospinal fluid, joint fluid), except blood;
  0.00   0.00   **FUD** XXX   N
  AMA: 2015,Jan,16; 2014,Jan,11; 2011,Sep,3-4

89051 with differential count
  0.00   0.00   **FUD** XXX   N
  AMA: 2015,Jan,16; 2014,Jan,11; 2011,Sep,3-4

89055 Leukocyte assessment, fecal, qualitative or semiquantitative
  0.00   0.00   **FUD** XXX   N
  AMA: 2015,Jan,16; 2014,Jan,11; 2011,Sep,3-4

89060 Crystal identification by light microscopy with or without polarizing lens analysis, tissue or any body fluid (except urine)
  Do not report for crystal identification on paraffin embedded tissue
  0.00   0.00   **FUD** XXX   N
  AMA: 2015,Jan,16; 2014,Jan,11; 2011,Sep,3-4

89125 Fat stain, feces, urine, or respiratory secretions
  0.00   0.00   **FUD** XXX   N
  AMA: 2015,Jan,16; 2014,Jan,11; 2011,Sep,3-4

89160 Meat fibers, feces
  0.00   0.00   **FUD** XXX   N
  AMA: 2015,Jan,16; 2014,Jan,11; 2011,Sep,3-4

89190 Nasal smear for eosinophils
  0.00   0.00   **FUD** XXX   N
  AMA: 2015,Jan,16; 2014,Jan,11; 2012,Jan,15-42; 2011,Sep,3-4; 2011,Jan,11

89220 Sputum, obtaining specimen, aerosol induced technique (separate procedure)
  0.44   0.44   **FUD** XXX   Q1 80 TC
  AMA: 2015,Jan,16; 2014,Jan,11; 2011,Sep,3-4

89230 Sweat collection by iontophoresis
  0.07   0.07   **FUD** XXX   Q1 80 TC
  AMA: 2015,Jan,16; 2014,Jan,11; 2011,Sep,3-4

89240 Unlisted miscellaneous pathology test
  0.00   0.00   **FUD** XXX   Q1 80
  AMA: 2015,Jan,16; 2014,Jan,11; 2012,Jan,15-42; 2011,Sep,3-4; 2011,Jan,11

Pathology and Laboratory

89250 — 89335

89250-89398 Infertility Treatment Services

CMS: 100-2,1,100 Treatment for Infertility

89250 **Culture of oocyte(s)/embryo(s), less than 4 days;**
🔧 0.00 ⚕ 0.00 **FUD** XXX [01]
AMA: 2015,Jan,16; 2014,Jan,11; 2012,Jan,15-42; 2011,Jan,11

89251 **with co-culture of oocyte(s)/embryos**
EXCLUDES *Extended culture of oocyte(s)/embryo(s) (89272)*
🔧 0.00 ⚕ 0.00 **FUD** XXX [01] 🖵
AMA: 2015,Jan,16; 2014,Jan,11; 2012,Jan,15-42; 2011,Jan,11

89253 **Assisted embryo hatching, microtechniques (any method)**
🔧 0.00 ⚕ 0.00 **FUD** XXX [01]
AMA: 2015,Jan,16; 2014,Jan,11; 2012,Jan,15-42; 2011,Jan,11

89254 **Oocyte identification from follicular fluid**
🔧 0.00 ⚕ 0.00 **FUD** XXX [01]
AMA: 2015,Jan,16; 2014,Jan,11; 2012,Jan,15-42; 2011,Jan,11

89255 **Preparation of embryo for transfer (any method)**
🔧 0.00 ⚕ 0.00 **FUD** XXX [01]
AMA: 2015,Jan,16; 2014,Jan,11; 2012,Jan,15-42; 2011,Jan,11

89257 **Sperm identification from aspiration (other than seminal fluid)**
EXCLUDES *Semen analysis (89300-89320)*
Sperm identification from testis tissue (89264)
🔧 0.00 ⚕ 0.00 **FUD** XXX [01] 🖵
AMA: 2015,Jan,16; 2014,Jan,11; 2012,Jan,15-42; 2011,Jan,11

89258 **Cryopreservation; embryo(s)**
🔧 0.00 ⚕ 0.00 **FUD** XXX [S]
AMA: 2015,Jan,16; 2014,Jan,11; 2012,Jan,15-42; 2011,Jan,11

89259 **sperm**
EXCLUDES *Cryopreservation of testicular reproductive tissue (89335)*
🔧 0.00 ⚕ 0.00 **FUD** XXX [01]
AMA: 2015,Jan,16; 2014,Jan,11; 2012,Jan,15-42; 2011,Jan,11

89260 **Sperm isolation; simple prep (eg, sperm wash and swim-up) for insemination or diagnosis with semen analysis**
🔧 0.00 ⚕ 0.00 **FUD** XXX [01] 🖵
AMA: 2015,Jan,16; 2014,Jan,11; 2012,Jan,15-42; 2011,Jan,11

89261 **complex prep (eg, Percoll gradient, albumin gradient) for insemination or diagnosis with semen analysis**
EXCLUDES *Semen analysis without sperm wash or swim-up (89320)*
🔧 0.00 ⚕ 0.00 **FUD** XXX [01] 🖵
AMA: 2015,Jan,16; 2014,Jan,11; 2012,Jan,15-42; 2011,Jan,11

89264 **Sperm identification from testis tissue, fresh or cryopreserved** ♂
EXCLUDES *Biopsy of testis (54500, 54505)*
Semen analysis (89300-89320)
Sperm identification from aspiration (89257)
🔧 0.00 ⚕ 0.00 **FUD** XXX [01] 🖵
AMA: 2015,Jan,16; 2014,Jan,11; 2012,Jan,15-42; 2011,Jan,11

89268 **Insemination of oocytes**
🔧 0.00 ⚕ 0.00 **FUD** XXX [01]
AMA: 2015,Jan,16; 2014,Jan,11; 2012,Jan,15-42; 2011,Jan,11

89272 **Extended culture of oocyte(s)/embryo(s), 4-7 days**
🔧 0.00 ⚕ 0.00 **FUD** XXX [S]
AMA: 2015,Jan,16; 2014,Jan,11; 2012,Jan,15-42; 2011,Jan,11

89280 **Assisted oocyte fertilization, microtechnique; less than or equal to 10 oocytes**
🔧 0.00 ⚕ 0.00 **FUD** XXX [S]
AMA: 2015,Jan,16; 2014,Jan,11; 2012,Jan,15-42; 2011,Jan,11

89281 **greater than 10 oocytes**
🔧 0.00 ⚕ 0.00 **FUD** XXX [01]
AMA: 2015,Jan,16; 2014,Jan,11; 2012,Jan,15-42; 2011,Jan,11

89290 **Biopsy, oocyte polar body or embryo blastomere, microtechnique (for pre-implantation genetic diagnosis); less than or equal to 5 embryos**
🔧 0.00 ⚕ 0.00 **FUD** XXX [01] [P0]
AMA: 2015,Jan,16; 2014,Jan,11; 2012,Jan,15-42; 2011,Jan,11

89291 **greater than 5 embryos**
🔧 0.00 ⚕ 0.00 **FUD** XXX [01] [P0]
AMA: 2015,Jan,16; 2014,Jan,11; 2012,Jan,15-42; 2011,Jan,11

89300 **Semen analysis; presence and/or motility of sperm including Huhner test (post coital)** ♀
🔧 0.00 ⚕ 0.00 **FUD** XXX [X] [N] 🖵
AMA: 2015,Jan,16; 2014,Jan,11; 2012,Jan,15-42; 2011,Jan,11

89310 **motility and count (not including Huhner test)** ♂
🔧 0.00 ⚕ 0.00 **FUD** XXX [N] 🖵
AMA: 2015,Jan,16; 2014,Jan,11; 2012,Jan,15-42; 2011,Jan,11

89320 **volume, count, motility, and differential** ♂
EXCLUDES *Skin testing (86485-86580, 95012-95199)*
🔧 0.00 ⚕ 0.00 **FUD** XXX [N] 🖵
AMA: 2015,Jan,16; 2014,Jan,11; 2012,Jan,15-42; 2011,Jan,11

89321 **sperm presence and motility of sperm, if performed** ♂
EXCLUDES *Hyaluronan binding assay (HBA) (89398)*
🔧 0.00 ⚕ 0.00 **FUD** XXX [X] [N] 🖵
AMA: 2015,Jan,16; 2014,Jan,11; 2012,Jan,15-42; 2011,Jan,11

89322 **volume, count, motility, and differential using strict morphologic criteria (eg, Kruger)** ♂
🔧 0.00 ⚕ 0.00 **FUD** XXX [N]
AMA: 2015,Jan,16; 2014,Jan,11; 2012,Jan,15-42; 2011,Jan,11

89325 **Sperm antibodies** ♂
EXCLUDES *Medicolegal identification of sperm (88125)*
🔧 0.00 ⚕ 0.00 **FUD** XXX [N] 🖵
AMA: 2015,Jan,16; 2014,Jan,11; 2012,Jan,15-42; 2011,Jan,11

89329 **Sperm evaluation; hamster penetration test** ♂
🔧 0.00 ⚕ 0.00 **FUD** XXX [N] 🖵
AMA: 2015,Jan,16; 2014,Jan,11; 2012,Jan,15-42; 2011,Jan,11

89330 **cervical mucus penetration test, with or without spinnbarkeit test** ♂
🔧 0.00 ⚕ 0.00 **FUD** XXX [N] 🖵
AMA: 2015,Jan,16; 2014,Jan,11; 2012,Jan,15-42; 2011,Jan,11

89331 **Sperm evaluation, for retrograde ejaculation, urine (sperm concentration, motility, and morphology, as indicated)** ♂
EXCLUDES *Detection of sperm in urine (81015)*
Code also semen analysis on concurrent sperm specimen (89300-89322)
🔧 0.00 ⚕ 0.00 **FUD** XXX [N]
AMA: 2015,Jan,16; 2014,Jan,11; 2012,Jan,15-42; 2011,Jan,11

89335 **Cryopreservation, reproductive tissue, testicular**
EXCLUDES *Cryopreservation of:*
Embryo(s) (89258)
Oocytes:
Immature ([0357T])
Mature (89337)
Ovarian tissue (0058T)
Sperm (89259)
🔧 0.00 ⚕ 0.00 **FUD** XXX [01]
AMA: 2015,Jan,16; 2014,Jan,11; 2012,Jan,15-42; 2011,Jan,11

89337	**Cryopreservation, mature oocyte(s)** ♀
	EXCLUDES *Cryopreservation of immature oocyte[s] ([0357T])*
	🚑 0.00 ⚕ 0.00 **FUD** XXX [01]
	AMA: 2015,Jan,16
89342	**Storage (per year); embryo(s)**
	🚑 0.00 ⚕ 0.00 **FUD** XXX [01]
	AMA: 2015,Jan,16; 2014,Jan,11; 2012,Jan,15-42; 2011,Jan,11
89343	**sperm/semen**
	🚑 0.00 ⚕ 0.00 **FUD** XXX [01]
	AMA: 2015,Jan,16; 2014,Jan,11; 2012,Jan,15-42; 2011,Jan,11
89344	**reproductive tissue, testicular/ovarian**
	🚑 0.00 ⚕ 0.00 **FUD** XXX [01]
	AMA: 2015,Jan,16; 2014,Jan,11; 2012,Jan,15-42; 2011,Jan,11
89346	**oocyte(s)**
	🚑 0.00 ⚕ 0.00 **FUD** XXX [01]
	AMA: 2015,Jan,16; 2014,Jan,11; 2012,Jan,15-42; 2011,Jan,11
89352	**Thawing of cryopreserved; embryo(s)**
	🚑 0.00 ⚕ 0.00 **FUD** XXX [01]
	AMA: 2015,Jan,16; 2014,Jan,11; 2012,Jan,15-42; 2011,Jan,11
89353	**sperm/semen, each aliquot**
	🚑 0.00 ⚕ 0.00 **FUD** XXX [01]
	AMA: 2015,Jan,16; 2014,Jan,11; 2012,Jan,15-42; 2011,Jan,11
89354	**reproductive tissue, testicular/ovarian**
	🚑 0.00 ⚕ 0.00 **FUD** XXX [01]
	AMA: 2015,Jan,16; 2014,Jan,11; 2012,Jan,15-42; 2011,Jan,11
89356	**oocytes, each aliquot**
	🚑 0.00 ⚕ 0.00 **FUD** XXX [01]
	AMA: 2015,Jan,16; 2014,Jan,11; 2012,Jan,15-42; 2011,Jan,11
89398	**Unlisted reproductive medicine laboratory procedure**
	🚑 0.00 ⚕ 0.00 **FUD** XXX [01]
	INCLUDES Hyaluronan binding assay (HBA)

90281-90399 Immunoglobulin Products

[INCLUDES] Immune globulin product only
Anti-infectives
Antitoxins
Isoantibodies
Monoclonal antibodies
Code also (96365-96372, 96374-96375)

90281 Immune globulin (Ig), human, for intramuscular use
[INCLUDES] Gamastan
🏥 0.00 🩺 0.00 **FUD** XXX [51] [E]
AMA: 2015,Jan,16; 2014,Jan,11; 2012,Jan,15-42; 2011,Jan,11

90283 Immune globulin (IgIV), human, for intravenous use
🏥 0.00 🩺 0.00 **FUD** XXX [51] [E]
AMA: 2015,Jan,16; 2014,Jan,11; 2012,Jan,15-42; 2011,Jan,11

90284 Immune globulin (SCIg), human, for use in subcutaneous infusions, 100 mg, each
🏥 0.00 🩺 0.00 **FUD** XXX [51] [E]
AMA: 2015,Jan,16; 2012,Jan,15-42; 2011,Jan,11

90287 Botulinum antitoxin, equine, any route
🏥 0.00 🩺 0.00 **FUD** XXX [51] [E]
AMA: 2015,Jan,16; 2014,Jan,11; 2012,Jan,15-42; 2011,Jan,11

90288 Botulism immune globulin, human, for intravenous use
🏥 0.00 🩺 0.00 **FUD** XXX [51] [E]
AMA: 2015,Jan,16; 2014,Jan,11; 2012,Jan,15-42; 2011,Jan,11

90291 Cytomegalovirus immune globulin (CMV-IgIV), human, for intravenous use
[INCLUDES] Cytogram
🏥 0.00 🩺 0.00 **FUD** XXX [51] [E]
AMA: 2015,Jan,16; 2014,Jan,11; 2012,Jan,15-42; 2011,Jan,11

90296 Diphtheria antitoxin, equine, any route
🏥 0.00 🩺 0.00 **FUD** XXX [51] [E]
AMA: 2015,Jan,16; 2014,Jan,11; 2012,Jan,15-42; 2011,Jan,11

90371 Hepatitis B immune globulin (HBIg), human, for intramuscular use
[INCLUDES] HBIG
🏥 0.00 🩺 0.00 **FUD** XXX [51] [K] [K2]
AMA: 2015,Jan,16; 2014,Jan,11; 2012,Jan,15-42; 2011,Jan,11

90375 Rabies immune globulin (RIg), human, for intramuscular and/or subcutaneous use
[INCLUDES] HyperRAB
🏥 0.00 🩺 0.00 **FUD** XXX [51] [K] [K2]
AMA: 2015,Jan,16; 2012,Jan,15-42; 2011,Jan,11

90376 Rabies immune globulin, heat-treated (RIg-HT), human, for intramuscular and/or subcutaneous use
🏥 0.00 🩺 0.00 **FUD** XXX [51] [K] [K2]
AMA: 2015,Jan,16; 2012,Jan,15-42; 2011,Jan,11

90378 Respiratory syncytial virus, monoclonal antibody, recombinant, for intramuscular use, 50 mg, each
[INCLUDES] Synagis
🏥 0.00 🩺 0.00 **FUD** XXX [51] [K] [K2]
AMA: 2015,Jan,16; 2014,Jan,11; 2012,Jan,15-42; 2011,Jan,11

90384 Rho(D) immune globulin (RhIg), human, full-dose, for intramuscular use
🏥 0.00 🩺 0.00 **FUD** XXX [51] [E]
AMA: 2015,Jan,16; 2014,Jan,11; 2012,Jan,15-42; 2011,Jan,11

90385 Rho(D) immune globulin (RhIg), human, mini-dose, for intramuscular use
🏥 0.00 🩺 0.00 **FUD** XXX [51] [N] [N1]
AMA: 2015,Jan,16; 2014,Jan,11; 2012,Jan,15-42; 2011,Jan,11

90386 Rho(D) immune globulin (RhIgIV), human, for intravenous use
🏥 0.00 🩺 0.00 **FUD** XXX [51] [E]
AMA: 2015,Jan,16; 2014,Jan,11; 2012,Jan,15-42; 2011,Jan,11

90389 Tetanus immune globulin (TIg), human, for intramuscular use
🏥 0.00 🩺 0.00 **FUD** XXX [51] [E]
AMA: 2015,Jan,16; 2014,Jan,11; 2012,Jan,15-42; 2011,Jan,11

90393 Vaccinia immune globulin, human, for intramuscular use
🏥 0.00 🩺 0.00 **FUD** XXX [51] [E]
AMA: 2015,Jan,16; 2014,Jan,11; 2012,Jan,15-42; 2011,Jan,11

90396 Varicella-zoster immune globulin, human, for intramuscular use
🏥 0.00 🩺 0.00 **FUD** XXX [51] [K] [K2]
AMA: 2015,Jan,16; 2014,Jan,11; 2012,Jan,15-42; 2011,Jan,11

90399 Unlisted immune globulin
🏥 0.00 🩺 0.00 **FUD** XXX [51] [E]
AMA: 2015,Jan,16; 2014,Jan,11; 2012,Jan,15-42; 2011,Jan,11

90460-90461 Injections Provided with Counseling

[INCLUDES] All components of influenza vaccine, report X 1 only
Combination vaccines which comprise multiple vaccine components
Components (all antigens) in vaccines to prevent disease due to specific organisms
Counseling by physician or other qualified health care professional
Multi-valent antigens or multiple antigen serotypes against single organisms are considered one component
Patient/family face-to-face counseling by doctor or qualified health care professional for patients 18 years of age and younger

[EXCLUDES] *Administration of influenza and pneumococcal vaccine for Medicare patients (G0008-G0009)*
Allergy testing (95004-95028)
Bacterial/viral/fungal skin tests (86485-86580)
Diagnostic or therapeutic injections (96365-96372, 96374-96375)
Vaccines provided without face-to-face counseling from a physician or qualified health care professional or to patients over the age of 18 (90471-90474)

Code also significant, separately identifiable E&M service when appropriate
Code also toxoid/vaccine (90476-90749 [90620, 90621, 90625, 90630, 90644, 90672, 90673])

90460 Immunization administration through 18 years of age via any route of administration, with counseling by physician or other qualified health care professional; first or only component of each vaccine or toxoid administered [A]
Code also each additional component in a vaccine (e.g., A 5-year-old receives DtaP-IPV IM administration, and MMR/Varicella vaccines SQ administration. Report initial component X 2, and additional components X 6)
🏥 0.71 🩺 0.71 **FUD** XXX [B] [80]
AMA: 2015,May,6; 2015,Apr,9; 2015,Apr,10; 2015,Jan,16; 2014,Mar,10; 2014,Jan,11; 2013,Aug,10; 2012,Jul,7; 2012,Jan,43; 2011,Mar,8; 2011,Mar,3-6

\+ **90461 each additional vaccine or toxoid component administered (List separately in addition to code for primary procedure)** [A]
Code also each additional component in a vaccine (e.g., A 5-year-old receives DtaP-IPV IM administration, and MMR/Varicella vaccines SQ administration. Report initial component X 2, and additional components X 6)
Code first the initial component in each vaccine provided (90460)
🏥 0.36 🩺 0.36 **FUD** ZZZ [B] [80]
AMA: 2015,May,6; 2015,Apr,10; 2015,Jan,16; 2014,Mar,10; 2014,Jan,11; 2013,Aug,10; 2012,Jul,7; 2012,Jan,43; 2011,Mar,8; 2011,Mar,3-6

90471-90474 Injections and Other Routes of Administration Without Physician Counseling

CMS: 100-4,18,10.4 CWF Edits for Influenza Virus and Pneumococcal Vaccinations

[EXCLUDES] *Administration of influenza and pneumococcal vaccine for Medicare patients (G0008-G0009)*
Administration of vaccine with counseling (90460-90461)
Allergy testing (95004-95028)
Bacterial/viral/fungal skin tests (86485-86580)
Diagnostic or therapeutic injections (96365-96371, 96374)
Patient/family face-to-face counseling

Code also significant, separately identifiable E&M service when appropriate
Code also toxoid/vaccine (90476-90749 [90620, 90621, 90625, 90630, 90644, 90672, 90673])

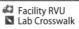

90471 **Immunization administration (includes percutaneous, intradermal, subcutaneous, or intramuscular injections); 1 vaccine (single or combination vaccine/toxoid)**

Do not report with intranasal/oral administration (90473)

💉 0.71　 ✂ 0.71　 **FUD** XXX　　　　 S 80 ▭

AMA: 2015,May,6; 2015,Apr,9; 2015,Apr,10; 2015,Jan,16; 2014,Mar,10; 2014,Jan,11; 2013,Aug,10; 2012,Jul,7; 2012,Jan,15-42; 2011,Mar,3-6; 2011,Jan,11

+ **90472** **each additional vaccine (single or combination vaccine/toxoid) (List separately in addition to code for primary procedure)**

EXCLUDES　 BCG vaccine, intravesical administration (51720, 90586)
Immune globulin administration (96365-96371, 96374)
Immune globulin product (90281-90399)
Code first initial vaccine (90460, 90471, 90473)

💉 0.36　 ✂ 0.36　 **FUD** ZZZ　　　　 N 80

AMA: 2015,May,6; 2015,Apr,9; 2015,Apr,10; 2015,Jan,16; 2014,Mar,10; 2014,Jan,11; 2013,Aug,10; 2012,Jul,7; 2012,Jan,15-42; 2011,Mar,3-6; 2011,Jan,11

90473 **Immunization administration by intranasal or oral route; 1 vaccine (single or combination vaccine/toxoid)**

Do not report with (90471)

💉 0.71　 ✂ 0.71　 **FUD** XXX　　　　 S 80 ▭

AMA: 2015,May,6; 2015,Jan,16; 2014,Mar,10; 2014,Jan,11; 2013,Aug,10; 2012,Jul,7; 2011,Mar,3-6

+ **90474** **each additional vaccine (single or combination vaccine/toxoid) (List separately in addition to code for primary procedure)**

Code first initial vaccine (90460, 90471, 90473)

💉 0.36　 ✂ 0.36　 **FUD** ZZZ　　　　 N 80

AMA: 2015,May,6; 2015,Apr,9; 2015,Jan,16; 2014,Mar,10; 2014,Jan,11; 2013,Aug,10; 2012,Jul,7; 2011,Mar,3-6

90476-90749 [90620, 90621, 90625, 90630, 90644, 90672, 90673] Vaccination Products

CMS: 100-2,15,50.4.4.2 Immunizations

INCLUDES　 Patient's age for coding purposes, not for product license
Vaccine product only

EXCLUDES　 Immune globulins and administration (90281-90399, 96365-96375)
Code also administration of vaccine (90460-90474)
Code also significant separately identifiable E&M service when appropriate
Do not report each component of a combination vaccine individually

90476 **Adenovirus vaccine, type 4, live, for oral use**

INCLUDES　 Adeno-4

💉 0.00　 ✂ 0.00　 **FUD** XXX　　　　 Ⓢ N N1

AMA: 2015,May,6; 2015,Jan,16; 2014,Jan,11; 2013,Aug,10; 2012,Jan,15-42; 2011,Mar,3-6; 2011,Jan,11

90477 **Adenovirus vaccine, type 7, live, for oral use**

INCLUDES　 Adeno-7

💉 0.00　 ✂ 0.00　 **FUD** XXX　　　　 Ⓢ E

AMA: 2015,May,6; 2015,Jan,16; 2014,Jan,11; 2013,Aug,10; 2012,Jan,15-42; 2011,Mar,3-6; 2011,Jan,11

90581 **Anthrax vaccine, for subcutaneous or intramuscular use**

INCLUDES　 BioThrax

💉 0.00　 ✂ 0.00　 **FUD** XXX　　　　 Ⓢ K K2 ▭

AMA: 2015,May,6; 2015,Jan,16; 2014,Jan,11; 2013,Aug,10; 2012,Jan,15-42; 2011,Mar,3-6; 2011,Jan,11

90585 **Bacillus Calmette-Guerin vaccine (BCG) for tuberculosis, live, for percutaneous use**

INCLUDES　 Mycobax

💉 0.00　 ✂ 0.00　 **FUD** XXX　　　　 Ⓢ K K2 ▭

AMA: 2015,May,6; 2015,Jan,16; 2014,Jan,11; 2013,Aug,10; 2012,Jan,15-42; 2011,Mar,3-6; 2011,Jan,11

90586 **Bacillus Calmette-Guerin vaccine (BCG) for bladder cancer, live, for intravesical use**

INCLUDES　 TheraCys
TICE BCG

💉 0.00　 ✂ 0.00　 **FUD** XXX　　　　 Ⓢ B

AMA: 2015,May,6; 2015,Jan,16; 2014,Jan,11; 2013,Aug,10; 2012,Jan,15-42; 2011,Mar,3-6; 2011,Jan,11

90620　 **Resequenced code. See code following 90734.**

90621　 **Resequenced code. See code following 90734.**

90625　 **Resequenced code. See code following 90723.**

90630　 **Resequenced code. See code following 90654.**

▲ **90632** **Hepatitis A vaccine (HepA), adult dosage, for intramuscular use** A

INCLUDES　 Havrix
Vaqta

💉 0.00　 ✂ 0.00　 **FUD** XXX　　　　 Ⓢ N N1 ▭

AMA: 2015,May,6; 2015,Jan,16; 2014,Jan,11; 2013,Aug,10; 2012,Jan,15-42; 2011,Mar,3-6; 2011,Jan,11

▲ **90633** **Hepatitis A vaccine (HepA), pediatric/adolescent dosage-2 dose schedule, for intramuscular use** A

INCLUDES　 Havrix
Vaqta

💉 0.00　 ✂ 0.00　 **FUD** XXX　　　　 Ⓢ N N1 ▭

AMA: 2015,May,6; 2015,Jan,16; 2014,Jan,11; 2013,Aug,10; 2012,Jan,15-42; 2011,Mar,3-6; 2011,Jan,11

▲ **90634** **Hepatitis A vaccine (HepA), pediatric/adolescent dosage-3 dose schedule, for intramuscular use** A

INCLUDES　 Havrix

💉 0.00　 ✂ 0.00　 **FUD** XXX　　　　 Ⓢ N N1 ▭

AMA: 2015,May,6; 2015,Jan,16; 2014,Jan,11; 2013,Aug,10; 2012,Jan,15-42; 2011,Mar,3-6; 2011,Jan,11

90636 **Hepatitis A and hepatitis B vaccine (HepA-HepB), adult dosage, for intramuscular use** A

INCLUDES　 Twinrix

💉 0.00　 ✂ 0.00　 **FUD** XXX　　　　 Ⓢ N N1 ▭

AMA: 2015,May,6; 2015,Jan,16; 2014,Jan,11; 2013,Aug,10; 2012,Jan,15-42; 2011,Mar,3-6; 2011,Jan,11

90644　 **Resequenced code. See code following 90732.**

90645 ~~Hemophilus influenza b vaccine (Hib), HbOC conjugate (4 dose schedule), for intramuscular use~~

90646 ~~Hemophilus influenza b vaccine (Hib), PRP-D conjugate, for booster use only, intramuscular use~~

▲ **90647** **Haemophilus influenzae type b vaccine (Hib), PRP-OMP conjugate, 3 dose schedule, for intramuscular use**

INCLUDES　 PedvaxHIB

💉 0.00　 ✂ 0.00　 **FUD** XXX　　　　 Ⓢ N N1 ▭

AMA: 2015,May,6; 2015,Jan,16; 2014,Jan,11; 2013,Aug,10; 2012,Jan,15-42; 2011,Mar,3-6; 2011,Jan,11

▲ **90648** **Haemophilus influenzae type b vaccine (Hib), PRP-T conjugate, 4 dose schedule, for intramuscular use**

INCLUDES　 ActHIB
Hiberix

💉 0.00　 ✂ 0.00　 **FUD** XXX　　　　 Ⓢ N N1 ▭

AMA: 2015,May,6; 2015,Jan,16; 2014,Jan,11; 2013,Aug,10; 2012,Jan,15-42; 2011,Mar,3-6; 2011,Jan,11

▲ **90649** **Human Papillomavirus vaccine, types 6, 11, 16, 18, quadrivalent (4vHPV), 3 dose schedule, for intramuscular use**

INCLUDES　 GARDASIL

💉 0.00　 ✂ 0.00　 **FUD** XXX　　　　 Ⓢ M

AMA: 2015,May,6; 2015,Jan,16; 2014,Jan,11; 2013,Aug,10; 2012,Jan,15-42; 2011,Mar,3-6; 2011,Jan,11

▲ **90650** **Human Papillomavirus vaccine, types 16, 18, bivalent (2vHPV), 3 dose schedule, for intramuscular use**

INCLUDES　 Cervarix

💉 0.00　 ✂ 0.00　 **FUD** XXX　　　　 Ⓢ M

AMA: 2015,May,6; 2015,Jan,16; 2014,Jan,11; 2013,Aug,10; 2012,Jan,15-42; 2011,Mar,3-6; 2011,Jan,11

▲ **90651** **Human Papillomavirus vaccine types 6, 11, 16, 18, 31, 33, 45, 52, 58, nonavalent (9vHPV), 3 dose schedule, for intramuscular use**
  INCLUDES GARDASIL 9
  🚑 0.00   👐 0.00   **FUD** XXX   ⑨ Ⓔ
  AMA: 2015,May,6; 2015,Jan,16

▲ **90653** **Influenza vaccine, inactivated (IIV), subunit, adjuvanted, for intramuscular use**
  🚑 0.00   👐 0.00   **FUD** XXX   ✗ ⑨ Ⓔ
  AMA: 2015,May,6; 2015,Jan,16; 2014,Jan,11; 2013,Aug,10

  90654 **Influenza virus vaccine, trivalent (IIV3), split virus, preservative-free, for intradermal use**
  INCLUDES Fluzone intradermal
  🚑 0.00   👐 0.00   **FUD** XXX   ⑨ Ⓛ Ⓛ⒤
  AMA: 2015,May,6; 2015,Apr,9; 2015,Jan,16; 2014,Jan,11; 2013,Aug,10; 2012,Jan,15-42; 2011,Mar,3-6; 2011,Jan,11

\# **90630** **Influenza virus vaccine, quadrivalent (IIV4), split virus, preservative free, for intradermal use**
  🚑 0.00   👐 0.00   **FUD** XXX   ⑨ Ⓔ
  AMA: 2015,May,6; 2015,Jan,16

▲ **90655** **Influenza virus vaccine, trivalent (IIV3), split virus, preservative free, when administered to children 6-35 months of age, for intramuscular use** Ⓐ
  INCLUDES Afluria
       Fluzone, no preservative, pediatric dose
  🚑 0.00   👐 0.00   **FUD** XXX   ⑨ Ⓛ Ⓛ⒤ ▱ Ⓟ⑨
  AMA: 2015,May,6; 2015,Jan,16; 2014,Jan,11; 2013,Aug,10; 2012,Jan,15-42; 2011,Mar,3-6; 2011,Jan,11

▲ **90656** **Influenza virus vaccine, trivalent (IIV3), split virus, preservative free, when administered to individuals 3 years and older, for intramuscular use** Ⓐ
  INCLUDES Afluria
       Fluvarix
       Fluvirin
       Fluzone, influenza virus vaccine, no preservative
  🚑 0.00   👐 0.00   **FUD** XXX   ⑨ Ⓛ Ⓛ⒤ ▱ Ⓟ⑨
  AMA: 2015,May,6; 2015,Jan,16; 2014,Jan,11; 2013,Aug,10; 2012,Jan,15-42; 2011,Mar,3-6; 2011,Jan,11

▲ **90657** **Influenza virus vaccine, trivalent (IIV3), split virus, when administered to children 6-35 months of age, for intramuscular use** Ⓐ
  INCLUDES Afluria
       Flulaval
       Fluvirin
       Fluzone (5 ml vial [0.25ml dose])
  🚑 0.00   👐 0.00   **FUD** XXX   ⑨ Ⓛ Ⓛ⒤ ▱ Ⓟ⑨
  AMA: 2015,May,6; 2015,Jan,16; 2014,Jan,11; 2013,Aug,10; 2012,Jan,15-42; 2011,Mar,3-6; 2011,Jan,11

▲ **90658** **Influenza virus vaccine, trivalent (IIV3), split virus, when administered to individuals 3 years of age and older, for intramuscular use** Ⓐ
  INCLUDES Afluria   Fluvirin
       Flulaval   Fluzone
  🚑 0.00   👐 0.00   **FUD** XXX   ⑨ Ⓔ ▱
  AMA: 2015,May,6; 2015,Jan,16; 2014,Jan,11; 2013,Aug,10; 2012,Jan,15-42; 2011,Mar,3-6; 2011,Jan,11

▲ **90660** **Influenza virus vaccine, trivalent, live (LAIV3), for intranasal use**
  INCLUDES FluMist
  🚑 0.00   👐 0.00   **FUD** XXX   ⑨ Ⓛ Ⓛ⒤ ▱ Ⓟ⑨
  AMA: 2015,May,6; 2015,Jan,16; 2014,Jan,11; 2013,Aug,10; 2012,Jan,15-42; 2011,Mar,3-6; 2011,Jan,11

▲ \# **90672** **Influenza virus vaccine, quadrivalent, live (LAIV4), for intranasal use**
  INCLUDES FluMist nasal spray
  🚑 0.00   👐 0.00   **FUD** XXX   ⑨ Ⓛ Ⓛ⒤
  AMA: 2015,May,6; 2015,Jan,16; 2014,Jan,11; 2013,Aug,10

▲ **90661** **Influenza virus vaccine (ccIIV3), derived from cell cultures, subunit, preservative and antibiotic free, for intramuscular use**
  INCLUDES Flucelvax
  🚑 0.00   👐 0.00   **FUD** XXX   ⑨ Ⓛ Ⓛ⒤ Ⓟ⑨
  AMA: 2015,May,6; 2015,Jan,16; 2014,Jan,11; 2013,Aug,10; 2012,Jan,15-42; 2011,Mar,3-6; 2011,Jan,11

▲ \# **90673** **Influenza virus vaccine, trivalent (RIV3), derived from recombinant DNA, hemagglutinin (HA) protein only, preservative and antibiotic free, for intramuscular use**
  INCLUDES Flublok (single dose vial)
  🚑 0.00   👐 0.00   **FUD** XXX   ⑨ Ⓛ Ⓛ⒤
  AMA: 2015,May,6; 2015,Jan,16; 2014,Mar,10; 2014,Jan,11

▲ **90662** **Influenza virus vaccine (IIV), split virus, preservative free, enhanced immunogenicity via increased antigen content, for intramuscular use**
  INCLUDES Fluzone high-dose
  🚑 0.00   👐 0.00   **FUD** XXX   ⑨ Ⓛ Ⓛ⒤ Ⓟ⑨
  AMA: 2015,May,6; 2015,Jan,16; 2014,Jan,11; 2013,Aug,10; 2012,Jan,15-42; 2011,Mar,3-6; 2011,Jan,11

▲ **90664** **Influenza virus vaccine, live (LAIV), pandemic formulation, for intranasal use**
  🚑 0.00   👐 0.00   **FUD** XXX   ⑨ Ⓔ Ⓟ⑨
  AMA: 2015,May,6; 2015,Jan,16; 2014,Jan,11; 2013,Aug,10; 2012,Jan,15-42; 2011,Mar,3-6; 2011,Jan,11

▲ **90666** **Influenza virus vaccine (IIV), pandemic formulation, split virus, preservative free, for intramuscular use**
  🚑 0.00   👐 0.00   **FUD** XXX   ✗ ⑨ Ⓔ Ⓟ⑨
  AMA: 2015,May,6; 2015,Jan,16; 2014,Jan,11; 2013,Aug,10; 2012,Jan,15-42; 2011,Mar,3-6; 2011,Jan,11

▲ **90667** **Influenza virus vaccine (IIV), pandemic formulation, split virus, adjuvanted, for intramuscular use**
  🚑 0.00   👐 0.00   **FUD** XXX   ✗ ⑨ Ⓔ Ⓟ⑨
  AMA: 2015,May,6; 2015,Jan,16; 2014,Jan,11; 2013,Aug,10; 2012,Jan,15-42; 2011,Mar,3-6; 2011,Jan,11

▲ **90668** **Influenza virus vaccine (IIV), pandemic formulation, split virus, for intramuscular use**
  🚑 0.00   👐 0.00   **FUD** XXX   ✗ ⑨ Ⓔ Ⓟ⑨
  AMA: 2015,May,6; 2015,Jan,16; 2014,Jan,11; 2013,Aug,10; 2012,Jan,15-42; 2011,Mar,3-6; 2011,Jan,11

  90669 ~~Pneumococcal conjugate vaccine, 7 valent (PCV7), for intramuscular use~~

▲ **90670** **Pneumococcal conjugate vaccine, 13 valent (PCV13), for intramuscular use**
  INCLUDES Prevnar 13
  🚑 0.00   👐 0.00   **FUD** XXX   ⑨ Ⓛ Ⓛ⒤
  AMA: 2015,May,6; 2015,Jan,16; 2014,Jan,11; 2013,Aug,10; 2012,Jan,15-42; 2011,Mar,8; 2011,Jan,11

  90672 **Resequenced code. See code following 90660.**

  90673 **Resequenced code. See code following 90661.**

  90675 **Rabies vaccine, for intramuscular use**
  INCLUDES Imovax
       RabAvert
  🚑 0.00   👐 0.00   **FUD** XXX   ⑨ Ⓚ Ⓚ② ▱
  AMA: 2015,May,6; 2015,Jan,16; 2014,Jan,11; 2013,Aug,10; 2012,Jan,15-42; 2011,Mar,3-6; 2011,Jan,11

  90676 **Rabies vaccine, for intradermal use**
  🚑 0.00   👐 0.00   **FUD** XXX   ⑨ Ⓚ Ⓚ② ▱
  AMA: 2015,May,6; 2015,Jan,16; 2014,Jan,11; 2013,Aug,10; 2012,Jul,7; 2012,Jan,15-42; 2011,Mar,3-6; 2011,Jan,11

▲ **90680** **Rotavirus vaccine, pentavalent (RV5), 3 dose schedule, live, for oral use**
  INCLUDES RotaTeq
  🚑 0.00   👐 0.00   **FUD** XXX   ⑨ Ⓝ Ⓝ①
  AMA: 2015,May,6; 2015,Jan,16; 2014,Jan,11; 2013,Aug,10; 2012,Jan,15-42; 2011,Mar,3-6; 2011,Jan,11

▲ 90681 Rotavirus vaccine, human, attenuated (RV1), 2 dose schedule, live, for oral use
INCLUDES Rotarix
📷 0.00   ⚬ 0.00   **FUD** XXX   Ⓢ Ⓔ
AMA: 2015,May,6; 2015,Jan,16; 2014,Jan,11; 2013,Aug,10; 2012,Jul,7; 2012,Jan,15-42; 2011,Mar,3-6; 2011,Mar,8; 2011,Jan,11

▲ 90685 Influenza virus vaccine, quadrivalent (IIV4), split virus, preservative free, when administered to children 6-35 months of age, for intramuscular use   Ⓐ
INCLUDES Fluzone Quadrivalent
📷 0.00   ⚬ 0.00   **FUD** XXX   Ⓢ Ⓛ
AMA: 2015,May,6; 2015,Jan,16; 2014,Mar,10; 2014,Jan,11; 2013,Aug,10

▲ 90686 Influenza virus vaccine, quadrivalent (IIV4), split virus, preservative free, when administered to individuals 3 years of age and older, for intramuscular use   Ⓐ
INCLUDES Fluarix Quadrivalent
         Fluzone Quadrivalent
📷 0.00   ⚬ 0.00   **FUD** XXX   Ⓢ Ⓛ Ⓛ¹
AMA: 2015,May,6; 2015,Jan,16; 2014,Mar,10; 2014,Jan,11; 2013,Aug,10

▲ 90687 Influenza virus vaccine, quadrivalent (IIV4), split virus, when administered to children 6-35 months of age, for intramuscular use   Ⓐ
📷 0.00   ⚬ 0.00   **FUD** XXX   Ⓢ Ⓛ Ⓛ¹
AMA: 2015,May,6; 2015,Jan,16; 2014,Mar,10; 2014,Jan,11; 2013,Aug,10

▲ 90688 Influenza virus vaccine, quadrivalent (IIV4), split virus, when administered to individuals 3 years of age and older, for intramuscular use   Ⓐ
INCLUDES FluLaval (multidose vial)
📷 0.00   ⚬ 0.00   **FUD** XXX   Ⓢ Ⓛ Ⓛ¹
AMA: 2015,May,6; 2015,Jan,16; 2014,Mar,10; 2014,Jan,11; 2013,Aug,10

90690 Typhoid vaccine, live, oral
INCLUDES Vivotif
📷 0.00   ⚬ 0.00   **FUD** XXX   Ⓢ Ⓝ Ⓝ¹
AMA: 2015,May,6; 2015,Jan,16; 2014,Jan,11; 2013,Aug,10; 2012,Jan,15-42; 2011,Mar,3-6; 2011,Jan,11

90691 Typhoid vaccine, Vi capsular polysaccharide (ViCPs), for intramuscular use
INCLUDES Typhim Vi
📷 0.00   ⚬ 0.00   **FUD** XXX   Ⓢ Ⓝ Ⓝ¹ 🖵
AMA: 2015,May,6; 2015,Jan,16; 2014,Jan,11; 2013,Aug,10; 2012,Jan,15-42; 2011,Mar,3-6; 2011,Jan,11

90692 Typhoid vaccine, heat- and phenol-inactivated (H-P), for subcutaneous or intradermal use

90693 Typhoid vaccine, acetone-killed, dried (AKD), for subcutaneous use (U.S. military)

▲ 90696 Diphtheria, tetanus toxoids, acellular pertussis vaccine and inactivated poliovirus vaccine (DTaP-IPV), when administered to children 4 through 6 years of age, for intramuscular use   Ⓐ
INCLUDES KINRIX
📷 0.00   ⚬ 0.00   **FUD** XXX   Ⓢ Ⓝ Ⓝ¹
AMA: 2015,May,6; 2015,Jan,16; 2014,Jan,11; 2013,Aug,10; 2012,Jan,15-42; 2011,Mar,3-6; 2011,Jan,11

▲ 90697 Diphtheria, tetanus toxoids, acellular pertussis vaccine, inactivated poliovirus vaccine, Haemophilus influenzae type b PRP-OMP conjugate vaccine, and hepatitis B vaccine (DTaP-IPV-Hib-HepB), for intramuscular use
📷 0.00   ⚬ 0.00   **FUD** XXX   ✎ Ⓢ Ⓔ
AMA: 2015,May,6; 2015,Jan,16

▲ 90698 Diphtheria, tetanus toxoids, acellular pertussis vaccine, Haemophilus influenzae type b, and inactivated poliovirus vaccine (DTaP-IPV/Hib), for intramuscular use
INCLUDES Pentacel
📷 0.00   ⚬ 0.00   **FUD** XXX   Ⓢ Ⓝ Ⓝ¹
AMA: 2015,May,6; 2015,Jan,16; 2014,Jan,11; 2013,Aug,10; 2012,Jan,15-42; 2011,Mar,3-6; 2011,Jan,11

90700 Diphtheria, tetanus toxoids, and acellular pertussis vaccine (DTaP), when administered to individuals younger than 7 years, for intramuscular use   Ⓐ
INCLUDES Daptacel
         Infanrix
📷 0.00   ⚬ 0.00   **FUD** XXX   Ⓢ Ⓝ Ⓝ¹ 🖵
AMA: 2015,May,6; 2015,Jan,16; 2014,Jan,11; 2013,Aug,10; 2012,Jul,7; 2012,Jan,15-42; 2011,Mar,8; 2011,Mar,3-6; 2011,Jan,11

▲ 90702 Diphtheria and tetanus toxoids adsorbed (DT) when administered to individuals younger than 7 years, for intramuscular use   Ⓐ
INCLUDES Diphtheria and Tetanus Toxoids Adsorbed USP (For Pediatric Use)
📷 0.00   ⚬ 0.00   **FUD** XXX   Ⓢ Ⓝ Ⓝ¹
AMA: 2015,May,6; 2015,Jan,16; 2014,Jan,11; 2013,Aug,10; 2012,Jan,15-42; 2011,Mar,3-6; 2011,Jan,11

90703 Tetanus toxoid adsorbed, for intramuscular use

90704 Mumps virus vaccine, live, for subcutaneous use

90705 Measles virus vaccine, live, for subcutaneous use

90706 Rubella virus vaccine, live, for subcutaneous use

90707 Measles, mumps and rubella virus vaccine (MMR), live, for subcutaneous use
INCLUDES M-M-R II
📷 0.00   ⚬ 0.00   **FUD** XXX   Ⓢ Ⓝ Ⓝ¹ 🖵
AMA: 2015,May,6; 2015,Jan,16; 2014,Jan,11; 2013,Aug,10; 2012,Jul,7; 2012,Jan,15-42; 2011,Mar,3-6; 2011,Jan,11

90708 Measles and rubella virus vaccine, live, for subcutaneous use

90710 Measles, mumps, rubella, and varicella vaccine (MMRV), live, for subcutaneous use
INCLUDES ProQuad
📷 0.00   ⚬ 0.00   **FUD** XXX   Ⓢ Ⓝ Ⓝ¹ 🖵
AMA: 2015,May,6; 2015,Jan,16; 2014,Jan,11; 2013,Aug,10; 2012,Jan,15-42; 2011,Mar,3-6; 2011,Jan,11

90712 Poliovirus vaccine, (any type[s]) (OPV), live, for oral use

90713 Poliovirus vaccine, inactivated (IPV), for subcutaneous or intramuscular use
INCLUDES IPOL
📷 0.00   ⚬ 0.00   **FUD** XXX   Ⓢ Ⓝ Ⓝ¹
AMA: 2015,May,6; 2015,Jan,16; 2014,Jan,11; 2013,Aug,10; 2012,Jan,15-42; 2011,Mar,8; 2011,Mar,3-6; 2011,Jan,11

▲ 90714 Tetanus and diphtheria toxoids adsorbed (Td), preservative free, when administered to individuals 7 years or older, for intramuscular use   Ⓐ
INCLUDES DECAVAC/TENIVAC
         Tetanus-diphtheria adult
📷 0.00   ⚬ 0.00   **FUD** XXX   Ⓢ Ⓝ Ⓝ¹
AMA: 2015,May,6; 2015,Jan,16; 2014,Jan,11; 2013,Aug,10; 2012,Jan,15-42; 2011,Mar,3-6; 2011,Jan,11

90715 Tetanus, diphtheria toxoids and acellular pertussis vaccine (Tdap), when administered to individuals 7 years or older, for intramuscular use   Ⓐ
INCLUDES Adacel
         Boostrix
📷 0.00   ⚬ 0.00   **FUD** XXX   Ⓢ Ⓝ Ⓝ¹
AMA: 2015,May,6; 2015,Jan,16; 2014,Jan,11; 2013,Aug,10; 2012,Jan,15-42; 2011,Mar,3-6; 2011,Jan,11

▲ **90716** Varicella virus vaccine (VAR), live, for subcutaneous use

INCLUDES Varivax

🔋 0.00 ⚗ 0.00 **FUD** XXX Ⓢ Ⓜ ▢

AMA: 2015,May,6; 2015,Mar,3; 2015,Jan,16; 2014,Jan,11; 2013,Aug,10; 2012,Jan,15-42; 2011,Mar,3-6; 2011,Jan,11

▲ **90717** Yellow fever vaccine, live, for subcutaneous use

INCLUDES YF-VAX

🔋 0.00 ⚗ 0.00 **FUD** XXX Ⓢ Ⓝ N1 ▢

AMA: 2015,May,6; 2015,Jan,16; 2014,Jan,11; 2013,Aug,10; 2012,Jan,15-42; 2011,Mar,3-6; 2011,Jan,11

~~90719~~ ~~Diphtheria toxoid, for intramuscular use~~

~~90720~~ ~~Diphtheria, tetanus toxoids, and whole cell pertussis vaccine and Haemophilus influenzae b vaccine (DTwP-Hib), for intramuscular use~~

~~90721~~ ~~Diphtheria, tetanus toxoids, and acellular pertussis vaccine and Haemophilus influenzae b vaccine (DTaP/Hib), for intramuscular use~~

▲ **90723** Diphtheria, tetanus toxoids, acellular pertussis vaccine, hepatitis B, and inactivated poliovirus vaccine (DTaP-HepB-IPV), for intramuscular use

INCLUDES PEDIARIX

🔋 0.00 ⚗ 0.00 **FUD** XXX Ⓢ Ⓔ

AMA: 2015,May,6; 2015,Jan,16; 2014,Jan,11; 2013,Aug,10; 2012,Jan,15-42; 2011,Mar,3-6; 2011,Jan,11

● # **90625** Cholera vaccine, live, adult dosage, 1 dose schedule, for oral use

🔋 0.00 ⚗ 0.00 **FUD** 000 ✗ Ⓢ

~~90725~~ ~~Cholera vaccine for injectable use~~

~~90727~~ ~~Plague vaccine, for intramuscular use~~

▲ **90732** Pneumococcal polysaccharide vaccine, 23-valent (PPSV23), adult or immunosuppressed patient dosage, when administered to individuals 2 years or older, for subcutaneous or intramuscular use Ⓐ

INCLUDES Pneumovax 23

🔋 0.00 ⚗ 0.00 **FUD** XXX Ⓢ Ⓛ L1 ▢

AMA: 2015,May,6; 2015,Jan,16; 2014,Jan,11; 2013,Aug,10; 2012,Jan,15-42; 2011,Mar,3-6; 2011,Jan,11

▲ # **90644** Meningococcal conjugate vaccine, serogroups C & Y and Haemophilus influenzae type b vaccine (Hib-MenCY), 4 dose schedule, when administered to children 2-18 months of age, for intramuscular use Ⓐ

INCLUDES 🔋 0.00 ⚗ 0.00 **FUD** XXX Ⓢ Ⓔ

AMA: 2015,May,6; 2015,Jan,16; 2014,Jan,11; 2013,Aug,10; 2012,Jan,15-42; 2011,Mar,3-6; 2011,Jan,11

▲ **90733** Meningococcal polysaccharide vaccine, serogroups A, C, Y, W-135, quadrivalent (MPSV4), for subcutaneous use

INCLUDES Menomune-A/C/Y/W-135

🔋 0.00 ⚗ 0.00 **FUD** XXX Ⓢ Ⓚ K2 ▢

AMA: 2015,May,6; 2015,Jan,16; 2014,Jan,11; 2013,Aug,10; 2012,Jan,15-42; 2011,Mar,3-6; 2011,Jan,11

▲ **90734** Meningococcal conjugate vaccine, serogroups A, C, Y and W-135, quadrivalent (MenACWY), for intramuscular use

INCLUDES Menactra
Menveo

🔋 0.00 ⚗ 0.00 **FUD** XXX Ⓢ Ⓝ N1 ▢

AMA: 2015,May,6; 2015,Jan,16; 2014,Jan,11; 2013,Aug,10; 2012,Jan,15-42; 2011,Mar,3-6; 2011,Jan,11

▲ # **90620** Meningococcal recombinant protein and outer membrane vesicle vaccine, serogroup B (MenB), 2 dose schedule, for intramuscular use

🔋 0.00 ⚗ 0.00 **FUD** XXX Ⓢ Ⓚ K2 ▢

AMA: 2015,May,6; 2015,Jan,16

▲ # **90621** Meningococcal recombinant lipoprotein vaccine, serogroup B (MenB), 3 dose schedule, for intramuscular use

🔋 0.00 ⚗ 0.00 **FUD** XXX Ⓢ Ⓚ K2

AMA: 2015,May,6; 2015,Jan,16

~~90735~~ ~~Japanese encephalitis virus vaccine, for subcutaneous use~~

▲ **90736** Zoster (shingles) vaccine (HZV), live, for subcutaneous injection

INCLUDES Zostavax

🔋 0.00 ⚗ 0.00 **FUD** XXX Ⓢ Ⓜ

AMA: 2015,May,6; 2015,Jan,16; 2014,Jan,11; 2013,Aug,10; 2012,Jan,15-42; 2011,Mar,3-6; 2011,Jan,11

▲ **90738** Japanese encephalitis virus vaccine, inactivated, for intramuscular use

INCLUDES Ixiaro

🔋 0.00 ⚗ 0.00 **FUD** XXX Ⓢ Ⓜ

AMA: 2015,May,6; 2015,Jan,16; 2014,Jan,11; 2013,Aug,10; 2012,Jan,15-42; 2011,Mar,3-6; 2011,Jan,11

▲ **90739** Hepatitis B vaccine (HepB), adult dosage, 2 dose schedule, for intramuscular use ✗ Ⓢ Ⓔ

🔋 0.00 ⚗ 0.00 **FUD** XXX

AMA: 2015,May,6; 2015,Jan,16; 2014,Jan,11; 2013,Aug,10

▲ **90740** Hepatitis B vaccine (HepB), dialysis or immunosuppressed patient dosage, 3 dose schedule, for intramuscular use

INCLUDES Recombivax dialysis

🔋 0.00 ⚗ 0.00 **FUD** XXX Ⓢ Ⓕ F4

AMA: 2015,May,6; 2015,Jan,16; 2014,Jan,11; 2013,Aug,10; 2012,Jan,15-42; 2011,Mar,3-6; 2011,Jan,11

▲ **90743** Hepatitis B vaccine (HepB), adolescent, 2 dose schedule, for intramuscular use Ⓐ

INCLUDES Energix-B
Recombivax HB

🔋 0.00 ⚗ 0.00 **FUD** XXX Ⓢ Ⓕ F4

AMA: 2015,May,6; 2015,Jan,16; 2014,Jan,11; 2013,Aug,10; 2012,Jan,15-42; 2011,Mar,3-6; 2011,Jan,11

▲ **90744** Hepatitis B vaccine (HepB), pediatric/adolescent dosage, 3 dose schedule, for intramuscular use Ⓐ

INCLUDES Energix-B
Recombivax HB

🔋 0.00 ⚗ 0.00 **FUD** XXX Ⓢ Ⓕ F4

AMA: 2015,May,6; 2015,Jan,16; 2014,Jan,11; 2013,Aug,10; 2012,Jan,15-42; 2011,Mar,3-6; 2011,Jan,11

▲ **90746** Hepatitis B vaccine (HepB), adult dosage, 3 dose schedule, for intramuscular use

INCLUDES Energix-B
Recombivax HB

🔋 0.00 ⚗ 0.00 **FUD** XXX Ⓢ Ⓕ F4

AMA: 2015,May,6; 2015,Jan,16; 2014,Jan,11; 2013,Aug,10; 2012,Jan,15-42; 2011,Mar,3-6; 2011,Jan,11

▲ **90747** Hepatitis B vaccine (HepB), dialysis or immunosuppressed patient dosage, 4 dose schedule, for intramuscular use

INCLUDES Energix-B
RECOMBIVAX dialysis

🔋 0.00 ⚗ 0.00 **FUD** XXX Ⓢ Ⓕ F4

AMA: 2015,May,6; 2015,Jan,16; 2014,Jan,11; 2013,Aug,10; 2012,Jan,15-42; 2011,Mar,3-6; 2011,Jan,11

▲ **90748** Hepatitis B and Haemophilus influenzae type b vaccine (Hib-HepB), for intramuscular use

INCLUDES COMVAX

🔋 0.00 ⚗ 0.00 **FUD** XXX Ⓢ Ⓔ

AMA: 2015,May,6; 2015,Jan,16; 2014,Jan,11; 2013,Aug,10; 2012,Jul,7; 2012,Jan,15-42; 2011,Mar,3-6; 2011,Mar,8; 2011,Jan,11

90749 Unlisted vaccine/toxoid

🔋 0.00 ⚗ 0.00 **FUD** XXX Ⓢ Ⓝ N1

AMA: 2015,May,6; 2015,Jan,16; 2014,Jan,11; 2012,Jan,15-42; 2011,Mar,3-6; 2011,Jan,11

90785 Complex Interactive Encounter

CMS: 100-2,15,160 Clinical Psychologist Services; 100-2,15,170 Clinical Social Worker (CSW) Services; 100-3,10.3 Inpatient Pain Rehabilitation Programs; 100-3,10.4 Outpatient Hospital Pain Rehabilitation Programs; 100-3,130.1 Inpatient Stays for Alcoholism Treatment; 100-4,12,100 Teaching Physician Services

[INCLUDES] At least one of the following activities:
Discussion of a sentinel event demanding third-party involvement (eg, abuse or neglect reported to a state agency)
Interference by the behavior or emotional state of caregiver to understand and assist in the plan of treatment
Managing discordant communication complicating care among participating members (eg, arguing, reactivity)
Use of nonverbal communication methods (eg, toys, other devices, or translator) to eliminate communication barriers
Complicated issues of communication affecting provision of the psychiatric service
Involved communication with:
Emotionally charged or dissonant family members
Patients wanting others present during the visit (e.g., family member, translator)
Patients with impaired or undeveloped verbal skills
Patients with third parties responsible for their care (eg, parents, guardians)
Third-party involvement (eg, schools, probation and parole officers, child protective agencies)
Do not report with E&M services codes when psychotherapy services are not also provided
Do not report with (90839-90840, 0364T-0367T, 0373T-0374T)

+ 90785 Interactive complexity (List separately in addition to the code for primary procedure)
Code first (99201-99255 [99224, 99225, 99226], 99304-99337, 99341-99350, 90791-90792, 90832-90834, 90836-90838, 90853)
🔧 0.40   ⚖ 0.40   **FUD** ZZZ   [N]
AMA: 2015,Jan,16; 2013,Jun,3-5; 2013,May,12

90791-90792 Psychiatric Evaluations

CMS: 100-2,15,170 Clinical Social Worker (CSW) Services; 100-2,15,270 Telehealth Services; 100-2,15,270.2 Medicare Telehealth Services; 100-2,15,270.4 Payment - Physician/Practitioner at a Distant Site; 100-3,10.3 Inpatient Pain Rehabilitation Programs; 100-3,130.1 Inpatient Stays for Alcoholism Treatment; 100-3,130.2 Outpatient Hospital Services for Alcoholism; 100-4,12,100 Teaching Physician Services; 100-4,12,190.3 Medicare Telehealth Services; 100-4,12,190.7 Contractor Editing of Telehealth Claims

[INCLUDES] Diagnostic assessment or reassessment without psychotherapy services
Code also interactive complexity services when applicable (90785)
Do not report with (99201-99337 [99224, 99225, 99226], 99341-99350, 99366-99368, 99401-99444, 90839-90840, 0364T-0367T, 0373T-0374T)

90791 Psychiatric diagnostic evaluation
🔧 3.56   ⚖ 3.67   **FUD** XXX   [Q3]
AMA: 2015,Jan,16; 2014,Jun,3; 2014,Jan,11; 2013,Dec,16; 2013,Jun,3-5; 2013,May,12

90792 Psychiatric diagnostic evaluation with medical services
🔧 4.00   ⚖ 4.12   **FUD** XXX   [Q3]
AMA: 2015,Jan,16; 2014,Jun,3; 2014,Jan,11; 2013,Dec,16; 2013,Jun,3-5

90832-90838 Psychotherapy Services

CMS: 100-2,15,160 Clinical Psychologist Services; 100-2,15,170 Clinical Social Worker (CSW) Services; 100-3,130.1 Inpatient Stays for Alcoholism Treatment; 100-3,130.2 Outpatient Hospital Services for Alcoholism; 100-3,130.3 Chemical Aversion Therapy for Treatment of Alcoholism; 100-4,12,100 Teaching Physician Services; 100-4,12,160 Independent Psychologist Services; 100-4,12,170 Clinical Psychologist Services; 100-4,12,190.3 Medicare Telehealth Services; 100-4,12,190.7 Contractor Editing of Telehealth Claims

[INCLUDES] Face-to-face time with patient (for part or all of the service) and/or family
Psychotherapy only (90832, 90834, 90837)
Psychotherapy with separately identifiable medical evaluation and management services includes add-on codes (90833, 90836, 90838)
Services provided in all settings
Therapeutic communication to:
Ameliorate the patient's mental and behavioral symptoms
Modify behavior
Support and encourage personality growth and development
Treatment for:
Behavior disturbances
Mental illness
[EXCLUDES] *Family psychotherapy without the patient (90846)*
Code also interactive complexity services with the time the provider spends performing the service reflected in the time for the appropriate psychotherapy code (90785)
Do not report time providing pharmacologic management with time allocated to psychotherapy service codes
Do not report with (90839-90840, 0364T-0367T, 0373T-0374T)

90832 Psychotherapy, 30 minutes with patient and/or family member
🔧 1.77   ⚖ 1.79   **FUD** XXX   [Q3]
AMA: 2015,Jan,16; 2014,Aug,5; 2014,Feb,3; 2013,Aug,13; 2013,Jun,3-5; 2013,May,12; 2013,Jan,3-5

+ 90833 Psychotherapy, 30 minutes with patient and/or family member when performed with an evaluation and management service (List separately in addition to the code for primary procedure)
Code first (99201-99255 [99224, 99225, 99226], 99304-99337, 99341-99350)
🔧 1.82   ⚖ 1.84   **FUD** ZZZ   [N]
AMA: 2015,Jan,16; 2014,Aug,5; 2014,Feb,3; 2013,Aug,13; 2013,Jun,3-5; 2013,May,12; 2013,Jan,3-5

90834 Psychotherapy, 45 minutes with patient and/or family member
🔧 2.35   ⚖ 2.37   **FUD** XXX   [Q3]
AMA: 2015,Jan,16; 2014,Jun,3; 2014,Feb,3; 2013,Aug,13; 2013,Jun,3-5; 2013,May,12; 2013,Jan,3-5

+ 90836 Psychotherapy, 45 minutes with patient and/or family member when performed with an evaluation and management service (List separately in addition to the code for primary procedure)
Code first (99201-99255 [99224, 99225, 99226], 99304-99337, 99341-99350)
🔧 2.32   ⚖ 2.33   **FUD** ZZZ   [N]
AMA: 2015,Jan,16; 2014,Feb,3; 2013,Aug,13; 2013,Jun,3-5; 2013,May,12; 2013,Jan,3-5

90837 Psychotherapy, 60 minutes with patient and/or family member
Code also prolonged service for psychotherapy performed without evaluation and management service face-to-face with the patient lasting 90 minutes or longer (99354-99357)
🔧 3.54   ⚖ 3.56   **FUD** XXX   [Q3]
AMA: 2015,Jan,16; 2014,Apr,6; 2014,Feb,3; 2013,Aug,13; 2013,Jun,3-5; 2013,May,12; 2013,Jan,3-5

+ 90838 Psychotherapy, 60 minutes with patient and/or family member when performed with an evaluation and management service (List separately in addition to the code for primary procedure)
Code first (99201-99255 [99224, 99225, 99226], 99304-99337, 99341-99350)
🔧 3.06   ⚖ 3.08   **FUD** ZZZ   [N]
AMA: 2015,Jan,16; 2014,Apr,6; 2014,Feb,3; 2013,Aug,13; 2013,Jun,3-5; 2013,May,12; 2013,Jan,3-5

Medicine

90839 — 90870

90839-90840 Services for Patients in Crisis

CMS: 100-2,15,170 Clinical Social Worker (CSW) Services; 100-3,130.1 Inpatient Stays for Alcoholism Treatment; 100-3,130.3 Chemical Aversion Therapy for Treatment of Alcoholism; 100-4,12,100 Teaching Physician Services; 100-4,12,160 Independent Psychologist Services; 100-4,12,160.1 Payment for Independent Psychologists' Services; 100-4,12,170 Clinical Psychologist Services

INCLUDES
- 30 minutes or more of face-to-face time with the patient (for all or part of the service) and/or family providing crisis psychotherapy
- All time spent exclusively with patient (for all or part of the service) and/or family, even if time is not continuous
- Emergent care to a patient in severe distress (eg, life threatening or complex)
- Institute interventions to minimize psychological trauma
- Measures to ease the crisis and reestablish safety
- Psychotherapy

EXCLUDES *Psychotherapy for crisis of less than 30 minutes (90832-90833)*

Do not report with (90785-90899, 0364T-0367T, 0373T-0374T)

90839   Psychotherapy for crisis; first 60 minutes

    INCLUDES   First 30-74 minutes of crisis psychotherapy per day

    Do not report more than one time per day, even when the service is not continuous on that date

    🖩 3.69   ⚕ 3.72   **FUD** XXX   03 80

    AMA: 2015,Jan,16; 2014,Aug,5; 2013,Jun,3-5

+ 90840   each additional 30 minutes (List separately in addition to code for primary service)

    INCLUDES   Up to 30 minutes of time beyond the initial 74 minutes

    Code first (90839)

    🖩 1.77   ⚕ 1.78   **FUD** ZZZ   N 80

    AMA: 2015,Jan,16; 2014,Aug,5; 2013,Jun,3-5

90845-90863 Additional Psychotherapy Services

CMS: 100-2,15,170 Clinical Social Worker (CSW) Services; 100-3,10.3 Inpatient Pain Rehabilitation Programs; 100-3,10.4 Outpatient Hospital Pain Rehabilitation Programs

EXCLUDES *Analysis/programming of neurostimulators for vagus nerve stimulation therapy (95970, 95974-95975)*

Do not report with (90839-90840, 0364T-0367T, 0373T-0374T)

90845   Psychoanalysis

    🖩 2.54   ⚕ 2.55   **FUD** XXX   03 80 PQ

    AMA: 2015,Jan,16; 2014,Jan,11; 2012,Jan,15-42; 2011,Jan,11; 2010,Mar,6-8

90846   Family psychotherapy (without the patient present)

    Do not report with (0368T-0371T)

    🖩 2.85   ⚕ 2.87   **FUD** XXX   03 80

    AMA: 2015,Jan,16; 2014,Jan,11; 2013,Dec,16; 2013,Jun,3-5; 2010,Mar,6-8

90847   Family psychotherapy (conjoint psychotherapy) (with patient present)

    Do not report with (0368T-0371T)

    🖩 2.97   ⚕ 2.99   **FUD** XXX   03 80

    AMA: 2015,Jan,16; 2014,Jan,11; 2013,Dec,16; 2013,Jun,3-5; 2010,Mar,6-8

90849   Multiple-family group psychotherapy

    🖩 0.89   ⚕ 0.99   **FUD** XXX   03 80 PQ

    AMA: 2015,Jan,16; 2014,Aug,14; 2014,Jan,11; 2010,Mar,6-8

90853   Group psychotherapy (other than of a multiple-family group)

    Code also group psychotherapy with interactive complexity (90785)

    Do not report with (0372T)

    🖩 0.71   ⚕ 0.72   **FUD** XXX   03 80 PQ

    AMA: 2015,Jan,16; 2014,Aug,14; 2014,Jun,3; 2014,Jan,11; 2013,Jun,3-5; 2010,Mar,6-8

+ 90863   Pharmacologic management, including prescription and review of medication, when performed with psychotherapy services (List separately in addition to the code for primary procedure)

    Code first (90832, 90834, 90837)

    Do not report time providing pharmacologic management with time allocated to psychotherapy service codes

    🖩 0.00   ⚕ 0.00   **FUD** XXX   E

    AMA: 2015,Jan,16; 2013,Jun,3-5

90865-90870 Other Psychiatric Treatment

EXCLUDES *Analysis/programming of neurostimulators for vagus nerve stimulation therapy (95970, 95974, 95975)*

Do not report with (90839-90840, 0364T-0367T, 0373T-0374T)

90865   Narcosynthesis for psychiatric diagnostic and therapeutic purposes (eg, sodium amobarbital (Amytal) interview)

    🖩 3.59   ⚕ 4.73   **FUD** XXX   03 80

    AMA: 2015,Jan,16; 2014,Jan,11

90867   Therapeutic repetitive transcranial magnetic stimulation (TMS) treatment; initial, including cortical mapping, motor threshold determination, delivery and management

    🖩 0.00   ⚕ 0.00   **FUD** 000   S

    INCLUDES   Evaluation and management services related directly to:
- Cortical mapping
- Delivery and management of TMS services
- Motor threshold determination

    EXCLUDES   *Medication management*

    Significant, separately identifiable evaluation and management service

    Significant, separately identifiable psychotherapy service

    Transcranial magnetic stimulation (TMS) motor function mapping for treatment planning, upper and lower extremity (0310T)

    Do not report more than one time for each course of treatment

    Do not report with (90868-90869, 95860, 95870, 95928-95929, [95939])

90868   subsequent delivery and management, per session

    🖩 0.00   ⚕ 0.00   **FUD** 000   S

    INCLUDES   Evaluation and management services related directly to:
- Cortical mapping
- Delivery and management of TMS services
- Motor threshold determination

    EXCLUDES   *Medication management*

    Significant, separately identifiable evaluation and management service

    Significant, separately identifiable psychotherapy service

    Transcranial magnetic stimulation (TMS) motor function mapping for treatment planning, upper and lower extremity (0310T)

90869   subsequent motor threshold re-determination with delivery and management

    🖩 0.00   ⚕ 0.00   **FUD** 000   S

    INCLUDES   Evaluation and management services related directly to:
- Cortical mapping
- Delivery and management of TMS services
- Motor threshold determination

    EXCLUDES   *Medication management*

    Significant, separately identifiable evaluation and management service

    Significant, separately identifiable psychotherapy service

    Transcranial magnetic stimulation (TMS) motor function mapping for treatment planning, upper and lower extremity (0310T)

    Do not report with (90867-90868, 95860-95870, 95928-95929, [95939])

90870   Electroconvulsive therapy (includes necessary monitoring)

    🖩 3.11   ⚕ 4.99   **FUD** 000   S 80

    AMA: 2015,Jan,16; 2014,Jan,11; 2010,Mar,6-8

| 26/TC PC/TC Comp Only | A2-Z3 ASC Pmt | 50 Bilateral | ♂ Male Only | ♀ Female Only | 🖩 Facility RVU | ⚕ Non-Facility RVU |
| **AMA:** CPT Asst | CMS: Pub 100 | A-Y OPPSI | ✎ Non-FDA Drug | | 🖵 Lab Crosswalk | 🖵 Radiology Crosswalk |

390   Medicare (Red Text)   CPT © 2015 American Medical Association. All Rights Reserved. (Black Text)   © 2015 Optum360, LLC (Blue Text)

90875-90880 Psychiatric Therapy with Biofeedback or Hypnosis

CMS: 100-2,15,170 Clinical Social Worker (CSW) Services; 100-4,12,160 Independent Psychologist Services; 100-4,12,160.1 Payment for Independent Psychologists' Services; 100-4,12,170 Clinical Psychologist Services

> *EXCLUDES* *Analysis/programming of neurostimulators for vagus nerve stimulation therapy (95970, 95974, 95975)*
> Do not report with (90839-90840, 0364T-0367T, 0373T-0374T)

90875 Individual psychophysiological therapy incorporating biofeedback training by any modality (face-to-face with the patient), with psychotherapy (eg, insight oriented, behavior modifying or supportive psychotherapy); 30 minutes

   1.73   1.73   **FUD** XXX   E

AMA: 2015,Jan,16; 2014,Jan,11; 2012,Jan,15-42; 2011,Jan,11

90876 45 minutes

   2.77   3.07   **FUD** XXX   E

AMA: 2015,Jan,16; 2014,Jan,11

90880 Hypnotherapy

   2.64   2.84   **FUD** XXX   03 80

AMA: 2015,Jan,16; 2014,Jan,11

90882-90899 Psychiatric Services without Patient Face-to-Face Contact

CMS: 100-4,12,160 Independent Psychologist Services; 100-4,12,160.1 Payment for Independent Psychologists' Services

> *EXCLUDES* *Analysis/programming of neurostimulators for vagus nerve stimulation therapy (95970, 95974, 95975)*
> Do not report with (90839-90840, 0364T-0367T, 0373T-0374T)

90882 Environmental intervention for medical management purposes on a psychiatric patient's behalf with agencies, employers, or institutions

   0.00   0.00   **FUD** XXX   E

AMA: 2015,Jan,16; 2014,Jan,11

90885 Psychiatric evaluation of hospital records, other psychiatric reports, psychometric and/or projective tests, and other accumulated data for medical diagnostic purposes

   1.40   1.40   **FUD** XXX   N

AMA: 2015,Jan,16; 2014,Jan,11; 2012,Jan,15-42; 2011,Jan,11

90887 Interpretation or explanation of results of psychiatric, other medical examinations and procedures, or other accumulated data to family or other responsible persons, or advising them how to assist patient

Do not report with (0368T-0371T)

   2.15   2.50   **FUD** XXX   N

AMA: 2015,Jan,16; 2014,Jan,11; 2012,Jan,15-42; 2011,Jan,11

90889 Preparation of report of patient's psychiatric status, history, treatment, or progress (other than for legal or consultative purposes) for other individuals, agencies, or insurance carriers

   0.00   0.00   **FUD** XXX   N

AMA: 2015,Jan,16; 2014,Jan,11

90899 Unlisted psychiatric service or procedure

   0.00   0.00   **FUD** XXX   03 80

AMA: 2015,Jan,16; 2014,Jan,11; 2012,Jan,15-42; 2011,Jan,11; 2010,Jan,11-12

90901-90911 Biofeedback Therapy

CMS: 100-5,5,40.7 Biofeedback Training for Urinary Incontinence

> *EXCLUDES* *Psychophysiological therapy utilizing biofeedback training (90875-90876)*

90901 Biofeedback training by any modality

   0.57   1.07   **FUD** 000   A 80

AMA: 2015,Jan,16; 2014,Jan,11; 2012,Jan,15-42; 2011,Jan,11

90911 Biofeedback training, perineal muscles, anorectal or urethral sphincter, including EMG and/or manometry

> *EXCLUDES* *Rectal sensation/tone/compliance testing (91120)*
> *Treatment for incontinence, pulsed magnetic neuromodulation (53899)*

   1.26   2.38   **FUD** 000   T 80

AMA: 2015,Jan,16; 2014,Sep,13; 2014,Jan,11; 2012,Jan,15-42; 2011,Jan,11

90935-90940 Hemodialysis Services: Inpatient ESRD and Outpatient Non-ESRD

CMS: 100-2,11,20 Renal Dialysis Items and Services ; 100-4,3,100.6 Inpatient Renal Services

> *EXCLUDES* *Attendance by physician or other qualified health care provider for a prolonged period of time (99354-99360 [99415, 99416])*
> *Blood specimen collection from partial/complete implantable venous access device (36591)*
> *Declotting of cannula (36831, 36833, 36860-36861)*
> *Hemodialysis home visit by non-physician health care professional (99512)*
> *Thrombolytic agent declotting of implanted vascular access device/catheter (36593)*
> Code also significant separately identifiable evaluation and management service not related to dialysis procedure or renal failure with modifier 25 (99201-99215, 99217-99223 [99224, 99225, 99226], 99231-99239, 99241-99245, 99281-99285, 99291-99292, 99304-99318, 99324-99337, 99341-99350, 99466-99467, 99468-99476, 99477-99480)

90935 Hemodialysis procedure with single evaluation by a physician or other qualified health care professional

> *INCLUDES* All evaluation and management services related to the patient's renal disease rendered on a day dialysis is performed
> Inpatient ESRD and non-ESRD procedures
> Only one evaluation of the patient related to hemodialysis procedure
> Outpatient non-ESRD dialysis

   2.05   2.05   **FUD** 000   S 80

AMA: 2015,Jan,16; 2014,Jan,11

90937 Hemodialysis procedure requiring repeated evaluation(s) with or without substantial revision of dialysis prescription

> *INCLUDES* All evaluation and management services related to the patient's renal disease rendered on a day dialysis is performed
> Inpatient ESRD and non-ESRD procedures
> Outpatient non-ESRD dialysis
> Re-evaluation of the patient during hemodialysis procedure

   2.94   2.94   **FUD** 000   B 80

AMA: 2015,Jan,16; 2014,Jan,11

90940 Hemodialysis access flow study to determine blood flow in grafts and arteriovenous fistulae by an indicator method

> *EXCLUDES* *Hemodialysis access duplex scan (93990)*

   0.00   0.00   **FUD** XXX   N

AMA: 2015,Jan,16; 2014,Jan,11; 2012,Jan,15-42; 2011,Jan,11

90945-90947 Dialysis Techniques Other Than Hemodialysis

CMS: 100-4,12,40.3 Global Surgery Review; 100-4,3,100.6 Inpatient Renal Services

> *INCLUDES* All evaluation and management services related to the patient's renal disease rendered on the day dialysis is performed
> Procedures other than hemodialysis:
> Continuous renal replacement therapies
> Hemofiltration
> Peritoneal dialysis

> *EXCLUDES* *Attendance by physician or other qualified health care provider for a prolonged period of time (99354-99360 [99415, 99416])*
> *Hemodialysis*
> *Tunneled intraperitoneal catheter insertion*
> *Open (49421)*
> *Percutaneous (49418)*
> Code also significant, separately identifiable evaluation and management service not related to dialysis procedure or renal failure with modifier 25 (99201-99215, 99217-99220 [99224, 99225, 99226], 99231-99239, 99241-99245, 99281-99285, 99291-99292, 99304-99318, 99324-99337, 99341-99350, 99466-99480 [99485, 99486])

90945 Dialysis procedure other than hemodialysis (eg, peritoneal dialysis, hemofiltration, or other continuous renal replacement therapies), with single evaluation by a physician or other qualified health care professional

> *INCLUDES* Only one evaluation of the patient related to the procedure
> *EXCLUDES* *Peritoneal dialysis home infusion (99601, 99602)*

   2.42   2.42   **FUD** 000   V 80 P0

AMA: 2015,Jan,16; 2014,Jan,11; 2012,Jan,15-42; 2011,Jan,11

90947 Dialysis procedure other than hemodialysis (eg, peritoneal dialysis, hemofiltration, or other continuous renal replacement therapies) requiring repeated evaluations by a physician or other qualified health care professional, with or without substantial revision of dialysis prescription

EXCLUDES *Re-evaluation during a procedure*

3.50 3.50 **FUD** 000 [B] [80] [PQ]

AMA: 2015,Jan,16; 2014,Jan,11; 2012,Jan,15-42; 2011,Jan,11

90951-90962 End-stage Renal Disease Monthly Outpatient Services

CMS: 100-2,11,20 Renal Dialysis Items and Services ; 100-4,8,140.1 ESRD-Related Services Under the Monthly Capitation Payment

INCLUDES Establishing dialyzing cycle
Management of dialysis visits
Outpatient evaluation and management of dialysis visits
Patient management during dialysis for a month
Telephone calls

EXCLUDES *Dialysis services provided during an inpatient hospitalization (90935-90937, 90945-90947)*
ESRD/non-ESRD dialysis services performed in an inpatient setting (90935-90937, 90945-90947)
Non-ESRD dialysis services performed in an outpatient setting (90935-90937, 90945-90947)
Non-ESRD related evaluation and management services that cannot be performed during the dialysis session
Do not report during the time transitional care management services are being provided (99495-99496)
Do not report in the same month with (99487-99489)

90951 End-stage renal disease (ESRD) related services monthly, for patients younger than 2 years of age to include monitoring for the adequacy of nutrition, assessment of growth and development, and counseling of parents; with 4 or more face-to-face visits by a physician or other qualified health care professional per month [A]

26.5 26.5 **FUD** XXX [M] [80] [PQ]

AMA: 2015,Jan,16; 2014,Oct,3; 2014,Jan,11; 2013,Nov,3; 2013,Apr,3-4

90952 with 2-3 face-to-face visits by a physician or other qualified health care professional per month [A]

0.00 0.00 **FUD** XXX [M] [80] [PQ]

AMA: 2015,Jan,16; 2014,Oct,3; 2014,Jan,11; 2013,Nov,3; 2013,Apr,3-4

90953 with 1 face-to-face visit by a physician or other qualified health care professional per month [A]

0.00 0.00 **FUD** XXX [M] [80] [PQ]

AMA: 2015,Jan,16; 2014,Oct,3; 2014,Jan,11; 2013,Nov,3; 2013,Apr,3-4

90954 End-stage renal disease (ESRD) related services monthly, for patients 2-11 years of age to include monitoring for the adequacy of nutrition, assessment of growth and development, and counseling of parents; with 4 or more face-to-face visits by a physician or other qualified health care professional per month [A]

23.0 23.0 **FUD** XXX [M] [80] [PQ]

AMA: 2015,Jan,16; 2014,Oct,3; 2014,Jan,11; 2013,Nov,3; 2013,Apr,3-4

90955 with 2-3 face-to-face visits by a physician or other qualified health care professional per month [A]

12.9 12.9 **FUD** XXX [M] [80] [PQ]

AMA: 2015,Jan,16; 2014,Oct,3; 2014,Jan,11; 2013,Nov,3; 2013,Apr,3-4

90956 with 1 face-to-face visit by a physician or other qualified health care professional per month [A]

9.04 9.04 **FUD** XXX [M] [80] [PQ]

AMA: 2015,Jan,16; 2014,Oct,3; 2014,Jan,11; 2013,Nov,3; 2013,Apr,3-4

90957 End-stage renal disease (ESRD) related services monthly, for patients 12-19 years of age to include monitoring for the adequacy of nutrition, assessment of growth and development, and counseling of parents; with 4 or more face-to-face visits by a physician or other qualified health care professional per month [A]

18.1 18.2 **FUD** XXX [M] [80] [PQ]

AMA: 2015,Jan,16; 2014,Oct,3; 2014,Jan,11; 2013,Nov,3; 2013,Apr,3-4

90958 with 2-3 face-to-face visits by a physician or other qualified health care professional per month [A]

12.2 12.2 **FUD** XXX [M] [80] [PQ]

AMA: 2015,Jan,16; 2014,Oct,3; 2014,Jan,11; 2013,Nov,3; 2013,Apr,3-4

90959 with 1 face-to-face visit by a physician or other qualified health care professional per month [A]

8.35 8.35 **FUD** XXX [M] [80] [PQ]

AMA: 2015,Jan,16; 2014,Oct,3; 2014,Jan,11; 2013,Nov,3; 2013,Apr,3-4

90960 End-stage renal disease (ESRD) related services monthly, for patients 20 years of age and older; with 4 or more face-to-face visits by a physician or other qualified health care professional per month [A]

8.01 8.01 **FUD** XXX [M] [80] [PQ]

AMA: 2015,Jan,16; 2014,Oct,3; 2014,Jan,11; 2013,Nov,3; 2013,Apr,3-4

90961 with 2-3 face-to-face visits by a physician or other qualified health care professional per month [A]

6.74 6.74 **FUD** XXX [M] [80] [PQ]

AMA: 2015,Jan,16; 2014,Oct,3; 2014,Jan,11; 2013,Nov,3; 2013,Apr,3-4

90962 with 1 face-to-face visit by a physician or other qualified health care professional per month [A]

5.19 5.19 **FUD** XXX [M] [80] [PQ]

AMA: 2015,Jan,16; 2014,Oct,3; 2014,Jan,11; 2013,Nov,3; 2013,Apr,3-4

90963-90966 End-stage Renal Disease Monthly Home Dialysis Services

CMS: 100-2,11,20 Renal Dialysis Items and Services ; 100-4,8,140.1 ESRD-Related Services Under the Monthly Capitation Payment; 100-4,8,140.1.1 Payment for Managing Patients on Home Dialysis

INCLUDES ESRD services for home dialysis patients
Services provided for a full month
Do not report during the time transitional care management services are being provided (99495-99496)
Do not report in the same month with (99487-99489)

90963 End-stage renal disease (ESRD) related services for home dialysis per full month, for patients younger than 2 years of age to include monitoring for the adequacy of nutrition, assessment of growth and development, and counseling of parents [A]

15.3 15.3 **FUD** XXX [M] [80] [PQ]

AMA: 2015,Jan,16; 2014,Oct,3; 2014,Jan,11; 2013,Nov,3; 2013,Apr,3-4

90964 End-stage renal disease (ESRD) related services for home dialysis per full month, for patients 2-11 years of age to include monitoring for the adequacy of nutrition, assessment of growth and development, and counseling of parents [A]

13.4 13.4 **FUD** XXX [M] [80] [PQ]

AMA: 2015,Jan,16; 2014,Oct,3; 2014,Jan,11; 2013,Nov,3; 2013,Apr,3-4

90965 End-stage renal disease (ESRD) related services for home dialysis per full month, for patients 12-19 years of age to include monitoring for the adequacy of nutrition, assessment of growth and development, and counseling of parents [A]

12.7 12.7 **FUD** XXX [M] [80] [PQ]

AMA: 2015,Jan,16; 2014,Oct,3; 2014,Jan,11; 2013,Nov,3; 2013,Apr,3-4

90966 End-stage renal disease (ESRD) related services for home dialysis per full month, for patients 20 years of age and older

    📋 6.71   ⚖ 6.71   **FUD** XXX   Ⓜ 80 PQ

    AMA: 2015,Jan,16; 2014,Oct,3; 2014,Jan,11; 2013,Nov,3; 2013,Apr,3-4

90967-90970 End-stage Renal Disease Services: Partial Month

CMS: 100-2,11,20 Renal Dialysis Items and Services

INCLUDES   ESRD services for less than a full month, such as:
    A patient who is transient, dies, recovers, or undergoes kidney transplant
    Outpatient ESRD-related services initiated prior to completion of assessment
    Patient spending part of the month as a hospital inpatient
    Services reported on a daily basis, less the days of hospitalization
Do not report during the time transitional care management services are being provided (99495-99496)
Do not report in the same month with (99487-99489)

90967 End-stage renal disease (ESRD) related services for dialysis less than a full month of service, per day; for patients younger than 2 years of age

    📋 0.51   ⚖ 0.51   **FUD** XXX   Ⓜ 80 PQ

    AMA: 2015,Jan,16; 2014,Oct,3; 2014,Jan,11; 2013,Nov,3; 2013,Apr,3-4

90968 for patients 2-11 years of age

    📋 0.44   ⚖ 0.44   **FUD** XXX   Ⓜ 80 PQ

    AMA: 2015,Jan,16; 2014,Oct,3; 2014,Jan,11; 2013,Nov,3; 2013,Apr,3-4

90969 for patients 12-19 years of age

    📋 0.43   ⚖ 0.43   **FUD** XXX   Ⓜ 80 PQ

    AMA: 2015,Jan,16; 2014,Oct,3; 2014,Jan,11; 2013,Nov,3; 2013,Apr,3-4

90970 for patients 20 years of age and older

    📋 0.22   ⚖ 0.22   **FUD** XXX   Ⓜ 80 PQ

    AMA: 2015,Jan,16; 2014,Oct,3; 2014,Jan,11; 2013,Nov,3; 2013,Apr,3-4

90989-90993 Dialysis Training Services

CMS: 100-4,3,100.6 Inpatient Renal Services

90989 Dialysis training, patient, including helper where applicable, any mode, completed course

    📋 0.00   ⚖ 0.00   **FUD** XXX   Ⓑ PQ

    AMA: 2015,Jan,16; 2014,Jan,11; 2012,Jan,15-42; 2011,Jan,11

90993 Dialysis training, patient, including helper where applicable, any mode, course not completed, per training session

    📋 0.00   ⚖ 0.00   **FUD** XXX   Ⓑ PQ

    AMA: 2015,Jan,16; 2014,Jan,11; 2012,Jan,15-42; 2011,Jan,11

90997-90999 Hemoperfusion and Unlisted Dialysis Procedures

CMS: 100-4,3,100.6 Inpatient Renal Services

90997 Hemoperfusion (eg, with activated charcoal or resin)

    📋 2.67   ⚖ 2.67   **FUD** 000   Ⓑ 80 PQ

    AMA: 1999,Nov,1; 1997,Nov,1

90999 Unlisted dialysis procedure, inpatient or outpatient

    📋 0.00   ⚖ 0.00   **FUD** XXX   Ⓑ 80 PQ

    AMA: 1999,Nov,1; 1997,Nov,1

91010-91022 Esophageal Manometry

91010 Esophageal motility (manometric study of the esophagus and/or gastroesophageal junction) study with interpretation and report;

    EXCLUDES   Esophageal motility studies with high-resolution esophageal pressure topography (91299)
    Code also for esophageal motility studies with stimulant or perfusion (91013)

    📋 5.03   ⚖ 5.03   **FUD** 000   Ⓢ 80

    AMA: 2005,May,3-6; 1997,Nov,1

+ **91013** with stimulation or perfusion (eg, stimulant, acid or alkali perfusion) (List separately in addition to code for primary procedure)

    📋 0.68   ⚖ 0.68   **FUD** ZZZ   Ⓝ 80

    EXCLUDES   Esophageal motility studies with high-resolution esophageal pressure topography (91299)
    Code first (91010)
    Do not report more than one time for each session

91020 Gastric motility (manometric) studies

    Do not report with (91112)

    📋 6.63   ⚖ 6.63   **FUD** 000   Ⓢ 80

    AMA: 2015,Jan,16; 2013,Sep,13-14

Gastric pertains to the stomach; peptic is a term for ulcers caused by digestive juices in the stomach, duodenum or jejunum; duodenal ulcers are more common in young people, gastric in the elderly

91022 Duodenal motility (manometric) study

    EXCLUDES   Fluoroscopy (76000)
    Gastric motility study (91020)
    Do not report with (91112)

    📋 4.82   ⚖ 4.82   **FUD** 000   Ⓢ 80

    AMA: 2015,Jan,16; 2013,Sep,13-14

91030-91040 Esophageal Reflux Tests

EXCLUDES   Duodenal intubation/aspiration (43756-43757)
    Esophagoscopy (43180-43233 [43211, 43212, 43213, 43214])
    Insertion of:
      Esophageal tamponade tube (43460)
      Miller-Abbott tube (44500)
    Radiologic services, gastrointestinal (74210-74363)
    Upper gastrointestinal endoscopy (43235-43259 [43233, 43266, 43270])

91030 Esophagus, acid perfusion (Bernstein) test for esophagitis

    📋 3.89   ⚖ 3.89   **FUD** 000   Ⓢ 80

91034 Esophagus, gastroesophageal reflux test; with nasal catheter pH electrode(s) placement, recording, analysis and interpretation

    📋 5.32   ⚖ 5.32   **FUD** 000   Ⓢ 80

    AMA: 2015,Jan,16; 2014,Feb,11; 2014,Jan,11

91035 with mucosal attached telemetry pH electrode placement, recording, analysis and interpretation

    INCLUDES   Endoscopy only to place device

    📋 13.7   ⚖ 13.7   **FUD** 000   Ⓢ 72 80

    AMA: 2015,Jan,16; 2014,Feb,11; 2014,Jan,11

91037 Esophageal function test, gastroesophageal reflux test with nasal catheter intraluminal impedance electrode(s) placement, recording, analysis and interpretation;

    📋 4.58   ⚖ 4.58   **FUD** 000   Ⓢ 80

    AMA: 2005,May,3-6

91038 prolonged (greater than 1 hour, up to 24 hours)

    📋 12.8   ⚖ 12.8   **FUD** 000   Ⓢ 80

    AMA: 2015,Jan,16; 2014,Feb,11

▲ **91040** Esophageal balloon distension study, diagnostic, with provocation when performed

    Do not report more than one time for each session

    📋 12.4   ⚖ 12.4   **FUD** 000   Ⓢ 80

    AMA: 2005,May,3-6

Medicine

91065 Breath Analysis

CMS: 100-3,100.5 Diagnostic Breath Analysis

EXCLUDES *H. pylori breath test analysis, radioactive (C-14) or nonradioactive (C-13) (78268, 83013)*
Code also each challenge administered

91065 **Breath hydrogen or methane test (eg, for detection of lactase deficiency, fructose intolerance, bacterial overgrowth, or oro-cecal gastrointestinal transit)**
     2.30   2.30   **FUD** 000   S 80
     AMA: 2015,Jan,16; 2014,Jan,11

91110-91299 Additional Gastrointestinal Diagnostic/Therapeutic Procedures

EXCLUDES *Abdominal paracentesis (49082-49084)*
Abdominal paracentesis with medication administration (96440, 96446)
Anoscopy (46600-46615)
Colonoscopy (45378-45393 [45388, 45390, 45398])
Duodenal intubation/aspiration (43756-43757)
Esophagoscopy (43180-43233 [43211, 43212, 43213, 43214])
Proctosigmoidoscopy (45300-45327)
Radiologic services, gastrointestinal (74210-74363)
Sigmoidoscopy (45330-45350 [45346])
Small intestine/stomal endoscopy (44360-44408 [44381, 44401])
Upper gastrointestinal endoscopy (43235-43259 [43233, 43266, 43270])

91110 **Gastrointestinal tract imaging, intraluminal (eg, capsule endoscopy), esophagus through ileum, with interpretation and report**
     Code also modifier 52 if ileum is not visualized
     Do not report with visualization of the colon separately
     Do not report with (91111, 0355T)
     25.3   25.3   **FUD** XXX   T 80
     AMA: 2015,Jan,16; 2014,Jan,11; 2013,Sep,13-14; 2012,Jan,15-42; 2011,Jan,11

91111 **Gastrointestinal tract imaging, intraluminal (eg, capsule endoscopy), esophagus with interpretation and report**
     EXCLUDES *Use of wireless capsule to measure transit times or pressure in gastrointestinal tract (91112)*
     Do not report with (91110, 0355T)
     20.7   20.7   **FUD** XXX   T 80
     AMA: 2015,Jan,16; 2013,Sep,13-14

91112 **Gastrointestinal transit and pressure measurement, stomach through colon, wireless capsule, with interpretation and report**
     Do not report with (83986, 91020, 91022, 91117)
     30.7   30.7   **FUD** XXX   T 80
     AMA: 2015,Jan,16; 2013,Sep,13-14

91117 **Colon motility (manometric) study, minimum 6 hours continuous recording (including provocation tests, eg, meal, intracolonic balloon distension, pharmacologic agents, if performed), with interpretation and report**
     EXCLUDES *Use of wireless capsule to measure transit times or pressure in gastrointestinal tract (91112)*
     Do not report more than one time regardless of the number of provocations
     Do not report with (91120, 91122)
     4.02   4.02   **FUD** 000   T 80
     AMA: 2015,Jan,16; 2013,Sep,13-14

91120 **Rectal sensation, tone, and compliance test (ie, response to graded balloon distention)**
     EXCLUDES *Anorectal manometry (91122)*
     Biofeedback training (90911)
     Do not report with (91117)
     12.2   12.2   **FUD** XXX   T 80
     AMA: 2015,Jan,16; 2014,Jan,11; 2013,Sep,13-14

91122 **Anorectal manometry**
     Do not report with (91117)
     6.38   6.38   **FUD** 000   T 80
     AMA: 2013,Sep,13-14

91132 **Electrogastrography, diagnostic, transcutaneous;**
     4.22   4.22   **FUD** XXX   S 80

91133 **with provocative testing**
     4.89   4.89   **FUD** XXX   S 80

91200 **Liver elastography, mechanically induced shear wave (eg, vibration), without imaging, with interpretation and report**
     1.01   1.01   **FUD** XXX   S Z3 80
     AMA: 2014,Dec,13

91299 **Unlisted diagnostic gastroenterology procedure**
     0.00   0.00   **FUD** XXX   S 80
     AMA: 2015,Jan,16; 2014,Jan,11

92002-92014 Ophthalmic Medical Services

CMS: 100-2,15,30.4 Optometrist's Services

INCLUDES Routine ophthalmoscopy
Services provided to established patients who have received professional services from the physician or other qualified health care provider or another physician or other qualified health care professional within the same group practice of the exact same specialty and subspecialty within the past three years
Services provided to new patients who have received no professional services from the physician or other qualified health care provider or another physician or other qualified health care professional within the same group practice of the exact same specialty and subspecialty within the past three years

EXCLUDES *Surgical procedures on the eye/ocular adnexa (65091-68899 [67810])*
Do not report with (99173-99174 [99177])

92002 **Ophthalmological services: medical examination and evaluation with initiation of diagnostic and treatment program; intermediate, new patient**
     INCLUDES Evaluation of new/existing condition complicated by new diagnostic or management problem
     Integrated services where medical decision making cannot be separated from examination methods
     Problems not related to primary diagnosis
     The following for intermediate services:
       External ocular/adnexal examination
       General medical observation
       History
     Other diagnostic procedures
       Biomicroscopy
       Mydriasis
       Ophthalmoscopy
       Tonometry
     1.35   2.28   **FUD** XXX   V 80 PQ
     AMA: 2015,Jan,16; 2014,Jan,11; 2012,Oct,9-11; 2012,Aug,9; 2012,Jan,15-42; 2011,Feb,6-7; 2011,Jan,11

92004 **comprehensive, new patient, 1 or more visits**
     INCLUDES General evaluation of complete visual system
     Integrated services where medical decision making cannot be separated from examination methods
     Single service that need not be performed at one session
     The following for comprehensive services:
       Basic sensorimotor examination
       Biomicroscopy
       Dilation (cycloplegia)
       External examinations
       General medical observation
       Gross visual fields
       History
       Initiation of diagnostic/treatment programs
       Mydriasis
       Ophthalmoscopic examinations
       Other diagnostic procedures
       Prescription of medication
       Special diagnostic/treatment services
       Tonometry
     2.81   4.17   **FUD** XXX   V 80 PQ
     AMA: 2015,Jan,16; 2014,Jan,11; 2012,Aug,9; 2012,Jan,15-42; 2011,Feb,6-7; 2011,Jan,9-10; 2011,Jan,11; 2010,Nov,8

92012 **Ophthalmological services: medical examination and evaluation, with initiation or continuation of diagnostic and treatment program; intermediate, established patient**

INCLUDES Evaluation of new/existing condition complicated by new diagnostic or management problem

Integrated services where medical decision making cannot be separated from examination methods

Problems not related to primary diagnosis

The following for intermediate services:
- External ocular/adnexal examination
- General medical observation
- History
- Other diagnostic procedures:
  - Biomicroscopy
  - Mydriasis
  - Ophthalmoscopy
  - Tonometry

1.48 2.40 **FUD** XXX   V 80 PQ

AMA: 2015,Jan,16; 2014,Jan,11; 2012,Aug,9; 2011,Feb,6-7

92014 **comprehensive, established patient, 1 or more visits**

INCLUDES General evaluation of complete visual system

Integrated services where medical decision making cannot be separated from examination methods

Single service that need not be performed at one session

The following for comprehensive services:
- Basic sensorimotor examination
- Biomicroscopy
- Dilation (cycloplegia)
- External examinations
- General medical observation
- Gross visual fields
- History
- Initiation of diagnostic/treatment programs
- Mydriasis
- Ophthalmoscopic examinations
- Other diagnostic procedures
- Prescription of medication
- Special diagnostic/treatment services
- Tonometry

2.25 3.47 **FUD** XXX   V 80 PQ

AMA: 2015,Jan,16; 2014,Jan,11; 2012,Oct,9-11; 2012,Aug,9; 2012,Jan,15-42; 2011,Feb,6-7; 2011,Jan,9-10; 2011,Jan,11; 2010,Nov,8

92015-92145 Ophthalmic Special Services

INCLUDES Routine ophthalmoscopy

EXCLUDES *Ocular screening that is instrument-based (99174 [99177])*
Surgical procedures on the eye/ocular adnexa (65091-68899 [67810])

Code also evaluation and management services, when performed

Code also general ophthalmological services, when performed (92002-92014)

92015 **Determination of refractive state**

INCLUDES Lens prescription
- Absorptive factor
- Axis
- Impact resistance
- Lens power
- Prism
- Specification of lens type:
  - Bifocal
  - Monofocal

EXCLUDES *Bilateral instrument based ocular screening (99174 [99177])*

Do not report with (99173-99174 [99177])

0.55 0.56 **FUD** XXX   E

AMA: 2015,Jan,16; 2014,Jan,11; 2013,Mar,6-7; 2012,Jan,15-42; 2011,Jan,11

92018 **Ophthalmological examination and evaluation, under general anesthesia, with or without manipulation of globe for passive range of motion or other manipulation to facilitate diagnostic examination; complete**

4.10 4.10 **FUD** XXX   T 80

AMA: 2015,Jan,16; 2014,Jan,11

92019 **limited**

2.03 2.03 **FUD** XXX   T 80

AMA: 2015,Jan,16; 2014,Jan,11

92020 **Gonioscopy (separate procedure)**

EXCLUDES *Gonioscopy under general anesthesia (92018)*

0.59 0.75 **FUD** XXX   01 80

AMA: 2015,Jan,16; 2014,Jan,11

92025 **Computerized corneal topography, unilateral or bilateral, with interpretation and report**

EXCLUDES *Manual keratoscopy*

Do not report with (65710-65771)

1.07 1.07 **FUD** XXX   Q1 80

AMA: 2015,Jan,16; 2014,Jan,11; 2012,Oct,9-11; 2012,Jan,15-42; 2011,Jan,11; 2010,Oct,9

92060 **Sensorimotor examination with multiple measurements of ocular deviation (eg, restrictive or paretic muscle with diplopia) with interpretation and report (separate procedure)**

1.83 1.83 **FUD** XXX   01 80

AMA: 2015,Jan,16; 2014,Jan,11

92065 **Orthoptic and/or pleoptic training, with continuing medical direction and evaluation**

1.51 1.51 **FUD** XXX   01 80

AMA: 2015,Jan,16; 2014,Jan,11; 2012,Jan,15-42; 2011,Jan,11

92071 **Fitting of contact lens for treatment of ocular surface disease**

Code also supply of lens with appropriate supply code or (99070)

Do not report with (92072)

0.95 1.07 **FUD** XXX   N N1 80 50

AMA: 2012,Aug,9

92072 **Fitting of contact lens for management of keratoconus, initial fitting**

EXCLUDES *Subsequent fittings (99211-99215, 92012-92014)*

Code also supply of lens with appropriate supply code or (99070)

Do not report with (92071)

2.90 3.79 **FUD** XXX   N N1 80

AMA: 2015,Jan,16; 2014,Jan,11; 2012,Aug,9

92081 **Visual field examination, unilateral or bilateral, with interpretation and report; limited examination (eg, tangent screen, Autoplot, arc perimeter, or single stimulus level automated test, such as Octopus 3 or 7 equivalent)**

0.96 0.96 **FUD** XXX   01 80

AMA: 2015,Jan,16; 2014,Jan,11; 2012,Oct,9-11; 2012,Jan,15-42; 2011,Jan,11; 2010,Sep,9

92082 **intermediate examination (eg, at least 2 isopters on Goldmann perimeter, or semiquantitative, automated suprathreshold screening program, Humphrey suprathreshold automatic diagnostic test, Octopus program 33)**

1.35 1.35 **FUD** XXX   01 80

AMA: 2015,Jan,16; 2014,Jan,11; 2012,Oct,9-11

92083 **extended examination (eg, Goldmann visual fields with at least 3 isopters plotted and static determination within the central 30°, or quantitative, automated threshold perimetry, Octopus program G-1, 32 or 42, Humphrey visual field analyzer full threshold programs 30-2, 24-2, or 30/60-2)**

EXCLUDES *Assessment of visual field by transmission of data by patient to a surveillance center (0378T-0379T)*

Do not report gross visual field testing/confrontation testing separately

1.81 1.81 **FUD** XXX   01 80

AMA: 2015,Jan,16; 2014,Jan,11; 2012,Oct,9-11

● New Code   ▲ Revised Code   ○ Reinstated   M Maternity   A Age Edit   Unlisted   Not Covered   # Resequenced
⊘ AMA Mod 51 Exempt   ⑤ Optum Mod 51 Exempt   ⑥ Mod 63 Exempt   ⊙ Mod Sedation   + Add-on   CCI   PQ PQRS   **FUD** Follow-up Days

© 2015 Optum360, LLC (Blue Text)   CPT © 2015 American Medical Association. All Rights Reserved. (Black Text)   Medicare (Red Text)   395
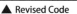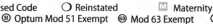

92100 Serial tonometry (separate procedure) with multiple measurements of intraocular pressure over an extended time period with interpretation and report, same day (eg, diurnal curve or medical treatment of acute elevation of intraocular pressure)

> EXCLUDES *Intraocular pressure monitoring for 24 hours or more (0329T)*
> *Ocular blood flow measurements (0198T)*
> *Single-episode tonometry (99201-99215, 92002-92004)*

0.96   2.26   **FUD** XXX   N 80

AMA: 2015,Jan,16; 2014,May,5; 2014,Jan,11; 2012,Oct,9-11; 2012,Aug,9; 2012,Jan,15-42; 2011,Jan,11

92132 Scanning computerized ophthalmic diagnostic imaging, anterior segment, with interpretation and report, unilateral or bilateral

> EXCLUDES *Imaging of anterior segment with specular microscopy and endothelial cell analysis (92286)*
> *Scanning computerized ophthalmic diagnostic imaging of optic nerve and retina (92133-92134)*
> *Tear film imaging (0330T)*

0.98   0.98   **FUD** XXX   Q1 80

AMA: 2015,Jan,16; 2014,May,5; 2014,Jan,11; 2013,Apr,7; 2013,Mar,6-7; 2012,Oct,9-11; 2011,Feb,6-7

92133 Scanning computerized ophthalmic diagnostic imaging, posterior segment, with interpretation and report, unilateral or bilateral; optic nerve

> Do not report with (92227-92228)
> Do not report with scanning computerized ophthalmic imaging of retina at same visit (92134)

1.24   1.24   **FUD** XXX   Q1 80

AMA: 2015,Jan,16; 2014,Nov,10; 2014,Jan,11; 2012,Oct,9-11; 2011,Feb,6-7

92134 retina

> Do not report with (92227-92228)
> Do not report with scanning computerized ophthalmic imaging of optic nerve at same visit (92133)

1.27   1.27   **FUD** XXX   Q1 80

AMA: 2015,Jan,16; 2014,Nov,10; 2014,Jan,11; 2012,Oct,9-11; 2011,Feb,6-7

92136 Ophthalmic biometry by partial coherence interferometry with intraocular lens power calculation

> EXCLUDES *Tear film imaging (0330T)*

2.54   2.54   **FUD** XXX   Q1 80

AMA: 2015,Jan,16; 2014,May,5; 2014,Jan,11; 2012,Jan,15-42; 2011,Jan,11

92140 Provocative tests for glaucoma, with interpretation and report, without tonography

0.75   1.77   **FUD** XXX   Q1 80

AMA: 2015,Jan,16; 2014,Jan,11; 2012,Oct,9-11

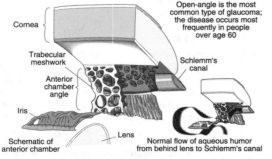

Open-angle is the most common type of glaucoma; the disease occurs most frequently in people over age 60

Cornea
Trabecular meshwork
Schlemm's canal
Anterior chamber angle
Iris
Lens
Schematic of anterior chamber
Normal flow of aqueous humor from behind lens to Schlemm's canal

Glaucoma is caused by excessive intraocular pressure and abnormal accumulation of aqueous humor in the anterior chamber of the eye; pressure reduces blood supply to the optic nerve and causes nerve damage

92145 Corneal hysteresis determination, by air impulse stimulation, unilateral or bilateral, with interpretation and report

0.44   0.44   **FUD** XXX   Q1 80

92225-92287 Other Ophthalmology Services

> EXCLUDES *Prescription, fitting, and/or medical supervision of ocular prosthesis adaptation by physician (99201-99215, 99241-99245, 92002-92014)*

92225 Ophthalmoscopy, extended, with retinal drawing (eg, for retinal detachment, melanoma), with interpretation and report; initial

> EXCLUDES *Ophthalmoscopy under general anesthesia (92018)*

0.60   0.76   **FUD** XXX   Q1 80

AMA: 2015,Jan,16; 2014,Jan,11; 2012,Oct,9-11; 2012,Jan,15-42; 2011,Feb,6-7; 2011,Jan,11

92226 subsequent

0.54   0.70   **FUD** XXX   Q1 80

AMA: 2015,Jan,16; 2014,Jan,11; 2011,Feb,6-7

92227 Remote imaging for detection of retinal disease (eg, retinopathy in a patient with diabetes) with analysis and report under physician supervision, unilateral or bilateral

> Do not report with E&M services as part of a single organ system or (92002-92014, 92133-92134, 92228, 92250)

0.41   0.41   **FUD** XXX   Q1 80 TC

AMA: 2015,Jan,16; 2014,Jan,11; 2012,Oct,9-11; 2012,Jan,15-42; 2011,May,9; 2011,Feb,6-7

92228 Remote imaging for monitoring and management of active retinal disease (eg, diabetic retinopathy) with physician review, interpretation and report, unilateral or bilateral

> Do not report with E&M services as part of a single organ system or (92002-92014, 92133-92134, 92227, 92250)

1.00   1.00   **FUD** XXX   Q1 80

AMA: 2015,Jan,16; 2014,Jan,11; 2012,Oct,9-11; 2012,Jan,15-42; 2011,May,9; 2011,Feb,6-7

92230 Fluorescein angioscopy with interpretation and report

0.94   1.63   **FUD** XXX   Q1 80

AMA: 2015,Jan,16; 2014,Jan,11; 2011,Feb,6-7

92235 Fluorescein angiography (includes multiframe imaging) with interpretation and report

3.09   3.09   **FUD** XXX   S 80

AMA: 2015,Jan,16; 2014,Jan,11; 2011,Feb,6-7

92240 Indocyanine-green angiography (includes multiframe imaging) with interpretation and report

7.17   7.17   **FUD** XXX   S 80

AMA: 2015,Jan,16; 2014,Jan,11; 2012,Oct,9-11; 2011,Feb,6-7

92250 Fundus photography with interpretation and report

2.22   2.22   **FUD** XXX   Q1 80

AMA: 2015,May,9; 2015,Jan,16; 2014,Dec,16; 2014,Dec,16; 2014,Nov,10; 2014,Jan,11; 2012,Oct,9-11; 2011,Feb,6-7

92260 Ophthalmodynamometry

> EXCLUDES *Ophthalmoscopy under general anesthesia (92018)*

0.31   0.52   **FUD** XXX   Q1 80

AMA: 2015,Jan,16; 2014,Jan,11; 2011,Feb,6-7

92265 Needle oculoelectromyography, 1 or more extraocular muscles, 1 or both eyes, with interpretation and report

2.42   2.42   **FUD** XXX   Q1 80

AMA: 2015,Jan,16; 2014,Jan,11; 2012,Oct,9-11

92270 Electro-oculography with interpretation and report

> EXCLUDES *Recording of saccadic eye movements (92700)*
> *Vestibular function testing (92537-92538, 92540-92542, 92544-92548)*
> Do not report with (92537-92538, 92540-92542, 92544-92548)

2.59   2.59   **FUD** XXX   Q1 80

AMA: 2015,Jan,16; 2014,Jan,11; 2012,Oct,9-11; 2012,Jan,15-42; 2011,Jan,11

92275 Electroretinography with interpretation and report

> EXCLUDES *Vestibular function tests/electronystagmography (92541-92548)*
> (76511-76529)

4.13   4.13   **FUD** XXX   S 80

AMA: 2015,Jan,16; 2014,Jan,11; 2012,Oct,9-11

92283 Color vision examination, extended, eg, anomaloscope or equivalent

EXCLUDES Color vision testing with pseudoisochromatic plates (e.g., HRR, Ishihara) (92002-92004, 92012-92014, 99172)

🔲 1.58   ⚖ 1.58   **FUD** XXX   📵 80 🖵

AMA: 2015,Jan,16; 2014,Jan,11; 2012,Oct,9-11

92284 Dark adaptation examination with interpretation and report

🔲 1.76   ⚖ 1.76   **FUD** XXX   📵 80 🖵

AMA: 2015,Jan,16; 2014,Jan,11; 2012,Oct,9-11

92285 External ocular photography with interpretation and report for documentation of medical progress (eg, close-up photography, slit lamp photography, goniophotography, stereo-photography)

EXCLUDES Tear film imaging (0330T)

🔲 0.58   ⚖ 0.58   **FUD** XXX   📵 80 🖵

AMA: 2015,Jan,16; 2014,May,5; 2014,Jan,11; 2012,Oct,9-11; 2012,Jan,15-42; 2011,Jan,11

92286 Anterior segment imaging with interpretation and report; with specular microscopy and endothelial cell analysis

🔲 1.08   ⚖ 1.08   **FUD** XXX   📵 80 🖵

AMA: 2015,Jan,16; 2014,Jan,11; 2013,Mar,6-7; 2012,Oct,9-11

92287 with fluorescein angiography

🔲 3.88   ⚖ 3.88   **FUD** XXX   📵 80 🖵

AMA: 2015,Jan,16; 2014,Jan,11; 2013,Mar,6-7

92310-92326 Services Related to Contact Lenses

CMS: 100-2,15,30.4 Optometrist's Services

INCLUDES Incidental revision of lens during training period
Patient training/instruction
Specification of optical/physical characteristics:
Curvature
Flexibility
Gas-permeability
Power
Size

EXCLUDES Extended wear lenses follow up (92012-92014)
General ophthalmological services
Therapeutic/surgical use of contact lens (68340, 92071-92072)

92310 Prescription of optical and physical characteristics of and fitting of contact lens, with medical supervision of adaptation; corneal lens, both eyes, except for aphakia

Code also modifier 52 for one eye

🔲 1.69   ⚖ 2.70   **FUD** XXX   E

AMA: 2015,Jan,16; 2014,Jan,11; 2012,Oct,9-11

92311 corneal lens for aphakia, 1 eye

🔲 1.57   ⚖ 2.84   **FUD** XXX   📵 80 🖵

AMA: 2015,Jan,16; 2014,Jan,11; 2012,Oct,9-11

92312 corneal lens for aphakia, both eyes

🔲 1.82   ⚖ 3.31   **FUD** XXX   📵 80 🖵

AMA: 2015,Jan,16; 2014,Jan,11; 2012,Oct,9-11

92313 corneoscleral lens

🔲 1.34   ⚖ 2.74   **FUD** XXX   📵 80 🖵

AMA: 2015,Jan,16; 2014,Jan,11; 2012,Oct,9-11

92314 Prescription of optical and physical characteristics of contact lens, with medical supervision of adaptation and direction of fitting by independent technician; corneal lens, both eyes except for aphakia

Code also modifier 52 for one eye

🔲 0.99   ⚖ 2.25   **FUD** XXX   E

AMA: 2015,Jan,16; 2014,Jan,11; 2012,Oct,9-11

92315 corneal lens for aphakia, 1 eye

🔲 0.61   ⚖ 2.05   **FUD** XXX   📵 80 🖵

AMA: 2015,Jan,16; 2014,Jan,11; 2012,Oct,9-11

92316 corneal lens for aphakia, both eyes

🔲 0.93   ⚖ 2.58   **FUD** XXX   📵 80 🖵

AMA: 2015,Jan,16; 2014,Jan,11; 2012,Oct,9-11

92317 corneoscleral lens

🔲 0.62   ⚖ 2.14   **FUD** XXX   📵 80 🖵

AMA: 2015,Jan,16; 2014,Jan,11

92325 Modification of contact lens (separate procedure), with medical supervision of adaptation

🔲 1.19   ⚖ 1.19   **FUD** XXX   📵 80 🖵

AMA: 2015,Jan,16; 2014,Jan,11; 2012,Oct,9-11

92326 Replacement of contact lens

🔲 0.99   ⚖ 0.99   **FUD** XXX   📵 80 🖵

AMA: 2015,Jan,16; 2014,Jan,11

92340-92499 Services Related to Eyeglasses

CMS: 100-2,15,30.4 Optometrist's Services

INCLUDES Anatomical facial characteristics measurement
Final adjustment of spectacles to visual axes/anatomical topography
Written laboratory specifications

EXCLUDES Supply of materials

92340 Fitting of spectacles, except for aphakia; monofocal

🔲 0.53   ⚖ 1.00   **FUD** XXX   E

AMA: 2015,Jan,16; 2014,Jan,11; 2013,Mar,6-7

92341 bifocal

🔲 0.68   ⚖ 1.14   **FUD** XXX   E

AMA: 2015,Jan,16; 2014,Jan,11; 2013,Mar,6-7

92342 multifocal, other than bifocal

🔲 0.76   ⚖ 1.23   **FUD** XXX   E

AMA: 2015,Jan,16; 2014,Jan,11; 2013,Mar,6-7

92352 Fitting of spectacle prosthesis for aphakia; monofocal

🔲 0.53   ⚖ 1.14   **FUD** XXX   📵

AMA: 2015,Jan,16; 2014,Jan,11; 2013,Mar,6-7

92353 multifocal

🔲 0.72   ⚖ 1.33   **FUD** XXX   📵

AMA: 2015,Jan,16; 2014,Jan,11; 2013,Mar,6-7

92354 Fitting of spectacle mounted low vision aid; single element system

🔲 0.38   ⚖ 0.38   **FUD** XXX   📵

AMA: 2015,Jan,16; 2014,Jan,11; 2013,Mar,6-7

92355 telescopic or other compound lens system

🔲 0.59   ⚖ 0.59   **FUD** XXX   📵

AMA: 2015,Jan,16; 2014,Jan,11; 2013,Mar,6-7

92358 Prosthesis service for aphakia, temporary (disposable or loan, including materials)

🔲 0.32   ⚖ 0.32   **FUD** XXX   📵

AMA: 2015,Jan,16; 2014,Jan,11; 2013,Mar,6-7

92370 Repair and refitting spectacles; except for aphakia

🔲 0.46   ⚖ 0.87   **FUD** XXX   E

AMA: 2015,Jan,16; 2014,Jan,11; 2013,Mar,6-7

92371 spectacle prosthesis for aphakia

🔲 0.33   ⚖ 0.33   **FUD** XXX   📵

AMA: 2015,Jan,16; 2014,Jan,11; 2013,Mar,6-7

92499 Unlisted ophthalmological service or procedure

🔲 0.00   ⚖ 0.00   **FUD** XXX   📵 80

AMA: 2015,Jan,16; 2014,Jan,11

92502-92526 Special Procedures of the Ears/Nose/Throat

INCLUDES Diagnostic/treatment services not generally included in an evaluation and management service

EXCLUDES Laryngoscopy with stroboscopy (31579)

Do not report anterior rhinoscopy, tuning fork testing, otoscopy, or removal of cerumen (non-impacted) separately

92502 Otolaryngologic examination under general anesthesia

🔲 2.75   ⚖ 2.75   **FUD** 000   T 80 🖵

AMA: 1997,Nov,1

92504 Binocular microscopy (separate diagnostic procedure)

🔲 0.27   ⚖ 0.85   **FUD** XXX   N 80 🖵

AMA: 2015,Jan,16; 2014,Jan,11; 2013,Oct,14; 2012,Jan,15-42; 2011,Oct,10; 2011,Jan,11

92507 **Treatment of speech, language, voice, communication, and/or auditory processing disorder; individual**
EXCLUDES   *Auditory rehabilitation:*
Postlingual hearing loss (92633)
Prelingual hearing loss (92630)
Programming of cochlear implant (92601-92604)
Do not report with (0364T-0365T, 0368T-0369T)
🚑 2.23   ⚕ 2.23   **FUD** XXX   A 80 💻 PQ
AMA: 2015,Jan,16; 2014,Jan,11; 2013,Oct,7

92508 **group, 2 or more individuals**
EXCLUDES   *Auditory rehabilitation:*
Postlingual hearing loss (92633)
Prelingual hearing loss (92630)
Programming of cochlear implant (92601-92604)
Do not report with (0366T-0367T, 0372T)
🚑 0.66   ⚕ 0.66   **FUD** XXX   A 80 💻 PQ
AMA: 2015,Jan,16; 2014,Jun,3; 2014,Jan,11; 2013,Oct,7

92511 **Nasopharyngoscopy with endoscope (separate procedure)**
Do not report with (43197-43198)
🚑 1.38   ⚕ 3.85   **FUD** 000   T 80 💻
AMA: 1997,Nov,1

92512 **Nasal function studies (eg, rhinomanometry)**
🚑 0.81   ⚕ 1.73   **FUD** XXX   S 80
AMA: 1997,Nov,1

92516 **Facial nerve function studies (eg, electroneuronography)**
🚑 0.64   ⚕ 1.99   **FUD** XXX   S 80
AMA: 1997,Nov,1; 1995,Win,1

92520 **Laryngeal function studies (ie, aerodynamic testing and acoustic testing)**
EXCLUDES   *Other laryngeal function testing (92700)*
Swallowing/laryngeal sensory testing with flexible fiberoptic endoscope (92611-92617)
Code also modifier 52 for single test
🚑 1.17   ⚕ 2.12   **FUD** XXX   Q1 80 💻
AMA: 2015,Jan,16; 2014,Jan,11

92521 **Evaluation of speech fluency (eg, stuttering, cluttering)**
INCLUDES   Ability to execute motor movements needed for speech
Comprehension of written and verbal expression
Determination of patient's ability to create and communicate expressive thought
Evaluation of the ability to produce speech sound
🚑 3.04   ⚕ 3.04   **FUD** XXX   A 80
AMA: 2015,Jan,16; 2014,Jun,3

92522 **Evaluation of speech sound production (eg, articulation, phonological process, apraxia, dysarthria);**
INCLUDES   Ability to execute motor movements needed for speech
Comprehension of written and verbal expression
Determination of patient's ability to create and communicate expressive thought
Evaluation of the ability to produce speech sound
🚑 2.60   ⚕ 2.60   **FUD** XXX   A 80
AMA: 2015,Jan,16; 2014,Jun,3

92523 **with evaluation of language comprehension and expression (eg, receptive and expressive language)**
INCLUDES   Ability to execute motor movements needed for speech
Comprehension of written and verbal expression
Determination of patient's ability to create and communicate expressive thought
Evaluation of the ability to produce speech sound
🚑 5.30   ⚕ 5.30   **FUD** XXX   A 80
AMA: 2015,Jan,16; 2014,Jun,3

92524 **Behavioral and qualitative analysis of voice and resonance**
INCLUDES   Ability to execute motor movements needed for speech
Comprehension of written and verbal expression
Determination of patient's ability to create and communicate expressive thought
Evaluation of the ability to produce speech sound
🚑 2.54   ⚕ 2.54   **FUD** XXX   A 80
AMA: 2015,Jan,16; 2014,Jun,3

92526 **Treatment of swallowing dysfunction and/or oral function for feeding**
🚑 2.42   ⚕ 2.42   **FUD** XXX   A 80 💻 PQ
AMA: 1997,Nov,1; 1995,Win,1

92531-92548 Vestibular Function Tests

92531 **Spontaneous nystagmus, including gaze**
Do not report with evaluation and management services (99201-99215, 99218-99223 [99224, 99225, 99226], 99231-99236, 99241-99245, 99304-99318, 99324-99337)
🚑 0.00   ⚕ 0.00   **FUD** XXX   N
AMA: 1997,Nov,1

92532 **Positional nystagmus test**
Do not report with evaluation and management services (99201-99215, 99218-99223 [99224, 99225, 99226], 99231-99236, 99241-99245, 99304-99318, 99324-99337)
🚑 0.00   ⚕ 0.00   **FUD** XXX   N
AMA: 2002,May,7; 1997,Nov,1

92533 **Caloric vestibular test, each irrigation (binaural, bithermal stimulation constitutes 4 tests)**
INCLUDES   Barany caloric test
🚑 0.00   ⚕ 0.00   **FUD** XXX   N
AMA: 2015,Jan,16; 2014,Jan,11

92534 **Optokinetic nystagmus test**
🚑 0.00   ⚕ 0.00   **FUD** XXX   N
AMA: 2002,May,7; 1997,Nov,1

● **92537** **Caloric vestibular test with recording, bilateral; bithermal (ie, one warm and one cool irrigation in each ear for a total of four irrigations)**
Code also modifier 52 when only three irrigations are performed
Do not report with (92270, 92537)

● **92538** **monothermal (ie, one irrigation in each ear for a total of two irrigations)**
Code also modifier 52 if only one irrigation is performed
Do not report with (92270, 92537)

92540 **Basic vestibular evaluation, includes spontaneous nystagmus test with eccentric gaze fixation nystagmus, with recording, positional nystagmus test, minimum of 4 positions, with recording, optokinetic nystagmus test, bidirectional foveal and peripheral stimulation, with recording, and oscillating tracking test, with recording**
Do not report with (92270, 92541-92542, 92544-92545)
🚑 2.87   ⚕ 2.87   **FUD** XXX   S 80 PQ
AMA: 2010,Jan,3-5

92541 **Spontaneous nystagmus test, including gaze and fixation nystagmus, with recording**
Do not report with (92270, 92540, 92542, 92544-92545)
🚑 0.63   ⚕ 0.63   **FUD** XXX   Q1 80 💻 PQ
AMA: 2015,Jan,16; 2014,Jan,11; 2012,Jan,15-42; 2011,May,9

92542 **Positional nystagmus test, minimum of 4 positions, with recording**
Do not report with (92270, 92540-92541, 92544-92545)
🚑 0.74   ⚕ 0.74   **FUD** XXX   Q1 80 PQ
AMA: 2015,Jan,16; 2014,Jan,11; 2012,Jan,15-42; 2011,Jan,11; 2010,Sep,9

92543 ~~Caloric vestibular test, each irrigation (binaural, bithermal stimulation constitutes 4 tests), with recording~~
To report, see ~92537-92538

92544   **Optokinetic nystagmus test, bidirectional, foveal or peripheral stimulation, with recording**
Do not report with (92270, 92540-92542, 92545)
📷 0.44   👤 0.44   **FUD** XXX   S 80 PQ
AMA: 2015,Jan,16; 2014,Jan,11

92545   **Oscillating tracking test, with recording**
Do not report with (92270, 92540-92542, 92544)
📷 0.41   👤 0.41   **FUD** XXX   S 80 PQ
AMA: 2015,Jan,16; 2014,Jan,11; 2012,Jan,15-42; 2011,May,9

92546   **Sinusoidal vertical axis rotational testing**
Do not report with (92270)
📷 2.90   👤 2.90   **FUD** XXX   S 80 PQ
AMA: 2015,Jan,16; 2014,Jan,11; 2013,Jun,13; 2012,Jan,15-42; 2011,May,9; 2011,Jan,11

+ 92547   **Use of vertical electrodes (List separately in addition to code for primary procedure)**
EXCLUDES   Unlisted vestibular tests (92700)
Code first (92540-92546)
Do not report with (92270)
📷 0.18   👤 0.18   **FUD** ZZZ   N 80 TC PQ
AMA: 2015,Jan,16; 2014,Jan,11; 2012,Jan,15-42; 2011,Jan,11

92548   **Computerized dynamic posturography**
Do not report with (92270)
📷 2.91   👤 2.91   **FUD** XXX   S 80 PQ
AMA: 2015,Jan,16; 2014,Jan,11; 2012,Jan,15-42; 2011,May,9

92550-92597 [92558] Hearing and Speech Tests

INCLUDES   Diagnostic/treatment services not generally included in a comprehensive otorhinolaryngologic evaluation or office visit
Testing of both ears
Use of calibrated electronic equipment, recording of results, and a report with interpretation
EXCLUDES   Evaluation of speech/language/hearing problems using observation/assessment of performance (92521-92524)
Code also modifier 52 for unilateral testing
Do not report tuning fork or whispered voice hearing tests separately

92550   **Tympanometry and reflex threshold measurements**
Do not report with (92567-92568)
📷 0.59   👤 0.59   **FUD** XXX   Q1 80 PQ
AMA: 2015,Jan,16; 2014,Aug,3; 2010,Jan,3-5

92551   **Screening test, pure tone, air only**
📷 0.34   👤 0.34   **FUD** XXX   E
AMA: 2015,Jan,16; 2014,Aug,3

92552   **Pure tone audiometry (threshold); air only**
EXCLUDES   Automated test (0208T)
📷 0.88   👤 0.88   **FUD** XXX   Q1 80 TC ▯ PQ
AMA: 2015,Jan,16; 2014,Aug,3

92553   **air and bone**
EXCLUDES   Automated test (0209T)
📷 1.04   👤 1.04   **FUD** XXX   Q1 80 TC ▯ PQ
AMA: 2015,Jan,16; 2014,Aug,3; 2014,Jan,11; 2011,Mar,8

92555   **Speech audiometry threshold;**
EXCLUDES   Automated test (0210T)
📷 0.65   👤 0.65   **FUD** XXX   Q1 80 TC ▯ PQ
AMA: 2015,Jan,16; 2014,Aug,3

92556   **with speech recognition**
EXCLUDES   Automated test (0211T)
📷 1.05   👤 1.05   **FUD** XXX   Q1 80 TC ▯
AMA: 2015,Jan,16; 2014,Aug,3; 2014,Jan,11; 2011,Mar,8

92557   **Comprehensive audiometry threshold evaluation and speech recognition (92553 and 92556 combined)**
EXCLUDES   Automated test (0208T-0212T)
Evaluation/selection of hearing aid (92590-92595)
📷 0.91   👤 1.05   **FUD** XXX   Q1 80 ▯ PQ
AMA: 2015,Jan,16; 2014,Aug,3; 2014,Jan,11; 2011,Mar,8

92558   **Resequenced code. See code following 92586.**

92559   **Audiometric testing of groups**
INCLUDES   For group testing, indicate tests performed
📷 0.00   👤 0.00   **FUD** XXX   E
AMA: 2015,Jan,16; 2014,Aug,3

92560   **Bekesy audiometry; screening**
📷 0.00   👤 0.00   **FUD** XXX   E
AMA: 2015,Jan,16; 2014,Aug,3

92561   **diagnostic**
📷 1.06   👤 1.06   **FUD** XXX   Q1 80 TC ▯ PQ
AMA: 2015,Jan,16; 2014,Aug,3

92562   **Loudness balance test, alternate binaural or monaural**
INCLUDES   ABLB test
📷 1.30   👤 1.30   **FUD** XXX   Q1 80 TC ▯ PQ
AMA: 2015,Jan,16; 2014,Aug,3

92563   **Tone decay test**
📷 0.87   👤 0.87   **FUD** XXX   Q1 80 TC ▯ PQ
AMA: 2015,Jan,16; 2014,Aug,3

92564   **Short increment sensitivity index (SISI)**
📷 0.80   👤 0.80   **FUD** XXX   Q1 80 TC ▯ PQ
AMA: 2015,Jan,16; 2014,Aug,3; 2014,Jan,11

92565   **Stenger test, pure tone**
📷 0.44   👤 0.44   **FUD** XXX   Q1 80 TC ▯ PQ
AMA: 2015,Jan,16; 2014,Aug,3

92567   **Tympanometry (impedance testing)**
📷 0.31   👤 0.41   **FUD** XXX   Q1 80 ▯ PQ
AMA: 2015,Jan,16; 2014,Aug,3; 2014,Jan,11

92568   **Acoustic reflex testing, threshold**
📷 0.43   👤 0.44   **FUD** XXX   Q1 80 ▯ PQ
AMA: 2015,Jan,16; 2014,Aug,3; 2014,Jan,11; 2012,Jan,15-42; 2011,Jan,11

92570   **Acoustic immittance testing, includes tympanometry (impedance testing), acoustic reflex threshold testing, and acoustic reflex decay testing**
Do not report with (92567-92568)
📷 0.84   👤 0.90   **FUD** XXX   Q1 80 PQ
AMA: 2015,Jan,16; 2014,Aug,3; 2010,Jan,3-5

92571   **Filtered speech test**
📷 0.77   👤 0.77   **FUD** XXX   Q1 80 TC ▯ PQ
AMA: 2015,Jan,16; 2014,Aug,3; 2014,Jan,11

92572   **Staggered spondaic word test**
📷 0.88   👤 0.88   **FUD** XXX   Q1 80 TC ▯ PQ
AMA: 2015,Jan,16; 2014,Aug,3; 2014,Jan,11

92575   **Sensorineural acuity level test**
📷 2.00   👤 2.00   **FUD** XXX   Q1 80 TC ▯ PQ
AMA: 2015,Jan,16; 2014,Aug,3

92576   **Synthetic sentence identification test**
📷 0.99   👤 0.99   **FUD** XXX   Q1 80 TC ▯ PQ
AMA: 2015,Jan,16; 2014,Aug,3; 2014,Jan,11

92577   **Stenger test, speech**
📷 0.45   👤 0.45   **FUD** XXX   Q1 80 TC ▯ PQ
AMA: 2015,Jan,16; 2014,Aug,3

92579   **Visual reinforcement audiometry (VRA)**
📷 1.07   👤 1.27   **FUD** XXX   Q1 80 ▯ PQ
AMA: 2015,Jan,16; 2014,Aug,3

92582   **Conditioning play audiometry**
📷 2.01   👤 2.01   **FUD** XXX   Q1 80 TC ▯ PQ
AMA: 2015,Jan,16; 2014,Aug,3

92583   **Select picture audiometry**
📷 1.43   👤 1.43   **FUD** XXX   Q1 80 TC ▯
AMA: 2015,Jan,16; 2014,Aug,3

92584   **Electrocochleography**
📷 2.08   👤 2.08   **FUD** XXX   S 80 TC ▯ PQ
AMA: 2015,Jan,16; 2014,Aug,3; 2014,Jan,11; 2012,Jan,15-42; 2011,Jul,16-17

92585 **Auditory evoked potentials for evoked response audiometry and/or testing of the central nervous system; comprehensive**

🚗 3.81   ⚕ 3.81   **FUD** XXX   S 80 ▣ PQ

AMA: 2015,Jan,16; 2014,Aug,3; 2013,May,8-10

92586 **limited**

🚗 2.35   ⚕ 2.35   **FUD** XXX   S 80 TC ▣ PQ

AMA: 2015,Jan,16; 2014,Aug,3

\# **92558** **Evoked otoacoustic emissions, screening (qualitative measurement of distortion product or transient evoked otoacoustic emissions), automated analysis**

🚗 0.00   ⚕ 0.00   **FUD** XXX   E

AMA: 2015,Jan,16; 2014,Aug,3

92587 **Distortion product evoked otoacoustic emissions; limited evaluation (to confirm the presence or absence of hearing disorder, 3-6 frequencies) or transient evoked otoacoustic emissions, with interpretation and report**

🚗 0.61   ⚕ 0.61   **FUD** XXX   S 80 ▣ PQ

AMA: 2015,Jan,16; 2014,Aug,3; 2014,Jan,11

92588 **comprehensive diagnostic evaluation (quantitative analysis of outer hair cell function by cochlear mapping, minimum of 12 frequencies), with interpretation and report**

EXCLUDES   *Evaluation of central auditory function (92620-92621)*

🚗 0.93   ⚕ 0.93   **FUD** XXX   S 80 ▣ PQ

AMA: 2015,Jan,16; 2014,Aug,3

92590 **Hearing aid examination and selection; monaural**

🚗 0.00   ⚕ 0.00   **FUD** XXX   E

AMA: 2015,Jan,16; 2014,Aug,3; 2014,Jul,4

92591 **binaural**

🚗 0.00   ⚕ 0.00   **FUD** XXX   E

AMA: 2015,Jan,16; 2014,Aug,3

92592 **Hearing aid check; monaural**

🚗 0.00   ⚕ 0.00   **FUD** XXX   E

AMA: 2015,Jan,16; 2014,Aug,3

92593 **binaural**

🚗 0.00   ⚕ 0.00   **FUD** XXX   E

AMA: 2015,Jan,16; 2014,Aug,3

92594 **Electroacoustic evaluation for hearing aid; monaural**

🚗 0.00   ⚕ 0.00   **FUD** XXX   E

AMA: 2015,Jan,16; 2014,Aug,3

92595 **binaural**

🚗 0.00   ⚕ 0.00   **FUD** XXX   E

AMA: 2015,Jan,16; 2014,Aug,3

92596 **Ear protector attenuation measurements**

🚗 1.18   ⚕ 1.18   **FUD** XXX   Q1 80 TC ▣

AMA: 2015,Jan,16; 2014,Aug,3

92597   Resequenced code. See code following 92604.

92601-92609 [92597, 92618] Services Related to Hearing and Speech Devices

INCLUDES   Diagnostic/treatment services not generally included in a comprehensive otorhinolaryngologic evaluation or office visit

92601 **Diagnostic analysis of cochlear implant, patient younger than 7 years of age; with programming**   A

INCLUDES   Connection to cochlear implant

Postoperative analysis/fitting of previously placed external devices

Stimulator programming

EXCLUDES   *Cochlear implant placement (69930)*

🚗 3.34   ⚕ 3.88   **FUD** XXX   Q1 80 ▣ PQ

AMA: 2015,Jan,16; 2014,Jul,4; 2014,Jan,11; 2013,Oct,7; 2012,Jan,15-42; 2011,Jul,16-17

92602 **subsequent reprogramming**   A

INCLUDES   Internal stimulator re-programming

Subsequent sessions for external transmitter measurements/adjustment

EXCLUDES   *Aural rehabilitation services after a cochlear implant (92626-92627, 92630-92633)*

Cochlear implant placement (69930)

Do not report with (92601)

🚗 1.92   ⚕ 2.52   **FUD** XXX   Q1 80 ▣ PQ

AMA: 2015,Jan,16; 2014,Jul,4; 2014,Jan,11; 2013,Oct,7; 2012,Jan,15-42; 2011,Jan,11

92603 **Diagnostic analysis of cochlear implant, age 7 years or older; with programming**   A

INCLUDES   Connection to cochlear implant

Post-operative analysis/fitting of previously placed external devices

Stimulator programming

EXCLUDES   *Cochlear implant placement (69930)*

🚗 3.45   ⚕ 4.21   **FUD** XXX   Q1 80 ▣ PQ

AMA: 2015,Jan,16; 2014,Jul,4; 2014,Jan,11; 2013,Oct,7; 2012,Jan,15-42; 2011,Jul,16-17

92604 **subsequent reprogramming**   A

INCLUDES   Internal stimulator re-programming

Subsequent sessions for external transmitter measurements/adjustment

EXCLUDES   *Cochlear implant placement (69930)*

Do not report with (92603)

🚗 1.91   ⚕ 2.50   **FUD** XXX   Q1 80 ▣ PQ

AMA: 2015,Jan,16; 2014,Jul,4; 2014,Jan,11; 2013,Oct,7; 2012,Jan,15-42; 2011,Jul,16-17; 2011,Jan,11

\# **92597** **Evaluation for use and/or fitting of voice prosthetic device to supplement oral speech**

EXCLUDES   *Augmentative or alternative communication device services (92605, [92618], 92607-92608)*

🚗 2.03   ⚕ 2.03   **FUD** XXX   A 80 ▣

AMA: 2015,Jan,16; 2014,Jan,11

92605 **Evaluation for prescription of non-speech-generating augmentative and alternative communication device, face-to-face with the patient; first hour**

EXCLUDES   *Prosthetic voice device fitting or use evaluation (92597)*

🚗 2.54   ⚕ 2.65   **FUD** XXX   A

AMA: 2015,Jan,16; 2014,Jan,11; 2013,Oct,7

+ \# **92618** **each additional 30 minutes (List separately in addition to code for primary procedure)**

🚗 0.94   ⚕ 0.96   **FUD** ZZZ   A

Code first (92605)

92606 **Therapeutic service(s) for the use of non-speech-generating device, including programming and modification**

🚗 2.04   ⚕ 2.37   **FUD** XXX   A

AMA: 2015,Jan,16; 2014,Jan,11

92607 **Evaluation for prescription for speech-generating augmentative and alternative communication device, face-to-face with the patient; first hour**

EXCLUDES   *Evaluation for prescription of non-speech generating device (92605)*

Evaluation for use/fitting of voice prosthetic (92597)

🚗 3.50   ⚕ 3.50   **FUD** XXX   A 80 ▣

AMA: 2015,Jan,16; 2014,Jan,11; 2013,Oct,7

+ **92608** **each additional 30 minutes (List separately in addition to code for primary procedure)**

Code first initial hour (92607)

🚗 1.50   ⚕ 1.50   **FUD** ZZZ   A 80 ▣

AMA: 2015,Jan,16; 2014,Jan,11; 2013,Oct,7

92609 **Therapeutic services for the use of speech-generating device, including programming and modification**

EXCLUDES   *Therapeutic services for use of non-speech generating device (92606)*

🚗 3.12   ⚕ 3.12   **FUD** XXX   A 80 ▣

AMA: 2015,Jan,16; 2014,Jan,11

92610-92618 Swallowing Evaluations

92610 **Evaluation of oral and pharyngeal swallowing function**

> EXCLUDES *Evaluation with flexible endoscope (92612-92617)*
> *Motion fluoroscopic evaluation of swallowing function (92611)*

> 🚑 2.05 ⚗ 2.39 **FUD** XXX   Ⓐ 80🗔 PQ

> **AMA:** 2015,Jan,16; 2014,Jan,11

92611 **Motion fluoroscopic evaluation of swallowing function by cine or video recording**

> EXCLUDES *Evaluation of oral/pharyngeal swallowing function (92610)*
> Do not report with diagnostic flexible fiberoptic laryngoscopy (31575)
> ⚕ (74230)

> 🚑 2.44 ⚗ 2.44 **FUD** XXX   Ⓐ 80🗔 PQ

> **AMA:** 2015,Jan,16; 2014,Jul,5; 2014,Jan,11

92612 **Flexible fiberoptic endoscopic evaluation of swallowing by cine or video recording;**

> EXCLUDES *Flexible fiberoptic endoscopic examination/testing without cine or video recording (92700)*
> Do not report with diagnostic flexible fiberoptic laryngoscopy (31575)

> 🚑 1.93 ⚗ 4.88 **FUD** XXX   Ⓐ 80🗔 PQ

> **AMA:** 2015,Jan,16; 2014,Jan,11; 2012,Jan,15-42; 2011,Jan,11

92613 **interpretation and report only**

> EXCLUDES *Oral/pharyngeal swallowing function examination (92610)*
> *Swallowing function motion fluoroscopic examination (92611)*
> Do not report with diagnostic flexible fiberoptic laryngoscopy (31575)

> 🚑 1.09 ⚗ 1.09 **FUD** XXX   Ⓑ 80🗔

> **AMA:** 2015,Jan,16; 2014,Jan,11

92614 **Flexible fiberoptic endoscopic evaluation, laryngeal sensory testing by cine or video recording;**

> EXCLUDES *Flexible fiberoptic endoscopic examination/testing without cine or video recording (92700)*
> Do not report with diagnostic flexible fiberoptic laryngoscopy (31575)

> 🚑 1.91 ⚗ 4.07 **FUD** XXX   Ⓐ 80🗔

> **AMA:** 2015,Jan,16; 2014,Jan,11

92615 **interpretation and report only**

> Do not report with diagnostic flexible fiberoptic laryngoscopy (31575)

> 🚑 0.95 ⚗ 0.95 **FUD** XXX   Ⓔ 80🗔

> **AMA:** 2015,Jan,16; 2014,Jan,11

92616 **Flexible fiberoptic endoscopic evaluation of swallowing and laryngeal sensory testing by cine or video recording;**

> EXCLUDES *Flexible fiberoptic endoscopic examination/testing without cine or video recording (92700)*
> Do not report with diagnostic flexible fiberoptic laryngoscopy (31575)

> 🚑 2.86 ⚗ 5.80 **FUD** XXX   Ⓐ 80🗔

> **AMA:** 2015,Jan,16; 2014,Jan,11

92617 **interpretation and report only**

> Do not report with diagnostic flexible fiberoptic laryngoscopy (31575)

> 🚑 1.18 ⚗ 1.18 **FUD** XXX   Ⓔ 80🗔

> **AMA:** 2015,Jan,16; 2014,Jan,11

92618 **Resequenced code. See code following 92605.**

92620-92700 Diagnostic Hearing Evaluations and Rehabilitation

> INCLUDES Diagnostic/treatment services not generally included in a comprehensive otorhinolaryngologic evaluation or office visit

92620 **Evaluation of central auditory function, with report; initial 60 minutes**

> Do not report with (92521-92524)

> 🚑 2.33 ⚗ 2.65 **FUD** XXX   Q1 80🗔 PQ

> **AMA:** 2015,Jan,16; 2014,Aug,3

+ 92621 **each additional 15 minutes (List separately in addition to code for primary procedure)**

> Code first (92620)
> Do not report with (92521-92524)

> 🚑 0.54 ⚗ 0.63 **FUD** ZZZ   Ⓝ 80🗔 PQ

> **AMA:** 2015,Jan,16; 2014,Aug,3

92625 **Assessment of tinnitus (includes pitch, loudness matching, and masking)**

> Code also modifier 52 for unilateral procedure
> Do not report with (92562)

> 🚑 1.76 ⚗ 1.97 **FUD** XXX   Q1 80🗔 PQ

> **AMA:** 2015,Jan,16; 2014,Aug,3

92626 **Evaluation of auditory rehabilitation status; first hour**

> INCLUDES Face-to-face time spent with the patient or family
> The ability of the patient to use residual hearing in order to identify acoustic characteristics of sounds associated with speech communication

> 🚑 2.15 ⚗ 2.53 **FUD** XXX   Q1 80🗔 PQ

> **AMA:** 2015,Jan,16; 2014,Jul,4; 2014,May,10; 2014,Jan,11

+ 92627 **each additional 15 minutes (List separately in addition to code for primary procedure)**

> INCLUDES Face-to-face time spent with the patient or family
> The ability of the patient to use residual hearing in order to identify acoustic characteristics of sounds associated with speech communication
> Code first initial hour (92626)

> 🚑 0.50 ⚗ 0.62 **FUD** ZZZ   Ⓝ 80 PQ

> **AMA:** 2015,Jan,16; 2014,Jul,4; 2014,Jan,11

92630 **Auditory rehabilitation; prelingual hearing loss**

> 🚑 0.00 ⚗ 0.00 **FUD** XXX   Ⓔ

> **AMA:** 2015,Jan,16; 2014,Jan,11; 2013,Oct,7

92633 **postlingual hearing loss**

> 🚑 0.00 ⚗ 0.00 **FUD** XXX   Ⓔ

> **AMA:** 2015,Jan,16; 2014,Jan,11; 2013,Oct,7

92640 **Diagnostic analysis with programming of auditory brainstem implant, per hour**

> 🚑 2.70 ⚗ 3.20 **FUD** XXX   Q1 80 PQ

> EXCLUDES *Nonprogramming services (cardiac monitoring)*

92700 **Unlisted otorhinolaryngological service or procedure**

> INCLUDES Lombard test

> 🚑 0.00 ⚗ 0.00 **FUD** XXX   Q1 80

> **AMA:** 2015,Jan,16; 2014,May,10; 2014,Jan,11; 2012,Jan,15-42; 2011,Jul,16-17; 2011,Mar,9; 2011,Jan,11

92920-92953 Emergency Cardiac Procedures

92920	**Resequenced code. See code following 92998.**
92921	**Resequenced code. See code following 92998.**
92924	**Resequenced code. See code following 92998.**
92925	**Resequenced code. See code following 92998.**
92928	**Resequenced code. See code following 92998.**
92929	**Resequenced code. See code following 92998.**
92933	**Resequenced code. See code following 92998.**
92934	**Resequenced code. See code following 92998.**
92937	**Resequenced code. See code following 92998.**
92938	**Resequenced code. See code following 92998.**
92941	**Resequenced code. See code following 92998.**
92943	**Resequenced code. See code following 92998.**
92944	**Resequenced code. See code following 92998.**

92950 **Cardiopulmonary resuscitation (eg, in cardiac arrest)**

> EXCLUDES *Critical care services (99291-99292)*

> 🚑 5.35 ⚗ 8.63 **FUD** 000   Ⓢ 80🗔

> **AMA:** 2015,Jan,16; 2014,Jan,11; 2012,Oct,14; 2012,Sep,16; 2012,Jul,12-14; 2012,Jan,15-42; 2011,Jan,11

● New Code   ▲ Revised Code   ○ Reinstated   Ⓜ Maternity   Ⓐ Age Edit   Unlisted   Not Covered   # Resequenced
Ⓢ AMA Mod 51 Exempt   Ⓢ Optum Mod 51 Exempt   🌑 Mod 63 Exempt   ☉ Mod Sedation   + Add-on   🗔 CCI   PQ PQRS   FUD Follow-up Days

© 2015 Optum360, LLC (Blue Text)   CPT © 2015 American Medical Association. All Rights Reserved. (Black Text)   Medicare (Red Text)   **401**

	92953	**Temporary transcutaneous pacing**
		EXCLUDES *Direction of ambulance/rescue personnel by physician or other qualified health care professional (99288)*
		🔧 0.32 ⚖ 0.32 **FUD** 000 ⊙ 03 80 💻
		AMA: 2015,Jan,16; 2014,May,4; 2014,Jan,11

92960-92961 Cardioversion

	92960	**Cardioversion, elective, electrical conversion of arrhythmia; external**
		🔧 3.49 ⚖ 5.84 **FUD** 000 ⊙ S 80 💻
		AMA: 2015,Jan,16; 2014,Jan,11; 2012,Jan,15-42; 2012,Jan,13-14; 2011,Jan,11
	92961	**internal (separate procedure)**
		Do not report with (93282-93284, 93287, 93289, 93295-93296, 93618-93624, 93631, 93640-93642, 93650, 93653-93657, 93662)
		🔧 7.54 ⚖ 7.54 **FUD** 000 ⊙ S 💻
		AMA: 2015,Feb,3; 2015,Jan,16; 2014,Jan,11

92970-92979 Circulatory Assist: External/Internal

EXCLUDES *Atrial septostomy, balloon (92992)*
Catheter placement for use in circulatory assist devices (intra-aortic balloon pump) (33970)

	92970	**Cardioassist-method of circulatory assist; internal**
		🔧 5.38 ⚖ 5.38 **FUD** 000 C 80 💻
		AMA: 1997,Nov,1
	92971	**external**
		🔧 2.92 ⚖ 2.92 **FUD** 000 C 80 💻
		AMA: 1997,Nov,1
	92973	**Resequenced code. See code following 92998.**
	92974	**Resequenced code. See code following 92998.**
	92975	**Resequenced code. See code following 92998.**
	92977	**Resequenced code. See code following 92998.**
	92978	**Resequenced code. See code following 92998.**
	92979	**Resequenced code. See code following 92998.**

92986-92993 Percutaneous Procedures of Heart Valves and Septum

	92986	**Percutaneous balloon valvuloplasty; aortic valve**
		🔧 38.6 ⚖ 38.6 **FUD** 090 ⊙ J 80 💻
		AMA: 2015,Feb,3; 2015,Jan,16; 2014,Jan,11; 2013,Jan,6-8
	92987	**mitral valve**
		🔧 39.8 ⚖ 39.8 **FUD** 090 ⊙ J 80 💻
		AMA: 2015,Feb,3
	92990	**pulmonary valve**
		🔧 31.5 ⚖ 31.5 **FUD** 090 J 80 💻
		AMA: 2015,Jul,10; 2015,Feb,3
	92992	**Atrial septectomy or septostomy; transvenous method, balloon (eg, Rashkind type) (includes cardiac catheterization)**
		🔧 0.00 ⚖ 0.00 **FUD** 090 C 80 💻
		AMA: 2015,Jan,16; 2014,Jan,11; 2012,Jan,15-42; 2011,Jan,11
	92993	**blade method (Park septostomy) (includes cardiac catheterization)**
		🔧 0.00 ⚖ 0.00 **FUD** 090 C 80 💻
		AMA: 2015,Jan,16; 2014,Jan,11

92997-92998 Percutaneous Angioplasty: Pulmonary Artery

	92997	**Percutaneous transluminal pulmonary artery balloon angioplasty; single vessel**
		🔧 19.2 ⚖ 19.2 **FUD** 000 J 80 💻
		AMA: 2015,Feb,3
+	92998	**each additional vessel (List separately in addition to code for primary procedure)**
		Code first single vessel (92997)
		🔧 9.41 ⚖ 9.41 **FUD** ZZZ N 80 💻
		AMA: 2015,Feb,3

[92920, 92921, 92924, 92925, 92928, 92929, 92933, 92934, 92937, 92938, 92941, 92943, 92944] Intravascular Coronary Procedures

INCLUDES Accessing the vessel
All procedures performed in all segments of branches of coronary arteries
    Branches of left anterior descending (diagonals), left circumflex (marginals), and right (posterior descending, posterolaterals)
    Distal, proximal, and mid segments
All procedures performed in all segments of major coronary arteries through the native vessels:
    Distal, proximal, and mid segments
    Left main, left anterior descending, left circumflex, right, and ramus intermedius arteries
All procedures performed in major coronary arteries or recognized coronary artery branches through a coronary artery bypass graft
    A sequential bypass graft with more than a single distal anastomosis as one graft
    Branching bypass grafts (eg, "Y" grafts) include a coronary vessel for the primary graft, with each branch off the primary graft making up an additional coronary vessel
    Each coronary artery bypass graft denotes a single coronary vessel
    Embolic protection devices when used
Arteriotomy closure through the access sheath
Atherectomy (eg, directional, laser, rotational)
Balloon angioplasty (eg, cryoplasty, cutting balloon, wired balloons)
Imaging once procedure is complete
Percutaneous coronary interventions (PCI) for disease of coronary vessels, native and bypass grafts
Radiological supervision and interpretation of intervention(s)
Reporting the most comprehensive treatment in a given vessel according to a hierarchy of intensity for the base and add-on codes:
    Add-on codes: 92944 = 92938 > 92934 > 92925 > 92929 > 92921
    Base codes: 92943 = 92941 > 92933 > 92924 > 92937 > 92928 > 92920
Selective vessel catheterization
Stenting (eg, balloon expandable, bare metal, covered, drug eluting, self-expanding)
Traversing of the lesion

EXCLUDES *Application of intravascular radioelements (77770-77772)*
Insertion of device for coronary intravascular brachytherapy (92974)
Reduction of septum (eg, alcohol ablation) (93799)

Code also add-on codes for procedures performed during the same session in additional recognized branches of the target vessel
Code also diagnostic angiography at the time of the interventional procedure when:
    A previous study is available, but documentation states the patient's condition has changed since the previous study or visualization of the anatomy/pathology is inadequate, or a change occurs during the procedure warranting additional evaluation of an area outside the current target area
    No previous catheter-based coronary angiography study is available, and a full diagnostic study is performed, with the decision to perform the intervention based on that study, or
Code also diagnostic angiography performed at a session separate from the interventional procedure
Code also individual base codes for treatment of a segment of a major native coronary artery and another segment of the same artery that requires treatment through a bypass graft when performed at the same time
Code also procedures for both vessels for a bifurcation lesion
Code also procedures performed in second branch of a major coronary artery
Do not report additional procedures performed in a third branch of a major coronary artery
Do not report more than one base code for percutaneous coronary revascularization of recognized branches of a major coronary artery
Do not report more than one code when a single lesion continues from one target vessel (major artery, branch, or bypass graft) to another and revascularization can be achieved with a single procedure
Do not report procedures in branches of the left main and ramus intermedius coronary arteries as they are unrecognized for purposes of reporting
Do not report separately when included in the coronary revascularization service (93454-93461, 93563-93564)

#	92920	**Percutaneous transluminal coronary angioplasty; single major coronary artery or branch**
		🔧 15.8 ⚖ 15.8 **FUD** 000 ⊙ J 80
		AMA: 2015,Jan,16; 2014,Dec,6; 2013,Jan,3-5

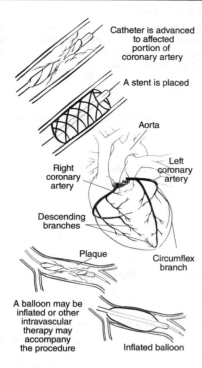

Catheter is advanced
to affected
portion of
coronary artery

A stent is placed

Aorta

Right
coronary
artery

Left
coronary
artery

Descending
branches

Plaque

Circumflex
branch

A balloon may be
inflated or other
intravascular
therapy may
accompany
the procedure

Inflated balloon

+ # **92921** **each additional branch of a major coronary artery (List separately in addition to code for primary procedure)**
Code first (92920, 92924, 92928, 92933, 92937, 92941, 92943)
0.00 0.00 **FUD** ZZZ ⊙ N
AMA: 2015,Jan,16; 2014,Dec,6; 2014,Sep,13; 2013,Jan,3-5

92924 **Percutaneous transluminal coronary atherectomy, with coronary angioplasty when performed; single major coronary artery or branch**
18.7 18.7 **FUD** 000 ⊙ J 80
AMA: 2015,Jan,16; 2014,Dec,6; 2013,Jan,3-5

+ # **92925** **each additional branch of a major coronary artery (List separately in addition to code for primary procedure)**
Code first (92924, 92928, 92933, 92937, 92941, 92943)
0.00 0.00 **FUD** ZZZ ⊙ N
AMA: 2015,Jan,16; 2014,Dec,6; 2014,Sep,13; 2013,Jan,3-5

92928 **Percutaneous transcatheter placement of intracoronary stent(s), with coronary angioplasty when performed; single major coronary artery or branch**
17.5 17.5 **FUD** 000 ⊙ J 80
AMA: 2015,Jan,16; 2014,Dec,6; 2014,Sep,13; 2014,Mar,13; 2014,Jan,3; 2013,Jan,3-5

+ # **92929** **each additional branch of a major coronary artery (List separately in addition to code for primary procedure)**
Code first (92928, 92933, 92937, 92941, 92943)
0.00 0.00 **FUD** ZZZ ⊙ N
AMA: 2015,Jan,16; 2014,Dec,6; 2014,Sep,13; 2013,Jan,3-5

92933 **Percutaneous transluminal coronary atherectomy, with intracoronary stent, with coronary angioplasty when performed; single major coronary artery or branch**
19.6 19.6 **FUD** 000 ⊙ J 80
AMA: 2015,Jan,16; 2014,Dec,6; 2013,Jan,3-5

+ # **92934** **each additional branch of a major coronary artery (List separately in addition to code for primary procedure)**
Code first (92933, 92937, 92941, 92943)
0.00 0.00 **FUD** ZZZ ⊙ N
AMA: 2015,Jan,16; 2014,Dec,6; 2014,Sep,13; 2013,Jan,3-5

92937 **Percutaneous transluminal revascularization of or through coronary artery bypass graft (internal mammary, free arterial, venous), any combination of intracoronary stent, atherectomy and angioplasty, including distal protection when performed; single vessel**
17.5 17.5 **FUD** 000 ⊙ J 80
AMA: 2015,Jan,16; 2014,Dec,6; 2014,Mar,13; 2013,Jan,3-5

+ # **92938** **each additional branch subtended by the bypass graft (List separately in addition to code for primary procedure)**
Code first (92937)
0.00 0.00 **FUD** ZZZ ⊙ N
AMA: 2015,Jan,16; 2014,Dec,6; 2014,Sep,13; 2014,Mar,13; 2013,Jan,3-5

92941 **Percutaneous transluminal revascularization of acute total/subtotal occlusion during acute myocardial infarction, coronary artery or coronary artery bypass graft, any combination of intracoronary stent, atherectomy and angioplasty, including aspiration thrombectomy when performed, single vessel**
INCLUDES Aspiration thrombectomy, when performed
Embolic protection
Rheolytic thrombectomy
Code also mechanical thrombectomy, when performed
Code also treatment of additional vessels, when appropriate (92920-92938, 92943-92944)
19.6 19.6 **FUD** 000 ⊙ J 80
AMA: 2015,Jan,16; 2014,Dec,6; 2014,Mar,13; 2014,Jan,3; 2013,Jan,3-5

92943 **Percutaneous transluminal revascularization of chronic total occlusion, coronary artery, coronary artery branch, or coronary artery bypass graft, any combination of intracoronary stent, atherectomy and angioplasty; single vessel**
INCLUDES Lack of antegrade flow with angiography and clinical criteria indicative of chronic total occlusion
19.6 19.6 **FUD** 000 ⊙ J 80
AMA: 2015,Jan,16; 2014,Dec,6; 2013,Jan,3-5

+ # **92944** **each additional coronary artery, coronary artery branch, or bypass graft (List separately in addition to code for primary procedure)**
EXCLUDES Application of intravascular radioelements (77770-77772)
Code first (92924, 92928, 92933, 92937, 92941, 92943)
0.00 0.00 **FUD** ZZZ ⊙ N
AMA: 2015,Jan,16; 2014,Dec,6; 2014,Sep,13; 2013,Jan,3-5

[92973, 92974, 92975, 92977, 92978, 92979] Additional Coronary Artery Procedures

+ # **92973** **Percutaneous transluminal coronary thrombectomy mechanical (List separately in addition to code for primary procedure)**
EXCLUDES Aspiration thrombectomy
Code first (92920, 92924, 92928, 92933, 92937, 92941, 92943, 92975, 93454-93461, 93563-93564)
5.15 5.15 **FUD** ZZZ ⊙ N 80 ⌷
AMA: 2015,Jan,16; 2014,Dec,6; 2014,Jan,11; 2012,Jan,15-42; 2011,Jan,11

+ # **92974** **Transcatheter placement of radiation delivery device for subsequent coronary intravascular brachytherapy (List separately in addition to code for primary procedure)**
EXCLUDES Application of intravascular radioelements (77770-77772)
Code first (92920, 92924, 92928, 92933, 92937, 92941, 92943, 93454-93461)
4.70 4.70 **FUD** ZZZ ⊙ N 80 ⌷
AMA: 2015,Jan,16; 2014,Dec,6; 2014,Jan,11

Medicine

92920 — 92974

Medicine (side tab)

 # 92975 Thrombolysis, coronary; by intracoronary infusion, including selective coronary angiography

     EXCLUDES   *Thrombolysis, cerebral (37195)*

         Thrombolysis other than coronary ([37211, 37212, 37213, 37214])

     🔧 11.3   ⚕ 11.3   **FUD** 000   ⊙ C 80 ▭

     AMA: 1997,Nov,1; 1991,Win,1

 # 92977 by intravenous infusion

     EXCLUDES   *Thrombolysis, cerebral (37195)*

         Thrombolysis other than coronary ([37211, 37212, 37213, 37214])

     🔧 1.62   ⚕ 1.62   **FUD** XXX   T 80 ▭

     AMA: 1997,Nov,1; 1991,Win,1

+ # 92978 Intravascular ultrasound (coronary vessel or graft) during diagnostic evaluation and/or therapeutic intervention including imaging supervision, interpretation and report; initial vessel (List separately in addition to code for primary procedure)

     Code first primary procedure (92920, 92924, 92928, 92933, 92937, 92941, 92943, 92975, 93454-93461, 93563-93564)

     🔧 0.00   ⚕ 0.00   **FUD** ZZZ   ⊙ N 80 ▭

     AMA: 2015,Jan,16; 2014,Dec,6; 2014,Jan,11; 2013,Dec,16; 2012,Jan,15-42; 2011,Jan,11

+ # 92979 each additional vessel (List separately in addition to code for primary procedure)

     INCLUDES   Transducer manipulations/repositioning in the vessel examined, before and after therapeutic intervention

     EXCLUDES   *Intravascular optic coherence tomography (0291T-0292T)*

         Intravascular spectroscopy (0205T)

     Code first initial vessel (92978)

     🔧 0.00   ⚕ 0.00   **FUD** ZZZ   ⊙ N 80

     AMA: 2015,Jan,16; 2014,Dec,6; 2014,Jan,11; 2013,Dec,16

93000-93010 Electrocardiographic Services

     INCLUDES   Specific order for the service, a separate written and signed report, and documentation of medical necessity

     EXCLUDES   *Acoustic cardiography (93799)*

         Echocardiography (93303-93350)

         ECG monitoring (99354-99360 [99415, 99416])

         ECG with 64 or more leads, graphic presentation, and analysis (0178T-0180T)

         Use of these codes for the review of telemetry monitoring strips

93000 Electrocardiogram, routine ECG with at least 12 leads; with interpretation and report

     🔧 0.48   ⚕ 0.48   **FUD** XXX   M 80 ▭

     AMA: 2015,Jan,16; 2014,Jan,11

93005 tracing only, without interpretation and report

     🔧 0.24   ⚕ 0.24   **FUD** XXX   01 80 TC ▭

     AMA: 2015,Jan,16; 2014,Jan,11

93010 interpretation and report only

     🔧 0.24   ⚕ 0.24   **FUD** XXX   B 80 26 ▭

     AMA: 2015,Jan,16; 2014,Jan,11

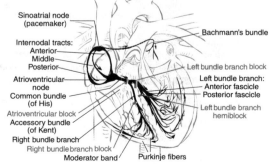

Sinoatrial node (pacemaker)
Internodal tracts: Anterior, Middle, Posterior
Atrioventricular node
Common bundle (of His)
Atrioventricular block
Accessory bundle (of Kent)
Right bundle branch
Right bundle branch block
Moderator band
Bachmann's bundle
Left bundle branch block
Left bundle branch: Anterior fascicle, Posterior fascicle
Left bundle branch hemiblock
Purkinje fibers

93015-93018 Stress Test

93015 Cardiovascular stress test using maximal or submaximal treadmill or bicycle exercise, continuous electrocardiographic monitoring, and/or pharmacological stress; with supervision, interpretation and report

     🔧 2.15   ⚕ 2.15   **FUD** XXX   B 80 ▭

     AMA: 2015,Jan,16; 2014,Jan,11; 2012,Jan,15-42; 2011,Jan,11; 2010,May,5-6; 2010,Jan,8-10

93016 supervision only, without interpretation and report

     🔧 0.63   ⚕ 0.63   **FUD** XXX   B 80 26 ▭

     AMA: 2015,Jan,16; 2014,Jan,11; 2012,Jan,15-42; 2011,Jan,11; 2010,May,5-6; 2010,Jan,8-10

93017 tracing only, without interpretation and report

     🔧 1.11   ⚕ 1.11   **FUD** XXX   01 80 TC ▭

     AMA: 2015,Jan,16; 2014,Jan,11; 2012,Jan,15-42; 2011,Jan,11; 2010,May,5-6; 2010,Jan,8-10

93018 interpretation and report only

     🔧 0.41   ⚕ 0.41   **FUD** XXX   B 80 26 ▭

     AMA: 2015,Jan,16; 2014,Jan,11; 2012,Jan,15-42; 2011,Jan,11; 2010,May,5-6; 2010,Jan,8-10

93024 Provocation Test for Coronary Vasospasm

93024 Ergonovine provocation test

     🔧 3.17   ⚕ 3.17   **FUD** XXX   S 80 ▭

93025 Microvolt T-Wave Alternans

     CMS: 100-3,20.30 Microvolt T-Wave Alternans (MTWA); 100-4,32,370 Microvolt T-wave Alternans; 100-4,32,370.1 Coding and Claims Processing for MTWA; 100-4,32,370.2 Messaging for MTWA

     INCLUDES   Specific order for the service, a separate written and signed report, and documentation of medical necessity

     EXCLUDES   *Echocardiography (93303-93350)*

         ECG with 64 or more leads, graphic presentation, and analysis (0178T-0180T)

         Use of these codes for the review of telemetry monitoring strips

93025 Microvolt T-wave alternans for assessment of ventricular arrhythmias

     🔧 4.61   ⚕ 4.61   **FUD** XXX   S 80 ▭

     AMA: 2015,Jan,16; 2014,Jan,11

93040-93042 Rhythm Strips

     INCLUDES   Specific order for the service, a separate written and signed report, and documentation of medical necessity

     EXCLUDES   *Echocardiography (93303-93350)*

         ECG with 64 or more leads, graphic presentation, and analysis (0178T-0180T)

         Use of these codes for the review of telemetry monitoring strips

     Do not report with (93260-93261, 93279-93289 [93260], 93291-93296, 93298-93299)

93040 Rhythm ECG, 1-3 leads; with interpretation and report

     🔧 0.36   ⚕ 0.36   **FUD** XXX   B 80 ▭

     AMA: 2015,Jan,16; 2014,Jan,11; 2012,Nov,6-9; 2012,Aug,6-8; 2012,Jan,15-42; 2010,Oct,9

93041 tracing only without interpretation and report

     🔧 0.16   ⚕ 0.16   **FUD** XXX   01 80 TC

     AMA: 2015,Jan,16; 2014,Jan,11; 2012,Aug,6-8; 2012,Jan,15-42; 2010,Oct,9

93042 interpretation and report only

     🔧 0.20   ⚕ 0.20   **FUD** XXX   B 80 26 ▭

     AMA: 2015,Jan,16; 2014,Jan,11; 2012,Aug,6-8; 2012,Jan,15-42; 2011,Oct,5-7; 2011,Jan,11; 2010,Oct,9

93050 Arterial Waveform Analysis

     Do not report with any intraarterial diagnostic or interventional procedure

● **93050 Arterial pressure waveform analysis for assessment of central arterial pressures, includes obtaining waveform(s), digitization and application of nonlinear mathematical transformations to determine central arterial pressures and augmentation index, with interpretation and report, upper extremity artery, non-invasive**

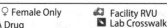

93224-93227 Holter Monitor

INCLUDES Cardiac monitoring using in-person as well as remote technology for the assessment of electrocardiographic data
Up to 48 hours of recording on a continuous basis
EXCLUDES *Echocardiography (93303-93355)*
ECG with 64 or more leads, graphic presentation, and analysis (0178T-0180T)
Implantable patient activated cardiac event recorders (33282, 93285, 93291, 93298)
More than 48 hours of monitoring (0295T-0298T)
Code also modifier 52 when less than 12 hours of continuous recording is provided

93224 **External electrocardiographic recording up to 48 hours by continuous rhythm recording and storage; includes recording, scanning analysis with report, review and interpretation by a physician or other qualified health care professional**
📷 2.59 ⚕ 2.59 **FUD** XXX M 80 ▭
AMA: 2015,Jan,16; 2014,Jan,11; 2012,Jan,15-42; 2011,Oct,5-7

93225 **recording (includes connection, recording, and disconnection)**
📷 0.76 ⚕ 0.76 **FUD** XXX 01 80 TC ▭
AMA: 2015,Jan,16; 2014,Jan,11; 2012,Jan,15-42; 2011,Oct,5-7

93226 **scanning analysis with report**
📷 1.07 ⚕ 1.07 **FUD** XXX 01 80 TC ▭
AMA: 2015,Jan,16; 2014,Jan,11; 2012,Jan,15-42; 2011,Oct,5-7

93227 **review and interpretation by a physician or other qualified health care professional**
📷 0.76 ⚕ 0.76 **FUD** XXX M 80 26 ▭
AMA: 2015,Jan,16; 2014,Jan,11; 2012,Jan,15-42; 2011,Oct,5-7

93228-93229 Remote Cardiovascular Telemetry

INCLUDES Cardiac monitoring using in-person as well as remote technology for the assessment of electrocardiographic data
Mobile telemetry monitors with the capacity to:
Detect arrhythmias
Real-time data analysis for the evaluation quality of the signal
Records ECG rhythm on a continuous basis using external electrodes on the patient
Transmit a tracing at any time
Transmit data to an attended surveillance center where a technician is available to respond to device or rhythm alerts and contact the physician or qualified health care professional if needed
Do not report more than one time in a 30-day period

93228 **External mobile cardiovascular telemetry with electrocardiographic recording, concurrent computerized real time data analysis and greater than 24 hours of accessible ECG data storage (retrievable with query) with ECG triggered and patient selected events transmitted to a remote attended surveillance center for up to 30 days; review and interpretation with report by a physician or other qualified health care professional**
Do not report with (93224, 93227)
📷 0.74 ⚕ 0.74 **FUD** XXX M 80 26
AMA: 2015,Jan,16; 2014,Jan,11; 2012,Jan,15-42; 2011,Oct,5-7

93229 **technical support for connection and patient instructions for use, attended surveillance, analysis and transmission of daily and emergent data reports as prescribed by a physician or other qualified health care professional**
EXCLUDES *Cardiovascular monitors that do not perform automatic ECG triggered transmissions to an attended surveillance center (93224-93227, 93268-93272)*
Do not report with (93224, 93226)
📷 19.0 ⚕ 19.0 **FUD** XXX S 80 TC
AMA: 2015,Jan,16; 2014,Jan,11; 2012,Jan,15-42; 2011,Oct,5-7

93260-93272 Event Monitors

INCLUDES ECG rhythm derived elements, which differ from physiologic data and include rhythm of the heart, rate, ST analysis, heart rate variability, T-wave alternans, among others
Event monitors that:
Record parts of ECGs in response to patient activation or an automatic detection algorithm (or both)
Require attended surveillance
Transmit data upon request (although not immediately when activated)
Do not report with (93279-93289 [93260], 93291-93296, 93298-93299)

93260 Resequenced code. See code following 93284.

93261 Resequenced code. See code following 93289.

93268 **External patient and, when performed, auto activated electrocardiographic rhythm derived event recording with symptom-related memory loop with remote download capability up to 30 days, 24-hour attended monitoring; includes transmission, review and interpretation by a physician or other qualified health care professional**
EXCLUDES *Implanted patient activated cardiac event recording (33282, 93285, 93291, 93298)*
📷 5.78 ⚕ 5.78 **FUD** XXX M 80 ▭
AMA: 2015,Jan,16; 2014,Jan,11; 2012,Jan,15-42; 2011,Oct,5-7

93270 **recording (includes connection, recording, and disconnection)**
📷 0.26 ⚕ 0.26 **FUD** XXX 01 80 TC ▭
AMA: 2015,Jan,16; 2014,Jan,11; 2012,Jan,15-42; 2011,Oct,5-7; 2011,Jan,11; 2010,Aug,12; 2010,Aug,12

93271 **transmission and analysis**
📷 4.80 ⚕ 4.80 **FUD** XXX S 80 TC ▭
AMA: 2015,Jan,16; 2014,Jan,11; 2012,Jan,15-42; 2011,Oct,5-7

93272 **review and interpretation by a physician or other qualified health care professional**
📷 0.72 ⚕ 0.72 **FUD** XXX M 80 26 ▭
AMA: 2015,Jan,16; 2014,Jan,11; 2012,Jan,15-42; 2011,Oct,5-7; 2011,Jan,11

93278 Signal-averaged Electrocardiography

EXCLUDES *Echocardiography (93303-93355)*
ECG with 64 or more leads, graphic presentation, and analysis (0178T-0180T)
Code also modifier 26 for the interpretation and report only

93278 **Signal-averaged electrocardiography (SAECG), with or without ECG**
📷 0.86 ⚕ 0.86 **FUD** XXX 01 80 ▭
AMA: 2015,Jan,16; 2014,Jan,11; 2012,Jan,15-42; 2011,Oct,5-7

93279-93299 [93260, 93261] Monitoring of Cardiovascular Devices

INCLUDES Implantable defibrillator interrogation:
Battery
Capture and sensing functions
Leads
Presence or absence of therapy for ventricular tachyarrhythmias
Programmed parameters
Underlying heart rhythm
Implantable cardiovascular monitor (ICM) interrogation:
Analysis of at least one recorded physiologic cardiovascular data element from either internal or external sensors
Programmed parameters
Implantable loop recorder (ILR) interrogation:
Heart rate and rhythm during recorded episodes from both patient-initiated and device detected events
Programmed parameters
Interrogation evaluation of device
Pacemaker interrogation:
Battery
Capture and sensing functions
Heart rhythm
Leads
Programmed parameters
Time period established by the initiation of remote monitoring or the 91st day of implantable defibrillator or pacemaker monitoring or the 31st day of ILR monitoring and extending for the succeeding 30- or 90-day period
EXCLUDES *Evaluation of subcutaneous implantable defibrillator device (93260, 93261)*
Wearable device monitoring (93224-93272)
Do not report in-person and remote interrogation of the same device during the same period
Do not report programming and in-person interrogation on the same day by the same physician

Medicine

93279 — 93293

93279 Programming device evaluation (in person) with iterative adjustment of the implantable device to test the function of the device and select optimal permanent programmed values with analysis, review and report by a physician or other qualified health care professional; single lead pacemaker system

Do not report with (93040-93042, 93268-93272, 93286, 93288)
🚑 1.40   ⚕ 1.40   **FUD** XXX   01 80

AMA: 2015,Jan,16; 2014,Nov,5; 2014,Jul,3; 2014,Jan,11; 2013,Jul,7-9; 2013,Jun,6-8

93280 dual lead pacemaker system

Do not report with (93040-93042, 93268-93272, 93286, 93288)
🚑 1.65   ⚕ 1.65   **FUD** XXX   01 80

AMA: 2015,Jan,16; 2014,Nov,5; 2014,Jul,3; 2014,Jan,11; 2013,Jul,7-9; 2013,Jun,6-8

93281 multiple lead pacemaker system

Do not report with (93040-93042, 93268-93272, 93286, 93288)
🚑 1.92   ⚕ 1.92   **FUD** XXX   01 80

AMA: 2015,Jan,16; 2014,Nov,5; 2014,Jul,3; 2014,Jan,11; 2013,Jul,7-9; 2013,Jun,6-8

93282 single lead transvenous implantable defibrillator system

Do not report with (93040-93042, 93260, 93268-93272, 93287, 93289, 93745)
🚑 1.79   ⚕ 1.79   **FUD** XXX   01 80

AMA: 2015,Jan,16; 2014,Nov,5; 2014,Jul,3; 2014,Jan,11; 2013,Jul,7-9; 2013,Jun,6-8

93283 dual lead transvenous implantable defibrillator system

Do not report with (93040-93042, 93268-93272, 93287, 93289)
🚑 2.30   ⚕ 2.30   **FUD** XXX   01 80

AMA: 2015,Jan,16; 2014,Nov,5; 2014,Jul,3; 2014,Jan,11; 2013,Jul,7-9; 2013,Jun,6-8

93284 multiple lead transvenous implantable defibrillator system

Do not report with (93040-93042, 93268-93272, 93287, 93289)
🚑 2.53   ⚕ 2.53   **FUD** XXX   01 80

AMA: 2015,Jan,16; 2014,Nov,5; 2014,Jul,3; 2014,Jan,11; 2013,Jul,7-9; 2013,Jun,6-8

\# **93260** implantable subcutaneous lead defibrillator system

Do not report with (33240, 33241, [33262], [33270, 33271, 33272, 33273], 93040-93042, 93261, 93268-93272, 93282, 93287)
🚑 1.89   ⚕ 1.89   **FUD** XXX   01 80

AMA: 2015,Jan,16; 2014,Nov,5

93285 implantable loop recorder system

Do not report with (33282, 93040-93042, 93268-93272, 93279-93284, 93291)
🚑 1.19   ⚕ 1.19   **FUD** XXX   01 80

AMA: 2015,Jan,16; 2014,Nov,5; 2014,Jul,3; 2014,Jan,11

93286 Peri-procedural device evaluation (in person) and programming of device system parameters before or after a surgery, procedure, or test with analysis, review and report by a physician or other qualified health care professional; single, dual, or multiple lead pacemaker system

INCLUDES   One evaluation and programming (if performed once before and once after, report as two units)

EXCLUDES   Subcutaneous implantable defibrillator peri-procedural device evaluation and programming (93260, 93261)

Do not report with (93040-93042, 93268-93272, 93279-93281, 93288)
🚑 0.77   ⚕ 0.77   **FUD** XXX   N 80

AMA: 2015,Jan,16; 2014,Nov,5; 2014,Jul,3; 2014,Jan,11; 2013,Jul,7-9; 2013,Jun,6-8

93287 single, dual, or multiple lead implantable defibrillator system

INCLUDES   One evaluation and programming (if performed once before and once after, report as two units)

EXCLUDES   Subcutaneous implantable defibrillator peri-procedural device evaluation and programming (93260, 93261)

Do not report with (93040-93042, 93260, 93261, 93268-93272, 93282-93284, 93289)
🚑 1.02   ⚕ 1.02   **FUD** XXX   N 80

AMA: 2015,Jan,16; 2014,Nov,5; 2014,Jul,3; 2014,Jan,11; 2013,Jul,7-9; 2013,Jun,6-8

93288 Interrogation device evaluation (in person) with analysis, review and report by a physician or other qualified health care professional, includes connection, recording and disconnection per patient encounter; single, dual, or multiple lead pacemaker system

Do not report with (93040-93042, 93268-93272, 93279-93281, 93286, 93294, 93296)
🚑 1.06   ⚕ 1.06   **FUD** XXX   01 80

AMA: 2015,Jan,16; 2014,Nov,5; 2014,Jul,3; 2014,Jan,11; 2013,Jul,7-9; 2013,Jun,6-8

93289 single, dual, or multiple lead transvenous implantable defibrillator system, including analysis of heart rhythm derived data elements

EXCLUDES   Monitoring physiologic cardiovascular data elements derived from an implantable defibrillator (93290)

Do not report with (93040-93042, 93261, 93268-93272, 93282-93284, 93287, 93295-93296)
🚑 1.84   ⚕ 1.84   **FUD** XXX   01 80

AMA: 2015,Jan,16; 2014,Nov,5; 2014,Jul,3; 2014,Jan,11; 2013,Jul,7-9; 2013,Jun,6-8

\# **93261** implantable subcutaneous lead defibrillator system

Do not report with (33240, 33241, [33262], [33270, 33271, 33272, 33273], 93040-93042, 93260, 93268-93272, 93287, 93289)
🚑 1.73   ⚕ 1.73   **FUD** XXX   01 80

AMA: 2015,Jan,16; 2014,Nov,5

93290 implantable cardiovascular monitor system, including analysis of 1 or more recorded physiologic cardiovascular data elements from all internal and external sensors

EXCLUDES   Heart rhythm derived data (93289)

Do not report with (93297, 93299)
🚑 0.87   ⚕ 0.87   **FUD** XXX   01 80

AMA: 2015,Jan,16; 2014,Nov,5; 2014,Jul,3; 2014,Jan,11; 2013,Apr,10-11; 2012,Jan,15-42; 2011,Jan,11; 2010,Jan,12-15

93291 implantable loop recorder system, including heart rhythm derived data analysis

Do not report with (33282, 93040-93042, 93268-93272, 93288-93290 [93261], 93298-93299)
🚑 1.01   ⚕ 1.01   **FUD** XXX   01 80

AMA: 2015,Jan,16; 2014,Nov,5; 2014,Jul,3; 2014,Jan,11

93292 wearable defibrillator system

Do not report with (93040-93042, 93268-93272, 93745)
🚑 0.91   ⚕ 0.91   **FUD** XXX   01 80

AMA: 2015,Jan,16; 2014,Nov,5; 2014,Jul,3; 2014,Jan,11

93293 Transtelephonic rhythm strip pacemaker evaluation(s) single, dual, or multiple lead pacemaker system, includes recording with and without magnet application with analysis, review and report(s) by a physician or other qualified health care professional, up to 90 days

EXCLUDES   In-person evaluation (93040-93042)

Do not report more than one time in a 90 day period
Do not report when monitoring period is less than 30 days
Do not report with (93040-93042, 93268-93272, 93294)
🚑 1.51   ⚕ 1.51   **FUD** XXX   01 80

AMA: 2015,Jan,16; 2014,Nov,5; 2014,Jul,3; 2014,Jan,11

93294   Interrogation device evaluation(s) (remote), up to 90 days; single, dual, or multiple lead pacemaker system with interim analysis, review(s) and report(s) by a physician or other qualified health care professional

> Do not report more than one time in a 90 day period
> Do not report when monitoring period is less than 30 days
> Do not report with (93040-93042, 93268-93272, 93288, 93293)
> 📖 0.96   ⚕ 0.96   **FUD** XXX   M 80 26
>
> **AMA:** 2015,Jan,16; 2014,Nov,5; 2014,Jul,3; 2014,Jan,11; 2012,Jun,3-9

93295   single, dual, or multiple lead implantable defibrillator system with interim analysis, review(s) and report(s) by a physician or other qualified health care professional

> **EXCLUDES**   *Remote monitoring of physiological cardiovascular data (93297)*
> Do not report more than one time in a 90 day period
> Do not report when monitoring period is less than 30 days
> Do not report with (93040-93042, 93268-93272, 93289)
> 📖 1.91   ⚕ 1.91   **FUD** XXX   M 80 26
>
> **AMA:** 2015,Jan,16; 2014,Nov,5; 2014,Jul,3; 2014,Jan,11

93296   single, dual, or multiple lead pacemaker system or implantable defibrillator system, remote data acquisition(s), receipt of transmissions and technician review, technical support and distribution of results

> Do not report more than one time in a 90-day period
> Do not report when monitoring period is less than 30 days
> Do not report with (93040-93042, 93268-93272, 93288-93289, 93299)
> 📖 0.73   ⚕ 0.73   **FUD** XXX   01 80 TC
>
> **AMA:** 2015,Jan,16; 2014,Nov,5; 2014,Jul,3; 2014,Jan,11

93297   Interrogation device evaluation(s), (remote) up to 30 days; implantable cardiovascular monitor system, including analysis of 1 or more recorded physiologic cardiovascular data elements from all internal and external sensors, analysis, review(s) and report(s) by a physician or other qualified health care professional

> **EXCLUDES**   *Heart rhythm derived data (93295)*
> Do not report more than one time in a 30 day period
> Do not report when monitoring period is less than 10 days
> Do not report with (93290, 93298)
> 📖 0.75   ⚕ 0.75   **FUD** XXX   M 80 26
>
> **AMA:** 2015,Jan,16; 2014,Nov,5; 2014,Jul,3; 2014,Jan,11; 2013,Apr,10-11

93298   implantable loop recorder system, including analysis of recorded heart rhythm data, analysis, review(s) and report(s) by a physician or other qualified health care professional

> Do not report more than one time in a 30 day period
> Do not report when monitoring period is less than 10 days
> Do not report with (33282, 93040-93042, 93268-93272, 93291, 93297)
> 📖 0.75   ⚕ 0.75   **FUD** XXX   M 80 26
>
> **AMA:** 2015,Jan,16; 2014,Nov,5; 2014,Jul,3; 2014,Jan,11

93299   implantable cardiovascular monitor system or implantable loop recorder system, remote data acquisition(s), receipt of transmissions and technician review, technical support and distribution of results

> Do not report more than one time in a 30 day period
> Do not report when monitoring period is less than 10 days
> Do not report with (93040-93042, 93268-93272, 93290-93291, 93296)
> 📖 0.00   ⚕ 0.00   **FUD** XXX   01 80 TC
>
> **AMA:** 2015,Jan,16; 2014,Nov,5; 2014,Jul,3; 2014,Jan,11; 2013,Apr,10-11

93303-93355 Echocardiography

> **INCLUDES**   Interpretation and report
> Obtaining ultrasonic signals from heart/great arteries
> Report of study which includes:
>   Description of recognized abnormalities
>   Documentation of all clinically relevant findings which includes obtained quantitative measurements
>   Interpretation of all information obtained
> Two-dimensional image/doppler ultrasonic signal documentation
> Ultrasound exam of:
>   Adjacent great vessels
>   Cardiac chambers/valves
>   Pericardium
>
> **EXCLUDES**   *Contrast agents and/or drugs used for pharmacological stress Echocardiography, fetal (76825-76828)*
> *Ultrasound with thorough examination of the organ(s) or anatomic region/documentation of the image/final written report*

93303   Transthoracic echocardiography for congenital cardiac anomalies; complete

> 📖 6.69   ⚕ 6.69   **FUD** XXX   S 80 🖵
>
> **AMA:** 2015,May,10; 2015,Jan,16; 2014,Jan,11; 2013,Dec,14; 2013,Aug,3; 2012,Jan,15-42; 2011,Jan,11; 2010,Dec,12; 2010,Jan,8-10

93304   follow-up or limited study

> 📖 4.36   ⚕ 4.36   **FUD** XXX   S 80 🖵
>
> **AMA:** 2015,May,10; 2015,Jan,16; 2014,Jan,11; 2013,Dec,14; 2013,Aug,3; 2010,Dec,12; 2010,Jan,8-10

93306   Echocardiography, transthoracic, real-time with image documentation (2D), includes M-mode recording, when performed, complete, with spectral Doppler echocardiography, and with color flow Doppler echocardiography

> **INCLUDES**   Doppler and color flow
> Two-dimensional and M-mode
> **EXCLUDES**   *Transthoracic without spectral and color doppler (93307)*
> 📖 6.40   ⚕ 6.40   **FUD** XXX   S 80
>
> **AMA:** 2015,May,10; 2015,Jan,16; 2013,Aug,3; 2010,Dec,12; 2010,Jan,8-10

93307   Echocardiography, transthoracic, real-time with image documentation (2D), includes M-mode recording, when performed, complete, without spectral or color Doppler echocardiography

> **INCLUDES**   Additional structures that may be viewed such as pulmonary vein or artery, pulmonic valve, inferior vena cava
> Obtaining/recording appropriate measurements
> Two-dimensional/selected M-mode exam of:
>   Adjacent portions of the aorta
>   Aortic/mitral/tricuspid valves
>   Left/right atria
>   Left/right ventricles
>   Pericardium
>   Using multiple views as required to obtain a complete functional/anatomic evaluation
> Do not report with (93320-93321, 93325)
> 📖 3.67   ⚕ 3.67   **FUD** XXX   S 80 🖵
>
> **AMA:** 2015,May,10; 2015,Jan,16; 2014,Jan,11; 2013,Aug,3; 2012,Jan,15-42; 2011,Jan,11; 2010,Dec,12; 2010,Jan,8-10

93308   Echocardiography, transthoracic, real-time with image documentation (2D), includes M-mode recording, when performed, follow-up or limited study

> **INCLUDES**   An exam that does not evaluate/document the attempt to evaluate all the structures that comprise the complete echocardiographic exam
> 📖 3.51   ⚕ 3.51   **FUD** XXX   S 80 🖵
>
> **AMA:** 2015,May,10; 2015,Jan,16; 2014,Jan,11; 2013,Aug,3; 2012,Mar,9-10; 2012,Jan,15-42; 2011,Jan,11; 2010,Dec,12; 2010,Jan,8-10

Medicine

93312 — **93355**

93312 Echocardiography, transesophageal, real-time with image documentation (2D) (with or without M-mode recording); including probe placement, image acquisition, interpretation and report

> Do not report with (93355)
> 🔧 8.62   ⚖ 8.62   **FUD** XXX   ⊙ Ⓢ 80 ▭
>
> **AMA:** 2015,Jan,16; 2014,Jul,8; 2014,Jan,11; 2013,Aug,3; 2012,Oct,14; 2012,Jan,15-42; 2011,Jan,11; 2010,Jan,8-10

93313 placement of transesophageal probe only

> Do not report when performed by same person as (93355)
> 🔧 0.64   ⚖ 0.64   **FUD** XXX   ⊙ Ⓢ 80 ▭
>
> **AMA:** 2015,Jan,16; 2014,Jul,8; 2014,Jan,11; 2013,Aug,3; 2010,Jan,8-10

93314 image acquisition, interpretation and report only

> Do not report with (93355)
> 🔧 8.28   ⚖ 8.28   **FUD** XXX   ⊙ Ⓝ 80 ▭
>
> **AMA:** 2015,Jan,16; 2014,Jul,8; 2014,Jan,11; 2013,Aug,3; 2010,Jan,8-10

93315 Transesophageal echocardiography for congenital cardiac anomalies; including probe placement, image acquisition, interpretation and report

> Do not report with (93355)
> 🔧 0.00   ⚖ 0.00   **FUD** XXX   ⊙ Ⓢ 80 ▭
>
> **AMA:** 2015,Jan,16; 2014,Jul,8; 2014,Jan,11; 2013,Dec,14; 2013,Aug,3; 2010,Jan,8-10

93316 placement of transesophageal probe only

> Do not report with (93355)
> 🔧 1.08   ⚖ 1.08   **FUD** XXX   ⊙ Ⓢ 80 ▭
>
> **AMA:** 2015,Jan,16; 2014,Jan,11; 2013,Dec,14; 2013,Aug,3; 2010,Jan,8-10

93317 image acquisition, interpretation and report only

> Do not report with (93355)
> 🔧 0.00   ⚖ 0.00   **FUD** XXX   ⊙ Ⓝ 80 ▭
>
> **AMA:** 2015,Jan,16; 2014,Jan,11; 2013,Dec,14; 2013,Aug,3; 2010,Jan,8-10

93318 Echocardiography, transesophageal (TEE) for monitoring purposes, including probe placement, real time 2-dimensional image acquisition and interpretation leading to ongoing (continuous) assessment of (dynamically changing) cardiac pumping function and to therapeutic measures on an immediate time basis

> Do not report with (93355)
> 🔧 0.00   ⚖ 0.00   **FUD** XXX   ⊙ Ⓢ 80 ▭
>
> **AMA:** 2015,Jan,16; 2014,Jan,11; 2013,Aug,3; 2010,Apr,6-8; 2010,Jan,8-10

+ 93320 Doppler echocardiography, pulsed wave and/or continuous wave with spectral display (List separately in addition to codes for echocardiographic imaging); complete

> Code first (93303-93304, 93312, 93314-93315, 93317, 93350-93351)
> Do not report with (93355)
> 🔧 1.54   ⚖ 1.54   **FUD** ZZZ   Ⓝ 80 ▭
>
> **AMA:** 2015,Jan,16; 2014,Jan,11; 2013,Aug,3; 2010,Jan,8-10

+ 93321 follow-up or limited study (List separately in addition to codes for echocardiographic imaging)

> Code first (93303-93304, 93308, 93312, 93314-93315, 93317, 93350-93351)
> Do not report with (93355)
> 🔧 0.78   ⚖ 0.78   **FUD** ZZZ   Ⓝ 80 ▭
>
> **AMA:** 2015,Jan,16; 2014,Jan,11; 2013,Aug,3; 2010,Jan,8-10

+ 93325 Doppler echocardiography color flow velocity mapping (List separately in addition to codes for echocardiography)

> Code first (76825-76828, 93303-93304, 93308, 93312, 93314-93315, 93317, 93350-93351)
> Do not report with (93355)
> 🔧 0.74   ⚖ 0.74   **FUD** ZZZ   Ⓝ 80 ▭
>
> **AMA:** 2015,Jan,16; 2014,Jan,11; 2013,Aug,3; 2010,Jan,8-10

93350 Echocardiography, transthoracic, real-time with image documentation (2D), includes M-mode recording, when performed, during rest and cardiovascular stress test using treadmill, bicycle exercise and/or pharmacologically induced stress, with interpretation and report;

> Code also exercise stress testing (93016-93018)
> Do not report with (93015)
> 🔧 6.78   ⚖ 6.78   **FUD** XXX   Ⓢ 80 ▭
>
> **AMA:** 2015,Jan,16; 2014,Jul,8; 2014,Jan,11; 2013,Aug,3; 2012,Jan,15-42; 2011,Jan,11; 2010,Dec,12; 2010,Jan,8-10

93351 including performance of continuous electrocardiographic monitoring, with supervision by a physician or other qualified health care professional

> **INCLUDES** Stress echocardiogram performed with a complete cardiovascular stress test
>
> **EXCLUDES** *Professional only components of complete stress test and stress echocardiogram performed in a facility by same physician, report with modifier 26*
>
> Code also components of cardiovascular stress test when professional services not performed by same physician performing stress echocardiogram (93016-93018)
> Do not report professional component with (93016, 93018, 93350)
> Do not report with (93015-93018, 93350)
> 🔧 7.62   ⚖ 7.62   **FUD** XXX   Ⓢ
>
> **AMA:** 2015,Jan,16; 2014,Jul,8; 2014,Jan,11; 2013,Aug,3; 2012,Jan,15-42; 2011,Jan,11; 2010,Jan,8-10

+ 93352 Use of echocardiographic contrast agent during stress echocardiography (List separately in addition to code for primary procedure)

> Code first (93350, 93351)
> Do not report more than one time for each stress echocardiogram
> 🔧 0.96   ⚖ 0.96   **FUD** ZZZ   Ⓜ 80
>
> **AMA:** 2015,Jan,16; 2014,Jan,11; 2013,Aug,3; 2012,Jan,15-42; 2011,Jan,11; 2010,Dec,12; 2010,Jan,8-10

93355 Echocardiography, transesophageal (TEE) for guidance of a transcatheter intracardiac or great vessel(s) structural intervention(s) (eg,TAVR, transcathether pulmonary valve replacement, mitral valve repair, paravlvular regurgitation repair, left atrial appendage occlusion/closure, ventricular septal defect closure) (peri-and intra-procedural), real-time image acquisition and documentation, guidance with quantitative measurements, probe manipulation, interpretation, and report, including diagnostic transesophageal echocardiography and, when performed, administration of ultrasound contrast, Doppler, color flow, and 3D

> 🔧 6.43   ⚖ 6.43   **FUD** XXX   Ⓝ 80
>
> **EXCLUDES** *Transesophageal probe positioning by different provider (93313)*
>
> Do not report with (76376-76377, 93312-93318, 93320-93321, 93325)

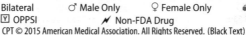

93451-93505 Heart Catheterization

INCLUDES Access site imaging and placement of closure device
Catheter insertion and positioning
Contrast injection (except as listed below)
Imaging and insertion of closure device
Radiology supervision and interpretation
Roadmapping angiography

EXCLUDES *Congenital cardiac cath procedures (93530-93533)*

Code also separately identifiable:
 Aortography (93567)
 Noncardiac angiography (see radiology and vascular codes)
 Pulmonary angiography (93568)
 Right ventricular or atrial injection (93566)

93451 **Right heart catheterization including measurement(s) of oxygen saturation and cardiac output, when performed**

 INCLUDES Cardiac output review
  Insertion catheter into 1+ right cardiac chambers or areas
  Obtaining samples for blood gas

 Code also administration of medication or exercise to repeat assessment of hemodynamic measurement (93463-93464)

 Do not report with (93453, 93456-93457, 93460-93461, 93503, 93561-93562, 93580, 0345T)

 Do not report with insertion of hemodynamic monitor unless done for a reason other than insertion or maintenance of hemodynamic monitoring system (0293T-0294T)

 🔁 22.2 ⚖ 22.2 **FUD** 000 🚫 ⊙ T 80

 AMA: 2015,Jan,16; 2014,Jul,3; 2014,Jan,11; 2013,May,12; 2012,Mar,9-10; 2011,Aug,3-5; 2011,Dec,9-12

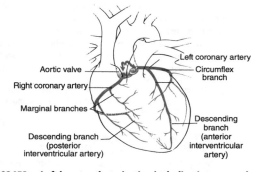

93452 **Left heart catheterization including intraprocedural injection(s) for left ventriculography, imaging supervision and interpretation, when performed**

 INCLUDES Insertion of catheter into left cardiac chambers

 Code also administration of medication or exercise to repeat assessment of hemodynamic measurement (93463-93464)

 Code also transapical or transseptal puncture (93462)

 Do not report with (93453, 93458-93461, 93503, 93561-93565, 93580)

 Do not report with insertion of hemodynamic monitor unless done for a reason other than insertion or maintenance of hemodynamic monitoring system (0293T-0294T)

 🔁 25.1 ⚖ 25.1 **FUD** 000 ⊙ T 80

 AMA: 2015,Jan,16; 2014,Jul,3; 2014,Jan,11; 2013,May,12; 2013,Jan,6-8; 2012,Mar,9-10; 2011,Aug,3-5; 2011,Dec,9-12

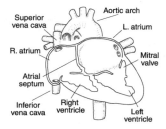

Left heart is catheterized

93453 **Combined right and left heart catheterization including intraprocedural injection(s) for left ventriculography, imaging supervision and interpretation, when performed**

 INCLUDES Cardiac output review
  Insertion catheter into 1+ right cardiac chambers or areas
  Insertion of catheter into left cardiac chambers
  Obtaining samples for blood gas

 Code also administration of medication or exercise to repeat assessment of hemodynamic measurement (93463-93464)

 Code also transapical or transseptal puncture (93462)

 Do not report with (93451-93452, 93456-93461, 93503, 93561-93565, 93580, 0345T)

 Do not report with insertion of hemodynamic monitor unless done for a reason other than insertion or maintenance of hemodynamic monitoring system (0293T-0294T)

 🔁 32.3 ⚖ 32.3 **FUD** 000 ⊙ T 80

 AMA: 2015,Jan,16; 2014,Jul,3; 2014,Jan,11; 2013,May,12; 2013,Jan,6-8; 2012,Mar,9-10; 2011,Aug,3-5; 2011,Dec,9-12

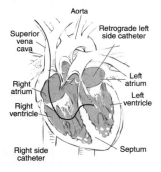

Both sides of the heart are catheterized

93454 **Catheter placement in coronary artery(s) for coronary angiography, including intraprocedural injection(s) for coronary angiography, imaging supervision and interpretation;**

 Do not report with (93503, 93561-93565, 0345T)

 🔁 25.4 ⚖ 25.4 **FUD** 000 ⊙ T 80

 AMA: 2015,Jan,16; 2014,Dec,6; 2014,Jul,3; 2014,Jan,11; 2013,May,12; 2012,Mar,9-10; 2011,Aug,3-5; 2011,Dec,9-12

93455 **with catheter placement(s) in bypass graft(s) (internal mammary, free arterial, venous grafts) including intraprocedural injection(s) for bypass graft angiography**

 Do not report with (93503, 93561-93565, 93580)

 🔁 29.5 ⚖ 29.5 **FUD** 000 ⊙ T 80

 AMA: 2015,Jan,16; 2014,Dec,6; 2014,Jul,3; 2014,Jan,11; 2013,May,12; 2012,Mar,9-10; 2011,Aug,3-5; 2011,Dec,9-12

93456 **with right heart catheterization**

 INCLUDES Cardiac output review
  Insertion catheter into 1+ right cardiac chambers or areas
  Obtaining samples for blood gas

 Code also administration of medication or exercise to repeat assessment of hemodynamic measurement (93463-93464)

 Do not report with (93503, 93561-93565, 93580, 0345T)

 🔁 31.8 ⚖ 31.8 **FUD** 000 🚫 ⊙ T 80

 AMA: 2015,Jan,16; 2014,Dec,6; 2014,Jul,3; 2014,Jan,11; 2013,May,12; 2012,Mar,9-10; 2011,Aug,3-5; 2011,Dec,9-12

93457 **with catheter placement(s) in bypass graft(s) (internal mammary, free arterial, venous grafts) including intraprocedural injection(s) for bypass graft angiography and right heart catheterization**

INCLUDES   Cardiac output review

Insertion catheter into 1+ right cardiac chambers or areas

Obtaining samples for blood gas

Code also administration of medication or exercise to repeat assessment of hemodynamic measurement (93463-93464)

Do not report with (93503, 93561-93565, 93580)

📋 35.9   ⚕ 35.9   **FUD** 000   ⊙ T 80

AMA: 2015,Jan,16; 2014,Dec,6; 2014,Jul,3; 2014,Jan,11; 2013,May,12; 2012,Mar,9-10; 2011,Aug,3-5; 2011,Dec,9-12

93458 **with left heart catheterization including intraprocedural injection(s) for left ventriculography, when performed**

INCLUDES   Insertion of catheter into left cardiac chambers

Code also administration of medication or exercise to repeat assessment of hemodynamic measurement (93463-93464)

Code also transapical or transseptal puncture (93462)

Do not report with (93503, 93561-93565, 93580)

📋 30.4   ⚕ 30.4   **FUD** 000   ⊙ T 80

AMA: 2015,Jan,16; 2014,Dec,6; 2014,Jul,3; 2014,Jan,11; 2013,May,12; 2013,Jan,6-8; 2012,Mar,9-10; 2011,Aug,3-5; 2011,Dec,9-12

93459 **with left heart catheterization including intraprocedural injection(s) for left ventriculography, when performed, catheter placement(s) in bypass graft(s) (internal mammary, free arterial, venous grafts) with bypass graft angiography**

INCLUDES   Insertion of catheter into left cardiac chambers

Code also administration of medication or exercise to repeat assessment of hemodynamic measurement (93463-93464)

Code also transapical or transseptal puncture (93462)

Do not report with (93503, 93561-93565, 93580)

📋 33.6   ⚕ 33.6   **FUD** 000   ⊙ T 80

AMA: 2015,Jan,16; 2014,Dec,6; 2014,Jul,3; 2014,Jan,11; 2013,May,12; 2013,Jan,6-8; 2012,Mar,9-10; 2011,Aug,3-5; 2011,Dec,9-12

93460 **with right and left heart catheterization including intraprocedural injection(s) for left ventriculography, when performed**

INCLUDES   Cardiac output review

Insertion catheter into 1+ right cardiac chambers or areas

Insertion of catheter into left cardiac chambers

Obtaining samples for blood gas

Code also administration of medication or exercise to repeat assessment of hemodynamic measurement (93463-93464)

Code also transapical or transseptal puncture (93462)

Do not report with (93503, 93561-93565, 93580)

📋 36.1   ⚕ 36.1   **FUD** 000   ⊙ T 80

AMA: 2015,Jan,16; 2014,Dec,6; 2014,Jul,3; 2014,Jan,11; 2013,May,12; 2013,Jan,6-8; 2012,Mar,9-10; 2011,Aug,3-5; 2011,Dec,9-12

93461 **with right and left heart catheterization including intraprocedural injection(s) for left ventriculography, when performed, catheter placement(s) in bypass graft(s) (internal mammary, free arterial, venous grafts) with bypass graft angiography**

INCLUDES   Cardiac output review

Insertion catheter into 1+ right cardiac chambers or areas

Insertion of catheter into left cardiac chambers

Obtaining samples for blood gas

Code also administration of medication or exercise to repeat assessment of hemodynamic measurement (93463-93464)

Code also transapical or transseptal puncture (93462)

Do not report with (93503, 93561-93565, 93580, 0345T)

📋 41.3   ⚕ 41.3   **FUD** 000   ⊙ T 80

AMA: 2015,Jan,16; 2014,Dec,6; 2014,Jul,3; 2014,Jan,11; 2013,May,12; 2013,Jan,6-8; 2012,Mar,9-10; 2011,Aug,3-5; 2011,Dec,9-12

+ 93462 **Left heart catheterization by transseptal puncture through intact septum or by transapical puncture (List separately in addition to code for primary procedure)**

INCLUDES   Insertion of catheter into left cardiac chambers

Code first (33477, 93452-93453, 93458-93461, 93582, 93653-93654)

Do not report with (93656, 0345T)

📋 6.03   ⚕ 6.03   **FUD** ZZZ   ⊙ N 80

AMA: 2015,Jan,16; 2014,Jul,3; 2014,Jan,11; 2013,Jun,6-8; 2013,May,12; 2012,Mar,9-10; 2011,Aug,3-5; 2011,Dec,9-12

+ 93463 **Pharmacologic agent administration (eg, inhaled nitric oxide, intravenous infusion of nitroprusside, dobutamine, milrinone, or other agent) including assessing hemodynamic measurements before, during, after and repeat pharmacologic agent administration, when performed (List separately in addition to code for primary procedure)**

Code first (33477, 93451-93453, 93456-93461, 93530-93533, 93580-93581)

Do not report more than one time per catheterization

Do not report with coronary interventional procedures (92920-92944, 92975, 92977)

📋 2.82   ⚕ 2.82   **FUD** ZZZ   ⊙ N 80

AMA: 2015,Jan,16; 2014,Dec,6; 2014,Jul,3; 2014,Jan,11; 2012,Mar,9-10; 2011,Aug,3-5; 2011,Dec,9-12

+ 93464 **Physiologic exercise study (eg, bicycle or arm ergometry) including assessing hemodynamic measurements before and after (List separately in addition to code for primary procedure)**

EXCLUDES   *Administration of pharmacologic agent (93463)*

Bundle of His recording (93600)

Code first (33477, 93451-93453, 93456-93461, 93530-93533)

Do not report more than one time per catheterization

📋 7.76   ⚕ 7.76   **FUD** ZZZ   ⊙ N 80

AMA: 2015,Jan,16; 2014,Jul,3; 2014,Jan,11; 2012,Mar,9-10; 2011,Aug,3-5; 2011,Dec,9-12

93503 **Insertion and placement of flow directed catheter (eg, Swan-Ganz) for monitoring purposes**

EXCLUDES   *Subsequent monitoring (99356-99357)*

Do not report with codes for diagnostic cardiac catheterization (93451-93461, 93530-93533)

📋 3.70   ⚕ 3.70   **FUD** 000   ⊘ T 80 🔲 P0

AMA: 2015,Jan,16; 2014,Jan,11; 2012,Jan,15-42; 2011,Aug,3-5; 2011,Dec,14-18

| 26/TC PC/TC Comp Only | A2-Z3 ASC Pmt | 50 Bilateral | ♂ Male Only | ♀ Female Only | 📋 Facility RVU | ⚕ Non-Facility RVU |
| AMA: CPT Asst | CMS: Pub 100 | A-Y OPPSI | ✎ Non-FDA Drug | | 🔲 Lab Crosswalk | 🔲 Radiology Crosswalk |

410   Medicare (Red Text)   CPT © 2015 American Medical Association. All Rights Reserved. (Black Text)   © 2015 Optum360, LLC (Blue Text)

93505 **Endomyocardial biopsy**

EXCLUDES *Intravascular brachytherapy radionuclide insertion (77770-77772)*

Transcatheter insertion of brachytherapy delivery device (92974)

21.6 21.6 **FUD** 000 ⊙ T 80 ☐ PQ

AMA: 2015,Jan,16; 2014,Jan,11; 2012,Jan,15-42; 2011,Aug,3-5; 2011,Jan,11

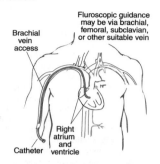

Fluroscopic guidance may be via brachial, femoral, subclavian, or other suitable vein

Brachial vein access

Right atrium and ventricle

Catheter

93530-93533 Congenital Heart Defect Catheterization

INCLUDES Access site imaging and placement of closure device
Cardiac output review
Insertion catheter into 1+ right cardiac chambers or areas
Obtaining samples for blood gas
Radiology supervision and interpretation
Roadmapping angiography

EXCLUDES *Cardiac cath on noncongenital heart (93451-93453, 93456-93461)*
Code also injection procedure (93563-93568)
Do not report with (93503, 93580)

93530 **Right heart catheterization, for congenital cardiac anomalies**

0.00 0.00 **FUD** 000 ⊙ T 80 ☐

AMA: 2015,Jan,16; 2014,Jul,3; 2014,Jan,11; 2013,May,12; 2012,Mar,9-10; 2012,Jan,15-42; 2011,Aug,3-5; 2011,Dec,9-12; 2011,Jan,11

93531 **Combined right heart catheterization and retrograde left heart catheterization, for congenital cardiac anomalies**

0.00 0.00 **FUD** 000 T 80 ☐

AMA: 2015,Jan,16; 2014,Jul,3; 2014,Jan,11; 2012,Mar,9-10; 2011,Aug,3-5; 2011,Dec,9-12

93532 **Combined right heart catheterization and transseptal left heart catheterization through intact septum with or without retrograde left heart catheterization, for congenital cardiac anomalies**

0.00 0.00 **FUD** 000 T 80 ☐

AMA: 2015,Jan,16; 2014,Jul,3; 2014,Jan,11; 2012,Mar,9-10; 2012,Jan,15-42; 2011,Aug,3-5; 2011,Dec,9-12; 2011,Jan,11

93533 **Combined right heart catheterization and transseptal left heart catheterization through existing septal opening, with or without retrograde left heart catheterization, for congenital cardiac anomalies**

0.00 0.00 **FUD** 000 T 80 ☐

AMA: 2015,Jan,16; 2014,Jul,3; 2014,Jan,11; 2012,Mar,9-10; 2011,Aug,3-5; 2011,Dec,9-12

93561-93568 Injection Procedures

INCLUDES Catheter repositioning
Radiology supervision and interpretation
Using automatic power injector

93561 **Indicator dilution studies such as dye or thermodilution, including arterial and/or venous catheterization; with cardiac output measurement (separate procedure)**

EXCLUDES *Cardiac output, radioisotope method (78472-78473, 78481)*

Do not report with (93451-93462, 93582)

0.00 0.00 **FUD** 000 ⊙ N 80 ☐

AMA: 2015,Jan,16; 2014,Jul,3; 2014,Jan,11; 2012,Jan,15-42; 2011,Aug,3-5; 2011,Jan,11

93562 **subsequent measurement of cardiac output**

EXCLUDES *Cardiac output, radioisotope method (78472-78473, 78481)*

Do not report with (93451-93462, 93582)

0.00 0.00 **FUD** 000 ⊙ N 80 ☐

AMA: 2015,Jan,16; 2014,Jul,3; 2014,May,4; 2014,Jan,11; 2011,Aug,3-5

+ **93563** **Injection procedure during cardiac catheterization including imaging supervision, interpretation, and report; for selective coronary angiography during congenital heart catheterization (List separately in addition to code for primary procedure)**

Code first (93530-93533)
Do not report with (93452-93461, 0345T)

1.71 1.71 **FUD** ZZZ ⊙ N 80

AMA: 2015,Jan,16; 2014,Dec,6; 2014,Jan,11; 2013,Jan,6-8; 2011,Aug,3-5; 2011,Dec,9-12

+ **93564** **for selective opacification of aortocoronary venous or arterial bypass graft(s) (eg, aortocoronary saphenous vein, free radial artery, or free mammary artery graft) to one or more coronary arteries and in situ arterial conduits (eg, internal mammary), whether native or used for bypass to one or more coronary arteries during congenital heart catheterization, when performed (List separately in addition to code for primary procedure)**

Code first (93530-93533)
Do not report with (93452-93461, 93580, 0345T)

1.79 1.79 **FUD** ZZZ ⊙ N 80

AMA: 2015,Jan,16; 2014,Dec,6; 2014,Jan,11; 2013,Jan,6-8; 2011,Aug,3-5; 2011,Dec,9-12

+ **93565** **for selective left ventricular or left atrial angiography (List separately in addition to code for primary procedure)**

Code first (93530-93533)
Do not report with (93452-93461, 93580)

1.34 1.34 **FUD** ZZZ ⊙ N 80 PQ

AMA: 2015,Jan,16; 2014,Jan,11; 2013,Jan,6-8; 2011,Aug,3-5; 2011,Dec,9-12

+ **93566** **for selective right ventricular or right atrial angiography (List separately in addition to code for primary procedure)**

Code first (93451, 93453, 93456-93457, 93460-93461, 93530-93533)
Do not report when right ventriculography is performed during insertion leadless pacemaker (0387T)
Do not report with (93580)

1.34 4.85 **FUD** ZZZ ⊙ N 80 PQ

AMA: 2015,May,3; 2015,Jan,16; 2014,Jan,11; 2013,Jan,6-8; 2011,Aug,3-5; 2011,Dec,9-12

+ **93567** **for supravalvular aortography (List separately in addition to code for primary procedure)**

EXCLUDES *Abdominal aortography or non-supravalvular thoracic aortography at same time as cardiac catheterization (36221, 75600-75630)*

Code first (93451-93461, 93530-93533)

1.52 4.02 **FUD** ZZZ ⊙ N 80 PQ

AMA: 2015,Jan,16; 2014,Jan,11; 2013,Jan,6-8; 2011,Aug,3-5; 2011,Dec,9-12

+ **93568** **for pulmonary angiography (List separately in addition to code for primary procedure)**

Code first (93451, 93453, 93456-93457, 93460-93461, 93530-93533)

1.37 4.36 **FUD** ZZZ ⊙ N 80 PQ

AMA: 2015,Jan,16; 2014,Jan,11; 2013,Jan,6-8; 2011,Aug,3-5; 2011,Dec,9-12

93571-93572 Coronary Artery Doppler Studies

> **INCLUDES** Doppler transducer manipulations/repositioning within the vessel examined, during coronary angiography/therapeutic intervention (angioplasty)

+ **93571** **Intravascular Doppler velocity and/or pressure derived coronary flow reserve measurement (coronary vessel or graft) during coronary angiography including pharmacologically induced stress; initial vessel (List separately in addition to code for primary procedure)**

  Code first (92920, 92924, 92928, 92933, 92937, 92941, 92943, 92975, 93454-93461, 93563-93564)

  🖩 0.00　　🖩 0.00　　**FUD** ZZZ　　　　⊙ N 80 ▭

  AMA: 2015,May,10; 2015,Jan,16; 2014,Dec,6; 2014,Jan,11; 2011,Aug,3-5

+ **93572** **each additional vessel (List separately in addition to code for primary procedure)**

  Code first initial vessel (93571)

  🖩 0.00　　🖩 0.00　　**FUD** ZZZ　　　　⊙ N 80

  AMA: 2015,May,10; 2015,Jan,16; 2014,Dec,6; 2014,Jan,11; 2011,Aug,3-5

93580-93583 Percutaneous Repair of Congenital Heart Defects

93580 **Percutaneous transcatheter closure of congenital interatrial communication (ie, Fontan fenestration, atrial septal defect) with implant**

> **INCLUDES** Injection of contrast for atrial/ventricular angiograms
> Right heart catheterization

  Code also echocardiography, when performed (93303-93317, 93662)

  Do not report with (93451-93453, 93455-93461, 93530-93533, 93564-93566)

  🖩 28.3　　🖩 28.3　　**FUD** 000　　　　J 80 ▭

  AMA: 2015,Jan,16; 2014,Jan,11; 2012,Jan,15-42; 2011,Jan,11

93581 **Percutaneous transcatheter closure of a congenital ventricular septal defect with implant**

> **INCLUDES** Injection of contrast for atrial/ventricular angiograms
> Right heart catheterization

  Code also echocardiography, when performed (93303-93317, 93662)

  Do not report with (93451-93453, 93455-93461, 93530-93533, 93564-93566)

  🖩 38.6　　🖩 38.6　　**FUD** 000　　　　J 80 ▭

  AMA: 2015,Jan,16; 2014,Jan,11; 2012,Jan,15-42; 2011,Jan,11

93582 **Percutaneous transcatheter closure of patent ductus arteriosus**

> **INCLUDES** Right and left heart catheterization, aorta catheter placement, and angiography of the aortic arch when performed

> **EXCLUDES** Intracardiac echocardiographic services (93662)
> Left heart catheterization performed via transapical puncture or transseptal puncture through intact septum (93462)
> Ligation repair (33820, 33822, 33824)
> Other cardiac angiographic procedures (93563-93566, 93568)
> Other echocardiographic services by different provider (93315-93317)

  Do not report with (36013-36014, 36200, 75600, 75605, 93451-93461, 93530-93533, 93567)

  🖩 19.5　　🖩 19.5　　**FUD** 000　　　　⊙ J 80

  AMA: 2015,Jan,16; 2014,Jul,3

93583 **Percutaneous transcatheter septal reduction therapy (eg, alcohol septal ablation) including temporary pacemaker insertion when performed**

  🖩 21.7　　🖩 21.7　　**FUD** 000　　　　⊙ ⊙ C 80

> **INCLUDES** Left anterior descending coronary angiography performed to guide the intervention through roadmapping
> Left heart catheterization
> Temporary pacemaker insertion

> **EXCLUDES** Intracardiac echocardiographic services when performed (93662)
> Myectomy (surgical ventriculomyotomy) to treat idiopathic hypertrophic subaortic stenosis (33416)
> Other echocardiographic services rendered by different provider (93312-93317)

  Code also diagnostic cardiac catheterization procedures if the patient's condition (clinical indication) has changed since the intervention or prior study, there is no available prior catheter-based diagnostic study of the treatment zone, or the prior study is not adequate (93451, 93454-93457, 93530, 93563-93564, 93566-93568)

  Do not report alcohol injection (93463)

  Do not report for coronary angiography during the procedure in order to roadmap, guide the intervention, measure the vessel, and complete the angiography (93454-93461, 93563)

  Do not report with (33210-33211, 93452-93453, 93458-93459, 93460-93461, 93531-93533, 93565)

93600-93603 Recording of Intracardiac Electrograms

> **INCLUDES** Unusual situations where there may be recording/pacing/attempt at arrhythmia induction from only one side of the heart

Do not report with (93619-93620, 93653-93654, 93656)

93600 **Bundle of His recording**

  🖩 0.00　　🖩 0.00　　**FUD** 000　　　　⊘ J 80 ▭

  AMA: 2015,Jan,16; 2014,Apr,3; 2014,Jan,11; 2013,Jul,7-9; 2013,Jun,6-8; 2012,Jan,15-42; 2011,Jan,11

93602 **Intra-atrial recording**

  🖩 0.00　　🖩 0.00　　**FUD** 000　　　　⊘ J 80 ▭

  AMA: 2015,Jan,16; 2014,Apr,3; 2014,Jan,11; 2013,Jul,7-9; 2013,Jun,6-8; 2012,Jan,15-42; 2011,Jan,11

93603 **Right ventricular recording**

  🖩 0.00　　🖩 0.00　　**FUD** 000　　　　⊘ J 80 ▭

  AMA: 2015,Jan,16; 2014,Apr,3; 2014,Jan,11; 2013,Jul,7-9; 2013,Jun,6-8

93609-93613 Intracardiac Mapping and Pacing

+ **93609** **Intraventricular and/or intra-atrial mapping of tachycardia site(s) with catheter manipulation to record from multiple sites to identify origin of tachycardia (List separately in addition to code for primary procedure)**

  Code first (93620, 93653, 93656)

  Do not report with (93613, 93654)

  🖩 0.00　　🖩 0.00　　**FUD** ZZZ　　　　⊙ N 80 ▭

  AMA: 2015,Jan,16; 2014,Apr,3; 2014,Jan,11; 2013,Jul,7-9; 2013,Jun,6-8

93610 **Intra-atrial pacing**

> **INCLUDES** Unusual situations where there may be recording/pacing/attempt at arrhythmia induction from only one side of the heart

  Do not report with (93619-93620, 93653-93654, 93656)

  🖩 0.00　　🖩 0.00　　**FUD** 000　　　　⊘ J 80 ▭

  AMA: 2015,Jan,16; 2014,Apr,3; 2014,Jan,11; 2013,Jul,7-9; 2013,Jun,6-8

93612 **Intraventricular pacing**

> **INCLUDES** Unusual situations where there may be recording/pacing/attempt at arrhythmia induction from only one side of the heart

  Do not report with (93619-93622, 93653-93654, 93656)

  🖩 0.00　　🖩 0.00　　**FUD** 000　　　　⊘ J 80 ▭

  AMA: 2015,Jan,16; 2014,Apr,3; 2014,Jan,11; 2013,Jul,7-9; 2013,Jun,6-8

26/TC PC/TC Comp Only	A2-Z3 ASC Pmt	50 Bilateral	♂ Male Only	♀ Female Only	🖩 Facility RVU	🖩 Non-Facility RVU
AMA: CPT Asst	CMS: Pub 100	A-Y OPPSI	⚡ Non-FDA Drug		🖩 Lab Crosswalk	🖩 Radiology Crosswalk

412　　Medicare (Red Text)　　CPT © 2015 American Medical Association. All Rights Reserved. (Black Text)　　© 2015 Optum360, LLC (Blue Text)

+ 93613 Intracardiac electrophysiologic 3-dimensional mapping (List separately in addition to code for primary procedure)

Code first (93620, 93653, 93656)
Do not report with (93609, 93654)

🚗 11.4   ⚖ 11.4   **FUD** ZZZ   ⊙ N 80▢

AMA: 2015,Jan,16; 2014,Apr,3; 2014,Jan,11; 2013,Jul,7-9; 2013,Jun,6-8

93615-93616 Recording and Pacing via Esophagus

93615 Esophageal recording of atrial electrogram with or without ventricular electrogram(s);

🚗 0.00   ⚖ 0.00   **FUD** 000   ⊘ ⊙ J 80▢

AMA: 2015,Jan,16; 2014,Jan,11

93616 with pacing

🚗 0.00   ⚖ 0.00   **FUD** 000   ⊘ ⊙ J 80▢

AMA: 2015,Jan,16; 2014,Jan,11

93618 Pacing to Produce an Arrhythmia

CMS: 100-3,20.12 Diagnostic Endocardial Electrical Stimulation (Pacing)

INCLUDES Unusual situations where there may be recording/pacing/attempt at arrhythmia induction from only one side of the heart

EXCLUDES Intracardiac phonocardiogram (93799)

Do not report with (93619-93622, 93653-93654, 93656)

93618 Induction of arrhythmia by electrical pacing

🚗 0.00   ⚖ 0.00   **FUD** 000   ⊘ ⊙ J 80▢

AMA: 2015,Jan,16; 2014,Apr,3; 2014,Jan,11; 2013,Jul,7-9; 2013,Jun,6-8; 2012,Jan,15-42; 2011,Jan,11

93619-93623 Comprehensive Electrophysiological Studies

CMS: 100-3,20.12 Diagnostic Endocardial Electrical Stimulation (Pacing)

93619 Comprehensive electrophysiologic evaluation with right atrial pacing and recording, right ventricular pacing and recording, His bundle recording, including insertion and repositioning of multiple electrode catheters, without induction or attempted induction of arrhythmia

INCLUDES Evaluation of sinus node/atrioventricular node/His-Purkinje conduction system without arrhythmia induction

Do not report with (93600, 93602-93603, 93610, 93612, 93618, 93620-93622, 93653-93657)

🚗 0.00   ⚖ 0.00   **FUD** 000   ⊙ J 80▢

AMA: 2015,Jan,16; 2014,Apr,3; 2014,Jan,11; 2013,Jul,7-9; 2013,Jun,6-8; 2012,Nov,6-9; 2012,Jan,15-42; 2011,Jan,11

93620 Comprehensive electrophysiologic evaluation including insertion and repositioning of multiple electrode catheters with induction or attempted induction of arrhythmia; with right atrial pacing and recording, right ventricular pacing and recording, His bundle recording

INCLUDES Recording/pacing/attempted arrhythmia induction from one or more site(s) in the heart

Do not report with (93600, 93602-93603, 93610, 93612, 93618-93619, 93653-93657)

🚗 0.00   ⚖ 0.00   **FUD** 000   ⊙ J 80▢

AMA: 2015,Jan,16; 2014,Apr,3; 2014,Jan,11; 2013,Jul,7-9; 2013,Jun,6-8; 2012,Nov,6-9; 2012,Jan,15-42; 2011,Jan,11

+ 93621 with left atrial pacing and recording from coronary sinus or left atrium (List separately in addition to code for primary procedure)

INCLUDES Recording/pacing/attempted arrhythmia induction from one or more site(s) in the heart

Code first (93620, 93653-93654)
Do not report with (93656)

🚗 0.00   ⚖ 0.00   **FUD** ZZZ   ⊙ N 80▢

AMA: 2015,Jan,16; 2014,Apr,3; 2014,Jan,11; 2013,Jul,7-9; 2013,Jun,6-8; 2012,Nov,6-9; 2012,Jan,15-42; 2011,Jan,11

+ 93622 with left ventricular pacing and recording (List separately in addition to code for primary procedure)

Code first (93620, 93653, 93656)
Do not report with (93654)

🚗 0.00   ⚖ 0.00   **FUD** ZZZ   ⊙ N 80▢

AMA: 2015,Jan,16; 2014,Apr,3; 2014,Jan,11; 2013,Jul,7-9; 2013,Jun,6-8; 2012,Nov,6-9; 2012,Jan,15-42; 2011,Jan,11

+ 93623 Programmed stimulation and pacing after intravenous drug infusion (List separately in addition to code for primary procedure)

INCLUDES Recording/pacing/attempted arrhythmia induction from one or more site(s) in the heart

Code first comprehensive electrophysiologic evaluation (93610, 93612, 93619-93620, 93653-93654, 93656)

🚗 0.00   ⚖ 0.00   **FUD** ZZZ   N 80▢

AMA: 2015,Jan,16; 2014,Apr,3; 2014,Jan,11; 2013,Jul,7-9; 2012,Jan,15-42; 2011,Jan,11

93624-93631 Followup and Intraoperative Electrophysiologic Studies

CMS: 100-3,20.12 Diagnostic Endocardial Electrical Stimulation (Pacing)

93624 Electrophysiologic follow-up study with pacing and recording to test effectiveness of therapy, including induction or attempted induction of arrhythmia

INCLUDES Recording/pacing/attempted arrhythmia induction from one or more site(s) in the heart

🚗 0.00   ⚖ 0.00   **FUD** 000   ⊙ J 80▢

AMA: 2015,Jan,16; 2014,Jan,11

93631 Intra-operative epicardial and endocardial pacing and mapping to localize the site of tachycardia or zone of slow conduction for surgical correction

EXCLUDES Operative ablation of an arrhythmogenic focus or pathway by a separate provider (33250-33261)

🚗 0.00   ⚖ 0.00   **FUD** 000   ⊘ N 80▢

AMA: 2015,Jan,16; 2014,Jan,11

93640-93644 Electrophysiologic Studies of Cardioverter-Defibrillators

INCLUDES Recording/pacing/attempted arrhythmia induction from one or more site(s) in the heart

93640 Electrophysiologic evaluation of single or dual chamber pacing cardioverter-defibrillator leads including defibrillation threshold evaluation (induction of arrhythmia, evaluation of sensing and pacing for arrhythmia termination) at time of initial implantation or replacement;

🚗 0.00   ⚖ 0.00   **FUD** 000   ⊙ N 80▢

AMA: 2015,Jan,16; 2014,Jan,11; 2012,Jun,3-9

93641 with testing of single or dual chamber pacing cardioverter-defibrillator pulse generator

EXCLUDES Single/dual chamber pacing cardioverter-defibrillators reprogramming/electronic analysis, subsequent/periodic (93282-93283, 93289, 93292, 93295, 93642)

🚗 0.00   ⚖ 0.00   **FUD** 000   ⊙ N 80▢

AMA: 2015,Jan,16; 2014,Apr,3; 2014,Jan,11; 2012,Jun,3-9

93642 Electrophysiologic evaluation of single or dual chamber transvenous pacing cardioverter-defibrillator (includes defibrillation threshold evaluation, induction of arrhythmia, evaluation of sensing and pacing for arrhythmia termination, and programming or reprogramming of sensing or therapeutic parameters)

🚗 12.1   ⚖ 12.1   **FUD** 000   ⊙ J 80▢

AMA: 2015,Jan,16; 2014,Apr,3; 2014,Jan,11; 2013,Jul,7-9; 2013,Jun,6-8

93644 Electrophysiologic evaluation of subcutaneous implantable defibrillator (includes defibrillation threshold evaluation, induction of arrhythmia, evaluation of sensing for arrhythmia termination, and programming or reprogramming of sensing or therapeutic parameters)

🚗 8.48   ⚖ 8.48   **FUD** 000   ⊙ N 80

EXCLUDES Subcutaneous cardioverter-defibrillator electrophysiologic evaluation, subsequent/periodic (93260-93261)

Do not report with ([33270])

93650-93657 Intracardiac Ablation

INCLUDES   Ablation services include selective delivery of cryo-energy or radiofrequency to targeted tissue
Electrophysiologic studies performed in the same session with ablation

93650   **Intracardiac catheter ablation of atrioventricular node function, atrioventricular conduction for creation of complete heart block, with or without temporary pacemaker placement**

🚑 17.4   ✂ 17.4   **FUD** 000   ⊙ J 80 ▢

AMA: 2015,Jan,16; 2014,Jan,11; 2012,May,14-15; 2012,Apr,17-18

93653   **Comprehensive electrophysiologic evaluation including insertion and repositioning of multiple electrode catheters with induction or attempted induction of an arrhythmia with right atrial pacing and recording, right ventricular pacing and recording (when necessary), and His bundle recording (when necessary) with intracardiac catheter ablation of arrhythmogenic focus; with treatment of supraventricular tachycardia by ablation of fast or slow atrioventricular pathway, accessory atrioventricular connection, cavo-tricuspid isthmus or other single atrial focus or source of atrial re-entry**

Do not report with (93600-93603, 93610, 93612, 93618-93620, 93642, 93654, 93656)

🚑 24.5   ✂ 24.5   **FUD** 000   ⊙ J 80

AMA: 2015,Jan,16; 2014,Apr,3; 2013,Jul,7-9; 2013,Jun,6-8

93654   **with treatment of ventricular tachycardia or focus of ventricular ectopy including intracardiac electrophysiologic 3D mapping, when performed, and left ventricular pacing and recording, when performed**

Do not report with (93279-93284, 93286-93289, 93600-93603, 93609-93610, 93612-93613, 93618-93620, 93622, 93642, 93653, 93656)

🚑 32.7   ✂ 32.7   **FUD** 000   ⊙ J 80 ▢

AMA: 2015,Jan,16; 2014,Apr,3; 2013,Jul,7-9; 2013,Jun,6-8

+ **93655**   **Intracardiac catheter ablation of a discrete mechanism of arrhythmia which is distinct from the primary ablated mechanism, including repeat diagnostic maneuvers, to treat a spontaneous or induced arrhythmia (List separately in addition to code for primary procedure)**

Code first (93653-93654, 93656)

🚑 12.2   ✂ 12.2   **FUD** ZZZ   ⊙ N 80

AMA: 2015,Jan,16; 2014,Apr,3; 2013,Jul,7-9; 2013,Jun,6-8

93656   **Comprehensive electrophysiologic evaluation including transseptal catheterizations, insertion and repositioning of multiple electrode catheters with induction or attempted induction of an arrhythmia including left or right atrial pacing/recording when necessary, right ventricular pacing/recording when necessary, and His bundle recording when necessary with intracardiac catheter ablation of atrial fibrillation by pulmonary vein isolation**

INCLUDES   His bundle recording when indicated
Left atrial pacing/recording
Right ventricular pacing/recording

Do not report with (93279-93284, 93286-93289, 93462, 93600, 93602-93603, 93610, 93612, 93618-93621, 93653-93654)

🚑 32.8   ✂ 32.8   **FUD** 000   ⊙ J 80

AMA: 2015,Jan,16; 2014,Apr,3; 2013,Jul,7-9; 2013,Jun,6-8

+ **93657**   **Additional linear or focal intracardiac catheter ablation of the left or right atrium for treatment of atrial fibrillation remaining after completion of pulmonary vein isolation (List separately in addition to code for primary procedure)**

Code first (93656)

🚑 12.2   ✂ 12.2   **FUD** ZZZ   ⊙ N 80

AMA: 2015,Jan,16; 2014,Apr,3; 2013,Jul,7-9; 2013,Jun,6-8

93660-93662 Other Tests for Cardiac Function

93660   **Evaluation of cardiovascular function with tilt table evaluation, with continuous ECG monitoring and intermittent blood pressure monitoring, with or without pharmacological intervention**

EXCLUDES   Autonomic nervous system function testing (95921, 95924, [95943])

🚑 4.46   ✂ 4.46   **FUD** 000   S 80 ▢

AMA: 2015,Jan,16; 2014,Jan,11; 2012,Nov,6-9

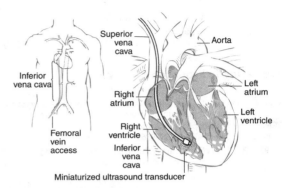

Superior vena cava
Aorta
Inferior vena cava
Right atrium
Left atrium
Left ventricle
Femoral vein access
Right ventricle
Inferior vena cava
Miniaturized ultrasound transducer

+ **93662**   **Intracardiac echocardiography during therapeutic/diagnostic intervention, including imaging supervision and interpretation (List separately in addition to code for primary procedure)**

Code first (as appropriate) (92987, 93453, 93460-93462, 93532, 93580-93581, 93620-93622, 93653-93654, 93656)

Do not report with internal cardioversion (92961)

🚑 0.00   ✂ 0.00   **FUD** ZZZ   N 80 ▢

AMA: 2015,Jan,16; 2014,Jan,11; 2012,Jan,15-42; 2011,Jan,11

93668 Rehabilitation Services: Peripheral Arterial Disease

INCLUDES   Monitoring:
Other cardiovascular limitations for adjustment of workload
Patient's claudication threshold
Motorized treadmill or track
Sessions lasting 45-60 minutes
Supervision by exercise physiologist/nurse
Code also appropriate evaluation and management service, when performed

93668   **Peripheral arterial disease (PAD) rehabilitation, per session**

🚑 0.54   ✂ 0.54   **FUD** XXX   E

AMA: 2008,Mar,4-5

93701-93702 Thoracic Electrical Bioimpedance

EXCLUDES   Bioelectrical impedance analysis whole body (0358T)
Indirect measurement of left ventricular filling pressure by computerized calibration of the arterial waveform response to Valsalva (93799)

93701   **Bioimpedance-derived physiologic cardiovascular analysis**

🚑 0.69   ✂ 0.69   **FUD** XXX   Q1 80 TC

AMA: 2015,Jan,16; 2014,Jan,11

93702   **Bioimpedance spectroscopy (BIS), extracellular fluid analysis for lymphedema assessment(s)**

🚑 3.20   ✂ 3.20   **FUD** XXX   S 80 TC

93724 Electronic Analysis of Pacemaker Function

93724   **Electronic analysis of antitachycardia pacemaker system (includes electrocardiographic recording, programming of device, induction and termination of tachycardia via implanted pacemaker, and interpretation of recordings)**

🚑 7.74   ✂ 7.74   **FUD** 000   S 80 ▢

AMA: 2015,Jan,16; 2014,Jan,11

93740 Temperature Gradient Assessment

93740   **Temperature gradient studies**

🚑 0.23   ✂ 0.23   **FUD** XXX   Q1

93745 Wearable Cardioverter-Defibrillator System Services

Do not report with (93282, 93292)

93745 **Initial set-up and programming by a physician or other qualified health care professional of wearable cardioverter-defibrillator includes initial programming of system, establishing baseline electronic ECG, transmission of data to data repository, patient instruction in wearing system and patient reporting of problems or events**

    🚑 0.00   ⚕ 0.00 **FUD** XXX   [S] [80] [▭]

    AMA: 2009,Mar,5-7; 2009,Feb,3-12

93750 Ventricular Assist Device (VAD) Interrogation

CMS: 100-3,20.9 Artificial Hearts and Related Devices; 100-3,20.9.1 Ventricular Assist Devices; 100-4,32,320.1 Artificial Hearts Prior to May 1, 2008; 100-4,32,320.2 Coding for Artificial Hearts After May 1, 2008; 100-4,32,320.3 Ventricular Assist Devices; 100-4,32,320.3.1 Post-cardiotomy; 100-4,32,320.3.2 Bridge- to -Transplantation
Do not report with (33975-33976, 33979, 33981-33983)

93750 **Interrogation of ventricular assist device (VAD), in person, with physician or other qualified health care professional analysis of device parameters (eg, drivelines, alarms, power surges), review of device function (eg, flow and volume status, septum status, recovery), with programming, if performed, and report**

    🚑 1.32   ⚕ 1.58 **FUD** XXX   [S] [80]

    AMA: 2015,Jan,16; 2014,Jan,11; 2010,Apr,6-8

93770 Peripheral Venous Blood Pressure Assessment

CMS: 100-3,20.19 Ambulatory Blood Pressure Monitoring (20.19)
   EXCLUDES   *Cannulization, central venous (36500, 36555-36556)*

93770 **Determination of venous pressure**

    🚑 0.23   ⚕ 0.23 **FUD** XXX   [N]

93784-93790 Ambulatory Blood Pressure Monitoring

CMS: 100-3,20.19 Ambulatory Blood Pressure Monitoring (20.19); 100-4,32,10.1 Ambulatory Blood Pressure Monitoring Billing Requirements

93784 **Ambulatory blood pressure monitoring, utilizing a system such as magnetic tape and/or computer disk, for 24 hours or longer; including recording, scanning analysis, interpretation and report**

    🚑 1.52   ⚕ 1.52 **FUD** XXX   [B] [80] [▭]

    AMA: 1991,Win,1

93786 **recording only**

    🚑 0.84   ⚕ 0.84 **FUD** XXX   [01] [80] [TC]

93788 **scanning analysis with report**

    🚑 0.15   ⚕ 0.15 **FUD** XXX   [01] [80] [TC]

93790 **review with interpretation and report**

    🚑 0.53   ⚕ 0.53 **FUD** XXX   [M] [80] [26]

93797-93799 Cardiac Rehabilitation

CMS: 100-2,15,232 Cardiac Rehabilitation and Intensive Cardiac Rehabilitation; 100-4,32,140.2 Cardiac Rehabilitation On or After January 1, 2010; 100-4,32,140.2.1 Coding Cardiac Rehabilitation Services On or After January 1, 2010; 100-4,32,140.2.2.2 Institutional Claims for CR and ICR Services; 100-4,32,140.2.2.4 CR Services Exceeding 36 Sessions; 100-4,32,140.3 Intensive Cardiac Rehabilitation On or After January 1, 2010

93797 **Physician or other qualified health care professional services for outpatient cardiac rehabilitation; without continuous ECG monitoring (per session)**

    🚑 0.25   ⚕ 0.46 **FUD** 000   [S] [80] [▭]

93798 **with continuous ECG monitoring (per session)**

    🚑 0.40   ⚕ 0.71 **FUD** 000   [S] [80] [▭]

    AMA: 2005,Nov,1-9

93799 **Unlisted cardiovascular service or procedure**

    🚑 0.00   ⚕ 0.00 **FUD** XXX   [S] [80]

    AMA: 2015,Jan,16; 2014,Jan,11; 2013,Dec,16; 2012,Jan,15-42; 2011,Oct,5-7; 2011,Jan,11; 2010,Jul,10

93880-93895 Noninvasive Tests Extracranial/Intracranial Arteries

   INCLUDES   Patient care required to perform/supervise studies and interpret results
Do not report for hand-held dopplers that do not provide a hard copy (See E&M codes)
Do not report for hand-held dopplers that do not permit vascular flow bidirectional analysis (see E&M codes)

93880 **Duplex scan of extracranial arteries; complete bilateral study**

    Do not report with (93895, 0126T)

    🚑 5.71   ⚕ 5.71 **FUD** XXX   [S] [80] [▭] [PQ]

    AMA: 2015,Jan,16; 2014,Jan,11

93882 **unilateral or limited study**

    Do not report with (93895, 0126T)

    🚑 3.64   ⚕ 3.64 **FUD** XXX   [S] [80] [▭] [PQ]

    AMA: 2015,Jan,16; 2014,Jan,11

93886 **Transcranial Doppler study of the intracranial arteries; complete study**

    INCLUDES   Complete transcranial doppler (TCD) study
         Ultrasound evaluation of right/left anterior circulation territories and posterior circulation territory

    🚑 8.12   ⚕ 8.12 **FUD** XXX   [S] [80] [▭]

    AMA: 2015,Jan,16; 2014,Jan,11

93888 **limited study**

    INCLUDES   Limited TCD study
         Ultrasound examination of two or fewer of these territories (right/left anterior circulation, posterior circulation)

    🚑 4.22   ⚕ 4.22 **FUD** XXX   [S] [80] [▭]

    AMA: 2015,Jan,16; 2014,Jan,11

93890 **vasoreactivity study**

    Do not report with limited TCD study (93888)

    🚑 8.22   ⚕ 8.22 **FUD** XXX   [S] [80] [▭]

    AMA: 2015,Jan,16; 2014,Jan,11

93892 **emboli detection without intravenous microbubble injection**

    Do not report with limited TCD study (93888)

    🚑 9.53   ⚕ 9.53 **FUD** XXX   [S] [80] [▭]

    AMA: 2015,Jan,16; 2014,Jan,11

93893 **emboli detection with intravenous microbubble injection**

    Do not report with limited TCD study (93888)

    🚑 9.78   ⚕ 9.78 **FUD** XXX   [S] [80] [▭]

    AMA: 2015,Jan,16; 2014,Jan,11

93895 **Quantitative carotid intima media thickness and carotid atheroma evaluation, bilateral**

    🚑 0.00   ⚕ 0.00 **FUD** XXX   [E] [80]

    Do not report with (93880, 93882, 0126T)

93922-93971 Noninvasive Vascular Studies: Extremities

INCLUDES Patient care required to perform/supervise studies and interpret results

Do not report for hand-held dopplers that do not permit vascular flow bidirectional analysis (see E&M codes)

Do not report for hand-held dopplers that do not provide a hard copy (See E&M codes)

93922 **Limited bilateral noninvasive physiologic studies of upper or lower extremity arteries, (eg, for lower extremity: ankle/brachial indices at distal posterior tibial and anterior tibial/dorsalis pedis arteries plus bidirectional, Doppler waveform recording and analysis at 1-2 levels, or ankle/brachial indices at distal posterior tibial and anterior tibial/dorsalis pedis arteries plus volume plethysmography at 1-2 levels, or ankle/brachial indices at distal posterior tibial and anterior tibial/dorsalis pedis arteries with, transcutaneous oxygen tension measurement at 1-2 levels)**

INCLUDES Evaluation of:
Doppler analysis of bidirectional blood flow
Nonimaging physiologic recordings of pressure
Oxygen tension measurements and/or plethysmography
Lower extremity (potential levels include high thigh, low thigh, calf, ankle, metatarsal and toes) limited study includes either:
Ankle/brachial indices at distal posterior tibial and anterior tibial/dorsalis pedis arteries plus bidirectional Doppler waveform recording and analysis as 1-2 levels; OR
Ankle/brachial indices at distal posterior tibial and anterior tibial/dorsalis pedis arteries plus volume plethysmography at 1-2 levels; OR
Ankle/brachial indices at distal posterior tibial and anterior tibial/dorsalis pedis arteries with transcutaneous oxygen tension measurements at 1-2 levels
Unilateral provocative functional measurement
Unilateral study of 3 or move levels
Upper extremity (potential levels include arm, forearm, wrist, and digits) limited study includes:
Doppler-determined systolic pressures and bidirectional waveform recording with analysis at 1-2 levels; OR
Doppler-determined systolic pressures and transcutaneous oxygen tension measurements at 1-2 levels; OR
Doppler-determined systolic pressures and volume plethysmography at 1-2 levels

EXCLUDES *Transcutaneous oxyhemoglobin measurement in wound of lower extremity by near infrared spectroscopy (0286T)*

Code also modifier 52 for unilateral study of 1-2 levels
Code also twice with modifier 59 for upper and lower extremity study
Do not report more than one time for the lower extremity(s)
Do not report more than one time for the upper extremity(s)
Do not report with (0337T)

🔧 2.53 ⚗ 2.53 **FUD** XXX   S 80 ▢

AMA: 2015,Jan,16; 2014,Jan,9; 2014,Jan,11; 2013,Jun,13; 2012,Jun,15-16

93923 **Complete bilateral noninvasive physiologic studies of upper or lower extremity arteries, 3 or more levels (eg, for lower extremity: ankle/brachial indices at distal posterior tibial and anterior tibial/dorsalis pedis arteries plus segmental blood pressure measurements with bidirectional Doppler waveform recording and analysis, at 3 or more levels, or ankle/brachial indices at distal posterior tibial and anterior tibial/dorsalis pedis arteries plus segmental volume plethysmography at 3 or more levels, or ankle/brachial indices at distal posterior tibial and anterior tibial/dorsalis pedis arteries plus segmental transcutaneous oxygen tension measurements at 3 or more levels), or single level study with provocative functional maneuvers (eg, measurements with postural provocative tests, or measurements with reactive hyperemia)**

INCLUDES Evaluation of:
Doppler analysis of bidirectional blood flow
Nonimaging physiologic recordings of pressures
Oxygen tension measurements
Lower extremity:
Ankle/brachial indices at distal posterior tibial and anterior tibial/dorsalis pedis arteries plus bidirectional Doppler waveform recording and analysis at 3 or more levels; OR
Ankle/brachial indices at distal posterior tibial and anterior tibial/dorsalis pedis arteries with transcutaneous oxygen tension measurements at 3 or more levels; OR
Ankle/brachial indices at distal posterior tibial and anterior tibial/dorsalis pedis arteries plus volume plethysmography at 3 or more levels; OR
Provocative functional maneuvers and measurement at a single level
Upper extremity complete study:
Doppler-determined systolic pressures and bidirectional waveform recording with analysis at 3 or more levels; OR
Doppler-determined systolic pressures and transcutaneous oxygen tension measurements at 3 or more levels; OR
Doppler-determined systolic pressures and volume plethysmography at 3 or more levels; OR
Provocative functional maneuvers and measurement at a single level

EXCLUDES *Transcutaneous oxyhemoglobin measurement in wound of lower extremity by near infrared spectroscopy (0286T)*
Unilateral study at 3 or more levels (93922)

Code also twice with modifier 59 for upper and lower extremity study
Do not report more than one time for the lower extremity(s)
Do not report more than one time for the upper extremity(s)
Do not report with (0337T)

🔧 3.92 ⚗ 3.92 **FUD** XXX   S 80 ▢

AMA: 2015,Jan,16; 2014,Jan,9; 2014,Jan,11; 2012,Jun,15-16; 2012,Jan,15-42; 2011,Jan,11

93924 **Noninvasive physiologic studies of lower extremity arteries, at rest and following treadmill stress testing, (ie, bidirectional Doppler waveform or volume plethysmography recording and analysis at rest with ankle/brachial indices immediately after and at timed intervals following performance of a standardized protocol on a motorized treadmill plus recording of time of onset of claudication or other symptoms, maximal walking time, and time to recovery) complete bilateral study**

INCLUDES Evaluation of:
Doppler analysis of bidirectional blood flow
Non-imaging physiologic recordings of pressures
Oxygen tension measurements
Plethysmography
Do not report this code for other types of exercise
Do not report with (93922-93923)

🔧 4.89 ⚗ 4.89 **FUD** XXX   S 80 ▢

AMA: 2015,Jan,16; 2014,Jan,9; 2014,Jan,11; 2012,Jun,15-16

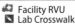
93922 — 93924

93925 Duplex scan of lower extremity arteries or arterial bypass grafts; complete bilateral study
7.37 · 7.37 **FUD** XXX · S 80 ▢
AMA: 2015,Jan,16; 2014,Jan,11

93926 unilateral or limited study
4.34 · 4.34 **FUD** XXX · S 80 ▢
AMA: 2015,Jan,16; 2014,Jan,11

93930 Duplex scan of upper extremity arteries or arterial bypass grafts; complete bilateral study
5.92 · 5.92 **FUD** XXX · S 80 ▢
AMA: 2015,Jan,16; 2014,Jan,11

93931 unilateral or limited study
3.68 · 3.68 **FUD** XXX · S 80 ▢
AMA: 2015,Jan,16; 2014,Jan,11

93965 Noninvasive physiologic studies of extremity veins, complete bilateral study (eg, Doppler waveform analysis with responses to compression and other maneuvers, phleborheography, impedance plethysmography)
INCLUDES Evaluation of:
Doppler analysis of bidirectional blood flow
Nonimaging physiologic recordings of pressures
Oxygen tension measurements
Plethysmography
3.41 · 3.41 **FUD** XXX · S 80 ▢
AMA: 2015,Jan,16; 2014,Jan,11

93970 Duplex scan of extremity veins including responses to compression and other maneuvers; complete bilateral study
Do not report with (36475-36476, 36478-36479)
5.58 · 5.58 **FUD** XXX · S 80 ▢
AMA: 2015,Jan,16; 2014,Oct,6; 2014,Jan,11; 2012,Feb,11; 2012,Jan,13-14

93971 unilateral or limited study
Do not report with (36475-36476, 36478-36479)
3.43 · 3.43 **FUD** XXX · S 80 ▢
AMA: 2015,Aug,8; 2015,Jan,16; 2014,Oct,6; 2014,Jan,11; 2012,Feb,11; 2012,Jan,13-14; 2012,Jan,15-42; 2011,Apr,12; 2011,Jan,11; 2010,Jul,6

93975-93982 Noninvasive Vascular Studies: Abdomen/Chest/Pelvis

93975 Duplex scan of arterial inflow and venous outflow of abdominal, pelvic, scrotal contents and/or retroperitoneal organs; complete study
7.97 · 7.97 **FUD** XXX · S 80 ▢
AMA: 2015,Mar,9; 2015,Jan,16; 2014,Jun,14; 2014,Jan,11; 2012,Jan,15-42; 2011,Jan,11

93976 limited study
4.62 · 4.62 **FUD** XXX · S 80 ▢
AMA: 2015,Mar,9; 2015,Jan,16; 2014,Jan,11; 2012,Jan,15-42; 2011,Jan,11

93978 Duplex scan of aorta, inferior vena cava, iliac vasculature, or bypass grafts; complete study
5.40 · 5.40 **FUD** XXX · S 80 ▢
AMA: 2015,Jan,16; 2014,Jan,11

93979 unilateral or limited study
3.41 · 3.41 **FUD** XXX · S 80 ▢
AMA: 2015,Jan,16; 2014,Jun,14; 2014,Jan,11

93980 Duplex scan of arterial inflow and venous outflow of penile vessels; complete study
3.38 · 3.38 **FUD** XXX · S 80 ▢
AMA: 2015,Jan,16; 2014,Jan,11

93981 follow-up or limited study
2.03 · 2.03 **FUD** XXX · S 80 ▢
AMA: 2015,Jan,16; 2014,Jan,11

93982 Noninvasive physiologic study of implanted wireless pressure sensor in aneurysmal sac following endovascular repair, complete study including recording, analysis of pressure and waveform tracings, interpretation and report
1.23 · 1.23 **FUD** XXX · S 80
Do not report with (34806)

93990-93998 Noninvasive Vascular Studies: Hemodialysis Access

93990 Duplex scan of hemodialysis access (including arterial inflow, body of access and venous outflow)
EXCLUDES Hemodialysis access flow measurement by indicator method (90940)
4.56 · 4.56 **FUD** XXX · S 80 ▢
AMA: 2015,Jan,16; 2014,Jan,11

93998 Unlisted noninvasive vascular diagnostic study
0.00 · 0.00 **FUD** XXX · Q1 80
AMA: 2015,Jan,16; 2014,Jan,9; 2012,Oct,13; 2012,Sep,9

94002-94005 Ventilator Management Services

94002 Ventilation assist and management, initiation of pressure or volume preset ventilators for assisted or controlled breathing; hospital inpatient/observation, initial day
Do not report with E&M services
2.63 · 2.63 **FUD** XXX · Q3 80
AMA: 2015,Jan,16; 2014,Oct,8; 2014,May,4; 2014,Jan,11; 2012,Jan,15-42; 2011,Jan,11

94003 hospital inpatient/observation, each subsequent day
Do not report with E&M services
1.90 · 1.90 **FUD** XXX · Q3 80
AMA: 2015,Jan,16; 2014,Oct,8; 2014,May,4; 2014,Jan,11

94004 nursing facility, per day
Do not report with E&M services
1.38 · 1.38 **FUD** XXX · B 80
AMA: 2015,Jan,16; 2014,Oct,8; 2014,Jan,11

94005 Home ventilator management care plan oversight of a patient (patient not present) in home, domiciliary or rest home (eg, assisted living) requiring review of status, review of laboratories and other studies and revision of orders and respiratory care plan (as appropriate), within a calendar month, 30 minutes or more
Code also when a different provider reports care plan oversight in the same 30 days (99339-99340, 99374-99378)
2.63 · 2.63 **FUD** XXX · M
AMA: 2015,Jan,16; 2014,Oct,8; 2014,Jan,11; 2012,Jan,15-42; 2011,Jan,11

94010-94799 Respiratory Services: Diagnostic and Therapeutic

INCLUDES Laboratory procedure(s)
Test results interpretation
EXCLUDES Separately identifiable E&M service

94010 Spirometry, including graphic record, total and timed vital capacity, expiratory flow rate measurement(s), with or without maximal voluntary ventilation
INCLUDES Measurement of expiratory airflow and volumes
EXCLUDES Diffusing capacity (94729)
Do not report with (94150, 94200, 94375, 94728)
1.02 · 1.02 **FUD** XXX · Q1 80 ▢
AMA: 2015,Jan,16; 2014,Mar,11; 2014,Jan,11; 2013,Dec,12; 2012,Nov,11-12; 2012,Nov,13-14; 2012,Aug,6-8; 2012,Jan,15-42; 2011,Jan,11; 2010,Dec,12

94011 Measurement of spirometric forced expiratory flows in an infant or child through 2 years of age
2.84 · 2.84 **FUD** XXX · ⊙ Q1 80
AMA: 2015,Jan,16; 2014,Jan,11; 2013,Dec,12; 2012,Aug,6-8; 2011,Jan,11; 2010,May,7

Medicine

93925 — 94011

94012 Measurement of spirometric forced expiratory flows, before and after bronchodilator, in an infant or child through 2 years of age
🚑 4.69   ⚕ 4.69   **FUD** XXX   ⊙ 🔢 🔢
AMA: 2015,Jan,16; 2014,Jan,11; 2013,Dec,12; 2012,Aug,6-8; 2011,Jan,11; 2010,May,7

94013 Measurement of lung volumes (ie, functional residual capacity [FRC], forced vital capacity [FVC], and expiratory reserve volume [ERV]) in an infant or child through 2 years of age
🚑 0.88   ⚕ 0.88   **FUD** XXX   ⊙ 🔢 🔢
AMA: 2015,Jan,16; 2014,Jan,11; 2013,Dec,12; 2012,Aug,6-8; 2011,Jan,11; 2010,May,7

94014 Patient-initiated spirometric recording per 30-day period of time; includes reinforced education, transmission of spirometric tracing, data capture, analysis of transmitted data, periodic recalibration and review and interpretation by a physician or other qualified health care professional
🚑 1.58   ⚕ 1.58   **FUD** XXX   🔢 🔢 🖵
AMA: 2015,Jan,16; 2014,Jan,11; 2013,Dec,12; 2012,Aug,6-8; 2011,Jan,11

94015 recording (includes hook-up, reinforced education, data transmission, data capture, trend analysis, and periodic recalibration)
🚑 0.86   ⚕ 0.86   **FUD** XXX   🔢 🔢 🆃�🅲 🖵
AMA: 2015,Jan,16; 2014,Jan,11; 2013,Dec,12; 2012,Aug,6-8; 2011,Jan,11

94016 review and interpretation only by a physician or other qualified health care professional
🚑 0.72   ⚕ 0.72   **FUD** XXX   🅰 🔢 🈴 🖵
AMA: 2015,Jan,16; 2014,Jan,11; 2013,Dec,12; 2012,Aug,6-8; 2011,Jan,11

94060 Bronchodilation responsiveness, spirometry as in 94010, pre- and post-bronchodilator administration
   INCLUDES   Spirometry performed prior to and after a bronchodilator has been administered
   EXCLUDES   Bronchospasm prolonged exercise test with pre- and post-spirometry (94620)
             Diffusing capacity (94729)
   Code also bronchodilator supply with appropriate supply code or (99070)
   Do not report with (94150, 94200, 94375, 94640, 94728)
🚑 1.72   ⚕ 1.72   **FUD** XXX   🆂 🔢 🖵
AMA: 2015,Jan,16; 2014,Mar,11; 2014,Jan,11; 2013,Dec,12; 2012,Aug,6-8; 2012,Jan,15-42; 2011,Jan,11

94070 Bronchospasm provocation evaluation, multiple spirometric determinations as in 94010, with administered agents (eg, antigen[s], cold air, methacholine)
   EXCLUDES   Diffusing capacity (94729)
   Code also antigen(s) administration with appropriate supply code or (99070)
   Do not report with (94640)
🚑 1.68   ⚕ 1.68   **FUD** XXX   🆂 🔢 🖵
AMA: 2015,Jan,16; 2014,Jan,11; 2013,Dec,12; 2012,Nov,11-12; 2012,Aug,6-8; 2011,Jan,11

94150 Vital capacity, total (separate procedure)
   EXCLUDES   Thoracic gas volumes (94726-94727)
   Do not report with (94010, 94060, 94728)
🚑 0.72   ⚕ 0.72   **FUD** XXX   🔢
AMA: 2015,Jan,16; 2014,Mar,11; 2014,Jan,11; 2013,Dec,12; 2012,Aug,6-8; 2012,Jan,15-42; 2011,Jan,11

94200 Maximum breathing capacity, maximal voluntary ventilation
   Do not report with (94010, 94060)
🚑 0.72   ⚕ 0.72   **FUD** XXX   🔢 🔢
AMA: 2015,Jan,16; 2014,Mar,11; 2014,Jan,11; 2013,Dec,12; 2012,Aug,6-8; 2012,Jan,15-42; 2011,Jan,11

94250 Expired gas collection, quantitative, single procedure (separate procedure)
🚑 0.74   ⚕ 0.74   **FUD** XXX   🔢 🔢
AMA: 2015,Jan,16; 2014,Jan,11; 2013,Dec,12; 2012,Aug,6-8; 2011,Jan,11

94375 Respiratory flow volume loop
   INCLUDES   Identification of obstruction patterns in central or peripheral airways (inspiratory and/or expiratory)
   EXCLUDES   Diffusing capacity (94729)
   Do not report with (94010, 94060, 94728)
🚑 1.11   ⚕ 1.11   **FUD** XXX   🔢 🔢 🖵
AMA: 2015,Jan,16; 2014,Mar,11; 2014,Jan,11; 2013,Dec,12; 2012,Aug,6-8; 2011,Jan,11

94400 Breathing response to CO2 (CO2 response curve)
   Do not report with (94640)
🚑 1.60   ⚕ 1.60   **FUD** XXX   🔢 🔢 🖵
AMA: 2015,Jan,16; 2014,Mar,11; 2014,Jan,11; 2013,Dec,12; 2012,Aug,6-8; 2012,Jan,15-42; 2011,Jan,11

94450 Breathing response to hypoxia (hypoxia response curve)
   EXCLUDES   HAST - high altitude simulation test (94452, 94453)
🚑 1.88   ⚕ 1.88   **FUD** XXX   🔢 🔢 🖵
AMA: 2015,Jan,16; 2014,Jan,11; 2013,Dec,12; 2012,Aug,6-8; 2011,Jan,11

94452 High altitude simulation test (HAST), with interpretation and report by a physician or other qualified health care professional;
   EXCLUDES   Obtaining arterial blood gases (36600)
   Do not report with (94453, 94760-94761)
🚑 1.63   ⚕ 1.63   **FUD** XXX   🔢 🔢 🖵
AMA: 2015,Jan,16; 2014,Jan,11; 2013,Dec,12; 2012,Aug,6-8; 2011,Jan,11

94453 with supplemental oxygen titration
   EXCLUDES   Obtaining arterial blood gases (36600)
   Do not report with (94452, 94760-94761)
🚑 2.26   ⚕ 2.26   **FUD** XXX   🔢 🔢 🖵
AMA: 2015,Jan,16; 2014,Jan,11; 2013,Dec,12; 2012,Aug,6-8; 2011,Jan,11

94610 Intrapulmonary surfactant administration by a physician or other qualified health care professional through endotracheal tube
   INCLUDES   Reporting once per dosing episode
   EXCLUDES   Intubation, endotracheal (31500)
   Do not report with (99468-99472)
🚑 1.60   ⚕ 1.60   **FUD** XXX   ⊘ 🔢 🔢
AMA: 2015,Jan,16; 2014,Jan,11; 2013,Dec,12; 2012,Aug,6-8; 2012,Jan,15-42; 2011,Jan,11

94620 Pulmonary stress testing; simple (eg, 6-minute walk test, prolonged exercise test for bronchospasm with pre- and post-spirometry and oximetry)
🚑 1.58   ⚕ 1.58   **FUD** XXX   🔢 🔢 🖵
AMA: 2015,Jan,16; 2014,Jan,11; 2013,Dec,12; 2012,Nov,13-14; 2012,Aug,6-8; 2012,Jan,15-42; 2011,Jan,11

94621 complex (including measurements of CO2 production, O2 uptake, and electrocardiographic recordings)
🚑 4.63   ⚕ 4.63   **FUD** XXX   🆂 🔢 🖵
AMA: 2015,Jan,16; 2014,Jan,11; 2013,Dec,12; 2012,Nov,13-14; 2012,Aug,6-8; 2012,Jan,15-42; 2011,Jan,11

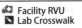

▲ 94640 Pressurized or nonpressurized inhalation treatment for acute airway obstruction for therapeutic purposes and/or for diagnostic purposes such as sputum induction with an aerosol generator, nebulizer, metered dose inhaler or intermittent positive pressure breathing (IPPB) device

    EXCLUDES 1 hour or more of continuous inhalation treatment (94644, 94645)
    Code also modifier 76 when more than 1 inhalation treatment is performed on the same date
    Do not report with (94060, 94070, 94400)
    ⚕ 0.52   0.52   **FUD** XXX   01 80

    AMA: 2015,Jan,16; 2014,Mar,11; 2014,Jan,11; 2013,Dec,12; 2012,Aug,6-8; 2012,Jan,15-42; 2011,Jan,11; 2010,Sep,3

94642 Aerosol inhalation of pentamidine for pneumocystis carinii pneumonia treatment or prophylaxis

    ⚕ 0.00   0.00   **FUD** XXX   01 80

    AMA: 2015,Jan,16; 2014,Jan,11; 2013,Dec,12; 2012,Aug,6-8; 2011,Jan,11

94644 Continuous inhalation treatment with aerosol medication for acute airway obstruction; first hour

    EXCLUDES Services that are less than 1 hour (94640)
    ⚕ 1.23   1.23   **FUD** XXX   01 80

    AMA: 2015,Jan,16; 2014,Mar,11; 2014,Jan,11; 2013,Dec,12; 2012,Aug,6-8; 2011,Jan,11

+ 94645 each additional hour (List separately in addition to code for primary procedure)

    Code first initial hour (94644)
    ⚕ 0.39   0.39   **FUD** XXX   N 80

    AMA: 2015,Jan,16; 2014,Mar,11; 2014,Jan,11; 2013,Dec,12; 2012,Aug,6-8; 2011,Jan,11

94660 Continuous positive airway pressure ventilation (CPAP), initiation and management

    ⚕ 1.07   1.77   **FUD** XXX   03 80

    AMA: 2015,Jan,16; 2014,Oct,8; 2014,May,4; 2014,Jan,11; 2013,Dec,12; 2012,Aug,6-8; 2012,Jan,15-42; 2011,Jan,11

94662 Continuous negative pressure ventilation (CNP), initiation and management

    ⚕ 0.97   0.97   **FUD** XXX   03 80

    AMA: 2015,Jan,16; 2014,May,4; 2014,Jan,11; 2013,Dec,12; 2012,Aug,6-8; 2012,Jan,15-42; 2011,Jan,11

94664 Demonstration and/or evaluation of patient utilization of an aerosol generator, nebulizer, metered dose inhaler or IPPB device

    INCLUDES Reporting only one time per day of service
    ⚕ 0.49   0.49   **FUD** XXX   01 80

    AMA: 2015,Jan,16; 2014,Jan,11; 2013,Dec,12; 2012,Aug,6-8; 2012,Jan,15-42; 2011,Jan,11; 2010,Sep,3

94667 Manipulation chest wall, such as cupping, percussing, and vibration to facilitate lung function; initial demonstration and/or evaluation

    ⚕ 0.74   0.74   **FUD** XXX   01 80

    AMA: 2015,Jan,16; 2014,Mar,11; 2014,Jan,11; 2013,Dec,12; 2012,Aug,6-8; 2012,Jan,15-42; 2011,Jan,11; 2010,Sep,3

94668 subsequent

    ⚕ 0.81   0.81   **FUD** XXX   01 80

    AMA: 2015,Jan,16; 2014,Mar,11; 2014,Jan,11; 2013,Dec,12; 2012,Aug,6-8; 2012,Jan,15-42; 2011,Jan,11; 2010,Sep,3

94669 Mechanical chest wall oscillation to facilitate lung function, per session

    INCLUDES Application of an external wrap or vest to provide mechanical oscillation
    ⚕ 1.00   1.00   **FUD** XXX   01 80

    AMA: 2015,Jan,16; 2014,Jan,11; 2013,Dec,12

94680 Oxygen uptake, expired gas analysis; rest and exercise, direct, simple

    ⚕ 1.62   1.62   **FUD** XXX   01 80

    AMA: 2015,Jan,16; 2014,Jan,11; 2013,Dec,12; 2012,Aug,6-8; 2011,Jan,11

94681 including CO2 output, percentage oxygen extracted

    ⚕ 1.51   1.51   **FUD** XXX   01 80

    AMA: 2015,Jan,16; 2014,Jan,11; 2013,Dec,12; 2012,Aug,6-8; 2011,Jan,11

94690 rest, indirect (separate procedure)

    EXCLUDES Arterial puncture (36600)
    ⚕ 1.40   1.40   **FUD** XXX   01 80

    AMA: 2015,Jan,16; 2014,Jan,11; 2013,Dec,12; 2012,Aug,6-8; 2011,Jan,11

94726 Plethysmography for determination of lung volumes and, when performed, airway resistance

    INCLUDES Airway resistance
    Determination of:
      Functional residual capacity
      Residual volume
      Total lung capacity
    EXCLUDES Bronchial provocation (94070)
    Diffusing capacity (94729)
    Spirometry (94010, 94060)
    Do not report with (94727-94728)
    ⚕ 1.49   1.49   **FUD** XXX   01 80

    AMA: 2015,Jan,16; 2014,Jan,11; 2013,Dec,12; 2013,May,11; 2012,Aug,6-8; 2012,Jan,3-5

94727 Gas dilution or washout for determination of lung volumes and, when performed, distribution of ventilation and closing volumes

    EXCLUDES Bronchial provocation (94070)
    Diffusing capacity (94729)
    Spirometry (94010, 94060)
    Do not report with (94726)
    ⚕ 1.19   1.19   **FUD** XXX   01 80

    AMA: 2015,Jan,16; 2014,Jan,11; 2013,Dec,12; 2013,May,11; 2012,Aug,6-8; 2012,Jan,3-5

94728 Airway resistance by impulse oscillometry

    EXCLUDES Diffusing capacity (94729)
    Gas dilution techniques
    Do not report with (94010, 94060, 94070, 94375, 94726)
    ⚕ 1.11   1.11   **FUD** XXX   01 80

    AMA: 2015,Jan,16; 2014,Mar,11; 2014,Jan,11; 2013,Dec,12; 2013,May,11; 2012,Aug,6-8; 2012,Jan,3-5

+ 94729 Diffusing capacity (eg, carbon monoxide, membrane) (List separately in addition to code for primary procedure)

    Code first (94010, 94060, 94070, 94375, 94726-94728)
    ⚕ 1.54   1.54   **FUD** ZZZ   N 80

    AMA: 2015,Jan,16; 2014,Jan,11; 2013,Dec,12; 2012,Aug,6-8; 2012,Jan,3-5

94750 Pulmonary compliance study (eg, plethysmography, volume and pressure measurements)

    ⚕ 2.29   2.29   **FUD** XXX   01 80

    AMA: 2015,Jan,16; 2014,Jan,11; 2013,Dec,12; 2012,Aug,6-8; 2011,Jan,11

94760 Noninvasive ear or pulse oximetry for oxygen saturation; single determination

    EXCLUDES Blood gases (82803-82810)
    ⚕ 0.09   0.09   **FUD** XXX   N 80 TC

    AMA: 2015,Jan,16; 2014,May,4; 2014,Jan,11; 2013,Dec,12; 2012,Aug,6-8; 2012,Jan,15-42; 2011,Jan,11

94761 multiple determinations (eg, during exercise)

    ⚕ 0.14   0.14   **FUD** XXX   N 80 TC

    AMA: 2015,Jan,16; 2014,May,4; 2014,Jan,11; 2013,Dec,12; 2012,Aug,6-8; 2012,Jan,15-42; 2011,Jan,11

94762 by continuous overnight monitoring (separate procedure)

    ⚕ 0.69   0.69   **FUD** XXX   03 80 TC

    AMA: 2015,Jan,16; 2014,May,4; 2014,Jan,11; 2013,Dec,12; 2012,Aug,6-8; 2011,Jan,11

Medicine

94770 — 95044

94770 **Carbon dioxide, expired gas determination by infrared analyzer**

> EXCLUDES Arterial catheterization/cannulation (36620)
> Arterial puncture (36600)
> Bronchoscopy (31622-31646)
> Flow directed catheter placement (93503)
> Needle biopsy of the lung (32405)
> Orotracheal/nasotracheal intubation (31500)
> Placement of central venous catheter (36555-36556)
> Therapeutic phlebotomy (99195)
> Thoracentesis (32554-32555)
> Venipuncture (36410)

> 🚑 0.21 ⚕ 0.21 **FUD** XXX [S] [80] ▢

> **AMA:** 2015,Jan,16; 2014,Mar,11; 2014,Jan,11; 2013,Dec,12; 2012,Aug,6-8; 2011,Jan,11

94772 **Circadian respiratory pattern recording (pediatric pneumogram), 12-24 hour continuous recording, infant** [A]

> EXCLUDES Electromyograms/EEG/ECG/respiration recordings
> 🚑 0.00 ⚕ 0.00 **FUD** XXX [S] [80] ▢

> **AMA:** 2015,Jan,16; 2014,Jan,11; 2013,Dec,12; 2012,Aug,6-8; 2011,Jan,11

94774 **Pediatric home apnea monitoring event recording including respiratory rate, pattern and heart rate per 30-day period of time; includes monitor attachment, download of data, review, interpretation, and preparation of a report by a physician or other qualified health care professional** [A]

> INCLUDES Oxygen saturation monitoring
> EXCLUDES Sleep testing (95805-95811 [95800, 95801])
> Do not report with (93224-93272, 94775-94777)
> 🚑 0.00 ⚕ 0.00 **FUD** YYY [B] [80]

> **AMA:** 2015,Jan,16; 2014,Jan,11; 2013,Dec,12; 2012,Aug,6-8; 2011,Jan,11

94775 **monitor attachment only (includes hook-up, initiation of recording and disconnection)** [A]

> INCLUDES Oxygen saturation monitoring
> EXCLUDES Sleep testing (95805-95811 [95800, 95801])
> Do not report with (93224-93272)
> 🚑 0.00 ⚕ 0.00 **FUD** YYY [S] [80] [TC]

> **AMA:** 2015,Jan,16; 2014,Jan,11; 2013,Dec,12; 2012,Aug,6-8; 2011,Jan,11

94776 **monitoring, download of information, receipt of transmission(s) and analyses by computer only** [A]

> INCLUDES Oxygen saturation monitoring
> EXCLUDES Sleep testing (95805-95811 [95800, 95801])
> Do not report with (93224-93272)
> 🚑 0.00 ⚕ 0.00 **FUD** YYY [S] [80] [TC]

> **AMA:** 2015,Jan,16; 2014,Jan,11; 2013,Dec,12; 2012,Aug,6-8; 2011,Jan,11

94777 **review, interpretation and preparation of report only by a physician or other qualified health care professional** [A]

> INCLUDES Oxygen saturation monitoring
> EXCLUDES Sleep testing (95805-95811 [95800, 95801])
> Do not report with (93224-93272)
> 🚑 0.00 ⚕ 0.00 **FUD** YYY [B] [80] [26]

> **AMA:** 2015,Jan,16; 2014,Jan,11; 2013,Dec,12; 2012,Aug,6-8; 2011,Jan,11

94780 **Car seat/bed testing for airway integrity, neonate, with continual nursing observation and continuous recording of pulse oximetry, heart rate and respiratory rate, with interpretation and report; 60 minutes** [A]

> Do not report for less than 60 minutes
> Do not report with (99468-99472, 99477-99480, 93040-93042, 94760-94761)
> 🚑 0.71 ⚕ 1.77 **FUD** XXX [01]

> **AMA:** 2015,May,10; 2015,Jan,16; 2014,Jan,11; 2013,Dec,12; 2012,Aug,6-8

+ 94781 **each additional full 30 minutes (List separately in addition to code for primary procedure)** [A]

> Code first (94780)
> 🚑 0.25 ⚕ 0.65 **FUD** ZZZ [N]

> **AMA:** 2015,May,10; 2015,Jan,16; 2014,Jan,11; 2013,Dec,12; 2012,Aug,6-8

94799 **Unlisted pulmonary service or procedure**

> 🚑 0.00 ⚕ 0.00 **FUD** XXX [01] [80]

> **AMA:** 2015,May,10; 2015,Jan,16; 2014,Jan,11; 2013,Dec,12; 2012,Nov,13-14; 2012,Aug,6-8; 2012,Jan,15-42; 2011,Jan,11; 2010,Dec,12

95004-95071 Allergy Tests

> EXCLUDES Drugs administered for intractable/severe allergic reaction (eg, antihistamines, epinephrine, steroids) (96372)
> Laboratory tests for allergies (86000-86999 [86152, 86153])

Code also medical conferences regarding use of equipment (eg, air filters, humidifiers, dehumidifiers), climate therapy, physical, occupational, and recreation therapy using appropriate evaluation and management codes

Code also significant, separately identifiable E&M services using modifier 25, when performed (99201-99215, 99217-99223 [99224, 99225, 99226], 99231-99233, 99241-99255, 99281-99285, 99304-99318, 99324-99337, 99341-99350, 99381-99429)

Do not report with codes for evaluation and management services when reporting test interpretation/report

95004 **Percutaneous tests (scratch, puncture, prick) with allergenic extracts, immediate type reaction, including test interpretation and report, specify number of tests**

> 🚑 0.18 ⚕ 0.18 **FUD** XXX [01] [80] ▢

> **AMA:** 2015,Jan,16; 2014,Jan,11; 2013,Jan,9-10; 2012,Jan,15-42; 2011,Jan,11; 2010,May,3-4

95012 **Nitric oxide expired gas determination**

> 🚑 0.55 ⚕ 0.55 **FUD** XXX [01] [80]

> **AMA:** 2015,Jan,16; 2014,Mar,11; 2014,Jan,11; 2013,Jan,9-10; 2012,Jan,15-42; 2011,Jan,11

95017 **Allergy testing, any combination of percutaneous (scratch, puncture, prick) and intracutaneous (intradermal), sequential and incremental, with venoms, immediate type reaction, including test interpretation and report, specify number of tests**

> 🚑 0.10 ⚕ 0.22 **FUD** XXX [01] [80]

> **AMA:** 2015,Jul,9; 2015,Jan,16; 2013,Jan,9-10

95018 **Allergy testing, any combination of percutaneous (scratch, puncture, prick) and intracutaneous (intradermal), sequential and incremental, with drugs or biologicals, immediate type reaction, including test interpretation and report, specify number of tests**

> 🚑 0.20 ⚕ 0.53 **FUD** XXX [01] [80]

> **AMA:** 2015,Jul,9; 2015,Jan,16; 2013,Jan,9-10

95024 **Intracutaneous (intradermal) tests with allergenic extracts, immediate type reaction, including test interpretation and report, specify number of tests**

> 🚑 0.03 ⚕ 0.22 **FUD** XXX [01] [80] ▢

> **AMA:** 2015,Jan,16; 2014,Jan,11; 2013,Jan,9-10; 2012,Jan,15-42; 2011,Jan,11; 2010,May,3-4

95027 **Intracutaneous (intradermal) tests, sequential and incremental, with allergenic extracts for airborne allergens, immediate type reaction, including test interpretation and report, specify number of tests**

> 🚑 0.13 ⚕ 0.13 **FUD** XXX [01] [80] ▢

> **AMA:** 2015,Jan,16; 2014,Jan,11; 2013,Jan,9-10; 2012,Jan,15-42; 2011,Jan,11; 2010,May,3-4

95028 **Intracutaneous (intradermal) tests with allergenic extracts, delayed type reaction, including reading, specify number of tests**

> 🚑 0.38 ⚕ 0.38 **FUD** XXX [01] [80] [TC]

> **AMA:** 2015,Jan,16; 2014,Jan,11; 2013,Jan,9-10; 2010,May,3-4

95044 **Patch or application test(s) (specify number of tests)**

> 🚑 0.16 ⚕ 0.16 **FUD** XXX [01] [80] ▢

> **AMA:** 2015,Jan,16; 2014,Jan,11; 2013,Jan,9-10

| 26/TC PC/TC Comp Only | A2-Z3 ASC Pmt | 50 Bilateral | ♂ Male Only | ♀ Female Only | 🚑 Facility RVU | ⚕ Non-Facility RVU |
| AMA: CPT Asst | CMS: Pub 100 | A-Y OPPSI | ✗ Non-FDA Drug | | 🔬 Lab Crosswalk | ⊕ Radiology Crosswalk |

420 Medicare (Red Text) CPT © 2015 American Medical Association. All Rights Reserved. (Black Text) © 2015 Optum360, LLC (Blue Text)

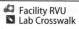

95052 **Photo patch test(s) (specify number of tests)**
 ⚕ 0.19   ⚗ 0.19   **FUD** XXX   [91] [80] [▭]
 AMA: 2015,Jan,16; 2014,Jan,11; 2013,Jan,9-10

95056 **Photo tests**
 ⚕ 1.25   ⚗ 1.25   **FUD** XXX   [91] [80] [▭]
 AMA: 2015,Jan,16; 2014,Jan,11; 2013,Jan,9-10

95060 **Ophthalmic mucous membrane tests**
 ⚕ 0.99   ⚗ 0.99   **FUD** XXX   [91] [80] [TC]
 AMA: 2015,Jan,16; 2014,Jan,11; 2013,Jan,9-10

95065 **Direct nasal mucous membrane test**
 ⚕ 0.71   ⚗ 0.71   **FUD** XXX   [91] [80] [TC] [▭]
 AMA: 2015,Jan,16; 2014,Jan,11; 2013,Jan,9-10

95070 **Inhalation bronchial challenge testing (not including necessary pulmonary function tests); with histamine, methacholine, or similar compounds**
 EXCLUDES   Pulmonary function tests (94060, 94070)
 ⚕ 0.85   ⚗ 0.85   **FUD** XXX   [S] [80] [TC] [▭]
 AMA: 2015,Jan,16; 2014,Jan,11; 2013,Jan,9-10; 2012,Nov,11-12

95071 **with antigens or gases, specify**
 EXCLUDES   Pulmonary function tests (94060, 94070)
 ⚕ 0.98   ⚗ 0.98   **FUD** XXX   [91] [80] [TC] [▭]
 AMA: 2015,Jan,16; 2014,Jan,11; 2013,Jan,9-10; 2012,Nov,11-12

95076-95079 Challenge Ingestion Testing

CMS: 100-3,110.12 Challenge Ingestion Food Testing
 INCLUDES   Assessment and monitoring for allergic reactions (eg, blood pressure, peak flow meter)
 Testing time until the test ends or to the point an E&M service is needed
Code also interventions when appropriate (eg, injection of epinephrine or steroid)
Do not report testing time less than 61 minutes, such as a positive challenge resulting in ending the test (use evaluation and management codes as appropriate)

95076 **Ingestion challenge test (sequential and incremental ingestion of test items, eg, food, drug or other substance); initial 120 minutes of testing**
 INCLUDES   First 120 minutes of testing time (not face-to-face time with physician)
 ⚕ 2.06   ⚗ 3.27   **FUD** XXX   [S] [80]
 AMA: 2015,Jan,16; 2013,Jan,9-10

+ 95079 **each additional 60 minutes of testing (List separately in addition to code for primary procedure)**
 INCLUDES   Includes each 60 minutes of additional testing time (not face-to-face time with physician)
 Code first (95076)
 ⚕ 1.89   ⚗ 2.33   **FUD** ZZZ   [N] [80]
 AMA: 2015,Jan,16; 2013,Jan,9-10

95115-95199 Allergy Immunotherapy

CMS: 100-3,110.9 Antigens Prepared for Sublingual Administration
 INCLUDES   Allergen immunotherapy professional services
 EXCLUDES   Bacterial/viral/fungal extracts skin testing (86485-86580, 95028)
 Special reports for allergy patients (99080)
 The following procedures for testing: (See Pathology/Immunology section or code:) (95199)
 Leukocyte histamine release (LHR)
 Lymphocytic transformation test (LTT)
 Mast cell degranulation test (MCDT)
 Migration inhibitory factor test (MIF)
 Nitroblue tetrazolium dye test (NTD)
 Radioallergosorbent testing (RAST)
 Rat mast cell technique (RMCT)
 Transfer factor test (TFT)
Code also significant separately identifiable E&M services, when performed

95115 **Professional services for allergen immunotherapy not including provision of allergenic extracts; single injection**
 ⚕ 0.25   ⚗ 0.25   **FUD** XXX   [S] [80] [▭]
 AMA: 2015,Jan,16; 2014,Jan,11; 2013,Jan,9-10

95117 **2 or more injections**
 ⚕ 0.29   ⚗ 0.29   **FUD** XXX   [S] [80] [▭]
 AMA: 2015,Jan,16; 2014,Jan,11; 2013,Jan,9-10; 2012,Jan,15-42; 2011,Jan,11

95120 **Professional services for allergen immunotherapy in the office or institution of the prescribing physician or other qualified health care professional, including provision of allergenic extract; single injection**
 ⚕ 0.00   ⚗ 0.00   **FUD** XXX   [E]
 AMA: 2015,Jan,16; 2014,Jan,11; 2013,Jan,9-10

95125 **2 or more injections**
 ⚕ 0.00   ⚗ 0.00   **FUD** XXX   [E]
 AMA: 2015,Jan,16; 2014,Jan,11; 2013,Jan,9-10; 2012,Jan,15-42; 2011,Jan,11

95130 **single stinging insect venom**
 ⚕ 0.00   ⚗ 0.00   **FUD** XXX   [E]
 AMA: 2015,Jan,16; 2014,Jan,11; 2013,Jan,9-10; 2012,Jan,15-42; 2011,Jan,11

95131 **2 stinging insect venoms**
 ⚕ 0.00   ⚗ 0.00   **FUD** XXX   [E]
 AMA: 2015,Jan,16; 2014,Jan,11; 2013,Jan,9-10; 2012,Jan,15-42; 2011,Jan,11

95132 **3 stinging insect venoms**
 ⚕ 0.00   ⚗ 0.00   **FUD** XXX   [E]
 AMA: 2015,Jan,16; 2014,Jan,11; 2013,Jan,9-10; 2012,Jan,15-42; 2011,Jan,11

95133 **4 stinging insect venoms**
 ⚕ 0.00   ⚗ 0.00   **FUD** XXX   [E]
 AMA: 2015,Jan,16; 2014,Jan,11; 2013,Jan,9-10; 2012,Jan,15-42; 2011,Jan,11

95134 **5 stinging insect venoms**
 ⚕ 0.00   ⚗ 0.00   **FUD** XXX   [E]
 AMA: 2015,Jan,16; 2014,Jan,11; 2013,Jan,9-10; 2012,Jan,15-42; 2011,Jan,11

95144 **Professional services for the supervision of preparation and provision of antigens for allergen immunotherapy, single dose vial(s) (specify number of vials)**
 INCLUDES   Single dose vial/single dose of antigen administered in one injection
 ⚕ 0.09   ⚗ 0.35   **FUD** XXX   [S] [80] [▭]
 AMA: 2015,Jan,16; 2014,Jan,11; 2013,Jan,9-10; 2012,Jan,15-42; 2011,Jan,11

95145 **Professional services for the supervision of preparation and provision of antigens for allergen immunotherapy (specify number of doses); single stinging insect venom**
 ⚕ 0.09   ⚗ 0.62   **FUD** XXX   [S] [80] [▭]
 AMA: 2015,Jan,16; 2014,Jan,11; 2013,Jan,9-10; 2012,Jan,15-42; 2011,Jan,11

95146 **2 single stinging insect venoms**
 ⚕ 0.09   ⚗ 1.10   **FUD** XXX   [S] [80] [▭]
 AMA: 2015,Jan,16; 2014,Jan,11; 2013,Jan,9-10

95147 **3 single stinging insect venoms**
 ⚕ 0.09   ⚗ 0.99   **FUD** XXX   [S] [80] [▭]
 AMA: 2015,Jan,16; 2014,Jan,11; 2013,Jan,9-10

95148 **4 single stinging insect venoms**
 ⚕ 0.09   ⚗ 1.48   **FUD** XXX   [S] [80] [▭]
 AMA: 2015,Jan,16; 2014,Jan,11; 2013,Jan,9-10

95149 **5 single stinging insect venoms**
 ⚕ 0.09   ⚗ 1.98   **FUD** XXX   [S] [80] [▭]
 AMA: 2015,Jan,16; 2014,Jan,11; 2013,Jan,9-10

95165 **Professional services for the supervision of preparation and provision of antigens for allergen immunotherapy; single or multiple antigens (specify number of doses)**
 ⚕ 0.09   ⚗ 0.36   **FUD** XXX   [S] [80] [▭]
 AMA: 2015,Jan,16; 2014,Jan,11; 2013,Jan,9-10; 2012,Jan,15-42; 2011,Jan,11

95170 whole body extract of biting insect or other arthropod (specify number of doses)

> INCLUDES A dose which is the amount of antigen(s) administered in a single injection from a multiple dose vial

🚑 0.09   ⚕ 0.27   **FUD** XXX   S 80 💻

AMA: 2015,Jan,16; 2014,Jan,11; 2013,Jan,9-10; 2012,Jan,15-42; 2011,Jan,11

95180 Rapid desensitization procedure, each hour (eg, insulin, penicillin, equine serum)

🚑 2.86   ⚕ 3.77   **FUD** XXX   01 80 💻

AMA: 2015,Jan,16; 2014,Jan,11; 2013,Jan,9-10

95199 Unlisted allergy/clinical immunologic service or procedure

🚑 0.00   ⚕ 0.00   **FUD** XXX   01 80

AMA: 2015,Jan,16; 2014,Jan,11; 2013,Jan,9-10

95250-95251 Glucose Monitoring By Subcutaneous Device

Do not report more than one time per month
Do not report with physiologic data collection/interpretation (99091)

95250 Ambulatory continuous glucose monitoring of interstitial tissue fluid via a subcutaneous sensor for a minimum of 72 hours; sensor placement, hook-up, calibration of monitor, patient training, removal of sensor, and printout of recording

🚑 4.44   ⚕ 4.44   **FUD** XXX   V 80 TC 💻

AMA: 2015,Jan,16; 2014,Jan,11; 2011,Jan,11; 2010,Jan,12-15

95251 interpretation and report

🚑 1.22   ⚕ 1.22   **FUD** XXX   B 80 26

AMA: 2015,Jan,16; 2014,Jan,11

95782-95811 [95782, 95783, 95800, 95801] Sleep Studies

> INCLUDES Assessment of sleep disorders in adults and children
> Continuous and simultaneous monitoring and recording of physiological sleep parameters of 6 hours or more
> Evaluation of patient's response to therapies
> Physician:
>   Interpretation
>   Recording
>   Report
> Recording sessions may be:
>   Attended studies that include the presence of a technologist or qualified health care professional to respond to the needs of the patient or technical issues at the bedside
>   Remote without the presence of a technologist or a qualified health professional
>   Unattended without the presence of a technologist or qualified health care professional
> Testing parameters include:
>   Actigraphy: Use of a noninvasive portable device to record gross motor movements to approximate periods of sleep and wakefulness
>   Electrooculogram (EOG): Records electrical activity associated with eye movements
>   Maintenance of wakefulness test (MWT): An attended study used to determine the patient's ability to stay awake
>   Multiple sleep latency test (MSLT): Attended study to determine the tendency of the patient to fall asleep
>   Peripheral arterial tonometry (PAT): Pulsatile volume changes in a digit are measured to determine activity in the sympathetic nervous system for respiratory analysis
>   Polysomnography: An attended continuous, simultaneous recording of physiological parameters of sleep for at least 6 hours in a sleep laboratory setting that also includes four or more of the following:
>   2. Bilateral anterior tibialis EMG
>   3. Electrocardiogram (ECG)
>   1. Airflow-oral and/or nasal
>   4. Oxyhemoglobin saturation, SpO2
>   5. Respiratory effort
>   Positive airway pressure (PAP): Noninvasive devices used to treat sleep-related disorders
>   Respiratory airflow (ventilation): Assessment of air movement during inhalation and exhalation as measured by nasal pressure sensors and thermistor
>   Respiratory analysis: Assessment of components of respiration obtained by other methods such as airflow or peripheral arterial tone
>   Respiratory effort: Use of the diaphragm and/or intercostal muscle for airflow is measured using transducers to estimate thoracic and abdominal motion
>   Respiratory movement: Measures the movement of the chest and abdomen during respiration
>   Sleep latency: Pertains to the time it takes to get to sleep
>   Sleep staging: Determination of the separate levels of sleep according to physiological measurements
>   Total sleep time: Determined by the use of actigraphy and other methods
> Use of portable and in-laboratory technology

> EXCLUDES *Evaluation and management services*

95782 Resequenced code. See code following 95811.

95783 Resequenced code. See code following 95811.

95800 Resequenced code. See code following 95806.

95801 Resequenced code. See code following 95806.

95803 Actigraphy testing, recording, analysis, interpretation, and report (minimum of 72 hours to 14 consecutive days of recording)

> Do not report more than one time in a 14 day period
> Do not report with (95806-95811 [95800, 95801])

🚑 3.99   ⚕ 3.99   **FUD** XXX   01 80

AMA: 2015,Jan,16; 2014,Jan,11

95805   **Multiple sleep latency or maintenance of wakefulness testing, recording, analysis and interpretation of physiological measurements of sleep during multiple trials to assess sleepiness**

> INCLUDES   Physiological sleep parameters as measured by:
> Frontal, central, and occipital EEG leads (3 leads)
> Left and right EOG
> Submental EMG lead
>
> EXCLUDES   *Polysomnography (95808-95811)*
> *Sleep study, not attended (95806)*
>
> Code also modifier 52 when less than four nap opportunities are recorded
> 11.8   11.8   **FUD** XXX   [S] [80][⬚]
>
> **AMA:** 2015,Jan,16; 2014,Jan,11; 2013,Feb,14-15

95806   **Sleep study, unattended, simultaneous recording of, heart rate, oxygen saturation, respiratory airflow, and respiratory effort (eg, thoracoabdominal movement)**

> EXCLUDES   *Unattended sleep study with measurement of a minimum heart rate, oxygen saturation, and respiratory analysis (95801)*
> *Unattended sleep study with measurement of heart rate, oxygen saturation, respiratory analysis, and sleep time (95800)*
>
> Code also modifier 52 for fewer than 6 hours of recording
> Do not report with (93041-93229, 93268-93272, 95800-95801)
> 4.74   4.74   **FUD** XXX   [S] [80][⬚]
>
> **AMA:** 2015,Jan,16; 2014,Jan,11; 2013,Jul,11-12; 2013,Feb,14-15; 2012,Jan,15-42; 2011,Jan,11; 2011,Jan,6-7

\#   95800   **Sleep study, unattended, simultaneous recording; heart rate, oxygen saturation, respiratory analysis (eg, by airflow or peripheral arterial tone), and sleep time**

> 5.07   5.07   **FUD** XXX   [S] [80]
>
> **AMA:** 2015,Jan,16; 2014,Jan,11; 2013,Feb,14-15; 2011,Jan,6-7

\#   95801   **minimum of heart rate, oxygen saturation, and respiratory analysis (eg, by airflow or peripheral arterial tone)**

> 2.59   2.59   **FUD** XXX   [S] [80]
>
> **AMA:** 2015,Jan,16; 2014,Jan,11; 2013,Feb,14-15; 2011,Jan,6-7

95807   **Sleep study, simultaneous recording of ventilation, respiratory effort, ECG or heart rate, and oxygen saturation, attended by a technologist**

> EXCLUDES   *Polysomnography (95808-95811)*
> *Sleep study, not attended (95806)*
>
> Code also modifier 52 for fewer than 6 hours of recording
> 13.2   13.2   **FUD** XXX   [S] [80][⬚]
>
> **AMA:** 2015,Jan,16; 2014,Jan,11; 2013,Feb,14-15

95808   **Polysomnography; any age, sleep staging with 1-3 additional parameters of sleep, attended by a technologist**

> EXCLUDES   *Sleep study, not attended (95806)*
> 16.9   16.9   **FUD** XXX   [S] [80][⬚]
>
> **AMA:** 2015,Jan,16; 2014,Jan,11; 2013,Feb,14-15; 2012,Jan,15-42; 2011,Jan,11

95810   **age 6 years or older, sleep staging with 4 or more additional parameters of sleep, attended by a technologist**   [A]

> EXCLUDES   *Sleep study, not attended (95806)*
> Code also modifier 52 for fewer than 6 hours of recording
> 17.5   17.5   **FUD** XXX   [S] [80][⬚]
>
> **AMA:** 2015,Jan,16; 2014,Jan,11; 2013,Feb,14-15

95811   **age 6 years or older, sleep staging with 4 or more additional parameters of sleep, with initiation of continuous positive airway pressure therapy or bilevel ventilation, attended by a technologist**   [A]

> EXCLUDES   *Sleep study, not attended (95806)*
> Code also modifier 52 for fewer than 6 hours of recording
> 18.3   18.3   **FUD** XXX   [S] [80][⬚]
>
> **AMA:** 2015,Jan,16; 2014,Oct,8; 2014,Jan,11; 2013,Feb,14-15

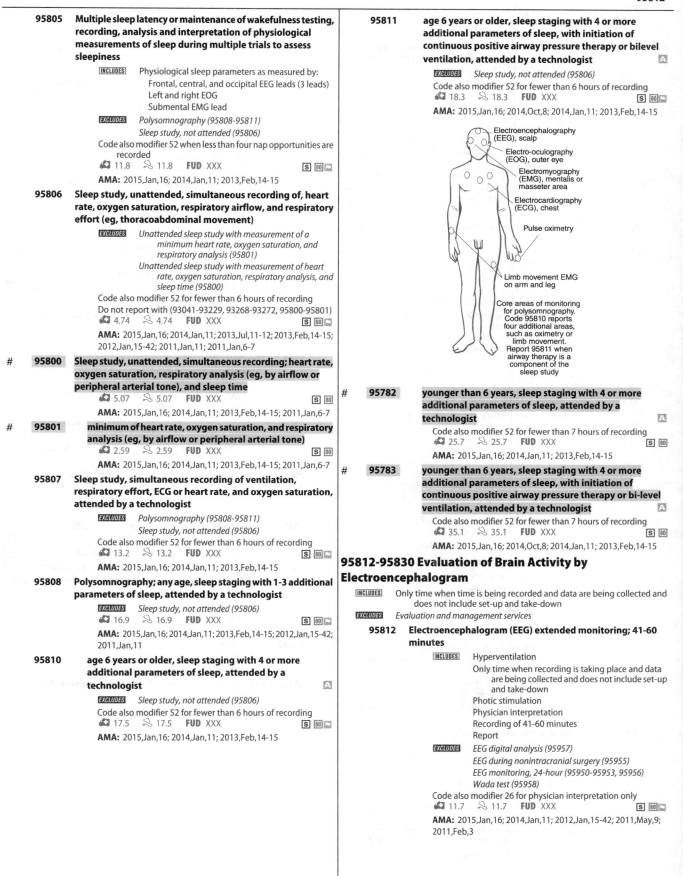

Electroencephalography (EEG), scalp
Electro-oculography (EOG), outer eye
Electromyography (EMG), mentalis or masseter area
Electrocardiography (ECG), chest
Pulse oximetry
Limb movement EMG on arm and leg

Core areas of monitoring for polysomnography. Code 95810 reports four additional areas, such as oximetry or limb movement. Report 95811 when airway therapy is a component of the sleep study

\#   95782   **younger than 6 years, sleep staging with 4 or more additional parameters of sleep, attended by a technologist**   [A]

> Code also modifier 52 for fewer than 7 hours of recording
> 25.7   25.7   **FUD** XXX   [S] [80]
>
> **AMA:** 2015,Jan,16; 2014,Jan,11; 2013,Feb,14-15

\#   95783   **younger than 6 years, sleep staging with 4 or more additional parameters of sleep, with initiation of continuous positive airway pressure therapy or bi-level ventilation, attended by a technologist**   [A]

> Code also modifier 52 for fewer than 7 hours of recording
> 35.1   35.1   **FUD** XXX   [S] [80]
>
> **AMA:** 2015,Jan,16; 2014,Oct,8; 2014,Jan,11; 2013,Feb,14-15

95812-95830 Evaluation of Brain Activity by Electroencephalogram

> INCLUDES   Only time when time is being recorded and data are being collected and does not include set-up and take-down
> EXCLUDES   *Evaluation and management services*

95812   **Electroencephalogram (EEG) extended monitoring; 41-60 minutes**

> INCLUDES   Hyperventilation
> Only time when recording is taking place and data are being collected and does not include set-up and take-down
> Photic stimulation
> Physician interpretation
> Recording of 41-60 minutes
> Report
>
> EXCLUDES   *EEG digital analysis (95957)*
> *EEG during nonintracranial surgery (95955)*
> *EEG monitoring, 24-hour (95950-95953, 95956)*
> *Wada test (95958)*
>
> Code also modifier 26 for physician interpretation only
> 11.7   11.7   **FUD** XXX   [S] [80][⬚]
>
> **AMA:** 2015,Jan,16; 2014,Jan,11; 2012,Jan,15-42; 2011,May,9; 2011,Feb,3

	95813	**greater than 1 hour**

INCLUDES   Hyperventilation
Only time when recording is taking place and data are being collected and does not include set-up and take-down
Photic stimulation
Physician interpretation
Recording of 61 minutes or more
Report

EXCLUDES   *EEG digital analysis (95957)*
EEG during nonintracranial surgery (95955)
EEG monitoring, 24-hour (95950-95953, 95956)
Wada test (95958)

Code also modifier 26 for physician interpretation only
📷 14.1   ⬦ 14.1   **FUD** XXX   [S] [80] ▭

AMA: 2015,Jan,16; 2014,Jan,11; 2012,Jan,15-42; 2011,May,9; 2011,Feb,3

95816   Electroencephalogram (EEG); including recording awake and drowsy

INCLUDES   Photic stimulation
Physician interpretation
Recording of 20-40 minutes
Report

EXCLUDES   *EEG digital analysis (95957)*
EEG during nonintracranial surgery (95955)
EEG monitoring, 24-hour (95950-95953, 95956)
Wada test (95958)

Code also modifier 26 for physician interpretation only
📷 10.1   ⬦ 10.1   **FUD** XXX   [S] [80] ▭

AMA: 2015,Jan,16; 2014,Jan,11; 2012,Jan,15-42; 2011,Feb,3; 2011,Jan,11

95819   including recording awake and asleep

INCLUDES   Hyperventilation
Photic stimulation
Physician interpretation
Recording of 20-40 minutes
Report

EXCLUDES   *EEG digital analysis (95957)*
EEG during nonintracranial surgery (95955)
EEG monitoring, 24-hour (95950-95953, 95956)
Wada test (95958)

Code also modifier 26 for interpretation only
📷 11.5   ⬦ 11.5   **FUD** XXX   [S] [80] ▭

AMA: 2015,Jan,16; 2014,Jan,11; 2011,Feb,3

95822   recording in coma or sleep only

INCLUDES   Hyperventilation
Photic stimulation
Physician interpretation
Recording of 20-40 minutes
Report

EXCLUDES   *EEG digital analysis (95957)*
EEG during nonintracranial surgery (95955)
EEG monitoring, 24-hour (95950-95953, 95956)
Wada test (95958)

Code also modifier 26 for interpretation only
📷 10.4   ⬦ 10.4   **FUD** XXX   [S] [80]

AMA: 2015,Jan,16; 2014,Dec,18; 2014,Jan,11; 2013,May,8-10; 2011,Feb,3

95824   cerebral death evaluation only

INCLUDES   Physician interpretation
Recording
Report

EXCLUDES   *EEG digital analysis (95957)*
EEG during nonintracranial surgery (95955)
EEG monitoring, 24-hour (95950-95953, 95956)
Wada test (95958)

Code also modifier 26 for physician interpretation only
📷 0.00   ⬦ 0.00   **FUD** XXX   [S] [80] ▭

AMA: 2003,Dec,4; 2001,Nov,4

95827   all night recording

INCLUDES   Physician interpretation
Recording
Report

EXCLUDES   *EEG digital analysis (95957)*
EEG during nonintracranial surgery (95955)
EEG monitoring, 24-hour (95950-95953, 95956)
Wada test (95958)

Code also modifier 26 for interpretation only
📷 22.1   ⬦ 22.1   **FUD** XXX   [S] [80] ▭

AMA: 2003,Dec,4; 2001,Nov,4

95829   Electrocorticogram at surgery (separate procedure)

INCLUDES   Physician interpretation
Recording
Report

Code also modifier 26 for interpretation only
📷 53.1   ⬦ 53.1   **FUD** XXX   [N] [80] ▭

AMA: 2003,Dec,4; 2001,Nov,4

95830   Insertion by physician or other qualified health care professional of sphenoidal electrodes for electroencephalographic (EEG) recording
📷 2.60   ⬦ 6.94   **FUD** XXX   [B] [80] ▭

AMA: 2003,Dec,4; 2001,Nov,4

95831-95857 Evaluation of Muscles and Range of Motion

CMS: 100-2,15,230.4 Services By a Physical/Occupational Therapist in Private Practice

EXCLUDES   *Evaluation and management services*

95831   Muscle testing, manual (separate procedure) with report; extremity (excluding hand) or trunk
📷 0.43   ⬦ 0.87   **FUD** XXX   [A] [80] ▭

AMA: 2015,Jan,16; 2014,Jan,11; 2013,Aug,7; 2012,Jan,15-42; 2011,Jan,11

95832   hand, with or without comparison with normal side
📷 0.46   ⬦ 0.86   **FUD** XXX   [A] [80] ▭

AMA: 2015,Jan,16; 2014,Jan,11; 2013,Aug,7; 2012,Jan,15-42; 2011,Jan,11

95833   total evaluation of body, excluding hands
📷 0.61   ⬦ 1.06   **FUD** XXX   [A] [80] ▭

AMA: 2015,Jan,16; 2014,Jan,11; 2013,Aug,7; 2012,Oct,14; 2012,Sep,16

95834   total evaluation of body, including hands
📷 0.89   ⬦ 1.43   **FUD** XXX   [A] [80] ▭

AMA: 2015,Jan,16; 2014,Jan,11; 2013,Aug,7

95851   Range of motion measurements and report (separate procedure); each extremity (excluding hand) or each trunk section (spine)
📷 0.22   ⬦ 0.52   **FUD** XXX   [A] [80]

AMA: 2015,Jan,16; 2014,Jan,11; 2013,Aug,7; 2012,Jan,15-42; 2011,Jan,11

95852   hand, with or without comparison with normal side
📷 0.17   ⬦ 0.46   **FUD** XXX   [A] [80]

AMA: 2015,Jan,16; 2014,Jan,11; 2013,Aug,7

95857   Cholinesterase inhibitor challenge test for myasthenia gravis
📷 0.83   ⬦ 1.52   **FUD** XXX   [S] [80] ▭

AMA: 2015,Jan,16; 2014,Jan,11; 2011,Feb,3

95860-95887 [95885, 95886, 95887] Evaluation of Nerve and Muscle Function: EMGs with/without Nerve Conduction Studies

INCLUDES Physician interpretation
Recording
Report
EXCLUDES *Evaluation and management services*

95860 **Needle electromyography; 1 extremity with or without related paraspinal areas**

INCLUDES Testing of five or more muscles per extremity
EXCLUDES *Dynamic electromyography during motion analysis studies (96002-96003)*
Do not report with (95873-95874, 96002-96003)
🔗 3.47 ⚕ 3.47 **FUD** XXX   [01] [80] [CCI]

AMA: 2015,Mar,6; 2015,Jan,16; 2014,Jan,11; 2013,May,8-10; 2013,Mar,3-5; 2012,Feb,8; 2012,Jan,15-42; 2011,Jan,11; 2010,Dec,12

95861 **2 extremities with or without related paraspinal areas**

INCLUDES Testing of five or more muscles per extremity
EXCLUDES *Dynamic electromyography during motion analysis studies (96002-96003)*
Do not report with (95873-95874, 96002-96003)
🔗 4.87 ⚕ 4.87 **FUD** XXX   [S] [80] [CCI]

AMA: 2015,Mar,6; 2015,Jan,16; 2014,Jan,11; 2013,May,8-10; 2013,Mar,3-5; 2012,Feb,8; 2012,Jan,15-42; 2011,Jan,11; 2010,Dec,12

95863 **3 extremities with or without related paraspinal areas**

INCLUDES Testing of five or more muscles per extremity
Do not report with (95873-95874, 96002-96003)
🔗 6.02 ⚕ 6.02 **FUD** XXX   [S] [80] [CCI]

AMA: 2015,Mar,6; 2015,Jan,16; 2014,Jan,11; 2013,May,8-10; 2013,Mar,3-5; 2012,Feb,8; 2012,Jan,15-42; 2011,Jan,11; 2010,Dec,12

95864 **4 extremities with or without related paraspinal areas**

INCLUDES Testing of five or more muscles per extremity
Do not report with (95873-95874, 96002-96003)
🔗 6.84 ⚕ 6.84 **FUD** XXX   [S] [80] [CCI]

AMA: 2015,Mar,6; 2015,Jan,16; 2014,Jan,11; 2013,May,8-10; 2013,Mar,3-5; 2012,Feb,8; 2012,Jan,15-42; 2011,Jan,11; 2010,Dec,12

95865 **larynx**

Code also modifier 52 for unilateral procedure
Do not report with (95873-95874, 96002-96003)
🔗 4.07 ⚕ 4.07 **FUD** XXX   [01] [80]

AMA: 2015,Mar,6; 2015,Jan,16; 2014,Jan,6; 2014,Jan,11; 2013,May,8-10; 2012,Jan,15-42; 2011,Jan,11

95866 **hemidiaphragm**

Do not report with (95873-95874, 96002-96003)
🔗 3.76 ⚕ 3.76 **FUD** XXX   [01] [80]

AMA: 2015,Mar,6; 2015,Jan,16; 2014,Jan,11; 2013,May,8-10; 2012,Jan,15-42; 2011,Jan,11

95867 **cranial nerve supplied muscle(s), unilateral**

Do not report with (95873-95874)
🔗 2.63 ⚕ 2.63 **FUD** XXX   [S] [80] [CCI]

AMA: 2015,Mar,6; 2015,Jan,16; 2014,Jan,11; 2013,May,8-10; 2013,Mar,3-5; 2012,Feb,8; 2012,Jan,15-42; 2011,Jan,11

95868 **cranial nerve supplied muscles, bilateral**

Do not report with (95873-95874)
🔗 3.73 ⚕ 3.73 **FUD** XXX   [S] [80] [CCI]

AMA: 2015,Mar,6; 2015,Jan,16; 2014,Jan,11; 2013,May,8-10; 2013,Mar,3-5; 2012,Feb,8; 2012,Jan,15-42; 2011,Jan,11

95869 **thoracic paraspinal muscles (excluding T1 or T12)**

Do not report with (95873-95874, 96002-96003)
🔗 2.30 ⚕ 2.30 **FUD** XXX   [01] [80] [CCI]

AMA: 2015,Mar,6; 2015,Jan,16; 2014,Jan,11; 2013,May,8-10; 2013,Mar,3-5; 2012,Feb,8; 2012,Jan,15-42; 2011,Jan,11; 2010,May,9

95870 **limited study of muscles in 1 extremity or non-limb (axial) muscles (unilateral or bilateral), other than thoracic paraspinal, cranial nerve supplied muscles, or sphincters**

INCLUDES Adson test
Testing of four or less muscles per extremity
EXCLUDES *Anal/urethral sphincter/detrusor/urethra/perineum musculature (51785-51792)*
Complete study of extremities (95860-95864)
Eye muscles (92265)
Do not report with (95873-95874, 96002-96003)
🔗 2.49 ⚕ 2.49 **FUD** XXX   [01] [80]

AMA: 2015,Mar,6; 2015,Jan,16; 2014,Jan,11; 2013,May,8-10; 2013,Mar,3-5; 2012,Feb,8; 2012,Jan,15-42; 2011,Jan,11

95872 **Needle electromyography using single fiber electrode, with quantitative measurement of jitter, blocking and/or fiber density, any/all sites of each muscle studied**

Do not report with motion analysis (96002-96003)
🔗 5.59 ⚕ 5.59 **FUD** XXX   [S] [80]

AMA: 2015,Mar,6; 2015,Jan,16; 2014,Jan,11; 2012,Jan,15-42; 2011,Jan,11

+ # **95885** **Needle electromyography, each extremity, with related paraspinal areas, when performed, done with nerve conduction, amplitude and latency/velocity study; limited (List separately in addition to code for primary procedure)**

INCLUDES Testing of four or less muscles per extremity
Code also, when applicable, for a combined maximum total of four units per patient if all four extremities are tested ([95886])
Code first nerve conduction tests (95907-95913)
Do not report more than one time per extremity
Do not report with (95860-95864, 95870, 95905, 96002-96003)
🔗 1.65 ⚕ 1.65 **FUD** ZZZ   [N] [80]

AMA: 2015,Mar,6; 2015,Jan,16; 2014,Jan,11; 2013,Sep,17; 2013,May,8-10; 2013,Mar,3-5; 2012,Feb,8; 2012,Jan,15-42

+ # **95886** **complete, five or more muscles studied, innervated by three or more nerves or four or more spinal levels (List separately in addition to code for primary procedure)**

INCLUDES Testing of five or more muscles per extremity
Code also, when applicable, for a combined maximum total of four units per patient if all four extremities are tested ([95885])
Code first nerve conduction tests (95907-95913)
Do not report more than one time per extremity
Do not report with (95860-95864, 95870, 95905, 96002-96003)
🔗 2.57 ⚕ 2.57 **FUD** ZZZ   [N] [80]

AMA: 2015,Mar,6; 2015,Jan,16; 2014,Jan,11; 2013,Sep,17; 2013,May,8-10; 2013,Mar,3-5; 2012,Feb,8; 2012,Jan,15-42

+ # **95887** **Needle electromyography, non-extremity (cranial nerve supplied or axial) muscle(s) done with nerve conduction, amplitude and latency/velocity study (List separately in addition to code for primary procedure)**

INCLUDES Nerve study of unilateral cranial nerve innervated muscles
EXCLUDES *Nerve study of extra-ocular or laryngeal nerves*
Code also modifier 50 when performed bilaterally
Code first nerve conduction tests (95907-95913)
Do not report more than once per anatomic site
Do not report with (95867-95870, 95874, 96002-96003)
🔗 2.30 ⚕ 2.30 **FUD** ZZZ   [N] [80]

AMA: 2015,Mar,6; 2015,Jan,16; 2014,Jan,8; 2014,Jan,11; 2013,Mar,3-5; 2012,Jul,12-14; 2012,Feb,8; 2012,Jan,15-42

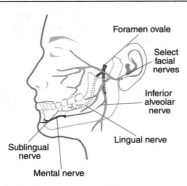

Foramen ovale

Select facial nerves

Inferior alveolar nerve

Lingual nerve

Sublingual nerve

Mental nerve

Cranial Nerves: trigeminal branches of lower face and select facial nerves

Needle EMG is performed to determine conduction, amplitude, and latency/velocity

+ **95873** **Electrical stimulation for guidance in conjunction with chemodenervation (List separately in addition to code for primary procedure)**

    Code first chemodenervation (64612, 64615-64616, 64642-64647)

    Do not report more than one guidance code for each code for chemodenervation.

    Do not report with (64617, 95860-95870, 95874)

    2.11   2.11   **FUD** ZZZ   N 80

    AMA: 2015,Mar,6; 2015,Jan,16; 2014,Jan,6; 2014,Jan,11; 2013,Apr,5-6; 2012,Jan,15-42; 2011,Jan,11

+ **95874** **Needle electromyography for guidance in conjunction with chemodenervation (List separately in addition to code for primary procedure)**

    Code first chemodenervation (64612, 64615-64616, 64642-64647)

    Do not report more than one guidance code for each code for chemodenervation

    Do not report with (64617, 95860-95870, 95873)

    2.03   2.03   **FUD** ZZZ   N 80

    AMA: 2015,Mar,6; 2015,Jan,16; 2014,Oct,14; 2014,Jan,6; 2014,Jan,11; 2013,Apr,5-6; 2012,Jan,15-42; 2011,Jan,11

95875 **Ischemic limb exercise test with serial specimen(s) acquisition for muscle(s) metabolite(s)**

    3.41   3.41   **FUD** XXX   S 80

    AMA: 2015,Mar,6; 2015,Jan,16; 2014,Jan,11; 2012,Jan,15-42; 2011,Jan,11

95885 **Resequenced code. See code following 95872.**

95886 **Resequenced code. See code following 95872.**

95887 **Resequenced code. See code before 95873.**

95905-95913 Evaluation of Nerve Function: Nerve Conduction Studies

CMS: 100-2,15,230.4 Services By a Physical/Occupational Therapist in Private Practice

INCLUDES Conduction studies of motor and sensory nerves

    Reports from on-site examiner including the work product of the interpretation of results using established methodologies, calculations, comparisons to normal studies, and interpretation by physician or other qualified health care professional

    Single conduction study comprising a sensory and motor conduction test with/without F or H wave testing, and all orthodromic and antidromic impulses

    Total number of tests performed indicate which code is appropriate

Code also electromyography performed with nerve conduction studies, as appropriate ([95885, 95886, 95887])

Do not report more than one study when multiple sites on the same nerve are tested

95905 **Motor and/or sensory nerve conduction, using preconfigured electrode array(s), amplitude and latency/velocity study, each limb, includes F-wave study when performed, with interpretation and report**

    INCLUDES Study with preconfigured electrodes that are customized to a specific body location

    Do not report this code more than one time for each limb studied

    Do not report with ([95885, 95886], 95907-95913)

    2.02   2.02   **FUD** XXX   ⃠ 01 80

    AMA: 2015,Jan,16; 2014,Jan,11; 2013,Mar,3-5; 2012,Feb,8

95907 **Nerve conduction studies; 1-2 studies**

    2.74   2.74   **FUD** XXX   S 80

    AMA: 2015,Jan,16; 2014,Jan,11; 2013,Sep,17; 2013,May,8-10; 2013,Mar,3-5

95908 **3-4 studies**

    3.52   3.52   **FUD** XXX   S 80

    AMA: 2015,Mar,6; 2015,Jan,16; 2014,Jan,11; 2013,Sep,17; 2013,May,8-10; 2013,Mar,3-5

95909 **5-6 studies**

    4.17   4.17   **FUD** XXX   S 80

    AMA: 2015,Jan,16; 2014,Jan,11; 2013,Sep,17; 2013,May,8-10; 2013,Mar,3-5

95910 **7-8 studies**

    5.54   5.54   **FUD** XXX   S 80

    AMA: 2015,Jan,16; 2014,Jan,11; 2013,Sep,17; 2013,May,8-10; 2013,Mar,3-5

95911 **9-10 studies**

    6.59   6.59   **FUD** XXX   S 80

    AMA: 2015,Jan,16; 2014,Jan,11; 2013,Sep,17; 2013,May,8-10; 2013,Mar,3-5

95912 **11-12 studies**

    7.35   7.35   **FUD** XXX   S 80

    AMA: 2015,Jan,16; 2014,Jan,11; 2013,Sep,17; 2013,May,8-10; 2013,Mar,3-5

95913 **13 or more studies**

    8.33   8.33   **FUD** XXX   S 80

    AMA: 2015,Jan,16; 2014,Jan,11; 2013,Sep,17; 2013,May,8-10; 2013,Mar,3-5

[95940, 95941] Intraoperative Neurophysiological Monitoring

INCLUDES Monitoring, testing, and data evaluation during surgical procedures by a monitoring professional dedicated only to performing the necessary testing and monitoring

EXCLUDES *Baseline neurophysiologic monitoring*
    EEG during nonintracranial surgery (95955)
    Electrocorticography (95829)
    Intraoperative cortical and subcortical mapping (95961-95962)
    Neurostimulator programming/analysis (95970-95975)
    Time required for set-up, recording, interpretation, and removal of electrodes

Code also baseline studies (eg, EMGs, NCVs), no more than one time per operative session

Code also services provided after midnight using the date when monitoring started and the total monitoring time

Code also standby time prior to procedure (99360)

Code first (92585, 95822, 95860-95870, 95907-95913, 95925-95937 [95938, 95939])

Do not report monitoring services provided by the anesthesiologist or surgeon separately

+ # 95940 Continuous intraoperative neurophysiology monitoring in the operating room, one on one monitoring requiring personal attendance, each 15 minutes (List separately in addition to code for primary procedure)

> INCLUDES 15 minute increments of monitoring service
> A total of all monitoring time for procedures overlapping midnight
> Based on time spent monitoring, regardless of number of tests or parameters monitored
> Continuous intraoperative neurophysiologic monitoring by a dedicated monitoring professional in the operating room providing one-on-one patient care
> Monitoring time may begin prior to the incision
> Monitoring time that is distinct from baseline neurophysiologic study/s time or other services (eg, mapping)
>
> EXCLUDES *Time spent in executing or interpreting the baseline neurophysiologic study or studies*
> Code also monitoring from outside of the operative room, when applicable ([95941])
>
> ⏢ 0.93　⚖ 0.93　**FUD** XXX　　　Ⓝ Ⓝ1 80
>
> **AMA:** 2015,Jan,16; 2014,Apr,10; 2014,Apr,5; 2013,May,8-10

+ # 95941 Continuous intraoperative neurophysiology monitoring, from outside the operating room (remote or nearby) or for monitoring of more than one case while in the operating room, per hour (List separately in addition to code for primary procedure)

> INCLUDES Based on time spent monitoring, regardless of number of tests or parameters monitored
> Monitoring time that is distinct from baseline neurophysiologic study/s time or other services (eg, mapping)
> One hour increments of monitoring service
>
> ⏢ 0.00　⚖ 0.00　**FUD** XXX　　　Ⓝ Ⓝ1
>
> **AMA:** 2015,Jan,16; 2014,Dec,18; 2014,Apr,10; 2014,Apr,5; 2014,Jan,11; 2013,May,8-10; 2013,Feb,16-17

95921-95924 [95943] Evaluation of Autonomic Nervous System

> INCLUDES Physician interpretation
> Recording
> Report
> Testing for autonomic dysfunction including site and autonomic subsystems

95921 Testing of autonomic nervous system function; cardiovagal innervation (parasympathetic function), including 2 or more of the following: heart rate response to deep breathing with recorded R-R interval, Valsalva ratio, and 30:15 ratio

> INCLUDES Display on a monitor
> Minimum of two of the following elements are performed:
> Cardiovascular function as indicated by a 30:15 ration (R/R interval at beat 30)/(R-R interval at beat 15)
> Heart rate response to deep breathing obtained by visual quantitative analysis of recordings with patient taking 5-6 breaths per minute
> Valsalva ratio (at least 2) obtained by dividing the highest heart rate by the lowest
> Monitoring of heart rate by electrocardiography of rate obtained from time between two successive R waves (R-R interval)
> Storage of data for waveform analysis
> Testing most usually in prone position
> Tilt table testing, when performed
> Do not report with (95922, 95924 [95943])
>
> ⏢ 2.47　⚖ 2.47　**FUD** XXX　　　Ⓢ 80 ▭
>
> **AMA:** 2015,Jan,16; 2014,Jan,11; 2012,Nov,6-9; 2012,Jan,15-42; 2011,Jan,11

95922 vasomotor adrenergic innervation (sympathetic adrenergic function), including beat-to-beat blood pressure and R-R interval changes during Valsalva maneuver and at least 5 minutes of passive tilt

> INCLUDES Must include all of the following elements:
> Beat-to-beat blood pressure and heart rate recording during at least 2 Valsalva maneuvers
> Constant beat-to-beat blood pressure and heart rate recording with EKG equipment that allows for a precise graphical quantitative measurement of R-R interval
> Rest period in supine position for at least 20 minutes before test
> Tilt table testing with recording of beat-to-beat blood pressure and heart rate recording for at least 5 minutes in the head-up position before tilt-back to supine position
> Do not report with (95921, 95924 [95943])
>
> ⏢ 2.83　⚖ 2.83　**FUD** XXX　　　Ⓠ1 80 ▭
>
> **AMA:** 2015,Jan,16; 2014,Jan,11; 2012,Nov,6-9; 2012,Jan,15-42; 2011,Jan,11

95923 sudomotor, including 1 or more of the following: quantitative sudomotor axon reflex test (QSART), silastic sweat imprint, thermoregulatory sweat test, and changes in sympathetic skin potential

> ⏢ 5.40　⚖ 5.40　**FUD** XXX　　　Ⓠ1 80 ▭
>
> **AMA:** 2015,Jan,16; 2014,Jan,11; 2012,Nov,6-9; 2012,Jan,15-42; 2011,Jan,11

95924 combined parasympathetic and sympathetic adrenergic function testing with at least 5 minutes of passive tilt

> INCLUDES Tilt table testing of adrenergic and parasympathetic function
> Do not report with (95921-95922, [95943])
>
> ⏢ 4.32　⚖ 4.32　**FUD** XXX　　　Ⓢ 80
>
> **AMA:** 2015,Jan,16; 2012,Nov,6-9

 # 95943 Simultaneous, independent, quantitative measures of both parasympathetic function and sympathetic function, based on time-frequency analysis of heart rate variability concurrent with time-frequency analysis of continuous respiratory activity, with mean heart rate and blood pressure measures, during rest, paced (deep) breathing, Valsalva maneuvers, and head-up postural change

> Do not report with (93040, 95921-95922, 95924)
>
> ⏢ 0.00　⚖ 0.00　**FUD** XXX　　　Ⓢ 80
>
> **AMA:** 2015,Jan,16; 2012,Nov,6-9

95925-95943 [95938, 95939] Neurotransmission Studies

95925 Short-latency somatosensory evoked potential study, stimulation of any/all peripheral nerves or skin sites, recording from the central nervous system; in upper limbs

> EXCLUDES *Auditory evoked potentials (92585)*
> Do not report with (95926, [95938])
>
> ⏢ 4.43　⚖ 4.43　**FUD** XXX　　　Ⓢ 80
>
> **AMA:** 2015,Jan,16; 2014,Jan,11; 2013,May,8-10; 2012,Apr,17-18

95926 in lower limbs

> EXCLUDES *Auditory evoked potentials (92585, [95938])*
> Do not report with (95925, [95938])
>
> ⏢ 4.06　⚖ 4.06　**FUD** XXX　　　Ⓢ 80
>
> **AMA:** 2015,Jan,16; 2014,Jan,11; 2013,May,8-10; 2012,Apr,17-18; 2012,Jan,15-42; 2011,Jan,11

 # 95938 in upper and lower limbs

> Do not report with (95925-95926)
>
> ⏢ 9.62　⚖ 9.62　**FUD** XXX　　　Ⓢ 80
>
> **AMA:** 2015,Jan,16; 2014,Jan,11; 2013,May,8-10; 2013,Feb,16-17; 2012,Apr,17-18

95927 in the trunk or head

> EXCLUDES *Auditory evoked potentials (92585)*
> Code also modifier 52 for unilateral test
>
> ⏢ 4.30　⚖ 4.30　**FUD** XXX　　　Ⓢ 80
>
> **AMA:** 2015,Jan,16; 2014,Jan,11; 2013,May,8-10

95928 **Central motor evoked potential study (transcranial motor stimulation); upper limbs**

Do not report with (95929)

🏥 7.30 🚶 7.30 **FUD** XXX [S] [80]

AMA: 2015,Jan,16; 2013,May,8-10

95929 **lower limbs**

Do not report with (95928)

🏥 7.29 🚶 7.29 **FUD** XXX [Q1] [80]

AMA: 2015,Jan,16; 2014,Dec,6; 2013,May,8-10

\# **95939** **in upper and lower limbs**

Do not report with (95928-95929)

🏥 14.1 🚶 14.1 **FUD** XXX [S] [80]

AMA: 2015,Jan,16; 2014,Jan,11; 2013,May,8-10; 2012,Apr,17-18

95930 **Visual evoked potential (VEP) testing central nervous system, checkerboard or flash**

[EXCLUDES] *Visual acuity screening using automated visual evoked potential devices (0333T)*

🏥 3.62 🚶 3.62 **FUD** XXX [S] [80]

AMA: 2015,Jan,16; 2014,Aug,8; 2013,May,8-10

95933 **Orbicularis oculi (blink) reflex, by electrodiagnostic testing**

🏥 2.37 🚶 2.37 **FUD** XXX [Q1] [80]

AMA: 2015,Jan,16; 2013,May,8-10

95937 **Neuromuscular junction testing (repetitive stimulation, paired stimuli), each nerve, any 1 method**

🏥 2.34 🚶 2.34 **FUD** XXX [S] [80]

AMA: 2015,Jan,16; 2014,Jan,11; 2013,May,8-10; 2013,Mar,3-5

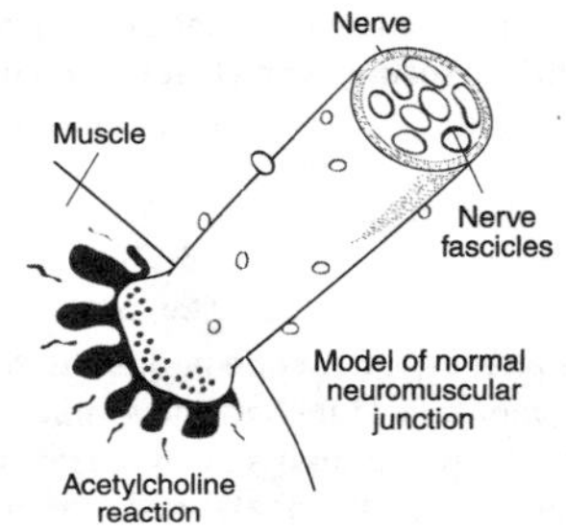
Nerve
Muscle
Nerve fascicles
Model of normal neuromuscular junction
Acetylcholine reaction

A selected neuromuscular junction is repeatedly stimulated. The test is useful to demonstrate reduced muscle action potential from fatique

95938 **Resequenced code. See code following 95926.**

95939 **Resequenced code. See code following 95929.**

95940 **Resequenced code. See code following 95913.**

95941 **Resequenced code. See code following 95913.**

95943 **Resequenced code. See code following 95924.**

95950-95962 Electroencephalography For Seizure Monitoring/Intraoperative Use

[EXCLUDES] *Evaluation and management services*

95950 **Monitoring for identification and lateralization of cerebral seizure focus, electroencephalographic (eg, 8 channel EEG) recording and interpretation, each 24 hours**

[INCLUDES] Only time when recording is taking place and data are being collected and does not include set-up and take-down

Recording for more than 12 hours up to 24 hours

Code also modifier 52 only when recording is 12 hours or less

Do not report more than one time per 24 hour period

🏥 9.26 🚶 9.26 **FUD** XXX [S] [80]

AMA: 2015,Jan,16; 2014,Jan,11; 2011,Feb,3

95951 **Monitoring for localization of cerebral seizure focus by cable or radio, 16 or more channel telemetry, combined electroencephalographic (EEG) and video recording and interpretation (eg, for presurgical localization), each 24 hours**

[INCLUDES] Interpretations during recording with changes to care of patient

Only time when recording is taking place and data are being collected and does not include set-up and take-down

Recording for more than 12 hours up to 24 hours

Code also modifier 52 only when recording is 12 hours or less

Do not report more than one time per 24 hour period

🏥 0.00 🚶 0.00 **FUD** XXX [S] [80]

AMA: 2015,Jan,16; 2014,Dec,16; 2014,Dec,16; 2014,Jan,11; 2013,Aug,13; 2012,Jan,15-42; 2011,Feb,3; 2011,Jan,11; 2010,Nov,6

95953 **Monitoring for localization of cerebral seizure focus by computerized portable 16 or more channel EEG, electroencephalographic (EEG) recording and interpretation, each 24 hours, unattended**

[INCLUDES] Only time when recording is taking place and data are being collected and does not include set-up and take-down

Recording for more than 12 hours up to 24 hours

Code also modifier 52 only when recording is 12 hours or less

Do not report more than one time per 24 hour period

🏥 11.8 🚶 11.8 **FUD** XXX [S] [80]

AMA: 2015,Jan,16; 2014,Dec,16; 2014,Dec,16; 2014,Jan,11; 2011,Feb,3

95954 **Pharmacological or physical activation requiring physician or other qualified health care professional attendance during EEG recording of activation phase (eg, thiopental activation test)**

🏥 12.9 🚶 12.9 **FUD** XXX [S] [80]

AMA: 2015,Jan,16; 2014,Jan,11

95955 **Electroencephalogram (EEG) during nonintracranial surgery (eg, carotid surgery)**

🏥 6.02 🚶 6.02 **FUD** XXX [N] [80]

AMA: 2015,Jan,16; 2014,Dec,18

95956 **Monitoring for localization of cerebral seizure focus by cable or radio, 16 or more channel telemetry, electroencephalographic (EEG) recording and interpretation, each 24 hours, attended by a technologist or nurse**

[INCLUDES] Only time when recording is taking place and data are being collected and does not include set-up and take-down

Recording for more than 12 hours up to 24 hours

Code also modifier 52 only when recording is 12 hours or less

Do not report more than one time per 24 hour period

🏥 47.0 🚶 47.0 **FUD** XXX [S] [80]

AMA: 2015,Jan,16; 2014,Jan,11; 2011,Feb,3

95957 **Digital analysis of electroencephalogram (EEG) (eg, for epileptic spike analysis)**

🏥 8.92 🚶 8.92 **FUD** XXX [N] [80]

AMA: 2015,Jan,16; 2014,Jan,11; 2010,Nov,6

95958 **Wada activation test for hemispheric function, including electroencephalographic (EEG) monitoring**

🏥 16.3 🚶 16.3 **FUD** XXX [S] [80]

AMA: 2000,Jul,1; 1998,Nov,1

95961 **Functional cortical and subcortical mapping by stimulation and/or recording of electrodes on brain surface, or of depth electrodes, to provoke seizures or identify vital brain structures; initial hour of attendance by a physician or other qualified health care professional**

INCLUDES One hour of attendance by physician or other qualified health care professional

Code also each additional hour of attendance by physician or other qualified health care professional, when appropriate (95962)

Code also modifier 52 for 30 minutes or less of attendance by physician or other qualified health care professional

8.18 ⚖ 8.18 **FUD** XXX [S] [80] 🖵

AMA: 2015,Jan,16; 2014,Jan,11; 2012,Jan,15-42; 2011,Feb,3; 2011,Jan,11; 2010,Aug,12; 2010,Aug,12; 2010,Apr,10

+ 95962 **each additional hour of attendance by a physician or other qualified health care professional (List separately in addition to code for primary procedure)**

INCLUDES One hour of attendance by physician or other qualified health care professional

Code first initial hour (95961)

7.23 ⚖ 7.23 **FUD** ZZZ [N] [80] 🖵

AMA: 2015,Jan,16; 2014,Jan,11; 2012,Jan,15-42; 2011,Feb,3; 2011,Jan,11; 2010,Aug,12; 2010,Aug,12; 2010,Apr,10

95965-95967 Magnetoencephalography

INCLUDES Physician interpretation
Recording
Report

EXCLUDES *CT provided along with magnetoencephalography (70450-70470, 70496)*
Electroencephalography provided along with magnetoencephalography (95812-95827)
Evaluation and management services
MRI provided along with magnetoencephalography (70551-70553)
Somatosensory evoked potentials/auditory evoked potentials/visual evoked potentials provided along with magnetic evoked field responses (92585, 95925, 95926, 95930)

95965 **Magnetoencephalography (MEG), recording and analysis; for spontaneous brain magnetic activity (eg, epileptic cerebral cortex localization)**

0.00 ⚖ 0.00 **FUD** XXX [S] [80] 🖵

AMA: 1997,Nov,1

95966 **for evoked magnetic fields, single modality (eg, sensory, motor, language, or visual cortex localization)**

0.00 ⚖ 0.00 **FUD** XXX [S] [80] 🖵

AMA: 1997,Nov,1

+ 95967 **for evoked magnetic fields, each additional modality (eg, sensory, motor, language, or visual cortex localization) (List separately in addition to code for primary procedure)**

Code first single modality (95966)

0.00 ⚖ 0.00 **FUD** ZZZ [N] [80]

AMA: 1997,Nov,1

95970-95982 Evaluation of Implanted Neurostimulator

INCLUDES Simple intraoperative or subsequent programming of neurostimulator (three or less of the following); or complex neurostimulator (three or more of the following):
8 or more electrode contacts
Alternating electrode polarities
Cycling
Dose time
More than 1 clinical feature
Number of channels
Number of programs
Pulse amplitude
Pulse duration
Pulse frequency
Rate
Stimulation train duration
Train spacing

EXCLUDES *Electronic analysis and reprogramming of peripheral subcutaneous field stimulation pulse generator (0285T)*
Evaluation and management services
Neurostimulator electrodes:
Implantation (43647, 43881, 61850-61870, 63650-63655, 64553-64580)
Revision/removal (43648, 43882, 61880, 63661-63664, 64585)
Neurostimulator pulse generator/receiver:
Insertion (61885, 63685, 64590)
Revision/removal (61888, 63688, 64595)

95970 **Electronic analysis of implanted neurostimulator pulse generator system (eg, rate, pulse amplitude, pulse duration, configuration of wave form, battery status, electrode selectability, output modulation, cycling, impedance and patient compliance measurements); simple or complex brain, spinal cord, or peripheral (ie, cranial nerve, peripheral nerve, sacral nerve, neuromuscular) neurostimulator pulse generator/transmitter, without reprogramming**

0.68 ⚖ 1.89 **FUD** XXX [01] [80] 🖵

AMA: 2015,Jan,16; 2014,Jan,11; 2012,Jan,15-42; 2011,Apr,10-11; 2011,Jan,11

95971 **simple spinal cord, or peripheral (ie, peripheral nerve, sacral nerve, neuromuscular) neurostimulator pulse generator/transmitter, with intraoperative or subsequent programming**

1.15 ⚖ 1.62 **FUD** XXX [S] [80] 🖵

AMA: 2015,Jan,16; 2014,Jan,11; 2012,Oct,14; 2012,Jan,15-42; 2011,Apr,10-11; 2011,Jan,11; 2010,Dec,12

95972 **complex spinal cord, or peripheral (ie, peripheral nerve, neuromuscular)(except cranial nerve) neurostimulator pulse generator/transmitter, with introperative or subsequent programming**

Code also modifier 52 for service less than 31 minutes

1.18 ⚖ 1.56 **FUD** XXX [S] [80] 🖵

AMA: 2015,Jan,16; 2014,Aug,5; 2014,Jan,11; 2011,Apr,10-11; 2011,Apr,9

95973 ~~complex spinal cord, or peripheral (ie, peripheral nerve, sacral nerve, neuromuscular) (except cranial nerve) neurostimulator pulse generator/transmitter, with intraoperative or subsequent programming, each additional 30 minutes after first hour (List separately in addition to code for primary procedure)~~

95974 **complex cranial nerve neurostimulator pulse generator/transmitter, with intraoperative or subsequent programming, with or without nerve interface testing, first hour**

Code also modifier 52 for service less than 31 minutes

4.67 ⚖ 5.89 **FUD** XXX [S] [80]

AMA: 2015,Jan,16; 2014,Aug,5; 2014,Jan,11; 2012,Jan,15-42; 2011,Apr,10-11; 2011,Jan,11

Medicine

95961 — 95974

+   95975   complex cranial nerve neurostimulator pulse generator/transmitter, with intraoperative or subsequent programming, each additional 30 minutes after first hour (List separately in addition to code for primary procedure)

Code first initial hour (95974)

🖩 2.64   ⚖ 3.16   **FUD** ZZZ   N 80

AMA: 2015,Jan,16; 2014,Jan,11; 2012,Jan,15-42; 2011,Apr,10-11; 2011,Jan,11

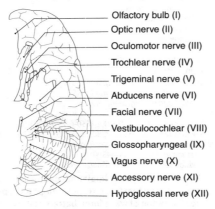

- Olfactory bulb (I)
- Optic nerve (II)
- Oculomotor nerve (III)
- Trochlear nerve (IV)
- Trigeminal nerve (V)
- Abducens nerve (VI)
- Facial nerve (VII)
- Vestibulocochlear (VIII)
- Glossopharyngeal (IX)
- Vagus nerve (X)
- Accessory nerve (XI)
- Hypoglossal nerve (XII)

Cranial nerves at base of brain

95978   Electronic analysis of implanted neurostimulator pulse generator system (eg, rate, pulse amplitude and duration, battery status, electrode selectability and polarity, impedance and patient compliance measurements), complex deep brain neurostimulator pulse generator/transmitter, with initial or subsequent programming; first hour

Code also modifier 52 for service less than 31 minutes

🖩 5.47   ⚖ 7.05   **FUD** XXX   S 80 ▭

AMA: 2015,Jan,16; 2014,Aug,5; 2014,Jan,11

+   95979   each additional 30 minutes after first hour (List separately in addition to code for primary procedure)

Code first initial hour (95978)

🖩 2.55   ⚖ 3.07   **FUD** ZZZ   N 80

AMA: 2015,Jan,16; 2014,Jan,11

95980   Electronic analysis of implanted neurostimulator pulse generator system (eg, rate, pulse amplitude and duration, configuration of wave form, battery status, electrode selectability, output modulation, cycling, impedance and patient measurements) gastric neurostimulator pulse generator/transmitter; intraoperative, with programming

INCLUDES   Gastric neurostimulator of lesser curvature

EXCLUDES   *Analysis, with programming when performed, of vagus nerve trunk stimulator for morbid obesity (0312T, 0317T)*

🖩 1.31   ⚖ 1.31   **FUD** XXX   N 80

AMA: 2015,Jan,16; 2014,Jan,11; 2012,Jan,15-42; 2011,Jan,11; 2010,Nov,8

95981   subsequent, without reprogramming

EXCLUDES   *Analysis, with programming when performed, of vagus nerve trunk stimulator for morbid obesity (0312T, 0317T)*

🖩 0.50   ⚖ 0.90   **FUD** XXX   Q1 80

AMA: 2015,Jan,16; 2014,Jan,11

95982   subsequent, with reprogramming

EXCLUDES   *Analysis, with programming when performed, of vagus nerve trunk stimulator for morbid obesity (0312T, 0317T)*

🖩 1.05   ⚖ 1.50   **FUD** XXX   Q1 80

AMA: 2015,Jan,16; 2014,Jan,11

95990-95991 Refill/Upkeep of Implanted Drug Delivery Pump to Central Nervous System

EXCLUDES   *Analysis/reprogramming of implanted pump for infusion (62367-62370)*
Evaluation and management services
Do not report with (62367-62370)

95990   Refilling and maintenance of implantable pump or reservoir for drug delivery, spinal (intrathecal, epidural) or brain (intraventricular), includes electronic analysis of pump, when performed;

🖩 2.54   ⚖ 2.54   **FUD** XXX   S 80 ▭

AMA: 2015,Jan,16; 2014,Jan,11; 2012,Aug,10-12; 2012,Jul,3-6; 2012,Jan,15-42; 2011,Jan,11

95991   requiring skill of a physician or other qualified health care professional

🖩 1.12   ⚖ 3.41   **FUD** XXX   S 80 ▭

AMA: 2015,Jan,16; 2014,Jan,11; 2012,Aug,10-12; 2012,Jul,3-6

95992-95999 Other and Unlisted Neurological Procedures

95992   Canalith repositioning procedure(s) (eg, Epley maneuver, Semont maneuver), per day

Do not report with (92531-92532)

🖩 1.05   ⚖ 1.20   **FUD** XXX   ⊘ A 80

AMA: 2015,Jan,16; 2014,Jan,11

95999   Unlisted neurological or neuromuscular diagnostic procedure

🖩 0.00   ⚖ 0.00   **FUD** XXX   Q1 80

AMA: 2015,Aug,8; 2015,Jan,16; 2014,Jan,11; 2012,Jan,15-42; 2011,Jan,11

96000-96004 Motion Analysis Studies

CMS: 100-2,15,230.4 Services By a Physical/Occupational Therapist in Private Practice

INCLUDES   Services provided as part of major therapeutic/diagnostic decision making
Services provided in a dedicated motion analysis department capable of:
3-D kinetics/dynamic electromyography
Computerized 3-D kinematics
Videotaping from the front/back/both sides

EXCLUDES   *Evaluation and management services*
Gait training (97116)
Needle electromyography (95860-95872 [95885, 95886, 95887])

96000   Comprehensive computer-based motion analysis by video-taping and 3D kinematics;

🖩 2.70   ⚖ 2.70   **FUD** XXX   S 80 ▭

AMA: 2015,Jan,16; 2014,Jan,11

96001   with dynamic plantar pressure measurements during walking

🖩 2.87   ⚖ 2.87   **FUD** XXX   S 80 ▭

AMA: 2015,Jan,16; 2014,Jan,11

96002   Dynamic surface electromyography, during walking or other functional activities, 1-12 muscles

Do not report with (95860-95866, 95869-95872, [95885, 95886, 95887])

🖩 0.62   ⚖ 0.62   **FUD** XXX   S 80 ▭

AMA: 2015,Aug,8; 2015,Jan,16; 2014,Jan,11

96003   Dynamic fine wire electromyography, during walking or other functional activities, 1 muscle

Do not report with (95860-95866, 95869-95872, [95885, 95886, 95887])

🖩 0.54   ⚖ 0.54   **FUD** XXX   Q1 80 ▭

AMA: 2015,Jan,16; 2014,Jan,11

96004   Review and interpretation by physician or other qualified health care professional of comprehensive computer-based motion analysis, dynamic plantar pressure measurements, dynamic surface electromyography during walking or other functional activities, and dynamic fine wire electromyography, with written report

🖩 3.33   ⚖ 3.33   **FUD** XXX   B 80 26 ▭

AMA: 2015,Aug,8; 2015,Jan,16; 2014,Jan,11

96020 Neurofunctional Brain Testing

INCLUDES | Selection/administration of testing of:
Cognition
Determination of validity of neurofunctional testing relative to separately
interpreted functional magnetic resonance images
Functional neuroimaging
Language
Memory
Monitoring performance of testing
Movement
Other neurological functions
Sensation

EXCLUDES | Clinical depression treatment by repetitive transcranial magnetic stimulation
(90867-90868)
Functional MRI of the brain (70555)
Do not report with (70554, 96101-96103, 96116-96120)
Do not report with E&M codes on the same date of service

96020 **Neurofunctional testing selection and administration during noninvasive imaging functional brain mapping, with test administered entirely by a physician or other qualified health care professional (ie, psychologist), with review of test results and report**
🚑 0.00   ⚕ 0.00   **FUD** XXX   N 80

AMA: 2015,Jan,16; 2014,Jan,11

96040 Genetic Counseling Services

INCLUDES | Analysis for genetic risk assessment
Counseling of patient/family
Counseling services
Face-to-face interviews
Obtaining structured family genetic history
Pedigree construction
Review of medical data/family information
Services provided by trained genetic counselor
Services provided during one or more sessions
Thirty minutes of face-to-face time and is reported one time for each 16-30
minutes of the service

EXCLUDES | Education/genetic counseling by a physician or other qualified health care
provider to a group (99078)
Education/genetic counseling by a physician or other qualified health care
provider to an individual; use appropriate E&M code
Education regarding genetic risks by a nonphysician to a group (98961, 98962)
Genetic counseling and/or risk factor reduction intervention from a physician
or other qualified health care provider provided to patients without
symptoms/diagnosis (99401-99412)
Do not report when 15 minutes or less of face-to-face time is provided

96040 **Medical genetics and genetic counseling services, each 30 minutes face-to-face with patient/family**
🚑 1.33   ⚕ 1.33   **FUD** XXX   B

AMA: 2015,Jan,16; 2014,Jan,11

96101-96127 Cognitive Capability Assessments

CMS: 100-2,15,80.2 Psychological and Neuropsychological Tests

INCLUDES | Cognitive function testing of the central nervous system
EXCLUDES | Cognitive skills development (97532, 97533)
Physician conducted mini-mental status examination; use appropriate
evaluation and management code

96101 **Psychological testing (includes psychodiagnostic assessment of emotionality, intellectual abilities, personality and psychopathology, eg, MMPI, Rorschach, WAIS), per hour of the psychologist's or physician's time, both face-to-face time administering tests to the patient and time interpreting these test results and preparing the report**

INCLUDES | Situations when more time is needed to assimilate
other clinical data sources including tests
administered by a technician or computer and
previously reported
Time spent face to face, interpretation, and preparing
report
Do not report less than 31 minutes of time
Do not report with (0364T-0367T, 0373T-0374T)
🚑 2.22   ⚕ 2.24   **FUD** XXX   03 80

AMA: 2015,Aug,5; 2015,Jan,16; 2014,Jun,3; 2014,Jan,11;
2012,Jan,15-42; 2011,Oct,3-4; 2011,Jan,11; 2010,Sep,9

96102 **Psychological testing (includes psychodiagnostic assessment of emotionality, intellectual abilities, personality and psychopathology, eg, MMPI and WAIS), with qualified health care professional interpretation and report, administered by technician, per hour of technician time, face-to-face**
Do not report less than 31 minutes of time
Do not report with (0364T-0367T, 0373T-0374T)
🚑 0.65   ⚕ 1.79   **FUD** XXX   03 80

AMA: 2015,Aug,5; 2015,Jan,16; 2014,Jan,11

96103 **Psychological testing (includes psychodiagnostic assessment of emotionality, intellectual abilities, personality and psychopathology, eg, MMPI), administered by a computer, with qualified health care professional interpretation and report**
Do not report with (0364T-0367T, 0373T-0374T)
🚑 0.75   ⚕ 0.77   **FUD** XXX   03 80

AMA: 2015,Aug,5; 2015,Jan,16; 2014,Jan,11; 2012,Jan,15-42;
2011,Oct,10

96105 **Assessment of aphasia (includes assessment of expressive and receptive speech and language function, language comprehension, speech production ability, reading, spelling, writing, eg, by Boston Diagnostic Aphasia Examination) with interpretation and report, per hour**
Do not report with (0364T-0367T, 0373T-0374T)
🚑 2.93   ⚕ 2.93   **FUD** XXX   A 80

AMA: 2015,Aug,5; 2015,Jan,16; 2014,Jan,11

96110 **Developmental screening (eg, developmental milestone survey, speech and language delay screen), with scoring and documentation, per standardized instrument**
Do not report with (0364T-0367T, 0373T-0374T)
🚑 0.27   ⚕ 0.27   **FUD** XXX   E

AMA: 2015,Aug,5; 2015,Jan,16; 2014,Jun,3; 2014,Jan,11

96111 **Developmental testing, (includes assessment of motor, language, social, adaptive, and/or cognitive functioning by standardized developmental instruments) with interpretation and report**
Do not report with (0364T-0367T, 0373T-0374T)
🚑 3.42   ⚕ 3.61   **FUD** XXX   03 80

AMA: 2015,Aug,5; 2015,Jan,16; 2014,Jan,11

96116 **Neurobehavioral status exam (clinical assessment of thinking, reasoning and judgment, eg, acquired knowledge, attention, language, memory, planning and problem solving, and visual spatial abilities), per hour of the psychologist's or physician's time, both face-to-face time with the patient and time interpreting test results and preparing the report**

INCLUDES | Time spent face to face, interpretation, and preparing
report
Do not report less than 31 minutes of time
Do not report with (0364T-0367T, 0373T-0374T)
🚑 2.45   ⚕ 2.62   **FUD** XXX   03 80 PQ

AMA: 2015,Aug,5; 2015,Jan,16; 2014,Jun,3; 2014,Jan,11;
2012,Jan,15-42; 2011,Oct,3-4; 2011,Jan,11

96118 **Neuropsychological testing (eg, Halstead-Reitan Neuropsychological Battery, Wechsler Memory Scales and Wisconsin Card Sorting Test), per hour of the psychologist's or physician's time, both face-to-face time administering tests to the patient and time interpreting these test results and preparing the report**

INCLUDES | Situations when more time is needed to assimilate
other clinical data sources including tests
administered by a technician or computer and
previously reported
Time spent face to face, interpretation, and preparing
report
Do not report less than 31 minutes of time
Do not report with (0364T-0367T, 0373T-0374T)
🚑 2.21   ⚕ 2.74   **FUD** XXX   03 80

AMA: 2015,Aug,5; 2015,Jan,16; 2014,Jun,3; 2014,Jan,11;
2012,Jan,15-42; 2011,Oct,3-4; 2011,Jan,11; 2010,Sep,9

96119 Neuropsychological testing (eg, Halstead-Reitan Neuropsychological Battery, Wechsler Memory Scales and Wisconsin Card Sorting Test), with qualified health care professional interpretation and report, administered by technician, per hour of technician time, face-to-face

> Do not report less than 31 minutes of time
> Do not report with (0364T-0367T, 0373T-0374T)
> 🚑 0.67 ⚕ 2.28 **FUD** XXX   Q3 80

> **AMA:** 2015,Aug,5; 2015,Jan,16; 2014,Jan,11

96120 Neuropsychological testing (eg, Wisconsin Card Sorting Test), administered by a computer, with qualified health care professional interpretation and report

> Do not report with (0364T-0367T, 0373T-0374T)
> 🚑 0.73 ⚕ 1.35 **FUD** XXX   Q3 80

> **AMA:** 2015,Aug,5; 2015,Jan,16; 2014,Jan,11; 2012,Jan,15-42; 2011,Jan,11

96125 Standardized cognitive performance testing (eg, Ross Information Processing Assessment) per hour of a qualified health care professional's time, both face-to-face time administering tests to the patient and time interpreting these test results and preparing the report

> INCLUDES Time spent face to face, interpretation, and preparing report
> EXCLUDES *Neuropsychological testing (96118-96120)*
> *Psychological testing (96101-96103)*
> Do not report less than 31 minutes of time
> Do not report with (0364T-0367T, 0373T-0374T)
> 🚑 3.30 ⚕ 3.30 **FUD** XXX   A 80

> **AMA:** 2015,Aug,5; 2015,Jan,16; 2014,Jan,11; 2012,Jan,15-42; 2011,Oct,3-4; 2011,Jan,11

96127 Brief emotional/behavioral assessment (eg, depression inventory, attention-deficit/hyperactivity disorder [ADHD] scale), with scoring and documentation, per standardized instrument

> 🚑 0.15 ⚕ 0.15 **FUD** XXX   Q1 80 TC

> **AMA:** 2015,Aug,5

96150-96155 Biopsychosocial Assessment/Intervention

INCLUDES Services for patients that have primary physical illnesses/diagnoses/symptoms who may benefit from assessments/interventions that focus on the biopsychosocial factors related to the patient's health status
Services used to identify the following factors which are important to the prevention/treatment/management of physical health problems:
Behavioral
Cognitive
Emotional
Psychological
Social
Do not report E&M codes on the same date of service
Do not report on same date of service with (99401-99412, 90785-90899)
Do not report with (0364T-0367T, 0373T-0374T)

96150 Health and behavior assessment (eg, health-focused clinical interview, behavioral observations, psychophysiological monitoring, health-oriented questionnaires), each 15 minutes face-to-face with the patient; initial assessment

> 🚑 0.60 ⚕ 0.61 **FUD** XXX   Q3 80 ▭ PQ

> **AMA:** 2015,Jan,16; 2014,Sep,13; 2014,Jun,3; 2014,Jan,11; 2013,May,12; 2012,Jan,15-42; 2011,Jan,11

96151 re-assessment

> 🚑 0.57 ⚕ 0.58 **FUD** XXX   Q3 80 ▭ PQ

> **AMA:** 2015,Jan,16; 2014,Sep,13; 2014,Jun,3; 2014,Jan,11; 2013,May,12; 2012,Jan,15-42; 2011,Jan,11

96152 Health and behavior intervention, each 15 minutes, face-to-face; individual

> 🚑 0.54 ⚕ 0.55 **FUD** XXX   Q3 80 ▭ PQ

> **AMA:** 2015,Jan,16; 2014,Sep,13; 2014,Jun,3; 2014,Jan,11; 2013,May,12; 2012,Jan,15-42; 2011,Jan,11

96153 group (2 or more patients)

> 🚑 0.12 ⚕ 0.13 **FUD** XXX   Q3 80 ▭

> **AMA:** 2015,Jan,16; 2014,Sep,13; 2014,Jun,3; 2014,Jan,11; 2013,May,12; 2012,Jan,15-42; 2011,Jan,11

96154 family (with the patient present)

> 🚑 0.53 ⚕ 0.54 **FUD** XXX   Q3 80 ▭

> **AMA:** 2015,Jan,16; 2014,Sep,13; 2014,Jun,3; 2014,Jan,11; 2013,May,12; 2012,Jan,15-42; 2011,Jan,11

96155 family (without the patient present)

> 🚑 0.64 ⚕ 0.64 **FUD** XXX   E

> **AMA:** 2015,Jan,16; 2014,Sep,13; 2014,Jun,3; 2014,Jan,11; 2013,May,12; 2012,Jan,15-42; 2011,Jan,11

96360-96361 Intravenous Fluid Infusion for Hydration (Nonchemotherapy)

CMS: 100-4,4,230.2 OPPS Drug Administration

INCLUDES Administration of prepackaged fluids and electrolytes
Coding hierarchy rules for facility reporting only:
Chemotherapy services are primary to diagnostic, prophylactic, and therapeutic services
Diagnostic, prophylactic, and therapeutic services are primary to hydration services
Infusions are primary to pushes
Pushes are primary to injections
Constant observance/attendance of person administering the drug or substance
Infusion of 15 minutes or less
Direct supervision by physician or other qualified health care provider:
Direction of personnel
Minimal supervision for:
Consent
Safety oversight
Supervision of personnel
Report the initial code for the primary reason for the visit regardless of the order in which the infusions or injections are given
The following if done to facilitate the injection/infusion:
Flush at the end of infusion
Indwelling IV, subcutaneous catheter/port access
Local anesthesia
Start of IV
Supplies/tubing/syringes
Treatment plan verification
EXCLUDES *Catheter/port declotting (36593)*
Drugs/other substances
Significant separately identifiable E&M service if performed
Do not report a second initial service on the same date for accessing a multi-lumen catheter or restarting an IV, or when two IV lines are needed to meet an infusion rate
Do not report for services provided by physicians or other qualified health care providers in facility settings
Do not report to keep the vein open or during other therapeutic infusions
Do not report with infusion for hydration that is 30 minutes or less

96360 Intravenous infusion, hydration; initial, 31 minutes to 1 hour

> Do not report hydration infusions of 31 minutes or less
> Do not report if performed as a concurrent infusion
> 🚑 1.62 ⚕ 1.62 **FUD** XXX   S 80

> **AMA:** 2015,Jan,16; 2014,May,10; 2014,Jan,11; 2013,Oct,3; 2011,Dec,3-5; 2011,Oct,3-4; 2011,May,7; 2010,May,8

+ **96361** each additional hour (List separately in addition to code for primary procedure)

> INCLUDES Hydration infusion of more than 30 minutes beyond 1 hour
> Hydration provided as a secondary or subsequent service after a different initial service via the same IV access site
> Code first (96360)
> 🚑 0.43 ⚕ 0.43 **FUD** ZZZ   S 80

> **AMA:** 2015,Jan,16; 2014,May,10; 2014,Jan,11; 2013,Oct,3; 2011,Dec,3-5; 2011,Oct,3-4; 2011,May,7; 2010,May,8

96365-96371 Infusions: Diagnostic/Preventive/Therapeutic

CMS: 100-4,4,230.2 OPPS Drug Administration

INCLUDES Administration of fluid
Administration of substances/drugs
An infusion of 16 minutes or more
Coding hierarchy rules for facility reporting:
Chemotherapy services are primary to diagnostic, prophylactic, and therapeutic services
Diagnostic, prophylactic, and therapeutic services are primary to hydration services
Infusions are primary to pushes
Pushes are primary to injections
Constant presence of health care professional administering the substance/drug
Direct supervision of physician or other qualified health care provider:
Consent
Direction of personnel
Patient assessment
Safety oversight
Supervision of personnel
The following if done to facilitate the injection/infusion:
Flush at the end of infusion
Indwelling IV, subcutaneous catheter/port access
Local anesthesia
Start of IV
Supplies/tubing/syringes
Training to assess patient and monitor vital signs
Training to prepare/dose/dispose
Treatment plan verification

EXCLUDES *Catheter/port declotting (36593)*
Significant separately identifiable E&M service, when performed
Code also drugs/materials
Do not report a second initial service on the same date for accessing a multi-lumen catheter or restarting an IV, or when two IV lines are needed to meet an infusion rate
Do not report for services provided by physicians or other qualified health care providers in facility settings
Do not report with codes for which IV push or infusion is an integral part of the procedure

96365 **Intravenous infusion, for therapy, prophylaxis, or diagnosis (specify substance or drug); initial, up to 1 hour**

Code also second initial service with modifier 59 when patient's condition or drug protocol mandates the use of two IV lines
🔌 1.96 ⚗ 1.96 **FUD** XXX [S] [80]
AMA: 2015,Jan,16; 2014,Jan,11; 2012,Jan,15-42; 2011,Dec,3-5; 2011,Oct,3-4; 2011,May,7; 2011,Jan,11; 2010,May,8

+ **96366** **each additional hour (List separately in addition to code for primary procedure)**

INCLUDES Additional hours of sequential infusion
Infusion intervals of more than 30 minutes beyond one hour
Second and subsequent infusions of the same drug or substance
Code also additional infusion, when appropriate (96367)
Code first (96365)
🔌 0.53 ⚗ 0.53 **FUD** ZZZ [S] [80]
AMA: 2015,Jan,16; 2014,Jan,11; 2012,Jan,15-42; 2011,Dec,3-5; 2011,May,7; 2011,Jan,11

+ **96367** **additional sequential infusion of a new drug/substance, up to 1 hour (List separately in addition to code for primary procedure)**

INCLUDES A secondary or subsequent service with a new drug or substance after a different initial service via the same IV access
Code first (96365, 96374, 96409, 96413)
Do not report more than one time per sequential infusion of the same mix
🔌 0.85 ⚗ 0.85 **FUD** ZZZ [S] [80]
AMA: 2015,Jan,16; 2014,Jan,11; 2012,Jan,15-42; 2011,Dec,3-5; 2011,May,7; 2011,Jan,11

+ **96368** **concurrent infusion (List separately in addition to code for primary procedure)**

Code first (96365, 96366, 96413, 96415, 96416)
Do not report more than one time per date of service
🔌 0.58 ⚗ 0.58 **FUD** ZZZ [N] [80]
AMA: 2015,Jan,16; 2014,Jan,11; 2011,Dec,3-5; 2011,May,7; 2010,May,8

96369 **Subcutaneous infusion for therapy or prophylaxis (specify substance or drug); initial, up to 1 hour, including pump set-up and establishment of subcutaneous infusion site(s)**

EXCLUDES *Infusions of 15 minutes or less (96372)*
Do not report more than one time per encounter
🔌 5.48 ⚗ 5.48 **FUD** XXX [S] [80]
AMA: 2015,Jan,16; 2014,Jan,11; 2011,Dec,3-5; 2011,May,7

+ **96370** **each additional hour (List separately in addition to code for primary procedure)**

INCLUDES Infusions of more than 30 minutes beyond one hour
Code first (96369)
🔌 0.43 ⚗ 0.43 **FUD** ZZZ [S] [80]
AMA: 2015,Jan,16; 2014,Jan,11; 2011,Dec,3-5; 2011,May,7

+ **96371** **additional pump set-up with establishment of new subcutaneous infusion site(s) (List separately in addition to code for primary procedure)**

Code first (96369)
Do not report more than one time per encounter
🔌 2.53 ⚗ 2.53 **FUD** ZZZ [N] [80]
AMA: 2015,Jan,16; 2014,Jan,11; 2011,Dec,3-5; 2011,May,7

96372-96379 Injections: Diagnostic/Preventive/Therapeutic

CMS: 100-4,4,230.2 OPPS Drug Administration

INCLUDES Administration of fluid
Administration of substances/drugs
Coding hierarchy rules for facility reporting:
Chemotherapy services are primary to diagnostic, prophylactic, and therapeutic services
Infusions are primary to pushes
Pushes are primary to injections
Constant presence of health care professional administering the substance/drug
Direct supervision by physician or other qualified health care provider:
Consent
Direction of personnel
Patient assessment
Safety oversight
Supervision of personnel
Infusion of 15 minutes or less
The following if done to facilitate the injection/infusion:
Flush at the end of infusion
Indwelling IV, subcutaneous catheter/port access
Local anesthesia
Start of IV
Supplies/tubing/syringes
Training to assess patient and monitor vital signs
Training to prepare/dose/dispose
Treatment plan verification

EXCLUDES *Catheter/port declotting (36593)*
Significant separately identifiable evaluation and management service, when performed
Code also drugs/materials
Do not report a second initial service on the same date for accessing a multi-lumen catheter or restarting an IV, or when two IV lines are needed to meet an infusion rate
Do not report services of physicians or other qualified health care providers provided in facility settings
Do not report with codes for which IV push or infusion is an integral part of the procedure

96372 Therapeutic, prophylactic, or diagnostic injection (specify substance or drug); subcutaneous or intramuscular

INCLUDES Direct supervision by physician or other qualified health care provider when reported by the physician/other qualified health care provider. When reported by a hospital, physician/other qualified health care provider need not be present.

Hormonal therapy injections (non-antineoplastic) (96372)

EXCLUDES *Administration of vaccines/toxoids (90460-90474)*
Allergen immunotherapy injections (95115-95117)
Antineoplastic hormonal injections (96402)
Antineoplastic nonhormonal injections (96401)
Injections administered without direct supervision by physician or other qualified health care provider (99211)

🚑 0.71 ⚖ 0.71 **FUD** XXX [S] [80]

AMA: 2015,Jan,16; 2014,Jan,9; 2014,Jan,11; 2013,Jan,9-10; 2012,Jan,15-42; 2011,Dec,3-5; 2011,May,7; 2011,Jan,11; 2010,May,9

96373 intra-arterial

🚑 0.55 ⚖ 0.55 **FUD** XXX [S] [80]

AMA: 2015,Jan,16; 2014,Jan,11; 2011,Dec,3-5; 2011,May,7

96374 intravenous push, single or initial substance/drug

Code also second initial service with modifier 59 when patient's condition or drug protocol mandates the use of two IV lines

🚑 1.60 ⚖ 1.60 **FUD** XXX [S] [80]

AMA: 2015,Jan,16; 2014,Jan,11; 2013,Jun,9-11; 2013,Feb,3-6; 2011,Dec,3-5; 2011,Oct,3-4; 2011,May,7; 2010,May,8; 2010,Jan,8-10

+ **96375** each additional sequential intravenous push of a new substance/drug (List separately in addition to code for primary procedure)

INCLUDES IV push of a new substance/drug provided as a secondary or subsequent service after a different initial service via same IV access site

Code first (96365, 96374, 96409, 96413)

🚑 0.63 ⚖ 0.63 **FUD** ZZZ [S] [80]

AMA: 2015,Jan,16; 2014,Jan,11; 2013,Feb,3-6; 2011,Dec,3-5; 2011,May,7; 2010,May,8

+ **96376** each additional sequential intravenous push of the same substance/drug provided in a facility (List separately in addition to code for primary procedure)

INCLUDES Facilities only

EXCLUDES *Services performed by any provider that is not a facility*

Code first (96365, 96374, 96409, 96413)

Do not report a push performed within 30 minutes of a reported push of the same substance or drug

🚑 0.00 ⚖ 0.00 **FUD** ZZZ [N]

AMA: 2015,Jan,16; 2014,Nov,14; 2014,Jan,11; 2011,Dec,3-5; 2011,May,7; 2010,May,8

96379 Unlisted therapeutic, prophylactic, or diagnostic intravenous or intra-arterial injection or infusion

🚑 0.00 ⚖ 0.00 **FUD** XXX [S] [80]

AMA: 2015,Jan,16; 2014,Jan,11; 2011,Dec,3-5; 2011,May,7

96401-96411 Chemotherapy and Other Complex Drugs, Biologicals: Injection and IV Push

CMS: 100-3,110.2 Certain Drugs Distributed by the National Cancer Institute; 100-3,110.6 Scalp Hypothermia During Chemotherapy, to Prevent Hair Loss; 100-4,4,230.2 OPPS Drug Administration

INCLUDES Highly complex services that require direct supervision for:
Consent
Patient assessment
Safety oversight
Supervision
More intense work and monitoring of clinical staff by physician or other qualified health care provider due to greater risk of severe patient reactions
Parenteral administration of:
→ Anti-neoplastic agents for noncancer diagnoses
Monoclonal antibody agents
Nonradionuclide antineoplastic drugs
Other biologic response modifiers
Do not report a second initial service on the same date for accessing a multi-lumen catheter or restarting an IV, or when two IV lines are needed to meet an infusion rate

96401 Chemotherapy administration, subcutaneous or intramuscular; non-hormonal anti-neoplastic

Do not report for services of physicians or other qualified health care providers in facility settings

🚑 2.10 ⚖ 2.10 **FUD** XXX [S] [80] [PQ]

AMA: 2015,Jan,16; 2014,Jan,11; 2012,Jan,15-42; 2011,Aug,9-10; 2011,Dec,3-5; 2011,Jan,11

96402 hormonal anti-neoplastic

Do not report for services by physician or other qualified health care provider in facility settings

🚑 0.91 ⚖ 0.91 **FUD** XXX [S] [80] [PQ]

AMA: 2015,Jan,16; 2014,Jan,11; 2012,Jan,15-42; 2011,Aug,9-10; 2011,Dec,3-5; 2011,Jan,11

96405 Chemotherapy administration; intralesional, up to and including 7 lesions

🚑 0.84 ⚖ 2.30 **FUD** 000 [S] [□] [PQ]

AMA: 2015,Jan,16; 2014,Jan,11; 2012,Jan,15-42; 2011,Aug,9-10; 2011,Jan,11

96406 intralesional, more than 7 lesions

🚑 1.31 ⚖ 3.34 **FUD** 000 [S] [□] [PQ]

AMA: 2015,Jan,16; 2014,Jan,11; 2012,Jan,15-42; 2011,Aug,9-10; 2011,Jan,11

96409 intravenous, push technique, single or initial substance/drug

INCLUDES Push technique includes:
Administration of injection directly into vessel or access line by health care professional; or
Infusion less than or equal to 15 minutes
Code also second initial service with modifier 59 when patient's condition or drug protocol mandates the use of two IV lines
Do not report for services by physicians or other qualified health care provider in facility settings
Do not report with (36823)

🚑 3.11 ⚖ 3.11 **FUD** XXX [S] [80] [PQ]

AMA: 2015,Jan,16; 2014,Jan,11; 2012,Jan,15-42; 2011,Aug,9-10; 2011,Dec,3-5; 2011,May,7; 2011,Jan,11; 2010,May,8

+ **96411** intravenous, push technique, each additional substance/drug (List separately in addition to code for primary procedure)

INCLUDES Push technique includes:
Administration of injection directly into vessel or access line by health care professional; or
Infusion less than or equal to 15 minutes
Code first initial substance/drug (96409, 96413)
Do not report for services of physicians or other qualified health care providers in facility settings
Do not report with (36823)

🚑 1.74 ⚖ 1.74 **FUD** ZZZ [S] [80] [PQ]

AMA: 2015,Jan,16; 2014,Jan,11; 2012,Jan,15-42; 2011,Aug,9-10; 2011,Dec,3-5; 2011,Jan,11

434

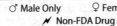
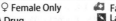
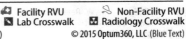

96413-96417 Chemotherapy and Complex Drugs, Biologicals: Intravenous Infusion

CMS: 100-3,110.2 Certain Drugs Distributed by the National Cancer Institute; 100-3,110.6 Scalp Hypothermia During Chemotherapy, to Prevent Hair Loss; 100-4,4,230.2 OPPS Drug Administration

INCLUDES Highly complex services that require direct supervision for:
  Consent
  Patient assessment
  Safety oversight
  Supervision
More intense work and monitoring of clinical staff by physician or other qualified health care provider due to greater risk of severe patient reactions
Parenteral administration of:
  Anti-neoplastic agents for noncancer diagnoses
  Monoclonal antibody agents
  Nonradionuclide antineoplastic drugs
  Other biologic response modifiers
The following in the administration:
  Access to IV/catheter/port
  Drug preparation
  Flushing at the completion of the infusion
  Hydration fluid
  Routine tubing/syringe/supplies
  Starting the IV
  Use of local anesthesia

EXCLUDES *Administration of nonchemotherapy agents such as antibiotics/steroids/analgesics*
  Declotting of catheter/port (36593)
  Home infusion (99601-99602)
Code also drug or substance
Code also significant separately identifiable evaluation and management service, when performed
Do not report a second initial service on the same date for accessing a multi-lumen catheter or restarting an IV, or when two IV lines are needed to meet an infusion rate
Do not report for services of physicians or other qualified health care providers in facility settings
Do not report with (36823)

96413 Chemotherapy administration, intravenous infusion technique; up to 1 hour, single or initial substance/drug

INCLUDES Push technique includes:
  Administration of injection directly into vessel or access line by health care professional; or
  Infusion less than or equal to 15 minutes
EXCLUDES *Hydration administered as secondary or subsequent service via same IV access site (96361)*
  Therapeutic/prophylactic/diagnostic drug infusion/injection through the same intravenous access (96366, 96367, 96375)
Code also second initial service with modifier 59 when patient's condition or drug protocol mandates the use of two IV lines
🔧 3.80 ⚕ 3.80 **FUD** XXX [S] [80] [PO]
AMA: 2015,Jan,16; 2014,Jan,11; 2012,Jan,15-42; 2011,Aug,9-10; 2011,Dec,3-5; 2011,Jan,11; 2011,May,7; 2011,Jan,11; 2010,May,8

+ 96415 each additional hour (List separately in addition to code for primary procedure)

INCLUDES Infusion intervals of more than 30 minutes past 1-hour increments
Code first initial hour (96413)
🔧 0.79 ⚕ 0.79 **FUD** ZZZ [S] [80] [PO]
AMA: 2015,Jan,16; 2014,Jan,11; 2012,Jan,15-42; 2011,Aug,9-10; 2011,Dec,3-5; 2011,Jan,11

96416 initiation of prolonged chemotherapy infusion (more than 8 hours), requiring use of a portable or implantable pump

EXCLUDES *Portable or implantable infusion pump/reservoir refilling/maintenance for drug delivery (96521-96523)*
🔧 3.94 ⚕ 3.94 **FUD** XXX [S] [80] [PO]
AMA: 2015,Jan,16; 2014,Jan,11; 2012,Jan,15-42; 2011,Aug,9-10; 2011,Dec,3-5; 2011,Jan,11

+ 96417 each additional sequential infusion (different substance/drug), up to 1 hour (List separately in addition to code for primary procedure)

INCLUDES Push technique includes:
  Administration of injection directly into vessel or access line by health care professional; or
  Infusion less than or equal to 15 minutes
EXCLUDES *Additional hour(s) of sequential infusion (96415)*
Code first initial substance/drug (96413)
Do not report more than one time per sequential infusion
🔧 1.76 ⚕ 1.76 **FUD** ZZZ [S] [80] [PO]
AMA: 2015,Jan,16; 2014,Jan,11; 2012,Jan,15-42; 2011,Aug,9-10; 2011,Dec,3-5; 2011,Jan,11

96420-96425 Chemotherapy and Complex Drugs, Biologicals: Intra-arterial

CMS: 100-3,110.2 Certain Drugs Distributed by the National Cancer Institute; 100-3,110.6 Scalp Hypothermia During Chemotherapy, to Prevent Hair Loss; 100-4,4,230.2 OPPS Drug Administration

INCLUDES Highly complex services that require direct supervision for:
  Consent
  Patient assessment
  Safety oversight
  Supervision
More intense work and monitoring of clinical staff by physician or other qualified health care provider due to greater risk of severe patient reactions
Parenteral administration of:
  Anti-neoplastic agents for noncancer diagnoses
  Monoclonal antibody agents
  Non-radionuclide antineoplastic drugs
  Other biologic response modifiers
The following in the administration:
  Access to IV/catheter/port
  Drug preparation
  Flushing at the completion of the infusion
  Hydration fluid
  Routine tubing/syringe/supplies
  Starting the IV
  Use of local anesthesia

EXCLUDES *Administration of non-chemotherapy agents such as antibiotics/steroids/analgesics*
  Declotting of catheter/port (36593)
  Home infusion (99601-99602)
Code also drug or substance
Code also significant separately identifiable evaluation and management service, when performed
Do not report a second initial service on the same date for accessing a multi-lumen catheter or restarting an IV, or when two IV lines are needed to meet an infusion rate
Do not report for services by physician or other qualified health care provider in facility settings

96420 Chemotherapy administration, intra-arterial; push technique

INCLUDES Push technique includes:
  Administration of injection directly into vessel or access line by health care professional; or
  Infusion less than or equal to 15 minutes
  Regional chemotherapy perfusion
EXCLUDES *Placement of intra-arterial catheter*
Do not report with (36823)
🔧 2.92 ⚕ 2.92 **FUD** XXX [S] [80] [▭] [PO]
AMA: 2015,Jan,16; 2014,Jan,11; 2013,Nov,6; 2012,Jan,15-42; 2011,Aug,9-10; 2011,Dec,3-5; 2011,Jan,11

96422 infusion technique, up to 1 hour

INCLUDES Push technique includes:
  Administration of injection directly into vessel or access line by health care professional; or
  Infusion less than or equal to 15 minutes
  Regional chemotherapy perfusion
EXCLUDES *Placement of intra-arterial catheter*
Do not report with (36823)
🔧 4.78 ⚕ 4.78 **FUD** XXX [S] [80] [▭] [PO]
AMA: 2015,Jan,16; 2014,Jan,11; 2012,Jan,15-42; 2011,Aug,9-10; 2011,Dec,3-5; 2011,Jan,11

Medicine

96423 — 96523

+ 96423 **infusion technique, each additional hour (List separately in addition to code for primary procedure)**

> INCLUDES: Infusion intervals of more than 30 minutes past 1-hour increments
> Regional chemotherapy perfusion
>
> EXCLUDES: *Arterial/venous cannula insertion with regional chemotherapy perfusion to an extremity (36823)*
> *Placement of intra-arterial catheter*

Code first initial hour (96422)
Do not report with (36823)

📋 2.22   ⚕ 2.22   **FUD** ZZZ   S 80 ▭ PQ

AMA: 2015,Jan,16; 2014,Jan,11; 2012,Jan,15-42; 2011,Aug,9-10; 2011,Dec,3-5; 2011,Jan,11

96425 **infusion technique, initiation of prolonged infusion (more than 8 hours), requiring the use of a portable or implantable pump**

> INCLUDES: Regional chemotherapy perfusion
>
> EXCLUDES: *Placement of intra-arterial catheter*
> *Portable or implantable infusion pump/reservoir refilling/maintenance for drug delivery (96521-96523)*

Do not report with (36823)

📋 5.07   ⚕ 5.07   **FUD** XXX   S 80 ▭ PQ

AMA: 2015,Jan,16; 2014,Jan,11; 2012,Jan,15-42; 2011,Aug,9-10; 2011,Dec,3-5; 2011,Jan,11

96440-96450 Chemotherapy Administration: Intrathecal/Peritoneal Cavity/Pleural Cavity

CMS: 100-3,110.2 Certain Drugs Distributed by the National Cancer Institute; 100-4,4,230.2 OPPS Drug Administration

96440 **Chemotherapy administration into pleural cavity, requiring and including thoracentesis**

📋 4.01   ⚕ 24.2   **FUD** 000   S 80 ▭ PQ

AMA: 2015,Jan,16; 2014,Jan,11; 2012,Jan,15-42; 2011,Jan,11

96446 **Chemotherapy administration into the peritoneal cavity via indwelling port or catheter**

📋 0.83   ⚕ 5.66   **FUD** XXX   S 80 PQ

AMA: 2015,Jan,16; 2014,Jan,11; 2012,Jan,15-42; 2011,Jan,11; 2010,Dec,12

96450 **Chemotherapy administration, into CNS (eg, intrathecal), requiring and including spinal puncture**

> EXCLUDES: *Chemotherapy administration, intravesical/bladder (51720)*
> *Insertion of catheter/reservoir:*
> *Intraventricular (61210, 61215)*
> *Subarachnoid (62350-62351, 62360-62362)*

📋 2.29   ⚕ 5.13   **FUD** 000   S 80 ▭ PQ

AMA: 2015,Jan,16; 2014,Jan,11; 2012,Jan,15-42; 2011,Jan,11

96521-96523 Refill/Upkeep of Drug Delivery Device

CMS: 100-4,4,230.2 OPPS Drug Administration

> INCLUDES: Highly complex services that require direct supervision for:
> Consent
> Patient assessment
> Safety oversight
> Supervision
> Parenteral administration of:
> Anti-neoplastic agents for noncancer diagnoses
> Monoclonal antibody agents
> Non-radionuclide antineoplastic drugs
> Other biologic response modifiers
> The following in the administration:
> Access to IV/catheter/port
> Drug preparation
> Flushing at the completion of the infusion
> Hydration fluid
> Routine tubing/syringe/supplies
> Starting the IV
> Use of local anesthesia
> Therapeutic drugs other than chemotherapy
>
> EXCLUDES: *Administration of non-chemotherapy agents such as antibiotics/steroids/analgesics*
> *Blood specimen collection from completely implantable venous access device (36591)*
> *Declotting of catheter/port (36593)*
> *Home infusion (99601-99602)*

Code also drug or substance
Code also significant separately identifiable evaluation and management service, when performed
Do not report for services by physician or other qualified health care provider in facility settings

96521 **Refilling and maintenance of portable pump**

📋 3.88   ⚕ 3.88   **FUD** XXX   S 80 PQ

AMA: 2015,Jan,16; 2014,Jan,11; 2011,Dec,3-5

96522 **Refilling and maintenance of implantable pump or reservoir for drug delivery, systemic (eg, intravenous, intra-arterial)**

> EXCLUDES: *Implantable infusion pump refilling/maintenance for spinal/brain drug delivery (95990-95991)*

📋 3.20   ⚕ 3.20   **FUD** XXX   S 80 PQ

AMA: 2015,Jan,16; 2014,Jan,11; 2012,Aug,10-12; 2011,Dec,3-5

96523 **Irrigation of implanted venous access device for drug delivery systems**

> EXCLUDES: *Direct supervision by physician or other qualified health care provider in facility settings*

Do not report with any other services on the same date of service

📋 0.70   ⚕ 0.70   **FUD** XXX   Q1 80 PQ

AMA: 2015,Jan,16; 2014,Jan,11; 2012,Jan,15-42; 2011,Dec,3-5; 2011,Jul,16-17

96542-96549 Chemotherapy Injection Into Brain

CMS: 100-4,4,230.2 OPPS Drug Administration

> INCLUDES: Highly complex services that require direct supervision for:
> Consent
> Patient assessment
> Safety oversight
> Supervision
> Parenteral administration of:
> Anti-neoplastic agents for noncancer diagnoses
> Monoclonal antibody agents
> Non-radionuclide antineoplastic drugs
> Other biologic response modifiers
> The following in the administration:
> Access to IV/catheter/port
> Drug preparation
> Flushing at the completion of the infusion
> Hydration fluid
> Routine tubing/syringe/supplies
> Starting the IV
> Use of local anesthesia
>
> EXCLUDES: *Administration of non-chemotherapy agents such as antibiotics/steroids/analgesics*
> *Blood specimen collection from completely implantable venous access device (36591)*
> *Declotting of catheter/port (36593)*
> *Home infusion (99601-99602)*

Code also drug or substance
Code also significant separately identifiable evaluation and management service, when performed

96542 Chemotherapy injection, subarachnoid or intraventricular via subcutaneous reservoir, single or multiple agents

EXCLUDES *Oral radioactive isotope therapy (79005)*

📟 1.19   ☈ 3.37   **FUD** XXX   [S] [80] 🖵 [PQ]

AMA: 2015,Jan,16; 2014,Jan,11

96549 Unlisted chemotherapy procedure

📟 0.00   ☈ 0.00   **FUD** XXX   [S] [80] [PQ]

AMA: 2015,Jan,16; 2014,Jan,11; 2012,Jan,15-42; 2011,Jan,11; 2010,Dec,12

96567-96571 Destruction of Lesions: Photodynamic Therapy

EXCLUDES *Ocular photodynamic therapy (67221)*

96567 Photodynamic therapy by external application of light to destroy premalignant and/or malignant lesions of the skin and adjacent mucosa (eg, lip) by activation of photosensitive drug(s), each phototherapy exposure session

📟 3.79   ☈ 3.79   **FUD** XXX   [T] [80] 🖵

AMA: 2015,Jan,16; 2014,Jan,11; 2012,Jan,15-42; 2011,Jan,11; 2010,Mar,9-11

\+ **96570** Photodynamic therapy by endoscopic application of light to ablate abnormal tissue via activation of photosensitive drug(s); first 30 minutes (List separately in addition to code for endoscopy or bronchoscopy procedures of lung and gastrointestinal tract)

Code also for 38-52 minutes (96571)
Code also modifier 52 when services with report are less than 23 minutes
Code first (31641, 43229)

📟 1.63   ☈ 1.63   **FUD** ZZZ   [N] 🖵

AMA: 2015,Jan,16; 2014,Jan,11; 2013,Apr,8-9; 2011,Oct,3-4

\+ **96571** each additional 15 minutes (List separately in addition to code for endoscopy or bronchoscopy procedures of lung and gastrointestinal tract)

EXCLUDES *23-37 minutes of service (96570)*
Code first (96570)
Code first when appropriate (31641, 43229)

📟 0.75   ☈ 0.75   **FUD** ZZZ   [N]

AMA: 2015,Jan,16; 2014,Jan,11; 2013,Apr,8-9; 2011,Oct,3-4

96900-96999 Diagnostic/Therapeutic Skin Procedures

EXCLUDES *Evaluation and management services*
Injection, intralesional (11900-11901)

96900 Actinotherapy (ultraviolet light)

EXCLUDES *Rhinophototherapy (30999)*
🔳 (88160-88161)

📟 0.58   ☈ 0.58   **FUD** XXX   [01] [80] 🖵

AMA: 2015,Jan,16; 2014,Jan,11; 2012,Jul,9; 2012,Jan,15-42; 2011,Jan,11

96902 Microscopic examination of hairs plucked or clipped by the examiner (excluding hair collected by the patient) to determine telogen and anagen counts, or structural hair shaft abnormality

🔳 (88160-88161)

📟 0.59   ☈ 0.61   **FUD** XXX   [N]

AMA: 1997,Nov,1

96904 Whole body integumentary photography, for monitoring of high risk patients with dysplastic nevus syndrome or a history of dysplastic nevi, or patients with a personal or familial history of melanoma

🔳 (88160-88161)

📟 1.77   ☈ 1.77   **FUD** XXX   [N] [80]

AMA: 2006,Dec,10-12

96910 Photochemotherapy; tar and ultraviolet B (Goeckerman treatment) or petrolatum and ultraviolet B

🔳 (88160-88161)

📟 2.01   ☈ 2.01   **FUD** XXX   [01] [80] 🖵

AMA: 2015,Jan,16; 2014,Jan,11; 2012,Jul,9

96912 psoralens and ultraviolet A (PUVA)

🔳 (88160-88161)

📟 2.58   ☈ 2.58   **FUD** XXX   [01] [80] 🖵

AMA: 2015,Jan,16; 2014,Jan,11; 2012,Jul,9

96913 Photochemotherapy (Goeckerman and/or PUVA) for severe photoresponsive dermatoses requiring at least 4-8 hours of care under direct supervision of the physician (includes application of medication and dressings)

🔳 (88160-88161)

📟 3.63   ☈ 3.63   **FUD** XXX   [T] [80] 🖵

AMA: 1997,Nov,1; 1995,Sum,5

96920 Laser treatment for inflammatory skin disease (psoriasis); total area less than 250 sq cm

EXCLUDES *Destruction by laser of:*
Benign lesions (17110-17111)
Cutaneous vascular proliferative lesions (17106-17108)
Malignant lesions (17260-17286)
Premalignant lesions (17000-17004)
🔳 (88160-88161)

📟 1.89   ☈ 4.37   **FUD** 000   [01] 🖵

AMA: 2015,Jan,16; 2014,Jan,11; 2013,May,12; 2012,Jul,9; 2012,Jan,15-42; 2011,Jan,11; 2010,Oct,9

96921 250 sq cm to 500 sq cm

EXCLUDES *Destruction by laser of:*
Benign lesions (17110-17111)
Cutaneous vascular proliferative lesions (17106-17108)
Malignant lesions (17260-17286)
Premalignant lesions (17000-17004)
🔳 (88160-88161)

📟 2.14   ☈ 4.83   **FUD** 000   [01] 🖵

AMA: 2015,Jan,16; 2014,Jan,11; 2013,May,12; 2012,Jul,9; 2012,Jan,15-42; 2011,Jan,11; 2010,Oct,9

96922 over 500 sq cm

EXCLUDES *Destruction by laser of:*
Benign lesions (17110-17111)
Cutaneous vascular proliferative lesions (17106-17108)
Malignant lesions (17260-17286)
Premalignant lesions (17000-17004)
🔳 (88160-88161)

📟 3.46   ☈ 6.68   **FUD** 000   [01] 🖵

AMA: 2015,Jan,16; 2014,Jan,11; 2013,May,12; 2012,Jul,9; 2012,Jan,15-42; 2011,Jan,11; 2010,Oct,9

● **96931** Reflectance confocal microscopy (RCM) for cellular and sub-cellular imaging of skin; image acquisition and interpretation and report, first lesion

● **96932** image acquisition only, first lesion

● **96933** interpretation and report only, first lesion

● \+ **96934** image acquisition and interpretation and report, each additional lesion (List separately in addition to code for primary procedure)

📟 0.00   ☈ 0.00   **FUD** 000

Code first (96931)

● \+ **96935** image acquisition only, each additional lesion (List separately in addition to code for primary procedure)

📟 0.00   ☈ 0.00   **FUD** 000

Code first (96932)

● \+ **96936** interpretation and report only, each additional lesion (List separately in addition to code for primary procedure)

📟 0.00   ☈ 0.00   **FUD** 000

Code first (96933)

96999 Unlisted special dermatological service or procedure

📟 0.00   ☈ 0.00   **FUD** XXX   [01] [80]

AMA: 2015,Jan,16; 2014,Jan,11; 2013,May,12; 2012,Jul,9

● New Code   ▲ Revised Code   ○ Reinstated   [M] Maternity   [A] Age Edit   Unlisted   Not Covered   # Resequenced
☈ AMA Mod 51 Exempt   [91] Optum Mod 51 Exempt   [63] Mod 63 Exempt   🖵 Mod Sedation   \+ Add-on   [C] CCI   [PQ] PQRS   **FUD** Follow-up Days

Medicine *(left margin)*

97001 — 97039 *(left margin)*

97001-97006 Physical Medicine Assessments

CMS: 100-2,15,230 Practice of Physical Therapy, Occupational Therapy, and Speech-Language Pathology; 100-2,15,230.1 Practice of Physical Therapy; 100-2,15,230.4 Services By a Physical/Occupational Therapist in Private Practice; 100-3,10.3 Inpatient Pain Rehabilitation Programs; 100-3,10.4 Outpatient Hospital Pain Rehabilitation Programs; 100-3,160.17 Payment for L-Dopa /Associated Inpatient Hospital Services; 100-4,5,10 Part B Outpatient Rehabilitation and Comprehensive Outpatient Rehabilitation Facility (CORF) Services - General; 100-4,5,20.2 Reporting Units of Service

EXCLUDES   Electromyography (95860-95872 [95885, 95886, 95887])
EMG biofeedback training (90901)
Muscle and range of motion tests (95831-95857)
Nerve conduction studies (95905-95913)
Transcutaneous nerve stimulation (TNS) (64550)

97001   **Physical therapy evaluation**
2.11   2.11   **FUD** XXX   ⑤ Ⓐ 80 🖵 PQ
AMA: 2015,Jun,10; 2015,Jan,16; 2014,Jan,11; 2012,Jan,15-42; 2011,Jan,11

97002   **Physical therapy re-evaluation**
1.18   1.18   **FUD** XXX   ⑤ Ⓐ 80 🖵 PQ
AMA: 2015,Jan,16; 2014,Jan,11; 2012,Jan,15-42; 2011,Jan,11

97003   **Occupational therapy evaluation**
2.39   2.39   **FUD** XXX   ⑤ Ⓐ 80 🖵 PQ
AMA: 2015,Jan,16; 2014,Jun,3; 2014,Jan,11; 2012,Jan,15-42; 2011,Jan,11

97004   **Occupational therapy re-evaluation**
1.48   1.48   **FUD** XXX   ⑤ Ⓐ 80 🖵 PQ
AMA: 2015,Jan,16; 2014,Jun,3; 2014,Jan,11; 2012,Jan,15-42; 2011,Jan,11

97005   **Athletic training evaluation**
0.00   0.00   **FUD** XXX   ⑤ Ⓔ
AMA: 2015,Jan,16; 2014,Jan,11

97006   **Athletic training re-evaluation**
0.00   0.00   **FUD** XXX   ⑤ Ⓔ
AMA: 2015,Jan,16; 2014,Jan,11

97010-97028 Physical Therapy Treatment Modalities: Supervised

CMS: 100-2,15,230 Practice of Physical Therapy, Occupational Therapy, and Speech-Language Pathology; 100-2,15,230.1 Practice of Physical Therapy; 100-2,15,230.2 Practice of Occupational Therapy; 100-2,15,230.4 Services By a Physical/Occupational Therapist in Private Practice; 100-3,10.3 Inpatient Pain Rehabilitation Programs; 100-3,10.4 Outpatient Hospital Pain Rehabilitation Programs; 100-3,160.17 Payment for L-Dopa /Associated Inpatient Hospital Services; 100-4,5,10.2 Financial Limitation for Outpatient Rehabilitation Services; 100-4,5,20.2 Reporting Units of Service

INCLUDES   Adding incremental intervals of treatment time for the same visit to calculate the total service time

EXCLUDES   Direct patient contact by the provider
Electromyography (95860-95872 [95885, 95886, 95887])
EMG biofeedback training (90901)
Muscle and range of motion tests (95831-95857)
Nerve conduction studies (95905-95913)
Transcutaneous nerve stimulation (TNS) (64550)

97010   **Application of a modality to 1 or more areas; hot or cold packs**
0.17   0.17   **FUD** XXX   ⑤ Ⓐ
AMA: 2015,Jan,16; 2014,Jan,11; 2012,Jan,15-42; 2011,Jan,11; 2010,Aug,12; 2010,Nov,8; 2010,Aug,12; 2010,Jun,8

97012   **traction, mechanical**
0.45   0.45   **FUD** XXX   ⑤ Ⓐ 80 🖵
AMA: 2015,Jan,16; 2014,Jan,11; 2012,Jan,15-42; 2011,Jan,11; 2010,Nov,8; 2010,Jun,8

97014   **electrical stimulation (unattended)**
EXCLUDES   Acupuncture with electrical stimulation (97813, 97814)
0.45   0.45   **FUD** XXX   ⑤ Ⓔ
AMA: 2015,Jan,16; 2014,Jan,11; 2012,Jan,15-42; 2011,Aug,6-7; 2011,Jan,11; 2010,Nov,8; 2010,Jun,8

97016   **vasopneumatic devices**
0.54   0.54   **FUD** XXX   ⑤ Ⓐ 80 🖵
AMA: 2015,Jan,16; 2014,Jan,11; 2012,Jan,15-42; 2011,Jan,11; 2010,Nov,8; 2010,Jun,8

97018   **paraffin bath**
0.31   0.31   **FUD** XXX   ⑤ Ⓐ 80 🖵
AMA: 2015,Jan,16; 2014,Jan,11; 2012,Jan,15-42; 2011,Jan,11; 2010,Nov,8; 2010,Jun,8

97022   **whirlpool**
0.66   0.66   **FUD** XXX   ⑤ Ⓐ 80 🖵
AMA: 2015,Jan,16; 2014,Jan,11; 2012,Jan,15-42; 2011,Jan,11; 2010,Nov,8; 2010,Jun,8

97024   **diathermy (eg, microwave)**
0.18   0.18   **FUD** XXX   ⑤ Ⓐ 80 🖵
AMA: 2015,Jan,16; 2014,Jan,11; 2012,Jan,15-42; 2011,Jan,11; 2010,Nov,8; 2010,Jun,8

97026   **infrared**
0.17   0.17   **FUD** XXX   ⑤ Ⓐ 80 🖵
AMA: 2015,Jan,16; 2014,Jan,11; 2012,Jan,15-42; 2011,Jan,11; 2010,Nov,8; 2010,Jun,8; 2010,Jan,12-15

97028   **ultraviolet**
0.21   0.21   **FUD** XXX   ⑤ Ⓐ 80 🖵
AMA: 2015,Jan,16; 2014,Jan,11; 2012,Jan,15-42; 2011,Jan,11; 2010,Nov,8; 2010,Jun,8

97032-97039 Physical Therapy Treatment Modalities: Constant Attendance

CMS: 100-2,15,230 Practice of Physical Therapy, Occupational Therapy, and Speech-Language Pathology; 100-2,15,230.1 Practice of Physical Therapy; 100-2,15,230.2 Practice of Occupational Therapy; 100-2,15,230.4 Services By a Physical/Occupational Therapist in Private Practice; 100-3,10.3 Inpatient Pain Rehabilitation Programs; 100-3,10.4 Outpatient Hospital Pain Rehabilitation Programs; 100-3,160.17 Payment for L-Dopa /Associated Inpatient Hospital Services; 100-4,5,20.2 Reporting Units of Service

INCLUDES   Adding incremental intervals of treatment time for the same visit to calculate the total service time
Direct patient contact by the provider

EXCLUDES   Electromyography (95860-95872 [95885, 95886, 95887])
EMG biofeedback training (90901)
Muscle and range of motion tests (95831-95857)
Nerve conduction studies (95905-95913)
Transcutaneous nerve stimulation (TNS) (64550)

97032   **Application of a modality to 1 or more areas; electrical stimulation (manual), each 15 minutes**
EXCLUDES   Transcutaneous electrical modulation pain reprocessing (TEMPR) (scrambler therapy) (0278T)
0.54   0.54   **FUD** XXX   ⑤ Ⓐ 80 🖵
AMA: 2015,Jan,16; 2014,Jan,11; 2012,Jan,15-42; 2011,Jan,11; 2010,Aug,12; 2010,Nov,8; 2010,Aug,12; 2010,Jun,8

97033   **iontophoresis, each 15 minutes**
0.92   0.92   **FUD** XXX   ⑤ Ⓐ 80 🖵
AMA: 2015,Jan,16; 2014,Jan,11; 2010,Aug,12; 2010,Nov,8; 2010,Aug,12; 2010,Jun,8

97034   **contrast baths, each 15 minutes**
0.51   0.51   **FUD** XXX   ⑤ Ⓐ 80 🖵
AMA: 2015,Jan,16; 2014,Jan,11; 2010,Aug,12; 2010,Nov,8; 2010,Aug,12; 2010,Jun,8

97035   **ultrasound, each 15 minutes**
0.36   0.36   **FUD** XXX   ⑤ Ⓐ 80 🖵
AMA: 2015,Jan,16; 2014,Jan,11; 2012,Jan,15-42; 2011,Jan,11; 2010,Aug,12; 2010,Nov,8; 2010,Aug,12; 2010,Jun,8

97036   **Hubbard tank, each 15 minutes**
0.94   0.94   **FUD** XXX   ⑤ Ⓐ 80 🖵
AMA: 2015,Jan,16; 2014,Jan,11; 2010,Aug,12; 2010,Nov,8; 2010,Aug,12; 2010,Jun,8

97039   **Unlisted modality (specify type and time if constant attendance)**
0.00   0.00   **FUD** XXX   Ⓐ 80 🖵
AMA: 2015,Jan,16; 2014,Jan,11; 2012,Jan,15-42; 2011,Jan,11; 2010,Aug,12; 2010,Nov,8; 2010,Aug,12; 2010,Jun,8; 2010,Jan,12-15

97110-97546 Other Therapeutic Techniques With Direct Patient Contact

CMS: 100-2,15,230 Practice of Physical Therapy, Occupational Therapy, and Speech-Language Pathology; 100-2,15,230.1 Practice of Physical Therapy; 100-2,15,230.2 Practice of Occupational Therapy; 100-2,15,230.4 Services By a Physical/Occupational Therapist in Private Practice; 100-3,10.3 Inpatient Pain Rehabilitation Programs; 100-3,10.4 Outpatient Hospital Pain Rehabilitation Programs; 100-4,5,10.2 Financial Limitation for Outpatient Rehabilitation Services; 100-4,5,20.2 Reporting Units of Service

[INCLUDES] Application of clinical skills/services to improve function
Direct patient contact by the provider

[EXCLUDES] *Electromyography (95860-95872 [95885, 95886, 95887])*
EMG biofeedback training (90901)
Muscle and range of motion tests (95831-95857)
Nerve conduction studies (95905-95913)
Transcutaneous nerve stimulation (TNS) (64550)

97110 **Therapeutic procedure, 1 or more areas, each 15 minutes; therapeutic exercises to develop strength and endurance, range of motion and flexibility**
🏢 0.91 ✂ 0.91 **FUD** XXX [51] [A] [80] ▣
AMA: 2015,Jan,16; 2014,Aug,5; 2014,Mar,13; 2014,Jan,11; 2012,Mar,9-10; 2012,Jan,15-42; 2011,Jan,11; 2010,May,9

97112 **neuromuscular reeducation of movement, balance, coordination, kinesthetic sense, posture, and/or proprioception for sitting and/or standing activities**
🏢 0.94 ✂ 0.94 **FUD** XXX [51] [A] [80] ▣
AMA: 2015,Jan,16; 2014,Mar,13; 2014,Jan,11; 2012,Mar,9-10; 2012,Jan,15-42; 2011,Jan,11; 2010,May,9

97113 **aquatic therapy with therapeutic exercises**
🏢 1.21 ✂ 1.21 **FUD** XXX [51] [A] [80] ▣
AMA: 2015,Jan,16; 2014,Mar,13; 2014,Jan,11; 2012,Jan,15-42; 2011,Jan,11; 2010,May,9

97116 **gait training (includes stair climbing)**
[EXCLUDES] *Comprehensive gait/motion analysis (96000-96003)*
🏢 0.80 ✂ 0.80 **FUD** XXX [51] [A] [80] ▣
AMA: 2015,Jan,16; 2014,Mar,13; 2014,Jan,11; 2012,Jan,15-42; 2011,Jan,11; 2010,May,9

97124 **massage, including effleurage, petrissage and/or tapotement (stroking, compression, percussion)**
[EXCLUDES] *Myofascial release (97140)*
🏢 0.75 ✂ 0.75 **FUD** XXX [51] [A] [80] ▣
AMA: 2015,Jan,16; 2014,Mar,13; 2014,Jan,11; 2012,Jan,15-42; 2011,Jan,11; 2010,May,9

97139 **Unlisted therapeutic procedure (specify)**
🏢 0.00 ✂ 0.00 **FUD** XXX [A] [80] ▣
AMA: 2015,Jan,16; 2014,Mar,13; 2014,Jan,11; 2012,Jan,15-42; 2011,Jan,11

97140 **Manual therapy techniques (eg, mobilization/ manipulation, manual lymphatic drainage, manual traction), 1 or more regions, each 15 minutes**
🏢 0.84 ✂ 0.84 **FUD** XXX [51] [A] [80] ▣
AMA: 2015,Mar,9; 2015,Jan,16; 2014,Mar,13; 2014,Jan,11; 2012,Jan,15-42; 2011,Jan,11

97150 **Therapeutic procedure(s), group (2 or more individuals)**
[INCLUDES] Constant attendance by the physician/therapist
Reporting this procedure for each member of group
[EXCLUDES] *Osteopathic manipulative treatment (98925-98929)*
Do not report with (0366T-0367T, 0372T)
🏢 0.49 ✂ 0.49 **FUD** XXX [51] [A] [80] ▣
AMA: 2015,Jan,16; 2014,Mar,13; 2014,Jan,11; 2012,Jan,15-42; 2011,Jan,11

97530 **Therapeutic activities, direct (one-on-one) patient contact (use of dynamic activities to improve functional performance), each 15 minutes**
🏢 0.98 ✂ 0.98 **FUD** XXX [51] [A] [80] ▣
AMA: 2015,Jan,16; 2014,Mar,13; 2014,Jan,11; 2012,Jan,15-42; 2011,Jan,11

97532 **Development of cognitive skills to improve attention, memory, problem solving (includes compensatory training), direct (one-on-one) patient contact, each 15 minutes**
🏢 0.75 ✂ 0.75 **FUD** XXX [51] [A] [80] ▣ [PQ]
AMA: 2015,Jan,16; 2014,Mar,13; 2014,Jan,11

97533 **Sensory integrative techniques to enhance sensory processing and promote adaptive responses to environmental demands, direct (one-on-one) patient contact, each 15 minutes**
🏢 0.82 ✂ 0.82 **FUD** XXX [51] [A] [80] ▣
AMA: 2015,Jan,16; 2014,Mar,13; 2014,Jan,11

97535 **Self-care/home management training (eg, activities of daily living (ADL) and compensatory training, meal preparation, safety procedures, and instructions in use of assistive technology devices/adaptive equipment) direct one-on-one contact, each 15 minutes**
🏢 0.98 ✂ 0.98 **FUD** XXX [51] [A] [80] ▣
AMA: 2015,Jun,10; 2015,Mar,9; 2015,Jan,16; 2014,Mar,13; 2014,Jan,11; 2012,Jan,15-42; 2011,Jan,11

97537 **Community/work reintegration training (eg, shopping, transportation, money management, avocational activities and/or work environment/modification analysis, work task analysis, use of assistive technology device/adaptive equipment), direct one-on-one contact, each 15 minutes**
[EXCLUDES] *Wheelchair management/propulsion training (97542)*
🏢 0.85 ✂ 0.85 **FUD** XXX [51] [A] [80] ▣
AMA: 2015,Jan,16; 2014,Mar,13; 2014,Jan,11

97542 **Wheelchair management (eg, assessment, fitting, training), each 15 minutes**
🏢 0.86 ✂ 0.86 **FUD** XXX [51] [A] [80] ▣
AMA: 2015,Jun,10; 2015,Jan,16; 2014,Mar,13; 2014,Jan,11

97545 **Work hardening/conditioning; initial 2 hours**
🏢 0.00 ✂ 0.00 **FUD** XXX [51] [A] [80] ▣
AMA: 2015,Jan,16; 2014,Mar,13; 2014,Jan,11; 2012,Jan,15-42; 2011,Jan,11

\+ **97546** **each additional hour (List separately in addition to code for primary procedure)**
Code first initial 2 hours (97545)
🏢 0.00 ✂ 0.00 **FUD** ZZZ [51] [A] [80]
AMA: 2015,Jan,16; 2014,Mar,13; 2014,Jan,11; 2012,Jan,15-42; 2011,Jan,11

97597-97610 Treatment of Wounds

CMS: 100-2,15,230.4 Services By a Physical/Occupational Therapist in Private Practice; 100-3,270.3 Blood-derived Products for Chronic Nonhealing Wounds; 100-4,4,200.9 Billing for "Sometimes Therapy" Services that May be Paid as Non-Therapy Services

[INCLUDES] Direct patient contact
Removing devitalized/necrotic tissue and promoting healing

[EXCLUDES] *Burn wound debridement (16020-16030)*

97597 **Debridement (eg, high pressure waterjet with/without suction, sharp selective debridement with scissors, scalpel and forceps), open wound, (eg, fibrin, devitalized epidermis and/or dermis, exudate, debris, biofilm), including topical application(s), wound assessment, use of a whirlpool, when performed and instruction(s) for ongoing care, per session, total wound(s) surface area; first 20 sq cm or less**
🏢 0.68 ✂ 2.15 **FUD** 000 [51] [T] [80] ▣ [PQ]
AMA: 2015,Jan,16; 2014,Jun,11; 2014,Jan,11; 2012,Oct,3-8; 2012,Mar,3; 2012,Jan,15-42; 2012,Jan,6-10; 2011,Sep,11-12; 2011,May,3-5; 2011,Jan,11; 2010,Nov,8; 2010,Jun,8

Wound may be washed, addressed with scissors, and/or tweezers and scalpel

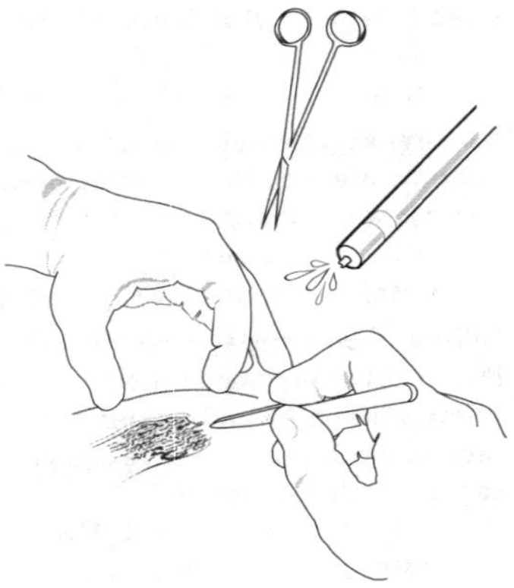

\+ **97598** **each additional 20 sq cm, or part thereof (List separately in addition to code for primary procedure)**

Code first (97597)

🏥 0.33 ⚕ 0.71 **FUD** ZZZ [51] [N] [80] ⚑ [PQ]

AMA: 2015,Jan,16; 2014,Jun,11; 2014,Jan,11; 2012,Mar,3; 2012,Jan,6-10; 2012,Jan,15-42; 2011,Sep,11-12; 2011,May,3-5

97602 **Removal of devitalized tissue from wound(s), non-selective debridement, without anesthesia (eg, wet-to-moist dressings, enzymatic, abrasion), including topical application(s), wound assessment, and instruction(s) for ongoing care, per session**

🏥 0.00 ⚕ 0.00 **FUD** XXX [51] [T]

AMA: 2015,Jan,16; 2014,Jun,11; 2014,Jan,11; 2012,Dec,12; 2012,Mar,3; 2012,Jan,6-10; 2012,Jan,15-42; 2011,Aug,6-7; 2011,May,3-5; 2011,Jan,11

97605 **Negative pressure wound therapy (eg, vacuum assisted drainage collection), utilizing durable medical equipment (DME), including topical application(s), wound assessment, and instruction(s) for ongoing care, per session; total wound(s) surface area less than or equal to 50 square centimeters**

Do not report with (97607-97608)

🏥 0.78 ⚕ 1.23 **FUD** XXX [51] [Q1] [80]

AMA: 2015,Jan,16; 2014,Nov,8; 2014,Jan,11; 2012,Jan,15-42; 2011,May,3-5; 2011,Jan,11; 2010,Jan,3-5

97606 **total wound(s) surface area greater than 50 square centimeters**

Do not report with (97607-97608)

🏥 0.86 ⚕ 1.46 **FUD** XXX [51] [T] [80]

AMA: 2015,Jan,16; 2014,Nov,8; 2014,Jan,11; 2012,Jan,15-42; 2011,May,3-5; 2011,Jan,11; 2010,Jan,3-5

97607 **Negative pressure wound therapy, (eg, vacuum assisted drainage collection), utilizing disposable, non-durable medical equipment including provision of exudate management collection system, topical application(s), wound assessment, and instructions for ongoing care, per session; total wound(s) surface area less than or equal to 50 square centimeters**

Do not report with (97605-97606)

🏥 0.00 ⚕ 0.00 **FUD** XXX [51] [T] [80]

AMA: 2015,Jan,16; 2014,Nov,8

97608 **total wound(s) surface area greater than 50 square centimeters**

Do not report with (97605-97606)

🏥 0.00 ⚕ 0.00 **FUD** XXX [51] [T] [80]

AMA: 2015,Jan,16; 2014,Nov,8

97610 **Low frequency, non-contact, non-thermal ultrasound, including topical application(s), when performed, wound assessment, and instruction(s) for ongoing care, per day**

🏥 0.51 ⚕ 3.43 **FUD** XXX [51] [T] [80]

AMA: 2015,Jan,16; 2014,Jun,11

97750-97799 Assessments and Training

CMS: 100-2,15,230.1 Practice of Physical Therapy; 100-2,15,230.2 Practice of Occupational Therapy; 100-2,15,230.4 Services By a Physical/Occupational Therapist in Private Practice

97750 **Physical performance test or measurement (eg, musculoskeletal, functional capacity), with written report, each 15 minutes**

[INCLUDES] Direct patient contact

[EXCLUDES] *Muscle/range of motion testing and electromyography/nerve velocity determination (95831-95857, 95860-95872, [95885, 95886, 95887], 95907-95913)*

🏥 0.93 ⚕ 0.93 **FUD** XXX [51] [A] [80] ⚑ [PQ]

AMA: 2015,Jan,16; 2014,Jan,11; 2013,Aug,7; 2012,Jan,15-42; 2011,Jan,11

97755 **Assistive technology assessment (eg, to restore, augment or compensate for existing function, optimize functional tasks and/or maximize environmental accessibility), direct one-on-one contact, with written report, each 15 minutes**

[INCLUDES] Direct patient contact

[EXCLUDES] *Augmentative/alternative communication device (92605, 92607)*

Muscle/range of motion testing and electromyography/nerve velocity determination (95831-95857, 95860-95872, [95885, 95886, 95887], 95907-95913)

🏥 1.01 ⚕ 1.01 **FUD** XXX [51] [A] [80] ⚑

AMA: 1996,Sep,7; 1995,Sum,5

97760 **Orthotic(s) management and training (including assessment and fitting when not otherwise reported), upper extremity(s), lower extremity(s) and/or trunk, each 15 minutes**

Do not report with gait training, if performed on the same extremity (97116)

🏥 1.07 ⚕ 1.07 **FUD** XXX [A] [80]

AMA: 2015,Jan,16; 2014,Jan,11

97761 **Prosthetic training, upper and/or lower extremity(s), each 15 minutes**

🏥 0.93 ⚕ 0.93 **FUD** XXX [A] [80]

AMA: 2015,Jan,16; 2014,Jan,11; 2012,Jan,15-42; 2011,Jan,11

97762 **Checkout for orthotic/prosthetic use, established patient, each 15 minutes**

🏥 1.35 ⚕ 1.35 **FUD** XXX [A] [80]

AMA: 2015,Jan,16; 2014,Jan,11

97799 **Unlisted physical medicine/rehabilitation service or procedure**

🏥 0.00 ⚕ 0.00 **FUD** XXX [A] [80]

AMA: 2015,Jan,16; 2014,Jan,11

97802-97804 Medical Nutrition Therapy Services

CMS: 100-2,15,270 Telehealth Services; 100-2,15,270.2 Medicare Telehealth Services; 100-2,15,270.4 Payment - Physician/Practitioner at a Distant Site; 100-3,180.1 Medical Nutrition Therapy; 100-4,12,190.3 Medicare Telehealth Services; 100-4,12,190.7 Contractor Editing of Telehealth Claims; 100-4,4,300 Medical Nutrition Therapy Services; 100-4,4,300.6 CWF Edits for MNT/DSMT; 100-4,9,182 Medical Nutrition Therapy (MNT) Services

[EXCLUDES] *Medical nutrition therapy assessment/intervention provided by physician or other qualified health care provider; use appropriate E&M codes*

97802 **Medical nutrition therapy; initial assessment and intervention, individual, face-to-face with the patient, each 15 minutes**

🏥 0.92 ⚕ 0.98 **FUD** XXX [A] [80] ⚑ [PQ]

AMA: 2015,Jan,16; 2014,Jan,11

97803 **re-assessment and intervention, individual, face-to-face with the patient, each 15 minutes**

🏥 0.77 ⚕ 0.84 **FUD** XXX [A] [80] ⚑ [PQ]

AMA: 2015,Jan,16; 2014,Jan,11

97804 group (2 or more individual(s)), each 30 minutes
    🚑 0.43   ✂ 0.45   **FUD** XXX   A 80 PQ
    AMA: 2015,Jan,16; 2014,Jan,11

97810-97814 Acupuncture

CMS: 100-2,15,230.4 Services By a Physical/Occupational Therapist in Private Practice; 100-3,10.3 Inpatient Pain Rehabilitation Programs; 100-3,10.4 Outpatient Hospital Pain Rehabilitation Programs; 100-3,30.3 Acupuncture; 100-3,30.3.1 Acupuncture for Fibromyalgia; 100-3,30.3.2 Acupuncture for Osteoarthritis

INCLUDES 15 minute increments of face-to-face contact with the patient
        Reporting only one code for each 15 minute increment
EXCLUDES *Time providing evaluation and management services*
Code also significant separately identifiable E&M service using modifier 25, when performed

97810 Acupuncture, 1 or more needles; without electrical stimulation, initial 15 minutes of personal one-on-one contact with the patient
    EXCLUDES *Electrical stimulation (97813-97814)*
    Do not report with (97813)
    🚑 0.87   ✂ 1.03   **FUD** XXX   E
    AMA: 2015,Jan,16; 2014,Jan,11; 2012,Jan,15-42; 2011,Jan,11

+ **97811** without electrical stimulation, each additional 15 minutes of personal one-on-one contact with the patient, with re-insertion of needle(s) (List separately in addition to code for primary procedure)
    EXCLUDES *Electrical stimulation (97813-97814)*
    Code first initial 15 minutes (97810, 97813)
    🚑 0.72   ✂ 0.77   **FUD** ZZZ   E
    AMA: 2015,Jan,16; 2014,Jan,11

97813 with electrical stimulation, initial 15 minutes of personal one-on-one contact with the patient
    INCLUDES Electrical stimulation
    Do not report with (97810)
    🚑 0.94   ✂ 1.10   **FUD** XXX   E
    AMA: 2015,Jan,16; 2014,Jan,11

+ **97814** with electrical stimulation, each additional 15 minutes of personal one-on-one contact with the patient, with re-insertion of needle(s) (List separately in addition to code for primary procedure)
    INCLUDES Electrical stimulation
    Code first initial 15 minutes (97810, 97813)
    🚑 0.79   ✂ 0.87   **FUD** ZZZ   E
    AMA: 2015,Jan,16; 2014,Jan,11

98925-98929 Osteopathic Manipulation

CMS: 100-3,150.1 Manipulation

INCLUDES Physician applied manual treatment done to eliminate/alleviate somatic dysfunction and related disorders using a variety of techniques
        The following body regions:
            Abdomen/visceral region
            Cervical region
            Head region
            Lower extremities
            Lumbar region
            Pelvic region
            Rib cage region
            Sacral region
            Thoracic region
            Upper extremities
Code also significant separately identifiable evaluation and management service using modifier 25, when performed

98925 Osteopathic manipulative treatment (OMT); 1-2 body regions involved
    🚑 0.67   ✂ 0.88   **FUD** 000   Q1 80 ▭
    AMA: 2015,Jan,16; 2014,Jan,11; 2012,Jan,15-42; 2011,Jan,11

98926 3-4 body regions involved
    🚑 1.01   ✂ 1.28   **FUD** 000   Q1 80 ▭
    AMA: 2015,Jan,16; 2014,Jan,11; 2012,Jan,15-42; 2011,Jan,11

98927 5-6 body regions involved
    🚑 1.34   ✂ 1.67   **FUD** 000   Q1 80 ▭
    AMA: 2015,Jan,16; 2014,Jan,11; 2012,Jan,15-42; 2011,Jan,11

98928 7-8 body regions involved
    🚑 1.69   ✂ 2.05   **FUD** 000   Q1 80 ▭
    AMA: 2015,Jan,16; 2014,Jan,11; 2012,May,14-15; 2012,Jan,15-42; 2011,Jan,11

98929 9-10 body regions involved
    🚑 2.03   ✂ 2.45   **FUD** 000   Q1 80 ▭
    AMA: 2015,Jan,16; 2014,Jan,11; 2012,Jan,15-42; 2011,Jan,11

98940-98943 Chiropractic Manipulation

CMS: 100-1,5,70.6 Chiropractors; 100-2,15,240 Chiropractic Services - General; 100-2,15,240.1.3 Necessity for Treatment; 100-2,15,30.5 Chiropractor's Services; 100-3,150.1 Manipulation

INCLUDES Form of manual treatment performed to influence joint/neurophysical function
        The following five extraspinal regions:
            Abdomen
            Head, including temporomandibular joint, excluding atlanto-occipital region
            Lower extremities
            Rib cage, not including costotransverse/costovertebral joints
            Upper extremities
        The following five spinal regions:
            Cervical region (atlanto-occipital joint)
            Lumbar region
            Pelvic region (sacro-iliac joint)
            Sacral region
            Thoracic region (costovertebral/costotransverse joints)
Code also significant separately identifiable E&M service using modifier 25 when performed

98940 Chiropractic manipulative treatment (CMT); spinal, 1-2 regions
    🚑 0.63   ✂ 0.79   **FUD** 000   Q1 80 ▭ PQ
    AMA: 2015,Jan,16; 2014,Jan,11; 2013,Dec,14; 2012,Jan,15-42; 2011,Jan,11; 2010,May,9

98941 spinal, 3-4 regions
    🚑 0.98   ✂ 1.15   **FUD** 000   Q1 80 ▭ PQ
    AMA: 2015,Jan,16; 2014,Jan,11; 2013,Dec,14; 2012,Jan,15-42; 2011,Jan,11; 2010,May,9

98942 spinal, 5 regions
    🚑 1.32   ✂ 1.50   **FUD** 000   Q1 80 ▭ PQ
    AMA: 2015,Jan,16; 2014,Jan,11; 2013,Dec,14; 2012,Jan,15-42; 2011,Jan,11; 2010,May,9

98943 extraspinal, 1 or more regions
    🚑 0.67   ✂ 0.77   **FUD** XXX   E
    AMA: 2015,Jan,16; 2014,Jan,11; 2013,Dec,14; 2012,Jan,15-42; 2011,Jan,11; 2010,May,9

98960-98962 Self-Management Training

INCLUDES Education/training services:
        Prescribed by a physician or other qualified health care professional
        Provided by a qualified nonphysician health care provider
        Standardized curriculum that may be modified as necessary for:
            Clinical needs
            Cultural norms
            Health literacy
        Teaching the patient how to manage the illness/delay the comorbidity(s)
EXCLUDES *Genetic counseling education services (96040, 98961-98962)*
    Health/behavior assessment (96150-96155)
    Medical nutrition therapy (97802-97804)
    The following services:
        Counseling/education to a group (99078)
        Counseling/education to individuals (99201-99215, 99217-99223 [99224, 99225, 99226], 99231-99233, 99241-99255, 99281-99285, 99304-99318, 99324-99337, 99341-99350, 99401-99429)
        Counseling/risk factor reduction without symptoms/established disease (99401-99412)

98960 Education and training for patient self-management by a qualified, nonphysician health care professional using a standardized curriculum, face-to-face with the patient (could include caregiver/family) each 30 minutes; individual patient
    🚑 0.79   ✂ 0.79   **FUD** XXX   E PQ
    AMA: 2015,Jan,16; 2014,Oct,3; 2014,Jan,11; 2013,Nov,3; 2013,Apr,3-4

98961 **2-4 patients**
[INCLUDES] Group education regarding genetic risks
Facility RVU 0.38 Non-Facility RVU 0.38 **FUD** XXX [E] [PQ]
AMA: 2015,Jan,16; 2014,Oct,3; 2014,Jan,11; 2013,Nov,3; 2013,Apr,3-4

98962 **5-8 patients**
[INCLUDES] Group education regarding genetic risks
Facility RVU 0.28 Non-Facility RVU 0.28 **FUD** XXX [E] [PQ]
AMA: 2015,Jan,16; 2014,Oct,3; 2014,Jan,11; 2013,Nov,3; 2013,Apr,3-4

98966-98968 Nonphysician Telephone Services

[INCLUDES] Assessment and management services provided by telephone by a qualified health care professional
Episode of care initiated by an established patient or his/her guardian
[EXCLUDES] *Call initiated by the qualified health care professional*
Calls during the postoperative period of a procedure
Decision to see the patient at the next available urgent care appointment
Decision to see the patient within 24 hours of the call
Telephone services provided by a physician (99441-99443)
Telephone services that are considered a part of a previous or subsequent service
Do not report if performed during the service time for (99495-99496)
Do not report if performed in the same month with (99487-99489)
Do not report when performed in the previous seven days as (98966-98969)

98966 **Telephone assessment and management service provided by a qualified nonphysician health care professional to an established patient, parent, or guardian not originating from a related assessment and management service provided within the previous 7 days nor leading to an assessment and management service or procedure within the next 24 hours or soonest available appointment; 5-10 minutes of medical discussion**
Facility RVU 0.37 Non-Facility RVU 0.40 **FUD** XXX [E]
AMA: 2015,Jan,16; 2014,Oct,3; 2014,Jan,11; 2013,Oct,11; 2013,Nov,3; 2013,Apr,3-4

98967 **11-20 minutes of medical discussion**
Facility RVU 0.72 Non-Facility RVU 0.76 **FUD** XXX [E]
AMA: 2015,Jan,16; 2014,Oct,3; 2014,Jan,11; 2013,Oct,11; 2013,Nov,3; 2013,Apr,3-4

98968 **21-30 minutes of medical discussion**
Facility RVU 1.09 Non-Facility RVU 1.13 **FUD** XXX [E]
AMA: 2015,Jan,16; 2014,Oct,3; 2014,Jan,11; 2013,Oct,11; 2013,Nov,3; 2013,Apr,3-4

98969 Nonphysician Online Service

[INCLUDES] On-line assessment and management service provided by a qualified health care professional
Timely reply to the patient as well as:
Ordering laboratory services
Permanent record of the service; either hard copy or electronic
Providing a prescription
Related telephone calls
[EXCLUDES] *On-line evaluation service:*
Provided during the postoperative period of a procedure
Provided more than once in a seven day period
Related to a service provided in the previous seven days
Do not report in same month with (99487-99489)
Do not report when performed during the service time for (99495-99496)
Do not report with (99339-99340, 99363-99364, 99374-99380)

98969 **Online assessment and management service provided by a qualified nonphysician health care professional to an established patient or guardian, not originating from a related assessment and management service provided within the previous 7 days, using the Internet or similar electronic communications network**
Facility RVU 0.00 Non-Facility RVU 0.00 **FUD** XXX [E]
AMA: 2015,Jan,16; 2014,Oct,3; 2014,Jan,11; 2013,Oct,11; 2013,Nov,3; 2013,Apr,3-4

99000-99091 Supplemental Services and Supplies

[INCLUDES] Supplemental reporting for services adjunct to the basic service provided

99000 **Handling and/or conveyance of specimen for transfer from the office to a laboratory**
Facility RVU 0.00 Non-Facility RVU 0.00 **FUD** XXX [E]
AMA: 2015,Jan,16; 2014,Jan,11; 2012,Jan,15-42; 2011,Jan,11

99001 **Handling and/or conveyance of specimen for transfer from the patient in other than an office to a laboratory (distance may be indicated)**
Facility RVU 0.00 Non-Facility RVU 0.00 **FUD** XXX [E]
AMA: 2015,Jan,16; 2014,Jan,11; 2012,Jan,15-42; 2011,Jan,11

99002 **Handling, conveyance, and/or any other service in connection with the implementation of an order involving devices (eg, designing, fitting, packaging, handling, delivery or mailing) when devices such as orthotics, protectives, prosthetics are fabricated by an outside laboratory or shop but which items have been designed, and are to be fitted and adjusted by the attending physician or other qualified health care professional**
[EXCLUDES] *Venous blood routine collection (36415)*
Facility RVU 0.00 Non-Facility RVU 0.00 **FUD** XXX [B]
AMA: 2015,Jan,16; 2014,Jan,11; 2012,Jan,15-42; 2011,Jan,11

99024 **Postoperative follow-up visit, normally included in the surgical package, to indicate that an evaluation and management service was performed during a postoperative period for a reason(s) related to the original procedure**
Facility RVU 0.00 Non-Facility RVU 0.00 **FUD** XXX [B]
AMA: 2015,Mar,3; 2015,Jan,16; 2014,Jan,11; 2012,Jan,15-42; 2011,Jan,11

99026 **Hospital mandated on call service; in-hospital, each hour**
[EXCLUDES] *Physician stand-by services with prolonged physician attendance (99360)*
Time spent providing procedures or services that may be separately reported
Facility RVU 0.00 Non-Facility RVU 0.00 **FUD** XXX [E]
AMA: 2015,Jan,16; 2014,Jan,11; 2012,Jan,15-42; 2011,Jan,11

99027 **out-of-hospital, each hour**
[EXCLUDES] *Physician stand-by services with prolonged physician attendance (99360)*
Time spent providing procedures or services that may be separately reported
Facility RVU 0.00 Non-Facility RVU 0.00 **FUD** XXX [E]
AMA: 2015,Jan,16; 2014,Jan,11; 2012,Jan,15-42; 2011,Jan,11

99050 **Services provided in the office at times other than regularly scheduled office hours, or days when the office is normally closed (eg, holidays, Saturday or Sunday), in addition to basic service**
Code also more than one adjunct code per encounter when appropriate
Code first basic service provided
Facility RVU 0.00 Non-Facility RVU 0.00 **FUD** XXX [51] [B]
AMA: 2015,Jan,16; 2014,Jan,11; 2012,Jan,15-42; 2011,Jan,11; 2010,Aug,9; 2010,Aug,8&15; 2010,Aug,3-7; 2010,Aug,9

99051 Service(s) provided in the office during regularly scheduled evening, weekend, or holiday office hours, in addition to basic service

    Code also more than one adjunct code per encounter when appropriate

    Code first basic service provided

    0.00   0.00   **FUD** XXX   [51] [B]

    AMA: 2015,Jan,16; 2014,Jan,11; 2012,Jan,15-42; 2011,Jan,11; 2010,Aug,9; 2010,Aug,8&15; 2010,Aug,3-7; 2010,Aug,9

99053 Service(s) provided between 10:00 PM and 8:00 AM at 24-hour facility, in addition to basic service

    Code also more than one adjunct code per encounter when appropriate

    Code first basic service provided

    0.00   0.00   **FUD** XXX   [51] [B]

    AMA: 2015,Jan,16; 2014,Jan,11; 2012,Jan,15-42; 2011,Jan,11

99056 Service(s) typically provided in the office, provided out of the office at request of patient, in addition to basic service

    Code also more than one adjunct code per encounter when appropriate

    Code first basic service provided

    0.00   0.00   **FUD** XXX   [51] [B]

    AMA: 2015,Jan,16; 2014,Jan,11; 2012,Jan,15-42; 2011,Jan,11

99058 Service(s) provided on an emergency basis in the office, which disrupts other scheduled office services, in addition to basic service

    Code also more than one adjunct code per encounter when appropriate

    Code first basic service provided

    0.00   0.00   **FUD** XXX   [51] [B]

    AMA: 2015,Jan,16; 2014,Jan,11; 2012,Jan,15-42; 2011,Jan,11; 2010,Aug,9; 2010,Aug,9

99060 Service(s) provided on an emergency basis, out of the office, which disrupts other scheduled office services, in addition to basic service

    Code also more than one adjunct code per encounter when appropriate

    Code first basic service provided

    0.00   0.00   **FUD** XXX   [51] [B]

    AMA: 2015,Jan,16; 2014,Jan,11; 2012,Jan,15-42; 2011,Jan,11

99070 Supplies and materials (except spectacles), provided by the physician or other qualified health care professional over and above those usually included with the office visit or other services rendered (list drugs, trays, supplies, or materials provided)

    EXCLUDES Spectacles supply

    0.00   0.00   **FUD** XXX   [B]

    AMA: 2015,Jan,16; 2014,Mar,11; 2014,Jan,11; 2013,Dec,12; 2013,Mar,6-7; 2012,Nov,11-12; 2012,Aug,9; 2012,Apr,10; 2012,Jan,15-42; 2011,Jan,11; 2010,Sep,3; 2010,Jun,8; 2010,May,9

99071 Educational supplies, such as books, tapes, and pamphlets, for the patient's education at cost to physician or other qualified health care professional

    0.00   0.00   **FUD** XXX   [B]

    AMA: 2015,Jan,16; 2014,Oct,3; 2014,Jan,11; 2013,Nov,3; 2013,Apr,3-4; 2012,Jan,15-42; 2011,Jan,11

99075 Medical testimony

    0.00   0.00   **FUD** XXX   [E]

    AMA: 2015,Jan,16; 2014,Jan,11; 2012,Jan,15-42; 2011,Jan,11

99078 Physician or other qualified health care professional qualified by education, training, licensure/regulation (when applicable) educational services rendered to patients in a group setting (eg, prenatal, obesity, or diabetic instructions)

    0.00   0.00   **FUD** XXX   [N] [P0]

    AMA: 2015,Jan,16; 2014,Oct,3; 2014,Jan,11; 2013,Nov,3; 2013,Apr,3-4; 2012,Jan,15-42; 2011,Jan,11

99080 Special reports such as insurance forms, more than the information conveyed in the usual medical communications or standard reporting form

    Do not report for completion of workmen's compensation forms (99455-99456)

    0.00   0.00   **FUD** XXX   [B]

    AMA: 2015,Jan,16; 2014,Oct,3; 2014,Jan,11; 2013,Nov,3; 2013,Apr,3-4; 2012,Jan,15-42; 2011,Jan,11

99082 Unusual travel (eg, transportation and escort of patient)

    0.00   0.00   **FUD** XXX   [B] [80]

    AMA: 2015,Jan,16; 2014,Jan,11; 2012,Jan,15-42; 2011,Jan,11

99090 Analysis of clinical data stored in computers (eg, ECGs, blood pressures, hematologic data)

    EXCLUDES Collection/interpretation by health care professional/physician of physiologic data stored/transmitted by patient or caregiver (99091)

    Do not report this service when a more specific CPT code exists for cardiographic services, glucose monitoring, or musculoskeletal function testing (93227, 93272, 95250, 97750, 0206T)

    0.00   0.00   **FUD** XXX   [B]

    AMA: 2015,Jan,16; 2014,Oct,3; 2014,May,4; 2014,Jan,11; 2013,Nov,3; 2013,Apr,3-4; 2012,Jan,15-42; 2011,Jan,11

99091 Collection and interpretation of physiologic data (eg, ECG, blood pressure, glucose monitoring) digitally stored and/or transmitted by the patient and/or caregiver to the physician or other qualified health care professional, qualified by education, training, licensure/regulation (when applicable) requiring a minimum of 30 minutes of time

    1.59   1.59   **FUD** XXX   [N]

    AMA: 2015,Jan,16; 2014,Oct,3; 2014,Jan,11; 2013,Nov,3; 2013,Apr,3-4; 2012,Jan,15-42; 2011,Jan,11

99100-99140 Modifying Factors for Anesthesia Services

CMS: 100-4,12,140.3 Payment for Qualified Nonphysician Anesthetists; 100-4,12,140.3.3 Billing Modifiers; 100-4,12,140.3.4 General Billing Instructions; 100-4,12,140.4.1 Anesthesiologist/Qualified Nonphysican Anesthetist; 100-4,12,140.4.2 Anesthetist and Anesthesiologist in a Single Procedure; 100-4,12,140.4.4 Conversion Factors for Anesthesia Services; 100-4,4,250.3.2 Anesthesia in a Hospital Outpatient Setting

    Code first primary anesthesia procedure

+ 99100 Anesthesia for patient of extreme age, younger than 1 year and older than 70 (List separately in addition to code for primary anesthesia procedure)   [A]

    EXCLUDES Anesthesia services for infants one year old or less at the time of surgery (00326, 00561, 00834, 00836)

    Do not report with (00561)

    0.00   0.00   **FUD** ZZZ   [B]

    AMA: 2015,Jan,16; 2014,Jan,11

+ 99116 Anesthesia complicated by utilization of total body hypothermia (List separately in addition to code for primary anesthesia procedure)

    Do not report with (00561)

    0.00   0.00   **FUD** ZZZ   [B]

    AMA: 2015,Jan,16; 2014,Jan,11

+ 99135 Anesthesia complicated by utilization of controlled hypotension (List separately in addition to code for primary anesthesia procedure)

    Do not report with (00561)

    0.00   0.00   **FUD** ZZZ   [B]

    AMA: 2015,Jan,16; 2014,Jan,11

+ 99140 Anesthesia complicated by emergency conditions (specify) (List separately in addition to code for primary anesthesia procedure)

    INCLUDES Circumstances where a delay in treatment would lead to a significant increase in the threat to life or body part

    0.00   0.00   **FUD** ZZZ   [B]

    AMA: 2015,Jan,16; 2014,Jan,11; 2012,Jan,15-42; 2011,Jan,11

99143-99150 Moderate Sedation Services

INCLUDES   Administration of medication
IV access
Maintenance of sedation
Monitoring of oxygen saturation/heart rate/blood pressure
Patient assessment
Recovery (not included in intraservice time)

EXCLUDES   *Minimal sedation/anxiolysis/deep sedation/monitored anesthesia care (00100-01999)*

Do not report with anesthesia for diagnostic or therapeutic injections and nerve blocks (01991-01992)

Do not report with pulse oximetry (94760-94762)

99143   **Moderate sedation services (other than those services described by codes 00100-01999) provided by the same physician or other qualified health care professional performing the diagnostic or therapeutic service that the sedation supports, requiring the presence of an independent trained observer to assist in the monitoring of the patient's level of consciousness and physiological status; younger than 5 years of age, first 30 minutes intra-service time**   A

🚑 0.00   ⚕ 0.00   **FUD** XXX   ⊘ N 80

AMA: 2015,Jan,16; 2014,Aug,5; 2014,Jan,11; 2013,May,12; 2013,Feb,3-6; 2012,Nov,3-5; 2012,Jan,15-42; 2011,Oct,3-4; 2011,Jan,11; 2010,Jan,6-7

99144   **age 5 years or older, first 30 minutes intra-service time**   A

🚑 0.00   ⚕ 0.00   **FUD** XXX   ⊘ N 80

AMA: 2015,Jan,16; 2014,Aug,5; 2014,Jan,11; 2013,May,12; 2013,Feb,3-6; 2012,Nov,3-5; 2012,Jul,12-14; 2012,Jan,15-42; 2011,Oct,3-4; 2011,Jul,16-17; 2011,Jan,11; 2010,Jan,6-7

+ 99145   **each additional 15 minutes intra-service time (List separately in addition to code for primary service)**
Code first initial 30 minutes (99143, 99144)

🚑 0.00   ⚕ 0.00   **FUD** ZZZ   N 80

AMA: 2015,Jan,16; 2014,Aug,5; 2014,Jan,11; 2013,May,12; 2013,Feb,3-6; 2012,Nov,3-5; 2012,Jan,15-42; 2011,Oct,3-4; 2011,Jul,16-17; 2011,Jan,11; 2010,Jan,6-7

99148   **Moderate sedation services (other than those services described by codes 00100-01999), provided by a physician or other qualified health care professional other than the health care professional performing the diagnostic or therapeutic service that the sedation supports; younger than 5 years of age, first 30 minutes intra-service time**   A

🚑 0.00   ⚕ 0.00   **FUD** XXX   N 80

AMA: 2015,Jan,16; 2014,Aug,5; 2014,Jan,11; 2013,May,12; 2013,Feb,3-6; 2012,Jan,15-42; 2011,Oct,3-4; 2011,Jan,11

99149   **age 5 years or older, first 30 minutes intra-service time**   A

🚑 0.00   ⚕ 0.00   **FUD** XXX   N 80

AMA: 2015,Jan,16; 2014,Aug,5; 2014,Jan,11; 2013,May,12; 2013,Feb,3-6; 2012,Jan,15-42; 2011,Oct,3-4; 2011,Jan,11

+ 99150   **each additional 15 minutes intra-service time (List separately in addition to code for primary service)**
Code first initial 30 minutes (99148, 99149)

🚑 0.00   ⚕ 0.00   **FUD** ZZZ   N 80

AMA: 2015,Jan,16; 2014,Aug,5; 2014,Jan,11; 2013,May,12; 2013,Feb,3-6; 2012,Jan,15-42; 2011,Oct,3-4; 2011,Jan,11

99170 Specialized Examination of Child

EXCLUDES   *Moderate sedation (99143-99150)*

99170   **Anogenital examination, magnified, in childhood for suspected trauma, including image recording when performed**   A

🚑 2.29   ⚕ 4.51   **FUD** 000   T ▭

AMA: 2015,Jan,16; 2014,Sep,7; 2014,Jan,11

99172-99173 Visual Acuity Screening Tests

INCLUDES   Graduated visual acuity stimuli that allow a quantitative determination/estimation of visual acuity

99172   **Visual function screening, automated or semi-automated bilateral quantitative determination of visual acuity, ocular alignment, color vision by pseudoisochromatic plates, and field of vision (may include all or some screening of the determination[s] for contrast sensitivity, vision under glare)**

Do not report with (99173, 99174 [99177])
Do not report with general ophthalmological service or E&M service

🚑 0.00   ⚕ 0.00   **FUD** XXX   E

AMA: 2015,Jan,16; 2014,Jan,11; 2012,Jan,15-42; 2011,Jan,11

99173   **Screening test of visual acuity, quantitative, bilateral**

Do not report with (99172, 99174, [99177])

🚑 0.09   ⚕ 0.09   **FUD** XXX   E

AMA: 2015,Jan,16; 2014,Jan,11

99174 [99177] Screening For Amblyogenic Factors

Do not report with (92002-92014, 99172-99173, [99177])

▲   **99174**   **Instrument-based ocular screening (eg, photoscreening, automated-refraction), bilateral; with remote analysis and report**

🚑 0.00   ⚕ 0.00   **FUD** XXX   E

AMA: 2015,Jan,16; 2014,Jan,11; 2013,Mar,6-7

● #   **99177**   **with on-site analysis**

🚑 0.00   ⚕ 0.00   **FUD** 000

99175-99177 Drug Administration to Induce Vomiting

EXCLUDES   *Diagnostic gastric lavage (43754-43755)*
Diagnostic gastric intubation (43754-43755)

99175   **Ipecac or similar administration for individual emesis and continued observation until stomach adequately emptied of poison**

🚑 0.48   ⚕ 0.48   **FUD** XXX   N 80

AMA: 1997,Nov,1

99177   **Resequenced code. See code following 99174.**

99183-99184 Hyperbaric Oxygen Therapy

CMS: 100-3,20.29 Hyperbaric Oxygen Therapy; 100-4,32,30.1 HBO Therapy for Lower Extremity Diabetic Wounds

EXCLUDES   *Evaluation and management services, when performed*
Other procedures such as wound debridement, when performed

99183   **Physician or other qualified health care professional attendance and supervision of hyperbaric oxygen therapy, per session**

proatech

🚑 3.15   ⚕ 3.15   **FUD** XXX   B 80 26

AMA: 2015,Jan,16; 2014,Jan,11; 2012,Jan,15-42; 2011,Jan,11

99184   **Initiation of selective head or total body hypothermia in the critically ill neonate, includes appropriate patient selection by review of clinical, imaging and laboratory data, confirmation of esophageal temperature probe location, evaluation of amplitude EEG, supervision of controlled hypothermia, and assessment of patient tolerance of cooling**   A

🚑 6.62   ⚕ 6.62   **FUD** XXX   C 80

Do not report more than one time per hospitalization

99188 Topical Fluoride Application

99188   **Application of topical fluoride varnish by a physician or other qualified health care professional**

🚑 0.00   ⚕ 0.00   **FUD** XXX   E 80

99190-99192 Assemble and Manage Pump with Oxygenator/Heat Exchange

99190   **Assembly and operation of pump with oxygenator or heat exchanger (with or without ECG and/or pressure monitoring); each hour**

🚑 0.00   ⚕ 0.00   **FUD** XXX   C ▭

AMA: 1997,Nov,1

99191	**45 minutes**				
	0.00	0.00	**FUD** XXX		C ▢
	AMA: 1997,Nov,1				

99192	**30 minutes**				
	0.00	0.00	**FUD** XXX		C ▢
	AMA: 1997,Nov,1				

99195-99199 Therapeutic Phlebotomy and Unlisted Procedures

99195 **Phlebotomy, therapeutic (separate procedure)**
2.83   2.83   **FUD** XXX   01 80 ▢
AMA: 2015,Jan,16; 2014,Jan,11; 2012,Jan,15-42; 2011,Jan,11

99199 **Unlisted special service, procedure or report**
0.00   0.00   **FUD** XXX   B 80
AMA: 2015,Jan,16; 2014,Jan,11; 2012,Oct,13; 2012,Sep,9; 2012,Jun,15-16

99500-99602 Home Visit By Non-Physician Professionals

INCLUDES Services performed by non-physician providers
Services provided in patient's:
  Assisted living apartment
  Custodial care facility
  Group home
  Non-traditional private home
  Residence
  School
EXCLUDES *Home visits performed by physicians (99341-99350)*
Other services/procedures provided by physicians to patients at home
Code also home visit E&M codes if health care provider is authorized to use (99341-99350)
Code also significant separately identifiable E&M service, when performed

99500 **Home visit for prenatal monitoring and assessment to include fetal heart rate, non-stress test, uterine monitoring, and gestational diabetes monitoring** M ♀
0.00   0.00   **FUD** XXX   E
AMA: 2015,Jan,16; 2014,Jan,11; 2012,Jan,15-42; 2011,Jan,11

99501 **Home visit for postnatal assessment and follow-up care** M ♀
0.00   0.00   **FUD** XXX   E
AMA: 2015,Jan,16; 2014,Jan,11

99502 **Home visit for newborn care and assessment** A
0.00   0.00   **FUD** XXX   E
AMA: 2015,Jan,16; 2014,Jan,11

99503 **Home visit for respiratory therapy care (eg, bronchodilator, oxygen therapy, respiratory assessment, apnea evaluation)**
0.00   0.00   **FUD** XXX   E
AMA: 2015,Jan,16; 2014,Jan,11

99504 **Home visit for mechanical ventilation care**
0.00   0.00   **FUD** XXX   E
AMA: 2015,Jan,16; 2014,Jan,11

99505 **Home visit for stoma care and maintenance including colostomy and cystostomy**
0.00   0.00   **FUD** XXX   E
AMA: 2015,Jan,16; 2014,Jan,11

99506 **Home visit for intramuscular injections**
0.00   0.00   **FUD** XXX   E
AMA: 2015,Jan,16; 2014,Jan,11

99507 **Home visit for care and maintenance of catheter(s) (eg, urinary, drainage, and enteral)**
0.00   0.00   **FUD** XXX   E
AMA: 2015,Jan,16; 2014,Jan,11

99509 **Home visit for assistance with activities of daily living and personal care**
EXCLUDES *Medical nutrition therapy/assessment home services (97802-97804)*
Self-care/home management training (97535)
Speech therapy home services (92507-92508)
0.00   0.00   **FUD** XXX   E
AMA: 2015,Jan,16; 2014,Jan,11

99510 **Home visit for individual, family, or marriage counseling**
0.00   0.00   **FUD** XXX   E
AMA: 2015,Jan,16; 2014,Jan,11

99511 **Home visit for fecal impaction management and enema administration**
0.00   0.00   **FUD** XXX   E
AMA: 2015,Jan,16; 2014,Jan,11

99512 **Home visit for hemodialysis**
EXCLUDES *Peritoneal dialysis home infusion (99601-99602)*
0.00   0.00   **FUD** XXX   E
AMA: 2015,Jan,16; 2014,Jan,11

99600 **Unlisted home visit service or procedure**
0.00   0.00   **FUD** XXX   E
AMA: 2015,Jan,16; 2014,Jan,11; 2012,Jan,15-42; 2011,Jan,11

99601 **Home infusion/specialty drug administration, per visit (up to 2 hours);**
0.00   0.00   **FUD** XXX   E
AMA: 2005,Nov,1-9; 2003,Oct,7

+ **99602** **each additional hour (List separately in addition to code for primary procedure)**
Code first (99601)
0.00   0.00   **FUD** XXX   E
AMA: 2005,Nov,1-9; 2003,Oct,7

99605-99607 Medication Management By Pharmacist

INCLUDES Direct (face-to-face) assessment and intervention by a pharmacist for the purpose of:
  Managing medication complications and/or interactions
  Maximizing the patient's response to drug therapy
  Documenting the following required elements:
    Advice given regarding improvement of treatment compliance and outcomes
    Profile of medications (prescription and nonprescription)
    Review of applicable patient history
EXCLUDES *Routine tasks associated with dispensing and related activities (e.g., providing product information)*

99605 **Medication therapy management service(s) provided by a pharmacist, individual, face-to-face with patient, with assessment and intervention if provided; initial 15 minutes, new patient**
0.00   0.00   **FUD** XXX   E
AMA: 2015,Jan,16; 2014,Oct,3; 2014,Jan,11; 2013,Nov,3; 2013,Apr,3-4; 2012,Jan,15-42

99606 **initial 15 minutes, established patient**
0.00   0.00   **FUD** XXX   E
AMA: 2015,Jan,16; 2014,Oct,3; 2014,Jan,11; 2013,Nov,3; 2013,Apr,3-4; 2012,Jan,15-42

+ **99607** **each additional 15 minutes (List separately in addition to code for primary service)**
Code first (99605, 99606)
0.00   0.00   **FUD** XXX   E
AMA: 2015,Jan,16; 2014,Oct,3; 2014,Jan,11; 2013,Nov,3; 2013,Apr,3-4; 2012,Jan,15-42; 2011,Jan,11

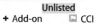

Evaluation and Management (E/M) Services Guidelines

In addition to the information presented in the Introduction, several other items unique to this section are defined or identified here.

Classification of Evaluation and Management (E/M) Services

The E/M section is divided into broad categories such as office visits, hospital visits, and consultations. Most of the categories are further divided into two or more subcategories of E/M services. For example, there are two subcategories of office visits (new patient and established patient) and there are two subcategories of hospital visits (initial and subsequent). The subcategories of E/M services are further classified into levels of E/M services that are identified by specific codes. This classification is important because the nature of work varies by type of service, place of service, and the patient's status.

The basic format of the levels of E/M services is the same for most categories. First, a unique code number is listed. Second, the place and/or type of service is specified, eg, office consultation. Third, the content of the service is defined, eg, comprehensive history and comprehensive examination. (See "Levels of E/M Services," for details on the content of E/M services.) Fourth, the nature of the presenting problem(s) usually associated with a given level is described. Fifth, the time typically required to provide the service is specified. (A detailed discussion of time is provided separately.)

Definitions of Commonly Used Terms

Certain key words and phrases are used throughout the E/M section. The following definitions are intended to reduce the potential for differing interpretations and to increase the consistency of reporting by physicians in differing specialties. E/M services may also be reported by other qualified health care professionals who are authorized to perform such services within the scope of their practice.

New and Established Patient

Solely for the purposes of distinguishing between new and established patients, professional services are those face-to-face services rendered by physicians and other qualified health care professionals who may report E/M services with a specific CPT® code or codes. A new patient is one who has not received any professional services from the physician/qualified health care professional or another physician/qualified health care professional of the exact same specialty and subspecialty who belongs to the same group practice, within the past three years.

An established patient is one who has received professional services from the physician/qualified health care professional or another physician/qualified health care professional of the exact same specialty and subspecialty who belongs to the same group practice, within the past three years. See the decision tree at right.

When a physician/qualified health care professional is on call or covering for another physician/qualified health care professional, the patient's encounter is classified as it would have been by the physician/qualified health care professional who is not available. When advanced practice nurses and physician assistants are working with physicians, they are considered as working in the exact same specialty and exact same subspecialties as the physician.

No distinction is made between new and established patients in the emergency department. E/M services in the emergency department category may be reported for any new or established patient who presents for treatment in the emergency department.

The decision tree in the next column is provided to aid in determining whether to report the E/M service provided as a new or an established patient encounter.

Coding Tip

Instructions for Use of the CPT Code Book

When advanced practice nurses and physician assistants are working with physicians they are considered as working in the exact same specialty and exact same subspecialties as the physician. A "physician or other qualified health care professional" is an individual who is qualified by education, training, licensure/regulation (when applicable), and facility privileging (when applicable) who performs a professional service within his or her scope of practice and independently reports that professional service. These professionals are distinct from "clinical staff." A clinical staff member is a person who works under the supervision of a physician or other qualified health care professional and who is allowed by law, regulation, and facility policy to perform or assist in the performance of a specific professional service but does not individually report that professional service. Other policies may also affect who may report specific services.

CPT Coding Guidelines, Introduction, Instructions for Use of the CPT Codebook

---

Chief Complaint

A chief complaint is a concise statement describing the symptom, problem, condition, diagnosis, or other factor that is the reason for the encounter, usually stated in the patient's words.

Concurrent Care and Transfer of Care

Concurrent care is the provision of similar services (e.g., hospital visits) to the same patient by more than one physician or other qualified health care professional on the same day. When concurrent care is provided, no special reporting is required. Transfer of care is the process whereby a physician or other qualified health care professional who is managing some or all of a patient's problems relinquishes this responsibility to another physician or other qualified health care professional who explicitly agrees to accept this responsibility and who, from the initial encounter, is not providing consultative services. The physician or other qualified health care professional transferring care is then no longer providing care for these problems though he or she may continue providing care for other conditions when appropriate. Consultation codes should not be reported by the physician or other qualified health care professional who has agreed to accept transfer of care before an initial evaluation, but they are appropriate to report if the decision to accept transfer of care cannot be made until after the initial consultation evaluation, regardless of site of service.

Decision Tree for New vs Established Patients

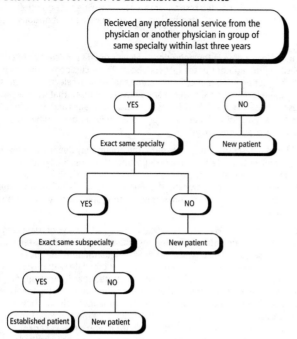

Counseling

Counseling is a discussion with a patient and/or family concerning one or more of the following areas:

- Diagnostic results, impressions, and/or recommended diagnostic studies

- Prognosis

- Risks and benefits of management (treatment) options

- Instructions for management (treatment) and/or follow-up

- Importance of compliance with chosen management (treatment) options

- Risk factor reduction

- Patient and family education
  (For psychotherapy, see 90832–90834, 90836–90840)

Family History

A review of medical events in the patient's family that includes significant information about:

- The health status or cause of death of parents, siblings, and children

- Specific diseases related to problems identified in the Chief Complaint or History of the Present Illness, and/or System Review

- Diseases of family members that may be hereditary or place the patient at risk

History of Present Illness

A chronological description of the development of the patient's present illness from the first sign and/or symptom to the present. This includes a description of location, quality, severity, timing, context, modifying factors, and associated signs and symptoms significantly related to the presenting problem(s).

Levels of E/M Services

Within each category or subcategory of E/M service, there are three to five levels of E/M services available for reporting purposes. Levels of E/M services are not interchangeable among the different categories or subcategories of service. For example, the first level of E/M services in the subcategory of office visit, new patient, does not have the same definition as the first level of E/M services in the subcategory of office visit, established patient.

The levels of E/M services include examinations, evaluations, treatments, conferences with or concerning patients, preventive pediatric and adult health supervision, and similar medical services, such as the determination of the need and/or location for appropriate care. Medical screening includes the history, examination, and medical decision-making required to determine the need and/or location for appropriate care and treatment of the patient (eg, office and other outpatient setting, emergency department, nursing facility). The levels of E/M services encompass the wide variations in skill, effort, time, responsibility, and medical knowledge required for the prevention or diagnosis and treatment of illness or injury and the promotion of optimal health. Each level of E/M services may be used by all physicians or other qualified health care professionals.

The descriptors for the levels of E/M services recognize seven components, six of which are used in defining the levels of E/M services. These components are:

- History

- Examination

- Medical decision making

- Counseling

- Coordination of care

- Nature of presenting problem

- Time

The first three of these components (history, examination, and medical decision making) are considered the key components in selecting a level of E/M services. (See "Determine the Extent of History Obtained.")

The next three components (counseling, coordination of care, and the nature of the presenting problem) are considered contributory factors in the majority of encounters. Although the first two of these contributory factors are important E/M services, it is not required that these services be provided at every patient encounter.

Coordination of care with other physicians, other qualified health care professionals, or agencies without a patient encounter on that day is reported using the case management codes.

The final component, time, is discussed in detail below.

Any specifically identifiable procedure (ie, identified with a specific CPT code) performed on or subsequent to the date of initial or subsequent E/M services should be reported separately.

The actual performance and/or interpretation of diagnostic tests/studies ordered during a patient encounter are not included in the levels of E/M services. Physician performance of diagnostic tests/studies for which specific CPT codes are available may be reported separately, in addition to the appropriate E/M code. The physician's interpretation of the results of diagnostic tests/studies (ie, professional component) with preparation of a separate distinctly identifiable signed written report may also be reported separately, using the appropriate CPT code with modifier 26 appended.

The physician or other health care professional may need to indicate that on the day a procedure or service identified by a CPT code was performed, the patient's condition required a significant separately identifiable E/M service above and beyond other services provided or beyond the usual preservice and postservice care associated with the procedure that was performed. The E/M service may be caused or prompted by the symptoms or condition for which the procedure and/or service was provided. This circumstance may be reported by adding modifier 25 to the appropriate level of E/M service. As such, different diagnoses are not required for reporting of the procedure and the E/M services on the same date.

Nature of Presenting Problem

A presenting problem is a disease, condition, illness, injury, symptom, sign, finding, complaint, or other reason for encounter, with or without a diagnosis being established at the time of the encounter. The E/M codes recognize five types of presenting problems that are defined as follows:

Minimal: A problem that may not require the presence of the physician or other qualified health care professional, but service is provided under the physician's or other qualified health care professional's supervision.

Self-limited or minor: A problem that runs a definite and prescribed course, is transient in nature, and is not likely to permanently alter health status OR has a good prognosis with management/compliance.

Low severity: A problem where the risk of morbidity without treatment is low; there is little to no risk of mortality without treatment; full recovery without functional impairment is expected.

Moderate severity: A problem where the risk of morbidity without treatment is moderate; there is moderate risk of mortality without treatment; uncertain prognosis OR increased probability of prolonged functional impairment.

High severity: A problem where the risk of morbidity without treatment is high to extreme; there is a moderate to high risk of mortality without treatment OR high probability of severe, prolonged functional impairment.

Past History

A review of the patient's past experiences with illnesses, injuries, and treatments that includes significant information about:

- Prior major illnesses and injuries
- Prior operations
- Prior hospitalizations
- Current medications
- Allergies (eg, drug, food)
- Age appropriate immunization status
- Age appropriate feeding/dietary status

Social History

An age appropriate review of past and current activities that includes significant information about:

- Marital status and/or living arrangements
- Current employment
- Occupational history
- Military history
- Use of drugs, alcohol, and tobacco
- Level of education
- Sexual history
- Other relevant social factors

System Review (Review of Systems)

An inventory of body systems obtained through a series of questions seeking to identify signs and/or symptoms that the patient may be experiencing or has experienced. For the purposes of the CPT codebook the following elements of a system review have been identified:

- Constitutional symptoms (fever, weight loss, etc)
- Eyes
- Ears, nose, mouth, throat
- Cardiovascular
- Respiratory
- Gastrointestinal
- Genitourinary
- Musculoskeletal
- Integumentary (skin and/or breast)
- Neurological
- Psychiatric
- Endocrine
- Hematologic/lymphatic
- Allergic/immunologic

The review of systems helps define the problem, clarify the differential diagnosis, identify needed testing, or serves as baseline data on other systems that might be affected by any possible management options.

Time

The inclusion of time in the definitions of levels of E/M services has been implicit in prior editions of the CPT codebook. The inclusion of time as an explicit factor beginning in *CPT 1992* is done to assist in selecting the most appropriate level of E/M services. It should be recognized that the specific times expressed in the visit code descriptors are averages and, therefore, represent a range of times that may be higher or lower depending on actual clinical circumstances.

Time is not a descriptive component for the emergency department levels of E/M services because emergency department services are typically provided on a variable intensity basis, often involving multiple encounters with several patients over an extended period of time. Therefore, it is often difficult to provide accurate estimates of the time spent face-to-face with the patient.

Studies to establish levels of E/M services employed surveys of practicing physicians to obtain data on the amount of time and work associated with typical E/M services. Since "work" is not easily quantifiable, the codes must rely on other objective, verifiable measures that correlate with physicians' estimates of their "work." It has been demonstrated that estimations of intraservice time, both within and across specialties, is a variable that is predictive of the "work" of E/M services. This same research has shown there is a strong relationship between intraservice time and total time for E/M services. Intraservice time, rather than total time, was chosen for inclusion with the codes because of its relative ease of measurement and because of its direct correlation with measurements of the total amount of time and work associated with typical E/M services.

Intraservice times are defined as face-to-face time for office and other outpatient visits and as unit/floor time for hospital and other inpatient visits. This distinction is necessary because most of the work of typical office visits takes place during the face-to-face time with the patient, while most of the work of typical hospital visits takes place during the time spent on the patient's floor or unit. When prolonged time occurs in either the office or the inpatient areas, the appropriate add-on code should be reported.

Face-to-face time (office and other outpatient visits and office consultations): For coding purposes, face-to-face time for these services is defined as only that time spent face-to-face with the patient and/or family. This includes the time spent performing such tasks as obtaining a history, performing an examination, and counseling the patient.

Time is also spent doing work before or after the face-to-face time with the patient, performing such tasks as reviewing records and tests, arranging for further services, and communicating further with other professionals and the patient through written reports and telephone contact.

This non-face-to-face time for office services—also called pre- and postencounter time—is not included in the time component described in the E/M codes. However, the pre- and post-non-face-to-face work associated with an encounter was included in calculating the total work of typical services in physician surveys.

Thus, the face-to-face time associated with the services described by any E/M code is a valid proxy for the total work done before, during, and after the visit.

Unit/floor time (hospital observation services, inpatient hospital care, initial inpatient hospital consultations, nursing facility): For reporting purposes, intraservice time for these services is defined as unit/floor time, which includes the time present on the patient's hospital unit and at the bedside rendering services for that patient. This includes the time to establish and/or review the patient's chart, examine the patient, write notes, and communicate with other professionals and the patient's family.

In the hospital, pre- and post-time includes time spent off the patient's floor performing such tasks as reviewing pathology and radiology findings in another part of the hospital.

This pre- and postvisit time is not included in the time component described in these codes. However, the pre- and postwork performed during the time spent off the floor or unit was included in calculating the total work of typical services in physician surveys.

Thus, the unit/floor time associated with the services described by any code is a valid proxy for the total work done before, during, and after the visit.

Unlisted Service

An E/M service may be provided that is not listed in this section of the CPT codebook. When reporting such a service, the appropriate unlisted code may be used to indicate the service, identifying it by "Special Report," as discussed in the following paragraph. The "Unlisted Services" and accompanying codes for the E/M section are as follows:

99429	**Unlisted preventive medicine service**
99499	**Unlisted evaluation and management service**

Special Report

An unlisted service or one that is unusual, variable, or new may require a special report demonstrating the medical appropriateness of the service. Pertinent information should include an adequate definition or description of the nature, extent, and need for the procedure and the time, effort, and equipment necessary to provide the service. Additional items that may be included are complexity of symptoms, final diagnosis, pertinent physical findings, diagnostic and therapeutic procedures, concurrent problems, and follow-up care.

Instructions for Selecting a Level of E/M Service

Review the Reporting Instructions for the Selected Category or Subcategory

Most of the categories and many of the subcategories of service have special guidelines or instructions unique to that category or subcategory. Where these are indicated, eg, "Inpatient Hospital Care," special instructions will be presented preceding the levels of E/M services.

Review the Level of E/M Service Descriptors and Examples in the Selected Category or Subcategory

The descriptors for the levels of E/M services recognize seven components, six of which are used in defining the levels of E/M services. These components are:

- History
- Examination
- Medical decision making
- Counseling
- Coordination of care
- Nature of presenting problem
- Time

The first three of these components (ie, history, examination, and medical decision making) should be considered the key components in selecting the level of E/M services. An exception to this rule is in the case of visits that consist predominantly of counseling or coordination of care.

The nature of the presenting problem and time are provided in some levels to assist the physician in determining the appropriate level of E/M service.

Determine the Extent of History Obtained

The extent of the history is dependent upon clinical judgment and on the nature of the presenting problem(s). The levels of E/M services recognize four types of history that are defined as follows:

Problem focused: Chief complaint; brief history of present illness or problem.

Expanded problem focused: Chief complaint; brief history of present illness; problem pertinent system review.

Detailed: Chief complaint; extended history of present illness; problem pertinent system review extended to include a review of a limited number of additional systems; pertinent past, family, and/or social history directly related to the patient's problems.

Comprehensive: Chief complaint; extended history of present illness; review of systems that is directly related to the problem(s) identified in the history of the present illness plus a review of all additional body systems; complete past, family, and social history.

The comprehensive history obtained as part of the preventive medicine E/M service is not problem-oriented and does not involve a chief complaint or present illness. It does, however, include a comprehensive system review and comprehensive or interval past, family, and social history as well as a comprehensive assessment/history of pertinent risk factors.

Determine the Extent of Examination Performed

The extent of the examination performed is dependent on clinical judgment and on the nature of the presenting problem(s). The levels of E/M services recognize four types of examination that are defined as follows:

Problem focused: A limited examination of the affected body area or organ system.

Expanded problem focused: A limited examination of the affected body area or organ system and other symptomatic or related organ system(s).

Detailed: An extended examination of the affected body area(s) and other symptomatic or related organ system(s).

Comprehensive: A general multisystem examination or a complete examination of a single organ system. Note: The comprehensive examination performed as part of the preventive medicine E/M service is multisystem, but its extent is based on age and risk factors identified.

For the purposes of these CPT definitions, the following body areas are recognized:

- Head, including the face
- Neck
- Chest, including breasts and axilla
- Abdomen
- Genitalia, groin, buttocks
- Back
- Each extremity

For the purposes of these CPT definitions, the following organ systems are recognized:

- Eyes
- Ears, nose, mouth, and throat
- Cardiovascular
- Respiratory
- Gastrointestinal
- Genitourinary
- Musculoskeletal
- Skin
- Neurologic
- Psychiatric
- Hematologic/lymphatic/immunologic

Determine the Complexity of Medical Decision Making

Medical decision making refers to the complexity of establishing a diagnosis and/or selecting a management option as measured by:

- The number of possible diagnoses and/or the number of management options that must be considered
- The amount and/or complexity of medical records, diagnostic tests, and/or other information that must be obtained, reviewed, and analyzed

• The risk of significant complications, morbidity, and/or mortality, as well as comorbidities associated with the patient's presenting problem(s), the diagnostic procedure(s), and/or the possible management options

Four types of medical decision making are recognized: straightforward, low complexity, moderate complexity, and high complexity. To qualify for a given type of decision making, two of the three elements in Table 1 must be met or exceeded.

Comorbidities and underlying diseases, in and of themselves, are not considered in selecting a level of E/M services unless their presence significantly increases the complexity of the medical decision making.

Select the Appropriate Level of E/M Services Based on the Following

For the following categories/subcategories, all of the key components, ie, history, examination, and medical decision making, must meet or exceed the stated requirements to qualify for a particular level of E/M service: office, new patient; hospital observation services; initial hospital care; office consultations; initial inpatient consultations; emergency department services; initial nursing facility care; domiciliary care, new patient; and home, new patient.

For the following categories/subcategories, two of the three key components (ie, history, examination, and medical decision making) must meet or exceed the stated requirements to qualify for a particular level of E/M services: office, established patient; subsequent hospital care; subsequent nursing facility care; domiciliary care, established patient; and home, established patient.

When counseling and/or coordination of care dominates (more than 50 percent) the encounter with the patient and/or family (face-to-face time in the office or other outpatient setting or floor/unit time in the hospital or nursing facility), then time shall be considered the key or controlling factor to qualify for a particular level of E/M services. This includes time spent with parties who have assumed responsibility for the care of the patient or decision making whether or not they are family members (e.g., foster parents, person acting in loco parentis, legal guardian). The extent of counseling and/or coordination of care must be documented in the medical record.

CONSULTATION CODES AND MEDICARE REIMBURSEMENT

The Centers for Medicare and Medicaid Services (CMS) no longer provides benefits for CPT consultation codes. CMS has, however, redistributed the value of the consultation codes across the other E/M codes for services which are covered by Medicare. CMS has retained codes 99241 - 99251 in the Medicare Physician Fee Schedule for those private payers that use this data for reimbursement. Note that private payers may choose to follow CMS or CPT guidelines, and the use of consultation codes should be verified with individual payers.

Table 1

Complexity of Medical Decision Making

Number of Diagnoses or Management Options	Amount and/or Complexity of Data to be Reviewed	Risk of Complications and/or Morbidity or Mortality	Type of Decision Making
minimal	minimal or none	minimal	straightforward
limited	limited	low	low complexity
multiple	moderate	moderate	moderate complexity
extensive	extensive	high	high complexity

99201-99215 Outpatient and Other Visits

CMS: 100-04,18,80.2 Contractor Billing Requirements; 100-2,15,270.2 Medicare Telehealth Services; 100-4,11,40.1.3 Independent Attending Physician Services; 100-4,12,100.1.1 Teaching Physicians E/M Services; 100-4,12,190.3 Medicare Telehealth Services; 100-4,12,190.7 Contractor Editing of Telehealth Claims; 100-4,12,230 Primary Care Incentive Payment Program; 100-4,12,230.1 Definition of Primary Care Practitioners and Services; 100-4,12,230.2 Coordination with Other Payments; 100-4,12,230.3 Claims Processing and Payment; 100-4,12,30.6.10 Consultation Services; 100-4,12,30.6.15.1 Prolonged Services With Direct Face-to-Face Patient Contact; 100-4,12,30.6.4 Services Furnished Incident to Physician's Service; 100-4,12,30.6.7 Payment for Office or Other Outpatient E&M Visits; 100-4,12,40.3 Global Surgery Review; 100-4,32,130.1 Billing and Payment of External counterpulsation (ECP)

INCLUDES Established patients: received prior professional services from the physician or qualified health care professional or another physician or qualified health care professional in the practice of the exact same specialty and subspecialty in the previous three years (99211-99215)
New patients: have not received professional services from the physician or qualified health care professional or any other physician or qualified health care professional in the same practice in the exact same specialty and subspecialty in the previous three years (99201-99205)
Office visits
Outpatient services (including services prior to a formal admission to a facility)

EXCLUDES Services provided in:
Emergency department (99281-99285)
Hospital observation (99217-99220 [99224, 99225, 99226])
Hospital observation or inpatient with same day admission and discharge (99234-99236)

99201 Office or other outpatient visit for the evaluation and management of a new patient, which requires these 3 key components: A problem focused history; A problem focused examination; Straightforward medical decision making. Counseling and/or coordination of care with other physicians, other qualified health care professionals, or agencies are provided consistent with the nature of the problem(s) and the patient's and/or family's needs. Usually, the presenting problem(s) are self limited or minor. Typically, 10 minutes are spent face-to-face with the patient and/or family.
🚑 0.75   ⚕ 1.23   **FUD** XXX   B 80 🖵 PQ

8;
un,3-5;
;
key
An
ward
medical decision making. Counseling and/or coordination of care with other physicians, other qualified health care professionals, or agencies are provided consistent with the nature of the problem(s) and the patient's and/or family's needs. Usually, the presenting problem(s) are of low to moderate severity. Typically, 20 minutes are spent face-to-face with the patient and/or family.
🚑 1.41   ⚕ 2.10   **FUD** XXX   B 80 🖵 PQ
AMA: 2015,Jan,12; 2015,Jan,16; 2014,Nov,14; 2014,Oct,8; 2014,Oct,3; 2014,Aug,3; 2014,Jan,11; 2013,Aug,13; 2013,Jun,3-5; 2013,Jan,9-10; 2012,Aug,3-5; 2012,Apr,10; 2012,Jan,3-5; 2012,Jan,15-42; 2011,Jun,3-7; 2011,Feb,6-7; 2011,Jan,11; 2011,Jan,3-5; 2010,Jul,3-5

99203 Office or other outpatient visit for the evaluation and management of a new patient, which requires these 3 key components: A detailed history; A detailed examination; Medical decision making of low complexity. Counseling and/or coordination of care with other physicians, other qualified health care professionals, or agencies are provided consistent with the nature of the problem(s) and the patient's and/or family's needs. Usually, the presenting problem(s) are of moderate severity. Typically, 30 minutes are spent face-to-face with the patient and/or family.
🚑 2.17   ⚕ 3.05   **FUD** XXX   B 80 🖵 PQ
AMA: 2015,Jan,12; 2015,Jan,16; 2014,Nov,14; 2014,Oct,8; 2014,Oct,3; 2014,Aug,3; 2014,Jan,11; 2013,Aug,13; 2013,Jun,3-5; 2013,Jan,9-10; 2012,Aug,3-5; 2012,Apr,10; 2012,Jan,3-5; 2012,Jan,15-42; 2011,Jun,3-7; 2011,Feb,6-7; 2011,Jan,11; 2011,Jan,3-5; 2010,Jul,3-5

99204 Office or other outpatient visit for the evaluation and management of a new patient, which requires these 3 key components: A comprehensive history; A comprehensive examination; Medical decision making of moderate complexity. Counseling and/or coordination of care with other physicians, other qualified health care professionals, or agencies are provided consistent with the nature of the problem(s) and the patient's and/or family's needs. Usually, the presenting problem(s) are of moderate to high severity. Typically, 45 minutes are spent face-to-face with the patient and/or family.
🚑 3.67   ⚕ 4.64   **FUD** XXX   B 80 🖵 PQ
AMA: 2015,Jan,12; 2015,Jan,16; 2014,Nov,14; 2014,Oct,8; 2014,Oct,3; 2014,Aug,3; 2014,Jan,11; 2013,Aug,13; 2013,Jun,3-5; 2013,Jan,9-10; 2012,Aug,3-5; 2012,Apr,10; 2012,Jan,3-5; 2012,Jan,15-42; 2011,Jun,3-7; 2011,Feb,6-7; 2011,Jan,11; 2011,Jan,3-5; 2010,Jul,3-5

99205 Office or other outpatient visit for the evaluation and management of a new patient, which requires these 3 key components: A comprehensive history; A comprehensive examination; Medical decision making of high complexity. Counseling and/or coordination of care with other physicians, other qualified health care professionals, or agencies are provided consistent with the nature of the problem(s) and the patient's and/or family's needs. Usually, the presenting problem(s) are of moderate to high severity. Typically, 60 minutes are spent face-to-face with the patient and/or family.
🚑 4.77   ⚕ 5.83   **FUD** XXX   B 80 🖵 PQ
AMA: 2015,Jan,12; 2015,Jan,16; 2014,Nov,14; 2014,Oct,8; 2014,Oct,3; 2014,Aug,3; 2014,Jan,11; 2013,Aug,13; 2013,Jun,3-5; 2013,Jan,9-10; 2012,Aug,3-5; 2012,Apr,10; 2012,Jan,3-5; 2012,Jan,15-42; 2011,Jun,3-7; 2011,Feb,6-7; 2011,Jan,11; 2011,Jan,3-5; 2010,Jul,3-5

99211 Office or other outpatient visit for the evaluation and management of an established patient, that may not require the presence of a physician or other qualified health care professional. Usually, the presenting problem(s) are minimal. Typically, 5 minutes are spent performing or supervising these services.
🚑 0.26   ⚕ 0.56   **FUD** XXX   B 80 🖵 PQ
AMA: 2015,Jan,12; 2015,Jan,16; 2014,Nov,14; 2014,Oct,8; 2014,Oct,3; 2014,Aug,3; 2014,Mar,13; 2014,Jan,11; 2013,Nov,3; 2013,Aug,13; 2013,Jun,3-5; 2013,Mar,13; 2013,Jan,9-10; 2012,Aug,3-5; 2012,Apr,10; 2012,Jan,3-5; 2012,Jan,15-42; 2011,Feb,6-7; 2011,Jan,3-5; 2011,Jan,11; 2010,Apr,10

Evaluation and Management

99212 — 99217

99212   Office or other outpatient visit for the evaluation and management of an established patient, which requires at least 2 of these 3 key components: A problem focused history; A problem focused examination; Straightforward medical decision making. Counseling and/or coordination of care with other physicians, other qualified health care professionals, or agencies are provided consistent with the nature of the problem(s) and the patient's and/or family's needs. Usually, the presenting problem(s) are self limited or minor. Typically, 10 minutes are spent face-to-face with the patient and/or family.

     🚑 0.72   ⚕ 1.23   **FUD** XXX   B 80 🖥 PQ

     AMA: 2015,Jan,16; 2015,Jan,12; 2014,Nov,14; 2014,Oct,8; 2014,Oct,3; 2014,Aug,3; 2014,Jan,11; 2013,Nov,3; 2013,Aug,13; 2013,Jun,3-5; 2013,Mar,13; 2013,Jan,9-10; 2012,Aug,3-5; 2012,Apr,10; 2012,Mar,4-7; 2012,Jan,15-42; 2012,Jan,3-5; 2011,Jun,3-7; 2011,Feb,6-7; 2011,Jan,11; 2011,Jan,3-5; 2010,Sep,4-5; 2010,Jul,3-5

99213   Office or other outpatient visit for the evaluation and management of an established patient, which requires at least 2 of these 3 key components: An expanded problem focused history; An expanded problem focused examination; Medical decision making of low complexity. Counseling and coordination of care with other physicians, other qualified health care professionals, or agencies are provided consistent with the nature of the problem(s) and the patient's and/or family's needs. Usually, the presenting problem(s) are of low to moderate severity. Typically, 15 minutes are spent face-to-face with the patient and/or family.

     🚑 1.43   ⚕ 2.04   **FUD** XXX   B 80 🖥 PQ

     AMA: 2015,Jan,16; 2015,Jan,12; 2014,Nov,14; 2014,Oct,8; 2014,Oct,3; 2014,Aug,3; 2014,Jan,11; 2013,Nov,3; 2013,Aug,13; 2013,Jun,3-5; 2013,Mar,13; 2013,Jan,9-10; 2012,Aug,3-5; 2012,Apr,10; 2012,Mar,4-7; 2012,Jan,15-42; 2012,Jan,3-5; 2011,Jun,3-7; 2011,Feb,6-7; 2011,Jan,11; 2011,Jan,3-5; 2010,Sep,4-5; 2010,Jul,3-5

99214   Office or other outpatient visit for the evaluation and management of an established patient, which requires at least 2 of these 3 key components: A detailed history; A detailed examination; Medical decision making of moderate complexity. Counseling and/or coordination of care with other physicians, other qualified health care professionals, or agencies are provided consistent with the nature of the problem(s) and the patient's and/or family's needs. Usually, the presenting problem(s) are of moderate to high severity. Typically, 25 minutes are spent face-to-face with the patient and/or family.

     🚑 2.21   ⚕ 3.03   **FUD** XXX   B 80 🖥 PQ

     AMA: 2015,Jan,12; 2015,Jan,16; 2014,Nov,14; 2014,Oct,8; 2014,Oct,3; 2014,Aug,3; 2014,Jan,11; 2013,Nov,3; 2013,Aug,13; 2013,Jun,3-5; 2013,Mar,13; 2013,Jan,9-10; 2012,Aug,3-5; 2012,Apr,10; 2012,Mar,4-7; 2012,Jan,3-5; 2012,Jan,15-42; 2011,Jun,3-7; 2011,Feb,6-7; 2011,Jan,11; 2011,Jan,3-5; 2010,Sep,4-5; 2010,Jul,3-5

99215   Office or other outpatient visit for the evaluation and management of an established patient, which requires at least 2 of these 3 key components: A comprehensive history; A comprehensive examination; Medical decision making of high complexity. Counseling and/or coordination of care with other physicians, other qualified health care professionals, or agencies are provided consistent with the nature of the problem(s) and the patient's and/or family's needs. Usually, the presenting problem(s) are of moderate to high severity. Typically, 40 minutes are spent face-to-face with the patient and/or family.

     🚑 3.14   ⚕ 4.09   **FUD** XXX   B 80 🖥 PQ

     AMA: 2015,Jan,12; 2015,Jan,16; 2014,Nov,14; 2014,Oct,8; 2014,Oct,3; 2014,Aug,3; 2014,Jan,11; 2013,Nov,3; 2013,Aug,13; 2013,Jun,3-5; 2013,Mar,13; 2013,Jan,9-10; 2012,Aug,3-5; 2012,Apr,10; 2012,Jan,3-5; 2012,Jan,15-42; 2011,Jun,3-7; 2011,Feb,6-7; 2011,Jan,11; 2011,Jan,3-5; 2010,Sep,4-5; 2010,Jul,3-5

99217-99220 Facility Observation Visits: Initial and Discharge

CMS: 100-4,11,40.1.3 Independent Attending Physician Services; 100-4,12,100.1.1 Teaching Physicians E/M Services; 100-4,12,30.6.4 Services Furnished Incident to Physician's Service; 100-4,12,30.6.8 Payment for Hospital Observation Services; 100-4,12,40.3 Global Surgery Review; 100-4,32,130.1 Billing and Payment of External counterpulsation (ECP)

   INCLUDES   Services provided on the same date in other settings or departments associated with the observation status admission (99201-99215, 99281-99285, 99304-99318, 99324-99337, 99341-99350, 99381-99429)
                    Services provided to new and established patients admitted to a hospital specifically for observation (not required to be a designated area of the hospital)

   EXCLUDES   *Services provided by physicians or another qualified health care professional other than the admitting physician ([99224, 99225, 99226], 99241-99245)*
                    Services provided to a patient admitted to the hospital following observation status (99221-99223)
                    Services provided to patients who are admitted and discharged from observation status on the same date (99234-99236)

   INCLUDES   Discussing the observation admission with the patient
                    Final patient evaluation:
                       Discharge instructions
                       Sign off on discharge medical records
                    Do not report with hospital discharge day management services (99238-99239)
                    Do not report with hospital inpatient care
                    Do not report with observation/inpatient admission/discharge on the same date (99234-99236)

     🚑 2.05   ⚕ 2.05   **FUD** XXX   B 80 🖥 PQ

     AMA: 2015,Jan,16; 2014,Nov,14; 2014,Oct,8; 2014,Jan,11; 2013,Jun,3-5; 2013,Jan,9-10; 2012,Jul,10-11; 2011,Jun,3-7; 2011,Feb,6-7; 2010,Sep,4-5

26/TC **PC/TC Comp Only**   A2-Z3 **ASC Pmt**   50 **Bilateral**   ♂ **Male Only**   ♀ **Female Only**   🚑 **Facility RVU**   ⚕ **Non-Facility RVU**

AMA: CPT Asst   **CMS:** Pub 100   A-Y **OPPSI**   80/80 **Surg Assist Allowed / w/Doc**   🔲 **Lab Crosswalk**   ✚ **Radiology Crosswalk**

452   Medicare (Red Text)   CPT © 2015 American Medical Association. All Rights Reserved. (Black Text)   © 2015 Optum360, LLC (Blue Text)

99218   Initial observation care, per day, for the evaluation and management of a patient which requires these 3 key components: A detailed or comprehensive history; A detailed or comprehensive examination; and Medical decision making that is straightforward or of low complexity. Counseling and/or coordination of care with other physicians, other qualified health care professionals, or agencies are provided consistent with the nature of the problem(s) and the patient's and/or family's needs. Usually, the problem(s) requiring admission to "observation status" are of low severity. Typically, 30 minutes are spent at the bedside and on the patient's hospital floor or unit.

2.83   2.83   **FUD** XXX   B 80 PQ

AMA: 2015,Jul,3; 2015,Mar,3; 2015,Jan,16; 2014,Nov,14; 2014,Oct,8; 2014,Jan,11; 2013,Aug,13; 2013,Jun,3-5; 2013,Jan,9-10; 2012,Aug,3-5; 2012,Jul,10-11; 2012,Jan,15-42; 2011,Jun,3-7; 2011,Feb,6-7; 2011,Jan,11; 2010,Sep,4-5

99219   Initial observation care, per day, for the evaluation and management of a patient, which requires these 3 key components: A comprehensive history; A comprehensive examination; and Medical decision making of moderate complexity. Counseling and/or coordination of care with other physicians, other qualified health care professionals, or agencies are provided consistent with the nature of the problem(s) and the patient's and/or family's needs. Usually, the problem(s) requiring admission to "observation status" are of moderate severity. Typically, 50 minutes are spent at the bedside and on the patient's hospital floor or unit.

3.83   3.83   **FUD** XXX   B 80 PQ

AMA: 2015,Jul,3; 2015,Jan,16; 2014,Nov,14; 2014,Oct,8; 2014,Jan,11; 2013,Aug,13; 2013,Jun,3-5; 2013,Jan,9-10; 2012,Aug,3-5; 2012,Jul,10-11; 2012,Jan,15-42; 2011,Jun,3-7; 2011,Feb,6-7; 2011,Jan,11; 2010,Sep,4-5

99220   Initial observation care, per day, for the evaluation and management of a patient which requires these 3 key components: A comprehensive history; A comprehensive examination; and Medical decision making of high complexity. Counseling and/or coordination of care with other physicians, other qualified health care professionals, or agencies are provided consistent with the nature of the problem(s) and the patient's and/or family's needs. Usually, the problem(s) requiring admission to "observation status" are of high severity. Typically, 70 minutes are spent at the bedside and on the patient's hospital floor or unit.

5.25   5.25   **FUD** XXX   B 80 PQ

AMA: 2015,Jul,3; 2015,Jan,16; 2014,Nov,14; 2014,Oct,8; 2014,Jan,11; 2013,Aug,13; 2013,Jun,3-5; 2013,Jan,9-10; 2012,Aug,3-5; 2012,Jul,10-11; 2012,Jan,15-42; 2011,Jun,3-7; 2011,Feb,6-7; 2011,Jan,11; 2010,Sep,4-5

[99224, 99225, 99226] Facility Observation Visits: Subsequent

CMS: 100-4,11,40.1.3 Independent Attending Physician Services; 100-4,12,100.1.1 Teaching Physicians E/M Services; 100-4,12,30.6.4 Services Furnished Incident to Physician's Service; 100-4,12,30.6.8 Payment for Hospital Observation Services; 100-4,12,30.6.9.1 Initial Hospital Care and Observation or Inpatient Care Services

INCLUDES Changes in patient's status (e.g., physical condition, history; response to medical management)
· Medical record review
· Review of diagnostic test results
· Services provided on the same date in other settings or departments associated with the observation status admission (99201-99215, 99281-99285, 99304-99318, 99324-99337, 99341-99350, 99381-99429)

EXCLUDES *Observation admission and discharge on the same day (99234-99236)*

\#   99224   Subsequent observation care, per day, for the evaluation and management of a patient, which requires at least 2 of these 3 key components: Problem focused interval history; Problem focused examination; Medical decision making that is straightforward or of low complexity. Counseling and/or coordination of care with other physicians, other qualified health care professionals, or agencies are provided consistent with the nature of the problem(s) and the patient's and/or family's needs. Usually, the patient is stable, recovering, or improving. Typically, 15 minutes are spent at the bedside and on the patient's hospital floor or unit.

1.11   1.11   **FUD** XXX   B 80 PQ

AMA: 2015,Jan,16; 2014,Nov,14; 2014,Oct,8; 2014,Jan,11; 2013,Aug,13; 2013,Jun,3-5; 2013,Jan,9-10; 2012,Aug,3-5; 2012,Jul,10-11; 2011,Aug,11; 2011,Jun,3-7; 2011,Feb,6-7

\#   99225   Subsequent observation care, per day, for the evaluation and management of a patient, which requires at least 2 of these 3 key components: An expanded problem focused interval history; An expanded problem focused examination; Medical decision making of moderate complexity. Counseling and/or coordination of care with other physicians, other qualified health care professionals, or agencies are provided consistent with the nature of the problem(s) and the patient's and/or family's needs. Usually, the patient is responding inadequately to therapy or has developed a minor complication. Typically, 25 minutes are spent at the bedside and on the patient's hospital floor or unit.

2.05   2.05   **FUD** XXX   B 80 PQ

AMA: 2015,Jan,16; 2014,Nov,14; 2014,Oct,8; 2014,Jan,11; 2013,Aug,13; 2013,Jun,3-5; 2013,Jan,9-10; 2012,Aug,3-5; 2012,Jul,10-11; 2011,Aug,11; 2011,Jun,3-7; 2011,Feb,6-7

\#   99226   Subsequent observation care, per day, for the evaluation and management of a patient, which requires at least 2 of these 3 key components: A detailed interval history; A detailed examination; Medical decision making of high complexity. Counseling and/or coordination of care with other physicians, other qualified health care professionals, or agencies are provided consistent with the nature of the problem(s) and the patient's and/or family's needs. Usually, the patient is unstable or has developed a significant complication or a significant new problem. Typically, 35 minutes are spent at the bedside and on the patient's hospital floor or unit.

2.97   2.97   **FUD** XXX   B 80 PQ

AMA: 2015,Jan,16; 2014,Nov,14; 2014,Oct,8; 2014,Jan,11; 2013,Aug,13; 2013,Jun,3-5; 2013,Jan,9-10; 2012,Aug,3-5; 2012,Jul,10-11; 2011,Aug,11; 2011,Jun,3-7; 2011,Feb,6-7

99221-99233 Inpatient Hospital Visits: Initial and Subsequent

CMS: 100-4,11,40.1.3 Independent Attending Physician Services; 100-4,12,100.1.1 Teaching Physicians E/M Services; 100-4,12,30.6.10 Consultation Services; 100-4,12,30.6.15.1 Prolonged Services With Direct Face-to-Face Patient Contact; 100-4,12,30.6.4 Services Furnished Incident to Physician's Service; 100-4,12,30.6.9 Hospital Visit and Critical Care on Same Day

INCLUDES Initial physician services provided to the patient in the hospital or "partial" hospital settings (99221-99223)
Services provided on the date of admission in other settings or departments associated with an observation status admission (99201-99215, 99281-99285, 99304-99318, 99324-99337, 99341-99350, 99381-99397)
Services provided to a new or established patient
EXCLUDES *Inpatient admission and discharge on the same date (99234-99236)*
Inpatient E&M services provided by other than the admitting physician

99221 Initial hospital care, per day, for the evaluation and management of a patient, which requires these 3 key components: A detailed or comprehensive history; A detailed or comprehensive examination; and Medical decision making that is straightforward or of low complexity. Counseling and/or coordination of care with other physicians, other qualified health care professionals, or agencies are provided consistent with the nature of the problem(s) and the patient's and/or family's needs. Usually, the problem(s) requiring admission are of low severity. Typically, 30 minutes are spent at the bedside and on the patient's hospital floor or unit.
 ⚕ 2.87   ⚕ 2.87   **FUD** XXX   B 80☐ PQ
AMA: 2015,Jul,3; 2015,Jan,16; 2014,Nov,14; 2014,Oct,8; 2014,Jan,11; 2013,Aug,13; 2013,Jun,3-5; 2013,Jan,9-10; 2012,Aug,3-5; 2012,Jul,10-11; 2012,Jul,12-14; 2012,Jan,15-42; 2011,Jun,3-7; 2011,Feb,6-7; 2011,Jan,11

99222 Initial hospital care, per day, for the evaluation and management of a patient, which requires these 3 key components: A comprehensive history; A comprehensive examination; and Medical decision making of moderate complexity. Counseling and/or coordination of care with other physicians, other qualified health care professionals, or agencies are provided consistent with the nature of the problem(s) and the patient's and/or family's needs. Usually, the problem(s) requiring admission are of moderate severity. Typically, 50 minutes are spent at the bedside and on the patient's hospital floor or unit.
 ⚕ 3.87   ⚕ 3.87   **FUD** XXX   B 80☐ PQ
AMA: 2015,Jul,3; 2015,Mar,3; 2015,Jan,16; 2014,Nov,14; 2014,Oct,8; 2014,Jan,11; 2013,Aug,13; 2013,Jun,3-5; 2013,Jan,9-10; 2012,Aug,3-5; 2012,Jul,12-14; 2012,Jul,10-11; 2012,Jan,15-42; 2011,Jun,3-7; 2011,Feb,6-7; 2011,Jan,11

99223 Initial hospital care, per day, for the evaluation and management of a patient, which requires these 3 key components: A comprehensive history; A comprehensive examination; and Medical decision making of high complexity. Counseling and/or coordination of care with other physicians, other qualified health care professionals, or agencies are provided consistent with the nature of the problem(s) and the patient's and/or family's needs. Usually, the problem(s) requiring admission are of high severity. Typically, 70 minutes are spent at the bedside and on the patient's hospital floor or unit.
 ⚕ 5.73   ⚕ 5.73   **FUD** XXX   B 80☐ PQ
AMA: 2015,Jul,3; 2015,Jan,16; 2014,Nov,14; 2014,Oct,8; 2014,Jan,11; 2013,Aug,13; 2013,Jun,3-5; 2013,Jan,9-10; 2012,Aug,3-5; 2012,Jul,10-11; 2012,Jul,12-14; 2012,Jan,15-42; 2011,Jun,3-7; 2011,Feb,6-7; 2011,Jan,11

99224 Resequenced code. See code following 99220.

99225 Resequenced code. See code following 99220.

99226 Resequenced code. See code before 99221.

99231 Subsequent hospital care, per day, for the evaluation and management of a patient, which requires at least 2 of these 3 key components: A problem focused interval history; A problem focused examination; Medical decision making that is straightforward or of low complexity. Counseling and/or coordination of care with other physicians, other qualified health care professionals, or agencies are provided consistent with the nature of the problem(s) and the patient's and/or family's needs. Usually, the patient is stable, recovering or improving. Typically, 15 minutes are spent at the bedside and on the patient's hospital floor or unit.
 ⚕ 1.10   ⚕ 1.10   **FUD** XXX   B 80☐ PQ
AMA: 2015,Jul,3; 2015,Jan,16; 2014,Nov,14; 2014,Oct,8; 2014,May,4; 2014,Jan,11; 2013,Sep,17; 2013,Aug,13; 2013,Jun,3-5; 2013,Jan,9-10; 2012,Aug,3-5; 2012,Jul,12-14; 2012,Jan,15-42; 2011,Aug,11; 2011,Jun,3-7; 2011,Feb,6-7; 2011,Jan,11

99232 Subsequent hospital care, per day, for the evaluation and management of a patient, which requires at least 2 of these 3 key components: An expanded problem focused interval history; An expanded problem focused examination; Medical decision making of moderate complexity. Counseling and/or coordination of care with other physicians, other qualified health care professionals, or agencies are provided consistent with the nature of the problem(s) and the patient's and/or family's needs. Usually, the patient is responding inadequately to therapy or has developed a minor complication. Typically, 25 minutes are spent at the bedside and on the patient's hospital floor or unit.
 ⚕ 2.04   ⚕ 2.04   **FUD** XXX   B 80☐ PQ
AMA: 2015,Jul,3; 2015,Jan,16; 2014,Nov,14; 2014,Oct,8; 2014,Jan,11; 2013,Aug,13; 2013,Jun,3-5; 2013,Jan,9-10; 2012,Aug,3-5; 2012,Jul,12-14; 2012,Jan,15-42; 2011,Aug,11; 2011,Jun,3-7; 2011,Feb,6-7; 2011,Jan,11

99233 Subsequent hospital care, per day, for the evaluation and management of a patient, which requires at least 2 of these 3 key components: A detailed interval history; A detailed examination; Medical decision making of high complexity. Counseling and/or coordination of care with other physicians, other qualified health care professionals, or agencies are provided consistent with the nature of the problem(s) and the patient's and/or family's needs. Usually, the patient is unstable or has developed a significant complication or a significant new problem. Typically, 35 minutes are spent at the bedside and on the patient's hospital floor or unit.
 ⚕ 2.94   ⚕ 2.94   **FUD** XXX   B 80☐ PQ
AMA: 2015,Jul,3; 2015,Jan,16; 2014,Nov,14; 2014,Oct,8; 2014,May,4; 2014,Jan,11; 2013,Aug,13; 2013,Jun,3-5; 2013,Jan,9-10; 2012,Aug,3-5; 2012,Jul,12-14; 2012,Jan,15-42; 2011,Aug,11; 2011,Jun,3-7; 2011,Feb,6-7; 2011,Jan,11

99234-99236 Observation/Inpatient Visits: Admitted/Discharged on Same Date

CMS: 100-4,11,40.1.3 Independent Attending Physician Services; 100-4,12,100.1.1 Teaching Physicians E/M Services; 100-4,12,30.6.4 Services Furnished Incident to Physician's Service; 100-4,12,30.6.8 Payment for Hospital Observation Services; 100-4,12,30.6.9 Payment for Inpatient Hospital Visits - General; 100-4,12,30.6.9.1 Initial Hospital Care and Observation or Inpatient Care Services; 100-4,12,30.6.9.2 Subsequent Hospital Visit and Discharge Management; 100-4,12,40.3 Global Surgery Review

INCLUDES Admission and discharge services on the same date in an observation or inpatient setting
All services provided by admitting physician or other qualified health care professional on same date of service, even when initiated in another setting (e.g., emergency department, nursing facility, office)

EXCLUDES Services provided to patients admitted to observation and discharged on a different date (99217-99220, [99224, 99225, 99226])

99234 Observation or inpatient hospital care, for the evaluation and management of a patient including admission and discharge on the same date, which requires these 3 key components: A detailed or comprehensive history; A detailed or comprehensive examination; and Medical decision making that is straightforward or of low complexity. Counseling and/or coordination of care with other physicians, other qualified health care professionals, or agencies are provided consistent with the nature of the problem(s) and the patient's and/or family's needs. Usually the presenting problem(s) requiring admission are of low severity. Typically, 40 minutes are spent at the bedside and on the patient's hospital floor or unit.
 ⚕ 3.78   ⚕ 3.78   **FUD** XXX   B 80☐ PQ
AMA: 2015,Jul,3; 2015,Jan,16; 2014,Oct,8; 2014,Jan,11; 2013,Jun,3-5; 2012,Jul,10-11; 2012,Jan,15-42; 2011,Jun,3-7; 2011,Feb,6-7; 2011,Jan,11; 2010,Sep,4-5

Left margin: Evaluation and Management
Left margin: 99221 — 99234

99235 Observation or inpatient hospital care, for the evaluation and management of a patient including admission and discharge on the same date, which requires these 3 key components: A comprehensive history; A comprehensive examination; and Medical decision making of moderate complexity. Counseling and/or coordination of care with other physicians, other qualified health care professionals, or agencies are provided consistent with the nature of the problem(s) and the patient's and/or family's needs. Usually the presenting problem(s) requiring admission are of moderate severity. Typically, 50 minutes are spent at the bedside and on the patient's hospital floor or unit.

     4.77   4.77   **FUD** XXX   B 80 PQ

     AMA: 2015,Jul,3; 2015,Jan,16; 2014,Oct,8; 2014,Jan,11; 2013,Jun,3-5; 2012,Jul,10-11; 2012,Jan,15-42; 2011,Jun,3-7; 2011,Feb,6-7; 2011,Jan,11; 2010,Sep,4-5

99236 Observation or inpatient hospital care, for the evaluation and management of a patient including admission and discharge on the same date, which requires these 3 key components: A comprehensive history; A comprehensive examination; and Medical decision making of high complexity. Counseling and/or coordination of care with other physicians, other qualified health care professionals, or agencies are provided consistent with the nature of the problem(s) and the patient's and/or family's needs. Usually the presenting problem(s) requiring admission are of high severity. Typically, 55 minutes are spent at the bedside and on the patient's hospital floor or unit.

     6.15   6.15   **FUD** XXX   B 80 PQ

     AMA: 2015,Jul,3; 2015,Jan,16; 2014,Oct,8; 2014,Jan,11; 2013,Jun,3-5; 2012,Jul,10-11; 2012,Jan,15-42; 2011,Jun,3-7; 2011,Feb,6-7; 2011,Jan,11; 2010,Sep,4-5

99241-99245 Consultations: Office and Outpatient

CMS: 100-2,15,270 Telehealth Services; 100-2,15,270.2 Medicare Telehealth Services; 100-2,15,270.4 Payment - Physician/Practitioner at a Distant Site; 100-4,11,40.1.3 Independent Attending Physician Services; 100-4,12,190.3 Medicare Telehealth Services; 100-4,12,190.7 Contractor Editing of Telehealth Claims; 100-4,12,30.6.10 Consultation Services; 100-4,12,30.6.15.1 Prolonged Services With Direct Face-to-Face Patient Contact; 100-4,12,30.6.4 Services Furnished Incident to Physician's Service; 100-4,12,30.6.9.1 Initial Hospital Care and Observation or Inpatient Care Services; 100-4,12,40.3 Global Surgery Review; 100-4,32,130.1 Billing and Payment of External counterpulsation (ECP); 100-4,4,160 Clinic and Emergency Visits Under OPPS

INCLUDES   A third-party mandated consultation

     All outpatient consultations provided in the office, outpatient or other ambulatory facility, domiciliary/rest home, emergency department, patient's home, and hospital observation

     Documentation of a request for a consultation from an appropriate source

     Documentation of the need for consultation in the patient's medical record

     One consultation per consultant

     Provision by a physician or qualified nonphysician practitioner whose advice, opinion, recommendation, suggestion, direction, or counsel, etc., is requested for evaluating/treating a patient since that individual's expertise in a specific medical area is beyond the scope of knowledge of the requesting physician

     Provision of a written report of findings/recommendations from the consultant to the referring physician

EXCLUDES   *Another appropriately requested and documented consultation pertaining to the same/new problem; repeat use of consultation codes*

     Any distinctly recognizable procedure/service provided on or following the consultation

     Assumption of care (all or partial); report subsequent codes as appropriate for the place of service (99211-99215, 99334-99337, 99347-99350)

     Consultation prompted by the patient/family; report codes for office, domiciliary/rest home, or home visits instead (99201-99215, 99324-99337, 99341-99350)

Do not report when services are provided to Medicare patients

99241 Office consultation for a new or established patient, which requires these 3 key components: A problem focused history; A problem focused examination; and Straightforward medical decision making. Counseling and/or coordination of care with other physicians, other qualified health care professionals, or agencies are provided consistent with the nature of the problem(s) and the patient's and/or family's needs. Usually, the presenting problem(s) are self limited or minor. Typically, 15 minutes are spent face-to-face with the patient and/or family.

     0.95   1.37   **FUD** XXX   E

     AMA: 2015,Jan,16; 2015,Jan,12; 2014,Nov,14; 2014,Oct,8; 2014,Sep,13; 2014,Aug,3; 2014,Jan,11; 2013,Jun,3-5; 2013,Jan,9-10; 2012,Aug,3-5; 2012,Apr,10; 2012,Jan,15-42; 2011,Jun,3-7; 2011,Feb,6-7; 2011,Jan,11; 2010,Jul,3-5; 2010,Jan,3-5

99242 Office consultation for a new or established patient, which requires these 3 key components: An expanded problem focused history; An expanded problem focused examination; and Straightforward medical decision making. Counseling and/or coordination of care with other physicians, other qualified health care professionals, or agencies are provided consistent with the nature of the problem(s) and the patient's and/or family's needs. Usually, the presenting problem(s) are of low severity. Typically, 30 minutes are spent face-to-face with the patient and/or family.

     1.98   2.57   **FUD** XXX   E

     AMA: 2015,Jan,16; 2015,Jan,12; 2014,Nov,14; 2014,Oct,8; 2014,Sep,13; 2014,Aug,3; 2014,Jan,11; 2013,Jun,3-5; 2013,Jan,9-10; 2012,Aug,3-5; 2012,Apr,10; 2012,Jan,15-42; 2011,Jun,3-7; 2011,Feb,6-7; 2011,Jan,11; 2010,Jul,3-5; 2010,Jan,3-5

A Age Edit   Unlisted   Not Covered   # Resequenced

Mod Sedation   + Add-on   CCI   PQ PQRS   **FUD** Follow-up Days

ights Reserved. (Black Text)   Medicare (Red Text)   **455**

99243   Office consultation for a new or established patient, which requires these 3 key components: A detailed history; A detailed examination; and Medical decision making of low complexity. Counseling and/or coordination of care with other physicians, other qualified health care professionals, or agencies are provided consistent with the nature of the problem(s) and the patient's and/or family's needs. Usually, the presenting problem(s) are of moderate severity. Typically, 40 minutes are spent face-to-face with the patient and/or family.

   🚑 2.76   ⚕ 3.51   **FUD** XXX   🅴 🖳

   AMA: 2015,Jan,16; 2015,Jan,12; 2014,Nov,14; 2014,Oct,8; 2014,Sep,13; 2014,Aug,3; 2014,Jan,11; 2013,Jun,3-5; 2013,Jan,9-10; 2012,Aug,3-5; 2012,Apr,10; 2012,Jan,15-42; 2011,Jun,3-7; 2011,Feb,6-7; 2011,Jan,11; 2010,Jul,3-5; 2010,Jan,3-5

99244   Office consultation for a new or established patient, which requires these 3 key components: A comprehensive history; A comprehensive examination; and Medical decision making of moderate complexity. Counseling and/or coordination of care with other physicians, other qualified health care professionals, or agencies are provided consistent with the nature of the problem(s) and the patient's and/or family's needs. Usually, the presenting problem(s) are of moderate to high severity. Typically, 60 minutes are spent face-to-face with the patient and/or family.

   🚑 4.37   ⚕ 5.19   **FUD** XXX   🅴 🖳

   AMA: 2015,Jan,16; 2015,Jan,12; 2014,Nov,14; 2014,Oct,8; 2014,Sep,13; 2014,Aug,3; 2014,Jan,11; 2013,Aug,12; 2013,Jun,3-5; 2013,Jan,9-10; 2012,Aug,3-5; 2012,Apr,10; 2012,Jan,15-42; 2011,Jun,3-7; 2011,Feb,6-7; 2011,Jan,11; 2010,Jul,3-5; 2010,Jan,3-5

99245   Office consultation for a new or established patient, which requires these 3 key components: A comprehensive history; A comprehensive examination; and Medical decision making of high complexity. Counseling and/or coordination of care with other physicians, other qualified health care professionals, or agencies are provided consistent with the nature of the problem(s) and the patient's and/or family's needs. Usually, the presenting problem(s) are of moderate to high severity. Typically, 80 minutes are spent face-to-face with the patient and/or family.

   🚑 5.43   ⚕ 6.35   **FUD** XXX   🅴 🖳

   AMA: 2015,Jan,16; 2015,Jan,12; 2014,Nov,14; 2014,Oct,8; 2014,Sep,13; 2014,Aug,3; 2014,Jan,11; 2013,Jun,3-5; 2013,Jan,9-10; 2012,Aug,3-5; 2012,Apr,10; 2012,Jan,15-42; 2011,Jun,3-7; 2011,Feb,6-7; 2011,Jan,11; 2010,Jul,3-5; 2010,Jan,3-5

99251-99255 Consultations: Inpatient

CMS: 100-2,15,270 Telehealth Services; 100-4,11,40.1.3 Independent Attending Physician Services; 100-4,12,190.3 Medicare Telehealth Services; 100-4,12,190.7 Contractor Editing of Telehealth Claims; 100-4,12,30.6.10 Consultation Services; 100-4,12,30.6.15.1 Prolonged Services With Direct Face-to-Face Patient Contact; 100-4,12,30.6.4 Services Furnished Incident to Physician's Service; 100-4,12,30.6.9.1 Initial Hospital Care and Observation or Inpatient Care Services; 100-4,12,40.3 Global Surgery Review

INCLUDES   A third-party mandated consultation
          All inpatient consultations include services provided in the hospital inpatient or partial hospital settings and nursing facilities
          Documentation of a request for a consultation from an appropriate source
          Documentation of the need for consultation in the patient's medical record
          One consultation by consultant per admission
          Provision by a physician or qualified nonphysician practitioner whose advice, opinion, recommendation, suggestion, direction, or counsel, etc. is requested for evaluating/treating a patient since that individual's expertise in a specific medical area is beyond the scope of knowledge of the requesting physician
          Provision of a written report of findings/recommendations from the consultant to the referring physician

EXCLUDES   *Another appropriately requested and documented consultation pertaining to the same/new problem: repeat use of consultation codes*
          Any distinctly recognizable procedure/service provided on or following the consultation
          Assumption of care (all or partial): report subsequent codes as appropriate for the place of service (99231-99233, 99307-99310)
          Consultation prompted by the patient/family: report codes for office, domiciliary/rest home, or home visits instead (99201-99215, 99324-99337, 99341-99350)

Do not report an outpatient consultation and an inpatient consultation for the same admission (99241-99245, 99251-99255)

Do not report when services are provided to Medicare patients

99251   Inpatient consultation for a new or established patient, which requires these 3 key components: A problem focused history; A problem focused examination; and Straightforward medical decision making. Counseling and/or coordination of care with other physicians, other qualified health care professionals,

99254 Inpatient consultation for a new or established patient, which requires these 3 key components: A comprehensive history; A comprehensive examination; and Medical decision making of moderate complexity. Counseling and/or coordination of care with other physicians, other qualified health care professionals, or agencies are provided consistent with the nature of the problem(s) and the patient's and/or family's needs. Usually, the presenting problem(s) are of moderate to high severity. Typically, 80 minutes are spent at the bedside and on the patient's hospital floor or unit.

⚒ 4.69 ⚖ 4.69 **FUD** XXX 🄴 ⬜

AMA: 2015,Jan,16; 2014,Nov,14; 2014,Oct,8; 2014,Jan,11; 2013,Jun,3-5; 2013,Jan,9-10; 2012,Aug,3-5; 2012,Jan,15-42; 2011,Feb,6-7; 2011,Jan,11; 2010,Jan,3-5

99255 Inpatient consultation for a new or established patient, which requires these 3 key components: A comprehensive history; A comprehensive examination; and Medical decision making of high complexity. Counseling and/or coordination of care with other physicians, other qualified health care professionals, or agencies are provided consistent with the nature of the problem(s) and the patient's and/or family's needs. Usually, the presenting problem(s) are of moderate to high severity. Typically, 110 minutes are spent at the bedside and on the patient's hospital floor or unit.

⚒ 5.67 ⚖ 5.67 **FUD** XXX 🄴 ⬜

AMA: 2015,Jan,16; 2014,Nov,14; 2014,Oct,8; 2014,Jan,11; 2013,Jun,3-5; 2013,Jan,9-10; 2012,Aug,3-5; 2012,Jan,15-42; 2011,Feb,6-7; 2011,Jan,11; 2010,Jan,3-5

99281-99288 Emergency Department Visits

CMS: 100-4,11,40.1.3 Independent Attending Physician Services; 100-4,12,30.6.11 Emergency Department Visits; 100-4,4,160 Clinic and Emergency Visits Under OPPS

INCLUDES Any amount of time spent with the patient, which usually involves a series of encounters while the patient is in the emergency department
Care provided to new and established patients

EXCLUDES Critical care services (99291-99292)
Observation services (99217-99220, 99234-99236)

99281 Emergency department visit for the evaluation and management of a patient, which requires these 3 key components: A problem focused history; A problem focused examination; and Straightforward medical decision making. Counseling and/or coordination of care with other physicians, other qualified health care professionals, or agencies are provided consistent with the nature of the problem(s) and the patient's and/or family's needs. Usually, the presenting problem(s) are self limited or minor.

⚒ 0.59 ⚖ 0.59 **FUD** XXX Ⓥ 80 ⬜ PQ

AMA: 2015,Jan,12; 2015,Jan,16; 2014,Nov,14; 2014,Oct,8; 2014,Jan,11; 2013,Jun,3-5; 2013,Jan,9-10; 2012,Jan,15-42; 2011,Feb,6-7; 2011,Jan,11

99282 Emergency department visit for the evaluation and management of a patient, which requires these 3 key components: An expanded problem focused history; An expanded problem focused examination; and Medical decision making of low complexity. Counseling and/or coordination of care with other physicians, other qualified health care professionals, or agencies are provided consistent with the nature of the problem(s) and the patient's and/or family's needs. Usually, the presenting problem(s) are of low to moderate severity.

⚒ 1.16 ⚖ 1.16 **FUD** XXX Ⓥ 80 ⬜ PQ

AMA: 2015,Jan,12; 2015,Jan,16; 2014,Nov,14; 2014,Oct,8;

99283 Emergency department visit for the evaluation and management of a patient, which requires these 3 key components: An expanded problem focused history; An expanded problem focused examination; and Medical decision making of moderate complexity. Counseling and/or coordination of care with other physicians, other qualified health care professionals, or agencies are provided consistent with the nature of the problem(s) and the patient's and/or family's needs. Usually, the presenting problem(s) are of moderate severity.

⚒ 1.75 ⚖ 1.75 **FUD** XXX Ⓥ 80 ⬜ PQ

AMA: 2015,Jan,12; 2015,Jan,16; 2014,Nov,14; 2014,Oct,8; 2014,Jan,11; 2013,Jun,3-5; 2013,Jan,9-10; 2012,Jan,15-42; 2011,Feb,6-7; 2011,Jan,11

99284 Emergency department visit for the evaluation and management of a patient, which requires these 3 key components: A detailed history; A detailed examination; and Medical decision making of moderate complexity. Counseling and/or coordination of care with other physicians, other qualified health care professionals, or agencies are provided consistent with the nature of the problem(s) and the patient's and/or family's needs. Usually, the presenting problem(s) are of high severity, and require urgent evaluation by the physician, or other qualified health care professionals but do not pose an immediate significant threat to life or physiologic function.

⚒ 3.33 ⚖ 3.33 **FUD** XXX Q3 80 ⬜ PQ

AMA: 2015,Jan,16; 2015,Jan,12; 2014,Nov,14; 2014,Oct,8; 2014,Jan,11; 2013,Jun,3-5; 2013,Jan,9-10; 2012,Jan,15-42; 2011,Feb,6-7; 2011,Jan,11

99285 Emergency department visit for the evaluation and management of a patient, which requires these 3 key components within the constraints imposed by the urgency of the patient's clinical condition and/or mental status: A comprehensive history; A comprehensive examination; and Medical decision making of high complexity. Counseling and/or coordination of care with other physicians, other qualified health care professionals, or agencies are provided consistent with the nature of the problem(s) and the patient's and/or family's needs. Usually, the presenting problem(s) are of high severity and pose an immediate significant threat to life or physiologic function.

⚒ 4.93 ⚖ 4.93 **FUD** XXX Q3 80 ⬜ PQ

AMA: 2015,Jan,12; 2015,Jan,16; 2014,Nov,14; 2014,Oct,8; 2014,Jan,11; 2013,Jun,3-5; 2013,Jan,9-10; 2012,Jan,15-42; 2011,Feb,6-7; 2011,Jan,11

99288 Physician or other qualified health care professional direction of emergency medical systems (EMS) emergency care, advanced life support

INCLUDES Management provided by an emergency/intensive care based physician or other qualified health care professional via voice contact to ambulance/rescue staff for services such as heart monitoring and drug administration

⚒ 0.00 ⚖ 0.00 **FUD** XXX Ⓑ

AMA: 2015,Jan,16; 2014,Oct,8; 2014,Jan,11; 2013,May,6-7; 2011,Feb,6-7

99291-99292 Critical Care Visits: Patients 72 Months of Age and Older

CMS: 100-4,11,40.1.3 Independent Attending Physician Services; 100-4,12,30.6.4 Services Furnished Incident to Physician's Service; 100-4,12,30.6.9 Swing Bed Visits; 100-4,12,40.3 Global Surgery Review; 100-4,4,160 Clinic and Emergency Visits Under OPPS; 100-4,4,160.1 Critical Care Services

INCLUDES 30 minutes or more of direct care provided by the physician or other qualified health care professional to a critically ill or injured patient, regardless of the location

All time spent exclusively with patient/family/caregivers on the nursing unit or elsewhere

Outpatient critical care provided to neonates and pediatric patients up through 71 months of age

Physician or other qualified health care professional presence during interfacility transfer for critically ill/injured patients over 24 months of age

Professional services for interpretation of:
Blood gases
Chest films (71010, 71015, 71020)
Measurement of cardiac output (93561-93562)
Other computer stored information (99090)
Pulse oximetry (94760-94762)

Professional services for:
Gastric intubation (43752-43753)
Transcutaneous pacing, temporary (92953)
Ventilation assistance and management, includes CPAP, CNP (94002-94004, 94660, 94662)
Venous access, arterial puncture (36000, 36410, 36415, 36591, 36600)

EXCLUDES *All services that are less than 30 minutes; report appropriate E&M code*

Critical care services provided via remote real-time interactive videoconferencing (0188T, 0189T)

Inpatient critical care services provided to child 2 through 5 years of age (99475-99476)

Inpatient critical care services provided to infants 29 days through 24 months of age (99471-99472)

Inpatient critical care services provided to neonates that are age 28 days or less (99468-99469)

Other procedures not listed as included performed by the physician or other qualified health care professional rendering critical care

Patients who are not critically ill but in the critical care department (report appropriate E&M code)

Physician or other qualified health care professional presence during interfacility transfer for critically ill/injured patients under 24 months of age (99466-99467)

Supervisory services of control physician during interfacility transfer for critically ill/injured patients under 24 months of age ([99485, 99486])

Do not report activities performed outside of the unit or off the floor

99291 Critical care, evaluation and management of the critically ill or critically injured patient; first 30-74 minutes

⚕ 6.33   ⚕ 7.77   **FUD** XXX   03 80 ▯ PQ

AMA: 2015,Jul,3; 2015,Feb,10; 2015,Jan,16; 2014,Oct,8; 2014,Oct,14; 2014,Aug,5; 2014,May,4; 2014,Jan,11; 2013,May,6-7; 2013,Feb,16-17; 2012,Oct,14; 2012,Sep,16; 2012,Jul,12-14; 2012,Jan,15-42; 2011,Aug,9-10; 2011,Sep,3-4; 2011,Feb,6-7; 2011,Jan,11

+   99292 each additional 30 minutes (List separately in addition to code for primary service)

Code first (99291)

⚕ 3.16   ⚕ 3.46   **FUD** ZZZ   N 80 ▯

AMA: 2015,Jul,3; 2015,Feb,10; 2015,Jan,16; 2014,Oct,8; 2014,Oct,14; 2014,Aug,5; 2014,May,4; 2014,Jan,11; 2013,May,6-7; 2013,Feb,16-17; 2012,Jan,15-42; 2011,Aug,9-10; 2011,Sep,3-4; 2011,Feb,6-7; 2011,Jan,11

99304-99310 Nursing Facility Visits

CMS: 100-4,11,40.1.3 Independent Attending Physician Services; 100-4,12,230 Primary Care Incentive Payment Program; 100-4,12,230.1 Definition of Primary Care Practitioners and Services; 100-4,12,230.2 Coordination with Other Payments; 100-4,12,230.3 Claims Processing and Payment; 100-4,12,30.6.10 Consultation Services; 100-4,12,30.6.13 Nursing Facility Visits; 100-4,12,30.6.15.1 Prolonged Services With Direct Face-to-Face Patient Contact; 100-4,12,30.6.4 Services Furnished Incident to Physician's Service; 100-4,12,30.6.9 Payment for Inpatient Hospital Visits - General

INCLUDES All E&M services provided by the admitting physician on the date of nursing facility admission in other locations (e.g., office, emergency department)

Initial care, subsequent care, discharge, and yearly assessments

Initial services include patient assessment and physician participation in developing a plan of care (99304-99306)

Services provided in a psychiatric residential treatment center

Services provided to new and established patients in a nursing facility (skilled, intermediate, and long-term care facilities)

Subsequent services include physician review of medical records, reassessment, and review of test results (99307-99310)

EXCLUDES *Care plan oversight services (99379-99380)*

Code also hospital discharge services on the same date of admission or readmission to the nursing home (99217, 99234-99236, 99238-99239)

99304 Initial nursing facility care, per day, for the evaluation and management of a patient, which requires these 3 key components: A detailed or comprehensive history; A detailed or comprehensive examination; and Medical decision making that is straightforward or of low complexity. Counseling and/or coordination of care with other physicians, other qualified health care professionals, or agencies are provided consistent with the nature of the problem(s) and the patient's and/or family's needs. Usually, the problem(s) requiring admission are of low severity. Typically, 25 minutes are spent at the bedside and on the patient's facility floor or unit.

⚕ 2.58   ⚕ 2.58   **FUD** XXX   B 80 PQ

AMA: 2015,Jan,16; 2014,Nov,14; 2014,Oct,8; 2014,Jan,11; 2013,Jun,3-5; 2013,Jan,9-10; 2012,Aug,3-5; 2012,Jul,12-14; 2012,Jan,3-5; 2011,Jun,3-7; 2011,Feb,6-7; 2011,Jan,3-5; 2010,Jul,3-5

99305 Initial nursing facility care, per day, for the evaluation and management of a patient, which requires these 3 key components: A comprehensive history; A comprehensive examination; and Medical decision making of moderate complexity. Counseling and/or coordination of care with other physicians, other qualified health care professionals, or agencies are provided consistent with the nature of the problem(s) and the patient's and/or family's needs. Usually, the problem(s) requiring admission are of moderate severity. Typically, 35 minutes are spent at the bedside and on the patient's facility floor or unit.

⚕ 3.68   ⚕ 3.68   **FUD** XXX   B 80 PQ

AMA: 2015,Jan,16; 2014,Nov,14; 2014,Oct,8; 2014,Jan,11; 2013,Jun,3-5; 2013,Jan,9-10; 2012,Aug,3-5; 2012,Jul,12-14; 2012,Jan,3-5; 2011,Jun,3-7; 2011,Feb,6-7; 2011,Jan,3-5; 2010,Jul,3-5

99306 Initial nursing facility care, per day, for the evaluation and management of a patient, which requires these 3 key components: A comprehensive history; A comprehensive examination; and Medical decision making of high complexity. Counseling and/or coordination of care with other physicians, other qualified health care professionals, or agencies are provided consistent with the nature of the problem(s) and the patient's and/or family's needs. Usually, the problem(s) requiring admission are of high severity. Typically, 45 minutes are spent at the bedside and on the patient's facility floor or unit.

⚕ 4.69   ⚕ 4.69   **FUD** XXX   B 80 PQ

AMA: 2015,Jan,16; 2014,Nov,14; 2014,Oct,8; 2014,Jan,11; 2013,Jun,3-5; 2013,Jan,9-10; 2012,Aug,3-5; 2012,Jul,12-14; 2012,Jan,3-5; 2011,Jun,3-7; 2011,Feb,6-7; 2011,Jan,3-5; 2010,Jul,3-5

26/TC PC/TC Comp Only	A2-Z3 ASC Pmt	50 Bilateral	♂ Male Only	♀ Female Only	⚕ Facility RVU	⚕ Non-Facility RVU
AMA: CPT Asst	**CMS:** Pub 100	A-Y OPPSI	80/80 Surg Assist Allowed / w/Doc		▣ Lab Crosswalk	▣ Radiology Crosswalk

458   Medicare (Red Text)   CPT © 2015 American Medical Association. All Rights Reserved. (Black Text)   © 2015 Optum360, LLC (Blue Text)

99307   Subsequent nursing facility care, per day, for the evaluation and management of a patient, which requires at least 2 of these 3 key components: A problem focused interval history; A problem focused examination; Straightforward medical decision making. Counseling and/or coordination of care with other physicians, other qualified health care professionals, or agencies are provided consistent with the nature of the problem(s) and the patient's and/or family's needs. Usually, the patient is stable, recovering, or improving. Typically, 10 minutes are spent at the bedside and on the patient's facility floor or unit.

🖐 1.25   ⚖ 1.25   **FUD** XXX   B 80 P0

AMA: 2015,Jan,16; 2014,Nov,14; 2014,Oct,8; 2014,Jan,11; 2013,Jun,3-5; 2013,Jan,9-10; 2012,Aug,3-5; 2012,Jul,12-14; 2012,Jan,3-5; 2012,Jan,15-42; 2011,Feb,6-7; 2011,Jan,3-5; 2011,Jan,11; 2010,Jul,3-5

99308   Subsequent nursing facility care, per day, for the evaluation and management of a patient, which requires at least 2 of these 3 key components: An expanded problem focused interval history; An expanded problem focused examination; Medical decision making of low complexity. Counseling and/or coordination of care with other physicians, other qualified health care professionals, or agencies are provided consistent with the nature of the problem(s) and the patient's and/or family's needs. Usually, the patient is responding inadequately to therapy or has developed a minor complication. Typically, 15 minutes are spent at the bedside and on the patient's facility floor or unit.

🖐 1.93   ⚖ 1.93   **FUD** XXX   B 80 P0

AMA: 2015,Jan,16; 2014,Nov,14; 2014,Oct,8; 2014,Jan,11; 2013,Jun,3-5; 2013,Jan,9-10; 2012,Aug,3-5; 2012,Jul,12-14; 2012,Jan,3-5; 2011,Feb,6-7; 2011,Jan,3-5; 2010,Jul,3-5

99309   Subsequent nursing facility care, per day, for the evaluation and management of a patient, which requires at least 2 of these 3 key components: A detailed interval history; A detailed examination; Medical decision making of moderate complexity. Counseling and/or coordination of care with other physicians, other qualified health care professionals, or agencies are provided consistent with the nature of the problem(s) and the patient's and/or family's needs. Usually, the patient has developed a significant complication or a significant new problem. Typically, 25 minutes are spent at the bedside and on the patient's facility floor or unit.

🖐 2.56   ⚖ 2.56   **FUD** XXX   B 80 P0

AMA: 2015,Jan,16; 2014,Nov,14; 2014,Oct,8; 2014,Jan,11; 2013,Jun,3-5; 2013,Jan,9-10; 2012,Aug,3-5; 2012,Jul,12-14; 2012,Jan,3-5; 2011,Feb,6-7; 2011,Jan,3-5; 2010,Jul,3-5

99310   Subsequent nursing facility care, per day, for the evaluation and management of a patient, which requires at least 2 of these 3 key components: A comprehensive interval history; A comprehensive examination; Medical decision making of high complexity. Counseling and/or coordination of care with other physicians, other qualified health care professionals, or agencies are provided consistent with the nature of the problem(s) and the patient's and/or family's needs. The patient may be unstable or may have developed a significant new problem requiring immediate physician attention. Typically, 35 minutes are spent at the bedside and on the patient's facility floor or unit.

🖐 3.81   ⚖ 3.81   **FUD** XXX   B 80 P0

AMA: 2015,Jan,16; 2014,Nov,14; 2014,Oct,8; 2014,Jan,11; 2013,Jun,3-5; 2013,Jan,9-10; 2012,Aug,3-5; 2012,Jul,12-14; 2012,Jan,3-5; 2012,Jan,15-42; 2011,Feb,6-7; 2011,Jan,3-5; 2011,Jan,11; 2010,Jul,3-5

99315-99316 Nursing Home Discharge

CMS: 100-4,11,40.1.3 Independent Attending Physician Services; 100-4,12,230 Primary Care Incentive Payment Program; 100-4,12,230.1 Definition of Primary Care Practitioners and Services; 100-4,12,230.2 Coordination with Other Payments; 100-4,12,230.3 Claims Processing and Payment; 100-4,12,30.6.13 Nursing Facility Visits; 100-4,12,30.6.4 Services Furnished Incident to Physician's Service; 100-4,12,40.3 Global Surgery Review

INCLUDES   Discharge services include all time spent by the physician or other qualified health care professional for:
Complete discharge records
Discharge instructions for patient and caregivers
Discussion regarding the stay in the facility
Final patient examination
Provide prescriptions and referrals as appropriate

99315   Nursing facility discharge day management; 30 minutes or less

🖐 2.05   ⚖ 2.05   **FUD** XXX   B 80 ▱ P0

AMA: 2015,Jan,16; 2014,Nov,14; 2014,Oct,8; 2014,Jan,11; 2013,Jun,3-5; 2013,Jan,9-10; 2012,Jul,12-14; 2012,Jan,3-5; 2012,Jan,15-42; 2011,Feb,6-7; 2011,Jan,3-5; 2011,Jan,11

99316   more than 30 minutes

🖐 2.96   ⚖ 2.96   **FUD** XXX   B 80 ▱ P0

AMA: 2015,Jan,16; 2014,Nov,14; 2014,Oct,8; 2014,Jan,11; 2013,Jun,3-5; 2013,Jan,9-10; 2012,Jul,12-14; 2012,Jan,3-5; 2012,Jan,15-42; 2011,Feb,6-7; 2011,Jan,3-5; 2011,Jan,11

99318 Annual Nursing Home Assessment

CMS: 100-4,12,230 Primary Care Incentive Payment Program; 100-4,12,230.1 Definition of Primary Care Practitioners and Services; 100-4,12,230.2 Coordination with Other Payments; 100-4,12,230.3 Claims Processing and Payment; 100-4,12,30.6.13 Nursing Facility Visits; 100-4,12,30.6.15.1 Prolonged Services With Direct Face-to-Face Patient Contact; 100-4,12,30.6.4 Services Furnished Incident to Physician's Service; 100-4,12,30.6.9 Hospital Visit and Critical Care on Same Day

Do not report on same date of service as (99304-99316)

99318   Evaluation and management of a patient involving an annual nursing facility assessment, which requires these 3 key components: A detailed interval history; A comprehensive examination; and Medical decision making that is of low to moderate complexity. Counseling and/or coordination of care with other physicians, other qualified health care professionals, or agencies are provided consistent with the nature of the problem(s) and the patient's and/or family's needs. Usually, the patient is stable, recovering, or improving. Typically, 30 minutes are spent at the bedside and on the patient's facility floor or unit.

🖐 2.70   ⚖ 2.70   **FUD** XXX   B 80 P0

AMA: 2015,Jan,16; 2014,Nov,14; 2014,Oct,8; 2014,Jan,11; 2013,Jun,3-5; 2013,Jan,9-10; 2012,Jan,3-5; 2011,Feb,6-7; 2011,Jan,3-5

99324-99337 Domiciliary Care, Rest Home, Assisted Living Visits

CMS: 100-4,11,40.1.3 Independent Attending Physician Services; 100-4,12,230 Primary Care Incentive Payment Program; 100-4,12,230.1 Definition of Primary Care Practitioners and Services; 100-4,12,230.2 Coordination with Other Payments; 100-4,12,230.3 Claims Processing and Payment; 100-4,12,30.6.14 Domiciliary Care, Rest Home, Assisted Living Visits; 100-4,12,30.6.15.1 Prolonged Services With Direct Face-to-Face Patient Contact; 100-4,12,30.6.4 Services Furnished Incident to Physician's Service

INCLUDES   E&M services for patients residing in assisted living, domiciliary care, and rest homes where medical care is not included
Services provided to new patients or established patients (99324-99328, 99334-99337)

EXCLUDES   Care plan oversight services provided to a patient in a rest home under the care of a home health agency (99374-99375)
Care plan oversight services provided to a patient under the care of a hospice agency (99377-99378)

Evaluation and Management

99324 Domiciliary or rest home visit for the evaluation and management of a new patient, which requires these 3 key components: A problem focused history; A problem focused examination; and Straightforward medical decision making. Counseling and/or coordination of care with other physicians, other qualified health care professionals, or agencies are provided consistent with the nature of the problem(s) and the patient's and/or family's needs. Usually, the presenting problem(s) are of low severity. Typically, 20 minutes are spent with the patient and/or family or caregiver.
   🚑 1.55   👐 1.55   **FUD** XXX   B 80 P0
   AMA: 2015,Jan,16; 2014,Nov,14; 2014,Oct,8; 2014,Oct,3; 2014,Jan,11; 2013,Jun,3-5; 2013,Jan,9-10; 2012,Aug,3-5; 2012,Apr,10; 2012,Jan,3-5; 2011,Feb,6-7; 2011,Jan,3-5

99325 Domiciliary or rest home visit for the evaluation and management of a new patient, which requires these 3 key components: An expanded problem focused history; An expanded problem focused examination; and Medical decision making of low complexity. Counseling and/or coordination of care with other physicians, other qualified health care professionals, or agencies are provided consistent with the nature of the problem(s) and the patient's and/or family's needs. Usually, the presenting problem(s) are of moderate severity. Typically, 30 minutes are spent with the patient and/or family or caregiver.
   🚑 2.26   👐 2.26   **FUD** XXX   B 80 P0
   AMA: 2015,Jan,16; 2014,Nov,14; 2014,Oct,8; 2014,Oct,3; 2014,Jan,11; 2013,Jun,3-5; 2013,Jan,9-10; 2012,Aug,3-5; 2012,Apr,10; 2012,Jan,3-5; 2011,Feb,6-7; 2011,Jan,3-5

99326 Domiciliary or rest home visit for the evaluation and management of a new patient, which requires these 3 key components: A detailed history; A detailed examination; and Medical decision making of moderate complexity. Counseling and/or coordination of care with other physicians, other qualified health care professionals, or agencies are provided consistent with the nature of the problem(s) and the patient's and/or family's needs. Usually, the presenting problem(s) are of moderate to high severity. Typically, 45 minutes are spent with the patient and/or family or caregiver.
   🚑 3.91   👐 3.91   **FUD** XXX   B 80 P0
   AMA: 2015,Jan,16; 2014,Nov,14; 2014,Oct,8; 2014,Oct,3; 2014,Jan,11; 2013,Jun,3-5; 2013,Jan,9-10; 2012,Aug,3-5; 2012,Apr,10; 2012,Jan,3-5; 2011,Feb,6-7; 2011,Jan,3-5

99327 Domiciliary or rest home visit for the evaluation and management of a new patient, which requires these 3 key components: A comprehensive history; A comprehensive examination; and Medical decision making of moderate complexity. Counseling and/or coordination of care with other physicians, other qualified health care professionals, or agencies are provided consistent with the nature of the problem(s) and the patient's and/or family's needs. Usually, the presenting problem(s) are of high severity. Typically, 60 minutes are spent with the patient and/or family or caregiver.
   🚑 5.22   👐 5.22   **FUD** XXX   B 80 P0
   AMA: 2015,Jan,16; 2014,Nov,14; 2014,Oct,8; 2014,Oct,3; 2014,Jan,11; 2013,Jun,3-5; 2013,Jan,9-10; 2012,Aug,3-5; 2012,Apr,10; 2012,Jan,3-5; 2011,Feb,6-7; 2011,Jan,3-5

99328 Domiciliary or rest home visit for the evaluation and management of a new patient, which requires these 3 key components: A comprehensive history; A comprehensive examination; and Medical decision making of high complexity. Counseling and/or coordination of care with other physicians, other qualified health care professionals, or agencies are provided consistent with the nature of the problem(s) and the patient's and/or family's needs. Usually, the patient is unstable or has developed a significant new problem requiring immediate physician attention. Typically, 75 minutes are spent with the patient and/or family or caregiver.
   🚑 6.11   👐 6.11   **FUD** XXX   B 80 P0
   AMA: 2015,Jan,16; 2014,Nov,14; 2014,Oct,8; 2014,Oct,3; 2014,Jan,11; 2013,Jun,3-5; 2013,Jan,9-10; 2012,Aug,3-5; 2012,Apr,10; 2012,Jan,3-5; 2011,Feb,6-7; 2011,Jan,3-5

99334 Domiciliary or rest home visit for the evaluation and management of an established patient, which requires at least 2 of these 3 key components: A problem focused interval history; A problem focused examination; Straightforward medical decision making. Counseling and/or coordination of care with other physicians, other qualified health care professionals, or agencies are provided consistent with the nature of the problem(s) and the patient's and/or family's needs. Usually, the presenting problem(s) are self-limited or minor. Typically, 15 minutes are spent with the patient and/or family or caregiver.
   🚑 1.69   👐 1.69   **FUD** XXX   B 80 P0
   AMA: 2015,Jan,16; 2014,Nov,14; 2014,Oct,8; 2014,Oct,3; 2014,Jan,11; 2013,Nov,3; 2013,Jun,3-5; 2013,Jan,9-10; 2012,Aug,3-5; 2012,Apr,10; 2012,Jan,3-5; 2011,Feb,6-7; 2011,Jan,3-5

99335 Domiciliary or rest home visit for the evaluation and management of an established patient, which requires at least 2 of these 3 key components: An expanded problem focused interval history; An expanded problem focused examination; Medical decision making of low complexity. Counseling and/or coordination of care with other physicians, other qualified health care professionals, or agencies are provided consistent with the nature of the problem(s) and the patient's and/or family's needs. Usually, the presenting problem(s) are of low to moderate severity. Typically, 25 minutes are spent with the patient and/or family or caregiver.
   🚑 2.67   👐 2.67   **FUD** XXX   B 80 P0
   AMA: 2015,Jan,16; 2014,Nov,14; 2014,Oct,8; 2014,Oct,3; 2014,Jan,11; 2013,Nov,3; 2013,Jun,3-5; 2013,Jan,9-10; 2012,Aug,3-5; 2012,Apr,10; 2012,Jan,3-5; 2011,Feb,6-7; 2011,Jan,3-5

99336 Domiciliary or rest home visit for the evaluation and management of an established patient, which requires at least 2 of these 3 key components: A detailed interval history; A detailed examination; Medical decision making of moderate complexity. Counseling and/or coordination of care with other physicians, other qualified health care professionals, or agencies are provided consistent with the nature of the problem(s) and the patient's and/or family's needs. Usually, the presenting problem(s) are of moderate to high severity. Typically, 40 minutes are spent with the patient and/or family or caregiver.
   🚑 3.78   👐 3.78   **FUD** XXX   B 80 P0
   AMA: 2015,Jan,16; 2014,Nov,14; 2014,Oct,8; 2014,Oct,3; 2014,Jan,11; 2013,Nov,3; 2013,Jun,3-5; 2013,Jan,9-10; 2012,Aug,3-5; 2012,Apr,10; 2012,Jan,3-5; 2011,Feb,6-7; 2011,Jan,3-5

99337 Domiciliary or rest home visit for the evaluation and management of an established patient, which requires at least 2 of these 3 key components: A comprehensive interval history; A comprehensive examination; Medical decision making of moderate to high complexity. Counseling and/or coordination of care with other physicians, other qualified health care professionals, or agencies are provided consistent with the nature of the problem(s) and the patient's and/or family's needs. Usually, the presenting problem(s) are of moderate to high severity. The patient may be unstable or may have developed a significant new problem requiring immediate physician attention. Typically, 60 minutes are spent with the patient and/or family or caregiver.

    5.41   5.41 **FUD** XXX   B 80 PQ

    AMA: 2015,Jan,16; 2014,Nov,14; 2014,Oct,8; 2014,Oct,3; 2014,Jan,11; 2013,Nov,3; 2013,Jun,3-5; 2013,Jan,9-10; 2012,Aug,3-5; 2012,Apr,10; 2012,Jan,3-5; 2011,Feb,6-7; 2011,Jan,3-5

99339-99340 Care Plan Oversight: Rest Home, Domiciliary Care, Assisted Living, and Home

CMS: 100-4,12,180 Payment of Care Plan Oversight (CPO); 100-4,12,180.1 Billing for Care Plan Oversight (CPO); 100-4,12,230 Primary Care Incentive Payment Program; 100-4,12,230.1 Definition of Primary Care Practitioners and Services; 100-4,12,230.2 Coordination with Other Payments; 100-4,12,230.3 Claims Processing and Payment; 100-4,12,30.6.14 Domiciliary Care, Rest Home, Assisted Living Visits; 100-4,12,30.6.4 Services Furnished Incident to Physician's Service

INCLUDES Care plan oversight for patients residing in assisted living, domiciliary care, private residences, and rest homes

EXCLUDES *Care plan oversight services furnished under a home health agency, nursing facility, or hospice (99374-99380)*

Do not report during the same period of time as (99441-99444, 99487, 99489, 99495-99496, 98966-98969)

99339 Individual physician supervision of a patient (patient not present) in home, domiciliary or rest home (eg, assisted living facility) requiring complex and multidisciplinary care modalities involving regular physician development and/or revision of care plans, review of subsequent reports of patient status, review of related laboratory and other studies, communication (including telephone calls) for purposes of assessment or care decisions with health care professional(s), family member(s), surrogate decision maker(s) (eg, legal guardian) and/or key caregiver(s) involved in patient's care, integration of new information into the medical treatment plan and/or adjustment of medical therapy, within a calendar month; 15-29 minutes

    2.20   2.20 **FUD** XXX   B

    AMA: 2015,Jan,16; 2014,Oct,8; 2014,Oct,3; 2014,Jan,11; 2013,Nov,3; 2013,Sep,15-16; 2013,Jun,3-5; 2013,Apr,3-4; 2012,Jan,3-5; 2012,Jan,15-42; 2011,Feb,6-7; 2011,Jan,11

99340 30 minutes or more

    3.07   3.07 **FUD** XXX   B PQ

    AMA: 2015,Jan,16; 2014,Oct,8; 2014,Oct,3; 2014,Jan,11; 2013,Nov,3; 2013,Sep,15-16; 2013,Jun,3-5; 2013,Apr,3-4; 2012,Jan,3-5; 2012,Jan,15-42; 2011,Feb,6-7; 2011,Jan,11

99341-99350 Home Visits

CMS: 100-4,11,40.1.3 Independent Attending Physician Services; 100-4,12,230 Primary Care Incentive Payment Program; 100-4,12,230.1 Definition of Primary Care Practitioners and Services; 100-4,12,230.2 Coordination with Other Payments; 100-4,12,230.3 Claims Processing and Payment; 100-4,12,30.6.14 Domiciliary Care, Rest Home, Assisted Living Visits; 100-4,12,30.6.14.1 Home Visits; 100-4,12,30.6.15.1 Prolonged Services With Direct Face-to-Face Patient Contact; 100-4,12,30.6.4 Services Furnished Incident to Physician's Service; 100-4,12,40.3 Global Surgery Review

INCLUDES Services for a new patient or an established patient (99341-99345, 99347-99350)

  Services provided to a patient in a private home

EXCLUDES *Services provided to patients under home health agency or hospice care (99374-99378)*

99341 Home visit for the evaluation and management of a new patient, which requires these 3 key components: A problem focused history; A problem focused examination; and Straightforward medical decision making. Counseling and/or coordination of care with other physicians, other qualified health care professionals, or agencies are provided consistent with the nature of the problem(s) and the patient's and/or family's needs. Usually, the presenting problem(s) are of low severity. Typically, 20 minutes are spent face-to-face with the patient and/or family.

    1.54   1.54 **FUD** XXX   B 80 PQ

    AMA: 2015,Jan,16; 2014,Nov,14; 2014,Oct,3; 2014,Jan,11; 2013,Jun,3-5; 2013,Jan,9-10; 2012,Aug,3-5; 2012,Apr,10; 2012,Jan,3-5; 2011,Feb,6-7; 2011,Jan,3-5

99342 Home visit for the evaluation and management of a new patient, which requires these 3 key components: An expanded problem focused history; An expanded problem focused examination; and Medical decision making of low complexity. Counseling and/or coordination of care with other physicians, other qualified health care professionals, or agencies are provided consistent with the nature of the problem(s) and the patient's and/or family's needs. Usually, the presenting problem(s) are of moderate severity. Typically, 30 minutes are spent face-to-face with the patient and/or family.

    2.24   2.24 **FUD** XXX   B 80 PQ

    AMA: 2015,Jan,16; 2014,Nov,14; 2014,Oct,3; 2014,Oct,8; 2014,Jan,11; 2013,Jun,3-5; 2013,Jan,9-10; 2012,Aug,3-5; 2012,Apr,10; 2012,Jan,3-5; 2011,Feb,6-7; 2011,Jan,3-5

99343 Home visit for the evaluation and management of a new patient, which requires these 3 key components: A detailed history; A detailed examination; and Medical decision making of moderate complexity. Counseling and/or coordination of care with other physicians, other qualified health care professionals, or agencies are provided consistent with the nature of the problem(s) and the patient's and/or family's needs. Usually, the presenting problem(s) are of moderate to high severity. Typically, 45 minutes are spent face-to-face with the patient and/or family.

    3.65   3.65 **FUD** XXX   B 80 PQ

    AMA: 2015,Jan,16; 2014,Nov,14; 2014,Oct,3; 2014,Oct,8; 2014,Jan,11; 2013,Jun,3-5; 2013,Jan,9-10; 2012,Aug,3-5; 2012,Apr,10; 2012,Jan,3-5; 2011,Feb,6-7; 2011,Jan,3-5

99344 Home visit for the evaluation and management of a new patient, which requires these 3 key components: A comprehensive history; A comprehensive examination; and Medical decision making of moderate complexity. Counseling and/or coordination of care with other physicians, other qualified health care professionals, or agencies are provided consistent with the nature of the problem(s) and the patient's and/or family's needs. Usually, the presenting problem(s) are of high severity. Typically, 60 minutes are spent face-to-face with the patient and/or family.

    5.12   5.12 **FUD** XXX   B 80 PQ

    AMA: 2015,Jan,16; 2014,Nov,14; 2014,Oct,3; 2014,Oct,8; 2014,Jan,11; 2013,Jun,3-5; 2013,Jan,9-10; 2012,Aug,3-5; 2012,Apr,10; 2012,Jan,3-5; 2011,Feb,6-7; 2011,Jan,3-5

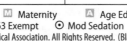

99345 Home visit for the evaluation and management of a new patient, which requires these 3 key components: A comprehensive history; A comprehensive examination; and Medical decision making of high complexity. Counseling and/or coordination of care with other physicians, other qualified health care professionals, or agencies are provided consistent with the nature of the problem(s) and the patient's and/or family's needs. Usually, the patient is unstable or has developed a significant new problem requiring immediate physician attention. Typically, 75 minutes are spent face-to-face with the patient and/or family.

    📊 6.20   ⚓ 6.20   **FUD** XXX   B 80 🖵 PQ

    AMA: 2015,Jan,16; 2014,Nov,14; 2014,Oct,3; 2014,Oct,8; 2014,Jan,11; 2013,Jun,3-5; 2013,Jan,9-10; 2012,Aug,3-5; 2012,Apr,10; 2012,Jan,3-5; 2011,Feb,6-7; 2011,Jan,3-5

99347 Home visit for the evaluation and management of an established patient, which requires at least 2 of these 3 key components: A problem focused interval history; A problem focused examination; Straightforward medical decision making. Counseling and/or coordination of care with other physicians, other qualified health care professionals, or agencies are provided consistent with the nature of the problem(s) and the patient's and/or family's needs. Usually, the presenting problem(s) are self limited or minor. Typically, 15 minutes are spent face-to-face with the patient and/or family.

    📊 1.56   ⚓ 1.56   **FUD** XXX   B 80 🖵 PQ

    AMA: 2015,Jan,16; 2014,Nov,14; 2014,Oct,8; 2014,Oct,3; 2014,Jan,11; 2013,Nov,3; 2013,Jun,3-5; 2013,Jan,9-10; 2012,Aug,3-5; 2012,Apr,10; 2012,Jan,3-5; 2011,Feb,6-7; 2011,Jan,3-5

99348 Home visit for the evaluation and management of an established patient, which requires at least 2 of these 3 key components: An expanded problem focused interval history; An expanded problem focused examination; Medical decision making of low complexity. Counseling and/or coordination of care with other physicians, other qualified health care professionals, or agencies are provided consistent with the nature of the problem(s) and the patient's and/or family's needs. Usually, the presenting problem(s) are of low to moderate severity. Typically, 25 minutes are spent face-to-face with the patient and/or family.

    📊 2.36   ⚓ 2.36   **FUD** XXX   B 80 🖵 PQ

    AMA: 2015,Jan,16; 2014,Nov,14; 2014,Oct,8; 2014,Oct,3; 2014,Jan,11; 2013,Nov,3; 2013,Jun,3-5; 2013,Jan,9-10; 2012,Aug,3-5; 2012,Apr,10; 2012,Jan,3-5; 2011,Feb,6-7; 2011,Jan,3-5

99349 Home visit for the evaluation and management of an established patient, which requires at least 2 of these 3 key components: A detailed interval history; A detailed examination; Medical decision making of moderate complexity. Counseling and/or coordination of care with other physicians, other qualified health care professionals, or agencies are provided consistent with the nature of the problem(s) and the patient's and/or family's needs. Usually, the presenting problem(s) are moderate to high severity. Typically, 40 minutes are spent face-to-face with the patient and/or family.

    📊 3.60   ⚓ 3.60   **FUD** XXX   B 80 🖵 PQ

    AMA: 2015,Jan,16; 2014,Nov,14; 2014,Oct,8; 2014,Oct,3; 2014,Jan,11; 2013,Nov,3; 2013,Jun,3-5; 2013,Jan,9-10; 2012,Aug,3-5; 2012,Apr,10; 2012,Jan,3-5; 2011,Feb,6-7; 2011,Jan,3-5

99350 Home visit for the evaluation and management of an established patient, which requires at least 2 of these 3 key components: A comprehensive interval history; A comprehensive examination; Medical decision making of moderate to high complexity. Counseling and/or coordination of care with other physicians, other qualified health care professionals, or agencies are provided consistent with the nature of the problem(s) and the patient's and/or family's needs. Usually, the presenting problem(s) are of moderate to high severity. The patient may be unstable or may have developed a significant new problem requiring immediate physician attention. Typically, 60 minutes are spent face-to-face with the patient and/or family.

    📊 4.98   ⚓ 4.98   **FUD** XXX   B 80 🖵 PQ

    AMA: 2015,Jan,16; 2014,Nov,14; 2014,Oct,8; 2014,Oct,3; 2014,Jan,11; 2013,Nov,3; 2013,Jun,3-5; 2013,Jan,9-10; 2012,Aug,3-5; 2012,Apr,10; 2012,Jan,3-5; 2011,Feb,6-7; 2011,Jan,3-5

99354-99357 Prolonged Services Direct Contact

CMS: 100-4,11,40.1.3 Independent Attending Physician Services; 100-4,12,30.6.15.1 Prolonged Services With Direct Face-to-Face Patient Contact; 100-4,12,30.6.4 Services Furnished Incident to Physician's Service

INCLUDES Personal contact with the patient by the physician or other qualified health professional

Services extending beyond the customary service provided in the inpatient or outpatient setting

Time spent providing additional indirect contact services on the floor or unit of the hospital or nursing facility during the same session as the direct contact

Time spent providing prolonged services on a date of service, even when the time is not continuous

EXCLUDES *Services provided independent of the date of personal contact with the patient (99358-99359)*

Code first E&M service code, as appropriate

Do not report any service of less than 30 minutes, or less than 15 minutes after the first hour or after the final 30 minutes

▲ + **99354** Prolonged evaluation and management or psychotherapy service(s) (beyond the typical service time of the primary procedure) in the office or other outpatient setting requiring direct patient contact beyond the usual service; first hour (List separately in addition to code for office or other outpatient Evaluation and Management or psychotherapy service)

    Code first (99201-99215, 99241-99245, 99324-99337, 99341-99350, 90837)

    Do not report more than one time per date of service

    Do not report with ([99415, 99416])

    📊 2.61   ⚓ 2.81   **FUD** ZZZ   N 80 🖵

    AMA: 2015,Jan,16; 2014,Oct,8; 2014,Jun,14; 2014,Apr,6; 2014,Jan,11; 2013,Oct,11; 2013,Jun,3-5; 2013,May,12; 2012,Aug,3-5; 2012,Apr,10

▲ + **99355** each additional 30 minutes (List separately in addition to code for prolonged service)

    Code first (99354)

    Do not report with ([99415, 99416])

    📊 2.52   ⚓ 2.73   **FUD** ZZZ   N 80 🖵

    AMA: 2015,Jan,16; 2014,Oct,8; 2014,Jun,14; 2014,Apr,6; 2014,Jan,11; 2013,Oct,11; 2013,Jun,3-5; 2013,May,12; 2012,Aug,3-5; 2012,Apr,10

+ **99356** Prolonged service in the inpatient or observation setting, requiring unit/floor time beyond the usual service; first hour (List separately in addition to code for inpatient Evaluation and Management service)

    Code first (99218-99223 [99224, 99225, 99226], 99231-99236, 99251-99255, 99304-99310, 90837)

    Do not report more than one time per date of service

    📊 2.59   ⚓ 2.59   **FUD** ZZZ   C 80 🖵 PQ

    AMA: 2015,Jan,16; 2014,Oct,8; 2014,Jun,14; 2014,Apr,6; 2014,Jan,11; 2013,Oct,11; 2013,Jun,3-5; 2013,May,12; 2012,Aug,3-5; 2012,Jul,10-11; 2011,Aug,11; 2011,Jun,3-7

| 26 TC PC/TC Comp Only | A2-Z9 ASC Pmt | 50 Bilateral | ♂ Male Only | ♀ Female Only | 📊 Facility RVU | ⚓ Non-Facility RVU |
| **AMA:** CPT Asst | **CMS:** Pub 100 | A-Y OPPSI | 80 / 80 Surg Assist Allowed / w/Doc | | 🖵 Lab Crosswalk | 🖥 Radiology Crosswalk |

462   Medicare (Red Text)   CPT © 2015 American Medical Association. All Rights Reserved. (Black Text)   © 2015 Optum360, LLC (Blue Text)

+ **99357**   **each additional 30 minutes (List separately in addition to code for prolonged service)**

Code first (99356)

📖 2.56   ⚕ 2.56   **FUD** ZZZ   [C] [80] [▯] [PQ]

AMA: 2015,Jan,16; 2014,Oct,8; 2014,Jun,14; 2014,Apr,6; 2014,Jan,11; 2013,Oct,11; 2013,Jun,3-5; 2013,May,12; 2012,Aug,3-5; 2012,Jul,10-11; 2011,Aug,11; 2011,Jun,3-7

99358-99359 Prolonged Services Indirect Contact

CMS: 100-4,11,40.1.3 Independent Attending Physician Services; 100-4,12,30.6.15.2 Prolonged Services Without Face to Face Service; 100-4,12,30.6.4 Services Furnished Incident to Physician's Service

INCLUDES   Services extending beyond the customary service
Time spent providing indirect contact services by the physician or other qualified health care professional in relation to patient management where face-to-face services have or will occur on a different date
Time spent providing prolonged services performed on a date of service (which may be other than the date of the primary service) that are not continuous

EXCLUDES   *Anticoagulation services (99363-99364)*
Any additional unit or floor time in the hospital or nursing facility during the same evaluation and management session
Care plan oversight (99339-99340, 99374-99380)
Online medical services (99444)
Other indirect services that have a more specific code and no upper time limit in the code
Time spent in medical team conference (99366-99368)

Code also E&M or other services provided
Do not report for services less than15 minutes after the first hour or beyond the final 30 minutes
Do not report in same month with (99487-99489)
Do not report during time-frame with (99495-99496)
Do not report services less than 30 minutes
Do not report with codes for other face-to-face services without an upper time limit

99358   **Prolonged evaluation and management service before and/or after direct patient care; first hour**

Do not report more than one time per date of service

📖 3.09   ⚕ 3.09   **FUD** XXX   [N]

AMA: 2015,Jan,16; 2014,Oct,3; 2014,Oct,8; 2014,Jan,11; 2013,Oct,11; 2013,Nov,3; 2013,Apr,3-4; 2012,Aug,3-5

+ **99359**   **each additional 30 minutes (List separately in addition to code for prolonged service)**

Code first (99358)

📖 1.48   ⚕ 1.48   **FUD** ZZZ   [N]

AMA: 2015,Jan,16; 2014,Oct,3; 2014,Oct,8; 2014,Jan,11; 2013,Oct,11; 2013,Nov,3; 2013,Apr,3-4; 2012,Aug,3-5

[99415, 99416] Prolonged Clinical Staff Services Under Supervision

INCLUDES   Time spent by clinical staff providing prolonged face-to-face services extending beyond the customary service under the supervision of a physician or other qualified health professional
Time spent by clinical staff providing prolonged services on a date of service, even when the time is not continuous

Code also E&M or other services provided
Do not report for more than two patients at the same time
Do not report services less than 45 minutes
Do not report with (99354-99357)

● + # **99415**   **Prolonged clinical staff service (the service beyond the typical service time) during an evaluation and management service in the office or outpatient setting, direct patient contact with physician supervision; first hour (List separately in addition to code for outpatient Evaluation and Management service)**

📖 0.00   ⚕ 0.00   **FUD** 000

Code first (99201-99215)
Do not report more than one time per date of service

● + # **99416**   **each additional 30 minutes (List separately in addition to code for prolonged service)**

📖 0.00   ⚕ 0.00   **FUD** 000

Code first ([99415])
Do not report services less than 15 minutes after the first hour or beyond the final 30 minutes

99360 Standby Services

CMS: 100-4,12,30.6.15.3 Standby Services; 100-4,12,30.6.4 Services Furnished Incident to Physician's Service

INCLUDES   Services requested by physician or qualified health care professional that involve no direct patient contact
Total standby time for the day

EXCLUDES   *On-call services mandated by the hospital (99026-99027)*

Code also as appropriate (99460, 99465)
Do not report less than 30 minutes of standby time
Do not report with (99464)

99360   **Standby service, requiring prolonged attendance, each 30 minutes (eg, operative standby, standby for frozen section, for cesarean/high risk delivery, for monitoring EEG)**

📖 1.73   ⚕ 1.73   **FUD** XXX   [B] [▯]

AMA: 2015,Jan,16; 2014,Oct,8; 2014,Apr,5; 2014,Jan,11; 2013,May,8-10; 2012,Jan,15-42; 2011,Feb,3; 2011,Jan,11

99363-99364 Supervision of Warfarin Therapy

CMS: 100-3,190.11 Home PT/INR Monitoring for Anticoagulation Management; 100-4,32,60.4.1 Anticoagulation Management: Covered Diagnosis Codes; 100-4,32,60.5.2 Anticoagulation Management: Carrier Diagnosis Codes

INCLUDES   Services provided on an outpatient basis only
Supervision of therapy with warfarin: ordering, dosage adjustments, analysis of International Normalized Ration (INR) tests, patient discussion

EXCLUDES   *Initial services provided/continued in the hospital or in observation: new period of subsequent therapy starts with discharge (99364)*
Services provided for less than 60 uninterrupted days
Services that fail to meet the required criteria (e.g., at least 8 INR tests/initial 90 days; 3 INR tests/each following 90 days
Warfarin therapy supervision accomplished online or via telephone contact (99441-99444, 98966-98969)

Do not report during the same time frame as (99495-99496)
Do not report in the same month with (99487-99489)
Do not report with (99217-99239 [99224, 99225, 99226], 99291-99292, 99304-99318, 99471-99476, 99477-99480)

99363   **Anticoagulant management for an outpatient taking warfarin, physician review and interpretation of International Normalized Ratio (INR) testing, patient instructions, dosage adjustment (as needed), and ordering of additional tests; initial 90 days of therapy (must include a minimum of 8 INR measurements)**

📖 2.39   ⚕ 3.60   **FUD** XXX   [B]

AMA: 2015,Jan,16; 2014,Oct,8; 2014,Oct,3; 2014,Jan,11; 2013,Nov,3; 2013,Apr,3-4

99364   **each subsequent 90 days of therapy (must include a minimum of 3 INR measurements)**

📖 0.91   ⚕ 1.22   **FUD** XXX   [B]

AMA: 2015,Jan,16; 2014,Oct,8; 2014,Oct,3; 2014,Jan,11; 2013,Nov,3; 2013,Apr,3-4

99366-99368 Interdisciplinary Conferences

CMS: 100-4,11,40.1.3 Independent Attending Physician Services; 100-4,12,30.6.16 Case Management Services (Codes 99362 and 99371 - 99373)

INCLUDES   Documentation of participation, contribution, and recommendations of the conference
Face-to-face participation by minimum of three qualified people from different specialties or disciplines
Only participants who have performed face-to-face evaluations or direct treatment to the patient within the previous 60 days
Start of the review of an individual patient and ends at conclusion of review

EXCLUDES   *Conferences of less than 30 minutes (not reportable)*
More than one individual from the same specialty at the same encounter
Time spent record keeping or writing a report

Do not report during the same time frame as (99495-99496)
Do not report in the same month with (99487-99489)

99366 Medical team conference with interdisciplinary team of health care professionals, face-to-face with patient and/or family, 30 minutes or more, participation by nonphysician qualified health care professional

> **INCLUDES** Team conferences of 30 minutes or more
> **EXCLUDES** *Team conferences by a physician with patient or family present, see appropriate evaluation and management service code*

📠 1.18　⚖ 1.21　**FUD** XXX　　　　　　N

AMA: 2015,Jan,16; 2014,Oct,8; 2014,Oct,3; 2014,Jun,3; 2014,Jan,11; 2013,Nov,3; 2013,Apr,3-4; 2012,Jan,15-42; 2011,Jan,11

99367 Medical team conference with interdisciplinary team of health care professionals, patient and/or family not present, 30 minutes or more; participation by physician

> **INCLUDES** Team conferences of 30 minutes or more

📠 1.59　⚖ 1.59　**FUD** XXX　　　　　　N

AMA: 2015,Jan,16; 2014,Oct,8; 2014,Jun,3; 2014,Jan,11; 2013,Nov,3; 2013,Apr,3-4

99368 participation by nonphysician qualified health care professional

> **INCLUDES** Team conferences of 30 minutes or more

📠 1.04　⚖ 1.04　**FUD** XXX　　　　　　N

AMA: 2015,Jan,16; 2014,Oct,8; 2014,Oct,3; 2014,Jun,3; 2014,Jan,11; 2013,Nov,3; 2013,Apr,3-4; 2012,Jan,15-42; 2011,Jan,11

99374-99380 Care Plan Oversight: Patient Under Care of HHA, Hospice, or Nursing Facility

CMS: 100-4,11,40.1.3 Independent Attending Physician Services; 100-4,12,180 Payment of Care Plan Oversight (CPO); 100-4,12,180.1 Billing for Care Plan Oversight (CPO); 100-4,12,30.6.4 Services Furnished Incident to Physician's Service

> **INCLUDES** Analysis of reports, diagnostic tests, treatment plans
> Discussions with other health care providers, outside of the practice, involved in the patient's care
> Establishment of and revisions to care plans within a 30-day period
> Payment to one physician per month for covered care plan oversight services (must be the same one who signed the plan of care)
> **EXCLUDES** *Care plan oversight services provided in a hospice agency (99377-99378)*
> *Care plan oversight services provided in assisted living, domiciliary care, or private residence, not under care of a home health agency or hospice (99339-99340)*
> *Routine postoperative care provided during a global surgery period*
> *Time discussing treatment with patient and/or caregivers*

Code also office/outpatient visits, hospital, home, nursing facility, domiciliary, or non-face-to-face services
Do not report during the same time frame as (99495-99496)
Do not report in same month with (99487-99489)
Do not report with (99441-99444, 98966-98969)

99374 Supervision of a patient under care of home health agency (patient not present) in home, domiciliary or equivalent environment (eg, Alzheimer's facility) requiring complex and multidisciplinary care modalities involving regular development and/or revision of care plans by that individual, review of subsequent reports of patient status, review of related laboratory and other studies, communication (including telephone calls) for purposes of assessment or care decisions with health care professional(s), family member(s), surrogate decision maker(s) (eg, legal guardian) and/or key caregiver(s) involved in patient's care, integration of new information into the medical treatment plan and/or adjustment of medical therapy, within a calendar month; 15-29 minutes

📠 1.59　⚖ 1.97　**FUD** XXX　　　　　　B

AMA: 2015,Jan,16; 2014,Oct,8; 2014,Oct,3; 2014,Jan,11; 2013,Nov,3; 2013,Sep,15-16; 2013,Jul,11-12; 2013,Apr,3-4

99375 30 minutes or more

📠 2.51　⚖ 2.97　**FUD** XXX　　　　　　E

AMA: 2015,Jan,16; 2014,Oct,8; 2014,Oct,3; 2014,Jan,11; 2013,Nov,3; 2013,Sep,15-16; 2013,Jul,11-12; 2013,Apr,3-4

99377 Supervision of a hospice patient (patient not present) requiring complex and multidisciplinary care modalities involving regular development and/or revision of care plans by that individual, review of subsequent reports of patient status, review of related laboratory and other studies, communication (including telephone calls) for purposes of assessment or care decisions with health care professional(s), family member(s), surrogate decision maker(s) (eg, legal guardian) and/or key caregiver(s) involved in patient's care, integration of new information into the medical treatment plan and/or adjustment of medical therapy, within a calendar month; 15-29 minutes

📠 1.59　⚖ 1.97　**FUD** XXX　　　　　　B

AMA: 2015,Jan,16; 2014,Oct,8; 2014,Oct,3; 2014,Jan,11; 2013,Nov,3; 2013,Sep,15-16; 2013,Jul,11-12; 2013,Apr,3-4

99378 30 minutes or more

📠 2.51　⚖ 2.97　**FUD** XXX　　　　　　E

AMA: 2015,Jan,16; 2014,Oct,8; 2014,Oct,3; 2014,Jan,11; 2013,Nov,3; 2013,Sep,15-16; 2013,Jul,11-12; 2013,Apr,3-4

99379 Supervision of a nursing facility patient (patient not present) requiring complex and multidisciplinary care modalities involving regular development and/or revision of care plans by that individual, review of subsequent reports of patient status, review of related laboratory and other studies, communication (including telephone calls) for purposes of assessment or care decisions with health care professional(s), family member(s), surrogate decision maker(s) (eg, legal guardian) and/or key caregiver(s) involved in patient's care, integration of new information into the medical treatment plan and/or adjustment of medical therapy, within a calendar month; 15-29 minutes

📠 1.59　⚖ 1.97　**FUD** XXX　　　　　　B

AMA: 2015,Jan,16; 2014,Oct,8; 2014,Oct,3; 2014,Jan,11; 2013,Nov,3; 2013,Sep,15-16; 2013,Jul,11-12; 2013,Apr,3-4

99380 30 minutes or more

📠 2.51　⚖ 2.97　**FUD** XXX　　　　　　B

AMA: 2015,Jan,16; 2014,Oct,8; 2014,Oct,3; 2014,Jan,11; 2013,Nov,3; 2013,Sep,15-16; 2013,Jul,11-12; 2013,Apr,3-4

99381-99397 Preventive Medicine Visits

CMS: 100-4,11,40.1.3 Independent Attending Physician Services; 100-4,12,30.6.2 Medically Necessary and Preventive Medicine Service on Same Date; 100-4,12,30.6.4 Services Furnished Incident to Physician's Service

> **INCLUDES** Care of a small problem or preexisting condition that requires no extra work
> New patients or established patients (99381-99387, 99391-99397)
> Regular preventive care (e.g., well-child exams) for all age groups
> **EXCLUDES** *Behavioral change interventions (99406-99409)*
> *Counseling/risk factor reduction interventions not provided with a preventive medical examination (99401-99412)*
> *Diagnostic tests and other procedures*

Code also immunization administration and product (90460-90461, 90471-90474, 90476-90749 [90620, 90621, 90625, 90630, 90644, 90672, 90673])
Code also significant, separately identifiable E&M service on the same date for substantial problems requiring additional work using modifier 25 and (99201-99215)

99381 Initial comprehensive preventive medicine evaluation and management of an individual including an age and gender appropriate history, examination, counseling/anticipatory guidance/risk factor reduction interventions, and the ordering of laboratory/diagnostic procedures, new patient; infant (age younger than 1 year)　　A

📠 2.17　⚖ 3.12　**FUD** XXX　　　　　　E

AMA: 2015,Jan,16; 2014,Oct,8; 2014,Jan,11; 2013,Jan,9-10; 2012,Jan,15-42; 2011,Jan,11

99382 early childhood (age 1 through 4 years)　　A

📠 2.32　⚖ 3.26　**FUD** XXX　　　　　　E

AMA: 2015,Jan,16; 2014,Oct,8; 2014,Jan,11; 2013,Jan,9-10

99383 late childhood (age 5 through 11 years)　　A

📠 2.46　⚖ 3.39　**FUD** XXX　　　　　　E

AMA: 2015,Jan,16; 2014,Oct,8; 2014,Jan,11; 2013,Jan,9-10

99384 **adolescent (age 12 through 17 years)** [A]
🔲 2.91 🔲 3.84 **FUD** XXX [E]
AMA: 2015,Jan,16; 2015,Jan,12; 2014,Oct,8; 2014,Jan,11; 2013,Jan,9-10

99385 **18-39 years** [A]
🔲 2.79 🔲 3.73 **FUD** XXX [E]
AMA: 2015,Jan,16; 2015,Jan,12; 2014,Oct,8; 2014,Jan,11; 2013,Jan,9-10

99386 **40-64 years** [A]
🔲 3.38 🔲 4.31 **FUD** XXX [E]
AMA: 2015,Jan,16; 2015,Jan,12; 2014,Oct,8; 2014,Jan,11; 2013,Jan,9-10

99387 **65 years and older** [A]
🔲 3.63 🔲 4.67 **FUD** XXX [E]
AMA: 2015,Jan,16; 2014,Oct,8; 2014,Jan,11; 2013,Jan,9-10

99391 **Periodic comprehensive preventive medicine reevaluation and management of an individual including an age and gender appropriate history, examination, counseling/anticipatory guidance/risk factor reduction interventions, and the ordering of laboratory/diagnostic procedures, established patient; infant (age younger than 1 year)** [A]
🔲 1.98 🔲 2.80 **FUD** XXX [E]
AMA: 2015,Jan,16; 2014,Oct,8; 2014,Jan,11; 2013,Jan,9-10

99392 **early childhood (age 1 through 4 years)** [A]
🔲 2.17 🔲 2.99 **FUD** XXX [E]
AMA: 2015,Jan,16; 2014,Oct,8; 2014,Jan,11; 2013,Jan,9-10

99393 **late childhood (age 5 through 11 years)** [A]
🔲 2.17 🔲 2.98 **FUD** XXX [E]
AMA: 2015,Jan,16; 2014,Oct,8; 2014,Jan,11; 2013,Jan,9-10

99394 **adolescent (age 12 through 17 years)** [A]
🔲 2.46 🔲 3.27 **FUD** XXX [E]
AMA: 2015,Jan,16; 2015,Jan,12; 2014,Oct,8; 2014,Jan,11; 2013,Jan,9-10

99395 **18-39 years** [A]
🔲 2.54 🔲 3.35 **FUD** XXX [E]
AMA: 2015,Jan,16; 2015,Jan,12; 2014,Oct,8; 2014,Jan,11; 2013,Jan,9-10

99396 **40-64 years** [A]
🔲 2.77 🔲 3.58 **FUD** XXX [E]
AMA: 2015,Jan,16; 2015,Jan,12; 2014,Oct,8; 2014,Jan,11; 2013,Jan,9-10; 2012,Mar,4-7

99397 **65 years and older** [A]
🔲 2.91 🔲 3.85 **FUD** XXX [E]
AMA: 2015,Jan,16; 2014,Oct,8; 2014,Jan,11; 2013,Jan,9-10; 2012,Jan,15-42; 2011,Jan,11

99401-99416 Counseling Services: Risk Factor and Behavioral Change Modification

[INCLUDES] Face-to-face services for new and established patients based on time increments of 15 to 60 minutes
Issues such as a healthy diet, exercise, alcohol and drug abuse
Services provided by a physician or other qualified healthcare professional for the purpose of promoting health and reducing illness and injury

← [EXCLUDES] *Counseling and risk factor reduction interventions included in preventive medicine services (99381-99397)*
Counseling services provided to patient groups with existing symptoms or illness (99078)
Code also significant, separately identifiable E&M services when performed and append modifier 25 to that service
Do not report with heath and behavioral services provided on the same day (96150-96155)

99401 **Preventive medicine counseling and/or risk factor reduction intervention(s) provided to an individual (separate procedure); approximately 15 minutes**
🔲 0.69 🔲 1.02 **FUD** XXX [E]
AMA: 2015,Jan,16; 2014,Oct,8; 2014,Aug,5; 2014,Jan,11; 2013,Jan,9-10; 2010,Dec,3-6

99402 **approximately 30 minutes**
🔲 1.41 🔲 1.74 **FUD** XXX [E]
AMA: 2015,Jan,16; 2014,Oct,8; 2014,Aug,5; 2014,Jan,11; 2013,Jan,9-10; 2010,Dec,3-6

99403 **approximately 45 minutes**
🔲 2.12 🔲 2.44 **FUD** XXX [E]
AMA: 2015,Jan,16; 2014,Oct,8; 2014,Aug,5; 2014,Jan,11; 2013,Jan,9-10; 2010,Dec,3-6

99404 **approximately 60 minutes**
🔲 2.84 🔲 3.16 **FUD** XXX [E]
AMA: 2015,Jan,16; 2014,Oct,8; 2014,Aug,5; 2014,Jan,11; 2013,Jan,9-10; 2010,Dec,3-6

99406 **Smoking and tobacco use cessation counseling visit; intermediate, greater than 3 minutes up to 10 minutes**
🔲 0.35 🔲 0.40 **FUD** XXX [S] [80]
AMA: 2015,Jan,16; 2014,Oct,8; 2014,Jan,11; 2013,Jan,9-10; 2012,Jan,15-42; 2011,Jan,11; 2010,Dec,3-6

99407 **intensive, greater than 10 minutes**
Do not report with (99406)
🔲 0.72 🔲 0.77 **FUD** XXX [S] [80]
AMA: 2015,Jan,16; 2014,Oct,8; 2014,Jan,11; 2013,Jan,9-10; 2012,Jan,15-42; 2011,Jan,11; 2010,Dec,3-6

99408 **Alcohol and/or substance (other than tobacco) abuse structured screening (eg, AUDIT, DAST), and brief intervention (SBI) services; 15 to 30 minutes**
[INCLUDES] Only initial screening and brief intervention Services of 15 minutes or more
Do not report with (99420)
🔲 0.94 🔲 0.99 **FUD** XXX [E]
AMA: 2015,Jan,16; 2014,Oct,8; 2014,Jan,11; 2013,Jan,9-10; 2010,Dec,3-6

99409 **greater than 30 minutes**
[INCLUDES] Only initial screening and brief intervention
Do not report with (99408, 99420)
🔲 1.89 🔲 1.94 **FUD** XXX [E]
AMA: 2015,Jan,16; 2014,Oct,8; 2014,Jan,11; 2013,Jan,9-10; 2010,Dec,3-6

99411 **Preventive medicine counseling and/or risk factor reduction intervention(s) provided to individuals in a group setting (separate procedure); approximately 30 minutes**
🔲 0.22 🔲 0.46 **FUD** XXX [E]
AMA: 2015,Jan,16; 2014,Oct,8; 2014,Jan,11; 2013,Jan,9-10; 2010,Dec,3-6

99412 **approximately 60 minutes**
🔲 0.37 🔲 0.61 **FUD** XXX [E]
AMA: 2015,Jan,16; 2014,Oct,8; 2014,Jan,11; 2013,Jan,9-10; 2010,Dec,3-6

99415 **Resequenced code. See code following 99359.**

99416 **Resequenced code. See code following 99359.**

99420-99429 Health Risk Assessment

CMS: 100-4,11,40.1.3 Independent Attending Physician Services

99420 **Administration and interpretation of health risk assessment instrument (eg, health hazard appraisal)**
🔲 0.31 🔲 0.31 **FUD** XXX [E]
AMA: 2015,Jan,16; 2014,Oct,8; 2014,Jan,11; 2013,Jan,9-10; 2010,Dec,3-6

99429 **Unlisted preventive medicine service**
🔲 0.00 🔲 0.00 **FUD** XXX [E]
AMA: 2015,Jan,16; 2014,Oct,8; 2014,Jan,11; 2013,Jan,9-10; 2010,Dec,3-6

99441-99443 Telephone Calls for Patient Management

CMS: 100-4,11,40.1.3 Independent Attending Physician Services

INCLUDES Episodes of care initiated by an established patient or the patient or guardian of an established patient

Non-face-to-face E&M services provided by a physician or other health care provider qualified to report E&M services

EXCLUDES *Services provided by a qualified nonphysician health care professional unable to report E&M codes (98966-98968)*

Do not report during the same time frame as (99495-99496)

Do not report in same month with (99487-99489)

Do not report with anticoagulation management reported with codes (99363-99364)

Do not report with a related E&M visit within the next 24 hours or as the next available urgent visit

Do not report with a related E&M service performed and reported within the previous seven days or within the postoperative period of a completed procedure

Do not report with the same call reported with codes (99339-99340, 99374-99380)

99441 Telephone evaluation and management service by a physician or other qualified health care professional who may report evaluation and management services provided to an established patient, parent, or guardian not originating from a related E/M service provided within the previous 7 days nor leading to an E/M service or procedure within the next 24 hours or soonest available appointment; 5-10 minutes of medical discussion

 0.37 0.40 **FUD** XXX E

AMA: 2015,Jan,16; 2014,Oct,8; 2014,Oct,3; 2014,Jan,11; 2013,Oct,11; 2013,Nov,3; 2013,Apr,3-4

99442 11-20 minutes of medical discussion

 0.72 0.76 **FUD** XXX E

AMA: 2015,Jan,16; 2014,Oct,8; 2014,Oct,3; 2014,Jan,11; 2013,Oct,11; 2013,Nov,3; 2013,Apr,3-4

99443 21-30 minutes of medical discussion

 1.09 1.13 **FUD** XXX E

AMA: 2015,Jan,16; 2014,Oct,8; 2014,Oct,3; 2014,Jan,11; 2013,Oct,11; 2013,Nov,3; 2013,Apr,3-4

99444 Online Patient Management Services

CMS: 100-4,11,40.1.3 Independent Attending Physician Services

INCLUDES All related communications such as related phone calls, prescription and lab orders

Permanent electronic or hardcopy storage

Physician evaluation and management services provided via the internet in response to a patient's on-line inquiry

The physician's personal timely response

EXCLUDES *Online medical evaluation by a qualified nonphysician health care professional (98969)*

Do not report during the same time frame as (99495-99496)

Do not report in same month with (99487-99489)

Do not report more than once per seven-day period for the same episode of care

Do not report when related to an E&M service performed and reported within the previous seven days or within the postoperative period of a completed procedure

Do not report with anticoagulation management reported with codes (99363-99364)

Do not report with (99339-99340, 99374-99380)

99444 Online evaluation and management service provided by a physician or other qualified health care professional who may report evaluation and management services provided to an established patient or guardian, not originating from a related E/M service provided within the previous 7 days, using the Internet or similar electronic communications network

 0.00 0.00 **FUD** XXX E

AMA: 2015,Jan,16; 2014,Oct,8; 2014,Oct,3; 2014,Jan,11; 2013,Oct,11; 2013,Nov,3; 2013,Apr,3-4; 2012,Nov,13-14

99446-99449 Online and Telephone Consultative Services

CMS: 100-4,11,40.1.3 Independent Attending Physician Services

INCLUDES Multiple telephone and/or internet contact needed to complete the consultation (e.g., test result(s) follow-up)

New or established patient with new problem or exacerbation of existing problem and not seen within the last 14 days

Review of pertinent lab, imaging and/or pathology studies, medical records, medications reported only once within a 7 day period

EXCLUDES *Communication with family with or without the patient present (99441-99444, 98966-98969)*

Online services

Physician to patient (99444)

Qualified health care professional to patient (98969)

Requesting physician's time 30 minutes over the typical E&M service and patient is not on-site (99358-99359)

Requesting physician's time 30 minutes over the typical E&M service and patient is on-site (99354-99357)

Telephone services

Physician to patient (99441-99443)

Qualified health care professional to patient (98966-98968)

Do not report if consultation is for transfer of care only

Do not report if consultation is less than 5 minutes

99446 Interprofessional telephone/Internet assessment and management service provided by a consultative physician including a verbal and written report to the patient's treating/requesting physician or other qualified health care professional; 5-10 minutes of medical consultative discussion and review

 0.00 0.00 **FUD** XXX E

AMA: 2015,Jan,16; 2014,Oct,8; 2014,Jun,14; 2013,Oct,11

99447 11-20 minutes of medical consultative discussion and review

 0.00 0.00 **FUD** XXX E

AMA: 2015,Jan,16; 2014,Oct,8; 2014,Jun,14; 2013,Oct,11

99448 21-30 minutes of medical consultative discussion and review

 0.00 0.00 **FUD** XXX E

AMA: 2015,Jan,16; 2014,Oct,8; 2014,Jun,14; 2013,Oct,11

99449 31 minutes or more of medical consultative discussion and review

 0.00 0.00 **FUD** XXX E

AMA: 2015,Jan,16; 2014,Oct,8; 2014,Jun,14; 2013,Oct,11

99450-99456 Life/Disability Insurance Eligibility Visits

CMS: 100-4,12,30.6.4 Services Furnished Incident to Physician's Service

INCLUDES Assessment services for insurance eligibility and work-related disability without medical management of the patient's illness/injury

Services provided to new/established patients at any site of service

EXCLUDES *Any additional E&M services or procedures performed on the same date of service: report with appropriate code*

99450 Basic life and/or disability examination that includes: Measurement of height, weight, and blood pressure; Completion of a medical history following a life insurance pro forma; Collection of blood sample and/or urinalysis complying with "chain of custody" protocols; and Completion of necessary documentation/certificates.

 0.00 0.00 **FUD** XXX E

AMA: 2015,Jan,16; 2014,Oct,8; 2014,Jan,11

99455 Work related or medical disability examination by the treating physician that includes: Completion of a medical history commensurate with the patient's condition; Performance of an examination commensurate with the patient's condition; Formulation of a diagnosis, assessment of capabilities and stability, and calculation of impairment; Development of future medical treatment plan; and Completion of necessary documentation/certificates and report.

Do not report with (99080)

 0.00 0.00 **FUD** XXX B 80 P0

AMA: 2015,Jan,16; 2014,Oct,8; 2014,Jan,11; 2013,Aug,13

| 26/TC PC/TC Comp Only | A2-Z3 ASC Pmt | 50 Bilateral | ♂ Male Only | ♀ Female Only | Facility RVU | Non-Facility RVU |
| AMA: CPT Asst | CMS: Pub 100 | A-Y OPPSI | 80/80 Surg Assist Allowed / w/Doc | Lab Crosswalk | Radiology Crosswalk |

466 Medicare (Red Text) CPT © 2015 American Medical Association. All Rights Reserved. (Black Text) © 2015 Optum360, LLC (Blue Text)

99456 Work related or medical disability examination by other than the treating physician that includes: Completion of a medical history commensurate with the patient's condition; Performance of an examination commensurate with the patient's condition; Formulation of a diagnosis, assessment of capabilities and stability, and calculation of impairment; Development of future medical treatment plan; and Completion of necessary documentation/certificates and report.

Do not report with (99080)

    0.00   0.00   **FUD** XXX   B 80 PQ

AMA: 2015,Jan,16; 2014,Oct,8; 2014,Jan,11; 2013,Aug,13

99460-99463 Evaluation and Management Services for Age 28 Days or Less

CMS: 100-4,12,30.6.4 Services Furnished Incident to Physician's Service

INCLUDES Family consultation
Healthy newborn history and physical
Medical record documentation
Ordering of diagnostic test and treatments
Services provided to healthy newborns age 28 days or less

EXCLUDES *Neonatal intensive and critical care services (99466-99469 [99485, 99486], 99477-99480)*
Newborn follow up services in an office or outpatient setting (99201-99215, 99381, 99391)
Newborn hospital discharge services if provided on a date subsequent to the admission date (99238-99239)
Nonroutine neonatal inpatient evaluation and management services (99221-99233)

Code also circumcision (54150)
Code also attendance at delivery (99464)
Code also emergency resuscitation services (99465)

99460 Initial hospital or birthing center care, per day, for evaluation and management of normal newborn infant A

    2.80   2.80   **FUD** XXX   V 80

AMA: 2015,Jan,16; 2014,Oct,8; 2014,Jan,11

99461 Initial care, per day, for evaluation and management of normal newborn infant seen in other than hospital or birthing center A

    1.77   2.53   **FUD** XXX   M 80

AMA: 2015,Jan,16; 2014,Oct,8; 2014,Jan,11

99462 Subsequent hospital care, per day, for evaluation and management of normal newborn A

    1.17   1.17   **FUD** XXX   C 80

AMA: 2015,Jan,16; 2014,Oct,8; 2014,Jan,11

99463 Initial hospital or birthing center care, per day, for evaluation and management of normal newborn infant admitted and discharged on the same date A

    3.38   3.38   **FUD** XXX   V 80

AMA: 2015,Jan,16; 2014,Oct,8; 2014,Jan,11

99464-99465 Newborn Delivery Attendance/Resuscitation

CMS: 100-4,12,30.6.4 Services Furnished Incident to Physician's Service

99464 Attendance at delivery (when requested by the delivering physician or other qualified health care professional) and initial stabilization of newborn A

Do not report with (99465)

    2.10   2.10   **FUD** XXX   N 80

AMA: 2015,Jan,16; 2014,Oct,8; 2014,Jan,11

99465 Delivery/birthing room resuscitation, provision of positive pressure ventilation and/or chest compressions in the presence of acute inadequate ventilation and/or cardiac output A

Code also any necessary procedures performed as part of the resuscitation
Do not report with (99464)

    4.25   4.25   **FUD** XXX   S 80

AMA: 2015,Jan,16; 2014,Oct,8; 2014,Jan,11

99466-99467 Critical Care Transport Age 24 Months or Younger

CMS: 100-4,12,30.6.4 Services Furnished Incident to Physician's Service

INCLUDES Face-to-face care starting when the physician assumes responsibility of the patient at the referring facility until the receiving facility accepts the patient
Physician presence during interfacility transfer of critically ill/injured patient 24 months of age or less
Services provided by the physician during transport:
  Blood gases
  Chest x-rays (71010, 71015, 71020)
  Data stored in computers (e.g., ECGs, blood pressures, hematologic data) (99090)
  Gastric intubation (43752-43753)
  Interpretation of cardiac output measurements (93562)
  Pulse oximetry (94760-94762)
  Routine monitoring:
    Heart rate
    Respiratory rate
  Temporary transcutaneous pacing (92953)
  Vascular access procedures (36000, 36400, 36405-36406, 36415, 36591, 36600)
  Ventilatory management (94002-94003, 94660, 94662)

EXCLUDES *Neonatal hypothermia (99184)*
Patient critical care transport services with personal contact with patient of less than 30 minutes
Physician directed emergency care via two-way voice communication with transporting staff (99288, [99485, 99486])
Services of the physician directing transport (control physician) ([99485, 99486])

Code also any services not designated as included in the critical care transport service
Do not report for services less than 30 minutes in duration (see E&M codes)
Do not report with non-face-to-face transport when performed by the same physician ([99485, 99486])

99466 Critical care face-to-face services, during an interfacility transport of critically ill or critically injured pediatric patient, 24 months of age or younger; first 30-74 minutes of hands-on care during transport A

    6.95   6.95   **FUD** XXX   N 80

AMA: 2015,Jan,16; 2014,Oct,8; 2014,Jan,11; 2013,May,6-7; 2011,Sep,3-4

+ **99467** each additional 30 minutes (List separately in addition to code for primary service) A

Code first (99466)

    3.49   3.49   **FUD** ZZZ   N 80

AMA: 2015,Jan,16; 2014,Oct,8; 2014,Jan,11; 2013,May,6-7; 2011,Sep,3-4

[99485, 99486] Critical Care Transport Supervision Age 24 Months or Younger

INCLUDES Advice for treatment to the transport team from the control physician
Non face-to-face care starts with first contact by the control physician with the transport team and ends when patient responsibility is assumed by the receiving facility

EXCLUDES *Emergency systems physician direction for pediatric patient older than 24 months (99288)*
Services provided by transport team

Do not report any other services performed by the control physician for the same time period
Do not report if done by same physician (99466-99467)
Do not report services less than 15 minutes

\# **99485** Supervision by a control physician of interfacility transport care of the critically ill or critically injured pediatric patient, 24 months of age or younger, includes two-way communication with transport team before transport, at the referring facility and during the transport, including data interpretation and report; first 30 minutes A

    2.17   2.17   **FUD** XXX   B

AMA: 2015,Jan,16; 2014,Oct,8; 2013,May,6-7

+ \# **99486** each additional 30 minutes (List separately in addition to code for primary procedure) A

Code first ([99485])

    1.89   1.89   **FUD** XXX   B

AMA: 2015,Jan,16; 2014,Oct,8; 2013,May,6-7

99468-99476 Critical Care Age 5 Years or Younger

CMS: 100-4,12,30.6.4 Services Furnished Incident to Physician's Service

INCLUDES   All services included in codes 99291-99292 as well as the following which may be reported by facilities only:
Administration of blood/blood components (36430, 36440)
Administration of intravenous fluids (96360-96361)
Administration of surfactant (94610)
Bladder aspiration, suprapubic (51100)
Bladder catheterization (51701, 51702)
Car seat evaluation (94780-94781)
Catheterization umbilical artery (36660)
Catheterization umbilical vein (36510)
Central venous catheter, centrally inserted (36555)
Endotracheal intubation (31500)
Lumbar puncture (62270)
Oral or nasogastric tube placement (43752)
Pulmonary function testing, performed at the bedside (94375)
Pulse or ear oximetry (94760-94762)
Vascular access, arteries (36140, 36620)
Vascular access, venous (36400-36406, 36420, 36600)
Ventilatory management (94002-94004, 94660)
Initial and subsequent care provided to a critically ill infant or child
Other hospital care or intensive care services by same group or individual done on same day that patient was transferred to initial neonatal/pediatric critical care
Readmission to critical unit on same day or during the same stay (subsequent care)

EXCLUDES   *Critical care services for patients 6 years of age or older (99291-99292)*
Critical care services provided by a second physician or physician of a different specialty (99291-99292)
Neonatal hypothermia (99184)
Services performed by transferring individual prior to transfer of patient to a different individual in a different group (99221-99233, 99291-99292, 99460-99462, 99477-99480)
Services provided by another individual in another group receiving a patient transferred to a lower level of care (99231-99233, 99478-99480)
Services provided by individual transferring a patient to a lower level of care (99231-99233, 99291-99292)

Code also normal newborn care if done on same day by same group or individual that provides critical care. Report modifier 25 with initial critical care code (99460-99462)
Do not report if performed by same or different individual in same group on same day (99291-99292)
Do not report with remote critical care (0188T-0189T)

99468   **Initial inpatient neonatal critical care, per day, for the evaluation and management of a critically ill neonate, 28 days of age or younger**   Ⓐ
    🔷 25.8   ⚖ 25.8   **FUD** XXX   Ⓒ 80
    AMA: 2015,Jul,3; 2015,Feb,10; 2015,Jan,16; 2014,Oct,8; 2014,May,4; 2014,Jan,11; 2012,Aug,6-8

99469   **Subsequent inpatient neonatal critical care, per day, for the evaluation and management of a critically ill neonate, 28 days of age or younger**   Ⓐ
    🔷 11.2   ⚖ 11.2   **FUD** XXX   Ⓒ 80
    AMA: 2015,Jul,3; 2015,Feb,10; 2015,Jan,16; 2014,Oct,8; 2014,May,4; 2014,Jan,11; 2012,Aug,6-8

99471   **Initial inpatient pediatric critical care, per day, for the evaluation and management of a critically ill infant or young child, 29 days through 24 months of age**   Ⓐ
    🔷 24.6   ⚖ 24.6   **FUD** XXX   Ⓒ 80
    AMA: 2015,Jul,3; 2015,Feb,10; 2015,Jan,16; 2014,Oct,8; 2014,Jan,11; 2012,Aug,6-8

99472   **Subsequent inpatient pediatric critical care, per day, for the evaluation and management of a critically ill infant or young child, 29 days through 24 months of age**   Ⓐ
    🔷 11.5   ⚖ 11.5   **FUD** XXX   Ⓒ 80
    AMA: 2015,Jul,3; 2015,Feb,10; 2015,Jan,16; 2014,Oct,8; 2014,Jan,11; 2012,Aug,6-8

99475   **Initial inpatient pediatric critical care, per day, for the evaluation and management of a critically ill infant or young child, 2 through 5 years of age**   Ⓐ
    🔷 16.2   ⚖ 16.2   **FUD** XXX   Ⓒ 80
    AMA: 2015,Jul,3; 2015,Feb,10; 2015,Jan,16; 2014,Oct,8; 2014,Jan,11

99476   **Subsequent inpatient pediatric critical care, per day, for the evaluation and management of a critically ill infant or young child, 2 through 5 years of age**   Ⓐ
    🔷 9.79   ⚖ 9.79   **FUD** XXX   Ⓒ 80
    AMA: 2015,Jul,3; 2015,Feb,10; 2015,Jan,16; 2014,Oct,8; 2014,Jan,11

99477-99486 Initial Inpatient Neonatal Intensive Care and Other Services

INCLUDES   All services included in codes 99291-99292 as well as the following that may be reported by facilities only:
Adjustments to enteral and/or parenteral nutrition
Airway and ventilator management (31500, 94002-94004, 94375, 94610, 94660)
Bladder catheterization (51701-51702)
Blood transfusion (36430, 36440)
Car seat evaluation (94780-94781)
Constant and/or frequent monitoring of vital signs
Continuous observation by the healthcare team
Heat maintenance
Intensive cardiac or respiratory monitoring
Oral or nasogastric tube insertion (43752)
Oxygen saturation (94760-94762)
Spinal puncture (62270)
Suprapubic catheterization (51100)
Vascular access procedures (36000, 36140, 36400, 36405-36406, 36420, 36510, 36555, 36600, 36620, 36660)

EXCLUDES   *Initial day intensive care provided by transferring individual same day neonate/infant transferred to a lower level of care (99477)*
Necessary resuscitation services done as part of delivery care prior to admission
Neonatal hypothermia (99184)
Services provided by receiving individual when patient is transferred for critical care (99468-99476)
Services for receiving provider when patient improves after the initial day and is transferred to a lower level of care (99231-99233, 99478-99480)
Subsequent care of a sick neonate, under 28 days of age, more than 5000 grams, not requiring critical or intensive care services (99231-99233)

Code also initial neonatal intensive care service when physician or other qualified health care professional is present for delivery and/or neonate requires resuscitation (99464-99465); append modifier 25 to (99477)
Code also care provided by receiving individual when patient is transferred to another individual in different group (99231-99233, 99462)
Do not report with critical care services for patient transferred after initial or subsequent intensive care is provided (99291-99292)
Do not report with inpatient neonatal/pediatric critical care services received on same day (99468-99476)

99477   **Initial hospital care, per day, for the evaluation and management of the neonate, 28 days of age or younger, who requires intensive observation, frequent interventions, and other intensive care services**   Ⓐ
    EXCLUDES   *Initiation of care of a critically ill neonate (99468)*
    Initiation of inpatient care of a normal newborn (99460)
    🔷 10.1   ⚖ 10.1   **FUD** XXX   Ⓒ 80
    AMA: 2015,Jul,3; 2015,Jan,16; 2014,Oct,8; 2014,Jan,11; 2012,Aug,6-8

99478   **Subsequent intensive care, per day, for the evaluation and management of the recovering very low birth weight infant (present body weight less than 1500 grams)**   Ⓐ
    🔷 3.99   ⚖ 3.99   **FUD** XXX   Ⓒ 80
    AMA: 2015,Jul,3; 2015,Jan,16; 2014,Oct,8; 2014,Jan,11; 2012,Aug,6-8

99479   **Subsequent intensive care, per day, for the evaluation and management of the recovering low birth weight infant (present body weight of 1500-2500 grams)**   Ⓐ
    🔷 3.51   ⚖ 3.51   **FUD** XXX   Ⓒ 80
    AMA: 2015,Jul,3; 2015,Jan,16; 2014,Oct,8; 2014,Jan,11; 2012,Aug,6-8

99480   **Subsequent intensive care, per day, for the evaluation and management of the recovering infant (present body weight of 2501-5000 grams)**   Ⓐ
    🔷 3.37   ⚖ 3.37   **FUD** XXX   Ⓒ 80
    AMA: 2015,Jul,3; 2015,Jan,16; 2014,Oct,8; 2014,Jan,11; 2012,Aug,6-8

99485   **Resequenced code. See code following 99467.**

99486   **Resequenced code. See code following 99467.**

| 26/TC PC/TC Comp Only | A2-Z3 ASC Pmt | 50 Bilateral | ♂ Male Only | ♀ Female Only | 🔷 Facility RVU | ⚖ Non-Facility RVU |
| **AMA:** CPT Asst | **CMS:** Pub 100 | A-Y OPPSI | 80/80 Surg Assist Allowed / w/Doc | | 🔲 Lab Crosswalk | 🔳 Radiology Crosswalk |

468   Medicare (Red Text)   CPT © 2015 American Medical Association. All Rights Reserved. (Black Text)   © 2015 Optum360, LLC (Blue Text)

[99490] Coordination of Services for Chronic Care

INCLUDES Case management services provided to patients that:
Have two or more conditions anticipated to endure more than 12 months or until the patient's death
Require at least 20 minutes of staff time monthly
Risk is high that conditions will result in decompensation, deterioration, or death
Do not report when performed during a postoperative surgical period
Do not report with (99339-99340, 99358-99359, 99363-99364, 99366-99368, 99374-99380, 99441-99444, 99495-99496, 90951-90970, 98960-98962, 98966-98969, 99071, 99078, 99080, 99090-99091, 99605-99607)

99490 **Chronic care management services, at least 20 minutes of clinical staff time directed by a physician or other qualified health care professional, per calendar month, with the following required elements: multiple (two or more) chronic conditions expected to last at least 12 months, or until the death of the patient; chronic conditions place the patient at significant risk of death, acute exacerbation/decompensation, or functional decline; comprehensive care plan established, implemented, revised, or monitored.**

0.92 1.20 **FUD** XXX V

AMA: 2015,Feb,3; 2015,Jan,16; 2014,Oct,3

99487-99490 Coordination of Complex Services for Chronic Care

INCLUDES All clinical non-face-to-face time with patient, family, and caregivers
Only services given by physician or other qualified health caregiver who has the role of care coordination for the patient for the month
Services provided to patients in a rest home, domiciliary, assisted living facility, or at home that include:
Caregiver education to family or patient, addressing independent living and self-management
Communication with patient and all caregivers and professionals regarding care
Determining which community and health resources would benefit the patient
Developing and maintaining a care plan
Health outcomes data and registry documentation
Providing communication with home health and other patient utilized services
Support for treatment and medication adherence
The facilitation of services and care
Services that address activities of daily living, psychosocial, and medical needs
Do not report in same month with (99339-99340, 99358-99359, 99363-99364, 99366-99368, 99374-99380, 99441-99444, 99495-99496, 90951-90970, 98960-98962, 98966-98969, 99071, 99078, 99080, 99090-99091, 99605-99607)

99487 **Complex chronic care management services, with the following required elements: multiple (two or more) chronic conditions expected to last at least 12 months, or until the death of the patient, chronic conditions place the patient at significant risk of death, acute exacerbation/decompensation, or functional decline, establishment or substantial revision of a comprehensive care plan, moderate or high complexity medical decision making; 60 minutes of clinical staff time directed by a physician or other qualified health care professional, per calendar month**

INCLUDES Clinical services, 60 to 74 minutes, during a calendar month

0.00 0.00 **FUD** XXX N 80

AMA: 2015,Jan,16; 2014,Oct,8; 2014,Oct,3; 2014,Jun,3; 2014,Feb,3; 2014,Jan,11; 2013,Nov,3; 2013,Sep,15-16; 2013,Apr,3-4; 2013,Jan,3-5

+ **99489** **each additional 30 minutes of clinical staff time directed by a physician or other qualified health care professional, per calendar month (List separately in addition to code for primary procedure)**

INCLUDES Each 30 additional minutes of clinical services in a calendar month
Code first (99487)
Do not report clinical services less than 30 minutes beyond the initial 60 minutes of care, per calendar month

0.00 0.00 **FUD** ZZZ N 80

AMA: 2015,Jan,16; 2014,Oct,8; 2014,Oct,3; 2014,Jun,3; 2014,Jan,11; 2013,Nov,3; 2013,Sep,15-16; 2013,Apr,3-4; 2013,Jan,3-5

99490 **Resequenced code. See code before 99487.**

99495-99496 Management of Transitional Care Services

CMS: 100-2,15,270.2 Medicare Telehealth Services; 100-4,12,190.3 Medicare Telehealth Services

INCLUDES First interaction (face-to-face, by telephone, or electronic) with patient or his/her caregiver and must be done within 2 working days of discharge
Initial face-to-face; must be done within code time frame and include medication management
New or established patient with moderate to high complexity medical decision making needs during care transitions
Services from discharge day up to 29 days post discharge
Subsequent discharge within 30 days
Without face-to-face patient care given by physician or other qualified health care professional includes:
Arrangement of follow-up and referrals with community resources and providers
Contacting qualified health care professionals for specific problems of patient
Discharge information review
Need for follow-up care review based on tests and treatments
Patient, family, and caregiver education
Without face-to-face patient care given by staff under the guidance of physician or other qualified health care professional includes:
Caregiver education to family or patient, addressing independent living and self-management
Communication with patient and all caregivers and professionals regarding care
Determining which community and health resources would benefit the patient
Providing communication with home health and other patient utilized services
Support for treatment and medication adherence
The facilitation of services and care
EXCLUDES *E&M services after the first face-to-face visit*
Do not report if done during same time frame (99339-99340, 99358-99359, 99363-99364, 99366-99368, 99374-99380, 99441-99444, 99487-99489, 90951-90970, 98960-98962, 98966-98969, 99071, 99078, 99080, 99090-99091, 99605-99607)

99495 **Transitional Care Management Services with the following required elements: Communication (direct contact, telephone, electronic) with the patient and/or caregiver within 2 business days of discharge Medical decision making of at least moderate complexity during the service period Face-to-face visit, within 14 calendar days of discharge**

3.13 4.63 **FUD** XXX V 80

AMA: 2015,Jan,16; 2014,Oct,8; 2014,Oct,3; 2014,Mar,13; 2014,Jan,11; 2013,Nov,3; 2013,Dec,11; 2013,Sep,15-16; 2013,Aug,13; 2013,Jul,11-12; 2013,Apr,3-4; 2013,Jan,3-5

99496 **Transitional Care Management Services with the following required elements: Communication (direct contact, telephone, electronic) with the patient and/or caregiver within 2 business days of discharge Medical decision making of high complexity during the service period Face-to-face visit, within 7 calendar days of discharge**

4.51 6.50 **FUD** XXX V 80

AMA: 2015,Jan,16; 2014,Oct,8; 2014,Oct,3; 2014,Mar,13; 2014,Jan,11; 2013,Nov,3; 2013,Sep,15-16; 2013,Aug,13; 2013,Jul,11-12; 2013,Apr,3-4; 2013,Jan,3-5

99497-99498 Advance Directive Guidance

EXCLUDES   *Treatment/management for an active problem (see appropriate E&M service)*
Do not report with (99291-99292, 99468-99469, 99471-99472, 99475-99476, 99477-99480)

99497   **Advance care planning including the explanation and discussion of advance directives such as standard forms (with completion of such forms, when performed), by the physician or other qualified health care professional; first 30 minutes, face-to-face with the patient, family member(s), and/or surrogate**
             0.00   0.00   **FUD** XXX   N 80
             AMA: 2015,Jan,16; 2014,Dec,11

+   99498   **each additional 30 minutes (List separately in addition to code for primary procedure)**
             Code first (99497)
             0.00   0.00   **FUD** ZZZ   N 80
             AMA: 2015,Jan,16; 2014,Dec,11

99499 Unlisted Evaluation and Management Services

CMS: 100-4,12,30.6.10 Consultation Services; 100-4,12,30.6.4 Services Furnished Incident to Physician's Service; 100-4,12,30.6.9.1 Initial Hospital Care and Observation or Inpatient Care Services

99499   **Unlisted evaluation and management service**
             0.00   0.00   **FUD** XXX   B 80
             AMA: 2015,Jan,16; 2014,Oct,8; 2014,Jan,11; 2012,Nov,13-14; 2012,Jul,10-11; 2012,Apr,10; 2012,Jan,15-42; 2011,May,7;

| 26/TC PC/TC Comp Only | A2-Z4 ASC Pmt | 50 Bilateral | ♂ Male Only | ♀ Female Only | Facility RVU | Non-Facility RVU |
| AMA: CPT Asst | CMS: Pub 100 | A-Y OPPSI | 80/80 Surg Assist Allowed / w/Doc | | Lab Crosswalk | Radiology Crosswalk |

470   Medicare (Red Text)   CPT © 2015 American Medical Association. All Rights Reserved. (Black Text)   © 2015 Optum360, LLC (Blue Text)

0001F-0015F Quality Measures with Multiple Components

INCLUDES   Several measures grouped within a single code descriptor to make possible reporting for clinical conditions when all of the components have been met

0001F   **Heart failure assessed (includes assessment of all the following components) (CAD): Blood pressure measured (2000F) Level of activity assessed (1003F) Clinical symptoms of volume overload (excess) assessed (1004F) Weight, recorded (2001F) Clinical signs of volume overload (excess) assessed (2002F)**

INCLUDES   Blood pressure measured (2000F)
Clinical signs of volume overload (excess) assessed (2002F)
Clinical symptoms of volume overload (excess) assessed (1004F)
Level of activity assessed (1003F)
Weight recorded (2001F)

🚗 0.00   ⚖ 0.00   **FUD** XXX   E

AMA: 2015,Jan,16; 2014,Jan,11

0005F   **Osteoarthritis assessed (OA) Includes assessment of all the following components: Osteoarthritis symptoms and functional status assessed (1006F) Use of anti-inflammatory or over-the-counter (OTC) analgesic medications assessed (1007F) Initial examination of the involved joint(s) (includes visual inspection, palpation, range of motion) (2004F)**

INCLUDES   Initial examination of the involved joint(s) (includes visual inspection/palpation/range of motion) (2004F)
Osteoarthritis symptoms and functional status assessed (1006F)
Use of anti-inflammatory or over-the-counter (OTC) analgesic medications assessed (1007F)

🚗 0.00   ⚖ 0.00   **FUD** XXX   E

AMA: 2005,Oct,1-5

0012F   **Community-acquired bacterial pneumonia assessment (includes all of the following components) (CAP): Co-morbid conditions assessed (1026F) Vital signs recorded (2010F) Mental status assessed (2014F) Hydration status assessed (2018F)**

🚗 0.00   ⚖ 0.00   **FUD** XXX   E

INCLUDES   Co-morbid conditions assessed (1026F)
Hydration status assessed (2018F)
Mental status assessed (2014F)
Vital signs recorded (2010F)

0014F   **Comprehensive preoperative assessment performed for cataract surgery with intraocular lens (IOL) placement (includes assessment of all of the following components) (EC): Dilated fundus evaluation performed within 12 months prior to cataract surgery (2020F) Pre-surgical (cataract) axial length, corneal power measurement and method of intraocular lens power calculation documented (must be performed within 12 months prior to surgery) (3073F) Preoperative assessment of functional or medical indication(s) for surgery prior to the cataract surgery with intraocular lens placement (must be performed within 12 months prior to cataract surgery) (3325F)**

INCLUDES   Evaluation of dilated fundus done within 12 months prior to surgery (2020F)
Preoperative assessment of functional or medical indications done within 12 months prior to surgery (3325F)
Presurgical measurement of axial length, corneal power, and IOL power calculation performed within 12 months prior to surgery (3073F)

🚗 0.00   ⚖ 0.00   **FUD** XXX   E

AMA: 2008,Mar,8-12

0015F   **Melanoma follow up completed (includes assessment of all of the following components) (ML): History obtained regarding new or changing moles (1050F) Complete physical skin exam performed (2029F) Patient counseled to perform a monthly self skin examination (5005F)**

INCLUDES   Complete physical skin exam (2029F)
Counseling to perform monthly skin self-examination (5005F)
History obtained of new or changing moles (1050F)

🚗 0.00   ⚖ 0.00   **FUD** XXX   E

AMA: 2008,Mar,8-12

0500F-0584F Care Provided According to Prevailing Guidelines

INCLUDES   Measures of utilization or patient care provided for certain clinical purposes

0500F   **Initial prenatal care visit (report at first prenatal encounter with health care professional providing obstetrical care. Report also date of visit and, in a separate field, the date of the last menstrual period [LMP]) (Prenatal)**   M ♀

🚗 0.00   ⚖ 0.00   **FUD** XXX   E

AMA: 2015,Jan,16; 2014,Jan,11

0501F   **Prenatal flow sheet documented in medical record by first prenatal visit (documentation includes at minimum blood pressure, weight, urine protein, uterine size, fetal heart tones, and estimated date of delivery). Report also: date of visit and, in a separate field, the date of the last menstrual period [LMP] (Note: If reporting 0501F Prenatal flow sheet, it is not necessary to report 0500F Initial prenatal care visit) (Prenatal)**   M ♀

🚗 0.00   ⚖ 0.00   **FUD** XXX   E

AMA: 2004,Nov,1

0502F   **Subsequent prenatal care visit (Prenatal) [Excludes: patients who are seen for a condition unrelated to pregnancy or prenatal care (eg, an upper respiratory infection; patients seen for consultation only, not for continuing care)]**   M ♀

EXCLUDES   Patients seen for an unrelated pregnancy/prenatal care condition (e.g., upper respiratory infection; patients seen for consultation only, not for continuing care)

🚗 0.00   ⚖ 0.00   **FUD** XXX   E

AMA: 2004,Nov,1

0503F   **Postpartum care visit (Prenatal)**   M ♀

🚗 0.00   ⚖ 0.00   **FUD** XXX   E

AMA: 2004,Nov,1

0505F   **Hemodialysis plan of care documented (ESRD, P-ESRD)**

🚗 0.00   ⚖ 0.00   **FUD** XXX   E

AMA: 2008,Mar,8-12

0507F   **Peritoneal dialysis plan of care documented (ESRD)**

🚗 0.00   ⚖ 0.00   **FUD** XXX   E

AMA: 2008,Mar,8-12

0509F   **Urinary incontinence plan of care documented (GER)**

🚗 0.00   ⚖ 0.00   **FUD** XXX   M PQ

0513F   **Elevated blood pressure plan of care documented (CKD)**

🚗 0.00   ⚖ 0.00   **FUD** XXX   M PQ

AMA: 2008,Mar,8-12

0514F   **Plan of care for elevated hemoglobin level documented for patient receiving Erythropoiesis-Stimulating Agent therapy (ESA) (CKD)**

🚗 0.00   ⚖ 0.00   **FUD** XXX   E

AMA: 2008,Mar,8-12

0516F   **Anemia plan of care documented (ESRD)**

🚗 0.00   ⚖ 0.00   **FUD** XXX   E

AMA: 2008,Mar,8-12

0517F   **Glaucoma plan of care documented (EC)**

🚗 0.00   ⚖ 0.00   **FUD** XXX   M PQ

AMA: 2008,Mar,8-12

0518F   Falls plan of care documented (GER)
🛏 0.00   ⚖ 0.00   **FUD** XXX   M PQ
AMA: 2008,Mar,8-12

0519F   Planned chemotherapy regimen, including at a minimum: drug(s) prescribed, dose, and duration, documented prior to initiation of a new treatment regimen (ONC)
🛏 0.00   ⚖ 0.00   **FUD** XXX   E
AMA: 2008,Mar,8-12

0520F   Radiation dose limits to normal tissues established prior to the initiation of a course of 3D conformal radiation for a minimum of 2 tissue/organ (ONC)
🛏 0.00   ⚖ 0.00   **FUD** XXX   M PQ
AMA: 2008,Mar,8-12

0521F   Plan of care to address pain documented (COA) (ONC)
🛏 0.00   ⚖ 0.00   **FUD** XXX   M PQ
AMA: 2008,Mar,8-12

0525F   Initial visit for episode (BkP)
🛏 0.00   ⚖ 0.00   **FUD** XXX   E
AMA: 2008,Mar,8-12

0526F   Subsequent visit for episode (BkP)
🛏 0.00   ⚖ 0.00   **FUD** XXX   M PQ
AMA: 2008,Mar,8-12

0528F   Recommended follow-up interval for repeat colonoscopy of at least 10 years documented in colonoscopy report (End/Polyp)
🛏 0.00   ⚖ 0.00   **FUD** XXX   M

0529F   Interval of 3 or more years since patient's last colonoscopy, documented (End/Polyp)
🛏 0.00   ⚖ 0.00   **FUD** XXX   M PQ

0535F   Dyspnea management plan of care, documented (Pall Cr)
🛏 0.00   ⚖ 0.00   **FUD** XXX   E

0540F   Glucorticoid Management Plan Documented (RA)
🛏 0.00   ⚖ 0.00   **FUD** XXX   M PQ

0545F   Plan for follow-up care for major depressive disorder, documented (MDD ADOL)
🛏 0.00   ⚖ 0.00   **FUD** XXX   E

0550F   Cytopathology report on routine nongynecologic specimen finalized within two working days of accession date (PATH)
🛏 0.00   ⚖ 0.00   **FUD** XXX   E

0551F   Cytopathology report on nongynecologic specimen with documentation that the specimen was non-routine (PATH)
🛏 0.00   ⚖ 0.00   **FUD** XXX   E

0555F   Symptom management plan of care documented (HF)
🛏 0.00   ⚖ 0.00   **FUD** XXX   E

0556F   Plan of care to achieve lipid control documented (CAD)
🛏 0.00   ⚖ 0.00   **FUD** XXX   E PQ

0557F   Plan of care to manage anginal symptoms documented (CAD)
🛏 0.00   ⚖ 0.00   **FUD** XXX   M PQ

0575F   HIV RNA control plan of care, documented (HIV)
🛏 0.00   ⚖ 0.00   **FUD** XXX   E PQ

0580F   Multidisciplinary care plan developed or updated (ALS)
🛏 0.00   ⚖ 0.00   **FUD** XXX   E

0581F   Patient transferred directly from anesthetizing location to critical care unit (Peri2)
🛏 0.00   ⚖ 0.00   **FUD** XXX   E

0582F   Patient not transferred directly from anesthetizing location to critical care unit (Peri2)
🛏 0.00   ⚖ 0.00   **FUD** XXX   E

0583F   Transfer of care checklist used (Peri2)
🛏 0.00   ⚖ 0.00   **FUD** XXX   E

0584F   Transfer of care checklist not used (Peri2)
🛏 0.00   ⚖ 0.00   **FUD** XXX   E

1000F-1505F Elements of History/Review of Systems

INCLUDES   Measures for specific aspects of patient history or review of systems

1000F   Tobacco use assessed (CAD, CAP, COPD, PV) (DM)
🛏 0.00   ⚖ 0.00   **FUD** XXX   E
AMA: 2015,Jan,16; 2014,Jan,11

1002F   Anginal symptoms and level of activity assessed (NMA-No Measure Associated)
🛏 0.00   ⚖ 0.00   **FUD** XXX   E
AMA: 2004,Nov,1

1003F   Level of activity assessed (NMA-No Measure Associated)
🛏 0.00   ⚖ 0.00   **FUD** XXX   E
AMA: 2006,Dec,10-12

1004F   Clinical symptoms of volume overload (excess) assessed (NMA-No Measure Associated)
🛏 0.00   ⚖ 0.00   **FUD** XXX   E
AMA: 2006,Dec,10-12

1005F   Asthma symptoms evaluated (includes documentation of numeric frequency of symptoms or patient completion of an asthma assessment tool/survey/questionnaire) (NMA-No Measure Associated)
🛏 0.00   ⚖ 0.00   **FUD** XXX   E

1006F   Osteoarthritis symptoms and functional status assessed (may include the use of a standardized scale or the completion of an assessment questionnaire, such as the SF-36, AAOS Hip & Knee Questionnaire) (OA) [Instructions: Report when osteoarthritis is addressed during the patient encounter]
🛏 0.00   ⚖ 0.00   **FUD** XXX   M PQ
INCLUDES   Osteoarthritis when it is addressed during the patient encounter

1007F   Use of anti-inflammatory or analgesic over-the-counter (OTC) medications for symptom relief assessed (OA)
🛏 0.00   ⚖ 0.00   **FUD** XXX   E PQ

1008F   Gastrointestinal and renal risk factors assessed for patients on prescribed or OTC non-steroidal anti-inflammatory drug (NSAID) (OA)
🛏 0.00   ⚖ 0.00   **FUD** XXX   E

1010F   Severity of angina assessed by level of activity (CAD)
🛏 0.00   ⚖ 0.00   **FUD** XXX   M PQ

1011F   Angina present (CAD)
🛏 0.00   ⚖ 0.00   **FUD** XXX   M PQ

1012F   Angina absent (CAD)
🛏 0.00   ⚖ 0.00   **FUD** XXX   M PQ

1015F   Chronic obstructive pulmonary disease (COPD) symptoms assessed (Includes assessment of at least 1 of the following: dyspnea, cough/sputum, wheezing), or respiratory symptom assessment tool completed (COPD)
🛏 0.00   ⚖ 0.00   **FUD** XXX   E

1018F   Dyspnea assessed, not present (COPD)
🛏 0.00   ⚖ 0.00   **FUD** XXX   E

1019F   Dyspnea assessed, present (COPD)
🛏 0.00   ⚖ 0.00   **FUD** XXX   E

1022F   Pneumococcus immunization status assessed (CAP, COPD)
🛏 0.00   ⚖ 0.00   **FUD** XXX   E
AMA: 2010,Jul,3-5

1026F   Co-morbid conditions assessed (eg, includes assessment for presence or absence of: malignancy, liver disease, congestive heart failure, cerebrovascular disease, renal disease, chronic obstructive pulmonary disease, asthma, diabetes, other co-morbid conditions) (CAP)
🛏 0.00   ⚖ 0.00   **FUD** XXX   E

1030F   Influenza immunization status assessed (CAP)
🛏 0.00   ⚖ 0.00   **FUD** XXX   E
AMA: 2008,Mar,8-12

1031F   Smoking status and exposure to second hand smoke in the home assessed (Asthma)
   0.00   0.00   **FUD** XXX   E PQ

1032F   Current tobacco smoker or currently exposed to secondhand smoke (Asthma)
   0.00   0.00   **FUD** XXX   E PQ

1033F   Current tobacco non-smoker and not currently exposed to secondhand smoke (Asthma)
   0.00   0.00   **FUD** XXX   E PQ

1034F   Current tobacco smoker (CAD, CAP, COPD, PV) (DM)
   0.00   0.00   **FUD** XXX   E
   AMA: 2008,Mar,8-12

1035F   Current smokeless tobacco user (eg, chew, snuff) (PV)
   0.00   0.00   **FUD** XXX   E
   AMA: 2008,Mar,8-12

1036F   Current tobacco non-user (CAD, CAP, COPD, PV) (DM) (IBD)
   0.00   0.00   **FUD** XXX   M PQ
   AMA: 2008,Mar,8-12

1038F   Persistent asthma (mild, moderate or severe) (Asthma)
   0.00   0.00   **FUD** XXX   M PQ
   AMA: 2015,Jan,16; 2014,Jan,11; 2010,Jul,3-5

1039F   Intermittent asthma (Asthma)
   0.00   0.00   **FUD** XXX   M PQ
   AMA: 2015,Jan,16; 2014,Jan,11; 2010,Jul,3-5

1040F   DSM-5 criteria for major depressive disorder documented at the initial evaluation (MDD, MDD ADOL)
   0.00   0.00   **FUD** XXX   E PQ
   AMA: 2008,Mar,8-12

1050F   History obtained regarding new or changing moles (ML)
   0.00   0.00   **FUD** XXX   E
   AMA: 2008,Mar,8-12

1052F   Type, anatomic location, and activity all assessed (IBD)
   0.00   0.00   **FUD** XXX   E

1055F   Visual functional status assessed (EC)
   0.00   0.00   **FUD** XXX   E

1060F   Documentation of permanent or persistent or paroxysmal atrial fibrillation (STR)
   0.00   0.00   **FUD** XXX   E

1061F   Documentation of absence of permanent and persistent and paroxysmal atrial fibrillation (STR)
   0.00   0.00   **FUD** XXX   E

1065F   Ischemic stroke symptom onset of less than 3 hours prior to arrival (STR)
   0.00   0.00   **FUD** XXX   E

1066F   Ischemic stroke symptom onset greater than or equal to 3 hours prior to arrival (STR)
   0.00   0.00   **FUD** XXX   E

1070F   Alarm symptoms (involuntary weight loss, dysphagia, or gastrointestinal bleeding) assessed; none present (GERD)
   0.00   0.00   **FUD** XXX   E

1071F   1 or more present (GERD)
   0.00   0.00   **FUD** XXX   E

1090F   Presence or absence of urinary incontinence assessed (GER)
   0.00   0.00   **FUD** XXX   M PQ

1091F   Urinary incontinence characterized (eg, frequency, volume, timing, type of symptoms, how bothersome) (GER)
   0.00   0.00   **FUD** XXX   E PQ

1100F   Patient screened for future fall risk; documentation of 2 or more falls in the past year or any fall with injury in the past year (GER)
   0.00   0.00   **FUD** XXX   M PQ
   AMA: 2008,Mar,8-12

1101F   documentation of no falls in the past year or only 1 fall without injury in the past year (GER)
   0.00   0.00   **FUD** XXX   M PQ
   AMA: 2008,Mar,8-12

1110F   Patient discharged from an inpatient facility (eg, hospital, skilled nursing facility, or rehabilitation facility) within the last 60 days (GER)
   0.00   0.00   **FUD** XXX   E PQ

1111F   Discharge medications reconciled with the current medication list in outpatient medical record (COA) (GER)
   0.00   0.00   **FUD** XXX   M PQ

1116F   Auricular or periauricular pain assessed (AOE)
   0.00   0.00   **FUD** XXX   E PQ
   AMA: 2008,Mar,8-12

1118F   GERD symptoms assessed after 12 months of therapy (GERD)
   0.00   0.00   **FUD** XXX   E
   AMA: 2008,Mar,8-12

1119F   Initial evaluation for condition (HEP C)(EPI, DSP)
   0.00   0.00   **FUD** XXX   E PQ
   AMA: 2008,Mar,8-12

1121F   Subsequent evaluation for condition (HEP C)(EPI)
   0.00   0.00   **FUD** XXX   E PQ
   AMA: 2008,Mar,8-12

1123F   Advance Care Planning discussed and documented advance care plan or surrogate decision maker documented in the medical record (DEM) (GER, Pall Cr)
   0.00   0.00   **FUD** XXX   M PQ
   AMA: 2008,Mar,8-12

1124F   Advance Care Planning discussed and documented in the medical record, patient did not wish or was not able to name a surrogate decision maker or provide an advance care plan (DEM) (GER, Pall Cr)
   0.00   0.00   **FUD** XXX   M PQ
   AMA: 2008,Mar,8-12

1125F   Pain severity quantified; pain present (COA) (ONC)
   0.00   0.00   **FUD** XXX   M PQ
   AMA: 2008,Mar,8-12

1126F   no pain present (COA) (ONC)
   0.00   0.00   **FUD** XXX   M PQ
   AMA: 2008,Mar,8-12

1127F   New episode for condition (NMA-No Measure Associated)
   0.00   0.00   **FUD** XXX   E
   AMA: 2008,Mar,8-12

1128F   Subsequent episode for condition (NMA-No Measure Associated)
   0.00   0.00   **FUD** XXX   E
   AMA: 2008,Mar,8-12

1130F   Back pain and function assessed, including all of the following: Pain assessment and functional status and patient history, including notation of presence or absence of "red flags" (warning signs) and assessment of prior treatment and response, and employment status (BkP)
   0.00   0.00   **FUD** XXX   E PQ
   AMA: 2008,Mar,8-12

1134F   Episode of back pain lasting 6 weeks or less (BkP)
   0.00   0.00   **FUD** XXX   E
   AMA: 2008,Mar,8-12

1135F   Episode of back pain lasting longer than 6 weeks (BkP)
   0.00   0.00   **FUD** XXX   E
   AMA: 2008,Mar,8-12

1136F   Episode of back pain lasting 12 weeks or less (BkP)
   0.00   0.00   **FUD** XXX   E
   AMA: 2008,Mar,8-12

1137F Episode of back pain lasting longer than 12 weeks (BkP)
🔲 0.00 ⚖ 0.00 **FUD** XXX E
AMA: 2008,Mar,8-12

1150F Documentation that a patient has a substantial risk of death within 1 year (Pall Cr)
🔲 0.00 ⚖ 0.00 **FUD** XXX E

1151F Documentation that a patient does not have a substantial risk of death within one year (Pall Cr)
🔲 0.00 ⚖ 0.00 **FUD** XXX E

1152F Documentation of advanced disease diagnosis, goals of care prioritize comfort (Pall Cr)
🔲 0.00 ⚖ 0.00 **FUD** XXX E

1153F Documentation of advanced disease diagnosis, goals of care do not prioritize comfort (Pall Cr)
🔲 0.00 ⚖ 0.00 **FUD** XXX E

1157F Advance care plan or similar legal document present in the medical record (COA)
🔲 0.00 ⚖ 0.00 **FUD** XXX E

1158F Advance care planning discussion documented in the medical record (COA)
🔲 0.00 ⚖ 0.00 **FUD** XXX M

1159F Medication list documented in medical record (COA)
🔲 0.00 ⚖ 0.00 **FUD** XXX E

1160F Review of all medications by a prescribing practitioner or clinical pharmacist (such as, prescriptions, OTCs, herbal therapies and supplements) documented in the medical record (COA)
🔲 0.00 ⚖ 0.00 **FUD** XXX E

1170F Functional status assessed (COA) (RA)
🔲 0.00 ⚖ 0.00 **FUD** XXX M PQ

1175F Functional status for dementia assessed and results reviewed (DEM)
🔲 0.00 ⚖ 0.00 **FUD** XXX M

1180F All specified thromboembolic risk factors assessed (AFIB)
🔲 0.00 ⚖ 0.00 **FUD** XXX E

1181F Neuropsychiatric symptoms assessed and results reviewed (DEM)
🔲 0.00 ⚖ 0.00 **FUD** XXX M

1182F Neuropsychiatric symptoms, one or more present (DEM)
🔲 0.00 ⚖ 0.00 **FUD** XXX E

1183F Neuropsychiatric symptoms, absent (DEM)
🔲 0.00 ⚖ 0.00 **FUD** XXX E

1200F Seizure type(s) and current seizure frequency(ies) documented (EPI)
🔲 0.00 ⚖ 0.00 **FUD** XXX E PQ

1205F Etiology of epilepsy or epilepsy syndrome(s) reviewed and documented (EPI)
🔲 0.00 ⚖ 0.00 **FUD** XXX E PQ

1220F Patient screened for depression (SUD)
🔲 0.00 ⚖ 0.00 **FUD** XXX E PQ

1400F Parkinson's disease diagnosis reviewed (Prkns)
🔲 0.00 ⚖ 0.00 **FUD** XXX M

1450F Symptoms improved or remained consistent with treatment goals since last assessment (HF)
🔲 0.00 ⚖ 0.00 **FUD** XXX E

1451F Symptoms demonstrated clinically important deterioration since last assessment (HF)
🔲 0.00 ⚖ 0.00 **FUD** XXX E

1460F Qualifying cardiac event/diagnosis in previous 12 months (CAD)
🔲 0.00 ⚖ 0.00 **FUD** XXX M PQ

1461F No qualifying cardiac event/diagnosis in previous 12 months (CAD)
🔲 0.00 ⚖ 0.00 **FUD** XXX M PQ

1490F Dementia severity classified, mild (DEM)
🔲 0.00 ⚖ 0.00 **FUD** XXX M

1491F Dementia severity classified, moderate (DEM)
🔲 0.00 ⚖ 0.00 **FUD** XXX M

1493F Dementia severity classified, severe (DEM)
🔲 0.00 ⚖ 0.00 **FUD** XXX M

1494F Cognition assessed and reviewed (DEM)
🔲 0.00 ⚖ 0.00 **FUD** XXX M

1500F Symptoms and signs of distal symmetric polyneuropathy reviewed and documented (DSP)
🔲 0.00 ⚖ 0.00 **FUD** XXX E

1501F Not initial evaluation for condition (DSP)
🔲 0.00 ⚖ 0.00 **FUD** XXX E

1502F Patient queried about pain and pain interference with function using a valid and reliable instrument (DSP)
🔲 0.00 ⚖ 0.00 **FUD** XXX E

1503F Patient queried about symptoms of respiratory insufficiency (ALS)
🔲 0.00 ⚖ 0.00 **FUD** XXX E

1504F Patient has respiratory insufficiency (ALS)
🔲 0.00 ⚖ 0.00 **FUD** XXX E

1505F Patient does not have respiratory insufficiency (ALS)
🔲 0.00 ⚖ 0.00 **FUD** XXX E

2000F-2060F Elements of Examination

INCLUDES Components of clinical assessment or physical exam

2000F Blood pressure measured (CKD)(DM)
🔲 0.00 ⚖ 0.00 **FUD** XXX M PQ
AMA: 2015,Jan,16; 2014,Jan,11

2001F Weight recorded (PAG)
🔲 0.00 ⚖ 0.00 **FUD** XXX E
AMA: 2006,Dec,10-12

2002F Clinical signs of volume overload (excess) assessed (NMA-No Measure Associated)
🔲 0.00 ⚖ 0.00 **FUD** XXX E
AMA: 2006,Dec,10-12

2004F Initial examination of the involved joint(s) (includes visual inspection, palpation, range of motion) (OA) [Instructions: Report only for initial osteoarthritis visit or for visits for new joint involvement]
INCLUDES Visits for initial osteoarthritis examination or new joint involvement
🔲 0.00 ⚖ 0.00 **FUD** XXX E
AMA: 2004,Feb,3; 2003,Aug,1

2010F Vital signs (temperature, pulse, respiratory rate, and blood pressure) documented and reviewed (CAP) (EM)
🔲 0.00 ⚖ 0.00 **FUD** XXX E PQ

2014F Mental status assessed (CAP) (EM)
🔲 0.00 ⚖ 0.00 **FUD** XXX E PQ

2015F Asthma impairment assessed (Asthma)
🔲 0.00 ⚖ 0.00 **FUD** XXX E PQ

2016F Asthma risk assessed (Asthma)
🔲 0.00 ⚖ 0.00 **FUD** XXX E PQ

2018F Hydration status assessed (normal/mildly dehydrated/severely dehydrated) (CAP)
🔲 0.00 ⚖ 0.00 **FUD** XXX E

2019F Dilated macular exam performed, including documentation of the presence or absence of macular thickening or hemorrhage and the level of macular degeneration severity (EC)
🔲 0.00 ⚖ 0.00 **FUD** XXX M PQ

2020F	Dilated fundus evaluation performed within 12 months prior to cataract surgery (EC)
	0.00 0.00 **FUD** XXX E
	AMA: 2008,Mar,8-12

2021F	Dilated macular or fundus exam performed, including documentation of the presence or absence of macular edema and level of severity of retinopathy (EC)
	0.00 0.00 **FUD** XXX E PQ

2022F	Dilated retinal eye exam with interpretation by an ophthalmologist or optometrist documented and reviewed (DM)
	0.00 0.00 **FUD** XXX M PQ
	AMA: 2008,Mar,8-12

2024F	7 standard field stereoscopic photos with interpretation by an ophthalmologist or optometrist documented and reviewed (DM)
	0.00 0.00 **FUD** XXX M PQ
	AMA: 2008,Mar,8-12

2026F	Eye imaging validated to match diagnosis from 7 standard field stereoscopic photos results documented and reviewed (DM)
	0.00 0.00 **FUD** XXX M PQ
	AMA: 2008,Mar,8-12

2027F	Optic nerve head evaluation performed (EC)
	0.00 0.00 **FUD** XXX M PQ

2028F	Foot examination performed (includes examination through visual inspection, sensory exam with monofilament, and pulse exam - report when any of the 3 components are completed) (DM)
	0.00 0.00 **FUD** XXX E PQ

2029F	Complete physical skin exam performed (ML)
	0.00 0.00 **FUD** XXX E
	AMA: 2008,Mar,8-12

2030F	Hydration status documented, normally hydrated (PAG)
	0.00 0.00 **FUD** XXX E

2031F	Hydration status documented, dehydrated (PAG)
	0.00 0.00 **FUD** XXX E

2035F	Tympanic membrane mobility assessed with pneumatic otoscopy or tympanometry (OME)
	0.00 0.00 **FUD** XXX E
	AMA: 2008,Mar,8-12

2040F	Physical examination on the date of the initial visit for low back pain performed, in accordance with specifications (BkP)
	0.00 0.00 **FUD** XXX E
	AMA: 2008,Mar,8-12

2044F	Documentation of mental health assessment prior to intervention (back surgery or epidural steroid injection) or for back pain episode lasting longer than 6 weeks (BkP)
	0.00 0.00 **FUD** XXX E
	AMA: 2008,Mar,8-12

2050F	Wound characteristics including size and nature of wound base tissue and amount of drainage prior to debridement documented (CWC)
	0.00 0.00 **FUD** XXX E

2060F	Patient interviewed directly on or before date of diagnosis of major depressive disorder (MDD ADOL)
	0.00 0.00 **FUD** XXX E

3006F-3776F Findings from Diagnostic or Screening Tests

INCLUDES   Results and medical decision making with regards to ordered tests:
    Clinical laboratory tests
    Other examination procedures
    Radiological examinations

3006F	Chest X-ray results documented and reviewed (CAP)
	0.00 0.00 **FUD** XXX E
	AMA: 2015,Jan,16; 2014,Jan,11

3008F	Body Mass Index (BMI), documented (PV)
	0.00 0.00 **FUD** XXX E

3011F	Lipid panel results documented and reviewed (must include total cholesterol, HDL-C, triglycerides and calculated LDL-C) (CAD)
	0.00 0.00 **FUD** XXX E

3014F	Screening mammography results documented and reviewed (PV)
	0.00 0.00 **FUD** XXX M PQ
	AMA: 2008,Mar,8-12

3015F	Cervical cancer screening results documented and reviewed (PV)
	0.00 0.00 **FUD** XXX ♀

3016F	Patient screened for unhealthy alcohol use using a systematic screening method (PV) (DSP)
	0.00 0.00 **FUD** XXX M PQ

3017F	Colorectal cancer screening results documented and reviewed (PV)
	0.00 0.00 **FUD** XXX M PQ
	AMA: 2008,Mar,8-12

3018F	Pre-procedure risk assessment and depth of insertion and quality of the bowel prep and complete description of polyp(s) found, including location of each polyp, size, number and gross morphology and recommendations for follow-up in final colonoscopy report documented (End/Polyp)
	0.00 0.00 **FUD** XXX E

3019F	Left ventricular ejection fraction (LVEF) assessment planned post discharge (HF)
	0.00 0.00 **FUD** XXX E

3020F	Left ventricular function (LVF) assessment (eg, echocardiography, nuclear test, or ventriculography) documented in the medical record (Includes quantitative or qualitative assessment results) (NMA-No Measure Associated)
	0.00 0.00 **FUD** XXX E
	AMA: 2006,Dec,10-12

3021F	Left ventricular ejection fraction (LVEF) less than 40% or documentation of moderately or severely depressed left ventricular systolic function (CAD, HF)
	0.00 0.00 **FUD** XXX M PQ

3022F	Left ventricular ejection fraction (LVEF) greater than or equal to 40% or documentation as normal or mildly depressed left ventricular systolic function (CAD, HF)
	0.00 0.00 **FUD** XXX M PQ

3023F	Spirometry results documented and reviewed (COPD)
	0.00 0.00 **FUD** XXX M PQ

3025F	Spirometry test results demonstrate FEV1/FVC less than 70% with COPD symptoms (eg, dyspnea, cough/sputum, wheezing) (CAP, COPD)
	0.00 0.00 **FUD** XXX E PQ

3027F	Spirometry test results demonstrate FEV1/FVC greater than or equal to 70% or patient does not have COPD symptoms (COPD)
	0.00 0.00 **FUD** XXX E PQ

3028F	Oxygen saturation results documented and reviewed (includes assessment through pulse oximetry or arterial blood gas measurement) (CAP, COPD) (EM)
	0.00 0.00 **FUD** XXX E PQ

3035F	Oxygen saturation less than or equal to 88% or a PaO2 less than or equal to 55 mm Hg (COPD)
	0.00 0.00 **FUD** XXX E

3037F Oxygen saturation greater than 88% or PaO2 greater than 55 mm Hg (COPD)
🔧 0.00   ⚖ 0.00   **FUD** XXX   E

3038F Pulmonary function test performed within 12 months prior to surgery (Lung/Esop Cx)
🔧 0.00   ⚖ 0.00   **FUD** XXX   E PQ

3040F Functional expiratory volume (FEV1) less than 40% of predicted value (COPD)
🔧 0.00   ⚖ 0.00   **FUD** XXX   E

3042F Functional expiratory volume (FEV1) greater than or equal to 40% of predicted value (COPD)
🔧 0.00   ⚖ 0.00   **FUD** XXX   E

3044F Most recent hemoglobin A1c (HbA1c) level less than 7.0% (DM)
🔧 0.00   ⚖ 0.00   **FUD** XXX   M PQ

3045F Most recent hemoglobin A1c (HbA1c) level 7.0-9.0% (DM)
🔧 0.00   ⚖ 0.00   **FUD** XXX   M PQ

3046F Most recent hemoglobin A1c level greater than 9.0% (DM)
🔧 0.00   ⚖ 0.00   **FUD** XXX   M PQ

> EXCLUDES *Levels of hemoglobin A1c less than or equal to 9.0% (3044F-3045F)*

3048F Most recent LDL-C less than 100 mg/dL (CAD) (DM)
🔧 0.00   ⚖ 0.00   **FUD** XXX   E PQ

3049F Most recent LDL-C 100-129 mg/dL (CAD) (DM)
🔧 0.00   ⚖ 0.00   **FUD** XXX   E PQ

3050F Most recent LDL-C greater than or equal to 130 mg/dL (CAD) (DM)
🔧 0.00   ⚖ 0.00   **FUD** XXX   E PQ

3055F Left ventricular ejection fraction (LVEF) less than or equal to 35% (HF)
🔧 0.00   ⚖ 0.00   **FUD** XXX   E

3056F Left ventricular ejection fraction (LVEF) greater than 35% or no LVEF result available (HF)
🔧 0.00   ⚖ 0.00   **FUD** XXX   E

3060F Positive microalbuminuria test result documented and reviewed (DM)
🔧 0.00   ⚖ 0.00   **FUD** XXX   M PQ

3061F Negative microalbuminuria test result documented and reviewed (DM)
🔧 0.00   ⚖ 0.00   **FUD** XXX   M PQ

3062F Positive macroalbuminuria test result documented and reviewed (DM)
🔧 0.00   ⚖ 0.00   **FUD** XXX   M PQ

3066F Documentation of treatment for nephropathy (eg, patient receiving dialysis, patient being treated for ESRD, CRF, ARF, or renal insufficiency, any visit to a nephrologist) (DM)
🔧 0.00   ⚖ 0.00   **FUD** XXX   M PQ

3072F Low risk for retinopathy (no evidence of retinopathy in the prior year) (DM)
🔧 0.00   ⚖ 0.00   **FUD** XXX   M PQ
AMA: 2008,Mar,8-12

3073F Pre-surgical (cataract) axial length, corneal power measurement and method of intraocular lens power calculation documented within 12 months prior to surgery (EC)
🔧 0.00   ⚖ 0.00   **FUD** XXX   E
AMA: 2008,Mar,8-12

3074F Most recent systolic blood pressure less than 130 mm Hg (DM), (HTN, CKD, CAD)
🔧 0.00   ⚖ 0.00   **FUD** XXX   E PQ
AMA: 2008,Mar,8-12

3075F Most recent systolic blood pressure 130 - 139 mm Hg (DM),(HTN, CKD, CAD)
🔧 0.00   ⚖ 0.00   **FUD** XXX   E PQ
AMA: 2008,Mar,8-12

3077F Most recent systolic blood pressure greater than or equal to 140 mm Hg (HTN, CKD, CAD) (DM)
🔧 0.00   ⚖ 0.00   **FUD** XXX   E PQ
AMA: 2008,Mar,8-12

3078F Most recent diastolic blood pressure less than 80 mm Hg (HTN, CKD, CAD) (DM)
🔧 0.00   ⚖ 0.00   **FUD** XXX   E PQ
AMA: 2008,Mar,8-12

3079F Most recent diastolic blood pressure 80-89 mm Hg (HTN, CKD, CAD) (DM)
🔧 0.00   ⚖ 0.00   **FUD** XXX   E PQ
AMA: 2008,Mar,8-12

3080F Most recent diastolic blood pressure greater than or equal to 90 mm Hg (HTN, CKD, CAD) (DM)
🔧 0.00   ⚖ 0.00   **FUD** XXX   E PQ
AMA: 2008,Mar,8-12

3082F Kt/V less than 1.2 (Clearance of urea [Kt]/volume [V]) (ESRD, P-ESRD)
🔧 0.00   ⚖ 0.00   **FUD** XXX   E
AMA: 2008,Mar,8-12

3083F Kt/V equal to or greater than 1.2 and less than 1.7 (Clearance of urea [Kt]/volume [V]) (ESRD, P-ESRD)
🔧 0.00   ⚖ 0.00   **FUD** XXX   E
AMA: 2008,Mar,8-12

3084F Kt/V greater than or equal to 1.7 (Clearance of urea [Kt]/volume [V]) (ESRD, P-ESRD)
🔧 0.00   ⚖ 0.00   **FUD** XXX   E
AMA: 2008,Mar,8-12

3085F Suicide risk assessed (MDD, MDD ADOL)
🔧 0.00   ⚖ 0.00   **FUD** XXX   E PQ

3088F Major depressive disorder, mild (MDD)
🔧 0.00   ⚖ 0.00   **FUD** XXX   E

3089F Major depressive disorder, moderate (MDD)
🔧 0.00   ⚖ 0.00   **FUD** XXX   E

3090F Major depressive disorder, severe without psychotic features (MDD)
🔧 0.00   ⚖ 0.00   **FUD** XXX   E

3091F Major depressive disorder, severe with psychotic features (MDD)
🔧 0.00   ⚖ 0.00   **FUD** XXX   E

3092F Major depressive disorder, in remission (MDD)
🔧 0.00   ⚖ 0.00   **FUD** XXX   E PQ

3093F Documentation of new diagnosis of initial or recurrent episode of major depressive disorder (MDD)
🔧 0.00   ⚖ 0.00   **FUD** XXX   E
AMA: 2008,Mar,8-12

3095F Central dual-energy X-ray absorptiometry (DXA) results documented (OP)(IBD)
🔧 0.00   ⚖ 0.00   **FUD** XXX   M PQ

3096F Central dual-energy X-ray absorptiometry (DXA) ordered (OP)(IBD)
🔧 0.00   ⚖ 0.00   **FUD** XXX   M PQ

3100F Carotid imaging study report (includes direct or indirect reference to measurements of distal internal carotid diameter as the denominator for stenosis measurement) (STR, RAD)
🔧 0.00   ⚖ 0.00   **FUD** XXX   M PQ
AMA: 2008,Mar,8-12

3110F Documentation in final CT or MRI report of presence or absence of hemorrhage and mass lesion and acute infarction (STR)

🔧 0.00 ⚖ 0.00 **FUD** XXX Ⓔ 🄿🄾

3111F CT or MRI of the brain performed in the hospital within 24 hours of arrival or performed in an outpatient imaging center, to confirm initial diagnosis of stroke, TIA or intracranial hemorrhage (STR)

🔧 0.00 ⚖ 0.00 **FUD** XXX Ⓔ 🄿🄾

3112F CT or MRI of the brain performed greater than 24 hours after arrival to the hospital or performed in an outpatient imaging center for purpose other than confirmation of initial diagnosis of stroke, TIA, or intracranial hemorrhage (STR)

🔧 0.00 ⚖ 0.00 **FUD** XXX Ⓔ 🄿🄾

3115F Quantitative results of an evaluation of current level of activity and clinical symptoms (HF)

🔧 0.00 ⚖ 0.00 **FUD** XXX Ⓔ

3117F Heart failure disease specific structured assessment tool completed (HF)

🔧 0.00 ⚖ 0.00 **FUD** XXX Ⓔ

3118F New York Heart Association (NYHA) Class documented (HF)

🔧 0.00 ⚖ 0.00 **FUD** XXX Ⓔ

3119F No evaluation of level of activity or clinical symptoms (HF)

🔧 0.00 ⚖ 0.00 **FUD** XXX Ⓔ

3120F 12-Lead ECG Performed (EM)

🔧 0.00 ⚖ 0.00 **FUD** XXX Ⓜ 🄿🄾

3126F Esophageal biopsy report with a statement about dysplasia (present, absent, or indefinite, and if present, contains appropriate grading) (PATH)

🔧 0.00 ⚖ 0.00 **FUD** XXX Ⓜ

3130F Upper gastrointestinal endoscopy performed (GERD)

🔧 0.00 ⚖ 0.00 **FUD** XXX Ⓔ

3132F Documentation of referral for upper gastrointestinal endoscopy (GERD)

🔧 0.00 ⚖ 0.00 **FUD** XXX Ⓔ

3140F Upper gastrointestinal endoscopy report indicates suspicion of Barrett's esophagus (GERD)

🔧 0.00 ⚖ 0.00 **FUD** XXX Ⓔ

3141F Upper gastrointestinal endoscopy report indicates no suspicion of Barrett's esophagus (GERD)

🔧 0.00 ⚖ 0.00 **FUD** XXX Ⓔ

3142F Barium swallow test ordered (GERD)

🔧 0.00 ⚖ 0.00 **FUD** XXX Ⓔ

INCLUDES Documentation of barium swallow test

3150F Forceps esophageal biopsy performed (GERD)

🔧 0.00 ⚖ 0.00 **FUD** XXX Ⓔ

3155F Cytogenetic testing performed on bone marrow at time of diagnosis or prior to initiating treatment (HEM)

🔧 0.00 ⚖ 0.00 **FUD** XXX Ⓜ 🄿🄾

AMA: 2008,Mar,8-12

3160F Documentation of iron stores prior to initiating erythropoietin therapy (HEM)

🔧 0.00 ⚖ 0.00 **FUD** XXX Ⓜ 🄿🄾

AMA: 2008,Mar,8-12

3170F Flow cytometry studies performed at time of diagnosis or prior to initiating treatment (HEM)

🔧 0.00 ⚖ 0.00 **FUD** XXX Ⓜ 🄿🄾

AMA: 2008,Mar,8-12

3200F Barium swallow test not ordered (GERD)

🔧 0.00 ⚖ 0.00 **FUD** XXX Ⓔ

3210F Group A Strep Test Performed (PHAR)

🔧 0.00 ⚖ 0.00 **FUD** XXX Ⓜ 🄿🄾

AMA: 2008,Mar,8-12

3215F Patient has documented immunity to Hepatitis A (HEP-C)

🔧 0.00 ⚖ 0.00 **FUD** XXX Ⓜ 🄿🄾

AMA: 2008,Mar,8-12

3216F Patient has documented immunity to Hepatitis B (HEP-C)(IBD)

🔧 0.00 ⚖ 0.00 **FUD** XXX Ⓔ 🄿🄾

AMA: 2008,Mar,8-12

3218F RNA testing for Hepatitis C documented as performed within 6 months prior to initiation of antiviral treatment for Hepatitis C (HEP-C)

🔧 0.00 ⚖ 0.00 **FUD** XXX Ⓔ 🄿🄾

AMA: 2008,Mar,8-12

3220F Hepatitis C quantitative RNA testing documented as performed at 12 weeks from initiation of antiviral treatment (HEP-C)

🔧 0.00 ⚖ 0.00 **FUD** XXX Ⓔ 🄿🄾

AMA: 2008,Mar,8-12

3230F Documentation that hearing test was performed within 6 months prior to tympanostomy tube insertion (OME)

🔧 0.00 ⚖ 0.00 **FUD** XXX Ⓔ

AMA: 2008,Mar,8-12

3250F Specimen site other than anatomic location of primary tumor (PATH)

🔧 0.00 ⚖ 0.00 **FUD** XXX Ⓜ 🄿🄾

3260F pT category (primary tumor), pN category (regional lymph nodes), and histologic grade documented in pathology report (PATH)

🔧 0.00 ⚖ 0.00 **FUD** XXX Ⓜ 🄿🄾

AMA: 2008,Mar,8-12

3265F Ribonucleic acid (RNA) testing for Hepatitis C viremia ordered or results documented (HEP C)

🔧 0.00 ⚖ 0.00 **FUD** XXX Ⓔ 🄿🄾

AMA: 2008,Mar,8-12

3266F Hepatitis C genotype testing documented as performed prior to initiation of antiviral treatment for Hepatitis C (HEP C)

🔧 0.00 ⚖ 0.00 **FUD** XXX Ⓔ 🄿🄾

AMA: 2008,Mar,8-12

3267F Pathology report includes pT category, pN category, Gleason score, and statement about margin status (PATH)

🔧 0.00 ⚖ 0.00 **FUD** XXX Ⓜ 🄿🄾

3268F Prostate-specific antigen (PSA), and primary tumor (T) stage, and Gleason score documented prior to initiation of treatment (PRCA)

🔧 0.00 ⚖ 0.00 **FUD** XXX Ⓔ

AMA: 2008,Mar,8-12

3269F Bone scan performed prior to initiation of treatment or at any time since diagnosis of prostate cancer (PRCA)

🔧 0.00 ⚖ 0.00 **FUD** XXX Ⓜ 🄿🄾

AMA: 2008,Mar,8-12

3270F Bone scan not performed prior to initiation of treatment nor at any time since diagnosis of prostate cancer (PRCA)

🔧 0.00 ⚖ 0.00 **FUD** XXX Ⓜ 🄿🄾

AMA: 2008,Mar,8-12

3271F Low risk of recurrence, prostate cancer (PRCA)

🔧 0.00 ⚖ 0.00 **FUD** XXX Ⓜ 🄿🄾

AMA: 2008,Mar,8-12

3272F Intermediate risk of recurrence, prostate cancer (PRCA)

🔧 0.00 ⚖ 0.00 **FUD** XXX Ⓔ 🄿🄾

AMA: 2008,Mar,8-12

3273F High risk of recurrence, prostate cancer (PRCA)

🔧 0.00 ⚖ 0.00 **FUD** XXX Ⓔ 🄿🄾

AMA: 2008,Mar,8-12

3274F Prostate cancer risk of recurrence not determined or neither low, intermediate nor high (PRCA)
🔧 0.00 ✂ 0.00 **FUD** XXX E P0
AMA: 2008,Mar,8-12

3278F Serum levels of calcium, phosphorus, intact Parathyroid Hormone (PTH) and lipid profile ordered (CKD)
🔧 0.00 ✂ 0.00 **FUD** XXX E
AMA: 2008,Mar,8-12

3279F Hemoglobin level greater than or equal to 13 g/dL (CKD, ESRD)
🔧 0.00 ✂ 0.00 **FUD** XXX E
AMA: 2008,Mar,8-12

3280F Hemoglobin level 11 g/dL to 12.9 g/dL (CKD, ESRD)
🔧 0.00 ✂ 0.00 **FUD** XXX E
AMA: 2008,Mar,8-12

3281F Hemoglobin level less than 11 g/dL (CKD, ESRD)
🔧 0.00 ✂ 0.00 **FUD** XXX E
AMA: 2008,Mar,8-12

3284F Intraocular pressure (IOP) reduced by a value of greater than or equal to 15% from the pre-intervention level (EC)
🔧 0.00 ✂ 0.00 **FUD** XXX M P0
AMA: 2008,Mar,8-12

3285F Intraocular pressure (IOP) reduced by a value less than 15% from the pre-intervention level (EC)
🔧 0.00 ✂ 0.00 **FUD** XXX M P0
AMA: 2008,Mar,8-12

3288F Falls risk assessment documented (GER)
🔧 0.00 ✂ 0.00 **FUD** XXX M P0
AMA: 2008,Mar,8-12

3290F Patient is D (Rh) negative and unsensitized (Pre-Cr)
🔧 0.00 ✂ 0.00 **FUD** XXX E
AMA: 2008,Mar,8-12

3291F Patient is D (Rh) positive or sensitized (Pre-Cr)
🔧 0.00 ✂ 0.00 **FUD** XXX E
AMA: 2008,Mar,8-12

3292F HIV testing ordered or documented and reviewed during the first or second prenatal visit (Pre-Cr)
🔧 0.00 ✂ 0.00 **FUD** XXX E
AMA: 2008,Mar,8-12

3293F ABO and Rh blood typing documented as performed (Pre-Cr)
🔧 0.00 ✂ 0.00 **FUD** XXX E
AMA: 2008,Mar,8-12

3294F Group B Streptococcus (GBS) screening documented as performed during week 35-37 gestation (Pre-Cr)
🔧 0.00 ✂ 0.00 **FUD** XXX E
AMA: 2008,Mar,8-12

3300F American Joint Committee on Cancer (AJCC) stage documented and reviewed (ONC)
🔧 0.00 ✂ 0.00 **FUD** XXX M P0
AMA: 2008,Mar,8-12

3301F Cancer stage documented in medical record as metastatic and reviewed (ONC)
EXCLUDES Cancer staging measures (3321F-3390F)
🔧 0.00 ✂ 0.00 **FUD** XXX M P0
AMA: 2008,Mar,8-12

3315F Estrogen receptor (ER) or progesterone receptor (PR) positive breast cancer (ONC)
🔧 0.00 ✂ 0.00 **FUD** XXX M P0
AMA: 2008,Mar,8-12

3316F Estrogen receptor (ER) and progesterone receptor (PR) negative breast cancer (ONC)
🔧 0.00 ✂ 0.00 **FUD** XXX M P0
AMA: 2008,Mar,8-12

3317F Pathology report confirming malignancy documented in the medical record and reviewed prior to the initiation of chemotherapy (ONC)
🔧 0.00 ✂ 0.00 **FUD** XXX E
AMA: 2008,Mar,8-12

3318F Pathology report confirming malignancy documented in the medical record and reviewed prior to the initiation of radiation therapy (ONC)
🔧 0.00 ✂ 0.00 **FUD** XXX E
AMA: 2008,Mar,8-12

3319F 1 of the following diagnostic imaging studies ordered: chest x-ray, CT, Ultrasound, MRI, PET, or nuclear medicine scans (ML)
🔧 0.00 ✂ 0.00 **FUD** XXX M P0
AMA: 2008,Mar,8-12

3320F None of the following diagnostic imaging studies ordered: chest X-ray, CT, Ultrasound, MRI, PET, or nuclear medicine scans (ML)
🔧 0.00 ✂ 0.00 **FUD** XXX M P0
AMA: 2008,Mar,8-12

3321F AJCC Cancer Stage 0 or IA Melanoma, documented (ML)
🔧 0.00 ✂ 0.00 **FUD** XXX M

3322F Melanoma greater than AJCC Stage 0 or IA (ML)
🔧 0.00 ✂ 0.00 **FUD** XXX M

3323F Clinical tumor, node and metastases (TNM) staging documented and reviewed prior to surgery (Lung/Esop Cx)
🔧 0.00 ✂ 0.00 **FUD** XXX E P0

3324F MRI or CT scan ordered, reviewed or requested (EPI)
🔧 0.00 ✂ 0.00 **FUD** XXX E

3325F Preoperative assessment of functional or medical indication(s) for surgery prior to the cataract surgery with intraocular lens placement (must be performed within 12 months prior to cataract surgery) (EC)
🔧 0.00 ✂ 0.00 **FUD** XXX E
AMA: 2008,Mar,8-12

3328F Performance status documented and reviewed within 2 weeks prior to surgery (Lung/Esop Cx)
🔧 0.00 ✂ 0.00 **FUD** XXX E P0

3330F Imaging study ordered (BkP)
🔧 0.00 ✂ 0.00 **FUD** XXX E

3331F Imaging study not ordered (BkP)
🔧 0.00 ✂ 0.00 **FUD** XXX E
AMA: 2008,Mar,8-12

3340F Mammogram assessment category of "incomplete: need additional imaging evaluation" documented (RAD)
🔧 0.00 ✂ 0.00 **FUD** XXX M P0
AMA: 2008,Mar,8-12

3341F Mammogram assessment category of "negative," documented (RAD)
🔧 0.00 ✂ 0.00 **FUD** XXX M P0
AMA: 2008,Mar,8-12

3342F Mammogram assessment category of "benign," documented (RAD)
🔧 0.00 ✂ 0.00 **FUD** XXX M P0
AMA: 2008,Mar,8-12

3343F Mammogram assessment category of "probably benign," documented (RAD)
🔧 0.00 ✂ 0.00 **FUD** XXX M P0
AMA: 2008,Mar,8-12

3344F Mammogram assessment category of "suspicious," documented (RAD)
🔧 0.00 ✂ 0.00 **FUD** XXX M P0
AMA: 2008,Mar,8-12

3345F Mammogram assessment category of "highly suggestive of malignancy," documented (RAD)

    🚗 0.00   🔧 0.00   **FUD** XXX   Ⓜ 🅿️

    AMA: 2008,Mar,8-12

3350F Mammogram assessment category of "known biopsy proven malignancy," documented (RAD)

    🚗 0.00   🔧 0.00   **FUD** XXX   Ⓜ 🅿️

    AMA: 2008,Mar,8-12

3351F Negative screen for depressive symptoms as categorized by using a standardized depression screening/assessment tool (MDD)

    🚗 0.00   🔧 0.00   **FUD** XXX   Ⓔ

3352F No significant depressive symptoms as categorized by using a standardized depression assessment tool (MDD)

    🚗 0.00   🔧 0.00   **FUD** XXX   Ⓔ

3353F Mild to moderate depressive symptoms as categorized by using a standardized depression screening/assessment tool (MDD)

    🚗 0.00   🔧 0.00   **FUD** XXX   Ⓔ

3354F Clinically significant depressive symptoms as categorized by using a standardized depression screening/assessment tool (MDD)

    🚗 0.00   🔧 0.00   **FUD** XXX   Ⓔ

3370F AJCC Breast Cancer Stage 0 documented (ONC)

    🚗 0.00   🔧 0.00   **FUD** XXX   Ⓜ 🅿️

3372F AJCC Breast Cancer Stage I: T1mic, T1a or T1b (tumor size ≤ 1 cm) documented (ONC)

    🚗 0.00   🔧 0.00   **FUD** XXX   Ⓜ 🅿️

3374F AJCC Breast Cancer Stage I: T1c (tumor size > 1 cm to 2 cm) documented (ONC)

    🚗 0.00   🔧 0.00   **FUD** XXX   Ⓜ 🅿️

3376F AJCC Breast Cancer Stage II documented (ONC)

    🚗 0.00   🔧 0.00   **FUD** XXX   Ⓜ 🅿️

3378F AJCC Breast Cancer Stage III documented (ONC)

    🚗 0.00   🔧 0.00   **FUD** XXX   Ⓜ 🅿️

3380F AJCC Breast Cancer Stage IV documented (ONC)

    🚗 0.00   🔧 0.00   **FUD** XXX   Ⓜ 🅿️

3382F AJCC colon cancer, Stage 0 documented (ONC)

    🚗 0.00   🔧 0.00   **FUD** XXX   Ⓜ 🅿️

3384F AJCC colon cancer, Stage I documented (ONC)

    🚗 0.00   🔧 0.00   **FUD** XXX   Ⓜ 🅿️

3386F AJCC colon cancer, Stage II documented (ONC)

    🚗 0.00   🔧 0.00   **FUD** XXX   Ⓜ 🅿️

3388F AJCC colon cancer, Stage III documented (ONC)

    🚗 0.00   🔧 0.00   **FUD** XXX   Ⓜ 🅿️

3390F AJCC colon cancer, Stage IV documented (ONC)

    🚗 0.00   🔧 0.00   **FUD** XXX   Ⓜ 🅿️

3394F Quantitative HER2 immunohistochemistry (IHC) evaluation of breast cancer consistent with the scoring system defined in the ASCO/CAP guidelines (PATH)

    🚗 0.00   🔧 0.00   **FUD** XXX   Ⓜ 🅿️

3395F Quantitative non-HER2 immunohistochemistry (IHC) evaluation of breast cancer (eg, testing for estrogen or progesterone receptors [ER/PR]) performed (PATH)

    🚗 0.00   🔧 0.00   **FUD** XXX   Ⓜ 🅿️

3450F Dyspnea screened, no dyspnea or mild dyspnea (Pall Cr)

    🚗 0.00   🔧 0.00   **FUD** XXX   Ⓔ

3451F Dyspnea screened, moderate or severe dyspnea (Pall Cr)

    🚗 0.00   🔧 0.00   **FUD** XXX   Ⓔ

3452F Dyspnea not screened (Pall Cr)

    🚗 0.00   🔧 0.00   **FUD** XXX   Ⓔ

3455F TB screening performed and results interpreted within six months prior to initiation of first-time biologic disease modifying anti-rheumatic drug therapy for RA (RA)

    🚗 0.00   🔧 0.00   **FUD** XXX   Ⓜ 🅿️

3470F Rheumatoid arthritis (RA) disease activity, low (RA)

    🚗 0.00   🔧 0.00   **FUD** XXX   Ⓜ 🅿️

3471F Rheumatoid arthritis (RA) disease activity, moderate (RA)

    🚗 0.00   🔧 0.00   **FUD** XXX   Ⓜ 🅿️

3472F Rheumatoid arthritis (RA) disease activity, high (RA)

    🚗 0.00   🔧 0.00   **FUD** XXX   Ⓜ 🅿️

3475F Disease prognosis for rheumatoid arthritis assessed, poor prognosis documented (RA)

    🚗 0.00   🔧 0.00   **FUD** XXX   Ⓜ 🅿️

3476F Disease prognosis for rheumatoid arthritis assessed, good prognosis documented (RA)

    🚗 0.00   🔧 0.00   **FUD** XXX   Ⓜ 🅿️

3490F History of AIDS-defining condition (HIV)

    🚗 0.00   🔧 0.00   **FUD** XXX   Ⓔ 🅿️

3491F HIV indeterminate (infants of undetermined HIV status born of HIV-infected mothers) (HIV)

    🚗 0.00   🔧 0.00   **FUD** XXX   Ⓔ

3492F History of nadir CD4+ cell count <350 cells/mm3 (HIV)

    🚗 0.00   🔧 0.00   **FUD** XXX   Ⓔ 🅿️

3493F No history of nadir CD4+ cell count <350 cells/mm3 and no history of AIDS-defining condition (HIV)

    🚗 0.00   🔧 0.00   **FUD** XXX   Ⓔ 🅿️

3494F CD4+ cell count <200 cells/mm3 (HIV)

    🚗 0.00   🔧 0.00   **FUD** XXX   Ⓜ 🅿️

3495F CD4+ cell count 200 - 499 cells/mm3 (HIV)

    🚗 0.00   🔧 0.00   **FUD** XXX   Ⓜ 🅿️

3496F CD4+ cell count ≥ 500 cells/mm3 (HIV)

    🚗 0.00   🔧 0.00   **FUD** XXX   Ⓜ 🅿️

3497F CD4+ cell percentage <15% (HIV)

    🚗 0.00   🔧 0.00   **FUD** XXX   Ⓔ

3498F CD4+ cell percentage ≥ 15% (HIV)

    🚗 0.00   🔧 0.00   **FUD** XXX   Ⓔ

3500F CD4+ cell count or CD4+ cell percentage documented as performed (HIV)

    🚗 0.00   🔧 0.00   **FUD** XXX   Ⓔ 🅿️

3502F HIV RNA viral load below limits of quantification (HIV)

    🚗 0.00   🔧 0.00   **FUD** XXX   Ⓔ 🅿️

3503F HIV RNA viral load not below limits of quantification (HIV)

    🚗 0.00   🔧 0.00   **FUD** XXX   Ⓔ 🅿️

3510F Documentation that tuberculosis (TB) screening test performed and results interpreted (HIV) (IBD)

    🚗 0.00   🔧 0.00   **FUD** XXX   Ⓜ

3511F Chlamydia and gonorrhea screenings documented as performed (HIV)

    🚗 0.00   🔧 0.00   **FUD** XXX   Ⓔ 🅿️

3512F Syphilis screening documented as performed (HIV)

    🚗 0.00   🔧 0.00   **FUD** XXX   Ⓔ 🅿️

3513F Hepatitis B screening documented as performed (HIV)

    🚗 0.00   🔧 0.00   **FUD** XXX   Ⓔ

3514F Hepatitis C screening documented as performed (HIV)

    🚗 0.00   🔧 0.00   **FUD** XXX   Ⓔ

3515F Patient has documented immunity to Hepatitis C (HIV)

    🚗 0.00   🔧 0.00   **FUD** XXX   Ⓔ

3517F Hepatitis B Virus (HBV) status assessed and results interpreted within one year prior to receiving a first course of anti-TNF (tumor necrosis factor) therapy (IBD)

    🚗 0.00   🔧 0.00   **FUD** XXX   Ⓜ

3520F	**Clostridium difficile testing performed (IBD)**
	0.00 0.00 **FUD** XXX E
3550F	**Low risk for thromboembolism (AFIB)**
	0.00 0.00 **FUD** XXX E
3551F	**Intermediate risk for thromboembolism (AFIB)**
	0.00 0.00 **FUD** XXX E
3552F	**High risk for thromboembolism (AFIB)**
	0.00 0.00 **FUD** XXX E
3555F	**Patient had International Normalized Ratio (INR) measurement performed (AFIB)**
	0.00 0.00 **FUD** XXX E
	AMA: 2010,Jul,3-5
3570F	**Final report for bone scintigraphy study includes correlation with existing relevant imaging studies (eg, x-ray, MRI, CT) corresponding to the same anatomical region in question (NUC_MED)**
	0.00 0.00 **FUD** XXX M PQ
3572F	**Patient considered to be potentially at risk for fracture in a weight-bearing site (NUC_MED)**
	0.00 0.00 **FUD** XXX E
3573F	**Patient not considered to be potentially at risk for fracture in a weight-bearing site (NUC_MED)**
	0.00 0.00 **FUD** XXX E
3650F	**Electroencephalogram (EEG) ordered, reviewed or requested (EPI)**
	0.00 0.00 **FUD** XXX E
3700F	**Psychiatric disorders or disturbances assessed (Prkns)**
	0.00 0.00 **FUD** XXX M
3720F	**Cognitive impairment or dysfunction assessed (Prkns)**
	0.00 0.00 **FUD** XXX M
3725F	**Screening for depression performed (DEM)**
	0.00 0.00 **FUD** XXX M
3750F	**Patient not receiving dose of corticosteroids greater than or equal to 10mg/day for 60 or greater consecutive days (IBD)**
	0.00 0.00 **FUD** XXX E
3751F	**Electrodiagnostic studies for distal symmetric polyneuropathy conducted (or requested), documented, and reviewed within 6 months of initial evaluation for condition (DSP)**
	0.00 0.00 **FUD** XXX E
3752F	**Electrodiagnostic studies for distal symmetric polyneuropathy not conducted (or requested), documented, or reviewed within 6 months of initial evaluation for condition (DSP)**
	0.00 0.00 **FUD** XXX E
3753F	**Patient has clear clinical symptoms and signs that are highly suggestive of neuropathy AND cannot be attributed to another condition, AND has an obvious cause for the neuropathy (DSP)**
	0.00 0.00 **FUD** XXX E
3754F	**Screening tests for diabetes mellitus reviewed, requested, or ordered (DSP)**
	0.00 0.00 **FUD** XXX E
3755F	**Cognitive and behavioral impairment screening performed (ALS)**
	0.00 0.00 **FUD** XXX E
3756F	**Patient has pseudobulbar affect, sialorrhea, or ALS-related symptoms (ALS)**
	0.00 0.00 **FUD** XXX E
3757F	**Patient does not have pseudobulbar affect, sialorrhea, or ALS-related symptoms (ALS)**
	0.00 0.00 **FUD** XXX E
3758F	**Patient referred for pulmonary function testing or peak cough expiratory flow (ALS)**
	0.00 0.00 **FUD** XXX E
3759F	**Patient screened for dysphagia, weight loss, and impaired nutrition, and results documented (ALS)**
	0.00 0.00 **FUD** XXX E
3760F	**Patient exhibits dysphagia, weight loss, or impaired nutrition (ALS)**
	0.00 0.00 **FUD** XXX E
3761F	**Patient does not exhibit dysphagia, weight loss, or impaired nutrition (ALS)**
	0.00 0.00 **FUD** XXX E
3762F	**Patient is dysarthric (ALS)**
	0.00 0.00 **FUD** XXX E
3763F	**Patient is not dysarthric (ALS)**
	0.00 0.00 **FUD** XXX E
3775F	**Adenoma(s) or other neoplasm detected during screening colonoscopy (SCADR)**
	0.00 0.00 **FUD** XXX M
3776F	**Adenoma(s) or other neoplasm not detected during screening colonoscopy (SCADR)**
	0.00 0.00 **FUD** XXX M

4000F-4563F Therapies Provided (Includes Preventive Services)

INCLUDES   Behavioral/pharmacologic/procedural therapies
Preventive services including patient education/counseling

4000F	**Tobacco use cessation intervention, counseling (COPD, CAP, CAD, Asthma) (DM) (PV)**
	0.00 0.00 **FUD** XXX E PQ
	AMA: 2015,Jan,16; 2014,Jan,11
4001F	**Tobacco use cessation intervention, pharmacologic therapy (COPD, CAD, CAP, PV, Asthma) (DM) (PV)**
	0.00 0.00 **FUD** XXX E PQ
	AMA: 2008,Mar,8-12; 2004,Nov,1
4003F	**Patient education, written/oral, appropriate for patients with heart failure, performed (NMA-No Measure Associated)**
	0.00 0.00 **FUD** XXX E
	AMA: 2004,Nov,1
4004F	**Patient screened for tobacco use and received tobacco cessation intervention (counseling, pharmacotherapy, or both), if identified as a tobacco user (PV, CAD)**
	0.00 0.00 **FUD** XXX M PQ
4005F	**Pharmacologic therapy (other than minerals/vitamins) for osteoporosis prescribed (OP) (IBD)**
	0.00 0.00 **FUD** XXX M PQ
4008F	**Beta-blocker therapy prescribed or currently being taken (CAD,HF)**
	0.00 0.00 **FUD** XXX M PQ
4010F	**Angiotensin Converting Enzyme (ACE) Inhibitor or Angiotensin Receptor Blocker (ARB) therapy prescribed or currently being taken (CAD, CKD, HF) (DM)**
	0.00 0.00 **FUD** XXX M PQ
4011F	**Oral antiplatelet therapy prescribed (CAD)**
	0.00 0.00 **FUD** XXX E
	AMA: 2004,Nov,1
4012F	**Warfarin therapy prescribed (NMA-No Measure Associated)**
	0.00 0.00 **FUD** XXX E
4013F	**Statin therapy prescribed or currently being taken (CAD)**
	0.00 0.00 **FUD** XXX E PQ
4014F	**Written discharge instructions provided to heart failure patients discharged home (Instructions include all of the following components: activity level, diet, discharge medications, follow-up appointment, weight monitoring, what to do if symptoms worsen) (NMA-No Measure Associated)**
	0.00 0.00 **FUD** XXX E

Category II Codes

3520F — 4014F

4015F Persistent asthma, preferred long term control medication or an acceptable alternative treatment, prescribed (NMA-No Measure Associated)

🚑 0.00   ✂ 0.00   **FUD** XXX

ⓔ

Code also modifier 2P for patient reasons for not prescribing
Do not report with modifier 1P

4016F Anti-inflammatory/analgesic agent prescribed (OA) (Use for prescribed or continued medication[s], including over-the-counter medication[s])

🚑 0.00   ✂ 0.00   **FUD** XXX

ⓔ

INCLUDES   Over-the-counter medication(s)
Prescribed/continued medication(s)

4017F Gastrointestinal prophylaxis for NSAID use prescribed (OA)

🚑 0.00   ✂ 0.00   **FUD** XXX

ⓔ

4018F Therapeutic exercise for the involved joint(s) instructed or physical or occupational therapy prescribed (OA)

🚑 0.00   ✂ 0.00   **FUD** XXX

ⓔ

4019F Documentation of receipt of counseling on exercise and either both calcium and vitamin D use or counseling regarding both calcium and vitamin D use (OP)

🚑 0.00   ✂ 0.00   **FUD** XXX

ⓔ

4025F Inhaled bronchodilator prescribed (COPD)

🚑 0.00   ✂ 0.00   **FUD** XXX

Ⓜ P0

4030F Long-term oxygen therapy prescribed (more than 15 hours per day) (COPD)

🚑 0.00   ✂ 0.00   **FUD** XXX

ⓔ

4033F Pulmonary rehabilitation exercise training recommended (COPD)

🚑 0.00   ✂ 0.00   **FUD** XXX

ⓔ

Code also dyspnea assessed, present (1019F)

4035F Influenza immunization recommended (COPD) (IBD)

🚑 0.00   ✂ 0.00   **FUD** XXX

ⓔ

AMA: 2008,Mar,8-12

4037F Influenza immunization ordered or administered (COPD, PV, CKD, ESRD)(IBD)

🚑 0.00   ✂ 0.00   **FUD** XXX

ⓔ

AMA: 2008,Mar,8-12

4040F Pneumococcal vaccine administered or previously received (COPD) (PV), (IBD)

🚑 0.00   ✂ 0.00   **FUD** XXX

Ⓜ P0

AMA: 2008,Mar,8-12

4041F Documentation of order for cefazolin OR cefuroxime for antimicrobial prophylaxis (PERI 2)

🚑 0.00   ✂ 0.00   **FUD** XXX

ⓔ P0

4042F Documentation that prophylactic antibiotics were neither given within 4 hours prior to surgical incision nor given intraoperatively (PERI 2)

🚑 0.00   ✂ 0.00   **FUD** XXX

Ⓜ P0

4043F Documentation that an order was given to discontinue prophylactic antibiotics within 48 hours of surgical end time, cardiac procedures (PERI 2)

🚑 0.00   ✂ 0.00   **FUD** XXX

ⓔ P0

4044F Documentation that an order was given for venous thromboembolism (VTE) prophylaxis to be given within 24 hours prior to incision time or 24 hours after surgery end time (PERI 2)

🚑 0.00   ✂ 0.00   **FUD** XXX

Ⓜ P0

4045F Appropriate empiric antibiotic prescribed (CAP), (EM)

🚑 0.00   ✂ 0.00   **FUD** XXX

ⓔ P0

4046F Documentation that prophylactic antibiotics were given within 4 hours prior to surgical incision or given intraoperatively (PERI 2)

🚑 0.00   ✂ 0.00   **FUD** XXX

Ⓜ P0

4047F Documentation of order for prophylactic parenteral antibiotics to be given within 1 hour (if fluoroquinolone or vancomycin, 2 hours) prior to surgical incision (or start of procedure when no incision is required) (PERI 2)

🚑 0.00   ✂ 0.00   **FUD** XXX

ⓔ P0

4048F Documentation that administration of prophylactic parenteral antibiotic was initiated within 1 hour (if fluoroquinolone or vancomycin, 2 hours) prior to surgical incision (or start of procedure when no incision is required) as ordered (PERI 2)

🚑 0.00   ✂ 0.00   **FUD** XXX

ⓔ P0

4049F Documentation that order was given to discontinue prophylactic antibiotics within 24 hours of surgical end time, non-cardiac procedure (PERI 2)

🚑 0.00   ✂ 0.00   **FUD** XXX

Ⓜ P0

4050F Hypertension plan of care documented as appropriate (NMA-No Measure Associated)

🚑 0.00   ✂ 0.00   **FUD** XXX

ⓔ P0

4051F Referred for an arteriovenous (AV) fistula (ESRD, CKD)

🚑 0.00   ✂ 0.00   **FUD** XXX

ⓔ

AMA: 2008,Mar,8-12

4052F Hemodialysis via functioning arteriovenous (AV) fistula (ESRD)

🚑 0.00   ✂ 0.00   **FUD** XXX

ⓔ

AMA: 2008,Mar,8-12

4053F Hemodialysis via functioning arteriovenous (AV) graft (ESRD)

🚑 0.00   ✂ 0.00   **FUD** XXX

ⓔ

AMA: 2008,Mar,8-12

4054F Hemodialysis via catheter (ESRD)

🚑 0.00   ✂ 0.00   **FUD** XXX

ⓔ

AMA: 2008,Mar,8-12

4055F Patient receiving peritoneal dialysis (ESRD)

🚑 0.00   ✂ 0.00   **FUD** XXX

ⓔ

AMA: 2008,Mar,8-12

4056F Appropriate oral rehydration solution recommended (PAG)

🚑 0.00   ✂ 0.00   **FUD** XXX

ⓔ

4058F Pediatric gastroenteritis education provided to caregiver (PAG)

🚑 0.00   ✂ 0.00   **FUD** XXX

ⓔ

4060F Psychotherapy services provided (MDD, MDD ADOL)

🚑 0.00   ✂ 0.00   **FUD** XXX

ⓔ

4062F Patient referral for psychotherapy documented (MDD, MDD ADOL)

🚑 0.00   ✂ 0.00   **FUD** XXX

ⓔ

4063F Antidepressant pharmacotherapy considered and not prescribed (MDD ADOL)

🚑 0.00   ✂ 0.00   **FUD** XXX

ⓔ

4064F Antidepressant pharmacotherapy prescribed (MDD, MDD ADOL)

🚑 0.00   ✂ 0.00   **FUD** XXX

ⓔ

4065F Antipsychotic pharmacotherapy prescribed (MDD)

🚑 0.00   ✂ 0.00   **FUD** XXX

ⓔ

4066F Electroconvulsive therapy (ECT) provided (MDD)

🚑 0.00   ✂ 0.00   **FUD** XXX

ⓔ

4067F Patient referral for electroconvulsive therapy (ECT) documented (MDD)

🚑 0.00   ✂ 0.00   **FUD** XXX

ⓔ

4069F Venous thromboembolism (VTE) prophylaxis received (IBD)

🚑 0.00   ✂ 0.00   **FUD** XXX

ⓔ

4070F Deep vein thrombosis (DVT) prophylaxis received by end of hospital day 2 (STR)
🖧 0.00 ⅋ 0.00 **FUD** XXX E PO

4073F Oral antiplatelet therapy prescribed at discharge (STR)
🖧 0.00 ⅋ 0.00 **FUD** XXX E

4075F Anticoagulant therapy prescribed at discharge (STR)
🖧 0.00 ⅋ 0.00 **FUD** XXX M PO

4077F Documentation that tissue plasminogen activator (t-PA) administration was considered (STR)
🖧 0.00 ⅋ 0.00 **FUD** XXX E

4079F Documentation that rehabilitation services were considered (STR)
🖧 0.00 ⅋ 0.00 **FUD** XXX E

4084F Aspirin received within 24 hours before emergency department arrival or during emergency department stay (EM)
🖧 0.00 ⅋ 0.00 **FUD** XXX E PO

4086F Aspirin or clopidogrel prescribed or currently being taken (CAD)
🖧 0.00 ⅋ 0.00 **FUD** XXX M PO

4090F Patient receiving erythropoietin therapy (HEM)
🖧 0.00 ⅋ 0.00 **FUD** XXX M PO
AMA: 2008,Mar,8-12

4095F Patient not receiving erythropoietin therapy (HEM)
🖧 0.00 ⅋ 0.00 **FUD** XXX E PO
AMA: 2008,Mar,8-12

4100F Bisphosphonate therapy, intravenous, ordered or received (HEM)
🖧 0.00 ⅋ 0.00 **FUD** XXX M PO
AMA: 2008,Mar,8-12

4110F Internal mammary artery graft performed for primary, isolated coronary artery bypass graft procedure (CABG)
🖧 0.00 ⅋ 0.00 **FUD** XXX M PO

4115F Beta blocker administered within 24 hours prior to surgical incision (CABG)
🖧 0.00 ⅋ 0.00 **FUD** XXX M PO

4120F Antibiotic prescribed or dispensed (URI, PHAR), (A-BRONCH)
🖧 0.00 ⅋ 0.00 **FUD** XXX M PO
AMA: 2008,Mar,8-12

4124F Antibiotic neither prescribed nor dispensed (URI, PHAR), (A-BRONCH)
🖧 0.00 ⅋ 0.00 **FUD** XXX M PO
AMA: 2008,Mar,8-12

4130F Topical preparations (including OTC) prescribed for acute otitis externa (AOE)
🖧 0.00 ⅋ 0.00 **FUD** XXX M PO
AMA: 2010,Jan,6-7

4131F Systemic antimicrobial therapy prescribed (AOE)
🖧 0.00 ⅋ 0.00 **FUD** XXX M PO
AMA: 2008,Mar,8-12

4132F Systemic antimicrobial therapy not prescribed (AOE)
🖧 0.00 ⅋ 0.00 **FUD** XXX M PO
AMA: 2008,Mar,8-12

4133F Antihistamines or decongestants prescribed or recommended (OME)
🖧 0.00 ⅋ 0.00 **FUD** XXX E
AMA: 2008,Mar,8-12

4134F Antihistamines or decongestants neither prescribed nor recommended (OME)
🖧 0.00 ⅋ 0.00 **FUD** XXX E
AMA: 2008,Mar,8-12

4135F Systemic corticosteroids prescribed (OME)
🖧 0.00 ⅋ 0.00 **FUD** XXX E
AMA: 2008,Mar,8-12

4136F Systemic corticosteroids not prescribed (OME)
🖧 0.00 ⅋ 0.00 **FUD** XXX E
AMA: 2008,Mar,8-12

4140F Inhaled corticosteroids prescribed (Asthma)
🖧 0.00 ⅋ 0.00 **FUD** XXX M PO

4142F Corticosteroid sparing therapy prescribed (IBD)
🖧 0.00 ⅋ 0.00 **FUD** XXX M

4144F Alternative long-term control medication prescribed (Asthma)
🖧 0.00 ⅋ 0.00 **FUD** XXX M PO

4145F Two or more anti-hypertensive agents prescribed or currently being taken (CAD, HTN)
🖧 0.00 ⅋ 0.00 **FUD** XXX E PO

4148F Hepatitis A vaccine injection administered or previously received (HEP-C)
🖧 0.00 ⅋ 0.00 **FUD** XXX M PO

4149F Hepatitis B vaccine injection administered or previously received (HEP-C, HIV) (IBD)
🖧 0.00 ⅋ 0.00 **FUD** XXX M PO

4150F Patient receiving antiviral treatment for Hepatitis C (HEP-C)
🖧 0.00 ⅋ 0.00 **FUD** XXX E PO
AMA: 2008,Mar,8-12

4151F Patient not receiving antiviral treatment for Hepatitis C (HEP-C)
🖧 0.00 ⅋ 0.00 **FUD** XXX M PO
AMA: 2008,Mar,8-12

4153F Combination peginterferon and ribavirin therapy prescribed (HEP-C)
🖧 0.00 ⅋ 0.00 **FUD** XXX E PO
AMA: 2008,Mar,8-12

4155F Hepatitis A vaccine series previously received (HEP-C)
🖧 0.00 ⅋ 0.00 **FUD** XXX E
AMA: 2008,Mar,8-12

4157F Hepatitis B vaccine series previously received (HEP-C)
🖧 0.00 ⅋ 0.00 **FUD** XXX E
AMA: 2008,Mar,8-12

4158F Patient counseled about risks of alcohol use (HEP-C)
🖧 0.00 ⅋ 0.00 **FUD** XXX E PO
AMA: 2008,Mar,8-12

4159F Counseling regarding contraception received prior to initiation of antiviral treatment (HEP-C)
🖧 0.00 ⅋ 0.00 **FUD** XXX E PO
AMA: 2008,Mar,8-12

4163F Patient counseling at a minimum on all of the following treatment options for clinically localized prostate cancer: active surveillance, and interstitial prostate brachytherapy, and external beam radiotherapy, and radical prostatectomy, provided prior to initiation of treatment (PRCA)
🖧 0.00 ⅋ 0.00 **FUD** XXX E
AMA: 2008,Mar,8-12

4164F Adjuvant (ie, in combination with external beam radiotherapy to the prostate for prostate cancer) hormonal therapy (gonadotropin-releasing hormone [GnRH] agonist or antagonist) prescribed/administered (PRCA)
🖧 0.00 ⅋ 0.00 **FUD** XXX M PO
AMA: 2008,Mar,8-12

4165F 3-dimensional conformal radiotherapy (3D-CRT) or intensity modulated radiation therapy (IMRT) received (PRCA)
🖧 0.00 ⅋ 0.00 **FUD** XXX E PO
AMA: 2008,Mar,8-12

4167F Head of bed elevation (30-45 degrees) on first ventilator day ordered (CRIT)

🚗 0.00   ⚕ 0.00   **FUD** XXX   E

AMA: 2008,Mar,8-12

4168F Patient receiving care in the intensive care unit (ICU) and receiving mechanical ventilation, 24 hours or less (CRIT)

🚗 0.00   ⚕ 0.00   **FUD** XXX   E

AMA: 2008,Mar,8-12

4169F Patient either not receiving care in the intensive care unit (ICU) OR not receiving mechanical ventilation OR receiving mechanical ventilation greater than 24 hours (CRIT)

🚗 0.00   ⚕ 0.00   **FUD** XXX   E

AMA: 2008,Mar,8-12

4171F Patient receiving erythropoiesis-stimulating agents (ESA) therapy (CKD)

🚗 0.00   ⚕ 0.00   **FUD** XXX   E PQ

AMA: 2008,Mar,8-12

4172F Patient not receiving erythropoiesis-stimulating agents (ESA) therapy (CKD)

🚗 0.00   ⚕ 0.00   **FUD** XXX   E PQ

AMA: 2008,Mar,8-12

4174F Counseling about the potential impact of glaucoma on visual functioning and quality of life, and importance of treatment adherence provided to patient and/or caregiver(s) (EC)

🚗 0.00   ⚕ 0.00   **FUD** XXX   E

AMA: 2008,Mar,8-12

4175F Best-corrected visual acuity of 20/40 or better (distance or near) achieved within the 90 days following cataract surgery (EC)

🚗 0.00   ⚕ 0.00   **FUD** XXX   M PQ

AMA: 2008,Mar,8-12

4176F Counseling about value of protection from UV light and lack of proven efficacy of nutritional supplements in prevention or progression of cataract development provided to patient and/or caregiver(s) (NMA-No Measure Associated)

🚗 0.00   ⚕ 0.00   **FUD** XXX   E

4177F Counseling about the benefits and/or risks of the Age-Related Eye Disease Study (AREDS) formulation for preventing progression of age-related macular degeneration (AMD) provided to patient and/or caregiver(s) (EC)

🚗 0.00   ⚕ 0.00   **FUD** XXX   M PQ

AMA: 2008,Mar,8-12

4178F Anti-D immune globulin received between 26 and 30 weeks gestation (Pre-Cr)   M

🚗 0.00   ⚕ 0.00   **FUD** XXX   E

AMA: 2008,Mar,8-12

4179F Tamoxifen or aromatase inhibitor (AI) prescribed (ONC)

🚗 0.00   ⚕ 0.00   **FUD** XXX   M PQ

AMA: 2008,Mar,8-12

4180F Adjuvant chemotherapy referred, prescribed, or previously received for Stage III colon cancer (ONC)

🚗 0.00   ⚕ 0.00   **FUD** XXX   E PQ

AMA: 2008,Mar,8-12

4181F Conformal radiation therapy received (NMA-No Measure Associated)

🚗 0.00   ⚕ 0.00   **FUD** XXX   E

4182F Conformal radiation therapy not received (NMA-No Measure Associated)

🚗 0.00   ⚕ 0.00   **FUD** XXX   E

4185F Continuous (12-months) therapy with proton pump inhibitor (PPI) or histamine H2 receptor antagonist (H2RA) received (GERD)

🚗 0.00   ⚕ 0.00   **FUD** XXX   E

AMA: 2008,Mar,8-12

4186F No continuous (12-months) therapy with either proton pump inhibitor (PPI) or histamine H2 receptor antagonist (H2RA) received (GERD)

🚗 0.00   ⚕ 0.00   **FUD** XXX   E

AMA: 2008,Mar,8-12

4187F Disease modifying anti-rheumatic drug therapy prescribed or dispensed (RA)

🚗 0.00   ⚕ 0.00   **FUD** XXX   M PQ

AMA: 2008,Mar,8-12

4188F Appropriate angiotensin converting enzyme (ACE)/angiotensin receptor blockers (ARB) therapeutic monitoring test ordered or performed (AM)

🚗 0.00   ⚕ 0.00   **FUD** XXX   E

AMA: 2008,Mar,8-12

4189F Appropriate digoxin therapeutic monitoring test ordered or performed (AM)

🚗 0.00   ⚕ 0.00   **FUD** XXX   E

AMA: 2008,Mar,8-12

4190F Appropriate diuretic therapeutic monitoring test ordered or performed (AM)

🚗 0.00   ⚕ 0.00   **FUD** XXX   E

AMA: 2008,Mar,8-12

4191F Appropriate anticonvulsant therapeutic monitoring test ordered or performed (AM)

🚗 0.00   ⚕ 0.00   **FUD** XXX   E

AMA: 2008,Mar,8-12

4192F Patient not receiving glucocorticoid therapy (RA)

🚗 0.00   ⚕ 0.00   **FUD** XXX   M PQ

4193F Patient receiving <10 mg daily prednisone (or equivalent), or RA activity is worsening, or glucocorticoid use is for less than 6 months (RA)

🚗 0.00   ⚕ 0.00   **FUD** XXX   M PQ

4194F Patient receiving ≥ 10 mg daily prednisone (or equivalent) for longer than 6 months, and improvement or no change in disease activity (RA)

🚗 0.00   ⚕ 0.00   **FUD** XXX   M PQ

4195F Patient receiving first-time biologic disease modifying anti-rheumatic drug therapy for rheumatoid arthritis (RA)

🚗 0.00   ⚕ 0.00   **FUD** XXX   M PQ

4196F Patient not receiving first-time biologic disease modifying anti-rheumatic drug therapy for rheumatoid arthritis (RA)

🚗 0.00   ⚕ 0.00   **FUD** XXX   M PQ

4200F External beam radiotherapy as primary therapy to prostate with or without nodal irradiation (PRCA)

🚗 0.00   ⚕ 0.00   **FUD** XXX   E PQ

AMA: 2008,Mar,8-12

4201F External beam radiotherapy with or without nodal irradiation as adjuvant or salvage therapy for prostate cancer patient (PRCA)

🚗 0.00   ⚕ 0.00   **FUD** XXX   E PQ

AMA: 2008,Mar,8-12

4210F Angiotensin converting enzyme (ACE) or angiotensin receptor blockers (ARB) medication therapy for 6 months or more (MM)

🚗 0.00   ⚕ 0.00   **FUD** XXX   E

AMA: 2008,Mar,8-12

4220F Digoxin medication therapy for 6 months or more (MM)

🚗 0.00   ⚕ 0.00   **FUD** XXX   E

AMA: 2008,Mar,8-12

4221F Diuretic medication therapy for 6 months or more (MM)

🚗 0.00   ⚕ 0.00   **FUD** XXX   E

AMA: 2008,Mar,8-12

4230F Anticonvulsant medication therapy for 6 months or more (MM)

🚗 0.00   ⚕ 0.00   **FUD** XXX   E

AMA: 2008,Mar,8-12

4240F Instruction in therapeutic exercise with follow-up provided to patients during episode of back pain lasting longer than 12 weeks (BkP)
0.00   0.00   **FUD** XXX   E
AMA: 2008,Mar,8-12

4242F Counseling for supervised exercise program provided to patients during episode of back pain lasting longer than 12 weeks (BkP)
0.00   0.00   **FUD** XXX   E
AMA: 2008,Mar,8-12

4245F Patient counseled during the initial visit to maintain or resume normal activities (BkP)
0.00   0.00   **FUD** XXX   E
AMA: 2008,Mar,8-12

4248F Patient counseled during the initial visit for an episode of back pain against bed rest lasting 4 days or longer (BkP)
0.00   0.00   **FUD** XXX   E
AMA: 2008,Mar,8-12

4250F Active warming used intraoperatively for the purpose of maintaining normothermia, or at least 1 body temperature equal to or greater than 36 degrees Centigrade (or 96.8 degrees Fahrenheit) recorded within the 30 minutes immediately before or the 15 minutes immediately after anesthesia end time (CRIT)
0.00   0.00   **FUD** XXX   M PQ
AMA: 2008,Mar,8-12

4255F Duration of general or neuraxial anesthesia 60 minutes or longer, as documented in the anesthesia record (CRIT) (Peri2)
0.00   0.00   **FUD** XXX   M PQ

4256F Duration of general or neuraxial anesthesia less than 60 minutes, as documented in the anesthesia record (CRIT) (Peri2)
0.00   0.00   **FUD** XXX   E PQ

4260F Wound surface culture technique used (CWC)
0.00   0.00   **FUD** XXX   E PQ

4261F Technique other than surface culture of the wound exudate used (eg, Levine/deep swab technique, semi-quantitative or quantitative swab technique) or wound surface culture technique not used (CWC)
0.00   0.00   **FUD** XXX   E PQ

4265F Use of wet to dry dressings prescribed or recommended (CWC)
0.00   0.00   **FUD** XXX   E PQ

4266F Use of wet to dry dressings neither prescribed nor recommended (CWC)
0.00   0.00   **FUD** XXX   E PQ

4267F Compression therapy prescribed (CWC)
0.00   0.00   **FUD** XXX   E PQ

4268F Patient education regarding the need for long term compression therapy including interval replacement of compression stockings received (CWC)
0.00   0.00   **FUD** XXX   E

4269F Appropriate method of offloading (pressure relief) prescribed (CWC)
0.00   0.00   **FUD** XXX   E

4270F Patient receiving potent antiretroviral therapy for 6 months or longer (HIV)
0.00   0.00   **FUD** XXX   E PQ

4271F Patient receiving potent antiretroviral therapy for less than 6 months or not receiving potent antiretroviral therapy (HIV)
0.00   0.00   **FUD** XXX   E PQ

4274F Influenza immunization administered or previously received (HIV) (P-ESRD)
0.00   0.00   **FUD** XXX   E

4276F Potent antiretroviral therapy prescribed (HIV)
0.00   0.00   **FUD** XXX   E PQ

4279F Pneumocystis jiroveci pneumonia prophylaxis prescribed (HIV)
0.00   0.00   **FUD** XXX   E

4280F Pneumocystis jiroveci pneumonia prophylaxis prescribed within 3 months of low CD4+ cell count or percentage (HIV)
0.00   0.00   **FUD** XXX   E PQ

4290F Patient screened for injection drug use (HIV)
0.00   0.00   **FUD** XXX   E PQ

4293F Patient screened for high-risk sexual behavior (HIV)
0.00   0.00   **FUD** XXX   E PQ

4300F Patient receiving warfarin therapy for nonvalvular atrial fibrillation or atrial flutter (AFIB)
0.00   0.00   **FUD** XXX   E

4301F Patient not receiving warfarin therapy for nonvalvular atrial fibrillation or atrial flutter (AFIB)
0.00   0.00   **FUD** XXX   E

4305F Patient education regarding appropriate foot care and daily inspection of the feet received (CWC)
0.00   0.00   **FUD** XXX   E

4306F Patient counseled regarding psychosocial and pharmacologic treatment options for opioid addiction (SUD)
0.00   0.00   **FUD** XXX   E

4320F Patient counseled regarding psychosocial and pharmacologic treatment options for alcohol dependence (SUD)
0.00   0.00   **FUD** XXX   E PQ

4322F Caregiver provided with education and referred to additional resources for support (DEM)
0.00   0.00   **FUD** XXX   M

4324F Patient (or caregiver) queried about Parkinson's disease medication related motor complications (Prkns)
0.00   0.00   **FUD** XXX   E

4325F Medical and surgical treatment options reviewed with patient (or caregiver) (Prkns)
0.00   0.00   **FUD** XXX   M

4326F Patient (or caregiver) queried about symptoms of autonomic dysfunction (Prkns)
0.00   0.00   **FUD** XXX   E

4328F Patient (or caregiver) queried about sleep disturbances (Prkns)
0.00   0.00   **FUD** XXX   M

4330F Counseling about epilepsy specific safety issues provided to patient (or caregiver(s)) (EPI)
0.00   0.00   **FUD** XXX   E

4340F Counseling for women of childbearing potential with epilepsy (EPI)
0.00   0.00   **FUD** XXX   M PQ

4350F Counseling provided on symptom management, end of life decisions, and palliation (DEM)
0.00   0.00   **FUD** XXX   E

4400F Rehabilitative therapy options discussed with patient (or caregiver) (Prkns)
0.00   0.00   **FUD** XXX   M

4450F Self-care education provided to patient (HF)
0.00   0.00   **FUD** XXX   E

4470F Implantable cardioverter-defibrillator (ICD) counseling provided (HF)
0.00   0.00   **FUD** XXX   E

4480F Patient receiving ACE inhibitor/ARB therapy and beta-blocker therapy for 3 months or longer (HF)
   0.00   0.00   FUD XXX   E

4481F Patient receiving ACE inhibitor/ARB therapy and beta-blocker therapy for less than 3 months or patient not receiving ACE inhibitor/ARB therapy and beta-blocker therapy (HF)
   0.00   0.00   FUD XXX   E

4500F Referred to an outpatient cardiac rehabilitation program (CAD)
   0.00   0.00   FUD XXX   M PQ

4510F Previous cardiac rehabilitation for qualifying cardiac event completed (CAD)
   0.00   0.00   FUD XXX   M PQ

4525F Neuropsychiatric intervention ordered (DEM)
   0.00   0.00   FUD XXX   M

4526F Neuropsychiatric intervention received (DEM)
   0.00   0.00   FUD XXX   M

4540F Disease modifying pharmacotherapy discussed (ALS)
   0.00   0.00   FUD XXX   E

4541F Patient offered treatment for pseudobulbar affect, sialorrhea, or ALS-related symptoms (ALS)
   0.00   0.00   FUD XXX   E

4550F Options for noninvasive respiratory support discussed with patient (ALS)
   0.00   0.00   FUD XXX   E

4551F Nutritional support offered (ALS)
   0.00   0.00   FUD XXX   E

4552F Patient offered referral to a speech language pathologist (ALS)
   0.00   0.00   FUD XXX   E

4553F Patient offered assistance in planning for end of life issues (ALS)
   0.00   0.00   FUD XXX   E

4554F Patient received inhalational anesthetic agent (Peri2)
   0.00   0.00   FUD XXX   E

4555F Patient did not receive inhalational anesthetic agent (Peri2)
   0.00   0.00   FUD XXX   E

4556F Patient exhibits 3 or more risk factors for post-operative nausea and vomiting (Peri2)
   0.00   0.00   FUD XXX   E

4557F Patient does not exhibit 3 or more risk factors for post-operative nausea and vomiting (Peri2)
   0.00   0.00   FUD XXX   E

4558F Patient received at least 2 prophylactic pharmacologic anti-emetic agents of different classes preoperatively and intraoperatively (Peri2)
   0.00   0.00   FUD XXX   E

4559F At least 1 body temperature measurement equal to or greater than 35.5 degrees Celsius (or 95.9 degrees Fahrenheit) recorded within the 30 minutes immediately before or the 15 minutes immediately after anesthesia end time (Peri2)
   0.00   0.00   FUD XXX   E

4560F Anesthesia technique did not involve general or neuraxial anesthesia (Peri2)
   0.00   0.00   FUD XXX   E

4561F Patient has a coronary artery stent (Peri2)
   0.00   0.00   FUD XXX   E

4562F Patient does not have a coronary artery stent (Peri2)
   0.00   0.00   FUD XXX   E

4563F Patient received aspirin within 24 hours prior to anesthesia start time (Peri2)
   0.00   0.00   FUD XXX   E

5005F-5250F Results Conveyed and Documented

INCLUDES   Patient's:
       Functional status
       Morbidity/mortality
       Satisfaction/experience with care
     Review/communication of test results to patients

5005F Patient counseled on self-examination for new or changing moles (ML)
   0.00   0.00   FUD XXX   E
   AMA: 2008,Mar,8-12

5010F Findings of dilated macular or fundus exam communicated to the physician or other qualified health care professional managing the diabetes care (EC)
   0.00   0.00   FUD XXX   M PQ

5015F Documentation of communication that a fracture occurred and that the patient was or should be tested or treated for osteoporosis (OP)
   0.00   0.00   FUD XXX   M PQ

5020F Treatment summary report communicated to physician(s) or other qualified health care professional(s) managing continuing care and to the patient within 1 month of completing treatment (ONC)
   0.00   0.00   FUD XXX   E
   AMA: 2008,Mar,8-12

5050F Treatment plan communicated to provider(s) managing continuing care within 1 month of diagnosis (ML)
   0.00   0.00   FUD XXX   M PQ
   AMA: 2008,Mar,8-12

5060F Findings from diagnostic mammogram communicated to practice managing patient's on-going care within 3 business days of exam interpretation (RAD)
   0.00   0.00   FUD XXX   E
   AMA: 2008,Mar,8-12

5062F Findings from diagnostic mammogram communicated to the patient within 5 days of exam interpretation (RAD)
   0.00   0.00   FUD XXX   E
   AMA: 2008,Mar,8-12

5100F Potential risk for fracture communicated to the referring physician or other qualified health care professional within 24 hours of completion of the imaging study (NUC_MED)
   0.00   0.00   FUD XXX   E

5200F Consideration of referral for a neurological evaluation of appropriateness for surgical therapy for intractable epilepsy within the past 3 years (EPI)
   0.00   0.00   FUD XXX   E

5250F Asthma discharge plan provided to patient (Asthma)
   0.00   0.00   FUD XXX   E

6005F-6150F Elements Related to Patient Safety Processes

INCLUDES   Patient safety practices

6005F Rationale (eg, severity of illness and safety) for level of care (eg, home, hospital) documented (CAP)
   0.00   0.00   FUD XXX   E
   AMA: 2015,Jan,16; 2014,Jan,11

6010F Dysphagia screening conducted prior to order for or receipt of any foods, fluids, or medication by mouth (STR)
   0.00   0.00   FUD XXX   E PQ

6015F Patient receiving or eligible to receive foods, fluids, or medication by mouth (STR)
   0.00   0.00   FUD XXX   E PQ

6020F NPO (nothing by mouth) ordered (STR)
   0.00   0.00   FUD XXX   E PQ

● New Code   ▲ Revised Code   ○ Reinstated   M Maternity   A Age Edit Edit   Unlisted   Not Covered   # Resequenced
⊘ AMA Mod 51 Exempt   51 Optum Mod 51 Exempt   63 Mod 63 Exempt   ⊙ Mod Sedation   + Add-on   CCI   PQ PQRS   FUD Follow-up Days

▲ **6030F** All elements of maximal sterile barrier technique, hand hygiene, skin preparation and, if ultrasound is used, sterile ultrasound techniques followed (CRIT)

   🔲 0.00   🔲 0.00   **FUD** XXX   M P0

   AMA: 2008,Mar,8-12

6040F Use of appropriate radiation dose reduction devices OR manual techniques for appropriate moderation of exposure, documented (RAD)

   🔲 0.00   🔲 0.00   **FUD** XXX   E

6045F Radiation exposure or exposure time in final report for procedure using fluoroscopy, documented (RAD)

   🔲 0.00   🔲 0.00   **FUD** XXX   M P0

   AMA: 2008,Mar,8-12

6070F Patient queried and counseled about anti-epileptic drug (AED) side effects (EPI)

   🔲 0.00   🔲 0.00   **FUD** XXX   E

6080F Patient (or caregiver) queried about falls (Prkns, DSP)

   🔲 0.00   🔲 0.00   **FUD** XXX   E

6090F Patient (or caregiver) counseled about safety issues appropriate to patient's stage of disease (Prkns)

   🔲 0.00   🔲 0.00   **FUD** XXX   E

6100F Timeout to verify correct patient, correct site, and correct procedure, documented (PATH)

   🔲 0.00   🔲 0.00   **FUD** XXX   E

6101F Safety counseling for dementia provided (DEM)

   🔲 0.00   🔲 0.00   **FUD** XXX   M

6102F Safety counseling for dementia ordered (DEM)

   🔲 0.00   🔲 0.00   **FUD** XXX   M

6110F Counseling provided regarding risks of driving and the alternatives to driving (DEM)

   🔲 0.00   🔲 0.00   **FUD** XXX   M

6150F Patient not receiving a first course of anti-TNF (tumor necrosis factor) therapy (IBD)

   🔲 0.00   🔲 0.00   **FUD** XXX   M

7010F-7025F Recall/Reminder System in Place

INCLUDES   Capabilities of the provider
       Measures that address the setting or system of care provided

7010F Patient information entered into a recall system that includes: target date for the next exam specified and a process to follow up with patients regarding missed or unscheduled appointments (ML)

   🔲 0.00   🔲 0.00   **FUD** XXX   M P0

   AMA: 2008,Mar,8-12

7020F Mammogram assessment category (eg, Mammography Quality Standards Act [MQSA], Breast Imaging Reporting and Data System [BI-RADS], or FDA approved equivalent categories) entered into an internal database to allow for analysis of abnormal interpretation (recall) rate (RAD)

   🔲 0.00   🔲 0.00   **FUD** XXX   E

   AMA: 2008,Mar,8-12

7025F Patient information entered into a reminder system with a target due date for the next mammogram (RAD)

   🔲 0.00   🔲 0.00   **FUD** XXX   M P0

   AMA: 2008,Mar,8-12

9001F-9007F No Measure Associated

INCLUDES   Aspects of care not associated with measures at the current time

9001F Aortic aneurysm less than 5.0 cm maximum diameter on centerline formatted CT or minor diameter on axial formatted CT (NMA-No Measure Associated)

   🔲 0.00   🔲 0.00   **FUD** XXX   E

9002F Aortic aneurysm 5.0 - 5.4 cm maximum diameter on centerline formatted CT or minor diameter on axial formatted CT (NMA-No Measure Associated)

   🔲 0.00   🔲 0.00   **FUD** XXX   E

9003F Aortic aneurysm 5.5 - 5.9 cm maximum diameter on centerline formatted CT or minor diameter on axial formatted CT (NMA-No Measure Associated)

   🔲 0.00   🔲 0.00   **FUD** XXX   M

9004F Aortic aneurysm 6.0 cm or greater maximum diameter on centerline formatted CT or minor diameter on axial formatted CT (NMA-No Measure Associated)

   🔲 0.00   🔲 0.00   **FUD** XXX   M

9005F Asymptomatic carotid stenosis: No history of any transient ischemic attack or stroke in any carotid or vertebrobasilar territory (NMA-No Measure Associated)

   🔲 0.00   🔲 0.00   **FUD** XXX   E

9006F Symptomatic carotid stenosis: Ipsilateral carotid territory TIA or stroke less than 120 days prior to procedure (NMA-No Measure Associated)

   🔲 0.00   🔲 0.00   **FUD** XXX   M

9007F Other carotid stenosis: Ipsilateral TIA or stroke 120 days or greater prior to procedure or any prior contralateral carotid territory or vertebrobasilar TIA or stroke (NMA-No Measure Associated)

   🔲 0.00   🔲 0.00   **FUD** XXX   M

0019T-0042T

0019T Extracorporeal shock wave involving musculoskeletal system, not otherwise specified, low energy

> **EXCLUDES** *High energy:*
> *Extracorporeal shock wave (0101T)*
> *Lateral humeral epicondyle extracorporeal shock wave (0102T)*

🔧 0.00   ⚖ 0.00   **FUD** XXX   A 80

AMA: 2006,Mar,1-5; 2005,Jun,6-8

0042T Cerebral perfusion analysis using computed tomography with contrast administration, including post-processing of parametric maps with determination of cerebral blood flow, cerebral blood volume, and mean transit time

🔧 0.00   ⚖ 0.00   **FUD** XXX   N N1 80 PQ

AMA: 2003,Nov,5

0051T-0053T

0051T Implantation of a total replacement heart system (artificial heart) with recipient cardiectomy

> **EXCLUDES** *Ventricular assist device implant (33975-33976)*

🔧 0.00   ⚖ 0.00   **FUD** XXX   C 80

AMA: 2004,Jun,7; 2003,Aug,1

0052T Replacement or repair of thoracic unit of a total replacement heart system (artificial heart)

> **EXCLUDES** *Exchange or repair of other artificial heart components (0053T)*

🔧 0.00   ⚖ 0.00   **FUD** XXX   C 80

AMA: 2015,Jan,16; 2014,Jan,11

0053T Replacement or repair of implantable component or components of total replacement heart system (artificial heart), excluding thoracic unit

> **EXCLUDES** *Exchange or repair of thoracic unit of artificial heart (0052T)*

🔧 0.00   ⚖ 0.00   **FUD** XXX   C 80

AMA: 2004,Jun,7; 2003,Aug,1

0054T-0055T

+ 0054T Computer-assisted musculoskeletal surgical navigational orthopedic procedure, with image-guidance based on fluoroscopic images (List separately in addition to code for primary procedure)

Code first primary procedure

🔧 0.00   ⚖ 0.00   **FUD** XXX   N 80

AMA: 2015,Jan,16; 2014,Jan,11; 2012,Jan,15-42; 2011,Jan,11

+ 0055T Computer-assisted musculoskeletal surgical navigational orthopedic procedure, with image-guidance based on CT/MRI images (List separately in addition to code for primary procedure)

> **INCLUDES** Performance of both CT and MRI in same session (1 unit)

Code first primary procedure

🔧 0.00   ⚖ 0.00   **FUD** XXX   N 80

AMA: 2015,Jan,16; 2014,Jan,11; 2012,Jan,15-42; 2011,Jan,11

0058T [0357T]

> **EXCLUDES** *Cryopreservation of:*
> *Embryos (89258)*
> *Oocyte(s), mature (89337)*
> *Sperm (89259)*
> *Testicular reproductive tissue (89335)*

0058T Cryopreservation; reproductive tissue, ovarian

🔧 0.00   ⚖ 0.00   **FUD** XXX   Q1 80

AMA: 2004,Apr,1; 2004,Jun,7

 # 0357T immature oocyte(s)   ♀

🔧 0.00   ⚖ 0.00   **FUD** XXX   Q1 80

0071T-0072T

Do not report with (51702, 77022)

0071T Focused ultrasound ablation of uterine leiomyomata, including MR guidance; total leiomyomata volume less than 200 cc of tissue   ♀

🔧 0.00   ⚖ 0.00   **FUD** XXX   S 80

AMA: 2005,Mar,1-6; 2005,Dec,3-6

0072T total leiomyomata volume greater or equal to 200 cc of tissue   ♀

🔧 0.00   ⚖ 0.00   **FUD** XXX   S 80

AMA: 2005,Mar,1-6; 2005,Dec,3-6

0075T-0076T

0075T Transcatheter placement of extracranial vertebral artery stent(s), including radiologic supervision and interpretation, open or percutaneous; initial vessel

> **INCLUDES** All diagnostic services for stenting
> Ipsilateral extracranial vertebral selective catheterization when confirming the need for stenting

> **EXCLUDES** *Selective catheterization and imaging when stenting is not required (report only selective catheterization codes)*

🔧 0.00   ⚖ 0.00   **FUD** XXX   C 80 PQ

AMA: 2015,Jan,16; 2014,Mar,8

+ 0076T each additional vessel (List separately in addition to code for primary procedure)

Code first (0075T)

🔧 0.00   ⚖ 0.00   **FUD** XXX   C 80

AMA: 2015,Jan,16; 2014,Mar,8

0085T

0085T Breath test for heart transplant rejection   E

🔧 0.00   ⚖ 0.00   **FUD** XXX

AMA: 2005,May,7-12

0095T-0098T

> **INCLUDES** Fluoroscopy

+ 0095T Removal of total disc arthroplasty (artificial disc), anterior approach, each additional interspace, cervical (List separately in addition to code for primary procedure)

> **EXCLUDES** *Lumbar disc (0164T)*
> *Revision of total disc arthroplasty, cervical (22861)*
> *Revision of total disc arthroplasty, lumbar (22862)*

Code first (22864)

🔧 0.00   ⚖ 0.00   **FUD** XXX   C 80

AMA: 2006,Feb,1-6; 2005,Jun,6-8

+ 0098T Revision including replacement of total disc arthroplasty (artificial disc), anterior approach, each additional interspace, cervical (List separately in addition to code for primary procedure)

> **EXCLUDES** *Spinal cord decompression (63001-63048)*

Code first (22861)
Do not report when performed at the same level with (22851)
Do not report with (0095T)

🔧 0.00   ⚖ 0.00   **FUD** XXX   C 80

AMA: 2006,Feb,1-6; 2005,Jun,6-8

0099T-0159T

0099T ~~Implantation of intrastromal corneal ring segments~~

To report, see ~65785

0100T Placement of a subconjunctival retinal prosthesis receiver and pulse generator, and implantation of intra-ocular retinal electrode array, with vitrectomy

🔧 0.00   ⚖ 0.00   **FUD** XXX   T G2 80

AMA: 2015,Jan,16; 2014,Jan,11; 2012,Jan,15-42

0101T Extracorporeal shock wave involving musculoskeletal system, not otherwise specified, high energy

> *EXCLUDES* *Extracorporeal shock wave therapy for healing of integumentary system wounds (0299T-0300T)*
> *Low energy extracorporeal shock wave (0019T)*
> Do not report for same area with (0299T-0300T)
> 0.00   0.00   **FUD** XXX   T 62 80
> **AMA:** 2015,Jan,16; 2014,Jan,11; 2012,Jan,15-42

0102T Extracorporeal shock wave, high energy, performed by a physician, requiring anesthesia other than local, involving lateral humeral epicondyle

> *EXCLUDES* *Low energy extracorporeal shock wave (0019T)*
> 0.00   0.00   **FUD** XXX   T 62 80
> **AMA:** 2015,Jan,16; 2014,Jan,11; 2012,Jan,15-42

0103T Holotranscobalamin, quantitative

> To report, see ~84999

0106T Quantitative sensory testing (QST), testing and interpretation per extremity; using touch pressure stimuli to assess large diameter sensation

> 0.00   0.00   **FUD** XXX   01 80
> **AMA:** 2015,Jan,16; 2014,Jan,11; 2012,Jan,15-42; 2011,May,9

0107T using vibration stimuli to assess large diameter fiber sensation

> 0.00   0.00   **FUD** XXX   01 80
> **AMA:** 2015,Jan,16; 2014,Jan,11; 2011,May,9

0108T using cooling stimuli to assess small nerve fiber sensation and hyperalgesia

> 0.00   0.00   **FUD** XXX   01 80
> **AMA:** 2015,Jan,16; 2014,Jan,11; 2011,May,9

0109T using heat-pain stimuli to assess small nerve fiber sensation and hyperalgesia

> 0.00   0.00   **FUD** XXX   01 80
> **AMA:** 2015,Jan,16; 2014,Jan,11; 2011,May,9

0110T using other stimuli to assess sensation

> 0.00   0.00   **FUD** XXX   01 80
> **AMA:** 2015,Jan,16; 2014,Jan,11; 2011,May,9

0111T Long-chain (C20-22) omega-3 fatty acids in red blood cell (RBC) membranes

> *EXCLUDES* *Very long chain fatty acids (82726)*
> 0.00   0.00   **FUD** XXX   A 80
> **AMA:** 2015,Jan,16; 2014,Jan,11

0123T Fistulization of sclera for glaucoma, through ciliary body

> To report, see ~66999

0126T Common carotid intima-media thickness (IMT) study for evaluation of atherosclerotic burden or coronary heart disease risk factor assessment

> Do not report with (93880, 93882, 93895)
> 0.00   0.00   **FUD** XXX   01 80
> **AMA:** 2015,Jan,16; 2014,Jan,11

+ **0159T** Computer-aided detection, including computer algorithm analysis of MRI image data for lesion detection/characterization, pharmacokinetic analysis, with further physician review for interpretation, breast MRI (List separately in addition to code for primary procedure)

> Code first (77058-77059)
> Do not report with (76376-76377)
> 0.00   0.00   **FUD** ZZZ   N 80
> **AMA:** 2015,Jan,16; 2014,Jan,11

0163T-0165T

CMS: 100-3,150.10 Lumbar Artificial Disc Replacement (LADR)

INCLUDES Fluoroscopy

EXCLUDES *Cervical disc procedures (22856)*
Decompression (63001-63048)
Do not report with these procedures when performed at the same level (22851, 49010)

+ **0163T** Total disc arthroplasty (artificial disc), anterior approach, including discectomy to prepare interspace (other than for decompression), each additional interspace, lumbar (List separately in addition to code for primary procedure)

> Code first (22857)
> 0.00   0.00   **FUD** YYY   C 80
> **AMA:** 2015,Jan,16; 2014,Jan,11

+ **0164T** Removal of total disc arthroplasty, (artificial disc), anterior approach, each additional interspace, lumbar (List separately in addition to code for primary procedure)

> Code first (22865)
> 0.00   0.00   **FUD** YYY   C 80
> **AMA:** 2015,Jan,16; 2014,Jan,11

+ **0165T** Revision including replacement of total disc arthroplasty (artificial disc), anterior approach, each additional interspace, lumbar (List separately in addition to code for primary procedure)

> Code first (22862)
> 0.00   0.00   **FUD** YYY   C 80
> **AMA:** 2015,Jan,16; 2014,Jan,11

0169T-0175T

0169T Stereotactic placement of infusion catheter(s) in the brain for delivery of therapeutic agent(s), including computerized stereotactic planning and burr hole(s)

> Do not report with (20660, 61107, 61781-61783)
> 0.00   0.00   **FUD** XXX   C 80
> **AMA:** 2015,Jan,16; 2014,Jan,11; 2012,Jan,15-42; 2011,Jan,11

0171T Insertion of posterior spinous process distraction device (including necessary removal of bone or ligament for insertion and imaging guidance), lumbar; single level

> 0.00   0.00   **FUD** XXX   J 80
> **AMA:** 2015,Jan,16; 2014,Oct,14; 2014,Jan,11; 2013,Dec,16

+ **0172T** each additional level (List separately in addition to code for primary procedure)

> Code first (0171T)
> 0.00   0.00   **FUD** XXX   N 80
> **AMA:** 2007,Jul,6-10; 2006,Dec,8-9

+ **0174T** Computer-aided detection (CAD) (computer algorithm analysis of digital image data for lesion detection) with further physician review for interpretation and report, with or without digitization of film radiographic images, chest radiograph(s), performed concurrent with primary interpretation (List separately in addition to code for primary procedure)

> Code first (71010, 71020-71022, 71030)
> 0.00   0.00   **FUD** XXX   N N1 80
> **AMA:** 2007,Jul,6-10; 2007,Mar,7-8

0175T Computer-aided detection (CAD) (computer algorithm analysis of digital image data for lesion detection) with further physician review for interpretation and report, with or without digitization of film radiographic images, chest radiograph(s), performed remote from primary interpretation

> Do not report with (71010, 71020-71022, 71030)
> 0.00   0.00   **FUD** XXX   N N1 80
> **AMA:** 2007,Jul,6-10; 2007,Mar,7-8

0178T-0180T

EXCLUDES *Separately performed 12-lead electrocardiogram (93000-93010)*

0178T Electrocardiogram, 64 leads or greater, with graphic presentation and analysis; with interpretation and report

> 0.00   0.00   **FUD** XXX   B 80

0179T tracing and graphics only, without interpretation and report

> 0.00   0.00   **FUD** XXX   S 80 TC

0180T interpretation and report only

> 0.00   0.00   **FUD** XXX   B 80 26

0182T-0184T

0182T ~~High dose rate electronic brachytherapy, per fraction~~

> To report, see ~0394T-0395T

0184T **Excision of rectal tumor, transanal endoscopic microsurgical approach (ie, TEMS), including muscularis propria (ie, full thickness)**

> INCLUDES Operating microscope (66990)
>
> EXCLUDES *Nonendoscopic excision of rectal tumor (45160, 45171-45172)*
>
> Do not report with (45300-45327)
>
> 🔲 0.00   🔲 0.00   **FUD** XXX   T 80
>
> **AMA:** 2015,Jan,16; 2014,Jan,11; 2010,Jun,3

0188T-0189T

> INCLUDES 30 minutes or more of direct medical care by a physician(s) or other qualified health care professional(s) to a critically ill or critically injured patient from an off-site location
> Additional on-site critical care services when a critically ill or injured patient requires critical care resources not available on-site
> Real time ability to:
>   Document the remote care services in the medical record
>   Enter orders electronically
>   Evaluate patients with high fidelity audio/video capabilities
>   Observe patient monitors, infusion pumps, ventilators
>   Talk to patients and family members
>   Videoconference with the health care team on-site in the patient's room
> Real-time access to the patient's:
>   Clinical laboratory test results
>   Diagnostic test results
>   Medical records
>   Radiographic images
> Review and/or interpretation of all diagnostic information
> Time spent with the patient, family, or surrogate decision makers to obtain a medical history, review the patient's condition/prognosis, or discuss treatment options from the remote site
> Do not report for same time period with other critical care services rendered by provider or other individual (99291-99292, 99468-99476)
> Do not report for time spent away from the remote site without real-time capabilities
> Do not report time spent for services that do not directly contribute to patient treatment

0188T **Remote real-time interactive video-conferenced critical care, evaluation and management of the critically ill or critically injured patient; first 30-74 minutes**

> INCLUDES First 30 to 74 minutes of remote critical care each day
> Do not report remote critical care less than 30 minutes total duration
>
> 🔲 0.00   🔲 0.00   **FUD** XXX   M
>
> **AMA:** 2015,Jan,16; 2014,Jan,11; 2012,Jan,15-42; 2011,Aug,9-10

+ **0189T** **each additional 30 minutes (List separately in addition to code for primary service)**

> INCLUDES Up to 30 minutes each beyond the first 74 minutes
> Code first (0188T)
>
> 🔲 0.00   🔲 0.00   **FUD** XXX   M
>
> **AMA:** 2015,Jan,16; 2014,Jan,11; 2012,Jan,15-42; 2011,Aug,9-10

0190T-0191T [0253T, 0376T]

+ **0190T** **Placement of intraocular radiation source applicator (List separately in addition to primary procedure)**

> EXCLUDES *Insertion of brachytherapy source by radiation oncologist (see Clinical Brachytherapy Section)*
> Code also brachytherapy source
> Code first (67036)
>
> 🔲 0.00   🔲 0.00   **FUD** XXX   N N1 80
>
> **AMA:** 2008,Jan,6-7

0191T **Insertion of anterior segment aqueous drainage device, without extracular reservoir, internal approach, into the trabecular meshwork; initial insertion**

> 🔲 0.00   🔲 0.00   **FUD** XXX   T G2 80
>
> **AMA:** 2015,Jan,16; 2014,Jan,11; 2012,Dec,12

+ # **0376T** **each additional device insertion (List separately in addition to code for primary procedure)**

> 🔲 0.00   🔲 0.00   **FUD** XXX   N 80
>
> Code first (0191T)

0253T **Insertion of anterior segment aqueous drainage device, without extracular reservoir, internal approach, into the suprachoroidal space**

> 🔲 0.00   🔲 0.00   **FUD** YYY   T G2 80
>
> EXCLUDES *Insertion aqueous drainage device, external approach (66183)*

0195T-0196T

> Do not report with (20930-20938, 22558, 22840, 22845, 22848, 22851, 72275, 76000, 76380, 76496-76497, 77002-77003, 77011-77012)

0195T **Arthrodesis, pre-sacral interbody technique, disc space preparation, discectomy, without instrumentation, with image guidance, includes bone graft when performed; L5-S1 interspace**

> 🔲 0.00   🔲 0.00   **FUD** XXX   C 80
>
> **AMA:** 2015,Jan,16; 2013,Jul,3-5; 2012,Apr,14-16

+ **0196T** **L4-L5 interspace (List separately in addition to code for primary procedure)**

> Code first (0195T)
>
> 🔲 0.00   🔲 0.00   **FUD** XXX   C 80
>
> **AMA:** 2015,Jan,16; 2013,Jul,3-5; 2012,Apr,14-16

0198T

0198T **Measurement of ocular blood flow by repetitive intraocular pressure sampling, with interpretation and report**

> 🔲 0.00   🔲 0.00   **FUD** XXX   Q1 80
>
> **AMA:** 2015,Jan,16; 2014,Jan,11; 2012,Aug,9; 2012,Jan,15-42; 2011,Mar,9

0200T-0201T

> Do not report at same level with (20225)

0200T **Percutaneous sacral augmentation (sacroplasty), unilateral injection(s), including the use of a balloon or mechanical device, when used, 1 or more needles, includes imaging guidance and bone biopsy, when performed**

> 🔲 0.00   🔲 0.00   **FUD** XXX   ⊙ T G2 80 50
>
> **AMA:** 2015,Apr,8; 2015,Jan,8

0201T **Percutaneous sacral augmentation (sacroplasty), bilateral injections, including the use of a balloon or mechanical device, when used, 2 or more needles, includes imaging guidance and bone biopsy, when performed**

> 🔲 0.00   🔲 0.00   **FUD** XXX   ⊙ T G2 80
>
> **AMA:** 2015,Apr,8; 2015,Jan,8

0202T-0207T

0202T **Posterior vertebral joint(s) arthroplasty (eg, facet joint[s] replacement), including facetectomy, laminectomy, foraminotomy, and vertebral column fixation, injection of bone cement, when performed, including fluoroscopy, single level, lumbar spine**

> 🔲 0.00   🔲 0.00   **FUD** XXX   C 80
>
> Do not report the following codes when performed at the same level: (22511, 22514, 22840, 22851, 22857, 63005, 63012, 63017, 63030, 63042, 63047, 63056)

+ **0205T** **Intravascular catheter-based coronary vessel or graft spectroscopy (eg, infrared) during diagnostic evaluation and/or therapeutic intervention including imaging supervision, interpretation, and report, each vessel (List separately in addition to code for primary procedure)**

> 🔲 0.00   🔲 0.00   **FUD** ZZZ   N 80
>
> Code first (92920, 92924, 92928, 92933, 92937, 92941, 92943, 92975, 93454-93461, 93563-93564)

0206T **Computerized database analysis of multiple cycles of digitized cardiac electrical data from two or more ECG leads, including transmission to a remote center, application of multiple nonlinear mathematical transformations, with coronary artery obstruction severity assessment**

> 🔲 0.00   🔲 0.00   **FUD** XXX   Q1 80 TC
>
> Code also 12-lead ECG when performed (93000-93010)

● New Code   ▲ Revised Code   ○ Reinstated   M Maternity   A Age Edit   Unlisted   Not Covered   # Resequenced
⊘ AMA Mod 51 Exempt   ⑤ Optum Mod 51 Exempt   ⑥ Mod 63 Exempt   ⊙ Mod Sedation   + Add-on   CCI   PQ PQRS   FUD Follow-up Days

0207T **Evacuation of meibomian glands, automated, using heat and intermittent pressure, unilateral**
   🛏 0.00   ⚕ 0.00   **FUD** XXX   01 80
   AMA: 2015,Jan,16; 2014,May,5

0208T-0212T

EXCLUDES   *Manual audiometric testing by a qualified health care professional, using audiometers (92551-92557)*

0208T **Pure tone audiometry (threshold), automated; air only**
   🛏 0.00   ⚕ 0.00   **FUD** XXX   01 80 TC
   AMA: 2015,Jan,16; 2014,Aug,3

0209T **air and bone**
   🛏 0.00   ⚕ 0.00   **FUD** XXX   01 80 TC
   AMA: 2015,Jan,16; 2014,Aug,3; 2014,Jan,11; 2011,Mar,8

0210T **Speech audiometry threshold, automated;**
   🛏 0.00   ⚕ 0.00   **FUD** XXX   01 80 TC
   AMA: 2014,Aug,3

0211T **with speech recognition**
   🛏 0.00   ⚕ 0.00   **FUD** XXX   01 80 TC
   AMA: 2015,Jan,16; 2014,Aug,3; 2014,Jan,11; 2011,Mar,8

0212T **Comprehensive audiometry threshold evaluation and speech recognition (0209T, 0211T combined), automated**
   🛏 0.00   ⚕ 0.00   **FUD** XXX   01 80 TC
   AMA: 2015,Jan,16; 2014,Aug,3; 2014,Jan,11; 2011,Mar,8

0213T-0215T

0213T **Injection(s), diagnostic or therapeutic agent, paravertebral facet (zygapophyseal) joint (or nerves innervating that joint) with ultrasound guidance, cervical or thoracic; single level**
   🛏 0.00   ⚕ 0.00   **FUD** XXX   T R2 80 50
   AMA: 2015,Jan,16; 2014,Jan,11; 2011,Jul,14; 2011,Feb,4-5; 2010,Jan,9-11

+ **0214T** **second level (List separately in addition to code for primary procedure)**
   Code first (0213T)
   🛏 0.00   ⚕ 0.00   **FUD** ZZZ   N N1 80 50
   AMA: 2015,Jan,16; 2014,Jan,11; 2011,Jul,14; 2011,Feb,4-5; 2010,Jan,9-11

+ **0215T** **third and any additional level(s) (List separately in addition to code for primary procedure)**
   Code first (0213T-0214T)
   Do not report more than one time per day
   🛏 0.00   ⚕ 0.00   **FUD** ZZZ   N N1 80 50
   AMA: 2015,Jan,16; 2014,Jan,11; 2011,Jul,14; 2011,Feb,4-5; 2010,Jan,9-11

0216T-0218T

EXCLUDES   *Injection with CT or fluoroscopic guidance (64490-64495)*

0216T **Injection(s), diagnostic or therapeutic agent, paravertebral facet (zygapophyseal) joint (or nerves innervating that joint) with ultrasound guidance, lumbar or sacral; single level**
   🛏 0.00   ⚕ 0.00   **FUD** XXX   T R2 80 50
   AMA: 2015,Jan,16; 2014,Jan,11; 2011,Jul,14; 2011,Feb,4-5; 2010,Jan,9-11

+ **0217T** **second level (List separately in addition to code for primary procedure)**
   Code first (0216T)
   🛏 0.00   ⚕ 0.00   **FUD** ZZZ   N N1 80 50
   AMA: 2015,Jan,16; 2014,Jan,11; 2011,Jul,14; 2011,Feb,4-5; 2010,Jan,9-11

+ **0218T** **third and any additional level(s) (List separately in addition to code for primary procedure)**
   Code first (0216T, 0217T)
   Do not report more than one time per day
   🛏 0.00   ⚕ 0.00   **FUD** ZZZ   N N1 80 50
   AMA: 2015,Jan,16; 2014,Jan,11; 2011,Jul,14; 2011,Feb,4-5; 2010,Jan,9-11

0219T-0222T

Do not report when performed at the same level (20930-20931, 22600-22614, 22840, 22851)
Do not report with any radiology service

0219T **Placement of a posterior intrafacet implant(s), unilateral or bilateral, including imaging and placement of bone graft(s) or synthetic device(s), single level; cervical**
   🛏 0.00   ⚕ 0.00   **FUD** XXX   C 80
   AMA: 2015,Jan,16; 2014,Jan,11; 2012,Jun,10-11; 2012,Jan,15-42; 2011,Jul,16-17; 2010,Nov,8

0220T **thoracic**
   🛏 0.00   ⚕ 0.00   **FUD** XXX   C 80
   AMA: 2015,Jan,16; 2014,Jan,11; 2012,Jun,10-11; 2012,Jan,15-42; 2011,Jul,16-17; 2010,Nov,8

0221T **lumbar**
   🛏 0.00   ⚕ 0.00   **FUD** XXX   T 80
   AMA: 2015,Jan,16; 2014,Jan,11; 2012,Jun,10-11; 2012,Jan,15-42; 2011,Jul,16-17; 2010,Nov,8

+ **0222T** **each additional vertebral segment (List separately in addition to code for primary procedure)**
   Code first (0219T-0221T)
   🛏 0.00   ⚕ 0.00   **FUD** ZZZ   N 80
   AMA: 2015,Jan,16; 2014,Jan,11; 2012,Jun,10-11; 2012,Jan,15-42; 2011,Jul,16-17; 2010,Nov,8

0223T-0225T

~~**0223T** **Acoustic cardiography, including automated analysis of combined acoustic and electrical intervals; single, with interpretation and report**~~
   To report, see ~93799

~~**0224T** **multiple, including serial trended analysis and limited reprogramming of device parameter, AV or VV delays only, with interpretation and report**~~
   To report, see ~93799

~~**0225T** **multiple, including serial trended analysis and limited reprogramming of device parameter, AV and VV delays, with interpretation and report**~~
   To report, see ~93799

0228T-0233T

0228T **Injection(s), anesthetic agent and/or steroid, transforaminal epidural, with ultrasound guidance, cervical or thoracic; single level**
   🛏 0.00   ⚕ 0.00   **FUD** XXX   T G2 50
   AMA: 2015,Jan,16; 2014,Jan,11; 2012,Jan,15-42; 2011,Jul,16-17; 2011,Feb,4-5

+ **0229T** **each additional level (List separately in addition to code for primary procedure)**
   Code first (0228T)
   🛏 0.00   ⚕ 0.00   **FUD** XXX   N N1 50
   AMA: 2015,Jan,16; 2014,Jan,11; 2012,Jan,15-42; 2011,Jul,16-17; 2011,Feb,4-5

0230T **Injection(s), anesthetic agent and/or steroid, transforaminal epidural, with ultrasound guidance, lumbar or sacral; single level**
   🛏 0.00   ⚕ 0.00   **FUD** XXX   T G2 50
   AMA: 2015,Jan,16; 2014,Jan,11; 2012,Jan,15-42; 2011,Jul,16-17; 2011,Feb,4-5

+ **0231T** each additional level (List separately in addition to code for primary procedure)

> EXCLUDES *Injection performed with CT or fluoroscopic guidance (64479-64484)*
> Code first (0230T)
> Do not report with (76942, 76998-76999)
> 🖫 0.00 ⬡ 0.00 **FUD** XXX ☐N☐ ☐N1☐ ☐50☐
>
> **AMA:** 2015,Jan,16; 2014,Jan,11; 2012,Jan,15-42; 2011,Jul,16-17; 2011,Feb,4-5

0232T Injection(s), platelet rich plasma, any site, including image guidance, harvesting and preparation when performed

> EXCLUDES *Aspiration of bone marrow for grafting, biopsy, harvesting for transplant (38220-38221, 38230)*
> Do not report with (20550-20551, 20600-20610, 20926, 76942, 77002, 77012, 77021, 86965)
> 🖫 0.00 ⬡ 0.00 **FUD** XXX ☐Q1☐ ☐N1☐
>
> **AMA:** 2015,Jan,16; 2014,Jan,11; 2012,Oct,14; 2012,May,11-12; 2010,Dec,7-10

~~0233T~~ ~~Skin advanced glycation endproducts (AGE) measurement by multi-wavelength fluorescent spectroscopy~~

> To report, see ~88749

0234T-0238T

> INCLUDES Atherectomy by any technique in arteries above the inguinal ligaments
> Radiology supervision and interpretation
> EXCLUDES *Accessing and catheterization of the vessel*
> *Atherectomy performed below the inguinal ligaments (37225, 37227, 37229, 37231, 37233, 37235)*
> *Closure of the arteriotomy by any technique*
> *Negotiating the lesion*
> *Other interventions to the same or different vessels*
> *Protection from embolism*

0234T Transluminal peripheral atherectomy, open or percutaneous, including radiological supervision and interpretation; renal artery

> 🖫 0.00 ⬡ 0.00 **FUD** YYY ☐J☐ ☐80☐ ☐PQ☐
>
> **AMA:** 2015,Jan,16; 2014,Jan,11; 2011,Jul,3-11

0235T visceral artery (except renal), each vessel

> 🖫 0.00 ⬡ 0.00 **FUD** YYY ☐C☐ ☐80☐ ☐PQ☐
>
> **AMA:** 2015,Jan,16; 2014,Jan,11; 2011,Jul,3-11

0236T abdominal aorta

> 🖫 0.00 ⬡ 0.00 **FUD** YYY ☐J☐ ☐80☐ ☐PQ☐
>
> **AMA:** 2015,Jan,16; 2014,Jan,11; 2011,Jul,3-11

0237T brachiocephalic trunk and branches, each vessel

> 🖫 0.00 ⬡ 0.00 **FUD** YYY ☐J☐ ☐80☐
>
> **AMA:** 2015,Jan,16; 2014,Jan,11; 2011,Jul,3-11

0238T iliac artery, each vessel

> 🖫 0.00 ⬡ 0.00 **FUD** YYY ☐J☐ ☐J8☐ ☐80☐ ☐PQ☐
>
> **AMA:** 2015,Jan,16; 2014,Jan,11; 2011,Jul,3-11

0240T-0241T

~~0240T~~ ~~Esophageal motility (manometric study of the esophagus and/or gastroesophageal junction) study with interpretation and report; with high resolution esophageal pressure topography~~

> To report, see ~91299

~~0241T~~ ~~with stimulation or perfusion during high resolution esophageal pressure topography study (eg, stimulant, acid or alkali perfusion) (List separately in addition to code for primary procedure)~~

> To report, see ~91299

0243T-0244T

~~0243T~~ ~~Intermittent measurement of wheeze rate for bronchodilator or bronchial-challenge diagnostic evaluation(s), with interpretation and report~~

> To report, see ~94799

~~0244T~~ ~~Continuous measurement of wheeze rate during treatment assessment or during sleep for documentation of nocturnal wheeze and cough for diagnostic evaluation 3 to 24 hours, with interpretation and report~~

> To report, see ~94799

0249T-0255T

0249T Ligation, hemorrhoidal vascular bundle(s), including ultrasound guidance

> Do not report with (46020, 46221, [46945, 46946], 46250-46262, 46600, 76872, 76942, 76998)
> 🖫 0.00 ⬡ 0.00 **FUD** YYY ☐T☐ ☐G2☐ ☐80☐
>
> **AMA:** 2015,Mar,9

0253T **Resequenced code, See code following 0191T.**

0254T Endovascular repair of iliac artery bifurcation (eg, aneurysm, pseudoaneurysm, arteriovenous malformation, trauma) using bifurcated endoprosthesis from the common iliac artery into both the external and internal iliac artery, unilateral;

> ☒ (0255T)
> 🖫 0.00 ⬡ 0.00 **FUD** YYY ☐C☐ ☐80☐
>
> **AMA:** 2015,Jan,16; 2014,Jan,11; 2013,Dec,8

0255T radiological supervision and interpretation

> 🖫 0.00 ⬡ 0.00 **FUD** YYY ☐C☐ ☐80☐
>
> **AMA:** 2015,Jan,16; 2014,Jan,11; 2013,Dec,8

0262T

~~0262T~~ ~~Implantation of catheter-delivered prosthetic pulmonary valve, endovascular approach~~

> To report, see ~33477

0263T-0265T

0263T Intramuscular autologous bone marrow cell therapy, with preparation of harvested cells, multiple injections, one leg, including ultrasound guidance, if performed; complete procedure including unilateral or bilateral bone marrow harvest

> 🖫 0.00 ⬡ 0.00 **FUD** XXX ☐S☐ ☐G2☐ ☐80☐
>
> Do not report with (38204-38242 [38243], 76942, 93925-93926)

0264T complete procedure excluding bone marrow harvest

> 🖫 0.00 ⬡ 0.00 **FUD** XXX ☐S☐ ☐G2☐ ☐80☐
>
> Do not report with (38204-38242 [38243], 76942, 93925-93926, 0265T)

0265T unilateral or bilateral bone marrow harvest only for intramuscular autologous bone marrow cell therapy

> 🖫 0.00 ⬡ 0.00 **FUD** XXX ☐S☐ ☐G2☐ ☐80☐
>
> EXCLUDES *Complete procedure (0263T)*
> Do not report with (38204-38242 [38243], 0264T)

0266T-0273T

0266T Implantation or replacement of carotid sinus baroreflex activation device; total system (includes generator placement, unilateral or bilateral lead placement, intra-operative interrogation, programming, and repositioning, when performed)

> 🖫 0.00 ⬡ 0.00 **FUD** YYY ☐C☐ ☐80☐

0267T lead only, unilateral (includes intra-operative interrogation, programming, and repositioning, when performed)

> 🖫 0.00 ⬡ 0.00 **FUD** YYY ☐T☐ ☐80☐
>
> Do not report with (0266T, 0269T-0273T)

Category III Codes

0268T — 0290T

0268T   pulse generator only (includes intra-operative interrogation, programming, and repositioning, when performed)

📋 0.00   ✂ 0.00   **FUD** YYY   J 80

Do not report with (0266T, 0269T-0273T)

0269T   Revision or removal of carotid sinus baroreflex activation device; total system (includes generator placement, unilateral or bilateral lead placement, intra-operative interrogation, programming, and repositioning, when performed)

📋 0.00   ✂ 0.00   **FUD** XXX   02 G2 80

Do not report with (0266T-0268T, 0270T-0273T)

0270T   lead only, unilateral (includes intra-operative interrogation, programming, and repositioning, when performed)

📋 0.00   ✂ 0.00   **FUD** XXX   02 G2 80

EXCLUDES   Removal of total carotid sinus baroreflex activation device (0269T)

Do not report with (0266T-0269T, 0271T-0273T)

0271T   pulse generator only (includes intra-operative interrogation, programming, and repositioning, when performed)

📋 0.00   ✂ 0.00   **FUD** XXX   02 G2 80

EXCLUDES   Removal and replacement (0266T-0268T)

Do not report with (0266T-0270T, 0272T-0273T)

0272T   Interrogation device evaluation (in person), carotid sinus baroreflex activation system, including telemetric iterative communication with the implantable device to monitor device diagnostics and programmed therapy values, with interpretation and report (eg, battery status, lead impedance, pulse amplitude, pulse width, therapy frequency, pathway mode, burst mode, therapy start/stop times each day);

📋 0.00   ✂ 0.00   **FUD** XXX   S 80

Do not report with (0266T-0271T, 0273T)

0273T   with programming

📋 0.00   ✂ 0.00   **FUD** XXX   S 80

Do not report with (0266T-0272T)

0274T-0275T

EXCLUDES   Laminotomy/hemilaminectomy by open and endoscopically assisted approach (63020-63035)
Percutaneous decompression of nucleus pulposus of intervertebral disc by needle-based technique (62287)

0274T   Percutaneous laminotomy/laminectomy (interlaminar approach) for decompression of neural elements, (with or without ligamentous resection, discectomy, facetectomy and/or foraminotomy), any method, under indirect image guidance (eg, fluoroscopic, CT), with or without the use of an endoscope, single or multiple levels, unilateral or bilateral; cervical or thoracic

📋 0.00   ✂ 0.00   **FUD** YYY   T G2 80

AMA: 2015,Jan,16; 2014,Jan,11; 2012,Jul,3-6; 2012,Jan,13-14

0275T   lumbar

📋 0.00   ✂ 0.00   **FUD** XXX   T G2

AMA: 2015,Jan,16; 2014,Jan,11; 2012,Jul,3-6; 2012,Jan,13-14

0278T-0281T

0278T   Transcutaneous electrical modulation pain reprocessing (eg, scrambler therapy), each treatment session (includes placement of electrodes)

📋 0.00   ✂ 0.00   **FUD** XXX   Q1 80

0281T   Percutaneous transcatheter closure of the left atrial appendage with implant, including fluoroscopy, transseptal puncture, catheter placement(s), left atrial angiography, left atrial appendage angiography, radiological supervision and interpretation

📋 0.00   ✂ 0.00   **FUD** XXX   C 80

Code also for right heart catheterization separately for reasons distinct from left atrial appendage closure (93451-93461, 93530-93533)

Code also for separately performed ventriculography with transseptal approach for reasons separate from the left atrial appendage closure. (93565)

Do not report with (93462)

Do not report with the following codes unless the catheterization of the left ventricle is done by a nontransseptal approach for reasons other than the left atrial appendage repair (93452-93453, 93458-93461, 93531-93533)

Do not report with the following codes unless the complete right heart catheterization is done for reasons other than the left atrial appendage repair (93451, 93453, 93456, 93460-93461, 93530-93533)

0282T-0285T

Do not report with (64550-64595, 77002-77003, 95970-95972)

0282T   Percutaneous or open implantation of neurostimulator electrode array(s), subcutaneous (peripheral subcutaneous field stimulation), including imaging guidance, when performed, cervical, thoracic or lumbar; for trial, including removal at the conclusion of trial period

📋 0.00   ✂ 0.00   **FUD** XXX   ⊙ J J8 80 50

0283T   permanent, with implantation of a pulse generator

📋 0.00   ✂ 0.00   **FUD** XXX   ⊙ J J8 80 50

0284T   Revision or removal of pulse generator or electrodes, including imaging guidance, when performed, including addition of new electrodes, when performed

📋 0.00   ✂ 0.00   **FUD** XXX   ⊙ 02 G2 80

0285T   Electronic analysis of implanted peripheral subcutaneous field stimulation pulse generator, with reprogramming when performed

📋 0.00   ✂ 0.00   **FUD** XXX   S 80

0286T-0287T

0286T   Near-infrared spectroscopy studies of lower extremity wounds (eg, for oxyhemoglobin measurement)

📋 0.00   ✂ 0.00   **FUD** XXX   N N1 80

AMA: 2015,Jan,16; 2014,Jan,11; 2012,Jun,15-16

0287T   Near-infrared guidance for vascular access requiring real-time digital visualization of subcutaneous vasculature for evaluation of potential access sites and vessel patency

📋 0.00   ✂ 0.00   **FUD** XXX   N N1 80

0288T

Do not report with (46600-46615)

0288T   Anoscopy, with delivery of thermal energy to the muscle of the anal canal (eg, for fecal incontinence)

📋 0.00   ✂ 0.00   **FUD** XXX   T G2 80

0289T-0290T

Code first (65710, 65730, 65750, 65755)

+   **0289T**   Corneal incisions in the donor cornea created using a laser, in preparation for penetrating or lamellar keratoplasty (List separately in addition to code for primary procedure)

📋 0.00   ✂ 0.00   **FUD** ZZZ   N N1 80

AMA: 2015,Jan,16; 2014,Jan,11; 2012,Aug,9

+   **0290T**   Corneal incisions in the recipient cornea created using a laser, in preparation for penetrating or lamellar keratoplasty (List separately in addition to code for primary procedure)

📋 0.00   ✂ 0.00   **FUD** ZZZ   N N1 80

AMA: 2015,Jan,16; 2014,Jan,11; 2012,Aug,9

 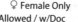

0291T-0292T

INCLUDES All manipulations and repositioning inside evaluated vessel including prior to and after the intervention

EXCLUDES Intravascular spectroscopy (0205T)

+ **0291T** Intravascular optical coherence tomography (coronary native vessel or graft) during diagnostic evaluation and/or therapeutic intervention, including imaging supervision, interpretation, and report; initial vessel (List separately in addition to primary procedure)

 0.00 0.00 **FUD** ZZZ   ⊙ N N1 80

Code first (92920, 92924, 92928, 92933, 92937, 92941, 92943, 92975, 93454-93461, 93563-93564)

+ **0292T** each additional vessel (List separately in addition to primary procedure)

 0.00 0.00 **FUD** ZZZ   ⊙ N N1 80

Code first (0291T)

0293T-0294T

Do not report with (93462, 93662)

Do not report with the following codes unless performed for separate clinical reason other than calibration or placement of left atrial hemodynamic monitoring system (33202-33249, 93451-93453) (33202-33249 [33221, 33227, 33228, 33229, 33230, 33231, 33262, 33263, 33264], 93451-93453)

0293T Insertion of left atrial hemodynamic monitor; complete system, includes implanted communication module and pressure sensor lead in left atrium including transseptal access, radiological supervision and interpretation, and associated injection procedures, when performed

 0.00 0.00 **FUD** XXX   ⊙ C 80

+ **0294T** pressure sensor lead at time of insertion of pacing cardioverter-defibrillator pulse generator including radiological supervision and interpretation and associated injection procedures, when performed (List separately in addition to code for primary procedure)

 0.00 0.00 **FUD** ZZZ   ⊙ C 80

Code first (33230-33231, 33240, [33262, 33263, 33264], 33249)

0295T-0298T

Do not report with (93224-93272)

0295T External electrocardiographic recording for more than 48 hours up to 21 days by continuous rhythm recording and storage; includes recording, scanning analysis with report, review and interpretation

 0.00 0.00 **FUD** XXX   M 80

AMA: 2015,Jan,16; 2014,Jan,11; 2013,Feb,16-17

0296T recording (includes connection and initial recording)

 0.00 0.00 **FUD** XXX   Q1 80

AMA: 2015,Jan,16; 2014,Jan,11; 2013,Feb,16-17

0297T scanning analysis with report

 0.00 0.00 **FUD** XXX   Q1 80

AMA: 2015,Jan,16; 2014,Jan,11; 2013,Feb,16-17

0298T review and interpretation

 0.00 0.00 **FUD** XXX   M 80

AMA: 2015,Jan,16; 2014,Jan,11; 2013,Feb,16-17

0299T-0301T

0299T Extracorporeal shock wave for integumentary wound healing, high energy, including topical application and dressing care; initial wound

 0.00 0.00 **FUD** XXX   T R2 80

+ **0300T** each additional wound (List separately in addition to code for primary procedure)

 0.00 0.00 **FUD** ZZZ   N N1 80

Code first (0299T)

Do not report with (0101T-0102T, 28890) when performed in the same area

0301T Destruction/reduction of malignant breast tumor with externally applied focused microwave, including interstitial placement of disposable catheter with combined temperature monitoring probe and microwave focusing sensocatheter under ultrasound thermotherapy guidance

 0.00 0.00 **FUD** XXX   ⊙ S G2 80

Do not report with (76641-76642, 76942, 76998, 77600-77615)

0302T-0304T

Do not report with (93000-93010)

0302T Insertion or removal and replacement of intracardiac ischemia monitoring system including imaging supervision and interpretation when performed and intra-operative interrogation and programming when performed; complete system (includes device and electrode)

 0.00 0.00 **FUD** YYY   ⊙ J J8

0303T electrode only

 0.00 0.00 **FUD** YYY   ⊙ J J8

0304T device only

 0.00 0.00 **FUD** YYY   ⊙ J J8

0305T-0307T

0305T Programming device evaluation (in person) of intracardiac ischemia monitoring system with iterative adjustment of programmed values, with analysis, review, and report

 0.00 0.00 **FUD** XXX   Q1 80

Do not report with (93000-93010, 0302T-0304T, 0306T)

0306T Interrogation device evaluation (in person) of intracardiac ischemia monitoring system with analysis, review, and report

 0.00 0.00 **FUD** XXX   Q1 80

Do not report with (93000-93010, 0302T-0305T)

0307T Removal of intracardiac ischemia monitoring device

 0.00 0.00 **FUD** YYY   ⊙ 02 G2

0308T-0311T

▲ **0308T** Insertion of ocular telescope prosthesis including removal of crystalline lens or intraocular lens prosthesis

INCLUDES Operating microscope (69990)

Do not report with (65800-65815, 66020, 66030, 66600-66635, 66761, 66825, 66982-66986)

 0.00 0.00 **FUD** YYY   ⊙ J J8 50

AMA: 2015,Jan,16; 2014,Jan,11; 2013,Mar,6-7

+ **0309T** Arthrodesis, pre-sacral interbody technique, including disc space preparation, discectomy, with posterior instrumentation, with image guidance, includes bone graft, when performed, lumbar, L4-L5 interspace (List separately in addition to code for primary procedure)

 0.00 0.00 **FUD** ZZZ   C 80

Code first (22586)

Do not report with (20930-20938, 22840, 22848, 72275, 77002-77003, 77011-77012)

0310T Motor function mapping using non-invasive navigated transcranial magnetic stimulation (nTMS) for therapeutic treatment planning, upper and lower extremity

 0.00 0.00 **FUD** XXX   S 80

Do not report with (95860-95870, 95928-95929, [95939])

~~**0311T** Non-invasive calculation and analysis of central arterial pressure waveforms with interpretation and report~~

To report, see ~93050

0312T-0317T

EXCLUDES Analysis and/or programming (or reprogramming) of vagus nerve stimulator (95970, 95974-95975)

Implantation, replacement, removal, and/or revision of vagus nerve neurostimulator (electrode array and/or pulse generator) for stimulation of vagus nerve other than at the esophagogastric junction (64568-64570)

Category III Codes

0312T — 0352T

0312T Vagus nerve blocking therapy (morbid obesity); laparoscopic implantation of neurostimulator electrode array, anterior and posterior vagal trunks adjacent to esophagogastric junction (EGJ), with implantation of pulse generator, includes programming

⚙ 0.00   ✂ 0.00   **FUD** XXX   C 80

AMA: 2015,Jan,16; 2013,Jan,11-12

0313T laparoscopic revision or replacement of vagal trunk neurostimulator electrode array, including connection to existing pulse generator

⚙ 0.00   ✂ 0.00   **FUD** XXX   T G2 80

AMA: 2015,Jan,16; 2013,Jan,11-12

0314T laparoscopic removal of vagal trunk neurostimulator electrode array and pulse generator

⚙ 0.00   ✂ 0.00   **FUD** XXX   Q2 G2 80

AMA: 2015,Jan,16; 2013,Jan,11-12

0315T removal of pulse generator

Do not report with (0316T)

⚙ 0.00   ✂ 0.00   **FUD** XXX   Q2 G2 80

AMA: 2015,Jan,16; 2013,Jan,11-12

0316T replacement of pulse generator

Do not report with (0315T)

⚙ 0.00   ✂ 0.00   **FUD** XXX   J J8 80

AMA: 2015,Jan,16; 2013,Jan,11-12

0317T neurostimulator pulse generator electronic analysis, includes reprogramming when performed

⚙ 0.00   ✂ 0.00   **FUD** XXX   Q1 80

AMA: 2015,Jan,16; 2013,Jan,11-12

0329T-0330T

0329T Monitoring of intraocular pressure for 24 hours or longer, unilateral or bilateral, with interpretation and report

⚙ 0.00   ✂ 0.00   **FUD** YYY   E

AMA: 2015,Jan,16; 2014,May,5

0330T Tear film imaging, unilateral or bilateral, with interpretation and report

⚙ 0.00   ✂ 0.00   **FUD** YYY   Q1

AMA: 2015,Jan,16; 2014,May,5

0331T-0332T

EXCLUDES *Myocardial infarction avid imaging (78466, 78468, 78469)*

0331T Myocardial sympathetic innervation imaging, planar qualitative and quantitative assessment;

⚙ 0.00   ✂ 0.00   **FUD** YYY   S Z2

AMA: 2015,Jan,16; 2014,Jun,14

0332T with tomographic SPECT

⚙ 0.00   ✂ 0.00   **FUD** YYY   S Z2

AMA: 2015,Jan,16; 2014,Jun,14

0333T-0337T

0333T Visual evoked potential, screening of visual acuity, automated

⚙ 0.00   ✂ 0.00   **FUD** YYY   E

AMA: 2015,Jan,16; 2014,Aug,8

0335T Extra-osseous subtalar joint implant for talotarsal stabilization

⚙ 0.00   ✂ 0.00   **FUD** YYY   ⊙ T G2

0336T Laparoscopy, surgical, ablation of uterine fibroid(s), including intraoperative ultrasound guidance and monitoring, radiofrequency   ♀

⚙ 0.00   ✂ 0.00   **FUD** YYY   T G2

Do not report with (76998, 0071T)

0337T Endothelial function assessment, using peripheral vascular response to reactive hyperemia, non-invasive (eg, brachial artery ultrasound, peripheral artery tonometry), unilateral or bilateral

⚙ 0.00   ✂ 0.00   **FUD** YYY   S

Do not report with (93922-93923)

0338T-0339T

Do not report with (36251-36254)

0338T Transcatheter renal sympathetic denervation, percutaneous approach including arterial puncture, selective catheter placement(s) renal artery(ies), fluoroscopy, contrast injection(s), intraprocedural roadmapping and radiological supervision and interpretation, including pressure gradient measurements, flush aortogram and diagnostic renal angiography when performed; unilateral

⚙ 0.00   ✂ 0.00   **FUD** YYY   S G2

0339T bilateral

⚙ 0.00   ✂ 0.00   **FUD** YYY   S G2

0340T-0342T

0340T Ablation, pulmonary tumor(s), including pleura or chest wall when involved by tumor extension, percutaneous, cryoablation, unilateral, includes imaging guidance

⚙ 0.00   ✂ 0.00   **FUD** YYY   ⊙ T G2

Do not report with (76940, 77013, 77022)

0341T Quantitative pupillometry with interpretation and report, unilateral or bilateral

⚙ 0.00   ✂ 0.00   **FUD** YYY   N N1

0342T Therapeutic apheresis with selective HDL delipidation and plasma reinfusion

⚙ 0.00   ✂ 0.00   **FUD** YYY   S G2

0345T-0347T

0345T Transcatheter mitral valve repair percutaneous approach via the coronary sinus

⚙ 0.00   ✂ 0.00   **FUD** YYY   C

EXCLUDES *Repair of mitral valve including transseptal puncture (33418-33419)*

Do not report with (93451-93454, 93456-93461, 93563-93564)

+ 0346T Ultrasound, elastography (List separately in addition to code for primary procedure)

⚙ 0.00   ✂ 0.00   **FUD** YYY   N N1

Code first (76536, 76604, 76641-76642, 76700, 76705, 76770, 76775, 76830, 76856-76857, 76870, 76872, 76881-76882)

0347T Placement of interstitial device(s) in bone for radiostereometric analysis (RSA)

⚙ 0.00   ✂ 0.00   **FUD** YYY   Q1

AMA: 2015,Jun,8

0348T-0350T

0348T Radiologic examination, radiostereometric analysis (RSA); spine, (includes cervical, thoracic and lumbosacral, when performed)

⚙ 0.00   ✂ 0.00   **FUD** YYY   Q1 N1

AMA: 2015,Jun,8

0349T upper extremity(ies), (includes shoulder, elbow, and wrist, when performed)

⚙ 0.00   ✂ 0.00   **FUD** YYY   Q1 N1

AMA: 2015,Jun,8

0350T lower extremity(ies), (includes hip, proximal femur, knee, and ankle, when performed)

⚙ 0.00   ✂ 0.00   **FUD** YYY   Q1 N1

AMA: 2015,Jun,8

0351T-0354T

0351T Optical coherence tomography of breast or axillary lymph node, excised tissue, each specimen; real-time intraoperative

⚙ 0.00   ✂ 0.00   **FUD** YYY   N

AMA: 2015,Apr,6

0352T interpretation and report, real-time or referred

Do not report if provided by same physician (0351T)

⚙ 0.00   ✂ 0.00   **FUD** YYY   B

AMA: 2015,Apr,6

0353T Optical coherence tomography of breast, surgical cavity; real-time intraoperative
Do not report more than one time per session
🔷 0.00   ⊘ 0.00   **FUD** YYY   [N]
AMA: 2015,Apr,6

0354T interpretation and report, real time or referred
Do not report when provided by same physician (0353T)
🔷 0.00   ⊘ 0.00   **FUD** YYY   [B]
AMA: 2015,Apr,6

0355T-0358T

0355T Gastrointestinal tract imaging, intraluminal (eg, capsule endoscopy), colon, with interpretation and report
🔷 0.00   ⊘ 0.00   **FUD** YYY   [T]

INCLUDES   Includes distal ileum imaging when performed
Do not report with (91110-91111)

0356T Insertion of drug-eluting implant (including punctal dilation and implant removal when performed) into lacrimal canaliculus, each
🔷 0.00   ⊘ 0.00   **FUD** YYY   [Q1] [N1]

0357T Resequenced code. See code following 0058T.

▲ **0358T** Bioelectrical impedance analysis whole body composition assessment, with interpretation and report
🔷 0.00   ⊘ 0.00   **FUD** YYY   [Q1]

0359T

INCLUDES   Evaluation of adaptive behavior
Provided by physician or other qualified health care professional with assistance of technician(s)
Do not report on same date of service with (90785-90899, 96101-96125, 96150-96155)

0359T Behavior identification assessment, by the physician or other qualified health care professional, face-to-face with patient and caregiver(s), includes administration of standardized and non-standardized tests, detailed behavioral history, patient observation and caregiver interview, interpretation of test results, discussion of findings and recommendations with the primary guardian(s)/caregiver(s), and preparation of report
🔷 0.00   ⊘ 0.00   **FUD** YYY   [V]
AMA: 2015,Jan,16; 2014,Jun,3

0360T-0363T

INCLUDES   Follow-up assessments
Provided to patients with destructive behaviors
Only the time of one technician when more than one is in attendance
Time reported during one day only
Do not report on same date of service with (90785-90899, 96101-96125, 96150-96155)

0360T Observational behavioral follow-up assessment, includes physician or other qualified health care professional direction with interpretation and report, administered by one technician; first 30 minutes of technician time, face-to-face with the patient
INCLUDES   Time based on face-to-face time provided by one technician and not the collective time of several technicians
Time spent by physician or other qualified health care professional involved in technician tasks is considered as technician time
Do not report less than 16 minutes of face-to-face technician time
🔷 0.00   ⊘ 0.00   **FUD** YYY   [V]
AMA: 2015,Jan,16; 2014,Jun,3

+ **0361T** each additional 30 minutes of technician time, face-to-face with the patient (List separately in addition to code for primary service)
Code first (0360T)
🔷 0.00   ⊘ 0.00   **FUD** ZZZ   [N]
AMA: 2015,Jan,16; 2014,Jun,3

0362T Exposure behavioral follow-up assessment, includes physician or other qualified health care professional direction with interpretation and report, administered by physician or other qualified health care professional with the assistance of one or more technicians; first 30 minutes of technician(s) time, face-to-face with the patient
INCLUDES   Time based on face-to-face time provided by one technician and not the collective time of several technicians
Time spent by physician or other qualified health care professional involved in technician tasks is considered as technician time
🔷 0.00   ⊘ 0.00   **FUD** YYY   [V]
AMA: 2015,Jan,16; 2014,Jun,3

+ **0363T** each additional 30 minutes of technician(s) time, face-to-face with the patient (List separately in addition to code for primary procedure)
Code first (0362T)
🔷 0.00   ⊘ 0.00   **FUD** ZZZ   [N]
AMA: 2015,Jan,16; 2014,Jun,3

0364T-0372T

0364T Adaptive behavior treatment by protocol, administered by technician, face-to-face with one patient; first 30 minutes of technician time
Do not report with (90785-90899, 92507, 96101-96155, 97532)
🔷 0.00   ⊘ 0.00   **FUD** YYY   [S]
AMA: 2015,Jan,16; 2014,Jun,3

+ **0365T** each additional 30 minutes of technician time (List separately in addition to code for primary procedure)
Code first (0364T)
Do not report with (90785-90899, 92507, 96101-96155, 97532)
🔷 0.00   ⊘ 0.00   **FUD** ZZZ   [N]
AMA: 2015,Jan,16; 2014,Jun,3

0366T Group adaptive behavior treatment by protocol, administered by technician, face-to-face with two or more patients; first 30 minutes of technician time
Do not report when group exceeds eight patients
Do not report with (90785-90899, 92508, 96101-96155, 97150)
🔷 0.00   ⊘ 0.00   **FUD** YYY   [S]
AMA: 2015,Jan,16; 2014,Jun,3

+ **0367T** each additional 30 minutes of technician time (List separately in addition to code for primary procedure)
Code first (0366T)
Do not report if group exceeds eight patients
Do not report with (90785-90899, 92508, 96101-96155, 97150)
🔷 0.00   ⊘ 0.00   **FUD** ZZZ   [N]
AMA: 2015,Jan,16; 2014,Jun,3

0368T Adaptive behavior treatment with protocol modification administered by physician or other qualified health care professional with one patient; first 30 minutes of patient face-to-face time
Do not report with (90791-90792, 90846-90847, 90887, 92507, 97532)
🔷 0.00   ⊘ 0.00   **FUD** YYY   [S]
AMA: 2015,Jan,16; 2014,Jun,3

+ **0369T** each additional 30 minutes of patient face-to-face time (List separately in addition to code for primary procedure)
Code first (0368T)
Do not report with (90791-90792, 90846-90847, 90887, 92507, 97532)
🔷 0.00   ⊘ 0.00   **FUD** ZZZ   [N]
AMA: 2015,Jan,16; 2014,Jun,3

0370T Family adaptive behavior treatment guidance, administered by physician or other qualified health care professional (without the patient present)
Do not report with (90791-90792, 90846-90847, 90887)
🔷 0.00   ⊘ 0.00   **FUD** YYY   [S]
AMA: 2015,Jan,16; 2014,Jun,3

0371T Multiple-family group adaptive behavior treatment guidance, administered by physician or other qualified health care professional (without the patient present)

> Do not report when group exceeds the families of more than eight patients
> Do not report with (90791-90792, 90846-90847, 90887)
> 🔧 0.00   ⚗ 0.00   **FUD** YYY   S
>
> **AMA:** 2015,Jan,16; 2014,Jun,3

0372T Adaptive behavior treatment social skills group, administered by physician or other qualified health care professional face-to-face with multiple patients

> Do not report if group exceeds eight patients
> Do not report with (90853, 92508, 97150)
> 🔧 0.00   ⚗ 0.00   **FUD** YYY   S
>
> **AMA:** 2015,Jan,16; 2014,Jun,3

0373T-0374T

Do not report with (90785-90899, 96101-96155)

0373T Exposure adaptive behavior treatment with protocol modification requiring two or more technicians for severe maladaptive behavior(s); first 60 minutes of technicians' time, face-to-face with patient

> 🔧 0.00   ⚗ 0.00   **FUD** YYY   S
>
> **AMA:** 2015,Jan,16; 2014,Jun,3

+ 0374T each additional 30 minutes of technicians' time face-to-face with patient (List separately in addition to code for primary procedure)

> Code first (0373T)
> 🔧 0.00   ⚗ 0.00   **FUD** ZZZ   N
>
> **AMA:** 2014,Jun,3

0375T

0375T Total disc arthroplasty (artificial disc), anterior approach, including discectomy with end plate preparation (includes osteophytectomy for nerve root or spinal cord decompression and microdissection), cervical, three or more levels

> Do not report at same level with (22851, 22856, [22858])
> 🔧 0.00   ⚗ 0.00   **FUD** XXX   C 80
>
> **AMA:** 2015,Apr,7

0376T-0377T

0376T Resequenced code. See code following 0191T.

0377T Anoscopy with directed submucosal injection of bulking agent for fecal incontinence

> 🔧 0.00   ⚗ 0.00   **FUD** XXX   T 62 80
>
> Do not report with (46600)

0378T-0380T

0378T Visual field assessment, with concurrent real time data analysis and accessible data storage with patient initiated data transmitted to a remote surveillance center for up to 30 days; review and interpretation with report by a physician or other qualified health care professional

> 🔧 0.00   ⚗ 0.00   **FUD** XXX   B 80
>
> **AMA:** 2015,Jan,10

0379T technical support and patient instructions, surveillance, analysis and transmission of daily and emergent data reports as prescribed by a physician or other qualified health care professional

> 🔧 0.00   ⚗ 0.00   **FUD** XXX   Q1 80
>
> **AMA:** 2015,Jan,10

0380T Computer-aided animation and analysis of time series retinal images for the monitoring of disease progression, unilateral or bilateral, with interpretation and report

> 🔧 0.00   ⚗ 0.00   **FUD** XXX   Q1 80

0381T-0386T

0381T External heart rate and 3-axis accelerometer data recording up to 14 days to assess changes in heart rate and to monitor motion analysis for the purposes of diagnosing nocturnal epilepsy seizure events; includes report, scanning analysis with report, review and interpretation by a physician or other qualified health care professional

> 🔧 0.00   ⚗ 0.00   **FUD** XXX   M 80
>
> Do not report with (0383T-0386T)

0382T review and interpretation only

> 🔧 0.00   ⚗ 0.00   **FUD** XXX   M 80
>
> Do not report with (0383T-0386T)

0383T External heart rate and 3-axis accelerometer data recording from 15 to 30 days to assess changes in heart rate and to monitor motion analysis for the purposes of diagnosing nocturnal epilepsy seizure events; includes report, scanning analysis with report, review and interpretation by a physician or other qualified health care professional

> 🔧 0.00   ⚗ 0.00   **FUD** XXX   M 80
>
> Do not report with (0381T-0382T, 0385T-0386T)

0384T review and interpretation only

> 🔧 0.00   ⚗ 0.00   **FUD** XXX   M 80
>
> Do not report with (0381T-0382T, 0385T-0386T)

0385T External heart rate and 3-axis accelerometer data recording more than 30 days to assess changes in heart rate and to monitor motion analysis for the purposes of diagnosing nocturnal epilepsy seizure events; includes report, scanning analysis with report, review and interpretation by a physician or other qualified health care professional

> 🔧 0.00   ⚗ 0.00   **FUD** XXX   M 80
>
> Do not report with (0381T-0384T)

0386T review and interpretation only

> 🔧 0.00   ⚗ 0.00   **FUD** XXX   M 80
>
> Do not report with (0381T-0384T)

0387T-0391T

0387T Transcatheter insertion or replacement of permanent leadless pacemaker, ventricular

> **INCLUDES** Fluoroscopy (76000)
>   Right ventriculography (93566)
>   Venography, femoral (75820)
> **EXCLUDES** *Procedures related to pacemaker systems with leads (33202-33203, 33206-33222 [33221], 33224-33226)*
> Do not report with (0388T-0391T)
> 🔧 0.00   ⚗ 0.00   **FUD** XXX   J J8 80
>
> **AMA:** 2015,May,3; 2015,Jan,16; 2014,Dec,16; 2014,Dec,16

0388T Transcatheter removal of permanent leadless pacemaker, ventricular

> **INCLUDES** Fluoroscopy (76000)
>   Right ventriculography (93566)
>   Venography, femoral (75820)
> **EXCLUDES** *Procedures related to removal of pacemaker systems with leads (33233-33238 [33227, 33228, 33229])*
> Do not report with (0387T)
> 🔧 0.00   ⚗ 0.00   **FUD** XXX   T 62 80
>
> **AMA:** 2015,May,3; 2015,Jan,16; 2014,Dec,16; 2014,Dec,16

0389T Programming device evaluation (in person) with iterative adjustment of the implantable device to test the function of the device and select optimal permanent programmed values with analysis, review and report, leadless pacemaker system

> **EXCLUDES** *Procedures to program pacemaker systems with leads (93279-93281, 0387T, 0390T-0391T)*
> Do not report with (0387T, 0390T-0391T)
> 🔧 0.00   ⚗ 0.00   **FUD** XXX   Q1 80
>
> **AMA:** 2015,May,3; 2015,Jan,16; 2014,Dec,16; 2014,Dec,16

0390T Peri-procedural device evaluation (in person) and programming of device system parameters before or after a surgery, procedure or test with analysis, review and report, leadless pacemaker system

> EXCLUDES *Procedures for peri-procedural evaluation and programming of pacemaker systems with leads (93286-93287)*
>
> Do not report with (0387T, 0389T, 0391T)
>
> 🔧 0.00   ✂ XXX   **FUD** XXX   N 80
>
> **AMA:** 2015,May,3; 2015,Jan,16; 2014,Dec,16; 2014,Dec,16

0391T Interrogation device evaluation (in person) with analysis, review and report, includes connection, recording and disconnection per patient encounter, leadless pacemaker system

> EXCLUDES *Procedures for interrogation device evaluation of pacemaker systems with leads (93288-93289)*
>
> Do not report with (0387T, 0389T-0390T)
>
> 🔧 0.00   ✂ 0.00   **FUD** XXX   Q1 80
>
> **AMA:** 2015,May,3

0392T-0393T

0392T Laparoscopy, surgical, esophageal sphincter augmentation procedure, placement of sphincter augmentation device (ie, magnetic band)

> 🔧 0.00   ✂ 0.00   **FUD** YYY   T G2 80

0393T Removal of esophageal sphincter augmentation device

> 🔧 0.00   ✂ 0.00   **FUD** YYY   Q2 G2 80
>
> Do not report with (43279-43282)

0394T-0395T

Do not report with (77261-77263, 77300, 77306-77307, 77316-77318, 77332-77334, 77336, 77427-77499, 77761-77772, 77778, 77789)

0394T High dose rate electronic brachytherapy, skin surface application, per fraction, includes basic dosimetry, when performed

> EXCLUDES *High dose radionuclide skin surface brachytherapy (77767-77768)*
>
> *Superficial non-brachytherapy radiation (77401)*

0395T High dose rate electronic brachytherapy, interstitial or intracavitary treatment, per fraction, includes basic dosimetry, when performed

> EXCLUDES *High dose rate skin surface application (0394T)*

0396T-0399T

+ 0396T Intra-operative use of kinetic balance sensor for implant stability during knee replacement arthroplasty (List separately in addition to code for primary procedure)

> 🔧 0.00   ✂ 0.00   **FUD** 000
>
> Code first (27445-27447, 27486-27488)

+ 0397T Endoscopic retrograde cholangiopancreatography (ERCP), with optical endomicroscopy (List separately in addition to code for primary procedure)

> 🔧 0.00   ✂ 0.00   **FUD** 000   ☉
>
> Code first (43260-43270 [43274, 43275, 43276, 43277, 43278])
> Do not report more than one time per operative session
> Do not report with (88375)

0398T Magnetic resonance image guided high intensity focused ultrasound (MRgFUS), stereotactic ablation lesion, intracranial for movement disorder including stereotactic navigation and frame placement when performed

> Do not report with (61781, 61800)

+ 0399T Myocardial strain imaging (quantitative assessment of myocardial mechanics using image-based analysis of local myocardial dynamics)

> 🔧 0.00   ✂ 0.00   **FUD** 000
>
> Code first (93303-93312, 93314-93315, 93317, 93350-93351, 93355)
> Do not report more than one time per session

0400T-0401T

0400T Multi-spectral digital skin lesion analysis of clinically atypical cutaneous pigmented lesions for detection of melanomas and high risk melanocytic atypia; one to five lesions

0401T six or more lesions

> Do not report with (0400T)

0402T-0405T

0402T Collagen cross-linking of cornea (including removal of the corneal epithelium and intraoperative pachymetry when performed)

> INCLUDES Operating microscope (69990)
> Do not report with (65435, 76514)

0403T Preventive behavior change, intensive program of prevention of diabetes using a standardized diabetes prevention program curriculum, provided to individuals in a group setting, minimum 60 minutes, per day

> **AMA:** 2015,Aug,4

0404T Transcervical uterine fibroid(s) ablation with ultrasound guidance, radiofrequency

0405T Oversight of the care of an extracorporeal liver assist system patient requiring review of status, review of laboratories and other studies, and revision of orders and liver assist care plan (as appropriate), within a calendar month, 30 minutes or more of non-face-to-face time

0406T-0407T

Do not report when performed on the same side (31200-31205, 31231, 31237, 31240, 31254-31255, 31288, 31290)

0406T Nasal endoscopy, surgical, ethmoid sinus, placement of drug eluting implant

0407T with biopsy, polypectomy or debridement

> Do not report when performed on the same side (0406T)

0408T-0418T

0408T Insertion or replacement of permanent cardiac contractility modulation system, including contractility evaluation when performed, and programming of sensing and therapeutic parameters; pulse generator with transvenous electrodes

> Code also removal of each electrode when pulse generator and electrodes are removed and replaced (0410T-0411T)
> Do not report with (93286-93287, 93452-93453, 93458-93461, 0415T, 0417T-0418T)

0409T pulse generator only

> Do not report with (93286-93287, 93452-93453, 93458-93461, 0417T-0418T)

0410T atrial electrode only

> INCLUDES Each atrial electrode inserted or replaced
> Do not report with (93286-93287, 93452-93453, 93458-93461, 0415T, 0417T-0418T)

0411T ventricular electrode only

> INCLUDES Each ventricular electrode inserted or replaced
> Do not report with (93261-93458 [93260, 93261], 93286-93287, 93452-93453, 0415T, 0417T-0418T)

0412T Removal of permanent cardiac contractility modulation system; pulse generator only

> Do not report with (0417T-0418T)

0413T transvenous electrode (atrial or ventricular)

> INCLUDES Each electrode removed
> Code also removal and replacement of electrode(s), as appropriate (0410T-0411T)
> Do not report with (0417T-0418T)

0414T Removal and replacement of permanent cardiac contractility modulation system pulse generator only

> Code also removal of each electrode when pulse generator and electrodes are removed and replaced (0412T-0413T)
> Do not report with (93286-93287, 93452-93453, 93458-93461, 0417T-0418T)

Category III Codes

0415T — 0436T

- **0415T** Repositioning of previously implanted cardiac contractility modulation transvenous electrode, (atrial or ventricular lead)

  Do not report with (93286-93287, 93452-93453, 93458-93461, 0408T, 0410T-0411T, 0417T-0418T)

- **0416T** Relocation of skin pocket for implanted cardiac contractility modulation pulse generator

- **0417T** Programming device evaluation (in person) with iterative adjustment of the implantable device to test the function of the device and select optimal permanent programmed values with analysis, including review and report, implantable cardiac contractility modulation system

  Do not report with (0408T-0415T, 0418T)

- **0418T** Interrogation device evaluation (in person) with analysis, review and report, includes connection, recording and disconnection per patient encounter; implantable cardiac contractility modulation system

  Do not report with (0408T-0415T, 0417T)

0419T-0420T

EXCLUDES *Neurofibroma excision (64792)*
Do not report more than one time for each session

- **0419T** Destruction neurofibromata, extensive, (cutaneous, dermal extending into subcutaneous); face, head and neck, greater than 50 neurofibromata

- **0420T** trunk and extremities, extensive, greater than 100 neurofibromata

0421T-0423T

- **0421T** Transurethral waterjet ablation of prostate, including control of post-operative bleeding, including ultrasound guidance, complete (vasectomy, meatotomy, cystourethroscopy, urethral calibration and/or dilation, and internal urethrotomy are included when performed)

  Do not report with (52500, 52630, 76872)

- **0422T** Tactile breast imaging by computer-aided tactile sensors, unilateral or bilateral

- **0423T** Secretory type II phospholipase A2 (sPLA2-IIA)

  EXCLUDES *Lipoprotein-associated phospholipase A2 [LpPLA2] (83698)*

0424T-0436T

INCLUDES Phrenic nerve stimulation system includes:
Pulse generator
Sensing lead (placed in azygos vein)
Stimulation lead (placed into right brachiocephalic vein or left periocardiophrenic vein)

- **0424T** Insertion or replacement of neurostimulator system for treatment of central sleep apnea; complete system (transvenous placement of right or left stimulation lead, sensing lead, implantable pulse generator)

  Code also when pulse generator and all leads are removed and replaced (0428T-0430T)
  Do not report with (0425T-0427T, 0432T-0436T)

- **0425T** sensing lead only

  Do not report with (0424T, 0432T-0436T)

- **0426T** stimulation lead only

  Do not report with (0424T, 0432T-0436T)

- **0427T** pulse generator only

  Do not report with (0424T, 0432T-0436T)

- **0428T** Removal of neurostimulator system for treatment of central sleep apnea; pulse generator only

  Code also when a lead is removed (0429T-0430T)
  Code also when complete system is removed and replaced (0424T, 0429T-0430T)
  Do not report with (0434T-0436T)

- **0429T** sensing lead only

  INCLUDES Removal of one sensing lead
  Do not report with (0434T-0436T)

- **0430T** stimulation lead only

  INCLUDES Removal of one stimulation lead
  Do not report with (0434T-0436T)
  AMA: 2015,Aug,4

- **0431T** Removal and replacement of neurostimulator system for treatment of central sleep apnea, pulse generator only

  EXCLUDES *Removal with replacement of pulse generator and all leads (0424T, 0428T-0430T)*
  Do not report with (0434T-0436T)

- **0432T** Repositioning of neurostimulator system for treatment of central sleep apnea; stimulation lead only

  Do not report with (0424T-0427T, 0434T-0436T)

- **0433T** sensing lead only

  Do not report with (0424T-0427T, 0434T-0436T)

- **0434T** Interrogation device evaluation implanted neurostimulator pulse generator system for central sleep apnea

  Do not report with (0424T-0433T)

- **0435T** Programming device evaluation of implanted neurostimulator pulse generator system for central sleep apnea; single session

  Do not report with (0424T-0433T, 0436T)

- **0436T** during sleep study

  Do not report more than one time for each sleep study
  Do not report with (0424T-0433T, 0435T)

Appendix A — Modifiers

CPT Modifiers

A modifier is a two-position alpha or numeric code appended to a CPT® code to clarify the services being billed. Modifiers provide a means by which a service can be altered without changing the procedure code. They add more information, such as the anatomical site, to the code. In addition, they help to eliminate the appearance of duplicate billing and unbundling. Modifiers are used to increase accuracy in reimbursement, coding consistency, editing, and to capture payment data.

22   Increased Procedural Services: When the work required to provide a service is substantially greater than typically required, it may be identified by adding modifier 22 to the usual procedure code. Documentation must support the substantial additional work and the reason for the additional work (ie, increased intensity, time, technical difficulty of procedure, severity of patient's condition, physical and mental effort required).
Note: This modifier should not be appended to an E/M service.

23   Unusual Anesthesia: Occasionally, a procedure, which usually requires either no anesthesia or local anesthesia, because of unusual circumstances must be done under general anesthesia. This circumstance may be reported by adding modifier 23 to the procedure code of the basic service.

24   Unrelated Evaluation and Management Service by the Same Physician or Other Qualified Health Care Professional During a Postoperative Period: The physician or other qualified health care professional may need to indicate that an evaluation and management service was performed during a postoperative period for a reason(s) unrelated to the original procedure. This circumstance may be reported by adding modifier 24 to the appropriate level of E/M service.

25   Significant, Separately Identifiable Evaluation and Management Service by the Same Physician or Other Qualified Health Care Professional on the Same Day of the Procedure or Other Service: It may be necessary to indicate that on the day a procedure or service identified by a CPT code was performed, the patient's condition required a significant, separately identifiable E/M service above and beyond the other service provided or beyond the usual preoperative and postoperative care associated with the procedure that was performed. A significant, separately identifiable E/M service is defined or substantiated by documentation that satisfies the relevant criteria for the respective E/M service to be reported (see Evaluation and Management Services Guidelines for instructions on determining level of E/M service). The E/M service may be prompted by the symptom or condition for which the procedure and/or service was provided. As such, different diagnoses are not required for reporting of the E/M services on the same date. This circumstance may be reported by adding modifier 25 to the appropriate level of E/M service.
Note: This modifier is not used to report an E/M service that resulted in a decision to perform surgery. See modifier 57. For significant, separately identifiable non-E/M services, see modifier 59.

26   Professional Component: Certain procedures are a combination of a physician or other qualified health care professional component and a technical component. When the physician or other qualified health care professional component is reported separately, the service may be identified by adding modifier 26 to the usual procedure number.

32   Mandated Services: Services related to mandated consultation and/or related services (eg, third-party payer, governmental, legislative or regulatory requirement) may be identified by adding modifier 32 to the basic procedure.

33   Preventive Services: When the primary purpose of the service is the delivery of an evidence-based service in accordance with a U.S. Preventive Services Task Force A or B rating in effect and other preventive services identified in preventive services mandates (legislative or regulatory), the service may be identified by adding 33 to the procedure. For separately reported services specifically identified as preventive, the modifier should not be used.

47   Anesthesia by Surgeon: Regional or general anesthesia provided by the surgeon may be reported by adding modifier 47 to the basic service. (This does not include local anesthesia.)
Note: Modifier 47 would not be used as a modifier for the anesthesia procedures 00100–01999.

50   Bilateral Procedure: Unless otherwise identified in the listings, bilateral procedures that are performed at the same session should be identified by adding modifier 50 to the appropriate 5-digit code.

51   Multiple Procedures: When multiple procedures, other than E/M services, Physical Medicine and Rehabilitation services or provision of supplies (e.g., vaccines), are performed at the same session by the same individual, the primary procedure or service may be reported as listed. The additional procedure(s) or service(s) may be identified by appending modifier 51 to the additional procedure or service code(s).
Note: This modifier should not be appended to designated "add-on" codes. See appendix E.

52   Reduced Services: Under certain circumstances a service or procedure is partially reduced or eliminated at the discretion of the physician or other qualified health care professional. Under these circumstances the service provided can be identified by its usual procedure number and the addition of modifier 52, signifying that the service is reduced. This provides a means of reporting reduced services without disturbing the identification of the basic service.
Note: For hospital outpatient reporting of a previously scheduled procedure/service that is partially reduced or cancelled as a result of extenuating circumstances or those that threaten the well-being of the patient prior to or after administration of anesthesia, see modifiers 73 and 74 (see modifiers approved for ASC hospital outpatient use).

53   Discontinued Procedure: Under certain circumstances, the physician or other qualified health care professional may elect to terminate a surgical or diagnostic procedure. Due to extenuating circumstances or those that threaten the well being of the patient, it may be necessary to indicate that a surgical or diagnostic procedure was started but discontinued. This circumstance may be reported by adding modifier 53 to the code reported by the physician for the discontinued procedure.
Note: This modifier is not used to report the elective cancellation of a procedure prior to the patient's anesthesia induction and/or surgical preparation in the operating suite. For outpatient hospital/ambulatory surgery center (ASC) reporting of a previously scheduled procedure/service that is partially reduced or cancelled as a result of extenuating circumstances or those that threaten the well being of the patient prior to or after administration of anesthesia, see modifiers 73 and 74 (see modifiers approved for ASC hospital outpatient use).

54   Surgical Care Only: When 1 physician or other qualified health care professional performs a surgical procedure and another provides preoperative and/or postoperative management, surgical services may be identified by adding modifier 54 to the usual procedure number.

55   Postoperative Management Only: When 1 physician or other qualified health care professional performed the postoperative management and another performed the surgical procedure, the postoperative component may be identified by adding modifier 55 to the usual procedure number.

56   Preoperative Management Only: When 1 physician or other qualified health care professional performed the preoperative care and evaluation and another performed the surgical procedure, the preoperative component may be identified by adding modifier 56 to the usual procedure number.

57   Decision for Surgery: An evaluation and management service that resulted in the initial decision to perform the surgery may be identified by adding modifier 57 to the appropriate level of E/M service.

58 **Staged or Related Procedure or Service by the Same Physician or Other Qualified Health Care Professional During the Postoperative Period:** It may be necessary to indicate that the performance of a procedure or service during the postoperative period was (a) planned or anticipated (staged); (b) more extensive than the original procedure; or (c) for therapy following a surgical procedure. This circumstance may be reported by adding modifier 58 to the staged or related procedure.
Note: For treatment of a problem that requires a return to the operating or procedure room (eg, unanticipated clinical condition), see modifier 78.

59 **Distinct Procedural Service:** Under certain circumstances, it may be necessary to indicate that a procedure or service was distinct or independent from other non-E/M services performed on the same day. Modifier 59 is used to identify procedures/services, other than E/M services, that are not normally reported together but are appropriate under the circumstances. Documentation must support a different session, different procedure or surgery, different site or organ system, separate incision/excision, separate lesion, or separate injury (or area of injury in extensive injuries) not ordinarily encountered or performed on the same day by the same individual. However, when another already established modifier is appropriate it should be used rather than modifier 59. Only if no more descriptive modifier is available and the use of modifier 59 best explains the circumstances, should modifier 59 be used.
Note: Modifier 59 should not be appended to an E/M service. To report a separate and distinct E/M service with a non-E/M service performed on the same date, see modifier 25. See also "Level II (HCPCS/National) Modifiers."

62 **Two Surgeons:** When 2 surgeons work together as primary surgeons performing distinct part(s) of a procedure, each surgeon should report his/her distinct operative work by adding modifier 62 to the procedure code and any associated add-on code(s) for that procedure as long as both surgeons continue to work together as primary surgeons. Each surgeon should report the cosurgery once using the same procedure code. If additional procedure(s) (including add-on procedure[s]) are performed during the same surgical session, separate code(s) may also be reported with modifier 62 added.
Note: If a cosurgeon acts as an assistant in the performance of additional procedure(s), other than those reported with the modifier 62, during the same surgical session, those services may be reported using separate procedure code(s) with modifier 80 or modifier 82 added, as appropriate.

63 **Procedure Performed on Infants less than 4 kg:** Procedures performed on neonates and infants up to a present body weight of 4 kg may involve significantly increased complexity and physician or other qualified health care professional work commonly associated with these patients. This circumstance may be reported by adding modifier 63 to the procedure number.
Note: Unless otherwise designated, this modifier may only be appended to procedures/services listed in the 20005-69990 code series. Modifier 63 should not be appended to any CPT codes listed in the Evaluation and Management Services, Anesthesia, Radiology, Pathology/Laboratory, or Medicine sections.

66 **Surgical Team:** Under some circumstances, highly complex procedures (requiring the concomitant services of several physicians or other qualified health care professionals, often of different specialties, plus other highly skilled, specially trained personnel, various types of complex equipment) are carried out under the "surgical team" concept. Such circumstances may be identified by each participating individual with the addition of modifier 66 to the basic procedure number used for reporting services.

76 **Repeat Procedure or Service by Same Physician or Other Qualified Health Care Professional:** It may be necessary to indicate that a procedure or service was repeated by the same physician or other qualified health care professional subsequent to the original procedure or service. This circumstance may be reported by adding modifier 76 to the repeated procedure or service.
Note: This modifier should not be appended to an E/M service.

77 **Repeat Procedure by Another Physician or Other Qualified Health Care Professional:** It may be necessary to indicate that a basic procedure or service was repeated by another physician or other qualified health care professional subsequent to the original procedure or service. This circumstance may be reported by adding modifier 77 to the repeated procedure or service.
Note: This modifier should not be appended to an E/M service.

78 **Unplanned Return to the Operating/Procedure Room by the Same Physician or Other Qualified Health Care Professional Following Initial Procedure for a Related Procedure During the Postoperative Period:** It may be necessary to indicate that another procedure was performed during the postoperative period of the initial procedure (unplanned procedure following initial procedure). When this procedure is related to the first, and requires the use of an operating/procedure room, it may be reported by adding modifier 78 to the related procedure. (For repeat procedures, see modifier 76.)

79 **Unrelated Procedure or Service by the Same Physician or Other Qualified Health Care Professional During the Postoperative Period:** The individual may need to indicate that the performance of a procedure or service during the postoperative period was unrelated to the original procedure. This circumstance may be reported by using modifier 79. (For repeat procedures on the same day, see modifier 76.)

80 **Assistant Surgeon:** Surgical assistant services may be identified by adding modifier 80 to the usual procedure number(s).

81 **Minimum Assistant Surgeon:** Minimum surgical assistant services are identified by adding modifier 81 to the usual procedure number.

82 **Assistant Surgeon (when qualified resident surgeon not available):** The unavailability of a qualified resident surgeon is a prerequisite for use of modifier 82 appended to the usual procedure code number(s).

90 **Reference (Outside) Laboratory:** When laboratory procedures are performed by a party other than the treating or reporting physician or other qualified health care professional, the procedure may be identified by adding modifier 90 to the usual procedure number.

91 **Repeat Clinical Diagnostic Laboratory Test:** In the course of treatment of the patient, it may be necessary to repeat the same laboratory test on the same day to obtain subsequent (multiple) test results. Under these circumstances, the laboratory test performed can be identified by its usual procedure number and the addition of modifier 91.
Note: This modifier may not be used when tests are rerun to confirm initial results; due to testing problems with specimens or equipment; or for any other reason when a normal, one-time, reportable result is all that is required. This modifier may not be used when another code(s) describes a series of test results (eg, glucose tolerance tests, evocative/suppression testing). This modifier may only be used for a laboratory test(s) performed more than once on the same day on the same patient.

92 **Alternative Laboratory Platform Testing** When laboratory testing is being performed using a kit or transportable instrument that wholly or in part consists of a single use, disposable analytical chamber, the service may be identified by adding modifier 92 to the usual laboratory procedure code (HIV testing 86701-86703, and 87389). The test does not require permanent dedicated space, hence by its design may be hand carried or transported to the vicinity of the patient for immediate testing at that site, although location of the testing is not in itself determinative of the use of this modifier.

99 **Multiple Modifiers:** Under certain circumstances 2 or more modifiers may be necessary to completely delineate a service. In such situations, modifier 99 should be added to the basic procedure and other applicable modifiers may be listed as part of the description of the service.

Anesthesia Physical Status Modifiers

All anesthesia services are reported by use of the five-digit anesthesia procedure code with the appropriate physical status modifier appended.

Under certain circumstances, when other modifier(s) are appropriate, they should be reported in addition to the physical status modifier.

P1 A normal healthy patient

P2 A patient with mild systemic disease

P3 A patient with severe systemic disease

P4 A patient with severe systemic disease that is a constant threat to life

P5 A moribund patient who is not expected to survive without the operation

P6 A declared brain-dead patient whose organs are being removed for donor purposes

Modifiers Approved for Ambulatory Surgery Center (ASC) Hospital Outpatient Use

CPT Level I Modifiers

25 **Significant, Separately Identifiable Evaluation and Management Service by the Same Physician or Other Qualified Health Care Professional on the Same Day of the Procedure or Other Service:** It may be necessary to indicate that on the day a procedure or service identified by a CPT code was performed, the patient's condition required a significant, separately identifiable E/M service above and beyond the other service provided or beyond the usual preoperative and postoperative care associated with the procedure that was performed. A significant, separately identifiable E/M service is defined or substantiated by documentation that satisfies the relevant criteria for the respective E/M service to be reported (see Evaluation and Management Services Guidelines for instructions on determining level of E/M service). The E/M service may be prompted by the symptom or condition for which the procedure and/or service was provided. As such, different diagnoses are not required for reporting of the E/M services on the same date. This circumstance may be reported by adding modifier 25 to the appropriate level of E/M service. **Note:** This modifier is not used to report an E/M service that resulted in a decision to perform surgery. See modifier 57. For significant, separately identifiable non-E/M services, see modifier 59.

27 **Multiple Outpatient Hospital E/M Encounters on the Same Date:** For hospital outpatient reporting purposes, utilization of hospital resources related to separate and distinct E/M encounters performed in multiple outpatient hospital settings on the same date may be reported by adding modifier 27 to each appropriate level outpatient and/or emergency department E/M code(s). This modifier provides a means of reporting circumstances involving evaluation and management services provided by a physician(s) in more than one (multiple) outpatient hospital setting(s) (eg, hospital emergency department, clinic). **Note:** This modifier is not to be used for physician reporting of multiple E/M services performed by the same physician on the same date. For physician reporting of all outpatient evaluation and management services provided by the same physician on the same date and performed in multiple outpatient settings (eg, hospital emergency department, clinic), see Evaluation and Management, Emergency Department, or Preventive Medicine Services codes.

50 **Bilateral Procedure:** Unless otherwise identified in the listings, bilateral procedures that are performed at the same session should be identified by adding modifier 50 to the appropriate 5-digit code.

52 **Reduced Services:** Under certain circumstances a service or procedure is partially reduced or eliminated at the discretion of the physician or other qualified health care professional. Under these circumstances the service provided can be identified by its usual procedure number and the addition of modifier 52, signifying that the service is reduced. This provides a means of reporting reduced services without disturbing the identification of the basic service. **Note:** For hospital outpatient reporting of a previously scheduled procedure/service that is partially reduced or cancelled as a result of extenuating circumstances or those that threaten the well-being of the patient prior to or after administration of anesthesia, see modifiers 73 and 74 (see modifiers approved for ASC hospital outpatient use).

58 **Staged or Related Procedure or Service by the Same Physician or Other Qualified Health Care Professional During the Postoperative Period:** It may be necessary to indicate that the performance of a procedure or service during the postoperative period was (a) planned or anticipated (staged); (b) more extensive than the original procedure; or (c) for therapy following a surgical procedure. This circumstance may be reported by adding modifier 58 to the staged or related procedure. **Note:** For treatment of a problem that requires a return to the operating or procedure room (eg, unanticipated clinical condition), see modifier 78.

59 **Distinct Procedural Service:** Under certain circumstances, it may be necessary to indicate that a procedure or service was distinct or independent from other non-E/M services performed on the same day. Modifier 59 is used to identify procedures/services, other than E/M services, that are not normally reported together but are appropriate under the circumstances. Documentation must support a different session, different procedure or surgery, different site or organ system, separate incision/excision, separate lesion, or separate injury (or area of injury in extensive injuries) not ordinarily encountered or performed on the same day by the same individual. However, when another already established modifier is appropriate it should be used rather than modifier 59. Only if no more descriptive modifier is available and the use of modifier 59 best explains the circumstances, should modifier 59 be used. **Note:** Modifier 59 should not be appended to an E/M service. To report a separate and distinct E/M service with a non-E/M service performed on the same date, see modifier 25. See also "Level II (HCPCS/National) Modifiers."

73 **Discontinued Out-Patient Hospital/Ambulatory Surgery Center (ASC) Procedure Prior to the Administration of Anesthesia:** Due to extenuating circumstances or those that threaten the well being of the patient, the physician may cancel a surgical or diagnostic procedure subsequent to the patient's surgical preparation (including sedation when provided, and being taken to the room where the procedure is to be performed), but prior to the administration of anesthesia (local, regional block(s), or general). Under these circumstances, the intended service that is prepared for but cancelled can be reported by its usual procedure number and the addition of modifier 73. **Note:** The elective cancellation of a service prior to the administration of anesthesia and/or surgical preparation of the patient should not be reported. For physician reporting of a discontinued procedure, see modifier 53.

74 **Discontinued Out-Patient Hospital/Ambulatory Surgery Center (ASC) Procedure After Administration of Anesthesia:** Due to extenuating circumstances or those that threaten the well being of the patient, the physician may terminate a surgical or diagnostic procedure after the administration of anesthesia (local, regional block(s), general) or after the procedure was started (incision made, intubation started, scope inserted, etc.). Under these circumstances, the procedure started but terminated can be reported by its usual procedure number and the addition of modifier 74. **Note:** The elective cancellation of a service prior to the administration of anesthesia and/or surgical preparation of the patient should not be reported. For physician reporting of a discontinued procedure, see modifier 53.

76 **Repeat Procedure or Service by Same Physician or Other Qualified Health Care Professional:** It may be necessary to indicate that a procedure or service was repeated by the same physician or other qualified health care professional subsequent to the original procedure or service. This circumstance may be reported by adding modifier 76 to the repeated procedure or service. **Note:** This modifier should not be appended to an E/M service.

77 **Repeat Procedure by Another Physician or Other Qualified Health Care Professional:** It may be necessary to indicate that a basic procedure or service was repeated by another physician or other qualified health care professional subsequent to the original procedure or service. This circumstance may be reported by adding modifier 77 to the repeated procedure or service. **Note:** This modifier should not be appended to an E/M service.

78 **Unplanned Return to the Operating/Procedure Room by the Same Physician or Other Qualified Health Care Professional Following Initial Procedure for a Related Procedure During the Postoperative Period:** It may be necessary to indicate that another procedure was performed during the postoperative period of the initial procedure (unplanned procedure following initial procedure). When this procedure is related to the first, and requires the use of an operating/procedure room, it may be reported by adding modifier 78 to the related procedure. (For repeat procedures, see modifier 76.)

79 Unrelated Procedure or Service by the Same Physician During the Postoperative Period: The individual may need to indicate that the performance of a procedure or service during the postoperative period was unrelated to the original procedure. This circumstance may be reported by using modifier 79. (For repeat procedures on the same day, see modifier 76.)

91 Repeat Clinical Diagnostic Laboratory Test: In the course of treatment of the patient, it may be necessary to repeat the same laboratory test on the same day to obtain subsequent (multiple) test results. Under these circumstances, the laboratory test performed can be identified by its usual procedure number and the addition of modifier 91.
Note: This modifier may not be used when tests are rerun to confirm initial results; due to testing problems with specimens or equipment; or for any other reason when a normal, one-time, reportable result is all that is required. This modifier may not be used when another code(s) describe a series of test results (eg, glucose tolerance tests, evocative/suppression testing). This modifier may only be used for a laboratory test(s) performed more than once on the same day on the same patient.

Level II (HCPCS/National) Modifiers

The HCPCS Level II modifiers included here are those most commonly used when coding procedures. See your 2016 HCPCS Level II book for a complete listing

Anatomical Modifiers

E1 Upper left, eyelid

E2 Lower left, eyelid

E3 Upper right, eyelid

E4 Lower right, eyelid

F1 Left hand, second digit

F2 Left hand, third digit

F3 Left hand, fourth digit

F4 Left hand, fifth digit

F5 Right hand, thumb

F6 Right hand, second digit

F7 Right hand, third digit

F8 Right hand, fourth digit

F9 Right hand, fifth digit

FA Left hand, thumb

LT Left side (used to identify procedures performed on the left side of the body)

RT Right side (used to identify procedures performed on the right side of the body)

T1 Left foot, second digit

T2 Left foot, third digit

T3 Left foot, fourth digit

T4 Left foot, fifth digit

T5 Right foot, great toe

T6 Right foot, second digit

T7 Right foot, third digit

T8 Right foot, fourth digit

T9 Right foot, fifth digit

TA Left foot, great toe

Anesthesia Modifiers

AA Anesthesia services performed personally by anesthesiologist

AD Medical supervision by a physician: more than four concurrent anesthesia procedures

G8 Monitored anesthesia care (MAC) for deep complex, complicated, or markedly invasive surgical procedure

G9 Monitored anesthesia care for patient who has history of severe cardiopulmonary condition

P1 A normal healthy patient

P2 A patient with mild systemic disease

P3 A patient with severe systemic disease

P4 A patient with severe systemic disease that is a constant threat to life

P5 A moribund patient who is not expected to survive without the operation

P6 A declared brain-dead patient whose organs are being removed for donor purposes

QK Medical direction of two, three, or four concurrent anesthesia procedures involving qualified individuals

QS Monitored anesthesia care service

QX CRNA service: with medical direction by a physician

QY Medical direction of one certified registered nurse anesthetist (CRNA) by an anesthesiologist

QZ CRNA service: without medical direction by a physician

Coronary Artery Modifiers

LC Left circumflex coronary artery

LD Left anterior descending coronary artery

LM Left main coronary artery

RC Right coronary artery

RI Ramus intermedius coronary artery

Ophthalmology Modifiers

AP Determination of refractive state was not performed in the course of diagnostic ophthalmological examination

LS FDA-monitored intraocular lens implant

PL Progressive addition lenses

VP Aphakic patient

Other Modifiers

AE Registered dietician

AF Specialty physician

AG Primary physician

AH Clinical psychologist

AI Principal physician of record

AJ Clinical social worker

AK Nonparticipating physician

AM Physician, team member service

AO Alternate payment method declined by provider of service

AQ Physician providing a service in an unlisted health professional shortage area (HPSA)

AR Physician provider services in a physician scarcity area

AS Physician assistant, nurse practitioner, or clinical nurse specialist services for assistant at surgery

AT Acute treatment (this modifier should be used when reporting service 98940, 98941, 98942)

CA Procedure payable only in the inpatient setting when performed emergently on an outpatient who expires prior to admission

CB Service ordered by a renal dialysis facility (RDF) physician as part of the ESRD beneficiary's dialysis benefit, is not part of the composite rate, and is separately reimbursable

CC Procedure code change (use 'CC' when the procedure code submitted was changed either for administrative reasons or because an incorrect code was filed)

CG Policy criteria applied

CR Catastrophe/disaster related

CS Item or service related, in whole or in part, to an illness, injury, or condition that was caused by or exacerbated by the effects, direct or indirect, of the 2010 oil spill in the gulf of Mexico, including but not limited to subsequent clean up activities

EA Erythropoetic stimulating agent (ESA) administered to treat anemia due to anticancer chemotherapy

EB Erythropoetic stimulating agent (ESA) administered to treat anemia due to anticancer radiotherapy

EC Erythropoetic stimulating agent (ESA) administered to treat anemia not due to anticancer radiotherapy or anticancer chemotherapy

EP Service provided as part of Medicaid early periodic screening diagnosis and treatment (EPSDT) program

ET Emergency services

EY No physician or other licensed health care provider order for this item or service

FB Item provided without cost to provider, supplier or practitioner, or full credit received for replaced device (examples, but not limited to covered under warranty, replaced due to defect, free samples)

FC Partial credit received for replacement device

FP Service provided as part of family planning program

G7 Pregnancy resulted from rape or incest or pregnancy certified by physician as life threatening

GA Waiver of liability statement issued as required by payer policy, individual case

GB Claim being resubmitted for payment because it is no longer covered under a global payment demonstration

GC This service has been performed in part by a resident under the direction of a teaching physician

GD Units of service exceeds medically unlikely edit value and represents reasonable and necessary services

GE This service has been performed by a resident without the presence of a teaching physician under the primary care exception

GF Non-physician (e.g. nurse practitioner (NP), certified registered nurse anesthetist (CRNA), certified registered nurse (CRN), clinical nurse specialist (CNS), physician assistant (PA)) services in a critical access hospital

GG Performance and payment of a screening mammogram and diagnostic mammogram on the same patient, same day

GH Diagnostic mammogram converted from screening mammogram on same day

GJ Opt out physician or practitioner emergency or urgent service

GK Reasonable and necessary item/service associated with GA or GZ modifier

GN Service delivered under an outpatient speech-language pathology plan of care

GO Service delivered an outpatient occupational therapy plan of care

GP Service delivered under an outpatient physical therapy plan of care

GQ Via asynchronous telecommunications system

GR This service was performed in whole or in part by a resident in a department of veterans affairs medical center or clinic, supervised in accordance with VA policy

GT Via interactive audio and video telecommunication systems

GU Waiver of liability statement issued as required by payer policy, routine notice

GV Attending physician not employed or paid under arrangement by the patient's hospice provider

GW Service not related to the hospice patient's terminal condition

GX Notice of liability issued, voluntary under payer policy

GY Item or service statutorily excluded, does not meet the definition of any Medicare benefit or for non-Medicare insurers, is not a contract benefit

GZ Item or service expected to be denied as not reasonable and necessary

H9 Court-ordered

HA Child/adolescent program

HB Adult program, nongeriatric

HC Adult program, geriatric

HD Pregnant/parenting women's program

HE Mental health program

HF Substance abuse program

HG Opioid addiction treatment program

HH Integrated mental health/substance abuse program

HI Integrated mental health and mental retardation/developmental disabilities program

HJ Employee assistance program

HK Specialized mental health programs for high-risk populations

HL Intern

HM Less than bachelor degree level

HN Bachelors degree level

HO Masters degree level

HP Doctoral level

HQ Group setting

HR Family/couple with client present

HS Family/couple without client present

HT Multi-disciplinary team

HU Funded by child welfare agency

HV Funded state addictions agency

HW Funded by state mental health agency

HX Funded by county/local agency

HY Funded by juvenile justice agency

HZ Funded by criminal justice agency

KB Beneficiary requested upgrade for ABN, more than four modifiers identified on claim

KX Requirements specified in the medical policy have been met

KZ New coverage not implemented by managed care

LR Laboratory round trip

M2 Medicare secondary payer (MSP)

PA Surgical or other invasive procedure on wrong body part

PB Surgical or other invasive procedure on wrong patient

PC Wrong surgery or other invasive procedure on patient

PD Diagnostic or related nondiagnostic item or service provided in a wholly owned or operated entity to a patient who is admitted as an inpatient within 3 days

PI Positron emission tomography (PET) or PET/computed tomography (CT) to inform the initial treatment strategy of tumors that are biopsy proven or strongly suspected of being cancerous based on other diagnostic testing

PM Post-mortem

PO Services, procedures and/or surgeries provided at off-campus provider-based outpatient departments

PS Positron emission tomography (PET) or PET/computed tomography (CT) to inform the subsequent treatment strategy of cancerous tumor when the beneficiary's treating physician determines that the PET study is needed to inform subsequent anti-tumor strategy

PT Colorectal cancer screening test; converted to diagnostic test or other procedure

Q0 Investigational clinical service provided in a clinical research study that is in an approved clinical research study

Q1 Routine clinical service provided in a clinical research study that is in an approved clinical research study

Q2 HCFA/ORD demonstration project procedure/service

Q4 Service for ordering/referring physician qualifies as a service exemption

Q5 Service furnished by a substitute physician under a reciprocal billing arrangement

Q6 Service furnished by a locum tenens physician

Q7 One Class A finding

Q8 Two Class B findings

Q9 One Class B and 2 Class C findings

QC Single channel monitoring

QD Recording and storage in solid state memory by a digital recorder

QJ Services/items provided to a prisoner or patient in state or local custody, however the state or local government, as applicable, meets the requirements in 42 CFR 411.4 (B)

QM Ambulance service provided under arrangement by a provider of services

QN Ambulance service furnished directly by a provider of services

QP Documentation is on file showing that the laboratory test(s) was ordered individually or ordered as a CPT-recognized panel other than automated profile codes

QT Recording and storage on tape by an analog tape recorder

QW CLIA waived test

RE Furnished in full compliance with FDA-mandated risk evaluation and mitigation strategy (REMS)

SA Nurse practitioner rendering service in collaboration with a physician

SB Nurse Midwife

SC Medically necessary service or supply

SD Services provided by registered nurse with specialized, highly technical home infusion training

SE State and/or federally funded programs/services

SF Second opinion ordered by a professional review organization (PRO) per section 9401, P.L.99-272 (100% reimbursement - no Medicare deductible or coinsurance)

SG Ambulatory surgical center (ASC) facility service

SH Second concurrently administered infusion therapy

SJ Third or more concurrently administered infusion therapy

SK Member of high risk population (use only with codes for immunization)

SL State supplied vaccine

SM Second surgical opinion

SN Third surgical opinion

SQ Item ordered by home health

SS Home infusion services provided in the infusion suite of the IV therapy provider

ST Related to trauma or injury

SU Procedure performed in physician's office (to denote use of facility and equipment)

SW Services provided by a certified diabetic educator

SY Persons who are in close contact with member of high-risk population (use only with codes for immunization)

TC Technical component. Under certain circumstances, a charge may be made for the technical component alone. Under those circumstances the technical component charge is identified by adding modifier 'TC' to the usual procedure number. Technical component charges are institutional charges and not billed separately by physicians. However, portable x-ray suppliers only bill for technical component and should utilize modifier TC. The charge data from portable x-ray suppliers will then be used to build customary and prevailing profiles.

TD RN

TE LPN/LVN

TF Intermediate level of care

TG Complex/high level of care

TH Obstetrical treatment/services, prenatal or postpartum

TJ Program group, child and/or adolescent

TK Extra patient or passenger, nonambulance

TL Early intervention/individualized family service plan (IFSP)

TM Individualized education program (IEP)

TN Rural/outside providers' customary service area

TR School-based individualized education program (IEP) services provided outside the public school district responsible for the student

TS Follow-up service

TT Individualized service provided to more than one patient in same setting

TU Special payment rate, overtime

TV Special payment rates, holidays/weekends

U1 Medicaid level of care 1, as defined by each state

U2 Medicaid level of care 2, as defined by each state

U3 Medicaid level of care 3, as defined by each state

U4 Medicaid level of care 4, as defined by each state

U5 Medicaid level of care 5, as defined by each state

U6 Medicaid level of care 6, as defined by each state

U7 Medicaid level of care 7, as defined by each state

U8 Medicaid level of care 8, as defined by each state

U9 Medicaid level of care 9, as defined by each state

UA Medicaid level of care 10, as defined by each state

UB Medicaid level of care 11, as defined by each state

UC Medicaid level of care 12, as defined by each state

UD Medicaid level of care 13, as defined by each state

UF Services provided in the morning

UG Services provided in the afternoon

UH Services provided in the evening

UJ Services provided at night

UK Services provided on behalf of the client to someone other than the client (collateral relationship)

UN Two patients served

UP Three patients served

UQ Four patients served

UR Five patients served

US Six or more patients served

V5 Vascular catheter (alone or with any other vascular access)

V6 Arteriovenous graft (or other vascular access not including a vascular catheter)

V7 Arteriovenous fistula only (in use with 2 needles)

* **XE** Separate encounter, a service that Is distinct because it occurred during a separate encounter

* **XP** Separate practitioner, a service that is distinct because it was performed by a different practitioner

* **XS** Separate structure, a service that is distinct because it was performed on a separate organ/structure

* **XU** Unusual non-overlapping service, the use of a service that is distinct because it does not overlap usual components of the main service

* CMS instituted additional HCPCS modifiers to define explicit subsets of modifier 59 Distinct Procedural Service.

Category II Modifiers

1P Performance measure exclusion modifier due to medical reasons

Includes:

- Not indicated (absence of organ/limb, already received/performed, other)

- Contraindicated (patient allergic history, potential adverse drug interaction, other)

- Other medical reasons

2P Performance measure exclusion modifier due to patient reasons

Includes:

- Patient declined

- Economic, social, or religious reasons

- Other patient reasons

3P Performance measure exclusion modifier due to system reasons
Includes:

- Resources to perform the services not available (eg, equipment, supplies)
- Insurance coverage or payer-related limitations
- Other reasons attributable to health care delivery system

8P Performance measure reporting modifier - action not performed, reason not otherwise specified

Dental Modifiers

AZ Physician providing a service in a dental health professional shortage area for the purpose of an electronic health record incentive payment

DA Oral health assessment by a licensed health professional other than a dentist

ET Emergency services (dental procedures performed in emergency situations should show the modifier ET)

ESRD Modifiers

AY Item or service furnished to an ESRD patient that is not for the treatment of ESRD

CD AMCC test has been ordered by an ESRD facility or MCP physician that is a part of the composite rate and is not separately billable

CE AMCC test has been ordered by an ESRD facility or MCP physician that is a composite rate test but is beyond the normal frequency

covered under the rate and is separately reimbursable based on medically necessary

CF AMCC test has been ordered by an ESRD facility or MCP physician that is not part of the composite rate and is separately billable

ED Hematocrit level has exceeded 39% (or hemoglobin level has exceeded 13.0 G/dl) for 3 or more consecutive billing cycles immediately prior to and including the current cycle

EE Hematocrit level has not exceeded 39% (or hemoglobin level has not exceeded 13.0 G/dl) for 3 or more consecutive billing cycles immediately prior to and including the current cycle

EJ Subsequent claims for a defined course of therapy, e.g., EPO, sodium hyaluronate, infliximab

EM Emergency reserve supply (for ESRD benefit only)

G1 Most recent URR reading of less than 60

G2 Most recent URR reading of 60 to 64.9

G3 Most recent URR reading of 65 to 69.9

G4 Most recent URR reading of 70 to 74.9

G5 Most recent URR reading of 75 or greater

G6 ESRD patient for whom less than 6 dialysis sessions have been provided in a month

GS Dosage of EPO or darbepoietin alfa has been reduced and maintained in response to hematocrit or hemoglobin level

JE Administered via dialysate

Q3 Live kidney donor surgery and related services

Appendix B — New, Changed and Deleted Codes

New Codes

0392T Laparoscopy, surgical, esophageal sphincter augmentation procedure, placement of sphincter augmentation device (ie, magnetic band)

0393T Removal of esophageal sphincter augmentation device

0394T High dose rate electronic brachytherapy, skin surface application, per fraction, includes basic dosimetry, when performed

0395T High dose rate electronic brachytherapy, interstitial or intracavitary treatment, per fraction, includes basic dosimetry, when performed

0396T Intra-operative use of kinetic balance sensor for implant stability during knee replacement arthroplasty (List separately in addition to code for primary procedure)

0397T Endoscopic retrograde cholangiopancreatography (ERCP), with optical endomicroscopy (List separately in addition to code for primary procedure)

0398T Magnetic resonance image guided high intensity focused ultrasound (MRgFUS), stereotactic ablation lesion, intracranial for movement disorder including stereotactic navigation and frame placement when performed

0399T Myocardial strain imaging (quantitative assessment of myocardial mechanics using image-based analysis of local myocardial dynamics)

0400T Multi-spectral digital skin lesion analysis of clinically atypical cutaneous pigmented lesions for detection of melanomas and high risk melanocytic atypia; one to five lesions

0401T Multi-spectral digital skin lesion analysis of clinically atypical cutaneous pigmented lesions for detection of melanomas and high risk melanocytic atypia; six or more lesions

0402T Collagen cross-linking of cornea (including removal of the corneal epithelium and intraoperative pachymetry when performed)

0403T Preventive behavior change, intensive program of prevention of diabetes using a standardized diabetes prevention program curriculum, provided to individuals in a group setting, minimum 60 minutes, per day

0404T Transcervical uterine fibroid(s) ablation with ultrasound guidance, radiofrequency

0405T Oversight of the care of an extracorporeal liver assist system patient requiring review of status, review of laboratories and other studies, and revision of orders and liver assist care plan (as appropriate), within a calendar month, 30 minutes or more of non-face-to-face time

0406T Nasal endoscopy, surgical, ethmoid sinus, placement of drug eluting implant

0407T Nasal endoscopy, surgical, ethmoid sinus, placement of drug eluting implant; with biopsy, polypectomy or debridement

0408T Insertion or replacement of permanent cardiac contractility modulation system, including contractility evaluation when performed, and programming of sensing and therapeutic parameters; pulse generator with transvenous electrodes

0409T Insertion or replacement of permanent cardiac contractility modulation system, including contractility evaluation when performed, and programming of sensing and therapeutic parameters; pulse generator only

0410T Insertion or replacement of permanent cardiac contractility modulation system, including contractility evaluation when performed, and programming of sensing and therapeutic parameters; atrial electrode only

0411T Insertion or replacement of permanent cardiac contractility modulation system, including contractility evaluation when performed, and programming of sensing and therapeutic parameters; ventricular electrode only

0412T Removal of permanent cardiac contractility modulation system; pulse generator only

0413T Removal of permanent cardiac contractility modulation system; transvenous electrode (atrial or ventricular)

0414T Removal and replacement of permanent cardiac contractility modulation system pulse generator only

0415T Repositioning of previously implanted cardiac contractility modulation transvenous electrode, (atrial or ventricular lead)

0416T Relocation of skin pocket for implanted cardiac contractility modulation pulse generator

0417T Programming device evaluation (in person) with iterative adjustment of the implantable device to test the function of the device and select optimal permanent programmed values with analysis, including review and report, implantable cardiac contractility modulation system

0418T Interrogation device evaluation (in person) with analysis, review and report, includes connection, recording and disconnection per patient encounter; implantable cardiac contractility modulation system

0419T Destruction neurofibromata, extensive, (cutaneous, dermal extending into subcutaneous); face, head and neck, greater than 50 neurofibromata

0420T Destruction neurofibromata, extensive, (cutaneous, dermal extending into subcutaneous); trunk and extremities, extensive, greater than 100 neurofibromata

0421T Transurethral waterjet ablation of prostate, including control of post-operative bleeding, including ultrasound guidance, complete (vasectomy, meatotomy, cystourethroscopy, urethral calibration and/or dilation, and internal urethrotomy are included when performed)

0422T Tactile breast imaging by computer-aided tactile sensors, unilateral or bilateral

0423T Secretory type II phospholipase A2 (sPLA2-IIA)

0424T Insertion or replacement of neurostimulator system for treatment of central sleep apnea; complete system (transvenous placement of right or left stimulation lead, sensing lead, implantable pulse generator)

0425T Insertion or replacement of neurostimulator system for treatment of central sleep apnea; sensing lead only

0426T Insertion or replacement of neurostimulator system for treatment of central sleep apnea; stimulation lead only

0427T Insertion or replacement of neurostimulator system for treatment of central sleep apnea; pulse generator only

0428T Removal of neurostimulator system for treatment of central sleep apnea; pulse generator only

0429T Removal of neurostimulator system for treatment of central sleep apnea; sensing lead only

0430T Removal of neurostimulator system for treatment of central sleep apnea; stimulation lead only

0431T Removal and replacement of neurostimulator system for treatment of central sleep apnea, pulse generator only

0432T Repositioning of neurostimulator system for treatment of central sleep apnea; stimulation lead only

0433T Repositioning of neurostimulator system for treatment of central sleep apnea; sensing lead only

0434T Interrogation device evaluation implanted neurostimulator pulse generator system for central sleep apnea

0435T Programming device evaluation of implanted neurostimulator pulse generator system for central sleep apnea; single session

0436T Programming device evaluation of implanted neurostimulator pulse generator system for central sleep apnea; during sleep study

10035 Placement of soft tissue localization device(s) (eg, clip, metallic pellet, wire/needle, radioactive seeds), percutaneous, including imaging guidance; first lesion

10036 Placement of soft tissue localization device(s) (eg, clip, metallic pellet, wire/needle, radioactive seeds), percutaneous, including imaging guidance; each additional lesion (List separately in addition to code for primary procedure)

31652 Bronchoscopy, rigid or flexible, including fluoroscopic guidance, when performed; with endobronchial ultrasound (EBUS) guided transtracheal and/or transbronchial sampling (eg, aspiration[s]/biopsy[ies]), one or two mediastinal and/or hilar lymph node stations or structures

31653 Bronchoscopy, rigid or flexible, including fluoroscopic guidance, when performed; with endobronchial ultrasound (EBUS) guided transtracheal and/or transbronchial sampling (eg, aspiration[s]/biopsy[ies]), 3 or more mediastinal and/or hilar lymph node stations or structures

31654 Bronchoscopy, rigid or flexible, including fluoroscopic guidance, when performed; with transendoscopic endobronchial ultrasound (EBUS) during bronchoscopic diagnostic or therapeutic intervention(s) for peripheral lesion(s) (List separately in addition to code for primary procedure[s])

33477 Transcatheter pulmonary valve implantation, percutaneous approach, including pre-stenting of the valve delivery site, when performed

37252 Intravascular ultrasound (noncoronary vessel) during diagnostic evaluation and/or therapeutic intervention, including radiological supervision and interpretation; initial noncoronary vessel (List separately in addition to code for primary procedure)

37253 Intravascular ultrasound (noncoronary vessel) during diagnostic evaluation and/or therapeutic intervention, including radiological supervision and interpretation; each additional noncoronary vessel (List separately in addition to code for primary procedure)

39401 Mediastinoscopy; includes biopsy(ies) of mediastinal mass (eg, lymphoma), when performed

39402 Mediastinoscopy; with lymph node biopsy(ies) (eg, lung cancer staging)

43210 Esophagogastroduodenoscopy, flexible, transoral; with esophagogastric fundoplasty, partial or complete, includes duodenoscopy when performed

47531 Injection procedure for cholangiography, percutaneous, complete diagnostic procedure including imaging guidance (eg, ultrasound and/or fluoroscopy) and all associated radiological supervision and interpretation; existing access

47532 Injection procedure for cholangiography, percutaneous, complete diagnostic procedure including imaging guidance (eg, ultrasound and/or fluoroscopy) and all associated radiological supervision and interpretation; new access (eg, percutaneous transhepatic cholangiogram)

47533 Placement of biliary drainage catheter, percutaneous, including diagnostic cholangiography when performed, imaging guidance (eg, ultrasound and/or fluoroscopy), and all associated radiological supervision and interpretation; external

47534 Placement of biliary drainage catheter, percutaneous, including diagnostic cholangiography when performed, imaging guidance (eg, ultrasound and/or fluoroscopy), and all associated radiological supervision and interpretation; internal-external

47535 Conversion of external biliary drainage catheter to internal-external biliary drainage catheter, percutaneous, including diagnostic cholangiography when performed, imaging guidance (eg, fluoroscopy), and all associated radiological supervision and interpretation

47536 Exchange of biliary drainage catheter (eg, external, internal-external, or conversion of internal-external to external only), percutaneous, including diagnostic cholangiography when performed, imaging guidance (eg, fluoroscopy), and all associated radiological supervision and interpretation

47537 Removal of biliary drainage catheter, percutaneous, requiring fluoroscopic guidance (eg, with concurrent indwelling biliary stents), including diagnostic cholangiography when performed, imaging guidance (eg, fluoroscopy), and all associated radiological supervision and interpretation

47538 Placement of stent(s) into a bile duct, percutaneous, including diagnostic cholangiography, imaging guidance (eg, fluoroscopy and/or ultrasound), balloon dilation, catheter exchange(s) and catheter removal(s) when performed, and all associated radiological supervision and interpretation, each stent; existing access

47539 Placement of stent(s) into a bile duct, percutaneous, including diagnostic cholangiography, imaging guidance (eg, fluoroscopy and/or ultrasound), balloon dilation, catheter exchange(s) and catheter removal(s) when performed, and all associated radiological supervision and interpretation, each stent; new access, without placement of separate biliary drainage catheter

47540 Placement of stent(s) into a bile duct, percutaneous, including diagnostic cholangiography, imaging guidance (eg, fluoroscopy and/or ultrasound), balloon dilation, catheter exchange(s) and catheter removal(s) when performed, and all associated radiological supervision and interpretation, each stent; new access, with placement of separate biliary drainage catheter (eg, external or internal-external)

47541 Placement of access through the biliary tree and into small bowel to assist with an endoscopic biliary procedure (eg, rendezvous procedure), percutaneous, including diagnostic cholangiography when performed, imaging guidance (eg, ultrasound and/or fluoroscopy), and all associated radiological supervision and interpretation, new access

47542 Balloon dilation of biliary duct(s) or of ampulla (sphincteroplasty), percutaneous, including imaging guidance (eg, fluoroscopy), and all associated radiological supervision and interpretation, each duct (List separately in addition to code for primary procedure)

47543 Endoluminal biopsy(ies) of biliary tree, percutaneous, any method(s) (eg, brush, forceps, and/or needle), including imaging guidance (eg, fluoroscopy), and all associated radiological supervision and interpretation, single or multiple (List separately in addition to code for primary procedure)

47544 Removal of calculi/debris from biliary duct(s) and/or gallbladder, percutaneous, including destruction of calculi by any method (eg, mechanical, electrohydraulic, lithotripsy) when performed, imaging guidance (eg, fluoroscopy), and all associated radiological supervision and interpretation (List separately in addition to code for primary procedure)

49185 Sclerotherapy of a fluid collection (eg, lymphocele, cyst, or seroma), percutaneous, including contrast injection(s), sclerosant injection(s), diagnostic study, imaging guidance (eg, ultrasound, fluoroscopy) and radiological supervision and interpretation when performed

50430 Injection procedure for antegrade nephrostogram and/or ureterogram, complete diagnostic procedure including imaging guidance (eg, ultrasound and fluoroscopy) and all associated radiological supervision and interpretation; new access

50431 Injection procedure for antegrade nephrostogram and/or ureterogram, complete diagnostic procedure including imaging guidance (eg, ultrasound and fluoroscopy) and all associated radiological supervision and interpretation; existing access

50432 Placement of nephrostomy catheter, percutaneous, including diagnostic nephrostogram and/or ureterogram when performed, imaging guidance (eg, ultrasound and/or fluoroscopy) and all associated radiological supervision and interpretation

50433 Placement of nephroureteral catheter, percutaneous, including diagnostic nephrostogram and/or ureterogram when performed, imaging guidance (eg, ultrasound and/or fluoroscopy) and all associated radiological supervision and interpretation, new access

50434 Convert nephrostomy catheter to nephroureteral catheter, percutaneous, including diagnostic nephrostogram and/or ureterogram when performed, imaging guidance (eg, ultrasound and/or fluoroscopy) and all associated radiological supervision and interpretation, via pre-existing nephrostomy tract

50435 Exchange nephrostomy catheter, percutaneous, including diagnostic nephrostogram and/or ureterogram when performed, imaging guidance (eg, ultrasound and/or fluoroscopy) and all associated radiological supervision and interpretation

50606 Endoluminal biopsy of ureter and/or renal pelvis, non-endoscopic, including imaging guidance (eg, ultrasound and/or fluoroscopy) and all associated radiological supervision and interpretation (List separately in addition to code for primary procedure)

50693 Placement of ureteral stent, percutaneous, including diagnostic nephrostogram and/or ureterogram when performed, imaging guidance (eg, ultrasound and/or fluoroscopy), and all associated radiological supervision and interpretation; pre-existing nephrostomy tract

50694 Placement of ureteral stent, percutaneous, including diagnostic nephrostogram and/or ureterogram when performed, imaging guidance (eg, ultrasound and/or fluoroscopy), and all associated radiological supervision and interpretation; new access, without separate nephrostomy catheter

50695 Placement of ureteral stent, percutaneous, including diagnostic nephrostogram and/or ureterogram when performed, imaging guidance (eg, ultrasound and/or fluoroscopy), and all associated radiological supervision and interpretation; new access, with separate nephrostomy catheter

50705 Ureteral embolization or occlusion, including imaging guidance (eg, ultrasound and/or fluoroscopy) and all associated radiological supervision and interpretation (List separately in addition to code for primary procedure)

50706 Balloon dilation, ureteral stricture, including imaging guidance (eg, ultrasound and/or fluoroscopy) and all associated radiological supervision and interpretation (List separately in addition to code for primary procedure)

54437 Repair of traumatic corporeal tear(s)

54438 Replantation, penis, complete amputation including urethral repair

61645 Percutaneous arterial transluminal mechanical thrombectomy and/or infusion for thrombolysis, intracranial, any method, including diagnostic angiography, fluoroscopic guidance, catheter placement, and intraprocedural pharmacological thrombolytic injection(s)

61650 Endovascular intracranial prolonged administration of pharmacologic agent(s) other than for thrombolysis, arterial, including catheter placement, diagnostic angiography, and imaging guidance; initial vascular territory

61651 Endovascular intracranial prolonged administration of pharmacologic agent(s) other than for thrombolysis, arterial, including catheter placement, diagnostic angiography, and imaging guidance; each additional vascular territory (List separately in addition to code for primary procedure)

64461 Paravertebral block (PVB) (paraspinous block), thoracic; single injection site (includes imaging guidance, when performed)

64462 Paravertebral block (PVB) (paraspinous block), thoracic; second and any additional injection site(s) (includes imaging guidance, when performed) (List separately in addition to code for primary procedure)

64463 Paravertebral block (PVB) (paraspinous block), thoracic; continuous infusion by catheter (includes imaging guidance, when performed)

65785 Implantation of intrastromal corneal ring segments

69209 Removal impacted cerumen using irrigation/lavage, unilateral

72081 Radiologic examination, spine, entire thoracic and lumbar, including skull, cervical and sacral spine if performed (eg, scoliosis evaluation); one view

72082 Radiologic examination, spine, entire thoracic and lumbar, including skull, cervical and sacral spine if performed (eg, scoliosis evaluation); 2 or 3 views

72083 Radiologic examination, spine, entire thoracic and lumbar, including skull, cervical and sacral spine if performed (eg, scoliosis evaluation); 4 or 5 views

72084 Radiologic examination, spine, entire thoracic and lumbar, including skull, cervical and sacral spine if performed (eg, scoliosis evaluation); minimum of 6 views

73501 Radiologic examination, hip, unilateral, with pelvis when performed; 1 view

73502 Radiologic examination, hip, unilateral, with pelvis when performed; 2-3 views

73503 Radiologic examination, hip, unilateral, with pelvis when performed; minimum of 4 views

73521 Radiologic examination, hips, bilateral, with pelvis when performed; 2 views

73522 Radiologic examination, hips, bilateral, with pelvis when performed; 3-4 views

73523 Radiologic examination, hips, bilateral, with pelvis when performed; minimum of 5 views

73551 Radiologic examination, femur; 1 view

73552 Radiologic examination, femur; minimum 2 views

74712 Magnetic resonance (eg, proton) imaging, fetal, including placental and maternal pelvic imaging when performed; single or first gestation

74713 Magnetic resonance (eg, proton) imaging, fetal, including placental and maternal pelvic imaging when performed; each additional gestation (List separately in addition to code for primary procedure)

77767 Remote afterloading high dose rate radionuclide skin surface brachytherapy, includes basic dosimetry, when performed; lesion diameter up to 2.0 cm or 1 channel

77768 Remote afterloading high dose rate radionuclide skin surface brachytherapy, includes basic dosimetry, when performed; lesion diameter over 2.0 cm and 2 or more channels, or multiple lesions

77770 Remote afterloading high dose rate radionuclide interstitial or intracavitary brachytherapy, includes basic dosimetry, when performed; 1 channel

77771 Remote afterloading high dose rate radionuclide interstitial or intracavitary brachytherapy, includes basic dosimetry, when performed; 2-12 channels

77772 Remote afterloading high dose rate radionuclide interstitial or intracavitary brachytherapy, includes basic dosimetry, when performed; over 12 channels

78265 Gastric emptying imaging study (eg, solid, liquid, or both); with small bowel transit

78266 Gastric emptying imaging study (eg, solid, liquid, or both); with small bowel and colon transit, multiple days

80081 Obstetric panel (includes HIV testing)

81162 *BRCA1, BRCA2 (breast cancer 1 and 2)* (eg, hereditary breast and ovarian cancer) gene analysis; full sequence analysis and full duplication/deletion analysis

81170 *ABL1 (ABL proto-oncogene 1, non-receptor tyrosine kinase)* (eg, acquired imatinib tyrosine kinase inhibitor resistance), gene analysis, variants in the kinase domain

81218 *CEBPA (CCAAT/enhancer binding protein [C/EBP], alpha)* (eg, acute myeloid leukemia), gene analysis, full gene sequence

81219 *CALR (calreticulin)* (eg, myeloproliferative disorders), gene analysis, common variants in exon 9

81272 *KIT (v-kit Hardy-Zuckerman 4 feline sarcoma viral oncogene homolog)* (eg, gastrointestinal stromal tumor [GIST], acute myeloid leukemia, melanoma), gene analysis, targeted sequence analysis (eg, exons 8, 11, 13, 17, 18)

81273 *KIT (v-kit Hardy-Zuckerman 4 feline sarcoma viral oncogene homolog)* (eg, mastocytosis), gene analysis, D816 variant

81276 *KRAS (Kirsten rat sarcoma viral oncogene homolog)* (eg, carcinoma) gene analysis; additional variant(s) (eg, codon 61, codon 146)

81311 *NRAS (neuroblastoma RAS viral [v-ras] oncogene homolog)* (eg, colorectal carcinoma), gene analysis, variants in exon 2 (eg, codons 12 and 13) and exon 3 (eg, codon 61)

81314 *PDGFRA (platelet-derived growth factor receptor, alpha polypeptide)* (eg, gastrointestinal stromal tumor [GIST]), gene analysis, targeted sequence analysis (eg, exons 12, 18)

81412 Ashkenazi Jewish associated disorders (eg, Bloom syndrome, Canavan disease, cystic fibrosis, familial dysautonomia, Fanconi anemia group C, Gaucher disease, Tay-Sachs disease), genomic sequence analysis panel, must include sequencing of at least 9 genes, including *ASPA, BLM, CFTR, FANCC, GBA, HEXA, IKBKAP, MCOLN1,* and *SMPD1*

81432 Hereditary breast cancer-related disorders (eg, hereditary breast cancer, hereditary ovarian cancer, hereditary endometrial cancer); genomic sequence analysis panel, must include sequencing of at least 14 genes, including *ATM, BRCA1, BRCA2, BRIP1, CDH1, MLH1, MSH2, MSH6, NBN, PALB2, PTEN, RAD51C, STK11,* and *TP53*

81433 Hereditary breast cancer-related disorders (eg, hereditary breast cancer, hereditary ovarian cancer, hereditary endometrial cancer); duplication/deletion analysis panel, must include analyses for *BRCA1, BRCA2, MLH1, MSH2,* and *STK11*

81434 Hereditary retinal disorders (eg, retinitis pigmentosa, Leber congenital amaurosis, cone-rod dystrophy), genomic sequence analysis panel, must include sequencing of at least 15 genes, including *ABCA4, CNGA1, CRB1, EYS, PDE6A, PDE6B, PRPF31, PRPH2, RDH12, RHO, RP1, RP2, RPE65, RPGR,* and *USH2A*

81437 Hereditary neuroendocrine tumor disorders (eg, medullary thyroid carcinoma, parathyroid carcinoma, malignant pheochromocytoma or paraganglioma); genomic sequence analysis panel, must include sequencing of at least 6 genes, including *MAX, SDHB, SDHC, SDHD, TMEM127,* and *VHL*

81438 Hereditary neuroendocrine tumor disorders (eg, medullary thyroid carcinoma, parathyroid carcinoma, malignant pheochromocytoma or paraganglioma); duplication/deletion analysis panel, must include analyses for *SDHB, SDHC, SDHD,* and *VHL*

81442 Noonan spectrum disorders (eg, Noonan syndrome, cardio-facio-cutaneous syndrome, Costello syndrome, LEOPARD syndrome, Noonan-like syndrome), genomic sequence analysis panel, must include sequencing of at least 12 genes, including *BRAF, CBL, HRAS, KRAS, MAP2K1, MAP2K2, NRAS, PTPN11, RAF1, RIT1, SHOC2,* and *SOS1*

81490 Autoimmune (rheumatoid arthritis), analysis of 12 biomarkers using immunoassays, utilizing serum, prognostic algorithm reported as a disease activity score

81493 Coronary artery disease, mRNA, gene expression profiling by real-time RT-PCR of 23 genes, utilizing whole peripheral blood, algorithm reported as a risk score

81525 Oncology (colon), mRNA, gene expression profiling by real-time RT-PCR of 12 genes (7 content and 5 housekeeping), utilizing formalin-fixed paraffin-embedded tissue, algorithm reported as a recurrence score

81528 Oncology (colorectal) screening, quantitative real-time target and signal amplification of 10 DNA markers (*KRAS* mutations, promoter methylation of *NDRG4* and *BMP3*) and fecal hemoglobin, utilizing stool, algorithm reported as a positive or negative result

81535 Oncology (gynecologic), live tumor cell culture and chemotherapeutic response by DAPI stain and morphology, predictive algorithm reported as a drug response score; first single drug or drug combination

81536 Oncology (gynecologic), live tumor cell culture and chemotherapeutic response by DAPI stain and morphology, predictive algorithm reported as a drug response score; each additional single drug or drug combination (List separately in addition to code for primary procedure)

81538 Oncology (lung), mass spectrometric 8-protein signature, including amyloid A, utilizing serum, prognostic and predictive algorithm reported as good versus poor overall survival

81540 Oncology (tumor of unknown origin), mRNA, gene expression profiling by real-time RT-PCR of 92 genes (87 content and 5 housekeeping) to classify tumor into main cancer type and subtype, utilizing formalin-fixed paraffin-embedded tissue, algorithm reported as a probability of a predicted main cancer type and subtype

81545 Oncology (thyroid), gene expression analysis of 142 genes, utilizing fine needle aspirate, algorithm reported as a categorical result (eg, benign or suspicious)

81595 Cardiology (heart transplant), mRNA, gene expression profiling by real-time quantitative PCR of 20 genes (11 content and 9 housekeeping), utilizing subfraction of peripheral blood, algorithm reported as a rejection risk score

88350 Immunofluorescence, per specimen; each additional single antibody stain procedure (List separately in addition to code for primary procedure)

90625 Cholera vaccine, live, adult dosage, 1 dose schedule, for oral use

92537 Caloric vestibular test with recording, bilateral; bithermal (ie, one warm and one cool irrigation in each ear for a total of four irrigations)

92538 Caloric vestibular test with recording, bilateral; monothermal (ie, one irrigation in each ear for a total of two irrigations)

93050 Arterial pressure waveform analysis for assessment of central arterial pressures, includes obtaining waveform(s), digitization and application of nonlinear mathematical transformations to determine central arterial pressures and augmentation index, with interpretation and report, upper extremity artery, non-invasive

96931 Reflectance confocal microscopy (RCM) for cellular and sub-cellular imaging of skin; image acquisition and interpretation and report, first lesion

96932 Reflectance confocal microscopy (RCM) for cellular and sub-cellular imaging of skin; image acquisition only, first lesion

96933 Reflectance confocal microscopy (RCM) for cellular and sub-cellular imaging of skin; interpretation and report only, first lesion

96934 Reflectance confocal microscopy (RCM) for cellular and sub-cellular imaging of skin; image acquisition and interpretation and report, each additional lesion (List separately in addition to code for primary procedure)

96935 Reflectance confocal microscopy (RCM) for cellular and sub-cellular imaging of skin; image acquisition only, each additional lesion (List separately in addition to code for primary procedure)

96936 Reflectance confocal microscopy (RCM) for cellular and sub-cellular imaging of skin; interpretation and report only, each additional lesion (List separately in addition to code for primary procedure)

99177 Instrument-based ocular screening (eg, photoscreening, automated-refraction), bilateral; with on-site analysis

99415 Prolonged clinical staff service (the service beyond the typical service time) during an evaluation and management service in the office or outpatient setting, direct patient contact with physician supervision; first hour (List separately in addition to code for outpatient Evaluation and Management service)

99416 Prolonged clinical staff service (the service beyond the typical service time) during an evaluation and management service in the office or outpatient setting, direct patient contact with physician supervision; each additional 30 minutes (List separately in addition to code for prolonged service)

Changed Codes

37184 Primary percutaneous transluminal mechanical thrombectomy, noncoronary, non-intracranial, arterial or arterial bypass graft, including fluoroscopic guidance and intraprocedural pharmacological thrombolytic injection(s); initial vessel

37185 second and all subsequent vessel(s) within the same vascular family (List separately in addition to code for primary mechanical thrombectomy procedure)

37186 Secondary percutaneous transluminal thrombectomy (eg, nonprimary mechanical, snare basket, suction technique), noncoronary, non-intracranial, arterial or arterial bypass graft, including fluoroscopic guidance and intraprocedural pharmacological thrombolytic injections, provided in conjunction with another percutaneous intervention other than primary mechanical thrombectomy (List separately in addition to code for primary procedure)

37211 Transcatheter therapy, arterial infusion for thrombolysis other than coronary or intracranial, any method, including radiological supervision and interpretation, initial treatment day

50387   Removal and replacement of externally accessible ~~transnephric ureteral stent~~ nephroureteral catheter (eg, external/internal stent) requiring fluoroscopic guidance, including radiological supervision and interpretation

65855   Trabeculoplasty by laser surgery ~~1 or more sessions (defined treatment series)~~

67101   Repair of retinal detachment, 1 or more sessions; cryotherapy or diathermy, ~~with or without~~ including drainage of subretinal fluid, when performed

67105   photocoagulation, ~~with or without~~ including drainage of subretinal fluid, when performed

67107   Repair of retinal detachment; scleral buckling (such as lamellar scleral dissection, imbrication or encircling procedure),~~with or without~~ including, when performed, implant, ~~with or without~~ cryotherapy, photocoagulation, and drainage of subretinal fluid

67108   with vitrectomy, any method, ~~with or without~~ including, when performed, air or gas tamponade, focal endolaser photocoagulation, cryotherapy, drainage of subretinal fluid, scleral buckling, and/or removal of lens by same technique

67113   Repair of complex retinal detachment (eg, proliferative vitreoretinopathy, stage C-1 or greater, diabetic traction retinal detachment, retinopathy of prematurity, retinal tear of greater than 90 degrees), with vitrectomy and membrane peeling, including, ~~may include~~ when performed, air, gas, or silicone oil tamponade, cryotherapy, endolaser photocoagulation, drainage of subretinal fluid, scleral buckling, and/or removal of lens

67227   Destruction of extensive or progressive retinopathy (eg, diabetic retinopathy),~~1 or more sessions,~~ cryotherapy, diathermy

67228   Treatment of extensive or progressive retinopathy (eg, ~~1 or more sessions~~ diabetic retinopathy), photocoagulation; ~~(eg, diabetic retinopathy), photocoagulation)~~

72080   Radiologic examination, spine; thoracolumbar junction, minimum of 2 views

74240   Radiologic examination, gastrointestinal tract, upper; with or without delayed ~~films~~ images, without KUB

74241   with or without delayed ~~films~~ images, with KUB

74245   with small intestine, includes multiple serial ~~films~~ images

74246   Radiological examination, gastrointestinal tract, upper, air contrast, with specific high density barium, effervescent agent, with or without glucagon; with or without delayed ~~films~~ images, without KUB

74247   with or without delayed ~~films~~ images, with KUB

74250   Radiologic examination, small intestine, includes multiple serial ~~films~~ images;

74251   Radiologic examination, small intestine, includes multiple serial ~~films~~ images; via enteroclysis tube

74340   Introduction of long gastrointestinal tube (eg, Miller-Abbott), including multiple fluoroscopies and ~~films~~ images, radiological supervision and interpretation

77057   Screening mammography, bilateral (2-view ~~film~~ study of each breast)

77417   Therapeutic radiology port ~~film~~ image(s)

77778   Interstitial radiation source application, complex, includes supervision, handling, loading of radiation source, when performed ;~~complex~~

77789   Surface application of ~~radiation~~ low dose rate radionuclide source

78264   Gastric emptying imaging study (eg, solid, liquid, or both);

81210   BRAF (~~vB-raf murine sarcoma viral~~ Raf proto-oncogene,~~homolog B1~~ serine/threonine kinase) (eg, colon cancer, melanoma), gene analysis, V600 ~~E~~ variant(s)

81275   KRAS (~~v-Ki-ras2~~ Kirsten rat sarcoma viral oncogene homolog) (eg, carcinoma) gene analysis; ~~variants in codons 12 and 13~~ variants in exon 2 (eg, codons 12 and 13)

81355   VKORC1 (vitamin K epoxide reductase complex, subunit 1) (eg, warfarin metabolism), gene analysis, common variants(s) (eg, ~~1639/3673~~ 1639G>A, c.173+1000C>T))

81401   Molecular pathology procedure, Level 2 (eg, 2-10 SNPs, 1 methylated variant, or 1 somatic variant [typically using nonsequencing target variant analysis], or detection of a dynamic mutation disorder/triplet repeat)

ABL1 (ABL ~~eproto~~ ~~abl~~ oncogene 1, non-receptor tyrosine kinase) (eg, acquired imatinib resistance), T315I variant

DEK/NUP214 (t(6;9)) (eg, acute myeloid leukemia), translocation analysis, qualitative, and quantitative, if performed

IGH@/BCL2 (t(14;18)) (eg, follicular lymphoma), translocation and analysis; single breakpoint (eg, major breakpoint region [MBR] or minor cluster region [mcr]), qualitative or quantitative

(When both MBR and mcr breakpoints are performed, use 81402)

81402   Molecular pathology procedure, Level 3 (eg, >10 SNPs, 2-10 methylated variants, or 2-10 somatic variants [typically using non-sequencing target variant analysis], immunoglobulin and T-cell receptor gene rearrangements, duplication/deletion variants of 1 exon, loss of heterozygosity [LOH], uniparental disomy [UPD])

~~KIT (v-kit-Hardy-Zuckerman 4 feline sarcoma viral oncogene homolog) (eg, mastocystosis), common variants (eg, D816V, D816Y, D816F)~~

81403   Molecular pathology procedure, Level 4 (eg, analysis of single exon by DNA sequence analysis, analysis of >10 amplicons using multiplex PCR in 2 or more independent reactions, mutation scanning or duplication/deletion variants of 2-5 exons)

~~ABL1 (c-abl oncogene 1, receptor tyrosine kinase) (eg, acquired imatinib tyrosine kinase inhibitor resistance), variants in the kinase domain~~

~~CEBPA (CCAAT/enhancer binding protein [C/EBP], alpha) (eg, acute myeloid leukemia), full gene sequence~~

~~KRAS (v-Ki-ras2-Kirsten rat sarcoma viral oncogene) (eg, carcinoma), gene analysis, variants(s) in exon 3 (eg, codon 61)~~

81404   Molecular pathology procedure, Level 5 (eg, analysis of 2-5 exons by DNA sequence analysis, mutation scanning or duplication/deletion variants of 6-10 exons, or characterization of a dynamic mutation disorder/triplet repeat by Southern blot analysis)

~~KIT (C-kit)(v-kit-Hardy-Zuckerman 4 feline sarcoma viral oncogene homolog) (eg, GIST, acute myeloid leukemia, melanoma), targeted gene analysis (eg, exons 8, 11, 13, 17, 18)~~

~~NRAS (neuroblastoma RAS viral oncogene homolog) (eg, colorectal carcinoma), exon 1 and exon 2 sequences~~

~~PDGFRA (platelet-derived growth factor receptor alpha polypeptide) (eg, gastrointestinal stromal tumor), targeted sequence analysis (eg, exons 12, 18)~~

81405   Molecular pathology procedure, Level 6 (eg, analysis of 6-10 exons by DNA sequence analysis, mutation scanning or duplication/deletion variants of 11-25 exons, regionally targeted cytogenomic array analysis)

KRAS (~~v-Ki-ras2~~ Kirsten rat sarcoma viral oncogene homolog) (eg, Noonan syndrome), full gene sequence

81406   Molecular pathology procedure, Level 7 (eg, analysis of 11-25 exons by DNA sequence analysis, mutation scanning or duplication/deletion variants of 26-50 exons, cytogenomic array analysis for neoplasia)

BRAF (~~v-B-raf murine sarcoma viral~~ Raf proto-oncogene ~~homolog B1~~, serine/threonine kinase) (eg, Noonan syndrome), full gene sequence

PCSK9 (proprotein convertase subtilisin/kexin type 9) (eg familial hypercholesterolemia), full gene sequence

81435   Hereditary colon cancer ~~syndromes~~ disorders (eg, Lynch syndrome, PTEN hamartoma syndrome, Cowden syndrome, familial adenomatosis polyposis); genomic sequence analysis panel, must include ~~analysis~~ sequencing of at least ~~7~~ 10 genes, including APC, BMPR1A, ~~CHEK2~~ CDH1, MLH1, MSH2, MSH6, MUTYH, PTEN, SMAD4, and ~~PMS2~~ STK11

81436   duplication/deletion ~~gene~~ analysis panel, must include analysis of at least ~~8~~ 5 genes, including APC ~~MLH1, MSH2, MSH6, PMS2~~ EPCAM, ~~CHEK2~~ SMAD4, and ~~MUTYH~~ STK11

81445 Targeted genomic sequence analysis panel, solid organ neoplasm, DNA analysis, and RNA analysis when performed, 5-50 genes (eg, *ALK, BRAF, CDKN2A, EGFR, ERBB2, KIT, KRAS, NRAS, MET, PDGFRA, PDGFRB, PGR, PIK3CA, PTEN, RET*), interrogation for sequence variants and copy number variants or rearrangements, if performed

81450 Targeted genomic sequence analysis panel, hematolymphoid neoplasm or disorder, DNA analysis, and RNA analysis when performed, 5-50 genes (eg, *BRAF, CEBPA, DNMT3A, EZH2, FLT3, IDH1, IDH2, JAK2, KRAS, KIT, MLL, NRAS, NPM1, NOTCH1*), interrogation for sequence variants, and copy number variants or rearrangements, or isoform expression or mRNA expression levels, if performed

81455 Targeted genomic sequence analysis panel, solid organ or hematolymphoid neoplasm, DNA analysis, and RNA analysis when performed, 51 or greater genes (eg, *ALK, BRAF, CDKN2A, CEBPA, DNMT3A, EGFR, ERBB2, EZH2, FLT3, IDH1, IDH2, JAK2, KIT, KRAS, MLL, NPM1, NRAS, MET, NOTCH1, PDGFRA, PDGFRB, PGR, PIK3CA, PTEN, RET*), interrogation for sequence variants and copy number variants or rearrangements, if performed

82542 Column chromatography/, includes mass spectrometry, if performed (eg, HPLC, LC, LC/MS, LC/MS-MS, GC, GC/MS-MS, or GC/MS, HPLC/MS), non-drug analyte(s) not elsewhere specified, qualitative or quantitative, each specimen; quantitative, single stationary and mobile phase

83789 Mass spectrometry and tandem mass spectrometry (eg, MS, MS/MS, MALDI, MS-TOF, QTOF), non-drug analyte(s) not elsewhere specified, qualitative or quantitative, each specimen; quantitative, each specimen

86708 Hepatitis A antibody (HAAb); total

86709 Hepatitis A antibody (HAAb), IgM antibody;IgM antibody

87301 Infectious agent antigen detection by immunoassay technique, (eg, enzyme immunoassay technique [EIA], enzyme-linked immunosorbent assay [ELISA], immunochemiluminometric assay [IMCA]) qualitative or semiquantitative, multiple-step method; adenovirus enteric types 40/41

87305 Aspergillus

87320 Chlamydia trachomatis

87324 Clostridium difficile toxin(s)

87327 Cryptococcus neoformans

87328 cryptosporidium

87329 giardia

87332 cytomegalovirus

87335 Escherichia coli 0157

87336 Entamoeba histolytica dispar group

87337 Entamoeba histolytica group

87338 Helicobacter pylori, stool

87339 Helicobacter pylori

87340 hepatitis B surface antigen (HBsAg)

87341 hepatitis B surface antigen (HBsAg) neutralization

87350 hepatitis Be antigen (HBeAg)

87380 hepatitis, delta agent

87385 Histoplasma capsulatum

87389 HIV-1 antigen(s), with HIV-1 and HIV-2 antibodies, single result

87390 HIV-1

87391 HIV-2

87400 Influenza, A or B, each

87420 respiratory syncytial virus

87425 rotavirus

87427 Shiga-like toxin

87430 Streptococcus, group A

87449 Infectious agent antigen detection by immunoassay technique, (eg, enzyme immunoassay technique [EIA], enzyme-linked immunosorbent assay [ELISA], immunochemiluminometric assay [IMCA]), qualitative or semiquantitative; multiple-step method, not otherwise specified, each organism

87450 single step method, not otherwise specified, each organism

87451 multiple step method, polyvalent for multiple organisms, each polyvalent antiserum

87502 Infectious agent detection by nucleic acid (DNA or RNA); influenza virus, for multiple types or sub-types, includes multiplex reverse transcription, when performed, and multiplex amplified probe technique, first 2 types or sub-types

87503 influenza virus, for multiple types or sub-types, includes multiplex reverse transcription, when performed, and multiplex amplified probe technique, each additional influenza virus type or sub-type beyond 2 (List separately in addition to code for primary procedure)

88346 Immunofluorescent study Immunofluorescence, each antibody per specimen; direct method initial single antibody stain procedure

90620 Meningococcal recombinant protein and outer membrane vesicle vaccine, serogroup B (MenB), 2 dose schedule, for intramuscular use

90621 Meningococcal recombinant lipoprotein vaccine, serogroup B (MenB), 3 dose schedule, for intramuscular use

90632 Hepatitis A vaccine (HepA), adult dosage, for intramuscular use

90633 Hepatitis A vaccine (HepA), pediatric/adolescent dosage-2 dose schedule, for intramuscular use

90634 Hepatitis A vaccine (HepA), pediatric/adolescent dosage-3 dose schedule, for intramuscular use

90644 Meningococcal conjugate vaccine, serogroups C & Y and Hemophilus influenza Haemophilus influenzae type b vaccine (Hib-MenCY), 4 dose schedule, when administered to children 2-15 18 months of age, for intramuscular use

90647 Hemophilus influenza Haemophilus influenzae type b vaccine (Hib), PRP-OMP conjugate, (3 dose schedule), for intramuscular use

90648 Hemophilus influenza Haemophilus influenzae type b vaccine (Hib), PRP-T conjugate, (4 dose schedule), for intramuscular use

90649 Human Papilloma virus (HPV) Papillomavirus vaccine, types 6, 11, 16, 18, (quadrivalent) quadrivalent (4vHPV), 3 dose schedule, for intramuscular use

90650 Human Papilloma virus (HPV) Papillomavirus vaccine, types 16, 18, bivalent (2vHPV), 3 dose schedule, for intramuscular use

90651 Human Papillomavirus vaccine types 6, 11, 16, 18, 31, 33, 45, 52, 58, nonavalent (HPV) (9vHPV), 3 dose schedule, for intramuscular use

90653 Influenza vaccine, inactivated (IIV), subunit, adjuvanted, for intramuscular use

90655 Influenza virus vaccine, trivalent (IIV3), split virus, preservative free, when administered to children 6-35 months of age, for intramuscular use

90656 Influenza virus vaccine, trivalent (IIV3), split virus, preservative free, when administered to individuals 3 years and older, for intramuscular use

90657 Influenza virus vaccine, trivalent (IIV3), split virus, when administered to children 6-35 months of age, for intramuscular use

90658 Influenza virus vaccine, trivalent (IIV3), split virus when administered to individuals 3 years of age and older, for intramuscular use

90660 Influenza virus vaccine, trivalent, live (LAIV3), for intranasal use

90661 Influenza virus vaccine (ccIIV3), derived from cell cultures, subunit, preservative and antibiotifree, for intramuscular use

90662 Influenza virus vaccine (IIV), split virus, preservative free, enhanced immunogenicity via increased antigen content, for intramuscular use

90664 Influenza virus vaccine, live (LAIV), pandemiformulation, live, for intranasal use

90666 Influenza virus vaccine (IIV), pandemiformulation, split virus, preservative free, for intramuscular use

90667 Influenza virus vaccine (IIV), pandemiformulation, split virus, adjuvanted, for intramuscular use

90668 Influenza virus vaccine (IIV), pandemiformulation, split virus for intramuscular use

90670 Pneumococcal conjugate vaccine, 13 valent (PCV13), for intramuscular use

90672 Influenza virus vaccine, quadrivalent, live (LAIV4), for intranasal use

90673　Influenza virus vaccine, trivalent (RIV3), derived from recombinant DNA (RIV3), hemagglutinin (HA) protein only, preservative and antibiotic free, for intramuscular use

90680　Rotavirus vaccine, pentavalent (RV5), 3 dose schedule, live, for oral use

90681　Rotavirus vaccine, human, attenuated (RV1), 2 dose schedule, live, for oral use

90685　Influenza virus vaccine, quadrivalent (IIV4), split virus, preservative free, when administered to children 6-35 months of age, for intramuscular use

90686　Influenza virus vaccine, quadrivalent (IIV4), split virus, preservative free, when administered to individuals 3 years of age and older, for intramuscular use

90687　Influenza virus vaccine, quadrivalent (IIV4), split virus, when administered to children 6-35 months of age, for intramuscular use

90688　Influenza virus vaccine, quadrivalent (IIV4), split virus, when administered to individuals 3 years of age and older, for intramuscular use

90696　Diphtheria, tetanus toxoids, acellular pertussis vaccine and inactivated poliovirus vaccine, inactivated (DTaP-IPV), when administered to children 4 through 6 years of age, for intramuscular use

90698　Diphtheria, tetanus toxoids, acellular pertussis vaccine, hHaemophilus influenza Type B, influenzae type b, and inactivated poliovirus vaccine (DTaP-IPV/Hib), for intramuscular use

90702　Diphtheria and tetanus toxoids adsorbed (DT) adsorbed when administered to individuals younger than 7 years, for intramuscular use

90714　Tetanus and diphtheria toxoids adsorbed (Td) adsorbed, preservative free, when administered to individuals 7 years or older, for intramuscular use

90716　Varicella virus vaccine (VAR), live, for subcutaneous use

90732　Pneumococcal polysaccharide vaccine, 23-valent (PPSV23), adult or immunosuppressed patient dosage, when administered to individuals 2 years or older, for subcutaneous or intramuscular use

90733　Meningococcal polysaccharide vaccine, (any group(s)) serogroups A, C, Y, W-135, quadrivalent (MPSV4), for subcutaneous use

90734　Meningococcal conjugate vaccine, serogroups A, C, Y and W-135, quadrivalent (MenACWY), for intramuscular use

90736　Zoster (shingles) vaccine (HZV), live, for subcutaneous injection

90739　Hepatitis B vaccine (HepB), adult dosage, 2 dose schedule, for intramuscular use

90740　Hepatitis B vaccine (HepB), dialysis or immunosuppressed patient dosage, (3 dose schedule), for intramuscular use

90743　Hepatitis B vaccine (HepB), adolescent, 2 dose schedule, for intramuscular use

90744　Hepatitis B vaccine (HepB), pediatric/adolescent dosage, (3 dose schedule), for intramuscular use

90746　Hepatitis B vaccine (HepB), adult dosage, (3 dose schedule), for intramuscular use

90747　Hepatitis B vaccine (HepB), dialysis or immunosuppressed patient dosage, (4 dose schedule), for intramuscular use

90748　Hepatitis B and Hemophilus influenza Haemophilus influenzae type b vaccine (HepB-Hib) (Hib-HepB), for intramuscular use

91040　Esophageal balloon distension study, diagnostic, with provocation study when performed

94640　Pressurized or nonpressurized inhalation treatment for acute airway obstruction or for sputum induction therapeutic purposes and/or for diagnostic purposes eg such as sputum induction with an aerosol generator, nebulizer, metered dose inhaler or intermittent positive pressure breathing [IPPB] (IPPB) device

95972　Electronic analysis of implanted neurostimulator pulse generator system (eg, rate, pulse amplitude, pulse duration, configuration of wave form, battery status, electrode selectability, output modulation, cycling, impedance and patient compliance measurements); complex spinal cord, or peripheral (ie, peripheral nerve, sacral nerve, neuromuscular) (except cranial nerve) neurostimulator pulse generator/transmitter, with intraoperative or subsequent programming up to 1 hour

99174　Instrument-based ocular screening (eg, photoscreening, automated-refraction), bilateral; with remote analysis and report

99354　Prolonged evaluation and management or psychotherapy service(s) (beyond the typical service time of the primary procedure) in the office or other outpatient setting requiring direct patient contact beyond the usual service; first hour (List separately in addition to code for office or other outpatient Evaluation and Management or psychotherapy service)

99355　each additional 30 minutes (List separately in addition to code for prolonged service)

6030F　All elements of maximal sterile barrier technique, followed including: cap and mask and sterile gown and sterile gloves and a large sterile sheet and hand hygiene, skin preparation and, if ultrasound is used, sterile ultrasound techniques followed and 2% chlorhexidine for cutaneous antisepsis (or acceptable alternative antiseptics, per current guideline) (CRIT)

0308T　Insertion of ocular telescope prosthesis including removal of crystalline lens or intraocular lens prosthesis

0358T　Bioelectrical impedance analysis whole body composition assessment, supine position with interpretation and report

Deleted Codes

21805	31620	37202	37250	37251	39400	47136
47500	47505	47510	47511	47525	47530	47560
47561	47630	50392	50393	50394	50398	64412
67112	70373	72010	72069	72090	73500	73510
73520	73530	73540	73550	74305	74320	74327
74475	74480	75896	75945	75946	75980	75982
77776	77777	77785	77786	77787	82486	82487
82488	82489	82491	82492	82541	82543	82544
83788	88347	90645	90646	90669	90692	90693
90703	90704	90705	90706	90708	90712	90719
90720	90721	90725	90727	90735	92543	95973
0099T	0103T	0123T	0182T	0223T	0224T	0225T
0233T	0240T	0241T	0243T	0244T	0262T	0311T

AMA Icon Changes

90630	90651	31632	31633	45399

Appendix C — Crosswalk of Deleted Codes

The deleted code crosswalk is meant to be used as a reference tool to find active codes that could be used in place of the deleted code. This will not always be an exact match. Please review the code descriptions and guidelines before selecting a code.

Code	Cross reference
31620	To report, see 31652-31654
37202	To report, see 61650-61651
37250	To report, see 37252
37251	To report, see 37253
39400	To report, see 39401-39402
47136	To report, see 47399
47500	To report, see 47531-47541
47505	To report, see 47531-47541
47510	To report, see 47531-47541
47511	To report, see 47531-47541
47525	To report, see 47531-47541
47530	To report, see 47531-47541
47560	To report, see 47579
47561	To report, see 47579
47630	To report, see 47544
50392	To report, see [50432]
50393	To report, see 50693-50695
50394	To report, see [50430, 50431]
50398	To report, see [50435]
64412	To report, see 64999
67112	To report, see 67107-67113
70373	To report, see 76499
72010	To report, see 72082
72069	To report, see 72081-72084
72090	To report, see 72081-72084
73500	To report, see 73501
73510	To report, see 73502-73503
73520	To report, see 73521-73523

Code	Cross reference
73530	To report, see 73501-73503
73540	To report, see 73501-73503
73550	To report, see 73551-73552
74305	To report, see 47531
74320	To report, see 47532
74327	To report, see 47544
74475	To report, see [50432, 50433, 50434, 50435], 50606, 50693-50695
74480	To report, see [50432, 50433, 50434, 50435], 50606, 50693-50695
75896	To report, see [37211, 37212, 37213, 37214], 61650-61651
75945	To report, see 37252-37253
75946	To report, see 37252-37253
75980	To report, see 47533-47537
75982	To report, see 47533-47540
77776	To report, see 77799
77777	To report, see 77799
77785	To report, see 77770-77772
77786	To report, see 77770-77772
77787	To report, see 77770-77772
82486	To report, see specific analyte or 82542
82487	To report, see specific analyte or 84999
82488	To report, see specific analyte or 84999
82489	To report, see specific analyte or 84999

Code	Cross reference
82491	To report, see specific analyte or 82542
82492	To report, see specific analytes or 82542
82541	To report, see specific analyte or 82542
82543	To report, see specific analyte or 82542
82544	To report, see specific analytes or 82542
83788	To report, see specific analyte or 83789
88347	To report, see 88346, [88350]
92543	To report, see 92537-92538
0099T	To report, see 65785
0103T	To report, see 84999
0123T	To report, see 66999
0182T	To report, see 0394T-0395T
0223T	To report, see 93799
0224T	To report, see 93799
0225T	To report, see 93799
0233T	To report, see 88749
0240T	To report, see 91299
0241T	To report, see 91299
0243T	To report, see 94799
0244T	To report, see 94799
0262T	To report, see 33477
0311T	To report, see 93050

Appendix D — Resequenced Codes

Code	Description	Reference
11045	Debridement, subcutaneous tissue (includes epidermis and dermis, if performed); each additional 20 sq cm, or part thereof (List separately in addition to code for primary procedure)	See code following 11042.
11046	Debridement, muscle and/or fascia (includes epidermis, dermis, and subcutaneous tissue, if performed); each additional 20 sq cm, or part thereof (List separately in addition to code for primary procedure)	See code following 11043.
21552	Excision, tumor, soft tissue of neck or anterior thorax, subcutaneous; 3 cm or greater	See code following 21555.
21554	Excision, tumor, soft tissue of neck or anterior thorax, subfascial (eg, intramuscular); 5 cm or greater	See code following 21556.
22858	Total disc arthroplasty (artificial disc), anterior approach, including discectomy with end plate preparation (includes osteophytectomy for nerve root or spinal cord decompression and microdissection); second level, cervical (List separately in addition to code for primary procedure)	See code following 22856.
23071	Excision, tumor, soft tissue of shoulder area, subcutaneous; 3 cm or greater	See code following 23075.
23073	Excision, tumor, soft tissue of shoulder area, subfascial (eg, intramuscular); 5 cm or greater	See code following 23076.
24071	Excision, tumor, soft tissue of upper arm or elbow area, subcutaneous; 3 cm or greater	See code following 24075
24073	Excision, tumor, soft tissue of upper arm or elbow area, subfascial (eg, intramuscular); 5 cm or greater	See code following 24076.
25071	Excision, tumor, soft tissue of forearm and/or wrist area, subcutaneous; 3 cm or greater	See code following 25075.
25073	Excision, tumor, soft tissue of forearm and/or wrist area, subfascial (eg, intramuscular); 3 cm or greater	See code following 25076.
26111	Excision, tumor or vascular malformation, soft tissue of hand or finger, subcutaneous; 1.5 cm or greater	See code following 26115.
26113	Excision, tumor, soft tissue, or vascular malformation, of hand or finger, subfascial (eg, intramuscular); 1.5 cm or greater	See code following 26116.
27043	Excision, tumor, soft tissue of pelvis and hip area, subcutaneous; 3 cm or greater	See code following 27047.
27045	Excision, tumor, soft tissue of pelvis and hip area, subfascial (eg, intramuscular); 5 cm or greater	See code following 27048.
27059	Radical resection of tumor (eg, sarcoma), soft tissue of pelvis and hip area; 5 cm or greater	See code following 27049.
27329	Radical resection of tumor (eg, sarcoma), soft tissue of thigh or knee area; less than 5 cm	See code following 27360.
27337	Excision, tumor, soft tissue of thigh or knee area, subcutaneous; 3 cm or greater	See code following 27327.
27339	Excision, tumor, soft tissue of thigh or knee area, subfascial (eg, intramuscular); 5 cm or greater	See code following 27328.
27632	Excision, tumor, soft tissue of leg or ankle area, subcutaneous; 3 cm or greater	See code following 27618.
27634	Excision, tumor, soft tissue of leg or ankle area, subfascial (eg, intramuscular); 5 cm or greater	See code following 27619.
28039	Excision, tumor, soft tissue of foot or toe, subcutaneous; 1.5 cm or greater	See code following 28043.
28041	Excision, tumor, soft tissue of foot or toe, subfascial (eg, intramuscular); 1.5 cm or greater	See code following 28045.
29914	Arthroscopy, hip, surgical; with femoroplasty (ie, treatment of cam lesion)	See code following 29863.
29915	Arthroscopy, hip, surgical; with acetabuloplasty (ie, treatment of pincer lesion)	See code following 29863.
29916	Arthroscopy, hip, surgical; with labral repair	See code before 29866.
31651	Bronchoscopy, rigid or flexible, including fluoroscopic guidance, when performed; with balloon occlusion, when performed, assessment of air leak, airway sizing, and insertion of bronchial valve(s), each additional lobe (List separately in addition to code for primary procedure[s])	See code following 31647.
33221	Insertion of pacemaker pulse generator only; with existing multiple leads	See code following 33213.
33227	Removal of permanent pacemaker pulse generator with replacement of pacemaker pulse generator; single lead system	See code following 33233.
33228	Removal of permanent pacemaker pulse generator with replacement of pacemaker pulse generator; dual lead system	See code following 33233.
33229	Removal of permanent pacemaker pulse generator with replacement of pacemaker pulse generator; multiple lead system	See code before 33234.
33230	Insertion of implantable defibrillator pulse generator only; with existing dual leads	See code following 33240.
33231	Insertion of implantable defibrillator pulse generator only; with existing multiple leads	See code before 33241.
33262	Removal of implantable defibrillator pulse generator with replacement of implantable defibrillator pulse generator; single lead system	See code following 33241.
33263	Removal of implantable defibrillator pulse generator with replacement of implantable defibrillator pulse generator; dual lead system	See code following 33241.
33264	Removal of implantable defibrillator pulse generator with replacement of implantable defibrillator pulse generator; multiple lead system	See code before 33243.
33270	Insertion or replacement of permanent subcutaneous implantable defibrillator system, with subcutaneous electrode, including defibrillation threshold evaluation, induction of arrhythmia, evaluation of sensing for arrhythmia termination, and programming or reprogramming of sensing or therapeutic parameters, when performed	See code following 33249.
33271	Insertion of subcutaneous implantable defibrillator electrode	See code following 33249.
33272	Removal of subcutaneous implantable defibrillator electrode	See code following 33249.
33273	Repositioning of previously implanted subcutaneous implantable defibrillator electrode	See code following 33249.
33962	Extracorporeal membrane oxygenation (ECMO)/extracorporeal life support (ECLS) provided by physician; reposition peripheral (arterial and/or venous) cannula(e), open, 6 years and older (includes fluoroscopic guidance, when performed)	See code following 33959.

Code	Description	Reference
33963	Extracorporeal membrane oxygenation (ECMO)/extracorporeal life support (ECLS) provided by physician; reposition of central cannula(e) by sternotomy or thoracotomy, birth through 5 years of age (includes fluoroscopic guidance, when performed)	See code following 33959.
33964	Extracorporeal membrane oxygenation (ECMO)/extracorporeal life support (ECLS) provided by physician; reposition central cannula(e) by sternotomy or thoracotomy, 6 years and older (includes fluoroscopic guidance, when performed)	See code following 33959.
33965	Extracorporeal membrane oxygenation (ECMO)/extracorporeal life support (ECLS) provided by physician; removal of peripheral (arterial and/or venous) cannula(e), percutaneous, birth through 5 years of age	See code following 33959.
33966	Extracorporeal membrane oxygenation (ECMO)/extracorporeal life support (ECLS) provided by physician; removal of peripheral (arterial and/or venous) cannula(e), percutaneous, 6 years and older	See code following 33959.
33969	Extracorporeal membrane oxygenation (ECMO)/extracorporeal life support (ECLS) provided by physician; removal of peripheral (arterial and/or venous) cannula(e), open, birth through 5 years of age	See code following 33959.
33984	Extracorporeal membrane oxygenation (ECMO)/extracorporeal life support (ECLS) provided by physician; removal of peripheral (arterial and/or venous) cannula(e), open, 6 years and older	See code following 33959.
33985	Extracorporeal membrane oxygenation (ECMO)/extracorporeal life support (ECLS) provided by physician; removal of central cannula(e) by sternotomy or thoracotomy, birth through 5 years of age	See code following 33959.
33986	Extracorporeal membrane oxygenation (ECMO)/extracorporeal life support (ECLS) provided by physician; removal of central cannula(e) by sternotomy or thoracotomy, 6 years and older	See code following 33959.
33987	Arterial exposure with creation of graft conduit (eg, chimney graft) to facilitate arterial perfusion for ECMO/ECLS (List separately in addition to code for primary procedure)	See code following 33959.
33988	Insertion of left heart vent by thoracic incision (eg, sternotomy, thoracotomy) for ECMO/ECLS	See code following 33959.
33989	Removal of left heart vent by thoracic incision (eg, sternotomy, thoracotomy) for ECMO/ECLS	See code following 33959.
37211	Transcatheter therapy, arterial infusion for thrombolysis other than coronary, any method, including radiological supervision and interpretation, initial treatment day	See code following 37200.
37212	Transcatheter therapy, venous infusion for thrombolysis, any method, including radiological supervision and interpretation, initial treatment day	See code following 37200.
37213	Transcatheter therapy, arterial or venous infusion for thrombolysis other than coronary, any method, including radiological supervision and interpretation, continued treatment on subsequent day during course of thrombolytic therapy, including follow-up catheter contrast injection, position change, or exchange, when performed;	See code following 37200.
37214	Transcatheter therapy, arterial or venous infusion for thrombolysis other than coronary, any method, including radiological supervision and interpretation, continued treatment on subsequent day during course of thrombolytic therapy, including follow-up catheter contrast injection, position change, or exchange, when performed; cessation of thrombolysis including removal of catheter and vessel closure by any method	See code following 37200.
38243	Hematopoietic progenitor cell (HPC); HPC boost	See code following 38241.
42310	Esophagogastroduodenoscopy, flexible, transoral; with esophagogastric fundoplasty, partial or complete, includes duodenoscopy when performed	See code following 43259.
43211	Esophagoscopy, flexible, transoral; with endoscopic mucosal resection	See code following 43217.
43212	Esophagoscopy, flexible, transoral; with placement of endoscopic stent (includes pre- and post-dilation and guide wire passage, when performed)	See code following 43217.
43213	Esophagoscopy, flexible, transoral; with dilation of esophagus, by balloon or dilator, retrograde (includes fluoroscopic guidance, when performed)	See code following 43220.
43214	Esophagoscopy, flexible, transoral; with dilation of esophagus with balloon (30 mm diameter or larger) (includes fluoroscopic guidance, when performed)	See code following 43220.
43233	Esophagogastroduodenoscopy, flexible, transoral; with dilation of esophagus with balloon (30 mm diameter or larger) (includes fluoroscopic guidance, when performed)	See code following 43249.
43266	Esophagogastroduodenoscopy, flexible, transoral; with placement of endoscopic stent (includes pre- and post-dilation and guide wire passage, when performed)	See code following 43255.
43270	Esophagogastroduodenoscopy, flexible, transoral; with ablation of tumor(s), polyp(s), or other lesion(s) (includes pre- and post-dilation and guide wire passage, when performed)	See code following 43257.
43274	Endoscopic retrograde cholangiopancreatography (ERCP); with placement of endoscopic stent into biliary or pancreatic duct, including pre- and post-dilation and guide wire passage, when performed, including sphincterotomy, when performed, each stent	See code following 43265.
43275	Endoscopic retrograde cholangiopancreatography (ERCP); with removal of foreign body(s) or stent(s) from biliary/pancreatic duct(s)	See code following 43265.
43276	Endoscopic retrograde cholangiopancreatography (ERCP); with removal and exchange of stent(s), biliary or pancreatic duct, including pre- and post-dilation and guide wire passage, when performed, including sphincterotomy, when performed, each stent exchanged	See code following 43265.
43277	Endoscopic retrograde cholangiopancreatography (ERCP); with trans-endoscopic balloon dilation of biliary/pancreatic duct(s) or of ampulla (sphincteroplasty), including sphincterotomy, when performed, each duct	See code before 43273.
43278	Endoscopic retrograde cholangiopancreatography (ERCP); with ablation of tumor(s), polyp(s), or other lesion(s), including pre- and post-dilation and guide wire passage, when performed	See code before 43273.
44381	Ileoscopy, through stoma; with transendoscopic balloon dilation	See code following 44382.
44401	Colonoscopy through stoma; with ablation of tumor(s), polyp(s), or other lesion(s) (includes pre-and post-dilation and guide wire passage, when performed)	See code following 44392.

© 2015 Optum360, LLC

Code	Description	Reference
45346	Sigmoidoscopy, flexible; with ablation of tumor(s), polyp(s), or other lesion(s) (includes pre- and post-dilation and guide wire passage, when performed)	See code following 45338.
45388	Colonoscopy, flexible; with ablation of tumor(s), polyp(s), or other lesion(s) (includes pre- and post-dilation and guide wire passage, when performed)	See code following 45382.
45390	Colonoscopy, flexible; with endoscopic mucosal resection	See code following 45392.
45398	Colonoscopy, flexible; with band ligation(s) (eg, hemorrhoids)	See code following 45393.
45399	Unlisted procedure, colon	See code before 45990.
46220	Excision of single external papilla or tag, anus	See code before 46230.
46320	Excision of thrombosed hemorrhoid, external	See code following 46230.
46945	Hemorrhoidectomy, internal, by ligation other than rubber band; single hemorrhoid column/group	See code following 46221.
46946	Hemorrhoidectomy, internal, by ligation other than rubber band; 2 or more hemorrhoid columns/groups	See code following 46221.
46947	Hemorrhoidopexy (eg, for prolapsing internal hemorrhoids) by stapling	See code following 46762.
50430	Injection procedure for antegrade nephrostogram and/or ureterogram, complete diagnostic procedure including imaging guidance (eg, ultrasound and fluoroscopy) and all associated radiological supervision and interpretation; new access	See code following 43259
50431	Injection procedure for antegrade nephrostogram and/or ureterogram, complete diagnostic procedure including imaging guidance (eg, ultrasound and fluoroscopy) and all associated radiological supervision and interpretation; existing access	See code following 43259.
50432	Placement of nephrostomy catheter, percutaneous, including diagnostic nephrostogram and/or ureterogram when performed, imaging guidance (eg, ultrasound and/or fluoroscopy) and all associated radiological supervision and interpretation	See code following 43259.
50433	Placement of nephroureteral catheter, percutaneous, including diagnostic nephrostogram and/or ureterogram when performed, imaging guidance (eg, ultrasound and/or fluoroscopy) and all associated radiological supervision and interpretation, new access	See code following 43259.
50434	Convert nephrostomy catheter to nephroureteral catheter, percutaneous, including diagnostic nephrostogram and/or ureterogram when performed, imaging guidance (eg, ultrasound and/or fluoroscopy) and all associated radiological supervision and interpretation, via pre-existing nephrostomy tract	See code following 43259.
50435	Exchange nephrostomy catheter, percutaneous, including diagnostic nephrostogram and/or ureterogram when performed, imaging guidance (eg, ultrasound and/or fluoroscopy) and all associated radiological supervision and interpretation	See code following 43259.
51797	Voiding pressure studies, intra-abdominal (ie, rectal, gastric, intraperitoneal) (List separately in addition to code for primary procedure)	See code following 51729.
52356	Cystourethroscopy, with ureteroscopy and/or pyeloscopy; with lithotripsy including insertion of indwelling ureteral stent (eg, Gibbons or double-J type)	See code following 52353.
64461	Paravertebral block (PVB) (paraspinous block), thoracic; single injection site (includes imaging guidance, when performed)	See code following 64484.
64462	Paravertebral block (PVB) (paraspinous block), thoracic; second and any additional injection site(s) (includes imaging guidance, when performed) (List separately in addition to code for primary procedure)	See code following 64484.
64463	Paravertebral block (PVB) (paraspinous block), thoracic; continuous infusion by catheter (includes imaging guidance, when performed)	See code following 64484.
64633	Destruction by neurolytic agent, paravertebral facet joint nerve(s), with imaging guidance (fluoroscopy or CT); cervical or thoracic, single facet joint	See code following 64620.
64634	Destruction by neurolytic agent, paravertebral facet joint nerve(s), with imaging guidance (fluoroscopy or CT); cervical or thoracic, each additional facet joint (List separately in addition to code for primary procedure)	See code following 64620.
64635	Destruction by neurolytic agent, paravertebral facet joint nerve(s), with imaging guidance (fluoroscopy or CT); lumbar or sacral, single facet joint	See code following 64620.
64636	Destruction by neurolytic agent, paravertebral facet joint nerve(s), with imaging guidance (fluoroscopy or CT); lumbar or sacral, each additional facet joint (List separately in addition to code for primary procedure)	See code before 64630.
67810	Incisional biopsy of eyelid skin including lid margin	See code following 67715.
77085	Dual-energy X-ray absorptiometry (DXA), bone density study, 1 or more sites; axial skeleton (eg, hips, pelvis, spine), including vertebral fracture assessment	See code following 77081.
77086	Vertebral fracture assessment via dual-energy X-ray absorptiometry (DXA)	See code before 77084.
77295	3-dimensional radiotherapy plan, including dose-volume histograms	See code before 77300.
77385	Intensity modulated radiation treatment delivery (IMRT), includes guidance and tracking, when performed; simple	See code following 77417.
77386	Intensity modulated radiation treatment delivery (IMRT), includes guidance and tracking, when performed; complex	See code following 77417.
77387	Guidance for localization of target volume for delivery of radiation treatment delivery, includes intrafraction tracking, when performed	See code following 77417.
77424	Intraoperative radiation treatment delivery, x-ray, single treatment session	See code before 77422.
77425	Intraoperative radiation treatment delivery, electrons, single treatment session	See code before 77422.
80081	Obstetric panel (includes HIV testing)	See code following 80055.
80164	Valproic acid (dipropylacetic acid); total	See code following 80201.
80165	Valproic acid (dipropylacetic acid); free	See code following 80201.

Code	Description	Reference
80171	Gabapentin, whole blood, serum, or plasma	See code following 80169.
80300	Drug screen, any number of drug classes from Drug Class List A; any number of non-TLC devices or procedures, (eg, immunoassay) capable of being read by direct optical observation, including instrumented-assisted when performed (eg, dipsticks, cups, cards, cartridges), per date of service	See code before 80150.
80301	Drug screen, any number of drug classes from Drug Class List A; single drug class method, by instrumented test systems (eg, discrete multichannel chemistry analyzers utilizing immunoassay or enzyme assay), per date of service	See code before 80150.
80302	Drug screen, presumptive, single drug class from Drug Class List B, by immunoassay (eg, ELISA) or non-TLC chromatography without mass spectrometry (eg, GC, HPLC), each procedure	See code before 80150.
80303	Drug screen, any number of drug classes, presumptive, single or multiple drug class method; thin layer chromatography procedure(s) (TLC) (eg, acid, neutral, alkaloid plate), per date of service	See code before 80150.
80304	Drug screen, any number of drug classes, presumptive, single or multiple drug class method; not otherwise specified presumptive procedure (eg, TOF, MALDI, LDTD, DESI, DART), each procedure	See code before 80150.
80320	Alcohols	See code before 80150.
80321	Alcohol biomarkers; 1 or 2	See code before 80150.
80322	Alcohol biomarkers; 3 or more	See code before 80150.
80323	Alkaloids, not otherwise specified	See code before 80150.
80324	Amphetamines; 1 or 2	See code before 80150.
80325	Amphetamines; 3 or 4	See code before 80150.
80326	Amphetamines; 5 or more	See code before 80150.
80327	Anabolic steroids; 1 or 2	See code before 80150.
80328	Anabolic steroids; 3 or more	See code before 80150.
80329	Analgesics, non-opioid; 1 or 2	See code before 80150.
80330	Analgesics, non-opioid; 3-5	See code before 80150.
80331	Analgesics, non-opioid; 6 or more	See code before 80150.
80332	Antidepressants, serotonergic class; 1 or 2	See code before 80150.
80333	Antidepressants, serotonergic class; 3-5	See code before 80150.
80334	Antidepressants, serotonergic class; 6 or more	See code before 80150.
80335	Antidepressants, tricyclic and other cyclicals; 1 or 2	See code before 80150.
80336	Antidepressants, tricyclic and other cyclicals; 3-5	See code before 80150.
80337	Antidepressants, tricyclic and other cyclicals; 6 or more	See code before 80150.
80338	Antidepressants, not otherwise specified	See code before 80150.
80339	Antiepileptics, not otherwise specified; 1-3	See code before 80150.
80340	Antiepileptics, not otherwise specified; 4-6	See code before 80150.
80341	Antiepileptics, not otherwise specified; 7 or more	See code before 80150.
80342	Antipsychotics, not otherwise specified; 1-3	See code before 80150.
80343	Antipsychotics, not otherwise specified; 4-6	See code before 80150.
80344	Antipsychotics, not otherwise specified; 7 or more	See code before 80150.
80345	Barbiturates	See code before 80150.
80346	Benzodiazepines; 1-12	See code before 80150.
80347	Benzodiazepines; 13 or more	See code following 80150.
80348	Buprenorphine	See code before 80150.
80349	Cannabinoids, natural	See code before 80150.
80350	Cannabinoids, synthetic; 1-3	See code before 80150.
80351	Cannabinoids, synthetic; 4-6	See code before 80150.
80352	Cannabinoids, synthetic; 7 or more	See code before 80150.
80353	Cocaine	See code before 80150.
80354	Fentanyl	See code before 80150.
80355	Gabapentin, non-blood	See code before 80150.
80356	Heroin metabolite	See code before 80150.
80357	Ketamine and norketamine	See code before 80150.
80358	Methadone	See code before 80150.
80359	Methylenedioxyamphetamines (MDA, MDEA, MDMA)	See code before 80150.
80360	Methylphenidate	See code before 80150.
80361	Opiates, 1 or more	See code before 80150.
80362	Opioids and opiate analogs; 1 or 2	See code before 80150.
80363	Opioids and opiate analogs; 3 or 4	See code before 80150.
80364	Opioids and opiate analogs; 5 or more	See code before 80150.
80365	Oxycodone	See code following 80364.
80366	Pregabalin	See code following 83992.

Code	Description	Reference
80367	Propoxyphene	See code following 80366.
80368	Sedative hypnotics (non-benzodiazepines)	See code following 80367.
80369	Skeletal muscle relaxants; 1 or 2	See code following 80368.
80370	Skeletal muscle relaxants; 3 or more	See code following 80369.
80371	Stimulants, synthetic	See code following 80370.
80372	Tapentadol	See code following 80371.
80373	Tramadol	See code following 80372.
80374	Stereoisomer (enantiomer) analysis, single drug class	See code following 80373.
80375	Drug(s) or substance(s), definitive, qualitative or quantitative, not otherwise specified; 1-3	See code following 80374.
80376	Drug(s) or substance(s), definitive, qualitative or quantitative, not otherwise specified; 4-6	See code following 80375.
80377	Drug(s) or substance(s), definitive, qualitative or quantitative, not otherwise specified; 7 or more	See code following 80376.
81161	DMD (dystrophin) (eg, Duchenne/Becker muscular dystrophy) deletion analysis, and duplication analysis, if performed	See code following 81229.
81162	BRCA1, BRCA2 (breast cancer 1 and 2) (eg, hereditary breast and ovarian cancer) gene analysis; full sequence analysis and full duplication/deletion analysis	See code following 81211.
81287	MGMT (O-6-methylguanine-DNA methyltransferase) (eg, glioblastoma multiforme), methylation analysis	See code following 81290.
81288	MLH1 (mutL homolog 1, colon cancer, nonpolyposis type 2) (eg, hereditary non-polyposis colorectal cancer, Lynch syndrome) gene analysis; promoter methylation analysis	See code following 81292.
81479	Unlisted molecular pathology procedure	See code following 81408.
82652	Vitamin D; 1, 25 dihydroxy, includes fraction(s), if performed	See code following 82306.
83992	Phencyclidine (PCP)	See code following 80365.
86152	Cell enumeration using immunologic selection and identification in fluid specimen (eg, circulating tumor cells in blood);	See code following 86147.
86153	Cell enumeration using immunologic selection and identification in fluid specimen (eg, circulating tumor cells in blood); physician interpretation and report, when required	See code before 86148.
87623	Infectious agent detection by nucleic acid (DNA or RNA); Human Papillomavirus (HPV), low-risk types (eg, 6, 11, 42, 43, 44)	See code following 87539.
87624	Infectious agent detection by nucleic acid (DNA or RNA); Human Papillomavirus (HPV), high-risk types (eg, 16, 18, 31, 33, 35, 39, 45, 51, 52, 56, 58, 59, 68)	See code following 87539.
87625	Infectious agent detection by nucleic acid (DNA or RNA); Human Papillomavirus (HPV), types 16 and 18 only, includes type 45, if performed	See code before 87540.
87806	Infectious agent antigen detection by immunoassay with direct optical observation; HIV-1 antigen(s), with HIV-1 and HIV-2 antibodies	See code following 87803.
87906	Infectious agent genotype analysis by nucleic acid (DNA or RNA); HIV-1, other region (eg, integrase, fusion)	See code following 87901.
87910	Infectious agent genotype analysis by nucleic acid (DNA or RNA); cytomegalovirus	See code following 87900.
87912	Infectious agent genotype analysis by nucleic acid (DNA or RNA); Hepatitis B virus	See code before 87902.
88177	Cytopathology, evaluation of fine needle aspirate; immediate cytohistologic study to determine adequacy for diagnosis, each separate additional evaluation episode, same site (List separately in addition to code for primary procedure)	See code following 88173.
88341	Immunohistochemistry or immunocytochemistry, per specimen; each additional single antibody stain procedure (List separately in addition to code for primary procedure)	See code following 88342.
88350	Immunofluorescence, per specimen; each additional single antibody stain procedure (List separately in addition to code for primary procedure)	See code following 88346.
88364	In situ hybridization (eg, FISH), per specimen; each additional single probe stain procedure (List separately in addition to code for primary procedure)	See code following 88365.
88373	Morphometric analysis, in situ hybridization (quantitative or semi-quantitative), using computer-assisted technology, per specimen; each additional single probe stain procedure (List separately in addition to code for primary procedure)	See code following 88367.
88374	Morphometric analysis, in situ hybridization (quantitative or semi-quantitative), using computer-assisted technology, per specimen; each multiplex probe stain procedure	See code following 88367.
88377	Morphometric analysis, in situ hybridization (quantitative or semi-quantitative), manual, per specimen; each multiplex probe stain procedure	See code following 88369.
90620	Meningococcal recombinant protein and outer membrane vesicle vaccine, serogroup B (MenB), 2 dose schedule, for intramuscular use	See code following 90734.
90621	Meningococcal recombinant lipoprotein vaccine, serogroup B (MenB), 3 dose schedule, for intramuscular use	See code following 90734.
90625	Cholera vaccine, live, adult dosage, 1 dose schedule, for oral use	See code following 90723.
90630	Influenza virus vaccine, quadrivalent (IIV4), split virus, preservative free, for intradermal use	See code following 90654.
90644	Meningococcal conjugate vaccine, serogroups C & Y and Haemophilus influenzae type b vaccine (Hib-MenCY), 4 dose schedule, when administered to children 2-18 months of age, for intramuscular use	See code following 90732.
90672	Influenza virus vaccine, quadrivalent, live, for intranasal use	See code following 90660.
90673	Influenza virus vaccine, trivalent, derived from recombinant DNA (RIV3), hemagglutinin (HA) protein only, preservative and antibiotic free, for intramuscular use	See code following 90661.

Code	Description	Reference
92558	Evoked otoacoustic emissions, screening (qualitative measurement of distortion product or transient evoked otoacoustic emissions), automated analysis	See code following 92586.
92597	Evaluation for use and/or fitting of voice prosthetic device to supplement oral speech	See code following 92604.
92618	Evaluation for prescription of non-speech-generating augmentative and alternative communication device, face-to-face with the patient; each additional 30 minutes (List separately in addition to code for primary procedure)	See code following 92605.
92920	Percutaneous transluminal coronary angioplasty; single major coronary artery or branch	See code following 92998.
92921	Percutaneous transluminal coronary angioplasty; each additional branch of a major coronary artery (List separately in addition to code for primary procedure)	See code following 92998.
92924	Percutaneous transluminal coronary atherectomy, with coronary angioplasty when performed; single major coronary artery or branch	See code following 92998.
92925	Percutaneous transluminal coronary atherectomy, with coronary angioplasty when performed; each additional branch of a major coronary artery (List separately in addition to code for primary procedure)	See code following 92998.
92928	Percutaneous transcatheter placement of intracoronary stent(s), with coronary angioplasty when performed; single major coronary artery or branch	See code following 92998.
92929	Percutaneous transcatheter placement of intracoronary stent(s), with coronary angioplasty when performed; each additional branch of a major coronary artery (List separately in addition to code for primary procedure)	See code following 92998.
92933	Percutaneous transluminal coronary atherectomy, with intracoronary stent, with coronary angioplasty when performed; single major coronary artery or branch	See code following 92998.
92934	Percutaneous transluminal coronary atherectomy, with intracoronary stent, with coronary angioplasty when performed; each additional branch of a major coronary artery (List separately in addition to code for primary procedure)	See code following 92998.
92937	Percutaneous transluminal revascularization of or through coronary artery bypass graft (internal mammary, free arterial, venous), any combination of intracoronary stent, atherectomy and angioplasty, including distal protection when performed; single vessel	See code following 92998.
92938	Percutaneous transluminal revascularization of or through coronary artery bypass graft (internal mammary, free arterial, venous), any combination of intracoronary stent, atherectomy and angioplasty, including distal protection when performed; each additional branch subtended by the bypass graft (List separately in addition to code for primary procedure)	See code following 92998.
92941	Percutaneous transluminal revascularization of acute total/subtotal occlusion during acute myocardial infarction, coronary artery or coronary artery bypass graft, any combination of intracoronary stent, atherectomy and angioplasty, including aspiration thrombectomy when performed, single vessel	See code following 92998.
92943	Percutaneous transluminal revascularization of chronic total occlusion, coronary artery, coronary artery branch, or coronary artery bypass graft, any combination of intracoronary stent, atherectomy and angioplasty; single vessel	See code following 92998.
92944	Percutaneous transluminal revascularization of chronic total occlusion, coronary artery, coronary artery branch, or coronary artery bypass graft, any combination of intracoronary stent, atherectomy and angioplasty; each additional coronary artery, coronary artery branch, or bypass graft (List separately in addition to code for primary procedure)	See code following 92998.
92973	Percutaneous transluminal coronary thrombectomy mechanical (List separately in addition to code for primary procedure)	See code following 92998.
92974	Transcatheter placement of radiation delivery device for subsequent coronary intravascular brachytherapy (List separately in addition to code for primary procedure)	See code following 92998.
92975	Thrombolysis, coronary; by intracoronary infusion, including selective coronary angiography	See code following 92998.
92977	Thrombolysis, coronary; by intravenous infusion	See code following 92998.
92978	Intravascular ultrasound (coronary vessel or graft) during diagnostic evaluation and/or therapeutic intervention including imaging supervision, interpretation and report; initial vessel (List separately in addition to code for primary procedure)	See code following 92998.
92979	Intravascular ultrasound (coronary vessel or graft) during diagnostic evaluation and/or therapeutic intervention including imaging supervision, interpretation and report; each additional vessel (List separately in addition to code for primary procedure)	See code following 92998.
93260	Programming device evaluation (in person) with iterative adjustment of the implantable device to test the function of the device and select optimal permanent programmed values with analysis, review and report by a physician or other qualified health care professional; implantable subcutaneous lead defibrillator system	See code following 93284.
93261	Interrogation device evaluation (in person) with analysis, review and report by a physician or other qualified health care professional, includes connection, recording and disconnection per patient encounter; implantable subcutaneous lead defibrillator system	See code following 93289.
95782	Polysomnography; younger than 6 years, sleep staging with 4 or more additional parameters of sleep, attended by a technologist	See code following 95811.
95783	Polysomnography; younger than 6 years, sleep staging with 4 or more additional parameters of sleep, with initiation of continuous positive airway pressure therapy or bi-level ventilation, attended by a technologist	See code following 95811.
95800	Sleep study, unattended, simultaneous recording; heart rate, oxygen saturation, respiratory analysis (eg, by airflow or peripheral arterial tone), and sleep time	See code following 95806.
95801	Sleep study, unattended, simultaneous recording; minimum of heart rate, oxygen saturation, and respiratory analysis (eg, by airflow or peripheral arterial tone)	See code following 95806.

Code	Description	Reference
95885	Needle electromyography, each extremity, with related paraspinal areas, when performed, done with nerve conduction, amplitude and latency/velocity study; limited (List separately in addition to code for primary procedure)	See code following 95872.
95886	Needle electromyography, each extremity, with related paraspinal areas, when performed, done with nerve conduction, amplitude and latency/velocity study; complete, five or more muscles studied, innervated by three or more nerves or four or more spinal levels (List separately in addition to code for primary procedure)	See code following 95872.
95887	Needle electromyography, non-extremity (cranial nerve supplied or axial) muscle(s) done with nerve conduction, amplitude and latency/velocity study (List separately in addition to code for primary procedure)	See code before 95873.
95938	Short-latency somatosensory evoked potential study, stimulation of any/all peripheral nerves or skin sites, recording from the central nervous system; in upper and lower limbs	See code following 95926.
95939	Central motor evoked potential study (transcranial motor stimulation); in upper and lower limbs	See code following 95929.
95940	Continuous intraoperative neurophysiology monitoring in the operating room, one on one monitoring requiring personal attendance, each 15 minutes (List separately in addition to code for primary procedure)	See code following 95913.
95941	Continuous intraoperative neurophysiology monitoring, from outside the operating room (remote or nearby) or for monitoring of more than one case while in the operating room, per hour (List separately in addition to code for primary procedure)	See code following 95913.
95943	Simultaneous, independent, quantitative measures of both parasympathetic function and sympathetic function, based on time-frequency analysis of heart rate variability concurrent with time-frequency analysis of continuous respiratory activity, with mean heart rate and blood pressure measures, during rest, paced (deep) breathing, Valsalva maneuvers, and head-up postural change	See code following 95924.
99177	Instrument-based ocular screening (eg, photoscreening, automated-refraction), bilateral; with on-site analysis	See code following 99174.
99224	Subsequent observation care, per day, for the evaluation and management of a patient, which requires at least 2 of these 3 key components: Problem focused interval history; Problem focused examination; Medical decision making that is straightforward or of low complexity. Counseling and/or coordination of care with other physicians, other qualified health care professionals, or agencies are provided consistent with the nature of the problem(s) and the patient's and/or family's needs. Usually, the patient is stable, recovering, or improving. Typically, 15 minutes are spent at the bedside and on the patient's hospital floor or unit.	See code following 99220.
99225	Subsequent observation care, per day, for the evaluation and management of a patient, which requires at least 2 of these 3 key components: An expanded problem focused interval history; An expanded problem focused examination; Medical decision making of moderate complexity. Counseling and/or coordination of care with other physicians, other qualified health care professionals, or agencies are provided consistent with the nature of the problem(s) and the patient's and/or family's needs. Usually, the patient is responding inadequately to therapy or has developed a minor complication. Typically, 25 minutes are spent at the bedside and on the patient's hospital floor or unit.	See code following 99220.
99226	Subsequent observation care, per day, for the evaluation and management of a patient, which requires at least 2 of these 3 key components: A detailed interval history; A detailed examination; Medical decision making of high complexity. Counseling and/or coordination of care with other physicians, other qualified health care professionals, or agencies are provided consistent with the nature of the problem(s) and the patient's and/or family's needs. Usually, the patient is unstable or has developed a significant complication or a significant new problem. Typically, 35 minutes are spent at the bedside and on the patient's hospital floor or unit.	See code before 99221.
99415	Prolonged clinical staff service (the service beyond the typical service time) during an evaluation and management service in the office or outpatient setting, direct patient contact with physician supervision; first hour (List separately in addition to code for outpatient Evaluation and Management service)	See code following 99359.
99416	Prolonged clinical staff service (the service beyond the typical service time) during an evaluation and management service in the office or outpatient setting, direct patient contact with physician supervision; each additional 30 minutes (List separately in addition to code for prolonged service)	See code following 99359.
99485	Supervision by a control physician of interfacility transport care of the critically ill or critically injured pediatric patient, 24 months of age or younger, includes two-way communication with transport team before transport, at the referring facility and during the transport, including data interpretation and report; first 30 minutes	See code following 99467.
99486	Supervision by a control physician of interfacility transport care of the critically ill or critically injured pediatric patient, 24 months of age or younger, includes two-way communication with transport team before transport, at the referring facility and during the transport, including data interpretation and report; each additional 30 minutes (List separately in addition to code for primary procedure)	See code following 99467.
99490	Chronic care management services, at least 20 minutes of clinical staff time directed by a physician or other qualified health care professional, per calendar month, with the following required elements: multiple (two or more) chronic conditions expected to last at least 12 months, or until the death of the patient; chronic conditions place the patient at significant risk of death, acute exacerbation/decompensation, or functional decline; comprehensive care plan established, implemented, revised, or monitored.	See code before 99487.
0253T	Insertion of anterior segment aqueous drainage device, without extracular reservoir, internal approach, into the suprachoroidal space	See code following 0191T.
0357T	Cryopreservation; immature oocyte(s)	See code following 0058T.
0376T	Insertion of anterior segment aqueous drainage device, without extracular reservoir, internal approach, into the trabecular meshwork; each additional device insertion (List separately in addition to code for primary procedure)	See code following 0191T.

Appendix E — Add-on Codes, Modifier 51 Exempt, Optum Modifier 51 Exempt, Modifier 63 Exempt, and Moderate Sedation Codes

Codes specified as add-on, exempt from modifier 51 and 63, and that include conscious sedation are listed. The lists are designed to be read left to right rather than vertically.

Add-on Codes

0054T	0055T	0076T	0095T	0098T	0159T	0163T
0164T	0165T	0172T	0174T	0189T	0190T	1953
1968	1969	0196T	0205T	0214T	0215T	0217T
0218T	0222T	0229T	0231T	0241T	0289T	0290T
0291T	0292T	0294T	0300T	0309T	0346T	0361T
0363T	0365T	0367T	0369T	0374T	0376T	0396T
0397T	0399T	10036	11001	11008	11045	11046
11047	11101	11201	11732	11922	13102	13122
13133	13153	14302	15003	15005	15101	15111
15116	15121	15131	15136	15151	15152	15156
15157	15201	15221	15241	15261	15272	15274
15276	15278	15777	15787	15847	16036	17003
17312	17314	17315	19001	19082	19084	19086
19126	19282	19284	19286	19288	19297	20930
20931	20936	20937	20938	20985	22103	22116
22208	22216	22226	22328	22512	22515	22527
22534	22552	22585	22614	22632	22634	22840
22841	22842	22843	22844	22845	22846	22847
22848	22851	22858	26125	26861	26863	27358
27692	29826	31620	31627	31632	31633	31637
31649	31651	31654	32501	32506	32507	32667
32668	32674	33141	33225	33257	33258	33259
33367	33368	33369	33419	33508	33517	33518
33519	33521	33522	33523	33530	33572	33768
33884	33924	33987	34806	34808	34813	34826
35306	35390	35400	35500	35572	35600	35681
35682	35683	35685	35686	35697	35700	36148
36218	36227	36228	36248	36476	36479	37185
37186	37222	37223	37232	37233	37234	37235
37237	37239	37250	37251	37252	37253	38102
38746	38747	38900	43273	43283	43338	43635
44015	44121	44128	44139	44203	44213	44701
44955	47001	47542	47543	47544	47550	48400
49326	49327	49412	49435	49568	49905	50606
50705	50706	51797	52442	56606	57267	58110
58611	59525	60512	61316	61517	61610	61611
61612	61641	61642	61651	61781	61782	61783
61797	61799	61800	61864	61868	62148	62160
63035	63043	63044	63048	63057	63066	63076
63078	63082	63086	63088	63091	63103	63295
63308	63621	64462	64480	64484	64491	64492
64494	64495	64634	64636	64643	64645	64727
64778	64783	64787	64832	64837	64859	64872
64874	64876	64901	64902	65757	66990	67225
67320	67331	67332	67334	67335	67340	69990
74301	74713	75565	75774	75946	75964	75968
76125	76802	76810	76812	76814	76937	77001
77051	77052	77063	77293	78020	78496	78730
81266	81416	81426	81536	82952	86826	87187
87503	87904	88155	88177	88185	88311	88314
88332	88334	88341	88350	88364	88369	88373
88388	90461	90472	90474	90785	90833	90836
90838	90840	90863	91013	92547	92608	92618
92621	92627	92921	92925	92929	92934	92938
92944	92973	92974	92978	92979	92998	93320
93321	93325	93352	93462	93463	93464	93563
93564	93565	93566	93567	93568	93571	93572
93609	93613	93621	93622	93623	93655	93657
93662	94645	94729	94781	95079	95873	95874
95885	95886	95887	95940	95941	95962	95967
95973	95975	95979	96361	96366	96367	96368
96370	96371	96375	96376	96411	96415	96417
96423	96570	96571	96934	96935	96936	97546
97598	97811	97814	99100	99116	99135	99140

99145	99150	99292	99354	99355	99356	99357
99359	99415	99416	99467	99486	99489	99498
99602	99607					

AMA Modifer 51 Exempt Codes

17004	20697	20974	20975	31500	36620	44500
61107	93451	93456	93503	93600	93602	93603
93610	93612	93615	93616	93618	93631	94610
95905	95992	99143	99144			

Modifier 63 Exempt Codes

30540	30545	31520	33401	33403	33470	33502
33503	33505	33506	33610	33611	33619	33647
33670	33690	33694	33730	33732	33735	33736
33750	33755	33762	33778	33786	33922	33946
33947	33948	33949	36415	36420	36450	36460
36510	36660	39503	43313	43314	43520	43831
44055	44126	44127	44128	46070	46705	46715
46716	46730	46735	46740	46742	46744	47700
47701	49215	49491	49492	49495	49496	49600
49605	49606	49610	49611	53025	54000	54150
54160	63700	63702	63704	63706	65820	

Moderate Sedation Codes

0200T	0201T	0282T	0283T	0284T	0291T	0292T
0293T	0294T	0301T	0302T	0303T	0304T	0307T
0308T	0335T	0340T	0397T	10030	19298	20982
20983	22510	22511	22512	22513	22514	22515
22526	22527	31615	31620	31622	31623	31624
31625	31626	31627	31628	31629	31632	31633
31634	31635	31645	31646	31647	31648	31649
31651	31652	31653	31654	31660	31661	31725
32405	32550	32551	32553	33010	33011	33206
33207	33208	33210	33211	33212	33213	33214
33216	33217	33218	33220	33221	33222	33223
33227	33228	33229	33230	33231	33233	33234
33235	33240	33241	33244	33249	33262	33263
33264	33282	33284	33990	33991	33992	33993
35471	35472	35475	35476	36010	36140	36147
36148	36200	36221	36222	36223	36224	36225
36226	36227	36228	36245	36246	36247	36248
36251	36252	36253	36254	36481	36555	36557
36558	36560	36561	36563	36565	36566	36568
36570	36571	36576	36578	36581	36582	36583
36585	36590	36870	37183	37184	37185	37186
37187	37188	37191	37192	37193	37197	37211
37212	37213	37214	37215	37216	37218	37220
37221	37222	37223	37224	37225	37226	37227
37228	37229	37230	37231	37232	37233	37234
37235	37236	37237	37238	37239	37241	37242
37243	37244	37252	37253	43200	43201	43202
43204	43205	43206	43211	43212	43213	43214
43215	43216	43217	43220	43226	43227	43229
43231	43232	43233	43235	43236	43237	43238
43239	43240	43241	43242	43243	43244	43245
43246	43247	43248	43249	43250	43251	43252
43253	43254	43255	43257	43259	43260	43261
43262	43263	43264	43265	43266	43270	43273
43274	43275	43276	43277	43278	43453	44360
44361	44363	44364	44365	44366	44369	44370
44372	44373	44376	44377	44378	44379	44380
44381	44382	44384	44385	44386	44388	44389
44390	44391	44392	44394	44401	44402	44403
44404	44405	44406	44407	44408	44500	45303
45305	45307	45308	45309	45315	45317	45320
45321	45327	45332	45333	45334	45335	45337

45338	45340	45341	45342	45346	45347	45349
45350	45378	45379	45380	45381	45382	45384
45385	45386	45388	45389	45390	45391	45392
45393	45398	47000	47382	47383	47525	47532
47533	47534	47535	47536	47538	47539	47540
47541	47542	47543	47544	49405	49406	49407
49411	49418	49440	49441	49442	49446	50200
50382	50384	50385	50386	50387	50430	50432
50433	50434	50592	50593	50606	50693	50694
50695	50705	50706	57155	66720	69300	77371
77600	77605	77610	77615	92920	92921	92924
92925	92928	92929	92933	92934	92937	92938
92941	92943	92944	92953	92960	92961	92973
92974	92975	92978	92979	92986	92987	93312
93313	93314	93315	93316	93317	93318	93451
93452	93453	93454	93455	93456	93457	93458
93459	93460	93461	93462	93463	93464	93505
93530	93561	93562	93563	93564	93565	93566
93567	93568	93571	93572	93582	93583	93609
93613	93615	93616	93618	93619	93620	93621
93622	93624	93640	93641	93642	93644	93650
93653	93654	93655	93656	93657	94011	94012
94013						

Optum Modifier 51 Exempt Codes

90281	90283	90284	90287	90288	90291	90296
90371	90375	90376	90378	90384	90385	90386
90389	90393	90396	90399	90476	90477	90581
90585	90586	90620	90621	90625	90630	90632
90633	90634	90636	90644	90647	90648	90649
90650	90651	90653	90654	90655	90656	90657
90658	90660	90661	90662	90664	90666	90667
90668	90670	90672	90673	90675	90676	90680
90681	90685	90686	90687	90688	90690	90691
90696	90697	90698	90700	90702	90707	90710
90713	90714	90715	90716	90717	90723	90732
90733	90734	90735	90736	90738	90739	90740
90743	90744	90746	90747	90748	90749	97001
97002	97003	97004	97005	97006	97010	97012
97014	97016	97018	97022	97024	97026	97028
97032	97033	97034	97035	97036	97110	97112
97113	97116	97124	97140	97150	97530	97532
97533	97535	97537	97542	97545	97546	97597
97598	97602	97605	97606	97607	97608	97610
97750	97755	99050	99051	99053	99056	99058
99060						

Appendix F — Pub 100 References

The Centers for Medicare and Medicaid Services restructured its paper-based manual system as a web-based system on October 1, 2003. Called the online CMS manual system, it combines all of the various program instructions into internet-only manuals (IOMs), which are used by all CMS programs and contractors. In many instances, the references from the online manuals in appendix F contain a mention of the old paper manuals from which the current information was obtained when the manuals were converted. This information is shown in the header of the text, in the following format, when applicable, as A3-3101, HO-210, and B3-2049. Complete versions of all of the manuals can be found at https://www.cms.gov/Regulations-and-Guidance/Guidance/Manuals/Internet-Only-Manuals-IOMs.html.

Effective with implementation of the IOMs, the former method of publishing program memoranda (PMs) to communicate program instructions was replaced by the following four templates:

* One-time notification
* Manual revisions
* Business requirements
* Confidential requirements

The web-based system has been organized by functional area (e.g., eligibility, entitlement, claims processing, benefit policy, program integrity) in an effort to eliminate redundancy within the manuals, simplify updating, and make CMS program instructions available more quickly. The web-based system contains the functional areas included below:

Pub. 100	Introduction
Pub. 100-1	Medicare General Information, Eligibility, and Entitlement Manual
Pub. 100-2	Medicare Benefit Policy Manual
Pub. 100-3	Medicare National Coverage Determinations (NCD) Manual
Pub. 100-4	Medicare Claims Processing Manual
Pub. 100-5	Medicare Secondary Payer Manual
Pub. 100-6	Medicare Financial Management Manual
Pub. 100-7	State Operations Manual
Pub. 100-8	Medicare Program Integrity Manual
Pub. 100-9	Medicare Contractor Beneficiary and Provider Communications Manual
Pub. 100-10	Quality Improvement Organization Manual
Pub. 100-11	Programs of All-Inclusive Care for the Elderly (PACE) Manual
Pub. 100-12	State Medicaid Manual (under development)
Pub. 100-13	Medicaid State Children's Health Insurance Program (under development)
Pub. 100-14	Medicare ESRD Network Organizations Manual
Pub. 100-15	Medicaid Integrity Program (MIP)
Pub. 100-16	Medicare Managed Care Manual
Pub. 100-17	CMS/Business Partners Systems Security Manual
Pub. 100-18	Medicare Prescription Drug Benefit Manual
Pub. 100-19	Demonstrations
Pub. 100-20	One-Time Notification
Pub. 100-21	Recurring Update Notification
Pub. 100-22	Medicare Quality Reporting Incentive Programs Manual
Pub. 100-24	State Buy-In Manual
Pub. 100-25	Information Security Acceptable Risk Safeguards Manual

A brief description of the Medicare manuals primarily used for *CPC Expert* follows:

The *National Coverage Determinations Manual* (NCD), is organized according to categories such as diagnostic services, supplies, and medical procedures. The table of contents lists each category and subject within that category. Revision transmittals identify any new or background material, recap the changes, and provide an effective date for the change.

When complete, the manual will contain two chapters. Chapter 1 currently includes a description of CMS's national coverage determinations. When available, chapter 2 will contain a list of HCPCS codes related to each coverage determination. The manual is organized in accordance with CPT category sequences.

The *Medicare Benefit Policy Manual* contains Medicare general coverage instructions that are not national coverage determinations. As a general rule, in the past these instructions have been found in chapter II of the *Medicare Carriers Manual,* the *Medicare Intermediary Manual*, other provider manuals, and program memoranda.

The *Medicare Claims Processing Manual* contains instructions for processing claims for contractors and providers.

The *Medicare Program Integrity Manual* communicates the priorities and standards for the Medicare integrity programs.

Medicare IOM references

100-1, 3, 20.5

Blood Deductibles (Part A and Part B)

Program payment may not be made for the first 3 pints of whole blood or equivalent units of packed red cells received under Part A and Part B combined in a calendar year. However, blood processing (e.g., administration, storage) is not subject to the deductible.

The blood deductibles are in addition to any other applicable deductible and coinsurance amounts for which the patient is responsible.

The deductible applies only to the first 3 pints of blood furnished in a calendar year, even if more than one provider furnished blood.

100-1, 5, 70.6

Chiropractors

A. General

A licensed chiropractor who meets uniform minimum standards (see subsection C) is a physician for specified services. Coverage extends only to treatment by means of manual manipulation of the spine to correct a subluxation demonstrated by X-ray, provided such treatment is legal in the State where performed. All other services furnished or ordered by chiropractors are not covered. An X-ray obtained by a chiropractor for his or her own diagnostic purposes before commencing treatment may suffice for claims documentation purposes. This means that if a chiropractor orders, takes, or interprets an X-ray to demonstrate a subluxation of the spine, the X-ray can be used for claims processing purposes. However, there is no coverage or payment for these services or for any other diagnostic or therapeutic service ordered or furnished by the chiropractor. In addition, in performing manual manipulation of the spine, some chiropractors use manual devices that are hand-held with the thrust of the force of the device being controlled manually. While such manual manipulation may be covered, there is no separate payment permitted for use of this device.

B. Licensure and Authorization to Practice

A chiropractor must be licensed or legally authorized to furnish chiropractic services by the State or jurisdiction in which the services are furnished.

C. Uniform Minimum Standards

I. Prior to July 1, 1974, Chiropractors licensed or authorized to practice prior to July 1, 1974, and those individuals who commenced their studies in a chiropractic college before that date must meet all of the following minimum standards to render payable services under the program:

    a. Preliminary education equal to the requirements for graduation from an accredited high school or other secondary school;

    b. Graduation from a college of chiropractic approved by the State's chiropractic examiners that included the completion of a course of study covering a period of not less than 3 school years of 6 months each year in actual continuous attendance covering adequate course of study in the subjects of anatomy, physiology, symptomatology and diagnosis, hygiene and sanitation, chemistry, histology, pathology, and principles and practice of chiropractic, including clinical instruction in vertebral palpation, nerve tracing and adjusting; and

    c. Passage of an examination prescribed by the State's chiropractic examiners covering the subjects listed in subsection b.

2. After June 30, 1974 - Individuals commencing their studies in a chiropractic college after June 30, 1974, must meet all of the following additional requirements:

   a. Satisfactory completion of 2 years of pre-chiropractic study at the college level;

   b. Satisfactory completion of a 4-year course of 8 months each year (instead of a 3-year course of 6 months each year) at a college or school of chiropractic that includes not less than 4,000 hours in the scientific and chiropractic courses specified in subsection1.b, plus courses in the use and effect of X-ray and chiropractic analysis; and

   c. The practitioner must be over 21 years of age.

100-2, 1, 90

Termination of Pregnancy

B3-4276.1,.2

Effective for services furnished on or after October 1, 1998, Medicare will cover abortions procedures in the following situations:

1. If the pregnancy is the result of an act or rape or incest; or

2. In the case where a woman suffers from a physical disorder, physical injury, or physical illness, including a life-endangering physical condition caused by the pregnancy itself that would, as certified by a physician, place the woman in danger of death unless an abortion is performed.

NOTE: The "G7" modifier must be used with the following CPT codes in order for these services to be covered when the pregnancy resulted from rape or incest, or the pregnancy is certified by a physician as life threatening to the mother:

   59840, 59841, 59850, 59851, 59852, 59855, 59856, 59857, 59866

100-2, 1, 100

Treatment for Infertility

A3-3101.13

Effective for services rendered on or after January 15, 1980, reasonable and necessary services associated with treatment for infertility are covered under Medicare. Like pregnancy (see Sec. 80 above), infertility is a condition sufficiently at variance with the usual state of health to make it appropriate for a person who normally would be expected to be fertile to seek medical consultation and treatment. Contractors should coordinate with QIOs to see that utilization guidelines are established for this treatment if inappropriate utilization or abuse is suspected.

100-2, 11, 20

Renal Dialysis Items and Services

Medicare provides payment under the ESRD PPS for all renal dialysis services for outpatient maintenance dialysis when they are furnished to Medicare ESRD patients for the treatment of ESRD by a Medicare certified ESRD facility or a special purpose dialysis facility. Renal dialysis services are the items and services included under the composite rate and the ESRD-related items and services that were separately paid as of December 31, 2010 that were used for the treatment of ESRD.

Renal dialysis services are furnished in various settings including hospital outpatient ESRD facilities, independent ESRD facilities, or in the patient's home. Renal dialysis items and services furnished at ESRD facilities differ according to the types of patients being treated, the types of equipment and supplies used, the preferences of the treating physician, and the capability and makeup of the staff. Although not all facilities provide an identical range of services, the most common elements of dialysis treatment include:

- Laboratory Tests;
- Drugs and Biologicals;
- Equipment and supplies - dialysis machine use and maintenance;
- Personnel services;
- Administrative services;
- Overhead costs;
- Monitoring access and related declotting or referring the patient, and
- Direct nursing services include registered nurses, licensed practical nurses, technicians, social workers, and dietitians.

100-2, 11, 20.2

Laboratory Services

All laboratory services furnished to individuals for the treatment of ESRD are included in the ESRD PPS as Part B services and are not paid separately as of January 1, 2011. The laboratory services include but are not limited to:

- Laboratory tests included under the composite rate as of December 31, 2010 (discussed below); and
- Former separately billable Part B laboratory tests that were billed by ESRD facilities and independent laboratories for ESRD patients.

Composite rate laboratory tests are listed in §20.2.E of this chapter. More information regarding composite rate laboratory tests can be found in Pub. 100-4, Medicare Claims Processing Manual, chapter 8, §50.1, §60.1, and §80. As discussed below, composite rate laboratory services should not be reported on claims.

The distinction of what is considered to be a renal dialysis laboratory test is a clinical decision determined by the ESRD patient's ordering practitioner. If a laboratory test is ordered for the treatment of ESRD, then the laboratory test is not paid separately.

Payment for all renal dialysis laboratory tests furnished under the ESRD PPS is made directly to the ESRD facility responsible for the patient's care. The ESRD facility must furnish the laboratory tests directly or under arrangement and report renal dialysis laboratory tests on the ESRD facility claim (with the exception of composite rate laboratory services).

An ESRD facility must report renal dialysis laboratory services on its claims in order for the laboratory tests to be included in the outlier payment calculation. Renal dialysis laboratory services that were or would have been paid separately under Medicare Part B prior to January 1, 2011, are priced for the outlier payment calculation using the Clinical Laboratory Fee Schedule. Further information regarding the outlier policy can be found in §60.D of this chapter.

Certain laboratory services will be subject to Part B consolidated billing requirements and will no longer be separately payable when provided to ESRD beneficiaries by providers other than the renal dialysis facility. The list below includes the renal dialysis laboratory tests that are routinely performed for the treatment of ESRD. Payment for the laboratory tests identified on this list is included in the ESRD PPS. The laboratory tests listed in the table are used to enforce consolidated billing edits to ensure that payment is not made for renal dialysis laboratory tests outside of the ESRD PPS. The list of renal dialysis laboratory tests is not an all-inclusive list. If any laboratory test is ordered for the treatment of ESRD, then the laboratory test is considered to be included in the ESRD PPS and is the responsibility of the ESRD facility. Additional renal dialysis laboratory tests may be added through administrative issuances in the future.

LABS SUBJECT TO ESRD CONSOLIDATED BILLING

CPT/ HCPCS	Short Description
80047	Basic Metabolic Panel (Calcium, ionized)
80048	Basic Metabolic Panel (Calcium, total)
80051	Electrolyte Panel
80053	Comprehensive Metabolic Panel
80061	Lipid Panel
80069	Renal Function Panel
80076	Hepatic Function Panel
82040	Assay of serum albumin
82108	Assay of aluminum
82306	Vitamin d, 25 hydroxy
82310	Assay of calcium
82330	Assay of calcium, Ionized
82374	Assay, blood carbon dioxide
82379	Assay of carnitine
82435	Assay of blood chloride
82565	Assay of creatinine
82570	Assay of urine creatinine
82575	Creatinine clearance test
82607	Vitamin B-12
82652	Vit d 1, 25-dihydroxy
82668	Assay of erythropoietin
82728	Assay of ferritin
82746	Blood folic acid serum
83540	Assay of iron
83550	Iron binding test
83735	Assay of magnesium
83970	Assay of parathormone
84075	Assay alkaline phosphatase
84100	Assay of phosphorus
84132	Assay of serum potassium
84134	Assay of prealbumin
84155	Assay of protein, serum
84157	Assay of protein by other source
84295	Assay of serum sodium
84466	Assay of transferrin
84520	Assay of urea nitrogen
84540	Assay of urine/urea-n
84545	Urea-N clearance test
85014	Hematocrit

CPT/ HCPCS	Short Description
85018	Hemoglobin
85025	Complete (cbc), automated (HgB, Hct, RBC, WBC, and Platelet count) and automated differential WBC count.
85027	Complete (cbc), automated (HgB, Hct, RBC, WBC, and Platelet count)
85041	Automated rbc count
85044	Manual reticulocyte count
85045	Automated reticulocyte count
85046	Reticyte/hgb concentrate
85048	Automated leukocyte count
86704	Hep b core antibody, total
86705	Hep b core antibody, igm
86706	Hep b surface antibody
87040	Blood culture for bacteria
87070	Culture, bacteria, other
87071	Culture bacteri aerobic othr
87073	Culture bacteria anaerobic
87075	Cultr bacteria, except blood
87076	Culture anaerobe ident, each
87077	Culture aerobic identify
87081	Culture screen only
87340	Hepatitis b surface ag, eia
G0306	CBC/diff wbc w/o platelet
G0307	CBC without platelet

A. Automated Multi-Channel Chemistry (AMCC) Tests

During the ESRD PPS transition period (see §70 of this chapter) ESRD facilities are required to report the renal dialysis AMCC tests with the appropriate modifiers (CD, CE, or CF) on their claims for purposes of applying the 50/50 rule under the composite rate portion of the blended payment. Refer to §70.B of this chapter for additional information regarding the composite rate portion of the blended payment during the transition.

The 50/50 rule is necessary for those ESRD facilities that chose to go through the transition period. If the 50/50 rule allows for separate payment, then the laboratory tests are priced using the clinical laboratory fee schedule. Information regarding the 50/50 rule can be found in §20.2.E of this chapter and in Pub. 100-4, Medicare Claims Processing Manual, chapter 16, §40.6.

NOTE: An ESRD facility billing a renal dialysis AMCC test must use the CF modifier when the AMCC is not in the composite rate but is a renal dialysis service. AMCC tests that are furnished to individuals for reasons other than for the treatment of ESRD should be billed with the AY modifier to Medicare directly by the entity furnishing the service with the AY modifier.

B. Laboratory Services Furnished for Reasons Other Than for the Treatment of ESRD

1. Independent Laboratory

A patient's physician or practitioner may order a laboratory test that is included on the list of items and services subject to consolidated billing edits for reasons other than for the treatment of ESRD. When this occurs, the patient's physician or practitioner should notify the independent laboratory or the ESRD facility (with the appropriate clinical laboratory certification in accordance with the Clinical Laboratory Improvement Act) that furnished the laboratory service that the test is not a renal dialysis service and that entity may bill Medicare separately using the AY modifier. The AY modifier serves as an attestation that the item or service is medically necessary for the patient but is not being used for the treatment of ESRD.

2. Hospital-Based Laboratory

Hospital outpatient clinical laboratories furnishing renal dialysis laboratory tests to ESRD patients for reasons other than for the treatment of ESRD may submit a claim for separate payment using the AY modifier. The AY modifier serves as an attestation that the item or service is medically necessary for the patient but is not being used for the treatment of ESRD.

C. Laboratory Services Performed in Emergency Rooms or Emergency Departments

In an emergency room or emergency department, the ordering physician or practitioner may not know at the time the laboratory test is being ordered, if it is being ordered as a renal dialysis service. Consequently, emergency rooms or emergency departments are not required to append an AY modifier to these laboratory tests when submitting claims with dates of service on or after January 1, 2012.

When a renal dialysis laboratory service is furnished to an ESRD patient in an emergency room or emergency department on a different date of service, hospitals can append an ET modifier to the laboratory tests furnished to ESRD patients to indicate that the laboratory test was furnished in conjunction with the emergency visit. Appending the ET modifier indicates that the laboratory service being furnished on a day other than the emergency visit is related to the emergency visit and at the time the ordering physician was unable to determine if the test was ordered for reasons of treating the patient's ESRD.

Allowing laboratory testing to bypass consolidated billing edits in the emergency room or department does not mean that ESRD facilities should send patients to other settings for routine laboratory testing for the purpose of not assuming financial responsibility of renal dialysis items and services. For additional information regarding laboratory services furnished in a variety of settings, see Pub. 100-4, Medicare Claims Processing Manual, chapter 16, §30.3 and §40.6.

D. Hepatitis B Laboratory Services for Transient Patients

Laboratory testing for hepatitis B is a renal dialysis service. Effective January 1, 2011, hepatitis B testing is included in the ESRD PPS and therefore cannot be billed separately to Medicare.

The Conditions for Coverage for ESRD facilities require routine hepatitis B testing (42 CFR §494.30(a)(1)). The ESRD facility is responsible for the payment of the laboratory test, regardless of frequency. If an ESRD patient wishes to travel, the patient's home ESRD facility should have systems in place for communicating hepatitis B test results to the destination ESRD facility.

E. Laboratory Services Included Under Composite Rate

Prior to the implementation of the ESRD PPS, the costs of certain ESRD laboratory services furnished for outpatient maintenance dialysis by either the ESRD facility's staff or an independent laboratory, were included in the composite rate calculations. Therefore, payment for all of these laboratory tests was included in the ESRD facility's composite rate and the tests could not have been billed separately to the Medicare program.

All laboratory services that were included under the composite rate are included under the ESRD PPS unless otherwise specified. Payments for these laboratory tests are included in the ESRD PPS and are not paid separately under the composite rate portion of the blended payment and are not eligible for outlier payments. Therefore, composite rate laboratory services should not be reported on the claim. Laboratory tests included in the composite payment rate are identified below.

1. Routinely Covered Tests Paid Under Composite Rate

The tests listed below are usually performed for dialysis patients and were routinely covered at the frequency specified in the absence of indications to the contrary, (i.e., no documentation of medical necessity was required other than knowledge of the patient's status as an ESRD beneficiary). When any of these tests were performed at a frequency greater than that specified, the additional tests were separately billable and were covered only if they were medically justified by accompanying documentation. A diagnosis of ESRD alone was not sufficient medical evidence to warrant coverage of the additional tests. The nature of the illness or injury (diagnosis, complaint, or symptom) requiring the performance of the test(s) must have been present, along with ICD diagnosis coding, on the claim for payment.

a. Hemodialysis, IPD, CCPD, and Hemofiltration

  – Per Treatment - All hematocrit, hemoglobin, and clotting time tests furnished incident to dialysis treatments;

  – Weekly - Prothrombin time for patients on anticoagulant therapy and Serum Creatinine;

  – Weekly or Thirteen Per Quarter - BUN;

  – Monthly - Serum Calcium, Serum Potassium, Serum Chloride, CBC, Serum Bicarbonate, Serum Phosphorous, Total Protein, Serum Albumin, Alkaline Phosphatase, aspartate amino transferase (AST) (SGOT) and LDH; and

  – Automated Multi-Channel Chemistry (AMCC) - If an automated battery of tests, such as the SMA-12, is performed and contains most of the tests listed in one of the weekly or monthly categories, it is not necessary to separately identify any tests in the battery that are not listed. Further information concerning automated tests and the "50 percent rule" can be found below and in Pub. 100-4, Medicare Claims Processing Manual, chapter 16, §40.6.1.

b. CAPD

  – Monthly – BUN, Creatinine, Sodium, Potassium, CO2, Calcium, Magnesium, Phosphate, Total Protein, Albumin, Alkaline Phosphatase, LDH, AST, SGOT, HCT, Hbg, and Dialysate Protein.

Under the ESRD PPS, frequency requirements do not apply for the purpose of payment. However, laboratory tests should be ordered as necessary and should not be restricted because of financial reasons.

2. Separately Billable Tests Under the Composite Rate

The following list identifies certain separately billable laboratory tests that were covered routinely and without documentation of medical necessity other than knowledge of the patient's status as an ESRD beneficiary, when furnished at specified frequencies. If they were performed at a frequency greater than that specified, they were covered only if accompanied by medical documentation. A diagnosis of ESRD alone was not sufficient documentation. The medical necessity of the test(s), the nature of the illness or injury (diagnosis, complaint or symptom) requiring the performance of the test(s) must have been furnished on claims using the ICD diagnosis coding system.

— Separately Billable Tests for Hemodialysis, IPD, CCPD, and Hemofiltration

  Serum Aluminum - one every 3 months

  Serum Ferritin - one every 3 months

— Separately Billable Tests for CAPD

WBC, RBC, and Platelet count – One every 3 months

Residual renal function and 24 hour urine volume – One every 6 months

Under the ESRD PPS frequency requirements do not apply for the purpose of payment. However, laboratory tests should be ordered as necessary and should not be restricted because of financial reasons.

3. Automated Multi-Channel Chemistry (AMCC) Tests Under the Composite Rate

Clinical diagnostic laboratory tests that comprise the AMCC (listed in Appendix A and B) could be considered to be composite rate and non-composite rate laboratory services. Composite rate payment was paid by the A/B MAC (A). To determine if separate payment was allowed for non-composite rate tests for a particular date of service, 50 percent or more of the covered tests must be non-composite rate tests. This policy also applies to the composite rate portion of the blended payment during the transition. Beginning January 1, 2014, the 50 percent rule will no longer apply and no separate payment will be made under the composite rate portion of the blended payment.

Medicare applied the following to AMCC tests for ESRD beneficiaries:

— Payment was the lowest rate for services performed by the same provider, for the same beneficiary, for the same date of service.

— The A/B MAC identified, for a particular date of service, the AMCC tests ordered that were included in the composite rate and those that were not included. The composite rate tests were defined for Hemodialysis, IPD, CCPD, and Hemofiltration (see Appendix A) and for CAPD (see Appendix B).

— If 50 percent or more of the covered tests were included under the composite rate payment, then all submitted tests were included within the composite payment. In this case, no separate payment in addition to the composite rate was made for any of the separately billable tests.

— If less than 50 percent of the covered tests were composite rate tests, all AMCC tests submitted for that Date of Service (DOS) were separately payable.

— A non-composite rate test was defined as any test separately payable outside of the composite rate or beyond the normal frequency covered under the composite rate that was reasonable and necessary.

Three pricing modifiers identify the different payment situations for ESRD AMCC tests. The physician who ordered the tests was responsible for identifying the appropriate modifier when ordering the tests.

— CD - AMCC test had been ordered by an ESRD facility or Medicare capitation payment (MCP) physician that was part of the composite rate and was not separately billable

— CE - AMCC test had been ordered by an ESRD facility or MCP physician that was a composite rate test but was beyond the normal frequency covered under the rate and was separately reimbursable based on medical necessity

— CF - AMCC test had been ordered by an ESRD facility or MCP physician that was not part of the composite rate and was separately billable

The ESRD clinical diagnostic laboratory tests identified with modifiers "CD", "CE" or "CF" may not have been billed as organ or disease panels. Effective October 1, 2003, all ESRD clinical diagnostic laboratory tests must be billed individually. See Pub. 100-4, Medicare Claims Processing Manual, chapter 16, §40.6.1, for additional billing and payment instructions as well as examples of the 50/50 rule.

For ESRD dialysis patients, CPT code 82330 Calcium; ionized shall be included in the calculation for the 50/50 rule (Pub. 100-4, Medicare Claims Processing Manual, chapter 16, §40.6.1). When CPT code 82330 is billed as a substitute for CPT code 82310, Calcium; total, it shall be billed with modifier CD or CE. When CPT code 82330 is billed in addition to CPT 82310, it shall be billed with CF modifier.

100-2, 15, 20.1

Physician Expense for Surgery, Childbirth, and Treatment for Infertility

B3-2005.I

A. Surgery and Childbirth

Skilled medical management is covered throughout the events of pregnancy, beginning with diagnosis, continuing through delivery and ending after the necessary postnatal care. Similarly, in the event of termination of pregnancy, regardless of whether terminated spontaneously or for therapeutic reasons (i.e., where the life of the mother would be endangered if the fetus were brought to term), the need for skilled medical management and/or medical services is equally important as in those cases carried to full term. After the infant is delivered and is a separate individual, items and services furnished to the infant are not covered on the basis of the mother's eligibility.

Most surgeons and obstetricians bill patients an all-inclusive package charge intended to cover all services associated with the surgical procedure or delivery of the child. All expenses for surgical and obstetrical care, including preoperative/prenatal examinations and tests and post-operative/postnatal services, are considered incurred on the date of surgery or delivery, as appropriate. This policy applies whether the physician bills on a package charge basis, or itemizes the bill separately for these items.

Occasionally, a physician's bill may include charges for additional services not directly related to the surgical procedure or the delivery. Such charges are considered incurred on the date the additional services are furnished.

The above policy applies only where the charges are imposed by one physician or by a clinic on behalf of a group of physicians. Where more than one physician imposes charges for surgical or obstetrical services, all preoperative/prenatal and post-operative/postnatal services performed by the physician who performed the surgery or delivery are considered incurred on the date of the surgery or delivery. Expenses for services rendered by other physicians are considered incurred on the date they were performed.

B. Treatment for Infertility

Reasonable and necessary services associated with treatment for infertility are covered under Medicare. Infertility is a condition sufficiently at variance with the usual state of health to make it appropriate for a person who normally is expected to be fertile to seek medical consultation and treatment.

100-2, 15, 30.4

Optometrist's Services

B3-2020.25

Effective April 1, 1987, a doctor of optometry is considered a physician with respect to all services the optometrist is authorized to perform under State law or regulation. To be covered under Medicare, the services must be medically reasonable and necessary for the diagnosis or treatment of illness or injury, and must meet all applicable coverage requirements. See the Medicare Benefit Policy Manual, Chapter 16, "General Exclusions from Coverage," for exclusions from coverage that apply to vision care services, and the Medicare Claims Processing Manual, Chapter 12, "Physician/Practitioner Billing," for information dealing with payment for items and services furnished by optometrists.

A. FDA Monitored Studies of Intraocular Lenses

Special coverage rules apply to situations in which an ophthalmologist is involved in a Food and Drug Administration (FDA) monitored study of the safety and efficacy of an investigational Intraocular Lens (IOL). The investigation process for IOLs is unique in that there is a core period and an adjunct period. The core study is a traditional, well-controlled clinical investigation with full record keeping and reporting requirements. The adjunct study is essentially an extended distribution phase for lenses in which only limited safety data are compiled. Depending on the lens being evaluated, the adjunct study may be an extension of the core study or may be the only type of investigation to which the lens may be subject.

All eye care services related to the investigation of the IOL must be provided by the investigator (i.e., the implanting ophthalmologist) or another practitioner (including a doctor of optometry) who provides services at the direction or under the supervision of the investigator and who has an agreement with the investigator that information on the patient is given to the investigator so that he or she may report on the patient to the IOL manufacturer. Eye care services furnished by anyone other than the investigator (or a practitioner who assists the investigator, as described in the preceding paragraph) are not covered during the period the IOL is being investigated, unless the services are not related to the investigation.

B. Concurrent Care

Where more than one practitioner furnishes concurrent care, services furnished to a beneficiary by both an ophthalmologist and another physician (including an optometrist) may be recognized for payment if it is determined that each practitioner's services were reasonable and necessary. (See Sec.30.E.)

100-2, 15, 30.5

Chiropractor's Services

B3-2020.26

A chiropractor must be licensed or legally authorized to furnish chiropractic services by the State or jurisdiction in which the services are furnished. In addition, a licensed chiropractor must meet the following uniform minimum standards to be considered a physician for Medicare coverage. Coverage extends only to treatment by means of manual manipulation of the spine to correct a subluxation provided such treatment is legal in the State where performed. All other services furnished or ordered by chiropractors are not covered. If a chiropractor orders, takes, or interprets an x-ray or other diagnostic procedure to demonstrate a subluxation of the spine, the x-ray can be used for documentation. However, there is no coverage or payment for these services or for any other diagnostic or therapeutic service ordered or furnished by the chiropractor. For detailed information on using x-rays to determine subluxation, see Sec.240.1.2. In addition, in performing manual manipulation of the spine, some chiropractors use manual devices that are hand-held with the thrust of the force of the device being controlled manually. While such manual manipulation may be covered, there is no separate payment permitted for use of this device.

A. Uniform Minimum Standards

Prior to July 1, 1974

Chiropractors licensed or authorized to practice prior to July 1, 1974, and those individuals who commenced their studies in a chiropractic college before that date must meet all of the following three minimum standards to render payable services under the program:

• Preliminary education equal to the requirements for graduation from an accredited high school or other secondary school;

- Graduation from a college of chiropractic approved by the State's chiropractic examiners that included the completion of a course of study covering a period of not less than 3 school years of 6 months each year in actual continuous attendance covering adequate course of study in the subjects of anatomy, physiology, symptomatology and diagnosis, hygiene and sanitation, chemistry, histology, pathology, and principles and practice of chiropractic, including clinical instruction in vertebral palpation, nerve tracing, and adjusting; and

- Passage of an examination prescribed by the State's chiropractic examiners covering the subjects listed above.

After June 30, 1974

Individuals commencing their studies in a chiropractic college after June 30, 1974, must meet all of the above three standards and all of the following additional requirements:

- Satisfactory completion of 2 years of pre-chiropractic study at the college level;

- Satisfactory completion of a 4-year course of 8 months each year (instead of a 3-year course of 6 months each year) at a college or school of chiropractic that includes not less than 4,000 hours in the scientific and chiropractic courses specified in the second bullet under "Prior to July 1, 1974" above, plus courses in the use and effect of x-ray and chiropractic analysis; and

- The practitioner must be over 21 years of age.

B. Maintenance Therapy

Under the Medicare program, Chiropractic maintenance therapy is not considered to be medically reasonable or necessary, and is therefore not payable. Maintenance therapy is defined as a treatment plan that seeks to prevent disease, promote health, and prolong and enhance the quality of life; or therapy that is performed to maintain or prevent deterioration of a chronic condition. When further clinical improvement cannot reasonably be expected from continuous ongoing care, and the chiropractic treatment becomes supportive rather than corrective in nature, the treatment is then considered maintenance therapy. For information on how to indicate on a claim a treatment is or is not maintenance, see Sec.240.1.3.

100-2, 15, 50.4.4.2

Immunizations

Vaccinations or inoculations are excluded as immunizations unless they are directly related to the treatment of an injury or direct exposure to a disease or condition, such as anti-rabies treatment, tetanus antitoxin or booster vaccine, botulin antitoxin, antivenin sera, or immune globulin. In the absence of injury or direct exposure, preventive immunization (vaccination or inoculation) against such diseases as smallpox, polio, diphtheria, etc., is not covered. However, pneumococcal, hepatitis B, and influenza virus vaccines are exceptions to this rule. (See items A, B, and C below.) In cases where a vaccination or inoculation is excluded from coverage, related charges are also not covered.

A. Pneumococcal Pneumonia Vaccinations

1. Background and History of Coverage:

   Section 1861(s)(10)(A) of the Social Security Act and regulations at 42 CFR 410.57 authorize Medicare coverage under Part B for pneumococcal vaccine and its administration.

   For services furnished on or after May 1, 1981 through September 18, 2014, the Medicare Part B program covered pneumococcal pneumonia vaccine and its administration when furnished in compliance with any applicable State law by any provider of services or any entity or individual with a supplier number. Coverage included an initial vaccine administered only to persons at high risk of serious pneumococcal disease (including all people 65 and older; immunocompetent adults at increased risk of pneumococcal disease or its complications because of chronic illness; and individuals with compromised immune systems), with revaccination administered only to persons at highest risk of serious pneumococcal infection and those likely to have a rapid decline in pneumococcal antibody levels, provided that at least 5 years had passed since the previous dose of pneumococcal vaccine.

   Those administering the vaccine did not require the patient to present an immunization record prior to administering the pneumococcal vaccine, nor were they compelled to review the patient's complete medical record if it was not available, relying on the patient's verbal history to determine prior vaccination status.

   Effective July 1, 2000, Medicare no longer required for coverage purposes that a doctor of medicine or osteopathy order the vaccine. Therefore, a beneficiary could receive the vaccine upon request without a physician's order and without physician supervision.

2. Coverage Requirements:

   Effective for claims with dates of service on and after September 19, 2014, an initial pneumococcal vaccine may be administered to all Medicare beneficiaries who have never received a pneumococcal vaccination under Medicare Part B. A different, second pneumococcal vaccine may be administered 1 year after the first vaccine was administered (i.e., 11 full months have passed following the month in which the last pneumococcal vaccine was administered).

   Those administering the vaccine should not require the patient to present an immunization record prior to administering the pneumococcal vaccine, nor should they feel compelled to review the patient's complete medical record if it is

not available. Instead, provided that the patient is competent, it is acceptable to rely on the patient's verbal history to determine prior vaccination status.

Medicare does not require for coverage purposes that a doctor of medicine or osteopathy order the vaccine. Therefore, the beneficiary may receive the vaccine upon request without a physician's order and without physician supervision.

B. Hepatitis B Vaccine

Effective for services furnished on or after September 1, 1984, P.L. 98-369 provides coverage under Part B for hepatitis B vaccine and its administration, furnished to a Medicare beneficiary who is at high or intermediate risk of contracting hepatitis B. High-risk groups currently identified include (see exception below):

- ESRD patients;

- Hemophiliacs who receive Factor VIII or IX concentrates;

- Clients of institutions for the mentally retarded;

- Persons who live in the same household as a Hepatitis B Virus (HBV) carrier;

- Homosexual men;

- Illicit injectable drug abusers; and

- Persons diagnosed with diabetes mellitus.

Intermediate risk groups currently identified include:

- Staff in institutions for the mentally retarded; and

- Workers in health care professions who have frequent contact with blood or blood-derived body fluids during routine work.

EXCEPTION: Persons in both of the above-listed groups in paragraph B, would not be considered at high or intermediate risk of contracting hepatitis B, however, if there were laboratory evidence positive for antibodies to hepatitis B. (ESRD patients are routinely tested for hepatitis B antibodies as part of their continuing monitoring and therapy.)

For Medicare program purposes, the vaccine may be administered upon the order of a doctor of medicine or osteopathy, by a doctor of medicine or osteopathy, or by home health agencies, skilled nursing facilities, ESRD facilities, hospital outpatient departments, and persons recognized under the incident to physicians' services provision of law.

A charge separate from the ESRD composite rate will be recognized and paid for administration of the vaccine to ESRD patients.

C. Influenza Virus Vaccine

Effective for services furnished on or after May 1, 1993, the Medicare Part B program covers influenza virus vaccine and its administration when furnished in compliance with any applicable State law by any provider of services or any entity or individual with a supplier number. Typically, these vaccines are administered once a flu season. Medicare does not require, for coverage purposes, that a doctor of medicine or osteopathy order the vaccine. Therefore, the beneficiary may receive the vaccine upon request without a physician's order and without physician supervision.

100-2, 15, 80.1

Clinical Laboratory Services

Section 1833 and 1861 of the Act provides for payment of clinical laboratory services under Medicare Part B. Clinical laboratory services involve the biological, microbiological, serological, chemical, immunohematological, hematological, biophysical, cytological, pathological, or other examination of materials derived from the human body for the diagnosis, prevention, or treatment of a disease or assessment of a medical condition. Laboratory services must meet all applicable requirements of the Clinical Laboratory Improvement Amendments of 1988 (CLIA), as set forth at 42 CFR part 493. Section 1862(a)(1)(A) of the Act provides that Medicare payment may not be made for services that are not reasonable and necessary. Clinical laboratory services must be ordered and used promptly by the physician who is treating the beneficiary as described in 42 CFR 410.32(a), or by a qualified nonphysician practitioner, as described in 42 CFR 410.32(a)(3).

See section 80.6 of this manual for related physician ordering instructions.

See the Medicare Claims Processing Manual Chapter 16 for related claims processing instructions.

100-2, 15, 80.2

Psychological Tests and Neuropsychological Tests

Medicare Part B coverage of psychological tests and neuropsychological tests is authorized under section 1861(s)(3) of the Social Security Act. Payment for psychological and neuropsychological tests is authorized under section 1842(b)(2)(A) of the Social Security Act. The payment amounts for the new psychological and neuropsychological tests (CPT codes 96102, 96103, 96119 and 96120) that are effective January 1, 2006, and are billed for tests administered by a technician or a computer reflect a site of service payment differential for the facility and non-facility settings.

Additionally, there is no authorization for payment for diagnostic tests when performed on an "incident to" basis.

Under the diagnostic tests provision, all diagnostic tests are assigned a certain level of supervision. Generally, regulations governing the diagnostic tests provision require that only physicians can provide the assigned level of supervision for diagnostic tests.

However, there is a regulatory exception to the supervision requirement for diagnostic psychological and neuropsychological tests in terms of who can provide the supervision.

That is, regulations allow a clinical psychologist (CP) or a physician to perform the general supervision assigned to diagnostic psychological and neuropsychological tests.

In addition, nonphysician practitioners such as nurse practitioners (NPs), clinical nurse specialists (CNSs) and physician assistants (PAs) who personally perform diagnostic psychological and neuropsychological tests are excluded from having to perform these tests under the general supervision of a physician or a CP. Rather, NPs and CNSs must perform such tests under the requirements of their respective benefit instead of the requirements for diagnostic psychological and neuropsychological tests. Accordingly, NPs and CNSs must perform tests in collaboration (as defined under Medicare law at section 1861(aa)(6) of the Act) with a physician. PAs perform tests under the general supervision of a physician as required for services furnished under the PA benefit.

Furthermore, physical therapists (PTs), occupational therapists (OTs) and speech language pathologists (SLPs) are authorized to bill three test codes as "sometimes therapy" codes. Specifically, CPT codes 96105, 96110 and 96111 may be performed by these therapists. However, when PTs, OTs and SLPs perform these three tests, they must be performed under the general supervision of a physician or a CP.

Who May Bill for Diagnostic Psychological and Neuropsychological Tests CPs - see qualifications under chapter 15, section 160 of the Benefits Policy Manual, Pub. 100-2.

- NPs -to the extent authorized under State scope of practice. See qualifications under chapter 15, section 200 of the Benefits Policy Manual, Pub. 100-2.

- CNSs -to the extent authorized under State scope of practice. See qualifications under chapter 15, section 210 of the Benefits Policy Manual, Pub. 100-2.

- PAs - to the extent authorized under State scope of practice. See qualifications under chapter 15, section 190 of the Benefits Policy Manual, Pub. 100-2.

- Independently Practicing Psychologists (IPPs) PTs, OTs and SLPs - see qualifications under chapter 15, sections 220-230.6 of the Benefits Policy Manual, Pub. 100-2.

Psychological and neuropsychological tests performed by a psychologist (who is not a CP) practicing independently of an institution, agency, or physician's office are covered when a physician orders such tests. An IPP is any psychologist who is licensed or certified to practice psychology in the State or jurisdiction where furnishing services or, if the jurisdiction does not issue licenses, if provided by any practicing psychologist. (It is CMS' understanding that all States, the District of Columbia, and Puerto Rico license psychologists, but that some trust territories do not. Examples of psychologists, other than CPs, whose psychological and neuropsychological tests are covered under the diagnostic tests provision include, but are not limited to, educational psychologists and counseling psychologists.)

The carrier must secure from the appropriate State agency a current listing of psychologists holding the required credentials to determine whether the tests of a particular IPP are covered under Part B in States that have statutory licensure or certification. In States or territories that lack statutory licensing or certification, the carrier checks individual qualifications before provider numbers are issued. Possible reference sources are the national directory of membership of the American Psychological Association, which provides data about the educational background of individuals and indicates which members are board-certified, the records and directories of the State or territorial psychological association, and the National Register of Health Service Providers. If qualification is dependent on a doctoral degree from a currently accredited program, the carrier verifies the date of accreditation of the school involved, since such accreditation is not retroactive. If the listed reference sources do not provide enough information (e.g., the psychologist is not a member of one of these sources), the carrier contacts the psychologist personally for the required information. Generally, carriers maintain a continuing list of psychologists whose qualifications have been verified.

NOTE: When diagnostic psychological tests are performed by a psychologist who is not practicing independently, but is on the staff of an institution, agency, or clinic, that entity bills for the psychological tests.

The carrier considers psychologists as practicing independently when:

- They render services on their own responsibility, free of the administrative and professional control of an employer such as a physician, institution or agency;

- The persons they treat are their own patients; and

- They have the right to bill directly, collect and retain the fee for their services.

A psychologist practicing in an office located in an institution may be considered an independently practicing psychologist when both of the following conditions exist:

- The office is confined to a separately-identified part of the facility which is used solely as the psychologist's office and cannot be construed as extending throughout the entire institution; and

- The psychologist conducts a private practice, i.e., services are rendered to patients from outside the institution as well as to institutional patients.

Payment for Diagnostic Psychological and Neuropsychological Tests

Expenses for diagnostic psychological and neuropsychological tests are not subject to the outpatient mental health treatment limitation, that is, the payment limitation on treatment services for mental, psychoneurotic and personality disorders as authorized under Section 1833(c) of the Act. The payment amount for the new

psychological and neuropsychological tests (CPT codes 96102, 96103, 96119 and 96120) that are billed for tests performed by a technician or a computer reflect a site of service payment differential for the facility and non-facility settings. CPs, NPs, CNSs and PAs are required by law to accept assigned payment for psychological and neuropsychological tests. However, while IPPs are not required by law to accept assigned payment for these tests, they must report the name and address of the physician who ordered the test on the claim form when billing for tests.

CPT Codes for Diagnostic Psychological and Neuropsychological Tests

The range of CPT codes used to report psychological and neuropsychological tests is 96101-96120. CPT codes 96101, 96102, 96103, 96105, 96110, and 96111 are appropriate for use when billing for psychological tests. CPT codes 96116, 96118, 96119 and 96120 are appropriate for use when billing for neuropsychological tests.

All of the tests under this CPT code range 96101-96120 are indicated as active codes under the physician fee schedule database and are covered if medically necessary.

Payment and Billing Guidelines for Psychological and Neuropsychological Tests

The technician and computer CPT codes for psychological and neuropsychological tests include practice expense, malpractice expense and professional work relative value units.

Accordingly, CPT psychological test code 96101 should not be paid when billed for the same tests or services performed under psychological test codes 96102 or 96103. CPT neuropsychological test code 96118 should not be paid when billed for the same tests or services performed under neuropsychological test codes 96119 or 96120. However, CPT codes 96101 and 96118 can be paid separately on the rare occasion when billed on the same date of service for different and separate tests from 96102, 96103, 96119 and 96120.

Under the physician fee schedule, there is no payment for services performed by students or trainees. Accordingly, Medicare does not pay for services represented by CPT codes 96102 and 96119 when performed by a student or a trainee. However, the presence of a student or a trainee while the test is being administered does not prevent a physician, CP, IPP, NP, CNS or PA from performing and being paid for the psychological test under 96102 or the neuropsychological test under 96119.

100-2, 15, 80.5.5

Frequency Standards

Medicare pays for a screening BMM once every 2 years (at least 23 months have passed since the month the last covered BMM was performed).

When medically necessary, Medicare may pay for more frequent BMMs. Examples include, but are not limited to, the following medical circumstances:

- Monitoring beneficiaries on long-term glucocorticoid (steroid) therapy of more than 3 months.

- Confirming baseline BMMs to permit monitoring of beneficiaries in the future.

100-2, 15, 150.1

Treatment of Temporomandibular Joint (TMJ) Syndrome

There are a wide variety of conditions that can be characterized as TMJ, and an equally wide variety of methods for treating these conditions. Many of the procedures fall within the Medicare program's statutory exclusion that prohibits payment for items and services that have not been demonstrated to be reasonable and necessary for the diagnosis and treatment of illness or injury (§1862(a)(1) of the Act). Other services and appliances used to treat TMJ fall within the Medicare program's statutory exclusion at 1862(a)(12), which prohibits payment "for services in connection with the care, treatment, filling, removal, or replacement of teeth or structures directly supporting teeth...." For these reasons, a diagnosis of TMJ on a claim is insufficient. The actual condition or symptom must be determined.

100-2, 15, 160

Clinical Psychologist Services

A. Clinical Psychologist (CP) Defined

To qualify as a clinical psychologist (CP), a practitioner must meet the following requirements: Hold a doctoral degree in psychology; Be licensed or certified, on the basis of the doctoral degree in psychology, by the State in which he or she practices, at the independent practice level of psychology to furnish diagnostic, assessment, preventive, and therapeutic services directly to individuals.

B. Qualified Clinical Psychologist Services Defined

Effective July 1, 1990, the diagnostic and therapeutic services of CPs and services and supplies furnished incident to such services are covered as the services furnished by a physician or as incident to physician's services are covered. However, the CP must be legally authorized to perform the services under applicable licensure laws of the State in which they are furnished.

C. Types of Clinical Psychologist Services

That May Be Covered Diagnostic and therapeutic services that the CP is legally authorized to perform in accordance with State law and/or regulation. Carriers pay all qualified CPs based on the physician fee schedule for the diagnostic and therapeutic services. (Psychological tests by practitioners who do not meet the requirements for a CP may be covered under the provisions for diagnostic tests as described in Sec. 80.2.)

Services and supplies furnished incident to a CP's services are covered if the requirements that apply to services incident to a physician's services, as described in Sec.60 are met. These services must be:

- Mental health services that are commonly furnished in CPs' offices;

- An integral, although incidental, part of professional services performed by the CP;

- Performed under the direct personal supervision of the CP; i.e., the CP must be physically present and immediately available;

- Furnished without charge or included in the CP's bill; and

- Performed by an employee of the CP (or an employee of the legal entity that employs the supervising CP) under the common law control test of the Act, as set forth in 20 CFR 404.1007 and Sec.RS 2101.020 of the Retirement and Survivors Insurance part of the Social Security Program Operations Manual System.

- Diagnostic psychological testing services when furnished under the general supervision of a CP.

Carriers are required to familiarize themselves with appropriate State laws and/or regulations governing a CP's scope of practice.

D. Noncovered Services

The services of CPs are not covered if the service is otherwise excluded from Medicare coverage even though a clinical psychologist is authorized by State law to perform them.

For example, Sec.1862(a)(1)(A) of the Act excludes from coverage services that are not "reasonable and necessary for the diagnosis or treatment of an illness or injury or to improve the functioning of a malformed body member." Therefore, even though the services are authorized by State law, the services of a CP that are determined to be not reasonable and necessary are not covered. Additionally, any therapeutic services that are billed by CPs under CPT psychotherapy codes that include medical evaluation and management services are not covered.

E. Requirement for Consultation

When applying for a Medicare provider number, a CP must submit to the carrier a signed Medicare provider/supplier enrollment form that indicates an agreement to the effect that, contingent upon the patient's consent, the CP will attempt to consult with the patient's attending or primary care physician in accordance with accepted professional ethical norms, taking into consideration patient confidentiality.

If the patient assents to the consultation, the CP must attempt to consult with the patient's physician within a reasonable time after receiving the consent. If the CP's attempts to consult directly with the physician are not successful, the CP must notify the physician within a reasonable time that he or she is furnishing services to the patient. Additionally, the CP must document, in the patient's medical record, the date the patient consented or declined consent to consultations, the date of consultation, or, if attempts to consult did not succeed, that date and manner of notification to the physician.

The only exception to the consultation requirement for CPs is in cases where the patient's primary care or attending physician refers the patient to the CP. Also, neither a CP nor a primary care nor attending physician may bill Medicare or the patient for this required consultation.

F. Outpatient Mental Health Services Limitation

All covered therapeutic services furnished by qualified CPs are subject to the outpatient mental health services limitation in Pub 100-1, Medicare General Information, Eligibility, and Entitlement Manual, Chapter 3, "Deductibles, Coinsurance Amounts, and Payment Limitations," Sec.30, (i.e., only 62 1/2 percent of expenses for these services are considered incurred expenses for Medicare purposes). The limitation does not apply to diagnostic services.

G. Assignment Requirement Assignment iSec. required.

100-2, 15, 170

Clinical Social Worker (CSW) Services

B3-2152

See the Medicare Claims Processing Manual Chapter 12, Physician/Nonphysician Practitioners, §150, "Clinical Social Worker Services," for payment requirements.

A. Clinical Social Worker Defined

Section 1861(hh) of the Act defines a "clinical social worker" as an individual who:

- Possesses a master's or doctor's degree in social work;

- Has performed at least two years of supervised clinical social work; and

- Is licensed or certified as a clinical social worker by the State in which the services are performed; or

- In the case of an individual in a State that does not provide for licensure or certification, has completed at least 2 years or 3,000 hours of post master's degree supervised clinical social work practice under the supervision of a master's level social worker in an appropriate setting such as a hospital, SNF, or clinic.

B. Clinical Social Worker Services Defined

Section 1861(hh)(2) of the Act defines "clinical social worker services" as those services that the CSW is legally authorized to perform under State law (or the State regulatory mechanism provided by State law) of the State in which such services are performed for the diagnosis and treatment of mental illnesses. Services furnished to an inpatient of a hospital or an inpatient of a SNF that the SNF is required to provide

as a requirement for participation are not included. The services that are covered are those that are otherwise covered if furnished by a physician or as incident to a physician's professional service.

C. Covered Services

Coverage is limited to the services a CSW is legally authorized to perform in accordance with State law (or State regulatory mechanism established by State law). The services of a CSW may be covered under Part B if they are:

- The type of services that are otherwise covered if furnished by a physician, or as incident to a physician's service. (See §30 for a description of physicians' services and §70 of Pub 100-1, the Medicare General Information, Eligibility, and Entitlement Manual, Chapter 5, for the definition of a physician.);

- Performed by a person who meets the definition of a CSW (See subsection A.); and

- Not otherwise excluded from coverage. Carriers should become familiar with the State law or regulatory mechanism governing a CSW's scope of practice in their service area.

D. Noncovered Services

Services of a CSW are not covered when furnished to inpatients of a hospital or to inpatients of a SNF if the services furnished in the SNF are those that the SNF is required to furnish as a condition of participation in Medicare. In addition, CSW services are not covered if they are otherwise excluded from Medicare coverage even though a CSW is authorized by State law to perform them. For example, the Medicare law excludes from coverage services that are not "reasonable and necessary for the diagnosis or treatment of an illness or injury or to improve the functioning of a malformed body member."

E. Outpatient Mental Health Services Limitation

All covered therapeutic services furnished by qualified CSWs are subject to the outpatient psychiatric services limitation in Pub 100-1, Medicare General Information, Eligibility, and Entitlement Manual, Chapter 3, "Deductibles, Coinsurance Amounts, and Payment Limitations," §30, (i.e., only 62 1/2 percent of expenses for these services are considered incurred expenses for Medicare purposes). The limitation does not apply to diagnostic services.

F. Assignment Requirement

Assignment is required.

100-2, 15, 180

Nurse-Midwife (CNM) Services

B3-2154

A. General

Effective on or after July 1, 1988, the services provided by a certified nurse-midwife or incident to the certified nurse-midwife's services are covered. Payment is made under assignment only. See the Medicare Claims Processing Manual, Chapter 12, "Physician and Nonphysician Practitioners," §130, for payment methodology for nurse midwife services.

B. Certified Nurse-Midwife Defined

A certified nurse-midwife is a registered nurse who has successfully completed a program of study and clinical experience in nurse-midwifery, meeting guidelines prescribed by the Secretary, or who has been certified by an organization recognized by the Secretary. The Secretary has recognized certification by the American College of Nurse-Midwives and State qualifying requirements in those States that specify a program of education and clinical experience for nurse-midwives for these purposes. A nurse-midwife must:

- Be currently licensed to practice in the State as a registered professional nurse; and

- Meet one of the following requirements:

  1. Be legally authorized under State law or regulations to practice as a nurse-midwife and have completed a program of study and clinical experience for nurse-midwives, as specified by the State; or

  2. If the State does not specify a program of study and clinical experience that nurse-midwives must complete to practice in that State, the nurse-midwife must:

     a. Be currently certified as a nurse-midwife by the American College of Nurse-Midwives.

     b. Have satisfactorily completed a formal education program (of at least one academic year) that, upon completion, qualifies the nurse to take the certification examination offered by the American College of Nurse-Midwives; or

     c. Have successfully completed a formal education program for preparing registered nurses to furnish gynecological and obstetrical care to women during pregnancy, delivery, and the postpartum period, and care to normal newborns, and have practiced as a nurse-midwife for a total of 12 months during any 18-month period from August 8, 1976, to July 16, 1982.

C. Covered Services

1. General - Effective January 1, 1988, through December 31, 1993, the coverage of nurse-midwife services was restricted to the maternity cycle. The maternity cycle is a period that includes pregnancy, labor, and the immediate postpartum period.

Beginning with services furnished on or after January 1, 1994, coverage is no longer limited to the maternity cycle. Coverage is available for services furnished by a nurse-midwife that he or she is legally authorized to perform in the State in which the services are furnished and that would otherwise be covered if furnished by a physician, including obstetrical and gynecological services.

2. Incident To- Services and supplies furnished incident to a nurse midwife's service are covered if they would have been covered when furnished incident to the services of a doctor of medicine or osteopathy, as described in §60.

D. Noncovered Services

The services of nurse-midwives are not covered if they are otherwise excluded from Medicare coverage even though a nurse-midwife is authorized by State law to perform them. For example, the Medicare program excludes from coverage routine physical checkups and services that are not reasonable and necessary for the diagnosis or treatment of an illness or injury or to improve the functioning of a malformed body member. Coverage of service to the newborn continues only to the point that the newborn is or would normally be treated medically as a separate individual. Items and services furnished the newborn from that point are not covered on the basis of the mother's eligibility.

E. Relationship With Physician

Most States have licensure and other requirements applicable to nurse-midwives. For example, some require that the nurse-midwife have an arrangement with a physician for the referral of the patient in the event a problem develops that requires medical attention. Others may require that the nurse-midwife function under the general supervision of a physician. Although these and similar State requirements must be met in order for the nurse-midwife to provide Medicare covered care, they have no effect on the nurse-midwife's right to personally bill for and receive direct Medicare payment. That is, billing does not have to flow through a physician or facility. See §60.2 for coverage of services performed by nurse-midwives incident to the service of physicians.

F. Place of Service

There is no restriction on place of service. Therefore, nurse-midwife services are covered if provided in the nurse-midwife's office, in the patient's home, or in a hospital or other facility, such as a clinic or birthing center owned or operated by a nurse-midwife.

G. Assignment Requirement

Assignment is required.

100-2, 15, 220

Coverage of Outpatient Rehabilitation Therapy Services (Physical Therapy, Occupational Therapy, and Speech-Language Pathology Services) Under Medical Insurance

A comprehensive knowledge of the policies that apply to therapy services cannot be obtained through manuals alone. The most definitive policies are Local Coverage Determinations found at the Medicare Coverage Database www.cms.hhs.gov/mcd. A list of Medicare contractors is found at the CMS Web site. Specific questions about all Medicare policies should be addressed to the contractors through the contact information supplied on their Web sites. General Medicare questions may be addressed to the Medicare regional offices http://www.cms.hhs.gov/RegionalOffices/.

A. Definitions

The following defines terms used in this section and §230:

ACTIVE PARTICIPATION of the clinician in treatment means that the clinician personally furnishes in its entirety at least 1 billable service on at least 1 day of treatment.

ASSESSMENT is separate from evaluation, and is included in services or procedures, (it is not separately payable). The term assessment as used in Medicare manuals related to therapy services is distinguished from language in Current Procedural Terminology (CPT) codes that specify assessment, e.g., 97755, Assistive Technology Assessment, which may be payable. Assessments shall be provided only by clinicians, because assessment requires professional skill to gather data by observation and patient inquiry and may include limited objective testing and measurement to make clinical judgments regarding the patient's condition(s). Assessment determines, e.g., changes in the patient's status since the last visit/treatment day and whether the planned procedure or service should be modified. Based on these assessment data, the professional may make judgments about progress toward goals and/or determine that a more complete evaluation or re-evaluation (see definitions below) is indicated. Routine weekly assessments of expected progression in accordance with the plan are not payable as re-evaluations.

CERTIFICATION is the physician's/nonphysician practitioner's (NPP) approval of the plan of care. Certification requires a dated signature on the plan of care or some other document that indicates approval of the plan of care.

The CLINICIAN is a term used in this manual and in Pub 100-4, chapter 5, section 10 or section 20, to refer to only a physician, nonphysician practitioner or a therapist (but not to an assistant, aide or any other personnel) providing a service within their scope of practice and consistent with state and local law. Clinicians make clinical judgments and are responsible for all services they are permitted to supervise. Services that require the skills of a therapist, may be appropriately furnished by clinicians, that is, by or under the supervision of qualified

physicians/NPPs when their scope of practice, state and local laws allow it and their personal professional training is judged by Medicare contractors as sufficient to provide to the beneficiary skills equivalent to a therapist for that service.

COMPLEXITIES are complicating factors that may influence treatment, e.g., they may influence the type, frequency, intensity and/or duration of treatment. Complexities may be represented by diagnoses (ICD codes), by patient factors such as age, severity, acuity, multiple conditions, and motivation, or by the patient's social circumstances such as the support of a significant other or the availability of transportation to therapy.

A DATE may be in any form (written, stamped or electronic). The date may be added to the record in any manner and at any time, as long as the dates are accurate. If they are different, refer to both the date a service was performed and the date the entry to the record was made. For example, if a physician certifies a plan and fails to date it, staff may add "Received Date" in writing or with a stamp. The received date is valid for certification/re-certification purposes. Also, if the physician faxes the referral, certification, or re-certification and forgets to date it, the date that prints out on the fax is valid. If services provided on one date are documented on another date, both dates should be documented.

The EPISODE of Outpatient Therapy – For the purposes of therapy policy, an outpatient therapy episode is defined as the period of time, in calendar days, from the first day the patient is under the care of the clinician (e.g., for evaluation or treatment) for the current condition(s) being treated by one therapy discipline (PT, or OT, or SLP) until the last date of service for that discipline in that setting.

During the episode, the beneficiary may be treated for more than one condition; including conditions with an onset after the episode has begun. For example, a beneficiary receiving PT for a hip fracture who, after the initial treatment session, develops low back pain would also be treated under a PT plan of care for rehabilitation of low back pain. That plan may be modified from the initial plan, or it may be a separate plan specific to the low back pain, but treatment for both conditions concurrently would be considered the same episode of PT treatment. If that same patient developed a swallowing problem during intubation for the hip surgery, the first day of treatment by the SLP would be a new episode of SLP care.

EVALUATION is a separately payable comprehensive service provided by a clinician, as defined above, that requires professional skills to make clinical judgments about conditions for which services are indicated based on objective measurements and subjective evaluations of patient performance and functional abilities. Evaluation is warranted e.g., for a new diagnosis or when a condition is treated in a new setting. These evaluative judgments are essential to development of the plan of care, including goals and the selection of interventions.

FUNCTIONAL REPORTING, which is required on claims for all outpatient therapy services pursuant to 42CFR410.59, 410.60, and 410.62, uses nonpayable G-codes and related modifiers to convey information about the patient's functional status at specified points during therapy. (See Pub 100-4, chapter 5, section 10.6)

RE-EVALUATION provides additional objective information not included in other documentation. Re-evaluation is separately payable and is periodically indicated during an episode of care when the professional assessment of a clinician indicates a significant improvement, or decline, or change in the patient's condition or functional status that was not anticipated in the plan of care. Although some state regulations and state practice acts require re-evaluation at specific times, for Medicare payment, reevaluations must also meet Medicare coverage guidelines. The decision to provide a reevaluation shall be made by a clinician.

INTERVAL of certified treatment (certification interval) consists of 90 calendar days or less, based on an individual's needs. A physician/NPP may certify a plan of care for an interval length that is less than 90 days. There may be more than one certification interval in an episode of care. The certification interval is not the same as a Progress Report period.

MAINTENANCE PROGRAM (MP) means a program established by a therapist that consists of activities and/or mechanisms that will assist a beneficiary in maximizing or maintaining the progress he or she has made during therapy or to prevent or slow further deterioration due to a disease or illness.

NONPHYSICIAN PRACTITIONERS (NPP) means physician assistants, clinical nurse specialists, and nurse practitioners, who may, if state and local laws permit it, and when appropriate rules are followed, provide, certify or supervise therapy services.

PHYSICIAN with respect to outpatient rehabilitation therapy services means a doctor of medicine, osteopathy (including an osteopathic practitioner), podiatric medicine, or optometry (for low vision rehabilitation only). Chiropractors and doctors of dental surgery or dental medicine are not considered physicians for therapy services and may neither refer patients for rehabilitation therapy services nor establish therapy plans of care.

PATIENT, client, resident, and beneficiary are terms used interchangeably to indicate enrolled recipients of Medicare covered services.

PROVIDERS of services are defined in §1861(u) of the Act, 42CFR400.202 and 42CFR485 Subpart H as participating hospitals, critical access hospitals (CAH), skilled nursing facilities (SNF), comprehensive outpatient rehabilitation facilities (CORF), home health agencies (HHA), hospices, participating clinics, rehabilitation agencies or outpatient rehabilitation facilities (ORF). Providers are also defined as public health agencies with agreements only to furnish outpatient therapy services, or community mental health centers with agreements only to furnish partial hospitalization services. To qualify as providers of services, these providers must meet certain conditions enumerated in the law and enter into an agreement with the Secretary in which they agree not to charge any beneficiary for covered services for which the program will pay and to refund any erroneous collections made. Note that the word PROVIDER in sections 220 and 230 is not used to mean a person who provides a service, but is used as in the statute to mean a facility or agency such as rehabilitation agency or home health agency.

QUALIFIED PROFESSIONAL means a physical therapist, occupational therapist, speech-language pathologist, physician, nurse practitioner, clinical nurse specialist, or physician's assistant, who is licensed or certified by the state to furnish therapy services, and who also may appropriately furnish therapy services under Medicare policies. Qualified professional may also include a physical therapist assistant (PTA) or an occupational therapy assistant (OTA) when furnishing services under the supervision of a qualified therapist, who is working within the state scope of practice in the state in which the services are furnished. Assistants are limited in the services they may furnish (see section 230.1 and 230.2) and may not supervise other therapy caregivers.

QUALIFIED PERSONNEL means staff (auxiliary personnel) who have been educated and trained as therapists and qualify to furnish therapy services only under direct supervision incident to a physician or NPP. See §230.5 of this chapter. Qualified personnel may or may not be licensed as therapists but meet all of the requirements for therapists with the exception of licensure.

SIGNATURE means a legible identifier of any type acceptable according to policies in Pub. 100-08, Medicare Program Integrity Manual, chapter 3, §3.3.2.4 concerning signatures.

SUPERVISION LEVELS for outpatient rehabilitation therapy services are the same as those for diagnostic tests defined in 42CFR410.32. Depending on the setting, the levels include personal supervision (in the room), direct supervision (in the office suite), and general supervision (physician/NPP is available but not necessarily on the premises).

SUPPLIERS of therapy services include individual practitioners such as physicians, NPPs, physical therapists and occupational therapists who have Medicare provider numbers. Regulatory references on physical therapists in private practice (PTPPs) and occupational therapists in private practice (OTPPs) are at 42CFR410.60 (C)(1), 485.701-729, and 486.150-163.

THERAPIST refers only to qualified physical therapists, occupational therapists and speech-language pathologists, as defined in §230. Qualifications that define therapists are in §§230.1, 230.2, and 230.3. Skills of a therapist are defined by the scope of practice for therapists in the state).

THERAPY (or outpatient rehabilitation services) includes only outpatient physical therapy (PT), occupational therapy (OT) and speech-language pathology (SLP) services paid using the Medicare Physician Fee Schedule or the same services when provided in hospitals that are exempt from the hospital Outpatient Prospective Payment System and paid on a reasonable cost basis, including critical access hospitals.

Therapy services referred to in this chapter are those skilled services furnished according to the standards and conditions in CMS manuals, (e.g., in this chapter and in Pub. 100-4, Medicare Claims Processing Manual, chapter 5), within their scope of practice by qualified professionals or qualified personnel, as defined in this section, represented by procedures found in the American Medical Association's "Current Procedural Terminology (CPT)." A list of CPT (HCPCS) codes is provided in Pub. 100-4, chapter 5, §20, and in Local Coverage Determinations developed by contractors.

TREATMENT DAY means a single calendar day on which treatment, evaluation and/or reevaluation is provided. There could be multiple visits, treatment sessions/encounters on a treatment day.

VISITS OR TREATMENT SESSIONS begin at the time the patient enters the treatment area (of a building, office, or clinic) and continue until all services (e.g., activities, procedures, services) have been completed for that session and the patient leaves that area to participate in a non-therapy activity. It is likely that not all minutes in the visits/treatment sessions are billable (e.g., rest periods). There may be two treatment sessions in a day, for example, in the morning and afternoon. When there are two visits/ treatment sessions in a day, plans of care indicate treatment amount of twice a day.

B. References

Paper Manuals. The following manuals, now outdated, were resources for the Internet Only Manuals:

- Part A Medicare Intermediary Manual, (Pub. 13)
- Part B Medicare Carrier Manual, (Pub. 14)
- Hospital Manual, (Pub. 10)
- Outpatient Physical Therapy/CORF Manual, (Pub. 9)

Regulation and Statute. The information in this section is based in part on the following current references:

- 42CFR refers to Title 42, Code of Federal Regulation (CFR).
- The Act refers to the Social Security Act.

Internet Only Manuals. Current Policies that concern providers and suppliers of therapy services are located in many places throughout CMS Manuals. Sites that may be of interest include:

- Pub.100-1 GENERAL INFORMATION, ELIGIBILITY, AND ENTITLEMENT
  — Chapter 1- General Overview
    – 10.1 - Hospital Insurance (Part A) for Inpatient Hospital, Hospice, Home Health and SNF Services - A Brief Description
    – 10.2 - Home Health Services
    – 10.3 - Supplementary Medical Insurance (Part B) - A Brief Description
    – 20.2 - Discrimination Prohibited
- Pub. 100-2, MEDICARE BENEFIT POLICY MANUAL
  — Ch 6 - Hospital Services Covered Under Part B
    – 10 - Medical and Other Health Services Furnished to Inpatients of Participating Hospitals
    – 20 - Outpatient Hospital Services
    – 20.2 - Outpatient Defined
    – 20.4.1 - Diagnostic Services Defined
    – 70 - Outpatient Hospital Psychiatric Services
  — Ch 8 - Coverage of Extended Care (SNF) Services Under Hospital Insurance
    – 30.4. - Direct Skilled Rehabilitation Services to Patients
    – 40 - Physician Certification and Recertification for Extended Care Services
    – 50.3 - Physical Therapy, Speech-Language Pathology, and Occupational Therapy Furnished by the Skilled Nursing Facility or by Others Under Arrangements with the Facility and Under Its Supervision
    – 70.3 - Inpatient Physical Therapy, Occupational Therapy, and Speech Pathology Services
  — Ch 12 - Comprehensive Outpatient Rehabilitation Facility (CORF) Coverage
    – 10 - Comprehensive Outpatient Rehabilitation Facility (CORF) Services Provided by Medicare
    – 20 - Required and Optional CORF Services
    – 20.1 - Required Services
    – 20.2 - Optional CORF Services
    – 30 - Rules for Provision of Services
    – 30.1 - Rules for Payment of CORF Services
    – 40 - Specific CORF Services
    – 40.1 - Physicians' Services
    – 40.2 - Physical Therapy Services
    – 40.3 - Occupational Therapy Services
    – 40.4 - Speech Language Pathology Services
- Pub. 100-3 MEDICARE NATIONAL COVERAGE DETERMINATIONS MANUAL
  — Part 1
    – 20.10 - Cardiac Rehabilitation Programs
    – 30.1 - Biofeedback Therapy
    – 30.1.1 - Biofeedback Therapy for the Treatment of Urinary Incontinence
    – 50.1 - Speech Generating Devices
    – 50.2 - Electronic Speech Aids
    – 50.4 - Tracheostomy Speaking Valve
  — Part 2
    – 150.2 - Osteogenic Stimulator
    – 160.7 - Electrical Nerve Stimulators
    – 160.12 - Neuromuscular Electrical Stimulation (NMES)
    – 160.13 - Supplies Used in the Delivery of Transcutaneous Electrical Nerve Stimulation (TENS) and Neuromuscular Electrical Stimulation (NMES)
    – 160.17 - L-Dopa
  — Part 3
    – 170.1 - Institutional and Home Care Patient Education Programs
    – 170.2 - Melodic Intonation Therapy
    – 170.3 - Speech Pathology Services for the Treatment of Dysphagia
    – 180 – Nutrition
  — Part 4
    – 230.8 - Non-implantable Pelvic Flood Electrical Stimulator
    – 240.7 - Postural Drainage Procedures and Pulmonary Exercises
    – 270.1 -Electrical Stimulation (ES) and Electromagnetic Therapy for the Treatment of Wounds
    – 270.4 - Treatment of Decubitus Ulcers
    – 280.3 - Mobility Assisted Equipment (MAE)

- 280.4 - Seat Lift
- 280.13 - Transcutaneous Electrical Nerve Stimulators (TENS)
- 290.1 - Home Health Visits to A Blind Diabetic
- Pub. 100-08 PROGRAM INTEGRITY MANUAL
  - Chapter 3 - Verifying Potential Errors and Taking Corrective Actions
    - 3.4.1.1 - Linking LCD and NCD ID Numbers to Edits
  - Chapter 13 - Local Coverage Determinations
    - 13.5.1 - Reasonable and Necessary Provisions in LCDs

Specific policies may differ by setting. Other policies concerning therapy services are found in other manuals. When a therapy service policy is specific to a setting, it takes precedence over these general outpatient policies. For special rules on:

- CORFs - See chapter 12 of this manual and also Pub. 100-4, chapter 5;
- SNF - See chapter 8 of this manual and also Pub. 100-4, chapter 6, for SNF claims/billing;
- HHA - See chapter 7 of this manual, and Pub. 100-4, chapter 10;
- GROUP THERAPY AND STUDENTS - See Pub. 100-2, chapter 15, §230;
- ARRANGEMENTS - Pub. 100-1, chapter 5, §10.3;
- COVERAGE is described in the Medicare Program Integrity Manual, Pub. 100-08, chapter 13, §13.5.1; and
- THERAPY CAPS - See Pub. 100-4, chapter 5, §10.2, for a complete description of this financial limitation.

C. General

Therapy services are a covered benefit in §§1861(g), 1861(p), and 1861(ll) of the Act. Therapy services may also be provided incident to the services of a physician/NPP under §§1861(s)(2) and 1862(a)(20) of the Act.

Covered therapy services are furnished by providers, by others under arrangements with and under the supervision of providers, or furnished by suppliers (e.g., physicians, NPP, enrolled therapists), who meet the requirements in Medicare manuals for therapy services.

Where a prospective payment system (PPS) applies, therapy services are paid when services conform to the requirements of that PPS. Reimbursement for therapy provided to Part A inpatients of hospitals or residents of SNFs in covered stays is included in the respective PPS rates.

Payment for therapy provided by an HHA under a plan of treatment is included in the home health PPS rate. Therapy may be billed by an HHA on bill type 34x if there are no home health services billed under a home health plan of care at the same time (e.g., the patient is not homebound), and there is a valid therapy plan of treatment.

In addition to the requirements described in this chapter, the services must be furnished in accordance with health and safety requirements set forth in regulations at 42CFR484, and 42CFR485.

When therapy services may be furnished appropriately in a community pool by a clinician in a physical therapist or occupational therapist private practice, physician office, outpatient hospital, or outpatient SNF, the practice/office or provider shall rent or lease the pool, or a specific portion of the pool. The use of that part of the pool during specified times shall be restricted to the patients of that practice or provider. The written agreement to rent or lease the pool shall be available for review on request. When part of the pool is rented or leased, the agreement shall describe the part of the pool that is used exclusively by the patients of that practice/office or provider and the times that exclusive use applies. Other providers, including rehabilitation agencies (previously referred to as OPTs and ORFs) and CORFs, are subject to the requirements outlined in the respective State Operations Manual regarding rented or leased community pools.

100-2, 15, 230

Practice of Physical Therapy, Occupational Therapy, and Speech-Language Pathology

A. Group Therapy Services.

Contractors pay for outpatient physical therapy services (which includes outpatient speech-language pathology services) and outpatient occupational therapy services provided simultaneously to two or more individuals by a practitioner as group therapy services (97150). The individuals can be, but need not be performing the same activity. The physician or therapist involved in group therapy services must be in constant attendance, but one-on-one patient contact is not required.

B. Therapy Students

1. General

   Only the services of the therapist can be billed and paid under Medicare Part B. The services performed by a student are not reimbursed even if provided under "line of sight" supervision of the therapist; however, the presence of the student "in the room" does not make the service unbillable. Pay for the direct (one-to-one) patient contact services of the physician or therapist provided to Medicare Part B patients. Group therapy services performed by a therapist or physician may be billed when a student is also present "in the room".

   EXAMPLES:

   Therapists may bill and be paid for the provision of services in the following scenarios:

- The qualified practitioner is present and in the room for the entire session. The student participates in the delivery of services when the qualified practitioner is directing the service, making the skilled judgment, and is responsible for the assessment and treatment.

- The qualified practitioner is present in the room guiding the student in service delivery when the therapy student and the therapy assistant student are participating in the provision of services, and the practitioner is not engaged in treating another patient or doing other tasks at the same time.

- The qualified practitioner is responsible for the services and as such, signs all documentation. (A student may, of course, also sign but it is not necessary since the Part B payment is for the clinician's service, not for the student's services).

2. Therapy Assistants as Clinical Instructors

   Physical therapist assistants and occupational therapy assistants are not precluded from serving as clinical instructors for therapy students, while providing services within their scope of work and performed under the direction and supervision of a licensed physical or occupational therapist to a Medicare beneficiary.

3. Services Provided Under Part A and Part B

   The payment methodologies for Part A and B therapy services rendered by a student are different. Under the MPFS (Medicare Part B), Medicare pays for services provided by physicians and practitioners that are specifically authorized by statute. Students do not meet the definition of practitioners under Medicare Part B. Under SNF PPS, payments are based upon the case mix or Resource Utilization Group (RUG) category that describes the patient. In the rehabilitation groups, the number of therapy minutes delivered to the patient determines the RUG category. Payment levels for each category are based upon the costs of caring for patients in each group rather than providing pecific payment for each therapy service as is done in Medicare Part B.

100-2, 15, 230.1

Practice of Physical Therapy

A. General

Physical therapy services are those services provided within the scope of practice of physical therapists and necessary for the diagnosis and treatment of impairments, functional limitations, disabilities or changes in physical function and health status. (See Pub. 100-3, the Medicare National Coverage Determinations Manual, for specific conditions or services.) For descriptions of aquatic therapy in a community center pool see section 220C of this chapter.

B. Qualified Physical Therapist Defined

Reference: 42CFR484.4

The new personnel qualifications for physical therapists were discussed in the 2008 Physician Fee Schedule. See the Federal Register of November 27, 2007, for the full text. See also the correction notice for this rule, published in the Federal Register on January 15, 2008.

The regulation provides that a qualified physical therapist (PT) is a person who is licensed, if applicable, as a PT by the state in which he or she is practicing unless licensure does not apply, has graduated from an accredited PT education program and passed a national examination approved by the state in which PT services are provided.

The phrase, "by the state in which practicing" includes any authorization to practice provided by the same state in which the service is provided, including temporary licensure, regardless of the location of the entity billing the services. The curriculum accreditation is provided by the Commission on Accreditation in Physical Therapy Education (CAPTE) or, for those who graduated before CAPTE, curriculum approval was provided by the American Physical Therapy Association (APTA). For internationally educated PTs, curricula are approved by a credentials evaluation organization either approved by the APTA or identified in 8 CFR 212.15(e) as it relates to PTs. For example, in 2007, 8 CFR 212.15(e) approved the credentials evaluation provided by the Federation of State Boards of Physical Therapy (FSBPT) and the Foreign Credentialing Commission on Physical Therapy (FCCPT). The requirements above apply to all PTs effective January 1, 2010, if they have not met any of the following requirements prior to January 1, 2010.

Physical therapists whose current license was obtained on or prior to December 31, 2009, qualify to provide PT services to Medicare beneficiaries if they:

- graduated from a CAPTE approved program in PT on or before December 31, 2009 (examination is not required); or,

- graduated on or before December 31, 2009, from a PT program outside the U.S. that is determined to be substantially equivalent to a U.S. program by a credentials evaluating organization approved by either the APTA or identified in 8 CFR 212.15(e) and also passed an examination for PTs approved by the state in which practicing.

Or, PTs whose current license was obtained before January 1, 2008, may meet the requirements in place on that date (i.e., graduation from a curriculum approved by either the APTA, the Committee on Allied Health Education and Accreditation of the American Medical Association, or both).

Or, PTs meet the requirements who are currently licensed and were licensed or qualified as a PT on or before December 31, 1977, and had 2 years appropriate experience as a PT, and passed a proficiency examination conducted, approved, or sponsored by the U.S. Public Health Service.

Or, PTs meet the requirements if they are currently licensed and before January 1, 1966, they were:

— admitted to membership by the APTA; or

— admitted to registration by the American Registry of Physical Therapists; or

— graduated from a 4-year PT curriculum approved by a State Department of Education; or

— licensed or registered and prior to January 1, 1970, they had 15 years of fulltime experience in PT under the order and direction of attending and referring doctors of medicine or osteopathy.

Or, PTs meet requirements if they are currently licensed and they were trained outside the U.S. before January 1, 2008, and after 1928 graduated from a PT curriculum approved in the country in which the curriculum was located, if that country had an organization that was a member of the World Confederation for Physical Therapy, and that PT qualified as a member of the organization.

For outpatient PT services that are provided incident to the services of physicians/NPPs, the requirement for PT licensure does not apply; all other personnel qualifications do apply. The qualified personnel providing PT services incident to the services of a physician/NPP must be trained in an accredited PT curriculum. For example, a person who, on or before December 31, 2009, graduated from a PT curriculum accredited by CAPTE, but who has not passed the national examination or obtained a license, could provide Medicare outpatient PT therapy services incident to the services of a physician/NPP if the physician assumes responsibility for the services according to the incident to policies. On or after January 1, 2010, although licensure does not apply, both education and examination requirements that are effective January 1, 2010, apply to qualified personnel who provide PT services incident to the services of a physician/NPP.

C. Services of Physical Therapy Support Personnel
Reference: 42CFR 484.4

Personnel Qualifications. The new personnel qualifications for physical therapist assistants (PTA) were discussed in the 2008 Physician Fee Schedule. See the Federal Register of November 27, 2007, for the full text. See also the correction notice for this rule, published in the Federal Register on January 15, 2008.

The regulation provides that a qualified PTA is a person who is licensed as a PTA unless licensure does not apply, is registered or certified, if applicable, as a PTA by the state in which practicing, and graduated from an approved curriculum for PTAs, and passed a national examination for PTAs. The phrase, "by the state in which practicing" includes any authorization to practice provided by the same state in which the service is provided, including temporary licensure, regardless of the location or the entity billing for the services. Approval for the curriculum is provided by CAPTE or, if internationally or military trained PTAs apply, approval will be through a credentialing body for the curriculum for PTAs identified by either the American Physical Therapy Association or identified in 8 CFR 212.15(e). A national examination for PTAs is, for example the one furnished by the Federation of State Boards of Physical Therapy. These requirements above apply to all PTAs effective January 1, 2010, if they have not met any of the following requirements prior to January 1, 2010.

Those PTAs also qualify who, on or before December 31, 2009, are licensed, registered or certified as a PTA and met one of the two following requirements:

1. Is licensed or otherwise regulated in the state in which practicing; or

2. In states that have no licensure or other regulations, or where licensure does not apply, PTAs have:

— graduated on or before December 31, 2009, from a 2-year college-level program approved by the APTA or CAPTE; and

— effective January 1, 2010, those PTAs must have both graduated from a CAPTE approved curriculum and passed a national examination for PTAs; or

— PTAs may also qualify if they are licensed, registered or certified as a PTA, if applicable and meet requirements in effect before January 1, 2008, that is,

– they have graduated before January 1, 2008, from a 2 year college level program approved by the APTA; or

– on or before December 31, 1977, they were licensed or qualified as a PTA and passed a proficiency examination conducted, approved, or sponsored by the U.S. Public Health Service.

Services. The services of PTAs used when providing covered therapy benefits are included as part of the covered service. These services are billed by the supervising physical therapist. PTAs may not provide evaluation services, make clinical judgments or decisions or take responsibility for the service. They act at the direction and under the supervision of the treating physical therapist and in accordance with state laws.

A physical therapist must supervise PTAs. The level and frequency of supervision differs by setting (and by state or local law). General supervision is required for PTAs in all settings except private practice (which requires direct supervision) unless state practice requirements are more stringent, in which case state or local requirements must be followed. See specific settings for details. For example, in clinics, rehabilitation services, either on or off the organization's premises, those services are supervised by a qualified physical therapist who makes an onsite supervisory visit at least once every 30 days or more frequently if required by state or local laws or regulation.

The services of a PTA shall not be billed as services incident to a physician/NPP's service, because they do not meet the qualifications of a therapist.

The cost of supplies (e.g., theraband, hand putty, electrodes) used in furnishing covered therapy care is included in the payment for the HCPCS codes billed by the physical therapist, and are, therefore, not separately billable. Separate coverage and billing provisions apply to items that meet the definition of brace in Sec.130.

Services provided by aides, even if under the supervision of a therapist, are not therapy services and are not covered by Medicare. Although an aide may help the therapist by providing unskilled services, those services that are unskilled are not covered by Medicare and shall be denied as not reasonable and necessary if they are billed as therapy services.

D. Application of Medicare Guidelines to PT Services
This subsection will be used in the future to illustrate the application of the above guidelines to some of the physical therapy modalities and procedures utilized in the treatment of patients.

100-2, 15, 230.2

Practice of Occupational Therapy

230.2 - Practice of Occupational Therapy (Rev. 88, Issued: 05-07-08, Effective: 01-01-08, Implementation: 06-09-08)

A. General

Occupational therapy services are those services provided within the scope of practice of occupational therapists and necessary for the diagnosis and treatment of impairments, functional disabilities or changes in physical function and health status. (See Pub. 100- 03, the Medicare National Coverage Determinations Manual, for specific conditions or services.)

Occupational therapy is medically prescribed treatment concerned with improving or restoring functions which have been impaired by illness or injury or, where function has been permanently lost or reduced by illness or injury, to improve the individual's ability to perform those tasks required for independent functioning. Such therapy may involve:

- The evaluation, and reevaluation as required, of a patient's level of function by administering diagnostic and prognostic tests;

- The selection and teaching of task-oriented therapeutic activities designed to restore physical function; e.g., use of woodworking activities on an inclined table to restore shoulder, elbow, and wrist range of motion lost as a result of burns;

- The planning, implementing, and supervising of individualized therapeutic activity programs as part of an overall "active treatment" program for a patient with a diagnosed psychiatric illness; e.g., the use of sewing activities which require following a pattern to reduce confusion and restore reality orientation in a schizophrenic patient;

- The planning and implementing of therapeutic tasks and activities to restore sensoryintegrative function; e.g., providing motor and tactile activities to increase sensory input and improve response for a stroke patient with functional loss resulting in a distorted body image;

- The teaching of compensatory technique to improve the level of independence in the activities of daily living, for example:

— Teaching a patient who has lost the use of an arm how to pare potatoes and chop vegetables with one hand;

— Teaching an upper extremity amputee how to functionally utilize a prosthesis;

— Teaching a stroke patient new techniques to enable the patient to perform feeding, dressing, and other activities as independently as possible; or

— Teaching a patient with a hip fracture/hip replacement techniques of standing tolerance and balance to enable the patient to perform such functional activities as dressing and homemaking tasks.

The designing, fabricating, and fitting of orthotics and self-help devices; e.g., making a hand splint for a patient with rheumatoid arthritis to maintain the hand in a functional position or constructing a device which would enable an individual to hold a utensil and feed independently; or Vocational and prevocational assessment and training, subject to the limitations specified in item B below.

Only a qualified occupational therapist has the knowledge, training, and experience required to evaluate and, as necessary, reevaluate a patient's level of function, determine whether an occupational therapy program could reasonably be expected to improve, restore, or compensate for lost function and, where appropriate, recommend to the physician/NPP a plan of treatment.

B. Qualified Occupational Therapist Defined
Reference: 42CFR484.4 The new personnel qualifications for occupational therapists (OT) were discussed in the 2008 Physician Fee Schedule. See the Federal Register of November 27, 2007, for the full text. See also the correction notice for this rule, published in the Federal Register on January 15, 2008.

The regulation provides that a qualified OT is an individual who is licensed, if licensure applies, or otherwise regulated, if applicable, as an OT by the state in which practicing, and graduated from an accredited education program for OTs, and is eligible to take or has passed the examination for OTs administered by the National Board for Certification in Occupational Therapy, Inc. (NBCOT). The phrase, "by the state in which practicing" includes any authorization to practice provided by the same state in which the service is provided, including temporary licensure, regardless of the location of the entity billing the services. The education program for U.S. trained OTs is accredited by the Accreditation Council for Occupational Therapy Education (ACOTE). The requirements above apply to all OTs effective January 1, 2010, if they have not met any of the following requirements prior to January 1, 2010.

The OTs may also qualify if on or before December 31, 2009:

- they are licensed or otherwise regulated as an OT in the state in which practicing (regardless of the qualifications they met to obtain that licensure or regulation); or
- when licensure or other regulation does not apply, OTs have graduated from an OT education program accredited by ACOTE and are eligible to take, or have successfully completed the NBCOT examination for OTs.

Also, those OTs who met the Medicare requirements for OTs that were in 42CFR484.4 prior to January 1, 2008, qualify to provide OT services for Medicare beneficiaries if:

- on or before January 1, 2008, they graduated from an OT program approved jointly by the American Medical Association and the AOTA, or
- they are eligible for the National Registration Examination of AOTA or the National Board for Certification in OT.

Also, they qualify who on or before December 31, 1977, had 2 years of appropriate experience as an occupational therapist, and had achieved a satisfactory grade on a proficiency examination conducted, approved, or sponsored by the U.S. Public Health Service.

Those educated outside the U.S. may meet the same qualifications for domestic trained OTs. For example, they qualify if they were licensed or otherwise regulated by the state in which practicing on or before December 31, 2009. Or they are qualified if they:

- graduated from an OT education program accredited as substantially equivalent to a U.S. OT education program by ACOTE, the World Federation of Occupational Therapists, or a credentialing body approved by AOTA; and
- passed the NBCOT examination for OT; and
- Effective January 1, 2010, are licensed or otherwise regulated, if applicable as an OT by the state in which practicing.

For outpatient OT services that are provided incident to the services of physicians/NPPs, the requirement for OT licensure does not apply; all other personnel qualifications do apply. The qualified personnel providing OT services incident to the services of a physician/NPP must be trained in an accredited OT curriculum. For example, a person who, on or before December 31, 2009, graduated from an OT curriculum accredited by ACOTE and is eligible to take or has successfully completed the entry-level certification examination for OTs developed and administered by NBCOT, could provide Medicare outpatient OT services incident to the services of a physician/NPP if the physician assumes responsibility for the services according to the incident to policies. On or after January 1, 2010, although licensure does not apply, both education and examination requirements that are effective January 1, 2010, apply to qualified personnel who provide OT services incident to the services of a physician/NPP.

C. Services of Occupational Therapy Support Personnel
Reference: 42CFR 484.4

The new personnel qualifications for occupational therapy assistants were discussed in the 2008 Physician Fee Schedule. See the Federal Register of November 27, 2007, for the full text. See also the correction notice for this rule, published in the Federal Register on January 15, 2008.

The regulation provides that an occupational therapy assistant is a person who is licensed, unless licensure does not apply, or otherwise regulated, if applicable, as an OTA by the state in which practicing, and graduated from an OTA education program accredited by ACOTE and is eligible to take or has successfully completed the NBCOT examination for OTAs. The phrase, "by the state in which practicing" includes any authorization to practice provided by the same state in which the service is provided, including temporary licensure, regardless of the location of the entity billing the services.

If the requirements above are not met, an OTA may qualify if, on or before December 31, 2009, the OTA is licensed or otherwise regulated as an OTA, if applicable, by the state in which practicing, or meets any qualifications defined by the state in which practicing.

Or, where licensure or other state regulation does not apply, OTAs may qualify if they have, on or before December 31, 2009:

- completed certification requirements to practice as an OTA established by a credentialing organization approved by AOTA; and
- after January 1, 2010, they have also completed an education program accredited by ACOTE and passed the NBCOT examination for OTAs.

OTAs who qualified under the policies in effect prior to January 1, 2008, continue to qualify to provide OT directed and supervised OTA services to Medicare beneficiaries.

Therefore, OTAs qualify who after December 31, 1977, and on or before December 31, 2007:

- completed certification requirements to practice as an OTA established by a credentialing organization approved by AOTA; or
- completed the requirements to practice as an OTA applicable in the state in which practicing.

Those OTAs who were educated outside the U.S. may meet the same requirements as domestically trained OTAs. Or, if educated outside the U.S. on or after January 1, 2008, they must have graduated from an OTA program accredited as substantially equivalent to OTA entry level education in the U.S. by ACOTE, its successor organization, or the World Federation of Occupational Therapists or a credentialing body approved by AOTA. In addition, they must have passed an exam for OTAs administered by NBCOT.

Services. The services of OTAs used when providing covered therapy benefits are included as part of the covered service. These services are billed by the supervising occupational therapist. OTAs may not provide evaluation services, make clinical judgments or decisions or take responsibility for the service. They act at the direction and under the supervision of the treating occupational therapist and in accordance with state laws.

An occupational therapist must supervise OTAs. The level and frequency of supervision differs by setting (and by state or local law). General supervision is required for OTAs in all settings except private practice (which requires direct supervision) unless state practice requirements are more stringent, in which case state or local requirements must be followed. See specific settings for details. For example, in clinics, rehabilitation agencies, and public health agencies, 42CFR485.713 indicates that when an OTA provides services, either on or off the organization's premises, those services are supervised by a qualified occupational therapist who makes an onsite supervisory visit at least once every 30 days or more frequently if required by state or local laws or regulation.

The services of an OTA shall not be billed as services incident to a physician/NPP's service, because they do not meet the qualifications of a therapist.

The cost of supplies (e.g., looms, ceramic tiles, or leather) used in furnishing covered therapy care is included in the payment for the HCPCS codes billed by the occupational therapist and are, therefore, not separately billable. Separate coverage and billing provisions apply to items that meet the definition of brace in Sec.130 of this manual.

Services provided by aides, even if under the supervision of a therapist, are not therapy services in the outpatient setting and are not covered by Medicare. Although an aide may help the therapist by providing unskilled services, those services that are unskilled are not covered by Medicare and shall be denied as not reasonable and necessary if they are billed as therapy services.

D. Application of Medicare Guidelines to Occupational Therapy Services
Occupational therapy may be required for a patient with a specific diagnosed psychiatric illness. If such services are required, they are covered assuming the coverage criteria are met. However, where an individual's motivational needs are not related to a specific diagnosed psychiatric illness, the meeting of such needs does not usually require an individualized therapeutic program. Such needs can be met through general activity programs or the efforts of other professional personnel involved in the care of the patient. Patient motivation is an appropriate and inherent function of all health disciplines, which is interwoven with other functions performed by such personnel for the patient. Accordingly, since the special skills of an occupational therapist are not required, an occupational therapy program for individuals who do not have a specific diagnosed psychiatric illness is not to be considered reasonable and necessary for the treatment of an illness or injury. Services furnished under such a program are not covered.

Occupational therapy may include vocational and prevocational assessment and training. When services provided by an occupational therapist are related solely to specific employment opportunities, work skills, or work settings, they are not reasonable or necessary for the diagnosis or treatment of an illness or injury and are not covered. However, carriers and intermediaries exercise care in applying this exclusion, because the assessment of level of function and the teaching of compensatory techniques to improve the level of function, especially in activities of daily living, are services which occupational therapists provide for both vocational and nonvocational purposes. For example, an assessment of sitting and standing tolerance might be nonvocational for a mother of young children or a retired individual living alone, but could also be a vocational test for a sales clerk. Training an amputee in the use of prosthesis for telephoning is necessary for everyday activities as well as for employment purposes. Major changes in life style may be mandatory for an individual with a substantial disability. The techniques of adjustment cannot be considered exclusively vocational or nonvocational.

100-2, 15, 230.4

Services Furnished by a Therapist in Private Practice

A. General
See section 220 of this chapter for definitions. Therapist refers only to a qualified physical therapist, occupational therapist or speech-language pathologist. TPP refers to therapists in private practice (qualified physical therapists, occupational therapists and speech-language pathologists).

In order to qualify to bill Medicare directly as a therapist, each individual must be enrolled as a private practitioner and employed in one of the following practice types: an unincorporated solo practice, unincorporated partnership, unincorporated group practice, physician/NPP group or groups that are not professional corporations, if allowed by state and local law. Physician/NPP group practices may employ TPP if state and local law permits this employee relationship.

For purposes of this provision, a physician/NPP group practice is defined as one or more physicians/NPPs enrolled with Medicare who may bill as one entity. For further details on issues concerning enrollment, see the provider enrollment Web site at www.cms.hhs.gov/MedicareProviderSupEnroll and Pub. 100-08, Medicare Program Integrity Manual, chapter15, section 15.4.4.9.

Private practice also includes therapists who are practicing therapy as employees of another supplier, of a professional corporation or other incorporated therapy practice. Private practice does not include individuals when they are working as employees of an institutional provider.

Services should be furnished in the therapist's or group's office or in the patient's home. The office is defined as the location(s) where the practice is operated, in the state(s) where the therapist (and practice, if applicable) is legally authorized to furnish services, during the hours that the therapist engages in the practice at that location. If services are furnished in a private practice office space, that space shall be owned, leased, or rented by the practice and used for the exclusive purpose of operating the practice. For descriptions of aquatic therapy in a community center pool see section 220C of this chapter.

Therapists in private practice must be approved as meeting certain requirements, but do not execute a formal provider agreement with the Secretary.

If therapists who have their own Medicare National Provider Identifier (NPI) are employed by therapist groups, physician/NPP groups, or groups that are not professional organizations, the requirement that therapy space be owned, leased, or rented may be satisfied by the group that employs the therapist. Each therapist employed by a group should enroll as a TPP.

When therapists with a Medicare NPI provide services in the physician's/NPP's office in which they are employed, and bill using their NPI for each therapy service, then the direct supervision requirement for enrolled staff apply.

When the therapist who has a Medicare NPI is employed in a physician's/NPP's office the services are ordinarily billed as services of the therapist, with the therapist identified on the claim as the supplier of services. However, services of the therapist who has a Medicare NPI may also be billed by the physician/NPP as services incident to the physician's/NPP's service. (See §230.5 for rules related to therapy services incident to a physician.) In that case, the physician/NPP is the supplier of service, the NPI of the supervising physician/NPP is reported on the claim with the service and all the rules for both therapy services and incident to services (§230.5) must be followed.

B. Private Practice Defined

Reference: Federal Register November, 1998, pages 58863-58869; 42CFR 410.38(b), 42CFR410.59, 42CFR410.60, 42CFR410.62

The contractor considers a therapist to be in private practice if the therapist maintains office space at his or her own expense and furnishes services only in that space or the patient's home. Or, a therapist is employed by another supplier and furnishes services in facilities provided at the expense of that supplier.

The therapist need not be in full-time private practice but must be engaged in private practice on a regular basis; i.e., the therapist is recognized as a private practitioner and for that purpose has access to the necessary equipment to provide an adequate program of therapy.

The therapy services must be provided either by or under the direct supervision of the TPP. Each TPP should be enrolled as a Medicare provider. If a therapist is not enrolled, the services of that therapist must be directly supervised by an enrolled therapist. Direct supervision requires that the supervising private practice therapist be present in the office suite at the time the service is performed. These direct supervision requirements apply only in the private practice setting and only for therapists and their assistants. In other outpatient settings, supervision rules differ. The services of support personnel must be included in the therapist's bill. The supporting personnel, including other therapists, must be W-2 or 1099 employees of the TPP or other qualified employer.

Coverage of outpatient therapy under Part B includes the services of a qualified TPP when furnished in the therapist's office or the beneficiary's home. For this purpose, "home" includes an institution that is used as a home, but not a hospital, CAH or SNF, (Federal Register Nov. 2, 1998, pg 58869).

C. Assignment

Reference: Nov. 2, 1998 Federal Register, pg. 58863

See also Pub. 100-4 chapter 1, §30.2.

When physicians, NPPs, or TPPs obtain provider numbers, they have the option of accepting assignment (participating) or not accepting assignment (nonparticipating). In contrast, providers, such as outpatient hospitals, SNFs, rehabilitation agencies, and CORFs, do not have the option. For these providers, assignment is mandatory.

If physicians/NPPs, or TPPs accept assignment (are participating), they must accept the Medicare Physician Fee Schedule amount as payment. Medicare pays 80% and the patient is responsible for 20%. In contrast, if they do not accept assignment, Medicare will only pay 95% of the fee schedule amount. However, when these services are not furnished on an assignment-related basis, the limiting charge applies. (See §1848(g)(2)(c) of the Act.)

NOTE: Services furnished by a therapist in the therapist's office under arrangements with hospitals in rural communities and public health agencies (or services provided in the beneficiary's home under arrangements with a provider of outpatient physical or occupational therapy services) are not covered under this provision. See section 230.6.

100-2, 15, 232

Cardiac Rehabilitation (CR) and Intensive Cardiac Rehabilitation (ICR) Services Furnished On or After January 1, 2010

Cardiac rehabilitation (CR) services mean a physician-supervised program that furnishes physician prescribed exercise, cardiac risk factor modification, including education, counseling, and behavioral intervention; psychosocial assessment, outcomes assessment, and other items/services as determined by the Secretary under certain conditions. Intensive cardiac rehabilitation (ICR) services mean a physician-supervised program that furnishes the same items/services under the same conditions as a CR program but must also demonstrate, as shown in peer-reviewed published research, that it improves patients' cardiovascular disease through specific outcome measurements described in 42 CFR 410.49(c). Effective January 1, 2010, Medicare Part B pays for CR/ICR programs and related items/services if specific criteria is met by the Medicare beneficiary, the CR/ICR program itself, the setting in which is it administered, and the physician administering the program, as outlined below:

CR/ICR Program Beneficiary Requirements:

Medicare covers CR/ICR program services for beneficiaries who have experienced one or more of the following:

- Acute myocardial infarction within the preceding 12 months;
- Coronary artery bypass surgery;
- Current stable angina pectoris;
- Heart valve repair or replacement;
- Percutaneous transluminal coronary angioplasty (PTCA) or coronary stenting;
- Heart or heart-lung transplant.

For cardiac rehabilitation only: Stable, chronic heart failure defined as patients with left ventricular ejection fraction of 35% or less and New York Heart Association (NYHA) class II to IV symptoms despite being on optimal heart failure therapy for at least 6 weeks. (Effective February 18, 2014.)

CR/ICR Program Component Requirements:

- Physician-prescribed exercise. This physical activity includes aerobic exercise combined with other types of exercise (i.e., strengthening, stretching) as determined to be appropriate for individual patients by a physician each day CR/ICR items/services are furnished.
- Cardiac risk factor modification. This includes education, counseling, and behavioral intervention, tailored to the patients' individual needs.
- Psychosocial assessment. This assessment means an evaluation of an individual's mental and emotional functioning as it relates to the individual's rehabilitation. It should include: (1) an assessment of those aspects of the individual's family and home situation that affects the individual's rehabilitation treatment, and, (2) a psychosocial evaluation of the individual's response to, and rate of progress under, the treatment plan.
- Outcomes assessment. These should include: (i) minimally, assessments from the commencement and conclusion of CR/ICR, based on patient-centered outcomes which must be measured by the physician immediately at the beginning and end of the program, and, (ii) objective clinical measures of the effectiveness of the CR/ICR program for the individual patient, including exercise performance and self-reported measures of exertion and behavior.
- Individualized treatment plan. This plan should be written and tailored to each individual patient and include (i) a description of the individual's diagnosis; (ii) the type, amount, frequency, and duration of the CR/ICR items/services furnished; and (iii) the goals set for the individual under the plan. The individualized treatment plan must be established, reviewed, and signed by a physician every 30 days.

As specified at 42 CFR 410.49(f)(1), CR sessions are limited to a maximum of 2 1-hour sessions per day for up to 36 sessions over up to 36 weeks with the option for an additional 36 sessions over an extended period of time if approved by the contractor under section 1862(a)(1)(A) of the Act. ICR sessions are limited to 72 1-hour sessions (as defined in section 1848(b)(5) of the Act), up to 6 sessions per day, over a period of up to 18 weeks.

CR/ICR Program Setting Requirements:

CR/ICR services must be furnished in a physician's office or a hospital outpatient setting (for ICR, the hospital outpatient setting must provide ICR using an approved ICR program). All settings must have a physician immediately available and accessible for medical consultations and emergencies at all times when items/services are being furnished under the program. This provision is satisfied if the physician meets the requirements for direct supervision of physician office services as specified at 42 CFR 410.26, and for hospital outpatient services as specified at 42 CFR 410.27.

ICR Program Approval Requirements:

All prospective ICR programs must be approved through the national coverage determination (NCD) process. To be approved as an ICR program, it must demonstrate through peer-reviewed, published research that it has accomplished one or more of the following for its patients: (i) positively affected the progression of coronary heart disease, (ii) reduced the need for coronary bypass surgery, or, (iii) reduced the need for percutaneous coronary interventions.

An ICR program must also demonstrate through peer-reviewed, published research that it accomplished a statistically significant reduction in five or more of the following measures for patients from their levels before CR services to after CR services: (i) low density lipoprotein, (ii) triglycerides, (iii) body mass index, (iv) systolic blood pressure, (v) diastolic blood pressure, and (vi) the need for cholesterol, blood pressure, and diabetes medications.

A list of approved ICR programs, identified through the NCD process, will be posted to the CMS Web site and listed in the Federal Register.

Once an ICR program is approved through the NCD process, all prospective ICR sites wishing to furnish ICR items/services via an approved ICR program may enroll with their local contractor to become an ICR program supplier using the designated forms as specified at 42 CFR 424.510, and report specialty code 31 to be identified as an enrolled ICR supplier. For purposes of appealing an adverse determination concerning site approval, an ICR site is considered a supplier (or prospective supplier) as defined in 42 CFR 498.2.

CR/ICR Program Physician Requirements:

Physicians responsible for CR/ICR programs are identified as medical directors who oversee or supervise the CR/ICR program at a particular site. The medical director, in consultation with staff, is involved in directing the progress of individuals in the program. The medical director, as well as physicians acting as the supervising physician, must possess all of the following: (1) expertise in the management of individuals with cardiac pathophysiology, (2) cardiopulmonary training in basic life support or advanced cardiac life support, and (3) licensed to practice medicine in the state in which the CR/ICR program is offered. Direct physician supervision may be provided by a supervising physician or the medical director.

(See Pub. 100-3, Medicare National Coverage Determinations Manual, Chapter 1, Part 1, section 20.10.1, Pub. 100-4, Medicare Claims Processing Manual, Chapter 32, section 140, Pub. 100-08, Medicare Program Integrity Manual, Chapter 15, section 15.4.2.8, for specific claims processing, coding, and billing requirements for CR/ICR program services.)

100-2, 15, 240

Chiropractic Services - General

B3-2250, B3-4118

The term "physician" under Part B includes a chiropractor who meets the specified qualifying requirements set forth in Sec.30.5 but only for treatment by means of manual manipulation of the spine to correct a subluxation.

Effective for claims with dates of services on or after January 1, 2000, an x-ray is not required to demonstrate the subluxation.

Implementation of the chiropractic benefit requires an appreciation of the differences between chiropractic theory and experience and traditional medicine due to fundamental differences regarding etiology and theories of the pathogenesis of disease. Judgments about the reasonableness of chiropractic treatment must be based on the application of chiropractic principles. So that Medicare beneficiaries receive equitable adjudication of claims based on such principles and are not deprived of the benefits intended by the law, carriers may use chiropractic consultation in carrier review of Medicare chiropractic claims.

Payment is based on the physician fee schedule and made to the beneficiary or, on assignment, to the chiropractor.

A. Verification of Chiropractor's Qualifications

Carriers must establish a reference file of chiropractors eligible for payment as physicians under the criteria in Sec.30.1. They pay only chiropractors on file. Information needed to establish such files is furnished by the CMS RO.

The RO is notified by the appropriate State agency which chiropractors are licensed and whether each meets the national uniform standards.

100-2, 15, 240.1.3

Necessity for Treatment

The patient must have a significant health problem in the form of a neuromusculoskeletal condition necessitating treatment, and the manipulative services rendered must have a direct therapeutic relationship to the patient's condition and provide reasonable expectation of recovery or improvement of function. The patient must have a subluxation of the spine as demonstrated by x-ray or physical exam, as described above.

Most spinal joint problems fall into the following categories:

* Acute subluxation-A patient's condition is considered acute when the patient is being treated for a new injury, identified by x-ray or physical exam as specified above. The result of chiropractic manipulation is expected to be an improvement in, or arrest of progression, of the patient's condition.

* Chronic subluxation-A patient's condition is considered chronic when it is not expected to significantly improve or be resolved with further treatment (as is the case with an acute condition), but where the continued therapy can be expected to result in some functional improvement. Once the clinical status has remained stable for a given condition, without expectation of additional objective clinical improvements, further manipulative treatment is considered maintenance therapy and is not covered.

For Medicare purposes, a chiropractor must place an AT modifier on a claim when providing active/corrective treatment to treat acute or chronic subluxation. However the presence of the AT modifier may not in all instances indicate that the service is reasonable and necessary. As always, contractors may deny if appropriate after medical review.

A. Maintenance Therapy

Maintenance therapy includes services that seek to prevent disease, promote health and prolong and enhance the quality of life, or maintain or prevent deterioration of a chronic condition. When further clinical improvement cannot reasonably be expected from continuous ongoing care, and the chiropractic treatment becomes supportive rather than corrective in nature, the treatment is then considered maintenance therapy. The AT modifier must not be placed on the claim when maintenance therapy has been provided. Claims without the AT modifier will be considered as maintenance therapy and denied. Chiropractors who give or receive from beneficiaries an ABN shall follow the instructions in Pub. 100-4, Medicare Claims Processing Manual, chapter 23, section 20.9.1.1 and include a GA (or in rare instances a GZ) modifier on the claim.

B. Contraindications

Dynamic thrust is the therapeutic force or maneuver delivered by the physician during manipulation in the anatomic region of involvement. A relative contraindication is a condition that adds significant risk of injury to the patient from dynamic thrust, but does not rule out the use of dynamic thrust. The doctor should discuss this risk with the patient and record this in the chart. The following are relative contraindications to dynamic thrust:

* Articular hyper mobility and circumstances where the stability of the joint is uncertain;

* Severe demineralization of bone;

* Benign bone tumors (spine);

* Bleeding disorders and anticoagulant therapy; and

* Radiculopathy with progressive neurological signs.

* Dynamic thrust is absolutely contraindicated near the site of demonstrated subluxation and proposed manipulation in the following:

* Acute arthropathies characterized by acute inflammation and ligamentous laxity and anatomic subluxation or dislocation; including acute rheumatoid arthritis and ankylosing spondylitis;

* Acute fractures and dislocations or healed fractures and dislocations with signs of instability;

* An unstable os odontoideum;

* Malignancies that involve the vertebral column;

* Infection of bones or joints of the vertebral column;

* Signs and symptoms of myelopathy or cauda equina syndrome;

* For cervical spinal manipulations, vertebrobasilar insufficiency syndrome; and

* A significant major artery aneurysm near the proposed manipulation.

100-2, 15, 270

Telehealth Services

Background

Section 223 of the Medicare, Medicaid and SCHIP Benefits Improvement and Protection Act of 2000 (BIPA) - Revision of Medicare Reimbursement for Telehealth Services amended §1834 of the Act to provide for an expansion of Medicare payment for telehealth services.

Effective October 1, 2001, coverage and payment for Medicare telehealth includes consultation, office visits, individual psychotherapy, and pharmacologic management delivered via a telecommunications system. Eligible geographic areas include rural health professional shortage areas (HPSA) and counties not classified as a metropolitan statistical area (MSA). Additionally, Federal telemedicine demonstration projects as of December 31, 2000, may serve as the originating site regardless of geographic location.

An interactive telecommunications system is required as a condition of payment; however, BIPA does allow the use of asynchronous "store and forward" technology in delivering these services when the originating site is a Federal telemedicine demonstration program in Alaska or Hawaii. BIPA does not require that a practitioner present the patient for interactive telehealth services.

With regard to payment amount, BIPA specified that payment for the professional service performed by the distant site practitioner (i.e., where the expert physician or practitioner is physically located at time of telemedicine encounter) is equal to what would have been paid without the use of telemedicine. Distant site practitioners include only a physician as described in §1861(r) of the Act and a medical practitioner as described in §1842(b)(18)(C) of the Act. BIPA also expanded payment under Medicare to include a $20 originating site facility fee (location of beneficiary).

Previously, the Balanced Budget Act of 1997 (BBA) limited the scope of Medicare telehealth coverage to consultation services and the implementing regulation prohibited the use of an asynchronous 'store and forward' telecommunications system. The BBA of 1997 also required the professional fee to be shared between the referring and consulting practitioners, and prohibited Medicare payment for facility fees and line charges associated with the telemedicine encounter.

The BIPA required that Medicare Part B (Supplementary Medical Insurance) pay for this expansion of telehealth services beginning with services furnished on October 1, 2001.

Section 149 of the Medicare Improvements for Patients and Providers Act of 2008 (MIPPA) amended §1834(m) of the Act to add certain entities as originating sites for payment of telehealth services. Effective for services furnished on or after January 1, 2009, eligible originating sites include a hospital-based or critical access hospital-based renal dialysis center (including satellites); a skilled nursing facility (as defined in §1819(a) of the Act); and a community mental health center (as defined in §1861(ff)(3)(B) of the Act). MIPPA also amended§1888(e)(2)(A)(ii) of the Act to exclude telehealth services furnished under §1834(m)(4)(C)(ii)(VII) from the consolidated billing provisions of the skilled nursing facility prospective payment system (SNF PPS).

NOTE: MIPPA did not add independent renal dialysis facilities as originating sites for payment of telehealth services.

The telehealth provisions authorized by §1834(m) of the Act are implemented in 42 CFR 410.78 and 414.65.

100-2, 15, 270.2
List of Medicare Telehealth Services
The use of a telecommunications system may substitute for an in-person encounter for professional consultations, office visits, office psychiatry services, and a limited number of other physician fee schedule (PFS) services. These services are listed below.

Consultations (Effective October 1, 2001- December 31, 2009)

Telehealth consultations, emergency department or initial inpatient (Effective January 1, 2010)

Follow-up inpatient telehealth consultations (Effective January 1, 2009)

Office or other outpatient visits

Subsequent hospital care services (with the limitation of one telehealth visit every 3 days) (Effective January 1, 2011)

Subsequent nursing facility care services (with the limitation of one telehealth visit every 30 days) (Effective January 1, 2011)

Individual psychotherapy

Pharmacologic management (Effective March 1, 2003)

Psychiatric diagnostic interview examination (Effective March 1, 2003)

End stage renal disease related services (Effective January 1, 2005)

Individual and group medical nutrition therapy (Individual effective January 1, 2006; group effective January 1, 2011)

Neurobehavioral status exam (Effective January 1, 2008)

Individual and group health and behavior assessment and intervention (Individual effective January 1, 2010; group effective January 1, 2011)

Individual and group kidney disease education (KDE) services (Effective January 1, 2011)

Individual and group diabetes self-management training (DSMT) services (with a minimum of 1 hour of in-person instruction to be furnished in the initial year training period to ensure effective injection training) (Effective January 1, 2011)

Smoking Cessation Services (Effective January 1, 2012)

Alcohol and/or substance (other than tobacco) abuse structured assessment and intervention services (Effective January 1, 2013)

Annual alcohol misuse screening (Effective January 1, 2013)

Brief face-to-face behavioral counseling for alcohol misuse (Effective January 1, 2013).

Annual Depression Screening (Effective January 1, 2013)

High-intensity behavioral counseling to prevent sexually transmitted infections (Effective January 1, 2013)

Annual, face-to-face Intensive behavioral therapy for cardiovascular disease (Effective January 1, 2013)

Face-to-face behavioral counseling for obesity (Effective January 1, 2013)

Transitional Care Management Services (Effective January 1, 2014)

NOTE: Beginning January 1, 2010, CMS eliminated the use of all consultation codes, except for inpatient telehealth consultation G-codes. CMS no longer recognizes office/outpatient or inpatient consultation CPT codes for payment of office/outpatient or inpatient visits. Instead, physicians and practitioners are instructed to bill a new or established patient office/outpatient visit CPT code or appropriate hospital or nursing facility care code, as appropriate to the particular patient, for all office/outpatient or inpatient visits. For detailed instructions regarding reporting these and other telehealth services, see Pub. 100-4, Medicare Claims Processing Manual, chapter 12, section 190.3.

The conditions of payment for Medicare telehealth services, including qualifying originating sites and the types of telecommunications systems recognized by Medicare, are subject to the provisions of 42 CFR 410.78. Payment for these services is subject to the provisions of 42 CFR 414.65.

100-2, 15, 270.4
Payment - Physician/Practitioner at a Distant Site
The term "distant site" means the site where the physician or practitioner providing the professional service is located at the time the service is provided via a telecommunications system.

The payment amount for the professional service provided via a telecommunications system by the physician or practitioner at the distant site is equal to the current physician fee schedule amount for the service. For telehealth services (see section 270.2 of this chapter) should be made at the same amount as when these services are furnished without the use of a telecommunications system. For Medicare payment to occur, the service must be within a practitioner's scope of practice under State law. The beneficiary is responsible for any unmet deductible amount and applicable coinsurance.

Medicare Practitioners Who May Receive Payment at the Distant Site (i.e., at a Site Other Than Where the Beneficiary is Located)

As a condition of Medicare Part B payment for telehealth services, the physician or practitioner at the distant site must be licensed to provide the service under State law. When the physician or practitioner at the distant site is licensed under State law to provide a covered telehealth service (see section 270.2 of this chapter) then he or she may bill for and receive payment for this service when delivered via a telecommunications system.

Medicare practitioners who may bill for a covered telehealth service are listed below (subject to State law):

- Physician;
- Nurse practitioner;
- Physician assistant;
- Nurse midwife;
- Clinical nurse specialist;
- Clinical psychologist;
- Clinical social worker; and
- Registered dietitian or nutrition professional.

* Clinical psychologists and clinical social workers cannot bill for psychotherapy services that include medical evaluation and management services under Medicare. These practitioners may not bill or receive payment for the following CPT codes: 90805, 90807, and 90809.

100-2, 15, 290
Foot Care

A. Treatment of Subluxation of Foot

Subluxations of the foot are defined as partial dislocations or displacements of joint surfaces, tendons ligaments, or muscles of the foot. Surgical or nonsurgical treatments undertaken for the sole purpose of correcting a subluxated structure in the foot as an isolated entity are not covered.

However, medical or surgical treatment of subluxation of the ankle joint (talo-crural joint) is covered. In addition, reasonable and necessary medical or surgical services, diagnosis, or treatment for medical conditions that have resulted from or are associated with partial displacement of structures is covered. For example, if a patient has osteoarthritis that has resulted in a partial displacement of joints in the foot, and the primary treatment is for the osteoarthritis, coverage is provided.

B. Exclusions from Coverage

The following foot care services are generally excluded from coverage under both Part A and Part B. (See Sec. 290.F and Sec. 290.G for instructions on applying foot care exclusions.)

1. Treatment of Flat Foot

   The term "flat foot" is defined as a condition in which one or more arches of the foot have flattened out. Services or devices directed toward the care or correction of such conditions, including the prescription of supportive devices, are not covered.

2. Routine Foot Care

   Except as provided above, routine foot care is excluded from coverage. Services that normally are considered routine and not covered by Medicare include the following:

   — The cutting or removal of corns and calluses;

   — The trimming, cutting, clipping, or debriding of nails; and

   — Other hygienic and preventive maintenance care, such as cleaning and soaking the feet, the use of skin creams to maintain skin tone of either ambulatory or bedfast patients, and any other service performed in the absence of localized illness, injury, or symptoms involving the foot.

3. Supportive Devices for Feet Orthopedic shoes and other supportive devices for the feet generally are not covered.

   However, this exclusion does not apply to such a shoe if it is an integral part of a leg brace, and its expense is included as part of the cost of the brace. Also, this exclusion does not apply to therapeutic shoes furnished to diabetics.

C. Exceptions to Routine Foot Care Exclusion

1. Necessary and Integral Part of Otherwise Covered Services

   In certain circumstances, services ordinarily considered to be routine may be covered if they are performed as a necessary and integral part of otherwise covered services, such as diagnosis and treatment of ulcers, wounds, or infections.

2. Treatment of Warts on Foot

   The treatment of warts (including plantar warts) on the foot is covered to the same extent as services provided for the treatment of warts located elsewhere on the body.

3. Presence of Systemic Condition

   The presence of a systemic condition such as metabolic, neurologic, or peripheral vascular disease may require scrupulous foot care by a professional that in the absence of such condition(s) would be considered routine (and, therefore, excluded from coverage). Accordingly, foot care that would otherwise be considered routine may be covered when systemic condition(s) result in severe circulatory embarrassment or areas of diminished sensation in the individual's legs or feet. (See subsection A.)

   In these instances, certain foot care procedures that otherwise are considered routine (e.g., cutting or removing corns and calluses, or trimming, cutting, clipping, or debriding nails) may pose a hazard when performed by a nonprofessional person on patients with such systemic conditions. (See Sec.290.G for procedural instructions.)

4. Mycotic Nails

   In the absence of a systemic condition, treatment of mycotic nails may be covered.

   The treatment of mycotic nails for an ambulatory patient is covered only when the physician attending the patient's mycotic condition documents that (1) there is clinical evidence of mycosis of the toenail, and (2) the patient has marked limitation of ambulation, pain, or secondary infection resulting from the thickening and dystrophy of the infected toenail plate.

   The treatment of mycotic nails for a nonambulatory patient is covered only when the physician attending the patient's mycotic condition documents that (1) there is clinical evidence of mycosis of the toenail, and (2) the patient suffers from pain or secondary infection resulting from the thickening and dystrophy of the infected toenail plate.

   For the purpose of these requirements, documentation means any written information that is required by the carrier in order for services to be covered. Thus, the information submitted with claims must be substantiated by information found in the patient's medical record. Any information, including that contained in a form letter, used for documentation purposes is subject to carrier verification in order to ensure that the information adequately justifies coverage of the treatment of mycotic nails.

D. Systemic Conditions That Might Justify Coverage

Although not intended as a comprehensive list, the following metabolic, neurologic, and peripheral vascular diseases (with synonyms in parentheses) most commonly represent the underlying conditions that might justify coverage for routine foot care.

Diabetes mellitus *

Arteriosclerosis obliterans (A.S.O., arteriosclerosis of the extremities, occlusive peripheral arteriosclerosis)

Buerger's disease (thromboangiitis obliterans)

Chronic thrombophlebitis *

Peripheral neuropathies involving the feet -

— Associated with malnutrition and vitamin deficiency *

    – Malnutrition (general, pellagra)

    – Alcoholism

    – Malabsorption (celiac disease, tropical sprue)

    – Pernicious anemia Associated with carcinoma *

— Associated with diabetes mellitus *

— Associated with drugs and toxins *

— Associated with multiple sclerosis *

— Associated with uremia (chronic renal disease) *

— Associated with traumatic injury

— Associated with leprosy or neurosyphilis

— Associated with hereditary disorders

    – Hereditary sensory radicular neuropathy

    – Angiokeratoma corporis diffusum (Fabry's)

    – Amyloid neuropathy

When the patient's condition is one of those designated by an asterisk (*), routine procedures are covered only if the patient is under the active care of a doctor of medicine or osteopathy who documents the condition.

E. Supportive Devices for Feet Orthopedic shoes and other supportive devices for the feet generally are not covered.

However, this exclusion does not apply to such a shoe if it is an integral part of a leg brace, and its expense is included as part of the cost of the brace. Also, this exclusion does not apply to therapeutic shoes furnished to diabetics.

F. Presumption of Coverage

In evaluating whether the routine services can be reimbursed, a presumption of coverage may be made where the evidence available discloses certain physical and/or clinical findings consistent with the diagnosis and indicative of severe peripheral involvement.

For purposes of applying this presumption the following findings are pertinent:

Class A Findings

Nontraumatic amputation of foot or integral skeletal portion thereof.

Class B Findings

Absent posterior tibial pulse;

Advanced trophic changes as: hair growth (decrease or absence) nail changes (thickening) pigmentary changes (discoloration) skin texture (thin, shiny) skin color (rubor or redness) (Three required); and

Absent dorsalis pedis pulse.

Class C Findings

Claudication;

Temperature changes (e.g., cold feet);

Edema;

Paresthesias (abnormal spontaneous sensations in the feet); and

Burning.

The presumption of coverage may be applied when the physician rendering the routine foot care has identified:

1. A Class A finding;

2. Two of the Class B findings; or

3. One Class B and two Class C findings.

Cases evidencing findings falling short of these alternatives may involve podiatric treatment that may constitute covered care and should be reviewed by the intermediary's medical staff and developed as necessary.

For purposes of applying the coverage presumption where the routine services have been rendered by a podiatrist, the contractor may deem the active care requirement met if the claim or other evidence available discloses that the patient has seen an M.D. or D.O. for treatment and/or evaluation of the complicating disease process during the 6-month period prior to the rendition of the routine-type services. The intermediary may also accept the podiatrist's statement that the diagnosing and treating M.D. or D.O. also concurs with the podiatrist's findings as to the severity of the peripheral involvement indicated.

Services ordinarily considered routine might also be covered if they are performed as a necessary and integral part of otherwise covered services, such as diagnosis and treatment of diabetic ulcers, wounds, and infections.

G. Application of Foot Care Exclusions to Physician's Services

The exclusion of foot care is determined by the nature of the service. Thus, payment for an excluded service should be denied whether performed by a podiatrist, osteopath, or a doctor of medicine, and without regard to the difficulty or complexity of the procedure.

When an itemized bill shows both covered services and noncovered services not integrally related to the covered service, the portion of charges attributable to the noncovered services should be denied. (For example, if an itemized bill shows surgery for an ingrown toenail and also removal of calluses not necessary for the performance of toe surgery, any additional charge attributable to removal of the calluses should be denied.) In reviewing claims involving foot care, the carrier should be alert to the following exceptional situations:

1. Payment may be made for incidental noncovered services performed as a necessary and integral part of, and secondary to, a covered procedure. For example, if trimming of toenails is required for application of a cast to a fractured foot, the carrier need not allocate and deny a portion of the charge for the trimming of the nails. However, a separately itemized charge for such excluded service should be disallowed. When the primary procedure is covered the administration of anesthesia necessary for the performance of such procedure is also covered.

2. Payment may be made for initial diagnostic services performed in connection with a specific symptom or complaint if it seems likely that its treatment would be covered even though the resulting diagnosis may be one requiring only noncovered care.

The name of the M.D. or D.O. who diagnosed the complicating condition must be submitted with the claim. In those cases, where active care is required, the approximate date the beneficiary was last seen by such physician must also be indicated.

NOTE: Section 939 of P.L. 96-499 removed "warts" from the routine foot care exclusion effective July 1, 1981.

Relatively few claims for routine-type care are anticipated considering the severity of conditions contemplated as the basis for this exception. Claims for this type of foot care should not be paid in the absence of convincing evidence that nonprofessional performance of the service would have been hazardous for the beneficiary because of an underlying systemic disease. The mere statement of a diagnosis such as those mentioned in Sec.D above does not of itself indicate the severity of the condition. Where development is indicated to verify diagnosis and/or severity the carrier should follow existing claims processing practices, which may include review of carrier's history and medical consultation as well as physician contacts.

The rules in Sec.290.F concerning presumption of coverage also apply.

Codes and policies for routine foot care and supportive devices for the feet are not exclusively for the use of podiatrists. These codes must be used to report foot care services regardless of the specialty of the physician who furnishes the services. Carriers must instruct physicians to use the most appropriate code available when billing for routine foot care.

100-2, 16, 10

General Exclusions From Coverage

A3-3150, HO-260, HHA-232, B3-2300

No payment can be made under either the hospital insurance or supplementary medicalinsurance program for certain items and services, when the following conditions exist:

- Not reasonable and necessary (§20);
- No legal obligation to pay for or provide (§40);
- Paid for by a governmental entity (§50);
- Not provided within United States (§60);
- Resulting from war (§70);
- Personal comfort (§80);
- Routine services and appliances (§90);
- Custodial care (§110);
- Cosmetic surgery (§120);
- Charges by immediate relatives or members of household (§130);
- Dental services (§140);
- Paid or expected to be paid under workers' compensation (§150);
- Nonphysician services provided to a hospital inpatient that were not provided directly or arranged for by the hospital (§170);
- Services Related to and Required as a Result of Services Which are not Covered Under Medicare (§180);
- Excluded foot care services and supportive devices for feet (§30); or
- Excluded investigational devices (See Chapter 14, §30).

100-2, 16, 100

Hearing Aids and Auditory Implants

Section 1862(a)(7) of the Social Security Act states that no payment may be made under part A or part B for any expenses incurred for items or services "where such expenses are for . . . hearing aids or examinations therefore. . . ." This policy is further reiterated at 42 CFR 411.15(d) which specifically states that "hearing aids or examination for the purpose of prescribing, fitting, or changing hearing aids" are excluded from coverage.

Hearing aids are amplifying devices that compensate for impaired hearing. Hearing aids include air conduction devices that provide acoustic energy to the cochlea via stimulation of the tympanic membrane with amplified sound. They also include bone conduction devices that provide mechanical energy to the cochlea via stimulation of the scalp with amplified mechanical vibration or by direct contact with the tympanic membrane or middle ear ossicles.

Certain devices that produce perception of sound by replacing the function of the middle ear, cochlea or auditory nerve are payable by Medicare as prosthetic devices. These devices are indicated only when hearing aids are medically inappropriate or cannot be utilized due to congenital malformations, chronic disease, severe sensorineural hearing loss or surgery. The following are prosthetic devices:

- Cochlear implants and auditory brainstem implants, i.e., devices that replace the function of cochlear structures or auditory nerve and provide electrical energy to auditory nerve fibers and other neural tissue via implanted electrode arrays.
- Osseointegrated implants, i.e., devices implanted in the skull that replace the function of the middle ear and provide mechanical energy to the cochlea via a mechanical transducer.

Medicare contractors deny payment for an item or service that is associated with any hearing aid as defined above. See Sec.180 for policy for the medically necessary treatment of complications of implantable hearing aids, such as medically necessary removals of implantable hearing aids due to infection.

100-2, 16, 120

Cosmetic Surgery

A3-3160, HO-260.11, B3-2329

Cosmetic surgery or expenses incurred in connection with such surgery is not covered. Cosmetic surgery includes any surgical procedure directed at improving appearance, except when required for the prompt (i.e., as soon as medically feasible) repair of accidental injury or for the improvement of the functioning of a malformed body member. For example, this exclusion does not apply to surgery in connection with treatment of severe burns or repair of the face following a serious automobile accident, or to surgery for therapeutic purposes which coincidentally also serves some cosmetic purpose.

100-2, 16, 180

Services Related to and Required as a Result of Services Which Are Not Covered Under Medicare

B3-2300.1, A3-3101.14, HO-210.12

Medical and hospital services are sometimes required to treat a condition that arises as a result of services that are not covered because they are determined to be not reasonable and necessary or because they are excluded from coverage for other reasons. Services "related to" noncovered services (e.g., cosmetic surgery, noncovered organ transplants, noncovered artificial organ implants, etc.), including services related to follow-up care and complications of noncovered services which require treatment during a hospital stay in which the noncovered service was performed, are not covered services under Medicare. Services "not related to" noncovered services are covered under Medicare. Following are examples of services "related to" and "not related to" noncovered services while the beneficiary is an inpatient:

- A beneficiary was hospitalized for a noncovered service and broke a leg while in the hospital. Services related to care of the broken leg during this stay is a clear example of "not related to" services and are covered under Medicare.
- A beneficiary was admitted to the hospital for covered services, but during the course of hospitalization became a candidate for a noncovered transplant or implant and actually received the transplant or implant during that hospital stay. When the original admission was entirely unrelated to the diagnosis that led to a recommendation for a noncovered transplant or implant, the services related to the admitting condition would be covered.
- A beneficiary was admitted to the hospital for covered services related to a condition which ultimately led to identification of a need for transplant and receipt of a transplant during the same hospital stay. If, on the basis of the nature of the services and a comparison of the date they are received with the date on which the beneficiary is identified as a transplant candidate, the services could reasonably be attributed to preparation for the noncovered transplant, the services would be "related to" noncovered services and would also be noncovered.

Following is an example of services received subsequent to a noncovered inpatient stay:

- After a beneficiary has been discharged from the hospital stay in which the beneficiary received noncovered services, medical and hospital services required to treat a condition or complication that arises as a result of the prior noncovered services may be covered when they are reasonable and necessary in all other respects. Thus, coverage could be provided for subsequent inpatient stays or outpatient treatment ordinarily covered by Medicare, even if the need for treatment arose because of a previous noncovered procedure. Some examples of services that may be found to be covered under this policy are the reversal of intestinal bypass surgery for obesity, repair of complications from transsexual surgery or from cosmetic surgery, removal of a noncovered bladder stimulator, or treatment of any infection at the surgical site of a noncovered transplant that occurred following discharge from the hospital.

However, any subsequent services that could be expected to have been incorporated into a global fee are considered to have been paid in the global fee, and may not be paid again. Thus, where a patient undergoes cosmetic surgery and the treatment regimen calls for a series of postoperative visits to the surgeon for evaluating the patient's progress, these visits are not paid.

100-3, 10.2

NCD for Transcutaneous Electrical Nerve Stimulation (TENS) for Acute Post-Operative Pain (10.2)

Indications and Limitations of Coverage

The use of Transcutaneous Electrical Nerve Stimulation (TENS) for the relief of acute post-operative pain is covered under Medicare. TENS may be covered whether used as an adjunct to the use of drugs, or as an alternative to drugs, in the treatment of acute pain resulting from surgery.

TENS devices, whether durable or disposable, may be used in furnishing this service. When used for the purpose of treating acute post-operative pain, TENS devices are considered supplies. As such they may be hospital supplies furnished inpatients covered under Part A, or supplies incident to a physician's service when furnished in connection with surgery done on an outpatient basis, and covered under Part B.

It is expected that TENS, when used for acute post-operative pain, will be necessary for relatively short periods of time, usually 30 days or less. In cases when TENS is used for longer periods, Medicare Administrative Contractors should attempt to ascertain whether TENS is no longer being used for acute pain but rather for chronic pain, in which case the TENS device may be covered as durable medical equipment as described in §160.27.

Cross-references:

Medicare Benefit Policy Manual, Chapter 1, "Inpatient Hospital Services," §40;

Medicare Benefit Policy Manual, Chapter 2, "Hospital Services Covered Under Part B," §§20, 20.4, and 80; Medicare Benefit Policy Manual, Chapter 15, "Covered Medical and other Health Services, §110."

100-3, 10.3

NCD for Inpatient Hospital Pain Rehabilitation Programs (10.3)

Since pain rehabilitation programs of a lesser scope than that described above would raise a question as to whether the program could be provided in a less intensive setting than on an inpatient hospital basis, carefully evaluate such programs to determine whether the program does, in fact, necessitate a hospital level of care. Some pain rehabilitation programs may utilize services and devices which are excluded from coverage, e.g., acupuncture (see 35-8), biofeedback (see 35-27), dorsal column stimulator (see 65-8), and family counseling services (see 35-I4). In determining whether the scope of a pain program does necessitate inpatient hospital care, evaluate only those services and devices which are covered. Although diagnostic tests may be an appropriate part of pain rehabilitation programs, such tests would be covered in an individual case only where they can be reasonably related to a patient's illness, complaint, symptom, or injury and where they do not represent an unnecessary duplication of tests previously performed.

An inpatient program of 4 weeks' duration is generally required to modify pain behavior. After this period it would be expected that any additional rehabilitation services which might be required could be effectively provided on an outpatient basis under an outpatient pain rehabilitation program (see 10.4 of the NCD Manual) or other outpatient program. The first 7-I0 days of such an inpatient program constitute, in effect, an evaluation period. If a patient is unable to adjust to the program within this period, it is generally concluded that it is unlikely that the program will be effective and the patient is discharged from the program. On occasions a program longer than 4 weeks may be required in a particular case. In such a case there should be documentation to substantiate that inpatient care beyond a 4-week period was reasonable and necessary. Similarly, where it appears that a patient participating in a program is being granted frequent outside passes, a question would exist as to whether an inpatient program is reasonable and necessary for the treatment of the patient's condition.

An inpatient hospital stay for the purpose of participating in a pain rehabilitation program would be covered as reasonable and necessary to the treatment of a patient's condition where the pain is attributable to a physical cause, the usual methods of treatment have not been successful in alleviating it, and a significant loss of ability to function independently has resulted from the pain. Chronic pain patients often have psychological problems which accompany or stem from the physical pain and it is appropriate to include psychological treatment in the multidisciplinary approach. However, patients whose pain symptoms result from a mental condition, rather than from any physical cause, generally cannot be succesfully treated in a pain rehabilitation program.

100-3, 10.4

NCD for Outpatient Hospital Pain Rehabilitation Programs (10.4)

Coverage of services furnished under outpatient hospital pain rehabilitation programs, including services furnished in group settings under individualized plans of treatment, is available if the patient's pain is attributable to a physical cause, the usual methods of treatment have not been successful in alleviating it, and a significant loss of ability by the patient to function independently has resulted from the pain. If a patient meets these conditions and the program provides services of the types discussed in §10.3, the services provided under the program may be covered. Non-covered services (e.g., vocational counseling, meals for outpatients, or acupuncture) continue to be excluded from coverage, and A/B Medicare Administrative Contractors would not be precluded from finding, in the case of particular patients, that the pain rehabilitation program is not reasonable and necessary under §1862(a)(1) of the Social Security Act for the treatment of their conditions.

100-3, 10.5

NCD for Autogenous Epidural Blood Graft (10.5)

Autogenous epidural blood grafts are considered a safe and effective remedy for severe headaches that may occur after performance of spinal anesthesia, spinal taps or myelograms, and are covered.

100-3, 10.6

NCD for Anesthesia in Cardiac Pacemaker Surgery (10.6)

The use of general or monitored anesthesia during transvenous cardiac pacemaker surgery may be reasonable and necessary and therefore covered under Medicare only if adequate documentation of medical necessity is provided on a case-by-case basis. The Medicare Adminstrative Contractor obtains advice from its medical consultants or from appropriate specialty physicians or groups in its locality

regarding the adequacy of documentation before deciding whether a particular claim should be covered.

A second type of pacemaker surgery that is sometimes performed involves the use of the thoracic method of implantation which requires open surgery. Where the thoracic method is employed, general anesthesia is always used and should not require special medical documentation.

100-3, 20.2

NCD for Extracranial-Intracranial (EC-IC) Arterial Bypass Surgery (20.2)

Extracranial-Intracranial (EC-IC) arterial bypass surgery is not a covered procedure when it is performed as a treatment for ischemic cerebrovascular disease of the carotid or middle cerebral arteries which includes the treatment or prevention of strokes. The premise that this procedure which bypasses narrowed arterial segments, improves the blood supply to the brain and reduces the risk of having a stroke has not been demonstrated to be any more effective than no surgical intervention. Accordingly, EC-IC arterial bypass surgery is not considered reasonable and necessary within the meaning of §1862(a)(1) of the Act when it is performed as a treatment for ischemic cerebrovascular disease of the carotid or middle cerebral arteries.

100-3, 20.12

NCD for Diagnostic Endocardial Electrical Stimulation (Pacing) (20.12)

Diagnostic endocardial electrical stimulation (EES), also called programmed electrical stimulation of the heart, is covered under Medicare when used for patients with severe cardiac arrhythmias.

100-3, 20.19

NCD for Ambulatory Blood Pressure Monitoring (20.19)

ABPM must be performed for at least 24 hours to meet coverage criteria.

ABPM is only covered for those patients with suspected white coat hypertension. Suspected white coat hypertension is defined as

1) office blood pressure > 140/90 mm Hg on at least three separate clinic/office visits with two separate measurements made at each visit;

2) at least two documented blood pressure measurements taken outside the office which are < 140/90 mm Hg; and

3) no evidence of end-organ damage.

The information obtained by ABPM is necessary in order to determine the appropriate management of the patient. ABPM is not covered for any other uses. In the rare circumstance that ABPM needs to be performed more than once in a patient, the qualifying criteria described above must be met for each subsequent ABPM test.

For those patients that undergo ABPM and have an ambulatory blood pressure of < 135/85 with no evidence of end-organ damage, it is likely that their cardiovascular risk is similar to that of normotensives. They should be followed over time. Patients for which ABPM demonstrates a blood pressure of > 135/85 may be at increased cardiovascular risk, and a physician may wish to consider antihypertensive therapy.

100-3, 20.26

NCD for Partial Ventriculectomy (20.26)

Since the mortality rate is high and there are no published scientific articles or clinical studies regarding partial ventriculectomy, this procedure cannot be considered reasonable and necessary within the meaning of Sec.1862(a)(1) of the Act. Therefore, partial ventriculectomy is not covered by Medicare.

100-3, 20.28

NCD for Therapeutic Embolization (20.28)

Therapeutic embolization is covered when done for hemorrhage, and for other conditions amenable to treatment by the procedure, when reasonable and necessary for the individual patient. Renal embolization for the treatment of renal adenocarcinoma continues to be covered, effective December 15, 1978, as one type of therapeutic embolization, to:

- Reduce tumor vascularity preoperatively;

- Reduce tumor bulk in inoperable cases; or

- Palliate specific symptoms.

100-3, 20.29

NCD for Hyperbaric Oxygen Therapy (20.29)

A. Covered Conditions

Program reimbursement for HBO therapy will be limited to that which is administered in a chamber (including the one man unit) and is limited to the following conditions:

1. Acute carbon monoxide intoxication,

2. Decompression illness,

3. Gas embolism,

4. Gas gangrene,

5. Acute traumatic peripheral ischemia. HBO therapy is a valuable adjunctive treatment to be used in combination with accepted standard therapeutic measures when loss of function, limb, or life is threatened.

6. Crush injuries and suturing of severed limbs. As in the previous conditions, HBO therapy would be an adjunctive treatment when loss of function, limb, or life is threatened.

7. Progressive necrotizing infections (necrotizing fasciitis),

8. Acute peripheral arterial insufficiency,

9. Preparation and preservation of compromised skin grafts (not for primary management of wounds),

10. Chronic refractory osteomyelitis, unresponsive to conventional medical and surgical management,

11. Osteoradionecrosis as an adjunct to conventional treatment,

12. Soft tissue radionecrosis as an adjunct to conventional treatment,

13. Cyanide poisoning,

14. Actinomycosis, only as an adjunct to conventional therapy when the disease process is refractory to antibiotics and surgical treatment,

14. Diabetic wounds of the lower extremities in patients who meet the following three criteria:

   a. Patient has type I or type II diabetes and has a lower extremity wound that is due to diabetes;

   b. Patient has a wound classified as Wagner grade III or higher; and

   c. Patient has failed an adequate course of standard wound therapy.

The use of HBO therapy is covered as adjunctive therapy only after there are no measurable signs of healing for at least 30 -days of treatment with standard wound therapy and must be used in addition to standard wound care. Standard wound care in patients with diabetic wounds includes: assessment of a patient's vascular status and correction of any vascular problems in the affected limb if possible, optimization of nutritional status, optimization of glucose control, debridement by any means to remove devitalized tissue, maintenance of a clean, moist bed of granulation tissue with appropriate moist dressings, appropriate off-loading, and necessary treatment to resolve any infection that might be present. Failure to respond to standard wound care occurs when there are no measurable signs of healing for at least 30 consecutive days. Wounds must be evaluated at least every 30 days during administration of HBO therapy. Continued treatment with HBO therapy is not covered if measurable signs of healing have not been demonstrated within any 30-day period of treatment.

B. Noncovered Conditions

All other indications not specified under Sec.270.4(A) are not covered under the Medicare program. No program payment may be made for any conditions other than those listed in Sec. 270.4(A).

No program payment may be made for HBO in the treatment of the following conditions:

1. Cutaneous, decubitus, and stasis ulcers.

2. Chronic peripheral vascular insufficiency.

3. Anaerobic septicemia and infection other than clostridial.

4. Skin burns (thermal).

5. Senility.

6. Myocardial infarction.

7. Cardiogenic shock.

8. Sickle cell anemia.

9. Acute thermal and chemical pulmonary damage, i.e., smoke inhalation with pulmonary insufficiency.

10. Acute or chronic cerebral vascular insufficiency.

11. Hepatic necrosis.

12. Aerobic septicemia.

13. Nonvascular causes of chronic brain syndrome (Pick's disease, Alzheimer's disease, Korsakoff's disease).

14. Tetanus.

15. Systemic aerobic infection.

16. Organ transplantation.

17. Organ storage.

18. Pulmonary emphysema.

19. Exceptional blood loss anemia.

20. Multiple Sclerosis.

21. Arthritic Diseases.

22. Acute cerebral edema.

C. Topical Application of Oxygen

This method of administering oxygen does not meet the definition of HBO therapy as stated above. Also, its clinical efficacy has not been established. Therefore, no Medicare reimbursement may be made for the topical application of oxygen.

100-3, 20.30

NCD for Microvolt T-Wave Alternans (MTWA) (20.30)

B. Nationally Covered Indications

Microvolt T-wave Alternans diagnostic testing is covered for the evaluation of patients at risk for SCD, only when the spectral analysis method is used.

C. Nationally Non-Covered Indications

Microvolt T-wave Alternans diagnostic test is non-covered for the evaluation of patients at risk for SCD if measurement is not performed employing the spectral analysis.

D. Other

N/A

100-3, 20.32

Transcatheter Aortic Valve Replacement (TAVR)

A. General

Transcatheter aortic valve replacement (TAVR - also known as TAVI or transcatheter aortic valve implantation) is used in the treatment of aortic stenosis. A bioprosthetic valve is inserted percutaneously using a catheter and implanted in the orifice of the aortic valve.

B. Nationally Covered Indications

The Centers for Medicare & Medicaid Services (CMS) covers transcatheter aortic valve replacement (TAVR) under Coverage with Evidence Development (CED) with the following conditions:

A. TAVR is covered for the treatment of symptomatic aortic valve stenosis when furnished according to a Food and Drug Administration (FDA)-approved indication and when all of the following conditions are met:

1. The procedure is furnished with a complete aortic valve and implantation system that has received FDA premarket approval (PMA) for that system's FDA approved indication.

2. Two cardiac surgeons have independently examined the patient face-to-face and evaluated the patient's suitability for open aortic valve replacement (AVR) surgery; and both surgeons have documented the rationale for their clinical judgment and the rationale is available to the heart team.

3. The patient (preoperatively and postoperatively) is under the care of a heart team: a cohesive, multi-disciplinary, team of medical professionals. The heart team concept embodies collaboration and dedication across medical specialties to offer optimal patient-centered care.

   TAVR must be furnished in a hospital with the appropriate infrastructure that includes but is not limited to:

   a. On-site heart valve surgery program,

   b. Cardiac catheterization lab or hybrid operating room/catheterization lab equipped with a fixed radiographic imaging system with flat-panel fluoroscopy, offering quality imaging,

   c. Non-invasive imaging such as echocardiography, vascular ultrasound, computed tomography (CT) and magnetic resonance (MR),

   d. Sufficient space, in a sterile environment, to accommodate necessary equipment for cases with and without complications,

   e. Post-procedure intensive care facility with personnel experienced in managing patients who have undergone open-heart valve procedures,

   f. Appropriate volume requirements per the applicable qualifications below.

There are two sets of qualifications; the first set outlined below is for hospital programs and heart teams without previous TAVR experience and the second set is for those with TAVR experience.

Qualifications to begin a TAVR program for hospitals without TAVR experience:

The hospital program must have the following:

   a. ≥ 50 total AVRs in the previous year prior to TAVR, including = 10 high-risk patients, and;

   b. ≥ 2 physicians with cardiac surgery privileges, and;

   c. ≥ 1000 catheterizations per year, including = 400 percutaneous coronary interventions (PCIs) per year.

Qualifications to begin a TAVR program for heart teams without TAVR experience:

The heart team must include:

   a. Cardiovascular surgeon with:

      i. ≥ 100 career AVRs including 10 high-risk patients; or,

ii. ≥ 25 AVRs in one year; or,

iii. ≥ 50 AVRs in 2 years; and which include at least 20 AVRs in the last year prior to TAVR initiation; and,

  b. Interventional cardiologist with:

    i. Professional experience with 100 structural heart disease procedures lifetime; or,

    ii. 30 left-sided structural procedures per year of which 60% should be balloon aortic valvuloplasty (BAV). Atrial septal defect and patent foramen ovale closure are not considered left-sided procedures; and,

  c. Additional members of the heart team such as echocardiographers, imaging specialists, heart failure specialists, cardiac anesthesiologists, intensivists, nurses, and social workers; and,

  d. Device-specific training as required by the manufacturer.

Qualifications for hospital programs with TAVR experience:

The hospital program must maintain the following:

  a. ≥ 20 AVRs per year or = 40 AVRs every 2 years; and,

  b. ≥ 2 physicians with cardiac surgery privileges; and,

  c. ≥ 1000 catheterizations per year, including = 400 percutaneous coronary interventions (PCIs) per year.

Qualifications for heart teams with TAVR experience:

The heart team must include:

  a. cardiovascular surgeon and an interventional cardiologist whose combined experience maintains the following:

    i. ≥ 20 TAVR procedures in the prior year, or,

    ii. ≥ 40 TAVR procedures in the prior 2 years; and,

  b. Additional members of the heart team such as echocardiographers, imaging specialists, heart failure specialists, cardiac anesthesiologists, intensivists, nurses, and social workers.

4. The heart team's interventional cardiologist(s) and cardiac surgeon(s) must jointly participate in the intra-operative technical aspects of TAVR.

5. The heart team and hospital are participating in a prospective, national, audited registry that: 1) consecutively enrolls TAVR patients; 2) accepts all manufactured devices; 3) follows the patient for at least one year; and, 4) complies with relevant regulations relating to protecting human research subjects, including 45 CFR Part 46 and 21 CFR Parts 50 & 56. The following outcomes must be tracked by the registry; and the registry must be designed to permit identification and analysis of patient, practitioner and facility level variables that predict each of these outcomes:

  i. Stroke;

  ii. All cause mortality;

  iii. Transient Ischemic Attacks (TIAs);

  iv. Major vascular events;

  v. Acute kidney injury;

  vi. Repeat aortic valve procedures;

  vii. Quality of Life (QoL).

The registry should collect all data necessary and have a written executable analysis plan in place to address the following questions (to appropriately address some questions, Medicare claims or other outside data may be necessary):

– When performed outside a controlled clinical study, how do outcomes and adverse events compare to the pivotal clinical studies?

– How do outcomes and adverse events in subpopulations compare to patients in the pivotal clinical studies?

– What is the long term (≥ 5 year) durability of the device?

– What are the long term (≥ 5 year) outcomes and adverse events?

– How do the demographics of registry patients compare to the pivotal studies?

Consistent with section 1142 of the Act, the Agency for Healthcare Research and Quality (AHRQ) supports clinical research studies that CMS determines meet the above-listed standards and address the above-listed research questions.

B. TAVR is covered for uses that are not expressly listed as an FDA-approved indication when performed within a clinical study that fulfills all of the following.

1. The heart team's interventional cardiologist(s) and cardiac surgeon(s) must jointly participate in the intra-operative technical aspects of TAVR.

2. As a fully-described, written part of its protocol, the clinical research study must critically evaluate not only each patient's quality of life pre- and post-TAVR (minimum of 1 year), but must also address at least one of the following questions: § What is the incidence of stroke?

– What is the rate of all cause mortality?

– What is the incidence of transient ischemic attacks (TIAs)?

– What is the incidence of major vascular events?

– What is the incidence of acute kidney injury?

– What is the incidence of repeat aortic valve procedures?

3. The clinical study must adhere to the following standards of scientific integrity and relevance to the Medicare population:

  a. The principal purpose of the research study is to test whether a particular intervention potentially improves the participants' health outcomes.

  b. The research study is well supported by available scientific and medical information or it is intended to clarify or establish the health outcomes of interventions already in common clinical use.

  c. The research study does not unjustifiably duplicate existing studies.

  d. The research study design is appropriate to answer the research question being asked in the study.

  e. The research study is sponsored by an organization or individual capable of executing the proposed study successfully.

  f. The research study is in compliance with all applicable Federal regulations concerning the protection of human subjects found in the Code of Federal Regulations (CFR) at 45 CFR Part 46. If a study is regulated by the Food and Drug Administration (FDA), it also must be in compliance with 21 CFR Parts 50 and 56. In particular, the informed consent includes a straightforward explanation of the reported increased risks of stroke and vascular complications that have been published for TAVR.

  g. All aspects of the research study are conducted according to appropriate standards of scientific integrity (see http://www.icmje.org).

  h. The research study has a written protocol that clearly addresses, or incorporates by reference, the standards listed as Medicare coverage requirements.

  i. The clinical research study is not designed to exclusively test toxicity or disease pathophysiology in healthy individuals. Trials of all medical technologies measuring therapeutic outcomes as one of the objectives meet this standard only if the disease or condition being studied is life threatening as defined in 21 CFR §312.81(a) and the patient has no other viable treatment options.

  j. The clinical research study is registered on the www.ClinicalTrials.gov website by the principal sponsor/investigator prior to the enrollment of the first study subject.

  k. The research study protocol specifies the method and timing of public release of all pre-specified outcomes to be measured including release of outcomes if outcomes are negative or study is terminated early. The results must be made public within 24 months of the end of data collection. If a report is planned to be published in a peer reviewed journal, then that initial release may be an abstract that meets the requirements of the International Committee of Medical Journal Editors (http://www.icmje.org). However a full report of the outcomes must be made public no later than three (3) years after the end of data collection.

  l. The research study protocol must explicitly discuss subpopulations affected by the treatment under investigation, particularly traditionally underrepresented groups in clinical studies, how the inclusion and exclusion criteria affect enrollment of these populations, and a plan for the retention and reporting of said populations on the trial. If the inclusion and exclusion criteria are expected to have a negative effect on the recruitment or retention of underrepresented populations, the protocol must discuss why these criteria are necessary.

  m. The research study protocol explicitly discusses how the results are or are not expected to be generalizable to the Medicare population to infer whether Medicare patients may benefit from the intervention. Separate discussions in the protocol may be necessary for populations eligible for Medicare due to age, disability or Medicaid eligibility. Consistent with section 1142 of the Act, AHRQ supports clinical research studies that CMS determines meet the above-listed standards and address the above-listed research questions.

4. The principal investigator must submit the complete study protocol, identify the relevant CMS research question(s) that will be addressed, and cite the location of the detailed analysis plan for those questions in the protocol, plus provide a statement addressing how the study satisfies each of the standards of scientific integrity (a. through m. listed above), as well as the investigator's contact information, to the address below. The information will be reviewed, and approved studies will be identified on the CMS Website.

  Director, Coverage and Analysis Group
  Re: TAVR CED
  Centers for Medicare & Medicaid Services (CMS)
  7500 Security Blvd., Mail Stop S3-02-01
  Baltimore, MD 21244-1850

C. Nationally Non-Covered Indications

TAVR is not covered for patients in whom existing co-morbidities would preclude the expected benefit from correction of the aortic stenosis.

D.

NA

(This NCD last reviewed May 2012.)

100-3, 20.9

Artificial Hearts and Related Devices (Various Effective Dates Below)

A. General

An artificial heart is a biventricular replacement device which requires removal of a substantial part of the native heart, including both ventricles. Removal of this device is not compatible with life, unless the patient has a heart transplant.

B. Nationally Covered Indications

1. Bridge-to-transplant (BTT) (effective for services performed on or after May 1, 2008)

   An artificial heart for bridge-to-transplantation (BTT) is covered when performed under coverage with evidence development (CED) when a clinical study meets all of the criteria listed below. The clinical study must address at least one of the following questions:

   — Were there unique circumstances such as expertise available in a particular facility or an unusual combination of conditions in particular patients that affected their outcomes?

   — What will be the average time to device failure when the device is made available to larger numbers of patients?

   — Do results adequately give a reasonable indication of the full range of outcomes (both positive and negative) that might be expected from more widespread use?

   The clinical study must meet all of the criteria stated in Section D of this policy. The above information should be mailed to: Director, Coverage and Analysis Group, Centers for Medicare & Medicaid Services (CMS), Re: Artificial Heart, Mailstop S3-02-01, 7500 Security Blvd, Baltimore, MD 21244-1850.

   Clinical studies that are determined by CMS to meet the above requirements will be listed on the CMS Web site at: http://www.cms.gov/Medicare/Coverage/Coverage-with-Evidence-Development /Artificial-Hearts.html.

2. Destination therapy (DT) (effective for services performed on or after May 1, 2008)

   An artificial heart for destination therapy (DT) is covered when performed under CED when a clinical study meets all of the criteria listed below. The clinical study must address at least one of the following questions:

   — Were there unique circumstances such as expertise available in a particular facility or an unusual combination of conditions in particular patients that affected their outcomes?

   — What will be the average time to device failure when the device is made available to larger numbers of patients?

   — Do results adequately give a reasonable indication of the full range of outcomes (both positive and negative) that might be expected from more widespread use?

   The clinical study must meet all of the criteria stated in Section D of this policy. The above information should be mailed to: Director, Coverage and Analysis Group, Centers for Medicare & Medicaid Services, Re: Artificial Heart, Mailstop S3-02-01, 7500 Security Blvd, Baltimore, MD 21244-1850.

   Clinical studies that are determined by CMS to meet the above requirements will be listed on the CMS Web site at: http://www.cms.gov/Medicare/Coverage/Coverage-with-Evidence-Development/Ar tificial-Hearts.html.

C. Nationally Non-Covered Indications

All other indications for the use of artificial hearts not otherwise listed remain non-covered, except in the context of Category B investigational device exemption clinical trials (42 CFR 405) or as a routine cost in clinical trials defined under section 310.1 of the National Coverage Determinations (NCD) Manual.

D. Other

Clinical study criteria:

- The study must be reviewed and approved by the Food and Drug Administration (FDA).

- The principal purpose of the research study is to test whether a particular intervention potentially improves the participants' health outcomes.

- The research study is well supported by available scientific and medical information, or it is intended to clarify or establish the health outcomes of interventions already in common clinical use.

- The research study does not unjustifiably duplicate existing studies.

- The research study design is appropriate to answer the research question being asked in the study.

- The research study is sponsored by an organization or individual capable of executing the proposed study successfully.

- The research study is in compliance with all applicable Federal regulations concerning the protection of human subjects found at 45 CFR Part 46. If a study is FDA-regulated it also must be in compliance with 21 CFR Parts 50 and 56.

- All aspects of the research study are conducted according to appropriate standards of scientific integrity (see http://www.icmje.org).

- The research study has a written protocol that clearly addresses, or incorporates by reference, the standards listed here as Medicare requirements for CED.

- The clinical research study is not designed to exclusively test toxicity or disease pathophysiology in healthy individuals. Trials of all medical technologies measuring therapeutic outcomes as one of the objectives meet this standard only if the disease or condition being studied is life threatening as defined in 21 CFR §312.81(a) and the patient has no other viable treatment options.

- The clinical research study is registered on the www.ClinicalTrials.gov Web site by the principal sponsor/investigator as demonstrated by having a Clinicaltrials.gov Identifier.

- The research study protocol specifies the method and timing of public release of all pre-specified outcomes to be measured including release of outcomes if outcomes are negative or study is terminated early. The results must be made public within 24 months of the end of data collection. If a report is planned to be published in a peer-reviewed journal, then that initial release may be an abstract that meets the requirements of the International Committee of Medical Journal Editors (ICMJE) (http://www.icmje.org). However a full report of the outcomes must be made public no later than three (3) years after the end of data collection.

- The research study protocol must explicitly discuss subpopulations affected by the treatment under investigation, particularly traditionally under-represented groups in clinical studies, how the inclusion and exclusion criteria effect enrollment of these populations, and a plan for the retention and reporting of said populations in the trial. If the inclusion and exclusion criteria are expected to have a negative effect on the recruitment or retention of under-represented populations, the protocol must discuss why these criteria are necessary.

- The research study protocol explicitly discusses how the results are or are not expected to be generalizable to the Medicare population to infer whether Medicare patients may benefit from the intervention. Separate discussions in the protocol may be necessary for populations eligible for Medicare due to age, disability, or Medicaid eligibility.

Consistent with section 1142 of the Social Security Act (the Act), the Agency for Healthcare Research and Quality (AHRQ) supports clinical research studies that CMS determines meet the above-listed standards and address the above-listed research questions.

The principal investigator of an artificial heart clinical study seeking Medicare payment should submit the following documentation to CMS and should expect to be notified when the CMS review is complete:

- Complete study protocol (must be dated or identified with a version number);

- Protocol summary;

- Statement that the submitted protocol version has been agreed upon by the FDA;

- Statement that the above study standards are met;

- Statement that the study addresses at least one of the above questions related to artificial hearts;

- Complete contact information (phone number, email address, and mailing address); and,

- Clinicaltrials.gov Identifier.

100-3, 20.9.1

Ventricular Assist Devices (Various Effective Dates Below)

A. General

A ventricular assist device (VAD) is surgically attached to one or both intact ventricles and is used to assist or augment the ability of a damaged or weakened native heart to pump blood. Improvement in the performance of the native heart may allow the device to be removed.

B. Nationally Covered Indications

1. Post-cardiotomy (effective for services performed on or after October 18, 1993) Post-cardiotomy is the period following open-heart surgery. VADs used for support of blood circulation post-cardiotomy are covered only if they have received approval from the Food and Drug Administration (FDA) for that purpose, and the VADs are used according to the FDA-approved labeling instructions.

2. Bridge-to-Transplant (effective for services performed on or after January 22, 1996)

   The VADs used for bridge to transplant are covered only if they have received approval from the FDA for that purpose, and the VADs are used according to FDA-approved labeling instructions. All of the following criteria must be fulfilled in order for Medicare coverage to be provided for a VAD used as a bridge to transplant:

   — The patient is approved for heart transplantation by a Medicare-approved heart transplant center and is active on the Organ Procurement and Transplantation Network (OPTN) heart transplant waitlist.

— The implanting site, if different than the Medicare-approved transplant center, must receive written permission from the Medicare-approved transplant center under which the patient is listed prior to implantation of the VAD.

3. Destination Therapy (DT) (effective for services performed on or after October 1, 2003)

Destination therapy (DT) is for patients that require mechanical cardiac support. The VADs used for DT are covered only if they have received approval from the FDA for that purpose.

Patient Selection (effective November 9, 2010):

The VADs are covered for patients who have chronic end-stage heart failure (New York Heart Association Class IV end-stage left ventricular failure) who are not candidates for heart transplantation at the time of VAD implant, and meet the following conditions:Have failed to respond to optimal medical management (including beta-blockers and ACE inhibitors if tolerated) for 45 of the last 60 days, or have been balloon pump-dependent for 7 days, or IV inotrope-dependent for 14 days; and,

— Have a left ventricular ejection fraction (LVEF) <25%; and,

— Have demonstrated functional limitation with a peak oxygen consumption of =14 ml/kg/min unless balloon pump- or inotrope-dependent or physically unable to perform the test. Facility Criteria (effective October 30, 2013):

Facilities currently credentialed by the Joint Commission for placement of VADs as DT may continue as Medicare-approved facilities until October 30, 2014. At the conclusion of this transition period, these facilities must be in compliance with the following criteria as determined by a credentialing organization. As of the effective date, new facilities must meet the following criteria as a condition of coverage of this procedure as DT under section 1862(a)(1)(A) of the Social Security Act (the Act):

Beneficiaries receiving VADs for DT must be managed by an explicitly identified cohesive, multidisciplinary team of medical professionals with the appropriate qualifications, training, and experience. The team embodies collaboration and dedication across medical specialties to offer optimal patient-centered care. Collectively, the team must ensure that patients and caregivers have the knowledge and support necessary to participate in shared decision making and to provide appropriate informed consent. The team members must be based at the facility and must include individuals with experience working with patients before and after placement of a VAD.

The team must include, at a minimum:

– At least one physician with cardiothoracic surgery privileges and individual experience implanting at least 10 durable, intracorporeal, left VADs as BTT or DT over the course of the previous 36 months with activity in the last year.

– At least one cardiologist trained in advanced heart failure with clinical competence in medical and device-based management including VADs, and clinical competence in the management of patients before and after heart transplant.

– A VAD program coordinator.

– A social worker.

– A palliative care specialist. Facilities must be credentialed by an organization approved by the Centers for Medicare & Medicaid Services.

C. Nationally Non-Covered Indications

All other indications for the use of VADs not otherwise listed remain non-covered, except in the context of Category B investigational device exemption clinical trials (42 CFR 405) or as a routine cost in clinical trials defined under section 310.1 of the National Coverage Determinations (NCD) Manual.

D. Other

This policy does not address coverage of VADs for right ventricular support, biventricular support, use in beneficiaries under the age of 18, use in beneficiaries with complex congenital heart disease, or use in beneficiaries with acute heart failure without a history of chronic heart failure. Coverage under section 1862(a)(1)(A) of the Act for VADs in these situations will be made by local Medicare Administrative Contractors within their respective jurisdictions.

100-3, 30.3

NCD for Acupuncture (30.3)

Although acupuncture has been used for thousands of years in China and for decades in parts of Europe, it is a new agent of unknown use and efficacy in the United States. Even in those areas of the world where it has been widely used, its mechanism is not known. Three units of the National Institutes of Health, the National Institute of General Medical Sciences, National Institute of Neurological Diseases and Stroke, and Fogarty International Center have been designed to assess and identify specific opportunities and needs for research attending the use of acupuncture for surgical anesthesia and relief of chronic pain. Until the pending scientific assessment of the technique has been completed and its efficacy has been established, Medicare reimbursement for acupuncture, as an anesthetic or as an analgesic or for other therapeutic purposes, may not be made. Accordingly, acupuncture is not considered reasonable and necessary within the meaning of §1862(a)(1) of the Act.

100-3, 30.3.1

NCD for Acupuncture for Fibromyalgia (30.3.1)

General

Although acupuncture has been used for thousands of years in China and for decades in parts of Europe, it is still a relatively new agent of unknown use and efficacy in the United States. Even in those areas of the world where it has been widely used, its mechanism is not known. Three units of the National Institutes of Health, the National Institute of General Medical Sciences, National Institute of Neurological Diseases and Stroke, and Fogarty International Center were designated to assess and identify specific opportunities and needs for research attending the use of acupuncture for surgical anesthesia and relief of chronic pain. Following thorough review, and pending completion of the scientific assessment and efficacy of the technique, CMS initially issued a national noncoverage determination for acupuncture in May 1980.

Nationally Covered Indications

Not applicable.

Nationally Noncovered Indications

After careful reconsideration of its initial noncoverage determination for acupuncture, CMS concludes that there is no convincing evidence for the use of acupuncture for pain relief in patients with fibromyalgia. Study design flaws presently prohibit assessing acupuncture's utility for improving health outcomes. Accordingly, CMS determines that acupuncture is not considered reasonable and necessary for the treatment of fibromyalgia within the meaning of §1862(a)(1) of the Social Security Act, and the national noncoverage determination for acupuncture continues.

(This NCD last reviewed April 2004.)

100-3, 30.3.2

NCD for Acupuncture for Osteoarthritis (30.3.2)

General

Although acupuncture has been used for thousands of years in China and for decades in parts of Europe, it is still a relatively new agent of unknown use and efficacy in the United States. Even in those areas of the world where it has been widely used, its mechanism is not known. Three units of the National Institutes of Health, the National Institute of General Medical Sciences, National Institute of Neurological Diseases and Stroke, and Fogarty International Center were designated to assess and identify specific opportunities and needs for research attending the use of acupuncture for surgical anesthesia and relief of chronic pain. Following thorough review, and pending completion of the scientific assessment and efficacy of the technique, CMS initially issued a national noncoverage determination for acupuncture in May 1980.

Nationally Covered Indications

Not applicable.

Nationally Noncovered Indications

After careful reconsideration of its initial noncoverage determination for acupuncture, CMS concludes that there is no convincing evidence for the use of acupuncture for pain relief in patients with osteoarthritis. Study design flaws presently prohibit assessing acupuncture's utility for improving health outcomes. Accordingly, CMS determines that acupuncture is not considered reasonable and necessary for the treatment of osteoarthritis within the meaning of §1862(a)(1) of the Social Security Act, and the national noncoverage determination for acupuncture continues.

(This NCD last reviewed April 2004.)

100-3, 80.7

NCD for Refractive Keratoplasty (80.7)

The correction of common refractive errors by eyeglasses, contact lenses or other prosthetic devices is specifically excluded from coverage. The use of radial keratotomy and/or keratoplasty for the purpose of refractive error compensation is considered a substitute or alternative to eye glasses or contact lenses, which are specifically excluded by Sec.1862(a)(7) of the Act (except in certain cases in connection with cataract surgery). In addition, many in the medical community consider such procedures cosmetic surgery, which is excluded by section Sec.1862(a)(10) of the Act. Therefore, radial keratotomy and keratoplasty to treat refractive defects are not covered.

Keratoplasty that treats specific lesions of the cornea, such as phototherapeutic keratectomy that removes scar tissue from the visual field, deals with an abnormality of the eye and is not cosmetic surgery. Such cases may be covered under Sec.1862(a)(1)(A) of the Act.

The use of lasers to treat ophthalmic disease constitutes opthalmalogic surgery. Coverage is restricted to practitioners who have completed an approved training program in ophthalmologic surgery.

100-3, 80.10

NCD for Phaco-Emulsification procedure - cataract extraction (80.10)

In view of recommendations of authoritative sources in the field of ophthalmology, the subject technique is viewed as an accepted procedure for removal of cataracts. Accordingly, program reimbursement may be made for necessary services furnished in connection with cataract extraction utilizing the phaco-emulsification procedure.

100-3, 80.12

NCD for Intraocular Lenses (IOLs) (80.12)

Intraocular lens implantation services, as well as the lens itself, may be covered if reasonable and necessary for the individual. Implantation services may include hospital, surgical, and other medical services, including pre-implantation ultrasound (A-scan) eye measurement of one or both eyes.

100-3, 100.1

100.1 - Bariatric Surgery for Treatment of Co-Morbid Conditions Related to Morbid Obesity

Please note, sections 40.5, 100.8, 100.11, and 100.14 have been removed from the National Coverage Determination (NCD) Manual and incorporated into NCD 100.1.

A. General

Obesity may be caused by medical conditions such as hypothyroidism, Cushing's disease, and hypothalamic lesions, or can aggravate a number of cardiac and respiratory diseases as well as diabetes and hypertension. Non-surgical services in connection with the treatment of obesity are covered when such services are an integral and necessary part of a course of treatment for one of these medical conditions.

In addition, supplemented fasting is a type of very low calorie weight reduction regimen used to achieve rapid weight loss. The reduced calorie intake is supplemented by a mixture of protein, carbohydrates, vitamins, and minerals. Serious questions exist about the safety of prolonged adherence for 2 months or more to a very low calorie weight reduction regimen as a general treatment for obesity, because of instances of cardiopathology and sudden death, as well as possible loss of body protein.

Bariatric surgery procedures are performed to treat comorbid conditions associated with morbid obesity. Two types of surgical procedures are employed. Malabsorptive procedures divert food from the stomach to a lower part of the digestive tract where the normal mixing of digestive fluids and absorption of nutrients cannot occur. Restrictive procedures restrict the size of the stomach and decrease intake. Surgery can combine both types of procedures.

The following are descriptions of bariatric surgery procedures:

1. Roux-en-Y Gastric Bypass (RYGBP)

   The RYGBP achieves weight loss by gastric restriction and malabsorption. Reduction of the stomach to a small gastric pouch (30 cc) results in feelings of satiety following even small meals. This small pouch is connected to a segment of the jejunum, bypassing the duodenum and very proximal small intestine, thereby reducing absorption. RYGBP procedures can be open or laparoscopic.

2. Biliopancreatic Diversion with Duodenal Switch (BPD/DS) or Gastric Reduction Duodenal Switch (BPD/GRDS)

   The BPD achieves weight loss by gastric restriction and malabsorption. The stomach is partially resected, but the remaining capacity is generous compared to that achieved with RYGBP. As such, patients eat relatively normal-sized meals and do not need to restrict intake radically, since the most proximal areas of the small intestine (i.e., the duodenum and jejunum) are bypassed, and substantial malabsorption occurs. The partial BPD/DS or BPD/GRDS is a variant of the BPD procedure. It involves resection of the greater curvature of the stomach, preservation of the pyloric sphincter, and transection of the duodenum above the ampulla of Vater with a duodeno-ileal anastomosis and a lower ileo-ileal anastomosis. BPD/DS or BPD/GRDS procedures can be open or laparoscopic.

3. Adjustable Gastric Banding (AGB)

   The AGB achieves weight loss by gastric restriction only. A band creating a gastric pouch with a capacity of approximately 15 to 30 cc's encircles the uppermost portion of the stomach. The band is an inflatable doughnut-shaped balloon, the diameter of which can be adjusted in the clinic by adding or removing saline via a port that is positioned beneath the skin. The bands are adjustable, allowing the size of the gastric outlet to be modified as needed, depending on the rate of a patient's weight loss. AGB procedures are laparoscopic only.

4. Sleeve Gastrectomy

   Sleeve gastrectomy is a 70%-80% greater curvature gastrectomy (sleeve resection of the stomach) with continuity of the gastric lesser curve being maintained while simultaneously reducing stomach volume. In the past, sleeve gastrectomy was the first step in a two-stage procedure when performing RYGBP, but more recently has been offered as a stand-alone surgery. Sleeve gastrectomy procedures can be open or laparoscopic.

5. Vertical Gastric Banding (VGB)

The VGB achieves weight loss by gastric restriction only. The upper part of the stomach is stapled, creating a narrow gastric inlet or pouch that remains connected with the remainder of the stomach. In addition, a non-adjustable band is placed around this new inlet in an attempt to prevent future enlargement of the stoma (opening). As a result, patients experience a sense of fullness after eating small meals. Weight loss from this procedure results entirely from eating less. VGB procedures are essentially no longer performed.

B. Nationally Covered Indications

Effective for services performed on and after February 21, 2006, Open and laparoscopic Roux-en-Y gastric bypass (RYGBP), open and laparoscopic Biliopancreatic Diversion with Duodenal Switch (BPD/DS) or Gastric Reduction Duodenal Switch (BPD/GRDS), and laparoscopic adjustable gastric banding (LAGB) are covered for Medicare beneficiaries who have a body-mass index = 35, have at least one co-morbidity related to obesity, and have been previously unsuccessful with medical treatment for obesity.

Effective for dates of service on and after February 21, 2006, these procedures are only covered when performed at facilities that are: (1) certified by the American College of Surgeons as a Level 1 Bariatric Surgery Center (program standards and requirements in effect on February 15, 2006); or (2) certified by the American Society for Bariatric Surgery as a Bariatric Surgery Center of Excellence (program standards and requirements in effect on February 15, 2006). Effective for dates of service on and after September 24, 2013, facilities are no longer required to be certified.

Effective for services performed on and after February 12, 2009, the Centers for Medicare & Medicaid Services (CMS) determines that Type 2 diabetes mellitus is a co-morbidity for purposes of this NCD.

A list of approved facilities and their approval dates are listed and maintained on the CMS Coverage Web site at http://www.cms.gov/Medicare/Medicare-General-Information/MedicareApprovedFacilitie/Bariatric-Surgery.html , and published in the Federal Register for services provided up to and including date of service September 23, 2013.

C. Nationally Non-Covered Indications

Treatments for obesity alone remain non-covered.

Supplemented fasting is not covered under the Medicare program as a general treatment for obesity (see section D. below for discretionary local coverage).

The following bariatric surgery procedures are non-covered for all Medicare beneficiaries:

- Open adjustable gastric banding;
- Open sleeve gastrectomy;
- Laparoscopic sleeve gastrectomy (prior to June 27, 2012);
- Open and laparoscopic vertical banded gastroplasty;
- Intestinal bypass surgery; and,
- Gastric balloon for treatment of obesity.

D. Other

Effective for services performed on and after June 27, 2012, Medicare Administrative Contractors (MACs) acting within their respective jurisdictions may determine coverage of stand-alone laparoscopic sleeve gastrectomy (LSG) for the treatment of co-morbid conditions related to obesity in Medicare beneficiaries only when all of the following conditions a.-c. are satisfied.

a. The beneficiary has a body-mass index (BMI) = 35 kg/m2,

b. The beneficiary has at least one co-morbidity related to obesity, and,

c. The beneficiary has been previously unsuccessful with medical treatment for obesity.

The determination of coverage for any bariatric surgery procedures that are not specifically identified in an NCD as covered or non-covered, for Medicare beneficiaries who have a body-mass index = 35, have at least one co-morbidity related to obesity, and have been previously unsuccessful with medical treatment for obesity, is left to the local MACs.

Where weight loss is necessary before surgery in order to ameliorate the complications posed by obesity when it coexists with pathological conditions such as cardiac and respiratory diseases, diabetes, or hypertension (and other more conservative techniques to achieve this end are not regarded as appropriate), supplemented fasting with adequate monitoring of the patient is eligible for coverage on a case-by-case basis or pursuant to a local coverage determination. The risks associated with the achievement of rapid weight loss must be carefully balanced against the risk posed by the condition requiring surgical treatment.

100-3, 100.5

NCD for Diagnostic Breath Analyses (100.5)

The Following Breath Test is Covered:

- Lactose breath hydrogen to detect lactose malabsorption.

The Following Breath Tests are Excluded from Coverage;

- Lactulose breath hydrogen for diagnosing small bowel bacterial overgrowth and measuring small bowel transit time.
- CO_2 for diagnosing bile acid malabsorption.
- CO_2 for diagnosing fat malabsorption.

100-3, 100.13

NCD for Laparoscopic Cholecystectomy (100.13)

Laparoscopic cholecystectomy is a covered surgical procedure in which a diseased gall bladder is removed through the use of instruments introduced via cannulae, with vision of the operative field maintained by use of a high-resolution television camera-monitor system (video laparoscope). For inpatient claims, use ICD-9-CM code 51.23, Laparoscopic cholecystectomy. For all other claims, use CPT codes 49310 for laparoscopy, surgical; cholecystectomy (any method), and 49311 for laparoscopy, surgical: cholecystectomy with cholangiography.

100-3, 110.1

NCD for Hyperthermia for Treatment of Cancer (110.1)

Local hyperthermia is covered under Medicare when used in connection with radiation therapy for the treatment of primary or metastatic cutaneous or subcutaneous superficial malignancies. It is not covered when used alone or in connection with chemotherapy.

100-3, 110.2

NCD for Certain Drugs Distributed by the National Cancer Institute (110.2)

Under its Cancer Therapy Evaluation, the Division of Cancer Treatment of the National Cancer Institute (NCI), in cooperation with the Food and Drug Administration, approves and distributes certain drugs for use in treating terminally ill cancer patients. One group of these drugs, designated as Group C drugs, unlike other drugs distributed by the NCI, is not limited to use in clinical trials for the purpose of testing their efficacy. Drugs are classified as Group C drugs only if there is sufficient evidence demonstrating their efficacy within a tumor type and that they can be safely administered.

A physician is eligible to receive Group C drugs from the Divison of Cancer Treatment only if the following requirements are met:

- A physician must be registered with the NCI as an investigator by having completed an FD-Form 1573;

- A written request for the drug, indicating the disease to be treated, must be submitted to the NCI;

- The use of the drug must be limited to indications outlined in the NCI's guidelines; and

- All adverse reactions must be reported to the Investigational Drug Branch of the Division of Cancer Treatment.

In view of these NCI controls on distribution and use of Group C drugs, A/B Medicare Adminstrative Contractors (MACs) may assume, in the absence of evidence to the contrary, that a Group C drug and the related hospital stay are covered if all other applicable coverage requirements are satisfied.

If there is reason to question coverage in a particular case, the matter should be resolved with the assistance of the Quality Improvement Organization (QIO), or if there is none, the assistance of the MAC's medical consultants.

Information regarding those drugs which are classified as Group C drugs may be obtained from:

Chief, Investigational Drug Branch
Cancer Therapy Evaluation Program
Executive Plaza North, Suite 7134
National Cancer Institute
Rockville, Maryland 20852-7426

100-3, 110.4

Extracorporeal Photopheresis

A. General

Extracorporeal photopheresis is a medical procedure in which a patient's white blood cells are exposed first to a drug called 8-methoxypsoralen (8-MOP) and then to ultraviolet A (UVA) light. The procedure starts with the removal of the patient's blood, which is centrifuged to isolate the white blood cells. The drug is typically administered directly to the white blood cells after they have been removed from the patient (referred to as ex vivo administration) but the drug can alternatively be administered directly to the patient before the white blood cells are withdrawn. After UVA light exposure, the treated white blood cells are then re-infused into the patient.

B. Nationally Covered Indications

The Centers for Medicare & Medicaid Services (CMS) has determined that extracorporeal photopheresis is reasonable and necessary under §1862(a)(1)(A) of the Social Security Act (the Act) under the following circumstances:

1. Effective April 8, 1988, Medicare provides coverage for:

   Palliative treatment of skin manifestations of cutaneous T-cell lymphoma that has not responded to other therapy.

2. Effective December 19, 2006, Medicare also provides coverage for:

   Patients with acute cardiac allograft rejection whose disease is refractory to standard immunosuppressive drug treatment; and,

Patients with chronic graft versus host disease whose disease is refractory to standard immunosuppressive drug treatment.

3. Effective April 30, 2012, Medicare also provides coverage for:

   Extracorporeal photopheresis for the treatment of bronchiolitis obliterans syndrome (BOS) following lung allograft transplantation only when extracorporeal photopheresis is provided under a clinical research study that meets the following conditions:

   The clinical research study meets the requirements specified below to assess the effect of extracorporeal photopheresis for the treatment of BOS following lung allograft transplantation. The clinical study must address one or more aspects of the following question:

   Prospectively, do Medicare beneficiaries who have received lung allografts, developed BOS refractory to standard immunosuppressive therapy, and received extracorporeal photopheresis , experience improved patient-centered health outcomes as indicated by:

   a. improved forced expiratory volume in one second (FEV1);

   b. improved survival after transplant; and/or,

   c. improved quality of life?

      The required clinical study must adhere to the following standards of scientific integrity and relevance to the Medicare population:

   a. The principal purpose of the research study is to test whether extracorporeal photopheresis potentially improves the participants' health outcomes.

   b. The research study is well supported by available scientific and medical information or it is intended to clarify or establish the health outcomes of interventions already in common clinical use.

   c. The research study does not unjustifiably duplicate existing studies.

   d. The research study design is appropriate to answer the research question being asked in the study.

   e. The research study is sponsored by an organization or individual capable of successfully executing the proposed study.

   f. The research study is in compliance with all applicable Federal regulations concerning the protection of human subjects found at 45 CFR Part 46. If a study is regulated by the Food and Drug Administration (FDA), it must also be in compliance with 21 CFR parts 50 and 56.

   g. All aspects of the research study are conducted according to appropriate standards of scientific integrity (see http://www.icmje.org).

   h. The research study has a written protocol that clearly addresses, or incorporates by reference, the standards listed here as Medicare requirements for coverage with evidence development.

   i. The clinical research study is not designed to exclusively test toxicity or disease pathophysiology in healthy individuals. Trials of all medical technologies measuring therapeutic outcomes as one of the objectives meet this standard only if the disease or condition being studied is life threatening as defined in 21 CFR § 312.81(a) and the patient has no other viable treatment options.

   j. The clinical research study is registered on the ClinicalTrials.gov website by the principal sponsor/investigator prior to the enrollment of the first study subject.

   k. The research study protocol specifies the method and timing of public release of all prespecified outcomes to be measured including release of outcomes if outcomes are negative or study is terminated early. The results must be made public within 24 months of the end of data collection. If a report is planned to be published in a peer-reviewed journal, then that initial release may be an abstract that meets the requirements of the International Committee of Medical Journal Editors (http://www.icmje.org).

   l. The research study protocol must explicitly discuss subpopulations affected by the treatment under investigation, particularly traditionally underrepresented groups in clinical studies, how the inclusion and exclusion criteria effect enrollment of these populations, and a plan for the retention and reporting of said populations on the trial. If the inclusion and exclusion criteria are expected to have a negative effect on the recruitment or retention of underrepresented populations, the protocol must discuss why these criteria are necessary.

   m. The research study protocol explicitly discusses how the results are or are not expected to be generalizable to the Medicare population to infer whether Medicare patients may benefit from the intervention. Separate discussions in the protocol may be necessary for populations eligible for Medicare due to age, disability or Medicaid eligibility.

Consistent with section 1142 of the Act, the Agency for Healthcare Research and Quality supports clinical research studies that CMS determines meet the above-listed standards and address the above-listed research questions.

Any clinical study under which there is coverage of extracorporeal photopheresis for this indication pursuant to this national coverage determination (NCD) must be approved by April 30, 2014. If there are no approved clinical studies on this date, this NCD will expire and coverage of extracorporeal photopheresis for BOS will revert to the coverage policy in effect prior to the issuance of the final decision memorandum for this NCD.

C. Nationally Non-Covered Indications

All other indications for extracorporeal photopheresis not otherwise indicated above as covered remain non-covered.

D. Other

Claims processing instructions can be found in chapter 32, section 190 of the Medicare Claims Processing Manual.

(This NCD last reviewed April 2012.)

100-3, 110.6

NCD for Scalp Hypothermia During Chemotherapy, to Prevent Hair Loss (110.6)

While ice-filled bags or bandages or other devices used for scalp hypothermia during chemotherapy may be covered as supplies of the kind commonly furnished without a separate charge, no separate charge for them would be recognized.

100-3, 110.7

NCD for Blood Transfusions (110.7)

B. Policy Governing Transfusions

For Medicare coverage purposes, it is important to distinguish between a transfusion itself and preoperative blood services; e.g., collection, processing, storage. Medically necessary transfusion of blood, regardless of the type, may generally be a covered service under both Part A and Part B of Medicare. Coverage does not make a distinction between the transfusion of homologous, autologous, or donor-directed blood. With respect to the coverage of the services associated with the preoperative collection, processing, and storage of autologous and donor-directed blood, the following policies apply.

1. Hospital Part A and B Coverage and Payment

   Under Sec.1862(a)(14) of the Act, non-physician services furnished to hospital patients are covered and paid for as hospital services. As provided in Sec.1886 of the Act, under the prospective [payment system (PPS), the diganosis related group (DRG) payment to the hospital includes all covered blood and blood processing expenses, whether or not the blood is eventually used.

   Under its provider agreement, a hospital is required to furnish or arrange for all covered services furnished to hospital patients. medicare payment is made to the hospital, under PPS or cost reimbursement, for covered inpatient services, and it is intended to reflect payment for all costs of furnishing those services.

2. Nonhospital Part B Coverage

   Under Part B, to be eligible for separate coverage, a service must fit the definition of one of the services authorized by Sec.1832 of the Act. These services are defined in 42 CFR 410.10 and do not include a separate category for a supplier's services associated with blood donation services, either autologous or donor-directed. That is, the collection, processing, and storage of blood for later transfusion into the beneficiary is not recognized as a separate service under Part B. Therefore, there is no avenue through which a blood supplier can receive direct payment under Part B for blood donation services.

C. Perioperative Blood Salvage

When the perioperative blood salvage process is used in surgery on a hospital patient, payment made to the hospital (under PPS or through cost reimbursement) for the procedure in which that process is used is intended to encompass payment for all costs relating to that process.

100-3, 110.8

NCD for Blood Platelet Transfusions (110.8)

Blood platelet transplants are safe and effective for the correction of thrombocytopenia and other blood defects. It is covered under Medicare when treatment is reasonable and necessary for the individual patient.

100-3, 110.8.1

NCD for Stem Cell Transplantation (110.8.1)

Indications and Limitations of Coverage

1. Allogeneic Hematopoietic Stem Cell Transplantation (HSCT)

   Allogeneic hematopoietic stem cell transplantation (HSCT) is a procedure in which a portion of a healthy donor's stem cell or bone marrow is obtained and prepared for intravenous infusion.

   a. Nationally Covered Indications

      The following uses of allogeneic HSCT are covered under Medicare:

      i. Effective for services performed on or after August 1, 1978, for the treatment of leukemia, leukemia in remission, or aplastic anemia when it is reasonable and necessary,

      ii. Effective for services performed on or after June 3, 1985, for the treatment of severe combined immunodeficiency disease (SCID) and for the treatment of Wiskott-Aldrich syndrome.

      iii. Effective for services performed on or after August 4, 2010, for the treatment of Myelodysplastic Syndromes (MDS) pursuant to Coverage with Evidence Development (CED) in the context of a Medicare-approved, prospective clinical study.

The MDS refers to a group of diverse blood disorders in which the bone marrow does not produce enough healthy, functioning blood cells. These disorders are varied with regard to clinical characteristics, cytologic and pathologic features, and cytogenetics. The abnormal production of blood cells in the bone marrow leads to low blood cell counts, referred to as cytopenias, which are a hallmark feature of MDS along with a dysplastic and hypercellular-appearing bone marrow.

Medicare payment for these beneficiaries will be restricted to patients enrolled in an approved clinical study. In accordance with the Stem Cell Therapeutic and Research Act of 2005 (US Public Law 109-129) a standard dataset is collected for all allogeneic transplant patients in the United States by the Center for International Blood and Marrow Transplant Research. The elements in this dataset, comprised of two mandatory forms plus one additional form, encompass the information we require for a study under CED.

A prospective clinical study seeking Medicare payment for treating a beneficiary with allogeneic HSCT for MDS pursuant to CED must meet one or more aspects of the following questions:

— Prospectively, compared to Medicare beneficiaries with MDS who do not receive HSCT, do Medicare beneficiaries with MDS who receive HSCT have improved outcomes as indicated by:

  – Relapse-free mortality,
  – progression free survival,
  – relapse, and
  – overall survival?

— Prospectively, in Medicare beneficiaries with MDS who receive HSCT, how do International Prognostic Scoring System (IPSS) score, patient age, cytopenias and comorbidities predict the following outcomes:

  – Relapse-free mortality,
  – progression free survival,
  – relapse, and
  – overall survival?

— Prospectively, in Medicare beneficiaries with MDS who receive HSCT, what treatment facility characteristics predict meaningful clinical improvement in the following outcomes:

  – Relapse-free mortality,
  – progression free survival,
  – relapse, and
  – overall survival?

In addition, the clinical study must adhere to the following standards of scientific integrity and relevance to the Medicare population:

a. The principal purpose of the research study is to test whether a particular intervention potentially improves the participants' health outcomes.

b. The research study is well supported by available scientific and medical information or it is intended to clarify or establish the health outcomes of interventions already in common clinical use.

c. The research study does not unjustifiably duplicate existing studies.

d. The research study design is appropriate to answer the research question being asked in the study.

e. The research study is sponsored by an organization or individual capable of executing the proposed study successfully.

f. The research study is in compliance with all applicable Federal regulations concerning the protection of human subjects found at 45 CFR Part 46.

g. All aspects of the research study are conducted according to appropriate standards of scientific integrity (see http://www.icmje.org).

h. The research study has a written protocol that clearly addresses, or incorporates by reference, the standards listed here as Medicare requirements for CED coverage.

i. The clinical research study is not designed to exclusively test toxicity or disease pathophysiology in healthy individuals. Trials of all medical technologies measuring therapeutic outcomes as one of the objectives meet this standard only if the disease or condition being studied is life threatening as defined in 21 CFR §312.81(a) and the patient has no other viable treatment options.

j. The clinical research study is registered on the ClinicalTrials.gov Web site by the principal sponsor/investigator prior to the enrollment of the first study subject.

k. The research study protocol specifies the method and timing of public release of all pre-specified outcomes to be measured including release of outcomes if outcomes are negative or study is terminated early. The results must be made public within 24 months of the end of data collection. If a report is planned to be published in a peer-reviewed journal, then that initial release may be an abstract that meets the requirements of the International Committee of Medical Journal Editors (http://www.icmje.org). However a full report of the outcomes must be made public no later than 3 years after the end of data collection.

l. The research study protocol must explicitly discuss subpopulations affected by the treatment under investigation, particularly traditionally underrepresented groups in clinical studies, how the inclusion and exclusion criteria effect enrollment of these populations, and a plan for the retention and reporting of said populations on the trial. If the inclusion and exclusion criteria are expected to have a negative effect on the recruitment or retention of underrepresented populations, the protocol must discuss why these criteria are necessary.

m. The research study protocol explicitly discusses how the results are or are not expected to be generalizable to the Medicare population to infer whether Medicare patients may benefit from the intervention. Separate discussions in the protocol may be necessary for populations eligible for Medicare due to age, disability or Medicaid eligibility.

Consistent with section 1142 of the Social Security Act, the Agency for Health Research and Quality (AHRQ) supports clinical research studies that CMS determines meet the above-listed standards and address the above-listed research questions.

The clinical research study should also have the following features:

— It should be a prospective, longitudinal study with clinical information from the period before HSCT and short- and long-term follow-up information.

— Outcomes should be measured and compared among pre-specified subgroups within the cohort.

— The study should be powered to make inferences in subgroup analyses.

— Risk stratification methods should be used to control for selection bias. Data elements to be used in risk stratification models should include:

Patient selection:

— Patient Age at diagnosis of MDS and at transplantation

— Date of onset of MDS

— Disease classification (specific MDS subtype at diagnosis prior to preparative/conditioning regimen using World Health Organization (WHO) classifications). Include presence/absence of refractory cytopenias

— Comorbid conditions

— IPSS score (and WHO-adapted Prognostic Scoring System (WPSS) score, if applicable) at diagnosis and prior to transplantation

— Score immediately prior to transplantation and one year post-transplantation

— Disease assessment at diagnosis at start of preparative regimen and last assessment prior to preparative regimen Subtype of MDS (refractory anemia with or without blasts, degree of blasts, etc.)

— Type of preparative/conditioning regimen administered (myeloabalative, non-myeloablative, reduced–intensity conditioning)

— Donor type

— Cell Source

— IPSS Score at diagnosis

Facilities must submit the required transplant essential data to the Stem Cell Therapeutics Outcomes Database.

b. Nationally Non-Covered Indications

Effective for services performed on or after May 24, 1996, allogeneic HSCT is not covered as treatment for multiple myeloma.

2. Autologous Stem Cell Transplantation (AuSCT)

Autologous stem cell transplantation (AuSCT) is a technique for restoring stem cells using the patient's own previously stored cells.

a. Nationally Covered Indications

i. Effective for services performed on or after April 28, 1989, AuSCT is considered reasonable and necessary under §I862(a)(1)(A) of the Social Security Act (the Act) for the following conditions and is covered under Medicare for patients with:

• Acute leukemia in remission who have a high probability of relapse and who have no human leucocyte antigens (HLA)-matched;

• Resistant non-Hodgkin's lymphomas or those presenting with poor prognostic features following an initial response;

• Recurrent or refractory neuroblastoma; or

• Advanced Hodgkin's disease who have failed conventional therapy and have no HLA-matched donor.

ii. Effective October 1, 2000, single AuSCT is only covered for Durie-Salmon Stage II or III patients that fit the following requirements:

• Newly diagnosed or responsive multiple myeloma. This includes those patients with previously untreated disease, those with at least a partial response to prior chemotherapy (defined as a 50% decrease either in measurable paraprotein [serum and/or urine] or in bone marrow infiltration, sustained for at least 1 month), and those in responsive relapse; and,

• Adequate cardiac, renal, pulmonary, and hepatic function.

iii. Effective for services performed on or after March 15, 2005, when recognized clinical risk factors are employed to select patients for transplantation, high dose melphalan (HDM) together with AuSCT is reasonable and necessary for Medicare beneficiaries of any age group with primary amyloid light chain (AL) amyloidosis who meet the following criteria:

• Amyloid deposition in 2 or fewer organs; and,

• Cardiac left ventricular ejection fraction (EF) greater than 45%.

b. Nationally Non-Covered Indications

Insufficient data exist to establish definite conclusions regarding the efficacy of AuSCT for the following conditions:

– Acute leukemia not in remission;

– Chronic granulocytic leukemia;

– Solid tumors (other than neuroblastoma);

– Up to October 1, 2000, multiple myeloma;

– Tandem transplantation (multiple rounds of AuSCT) for patients with multiple myeloma;

– Effective October 1, 2000, non primary AL amyloidosis; and,

– Effective October 1, 2000, thru March 14, 2005, primary AL amyloidosis for Medicare beneficiaries age 64 or older.

In these cases, AuSCT is not considered reasonable and necessary within the meaning of §I862(a)(1)(A) of the Act and is not covered under Medicare.

B. Other

All other indications for stem cell transplantation not otherwise noted above as covered or non-covered nationally remain at Medicare Administrative Contractor discretion.

100-3, 110.9

NCD for Antigens Prepared for Sublingual Administration (110.9)

For antigens provided to patients on or after November 17, 1996, Medicare does not cover such antigens if they are to be administered sublingually, i.e., by placing drops under the patient's tongue. This kind of allergy therapy has not been proven to be safe and effective. Antigens are covered only if they are administered by injection.

100-3, 110.12

NCD for Challenge Ingestion Food Testing (110.12)

This procedure is covered when it is used on an outpatient basis if it is reasonable and necessary for the individual patient.

Challenge ingestion food testing has not been proven to be effective in the diagnosis of rheumatoid arthritis, depression, or respiratory disorders. Accordingly, its use in the diagnosis of these conditions is not reasonable and necessary within the meaning of section 1862(a)(1) of the Medicare law, and no program payment is made for this procedure when it is so used.

100-3, 110.14

NCD for Apheresis (Therapeutic Pheresis) (110.14)

B. Indications

Apheresis is covered for the following indications:

• Plasma exchange for acquired myasthenia gravis;

• Leukapheresis in the treatment of leukemekia

• Plasmapheresis in the treatment of primary macroglobulinemia (Waldenstrom);

• Treatment of hyperglobulinemias, including (but not limited to) multiple myelomas, cryoglobulinemia and hyperviscosity syndromes;

• Plasmapheresis or plasma exchange as a last resort treatment of thromobotic thrombocytopenic purpura (TTP);

• Plasmapheresis or plasma exchange in the last resort treatment of life threatening rheumatoid vasculitis;

• Plasma perfusion of charcoal filters for treatment of pruritis of cholestatic liver disease;

• Plasma exchange in the treatment of Goodpasture's Syndrome;

• Plasma exchange in the treatment of glomerulonephritis associated with antiglomerular basement membrane antibodies and advancing renal failure or pulmonary hemorrhage;

- Treatment of chronic relapsing polyneuropathy for patients with severe or life threatening symptoms who have failed to respond to conventional therapy;

- Treatment of life threatening scleroderma and polymyositis when the patient is unresponsive to conventional therapy;

- Treatment of Guillain-Barre Syndrome; and

- Treatment of last resort for life threatening systemic lupus erythematosus (SLE) when conventional therapy has failed to prevent clinical deterioration.

C. Settings

Apheresis is covered only when performed in a hospital setting (either inpatient or outpatient). or in a nonhospital setting. e.g. physician directed clinic when the following conditions are met:

- A physician (or a number of physicians) is present to perform medical services and to respond to medical emergencies at all times during patient care hours;

- Each patient is under the care of a physician; and

- All nonphysician services are furnished under the direct, personal supervision of a physician.

100-3, 110.16

NCD for Nonselective (Random) Transfusions and Living Related Donor Specific Transfusions (DST) in Kidney Transplantation (110.16)

These pretransplant transfusions are covered under Medicare without a specific limitation on the number of transfusions, subject to the normal Medicare blood deductible provisions. Where blood is given directly to the transplant patient; e.g., in the case of donor specific transfusions, the blood is considered replaced for purposes of the blood deductible provisions.

100-3, 130.1

NCD for Inpatient Hospital Stays for Treatment of Alcoholism (130.1)

A. Inpatient Hospital Stay for Alcohol Detoxification

Many hospitals provide detoxification services during the more acute stages of alcoholism or alcohol withdrawal. When the high probability or occurrence of medical complications (e.g., delirium, confusion, trauma, or unconsciousness) during detoxification for acute alcoholism or alcohol withdrawal necessitates the constant availability of physicians and/or complex medical equipment found only in the hospital setting, inpatient hospital care during this period is considered reasonable and necessary and is therefore covered under the program. Generally, detoxification can be accomplished within two to three days with an occasional need for up to five days where the patient's condition dictates. This limit (five days) may be extended in an individual case where there is a need for a longer period for detoxification for a particular patient.

In such cases, however, there should be documentation by a physician which substantiates that a longer period of detoxification was reasonable and necessary. When the detoxification needs of an individual no longer require an inpatient hospital setting, coverage should be denied on the basis that inpatient hospital care is not reasonable and necessary as required by §1862(a)(l) of the Social Security Act (the Act). Following detoxification a patient may be transferred to an inpatient rehabilitation unit or discharged to a residential treatment program or outpatient treatment setting.

B. Inpatient Hospital Stay for Alcohol Rehabilitation

Hospitals may also provide structured inpatient alcohol rehabilitation programs to the chronic alcoholic. These programs are composed primarily of coordinated educational and psychotherapeutic services provided on a group basis. Depending on the subject matter, a series of lectures, discussions, films, and group therapy sessions are led by either physicians, psychologists, or alcoholism counselors from the hospital or various outside organizations. In addition, individual psychotherapy and family counseling (see §70.1) may be provided in selected cases. These programs are conducted under the supervision and direction of a physician. Patients may directly enter an inpatient hospital rehabilitation program after having undergone detoxification in the same hospital or in another hospital or may enter an inpatient hospital rehabilitation program without prior hospitalization for detoxification.

Alcohol rehabilitation can be provided in a variety of settings other than the hospital setting. In order for an inpatient hospital stay for alcohol rehabilitation to be covered under Medicare it must be medically necessary for the care to be provided in the inpatient hospital setting rather than in a less costly facility or on an outpatient basis. Inpatient hospital care for receipt of an alcohol rehabilitation program would generally be medically necessary where either (l) there is documentation by the physician that recent alcohol rehabilitation services in a less intensive setting or on an outpatient basis have proven unsuccessful and, as a consequence, the patient requires the supervision and intensity of services which can only be found in the controlled environment of the hospital, or (2) only the hospital environment can assure the medical management or control of the patient's concomitant conditions during the course of alcohol rehabilitation. (However, a patient's concomitant condition may make the use of certain alcohol treatment modalities medically inappropriate.)

In addition, the "active treatment" criteria (see the Medicare Benefit Policy Manual, Chapter 2, "Inpatient Psychiatric Hospital Services," §20) should be applied to psychiatric care in the general hospital as well as to psychiatric care in a psychiatric hospital. Since alcoholism is classifiable as a psychiatric condition the "active treatment" criteria must also be met in order for alcohol rehabilitation services to be covered under Medicare. (Thus, it is the combined need for "active treatment" and for covered care which can only be provided in the inpatient hospital setting, rather than the fact that rehabilitation immediately follows a period of detoxification which provides the basis for coverage of inpatient hospital alcohol rehabilitation programs.)

Generally 16-19 days of rehabilitation services are sufficient to bring a patient to a point where care could be continued in other than an inpatient hospital setting. An inpatient hospital stay for alcohol rehabilitation may be extended beyond this limit in an individual case where a longer period of alcohol rehabilitation is medically necessary. In such cases, however, there should be documentation by a physician which substantiates the need for such care. Where the rehabilitation needs of an individual no longer require an inpatient hospital setting, coverage should be denied on the basis that inpatient hospital care is not reasonable and necessary as required by §1862 (a)(l) of the Act.

Subsequent admissions to the inpatient hospital setting for alcohol rehabilitation follow-up, reinforcement, or "recap" treatments are considered to be readmissions (rather than an extension of the original stay) and must meet the requirements of this section for coverage under Medicare. Prior admissions to the inpatient hospital setting - either in the same hospital or in a different hospital - may be an indication that the "active treatment" requirements are not met (i.e., there is no reasonable expectation of improvement) and the stay should not be covered. Accordingly, there should be documentation to establish that "readmission" to the hospital setting for alcohol rehabilitation services can reasonably be expected to result in improvement of the patient's condition. For example, the documentation should indicate what changes in the patient's medical condition, social or emotional status, or treatment plan make improvement likely, or why the patient's initial hospital treatment was not sufficient.

C. Combined Alcohol Detoxification/Rehabilitation Programs

Medicare Administrative Contractors (MACs) should apply the guidelines in A. and B. above to both phases of a combined inpatient hospital alcohol detoxification/rehabilitation program. Not all patients who require the inpatient hospital setting for detoxification also need the inpatient hospital setting for rehabilitation. (See §130.1 for coverage of outpatient hospital alcohol rehabilitation services.) Where the inpatient hospital setting is medically necessary for both alcohol detoxification and rehabilitation, generally a 3-week period is reasonable and necessary to bring the patient to the point where care can be continued in other than an inpatient hospital setting.

Decisions regarding reasonableness and necessity of treatment, the need for an inpatient hospital level of care, and length of treatment should be made by A/B MAC (A) based on accepted medical practice with the advice of their medical consultant. (In hospitals under PSRO review, PSRO determinations of medical necessity of services and appropriateness of the level of care at which services are provided are binding on A/B MAC (A) for purposes of adjudicating claims for payment.)

100-3, 130.2

NCD for Outpatient Hospital Services for Treatment of Alcoholism (130.2)

Coverage is available for both diagnostic and therapeutic services furnished for the treatment of alcoholism by the hospital to outpatients subject to the same rules applicable to outpatient hospital services in general. While there is no coverage for day hospitalization programs, per se, individual services which meet the requirements in the Medicare Benefit Policy Manual, Chapter 6, Sec.20 may be covered. (Meals, transportation and recreational and social activities do not fall within the scope of covered outpatient hospital services under Medicare.)

All services must be reasonable and necessary for diagnosis or treatment of the patient's condition (see the Medicare Benefit Policy Manual, chapter 16 Sec.20). Thus, educational services and family counseling would only be covered where they are directly related to treatment of the patient's condition. The frequency of treatment and period of time over which it occurs must also be reasonable and necessary.

100-3, 130.3

NCD for Chemical AversionTherapy for Treatment of Alcoholism (130.3)

Chemical aversion therapy is a behavior modification technique that is used in the treatment of alcoholism. Chemical aversion therapy facilitates alcohol abstinence through the development of conditioned aversions to the taste, smell, and sight of alcohol beverages. This is accomplished by repeatedly pairing alcohol with unpleasant symptoms (e.g., nausea) which have been induced by one of several chemical agents. While a number of drugs have been employed in chemical aversion therapy, the three most commonly used are emetine, apomorphine, and lithium. None of the drugs being used, however, have yet been approved by the Food and Drug Administration specifically for use in chemical aversion therapy for alcoholism. Accordingly, when these drugs are being employed in conjunction with this therapy, patients undergoing this treatment need to be kept under medical observation.

Available evidence indicates that chemical aversion therapy may be an effective component of certain alcoholism treatment programs, particularly as part of multi-modality treatment programs which include other behavioral techniques and therapies, such as psychotherapy. Based on this evidence, the Centers for Medicare & Medicaid Services' medical consultants have recommended that chemical aversion therapy be covered under Medicare. However, since chemical aversion therapy is a demanding therapy which may not be appropriate for all Medicare beneficiaries needing treatment for alcoholism, a physician should certify to the appropriateness of chemical aversion therapy in the individual case. Therefore, if chemical aversion therapy for treatment of alcoholism is determined to be reasonable and necessary for an individual patient, it is covered under Medicare.

When it is medically necessary for a patient to receive chemical aversion therapy as a hospital inpatient, coverage for care in that setting is available. (See §130.1 regarding coverage of multi-modality treatment programs.) Follow-up treatments for chemical aversion therapy can generally be provided on an outpatient basis. Thus, where a patient is admitted as an inpatient for receipt of chemical aversion therapy, there must be documentation by the physician of the need in the individual case for the inpatient hospital admission.

Decisions regarding reasonableness and necessity of treatment and the need for an inpatient hospital level of care should be made by the A/B MAC (A) based on accepted medical practice with the advice of their medical consultant. (In hospitals under Quality Improvement Organization (QIO) review, QIO determinations of medical necessity of services and appropriateness of the level of care at which services are provided are binding on the A/B MAC (A) for purposes of adjudicating claims for payment.)

100-3, 140.1

NCD for Abortion (140.1)

Abortions are not covered Medicare procedures except:

1. If the pregnancy is the result of an act of rape or incest; or

2. In the case where a woman suffers from a physical disorder, physical injury, or physical illness, including a life-endangering physical condition caused by or arising from the pregnancy itself, that would, as certified by a physician, place the woman in danger of death unless an abortion is performed.

100-3, 140.2

NCD for Breast Reconstruction Following Mastectomy (140.2)

Reconstruction of the affected and the contralateral unaffected breast following a medically necessary mastectomy is considered a relatively safe and effective noncosmetic procedure. Accordingly, program payment may be made for breast reconstruction surgery following removal of a breast for any medical reason.

Program payment may not be made for breast reconstruction for cosmetic reasons. (Cosmetic surgery is excluded from coverage under Sec.1862(a)(l0) of the Social Security Act.)

100-3, 140.5

NCD for Laser Procedures (140.5)

Medicare recognizes the use of lasers for many medical indications. Procedures performed with lasers are sometimes used in place of more conventional techniques. In the absence of a specific noncoverage instruction, and where a laser has been approved for marketing by the Food and Drug Administration, Medicare Administrative Contractor discretion may be used to determine whether a procedure performed with a laser is reasonable and necessary and, therefore, covered.

The determination of coverage for a procedure performed using a laser is made on the basis that the use of lasers to alter, revise, or destroy tissue is a surgical procedure. Therefore, coverage of laser procedures is restricted to practitioners with training in the surgical management of the disease or condition being treated.

100-3, 150.1

NCD for Manipulation (150.1)

Manipulation of the Rib Cage.--Manual manipulation of the rib cage contributes to the treatment of respiratory conditions such as bronchitis, emphysema, and asthma as part of a regimen which includes other elements of therapy, and is covered only under such circumstances.

Manipulation of the Head.--Manipulation of the occipitocervical or temporomandibular regions of the head when indicated for conditions affecting those portions of the head and neck is a covered service.

100-3, 150.2

NCD for Osteogenic Stimulators (150.2)

Electrical Osteogenic Stimulators

B. Nationally Covered Indications

1. Noninvasive Stimulator.

    The noninvasive stimulator device is covered only for the following indications:

    — Nonunion of long bone fractures;

    — Failed fusion, where a minimum of nine months has elapsed since the last surgery;

    — Congenital pseudarthroses; and

— Effective July 1, 1996, as an adjunct to spinal fusion surgery for patients at high risk of pseudarthrosis due to previously failed spinal fusion at the same site or for those undergoing multiple level fusion. A multiple level fusion involves 3 or more vertebrae (e.g., L3-L5, L4-S1, etc.).

— Effective September 15, 1980, nonunion of long bone fractures is considered to exist only after 6 or more months have elapsed without healing of the fracture.

— Effective April 1, 2000, nonunion of long bone fractures is considered to exist only when serial radiographs have confirmed that fracture healing has ceased for 3 or more months prior to starting treatment with the electrical osteogenic stimulator. Serial radiographs must include a minimum of 2 sets of radiographs, each including multiple views of the fracture site, separated by a minimum of 90 days.

2. Invasive (Implantable) Stimulator.

    The invasive stimulator device is covered only for the following indications:

    — Nonunion of long bone fractures

    — Effective July 1, 1996, as an adjunct to spinal fusion surgery for patients at high risk of pseudarthrosis due to previously failed spinal fusion at the same site or for those undergoing multiple level fusion. A multiple level fusion involves 3 or more vertebrae (e.g., L3-5, L4-S1, etc.)

    — Effective September 15, 1980, nonunion of long bone fractures is considered to exist only after 6 or more months have elapsed without healing of the fracture.

    — Effective April 1, 2000, non union of long bone fractures is considered to exist only when serial radiographs have confirmed that fracture healing has ceased for 3 or more months prior to starting treatment with the electrical osteogenic stimulator. Serial radiographs must include a minimum of 2 sets of radiographs, each including multiple views of the fracture site, separated by a minimum of 90 days.

    — Effective for services performed on or after January 1, 2001, ultrasonic osteogenic stimulators are covered as medically reasonable and necessary for the treatment of non-union fractures. In demonstrating nonunion of fractures, we would expect:

        – A minimum of two sets of radiographs obtained prior to starting treatment with the osteogenic stimulator, separated by a minimum of 90 days. Each radiograph must include multiple views of the fracture site accompanied with a written interpretation by a physician stating that there has been no clinically significant evidence of fracture healing between the two sets of radiographs.

        – Indications that the patient failed at least one surgical intervention for the treatment of the fracture.

    — Effective April 27, 2005, upon the recommendation of the ultrasound stimulation for nonunion fracture healing, CMS determins that the evidence is adequate to conclude that noninvasive ultrasound stimulation for the treatment of nonunion bone fractures prior to surfical intervention is reasonable and necessary. In demonstrating non-union fracturs, CMS expects:

        – A minimum of 2 sets of radiographs, obtained prior to starting treating with the osteogenic stimulator, separated by a minimum of 90 days. Each radiograph set must include multiple views of the fracture site accompanied with a written interpretation by a physician stating that there has been no clinically significant evidence of fracture healing between the 2 sets of radiographs.

C. Nationally Non-Covered Indications

Nonunion fractures of the skull, vertebrae and those that are tumor-related are excluded from coverage.

Ultrasonic osteogenic stimulators may not be used concurrently with other non-invasive osteogenic devices.

Ultrasonic osteogenic stimulators for fresh fractures and delayed unions remain non-covered.

(This NCD last reviewed June 2005)

100-3, 150.7

NCD for Prolotherapy, Joint Sclerotherapy, and Ligamentous Injections with Sclerosing Agents (150.7)

The medical effectiveness of the above therapies has not been verified by scientifically controlled studies. Accordingly, reimbursement for these modalities should be denied on the ground that they are not reasonable and necessary as required by Sec.1862(a)(1) of the Act.

100-3, 150.10

NCD for Lumbar Artificial Disc Replacement (LADR) (150.10)

A. General

The lumbar artificial disc replacement (LADR) is a surgical procedure on the lumbar spine that involves complete removal of the damaged or diseased lumbar intervertebral disc and implantation of an artificial disc. The procedure may be done as an alternative to lumbar spinal fusion and is intended to reduce pain, increase movement at the site of surgery and restore intervertebral disc height. The Food and Drug Administration has approved the use of LADR for spine arthroplasty in skeletally mature patients with degenerative or discogenic disc disease at one level for L3 to S1.

B. Nationally Covered Indications
N/A

C. Nationally Non-Covered Indications
Effective for services performed from May 16, 2006 through August 13, 2007, the Centers for Medicare and Medicaid Services (CMS) has found that LADR with the ChariteTM lumbar artificial disc is not reasonable and necessary for the Medicare population over 60 years of age; therefore, LADR with the ChariteTM lumbar artificial disc is non-covered for Medicare beneficiaries over 60 years of age.

Effective for services performed on or after August 14, 2007, CMS has found that LADR is not reasonable and necessary for the Medicare population over 60 years of age; therefore, LADR is non-covered for Medicare beneficiaries over 60 years of age.

D. Other
For Medicare beneficiaries 60 years of age and younger, there is no national coverage determination for LADR, leaving such determinations to continue to be made by the local Medicare Administrative Contractors.

For dates of service May 16, 2006 through August 13, 2007, Medicare coverage under the investigational device exemption (IDE) for LADR with a disc other than the ChariteTM lumbar disc in eligible clinical trials is not impacted.

100-3, 160.8

NCD for Electroencephalographic (EEG) Monitoring During Surgical Procedures Involving the Cerebral Vasculature (160.8)
CIM 35-57

Electroencephalographic (EEG) monitoring is a safe and reliable technique for the assessment of gross cerebral blood flow during general anesthesia and is covered under Medicare. Very characteristic changes in the EEG occur when cerebral perfusion is inadequate for cerebral function. EEG monitoring as an indirect measure of cerebral perfusion requires the expertise of an electroencephalographer, a neurologist trained in EEG, or an advanced EEG technician for its proper interpretation.

The EEG monitoring may be covered routinely in carotid endarterectomies and in other neurological procedures where cerebral perfusion could be reduced. Such other procedures might include aneurysm surgery where hypotensive anesthesia is used or other cerebral vascular procedures where cerebral blood flow may be interrupted.

100-3, 160.17

NCD for L-DOPA (160.17)

A. Part A Payment for L-Dopa and Associated Inpatient Hospital Services
A hospital stay and related ancillary services for the administration of L-Dopa are covered if medically required for this purpose. Whether a drug represents an allowable inpatient hospital cost during such stay depends on whether it meets the definition of a drug in Sec.1861(t) of the Act; i.e., on its inclusion in the compendia named in the Act or approval by the hospital's pharmacy and drug therapeutics (P&DT) or equivalent committee. (Levodopa (L-Dopa) has been favorably evaluated for the treatment of Parkinsonism by A.M.A. Drug Evaluations, First Edition 1971, the replacement compendia for "New Drugs.")

Inpatient hospital services are frequently not required in many cases when L-Dopa therapy is initiated. Therefore, determine the medical need for inpatient hospital services on the basis of medical facts in the individual case. It is not necessary to hospitalize the typical, well-functioning, ambulatory Parkinsonian patient who has no concurrent disease at the start of L-Dopa treatment. It is reasonable to provide inpatient hospital services for Parkinsonian patients with concurrent diseases, particularly of the cardiovascular, gastrointestinal, and neuropsychiatric systems. Although many patients require hospitalization for a period of under 2 weeks, a 4-week period of inpatient care is not unreasonable.

Laboratory tests in connection with the administration of L-Dopa - The tests medically warranted in connection with the achievement of optimal dosage and the control of the side effects of L-Dopa include a complete blood count, liver function tests such as SGOT, SGPT, and/or alkaline phosphatase, BUN or creatinine and urinalysis, blood sugar, and electrocardiogram.

Whether or not the patient is hospitalized, laboratory tests in certain cases are reasonable at weekly intervals although some physicians prefer to perform the tests much less frequently.

Physical therapy furnished in connection with administration of L-Dopa - Where, following administration of the drug, the patient experiences a reduction of rigidity which permits the reestablishment of a restorative goal for him/her, physical therapy services required to enable him/her to achieve this goal are payable provided they require the skills of a qualified physical therapist and are furnished by or under the supervision of such a therapist. However, once the individual's restoration potential has been achieved, the services required to maintain him/her at this level do not generally require the skills of a qualified physical therapist. In such situations, the role of the therapist is to evaluate the patient's needs in consultation with his/her physician and design a program of exercise appropriate to the capacity and tolerance of the patient and treatment objectives of the physician, leaving to others the actual carrying out of the program. While the evaluative services rendered by a qualified physical therapist are payable as physical therapy, services furnished by others in connection with the carrying out of the maintenance program established by the therapist are not.

B. Part A Reimbursement for L-Dopa Therapy in SNFs
Initiation of L-Dopa therapy can be appropriately carried out in the SNF setting, applying the same guidelines used for initiation of L-Dopa therapy in the hospital, including the types of patients who should be covered for inpatient services, the role of physical therapy, and the use of laboratory tests. (See subsection A.) Where inpatient care is required and L-Dopa therapy is initiated in the SNF, limit the stay to a maximum of 4 weeks; but in many cases the need may be no longer than 1 or 2 weeks, depending upon the patient's condition. However, where L-Dopa therapy is begun in the hospital and the patient is transferred to an SNF for continuation of the therapy, a combined length of stay in hospital and SNF of no longer than 4 weeks is reasonable (i.e., 1 week hospital stay followed by 3 weeks SNF stay; or 2 weeks hospital stay followed by 2 weeks SNF stay; etc.). Medical need must be demonstrated in cases where the combined length of stay in hospital and SNF is longer than 4 weeks. The choice of hospital or SNF, and the decision regarding the relative length of time spent in each, should be left to the medical judgment of the treating physician.

C. L-Dopa Coverage Under Part B
Part B reimbursement may not be made for the drug L-Dopa since it is a self-administrable drug. However, physician services rendered in connection with its administration and control of its side effects are covered if determined to be reasonable and necessary. Initiation of L-Dopa therapy on an outpatient basis is possible in most cases. Visit frequency ranging from every week to every 2 or 3 months is acceptable. However, after half a year of therapy, visits more frequent than every month would usually not be reasonable.

100-3, 180.1

NCD for Medical Nutrition Therapy (180.1)
Effective October 1, 2002, basic coverage of MNT for the first year a beneficiary receives MNT with either a diagnosis of renal disease or diabetes as defined at 42 CFR Sec.410.130 is 3 hours. Also effective October 1, 2002, basic coverage in subsequent years for renal disease or diabetes is 2 hours. The dietitian/nutritionist may choose how many units are performed per day as long as all of the other requirements in this NCD and 42 CFR Secs.410.130-410.134 are met. Pursuant to the exception at 42 CFR Sec.410.132(b)(5), additional hours are considered to be medically necessary and covered if the treating physician determines that there is a change in medical condition, diagnosis, or treatment regimen that requires a change in MNT and orders additional hours during that episode of care.

Effective October 1, 2002, if the treating physician determines that receipt of both MNT and DSMT is medically necessary in the same episode of care, Medicare will cover both DSMT and MNT initial and subsequent years without decreasing either benefit as long as DSMT and MNT are not provided on the same date of service. The dietitian/nutritionist may choose how many units are performed per day as long as all of the other requirements in the NCD and 42 CFR Secs.410.130-410.134 are met. Pursuant to the exception at 42 CFR 410.132(b)(5), additional hours are considered to be medically necessary and covered if the treating physician determines that there is a change in medical condition, diagnosis, or treatment regimen that requires a change in MNT and orders additional hours during that episode of care.

100-3, 190.1

NCD for Histocompatibility Testing (190.1)
This testing is safe and effective when it is performed on patients:

- In preparation for a kidney transplant;
- In preparation for bone marrow transplantation;
- In preparation for blood platelet transfusions (particularly where multiple infusions are involved); or
- Who are suspected of having ankylosing spondylitis.

This testing is covered under Medicare when used for any of the indications listed in A, B, and C and if it is reasonable and necessary for the patient.

It is covered for ankylosing spondylitis in cases where other methods of diagnosis would not be appropriate or have yielded inconclusive results. Request documentation supporting the medical necessity of the test from the physician in all cases where ankylosing spondylitis is indicated as the reason for the test.

100-3, 190.8

NCD for Lymphocyte Mitogen Response Assays (190.8)
It is a covered test under Medicare when it is medically necessary to assess lymphocytic function in diagnosed immunodeficiency diseases and to monitor immunotherapy.

It is not covered when it is used to monitor the treatment of cancer, because its use for that purpose is experimental.

100-3, 190.9

NCD for Serologic Testing for Acquired Immunodeficiency Syndrome (AIDS) (190.9)

These tests may be covered when performed to help determine a diagnosis for symptomatic patients. They are not covered when furnished as part of a screening program for asymptomatic persons.

Note: Two enzyme-linked immunosorbent assay (ELISA) tests that were conducted on the same specimen must both be positive before Medicare will cover the Western blot test.

100-3, 190.11

NCD for Home Prothrombin Time International Normalized Ratio (INR) Monitoring for Anticoagulation Management (190.11)

A. General

Use of the International Normalized Ratio (INR) or prothrombin time (PT) - standard measurement for reporting the blood's clotting time - allows physicians to determine the level of anticoagulation in a patient independent of the laboratory reagents used. The INR is the ratio of the patient's PT (extrinsic or tissue-factor dependent coagulation pathway) compared to the mean PT for a group of normal individuals. Maintaining patients within his/her prescribed therapeutic range minimizes adverse events associated with inadequate or excessive anticoagulation such as serious bleeding or thromboembolic events. Patient self-testing and self-management through the use of a home INR monitor may be used to improve the time in therapeutic rate (TTR) for select groups of patients. Increased TTR leads to improved clinical outcomes and reductions in thromboembolic and hemorrhagic events.

Warfarin (also prescribed under other trade names, e.g., Coumadin(R)) is a self-administered, oral anticoagulant (blood thinner) medication that affects the vitamin K- dependent clotting factors II, VII, IX and X. It is widely used for various medical conditions, and has a narrow therapeutic index, meaning it is a drug with less than a 2-fold difference between median lethal dose and median effective dose. For this reason, since October 4, 2006, it falls under the category of a Food and Drug dministration (FDA) "black-box" drug whose dosage must be closely monitored to avoid serious complications. A PT/INR monitoring system is a portable testing device that includes a finger-stick and an FDA-cleared meter that measures the time it takes for a person's blood plasma to clot.

B. Nationally Covered Indications

For services furnished on or after March 19, 2008, Medicare will cover the use of home PT/INR monitoring for chronic, oral anticoagulation management for patients with mechanical heart valves, chronic atrial fibrillation, or venous thromboembolism (inclusive of deep venous thrombosis and pulmonary embolism) on warfarin. The monitor and the home testing must be prescribed by a treating physician as provided at 42 CFR 410.32(a), and all of the following requirements must be met:

1. The patient must have been anticoagulated for at least 3 months prior to use of the home INR device; and,

2. The patient must undergo a face-to-face educational program on anticoagulation anagement and must have demonstrated the correct use of the device prior to its use in the home; and,

3. The patient continues to correctly use the device in the context of the management of the anticoagulation therapy following the initiation of home monitoring; and,

4. Self-testing with the device should not occur more frequently than once a week.

C. Nationally Non-Covered Indications
N/A

D. Other
1. All other indications for home PT/INR monitoring not indicated as nationally covered above remain at local Medicare contractor discretion.

2. This national coverage determination (NCD) is distinct from, and makes no changes to, the PT clinical laboratory NCD at section 190.17 of Publication 100-3 of the NCD Manual.

100-3, 190.14

NCD for Human Immunodeficiency Virus (HIV) Testing (Diagnosis) (190.14)

Indications and Limitations of Coverage

Indications

Diagnostic testing to establish HIV infection may be indicated when there is a strong clinical suspicion supported by one or more of the following clinical findings:

- The patient has a documented, otherwise unexplained, AIDS-defining or AIDS-associated opportunistic infection.

- The patient has another documented sexually transmitted disease which identifies significant risk of exposure to HIV and the potential for an early or subclinical infection.

- The patient has documented acute or chronic hepatitis B or C infection that identifies a significant risk of exposure to HIV and the potential for an early or subclinical infection.

- The patient has a documented AIDS-defining or AIDS-associated neoplasm.

- The patient has a documented AIDS-associated neurologic disorder or otherwise unexplained dementia.

- The patient has another documented AIDS-defining clinical condition, or a history of other severe, recurrent, or persistent conditions which suggest an underlying immune deficiency (for example, cutaneous or mucosal disorders).

- The patient has otherwise unexplained generalized signs and symptoms suggestive of a chronic process with an underlying immune deficiency (for example, fever, weight loss, malaise, fatigue, chronic diarrhea, failure to thrive, chronic cough, hemoptysis, shortness of breath, or lymphadenopathy).

- The patient has otherwise unexplained laboratory evidence of a chronic disease process with an underlying immune deficiency (for example, anemia, leukopenia, pancytopenia, lymphopenia, or low CD4+ lymphocyte count).

- The patient has signs and symptoms of acute retroviral syndrome with fever, malaise, lymphadenopathy, and skin rash.

- The patient has documented exposure to blood or body fluids known to be capable of transmitting HIV (for example, needlesticks and other significant blood exposures) and antiviral therapy is initiated or anticipated to be initiated.

- The patient is undergoing treatment for rape. (HIV testing is a part of the rape treatment protocol.)

Limitations

HIV antibody testing in the United States is usually performed using HIV-1 or HIV-½ combination tests. HIV-2 testing is indicated if clinical circumstances suggest HIV-2 is likely (that is, compatible clinical findings and HIV-1 test negative). HIV-2 testing may also be indicated in areas of the country where there is greater prevalence of HIV-2 infections.

The Western Blot test should be performed only after documentation that the initial EIA tests are repeatedly positive or equivocal on a single sample.

- The HIV antigen tests currently have no defined diagnostic usage.

- Direct viral RNA detection may be performed in those situations where serologic testing does not establish a diagnosis but strong clinical suspicion persists (for example, acute retroviral syndrome, nonspecific serologic evidence of HIV, or perinatal HIV infection).

- If initial serologic tests confirm an HIV infection, repeat testing is not indicated.

- If initial serologic tests are HIV EIA negative and there is no indication for confirmation of infection by viral RNA detection, the interval prior to retesting is 3-6 months.

- Testing for evidence of HIV infection using serologic methods may be medically appropriate in situations where there is a risk of exposure to HIV. However, in the absence of a documented AIDS defining or HIV- associated disease, an HIV associated sign or symptom, or documented exposure to a known HIV-infected source, the testing is considered by Medicare to be screening and thus is not covered by Medicare (for example, history of multiple blood component transfusions, exposure to blood or body fluids not resulting in consideration of therapy, history of transplant, history of illicit drug use, multiple sexual partners, same-sex encounters, prostitution, or contact with prostitutes).

- The CPT Editorial Panel has issued a number of codes for infectious agent detection by direct antigen or nucleic acid probe techniques that have not yet been developed or are only being used on an investigational basis. Laboratory providers are advised to remain current on FDA-approval status for these tests.

100-3, 190.15

NCD for Blood Counts (190.15)

Indications

Indications for a CBC or hemogram include red cell, platelet, and white cell disorders. Examples of these indications are enumerated individually below.

1. Indications for a CBC generally include the evaluation of bone marrow dysfunction as a result of neoplasms, therapeutic agents, exposure to toxic substances, or pregnancy. The CBC also is useful in assessing peripheral destruction of blood cells, suspected bone marrow failure or bone marrow infiltrate, suspected myeloproliferative, myelodysplastic, or lymphoproliferative processes, and immune disorders.

2. Indications for hemogram or CBC related to red cell (RBC) parameters of the hemogram include signs, symptoms, test results, illness, or disease that can be associated with anemia or other red blood cell disorder (e.g., pallor, weakness, fatigue, weight loss, bleeding, acute injury associated with blood loss or suspected blood loss, abnormal menstrual bleeding, hematuria, hematemesis, hematochezia, positive fecal occult blood test, malnutrition, vitamin deficiency, malabsorption, neuropathy, known malignancy, presence of acute or chronic disease that may have associated anemia, coagulation or hemostatic disorders, postural dizziness, syncope, abdominal pain, change in bowel habits, chronic marrow hypoplasia or decreased RBC production, tachycardia, systolic heart murmur, congestive heart failure, dyspnea, angina, nailbed deformities, growth

retardation, jaundice, hepatomegaly, splenomegaly, lymphadenopathy, ulcers on the lower extremities).

3. Indications for hemogram or CBC related to red cell (RBC) parameters of the hemogram include signs, symptoms, test results, illness, or disease that can be associated with polycythemia (for example, fever, chills, ruddy skin, conjunctival redness, cough, wheezing, cyanosis, clubbing of the fingers, orthopnea, heart murmur, headache, vague cognitive changes including memory changes, sleep apnea, weakness, pruritus, dizziness, excessive sweating, visual symptoms, weight loss, massive obesity, gastrointestinal bleeding, paresthesias, dyspnea, joint symptoms, epigastric distress, pain and erythema of the fingers or toes, venous or arterial thrombosis, thromboembolism, myocardial infarction, stroke, transient ischemic attacks, congenital heart disease, chronic obstructive pulmonary disease, increased erythropoietin production associated with neoplastic, renal or hepatic disorders, androgen or diuretic use, splenomegaly, hepatomegaly, diastolic hypertension.)

4. Specific indications for CBC with differential count related to the WBC include signs, symptoms, test results, illness, or disease associated with leukemia, infections or inflammatory processes, suspected bone marrow failure or bone marrow infiltrate, suspected myeloproliferative, myelodysplastic or lymphoproliferative disorder, use of drugs that may cause leukopenia, and immune disorders (e.g., fever, chills, sweats, shock, fatigue, malaise, tachycardia, tachypnea, heart murmur, seizures, alterations of consciousness, meningismus, pain such as headache, abdominal pain, arthralgia, odynophagia, or dysuria, redness or swelling of skin, soft tissue bone, or joint, ulcers of the skin or mucous membranes, gangrene, mucous membrane discharge, bleeding, thrombosis, respiratory failure, pulmonary infiltrate, jaundice, diarrhea, vomiting, hepatomegaly, splenomegaly, lymphadenopathy, opportunistic infection such as oral candidiasis.)

5. Specific indications for CBC related to the platelet count include signs, symptoms, test results, illness, or disease associated with increased or decreased platelet production and destruction, or platelet dysfunction (e.g., gastrointestinal bleeding, genitourinary tract bleeding, bilateral epistaxis, thrombosis, ecchymosis, purpura, jaundice, petechiae, fever, heparin therapy, suspected DIC, shock, pre-eclampsia, neonate with maternal ITP, massive transfusion, recent platelet transfusion, cardiopulmonary bypass, hemolytic uremic syndrome, renal diseases, lymphadenopathy, hepatomegaly, splenomegaly, hypersplenism, neurologic abnormalities, viral or other infection, myeloproliferative, myelodysplastic, or lymphoproliferative disorder, thrombosis, exposure to toxic agents, excessive alcohol ingestion, autoimmune disorders (SLE, RA and other).

6. Indications for hemogram or CBC related to red cell (RBC) parameters of the hemogram include, in addition to those already listed, thalassemia, suspected hemoglobinopathy, lead poisoning, arsenic poisoning, and spherocytosis.

7. Specific indications for CBC with differential count related to the WBC include, in addition to those already listed, storage diseases; mucopolysaccharidoses, and use of drugs that cause leukocytosis such as G-CSF or GM-CSF.

8. Specific indications for CBC related to platelet count include, in addition to those already listed, May-Hegglin syndrome and Wiskott-Aldrich syndrome.

Limitations:

1. Testing of patients who are asymptomatic, or who do not have a condition that could be expected to result in a hematological abnormality, is screening and is not a covered service.

2. In some circumstances it may be appropriate to perform only a hemoglobin or hematocrit to assess the oxygen carrying capacity of the blood. When the ordering provider requests only a hemoglobin or hematocrit, the remaining components of the CBC are not covered.

3. When a blood count is performed for an end-stage renal disease (ESRD) patient, and is billed outside the ESRD rate, documentation of the medical necessity for the blood count must be submitted with the claim.

4. In some patients presenting with certain signs, symptoms or diseases, a single CBC may be appropriate. Repeat testing may not be indicated unless abnormal results are found, or unless there is a change in clinical condition. If repeat testing is performed, a more descriptive diagnosis code (e.g., anemia) should be reported to support medical necessity. However, repeat testing may be indicated where results are normal in patients with conditions where there is a continued risk for the development of hematologic abnormality.

100-3, 190.18

Serum Iron Studies

Indications:

1. Ferritin (82728), iron (83540) and either iron binding capacity (83550) or transferrin (84466) are useful in the differential diagnosis of iron deficiency, anemia, and for iron overload conditions.

   a. The following presentations are examples that may support the use of these studies for evaluating iron deficiency:

   – Certain abnormal blood count values (i.e., decreased mean corpuscular volume (MCV), decreased hemoglobin/hematocrit when the MCV is low or normal, or increased red cell distribution width (RDW) and low or normal MCV);

   – Abnormal appetite (pica);

   – Acute or chronic gastrointestinal blood loss;

   – Hematuria;

   – Menorrhagia;

   – Malabsorption;

   – Status post-gastrectomy;

   – Status post-gastrojejunostomy;

   – Malnutrition;

   – Preoperative autologous blood collection(s);

   – Malignant, chronic inflammatory and infectious conditions associated with anemia which may present in a similar manner to iron deficiency anemia;

   – Following a significant surgical procedure where blood loss had occurred and had not been repaired with adequate iron replacement.

   b. The following presentations are examples that may support the use of these studies for evaluating iron overload:

   – Chronic Hepatitis;

   – Diabetes;

   – Hyperpigmentation of skin;

   – Arthropathy;

   – Cirrhosis;

   – Hypogonadism;

   – Hypopituitarism;

   – Impaired porphyrin metabolism;

   – Heart failure;

   – Multiple transfusions;

   – Sideroblastic anemia;

   – Thalassemia major;

   – Cardiomyopathy, cardiac dysrhythmias and conduction disturbances.

2. Follow-up testing may be appropriate to monitor response to therapy, e.g., oral or parenteral iron, ascorbic acid, and erythropoietin.

3. Iron studies may be appropriate in patients after treatment for other nutritional deficiency anemias, such as folate and vitamin B12, because iron deficiency may not be revealed until such a nutritional deficiency is treated.

4. Serum ferritin may be appropriate for monitoring iron status in patients with chronic renal disease with or without dialysis.

5. Serum iron may also be indicated for evaluation of toxic effects of iron and other metals (e.g., nickel, cadmium, aluminum, lead) whether due to accidental, intentional exposure or metabolic causes.

Limitations:

1. Iron studies should be used to diagnose and manage iron deficiency or iron overload states. These tests are not to be used solely to assess acute phase reactants where disease management will be unchanged. For example, infections and malignancies are associated with elevations in acute phase reactants such as ferritin, and decreases in serum iron concentration, but iron studies would only be medically necessary if results of iron studies might alter the management of the primary diagnosis or might warrant direct treatment of an iron disorder or condition.

2. If a normal serum ferritin level is documented, repeat testing would not ordinarily be medically necessary unless there is a change in the patient's condition, and ferritin assessment is needed for the ongoing management of the patient. For example, a patient presents with new onset insulin-dependent diabetes mellitus and has a serum ferritin level performed for the suspicion of hemochromatosis. If the ferritin level is normal, the repeat ferritin for diabetes mellitus would not be medically necessary.

3. When an End Stage Renal Disease (ESRD) patient is tested for ferritin, testing more frequently than every three months (the frequency authorized by 3167.3, Fiscal Intermediary manual) requires documentation of medical necessity [e.g., other than "Chronic Renal Failure" (ICD-9-CM 585) or "Renal Failure, Unspecified" (ICD-9-CM 586)].

4. It is ordinarily not necessary to measure both transferrin and TIBC at the same time because TIBC is an indirect measure of transferrin. When transferrin is ordered as part of the nutritional assessment for evaluating malnutrition, it is not necessary to order other iron studies unless iron deficiency or iron overload is suspected as well.

5. It is not ordinarily necessary to measure both iron/TIBC (or transferrin) and ferritin in initial patient testing. If clinically indicated after evaluation of the initial iron studies, it may be appropriate to perform additional iron studies either on the initial specimen or on a subsequently obtained specimen. After a diagnosis of iron deficiency or iron overload is established, either iron/TIBC (or transferrin) or ferritin may be medically necessary for monitoring, but not both.

6. It would not ordinarily be considered medically necessary to do a ferritin as a preoperative test except in the presence of anemia or recent autologous blood collections prior to the surgery.

100-3, 190.19
Collagen Crosslinks, Any Method

Indications:

Generally speaking, collagen crosslink testing is useful mostly in "fast losers" of bone. The age when these bone markers can help direct therapy is often pre-Medicare. By the time a fast loser of bone reaches age 65, she will most likely have been stabilized by appropriate therapy or have lost so much bone mass that further testing is useless. Coverage for bone marker assays may be established, however, for younger Medicare beneficiaries and for those men and women who might become fast losers because of some other therapy such as glucocorticoids. Safeguards should be incorporated to prevent excessive use of tests in patients for whom they have no clinical relevance.

Collagen crosslinks testing is used to:

- Identify individuals with elevated bone resorption, who have osteoporosis in whom response to treatment is being monitored;

- Predict response (as assessed by bone mass measurements) to FDA approved antiresorptive therapy in postmenopausal women; and

- Assess response to treatment of patients with osteoporosis, Paget's disease of the bone, or risk for osteoporosis where treatment may include FDA approved antiresorptive agents, anti-estrogens or selective estrogen receptor moderators.

Limitations:

Because of significant specimen to specimen collagen crosslink physiologic variability (15-20%), current recommendations for appropriate utilization include: one or two base-line assays from specified urine collections on separate days; followed by a repeat assay about three months after starting anti-resorptive therapy; followed by a repeat assay in 12 months after the three-month assay; and thereafter not more than annually, unless there is a change in therapy in which circumstance an additional test may be indicated three months after the initiation of new therapy.

Some collagen crosslink assays may not be appropriate for use in some disorders, according to FDA labeling restrictions.

Note: Scroll down for links to the quarterly Covered Code Lists (including narrative).

100-3, 190.20
NCD for Blood Glucose Testing (190.20)

Indications:

Blood glucose values are often necessary for the management of patients with diabetes mellitus, where hyperglycemia and hypoglycemia are often present. They are also critical in the determination of control of blood glucose levels in the patient with impaired fasting glucose (FPG 110-125 mg/dL), the patient with insulin resistance syndrome and/or carbohydrate intolerance (excessive rise in glucose following ingestion of glucose or glucose sources of food), in the patient with a hypoglycemia disorder such as nesidioblastosis or insulinoma, and in patients with a catabolic or malnutrition state. In addition to those conditions already listed, glucose testing may be medically necessary in patients with tuberculosis, unexplained chronic or recurrent infections, alcoholism, coronary artery disease (especially in women), or unexplained skin conditions (including pruritis, local skin infections, ulceration and gangrene without an established cause).

Many medical conditions may be a consequence of a sustained elevated or depressed glucose level. These include comas, seizures or epilepsy, confusion, abnormal hunger, abnormal weight loss or gain, and loss of sensation. Evaluation of glucose may also be indicated in patients on medications known to affect carbohydrate metabolism.

Effective January 1, 2005, the Medicare law expanded coverage to diabetic screening services. Some forms of blood glucode testing covered under this national coverage determination may be covered for screening purposes subject to specified frequencies. See 42 CFR 410.18 and section 90, chapter 18 of the Claims Processing Manual, for a full description of this screening benefit.

Limitations:

Frequent home blood glucose testing by diabetic patients should be encouraged. In stable, non-hospitalized patients who are unable or unwilling to do home monitoring, it may be reasonable and necessary to measure quantitative blood glucose up to four times annually.

Depending upon the age of the patient, type of diabetes, degree of control, complications of diabetes, and other co-morbid conditions, more frequent testing than four times annually may be reasonable and necessary.

In some patients presenting with nonspecific signs, symptoms, or diseases not normally associated with disturbances in glucose metabolism, a single blood glucose test may be medically necessary. Repeat testing may not be indicated unless abnormal results are found or unless there is a change in clinical condition. If repeat testing is performed, a specific diagnosis code (e.g., diabetes) should be reported to support medical necessity. However, repeat testing may be indicated where results are normal in patients with conditions where there is a confirmed continuing risk of glucose metabolism abnormality (e.g., monitoring glucocorticoid therapy).

100-3, 190.22
NCD for Thyroid Testing (190.22)

Indications

Thyroid function tests are used to define hyper function, euthyroidism, or hypofunction of thyroid disease. Thyroid testing may be reasonable and necessary to:

- Distinguish between primary and secondary hypothyroidism;

- Confirm or rule out primary hypothyroidism;

- Monitor thyroid hormone levels (for example, patients with goiter, thyroid nodules, or thyroid cancer);

- Monitor drug therapy in patients with primary hypothyroidism;

- Confirm or rule out primary hyperthyroidism; and

- Monitor therapy in patients with hyperthyroidism.

Thyroid function testing may be medically necessary in patients with disease or neoplasm of the thyroid and other endocrine glands. Thyroid function testing may also be medically necessary in patients with metabolic disorders; malnutrition; hyperlipidemia; certain types of anemia; psychosis and non-psychotic personality disorders; unexplained depression; ophthalmologic disorders; various cardiac arrhythmias; disorders of menstruation; skin conditions; myalgias; and a wide array of signs and symptoms, including alterations in consciousness; malaise; hypothermia; symptoms of the nervous and musculoskeletal system; skin and integumentary system; nutrition and metabolism; cardiovascular; and gastrointestinal system.

It may be medically necessary to do follow-up thyroid testing in patients with a personal history of malignant neoplasm of the endocrine system and in patients on long-term thyroid drug therapy.

Limitations

Testing may be covered up to two times a year in clinically stable patients; more frequent testing may be reasonable and necessary for patients whose thyroid therapy has been altered or in whom symptoms or signs of hyperthyroidism or hypothyroidism are noted.

100-3, 190.23
NCD for Lipid Testing (190.23)

Indications and Limitations of Coverage

Indications

The medical community recognizes lipid testing as appropriate for evaluating atherosclerotic cardiovascular disease. Conditions in which lipid testing may be indicated include:

- Assessment of patients with atherosclerotic cardiovascular disease.

- Evaluation of primary dyslipidemia.

- Any form of atherosclerotic disease, or any disease leading to the formation of atherosclerotic disease.

- Diagnostic evaluation of diseases associated with altered lipid metabolism, such as: nephrotic syndrome, pancreatitis, hepatic disease, and hypo and hyperthyroidism.

- Secondary dyslipidemia, including diabetes mellitus, disorders of gastrointestinal absorption, chronic renal failure.

- Signs or symptoms of dyslipidemias, such as skin lesions.

- As follow-up to the initial screen for coronary heart disease (total cholesterol + HDL cholesterol) when total cholesterol is determined to be high (>240 mg/dL), or borderline-high (200-240 mg/dL) plus two or more coronary heart disease risk factors, or an HDL cholesterol, <35 mg/dl.

To monitor the progress of patients on anti-lipid dietary management and pharmacologic therapy for the treatment of elevated blood lipid disorders, total cholesterol, HDL cholesterol and LDL cholesterol may be used. Triglycerides may be obtained if this lipid fraction is also elevated or if the patient is put on drugs (for example, thiazide diuretics, beta blockers, estrogens, glucocorticoids, and tamoxifen) which may raise the triglyceride level.

When monitoring long term anti-lipid dietary or pharmacologic therapy and when following patients with borderline high total or LDL cholesterol levels, it may be reasonable to perform the lipid panel annually. A lipid panel at a yearly interval will usually be adequate while measurement of the serum total cholesterol or a measured LDL should suffice for interim visits if the patient does not have hypertriglyceridemia.

Any one component of the panel or a measured LDL may be reasonable and necessary up to six times the first year for monitoring dietary or pharmacologic therapy. More frequent total cholesterol HDL cholesterol, LDL cholesterol and triglyceride testing may be indicated for marked elevations or for changes to anti-lipid therapy due to inadequate initial patient response to dietary or pharmacologic therapy. The LDL cholesterol or total cholesterol may be measured three times yearly after treatment goals have been achieved.

Electrophoretic or other quantitation of lipoproteins may be indicated if the patient has a primary disorder of lipoid metabolism.

Effective January 1, 2005, the Medicare law expanded coverage to cardiovascular screening services. Several of the procedures included in this NCD may be covered for screening purposes subject to specified frequencies. See 42 CFR 410.17 and section 100, chapter 18, of the Claims Processing Manual, for a full description of this benefit.

Limitations

Lipid panel and hepatic panel testing may be used for patients with severe psoriasis which has not responded to conventional therapy and for which the retinoid etretinate has been prescribed and who have developed hyperlipidemia or hepatic toxicity. Specific examples include erythrodermia and generalized pustular type and psoriasis associated with arthritis.

Routine screening and prophylactic testing for lipid disorder are not covered by Medicare. While lipid screening may be medically appropriate, Medicare by statute does not pay for it. Lipid testing in asymptomatic individuals is considered to be screening regardless of the presence of other risk factors such as family history, tobacco use, etc.

Once a diagnosis is established, one or several specific tests are usually adequate for monitoring the course of the disease. Less specific diagnoses (for example, other chest pain) alone do not support medical necessity of these tests.

When monitoring long term anti-lipid dietary or pharmacologic therapy and when following patients with borderline high total or LDL cholesterol levels, it is reasonable to perform the lipid panel annually. A lipid panel at a yearly interval will usually be adequate while measurement of the serum total cholesterol or a measured LDL should suffice for interim visits if the patient does not have hypertriglyceridemia.

Any one component of the panel or a measured LDL may be medically necessary up to six times the first year for monitoring dietary or pharmacologic therapy. More frequent total cholesterol HDL cholesterol, LDL cholesterol and triglyceride testing may be indicated for marked elevations or for changes to anti-lipid therapy due to inadequate initial patient response to dietary or pharmacologic therapy. The LDL cholesterol or total cholesterol may be measured three times yearly after treatment goals have been achieved.

If no dietary or pharmacological therapy is advised, monitoring is not necessary.

When evaluating non-specific chronic abnormalities of the liver (for example, elevations of transaminase, alkaline phosphatase, abnormal imaging studies, etc.), a lipid panel would generally not be indicated more than twice per year.

100-3, 190.26

NCD for Carcinoembryonic Antigen (CEA)

Carcinoembryonic antigen (CEA) is a protein polysaccharide found in some carcinomas. It is effective as a biochemical marker for monitoring the response of certain malignancies to therapy.

Indications

CEA may be medically necessary for follow-up of patients with colorectal carcinoma. It would however only be medically necessary at treatment decision-making points. In some clinical situations (e.g. adenocarcinoma of the lung, small cell carcinoma of the lung, and some gastrointestinal carcinomas) when a more specific marker is not expressed by the tumor, CEA may be a medically necessary alternative marker for monitoring. Preoperative CEA may also be helpful in determining the post-operative adequacy of surgical resection and subsequent medical management. In general, a single tumor marker will suffice in following patients with colorectal carcinoma or other malignancies that express such tumor markers.

In following patients who have had treatment for colorectal carcinoma, ASCO guideline suggests that if resection of liver metastasis would be indicated, it is recommended that post-operative CEA testing be performed every two to three months in patients with initial stage II or stage III disease for at least two years after diagnosis.

For patients with metastatic solid tumors which express CEA, CEA may be measured at the start of the treatment and with subsequent treatment cycles to assess the tumor's response to therapy.

Limitations:

Serum CEA determinations are generally not indicated more frequently than once per chemotherapy treatment cycle for patients with metastatic solid tumors which express CEA or every two months post-surgical treatment for patients who have had colorectal carcinoma. However, it may be proper to order the test more frequently in certain situations, for example, when there has been a significant change from prior CEA level or a significant change in patient status which could reflect disease progression or recurrence.

Testing with a diagnosis of an in situ carcinoma is not reasonably done more frequently than once, unless the result is abnormal, in which case the test may be repeated once.

100-3, 190.3

NCD for Cytogenetic Studies (190.3)

Medicare covers these tests when they are reasonable and necessary for the diagnosis or treatment of the following conditions:

- Genetic disorders (e.g., mongolism) in a fetus (See Medicare Benefit Policy Manual, Chapter 15, "Covered medical and Other health Services," Sec. 20.1)
- Failure of sexual development;
- Chronic myelogenous leukemia;
- Acute leukemias lymphoid (FAB L1-L3), myeloid (FAB M0-M7), and unclassified; or

- Mylodysplasia

100-3, 190.31

NCD for Prostate Specific Antigen (PSA) (190.31)

Indications:

PSA is of proven value in differentiating benign from malignant disease in men with lower urinary tract signs and symptoms (e.g., hematuria, slow urine stream, hesitancy, urgency, frequency, nocturia and incontinence) as well as with patients with palpably abnormal prostate glands on physician exam, and in patients with other laboratory or imaging studies that suggest the possibility of a malignant prostate disorder. PSA is also a marker used to follow the progress of prostate cancer once a diagnosis has been established, such as in detecting metastatic or persistent disease in patients who may require additional treatment. PSA testing may also be useful in the differential diagnosis of men presenting with as yet undiagnosed disseminated metastatic disease.

Limitations:

Generally, for patients with lower urinary tract signs or symptoms, the test is performed only once per year unless there is a change in the patient's medical condition.

Testing with a diagnosis of in situ carcinoma is not reasonably done more frequently than once, unless the result is abnormal, in which case the test may be repeated once.

100-3, 210.1

NCD for Prostate Cancer Screening Tests (210.1)

Indications and Limitations of Coverage

CIM 50-55

Covered

A. General

Section 4103 of the Balanced Budget Act of 1997 provides for coverage of certain prostate cancer screening tests subject to certain coverage, frequency, and payment limitations. Medicare will cover prostate cancer screening tests/procedures for the early detection of prostate cancer. Coverage of prostate cancer screening tests includes the following procedures furnished to an individual for the early detection of prostate cancer:

- Screening digital rectal examination; and
- Screening prostate specific antigen blood test

B. Screening Digital Rectal Examinations

Screening digital rectal examinations are covered at a frequency of once every 12 months for men who have attained age 50 (at least 11 months have passed following the month in which the last Medicare-covered screening digital rectal examination was performed). Screening digital rectal examination means a clinical examination of an individual's prostate for nodules or other abnormalities of the prostate. This screening must be performed by a doctor of medicine or osteopathy (as defined in §1861(r)(1) of the Act), or by a physician assistant, nurse practitioner, clinical nurse specialist, or certified nurse midwife (as defined in §1861(aa) and §1861(gg) of the Act) who is authorized under State law to perform the examination, fully knowledgeable about the beneficiary's medical condition, and would be responsible for using the results of any examination performed in the overall management of the beneficiary's specific medical problem.

C. Screening Prostate Specific Antigen Tests

Screening prostate specific antigen tests are covered at a frequency of once every 12 months for men who have attained age 50 (at least 11 months have passed following the month in which the last Medicare-covered screening prostate specific antigen test was performed). Screening prostate specific antigen tests (PSA) means a test to detect the marker for adenocarcinoma of prostate. PSA is a reliable immunocytochemical marker for primary and metastatic adenocarcinoma of prostate. This screening must be ordered by the beneficiary's physician or by the beneficiary's physician assistant, nurse practitioner, clinical nurse specialist, or certified nurse midwife (the term "attending physician"; is defined in §1861(r)(1) of the Act to mean a doctor of medicine or osteopathy and the terms ";physician assistant, nurse practitioner, clinical nurse specialist, or certified nurse midwife"; are defined in §1861(aa) and §1861(gg) of the Act) who is fully knowledgeable about the beneficiary's medical condition, and who would be responsible for using the results of any examination (test) performed in the overall management of the beneficiary's specific medical problem.

100-3, 210.2

NCD for Screening Pap Smears and Pelvic Examinations for Early Detection of Cervical or Vaginal Cancer (210.2)

Screening Pap Smear

A screening pap smear and related medically necessary services provided to a woman for the early detection of cervical cancer (including collection of the sample of cells and a physician's interpretation of the test results) and pelvic examination (including clinical breast examination) are covered under Medicare Part B when ordered by a physician (or authorized practitioner) under one of the following conditions:

- She has not had such a test during the preceding two years or is a woman of childbearing age (§1861(nn) of the Social Security Act (the Act).

- There is evidence (on the basis of her medical history or other findings) that she is at high risk of developing cervical cancer and her physician (or authorized practitioner) recommends that she have the test performed more frequently than every two years.

High risk factors for cervical and vaginal cancer are:

- Early onset of sexual activity (under 16 years of age)

- Multiple sexual partners (five or more in a lifetime)

- History of sexually transmitted disease (including HIV infection)

- Fewer than three negative or any pap smears within the previous seven years; and

- DES (diethylstilbestrol) - exposed daughters of women who took DES during pregnancy.

NOTE: Claims for pap smears must indicate the beneficiary's low or high risk status by including the appropriate diagnosis code on the line item (Item 24E of the Form CMS-1500).

Definitions

A woman as described in §1861(nn) of the Act is a woman who is of childbearing age and has had a pap smear test during any of the preceding 3 years that indicated the presence of cervical or vaginal cancer or other abnormality, or is at high risk of developing cervical or vaginal cancer.

A woman of childbearing age is one who is premenopausal and has been determined by a physician or other qualified practitioner to be of childbearing age, based upon the medical history or other findings.

Other qualified practitioner, as defined in 42 CFR 410.56(a) includes a certified nurse midwife (as defined in §1861(gg) of the Act), or a physician assistant, nurse practitioner, or clinical nurse specialist (as defined in §1861(aa) of the Act) who is authorized under State law to perform the examination.

Screening Pelvic Examination

Section 4102 of the Balanced Budget Act of 1997 provides for coverage of screening pelvic examinations (including a clinical breast examination) for all female beneficiaries, subject to certain frequency and other limitations. A screening pelvic examination (including a clinical breast examination) should include at least seven of the following eleven elements:

- Inspection and palpation of breasts for masses or lumps, tenderness, symmetry, or nipple discharge.

- Digital rectal examination including sphincter tone, presence of hemorrhoids, and rectal masses. Pelvic examination (with or without specimen collection for smears and cultures) including:

- External genitalia (for example, general appearance, hair distribution, or lesions).

- Urethral meatus (for example, size, location, lesions, or prolapse).

- Urethra (for example, masses, tenderness, or scarring).

- Bladder (for example, fullness, masses, or tenderness).

- Vagina (for example, general appearance, estrogen effect, discharge lesions, pelvic support, cystocele, or rectocele).

- Cervix (for example, general appearance, lesions, or discharge).

- Uterus (for example, size, contour, position, mobility, tenderness, consistency, descent, or support).

- Adnexa/parametria (for example, masses, tenderness, organomegaly, or nodularity).

- Anus and perineum.

This description is from Documentation Guidelines for Evaluation and Management Services, published in May 1997 and was developed by the Centers for Medicare & Medicaid Services and the American Medical Association.

100-3, 220.6.9

NCD for PET (FDG) for Refractory Seizures (220.6.9)

Beginning July 1, 2001, Medicare covers FDG PET for pre-surgical evaluation for the purpose of localization of a focus of refractory seizure activity.

Limitations: Covered only for pre-surgical evaluation.

Documentation that these conditions are met should be maintained by the referring physician in the beneficiary's medical record, as is normal business practice.

(This NCD last reviewed June 2001.)

100-3, 220.6.17

NCD for Positron Emission Tomography (FDG) for Oncologic Conditions (220.6.17)

A. General

FDG (2-[F18] fluoro-2-deoxy-D-glucose) Positron Emission Tomography (PET) is a minimally-invasive diagnostic imaging procedure used to evaluate glucose metabolism in normal tissue as well as in diseased tissues in conditions such as

cancer, ischemic heart disease, and some neurologic disorders. FDG is an injected radionuclide (or radiopharmaceutical) that emits sub-atomic particles, known as positrons, as it decays. FDG PET uses a positron camera (tomograph) to measure the decay of FDG. The rate of FDG decay provides biochemical information on glucose metabolism in the tissue being studied. As malignancies can cause abnormalities of metabolism and blood flow, FDG PET evaluation may indicate the probable presence or absence of a malignancy based upon observed differences in biologic activity compared to adjacent tissues.

The Centers for Medicare and Medicaid Services (CMS) was asked by the National Oncologic PET Registry (NOPR) to reconsider section 220.6 of the National Coverage Determinations (NCD) Manual to end the prospective data collection requirements under Coverage with Evidence Development (CED) across all oncologic indications of FDG PET imaging. The CMS received public input indicating that the current coverage framework of prospective data collection under CED be ended for all oncologic uses of FDG PET imaging.

1. Framework

   Effective for claims with dates of service on and after June 11, 2013, CMS is adopting a coverage framework that ends the prospective data collection requirements by NOPR under CED for all oncologic uses of FDG PET imaging. CMS is making this change for all NCDs that address coverage of FDG PET for oncologic uses addressed in this decision. This decision does not change coverage for any use of PET imaging using radiopharmaceuticals NaF-18 (fluorine-18 labeled sodium fluoride), ammonia N-13, or rubidium-82 (Rb-82).

2. Initial Anti-Tumor Treatment Strategy

   CMS continues to believe that the evidence is adequate to determine that the results of FDG PET imaging are useful in determining the appropriate initial anti-tumor treatment strategy for beneficiaries with suspected cancer and improve health outcomes and thus are reasonable and necessary under §1862(a)(1)(A) of the Social Security Act (the Act).

   Therefore, CMS continues to nationally cover one FDG PET study for beneficiaries who have cancers that are biopsy proven or strongly suspected based on other diagnostic testing when the beneficiary's treating physician determines that the FDG PET study is needed to determine the location and/or extent of the tumor for the following therapeutic purposes related to the initial anti-tumor treatment strategy:

   — To determine whether or not the beneficiary is an appropriate candidate for an invasive diagnostic or therapeutic procedure; or

   — To determine the optimal anatomic location for an invasive procedure; or

   — To determine the anatomic extent of tumor when the recommended antitumor treatment reasonably depends on the extent of the tumor.

   See the table at the end of this section for a synopsis of all nationally covered and noncovered oncologic uses of FDG PET imaging.

   B.1. Initial Anti-Tumor Treatment Strategy Nationally Covered Indications

   a. CMS continues to nationally cover FDG PET imaging for the initial anti-tumor treatment strategy for male and female breast cancer only when used in staging distant metastasis.

   b. CMS continues to nationally cover FDG PET to determine initial anti-tumor treatment strategy for melanoma other than for the evaluation of regional lymph nodes.

   c. CMS continues to nationally cover FDG PET imaging for the detection of pre-treatment metastasis (i.e., staging) in newly diagnosed cervical cancers following conventional imaging.

   C.1. Initial Anti-Tumor Treatment Strategy Nationally Non-Covered Indications

   a. CMS continues to nationally non-cover initial anti-tumor treatment strategy in Medicare beneficiaries who have adenocarcinoma of the prostate.

   b. CMS continues to nationally non-cover FDG PET imaging for diagnosis of breast cancer and initial staging of axillary nodes.

   c. CMS continues to nationally non-cover FDG PET imaging for initial anti-tumor treatment strategy for the evaluation of regional lymph nodes in melanoma.

   d. CMS continues to nationally non-cover FDG PET imaging for the diagnosis of cervical cancer related to initial anti-tumor treatment strategy.

3. Subsequent Anti-Tumor Treatment Strategy

   B.2. Subsequent Anti-Tumor Treatment Strategy Nationally Covered Indications

   Three FDG PET scans are nationally covered when used to guide subsequent management of anti-tumor treatment strategy after completion of initial anti-cancer therapy. Coverage of more than three FDG PET scans to guide subsequent management of anti-tumor treatment strategy after completion of initial anti-cancer therapy shall be determined by the local Medicare Administrative Contractors.

4. Synopsis of Coverage of FDG PET for Oncologic Conditions

Effective for claims with dates of service on and after June 11, 2013, the chart below summarizes national FDG PET coverage for oncologic conditions:

FDG PET for Cancers Tumor Type	Initial Treatment Strategy (formerly "diagnosis" & "staging")	Subsequent Treatment Strategy (formerly "restaging" & "monitoring response to treatment")
Colorectal	Cover	Cover
Esophagus	Cover	Cover
Head & Neck (not Thyroid, CNS)	Cover	Cover
Lymphoma	Cover	Cover
Non-Small Cell Lung	Cover	Cover
Ovary	Cover	Cover
Brain	Cover	Cover
Cervix	Cover w/exception*	Cover
Small Cell Lung	Cover	Cover
Soft Tissue Sarcoma	Cover	Cover
Pancreas	Cover	Cover
Testes	Cover	Cover
Prostate	Non-cover	Cover
Thyroid	Cover	Cover
Breast (male and female)	Cover w/exception*	Cover
Melanoma	Cover w/exception*	Cover
All Other Solid Tumors	Cover	Cover
Myeloma	Cover	Cover
All other cancers not listed	Cover	Cover

* Cervix: Nationally non-covered for the initial diagnosis of cervical cancer related to initial anti-tumor treatment strategy. All other indications for initial anti-tumor treatment strategy for cervical cancer are nationally covered.

* Breast: Nationally non-covered for initial diagnosis and/or staging of axillary lymph nodes. Nationally covered for initial staging of metastatic disease. All other indications for initial anti-tumor treatment strategy for breast cancer are nationally covered.

* Melanoma: Nationally non-covered for initial staging of regional lymph nodes. All other indications for initial anti-tumor treatment strategy for melanoma are nationally covered.

D. Other

N/A

100-3, 220.6.19

Positron Emission Tomography NaF-18 (NaF-18 PET) to Identify Bone Metastasis of Cancer (Effective February 26, 2010)

A. General

Positron Emission Tomography (PET) is a non-invasive, diagnostic imaging procedure that assesses the level of metabolic activity and perfusion in various organ systems of the body. A positron camera (tomograph) is used to produce cross-sectional tomographic images, which are obtained from positron-emitting radioactive tracer substances (radiopharmaceuticals) such as F-18 sodium fluoride. NaF-18 PET has been recognized as an excellent technique for imaging areas of altered osteogenic activity in bone. The clinical value of detecting and assessing the initial extent of metastatic cancer in bone is attested by a number of professional guidelines for oncology. Imaging to detect bone metastases is also recommended when a patient, following completion of initial treatment, is symptomatic with bone pain suspicious for metastases from a known primary tumor.

B. Nationally Covered Indications

Effective February 26, 2010, the Centers for Medicare & Medicaid Services (CMS) will cover NaF-18 PET imaging when the beneficiary's treating physician determines that the NaF-18 PET study is needed to inform the initial antitumor treatment strategy or to guide subsequent antitumor treatment strategy after the completion of initial treatment, and when the beneficiary is enrolled in, and the NaF-18 PET provider is participating in, the following type of prospective clinical study:

A NaF-18 PET clinical study that is designed to collect additional information at the time of the scan to assist in initial antitumor treatment planning or to guide subsequent treatment strategy by the identification, location and quantification of bone metastases in beneficiaries in whom bone metastases are strongly suspected based on clinical symptoms or the results of other diagnostic studies. Qualifying clinical studies must ensure that specific hypotheses are addressed; appropriate data elements are collected; hospitals and providers are qualified to provide the PET scan and interpret the results; participating hospitals and providers accurately report data on all enrolled patients not included in other qualifying trials through adequate auditing mechanisms; and all patient confidentiality, privacy, and other Federal laws must be followed.

The clinical studies for which Medicare will provide coverage must answer one or more of the following questions:

Prospectively, in Medicare beneficiaries whose treating physician determines that the NaF-18 PET study results are needed to inform the initial antitumor treatment strategy or to guide subsequent antitumor treatment strategy after the completion of initial treatment, does the addition of NaF-18 PET imaging lead to:

- A change in patient management to more appropriate palliative care; or
- A change in patient management to more appropriate curative care; or
- Improved quality of life; or Improved survival?

The study must adhere to the following standards of scientific integrity and relevance to the Medicare population:

a. The principal purpose of the research study is to test whether a particular intervention potentially improves the participants' health outcomes.

b. The research study is well-supported by available scientific and medical information or it is intended to clarify or establish the health outcomes of interventions already in common clinical use.

c. The research study does not unjustifiably duplicate existing studies.

d. The research study design is appropriate to answer the research question being asked in the study.

e. The research study is sponsored by an organization or individual capable of executing the proposed study successfully.

f. The research study is in compliance with all applicable Federal regulations concerning the protection of human subjects found in the Code of Federal Regulations (CFR) at 45 CFR Part 46. If a study is regulated by the Food and Drug Administration (FDA), it also must be in compliance with 21 CFR Parts 50 and 56.

g. All aspects of the research study are conducted according to the appropriate standards of scientific integrity.

h. The research study has a written protocol that clearly addresses, or incorporates by reference, the Medicare standards.

i. The clinical research study is not designed to exclusively test toxicity or disease pathophysiology in healthy individuals. Trials of all medical technologies measuring therapeutic outcomes as one of the objectives meet this standard only if the disease or condition being studied is life-threatening as defined in 21 CFR Sec.312.81(a) and the patient has no other viable treatment options.

j. The clinical research study is registered on the www.ClinicalTrials.gov Web site by the principal sponsor/investigator prior to the enrollment of the first study subject.

k. The research study protocol specifies the method and timing of public release of all pre-specified outcomes to be measured including release of outcomes if outcomes are negative or study is terminated early. The results must be made public within 24 months of the end of data collection. If a report is planned to be published in a peer-reviewed journal, then that initial release may be an abstract that meets the requirements of the International Committee of Medical Journal Editors. However, a full report of the outcomes must be made public no later than three (3) years after the end of data collection.

l. The research study protocol must explicitly discuss subpopulations affected by the treatment under investigation, particularly traditionally underrepresented groups in clinical studies, how the inclusion and exclusion criteria affect enrollment of these populations, and a plan for the retention and reporting of said populations on the trial. If the inclusion and exclusion criteria are expected to have a negative effect on the recruitment or retention of underrepresented populations, the protocol must discuss why these criteria are necessary.

m. The research study protocol explicitly discusses how the results are or are not expected to be generalizable to the Medicare population to infer whether Medicare patients may benefit from the intervention. Separate discussions in the protocol may be necessary for populations eligible for Medicare due to age, disability or Medicaid eligibility.

Consistent with section 1142 of the Social Security Act (the Act), the Agency for Healthcare Research and Quality (AHRQ) supports clinical research studies that the Centers for Medicare and Medicaid Services (CMS) determines meet the above-listed standards and address the above-listed research questions.

C. Nationally Non-Covered Indications

Effective February 26, 2010, CMS determines that the evidence is not sufficient to determine that the results of NaF-18 PET imaging to identify bone metastases improve health outcomes of beneficiaries with cancer and is not reasonable and necessary under Sec.1862(a)(1)(A) of the Act unless it is to inform initial antitumor treatment strategy or to guide subsequent antitumor treatment strategy after completion of initial treatment, and then only under CED. All other uses and clinical indications of NaF-18 PET are nationally non-covered.

D. Other

The only radiopharmaceutical diagnostic imaging agents covered by Medicare for PET cancer imaging are 2-[F-18] Fluoro-D-Glucose (FDG) and NaF-18 (sodium fluoride-18). All other PET radiopharmaceutical diagnostic imaging agents are non-covered for this indication.

(This NCD was last reviewed in February 2010.)

100-3, 220.13

NCD for Percutaneous Image-Guided Breast Biopsy (220.13)

Percutaneous image-guided breast biopsy is a method of obtaining a breast biopsy through a percutaneous incision by employing image guidance systems. Image guidance systems may be either ultrasound or stereotactic.

The Breast Imaging Reporting and Data System (or BIRADS system) employed by the American College of Radiology provides a standardized lexicon with which radiologists may report their interpretation of a mammogram. The BIRADS grading of mammograms is as follows: Grade I-Negative, Grade II-Benign finding, Grade III-Probably benign, Grade IV-Suspicious abnormality, and Grade V-Highly suggestive of malignant neoplasm.

A. Non-Palpable Breast Lesions

Effective January 1, 2003, Medicare covers percutaneous image-guided breast biopsy using stereotactic or ultrasound imaging for a radiographic abnormality that is non-palpable and is graded as a BIRADS III, IV, or V.

B. Palpable Breast Lesions

Effective January 1, 2003, Medicare covers percutaneous image guided breast biopsy using stereotactic or ultrasound imaging for palpable lesions that are difficult to biopsy using palpation alone. Medicare Administrative Contractors have the discretion to decide what types of palpable lesions are difficult to biopsy using palpation.

100-3, 230.1

NCD for Treatment of Kidney Stones (230.1)

In addition to the traditional surgical/endoscopic techniques for the treatment of kidney stones, the following lithotripsy techniques are also covered for services rendered on or after March I5, I985.

Extracorporeal Shock Wave Lithotripsy.--Extracorporeal Shock Wave Lithotripsy (ESWL) is a non-invasive method of treating kidney stones using a device called a lithotriptor. The lithotriptor uses shock waves generated outside of the body to break up upper urinary tract stones. It focuses the shock waves specifically on stones under X-ray visualization, pulverizing them by repeated shocks. ESWL is covered under Medicare for use in the treatment of upper urinary tract kidney stones.

Percutaneous Lithotripsy.--Percutaneous lithotripsy (or nephrolithotomy) is an invasive method of treating kidney stones by using ultrasound, electrohydraulic or mechanical lithotripsy. A probe is inserted through an incision in the skin directly over the kidney and applied to the stone. A form of lithotripsy is then used to fragment the stone. Mechanical or electrohydraulic lithotripsy may be used as an alternative or adjunct to ultrasonic lithotripsy. Percutaneous lithotripsy of kidney stones by ultrasound or by the related techniques of electrohydraulic or mechanical lithotripsy is covered under Medicare.

The following is covered for services rendered on or after January 16, 1988.

Transurethral Ureteroscopic Lithotripsy.--Transurethral ureteroscopic lithotripsy is a method of fragmenting and removing ureteral and renal stones through a cystoscope. The cystoscope is inserted through the urethra into the bladder. Catheters are passed through the scope into the opening where the ureters enter the bladder. Instruments passed through this opening into the ureters are used to manipulate and ultimately disintegrate stones, using either mechanical crushing, transcystoscopic electrohydraulic shock waves, ultrasound or laser. Transurethral ureteroscopic lithotripsy for the treatment of urinary tract stones of the kidney or ureter is covered under Medicare.

100-3, 230.3

NCD for Sterilization (230.3)

A. Nationally Covered Conditions

Payment may be made only where sterilization is a necessary part of the treatment of an illness or injury, e.g., removal of a uterus because of a tumor, removal of diseased ovaries.

Sterilization of a mentally challenged beneficiary is covered if it is a necessary part of the treatment of an illness or injury (bilateral oophorectomy or bilateral orchidectomy in a case of cancer of the prostate). The Medicare Administrative Contractor denies claims when the pathological evidence of the necessity to perform any such procedures to treat an illness or injury is absent; and

Monitor such surgeries closely and obtain the information needed to determine whether in fact the surgery was performed as a means of treating an illness or injury or only to achieve sterilization.

B. Nationally Non-Covered Conditions

- Elective hysterectomy, tubal ligation, and vasectomy, if the primary indication for these procedures is sterilization;

- A sterilization that is performed because a physician believes another pregnancy would endanger the overall general health of the woman is not considered to be reasonable and necessary for the diagnosis or treatment of illness or injury within the meaning of §1862(a)(1) of the Social Security Act. The same conclusion would apply where the sterilization is performed only as a measure to prevent the possible development of, or effect on, a mental condition should the individual become pregnant; and sterilization of a mentally retarded person where the purpose is to prevent conception, rather than the treatment of an illness or injury.

100-3, 230.4

NCD for Diagnosis and Treatment of Impotence (230.4)

Program payment may be made for diagnosis and treatment of sexual impotence. Impotence is a failure of a body part for which the diagnosis, and frequently the treatment, require medical expertise. Depending on the cause of the condition, treatment may be surgical; e.g., implantation of a penile prosthesis, or nonsurgical; e.g., medical or psychotherapeutic treatment. Since causes and, therefore, appropriate treatment vary, if abuse is suspected it may be necessary to request documentation of appropriateness in individual cases. If treatment is furnished to patients (other than hospital inpatients) in connection with a mental condition, apply the psychiatric service limitation described in the Medicare General Information, Eligibility, and Entitlement Manual, Chapter 3.

100-3, 230.10

NCD for Incontinence Control Devices (230.10)

A - Mechanical/Hydraulic Incontinence Control Devices

Mechanical/hydraulic incontinence control devices are accepted as safe and effective in the management of urinary incontinence in patients with permanent anatomic and neurologic dysfunctions of the bladder. This class of devices achieves control of urination by compression of the urethra. The materials used and the success rate may vary somewhat from device to device. Such a device is covered when its use is reasonable and necessary for the individual patient.

B - Collagen Implant

A collagen implant, which is injected into the submucosal tissues of the urethra and/or the bladder neck and into tissues adjacent to the urethra, is a prosthetic device used in the treatment of stress urinary incontinence resulting from intrinsic sphincter deficiency (ISD). ISD is a cause of stress urinary incontinence in which the urethral sphincter is unable to contract and generate sufficient resistance in the bladder, especially during stress maneuvers.

Prior to collagen implant therapy, a skin test for collagen sensitivity must be administered and evaluated over a 4 week period.

In male patients, the evaluation must include a complete history and physical examination and a simple cystometrogram to determine that the bladder fills and stores properly. The patient then is asked to stand upright with a full bladder and to cough or otherwise exert abdominal pressure on his bladder. If the patient leaks, the diagnosis of ISD is established.

In female patients, the evaluation must include a complete history and physical examination (including a pelvic exam) and a simple cystometrogram to rule out abnormalities of bladder compliance and abnormalities of urethral support. Following that determination, an abdominal leak point pressure (ALLP) test is performed. Leak point pressure, stated in cm H2O, is defined as the intra-abdominal pressure at which leakage occurs from the bladder (around a catheter) when the bladder has been filled with a minimum of 150 cc fluid. If the patient has an ALLP of less than 100 cm H_2O, the diagnosis of ISD is established.

To use a collagen implant, physicians must have urology training in the use of a cystoscope and must complete a collagen implant training program.

Coverage of a collagen implant, and the procedure to inject it, is limited to the following types of patients with stress urinary incontinence due to ISD:

- Male or female patients with congenital sphincter weakness secondary to conditions such as myelomeningocele or epispadias;

- Male or female patients with acquired sphincter weakness secondary to spinal cord lesions;

- Male patients following trauma, including prostatectomy and/or radiation; and

- Female patients without urethral hypermobility and with abdominal leak point pressures of 100 cm H2O or less.

Patients whose incontinence does not improve with 5 injection procedures (5 separate treatment sessions) are considered treatment failures, and no further treatment of urinary incontinence by collagen implant is covered. Patients who have a reoccurrence of incontinence following successful treatment with collagen implants in the past (e.g., 6-12 months previously) may benefit from additional treatment sessions. Coverage of additional sessions may be allowed but must be supported by medical justification.

100-3, 260.1

Adult Liver Transplantation

A. General

Liver transplantation, which is in situ replacement of a patient's liver with a donor liver, in certain circumstances, may be an accepted treatment for patients with end-stage liver disease due to a variety of causes. The procedure is used in selected patients as a treatment for malignancies, including primary liver tumors and certain metastatic tumors, which are typically rare but lethal with very limited treatment options. It has also been used in the treatment of patients with extrahepatic perihilar malignancies. Examples of malignancies include extrahepatic unresectable cholangiocarcinoma (CCA), liver metastases due to a neuroendocrine tumor (NET), and, hemangioendothelioma (HAE). Despite potential short- and long-term complications, transplantation may offer the only chance of cure for selected patients while providing meaningful palliation for some others.

B. Nationally Covered Indications

Effective July 15, 1996, adult liver transplantation when performed on beneficiaries with end- stage liver disease other than hepatitis B or malignancies is covered under Medicare when performed in a facility which is approved by the Centers for Medicare & Medicaid Services (CMS) as meeting institutional coverage criteria.

Effective December 10, 1999, adult liver transplantation when performed on beneficiaries with end-stage liver disease other than malignancies is covered under Medicare when performed in a facility which is approved by CMS as meeting institutional coverage criteria.

Effective September 1, 2001, Medicare covers adult liver transplantation for hepatocellular carcinoma when the following conditions are met:

- The patient is not a candidate for subtotal liver resection;

- The patient's tumor(s) is less than or equal to 5 cm in diameter;

- There is no macrovascular involvement;

- There is no identifiable extrahepatic spread of tumor to surrounding lymph nodes, lungs, abdominal organs or bone; and,

- The transplant is furnished in a facility that is approved by CMS as meeting institutional coverage criteria for liver transplants (see 65 FR 15006).

Effective June 21, 2012, Medicare Adminstrative Contractors acting within their respective jurisdictions may determine coverage of adult liver transplantation for the following malignancies: (1) extrahepatic unresectable cholangiocarcinoma (CCA); (2) liver metastases due to a neuroendocrine tumor (NET); and, (3) hemangioendothelioma (HAE).

1. Follow-Up Care

   Follow-up care or re-transplantation required as a result of a covered liver transplant is covered, provided such services are otherwise reasonable and necessary. Follow-up care is also covered for patients who have been discharged from a hospital after receiving non-covered liver transplant. Coverage for follow-up care is for items and services that are reasonable and necessary as determined by Medicare guidelines.

2. Immunosuppressive Drugs

   See the Medicare Benefit Policy Manual, Chapter 15, "Covered Medical and Other Health Services," §50.5.1 and the Medicare Claims Processing Manual, Chapter 17, "Drugs and Biologicals," §80.3.

C. Nationally Non-Covered Indications

Adult liver transplantation for other malignancies remains excluded from coverage.

D. Other

Coverage of adult liver transplantation is effective as of the date of the facility's approval, but for applications received before July 13, 1991, can be effective as early as March 8, 1990. (See 56 FR 15006 dated April 12, 1991.)

(This NCD last reviewed June 2012.)

100-3, 260.2

NCD for Pediatric Liver Transplantation (260.2)

Liver transplantation is covered for children (under age 18) with extrahepatic biliary atresia or any other form of end stage liver disease, except that coverage is not provided for children with a malignancy extending beyond the margins of the liver or those with persistent viremia.

Liver transplantation is covered for Medicare beneficiaries when performed in a pediatric hospital that performs pediatric liver transplants if the hospital submits an application which CMS approves documenting that:

- The hospital's pediatric liver transplant program is operated jointly by the hospital and another facility that has been found by CMS to meet the institutional coverage criteria in the "Federal Register" notice of April 12, 1991;

- The unified program shares the same transplant surgeons and quality assurance program (including oversight committee, patient protocol, and patient selection criteria); and

- The hospital is able to provide the specialized facilities, services, and personnel that are required by pediatric liver transplant patients.

100-3, 260.3

NCD for Pancreas Transplants (260.3)

B. Nationally Covered Indications

Effective for services performed on or after July 1, 1999, whole organ pancreas transplantation is nationally covered by Medicare when performed simultaneous with or after a kidney transplant. If the pancreas transplant occurs after the kidney transplant, immunosuppressive therapy begins with the date of discharge from the inpatient stay for the pancreas transplant.

Effective for services performed on or after April 26, 2006, pancreas transplants alone (PA) are reasonable and necessary for Medicare beneficiaries in the following limited circumstances:

1. PA will be limited to those facilities that are Medicare-approved for kidney transplantation. (Approved centers can be found at http://www.cms.hhs.gov/ESRDGeneralInformation/02_Data.asp#TopOfPage

2. Patients must have a diagnosis of type I diabetes:

   — Patient with diabetes must be beta cell autoantibody positive; or

   — Patient must demonstrate insulinopenia defined as a fasting C-peptide level that is less than or equal to 110% of the lower limit of normal of the laboratory's measurement method. Fasting C-peptide levels will only be considered valid with a concurrently obtained fasting glucose <225 mg/dL;

3. Patients must have a history of medically-uncontrollable labile (brittle) insulin-dependent diabetes mellitus with documented recurrent, severe, acutely life-threatening metabolic complications that require hospitalization. Aforementioned complications include frequent hypoglycemia unawareness or recurring severe ketoacidosis, or recurring severe hypoglycemic attacks;

4. Patients must have been optimally and intensively managed by an endocrinologist for at least 12 months with the most medically-recognized advanced insulin formulations and delivery systems;

5. Patients must have the emotional and mental capacity to understand the significant risks associated with surgery and to effectively manage the lifelong need for immunosuppression; and,

6. Patients must otherwise be a suitable candidate for transplantation.

C. Nationally Non-Covered Indications

The following procedure is not considered reasonable and necessary within the meaning of section 1862(a)(1)(A) of the Social Security Act:

1. Transplantation of partial pancreatic tissue or islet cells (except in the context of a clinical trial (see section 260.3.1 of the National Coverage Determinations Manual).

D. Other

Not applicable.

(This NCD last reviewed April 2006.)

100-3, 260.5

NCD for Intestinal and Multi-Visceral Transplantation (260.5)

A. General

Medicare covers intestinal and multi-visceral transplantation for the purpose of restoring intestinal function in patients with irreversible intestinal failure. Intestinal failure is defined as the loss of absorptive capacity of the small bowel secondary to severe primary gastrointestinal disease or surgically induced short bowel syndrome. It may be associated with both mortality and profound morbidity. Multi-visceral transplantation includes organs in the digestive system (stomach, duodenum, pancreas, liver and intestine).

The evidence supports the fact that aged patients generally do not survive as well as younger patients receiving intestinal transplantation. Nonetheless, some older patients who are free from other contraindications have received the procedure and are progressing well, as evidenced by the United Network for Organ Sharing (UNOS) data. Thus, it is not appropriate to include specific exclusions from coverage, such as an age limitation, in the national coverage policy.

B. Nationally Covered Indications

Effective for services performed on or after April 1, 2001, this procedure is covered only when performed for patients who have failed total parenteral nutrition (TPN) and only when performed in centers that meet approval criteria.

1. Failed TPN

   The TPN delivers nutrients intravenously, avoiding the need for absorption through the small bowel. TPN failure includes the following:

   — Impending or overt liver failure due to TPN induced liver injury. The clinical manifestations include elevated serum bilirubin and/or liver enzymes, splenomegaly, thrombocytopenia, gastroesophageal varices, coagulopathy, stomal bleeding or hepatic fibrosis/cirrhosis.

   — Thrombosis of the major central venous channels; jugular, subclavian, and femoral veins. Thrombosis of two or more of these vessels is considered a life threatening complication and failure of TPN therapy. The sequelae of central venous thrombosis are lack of access for TPN infusion, fatal sepsis due to infected thrombi, pulmonary embolism, Superior Vena Cava syndrome, or chronic venous insufficiency.

   — Frequent line infection and sepsis. The development of two or more episodes of systemic sepsis secondary to line infection per year that requires hospitalization indicates failure of TPN therapy. A single episode of line related fungemia, septic shock and/or Acute Respiratory Distress Syndrome are considered indicators of TPN failure.

   — Frequent episodes of severe dehydration despite intravenous fluid supplement in addition to TPN. Under certain medical conditions such as secretory diarrhea and non-constructable gastrointestinal tract, the loss of the gastrointestinal and pancreatobiliary secretions exceeds the maximum intravenous infusion rates that can be tolerated by the cardiopulmonary system. Frequent episodes of dehydration are deleterious to all body organs particularly kidneys and the central nervous system with the development of multiple kidney stones, renal failure, and permanent brain damage.

2. Approved Transplant Facilities

Intestinal transplantation is covered by Medicare if performed in an approved facility. The criteria for approval of centers will be based on a volume of 10 intestinal transplants per year with a 1-year actuarial survival of 65 percent using the Kaplan-Meier technique.

C. Nationally Non-covered Indications

All other indications remain non-covered.

D. Other

NA.

(This NCD last reviewed May 2006.)

100-3, 260.9

NCD for Heart Transplants (260.9)

A. General

Cardiac transplantation is covered under Medicare when performed in a facility which is approved by Medicare as meeting institutional coverage criteria. (See CMS Ruling 87-1.)

B. Exceptions

In certain limited cases, exceptions to the criteria may be warranted if there is justification and if the facility ensures our objectives of safety and efficacy. Under no circumstances will exceptions be made for facilities whose transplant programs have been in existence for less than two years, and applications from consortia will not be approved.

Although consortium arrangements will not be approved for payment of Medicare heart transplants, consideration will be given to applications from heart transplant facilities that consist of more than one hospital where all of the following conditions exist:

- The hospitals are under the common control or have a formal affiliation arrangement with each other under the auspices of an organization such as a university or a legally-constituted medical research institute; and

- The hospitals share resources by routinely using the same personnel or services in their transplant programs. The sharing of resources must be supported by the submission of operative notes or other information that documents the routine use of the same personnel and services in all of the individual hospitals. At a minimum, shared resources means:

- The individual members of the transplant team, consisting of the cardiac transplant surgeons, cardiologists and pathologists, must practice in all the hospitals and it can be documented that they otherwise function as members of the transplant team;

- The same organ procurement organization, immunology, and tissue-typing services must be used by all the hospitals;

- The hospitals submit, in the manner required (Kaplan-Meier method) their individual and pooled experience and survival data; and

- The hospitals otherwise meet the remaining Medicare criteria for heart transplant facilities; that is, the criteria regarding patient selection, patient management, program commitment, etc.

C. Pediatric Hospitals

Cardiac transplantation is covered for Medicare beneficiaries when performed in a pediatric hospital that performs pediatric heart transplants if the hospital submits an application which CMS approves as documenting that:

- The hospital's pediatric heart transplant program is operated jointly by the hospital and another facility that has been found by CMS to meet the institutional coverage criteria in CMS Ruling 87-1;

- The unified program shares the same transplant surgeons and quality assurance program (including oversight committee, patient protocol, and patient selection criteria); and

- The hospital is able to provide the specialized facilities, services, and personnel that are required by pediatric heart transplant patients.

D. Follow-Up Care

Follow-up care required as a result of a covered heart transplant is covered, provided such services are otherwise reasonable and necessary. Follow-up care is also covered for patients who have been discharged from a hospital after receiving a noncovered heart transplant. Coverage for follow-up care would be for items and services that are reasonable and necessary, as determined by Medicare guidelines. (See the Medicare Benefit Policy Manual, Chapter 16, "General Exclusions from Coverage," Sec.180.)

E. Immunosuppressive Drugs

See the Medicare Claims Processing Manual, Chapter 17, "Drugs and Biologicals," Sec.80.3.1, and Chapter 8, "Outpatient ESRD Hospital, Independent Facility, and Physician/Supplier Claims," Sec.120.1.

F. Artificial Hearts

Medicare does not cover the use of artificial hearts as a permanent replacement for a human heart or as a temporary life-support system until a human heart becomes available for transplant (often referred to as a "bridge to transplant"). Medicare does cover a ventricular assist device (VAD) when used in conjunction with specific criteria listed in Sec.20.9 of the NCD Manual.

100-3, 270.3

NCD for Blood-Derived Products for Chronic Non-Healing Wounds (270.3)

A. General

Wound healing is a dynamic, interactive process that involves multiple cells and proteins. There are three progressive stages of normal wound healing, and the typical wound healing duration is about 4 weeks. While cutaneous wounds are a disruption of the normal, anatomic structure and function of the skin, subcutaneous wounds involve tissue below the skin's surface. Wounds are categorized as either acute, in where the normal wound healing stages are not yet completed but it is presumed they will be, resulting in orderly and timely wound repair, or chronic, in where a wound has failed to progress through the normal wound healing stages and repair itself within a sufficient time period.

Platelet-rich plasma (PRP) is produced in an autologous or homologous manner. Autologous PRP is comprised of blood from the patient who will ultimately receive the PRP. Alternatively, homologous PRP is derived from blood from multiple donors.

Blood is donated by the patient and centrifuged to produce an autologous gel for treatment of chronic, non-healing cutaneous wounds that persists for 30 days or longer and fail to properly complete the healing process. Autologous blood derived products for chronic, non-healing wounds includes both: (1) platelet derived growth factor (PDGF) products (such as Procuren), and (2) PRP (such as AutoloGel).

The PRP is different from previous products in that it contains whole cells including white cells, red cells, plasma, platelets, fibrinogen, stem cells, macrophages, and fibroblasts.

The PRP is used by physicians in clinical settings in treating chronic, non-healing wounds, open, cutaneous wounds, soft tissue, and bone. Alternatively, PDGF does not contain cells and was previously marketed as a product to be used by patients at home.

B. Nationally Covered Indications

Effective August 2, 2012, upon reconsideration, The Centers for Medicare and Medicaid Services (CMS) has determined that platelet-rich plasma (PRP) – an autologous blood-derived product, will be covered only for the treatment of chronic non-healing diabetic, venous and/or pressure wounds and only when the following conditions are met:

The patient is enrolled in a clinical trial that addresses the following questions using validated and reliable methods of evaluation. Clinical study applications for coverage pursuant to this National coverage Determination (NCD) must be received by August 2, 2014.

The clinical research study must meet the requirements specified below to assess the effect of PRP for the treatment of chronic non-healing diabetic, venous and/or pressure wounds. The clinical study must address:

Prospectively, do Medicare beneficiaries that have chronic non-healing diabetic, venous and/or pressure wounds who receive well-defined optimal usual care along with PRP therapy, experience clinically significant health outcomes compared to patients who receive well-defined optimal usual care for chronic non-healing diabetic, venous and/or pressure wounds as indicated by addressing at least one of the following:

a. Complete wound healing?

b. Ability to return to previous function and resumption of normal activities?

c. Reduction of wound size or healing trajectory which results in the patient's ability to return to previous function and resumption of normal activities?

The required clinical trial of PRP must adhere to the following standards of scientific integrity and relevance to the Medicare population:

a. The principal purpose of the CLINICAL STUDY is to test whether PRP improves the participants' health outcomes.

b. The CLINICAL STUDY is well supported by available scientific and medical information or it is intended to clarify or establish the health outcomes of interventions already in common clinical use.

c. The CLINICAL STUDY does not unjustifiably duplicate existing studies.

d. The CLINICAL STUDY design is appropriate to answer the research question being asked in the study.

e. The CLINICAL STUDY is sponsored by an organization or individual capable of executing the proposed study successfully.

f. The CLINICAL STUDY is in compliance with all applicable Federal regulations concerning the protection of human subjects found at 45 CFR Part 46.

g. All aspects of the CLINICAL STUDY are conducted according to appropriate standards of scientific integrity set by the International Committee of Medical Journal Editors (http://www.icmje.org).

h. The CLINICAL STUDY has a written protocol that clearly addresses, or incorporates by reference, the standards listed here as Medicare requirements for coverage with evidence development (CED).

i. The CLINICAL STUDY is not designed to exclusively test toxicity or disease pathophysiology in healthy individuals. Trials of all medical technologies measuring therapeutic outcomes as one of the objectives meet this standard only if the disease or condition being studied is life threatening as defined in 21 CFR §312.81(a) and the patient has no other viable treatment options.

j. The CLINICAL STUDY is registered on the ClinicalTrials.gov website by the principal sponsor/investigator prior to the enrollment of the first study subject.

k. The CLINICAL STUDY protocol specifies the method and timing of public release of all pre-specified outcomes to be measured including release of outcomes if outcomes are negative or study is terminated early. The results must be made public within 24 months of the end of data collection. If a report is planned to be published in a peer reviewed journal, then that initial release may be an abstract that meets the requirements of the International Committee of Medical Journal Editors (http://www.icmje.org). However a full report of the outcomes must be made public no later than three (3) years after the end of data collection.

l. The CLINICAL STUDY protocol must explicitly discuss subpopulations affected by the treatment under investigation, particularly traditionally underrepresented groups in clinical studies, how the inclusion and exclusion criteria effect enrollment of these populations, and a plan for the retention and reporting of said populations on the trial. If the inclusion and exclusion criteria are expected to have a negative effect on the recruitment or retention of underrepresented populations, the protocol must discuss why these criteria are necessary.

m. The CLINICAL STUDY protocol explicitly discusses how the results are or are not expected to be generalizable to the Medicare population to infer whether Medicare patients may benefit from the intervention. Separate discussions in the protocol may be necessary for populations eligible for Medicare due to age, disability or Medicaid eligibility. Consistent with §1142 of the Social Security Act (the Act), the Agency for Healthcare Research and Quality (AHRQ) supports clinical research studies that CMS determines meet the above-listed standards and address the above-listed research questions.

Any clinical study undertaken pursuant to this NCD must be approved no later than August 2, 2014. If there are no approved clinical studies on or before August 2, 2014, this CED will expire. Any clinical study approved will adhere to the timeframe designated in the approved clinical study protocol.

C. Nationally Non-Covered Indications
1. Effective December 28, 1992, the Centers for Medicare & Medicaid Services (CMS) issued a national non-coverage determination for platelet-derived wound-healing formulas intended to treat patients with chronic, non-healing wounds. This decision was based on a lack of sufficient published data to determine safety and efficacy, and a public health service technology assessment.

100-4, 3, 90.1
Kidney Transplant - General
A3-3612, HO-E414

A major treatment for patients with ESRD is kidney transplantation. This involves removing a kidney, usually from a living relative of the patient or from an unrelated person who has died, and surgically placing the kidney into the patient. After the beneficiary receives a kidney transplant, Medicare pays the transplant hospital for the transplant and appropriate standard acquisition charges. Special provisions apply to payment. For the list of approved Medicare certified transplant facilities, refer to the following Web site:
http://www.cms.hhs.gov/CertificationandComplianc/20_Transplant.asp#TopOfPage

A transplant hospital may acquire cadaver kidneys by:
- Excising kidneys from cadavers in its own hospital; and
- Arrangements with a freestanding organ procurement organization (OPO) that provides cadaver kidneys to any transplant hospital or by a hospital based OPO.

A transplant hospital that is also a certified organ procurement organization may acquire cadaver kidneys by:
- Having its organ procurement team excise kidneys from cadavers in other hospitals;
- Arrangements with participating community hospitals, whether they excise kidneys on a regular or irregular basis; and
- Arrangements with an organ procurement organization that services the transplant hospital as a member of a network.

When the transplant hospital also excises the cadaver kidney, the cost of the procedure is included in its kidney acquisition costs and is considered in arriving at its standard cadaver kidney acquisition charge. When the transplant hospital excises a kidney to provide another hospital, it may use its standard cadaver kidney acquisition charge or its standard detailed departmental charges to bill that hospital.

When the excising hospital is not a transplant hospital, it bills its customary charges for services used in excising the cadaver kidney to the transplant hospital or organ procurement agency.

If the transplanting hospital's organ procurement team excises the cadaver kidney at another hospital, the cost of operating such a team is included in the transplanting hospital's kidney acquisition costs, along with the reasonable charges billed by the other hospital of its services.

100-4, 3, 90.1.1
The Standard Kidney Acquisition Charge
There are two basic standard charges that must be developed by transplant hospitals from costs expected to be incurred in the acquisition of kidneys:
- The standard charge for acquiring a live donor kidney; and
- The standard charge for acquiring a cadaver kidney.

The standard charge is not a charge representing the acquisition cost of a specific kidney; rather, it is a charge that reflects the average cost associated with each type of kidney acquisition.

When the transplant hospital bills the program for the transplant, it shows its standard kidney acquisition charge on revenue code 081X. Kidney acquisition charges are not considered for the IPPS outlier calculation.

Acquisition services are billed from the excising hospital to the transplant hospital. A billing form is not submitted from the excising hospital to the FI. The transplant hospital keeps an itemized statement that identifies the services furnished, the charges, the person receiving the service (donor/recipient), and whether this is a potential transplant donor or recipient. These charges are reflected in the transplant hospital's kidney acquisition costcenter and are used in determining the hospital's standard charge for acquiring a live donor's kidney or a cadaver's kidney. The standard charge is not a charge representing the acquisition cost of a specific kidney. Rather, it is a charge that reflects the average cost associated with each type of kidney acquisition. Also, it is an all-inclusive charge for all services required in acquisition of a kidney, i.e., tissue typing, post-operative evaluation.

A. Billing For Blood And Tissue Typing of the Transplant Recipient Whether or Not Medicare Entitlement Is Established
Tissue typing and pre-transplant evaluation can be reflected only through the kidney acquisition charge of the hospital where the transplant will take place. The transplant hospital includes in its kidney acquisition cost center the reasonable charges it pays to the independent laboratory or other hospital which typed the potential transplant recipient, either before or after his entitlement. It also includes reasonable charges paid for physician tissue typing services, applicable to live donors and recipients (during the preentitlement period and after entitlement, but prior to hospital admission for transplantation).

B. Billing for Blood and Tissue Typing and Other Pre-Transplant Evaluation of Live Donors
The entitlement date of the beneficiary who will receive the transplant is not a consideration in reimbursing for the services to donors, since no bill is submitted directly to Medicare. All charges for services to donors prior to admission into the hospital for excision are "billed" indirectly to Medicare through the live donor acquisition charge of transplanting hospitals.

C. Billing Donor And Recipient Pre-Transplant Services (Performed by Transplant Hospitals or Other Providers) to the Kidney Acquisition Cost Center
The transplant hospital prepares an itemized statement of the services rendered for submittal to its cost accounting department. Regular Medicare billing forms are not necessary for this purpose, since no bills are submitted to the A/B MAC (A) at this point.

The itemized statement should contain information that identifies the person receiving the service (donor/recipient), the health care insurance number, the service rendered and the charge for the service, as well as a statement as to whether this is a potential transplant donor or recipient. If it is a potential donor, the provider must identify the prospective recipient.

EXAMPLE:

Mary Jones
Health care insurance number
200 Adams St.
Anywhere, MS

Transplant donor evaluation services for recipient:

John Jones
Health care insurance number
200 Adams St.
Anywhere, MS

Services performed in a hospital other than the potential transplant hospital or by an independent laboratory are billed by that facility to the potential transplant hospital. This holds true regardless of where in the United States the service is performed. For example, if the donor services are performed in a Florida hospital and the transplant is to take place in a California hospital, the Florida hospital bills the California hospital (as described in above). The Florida hospital is paid by the California hospital, which recoups the monies through the kidney acquisition cost center.

D. Billing for Cadaveric Donor Services
Normally, various tests are performed to determine the type and suitability of a cadaver kidney. Such tests may be performed by the excising hospital (which may also be a transplant hospital) or an independent laboratory. When the excising-only hospital performs the tests, it includes the related charges on its bill to the transplant hospital or to the organ procurement agency. When the tests are performed by the transplant hospital, it uses the related costs in establishing the standard charge for acquiring the cadaver kidney. The transplant hospital includes the costs and charges in the appropriate departments for final cost settlement purposes. When the tests are performed by an independent laboratory for the excising-only hospital or the

transplant hospital, the laboratory bills the hospital that engages its services or the organ procurement agency. The excising-only hospital includes such charges in its charges to the transplant hospital, which then includes the charges in developing its standard charge for acquiring the cadaver kidney. It is the transplant hospitals' responsibility to assure that the independent laboratory does not bill both hospitals. The cost of these services cannot be billed directly to the program, since such tests and other procedures performed on a cadaver are not identifiable to a specific patient.

E. Billing For Physicians' Services Prior to Transplantation

Physicians' services applicable to kidney excisions involving live donors and recipients (during the pre-entitlement period and after entitlement, but prior to entrance into the hospital for transplantation) as well as all physicians' services applicable to cadavers are considered Part A hospital services (kidney acquisition costs).

F. Billing for Physicians' Services After Transplantation

All physicians' services rendered to the living donor and all physicians' services rendered to the transplant recipient are billed to the Medicare program in the same manner as all Medicare Part B services are billed. All donor physicians' services must be billed to the account of the recipient (i.e., the recipient's Medicare number).

G. Billing For Physicians' Renal Transplantation Services

To ensure proper payment when submitting a Part B bill for the renal surgeon's services to the recipient, the appropriate HCPCS codes must be submitted, including HCPCS codes for concurrent surgery, as applicable.

The bill must include all living donor physicians' services, e.g., Revenue Center code 081X.

100-4, 3, 90.1.2

Billing for Kidney Transplant and Acquisition Services

Applicable standard kidney acquisition charges are identified separately by revenue code 0811 (Living Donor Kidney Acquisition) or 0812 (Cadaver Donor Kidney Acquisition). Where interim bills are submitted, the standard acquisition charge appears on the billing form for the period during which the transplant took place. This charge is in addition to the hospital's charges for services rendered directly to the Medicare recipient.

The contractor deducts kidney acquisition charges for PPS hospitals for processing through Pricer. These costs, incurred by approved kidney transplant hospitals, are not included in the kidney transplant prospective payment. They are paid on a reasonable cost basis. Interim payment is paid as a "pass through" item. (See the Provider Reimbursement Manual, Part 1, §2802 B.8.) The contractor includes kidney acquisition charges under the appropriate revenue code in CWF.

Bill Review Procedures

The Medicare Code Editor (MCE) creates a Limited Coverage edit for kidney transplant procedure codes. Where these procedure codes are identified by MCE, the contractor checks the provider number to determine if the provider is an approved transplant center, and checks the effective approval date. The contractor shall also determine if the facility is certified for adults and/or pediatric transplants dependent upon the patient's age. If payment is appropriate (i.e., the center is approved and the service is on or after the approval date) it overrides the limited coverage edit.

100-4, 3, 90.2

Heart Transplants

Cardiac transplantation is covered under Medicare when performed in a facility which is approved by Medicare as meeting institutional coverage criteria. On April 6, 1987, CMS Ruling 87-1, "Criteria for Medicare Coverage of Heart Transplants" was published in the "Federal Register." For Medicare coverage purposes, heart transplants are medically reasonable and necessary when performed in facilities that meet these criteria. If a hospital wishes to bill Medicare for heart transplants, it must submit an application and documentation, showing its ongoing compliance with each criterion.

If a contractor has any questions concerning the effective or approval dates of its hospitals, it should contact its RO.

For a complete list of approved transplant centers, visit:

http://www.cms.hhs.gov/CertificationandCompliance/20_Transplant.asp#TopOfPage

A. Effective Dates

The effective date of coverage for heart transplants performed at facilities applying after July 6, 1987, is the date the facility receives approval as a heart transplant facility. Coverage is effective for discharges October 17, 1986 for facilities that would have qualified and that applied by July 6, 1987. All transplant hospitals will be recertified under the final rule, Federal Register / Vol. 72, No. 61 / Friday, March 30, 2007, / Rules and Regulations.

The CMS informs each hospital of its effective date in an approval letter.

B. Drugs

Medicare Part B covers immunosuppressive drugs following a covered transplant in an approved facility.

C. Noncovered Transplants

Medicare will not cover transplants or re-transplants in facilities that have not been approved as meeting the facility criteria. If a beneficiary is admitted for and receives a heart transplant from a hospital that is not approved, physicians' services, and inpatient services associated with the transplantation procedure are not covered.

If a beneficiary received a heart transplant from a hospital while it was not an approved facility and later requires services as a result of the noncovered transplant, the services are covered when they are reasonable and necessary in all other respects.

D. Charges for Heart Acquisition Services

The excising hospital bills the OPO, who in turn bills the transplant (implant) hospital for applicable services. It should not submit a bill to its contractor. The transplant hospital must keep an itemized statement that identifies the services rendered, the charges, the person receiving the service (donor/recipient), and whether this person is a potential transplant donor or recipient. These charges are reflected in the transplant hospital's heart acquisition cost center and are used in determining its standard charge for acquiring a donor's heart. The standard charge is not a charge representing the acquisition cost of a specific heart; rather, it reflects the average cost associated with each type of heart acquisition. Also, it is an all inclusive charge for all services required in acquisition of a heart, i.e., tissue typing, post-operative evaluation, etc.

E. Bill Review Procedures

The contractor takes the following actions to process heart transplant bills. It may accomplish them manually or modify its MCE and Grouper interface programs to handle the processing.

1. MCE Interface

    The MCE creates a Limited Coverage edit for heart transplant procedure codes. Where these procedure codes are identified by MCE, the contractor checks the provider number to determine if the provider is an approved transplant center, and checks the effective approval date. The contractor shall also determine if the facility is certified for adults and/or pediatric transplants dependent upon the patient's age. If payment is appropriate (i.e., the center is approved and the service is on or after the approval date) it overrides the limited coverage edit.

2. Handling Heart Transplant Billings From Nonapproved Hospitals

    Where a heart transplant and covered services are provided by a nonapproved hospital, the bill data processed through Grouper and Pricer must exclude transplant procedure codes and related charges.

100-4, 3, 90.3

Stem Cell Transplantation

Stem cell transplantation is a process in which stem cells are harvested from either a patient's or donor's bone marrow or peripheral blood for intravenous infusion. Autologous stem cell transplants (AuSCT) must be used to effect hematopoietic reconstitution following severely myelotoxic doses of chemotherapy (HDCT) and/or radiotherapy used to treat various malignancies. Allogeneic stem cell transplant may also be used to restore function in recipients having an inherited or acquired deficiency or defect.

Bone marrow and peripheral blood stem cell transplantation is a process which includes mobilization, harvesting, and transplant of bone marrow or peripheral blood stem cells and the administration of high dose chemotherapy or radiotherapy prior to the actual transplant. When bone marrow or peripheral blood stem cell transplantation is covered, all necessary steps are included in coverage. When bone marrow or peripheral blood stem cell transplantation is non-covered, none of the steps are covered.

Allogeneic and autologous stem cell transplants are covered under Medicare for specific diagnoses. Effective October 1, 1990, these cases were assigned to MS-DRG 009, Bone Marrow Transplant.

The A/B MAC (A)'s Medicare Code Editor (MCE) will edit stem cell transplant procedure codes 4101, 4102, 4103, 4104, 4105, 4107, 4108, and 4109 against diagnosis codes to determine which cases meet specified coverage criteria. Cases with a diagnosis code for a covered condition will pass (as covered) the MCE noncovered procedure edit. When a stem cell transplant case is selected for review based on the random selection of beneficiaries, the QIO will review the case on a post-payment basis to assure proper coverage decisions.

Bone marrow transplant codes that are reported with an ICD-9-CM that is "not otherwise specified" are returned to the hospital for a more specific procedure code. ICD-10-PCS codes are more precise and clearly identify autologous and nonautologous stem cells.

The A/B MAC (A) may choose to review if data analysis deems it a priority.

100-4, 3, 90.3.1

Allogeneic Stem Cell Transplantation

A. General

Allogeneic stem cell transplantation (ICD-9-CM Procedure Codes 41.02, 41.03, 41.05, and 41.08, CPT-4 Code 38240) is a procedure in which a portion of a healthy donor's stem cells are obtained and prepared for intravenous infusion to restore normal hematopoietic function in recipients having an inherited or acquired hematopoietic deficiency or defect. See Pub. 100-3, National Coverage Determinations Manual, chapter 1, section 110.8.1, for more information.

Expenses incurred by a donor are a covered benefit to the recipient/beneficiary but, except for physician services, are not paid separately. Services to the donor include physician services, hospital care in connection with screening the stem cell, and ordinary follow-up care.

B. Covered Conditions
1. Effective for services performed on or after August 1, 1978:
   — For the treatment of leukemia, leukemia in remission (ICD-9-CM codes 204.00 through 208.91), or aplastic anemia (ICD-9-CM codes 284.0 through 284.9) when it is reasonable and necessary; and
2. Effective for services performed on or after June 3, 1985:
   — For the treatment of severe combined immunodeficiency disease (SCID) (ICD-9-CM code 279.2), and for the treatment of Wiskott-Aldrich syndrome (ICD-9-CM 279.12).

C. Non-Covered Conditions
1. Effective for services performed on or after May 24, 1996:
   — Allogeneic stem cell transplantation is not covered as treatment for multiple myeloma (ICD-9-CM codes 203.00 and 203.01).
2. Effective for services performed on or after August 4, 2010:

The Centers for Medicare & Medicaid Services (CMS) issued an NCD stating that it believes the evidence does not demonstrate that the use of allogeneic hematopoietic stem cell transplantation (HSCT) improves health outcomes in Medicare beneficiaries with Myelodysplastic Syndrome (MDS). Therefore, allogeneic HSCT for MDS is not reasonable and necessary under §1862(a)(1)(A) of the Social Security Act (the Act).

However, allogeneic HSCT for MDS is reasonable and necessary under §1862(a)(1)(E) of the Act and therefore covered by Medicare ONLY if provided pursuant to a Medicare-approved clinical study under Coverage with Evidence Development (CED). These services are covered in both the inpatient and outpatient hospital setting. Refer to Pub. 100-3, NCD Manual, chapter 1, section 110.8.1, for further information about this policy, and Pub. 100-4, MCP Manual, chapter 32, section 90.6, for information on CED.

For inpatient hospital claims, TOB 11x, if ICD-9-CM is applicable, diagnoses are 238.75 and V70.7. If ICD-10-CM is applicable, the diagnosis codes are D46.9, D46.Z, and Z00.6.

NOTE: Coverage for conditions other than these specifically designated as covered or non-covered in the CP or NCD Manuals are left to local Medicare contractor discretion.

100-4, 3, 90.3.2
Autologous Stem Cell Transplantation (AuSCT)
Autologous Stem Cell Transplantation (AuSCT)

A. General
Autologous stem cell transplantation (AuSCT) (ICD-9-CM procedure code 41.01, 41.04, 41.07, and 41.09 and CPT-4 code 38241) is a technique for restoring stem cells using the patient's own previously stored cells. AuSCT must be used to effect hematopoietic reconstitution following severely myelotoxic doses of chemotherapy (high dose chemotherapy (HDCT)) and/or radiotherapy used to treat various malignancies.

If ICD-9-CM is applicable, use the following Procedure Codes and Descriptions

ICD-9-CM Code	Description
41.01	Autologous bone marrow transplant without purging
41.04	Autologous hematopoietic stem cell transplant without purging
41.07	Autologous hematopoietic stem cell transplant with purging
41.09	Autologous bone marrow transplant with purging

If ICD-10-PCS is applicable, use the following Procedure Codes and Descriptions

ICD-10-PCS Code	Description
30230AZ	Transfusion of Embryonic Stem Cells into Peripheral Vein, Open Approach
30230G0	Transfusion of Autologous Bone Marrow into Peripheral Vein, Open Approach
30230Y0	Transfusion of Autologous Hematopoietic Stem Cells into Peripheral Vein, Open Approach
30233G0	Transfusion of Autologous Bone Marrow into Peripheral Vein, Percutaneous Approach
30233Y0	Transfusion of Autologous Hematopoietic Stem Cells into Peripheral Vein, Percutaneous Approach
30240G0	Transfusion of Autologous Bone Marrow into Central Vein, Open Approach
30240Y0	Transfusion of Autologous Bone Marrow into Central Vein, Open Approach
30243G0	Transfusion of Autologous Bone Marrow into Central Vein, Percutaneous Approach
30243Y0	Transfusion of Autologous Hematopoietic Stem Cells into Central Vein, Percutaneous Approach

ICD-10-PCS Code	Description
30250G0	Transfusion of Autologous Bone Marrow into Peripheral Artery, Open Approach
30250Y0	Transfusion of Autologous Hematopoietic Stem Cells into Peripheral Artery, Open Approach
30253G0	Transfusion of Autologous Bone Marrow into Peripheral Artery, Percutaneous Approach
30253Y0	Transfusion of Autologous Hematopoietic Stem Cells into Peripheral Artery, Percutaneous Approach
30260G0	Transfusion of Autologous Bone Marrow into Central Artery, Open Approach
30260Y0	Transfusion of Autologous Hematopoietic Stem Cells into Central Artery, Open Approach
30263G0	Transfusion of Autologous Bone Marrow into Central Artery, Percutaneous Approach
30263Y0	Transfusion of Autologous Hematopoietic Stem Cells into Central Artery, Percutaneous Approach

B. Covered Conditions
1. Effective for services performed on or after April 28, 1989:

For acute leukemia in remission for patients who have a high probability of relapse and who have no human leucocyte antigens (HLA)-matched the following diagnosis codes are reported:

If ICD-9-CM is applicable, use the following Diagnosis Codes and Descriptions

Diagnosis Code	Description
204.01	Lymphoid leukemia, acute, in remission
205.01	Myeloid leukemia, acute, in remission
206.01	Monocytic leukemia, acute, in remission
207.01	Acute erythremia and erythroleukemia, in remission
208.01	Leukemia of unspecified cell type, acute, in remission

If ICD-10-CM is applicable, use the following Diagnosis Codes and Descriptions

Diagnosis Code	Description
C91.01	Acute lymphoblastic leukemia, in remission
C92.01	Acute myeloblastic leukemia, in remission
C92.41	Acute promyelocytic leukemia, in remission
C92.51	Acute myelomonocytic leukemia, in remission
C92.61	Acute myeloid leukemia with 11q23-abnormality in remission
C92.A1	Acute myeloid leukemia with multilineage dysplasia, in remission
C93.01	Acute monoblastic/monocytic leukemia, in remission
C94.01	Acute erythroid leukemia, in remission
C94.21	Acute megakaryoblastic leukemia, in remission
C94.41	Acute parmyelosis with myelofibrosis, in remission
C95.01	Acute leukemia of unspecified cell type, in remission

For resistant non-Hodgkin's lymphomas (or those presenting with poor prognostic features following an initial response the following diagnosis codes are reported:

If ICD-9-CM is applicable, use the following code ranges:
200.00 - 200.08,

200.10 - 00.18,

200.20 - 200.28,

200.80 - 200.88,

202.00 - 202.08,

202.80 - 202.88, and

202.90 - 202.98.

If ICD-10-CM is applicable use the following code ranges:
C82.00 - C85.29,

C85.80 - C86.6,

C96.4, and

C96.Z - C96.9.

For recurrent or refractory neuroblastoma (see ICD-9-CM Neoplasm by site, malignant for the appropriate diagnosis code)

If ICD-10-CM is applicable the following ranges are reported:

C00 - C96, and

D00 - D09 Resistant non-Hodgkin's lymphomas

For advanced Hodgkin's disease patients who have failed conventional therapy and have no HLA-matched donor the following diagnosis codes are reported:

If ICD-9-CM is applicable, 201.00-201.98.

If ICD-10-CM is applicable, C81.00 – C81.99.

2. Effective for services performed on or after October 1, 2000:

Durie-Salmon Stage II or III that fit the following requirement are covered: Newly diagnosed or responsive multiple myeloma (if ICD-9-CM is applicable, diagnosis codes 203.00 and 238.6, and, if ICD-10-CM is applicable, diagnosis codes C90.00 and D47.Z9). This includes those patients with previously untreated disease, those with at least a partial response to prior chemotherapy (defined as a 50% decrease either in measurable paraprotein [serum and/or urine] or in bone marrow infiltration, sustained for at least 1 month), and those in responsive relapse, and adequate cardiac, renal, pulmonary, and hepatic function.

3. Effective for Services On or After March 15, 2005

Effective for services performed on or after March 15, 2005 when recognized clinical risk factors are employed to select patients for transplantation, high-dose melphalan (HDM), together with AuSCT, in treating Medicare beneficiaries of any age group with primary amyloid light-chain (AL) amyloidosis who meet the following criteria:

Amyloid deposition in 2 or fewer organs; and,

Cardiac left ventricular ejection fraction (EF) of 45% or greater.

C. Noncovered Conditions

Insufficient data exist to establish definite conclusions regarding the efficacy of autologous stem cell transplantation for the following conditions:

- Acute leukemia not in remission:
  — If ICD-9-CM is applicable, diagnosis codes 204.00, 205.00, 206.00, 207.00 and 208.00 are noncovered;
  — If ICD-10-CM is applicable, diagnosis codes C91.00, C92.00, C92.40, C92.50, C92.60, C92.A0, C93.00, C94.00, and C95.00 are noncovered.
- Chronic granulocytic leukemia:
  — If ICD-9-CM is applicable, diagnosis codes 205.10 and 205.11;
  — If ICD-10-CM is applicable, diagnosis codes C92.10 and C92.11.
- Solid tumors (other than neuroblastoma):
  — If ICD-9-CM is applicable, diagnosis codes 140.0-199.1;
  — If ICD-10-CM is applicable, diagnosis codes C00.0 - C80.2 and D00.0 - D09.9. Multiple myeloma (ICD-9-CM codes 203.00 and 238.6), through September 30, 2000.
- Tandem transplantation (multiple rounds of autologous stem cell transplantation) for patients with multiple myeloma
  — If ICD-9-CM is applicable, diagnosis codes 203.00 and 238.6 and,
  — If ICD-10-CM is applicable, diagnosis codes C90.00 and D47.Z9)
- Non-primary (AL) amyloidosis,
  — If ICD-9-CM is applicable, diagnosis code 277.3. Effective October 1, 2000; ICD-9-CM code 277.3 was expanded to codes 277.30, 277.31, and 277.39 effective October 1, 2006.
  — If ICD-10-CM is applicable, diagnosis codes are E85.0 – E85.9. or
- Primary (AL) amyloidosis
  — If ICD-9-CM is applicable, diagnosis codes 277.30, 277.31, and 277.39 and for Medicare beneficiaries age 64 or older, effective October 1, 2000, through March 14, 2005.
  — If ICD-10-CM is applicable, diagnosis codes are E85.0 - E85.9.

NOTE: Coverage for conditions other than these specifically designated as covered or non-covered is left to the discretion of the A/B MAC (A).

100-4, 3, 90.3.3

Billing for Stem Cell Transplantation

A. Billing for Allogeneic Stem Cell Transplants

1. Definition of Acquisition Charges for Allogeneic Stem Cell Transplants

Acquisition charges for allogeneic stem cell transplants include, but are not limited to, charges for the costs of the following services:

- National Marrow Donor Program fees, if applicable, for stem cells from an unrelated donor;
- Tissue typing of donor and recipient;
- Donor evaluation;
- Physician pre-admission/pre-procedure donor evaluation services;
- Costs associated with harvesting procedure (e.g., general routine and special care services, procedure/operating room and other ancillary services, apheresis services, etc.);
- Post-operative/post-procedure evaluation of donor; and
- Preparation and processing of stem cells.

Payment for these acquisition services is included in the MS-DRG payment for the allogeneic stem cell transplant when the transplant occurs in the inpatient setting, and in the OPPS APC payment for the allogeneic stem cell transplant when the transplant occurs in the outpatient setting. The Medicare contractor does not make separate payment for these acquisition services, because hospitals may bill and receive payment only for services provided to the Medicare beneficiary who is the recipient of the stem cell transplant and whose illness is being treated with the stem cell transplant. Unlike the acquisition costs of solid organs for transplant (e.g., hearts and kidneys), which are paid on a reasonable cost basis, acquisition costs for allogeneic stem cells are included in prospective payment.

Acquisition charges for stem cell transplants apply only to allogeneic transplants, for which stem cells are obtained from a donor (other than the recipient himself or herself). Acquisition charges do not apply to autologous transplants (transplanted stem cells are obtained from the recipient himself or herself), because autologous transplants involve services provided to the beneficiary only (and not to a donor), for which the hospital may bill and receive payment (see Pub. 100-4, chapter 4, §231.10 and paragraph B of this section for information regarding billing for autologous stem cell transplants).

2. Billing for Acquisition Services

The hospital bills and shows acquisition charges for allogeneic stem cell transplants based on the status of the patient (i.e., inpatient or outpatient) when the transplant is furnished. See Pub. 100-4, chapter 4, §231.11 for instructions regarding billing for acquisition services for allogeneic stem cell transplants that are performed in the outpatient setting.

When the allogeneic stem cell transplant occurs in the inpatient setting, the hospital identifies stem cell acquisition charges for allogeneic bone marrow/stem cell transplants separately in FL 42 of Form CMS-1450 (or electronic equivalent) by using revenue code 0819 (Other Organ Acquisition). Revenue code 0819 charges should include all services required to acquire stem cells from a donor, as defined above.

On the recipient's transplant bill, the hospital reports the acquisition charges, cost report days, and utilization days for the donor's hospital stay (if applicable) and/or charges for other encounters in which the stem cells were obtained from the donor. The donor is covered for medically necessary inpatient hospital days of care or outpatient care provided in connection with the allogeneic stem cell transplant under Part A. Expenses incurred for complications are paid only if they are directly and immediately attributable to the stem cell donation procedure. The hospital reports the acquisition charges on the billing form for the recipient, as described in the first paragraph of this section. It does not charge the donor's days of care against the recipient's utilization record. For cost reporting purposes, it includes the covered donor days and charges as Medicare days and charges.

The transplant hospital keeps an itemized statement that identifies the services furnished, the charges, the person receiving the service (donor/recipient), and whether this is a potential transplant donor or recipient. These charges will be reflected in the transplant hospital's stem cell/bone marrow acquisition cost center. For allogeneic stem cell acquisition services in cases that do not result in transplant, due to death of the intended recipient or other causes, hospitals include the costs associated with the acquisition services on the Medicare cost report.

The hospital shows charges for the transplant itself in revenue center code 0362 or another appropriate cost center. Selection of the cost center is up to the hospital.

B. Billing for Autologous Stem Cell Transplants

The hospital bills and shows all charges for autologous stem cell harvesting, processing, and transplant procedures based on the status of the patient (i.e., inpatient or outpatient) when the services are furnished. It shows charges for the actual transplant, described by the appropriate ICD-9-CM procedure or CPT codes, in revenue center code 0362 or another appropriate cost center. ICD-9-CM or ICD-10-PCS codes are used to identify inpatient procedures.

The CPT codes describing autologous stem cell harvesting procedures may be billed and are separately payable under the OPPS when provided in the hospital outpatient setting of care. Autologous harvesting procedures are distinct from the acquisition services described in Pub. 100-4, chapter 4, §231.11 and section A. above for allogeneic stem cell transplants, which include services provided when stem cells are obtained from a donor and not from the patient undergoing the stem cell transplant. The CPT codes describing autologous stem cell processing procedures also may be billed and are separately payable under the OPPS when provided to hospital outpatients.

Payment for autologous stem cell harvesting procedures performed in the hospital inpatient setting of care, with transplant also occurring in the inpatient setting of care, is included in the MS-DRG payment for the autologous stem cell transplant.

100-4, 3, 90.4

Liver Transplants

A. Background

For Medicare coverage purposes, liver transplants are considered medically reasonable and necessary for specified conditions when performed in facilities that meet specific criteria. Coverage guidelines may be found in Publication 100-3, Section 260.1.

Effective for claims with dates of service June 21, 2012 and later, contractors may, at their discretion cover adult liver transplantation for patients with extrahepatic unresectable cholangiocarcinoma (CCA), (2) liver metastases due to a neuroendocrine tumor (NET) or (3) hemangioendothelimo (HAE) when furnished in an approved Liver Transplant Center (below). All other nationally non-covered malignancies continue to remain nationally non-covered.

To review the current list of approved Liver Transplant Centers, see http://www.cms.hhs.gov/CertificationandComplianc/20_Transplant.asp#TopOfPage

100-4, 3, 90.4.1

Standard Liver Acquisition Charge

A3-3615.1, A3-3615.3

Each transplant facility must develop a standard charge for acquiring a cadaver liver from costs it expects to incur in the acquisition of livers.

This standard charge is not a charge that represents the acquisition cost of a specific liver. Rather, it is a charge that reflects the average cost associated with a liver acquisition.

Services associated with liver acquisition are billed from the organ procurement organization or, in some cases, the excising hospital to the transplant hospital. The excising hospital does not submit a billing form to the FI. The transplant hospital keeps an itemized statement that identifies the services furnished, the charges, the person receiving the service (donor/recipient), and the potential transplant donor. These charges are reflected in the transplant hospital's liver acquisition cost center and are used in determining the hospital's standard charge for acquiring a cadaver's liver. The standard charge is not a charge representing the acquisition cost of a specific liver. Rather, it is a charge that reflects the average cost associated with liver acquisition. Also, it is an all inclusive charge for all services required in acquisition of a liver, e.g., tissue typing, transportation of organ, and surgeons' retrieval fees.

100-4, 3, 90.4.2

Billing for Liver Transplant and Acquisition Services

The inpatient claim is completed in accordance with instructions in chapter 25 for the beneficiary who receives a covered liver transplant. Applicable standard liver acquisition charges are identified separately in FL 42 by revenue code 0817 (Donor-Liver). Where interim bills are submitted, the standard acquisition charge appears on the billing form for the period during which the transplant took place. This charge is in addition to the hospital's charge for services furnished directly to the Medicare recipient.

The contractor deducts liver acquisition charges for IPPS hospitals prior to processing through Pricer. Costs of liver acquisition incurred by approved liver transplant facilities are not included in prospective payment DRG 480 (Liver Transplant). They are paid on a reasonable cost basis. This item is a "pass-through" cost for which interim payments are made. (See the Provider Reimbursement Manual, Part 1, §2802 B.8.) The contractor includes liver acquisition charges under revenue code 0817 in the HUIP record that it sends to CWF and the QIO.

A. Bill Review Procedures

The contractor takes the following actions to process liver transplant bills.

1. Operative Report

    The contractor requires the operative report with all claims for liver transplants, or sends a development request to the hospital for each liver transplant with a diagnosis code for a covered condition.

2. MCE Interface

    The MCE contains a limited coverage edit for liver transplant procedures using ICD-9-CM code 50.59 if ICD-9 is applicable, and, if ICD-10 is applicable, using ICD-10-PCS codes 0FY00Z0, 0FY00Z1, and 0FY00Z2.

    Where a liver transplant procedure code is identified by the MCE, the contractor shall check the provider number and effective date to determine if the provider is an approved liver transplant facility at the time of the transplant, and the contractor shall also determine if the facility is certified for adults and/or pediatric transplants dependent upon the patient's age. If yes, the claim is suspended for review of the operative report to determine whether the beneficiary has at least one of the covered conditions when the diagnosis code is for a covered condition. If payment is appropriate (i.e., the facility is approved, the service is furnished on or after the approval date, and the beneficiary has a covered condition), the contractor sends the claim to Grouper and Pricer.

    If none of the diagnoses codes are for a covered condition, or if the provider is not an approved liver transplant facility, the contractor denies the claim.

    NOTE: Some noncovered conditions are included in the covered diagnostic codes. (The diagnostic codes are broader than the covered conditions. Do not pay for noncovered conditions.)

3. Grouper

    If the bill shows a discharge date before March 8, 1990, the liver transplant procedure is not covered. If the discharge date is March 8, 1990 or later, the contractor processes the bill through Grouper and Pricer. If the discharge date is after March 7, 1990, and before October 1, 1990, Grouper assigned CMS DRG 191 or 192. The contractor sent the bill to Pricer with review code 08. Pricer would then overlay CMS DRG 191 or 192 with CMS DRG 480 and the weights and thresholds for CMS DRG 480 to price the bill. If the discharge date is after September 30, 1990, Grouper assigns CMS DRG 480 and Pricer is able to price without using review code 08. If the discharge date is after September 30, 2007, Grouper assigns MS-DRG 005 or 006 (Liver transplant with MCC or Intestinal

Transplant or Liver transplant without MCC, respectively) and Pricer is able to price without using review code 08.

4. Liver Transplant Billing From Non-approved Hospitals

    Where a liver transplant and covered services are provided by a non-approved hospital, the bill data processed through Grouper and Pricer must exclude transplant procedure codes and related charges.

    When CMS approves a hospital to furnish liver transplant services, it informs the hospital of the effective date in the approval letter. The contractor will receive a copy of the letter.

100-4, 3, 90.5

Pancreas Transplants Kidney Transplants

A. Background

Effective July 1, 1999, Medicare covered pancreas transplantation when performed simultaneously with or following a kidney transplant if ICD-9 is applicable, ICD-9-CM procedure code 55.69. If ICD-10 is applicable, the following ICD-10-PCS codes will be used: T

ØTY00ZØ,

ØTY00Z1,

ØTY00Z2,

ØTY10ZØ,

ØTY10Z1, and

ØTY10Z2.

Pancreas transplantation is performed to induce an insulin independent, euglycemic state in diabetic patients. The procedure is generally limited to those patients with severe secondary complications of diabetes including kidney failure. However, pancreas transplantation is sometimes performed on patients with labile diabetes and hypoglycemic unawareness.

Medicare has had a policy of not covering pancreas transplantation. The Office of Health Technology Assessment performed an assessment on pancreas-kidney transplantation in 1994. They found reasonable graft survival outcomes for patients receiving either simultaneous pancreas-kidney (SPK) transplantation or pancreas after kidney (PAK) transplantation. For a list of facilities approved to perform SPK or PAK, refer to the following Web site: http://www.cms.hhs.gov/CertificationandComplianc/20_Transplant.asp#TopOfPage

B. Billing for Pancreas Transplants

There are no special provisions related to managed care participants. Managed care plans are required to provide all Medicare covered services. Medicare does not restrict which hospitals or physicians may perform pancreas transplantation.

The transplant procedure and revenue code 0360 for the operating room are paid under these codes. Procedures must be reported using the current ICD-9-CM procedure codes for pancreas and kidney transplants. Providers must place at least one of the following transplant procedure codes on the claim:

If ICD-9 Is Applicable

52.80   Transplant of pancreas

52.82   Homotransplant of pancreas

The Medicare Code Editor (MCE) has been updated to include 52.80 and 52.82 as limited coverage procedures. The contractor must determine if the facility is approved for the transplant and certified for either pediatric or adult transplants dependent upon the age of the patient.

Effective October 1, 2000, ICD-9-CM code 52.83 was moved in the MCE to non-covered. The contractor must override any deny edit on claims that came in with 52.82 prior to October 1, 2000 and adjust, as 52.82 is the correct code.

If the discharge date is July 1, 1999, or later: the contractor processes the bill through Grouper and Pricer.

If ICD-10 is applicable, the following procedure codes (ICD-10-PCS) are:

ØFYGØZØ Transplantation of Pancreas, Allogeneic, Open Approach

ØFYGØZ1 Transplantation of Pancreas, Syngeneic, Open Approach

Pancreas transplantation is reasonable and necessary for the following diagnosis codes. However, since this is not an all-inclusive list, the contractor is permitted to determine if any additional diagnosis codes are covered for this procedure.

If ICD-9-CM is applicable, Diabetes Diagnosis Codes and Descriptions

ICD-9-CM Code	Description
250.00	Diabetes mellitus without mention of complication, type II (non-insulin dependent) (NIDDM) (adult onset) or unspecified type, not stated as uncontrolled.
250.01	Diabetes mellitus without mention of complication, type I (insulin dependent) (IDDM) (juvenile), not stated as uncontrolled.
250.02	Diabetes mellitus without mention of complication, type II (non-insulin dependent) (NIDDM) (adult onset) or unspecified type, uncontrolled.

ICD-9-CM Code	Description
250.03	Diabetes mellitus without mention of complication, type I (insulin dependent) (IDDM) (juvenile), uncontrolled.
250.1X	Diabetes with ketoacidosis
250.2X	Diabetes with hyperosmolarity
250.3X	Diabetes with coma
250.4X	Diabetes with renal manifestations
250.5X	Diabetes with ophthalmic manifestations
250.6X	Diabetes with neurological manifestations
250.7X	Diabetes with peripheral circulatory disorders
250.8X	Diabetes with other specified manifestations
250.9X	Diabetes with unspecified complication

NOTE: X=0-3

If ICD-10-CM is applicable, the diagnosis codes are: E10.10 - E10.9

Hypertensive Renal Diagnosis Codes and Descriptions if ICD-9-CM is applicable :

ICD-9-CM Code	Description
403.01	Malignant hypertensive renal disease, with renal failure
403.11	Benign hypertensive renal disease, with renal failure
403.91	Unspecified hypertensive renal disease, with renal failure
404.02	Malignant hypertensive heart and renal disease, with renal failure
404.03	Malignant hypertensive heart and renal disease, with congestive heart failure or renal failure
404.12	Benign hypertensive heart and renal disease, with renal failure
404.13	Benign hypertensive heart and renal disease, with congestive heart failure or renal failure
404.92	Unspecified hypertensive heart and renal disease, with renal failure
404.93	Unspecified hypertensive heart and renal disease, with congestive heart failure or renal failure
585.1–585.6, 585.9	Chronic Renal Failure Code

If ICD-10-CM is applicable, diagnosis codes and descriptions are:

ICD-10-CM code	Description
I12.0	Hypertensive chronic kidney disease with stage 5 chronic kidney disease or end stage renal disease
I13.11	Hypertensive heart and chronic kidney disease without heart failure, with stage 5 chronic kidney disease, or end stage renal disease
I13.2	Hypertensive heart and chronic kidney disease with heart failure and with stage 5 chronic kidney disease, or end stage renal disease
N18.1	Chronic kidney disease, stage 1
N18.2	Chronic kidney disease, stage 2 (mild)
N18.3	Chronic kidney disease, stage 3 (moderate)
N18.4	Chronic kidney disease, stage 4 (severe)
N18.5	Chronic kidney disease, stage 5
N18.6	End stage renal disease
N18.9	Chronic kidney disease, unspecified

NOTE: If a patient had a kidney transplant that was successful, the patient no longer has chronic kidney failure, therefore it would be inappropriate for the provider to bill ICD-9-CM codes 585.1 - 585.6, 585.9 or, if ICD-10-CM is applicable, the diagnosis codes N18.1 - N18.9 on such a patient. In these cases one of the following codes should be present on the claim or in the beneficiary's history.

The provider uses the following ICD-9-CM status codes only when a kidney transplant was performed before the pancreas transplant and ICD-9 is applicable:

ICD-9-CM code	Description
V42.0	Organ or tissue replaced by transplant kidney
V43.89	Organ tissue replaced by other means, kidney or pancreas

If ICD-10-CM is applicable, the following ICD-10-CM status codes will be used:

ICD-10-CM code	Description
Z48.22	Encounter for aftercare following kidney transplant
Z94.0	Kidney transplant status

NOTE: If a kidney and pancreas transplants are performed simultaneously, the claim should contain a diabetes diagnosis code and a renal failure code or one of the

hypertensive renal failure diagnosis codes. The claim should also contain two transplant procedure codes. If the claim is for a pancreas transplant only, the claim should contain a diabetes diagnosis code and a status code to indicate a previous kidney transplant. If the status code is not on the claim for the pancreas transplant, the contractor will search the beneficiary's claim history for a status code indicating a prior kidney transplant.

C. Drugs

If the pancreas transplant occurs after the kidney transplant, immunosuppressive therapy will begin with the date of discharge from the inpatient stay for the pancreas transplant.

D. Charges for Pancreas Acquisition Services

A separate organ acquisition cost center has been established for pancreas transplantation. The Medicare cost report will include a separate line to account for pancreas transplantation costs. The 42 CFR 412.2(e)(4) was changed to include pancreas in the list of organ acquisition costs that are paid on a reasonable cost basis.

Acquisition costs for pancreas transplantation as well as kidney transplants will occur in Revenue Center 081X. The contractor overrides any claims that suspend due to repetition of revenue code 081X on the same claim if the patient had a simultaneous kidney/pancreas transplant. It pays for acquisition costs for both kidney and pancreas organs if transplants are performed simultaneously. It will not pay for more than two organ acquisitions on the same claim.

E. Medicare Summary Notices (MSN) and Remittance Advice Messages

If the provider submits a claim for simultaneous pancreas kidney transplantation or pancreas transplantation following a kidney transplant, and omits one of the appropriate diagnosis/procedure codes, the contractor rejects the claim, using the following MSN:

- MSN 16.32, "Medicare does not pay separately for this service."

- Claim adjustment reason code B15, This service/procedure requires that a qualifying service/procedure be received and covered. The qualifying other service/procedure has not been received/adjudicated.

- If a claim is denied because no evidence of a prior kidney transplant is presented, use the following MSN message:

MSN 15.4, "The information provided does not support the need for this service or item."

The contractor uses the following Remittance Advice Message:

Claim adjustment reason code 50, These are non-covered services because this is not deemed a 'medical necessity' by the payer.

To further clarify the situation, the contractor should also use claim level remark code MA 126, "Pancreas transplant not covered unless kidney transplant performed."

100-4, 3, 90.5.1

Pancreas Transplants Alone (PA)

A. General

Pancreas transplantation is performed to induce an insulin-independent, euglycemic state in diabetic patients. The procedure is generally limited to those patients with severe secondary complications of diabetes, including kidney failure. However, pancreas transplantation is sometimes performed on patients

with labile diabetes and hypoglycemic unawareness. Medicare has had a long-standing policy of not covering pancreas transplantation, as the safety and effectiveness of the procedure had not been demonstrated. The Office of Health Technology Assessment performed an assessment of pancreas-kidney transplantation in 1994. It found reasonable graft survival outcomes for patients receiving either simultaneous pancreas-kidney transplantation or pancreas-after-kidney transplantation.

B. Nationally Covered Indications

CMS determines that whole organ pancreas transplantation will be nationally covered by Medicare when performed simultaneous with or after a kidney transplant. If the pancreas transplant occurs after the kidney transplant, immunosuppressive therapy will begin with the date of discharge from the inpatient stay for the pancreas transplant.

C. Billing and Claims Processing

Contractors shall pay for Pancreas Transplantation Alone (PA) effective for services on or after April 26, 2006 when performed in those facilities that are Medicare-approved for kidney transplantation. Approved facilities are located at the following address: https://www.cms.gov/Medicare/Provider-Enrollment-and-Certification/Certificationa ndComplianc/downloads/ApprovedTransplantPrograms.pdf

Contractors who receive claims for PA services that were performed in an unapproved facility, should reject such claims. Contractors should use the following messages upon the reject or denial:

- Medicare Summary Notice MSN Message - MSN code 16.2 (This service cannot be paid when provided in this location/facility)

- Remittance Advice Message - Claim Adjustment Reason Code 58. Treatment was deemed by the payer to have been rendered in an inappropriate or invalid place of service. Note: Refer to the 835 Healthcare Policy Identification Segment (loop 2110 Service Payment Information REF), if present.

Payment will be made for a PA service performed in an approved facility, and which meets the coverage guidelines mentioned above for beneficiaries with type I diabetes.

All-Inclusive List of Covered Diagnosis Codes for PA if ICD-9-CM is applicable
(NOTE: "X" = 1 and 3 only)

ICD-9-CM code	Description
250.0X	Diabetes mellitus without mention of complication, type I (insulin dependent) (IDDM) (juvenile), not stated as uncontrolled.
250.1X	Diabetes with ketoacidosis
250.2X	Diabetes with hyperosmolarity
250.3X	Diabetes with coma
250.4X	Diabetes with renal manifestations
250.5X	Diabetes with ophthalmic manifestations
250.6X	Diabetes with neurological manifestations
250.7X	Diabetes with peripheral circulatory disorders
250.8X	Diabetes with other specified manifestations
250.9X	Diabetes with unspecified complication

If ICD-10-CM is applicable, the provider uses the following range of ICD-10-CM codes:
    E10.10 – E10.9.

Procedure Codes

If ICD-9 CM is applicable
    52.80 - Transplant of pancreas

    52.82 - Homotransplant of pancreas

If ICD-10 is applicable, the provider uses the following ICD-10-PCS codes:
    ØFYGØZØ Transplantation of Pancreas, Allogeneic, Open Approach

    ØFYGØZ1 Transplantation of Pancreas, Syngeneic, Open Approach

Contractors who receive claims for PA that are not billed using the covered diagnosis/procedure codes listed above shall reject such claims. The MCE edits to ensure that the transplant is covered based on the diagnosis. The MCE also considers ICD-9-CM codes 52.80 and 52.82 and ICD-10-PCS codes ØFYGØZØ and ØFYGØZ1 as limited coverage dependent upon whether the facility is approved to perform the transplant and is certified for the age of the patient.

Contractors should use the following messages upon the reject or denial:

    Medicare Summary Notice MSN Message - MSN code 15.4 The information provided does not support the need for this service or item

    Remittance Advice Message - Claim Adjustment Reason Code 50 These are non-covered services because this is not deemed a 'medical necessity' by the payer. Note: Refer to the 835 Healthcare Policy Identification Segment (loop 2110 Service Payment Information REF), if present.

Contractors shall hold the provider liable for denied\rejected claims unless the hospital issues a Hospital Issued Notice of Non-coverage (HINN) or a physician issues an Advanced Beneficiary Notice (ABN) for Part-B for physician services.

D. Charges for Pancreas Alone Acquisition Services
A separate organ acquisition cost center has been established for pancreas transplantation. The Medicare cost report will include a separate line to account for pancreas transplantation costs. The 42 CFR 412.2(e)(4) was changed to include PA in the list of organ acquisition costs that are paid on a reasonable cost basis.

Acquisition costs for PA transplantation are billed in Revenue Code 081X. The contractor removes acquisition charges prior to sending the claims to Pricer so such charges are not included in the outlier calculation.

100-4, 3, 90.6

Intestinal and Multi-Visceral Transplants

A. Background
Effective for services on or after April 1, 2001, Medicare covers intestinal and multi-visceral transplantation for the purpose of restoring intestinal function in patients with irreversible intestinal failure. Intestinal failure is defined as the loss of absorptive capacity of the small bowel secondary to severe primary gastrointestinal disease or surgically induced short bowel syndrome. Intestinal failure prevents oral nutrition and may be associated with both mortality and profound morbidity. Multi-Visceral transplantation includes organs in the digestive system (stomach, duodenum, liver, and intestine). See §260.5 of the National Coverage Determinations Manual for further information.

B. Approved Transplant Facilities
Medicare will cover intestinal transplantation if performed in an approved facility. The approved facilities are located at:
https://www.cms.gov/Medicare/Provider-Enrollment-and-Certification/Certificationa ndComplianc/downloads/ApprovedTransplantPrograms.pdf

C. Billing
If ICD-9-CM is applicable, ICD-9-CM procedure code 46.97 is effective for discharges on or after April 1, 2001. If ICD-10 is applicable, the ICD-10-PCS procedure codes are ØDY80ZØ, ØDY80Z1, ØDY80Z2, ØDYEØZØ, ØDYEØZ1, and ØDYEØZ2. The Medicare Code Editor (MCE) lists these codes as limited coverage procedures. The contractor shall override the MCE when this procedure code is listed and the coverage criteria are met in an approved transplant facility, and also determine if the facility is certified for adults and/or pediatric transplants dependent upon the patient's age.

For these procedures where the provider is approved as transplant facility and certified for the adult and/or pediatric population, and the service is performed on or after the transplant approval date, the contractor must suspend the claim for clerical review of the operative report to determine whether the beneficiary has at least one of the covered conditions listed when the diagnosis code is for a covered condition.

This review is not part of the contractor's medical review workload. Instead, the contractor should complete this review as part of its claims processing workload.

If ICD-9-CM is applicable, charges for ICD-9-CM procedure code 46.97, and, if ICD-10 is applicable, the ICD-10-PCS procedure codes ØDY80ZØ, ØDY80Z1, ØDY80Z2, ØDYEØZØ, ØDYEØZ1, or ØDYEØZ2 should be billed under revenue code 0360, Operating Room Services.

For discharge dates on or after October 1, 2001, acquisition charges are billed under revenue code 081X, Organ Acquisition. For discharge dates between April 1, 2001, and September 30, 2001, hospitals were to report the acquisition charges on the claim, but there was no interim pass-through payment made for these costs.

Bill the procedure used to obtain the donor's organ on the same claim, using appropriate ICD procedure codes.

The 11X bill type should be used when billing for intestinal transplants.

Immunosuppressive therapy for intestinal transplantation is covered and should be billed consistent with other organ transplants under the current rules.

If ICD-9-CM is applicable, there is no specific ICD-9-CM diagnosis code for intestinal failure. Diagnosis codes exist to capture the causes of intestinal failure. Some examples of intestinal failure include but are not limited to the following conditions and their associated ICD-9-CM codes:

- Volvulus 560.2,
- Volvulus gastroschisis 756.79, other [congenital] anomalies of abdominal wall,
- Volvulus gastroschisis 569.89, other specified disorders of intestine,
- Necrotizing enterocolitis 777.5, necrotizing enterocolitis in fetus or newborn,
- Necrotizing enterocolitis 014.8, other tuberculosis of intestines, peritoneum, and mesenteric,
- Necrotizing enterocolitis and splanchnic vascular thrombosis 557.0, acute vascular insufficiency of intestine,
- Inflammatory bowel disease 569.9, unspecified disorder of intestine,
- Radiation enteritis 777.5, necrotizing enterocolitis in fetus or newborn, and
- Radiation enteritis 558.1.

If ICD-10-CM is applicable, some diagnosis codes that may be used for intestinal failure are:

- Volvulus K56.2,
- Enteroptosis K63.4,
- Other specified diseases of intestine K63.89,
- Other specified diseases of the digestive system K92.89,
- Postsurgical malabsorption, not elsewhere classified K91.2,
- Other congenital malformations of abdominal wall Q79.59,
- Necrotizing enterocolitis in newborn, unspecified P77.9,
- Stage 1 necrotizing enterocolitis in newborn P77.1,
- Stage 2 necrotizing enterocolitis in newborn P77.2, and
- Stage 3 necrotizing enterocolitis in newborn P77.3

Other specified diseases of intestine K63.89, Other specified diseases of the digestive system K92.89, Postsurgical malabsorption, not elsewhere classified K91.2, Other congenital malformations of abdominal wall Q79.59, Necrotizing enterocolitis in newborn, unspecified P77.9, Stage 1 necrotizing enterocolitis in newborn P77.1, Stage 2 necrotizing enterocolitis in newborn P77.2, and Stage 3 necrotizing enterocolitis in newborn P77.3.

D. Acquisition Costs
A separate organ acquisition cost center was established for acquisition costs incurred on or after October 1, 2001. The Medicare Cost Report will include a separate line to account for these transplantation costs. For intestinal and multi-visceral transplants performed between April 1, 2001, and October 1, 2001, the DRG payment was payment in full for all hospital services related to this procedure.

E. Medicare Summary Notices (MSN), Remittance Advice Messages, and Notice of Utilization Notices (NOU)
If an intestinal transplant is billed by an unapproved facility after April 1, 2001, the contractor shall deny the claim and use MSN message 21.6, "This item or service is not covered when performed, referred, or ordered by this provider;" 21.18, "This item or service is not covered when performed or ordered by this provider;" or, 16.2, "This service cannot be paid when provided in this location/facility;" and Remittance

Advice Message, Claim Adjustment Reason Code 52, "The referring/prescribing/rendering provider is not eligible to refer/prescribe/order/perform the service billed."

100-4, 3, 100.1

Billing for Abortion Services

Effective October 1, 1998, abortions are not covered under the Medicare program except for instances where the pregnancy is a result of an act of rape or incest; or the woman suffers from a physical disorder, physical injury, or physical illness, including a life endangering physical condition caused by the pregnancy itself that would, as certified by a physician, place the woman in danger of death unless an abortion is performed.

A. "G" Modifier

The "G7" modifier is defined as "the pregnancy resulted from rape or incest, or pregnancy certified by physician as life threatening."

Beginning July 1, 1999, providers should bill for abortion services using the new Modifier G7. This modifier can be used on claims with dates of services October 1, 1998, and after. CWF will be able to recognize the modifier beginning July 1, 1999.

B. A/B MAC (A) Billing Instructions

1. Hospital Inpatient Billing

    Hospitals use bill type 11X. Medicare will pay only when one of the following condition codes is reported:

Condition Code	Description
AA	Abortion Performed due to Rape
AB	Abortion Performed due to Incest
AD	Abortion Performed due to life endangering physical condition

With one of the following:

If ICD-9-CM Is Applicable:

*   an appropriate ICD principal diagnosis code that will group to DRG 770 (Abortion W D&C, Aspiration Curettage Or Hysterotomy) or
*   an appropriate ICD principal diagnosis code and one of the following ICD-9-CM operating room procedure that will group to DRG 779 (Abortion W/O D&C):69.01, 69.02, 69.51, 74.91.

If ICD-10-CM is applicable, one of the following ICD-10-PCS codes are used:

ICD-10-PCS code	Description
10A07ZZ	Abortion of Products of Conception, Via Natural or Artificial Opening
10A08ZZ	Abortion of Products of Conception, Via Natural or Artificial Opening Endoscopic
10D17ZZ	Extraction of Products of Conception, Retained, Via Natural or Artificial Opening
10D18ZZ	Extraction of Products of Conception, Retained, Via Natural or Artificial Opening Endoscopic
10A07ZZ	Abortion of Products of Conception, Via Natural or Artificial Opening
10A08ZZ	Abortion of Products of Conception, Via Natural or Artificial Opening Endoscopic
10A00ZZ	Abortion of Products of Conception, Open Approach
10A03ZZ	Abortion of Products of Conception, Percutaneous Approach
10A04ZZ	Abortion of Products of Conception, Percutaneous Endoscopic Approach

Providers must use ICD-9-CM codes 69.01 and 69.02 if ICD-9-CM is applicable, or, if ICD-10-CM is applicable, the related 1CD-10-PCS codes to describe exactly the procedure or service performed.

The A/B MAC (A) must manually review claims with the above ICD-9-CM/ICD-10-PCS procedure codes to verify that all of the above conditions are met.

2. Outpatient Billing

    Hospitals will use bill type 13X and 85X. Medicare will pay only if one of the following CPT codes is used with the "G7" modifier.

59840	59851	59856	59841	59852
59857	59850	59855	59866	

C. Common Working File (CWF) Edits

For hospital outpatient claims, CWF will bypass its edits for a managed care beneficiary who is having an abortion outside their plan and the claim is submitted with the "G7" modifier and one of the above CPT codes.

For hospital inpatient claims, CWF will bypass its edits for a managed care beneficiary who is having an abortion outside their plan and the claim is submitted with one of the above inpatient procedure codes.

D. Medicare Summary Notices (MSN)/Explanation of Your Medicare Benefits Remittance Advice Message

If a claim is submitted with one of the above CPT procedure codes but no "G7" modifier, the claim is denied. The A/B MAC (A) states on the MSN the following message:

This service was denied because Medicare covers this service only under certain circumstances." (MSN Message 21.21).

For the remittance advice the A/B MAC (A) uses existing ASC X12-835 claim adjustment reason code B5, "Claim/service denied/reduced because coverage guidelines were not met or were exceeded."

100-4, 3, 100.6

Inpatient Renal Services

HO-E400

Section 405.103I of Subpart J of Regulation 5 stipulates that only approved hospitals may bill for ESRD services. Hence, to allow hospitals to bill and be reimbursed for inpatient dialysis services furnished under arrangements, both facilities participating in the arrangement must meet the conditions of 405.2120 and 405.2160 of Subpart U of Regulation 5. In order for renal dialysis facilities to have a written arrangement with each other to provide inpatient dialysis care both facilities must meet the minimum utilization rate requirement, i.e., two dialysis stations with a performance capacity of at least four dialysis treatments per week.

Dialysis may be billed by an SNF as a service if: (a) it is provided by a hospital with which the facility has a transfer agreement in effect, and that hospital is approved to provide staff-assisted dialysis for the Medicare program; or (b) it is furnished directly by an SNF meeting all nonhospital maintenance dialysis facility requirements, including minimum utilization requirements. (See 1861(h)(6), 1861(h)(7), title XVIII.)

100-4, 4, 160

Clinic and Emergency Visits

CMS has acknowledged from the beginning of the OPPS that CMS believes that CPT Evaluation and Management (E/M) codes were designed to reflect the activities of physicians and do not describe well the range and mix of services provided by hospitals during visits of clinic and emergency department patients. While awaiting the development of a national set of facility-specific codes and guidelines, providers should continue to apply their current internal guidelines to the existing CPT codes. Each hospital's internal guidelines should follow the intent of the CPT code descriptors, in that the guidelines should be designed to reasonably relate the intensity of hospital resources to the different levels of effort represented by the codes. Hospitals should ensure that their guidelines accurately reflect resource distinctions between the five levels of codes.

Effective January 1, 2007, CMS is distinguishing between two types of emergency departments: Type A emergency departments and Type B emergency departments.

A Type A emergency department is defined as an emergency department that is available 24 hours a day, 7 days a week and is either licensed by the State in which it is located under applicable State law as an emergency room or emergency department or it is held out to the public (by name, posted signs, advertising, or other means) as a place that provides care for emergency medical conditions on an urgent basis without requiring a previously scheduled appointment.

A Type B emergency department is defined as an emergency department that meets the definition of a "dedicated emergency department" as defined in 42 CFR 489.24 under the EMTALA regulations. It must meet at least one of the following requirements: (1) It is licensed by the State in which it is located under applicable State law as an emergency room or emergency department; (2) It is held out to the public (by name, posted signs, advertising, or other means) as a place that provides care for emergency medical conditions on an urgent basis without requiring a previously scheduled appointment; or (3) During the calendar year immediately preceding the calendar year in which a determination under 42 CFR 489.24 is being made, based on a representative sample of patient visits that occurred during that calendar year, it provides at least one-third of all of its outpatient visits for the treatment of emergency medical conditions on an urgent basis without requiring a previously scheduled appointment.

Hospitals must bill for visits provided in Type A emergency departments using CPT emergency department E/M codes. Hospitals must bill for visits provided in Type B emergency departments using the G-codes that describe visits provided in Type B emergency departments.

Hospitals that will be billing the new Type B ED visit codes may need to update their internal guidelines to report these codes.

Emergency department and clinic visits are paid in some cases separately and in other cases as part of a composite APC payment. See section 10.2.1 of this chapter for further details.

100-4, 8, 140.1

Payment for ESRD-Related Services Under the Monthly Capitation Payment (Center Based Patients)

Physicians and practitioners managing center based patients on dialysis are paid a monthly rate for most outpatient dialysis-related physician services furnished to a Medicare ESRD beneficiary. The payment amount varies based on the number of visits provided within each month and the age of the ESRD beneficiary. Under this methodology, separate codes are billed for providing one visit per month, two to three visits per month and four or more visits per month. The lowest payment amount applies when a physician provides one visit per month; a higher payment is provided for two to three visits per month. To receive the highest payment amount, a physician or practitioner would have to provide at least four ESRD-related visits per month. The MCP is reported once per month for services performed in an outpatient setting that are related to the patients' ESRD.

The physician or practitioner who provides the complete assessment, establishes the patient's plan of care, and provides the ongoing management is the physician or practitioner who submits the bill for the monthly service.

a. Month defined.

For purposes of billing for physician and practitioner ESRD related services, the term 'month' means a calendar month. The first month the beneficiary begins dialysis treatments is the date the dialysis treatments begin through the end of the calendar month. Thereafter, the term 'month' refers to a calendar month.

b. Determination of the age of beneficiary.

The beneficiary's age at the end of the month is the age of the patient for determining the appropriate age related ESRD-related services code.

c. Qualifying Visits Under the MCP

- General policy.

Visits must be furnished face-to-face by a physician, clinical nurse specialist, nurse practitioner, or physician's assistant.

- Visits furnished by another physician or practitioner (who is not the MCP physician or practitioner).

The MCP physician or practitioner may use other physicians or qualified nonphysician practitioners to provide some of the visits during the month. The MCP physician or practitioner does not have to be present when these other physicians or practitioners provide visits. In this instance, the rules are consistent with the requirements for hospital split/shared evaluation and management visits. The non-MCP physician or practitioner must be a partner, an employee of the same group practice, or an employee of the MCP physician or practitioner. For example, the physician or practitioner furnishing visits under the MCP may be either a W-2 employee or 1099 independent contractor.

When another physician is used to furnish some of the visits during the month, the physician who provides the complete assessment, establishes the patient's plan of care, and provides the ongoing management should bill for the MCP service.

If the nonphysician practitioner is the practitioner who performs the complete assessment and establishes the plan of care, then the MCP service should be billed under the PIN of the clinical nurse specialist, nurse practitioner, or physician assistant.

- Residents, interns and fellows.

Patient visits by residents, interns and fellows enrolled in an approved Medicare graduate medical education (GME) program may be counted towards the MCP visits if the teaching MCP physician is present during the visit.

- Patients designated/admitted as hospital observation status.

ESRD-related visits furnished to patients in hospital observation status that occur on or after January 1, 2005, should be counted for purposes of billing the MCP codes. Visits furnished to patients in hospital observation status are included when submitting MCP claims for ESRD-related services.

- ESRD-related visits furnished to beneficiaries residing in a SNF.

ESRD-related visits furnished to beneficiaries residing in a SNF should be counted for purposes of billing the MCP codes.

- SNF residents admitted as an inpatient.

Inpatient visits are not counted for purposes of the MCP service. If the beneficiary residing in a SNF is admitted to the hospital as an inpatient, the appropriate inpatient visit code should be billed.

- ESRD Related Visits as a Telehealth Service

ESRD-related services with 2 or 3 visits per month and ESRD-related services with 4 or more visits per month may be furnished as a telehealth service. However, at least one visit per month is required in person to examine the vascular access site. A clinical examination of the vascular access site must be furnished face-to-face (not as a telehealth service) by a physician, nurse practitioner or physician's assistant. For more information on how ESRD-related visits may be furnished as a Medicare telehealth service and for general Medicare telehealth policy see Pub. 100-2, Medicare Benefit Policy manual, chapter 15, section 270. For claims processing instructions see Pub. 100-4, Medicare Claims Processing manual chapter 12, section 190.

100-4, 8, 140.1.1

Payment for Managing Patients on Home Dialysis

Physicians and practitioners managing ESRD patients who dialyze at home are paid a single monthly rate based on the age of the beneficiary. The MCP physician (or

practitioner) must furnish at least one face-to-face patient visit per month for the home dialysis MCP service. Documentation by the MCP physician (or practitioner) should support at least one face-to-face encounter per month with the home dialysis patient. Medicare contractors may waive the requirement for a monthly face-to-face visit for the home dialysis MCP service on a case by case basis, for example, when the nephrologist's notes indicate that the physician actively and adequately managed the care of the home dialysis patient throughout the month. The management of home dialysis patients who remain a home dialysis patient the entire month should be coded using the ESRD-related services for home dialysis patients HCPCS codes.

When another physician is used to furnish some of the visits during the month, the physician who provides the complete assessment, establishes the patient's plan of care, and provides the ongoing management should bill for the MCP service.

If the nonphysician practitioner is the practitioner who performs the complete assessment and establishes the plan of care, then the MCP service should be billed under the PIN of the clinical nurse specialist, nurse practitioner, or physician assistant.

Residents, interns and fellows. Patient visits by residents, interns and fellows enrolled in an approved Medicare graduate medical education (GME) program may be counted towards the MCP visits if the teaching MCP physician is present during the visit.

a. Month defined.

For purposes of billing for physician and practitioner ESRD related services, the term 'month' means a calendar month. The first month the beneficiary begins dialysis treatments is the date the dialysis treatments begin through the end of the calendar month. Thereafter, the term 'month' refers to a calendar month.

b. Qualifying Visits under the MCP

- General policy.

Visits must be furnished face-to-face by a physician, clinical nurse specialist, nurse practitioner, or physician's assistant.

- Visits furnished by another physician or practitioner (who is not the MCP physician or practitioner).

The MCP physician or practitioner may use other physicians or qualified nonphysician practitioners to provide the visit(s) during the month. The MCP physician or practitioner does not have to be present when these other physicians or practitioners provide visit(s). The non-MCP physician or practitioner must be a partner, an employee of the same group practice, or an employee of the MCP physician or practitioner. For example, the physician or practitioner furnishing visits under the MCP may be either a W-2 employee or 1099 independent contractor.

When another physician is used to furnish some of the visits during the month, the physician who provides the complete assessment, establishes the patient's plan of care, and provides the ongoing management should bill for the MCP service.

If the nonphysician practitioner is the practitioner who performs the complete assessment and establishes the plan of care, then the MCP service should be billed under the PIN of the clinical nurse specialist, nurse practitioner, or physician assistant.

- Residents, interns and fellows.

Patient visits by residents, interns and fellows enrolled in an approved Medicare graduate medical education (GME) program may be counted towards the MCP visits if the teaching MCP physician is present during the visit.

100-4, 9, 182

Medical Nutrition Therapy (MNT) Services

A - FQHCs

Previously, MNT type services were considered incident to services under the FQHC benefit, if all relevant program requirements were met. Therefore, separate all-inclusive encounter rate payment could not be made for the provision of MNT services. With passage of DRA, effective January 1, 2006, FQHCs are eligible for a separate payment under Part B for these services provided they meet all program requirements. Payment is made at the all-inclusive encounter rate to the FQHC. This payment can be in addition to payment for any other qualifying visit on the same date of service as the beneficiary received qualifying MNT services.

For FQHCs to qualify for a separate visit payment for MNT services, the services must be a one-on-one face-to-face encounter. Group sessions don't constitute a billable visit for any FQHC services. Rather, the cost of group sessions is included in the calculation of the all-inclusive FQHC visit rate. To receive payment for MNT services, the MNT services must be billed on TOB 73X with the appropriate individual MNT HCPCS code (codes 97802, 97803, or G0270) and with the appropriate site of service revenue code in the 052X revenue code series. This payment can be in addition to payment for any other qualifying visit on the same date of service as the beneficiary received qualifying MNT services as long as the claim for MNT services contain the appropriate coding specified above.

NOTE: MNT is not a qualifying visit on the same day that DSMT is provided.

Additional information on MNT can be found in Chapter 4, section 300 of this manual.

Group services (HCPCS 97804 or G0271) do not meet the criteria for a separate qualifying encounter. All line items billed on TOB 73x with HCPCS code 97804 or G0271 will be denied.

B - RHCs

Separate payment to RHCs for these practitioners/services continues to be precluded as these services are not within the scope of Medicare-covered RHC benefits. All line items billed on TOB 71x with HCPCS codes for MNT services will be denied.

100-4, 11, 40.1.3

Independent Attending Physician Services

When hospice coverage is elected, the beneficiary waives all rights to Medicare Part B payments for professional services that are related to the treatment and management of his/her terminal illness during any period his/her hospice benefit election is in force, except for professional services of an independent attending physician, who is not an employee of the designated hospice nor receives compensation from the hospice for those services. For purposes of administering the hospice benefit provisions, an "attending physician" means an individual who:

- Is a doctor of medicine or osteopathy or

- A nurse practitioner (for professional services related to the terminal illness that are furnished on or after December 8, 2003); and

- Is identified by the individual, at the time he/she elects hospice coverage, as having the most significant role in the determination and delivery of their medical care.

Hospices should reiterate with patients that they must not see independent physicians for care related to their terminal illness other than their independent attending physician unless the hospice arranges it.

Even though a beneficiary elects hospice coverage, he/she may designate and use an independent attending physician, who is not employed by nor receives compensation from the hospice for professional services furnished, in addition to the services of hospice-employed physicians. The professional services of an independent attending physician, who may be a nurse practitioner as defined in Chapter 9, that are reasonable and necessary for the treatment and management of a hospice patient's terminal illness are not considered Medicare Part A hospice services.

Where the service is related to the hospice patient's terminal illness but was furnished by someone other than the designated "attending physician" [or a physician substituting for the attending physician]) the physician or other provider must look to the hospice for payment.

Professional services related to the hospice patient's terminal condition that were furnished by an independent attending physician, who may be a nurse practitioner, are billed to the Medicare contractor through Medicare Part B. When the independent attending physician furnishes a terminal illness related service that includes both a professional and technical component (e.g., x-rays), he/she bills the professional component of such services to the Medicare contractor on a professional claim and looks to the hospice for payment for the technical component. Likewise, the independent attending physician, who may be a nurse practitioner, would look to the hospice for payment for terminal illness related services furnished that have no professional component (e.g., clinical lab tests). The remainder of this section explains this in greater detail.

When a Medicare beneficiary elects hospice coverage he/she may designate an attending physician, who may be a nurse practitioner, not employed by the hospice, in addition to receiving care from hospice-employed physicians. The professional services of a non-hospice affiliated attending physician for the treatment and management of a hospice patient's terminal illness are not considered Medicare Part A "hospice services." These independent attending physician services are billed through Medicare Part B to the Medicare contractor, provided they were not furnished under a payment arrangement with the hospice. The independent attending physician codes services with the GV modifier "Attending physician not employed or paid under agreement by the patient's hospice provider" when billing his/her professional services furnished for the treatment and management of a hospice patient's terminal condition. The Medicare contractor makes payment to the independent attending physician or beneficiary, as appropriate, based on the payment and deductible rules applicable to each covered service.

Payments for the services of an independent attending physician are not counted in determining whether the hospice cap amount has been exceeded because Part B services provided by an independent attending physician are not part of the hospice's care.

Services provided by an independent attending physician who may be a nurse practitioner must be coordinated with any direct care services provided by hospice physicians.

Only the direct professional services of an independent attending physician, who may be a nurse practitioner, to a patient may be billed; the costs for services such as lab or x-rays are not to be included in the bill.

If another physician covers for a hospice patient's designated attending physician, the services of the substituting physician are billed by the designated attending physician under the reciprocal or locum tenens billing instructions. In such instances, the attending physician bills using the GV modifier in conjunction with either the Q5 or Q6 modifier.

When services related to a hospice patient's terminal condition are furnished under a payment arrangement with the hospice by the designated attending physician who

may be a nurse practitioner (i.e., by a non-independent physician/nurse practitioner), the physician must look to the hospice for payment. In this situation the physicians' services are Part A hospice services and are billed by the hospice to its Medicare contractor.

Medicare contractors must process and pay for covered, medically necessary Part B services that physicians furnish to patients after their hospice benefits are revoked even if the patient remains under the care of the hospice. Such services are billed without the GV or GW modifiers. Make payment based on applicable Medicare payment and deductible rules for each covered service even if the beneficiary continues to be treated by the hospice after hospice benefits are revoked.

The CWF response contains the periods of hospice entitlement. This information is a permanent part of the notice and is furnished on all CWF replies and automatic notices. Medicare contractor use the CWF reply for validating dates of hospice coverage and to research, examine and adjudicate services coded with the GV or GW modifiers.

100-4, 12, 30.1

Digestive System (Codes 40000 - 49999)

B3-15100

A. Upper Gastrointestinal Endoscopy Including Endoscopic Ultrasound (EUS) (Code 43259)

If the person performing the original diagnostic endoscopy has access to the EUS and the clinical situation requires an EUS, the EUS may be done at the same time. The procedure, diagnostic and EUS, is reported under the same code, CPT 43259. This code conforms to CPT guidelines for the indented codes. The service represented by the indented code, in this case code 43259 for EUS, includes the service represented by the unintended code preceding the list of indented codes. Therefore, when a diagnostic examination of the upper gastrointestinal tract "including esophagus, stomach, and either the duodenum or jejunum as appropriate," includes the use of endoscopic ultrasonography, the service is reported by a single code, namely 43259.

Interpretation, whether by a radiologist or endoscopist, is reported under CPT code 76975-26. These codes may both be reported on the same day.

B. Incomplete Colonoscopies (Codes 45330 and 45378)

An incomplete colonoscopy, e.g., the inability to extend beyond the splenic flexure, is billed and paid using colonoscopy code 45378 with modifier "-53." The Medicare physician fee schedule database has specific values for code 45378-53. These values are the same as for code 45330, sigmoidoscopy, as failure to extend beyond the splenic flexure means that a sigmoidoscopy rather than a colonoscopy has been performed.

However, code 45378-53 should be used when an incomplete colonoscopy has been done because other MPFSDB indicators are different for codes 45378 and 45330.

100-4, 12, 30.6.2

Billing for Medically Necessary Visit on Same Occasion as Preventive Medicine Service

See Chapter 18 for payment for covered preventive services.

When a physician furnishes a Medicare beneficiary a covered visit at the same place and on the same occasion as a noncovered preventive medicine service (CPT codes 99381- 99397), consider the covered visit to be provided in lieu of a part of the preventive medicine service of equal value to the visit. A preventive medicine service (CPT codes 99381-99397) is a noncovered service. The physician may charge the beneficiary, as a charge for the noncovered remainder of the service, the amount by which the physician's current established charge for the preventive medicine service exceeds his/her current established charge for the covered visit. Pay for the covered visit based on the lesser of the fee schedule amount or the physician's actual charge for the visit. The physician is not required to give the beneficiary written advance notice of noncoverage of the part of the visit that constitutes a routine preventive visit. However, the physician is responsible for notifying the patient in advance of his/her liability for the charges for services that are not medically necessary to treat the illness or injury.

There could be covered and noncovered procedures performed during this encounter (e.g., screening x-ray, EKG, lab tests.). These are considered individually. Those procedures which are for screening for asymptomatic conditions are considered noncovered and, therefore, no payment is made. Those procedures ordered to diagnose or monitor a symptom, medical condition, or treatment are evaluated for medical necessity and, if covered, are paid.

100-4, 12, 30.6.4

Evaluation and Management (E/M) Services Furnished Incident to Physician's Service by Nonphysician Practitioners

When evaluation and management services are furnished incident to a physician's service by a nonphysician practitioner, the physician may bill the CPT code that describes the evaluation and management service furnished.

When evaluation and management services are furnished incident to a physician's service by a nonphysician employee of the physician, not as part of a physician service, the physician bills code 99211 for the service.

A physician is not precluded from billing under the "incident to" provision for services provided by employees whose services cannot be paid for directly under the Medicare program. Employees of the physician may provide services incident to the physician's service, but the physician alone is permitted to bill Medicare.

Services provided by employees as "incident to" are covered when they meet all the requirements for incident to and are medically necessary for the individual needs of the patient.

100-4, 12, 30.6.7

Payment for Office or Other Outpatient Evaluation and Management (E/M) Visits (Codes 99201 - 99215)

A. Definition of New Patient for Selection of E/M Visit Code

Interpret the phrase "new patient" to mean a patient who has not received any professional services, i.e., E/M service or other face-to-face service (e.g., surgical procedure) from the physician or physician group practice (same physician specialty) within the previous 3 years. For example, if a professional component of a previous procedure is billed in a 3 year time period, e.g., a lab interpretation is billed and no E/M service or other face-to-face service with the patient is performed, then this patient remains a new patient for the initial visit. An interpretation of a diagnostic test, reading an x-ray or EKG etc., in the absence of an E/M service or other face-to-face service with the patient does not affect the designation of a new patient.

B. Office/Outpatient E/M Visits Provided on Same Day for Unrelated Problems

As for all other E/M services except where specifically noted, carriers may not pay two E/M office visits billed by a physician (or physician of the same specialty from the same group practice) for the same beneficiary on the same day unless the physician documents that the visits were for unrelated problems in the office or outpatient setting which could not be provided during the same encounter (e.g., office visit for blood pressure medication evaluation, followed five hours later by a visit for evaluation of leg pain following an accident).

C. Office/Outpatient or Emergency Department E/M Visit on Day of Admission to Nursing Facility

Carriers may not pay a physician for an emergency department visit or an office visit and a comprehensive nursing facility assessment on the same day. Bundle E/M visits on the same date provided in sites other than the nursing facility into the initial nursing facility care code when performed on the same date as the nursing facility admission by the same physician.

D. Drug Administration Services and E/M Visits Billed on Same Day of Service

Carriers must advise physicians that CPT code 99211 cannot be paid if it is billed with a drug administration service such as a chemotherapy or nonchemotherapy drug infusion code (effective January 1, 2004). This drug administration policy was expanded in the Physician Fee Schedule Final Rule, November 15, 2004, to also include a therapeutic or diagnostic injection code (effective January 1, 2005). Therefore, when a medically necessary, significant and separately identifiable E/M service (which meets a higher complexity level than CPT code 99211) is performed, in addition to one of these drug administration services, the appropriate E/M CPT code should be reported with modifier -25. Documentation should support the level of E/M service billed. For an E/M service provided on the same day, a different diagnosis is not required.

100-4, 12, 30.6.8

Payment for Hospital Observation Services (Codes 99217– 99220) and Observation or Inpatient Care Services (Including Admission and Discharge Services – (Codes 99234 – 99236))

A. Who May Bill Observation Care Codes

Observation care is a well-defined set of specific, clinically appropriate services, which include ongoing short term treatment, assessment, and reassessment, that are furnished while a decision is being made regarding whether patients will require further treatment as hospital inpatients or if they are able to be discharged from the hospital. Observation services are commonly ordered for patients who present to the emergency department and who then require a significant period of treatment or monitoring in order to make a decision concerning their admission or discharge.

In only rare and exceptional cases do reasonable and necessary outpatient observation services span more than 48 hours. In the majority of cases, the decision whether to discharge a patient from the hospital following resolution of the reason for the observation care or to admit the patient as an inpatient can be made in less than 48 hours, usually in less than 24 hours.

Contractors pay for initial observation care billed by only the physician who ordered hospital outpatient observation services and was responsible for the patient during his/her observation care. A physician who does not have inpatient admitting privileges but who is authorized to furnish hospital outpatient observation services may bill these codes.

For a physician to bill observation care codes, there must be a medical observation record for the patient which contains dated and timed physician's orders regarding the observation services the patient is to receive, nursing notes, and progress notes prepared by the physician while the patient received observation services. This record must be in addition to any record prepared as a result of an emergency department or outpatient clinic encounter.

Payment for an initial observation care code is for all the care rendered by the ordering physician on the date the patient's observation services began. All other physicians who furnish consultations or additional evaluations or services while the patient is receiving hospital outpatient observation services must bill the appropriate outpatient service codes.

For example, if an internist orders observation services and asks another physician to additionally evaluate the patient, only the internist may bill the initial and subsequent observation care codes. The other physician who evaluates the patient must bill the new or established office or other outpatient visit codes as appropriate.

For information regarding hospital billing of observation services, see Chapter 4, §290.

B. Physician Billing for Observation Care Following Initiation of Observation Services

Similar to initial observation codes, payment for a subsequent observation care code is for all the care rendered by the treating physician on the day(s) other than the initial or discharge date. All other physicians who furnish consultations or additional evaluations or services while the patient is receiving hospital outpatient observation services must bill the appropriate outpatient service codes.

When a patient receives observation care for less than 8 hours on the same calendar date, the Initial Observation Care, from CPT code range 99218 – 99220, shall be reported by the physician. The Observation Care Discharge Service, CPT code 99217, shall not be reported for this scenario.

When a patient is admitted for observation care and then is discharged on a different calendar date, the physician shall report Initial Observation Care, from CPT code range 99218 – 99220, and CPT observation care discharge CPT code 99217. On the rare occasion when a patient remains in observation care for 3 days, the physician shall report an initial observation care code (99218-99220) for the first day of observation care, a subsequent observation care code (99224-99226) for the second day of observation care, and an observation care discharge CPT code 99217 for the observation care on the discharge date. When observation care continues beyond 3 days, the physician shall report a subsequent observation care code (99224-99226) for each day between the first day of observation care and the discharge date.

When a patient receives observation care for a minimum of 8 hours, but less than 24 hours, and is discharged on the same calendar date, Observation or Inpatient Care Services (Including Admission and Discharge Services) from CPT code range 99234 – 99236 shall be reported. The observation discharge, CPT code 99217, cannot also be reported for this scenario.

C. Documentation Requirements for Billing Observation or Inpatient Care Services (Including Admission and Discharge Services)

The physician shall satisfy the E/M documentation guidelines for furnishing observation care or inpatient hospital care. In addition to meeting the documentation requirements for history, examination, and medical decision making, documentation in the medical record shall include:

- Documentation stating the stay for observation care or inpatient hospital care involves 8 hours, but less than 24 hours;

- Documentation identifying the billing physician was present and personally performed the services; and

- Documentation identifying the order for observation services, progress notes, and discharge notes were written by the billing physician.

In the rare circumstance when a patient receives observation services for more than 2 calendar dates, the physician shall bill observation services furnished on day(s) other than the initial or discharge date using subsequent observation care codes. The physician may not use the subsequent hospital care codes since the patient is not an inpatient of the hospital.

D. Admission to Inpatient Status Following Observation Care

If the same physician who ordered hospital outpatient observation services also admits the patient to inpatient status before the end of the date on which the patient began receiving hospital outpatient observation services, pay only an initial hospital visit for the evaluation and management services provided on that date. Medicare payment for the initial hospital visit includes all services provided to the patient on the date of admission by that physician, regardless of the site of service. The physician may not bill an initial or subsequent observation care code for services on the date that he or she admits the patient to inpatient status. If the patient is admitted to inpatient status from hospital outpatient observation care subsequent to the date of initiation of observation services, the physician must bill an initial hospital visit for the services provided on that date. The physician may not bill the hospital observation discharge management code (code 99217) or an outpatient/office visit for the care provided while the patient received hospital outpatient observation services on the date of admission to inpatient status.

E. Hospital Observation Services During Global Surgical Period

The global surgical fee includes payment for hospital observation (codes 99217, 99218, 99219, 99220, 99224, 99225, 99226, 99234, 99235, and 99236) services unless the criteria for use of CPT modifiers "-24," "-25," or "-57" are met. Contractors must pay for these services in addition to the global surgical fee only if both of the following requirements are met:

- The hospital observation service meets the criteria needed to justify billing it with CPT modifiers "-24," "-25," or "-57" (decision for major surgery); and

- The hospital observation service furnished by the surgeon meets all of the criteria for the hospital observation code billed.

Examples of the decision for surgery during a hospital observation period are:

- An emergency department physician orders hospital outpatient observation services for a patient with a head injury. A neurosurgeon is called in to evaluate the need for surgery while the patient is receiving observation services and decides that the patient requires surgery. The surgeon would bill a new or established office or other outpatient visit code as appropriate with the "-57" modifier to indicate that the decision for surgery was made during the evaluation. The surgeon must bill the office or other outpatient visit code because the patient receiving hospital outpatient observation services is not an inpatient of the hospital. Only the physician who ordered hospital outpatient observation services may bill for observation care.

- A neurosurgeon orders hospital outpatient observation services for a patient with a head injury. During the observation period, the surgeon makes the decision for surgery. The surgeon would bill the appropriate level of hospital observation code with the "-57" modifier to indicate that the decision for surgery was made while the surgeon was providing hospital observation care.

Examples of hospital observation services during the postoperative period of a surgery are:

- A surgeon orders hospital outpatient observation services for a patient with abdominal pain from a kidney stone on the 80th day following a TURP (performed by that surgeon). The surgeon decides that the patient does not require surgery. The surgeon would bill the observation code with CPT modifier "-24" and documentation to support that the observation services are unrelated to the surgery.

- A surgeon orders hospital outpatient observation services for a patient with abdominal pain on the 80th day following a TURP (performed by that surgeon). While the patient is receiving hospital outpatient observation services, the surgeon decides that the patient requires kidney surgery. The surgeon would bill the observation code with HCPCS modifier "-57" to indicate that the decision for surgery was made while the patient was receiving hospital outpatient observation services. The subsequent surgical procedure would be reported with modifier "-79."

- A surgeon orders hospital outpatient observation services for a patient with abdominal pain on the 20th day following a resection of the colon (performed by that surgeon). The surgeon determines that the patient requires no further colon surgery and discharges the patient. The surgeon may not bill for the observation services furnished during the global period because they were related to the previous surgery.

An example of a billable hospital observation service on the same day as a procedure is when a physician repairs a laceration of the scalp in the emergency department for a patient with a head injury and then subsequently orders hospital outpatient observation services for that patient. The physician would bill the observation code with a CPT modifier 25 and the procedure code.

100-4, 12, 30.6.9

Payment for Inpatient Hospital Visits - General (Codes 99221 - 99239)

A. Hospital Visit and Critical Care on Same Day

When a hospital inpatient or office/outpatient evaluation and management service (E/M) are furnished on a calendar date at which time the patient does not require critical care and the patient subsequently requires critical care both the critical Care Services (CPT codes 99291 and 99292) and the previous E/M service may be paid on the same date of service. Hospital emergency department services are not paid for the same date as critical care services when provided by the same physician to the same patient.

During critical care management of a patient those services that do not meet the level of critical care shall be reported using an inpatient hospital care service with CPT Subsequent Hospital Care using a code from CPT code range 99231 – 99233.

Both Initial Hospital Care (CPT codes 99221 – 99223) and Subsequent Hospital Care codes are "per diem" services and may be reported only once per day by the same physician or physicians of the same specialty from the same group practice.

Physicians and qualified nonphysician practitioners (NPPs) are advised to retain documentation for discretionary contractor review should claims be questioned for both hospital care and critical care claims. The retained documentation shall support claims for critical care when the same physician or physicians of the same specialty in a group practice report critical care services for the same patient on the same calendar date as other E/M services.

B. Two Hospital Visits Same Day

Contractors pay a physician for only one hospital visit per day for the same patient, whether the problems seen during the encounters are related or not. The inpatient hospital visit descriptors contain the phrase "per day" which means that the code and the payment established for the code represent all services provided on that date. The physician should select a code that reflects all services provided during the date of the service.

C. Hospital Visits Same Day But by Different Physicians

In a hospital inpatient situation involving one physician covering for another, if physician A sees the patient in the morning and physician B, who is covering for A, sees the same patient in the evening, contractors do not pay physician B for the second visit. The hospital visit descriptors include the phrase "per day" meaning care for the day.

If the physicians are each responsible for a different aspect of the patient's care, pay both visits if the physicians are in different specialties and the visits are billed with different diagnoses. There are circumstances where concurrent care may be billed by physicians of the same specialty.

D. Visits to Patients in Swing Beds

If the inpatient care is being billed by the hospital as inpatient hospital care, the hospital care codes apply. If the inpatient care is being billed by the hospital as nursing facility care, then the nursing facility codes apply.

100-4, 12, 30.6.9.1

Payment for Initial Hospital Care Services (Codes 99221 – 99223 and Observation or Inpatient Care Services (Including Admission and Discharge Services) (Codes 99234 – 99236)

A. Initial Hospital Care From Emergency Room

Contractors pay for an initial hospital care service if a physician sees a patient in the emergency room and decides to admit the person to the hospital. They do not pay for both E/M services. Also, they do not pay for an emergency department visit by the same physician on the same date of service. When the patient is admitted to the hospital via another site of service (e.g., hospital emergency department, physician's office, nursing facility), all services provided by the physician in conjunction with that admission are considered part of the initial hospital care when performed on the same date as the admission.

B. Initial Hospital Care on Day Following Visit

Contractors pay both visits if a patient is seen in the office on one date and admitted to the hospital on the next date, even if fewer than 24 hours has elapsed between the visit and the admission.

C. Initial Hospital Care and Discharge on Same Day

When the patient is admitted to inpatient hospital care for less than 8 hours on the same date, then Initial Hospital Care, from CPT code range 99221 – 99223, shall be reported by the physician. The Hospital Discharge Day Management service, CPT codes 99238 or 99239, shall not be reported for this scenario.

When a patient is admitted to inpatient initial hospital care and then discharged on a different calendar date, the physician shall report an Initial Hospital Care from CPT code range 99221 – 99223 and a Hospital Discharge Day Management service, CPT code 99238 or 99239.

When a patient has been admitted to inpatient hospital care for a minimum of 8 hours but less than 24 hours and discharged on the same calendar date, Observation or Inpatient Hospital Care Services (Including Admission and Discharge Services), from CPT code range 99234 – 99236, shall be reported.

D. Documentation Requirements for Billing Observation or Inpatient Care Services (Including Admission and Discharge Services)

The physician shall satisfy the E/M documentation guidelines for admission to and discharge from inpatient observation or hospital care. In addition to meeting the documentation requirements for history, examination and medical decision making documentation in the medical record shall include:

- Documentation stating the stay for hospital treatment or observation care status involves 8 hours but less than 24 hours;

- Documentation identifying the billing physician was present and personally performed the services; and

- Documentation identifying the admission and discharge notes were written by the billing physician.

E. Physician Services Involving Transfer From One Hospital to Another; Transfer Within Facility to Prospective Payment System (PPS) Exempt Unit of Hospital; Transfer From One Facility to Another Separate Entity Under Same Ownership and/or Part of Same Complex; or Transfer From One Department to Another Within Single Facility

Physicians may bill both the hospital discharge management code and an initial hospital care code when the discharge and admission do not occur on the same day if the transfer is between:

- Different hospitals;

- Different facilities under common ownership which do not have merged records; or

- Between the acute care hospital and a PPS exempt unit within the same hospital when there are no merged records.

In all other transfer circumstances, the physician should bill only the appropriate level of subsequent hospital care for the date of transfer.

F. Initial Hospital Care Service History and Physical That Is Less Than Comprehensive

When a physician performs a visit that meets the definition of a Level 5 office visit several days prior to an admission and on the day of admission performs less than a comprehensive history and physical, he or she should report the office visit that reflects the services furnished and also report the lowest level initial hospital care code (i.e., code 99221) for the initial hospital admission. Contractors pay the office visit as billed and the Level 1 initial hospital care code.

Physicians who provide an initial visit to a patient during inpatient hospital care that meets the minimum key component work and/or medical necessity requirements shall report an initial hospital care code (99221-99223). The principal physician of record shall append modifier "-AI" (Principal Physician of Record) to the claim for the initial hospital care code. This modifier will identify the physician who oversees the patient's care from all other physicians who may be furnishing specialty care.

Physicians may bill initial hospital care service codes (99221-99223), for services that were reported with CPT consultation codes (99241 – 99255) prior to January 1, 2010, when the furnished service and documentation meet the minimum key component work and/or medical necessity requirements. Physicians must meet all the requirements of the initial hospital care codes, including "a detailed or comprehensive history" and "a detailed or comprehensive examination" to report CPT code 99221, which are greater than the requirements for consultation codes 99251 and 99252.

Subsequent hospital care CPT codes 99231 and 99232, respectively, require "a problem focused interval history" and "an expanded problem focused interval history." An E/M service that could be described by CPT consultation code 99251 or 99252 could potentially meet the component work and medical necessity requirements to report 99231 or 99232. Physicians may report a subsequent hospital care CPT code for services that were reported as CPT consultation codes (99241 – 99255) prior to January 1, 2010, where the medical record appropriately demonstrates that the work and medical necessity requirements are met for reporting a subsequent hospital care code (under the level selected), even though the reported code is for the provider's first E/M service to the inpatient during the hospital stay.

Reporting CPT code 99499 (Unlisted evaluation and management service) should be limited to cases where there is no other specific E/M code payable by Medicare that describes that service.

Reporting CPT code 99499 requires submission of medical records and contractor manual medical review of the service prior to payment. Contractors shall expect reporting under these circumstances to be unusual.

G. Initial Hospital Care Visits by Two Different M.D.s or D.O.s When They Are Involved in Same Admission

In the inpatient hospital setting all physicians (and qualified nonphysician practitioners where permitted) who perform an initial evaluation may bill the initial hospital care codes (99221 – 99223) or nursing facility care codes (99304 – 99306). Contractors consider only one M.D. or D.O. to be the principal physician of record (sometimes referred to as the admitting physician.) The principal physician of record is identified in Medicare as the physician who oversees the patient's care from other physicians who may be furnishing specialty care. Only the principal physician of record shall append modifier "-AI" (Principal Physician of Record) in addition to the E/M code. Follow-up visits in the facility setting shall be billed as subsequent hospital care visits and subsequent nursing facility care visits.

100-4, 12, 30.6.9.2

Subsequent Hospital Visit and Hospital Discharge Day Management (Codes 99231 - 99239)

A. Subsequent Hospital Visits During the Global Surgery Period

(Refer to Secs.40-40.4 on global surgery) The Medicare physician fee schedule payment amount for surgical procedures includes all services (e.g., evaluation and management visits) that are part of the global surgery payment; therefore, contractors shall not pay more than that amount when a bill is fragmented for staged procedures.

B. Hospital Discharge Day Management Service Hospital Discharge Day

Management Services, CPT code 99238 or 99239 is a face-to-face evaluation and management (E/M) service between the attending physician and the patient. The E/M discharge day management visit shall be reported for the date of the actual visit by the physician or qualified nonphysician practitioner even if the patient is discharged from the facility on a different calendar date. Only one hospital discharge day management service is payable per patient per hospital stay.

Only the attending physician of record reports the discharge day management service. Physicians or qualified nonphysician practitioners, other than the attending physician, who have been managing concurrent health care problems not primarily managed by the attending physician, and who are not acting on behalf of the attending physician, shall use Subsequent Hospital Care (CPT code range 99231 - 99233) for a final visit.

Medicare pays for the paperwork of patient discharge day management through the pre- and post- service work of an E/M service.

C. Subsequent Hospital Visit and Discharge Management on Same Day

Pay only the hospital discharge management code on the day of discharge (unless it is also the day of admission, in which case, refer to Sec.30.6.9.1 C for the policy on Observation or Inpatient Care Services (Including Admission and Discharge Services CPT Codes 99234 - 99236). Contractors do not pay both a subsequent hospital visit in addition to hospital discharge day management service on the same day by the same physician. Instruct physicians that they may not bill for both a hospital visit and hospital discharge management for the same date of service.

D. Hospital Discharge Management (CPT Codes 99238 and 99239) and Nursing Facility Admission Code When Patient Is Discharged From Hospital and Admitted to Nursing Facility on Same Day

Contractors pay the hospital discharge code (codes 99238 or 99239) in addition to a nursing facility admission code when they are billed by the same physician with the same date of service.

If a surgeon is admitting the patient to the nursing facility due to a condition that is not as a result of the surgery during the postoperative period of a service with the global surgical period, he/she bills for the nursing facility admission and care with a modifier "-24" and provides documentation that the service is unrelated to the surgery (e.g., return of an elderly patient to the nursing facility in which he/she has resided for five years following discharge from the hospital for cholecystectomy).

Contractors do not pay for a nursing facility admission by a surgeon in the postoperative period of a procedure with a global surgical period if the patient's admission to the nursing facility is to receive post operative care related to the surgery (e.g., admission to a nursing facility to receive physical therapy following a hip replacement). Payment for the nursing facility admission and subsequent nursing facility services are included in the global fee and cannot be paid separately.

E. Hospital Discharge Management and Death Pronouncement

Only the physician who personally performs the pronouncement of death shall bill for the face-to-face Hospital Discharge Day Management Service, CPT code 99238 or 99239. The date of the pronouncement shall reflect the calendar date of service on the day it was performed even if the paperwork is delayed to a subsequent date.

100-4, 12, 30.6.10

Consultation Services

Consultation Services versus Other Evaluation and Management (E/M) Visits

Effective January 1, 2010, the consultation codes are no longer recognized for Medicare Part B payment. Physicians shall code patient evaluation and management visits with E/M codes that represent where the visit occurs and that identify the complexity of the visit performed.

In the inpatient hospital setting and the nursing facility setting, physicians (and qualified nonphysician practitioners where permitted) may bill the most appropriate initial hospital care code (99221-99223), subsequent hospital care code (99231 and 99232), initial nursing facility care code (99304-99306), or subsequent nursing facility care code (99307-99310) that reflects the services the physician or practitioner furnished. Subsequent hospital care codes could potentially meet the component work and medical necessity requirements to be reported for an E/M service that could be described by CPT consultation code 99251 or 99252. Contractors shall not find fault in cases where the medical record appropriately demonstrates that the work and medical necessity requirements are met for reporting a subsequent hospital care code (under the level selected), even though the reported code is for the provider's first E/M service to the inpatient during the hospital stay. Unlisted evaluation and management service (code 99499) shall only be reported for consultation services when an E/M service that could be described by codes 99251 or 99252 is furnished, and there is no other specific E/M code payable by Medicare that describes that service. Reporting code 99499 requires submission of medical records and contractor manual medical review of the service prior to payment. CMS expects reporting under these circumstances to be unusual. T he principal physician of record is identified in Medicare as the physician who oversees the patient's care from other physicians who may be furnishing specialty care. The principal physician of record shall append modifier "-AI" (Principal Physician of Record), in addition to the E/M code. Follow-up visits in the facility setting shall be billed as subsequent hospital care visits and subsequent nursing facility care visits.

In the CAH setting, those CAHs that use method II shall bill the appropriate new or established visit code for those physician and non-physician practitioners who have reassigned their billing rights, depending on the relationship status between the physician and patient.

In the office or other outpatient setting where an evaluation is performed, physicians and qualified nonphysician practitioners shall use the CPT codes (99201 – 99215) depending on the complexity of the visit and whether the patient is a new or established patient to that physician. All physicians and qualified nonphysician practitioners shall follow the E/M documentation guidelines for all E/M services. These rules are applicable for Medicare secondary payer claims as well as for claims in which Medicare is the primary payer.

100-4, 12, 30.6.11

Emergency Department Visits (Codes 99281 - 99288)

A. Use of Emergency Department Codes by Physicians Not Assigned to Emergency Department

Any physician seeing a patient registered in the emergency department may use emergency department visit codes (for services matching the code description). It is not required that the physician be assigned to the emergency department.

B. Use of Emergency Department Codes In Office

Emergency department coding is not appropriate if the site of service is an office or outpatient setting or any sight of service other than an emergency department. The emergency department codes should only be used if the patient is seen in the emergency department and the services described by the HCPCS code definition are provided. The emergency department is defined as an organized hospital-based facility for the provision of unscheduled or episodic services to patients who present for immediate medical attention.

C. Use of Emergency Department Codes to Bill Nonemergency Services

Services in the emergency department may not be emergencies. However the codes (99281 - 99288) are payable if the described services are provided.

However, if the physician asks the patient to meet him or her in the emergency department as an alternative to the physician's office and the patient is not registered as a patient in the emergency department, the physician should bill the appropriate office/outpatient visit codes. Normally a lower level emergency department code would be reported for a nonemergency condition.

D. Emergency Department or Office/Outpatient Visits on Same Day As Nursing Facility Admission

Emergency department visit provided on the same day as a comprehensive nursing facility assessment are not paid. Payment for evaluation and management services on the same date provided in sites other than the nursing facility are included in the payment for initial nursing facility care when performed on the same date as the nursing facility admission.

E. Physician Billing for Emergency Department Services Provided to Patient by Both Patient's Personal Physician and Emergency Department Physician

If a physician advises his/her own patient to go to an emergency department (ED) of a hospital for care and the physician subsequently is asked by the ED physician to come to the hospital to evaluate the patient and to advise the ED physician as to whether the patient should be admitted to the hospital or be sent home, the physicians should bill as follows:

If the patient is admitted to the hospital by the patient's personal physician, then the patient's regular physician should bill only the appropriate level of the initial hospital care (codes 99221 - 99223) because all evaluation and management services provided by that physician in conjunction with that admission are considered part of the initial hospital care when performed on the same date as the admission. The ED physician who saw the patient in the emergency department should bill the appropriate level of the ED codes.

If the ED physician, based on the advice of the patient's personal physician who came to the emergency department to see the patient, sends the patient home, then the ED physician should bill the appropriate level of emergency department service. The patient's personal physician should also bill the level of emergency department code that describes the service he or she provided in the emergency department. If the patient's personal physician does not come to the hospital to see the patient, but only advises the emergency department physician by telephone, then the patient's personal physician may not bill.

F. Emergency Department Physician Requests Another Physician to See the Patient in Emergency Department or Office/Outpatient Setting

If the emergency department physician requests that another physician evaluate a given patient, the other physician should bill an emergency department visit code. If the patient is admitted to the hospital by the second physician performing the evaluation, he or she should bill an initial hospital care code and not an emergency department visit code.

100-4, 12, 30.6.13

Nursing Facility Services

A. Visits to Perform the Initial Comprehensive Assessment and Annual Assessments

The distinction made between the delegation of physician visits and tasks in a skilled nursing facility (SNF) and in a nursing facility (NF) is based on the Medicare Statute. Section 1819 (b) (6) (A) of the Social Security Act (the Act) governs SNFs while section 1919 (b) (6) (A) of the Act governs NFs. For further information refer to Medlearn Matters article number SE0418 at www.cms.hhs.gov/medlearn/matters.

The federally mandated visits in a SNF and NF must be performed by the physician except as otherwise permitted (42 CFR 483.40 (c) (4) and (f)). The principal physician of record must append the modifier "-AI", (Principal Physician of Record), to the initial nursing facility care code. This modifier will identify the physician who oversees the patient's care from other physicians who may be furnishing specialty care. All other physicians or qualified NPPs who perform an initial evaluation in the NF or SNF may bill the initial nursing facility care code. The initial federally mandated visit is defined in S&C-04-08 (see www.cms.hhs.gov/medlearn/matters) as the initial comprehensive visit during which the physician completes a thorough assessment, develops a plan of care, and writes or verifies admitting orders for the nursing facility resident. For Survey and Certification requirements, a visit must occur no later than 30 days after admission.

Further, per the Long Term Care regulations at 42 CFR 483.40 (c) (4) and (e) (2), in a SNF the physician may not delegate a task that the physician must personally perform. Therefore, as stated in S&C-04-08 the physician may not delegate the initial federally mandated comprehensive visit in a SNF.

The only exception, as to who performs the initial visit, relates to the NF setting. In the NF setting, a qualified NPP (i.e., a nurse practitioner (NP), physician assistant (PA), or a clinical nurse specialist (CNS)), who is not employed by the facility, may perform the initial visit when the State law permits. The evaluation and management (E/M) visit shall be within the State scope of practice and licensure requirements where the E/M visit is performed and the requirements for physician collaboration and physician supervision shall be met.

Under Medicare Part B payment policy, other medically necessary E/M visits may be performed prior to and after the initial visit, if the medical needs of the patient require an E/M visit. A qualified NPP may perform medically necessary E/M visits prior to and after the initial visit if all the requirements for collaboration, general physician supervision, licensure, and billing are met.

The CPT Nursing Facility Services codes shall be used with place of service (POS) 31 (SNF) if the patient is in a Part A SNF stay. They shall be used with POS 32 (nursing facility) if the patient does not have Part A SNF benefits or if the patient is in a NF or in a non-covered SNF stay (e.g., there was no preceding 3-day hospital stay). The CPT Nursing Facility code definition also includes POS 54 (Intermediate Care Facility/Mentally Retarded) and POS 56 (Psychiatric Residential Treatment Center). For further guidance on POS codes and associated CPT codes refer to §30.6.14.

Effective January 1, 2006, the Initial Nursing Facility Care codes 99301– 99303 are deleted.

Beginning January 1, 2006, the new CPT codes, Initial Nursing Facility Care, per day, (99304 – 99306) shall be used to report the initial federally mandated visit. Only a physician may report these codes for an initial federally mandated visit performed in a SNF or NF (with the exception of the qualified NPP in the NF setting who is not employed by the facility and when State law permits, as explained above).

A readmission to a SNF or NF shall have the same payment policy requirements as an initial admission in both the SNF and NF settings.

A physician who is employed by the SNF/NF may perform the E/M visits and bill independently to Medicare Part B for payment. An NPP who is employed by the SNF or NF may perform and bill Medicare Part B directly for those services where it is permitted as discussed above. The employer of the PA shall always report the visits performed by the PA. A physician, NP or CNS has the option to bill Medicare directly or to reassign payment for his/her professional service to the facility.

As with all E/M visits for Medicare Part B payment policy, the E/M documentation guidelines apply.

Medically Necessary Visits

Qualified NPPs may perform medically necessary E/M visits prior to and after the physician's initial federally mandated visit in both the SNF and NF. Medically necessary E/M visits for the diagnosis or treatment of an illness or injury or to improve the functioning of a malformed body member are payable under the physician fee schedule under Medicare Part B. A physician or NPP may bill the most appropriate initial nursing facility care code (CPT codes 99304-99306) or subsequent nursing facility care code (CPT codes 99307-99310), even if the E/M service is provided prior to the initial federally mandated visit.

SNF Setting--Place of Service Code 31

Following the initial federally mandated visit by the physician, the physician may delegate alternate federally mandated physician visits to a qualified NPP who meets collaboration and physician supervision requirements and is licensed as such by the State and performing within the scope of practice in that State.

NF Setting--Place of Service Code 32

Per the regulations at 42 CFR 483.40 (f), a qualified NPP, who meets the collaboration and physician supervision requirements, the State scope of practice and licensure requirements, and who is not employed by the NF, may at the option of the State, perform the initial federally mandated visit in a NF, and may perform any other federally mandated physician visit in a NF in addition to performing other medically necessary E/M visits.

Questions pertaining to writing orders or certification and recertification issues in the SNF and NF settings shall be addressed to the appropriate State Survey and Certification Agency departments for clarification.

B. Visits to Comply With Federal Regulations (42 CFR 483.40 (c) (1)) in the SNF and NF

Payment is made under the physician fee schedule by Medicare Part B for federally mandated visits. Following the initial federally mandated visit by the physician or qualified NPP where permitted, payment shall be made for federally mandated visits that monitor and evaluate residents at least once every 30 days for the first 90 days after admission and at least once every 60 days thereafter.

Effective January 1, 2006, the Subsequent Nursing Facility Care, per day, codes 99311– 99313 are deleted.

Beginning January 1, 2006, the new CPT codes, Subsequent Nursing Facility Care, per day, (99307 – 99310) shall be used to report federally mandated physician E/M visits and medically necessary E/M visits.

Carriers shall not pay for more than one E/M visit performed by the physician or qualified NPP for the same patient on the same date of service. The Nursing Facility Services codes represent a "per day" service.

The federally mandated E/M visit may serve also as a medically necessary E/M visit if the situation arises (i.e., the patient has health problems that need attention on the day the scheduled mandated physician E/M visit occurs). The physician/qualified NPP shall bill only one E/M visit.

Beginning January 1, 2006, the new CPT code, Other Nursing Facility Service (99318), may be used to report an annual nursing facility assessment visit on the required schedule of visits on an annual basis. For Medicare Part B payment policy, an annual nursing facility assessment visit code may substitute as meeting one of the federally mandated physician visits if the code requirements for CPT code 99318 are fully met and in lieu of reporting a Subsequent Nursing Facility Care, per day, service (codes 99307 – 99310). It shall not be performed in addition to the required number of federally mandated physician visits. The new CPT annual assessment code does not represent a new benefit service for Medicare Part B physician services.

Qualified NPPs, whether employed or not by the SNF, may perform alternating federally mandated physician visits, at the option of the physician, after the initial federally mandated visit by the physician in a SNF.

Qualified NPPs in the NF setting, who are not employed by the NF and who are working in collaboration with a physician, may perform federally mandated physician visits, at the option of the State.

Medicare Part B payment policy does not pay for additional E/M visits that may be required by State law for a facility admission or for other additional visits to satisfy facility or other administrative purposes. E/M visits, prior to and after the initial federally mandated physician visit, that are reasonable and medically necessary to meet the medical needs of the individual patient (unrelated to any State requirement or administrative purpose) are payable under Medicare Part B.

C. Visits by Qualified Nonphysician Practitioners

All E/M visits shall be within the State scope of practice and licensure requirements where the visit is performed and all the requirements for physician collaboration and physician supervision shall be met when performed and reported by qualified NPPs. General physician supervision and employer billing requirements shall be met for PA services in addition to the PA meeting the State scope of practice and licensure requirements where the E/M visit is performed.

Medically Necessary Visits

Qualified NPPs may perform medically necessary E/M visits prior to and after the physician's initial visit in both the SNF and NF. Medically necessary E/M visits for the diagnosis or treatment of an illness or injury or to improve the functioning of a malformed body member are payable under the physician fee schedule under Medicare Part B. A physician or NPP may bill the most appropriate initial nursing facility care code (CPT codes 99304-99306) or subsequent nursing facility care code (CPT codes 99307-99310), even if the E/M service is provided prior to the initial federally mandated visit.

SNF Setting--Place of Service Code 31

Following the initial federally mandated visit by the physician, the physician may delegate alternate federally mandated physician visits to a qualified NPP who meets collaboration and physician supervision requirements and is licensed as such by the State and performing within the scope of practice in that State.

NF Setting--Place of Service Code 32

Per the regulations at 42 CFR 483.40 (f), a qualified NPP, who meets the collaboration and physician supervision requirements, the State scope of practice and licensure requirements, and who is not employed by the NF, may at the option of the State, perform the initial federally mandated visit in a NF, and may perform any other federally mandated physician visit in a NF in addition to performing other medically necessary E/M visits.

Questions pertaining to writing orders or certification and recertification issues in the SNF and NF settings shall be addressed to the appropriate State Survey and Certification Agency departments for clarification.

D. Medically Complex Care

Payment is made for E/M visits to patients in a SNF who are receiving services for medically complex care upon discharge from an acute care facility when the visits are reasonable and medically necessary and documented in the medical record. Physicians and qualified NPPs shall report initial nursing facility care codes for their first visit with the patient. The principal physician of record must append the modifier "-AI" (Principal Physician of Record), to the initial nursing facility care code when billed to identify the physician who oversees the patient's care from other physicians who may be furnishing specialty care. Follow-up visits shall be billed as subsequent nursing facility care visits.

E. Incident to Services

Where a physician establishes an office in a SNF/NF, the "incident to" services and requirements are confined to this discrete part of the facility designated as his/her office. "Incident to" E/M visits, provided in a facility setting, are not payable under the Physician Fee Schedule for Medicare Part B. Thus, visits performed outside the designated "office" area in the SNF/NF would be subject to the coverage and payment rules applicable to the SNF/NF setting and shall not be reported using the CPT codes for office or other outpatient visits or use place of service code 11.

F. Use of the Prolonged Services Codes and Other Time-Related Services

Beginning January 1, 2008, typical/average time units for E/M visits in the SNF/NF settings are reestablished. Medically necessary prolonged services for E/M visits (codes 99356 and 99357) in a SNF or NF may be billed with the Nursing Facility Services in the code ranges (99304 – 99306, 99307 – 99310 and 99318).

Counseling and Coordination of Care Visits

With the reestablishment of typical/average time units, medically necessary E/M visits for counseling and coordination of care, for Nursing Facility Services in the code ranges (99304 – 99306, 99307 – 99310 and 99318) that are time-based services, may be billed with the appropriate prolonged services codes (99356 and 99357).

G. Multiple Visits

The complexity level of an E/M visit and the CPT code billed must be a covered and medically necessary visit for each patient (refer to §§1862 (a)(1)(A) of the Act). Claims for an unreasonable number of daily E/M visits by the same physician to multiple patients at a facility within a 24-hour period may result in medical review to

determine medical necessity for the visits. The E/M visit (Nursing Facility Services) represents a "per day" service per patient as defined by the CPT code. The medical record must be personally documented by the physician or qualified NPP who performed the E/M visit and the documentation shall support the specific level of E/M visit to each individual patient.

H. Split/Shared E/M Visit

A split/shared E/M visit cannot be reported in the SNF/NF setting. A split/shared E/M visit is defined by Medicare Part B payment policy as a medically necessary encounter with a patient where the physician and a qualified NPP each personally perform a substantive portion of an E/M visit face-to-face with the same patient on the same date of service. A substantive portion of an E/M visit involves all or some portion of the history, exam or medical decision making key components of an E/M service. The physician and the qualified NPP must be in the same group practice or be employed by the same employer. The split/shared E/M visit applies only to selected E/M visits and settings (i.e., hospital inpatient, hospital outpatient, hospital observation, emergency department, hospital discharge, office and non facility clinic visits, and prolonged visits associated with these E/M visit codes). The split/shared E/M policy does not apply to critical care services or procedures.

I. SNF/NF Discharge Day Management Service

Medicare Part B payment policy requires a face-to-face visit with the patient provided by the physician or the qualified NPP to meet the SNF/NF discharge day management service as defined by the CPT code. The E/M discharge day management visit shall be reported for the date of the actual visit by the physician or qualified NPP even if the patient is discharged from the facility on a different calendar date. The CPT codes 99315 – 99316 shall be reported for this visit. The Discharge Day Management Service may be reported using CPT code 99315 or 99316, depending on the code requirement, for a patient who has expired, but only if the physician or qualified NPP personally performed the death pronouncement.

100-4, 12, 30.6.14

Home Care and Domiciliary Care Visits (Codes 99324- 99350)

Physician Visits to Patients Residing in Various Places of Service

The American Medical Association's Current Procedural Terminology (CPT) 2006 new patient codes 99324 - 99328 and established patient codes 99334 - 99337(new codes beginning January 2006), for Domiciliary, Rest Home (e.g., Boarding Home), or Custodial Care Services, are used to report evaluation and management (E/M) services to residents residing in a facility which provides room, board, and other personal assistance services, generally on a long-term basis. These CPT codes are used to report E/M services in facilities assigned places of service (POS) codes 13 (Assisted Living Facility), 14 (Group Home), 33 (Custodial Care Facility) and 55 (Residential Substance Abuse Facility). Assisted living facilities may also be known as adult living facilities.

Physicians and qualified nonphysician practitioners (NPPs) furnishing E/M services to residents in a living arrangement described by one of the POS listed above must use the level of service code in the CPT code range 99324 - 99337 to report the service they provide. The CPT codes 99321 - 99333 for Domiciliary, Rest Home (e.g., Boarding Home), or Custodial Care Services are deleted beginning January, 2006.

Beginning in 2006, reasonable and medically necessary, face-to-face, prolonged services, represented by CPT codes 99354 - 99355, may be reported with the appropriate companion E/M codes when a physician or qualified NPP, provides a prolonged service involving direct (face-to-face) patient contact that is beyond the usual E/M visit service for a Domiciliary, Rest Home (e.g., Boarding Home) or Custodial Care Service. All the requirements for prolonged services at Sec.30.6.15.1 must be met.

The CPT codes 99341 through 99350, Home Services codes, are used to report E/M services furnished to a patient residing in his or her own private residence (e.g., private home, apartment, town home) and not residing in any type of congregate/shared facility living arrangement including assisted living facilities and group homes. The Home Services codes apply only to the specific 2-digit POS 12 (Home). Home Services codes may not be used for billing E/M services provided in settings other than in the private residence of an individual as described above.

Beginning in 2006, E/M services provided to patients residing in a Skilled Nursing Facility (SNF) or a Nursing Facility (NF) must be reported using the appropriate CPT level of service code within the range identified for Initial Nursing Facility Care (new CPT codes 99304 - 99306) and Subsequent Nursing Facility Care (new CPT codes 99307 - 99310). Use the CPT code, Other Nursing Facility Services (new CPT code 99318), for an annual nursing facility assessment. Use CPT codes 99315 - 99316 for SNF/NF discharge services. The CPT codes 99301 - 99303 and 99311 - 99313 are deleted beginning January, 2006. The Home Services codes should not be used for these places of service.

The CPT SNF/NF code definition includes intermediate care facilities (ICFs) and long term care facilities (LTCFs). These codes are limited to the specific 2-digit POS 31 (SNF), 32 (Nursing Facility), 54 (Intermediate Care Facility/Mentally Retarded) and 56 (Psychiatric Residential Treatment Center).

The CPT nursing facility codes should be used with POS 31 (SNF) if the patient is in a Part A SNF stay and POS 32 (nursing facility) if the patient does not have Part A SNF benefits. There is no longer a different payment amount for a Part A or Part B benefit period in these POS settings.

100-4, 12, 30.6.14.1

Home Services (Codes 99341 - 99350)

B3-15515, B3-15066

A. Requirement for Physician Presence

Home services codes 99341-99350 are paid when they are billed to report evaluation and management services provided in a private residence. A home visit cannot be billed by a physician unless the physician was actually present in the beneficiary's home.

B. Homebound Status

Under the home health benefit the beneficiary must be confined to the home for services to be covered. For home services provided by a physician using these codes, the beneficiary does not need to be confined to the home. The medical record must document the medical necessity of the home visit made in lieu of an office or outpatient visit.

C. Fee Schedule Payment for Services to Homebound

Patients under General Supervision Payment may be made in some medically underserved areas where there is a lack of medical personnel and home health services for injections, EKGs, and venipunctures that are performed for homebound patients under general physician supervision by nurses and paramedical employees of physicians or physician-directed clinics. Section 10 provides additional information on the provision of services to homebound Medicare patients.

100-4, 12, 30.6.15.1

Prolonged Services With Direct Face-to-Face Patient Contact Service (Codes 99354 - 99357) (ZZZ codes)

A. Definition

Prolonged physician services (CPT code 99354) in the office or other outpatient setting with direct face-to-face patient contact which require 1 hour beyond the usual service are payable when billed on the same day by the same physician or qualified nonphysician practitioner (NPP) as the companion evaluation and management codes. The time for usual service refers to the typical/average time units associated with the companion evaluation and management service as noted in the CPT code. Each additional 30 minutes of direct face-to-face patient contact following the first hour of prolonged services may be reported by CPT code 99355.

Prolonged physician services (code 99356) in the inpatient setting, with direct face-to-face patient contact which require 1 hour beyond the usual service are payable when they are billed on the same day by the same physician or qualified NPP as the companion evaluation and management codes. Each additional 30 minutes of direct face-to-face patient contact following the first hour of prolonged services may be reported by CPT code 99357.

Prolonged service of less than 30 minutes total duration on a given date is not separately reported because the work involved is included in the total work of the evaluation and management codes.

Code 99355 or 99357 may be used to report each additional 30 minutes beyond the first hour of prolonged services, based on the place of service. These codes may be used to report the final 15 – 30 minutes of prolonged service on a given date, if not otherwise billed. Prolonged service of less than 15 minutes beyond the first hour or less than 15 minutes beyond the final 30 minutes is not reported separately.

B. Required Companion Codes

- The companion evaluation and management codes for 99354 are the Office or Other Outpatient visit codes (99201 - 99205, 99212 – 99215), the Domiciliary, Rest Home, or Custodial Care Services codes (99324 – 99328, 99334 – 99337), the Home Services codes (99341 - 99345, 99347 – 99350);

- The companion codes for 99355 are 99354 and one of the evaluation and management codes required for 99354 to be used;

- The companion evaluation and management codes for 99356 are the Initial Hospital Care codes and Subsequent Hospital Care codes (99221 - 99223, 99231 – 99233); Nursing Facility Services codes (99304 -99318); or

- The companion codes for 99357 are 99356 and one of the evaluation and management codes required for 99356 to be used.

Prolonged services codes 99354 – 99357 are not paid unless they are accompanied by the companion codes as indicated.

C. Requirement for Physician Presence

Physicians may count only the duration of direct face-to-face contact between the physician and the patient (whether the service was continuous or not) beyond the typical/average time of the visit code billed to determine whether prolonged services can be billed and to determine the prolonged services codes that are allowable. In the case of prolonged office services, time spent by office staff with the patient, or time the patient remains unaccompanied in the office cannot be billed. In the case of prolonged hospital services, time spent reviewing charts or discussion of a patient with house medical staff and not with direct face-to-face contact with the patient, or waiting for test results, for changes in the patient's condition, for end of a therapy, or for use of facilities cannot be billed as prolonged services.

D. Documentation

Documentation is not required to accompany the bill for prolonged services unless the physician has been selected for medical review. Documentation is required in the medical record about the duration and content of the medically necessary evaluation and management service and prolonged services billed. The medical record must be appropriately and sufficiently documented by the physician or qualified NPP to show that the physician or qualified NPP personally furnished the direct face-to-face time with the patient specified in the CPT code definitions. The start and end times of the visit shall be documented in the medical record along with the date of service.

E. Use of the Codes

Prolonged services codes can be billed only if the total duration of the physician or qualified NPP direct face-to-face service (including the visit) equals or exceeds the threshold time for the evaluation and management service the physician or qualified NPP provided (typical/average time associated with the CPT E/M code plus 30 minutes). If the total duration of direct face-to-face time does not equal or exceed the threshold time for the level of evaluation and management service the physician or qualified NPP provided, the physician or qualified NPP may not bill for prolonged services.

F. Threshold Times for Codes 99354 and 99355 (Office or Other Outpatient Setting)

If the total direct face-to-face time equals or exceeds the threshold time for code 99354, but is less than the threshold time for code 99355, the physician should bill the evaluation and management visit code and code 99354. No more than one unit of 99354 is acceptable. If the total direct face-to-face time equals or exceeds the threshold time for code 99355 by no more than 29 minutes, the physician should bill the visit code 99354 and one unit of code 99355. One additional unit of code 99355 is billed for each additional increment of 30 minutes extended duration. Contractors use the following threshold times to determine if the prolonged services codes 99354 and/or 99355 can be billed with the office or other outpatient settings including domiciliary, rest home, or custodial care services and home services codes.

Threshold Time for Prolonged Visit Codes 99354 and/or 99355 Billed with Office/Outpatient Code

Code	Typical Time for Code	Threshold Time to Bill Code 99354	Threshold Time to Bill Codes 99354 and 99355
99201	10	40	85
99202	20	50	95
99203	30	60	105
99204	45	75	120
99205	60	90	135
99212	10	40	85
99213	15	45	90
99214	25	55	100
99215	40	70	115
99324	20	50	95
99325	30	60	105
99326	45	75	120
99327	60	90	135
99328	75	105	150
99334	15	45	90
99335	25	55	100
99336	40	70	115
99337	60	90	135
99341	20	50	95
99342	30	60	105
99343	45	75	120
99344	60	90	135
99345	75	105	150
99347	15	45	90
99348	25	55	100
99349	40	70	115
99350	60	90	135

G. Threshold Times for Codes 99356 and 99357

(Inpatient Setting) If the total direct face-to-face time equals or exceeds the threshold time for code 99356, but is less than the threshold time for code 99357, the physician should bill the visit and code 99356. Contractors do not accept more than one unit of code 99356. If the total direct face-to-face time equals or exceeds the threshold time for code 99356 by no more than 29 minutes, the physician bills the visit code 99356 and one unit of code 99357. One additional unit of code 99357 is billed for each additional increment of 30 minutes extended duration. Contractors use the following threshold times to determine if the prolonged services codes 99356 and/or 99357 can be billed with the inpatient setting codes.

Threshold Time for Prolonged Visit Codes 99356 and/or 99357 Billed with Inpatient Setting Codes Code

Code	Typical Time for Code	Threshold Time to Bill Code 99356	Threshold Time to Bill Codes 99356 and 99357
99221	30	60	105
99222	50	80	125
99223	70	100	145
99231	15	45	90
99232	25	55	100
99233	35	65	110
99304	25	55	100
99305	35	65	110
99306	45	75	120
99307	10	40	85
99308	15	45	90
99309	25	55	100
99310	35	65	110
99318	30	60	10

Add 30 minutes to the threshold time for billing codes 99356 and 99357 to get the threshold time for billing code 99356 and two units of 99357.

H. Prolonged Services Associated With Evaluation and Management Services Based on Counseling and/or Coordination of Care (Time-Based)

When an evaluation and management service is dominated by counseling and/or coordination of care (the counseling and/or coordination of care represents more than 50% of the total time with the patient) in a face-to-face encounter between the physician or qualified NPP and the patient in the office/clinic or the floor time (in the scenario of an inpatient service), then the evaluation and management code is selected based on the typical/average time associated with the code levels. The time approximation must meet or exceed the specific CPT code billed (determined by the typical/average time associated with the evaluation and management code) and should not be "rounded" to the next higher level.

In those evaluation and management services in which the code level is selected based on time, prolonged services may only be reported with the highest code level in that family of codes as the companion code.

I. Examples of Billable Prolonged Services

EXAMPLE 1

A physician performed a visit that met the definition of an office visit code 99213 and the total duration of the direct face-to-face services (including the visit) was 65 minutes. The physician bills code 99213 and one unit of code 99354.

EXAMPLE 2

A physician performed a visit that met the definition of a domiciliary, rest home care visit code 99327 and the total duration of the direct face-to-face contact (including the visit) was 140 minutes. The physician bills codes 99327, 99354, and one unit of code 99355.

EXAMPLE 3

A physician performed an office visit to an established patient that was predominantly counseling, spending 75 minutes (direct face-to-face) with the patient. The physician should report CPT code 99215 and one unit of code 99354.

J. Examples of Nonbillable Prolonged Services

EXAMPLE 1

A physician performed a visit that met the definition of visit code 99212 and the total duration of the direct face-to-face contact (including the visit) was 35 minutes. The physician cannot bill prolonged services because the total duration of direct face-to-face service did not meet the threshold time for billing prolonged services.

EXAMPLE 2

A physician performed a visit that met the definition of code 99213 and, while the patient was in the office receiving treatment for 4 hours, the total duration of the direct face-to-face service of the physician was 40 minutes. The physician cannot bill prolonged services because the total duration of direct face-to-face service did not meet the threshold time for billing prolonged services.

EXAMPLE 3

A physician provided a subsequent office visit that was predominantly counseling, spending 60 minutes (face-to-face) with the patient. The physician cannot code 99214, which has a typical time of 25 minutes, and one unit of code 99354. The physician must bill the highest level code in the code family (99215 which has 40 minutes typical/average time units associated with it). The additional time spent beyond this code is 20 minutes and does not meet the threshold time for billing prolonged services.

100-4, 12, 30.6.15.2

Prolonged Services Without Face to Face Service (Codes 99358 - 99359)

Contractors may not pay prolonged services codes 99358 and 99359, which do not require any direct patient face-to-face contact (e.g., telephone calls). Payment for these services is included in the payment for direct face-to-face services that

physicians bill. The physician cannot bill the patient for these services since they are Medicare covered services and payment is included in the payment for other billable services.

100-4, 12, 30.6.15.3

Physician Standby Service (Code 99360)

Standby services are not payable to physicians. Physicians may not bill Medicare or beneficiaries for standby services. Payment for standby services is included in the Part A payment to the facility. Such services are a part of hospital costs to provide quality care.

If hospitals pay physicians for standby services, such services are part of hospital costs to provide quality care.

100-4, 12, 30.6.16

Case Management Services (Codes 99362 and 99371 - 99373)

A. Team Conferences

Team conferences (codes 99361-99362) may not be paid separately. Payment for these services is included in the payment for the services to which they relate.

B. Telephone Calls

Telephone calls (codes 99371-99373) may not be paid separately. Payment for telephone calls is included in payment for billable services (e.g., visit, surgery, diagnostic procedure results).

100-4, 12, 40.3

Claims Review for Global Surgeries

A. Relationship to Correct Coding Initiative (CCI)

The CCI policy and computer edits allow A/B MACs (B) to detect instances of fragmented billing for certain intra-operative services and other services furnished on the same day as the surgery that are considered to be components of the surgical procedure and, therefore, included in the global surgical fee. When both correct coding and global surgery edits apply to the same claim, A/B MACs (B) first apply the correct coding edits, then, apply the global surgery edits to the correctly coded services.

B. Prepayment Edits to Detect Separate Billing of Services Included in the Global Package

In addition to the correct coding edits, A/B MACs (B) must be capable of detecting certain other services included in the payment for a major or minor surgery or for an endoscopy. On a prepayment basis, A/B MACs (B) identify the services that meet the following conditions:

- Preoperative services that are submitted on the same claim or on a subsequent claim as a surgical procedure; or

- Same day or postoperative services that are submitted on the same claim or on a subsequent claim as a surgical procedure or endoscopy;

  and -

- Services that were furnished within the prescribed global period of the surgical procedure;

- Services that are billed without modifier "-78," "-79," "-24," "25," or "-57" or are billed with modifier "-24" but without the required documentation; and

- Services that are billed with the same provider or group number as the surgical procedure or endoscopy. Also, edit for any visits billed separately during the postoperative period without modifier "-24" by a physician who billed for the postoperative care only with modifier "-55."

A/B MACs (B) use the following evaluation and management codes in establishing edits for visits included in the global package. CPT codes 99241, 99242, 99243, 99244, 99245, 99251, 99252, 99253, 99254, 99255, 99271, 99272, 99273, 99274, and 99275 have been transferred from the excluded category and are now included in the global surgery edits.

Evaluation and Management Codes for A/B MAC (B) Edits

92012	92014	99211	99212	99213	99214	99215
99217	99218	99219	99220	99221	99222	99223
99231	99232	99233	99234	99235	99236	99238
99239	99241	99242	99243	99244	99245	99251
99252	99253	99254	99255	99261	99262	99263
99271	99272	99273	99274	99275	99291	99292
99301	99302	99303	99311	99312	99313	99315
99316	99331	99332	99333	99347	99348	99349
99350	99374	99375	99377	99378		

NOTE: In order for codes 99291 or 99292 to be paid for services furnished during the preoperative or postoperative period, modifier "-25" or "-24," respectively, must be used to indicate that the critical care was unrelated to the specific anatomic injury or general surgical procedure performed.

If a surgeon is admitting a patient to a nursing facility for a condition not related to the global surgical procedure, the physician should bill for the nursing facility admission and care with a "-24" modifier and appropriate documentation. If a surgeon is admitting a patient to a nursing facility and the patient's admission to that facility relates to the global surgical procedure, the nursing facility admission and any services related to the global surgical procedure are included in the global surgery fee.

C. Exclusions from Prepayment Edits

A/B MACs (B) exclude the following services from the prepayment audit process and allow separate payment if all usual requirements are met:

- Services listed in §40.1.B; and
- Services billed with the modifier "-25," "-57," "-58," "-78," or "-79."

Exceptions

See §§40.2.A.8, 40.2.A.9, and 40.4.A for instances where prepayment review is required for modifier "-25." In addition, prepayment review is necessary for CPT codes 90935, 90937, 90945, and 90947 when a visit and modifier "-25" are billed with these services.

Exclude the following codes from the prepayment edits required in §40.3.B.

92002	92004	99201	99202	99203	99204	99205
99281	99282	99283	99284	99285	99321	99322
99323	99341	99342	99343	99344	99345	

100-4, 12, 40.7

Claims for Bilateral Surgeries

B3-4827, B3-15040

A. General

Bilateral surgeries are procedures performed on both sides of the body during the same operative session or on the same day.

The terminology for some procedure codes includes the terms "bilateral" (e.g., code 27395; Lengthening of the hamstring tendon; multiple, bilateral.) or "unilateral or bilateral" (e.g., code 52290; cystourethroscopy; with ureteral meatotomy, unilateral or bilateral). The payment adjustment rules for bilateral surgeries do not apply to procedures identified by CPT as "bilateral" or "unilateral or bilateral" since the fee schedule reflects any additional work required for bilateral surgeries.

Field 22 of the MFSDB indicates whether the payment adjustment rules apply to a surgical procedure.

B. Billing Instructions for Bilateral Surgeries

If a procedure is not identified by its terminology as a bilateral procedure (or unilateral or bilateral), physicians must report the procedure with modifier "-50." They report such procedures as a single line item. (NOTE: This differs from the CPT coding guidelines which indicate that bilateral procedures should be billed as two line items.)

If a procedure is identified by the terminology as bilateral (or unilateral or bilateral), as in codes 27395 and 52290, physicians do not report the procedure with modifier "-50."

C. Claims Processing System Requirements

Carriers must be able to:

1. Identify bilateral surgeries by the presence on the claim form or electronic submission of the "-50" modifier or of the same code on separate lines reported once with modifier "-LT" and once with modifier "-RT";

2. Access Field 34 or 35 of the MFSDB to determine the Medicare payment amount;

3. Access Field 22 of the MFSDB:

   — If Field 22 contains an indicator of "0," "2," or "3," the payment adjustment rules for bilateral surgeries do not apply. Base payment on the lower of the billed amount or 100 percent of the fee schedule amount (Field 34 or 35) unless other payment adjustment rules apply.

   NOTE: Some codes which have a bilateral indicator of "0" in the MFSDB may be performed more than once on a given day. These are services that would never be considered bilateral and thus should not be billed with modifier "-50." Where such a code is billed on multiple line tems or with more than 1 in the units field and carriers have determined that the code may be reported more than once, bypass the "0" bilateral indicator and refer to the multiple surgery field for pricing;

   — If Field 22 contains an indicator of "1," the standard adjustment rules apply. Base payment on the lower of the billed amount or 150 percent of the fee schedule amount (Field 34 or 35). (Multiply the payment amount in Field 34 or 35 for the surgery by 150 percent and round to the nearest cent.)

4. Apply the requirements 40 - 40.4 on global surgeries to bilateral surgeries; and

5. Retain the "-50" modifier in history for any bilateral surgeries paid at the adjusted amount.

   (NOTE: The "-50" modifier is not retained for surgeries which are bilateral by definition such as code 27395.)

100-4, 12, 40.8

Claims for Co-Surgeons and Team Surgeons

B3-4828, B3-15046

A. General

Under some circumstances, the individual skills of two or more surgeons are required to perform surgery on the same patient during the same operative session. This may be required because of the complex nature of the procedure(s) and/or the patient's condition.

In these cases, the additional physicians are not acting as assistants-at-surgery.

B. Billing Instructions

The following billing procedures apply when billing for a surgical procedure or procedures that required the use of two surgeons or a team of surgeons:

- If two surgeons (each in a different specialty) are required to perform a specific procedure, each surgeon bills for the procedure with a modifier "-62. " Co-surgery also refers to surgical procedures involving two surgeons performing the parts of the procedure simultaneously, i.e., heart transplant or bilateral knee replacements. Documentation of the medical necessity for two surgeons is required for certain services identified in the MFSDB. (See 40.8.C.5.);

- If a team of surgeons (more than 2 surgeons of different specialties) is required to perform a specific procedure, each surgeon bills for the procedure with a modifier "-66." Field 25 of the MFSDB identifies certain services submitted with a "-66" modifier which must be sufficiently documented to establish that a team was medically necessary. All claims for team surgeons must contain sufficient information to allow pricing "by report."

- If surgeons of different specialties are each performing a different procedure (with specific CPT codes), neither co-surgery nor multiple surgery rules apply (even if the procedures are performed through the same incision). If one of the surgeons performs multiple procedures, the multiple procedure rules apply to that surgeon's services. (See 40.6 for multiple surgery payment rules.)

For co-surgeons (modifier 62), the fee schedule amount applicable to the payment for each co-surgeon is 62.5 percent of the global surgery fee schedule amount. Team surgery (modifier 66) is paid for on a "By Report" basis.

C. Claims Processing System Requirements

Carriers must be able to:

1. Identify a surgical procedure performed by two surgeons or a team of surgeons by the presence on the claim form or electronic submission of the "-62" or "-66" modifier;

2. Access Field 34 or 35 of the MFSDB to determine the fee schedule payment amount for the surgery;

3. Access Field 24 or 25, as appropriate, of the MFSDB. These fields provide guidance on whether two or team surgeons are generally required for the surgical procedure;

4. If the surgery is billed with a "-62" or "-66" modifier and Field 24 or 25 contains an indicator of "0," payment adjustment rules for two or team surgeons do not apply:

   — Carriers pay the first bill submitted, and base payment on the lower of the billed amount or 100 percent of the fee schedule amount (Field 34 or 35) unless other payment adjustment rules apply;

   — Carriers deny bills received subsequently from other physicians and use the appropriate MSN message in 40.8.D. As these are medical necessity denials, the instructions in the Program Integrity Manual regarding denial of unassigned claims for medical necessity are applied;

5. If the surgery is billed with a "-62" modifier and Field 24 contains an indicator of "1," suspend the claim for manual review of any documentation submitted with the claim. If the documentation supports the need for co-surgeons, base payment for each physician on the lower of the billed amount or 62.5 percent of the fee schedule amount (Field 34 or 35);

6. If the surgery is billed with a "-62" modifier and Field 24 contains an indicator of "2," payment rules for two surgeons apply. Carriers base payment for each physician on the lower of the billed amount or 62.5 percent of the fee schedule amount (Field 34 or 35);

7. If the surgery is billed with a "-66" modifier and Field 25 contains an indicator of "1," carriers suspend the claim for manual review. If carriers determine that team surgeons were medically necessary, each physician is paid on a "by report" basis;

8. If the surgery is billed with a "-66" modifier and Field 25 contains an indicator of "2," carriers pay "by report";

   NOTE: A Medicare fee may have been established for some surgical procedures that are billed with the "-66" modifier. In these cases, all physicians on the team must agree on the percentage of the Medicare payment amount each is to receive.

   If carriers receive a bill with a "-66" modifier after carriers have paid one surgeon the full Medicare payment amount (on a bill without the modifier), deny the subsequent claim.

9. Apply the rules global surgical packages to each of the physicians participating in a co- or team surgery; and

10. Retain the "-62" and "-66" modifiers in history for any co- or team surgeries.

D. Beneficiary Liability on Denied Claims for Assistant, Co- surgeon and Team Surgeons

MSN message 23.10 which states "Medicare does not pay for a surgical assistant for this kind of surgery," was established for denial of claims for assistant surgeons. Where such payment is denied because the procedure is subject to the statutory restriction against payment for assistants-at-surgery. Carriers include the following statement in the MSN:

"You cannot be charged for this service." (Unnumbered add-on message.)

Carriers use Group Code CO on the remittance advice to the physician to signify that the beneficiary may not be billed for the denied service and that the physician could be subject to penalties if a bill is issued to the beneficiary.

If Field 23 of the MFSDB contains an indicator of "0" or "1" (assistant-at-surgery may not be paid) for procedures CMS has determined that an assistant surgeon is not generally medically necessary.

For those procedures with an indicator of "0," the limitation on liability provisions described in Chapter 30 apply to assigned claims. Therefore, carriers include the appropriate limitation of liability language from Chapter 21. For unassigned claims, apply the rules in the Program Integrity Manual concerning denial for medical necessity.

Where payment may not be made for a co- or team surgeon, use the following MSN message (MSN message number 15.13):

Medicare does not pay for team surgeons for this procedure.

Where payment may not be made for a two surgeons, use the following MSN message (MSN message number 15.12):

Medicare does not pay for two surgeons for this procedure.

Also see limitation of liability remittance notice REF remark codes M25, M26, and M27.

Use the following message on the remittance notice:

Multiple physicians/assistants are not covered in this case. (Reason code 54.)

100-4, 12, 100

Teaching Physician Services

Definitions

For purposes of this section, the following definitions apply.

Resident -An individual who participates in an approved graduate medical education (GME) program or a physician who is not in an approved GME program but who is authorized to practice only in a hospital setting. The term includes interns and fellows in GME programs recognized as approved for purposes of direct GME payments made by the FI. Receiving a staff or faculty appointment or participating in a fellowship does not by itself alter the status of "resident". Additionally, this status remains unaffected regardless of whether a hospital includes the physician in its full time equivalency count of residents.

Student- An individual who participates in an accredited educational program (e.g., a medical school) that is not an approved GME program. A student is never considered to be an intern or a resident. Medicare does not pay for any service furnished by a student. See 100.1.1B for a discussion concerning E/M service documentation performed by students.

Teaching Physician -A physician (other than another resident) who involves residents in the care of his or her patients.

Direct Medical and Surgical Services -Services to individual beneficiaries that are either personally furnished by a physician or furnished by a resident under the supervision of a physician in a teaching hospital making the reasonable cost election for physician services furnished in teaching hospitals. All payments for such services are made by the FI for the hospital.

Teaching Hospital -A hospital engaged in an approved GME residency program in medicine, osteopathy, dentistry, or podiatry.

Teaching Setting -Any provider, hospital-based provider, or nonprovider setting in which Medicare payment for the services of residents is made by the FI under the direct graduate medical education payment methodology or freestanding SNF or HHA in which such payments are made on a reasonable cost basis.

Critical or Key Portion- That part (or parts) of a service that the teaching physician determines is (are) a critical or key portion(s). For purposes of this section, these terms are interchangeable.

Documentation- Notes recorded in the patient's medical records by a resident, and/or teaching physician or others as outlined in the specific situations below regarding the service furnished. Documentation may be dictated and typed or hand-written, or computer-generated and typed or handwritten. Documentation must be dated and include a legible signature or identity. Pursuant to 42 CFR 415.172 (b), documentation must identify, at a minimum, the service furnished, the participation of the teaching physician in providing the service, and whether the teaching physician was physically present. In the context of an electronic medical record, the term 'macro' means a command in a computer or dictation application that automatically generates predetermined text that is not edited by the user.

When using an electronic medical record, it is acceptable for the teaching physician to use a macro as the required personal documentation if the teaching physician adds it personally in a secured (password protected) system. In addition to the

teaching physician's macro, either the resident or the teaching physician must provide customized information that is sufficient to support a medical necessity determination. The note in the electronic medical record must sufficiently describe the specific services furnished to the specific patient on the specific date. It is insufficient documentation if both the resident and the teaching physician use macros only.

Physically Present- The teaching physician is located in the same room (or partitioned or curtained area, if the room is subdivided to accommodate multiple patients) as the patient and/or performs a face-to-face service.

100-4, 12, 100.1.1

Evaluation and Management (E/M) Services

A. General Documentation Instructions and Common Scenarios

Evaluation and Management (E/M) Services -- For a given encounter, the selection of the appropriate level of E/M service should be determined according to the code definitions in the American Medical Association's Current Procedural Terminology (CPT) and any applicable documentation guidelines.

For purposes of payment, E/M services billed by teaching physicians require that they personally document at least the following:

- That they performed the service or were physically present during the key or critical portions of the service when performed by the resident; and
- The participation of the teaching physician in the management of the patient.

When assigning codes to services billed by teaching physicians, reviewers will combine the documentation of both the resident and the teaching physician.

Documentation by the resident of the presence and participation of the teaching physician is not sufficient to establish the presence and participation of the teaching physician.

On medical review, the combined entries into the medical record by the teaching physician and the resident constitute the documentation for the service and together must support the medical necessity of the service.

Following are four common scenarios for teaching physicians providing E/M services:

Scenario 1:

The teaching physician personally performs all the required elements of an E/M service without a resident. In this scenario the resident may or may not have performed the E/M service independently.

In the absence of a note by a resident, the teaching physician must document as he/she would document an E/M service in a nonteaching setting.

Where a resident has written notes, the teaching physician's note may reference the resident's note. The teaching physician must document that he/she performed the critical or key portion(s) of the service, and that he/she was directly involved in the management of the patient. For payment, the composite of the teaching physician's entry and the resident's entry together must support the medical necessity of the billed service and the level of the service billed by the teaching physician.

Scenario 2:

The resident performs the elements required for an E/M service in the presence of, or jointly with, the teaching physician and the resident documents the service. In this case, the teaching physician must document that he/she was present during the performance of the critical or key portion(s) of the service and that he/she was directly involved in the management of the patient. The teaching physician's note should reference the resident's note. For payment, the composite of the teaching physician's entry and the resident's entry together must support the medical necessity and the level of the service billed by the teaching physician.

Scenario 3:

The resident performs some or all of the required elements of the service in the absence of the teaching physician and documents his/her service. The teaching physician independently performs the critical or key portion(s) of the service with or without the resident present and, as appropriate, discusses the case with the resident. In this instance, the teaching physician must document that he/she personally saw the patient, personally performed critical or key portions of the service, and participated in the management of the patient. The teaching physician's note should reference the resident's note. For payment, the composite of the teaching physician's entry and the resident's entry together must support the medical necessity of the billed service and the level of the service billed by the teaching physician.

Scenario 4:

When a medical resident admits a patient to a hospital late at night and the teaching physician does not see the patient until later, including the next calendar day:

- The teaching physician must document that he/she personally saw the patient and participated in the management of the patient. The teaching physician may reference the resident's note in lieu of re-documenting the history of present illness, exam, medical decision-making, review of systems and/or past family/social history provided that the patient's condition has not changed, and the teaching physician agrees with the resident's note.
- The teaching physician's note must reflect changes in the patient's condition and clinical course that require that the resident's note be amended with further information to address the patient's condition and course at the time the patient is seen personally by the teaching physician.

- The teaching physician's bill must reflect the date of service he/she saw the patient and his/her personal work of obtaining a history, performing a physical, and participating in medical decision-making regardless of whether the combination of the teaching physician's and resident's documentation satisfies criteria for a higher level of service. For payment, the composite of the teaching physician's entry and the resident's entry together must support the medical necessity of the billed service and the level of the service billed by the teaching physician.

Following are examples of minimally acceptable documentation for each of these scenarios:

Scenario 1:

Admitting Note: "I performed a history and physical examination of the patient and discussed his management with the resident. I reviewed the resident's note and agree with the documented findings and plan of care."

Follow-up Visit: "Hospital Day #3. I saw and evaluated the patient. I agree with the findings and the plan of care as documented in the resident's note."

Follow-up Visit: "Hospital Day #5. I saw and examined the patient. I agree with the resident's note except the heart murmur is louder, so I will obtain an echo to evaluate."

(NOTE: In this scenario if there are no resident notes, the teaching physician must document as he/she would document an E/M service in a non-teaching setting.)

Scenario 2:

Initial or Follow-up Visit: "I was present with the resident during the history and exam. I discussed the case with the resident and agree with the findings and plan as documented in the resident's note."

Follow-up Visit: "I saw the patient with the resident and agree with the resident's findings and plan."

Scenarios 3 and 4:

Initial Visit: "I saw and evaluated the patient. I reviewed the resident's note and agree, except that picture is more consistent with pericarditis than myocardial ischemia. Will begin NSAIDs."

Initial or Follow-up Visit: "I saw and evaluated the patient. Discussed with resident and agree with resident's findings and plan as documented in the resident's note."

Follow-up Visit: "See resident's note for details. I saw and evaluated the patient and agree with the resident's finding and plans as written."

Follow-up Visit: "I saw and evaluated the patient. Agree with resident's note but lower extremities are weaker, now 3/5; MRI of L/S Spine today."

Following are examples of unacceptable documentation:

- "Agree with above." followed by legible countersignature or identity;
- "Rounded, Reviewed, Agree." followed by legible countersignature or identity;
- "Discussed with resident. Agree." followed by legible countersignature or identity;

- "Seen and agree." followed by legible countersignature or identity;
- "Patient seen and evaluated." followed by legible countersignature or identity; and
- A legible countersignature or identity alone.

Such documentation is not acceptable, because the documentation does not make it possible to determine whether the teaching physician was present, evaluated the patient, and/or had any involvement with the plan of care.

B. E/M Service Documentation Provided By Students

Any contribution and participation of a student to the performance of a billable service (other than the review of systems and/or past family/social history which are not separately billable, but are taken as part of an E/M service) must be performed in the physical presence of a teaching physician or physical presence of a resident in a service meeting the requirements set forth in this section for teaching physician billing.

Students may document services in the medical record. However, the documentation of an E/M service by a student that may be referred to by the teaching physician is limited to documentation related to the review of systems and/or past family/social history. The teaching physician may not refer to a student's documentation of physical exam findings or medical decision making in his or her personal note. If the medical student documents E/M services, the teaching physician must verify and redocument the history of present illness as well as perform and redocument the physical exam and medical decision making activities of the service.

C. Exception for E/M Services Furnished in Certain Primary Care Centers

Teaching physicians providing E/M services with a GME program granted a primary care exception may bill Medicare for lower and mid-level E/M services provided by residents. For the E/M codes listed below, teaching physicians may submit claims for services furnished by residents in the absence of a teaching physician:

New Patient	Established Patient
99201	99211
99202	99212
99203	99213

Effective January 1, 2005, the following code is included under the primary care exception: HCPCS code G0402 (Initial preventive physical examination; face-to-face visit services limited to new beneficiary during the first 12 months of Medicare enrollment).

Effective January 1, 2011, the following codes are included under the primary care exception: HCPCS codes G0438 (Annual wellness visit, including personal preventive plan service, first visit) and G0439 (Annual wellness visit, including personal preventive plan service, subsequent visit).

If a service other than those listed above needs to be furnished, then the general teaching physician policy set forth in §100.1 applies. For this exception to apply, a center must attest in writing that all the following conditions are met for a particular residency program. Prior approval is not necessary, but centers exercising the primary care exception must maintain records demonstrating that they qualify for the exception.

The services must be furnished in a center located in the outpatient department of a hospital or another ambulatory care entity in which the time spent by residents in patient care activities is included in determining direct GME payments to a teaching hospital by the hospital's FI. This requirement is not met when the resident is assigned to a physician's office away from the center or makes home visits. In the case of a nonhospital entity, verify with the FI that the entity meets the requirements of a written agreement between the hospital and the entity set forth at 42 CFR 413.78(e)(3)(ii).

Under this exception, residents providing the billable patient care service without the physical presence of a teaching physician must have completed at least 6 months of a GME approved residency program. Centers must maintain information under the provisions at 42 CFR 413.79(a)(6).

Teaching physicians submitting claims under this exception may not supervise more than four residents at any given time and must direct the care from such proximity as to constitute immediate availability. Teaching physicians may include residents with less than 6 months in a GME approved residency program in the mix of four residents under the teaching physician's supervision. However, the teaching physician must be physically present for the critical or key portions of services furnished by the residents with less than 6 months in a GME approved residency program. That is, the primary care exception does not apply in the case of residents with less than 6 months in a GME approved residency program.

Teaching physicians submitting claims under this exception must:

- Not have other responsibilities (including the supervision of other personnel) at the time the service was provided by the resident;
- Have the primary medical responsibility for patients cared for by the residents;
- Ensure that the care provided was reasonable and necessary;
- Review the care provided by the resident during or immediately after each visit. This must include a review of the patient's medical history, the resident's findings on physical examination, the patient's diagnosis, and treatment plan (i.e., record of tests and therapies); and
- Document the extent of his/her own participation in the review and direction of the services furnished to each patient.

Patients under this exception should consider the center to be their primary location for health care services. The residents must be expected to generally provide care to the same group of established patients during their residency training. The types of services furnished by residents under this exception include:

- Acute care for undifferentiated problems or chronic care for ongoing conditions including chronic mental illness;
- Coordination of care furnished by other physicians and providers; and,
- Comprehensive care not limited by organ system or diagnosis.

Residency programs most likely qualifying for this exception include family practice, general internal medicine, geriatric medicine, pediatrics, and obstetrics/gynecology.

Certain GME programs in psychiatry may qualify in special situations such as when the program furnishes comprehensive care for chronically mentally ill patients. These would be centers in which the range of services the residents are trained to furnish, and actually do furnish, include comprehensive medical care as well as psychiatric care. For example, antibiotics are being prescribed as well as psychotropic drugs.

100-4, 12, 140.1

Qualified Nonphysician Anesthetists

For payment purposes, qualified nonphysician anesthetists include both CRNAs and AAs. Thus, the term qualified nonphysician anesthetist will be used to refer to both CRNAs and AAs unless it is necessary to separately discuss these provider groups.

An AA is a person who:

- Is permitted by State law to administer anesthesia; and who
- Has successfully completed a six-year program for AAs of which two years consist of specialized academic and clinical training in anesthesia.

In contrast, a CRNA is a registered nurse who is licensed by the State in which the nurse practices and who:

- Is currently certified by the Council on Certification of Nurse Anesthetists or the Council on Recertification of Nurse Anesthetists, or
- Has graduated within the past 18 months from a nurse anesthesia program that meets the standards of the Council of Accreditation of Nurse Anesthesia Educational Programs and is awaiting initial certification.

100-4, 12, 140.3

Anesthesia Fee Schedule Payment for Qualified Nonphysician Anesthetists

Pay for the services of a qualified nonphysician anesthetist only on an assignment basis. The assignment agreed to by the qualified nonphysician anesthetist is binding upon any other person or entity claiming payment for the service. Except for deductible and coinsurance amounts, any person who knowingly and willfully presents or causes to be presented to a Medicare beneficiary a bill or request for payment for services of a qualified nonphysician anesthetist for which payment may be made on an assignment-related basis is subject to civil monetary penalties.

Services furnished by qualified nonphysician anesthetists are subject to the Part B deductible and coinsurance. If the Part B deductible has been satisfied, the fee schedule for anesthesia services prior to January 1, 1996, is the least of 80 percent of:

- The actual charge;
- The applicable CRNA conversion factor multiplied by the sum of allowable base and time units; or
- The applicable locality participating anesthesiologist's conversion factor multiplied by the sum of allowable base and time units.

For services furnished on or after January 1, 1996, the fee schedule for anesthesia services furnished by qualified nonphysician anesthetists is the least of 80 percent of:

- The actual charge;
- The applicable locality anesthesia conversion factor multiplied by the sum of allowable base and time units.

100-4, 12, 140.3.3

Billing Modifiers

The following modifiers are used when billing for anesthesia services:

- QX - Qualified nonphysician anesthetist with medical direction by a physician.
- QZ - CRNA without medical direction by a physician.
- QS - Monitored anesthesiology care services (can be billed by a qualified nonphysician anesthetist or a physician).
- QY - Medical direction of one qualified nonphysician anesthetist by an anesthesiologist. This modifier is effective for anesthesia services furnished by a qualified nonphysician anesthetist on or after January 1, 1998.

100-4, 12, 140.3.4

General Billing Instructions

Claims for reimbursement for qualified nonphysician anesthetist services should be completed in accord with existing billing instructions for anesthesiologists with the following additions.

- If an employer-physician furnishes concurrent medical direction for a procedure involving CRNAs and the medical direction service is unassigned, the physician should bill on an assigned basis on a separate claim for the qualified nonphysician anesthetist service. If the physician is participating or takes assignment, both services should be billed on one claim but as separate line items.
- All claims forms must have the provider billing number of the CRNA, AA and/or the employer of the qualified nonphysician anesthetist performing the service in either block 24.H of the Form CMS-1500 and/or block 31 as applicable. Verify that the billing number is valid before making payment.

Payments should be calculated in accordance with Medicare payment rules in §140.3. Contractors must institute all necessary payment edits to assure that duplicate payments are not made to physicians for CRNA or AA services or to a CRNA or AA directly for bills submitted on their behalf by qualified billers.

CRNAs are identified on the provider file by specialty code 43. AAs are identified on the provider file by specialty code 32.

100-4, 12, 140.4.1

An Anesthesiologist and Qualified Nonphysician Anesthetist Work Together

Contractors will distribute educational releases and use other established means to ensure that anesthesiologists understand the requirements for medical direction of qualified nonphysician anesthetists.

Contractors will perform reviews of payments for anesthesiology services to identify situations in which an excessive number of concurrent anesthesiology services may have been performed. They will use peer practice and their experience in developing review criteria. They will also periodically review a sample of claims for medical direction of four or fewer concurrent anesthesia procedures. During this process physicians may be requested to submit documentation of the names of procedures performed and the names of the anesthetists directed.

Physicians who cannot supply the necessary documentation for the sample claims must submit documentation with all subsequent claims before payment will be made.

100-4, 12, 140.4.2

Qualified Nonphysician Anesthetist and an Anesthesiologist in a Single Anesthesia Procedure

Where a single anesthesia procedure involves both a physician medical direction service and the service of the medically directed qualified nonphysician anesthetist, and the service is furnished on or after January 1, 1998, the payment amount for the service of each is 50 percent of the allowance otherwise recognized had the service been furnished by the anesthesiologist alone. The modifier to be used for current procedure identification is QX.

Beginning on or after January 1, 1998, where the qualified nonphysician anesthetist and the anesthesiologist are involved in a single anesthesia case, and the physician is performing medical direction, the service is billed in accordance with the following procedures:

- For the single medically directed service, the physician will use the modifier "QY" (MEDICAL DIRECTION OF ONE QUALIFIED NONPHYSICIAN ANESTHETIST BY AN ANESTHESIOLOGIST). This modifier is effective for claims for dates of service on or after January 1, 1998, and
- For the anesthesia service furnished by the medically directed qualified nonphysician anesthetist, the qualified nonphysician anesthetist will use the current modifier "QX."

In unusual circumstances when it is medically necessary for both the CRNA and the anesthesiologist to be completely and fully involved during a procedure, full payment for the services of each provider is allowed. The physician would report using the "AA" modifier and the CRNA would use "QZ," or the modifier for a nonmedically directed case.

Documentation must be submitted by each provider to support payment of the full fee.

100-4, 12, 140.4.3

Payment for Medical or Surgical Services Furnished by CRNAs

Payment shall be made for reasonable and necessary medical or surgical services furnished by CRNAs if they are legally authorized to perform these services in the state in which services are furnished. Payment is determined under the physician fee schedule on the basis of the national physician fee schedule conversion factor, the geographic adjustment factor, and the resource-based relative value units for the medical or surgical service.

100-4, 12, 140.4.4

Conversion Factors for Anesthesia Services of Qualified Nonphysician Anesthetists Furnished on or After January 1, 1992

Conversion factors used to determine fee schedule payments for anesthesia services furnished by qualified nonphysician anesthetists on or after January 1, 1992, are determined based on a statutory methodology.

For example, for anesthesia services furnished by a medically directed qualified nonphysician anesthetist in 1994, the medically directed allowance is 60 percent of the allowance that would be recognized for the anesthesia service if the physician personally performed the service without an assistant, i.e., alone. For subsequent years, the medically directed allowance is the following percent of the personally performed allowance.

Services furnished in 1995	57.5 percent
Services furnished in 1996	55.0 percent
Services furnished in 1997	52.5 percent
Services furnished in 1998 and after	50.0 percent

100-4, 12, 160

Independent Psychologist Services

B3-2150, B3-2070.2 See the Medicare Benefit Policy Manual, Chapter 15, for coverage requirements.

There are a number of types of psychologists. Educational psychologists engage in identifying and treating education-related issues. In contrast, counseling psychologists provide services that include a broader realm including phobias, familial issues, etc.

Psychometrists are psychologists who have been trained to administer and interpret tests.

However, clinical psychologists are defined as a provider of diagnostic and therapeutic services. Because of the differences in services provided, services provided by psychologists who do not provide clinical services are subject to different billing guidelines. One service often provided by nonclinical psychologist is diagnostic testing.

NOTE: Diagnostic psychological testing services performed by persons who meet these requirements are covered as other diagnostic tests. When, however, the psychologist is not practicing independently, but is on the staff of an institution, agency, or clinic, that entity bills for the diagnostic services.

Expenses for such testing are not subject to the payment limitation on treatment for mental, psychoneurotic, and personality disorders. Independent psychologists are not required by law to accept assignment when performing psychological tests. However, regardless of whether the psychologist accepts assignment, he or she must report on the claim form the name and address of the physician who ordered the test.

100-4, 12, 160.1

Payment

Diagnostic testing services are not subject to the outpatient mental health limitation. Refer to §210, below, for a discussion of the outpatient mental health limitation. The diagnostic testing services performed by a psychologist (who is not a clinical psychologist) practicing independently of an institution, agency, or physician's office are covered as other diagnostic tests if a physician orders such testing. Medicare covers this type of testing as an outpatient service if furnished by any psychologist who is licensed or certified to practice psychology in the State or jurisdiction where he or she is furnishing services or, if the jurisdiction does not issue licenses, if provided by any practicing psychologist. (It is CMS' understanding that all States, the District of Columbia, and Puerto Rico license psychologists, but that some trust territories do not. Examples of psychologists, other than clinical psychologists, whose services are covered under this provision include, but are not limited to, educational psychologists and counseling psychologists.)

To determine whether the diagnostic psychological testing services of a particular independent psychologist are covered under Part B in States which have statutory licensure or certification, carriers must secure from the appropriate State agency a current listing of psychologists holding the required credentials. In States or territories which lack statutory licensing and certification, carriers must check individual qualifications as claims are submitted. Possible reference sources are the national directory of membership of the American Psychological Association, which provides data about the educational background of individuals and indicates which members are board-certified, and records and directories of the State or territorial psychological association. If qualification is dependent on a doctoral degree from a currently accredited program, carriers must verify the date of accreditation of the school involved, since such accreditation is not retroactive. If the reference sources listed above do not provide enough information (e.g., the psychologist is not a member of the association), carriers must contact the psychologist personally for the required information. Carriers may wish to maintain a continuing list of psychologists whose qualifications have been verified.

Medicare excludes expenses for diagnostic testing from the payment limitation on treatment for mental/psychoneurotic/personality disorders.

Carriers must identify the independent psychologist's choice whether or not to accept assignment when performing psychological tests.

Carriers must accept an independent psychologist claim only if the psychologist reports the name/UPIN of the physician who ordered a test.

Carriers pay nonparticipating independent psychologists at 95 percent of the physician fee schedule allowed amount.

Carriers pay participating independent psychologists at 100 percent of the physician fee schedule allowed amount. Independent psychologists are identified on the provider file by specialty code 62 and provider type 35.

100-4, 12, 170

Clinical Psychologist Services

B3-2150 See Medicare Benefit Policy Manual, Chapter 15, for general coverage requirements.

Direct payment may be made under Part B for professional services. However, services furnished incident to the professional services of CPs to hospital patients remain bundled.

Therefore, payment must continue to be made to the hospital (by the FI) for such "incident to" services.

100-4, 12, 180

Care Plan Oversight Services

The Medicare Benefit Policy Manual, Chapter 15, contains requirements for coverage for medical and other health services including those of physicians and non-physician practitioners.

Care plan oversight (CPO) is the physician supervision of a patient receiving complex and/or multidisciplinary care as part of Medicare-covered services provided by a participating home health agency or Medicare approved hospice.

CPO services require complex or multidisciplinary care modalities involving:

- Regular physician development and/or revision of care plans;
- Review of subsequent reports of patient status;
- Review of related laboratory and other studies;
- Communication with other health professionals not employed in the same practice who are involved in the patient's care;
- Integration of new information into the medical treatment plan; and/or
- Adjustment of medical therapy.

The CPO services require recurrent physician supervision of a patient involving 30 or more minutes of the physician's time per month. Services not countable toward the

30 minutes threshold that must be provided in order to bill for CPO include, but are not limited to:

- Time associated with discussions with the patient, his or her family or friends to adjust medication or treatment;
- Time spent by staff getting or filing charts;
- Travel time; and/or Physician's time spent telephoning prescriptions into the pharmacist unless the telephone conversation involves discussions of pharmaceutical therapies.

Implicit in the concept of CPO is the expectation that the physician has coordinated an aspect of the patient's care with the home health agency or hospice during the month for which CPO services were billed. The physician who bills for CPO must be the same physician who signs the plan of care.

Nurse practitioners, physician assistants, and clinical nurse specialists, practicing within the scope of State law, may bill for care plan oversight. These non-physician practitioners must have been providing ongoing care for the beneficiary through evaluation and management services. These non-physician practitioners may not bill for CPO if they have been involved only with the delivery of the Medicare-covered home health or hospice service.

A. Home Health CPO

Non-physician practitioners can perform CPO only if the physician signing the plan of care provides regular ongoing care under the same plan of care as does the NPP billing for CPO and either:

- The physician and NPP are part of the same group practice; or
- If the NPP is a nurse practitioner or clinical nurse specialist, the physician signing the plan of care also has a collaborative agreement with the NPP; or
- If the NPP is a physician assistant, the physician signing the plan of care is also the physician who provides general supervision of physician assistant services for the practice.

Billing may be made for care plan oversight services furnished by an NPP when:

- The NPP providing the care plan oversight has seen and examined the patient;
- The NPP providing care plan oversight is not functioning as a consultant whose participation is limited to a single medical condition rather than multidisciplinary coordination of care; and
- The NPP providing care plan oversight integrates his or her care with that of the physician who signed the plan of care.

NPPs may not certify the beneficiary for home health care.

B. Hospice CPO

The attending physician or nurse practitioner (who has been designated as the attending physician) may bill for hospice CPO when they are acting as an "attending physician".

An "attending physician" is one who has been identified by the individual, at the time he/she elects hospice coverage, as having the most significant role in the determination and delivery of their medical care. They are not employed nor paid by the hospice. The care plan oversight services are billed using Form CMS-1500 or electronic equivalent.

For additional information on hospice CPO, see Chapter 11, 40.1.3.1 of this manual.

100-4, 12, 180.1

Care Plan Oversight Billing Requirements

A. Codes for Which Separate Payment May Be Made

Effective January 1, 1995, separate payment may be made for CPO oversight services for 30 minutes or more if the requirements specified in the Medicare Benefits Policy Manual, Chapter 15 are met.

Providers billing for CPO must submit the claim with no other services billed on that claim and may bill only after the end of the month in which the CPO services were rendered. CPO services may not be billed across calendar months and should be submitted (and paid) only for one unit of service.

Physicians may bill and be paid separately for CPO services only if all the criteria in the Medicare Benefit Policy Manual, Chapter 15 are met.

B. Physician Certification and Recertification of Home Health Plans of Care

Effective 2001, two new HCPCS codes for the certification and recertification and development of plans of care for Medicare-covered home health services were created.

See the Medicare General Information, Eligibility, and Entitlement Manual, Pub. 100-1, Chapter 4, "Physician Certification and Recertification of Services," 10-60, and the Medicare Benefit Policy Manual, Pub. 100-2, Chapter 7, "Home Health Services", 30.

The home health agency certification code can be billed only when the patient has not received Medicare-covered home health services for at least 60 days. The home health agency recertification code is used after a patient has received services for at least 60 days (or one certification period) when the physician signs the certification after the initial certification period. The home health agency recertification code will be reported only once every 60 days, except in the rare situation when the patient starts a new episode before 60 days elapses and requires a new plan of care to start a new episode.

C. Provider Number of Home Health Agency (HHA) or Hospice

For claims for CPO submitted on or after January 1, 1997, physicians must enter on the Medicare claim form the 6-character Medicare provider number of the HHA or hospice providing Medicare-covered services to the beneficiary for the period during which CPO services was furnished and for which the physician signed the plan of care. Physicians are responsible for obtaining the HHA or hospice Medicare provider numbers.

Additionally, physicians should provide their UPIN to the HHA or hospice furnishing services to their patient.

NOTE: There is currently no place on the HIPAA standard ASC X12N 837 professional format to specifically include the HHA or hospice provider number required for a care plan oversight claim. For this reason, the requirement to include the HHA or hospice provider number on a care plan oversight claim is temporarily waived until a new version of this electronic standard format is adopted under HIPAA and includes a place to provide the HHA and hospice provider numbers for care plan oversight claims.

100-4, 12, 190.3

List of Medicare Telehealth Services

The use of a telecommunications system may substitute for an in-person encounter for professional consultations, office visits, office psychiatry services, and a limited number of other physician fee schedule (PFS) services. The various services and corresponding current procedure terminology (CPT) or Healthcare Common Procedure Coding System (HCPCS) codes are listed below.

- Consultations (CPT codes 99241 - 99275) - Effective October 1, 2001 – December 31, 2005;

- Consultations (CPT codes 99241 - 99255) - Effective January 1, 2006 – December 31, 2005;

- Telehealth consultations, emergency department or initial inpatient (HCPCS codes G0425 – G0427) - Effective January 1, 2010;

- Follow-up inpatient telehealth consultations (HCPCS codes G0406, G0407, and G0408) - Effective January 1, 2009;

- Office or other outpatient visits (CPT codes 99201 - 99215);

- Subsequent hospital care services, with the limitation of one telehealth visit every 3 days (CPT codes 99231, 99232, and 99233) – Effective January 1, 2011;

- Subsequent nursing facility care services, with the limitation of one telehealth visit every 30 days (CPT codes 99307, 99308, 99309, and 99310) – Effective January 1, 2011;

- Pharmacologic management (CPT code 90862) – Effective March 1, 2003 – December 31, 2012; – Effective March 1, 2003 – December 31, 2012; (HCPCS code G0459) – Effective January 1, 2013;

- Individual psychotherapy (CPT codes 90804 - 90809); Psychiatric diagnostic interview examination (CPT code 90801) – Effective March 1, 2003 – December 31, 2012;

- Individual psychotherapy (CPT codes 90832 – 90834, 90836 – 90838); Psychiatric diagnostic interview examination (CPT codes 90791 -- 90792) – Effective January 1, 2013.

- Neurobehavioral status exam (CPT code 96116) - Effective January 1, 2008;

- End Stage Renal Disease (ESRD) related services (HCPCS codes G0308, G0309, G0311, G0312, G0314, G0315, G0317, and G0318) – Effective January 1, 2005 – December 31, 2008;

- End Stage Renal Disease (ESRD) related services (CPT codes 90951, 90952, 90954, 90955, 90957, 90958, 90960, and 90961) – Effective January 1, 2009;

- Individual and group medical nutrition therapy (HCPCS codes G0270, 97802, 97803, and 97804) – Individual effective January 1, 2006; group effective January 1, 2011;

- Individual and group health and behavior assessment and intervention (CPT codes 96150 – 96154) – Individual effective January 1, 2010; group effective January 1, 2011.

- Individual and group kidney disease education (KDE) services (HCPCS codes G0420 and G0421) – Effective January 1, 2011; and

- Individual and group diabetes self-management training (DSMT) services, with a minimum of 1 hour of in-person instruction to be furnished in the initial year training period to ensure effective injection training (HCPCS codes G0108 and G0109) - Effective January 1, 2011.

- Smoking Cessation Services (CPT codes 99406 and 99407and HCPCS codes G0436 and G0437) – Effective January 1, 2012.

- Alcohol and/or substance (other than tobacco) abuse structured assessment and intervention services (HCPCS codes G0396 and G0397) – Effective January 1, 2013.

- Annual alcohol misuse screening (HCPCS code G0442) – Effective January 1, 2013.

- Brief face-to-face behavioral counseling for alcohol misuse (HCPCS code G0443) – Effective January 1, 2013.

- Annual Depression Screening (HCPCS code G0444) – Effective January 1, 2013.

- High-intensity behavioral counseling to prevent sexually transmitted infections (HCPCS code G0445) – Effective January 1, 2013.

- Annual, face-to-face Intensive behavioral therapy for cardiovascular disease (HCPCS code G0446) – Effective January 1, 2013.

- Face-to-face behavioral counseling for obesity (HCPCS code G0447) – Effective January 1, 2013.

- Transitional Care Management Services (CPT codes 99495 -99496) – Effective January 1, 2014.

NOTE: Beginning January 1, 2010, CMS eliminated the use of all consultation codes, except for inpatient telehealth consultation G-codes. CMS no longer recognizes office/outpatient or inpatient consultation CPT codes for payment of office/outpatient or inpatient visits. Instead, physicians and practitioners are instructed to bill a new or established patient office/outpatient visit CPT code or appropriate hospital or nursing facility care code, as appropriate to the particular patient, for all office/outpatient or inpatient visits.

100-4, 12, 190.7

Contractor Editing of Telehealth Claims

Medicare telehealth services (as listed in section 190.3) are billed with either the "GT" or "GQ" modifier. The contractor shall approve covered telehealth services if the physician or practitioner is licensed under State law to provide the service. Contractors must familiarize themselves with licensure provisions of States for which they process claims and disallow telehealth services furnished by physicians or practitioners who are not authorized to furnish the applicable telehealth service under State law. For example, if a nurse practitioner is not licensed to provide individual psychotherapy under State law, he or she would not be permitted to receive payment for individual psychotherapy under Medicare. The contractor shall install edits to ensure that only properly licensed physicians and practitioners are paid for covered telehealth services.

If a contractor receives claims for professional telehealth services coded with the "GQ" modifier (representing "via asynchronous telecommunications system"), it shall approve/pay for these services only if the physician or practitioner is affiliated with a Federal telemedicine demonstration conducted in Alaska or Hawaii. The contractor may require the physician or practitioner at the distant site to document his or her participation in a Federal telemedicine demonstration program conducted in Alaska or Hawaii prior to paying for telehealth services provided via asynchronous, store and forward technologies.

If a contractor denies telehealth services because the physician or practitioner may not bill for them, the contractor uses MSN message 21.18: "This item or service is not covered when performed or ordered by this practitioner." The contractor uses remittance advice message 52 when denying the claim based upon MSN message 21.18.

If a service is billed with one of the telehealth modifiers and the procedure code is not designated as a covered telehealth service, the contractor denies the service using MSN message 9.4: "This item or service was denied because information required to make payment was incorrect." The remittance advice message depends on what is incorrect, e.g., B18 if procedure code or modifier is incorrect, 125 for submission billing errors, 4-12 for difference inconsistencies. The contractor uses B18 as the explanation for the denial of the claim.

The only claims from institutional facilities that FIs shall pay for telehealth services at the distant site, except for MNT services, are for physician or practitioner services when the distant site is located in a CAH that has elected Method II, and the physician or practitioner has reassigned his/her benefits to the CAH. The CAH bills its regular FI for the professional services provided at the distant site via a telecommunications system, in any of the revenue codes 096x, 097x or 098x. All requirements for billing distant site telehealth services apply.

Claims from hospitals or CAHs for MNT services are submitted to the hospital's or CAH's regular FI. Payment is based on the non-facility amount on the Medicare Physician Fee Schedule for the particular HCPCS codes.

100-4, 12, 230

Primary Care Incentive Payment Program (PCIP)

Section 5501(a) of the Affordable Care Act revises Section 1833 of the Social Security Act (the Act) by adding a new paragraph, (x), "Incentive Payments for Primary Care Services." Section 1833(x) of the Act states that in the case of primary care services furnished on or after January 1, 2011, and before January 1, 2016, there shall be a 10 percent incentive payment for such services under Part B when furnished by a primary care practitioner.

Information regarding Primary Care Incentive Payment Program (PCIP) payments made to critical access hospitals (CAHs) paid under the optional method can be found in Pub. 100-4, Chapter 4, §250.12 of this manual.

100-4, 12, 230.1

Definition of Primary Care Practitioners and Primary Care Services

Primary care practitioners are defined as:

1. A physician who has a primary specialty designation of family medicine, internal medicine, geriatric medicine, or pediatric medicine for whom primary care

services accounted for at least 60 percent of the allowed charges under Part B for the practitioner in a prior period as determined appropriate by the Secretary; or

2. A nurse practitioner, clinical nurse specialist, or physician assistant for whom primary care services accounted for at least 60 percent of the allowed charges under Part B for the practitioner in a prior period as determined appropriate by the Secretary.

Primary care services are defined as HCPCS Codes:

1. 99201 through 99215 for new and established patient office or outpatient evaluation and management (E/M) visits;

2. 99304 through 99340 for initial, subsequent, discharge, and other nursing facility E/M services; new and established patient domiciliary, rest home or custodial care E/M services; and domiciliary, rest home or home care plan oversight services; and

3. 99341 through 99350 for new and established patient home E/M visits.

Practitioner Identification

Eligible practitioners will be identified on claims by the National Provider Identifier (NPI) number of the rendering practitioner. If the claim is submitted by a practitioner's group practice, the rendering practitioner's NPI must be included on the line-item for the primary care service and reflect an eligible HCPCS as identified. In order to be eligible for the PCIP, physician assistants, clinical nurse specialists, and nurse practitioners must be billing for their services under their own NPI and not furnishing services incident to physicians' services. Regardless of the specialty area in which they may be practicing, the specific nonphysician practitioners are eligible for the PCIP based on their profession and historical percentage of allowed charges as primary care services that equals or exceeds the 60 percent threshold.

Beginning in calendar year (CY) 2011, primary care practitioners will be identified based on their primary specialty of enrollment in Medicare and percentage of allowed charges for primary care services that equals or exceeds the 60 percent threshold from Medicare claims data 2 years prior to the bonus payment year.

Eligible practitioners for PCIP payments in a given calendar year (CY) will be listed by eligible NPI in the Primary Care Incentive Payment Program Eligibility File, available after January 31, of the payment year on their Medicare contractor's website. Practitioners should contact their contractor with any questions regarding their eligibility for the PCIP.

100-4, 12, 230.2

Coordination with Other Payments

Section 5501(a)(3) of the Affordable Care Act provides payment under the PCIP as an additional payment amount for specified primary care services without regard to any additional payment for the service under Section 1833(m) of the Act. Therefore, an eligible primary care physician furnishing a primary care service in a health professional shortage area (HPSA) may receive both a HPSA physician bonus payment (as described in the Medicare Claims Processing Manual, Pub. 100-4, Chapter 12, §90.4) under the HPSA physician bonus program and a PCIP incentive payment under the new program beginning in CY 2011.

100-4, 12, 230.3

Claims Processing and Payment

A. General Overview

Incentive payments will be made on a quarterly basis and shall be equal to 10 percent of the amount paid for such services under the Medicare Physician Fee Schedule (PFS) for those services furnished during the bonus payment year. For information on PCIP payments to CAHs paid under the optional method, see the Medicare Claims Processing Manual, Pub. 100-4, Chapter 4, §250.12.

On an annual basis Medicare contractors shall receive a Primary Care Incentive Payment Program Eligibility File that they shall post to their website. The file will list the NPIs of all practitioners who are eligible to receive PCIP payments for the upcoming CY.

B. Method of Payment

- Calculate and pay qualifying primary care practitioners an additional 10 percent incentive payment;

- Calculate the payment based on the amount actually paid for the services, not the Medicare approved amounts;

- Combine the PCIP incentive payments, when appropriate, with other incentive payments, including the HPSA physician bonus payment, and the HPSA Surgical Incentive Payment Program (HSIP) payment;

- Provide a special remittance form that is forwarded with the incentive payment so that physicians and practitioners can identify which type of incentive payment (HPSA physician and/or PCIP) was paid for which services.

- Practitioners should contact their contractor with any questions regarding PCIP payments.

C. Changes for Contractor Systems

The Medicare Carrier System, (MCS), Common Working File (CWF) and the National Claims History (NCH) shall be modified to accept a new PCIP indicator on the claim line. Once the type of incentive payment has been identified by the shared systems, the shared system shall modify their systems to set the indicator on the claim line as follows:

1 = HPSA;

2 = PSA;

3 = HPSA and PSA;

4 = HSIP;

5 = HPSA and HSIP;

6 = PCIP;

7 = HPSA and PCIP; and

Space = Not Applicable.

The contractor shared system shall send the HIGLAS 810 invoice for incentive payment invoices, including the new PCIP payment. The contractor shall also combine the provider's HPSA physician bonus, physician scarcity (PSA) bonus (if it should become available at a later date), HSIP payment and/or PCIP payment invoice per provider. The contractor shall receive the HIGLAS 835 payment file from HIGLAS showing a single incentive payment per provider

100-4, 13, 30.1.3.1

A/B MAC (A) Payment for Low Osmolar Contrast Material (LOCM) (Radiology)

The LOCM is paid on a reasonable cost basis when rendered by a SNF to its Part B patients (in addition to payment for the radiology procedure) when it is used in one of the situations listed below.

The following HCPCS are used when billing for LOCM.

HCPCS Code	Description (January 1. 1994, and later)
A4644	Supply of low osmolar contrast material (100-199 mgs of iodine);
A4645	Supply of low osmolar contrast material (200-299 mgs of iodine); or
A4646	Supply of low osmolar contrast material (300-399 mgs of iodine).

When billing for LOCM, SNFs use revenue code 0636. If the SNF charge for the radiology procedure includes a charge for contrast material, the SNF must adjust the charge for the radiology procedure to exclude any amount for the contrast material.

NOTE: LOCM is never billed with revenue code 0255 or as part of the radiology procedure.

The A/B MAC (A) will edit for the intrathecal procedure codes and the following codes to determine if payment for LOCM is to be made. If an intrathecal procedure code is not present, or one of the ICD codes is not present to indicate that a required medical condition is met, the A/B MAC (A) will deny payment for LOCM. In these instances, LOCM is not covered and should not be billed to Medicare.

When LOCM Is Separately Billable and Related Coding Requirements

- In all intrathecal injections. HCPCS codes that indicate intrathecal injections are:

  70010, 70015, 72240, 72255, 72265, 72270, 72285, 72295

  One of these must be included on the claim; or

- In intravenous and intra-arterial injections only when certain medical conditions are present in an outpatient. The SNF must verify the existence of at least one of the following medical conditions, and report the applicable diagnosis code(s) either as a principal diagnosis code or other diagnosis codes on the claim:

  — A history of previous adverse reaction to contrast material. The applicable ICD-9-CM codes are V14.8 and V14.9. The applicable ICD-10-CM codes are Z88.8 and Z88.9. The conditions which should not be considered adverse reactions are a sensation of heat, flushing, or a single episode of nausea or vomiting. If the adverse reaction occurs on that visit with the induction of contrast material, codes describing hives, urticaria, etc. should also be present, as well as a code describing the external cause of injury and poisoning, ICD-9-CM code E947.8. The applicable ICD-10 CM codes are: T50.8X5A Adverse effect of diagnostic agents, initial encounter, T50.8X5S Adverse effect of diagnostic agents, sequela , T50.995A Adverse effect of other drugs, medicaments and biological substances, initial encounter, or T50.995S Adverse effect of other drugs, medicaments and biological substances, sequela;

  — A history or condition of asthma or allergy. The applicable ICD-9-CM codes are V07.1, V14.0 through V14.9, V15.0, 493.00, 493.01, 493.10, 493.11, 493.20, 493.21, 493.90, 493.91, 495.0, 495.1, 495.2, 495.3, 495.4, 495.5, 495.6, 495.7, 495.8, 495.9, 995.0, 995.1, 995.2, and 995.3. The applicable ICD-10-CM codes are in the table below:

ICD-10-CM Codes

J44.0	J44.9	J45.20	J45.22	J45.30	J45.32	J45.40
J45.42	J45.50	J45.52	J45.902	J45.909	J45.998	J67.0
J67.1	JJ67.2	J67.3	J67.4	J67.5	J67.6	J67.7
J67.8	J67.9	J96.00	J96.01	J96.02	J96.90	J96.91
J96.92	T36.0X5A	T36.1X5A	T36.2X5A	T36.3X5A	T36.4X5A	T36.5X5A
T36.6X5A	T36.7X5A	T36.8X5A	T36.95XA	T37.0X5A	T37.1X5A	T37.2X5A

T37.3X5A	T37.8X5A	T37.95XA	T38.0X5A	T38.1X5A	T38.2X5A	T38.3X5A
T38.4X5A	T38.6X5A	T38.7X5A	T38.805A	T38.815A	T38.895A	T38.905A
T38.995A	T39.015A	T39.095A	T39.1X5A	T39.2X5A	T39.2X5A	T39.315A
T39.395A	T39.4X5A	T39.8X5A	T39.95XA	T40.0X5A	T40.1X5A	T40.2X5A
T40.3X5A	T40.4X5A	T40.5X5A	T40.605A	T40.695A	T40.7X5A	T40.8X5A
T40.905A	T40.995A	T41.0X5A	T41.1X5A	T41.205A	T41.295A	T41.3X5A
T41.4X5A	T41.X5A	T41.5X5A	T42.0X5A	T42.1X5A	T42.2X5A	T42.3X5A
T42.4X5A	T42.5X5A	T42.6X5A	427.5XA	428.X5A	T43.015A	T43.025A
T43.1X5A	T43.205A	T43.215A	T43.225A	T43.295A	T43.3X5A	T43.4X5A
T43.505A	T43.595A	T43.605A	T43.615A	T43.625A	T43.635A	T43.695A
T43.8X5A	T43.95XA	T44.0X5A	T44.1X5A	T44.2X5A	T44.3X5A	T44.6X5A
T44.7X5A	T44.8X5A	T44.905A	T44.995A	T45.0X5A	T45.1X5A	T45.2X5A
T45.3X5A	T45.4X5A	T45.515A	T45.525A	T45.605A	T45.615A	T45.625A
T45.695A	T45.7X5A	T45.8X5A	T45.95XA	T46.0X5A	T46.1X5A	T46.2X5A
T46.3X5A	T46.4X5A	T46.5X5A	T46.6X5A	T46.7X5A	T46.8X5A	T46.905A
T46.995A	T47.0X5A	T47.1X5A	T47.2X5A	T47.3X5A	T47.4X5A	T47.5X5A
T47.6X5A	T47.7X5A	T47.8X5A	T47.95XA	T48.0X5A	T48.1X5A	T48.205A
T48.295A	T48.3X5A	T48.4X5A	T48.5X5A	T48.6X5A	T48.905A	T48.995A
T49.0X5A	T49.1X5A	T49.2X5A	T49.3X5A	T49.4X5A	T49.5X5A	T49.6X5A
T49.6X5A	T47.X5A9	T49.8X5A	T49.95XA	T50.0X5A	T50.1X5A	T50.2X5A
T50.3X5A	T50.4X5A	T50.5X5A	T50.6X5A	T50.7X5A	T50.8X5A	T50.905a
T50.995A	T50.A15A	T50.A25A	T50.A95A	T50.B15A	T50.B95A	T50.Z15A
T50.Z95A	T78.2XXA	T78.3XXA	T78.40XA	T78.41XA	T88.52XA	T88.59XA
T88.6XXA	Z51.89	Z88.0	Z88.1	Z88.2	Z88.3	Z88.4
Z88.5	Z88.6	Z88.7	Z88.8	Z88.9	Z91.010	

— Significant cardiac dysfunction including recent or imminent cardiac decompensation, severe arrhythmia, unstable angina pectoris, recent myocardial infarction, and pulmonary hypertension. The applicable ICD-9-CM codes are:

ICD-9-CM

402.00	402.01	402.10	402.11	402.90	402.91	404.00
404.01	404.02	404.03	404.10	404.11	404.12	404.13
404.90	404.91	404.92	404.93	410.00	410.01	410.02
410.10	410.11	410.12	410.20	410.21	410.22	410.30
410.31	410.32	410.40	410.41	410.42	410.50	410.51
410.52	410.60	410.61	410.62	410.70	410.71	410.72
410.80	410.81	410.82	410.90	410.91	410.92	411.1
415.0	416.0	416.1	416.8	416.9	420.0	420.90
420.91	420.99	424.90	424.91	424.99	427.0	427.1
427.2	427.31	427.32	427.41	427.42	427.5	427.60
427.61	427.69	427.81	427.89	427.9	428.0	428.1
428.9	429.0	429.1	429.2	429.3	429.4	429.5
429.6	429.71	429.79	429.81	429.82	429.89	429.9
785.50	785.51	785.59				

— The applicable ICD-10-CM codes are in the table below:

ICD-10-CM Codes

A18.84	I11.0	I11.9	I13.0	I13.10	I13.11	I13.2
I20.0	I21.01	I21.02	I21.09	I21.11	I21.19	I21.21
I21.29	I21.3	I21.4	I22.1	I22.2	I22.8	I23.0
I23.1	I23.2	I23.3	I23.4	I23.5	I23.6	I23.7
I23.8	I25.10	I25.110	I25.700	I25.710	I25.720	I25.730
I25.750	I25.760	I25.790	I26.01	I26.02	I26.09	I27.0
I27.1	I27.2	I27.81	I27.89	I27.9	I30.0	I30.1
I30.8	I30.9	I32	I38	I39	I46.2	I46.8
I46.9	I47.0	I471	I472	I47.9	I48.0	I48.1
I48.1	I48.2	I48.3	I48.4	I48.91	I48.92	I49.01
I49.02	I49.1	I49.2	I49.3	I49.40	I49.49	I49.5
I49.8	I49.9	I50.1	I50.20	I50.21	I50.22	I50.23
I50.30	I50.31	I50.32	I50.33	I50.40	I50.41	I50.42
I50.43	I50.9	I51	I51.0	I51.1	I51.2	I51.3
I51.4	I51.5	I51.7	I51.89	I51.9	I52	I97.0
I97.110	I97.111	I97.120	I97.121	I97.130	I97.131	I97.190
I97.191	M32.11	M32.12	R00.1	R57.0	R57.8	R57.9

— Generalized severe debilitation. The applicable ICD-9-CM codes are: 203.00, 203.01, all codes for diabetes mellitus, 518.81, 585, 586, 799.3, 799.4, and V46.1. The applicable ICD-10-CM codes are: J96.850, J96.00 through J96.02, J96.90 through J96.91, N18.1 through N19, R53.81, R64, and Z99.11 through Z99.12. Or

— Sickle Cell disease. The applicable ICD-9-CM codes are 282.4, 282.60, 282.61, 282.62, 282.63, and 282.69. The applicable ICD-10-CM codes are D56.0 through D56.3, D56.5 through D56.9, D57.00 through D57.1, D57.20, D57.411 through D57.419, and D57.811 through D57.819.

100-4, 13, 40.1.1

Magnetic Resonance Angiography (MRA) Coverage Summary

Section 1861(s)(2)(C) of the Social Security Act provides for coverage of diagnostic testing. Coverage of magnetic resonance angiography (MRA) of the head and neck, and MRA of the peripheral vessels of the lower extremities is limited as described in Publication (Pub.) 100-3, the Medicare National Coverage Determinations (NCD) Manual. This instruction has been revised as of July 1, 2003, based on a determination that coverage is reasonable and necessary in additional circumstances. Under that instruction, MRA is generally covered only to the extent that it is used as a substitute for contrast angiography, except to the extent that there are documented circumstances consistent with that instruction that demonstrates the medical necessity of both tests. Prior to June 3, 2010, there was no coverage of MRA outside of the indications and circumstances described in that instruction.

Effective for claims with dates of service on or after June 3, 2010, contractors have the discretion to cover or not cover all indications of MRA (and magnetic resonance imaging (MRI)) that are not specifically nationally covered or nationally non-covered as stated in section 220.2 of the NCD Manual.

Because the status codes for HCPCS codes 71555, 71555-TC, 71555-26, 74185, 74185-TC, and 74185-26 were changed in the Medicare Physician Fee Schedule Database from 'N' to 'R' on April 1, 1998, any MRA claims with those HCPCS codes with dates of service between April 1, 1998, and June 30, 1999, are to be processed according to the contractor's discretionary authority to determine payment in the absence of national policy.

Effective for claims with dates of service on or after February 24, 2011, Medicare will provide coverage for MRIs for beneficiaries with implanted cardiac pacemakers or implantable cardioverter defibrillators if the beneficiary is enrolled in an approved clinical study under the Coverage with Study Participation form of Coverage with Evidence Development that meets specific criteria per Pub. 100-3, the NCD Manual, chapter 1, section 220.2.C.1

100-4, 13, 40.1.2

HCPCS Coding Requirements

Providers must report HCPCS codes when submitting claims for MRA of the chest, abdomen, head, neck or peripheral vessels of lower extremities. The following HCPCS codes should be used to report these services:

MRA of head	70544, 70544-26, 70544-TC
MRA of head	70545, 70545-26, 70545-TC
MRA of head	70546, 70546-26, 70546-TC
MRA of neck	70547, 70547-26, 70547-TC
MRA of neck	70548, 70548-26, 70548-TC
MRA of neck	70549, 70549-26, 70549-TC
MRA of chest	71555, 71555-26, 71555-TC
MRA of pelvis	72198, 72198-26, 72198-TC
MRA of abdomen (dates of service on or after July 1, 2003) – see below.	74185, 74185-26, 74185-TC
MRA of peripheral vessels of lower extremities	73725, 73725-26, 73725-TC

100-4, 13, 60

Positron Emission Tomography (PET) Scans - General Information

Positron emission tomography (PET) is a noninvasive imaging procedure that assesses perfusion and the level of metabolic activity in various organ systems of the human body. A positron camera (tomograph) is used to produce cross-sectional tomographic images which are obtained by detecting radioactivity from a radioactive tracer substance radiopharmaceutical) that emits a radioactive tracer substance (radiopharmaceutical FDG) such as 2 -[F-18] flouro-D-glucose FDG, that is administered intravenously to the patient.

The Medicare National Coverage Determinations (NCD) Manual, Chapter 1, Sec.220.6, contains additional coverage instructions to indicate the conditions under which a PET scan is performed.

A. Definitions

For all uses of PET, excluding Rubidium 82 for perfusion of the heart, myocardial viability and refractory seizures, the following definitions apply:

- **Diagnosis:** PET is covered only in clinical situations in which the PET results may assist in avoiding an invasive diagnostic procedure, or in which the PET results may assist in determining the optimal anatomical location to perform an invasive diagnostic procedure. In general, for most solid tumors, a tissue diagnosis is made prior to the performance of PET scanning. PET scans following a tissue diagnosis are generally performed for the purpose of staging, rather than diagnosis. Therefore, the use of PET in the diagnosis of lymphoma, esophageal and colorectal cancers, as well as in melanoma, should be rare. PET is not covered for other diagnostic uses, and is not covered for screening (testing of patients without specific signs and symptoms of disease).

- **Staging:** PET is covered in clinical situations in which (1) (a) the stage of the cancer remains in doubt after completion of a standard diagnostic workup, including conventional imaging (computed tomography, magnetic resonance imaging, or ultrasound) or, (b) the use of PET would also be considered reasonable and necessary if it could potentially replace one or more conventional imaging studies when it is expected that conventional study information is insufficient for the clinical management of the patient and, (2) clinical management of the patient would differ depending on the stage of the cancer identified.

  NOTE: Effective for services on or after April 3, 2009, the terms "diagnosis" and "staging" will be replaced with "Initial Treatment Strategy." For further information on this new term, refer to Pub. 100-3, NCD Manual, section 220.6.17.

- **Restaging:** PET will be covered for restaging: (1) after the completion of treatment for the purpose of detecting residual disease, (2) for detecting suspected recurrence, or metastasis, (3) to determine the extent of a known recurrence, or (4) if it could potentially replace one or more conventional imaging studies when it is expected that conventional study information is to determine the extent of a known recurrence, or if study information is insufficient for the clinical management of the patient. Restaging applies to testing after a course of treatment is completed and is covered subject to the conditions above.

- **Monitoring:** Use of PET to monitor tumor response to treatment during the planned course of therapy (i.e., when a change in therapy is anticipated).

  NOTE: Effective for services on or after April 3, 2009, the terms "restaging" and "monitoring" will be replaced with "Subsequent Treatment Strategy." For further information on this new term, refer to Pub. 100-3, NCD Manual, section 220.6.17.

B. Limitations

For staging and restaging: PET is covered in either/or both of the following circumstances:

- The stage of the cancer remains in doubt after completion of a standard diagnostic workup, including conventional imaging (computed tomography, magnetic resonance imaging, or ultrasound); and/or

- The clinical management of the patient would differ depending on the stage of the cancer identified. PET will be covered for restaging after the completion of treatment for the purpose of detecting residual disease, for detecting suspected recurrence, or to determine the extent of a known recurrence. Use of PET would also be considered reasonable and necessary if it could potentially replace one or more conventional imaging studies when it is expected that conventional study information is insufficient for the clinical management of the patient.

The PET is not covered for other diagnostic uses, and is not covered for screening (testing of patients without specific symptoms). Use of PET to monitor tumor response during the planned course of therapy (i.e. when no change in therapy is being contemplated) is not covered.

100-4, 13, 60.13

Billing Requirements for PET Scans for Specific Indications of Cervical Cancer for Services Performed on or After January 28, 2005

Contractors shall accept claims for these services with the appropriate CPT code listed in section 60.3.1. Refer to Pub. 100-3, section 220.6.17, for complete coverage guidelines for this new PET oncology indication. The implementation date for these CPT codes will be April 18, 2005. Also see section 60.17, of this chapter for further claims processing instructions for cervical cancer indications.

100-4, 13, 60.15

Billing Requirements for CMS - Approved Clinical Trials and Coverage With Evidence Development Claims for PET Scans for Neurodegenerative Diseases, Previously Specified Cancer Indications, and All Other Cancer Indications Not Previously Specified

A/B MACs (A and B)

Effective for services on or after January 28, 2005, contractors shall accept and pay for claims for Positron Emission Tomography (PET) scans for lung cancer, esophageal cancer, colorectal cancer, lymphoma, melanoma, head & neck cancer, breast cancer, thyroid cancer, soft tissue sarcoma, brain cancer, ovarian cancer, pancreatic cancer, small cell lung cancer, and testicular cancer, as well as for neurodegenerative diseases and all other cancer indications not previously mentioned in this chapter, if these scans were performed as part of a Centers for Medicare & Medicaid (CMS)-approved clinical trial. (See Pub. 100-3, National Coverage Determinations (NCD) Manual, sections 220.6.13 and 220.6.17.)

Contractors shall also be aware that PET scans for all cancers not previously specified at Pub. 100-3, NCD Manual, section 220.6.17, remain nationally non-covered unless performed in conjunction with a CMS-approved clinical trial.

Effective for dates of service on or after June 11, 2013, Medicare has ended the coverage with evidence development (CED) requirement for FDG (2-[F18] fluoro-2-deoxy-D-glucose) PET and PET/computed tomography (CT) and PET/magnetic resonance imaging (MRI) for all oncologic indications contained in section 220.6.17 of the NCD Manual. Modifier -Q0 (Investigational clinical service provided in a clinical research study that is in an approved clinical research study) or -Q1 (routine clinical service

provided in a clinical research study that is in an approved clinical research study) is no longer mandatory for these services when performed on or after June 11, 2013.

A/B MACs (B) Only

A/B MACs (B) shall pay claims for PET scans for beneficiaries participating in a CMS-approved clinical trial submitted with an appropriate current procedural terminology (CPT) code from section 60.3.1 of this chapter and modifier Q0/Q1 for services performed on or after January 1, 2008, through June 10, 2013. (NOTE: Modifier QR (Item or service provided in a Medicare specified study) and QA (FDA investigational device exemption) were replaced by modifier Q0 effective January 1, 2008.) Modifier QV (item or service provided as routine care in a Medicare qualifying clinical trial) was replaced by modifier Q1 effective January 1, 2008.) Beginning with services performed on or after June 11, 2013, modifier Q0/Q1 is no longer required for PET FDG services.

A/B MACs (A) Only

In order to pay claims for PET scans on behalf of beneficiaries participating in a CMS-approved clinical trial, A/B MACs (A) require providers to submit claims with, if ICD-9-CM is applicable, ICD-9 code V70.7; if ICD-10-CM is applicable, ICD-10 code Z00.6 in the primary/secondary diagnosis position using the ASC X12 837 institutional claim format or on Form CMS-1450, with the appropriate principal diagnosis code and an appropriate CPT code from section 60.3.1. Effective for PET scan claims for dates of service on or after January 28, 2005, through December 31, 2007, A/B MACs (A) shall accept claims with the QR, QV, or QA modifier on other than inpatient claims. Effective for services on or after January 1, 2008, through June 10, 2013, modifier Q0 replaced the-QR and QA modifier, modifier Q1 replaced the QV modifier. Modifier Q0/Q1 is no longer required for services performed on or after June 11, 2013.

100-4, 13, 60.16

Billing and Coverage Changes for PET Scans Effective for Services on or After April 3, 2009

A. Summary of Changes

Effective for services on or after April 3, 2009, Medicare will not cover the use of FDG PET imaging to determine initial treatment strategy in patients with adenocarcinoma of the prostate.

Medicare will also not cover FDG PET imaging for subsequent treatment strategy for tumor types other than breast, cervical, colorectal, esophagus, head and neck (non-CNS/thyroid), lymphoma, melanoma, myeloma, non-small cell lung, and ovarian, unless the FDG PET is provided under the coverage with evidence development (CED) paradigm (billed with modifier -Q0/-Q1, see section 60.15 of this chapter).

Medicare will cover FDG PET imaging for initial treatment strategy for myeloma.

Effective for services performed on or after June 11, 2013, Medicare has ended the CED requirement for FDG PET and PET/CT and PET/MRI for all oncologic indications contained in section 220.6.17 of the NCD Manual. Effective for services on or after June 11, 2013, the Q0/Q1 modifier is no longer required.

Beginning with services performed on or after June 11, 2013, contractors shall pay for up to three (3) FDG PET scans when used to guide subsequent management of anti-tumor treatment strategy (modifier PS) after completion of initial anti-cancer therapy (modifier PI) for the exact same cancer diagnosis.

Coverage of any additional FDG PET scans (that is, beyond 3) used to guide subsequent management of anti-tumor treatment strategy after completion of initial anti-tumor therapy for the same cancer diagnosis will be determined by the A/B MACs (A or B). Claims will include the KX modifier indicating the coverage criteria is met for coverage of four or more FDG PET scans for subsequent treatment strategy for the same cancer diagnosis under this NCD.

A different cancer diagnosis whether submitted with a PI or a PS modifier will begin the count of one initial and three subsequent FDG PET scans not requiring the KX modifier and four or more FDG PET scans for subsequent treatment strategy for the same cancer diagnosis requiring the KX modifier.

NOTE: The presence or absence of an initial treatment strategy claim in a beneficiary's record does not impact the frequency criteria for subsequent treatment strategy claims for the same cancer diagnosis.

NOTE: Providers please refer to the following link for a list of appropriate diagnosis codes,
http://cms.gov/medicare/coverage/determinationprocess/downloads/petforsolidtumorsoncologicdxcodesattachment_NCD220_6_17.pdf

For further information regarding the changes in coverage, refer to Pub.100-3, NCD Manual, section 220.6.17.

B. Modifiers for PET Scans

Effective for claims with dates of service on or after April 3, 2009, the following modifiers have been created for use to inform for the initial treatment strategy of biopsy-proven or strongly suspected tumors or subsequent treatment strategy of cancerous tumors:

PI Positron Emission Tomography (PET) or PET/Computed Tomography (CT) to inform the initial treatment strategy of tumors that are biopsy proven or strongly suspected of being cancerous based on other diagnostic testing.

Short descriptor: PET tumor init tx strat

PS Positron Emission Tomography (PET) or PET/Computed Tomography (CT) to inform the subsequent treatment strategy of cancerous tumors when the beneficiary's treatment physician determines that the PET study is needed to inform subsequent anti-tumor strategy.

Short descriptor: PS - PET tumor subsq tx strategy

C. Billing for A/B MACs (A and B)

Effective for claims with dates of service on or after April 3, 2009, contractors shall accept FDG PET claims billed to inform initial treatment strategy with the following CPT codes AND modifier PI: 78608, 78811, 78812, 78813, 78814, 78815, 78816.

Effective for claims with dates of service on or after April 3, 2009, contractors shall accept FDG PET claims with modifier PS for the subsequent treatment strategy for solid tumors using a CPT code above AND a cancer diagnosis code.

Contractors shall also accept FDG PET claims billed to inform initial treatment strategy or subsequent treatment strategy when performed under CED with one of the PET or PET/CT CPT codes above AND modifier PI OR modifier PS AND a cancer diagnosis code AND modifier Q0/Q1. Effective for services performed on or after June 11, 2013, the CED requirement has ended and modifier Q0/Q1, along with condition code 30 (institutional claims only), or ICD-9 code V70.7, (both institutional and practitioner claims) are no longer required.

D. Medicare Summary Notices, Remittance Advice Remark Codes, and Claim Adjustment Reason Codes

Effective for dates of service on or after April 3, 2009, contractors shall return as unprocessable/return to provider claims that do not include the PI modifier with one of the PET/PET/CT CPT codes listed in subsection C. above when billing for the initial treatment strategy for solid tumors in accordance with Pub.100-3, NCD Manual, section 220.6.17.

In addition, contractors shall return as unprocessable/return to provider claims that do not include the PS modifier with one of the CPT codes listed in subsection C. above when billing for the subsequent treatment strategy for solid tumors in accordance with Pub.100-3, NCD Manual, section 220.6.17.

The following messages apply:

- Claim Adjustment Reason Code (CARC) 4 - The procedure code is inconsistent with the modifier used or a required modifier is missing.
- Remittance Advice Remark Code (RARC) MA-130 - Your claim contains incomplete and/or invalid information, and no appeal rights are afforded because the claim is unprocessable. Submit a new claim with the complete/correct information.
- RARC M16 - Alert: See our Web site, mailings, or bulletins for more details concerning this policy/procedure/decision.

Effective for claims with dates of service on or after April 3, 2009, through June 10, 2013, contractors shall return as unprocessable/return to provider FDG PET claims billed to inform initial treatment strategy or subsequent treatment strategy when performed under CED without one of the PET/PET/CT CPT codes listed in subsection C. above AND modifier PI OR modifier PS AND a cancer diagnosis code AND modifier Q0/Q1.

The following messages apply to return as unprocessable claims:

- CARC 4 - The procedure code is inconsistent with the modifier used or a required modifier is missing.
- RARC MA-130 - Your claim contains incomplete and/or invalid information, and no appeal rights are afforded because the claim is unprocessable. Submit a new claim with the complete/correct information.
- RARC M16 - Alert: See our Web site, mailings, or bulletins for more details concerning this policy/procedure/decision.

Effective April 3, 2009, contractors shall deny claims with ICD-9/ICD-10 diagnosis code 185/C61 for FDG PET imaging for the initial treatment strategy of patients with adenocarcinoma of the prostate.

For dates of service prior to June 11, 2013, contractors shall also deny claims for FDG PET imaging for subsequent treatment strategy for tumor types other than breast, cervical, colorectal, esophagus, head and neck (non-CNS/thyroid), lymphoma, melanoma, myeloma, non-small cell lung, and ovarian, unless the FDG PET is provided under CED (submitted with the Q0/Q1 modifier) and use the following messages:

- Medicare Summary Notice 15.4 - Medicare does not support the need for this service or item
- CARC 50 - These are non-covered services because this is not deemed a 'medical necessity' by the payer.
- Contractors shall use Group Code CO (Contractual Obligation)

If the service is submitted with a GA modifier indicating there is a signed Advance Beneficiary Notice (ABN) on file, the liability falls to the beneficiary. However, if the service is submitted with a GZ modifier indicating no ABN was provided, the liability falls to the provider.

Effective for dates of service on or after June 11, 2013, contractors shall use the following messages when denying claims in excess of three for PET FDG scans for subsequent treatment strategy when the KX modifier is not included, identified by CPT codes 78608, 78811, 78812, 78813, 78814, 78815, or 78816, modifier PS, HCPCS A9552, and the same cancer diagnosis code.

- CARC 96: "Non-Covered Charge(s). Note: Refer to the 835 Healthcare Policy Identification Segment (loop 2110 Service Payment Information REF), if present."
- RARC N435: "Exceeds number/frequency approved/allowed within time period without support documentation."
- MSN 23.17: "Medicare won't cover these services because they are not considered medically necessary."

Spanish Version: "Medicare no cubrirá estos servicios porque no son considerados necesarios por razones médicas."

Contractors shall use Group Code PR assigning financial liability to the beneficiary, if a claim is received with a GA modifier indicating a signed ABN is on file.

Contractors shall use Group Code CO assigning financial liability to the provider, if a claim is received with a GZ modifier indicating no signed ABN is on file.

100-4, 13, 60.17

Billing and Coverage Changes for PET Scans for Cervical Cancer Effective for Services on or After November 10, 2009

A. Billing Changes for A/B MACs (A and B)

Effective for claims with dates of service on or after November 10, 2009, contractors shall accept FDG PET oncologic claims billed to inform initial treatment strategy; specifically for staging in beneficiaries who have biopsy-proven cervical cancer when the beneficiary's treating physician determines the FDG PET study is needed to determine the location and/or extent of the tumor as specified in Pub. 100-3, section 220.6.17.

EXCEPTION: CMS continues to non-cover FDG PET for initial diagnosis of cervical cancer related to initial treatment strategy.

NOTE: Effective for claims with dates of service on and after November 10, 2009, the –Q0 modifier is no longer necessary for FDG PET for cervical cancer.

B. Medicare Summary Notices, Remittance Advice Remark Codes, and Claim Adjustment Reason Codes

Additionally, contractors shall return as unprocessable /return to provider for FDG PET for cervical cancer for initial treatment strategy billed without the following: one of the PET/PET/ CT CPT codes listed in 60.16 C above AND modifier –PI AND a cervical cancer diagnosis code.

Use the following messages:

- Claim Adjustment Reason Code 4 – the procedure code is inconsistent with the modifier used or a required modifier is missing.
- Remittance Advice Remark Code MA-130 - Your claim contains incomplete and/or invalid information, and no appeal rights are afforded because the claim is unprocessable. Submit a new claim with the complete/correct information.
- Remittance Advice Remark Code M16 - Alert: See our Web site, mailings, or bulletins for more details concerning this policy/procedure/decision.

100-4, 13, 60.18

Billing and Coverage Changes for PET (NaF-18) Scans to Identify Bone Metastasis of Cancer Effective for Claims With Dates of Services on or After February 26, 2010

Billing and Coverage Changes for PET (NaF-18) Scans to Identify Bone Metastasis of Cancer Effective for Claims With Dates of Services on or After February 26, 2010

A. Billing Changes for A/B MACs (A and B)

Effective for claims with dates of service on and after February 26, 2010, contractors shall pay for NaF-18 PET oncologic claims to inform of initial treatment strategy (PI) or subsequent treatment strategy (PS) for suspected or biopsy proven bone metastasis ONLY in the context of a clinical study and as specified in Pub. 100-3, section 220.6. All other claims for NaF-18 PET oncology claims remain non-covered.

B. Medicare Summary Notices, Remittance Advice Remark Codes, and Claim Adjustment Reason Codes

Effective for claims with dates of service on or after February 26, 2010, contractors shall return as unprocessable NaF-18 PET oncologic claims billed with modifier TC or globally (for A/B MACs (A) modifier TC or globally does not apply) and HCPCS A9580 to inform the initial treatment strategy or subsequent treatment strategy for bone metastasis that do not include ALL of the following:

- PI or –PS modifier AND
- PET or PET/CT CPT code (78811, 78812, 78813, 78814, 78815, 78816) AND
- Cancer diagnosis code AND

- Q0 modifier – Investigational clinical service provided in a clinical research study, are present on the claim.

NOTE: For institutional claims, continue to include ICD-9 diagnosis code V70.7 or ICD-10 diagnosis code Z00.6 and condition code 30 to denote a clinical study.

Use the following messages:

- Claim Adjustment Reason Code 4 – The procedure code is inconsistent with the modifier used or a required modifier is missing. Note: Refer to the 835 Healthcare Policy Identification Segment (loop 2110 Service Payment Information REF), if present.

- Remittance Advice Remark Code MA-130 - Your claim contains incomplete and/or invalid information, and no appeal rights are afforded because the claim is unprocessable. Submit a new claim with the complete/correct information.

- Remittance Advice Remark Code M16 - Alert: See our Web site, mailings, or bulletins for more details concerning this policy/procedure/decision.

- Claim Adjustment Reason Code 167 – This (these) diagnosis(es) is (are) not covered.

Effective for claims with dates of service on or after February 26, 2010, contractors shall accept PET oncologic claims billed with modifier 26 and modifier KX to inform the initial treatment strategy or strategy or subsequent treatment strategy for bone metastasis that include the following:

- PI or –PS modifier AND

- PET or PET/CT CPT code (78811, 78812, 78813, 78814, 78815, 78816) AND

- Cancer diagnosis code AND

- Q0 modifier – Investigational clinical service provided in a clinical research study, are present on the claim.

NOTE: If modifier KX is present on the professional component service, Contractors shall process the service as PET NaF-18 rather than PET with FDG.

Contractors shall also return as unprocessable NaF-18 PET oncologic professional component claims (i.e., claims billed with modifiers 26 and KX) to inform the initial treatment strategy or strategy or subsequent treatment strategy for bone metastasis billed with HCPCS A9580 and use the following message:

Claim Adjustment Reason Code 97 – The benefit for this service is included in the payment/allowance for another service/procedure that has already been adjudicated.

NOTE: Refer to the 835 Healthcare Policy identification Segment (loop 2110 Service Payment Information REF), if present.

100-4, 13, 60.2

Use of Gamma Cameras and Full Ring and Partial Ring PET Scanners for PET Scans

See the Medicare NCD Manual, Section 220.6, concerning 2-[F-18] Fluoro-D-Glucose (FDG) PET scanners and details about coverage.

On July 1, 2001, HCPCS codes G0210 - G0230 were added to allow billing for all currently covered indications for FDG PET. Although the codes do not indicate the type of PET scanner, these codes were used until January 1, 2002, by providers to bill for services in a manner consistent with the coverage policy.

Effective January 1, 2002, HCPCS codes G0210 - G0230 were updated with new descriptors to properly reflect the type of PET scanner used. In addition, four new HCPCS codes became effective for dates of service on and after January 1, 2002, (G0231, G0232, G0233, G0234) for covered conditions that may be billed if a gamma camera is used for the PET scan. For services performed from January 1, 2002, through January 27, 2005, providers should bill using the revised HCPCS codes G0210 - G0234.

Beginning January 28, 2005 providers should bill using the appropriate CPT code.

100-4, 13, 60.3

PET Scan Qualifying Conditions and HCPCS Code Chart

Below is a summary of all covered PET scan conditions, with effective dates.

NOTE: The G codes below except those a # can be used to bill for PET Scan services through January 27, 2005. Effective for dates of service on or after January 28, 2005, providers must bill for PET Scan services using the appropriate CPT codes. See section 60.3.1. The G codes with a # can continue to be used for billing after January 28, 2005 and these remain non-covered by Medicare. (NOTE: PET Scanners must be FDA-approved.)

Conditions	Coverage Effective Date	**** HCPCS/CPT
*Myocardial perfusion imaging (following previous PET G0030-G0047) single study, rest or stress (exercise and/or pharmacologic)	3/14/95	G0030
*Myocardial perfusion imaging (following previous PET G0030-G0047) multiple studies, rest or stress (exercise and/or pharmacologic)	3/14/95	G0031

Conditions	Coverage Effective Date	**** HCPCS/CPT
*Myocardial perfusion imaging (following rest SPECT, 78464); single study, rest or stress (exercise and/or pharmacologic)	3/14/95	G0032
*Myocardial perfusion imaging (following rest SPECT 78464); multiple studies, rest or stress (exercise and/or pharmacologic)	3/14/95	G0033
*Myocardial perfusion (following stress SPECT 78465); single study, rest or stress (exercise and/or pharmacologic)	3/14/95	G0034
*Myocardial Perfusion Imaging (following stress SPECT 78465); multiple studies, rest or stress (exercise and/or pharmacologic)	3/14/95	G0035
*Myocardial Perfusion Imaging (following coronary angiography 93510-93529); single study, rest or stress (exercise and/or pharmacologic)	3/14/95	G0036
*Myocardial Perfusion Imaging, (following coronary angiography), 93510-93529); multiple studies, rest or stress (exercise and/or pharmacologic)	3/14/95	G0037
*Myocardial Perfusion Imaging (following stress planar myocardial perfusion, 78460); single study, rest or stress (exercise and/or pharmacologic)	3/14/95	G0038
*Myocardial Perfusion Imaging (following stress planar myocardial perfusion, 78460); multiple studies, rest or stress (exercise and/or pharmacologic)	3/14/95	G0039
*Myocardial Perfusion Imaging (following stress echocardiogram 93350); single study, rest or stress (exercise and/or pharmacologic)	3/14/95	G0040
*Myocardial Perfusion Imaging (following stress echocardiogram, 93350); multiple studies, rest or stress (exercise and/or pharmacologic)	3/14/95	G0041
*Myocardial Perfusion Imaging (following stress nuclear ventriculogram 78481 or 78483); single study, rest or stress (exercise and/or pharmacologic)	3/14/95	G0042
*Myocardial Perfusion Imaging (following stress nuclear ventriculogram 78481 or 78483); multiple studies, rest or stress (exercise and/or pharmacologic)	3/14/95	G0043
*Myocardial Perfusion Imaging (following stress ECG, 93000); single study, rest or stress (exercise and/or pharmacologic)	3/14/95	G0044
*Myocardial perfusion (following stress ECG, 93000), multiple studies; rest or stress (exercise and/or pharmacologic)	3/14/95	G0045
*Myocardial perfusion (following stress ECG, 93015), single study; rest or stress (exercise and/or pharmacologic)	3/14/95	G0046
*Myocardial perfusion (following stress ECG, 93015); multiple studies, rest or stress (exercise and/or pharmacologic)	3/14/95	G0047
PET imaging regional or whole body; single pulmonary nodule	1/1/98	G0125
Lung cancer, non-small cell (PET imaging whole body) Diagnosis, Initial Staging, Restaging	7/1/01	G0210 G0211 G0212
Colorectal cancer (PET imaging whole body) Diagnosis, Initial Staging, Restaging	7/1/01	G0213 G0214 G0215
Melanoma (PET imaging whole body) Diagnosis, Initial Staging, Restaging	7/1/01	G0216 G0217 G0218
Melanoma for non-covered indications	7/1/01	#G0219
Lymphoma (PET imaging whole body) Diagnosis, Initial Staging, Restaging	7/1/01	G0220 G0221 G0222
Head and neck cancer; excluding thyroid and CNS cancers (PET imaging whole body or regional) Diagnosis, Initial Staging, Restaging	7/1/01	G0223 G0224 G0225
Esophageal cancer (PET imaging whole body) Diagnosis, Initial Staging, Restaging	7/1/01	G0226 G0227 G0228

Conditions	Coverage Effective Date	**** HCPCS/CPT
Metabolic brain imaging for pre-surgical evaluation of refractory seizures	7/1/01	G0229
Metabolic assessment for myocardial viability following inconclusive SPECT study	7/1/01	G0230
Recurrence of colorectal or colorectal metastatic cancer (PET whole body, gamma cameras only)	1/1/02	G0231
Staging and characterization of lymphoma (PET whole body, gamma cameras only)	1/1/02	G0232
Recurrence of melanoma or melanoma metastatic cancer (PET whole body, gamma cameras only)	1/1/02	G0233
Regional or whole body, for solitary pulmonary nodule following CT, or for initial staging of nonsmall cell lung cancer (gamma cameras only)	1/1/02	G0234
Non-Covered Service PET imaging, any site not otherwise specified	1/28/05	#G0235
Non-Covered Service Initial diagnosis of breast cancer and/or surgical planning for breast cancer (e.g., initial staging of axillary lymph nodes), not covered (full- and partialring PET scanners only)	10/1/02	#G0252
Breast cancer, staging/restaging of local regional recurrence or distant metastases, i.e., staging/restaging after or prior to course of treatment (full- and partial-ring PET scanners only)	10/1/02	G0253
Breast cancer, evaluation of responses to treatment, performed during course of treatment (full- and partial-ring PET scanners only)	10/1/02	G0254
Myocardial imaging, positron emission tomography (PET), metabolic evaluation	10/1/02	78459
Restaging or previously treated thyroid cancer of follicular cell origin following negative I-131 whole body scan (full- and partial-ring PET scanner only)	10/1/03	G0296
Tracer Rubidium**82 (Supply of Radiopharmaceutical Diagnostic Imaging Agent) (This is only billed through Outpatient Perspective Payment System, OPPS.) (Carriers must use HCPCS Code A4641).	10/1/03	Q3000
Supply of Radiopharmaceutical Diagnostic Imaging Agent, Ammonia N-13	01/1/04	A9526
PET imaging, brain imaging for the differential diagnosis of Alzheimer's disease with aberrant features vs. fronto-temporal dementia	09/15/04	Appropriate CPT Code from section 60.3.1
PET Cervical Cancer Staging as adjunct to conventional imaging, other staging, diagnosis, restaging, monitoring	1/28/05	Appropriate CPT Code from section 60.3.1

* NOTE: Carriers must report A4641 for the tracer Rubidium 82 when used with PET scan codes G0030 through G0047 for services performed on or before January 27, 2005

** NOTE: Not FDG PET

*** NOTE: For dates of service October 1, 2003, through December 31, 2003, use temporary code Q4078 for billing this radiopharmaceutical.

100-4, 13, 60.3.1

Appropriate CPT Codes Effective for PET Scans for Services Performed on or After January 28, 2005

NOTE: All PET scan services require the use of a radiopharmaceutical diagnostic imaging agent (tracer). The applicable tracer code should be billed when billing for a PET scan service. See section 60.3.2 below for applicable tracer codes.

CPT Code	Description
78459	Myocardial imaging, positron emission tomography (PET), metabolic evaluation
78491	Myocardial imaging, positron emission tomography (PET), perfusion, single study at rest or stress
78492	Myocardial imaging, positron emission tomography (PET), perfusion, multiple studies at rest and/or stress
78608	Brain imaging, positron emission tomography (PET); metabolic evaluation
78811	Tumor imaging, positron emission tomography (PET); limited area (eg, chest, head/neck)

CPT Code	Description
78812	Tumor imaging, positron emission tomography (PET); skull base to mid-thigh
78813	Tumor imaging, positron emission tomography (PET); whole body
78814	Tumor imaging, positron emission tomography (PET) with concurrently acquired computed tomography (CT) for attenuation correction and anatomical localization; limited area (eg, chest, head/neck)
78815	Tumor imaging, positron emission tomography (PET) with concurrently acquired computed tomography (CT) for attenuation correction and anatomical localization; skull base to mid-thigh
78816	Tumor imaging, positron emission tomography (PET) with concurrently acquired computed tomography (CT) for attenuation correction and anatomical localization; whole body

100-4, 13, 60.3.2

Tracer Codes Required for PET Scans

The following tracer codes are applicable only to CPT 78491 and 78492. They can not be reported with any other code.

Institutional providers billing the fiscal intermediary

HCPCS	Description
*A9555	Rubidium Rb-82, Diagnostic, Per study dose, Up To 60 Millicuries
* Q3000 (Deleted effective 12/31/05)	Supply of Radiopharmaceutical Diagnostic Imaging Agent, Rubidium Rb-82, per dose
A9526	Nitrogen N-13 Ammonia, Diagnostic, Per study dose, Up To 40 Millicuries

* NOTE: For claims with dates of service prior to 1/01/06, providers report Q3000 for supply of radiopharmaceutical diagnostic imaging agent, Rubidium Rb-82. For claims with dates of service 1/01/06 and later, providers report A9555 for radiopharmaceutical diagnostic imaging agent, Rubidium Rb-82 in place of Q3000.

Physicians / practitioners billing the carrier:

*A4641	Supply of Radiopharmaceutical Diagnostic Imaging Agent, Not Otherwise Classified
A9526	Nitrogen N-13 Ammonia, Diagnostic, Per study dose, Up To 40 Millicuries
A9555	Rubidium Rb-82, Diagnostic, Per study dose, Up To 60 Millicuries

* NOTE: Effective January 1, 2008, tracer code A4641 is not applicable for PET Scans.

The following tracer codes are applicable only to CPT 78459, 78608, 78811-78816. They can not be reported with any other code.

Institutional providers billing the fiscal intermediary:

* A9552	Fluorodeoxyglucose F18, FDG, Diagnostic, Per study dose, Up to 45 Millicuries
* C1775 (Deleted effective 12/31/05)	Supply of Radiopharmaceutical Diagnostic Imaging Agent, Fluorodeoxyglucose F18, (2-Deoxy-2-18F Fluoro-D-Glucose), Per dose (4-40 Mci/Ml)
**A4641	Supply of Radiopharmaceutical Diagnostic Imaging Agent, Not Otherwise Classified
A9580	Sodium Fluoride F-18, Diagnostic, per study dose, up to 30 Millicuries

* NOTE: For claims with dates of service prior to 1/01/06, OPPS hospitals report C1775 for supply of radiopharmaceutical diagnostic imaging agent, Fluorodeoxyglucose F18. For claims with dates of service January 1, 2006 and later, providers report A9552 for radiopharmaceutical diagnostic imaging agent, Fluorodeoxyglucose F18 in place of C1775.

** NOTE: Effective January 1, 2008, tracer code A4641 is not applicable for PET Scans.

*** NOTE: Effective for claims with dates of service February 26, 2010 and later, tracer code A9580 is applicable for PET Scans.

Physicians / practitioners billing the carrier:

A9552	Fluorodeoxyglucose F18, FDG, Diagnostic, Per study dose, Up to 45 Millicuries
*A4641	Supply of Radiopharmaceutical Diagnostic Imaging Agent, Not Otherwise Classified
A9580	Sodium Fluoride F-18, Diagnostic, per study dose, up to 30 Millicuries

* NOTE: Effective January 1, 2008, tracer code A4641 is not applicable for PET Scans.

*** NOTE: Effective for claims with dates of service February 26, 2010 and later, tracer code A9580 is applicable for PET Scans.

Positron Emission Tomography Reference Table

CPT	Short Descriptor	Tracer/Code	or	Tracer/Code	Comment
78459	Myocardial imaging, positron emission tomography (PET), metabolic imaging	FDG A9552	--	--	N/A
78491	Myocardial imaging, positron emission tomography (PET), perfusion; single study at rest or stress	N-13 A9526	or	Rb-82 A9555	N/A
78492	Myocardial imaging, positron emission tomography (PET), perfusion; multiple studies at rest and/or stress	N-13 A9526	or	Rb-82 A9555	N/A
78608	Brain imaging, positron emission tomography (PET); metabolic evaluation	FDG A9552	--	--	Covered indications: Alzheimer's disease/dementias, intractable seizures. Note: This code is also covered for dedicated PET brain tumor imaging.
78609	Brain imaging, positron emission tomography (PET); perfusion evaluation	--	--	--	Nationally noncovered
78811	Positron emission tomography (PET) imaging; limited area (e.g, chest, head/neck)	FDG A9552	or	NaF-18 A9580	NaF-18 PET is covered only to identify bone metastasis of cancer.
78812	Positron emission tomography (PET) imaging, skull base to mid-thigh	FDG A9552	or	NaF-18 A9580	NaF-18 PET is covered only to identify bone metastasis of cancer.
78813	Positron emission tomography (PET) imaging, whole body	FDG A9552	or	NaF-18 A9580	NaF-18 PET is covered only to identify bone metastasis of cancer.
78814	PET/CT imaging, limited area (e.g., chest, head/neck)	FDG A9552	or	NaF-18 A9580	NaF-18 PET is covered only to identify bone metastasis of cancer.
78815	PET/CT imaging skull base to mid-thigh	FDG A9552	or	NaF-18 A9580	NaF-18 PET is covered only to identify bone metastasis of cancer.
78816	PET/CT imaging, whole body	FDG A9552	or	NaF-18 A9580	NaF-18 PET is covered only to identify bone metastasis of cancer.

100-4, 13, 70.3

Radiation Treatment Delivery (CPT 77401 - 77417)

Carriers pay for these TC services on a daily basis under CPT codes 77401-77416 for radiation treatment delivery. They do not use local codes and RVUs in paying for the TC of radiation oncology services. Multiple treatment sessions on the same day are payable as long as there has been a distinct break in therapy services, and the individual sessions are of the character usually furnished on different days. Carriers pay for CPT code 77417 (Therapeutic radiology port film(s)) on a weekly (five fractions) basis.

100-4, 13, 70.4

Clinical Brachytherapy (CPT Codes 77750 - 77799)

Carriers must apply the bundled services policy to procedures in this family of codes other than CPT code 77776. For procedures furnished in settings in which TC payments are made, carriers must pay separately for the expendable source associated with these procedures under CPT code 79900 except in the case of remote after-loading high intensity brachytherapy procedures (CPT codes 77781-77784). In the four codes cited, the expendable source is included in the RVUs for the TC of the procedures.

100-4, 13, 70.5

Radiation Physics Services (CPT Codes 77300 - 77399)

Carriers pay for the PC and TC of CPT codes 77300-77334 and 77399 on the same basis as they pay for radiologic services generally. For professional component billings in all settings, carriers presume that the radiologist participated in the provision of the service, e.g., reviewed/validated the physicist's calculation. CPT codes 77336 and 77370 are technical services only codes that are payable by carriers in settings in which only technical component is are payable.

100-4, 13, 80.1

Physician Presence

Radiologic supervision and interpretation (S&I) codes are used to describe the personal supervision of the performance of the radiologic portion of a procedure by one or more physicians and the interpretation of the findings. In order to bill for the supervision aspect of the procedure, the physician must be present during its performance. This kind of personal supervision of the performance of the procedure is a service to an individual beneficiary and differs from the type of general supervision of the radiologic procedures performed in a hospital for which FIs pay the costs as physician services to the hospital. The interpretation of the procedure may be performed later by another physician. In situations in which a cardiologist, for example, bills for the supervision (the "S") of the S&I code, and a radiologist bills for the interpretation (the "I") of the code, both physicians should use a "-52" modifier indicating a reduced service, e.g., only one of supervision and/or interpretation. Payment for the fragmented S&I code is no more than if a single physician furnished both aspects of the procedure.

100-4, 13, 80.2

Multiple Procedure Reduction

Carriers make no multiple procedure reductions in the S&I or primary non-radiologic codes in these types of procedures, or in any procedure codes for which the descriptor and RVUs reflect a multiple service reduction. For additional procedure codes that do not reflect such a reduction, carriers apply the multiple procedure reductions.

100-4, 16, 40.6.1

Automated Multi-Channel Chemistry (AMCC) Tests for ESRDBeneficiaries - FIs

Instructions for Services Provided on and After January 1, 2011

Section 153b of the MIPPA requires that all ESRD-related laboratory tests must be reported by the ESRD facility whether provided directly or under arrangements with an independent laboratory. When laboratory services are billed by providers other than the ESRD facility and the laboratory test furnished is designated as a laboratory test that is included in the ESRD PPS (ESRD-related), the claim will be rejected or denied. In the event that an ESRD-related laboratory test was furnished to an ESRD beneficiary for reasons other than for the treatment of ESRD, the provider may submit a claim for separate payment using modifier AY. The AY modifier serves as an attestation that the item or service is medically necessary for the dialysis patient but is not being used for the treatment of ESRD. The items and services subject to consolidated billing located on the CMS website includes the list of ESRD-related laboratory tests that are routinely performed for the treatment of ESRD.

For services provided on or after January 1, 2011, the 50/50 rule no longer applies to independent laboratory claims for AMCC tests furnished to ESRD beneficiaries. The 50/50 rule modifiers (CD, CE, and CF) are no longer required for independent laboratories effective for dates of service on and after January 1, 2011. However, for services provided between January 1, 2011 and March 31, 2015, the 50/50 rule modifiers are still required for use by ESRD facilities that are receiving the transitional blended payment amount (the transition ends in CY 2014). For services provided on or after April 1, 2015, the 50/50 rule modifiers are no longer required for use by ESRD facilities.

Effective for dates of service on and after January 1, 2012, contractors shall allow organ disease panel codes (i.e., HCPCS codes 80047, 80048, 80051, 80053, 80061, 80069, and 80076) to be billed by independent laboratories for AMCC panel tests furnished to ESRD eligible beneficiaries if:

- The beneficiary is not receiving dialysis treatment for any reason (e.g., post-transplant beneficiaries), or

- The test is not related to the treatment of ESRD, in which case the supplier would append modifier "AY".

Contractors shall make payment for organ disease panels according to the Clinical Laboratory Fee Schedule and shall apply the normal ESRD PPS editing rules for independent laboratory claims. The aforementioned organ disease panel codes were added to the list of bundled ESRD PPS laboratory tests in January 2012.

Effective for dates of service on and after April 1, 2015, contractors shall allow organ disease panel codes (i.e., HCPCS codes 80047, 80048, 80051, 80053, 80061, 80069, and 80076) to be billed by ESRD facilities for AMCC panel tests furnished to ESRD eligible beneficiaries if:

- These codes best describe the laboratory services provided to the beneficiary, which are paid under the ESRD PPS, or

- The test is not related to the treatment of ESRD, in which case the ESRD facility would append modifier "AY" and the service may be paid separately from the ESRD PPS.

Instructions for Services Provided Prior to January 1, 2011

For claims with dates of service prior to January 1, 2011, Medicare will apply the following rules to Automated Multi-Channel Chemistry (AMCC) tests for ESRD beneficiaries:

- Payment is at the lowest rate for tests performed by the same provider, for the same beneficiary, for the same date of service.

- The facility/laboratory must identify, for a particular date of service, the AMCC tests ordered that are included in the composite rate and those that are not included. See Publication 100-2, Chapter 11, Section 30.2.2 for the chart detailing the composite rate tests for Hemodialysis, Intermittent Peritoneal Dialysis (IPD), Continuous Cycling Peritoneal Dialysis (CCPD), and Hemofiltration as well as a second chart detailing the composite rate tests for Continuous Ambulatory Peritoneal Dialysis (CAPD).

- If 50 percent or more of the covered tests are included under the composite rate payment, then all submitted tests are included within the composite payment. In this case, no separate payment in addition to the composite rate is made for any of the separately billable tests.

- If less than 50 percent of the covered tests are composite rate tests, all AMCC tests submitted for that Date of Service (DOS) for that beneficiary are separately payable.

- A noncomposite rate test is defined as any test separately payable outside of the composite rate or beyond the normal frequency covered under the composite rate that is reasonable and necessary.

- For carrier processed claims, all chemistries ordered for beneficiaries with chronic dialysis for ESRD must be billed individually and must be rejected when billed as a panel.

(See §100.6UH for details regarding pricing modifiers.)

Implementation of this Policy:

ESRD facilities when ordering an ESRD-related AMCC must specify for each test within the AMCC whether the test:

a. Is part of the composite rate and not separately payable;

b. Is a composite rate test but is, on the date of the order, beyond the frequency covered under the composite rate and thus separately payable; or

c. Is not part of the ESRD composite rate and thus separately payable.

Laboratories must:

a. Identify which tests, if any, are not included within the ESRD facility composite rate payment

b. Identify which tests ordered for chronic dialysis for ESRD as follows:

   1) Modifier CD: AMCC Test has been ordered by an ESRD facility or MCP physician that is part of the composite rate and is not separately billable.

   2) Modifier CE: AMCC Test has been ordered by an ESRD facility or MCP physician that is a composite rate test but is beyond the normal frequency covered under the rate and is separately reimbursable based on medical necessity.

   3) Modifier CF: AMCC Test has been ordered by an ESRD facility or MCP physician that is not part of the composite rate and is separately billable.

c. Bill all tests ordered for a chronic dialysis ESRD beneficiary individually and not as a panel.

The shared system must calculate the number of AMCC tests provided for any given date of service. Sum all AMCC tests with a CD modifier and divide the sum of all tests with a CD, CE, and CF modifier for the same beneficiary and provider for any given date of service.

If the result of the calculation for a date of service is 50 percent or greater, do not pay for the tests.

If the result of the calculation for a date of service is less than 50 percent, pay for all of the tests.

For FI processed claims, all tests for a date of service must be billed on the monthly ESRD bill. Providers that submit claims to a FI must send in an adjustment if they identify additional tests that have not been billed.

Carrier standard systems shall adjust the previous claim when the incoming claim for a date of service is compared to a claim on history and the action is adjust payment. Carrier standard systems shall spread the payment amount over each line item on both claims (the claim on history and the incoming claim).

The organ and disease oriented panels (80048, 80051, 80053, and 80076) are subject to the 50 percent rule. However, clinical diagnostic laboratories shall not bill these services as panels, they must be billed individually. Laboratory tests that are not covered under the composite rate and that are furnished to CAPD end stage renal disease (ESRD) patients dialyzing at home are billed in the same way as any other test furnished home patients.

FI Business Requirements for ESRD Reimbursement of AMCC Tests:

Requirement #	Requirements	Responsibility
1.1	The FI shared system must RTP a claim for AMCC tests when a claim for that date of service has already been submitted.	Shared system
1.2	Based upon the presence of the CD, CE and CF payment modifiers, identify the AMCC tests ordered that are included and not included in the composite rate payment.	Shared System
1.3	Based upon the determination of requirement 1.2, if 50 percent or more of the covered tests are included under the composite rate payment, no separate payment is made.	Shared System
1.4	Based upon the determination of requirement 1.2, if less than 50 percent are covered tests included under the composite rate, all AMCC tests for that date of service are payable.	Shared System
1.5	Effective for claims with dates of service on or after January 1, 2006, include any line items with a modifier 91 used in conjunction with the "CD," "CE," or "CF" modifier in the calculation of the 50/50 rule.	Shared System
1.6	FIs must return any claims for additional tests for any date of service within the billing period when the provider has already submitted a claim. Instruct the provider to adjust the first claim.	FI or Shared System
1.7	After the calculation of the 50/50 rule, services used to determine the payment amount may never exceed 22. Effective for claims with dates of service on or after January 1, 2006, accept all valid line items submitted for the date of service and pay a maximum of the ATP 22 rate.	Shared System

Carrier Business Requirements for ESRD Reimbursement of AMCC Tests:

Requirement #	Requirements	Responsibility
1	The standard systems shall calculate payment at the lowest rate for these automated tests even if reported on separate claims for services performed by the same provider, for the same beneficiary, for the same date of service.	Standard Systems
2	Standard Systems shall identify the AMCC tests ordered that are included and are not included in the composite rate payment based upon the presence of the "CD," "CE" and "CF" modifiers.	Standard Systems
3	Based upon the determination of requirement 2 if 50 percent or more of the covered services are included under the composite rate payment, Standard Systems shall indicate that no separate payment is provided for the services submitted for that date of service.	Standard Systems
4	Based upon the determination of requirement 2 if less than 50 percent are covered services included under the composite rate, Standard Systems shall indicate that all AMCC tests for that date of service are payable under the 50/50 rule.	Standard Systems
5	Effective for claims with dates of service on or after January 1, 2006, include any line items with a modifier 91 used in conjunction with the "CD," "CE," or "CF" modifier in the calculation of the 50/50 rule.	Standard Systems
6	Standard Systems shall adjust the previous claim when the incoming claim is compared to the claim on history and the action is to deny the previous claim. Spread the payment amount over each line item on both claims (the adjusted claim and the incoming claim).	Standard Systems
7	Standard Systems shall spread the adjustment across the incoming claim unless the adjusted amount would exceed the submitted amount of the services on the claim.	Standard System

Requirement #	Requirements	Responsibility
8	After the calculation of the 50/50 rule, services used to determine the payment amount may never exceed 22. Accept all valid line items for the date of service and pay a maximum of the ATP 22 rate.	Standard Systems

Examples of the Application of the 50/50 Rule

The following examples are to illustrate how claims should be paid. The percentages in the action section represent the number of composite rate tests over the total tests. If this percentage is 50 percent or greater, no payment should be made for the claim.

Example 1:
Provider Name: Jones Hospital
DOS 2/1/02

Claim/Services
82040 Mod CD
82310 Mod CD
82374 Mod CD
82435 Mod CD
82947 Mod CF
84295 Mod CF
82040 Mod CD (Returned as duplicate)
84075 Mod CE
82310 Mod CE
84155 Mod CE

ACTION: 9 services total, 2 non-composite rate tests, 3 composite rate tests beyond the frequency, 4 composite rate tests; 4/9 = 44.4%<50% pay at ATP 09

Example 2:
Provider Name: Bon Secours Renal Facility
DOS 2/15/02

Claim/Services
82040 Mod CE and Mod 91
84450 Mod CE
82310 Mod CE
82247 Mod CF
82465 No modifier present
82565 Mod CE
84550 Mod CF
82040 Mod CD
84075 Mod CE
82435 Mod CE
82550 Mod CF
82947 Mod CF
82977 Mod CF

ACTION: 12 services total, 5 non-composite rate tests, 6 composite rate tests beyond the frequency, 1 composite rate test; 1/12 = 8.3%<50% pay at ATP 12

Example 3:
Provider Name: Sinai Hospital Renal Facility
DOS 4/02/02

Claim/Services
82565 Mod CD
83615 Mod CD
82247 Mod CF
82248 Mod CF
82040 Mod CD
84450 Mod CD
82565 Mod CE

100-4, 16, 70.8

Certificate of Waiver

Effective September 1, 1992, all laboratory testing sites (except as provided in 42 CFR 493.3(b)) must have either a CLIA certificate of waiver, certificate for provider-performed microscopy procedures, certificate of registration, certificate of compliance, or certificate of accreditation to legally perform clinical laboratory testing on specimens from individuals in the United States.

The Food and Drug Administration approves CLIA waived tests on a flow basis. The CMS identifies CLIA waived tests by providing an updated list of waived tests to the Medicare contractors on a quarterly basis via a Recurring Update Notification. To be recognized as a waived test, some CLIA waived tests have unique HCPCS procedure codes and some must have a QW modifier included with the HCPCS code.

For a list of specific HCPCS codes subject to CLIA see

http://www.cms.hhs.gov/CLIA/downloads/waivetbl.pdf

100-4, 18, 10.2.2.1

FI Payment for Pneumococcal Pneumonia Virus, Influenza Virus, and Hepatitis B Virus Vaccines and Their Administration

Payment for Vaccines

Payment for all of these vaccines is on a reasonable cost basis for hospitals, home health agencies (HHAs), skilled nursing facilities (SNFs), critical access hospitals (CAHs), and hospital-based renal dialysis facilities (RDFs). Payment for comprehensive outpatient rehabilitation facilities (CORFs), Indian Health Service hospitals (IHS), IHS

CAHs and independent RDFs is based on 95 percent of the average wholesale price (AWP). Section 10.2.4 of this chapter contains information on payment of these vaccines when provided by RDFs or hospices. See §10.2.2.2 for payment to independent and provider- based Rural Health Centers and Federally Qualified Health Clinics.

Payment for these vaccines is as follows:

Facility	Type of Bill	Payment
Hospitals, other than Indian Health Service (IHS) Hospitals and Critical Access Hospitals (CAHs)	12x, 13x	Reasonable cost
IHS Hospitals	12x, 13x, 83x	95% of AWP
IHS CAHs	85x	95% of AWP
CAHs Method I and Method II	85x	Reasonable cost
Skilled Nursing Facilities	22x, 23x	Reasonable cost
Home Health Agencies	34x	Reasonable cost
Comprehensive Outpatient Rehabilitation Facilities	75x	95% of the AWP
Independent Renal Dialysis Facilities	72x	95% of the AWP
Hospital-based Renal Dialysis Facilities	72x	Reasonable cost

Payment for Vaccine Administration

Payment for the administration of Influenza Virus and PPV vaccines is as follows:

Facility	Type of Bill	Payment
Hospitals, other than IHS Hospitals and CAHs	12x, 13x	Outpatient Prospective Payment System (OPPS) for hospitals subject to OPPS Reasonable cost for hospitals not subject to OPPS
IHS Hospitals	12x, 13x, 83x	MPFS as indicated in guidelines below.
IHS CAHs	85x	MPFS as indicated in guidelines below.
CAHs Method I and II	85x	Reasonable cost
Skilled Nursing Facilities	22x, 23x	MPFS as indicated in the guidelines below
Home Health Agencies	34x	OPPS
Comprehensive Outpatient Rehabilitation Facilities	75x	MPFS as indicated in the guidelines below
Independent RDFs	72x	MPFS as indicated in the guidelines below
Hospital-based RDFs	72x	Reasonable cost

Guidelines for pricing PPV and Influenza vaccine administration under the MPFS.

Make reimbursement based on the rate in the MPFS associated with the CPT code 90782 or 90471 as follows:

HCPCS code	Effective prior to March 1, 2003	Effective on and after March 1, 2003
G0008	90782	90471
G0009	90782	90471

See §10.2.2.2 for payment to independent and provider based Rural Health Centers and Federally Qualified Health Clinics.

Payment for the administration of Hepatitis B vaccine is as follows:

Facility	Type of Bill	Payment
Hospitals other than IHS hospitals and CAHs	12x, 13x	Outpatient Prospective Payment System (OPPS) for hospitals subject to OPPS Reasonable cost for hospitals not subject to OPPS
IHS Hospitals	12x, 13x, 83x	MPFS as indicated in the guidelines below
CAHs	85x	Reasonable cost
Method I and II		
IHS CAHs	85x	MPFS as indicated in guidelines below.
Skilled Nursing Facilities	22x, 23x	MPFS as indicated in the chart below
Home Health Agencies	34x	OPPS

Facility	Type of Bill	Payment
Comprehensive Outpatient Rehabilitation Facilities	75x	MPFS as indicated in the guidelines below
Independent RDFs	72x	MPFS as indicated in the chart below
Hospital-based RDFs	72x	Reasonable cost

Guidelines for pricing Hepatitis B vaccine administration under the MPFS.

Make reimbursement based on the rate in the MPFS associated with the CPT code 90782 or 90471 as follows:

HCPCS code	Effective prior to March 1, 2003	Effective on and after March 1, 2003
G0010	90782	90471

See §10.2.2.2 for payment to independent and provider based Rural Health Centers and Federally Qualified Health Clinics.

100-4, 18, 10.4

CWF Edits

In order to prevent duplicate payments for influenza virus and pneumococcal vaccination claims by the local contractor/AB MAC and the centralized billing contractor, effective for claims received on or after July 1, 2002, CWF has implemented a number of edits.

NOTE: 90659 was discontinued December 31, 2003.

CWF returns information in Trailer 13 information from the history claim. The following fields are returned to the contractor:

- Trailer Code;
- Contractor Number;
- Document Control Number;
- First Service Date;
- Last Service Date;
- Provider, Physician, Supplier Number;
- Claim Type; Procedure code;
- Alert Code (where applicable); and,
- More history (where applicable.)

100-4, 18, 80.2

A/B Medicare Administrative Contractor (MAC) (B) Billing Requirements

Effective for dates of service on and after January 1, 2005, through December 31, 2008, contractors shall recognize the HCPCS codes G0344, G0366, G0367, and G0368 shown above in §80.1 for an IPPE. The type of service (TOS) for each of these codes is as follows:

G0344: TOS = 1

G0366: TOS = 5

G0367: TOS = 5

G0368: TOS = 5

Contractors shall pay physicians or qualified nonphysician practitioners for only one IPPE performed not later than 6 months after the date the individual's first coverage begins under Medicare Part B, but only if that coverage period begins on or after January 1, 2005.

Effective for dates of service on and after January 1, 2009, contractors shall recognize the HCPCS codes G0402, G0403, G0404, and G0405 shown above in §80.1 for an IPPE. The TOS for each of these codes is as follows:

G0402: TOS = 1

G0403: TOS = 5

G0404: TOS = 5

G0405: TOS = 5

Under the MIPPA of 2008, contractors shall pay physicians or qualified nonphysician practitioners for only one IPPE performed not later than 12 months after the date the individual's first coverage begins under Medicare Part B only if that coverage period begins on or after January 1, 2009.

Contractors shall allow payment for a medically necessary Evaluation and Management (E/M) service at the same visit as the IPPE when it is clinically appropriate. Physicians and qualified nonphysician practitioners shall use CPT codes 99201-99215 to report an E/M with CPT modifier 25 to indicate that the E/M is a significant, separately identifiable service from the IPPE code reported (G0344 or G0402, whichever applies based on the date the IPPE is performed). Refer to chapter 12, § 30.6.1.1, of this manual for the physician/practitioner billing correct coding and payment policy regarding E/M services.

If the EKG performed as a component of the IPPE is not performed by the primary physician or qualified NPP during the IPPE visit, another physician or entity may perform and/or interpret the EKG. The referring physician or qualified NPP needs to make sure that the performing physician or entity bills the appropriate G code for the screening EKG, and not a CPT code in the 93000 series. **Both the IPPE and the EKG should be billed in order for the beneficiary to receive the complete IPPE service.** Effective for dates of service on and after January 1, 2009, the screening EKG is optional and is no longer a mandated service of an IPPE if performed as a result of a referral from an IPPE.

Should the same physician or NPP need to perform an additional medically necessary EKG in the 93000 series on the same day as the IPPE, report the appropriate EKG CPT code(s) with modifier 59, indicating that the EKG is a distinct procedural service.

Physicians or qualified nonphysician practitioners shall bill the contractor the appropriate HCPCS codes for IPPE on the Form CMS-1500 claim or an approved electronic format. The HCPCS codes for an IPPE and screening EKG are paid under the Medicare Physician Fee Schedule (MPFS).

See §1.3 of this chapter for waiver of cost sharing requirements of coinsurance, copayment and deductible for furnished preventive services available in Medicare.

100-4, 32, 10.1

Ambulatory Blood Pressure Monitoring (ABPM) Billing Requirements

A. Coding Applicable to A/B MACs (A and B)

Effective April 1, 2002, a National Coverage Decision was made to allow for Medicare coverage of ABPM for those beneficiaries with suspected "white coat hypertension" (WCH). ABPM involves the use of a non-invasive device, which is used to measure blood pressure in 24-hour cycles. These 24-hour measurements are stored in the device and are later interpreted by a physician. Suspected "WCH" is defined as: (1) Clinic/office blood pressure >140/90 mm Hg on at least three separate clinic/office visits with two separate measurements made at each visit; (2) At least two documented separate blood pressure measurements taken outside the clinic/office which are < 140/90 mm Hg; and (3) No evidence of end-organ damage. ABPM is not covered for any other uses. Coverage policy can be found in Medicare National Coverage Determinations Manual, Chapter 1, Part 1, §20.19. (http://www.cms.hhs.gov/manuals/103_cov_determ/ncd103index.asp).

The ABPM must be performed for at least 24 hours to meet coverage criteria. Payment is not allowed for institutionalized beneficiaries, such as those receiving Medicare covered skilled nursing in a facility. In the rare circumstance that ABPM needs to be performed more than once for a beneficiary, the qualifying criteria described above must be met for each subsequent ABPM test.

Effective dates for applicable Common Procedure Coding System (HCPCS) codes for ABPM for suspected WCH and their covered effective dates are as follows:

HCPCS	Definition	Effective Date
93784	ABPM, utilizing a system such as magnetic tape and/or computer disk, for 24 hours or longer; including recording, scanning analysis, interpretation and report.	04/01/2002
93786	ABPM, utilizing a system such as magnetic tape and/or computer disk, for 24 hours or longer; recording only.	04/01/2002
93788	ABPM, utilizing a system such as magnetic tape and/or computer disk, for 24 hours or longer; scanning analysis with report.	01/01/2004
93790	ABPM, utilizing a system such as magnetic tape and/or computer disk, for 24 hours or longer; physician review with interpretation and report.	04/01/2002

In addition, one of the following diagnosis codes must be present:

	Diagnosis Code	Description
If ICD-9-CM is applicable	796.2	Elevated blood pressure reading without diagnosis of hypertension.
If ICD-10-CM is applicable	R03.0	Elevated blood pressure reading without diagnosis of hypertension

B. A/B MAC (A) Billing Instructions

The applicable types of bills acceptable when billing for ABPM services are 13X, 23X, 71X, 73X, 75X, and 85X. Chapter 25 of this manual provides general billing instructions that must be followed for bills submitted to A/B MACs (A). The A/B MACs (A) pay for hospital outpatient ABPM services billed on a 13X type of bill with HCPCS 93786 and/or 93788 as follows: (1) Outpatient Prospective Payment System (OPPS) hospitals pay based on the Ambulatory Payment Classification (APC); (2) non-OPPS hospitals (Indian Health Services Hospitals, Hospitals that provide Part B services only, and hospitals located in American Samoa, Guam, Saipan and the Virgin Islands) pay based on reasonable cost, except for Maryland Hospitals which are paid based on a percentage of cost. Effective 4/1/06, type of bill 14X is for non-patient laboratory specimens and is no longer applicable for ABPM.

The A/B MACs (A) pay for comprehensive outpatient rehabilitation facility (CORF) ABPM services billed on a 75x type of bill with HCPCS code 93786 and/or 93788 based on the Medicare Physician Fee Schedule (MPFS) amount for that HCPCS code.

The A/B MACs (A) pay for ABPM services for critical access hospitals (CAHs) billed on a 85x type of bill as follows: (1) for CAHs that elected the Standard Method and billed HCPCS code 93786 and/or 93788, pay based on reasonable cost for that HCPCS code; and (2) for CAHs that elected the Optional Method and billed any combination of HCPCS codes 93786, 93788 and 93790 pay based on reasonable cost for HCPCS 93786 and 93788 and pay 115% of the MPFS amount for HCPCS 93790.

The A/B MACs (A) pay for ABPM services for skilled nursing facility (SNF) outpatients billed on a 23x type of bill with HCPCS code 93786 and/or 93788, based on the MPFS.

The A/B MACs (A) accept independent and provider-based rural health clinic (RHC) bills for visits under the all-inclusive rate when the RHC bills on a 71x type of bill with revenue code 052x for providing the professional component of ABPM services. The A/B MACs (A) should not make a separate payment to a RHC for the professional component of ABPM services in addition to the all-inclusive rate. RHCs are not required to use ABPM HCPCS codes for professional services covered under the all-inclusive rate.

The A/B MACs (A) accept free-standing and provider-based federally qualified health center (FQHC) bills for visits under the all-inclusive rate when the FQHC bills on a 73x type of bill with revenue code 052x for providing the professional component of ABPM services.

The A/B MACs (A) should not make a separate payment to a FQHC for the professional component of ABPM services in addition to the all-inclusive rate. FQHCs are not required to use ABPM HCPCS codes for professional services covered under the all-inclusive rate.

The A/B MACs (A) pay provider-based RHCs/FQHCs for the technical component of ABPM services when billed under the base provider's number using the above requirements for that particular base provider type, i.e., a OPPS hospital based RHC would be paid for the ABPM technical component services under the OPPS using the APC for code 93786 and/or 93788 when billed on a 13x type of bill.

Independent and free-standing RHC/FQHC practitioners are only paid for providing the technical component of ABPM services when billed to the A/B MAC (B) following the MAC's instructions.

C. A/B MAC (B) Claims

A/B MACs (B) pay for ABPM services billed with ICD-9-CM diagnosis code 796.2 (if ICD-9 is applicable) or, if ICD-10 is applicable, ICD-10-CM diagnosis code R03.0 and HCPCS codes 93784 or for any combination of 93786, 93788 and 93790, based on the MPFS for the specific HCPCS code billed.

D. Coinsurance and Deductible

The A/B MACs (A and B) shall apply coinsurance and deductible to payments for ABPM services except for services billed to the A/B MAC (A) by FQHCs. For FQHCs only co-insurance applies.

100-4, 32, 30.1

Billing Requirements for HBO Therapy for the Treatment of Diabetic Wounds of the Lower Extremities

Hyperbaric Oxygen Therapy is a modality in which the entire body is exposed to oxygen under increased atmospheric pressure. Effective April 1, 2003, a National Coverage Decision expanded the use of HBO therapy to include coverage for the treatment of diabetic wounds of the lower extremities. For specific coverage criteria for HBO Therapy, refer to the National Coverage Determinations Manual, Chapter 1, section 20.29.

NOTE: Topical application of oxygen does not meet the definition of HBO therapy as stated above. Also, its clinical efficacy has not been established. Therefore, no Medicare reimbursement may be made for the topical application of oxygen.

I.   Billing Requirements for A/B MACs (A)

Claims for HBO therapy should be submitted using the ASC X12 837 institutional claim format or, in rare cases, on Form CMS-1450.

a. Applicable Bill Types

The applicable hospital bill types are 11X, 13X and 85X.

b. Procedural Coding

99183– Physician attendance and supervision of hyperbaric oxygen therapy, per session.

C1300 – Hyperbaric oxygen under pressure, full body chamber, per 30-minute interval.

NOTE: Code C1300 is not available for use other than in a hospital outpatient department. In skilled nursing facilities (SNFs), HBO therapy is part of the SNF PPS payment for beneficiaries in covered Part A stays.

For hospital inpatients and critical access hospitals (CAHs) not electing Method I, HBO therapy is reported under revenue code 940 without any HCPCS code. For inpatient services, if ICD-9-is applicable, show ICD-9-CM procedure code 93.59. If ICD-10 is applicable, show ICD-10-PCS code 5A05121.

For CAHs electing Method I, HBO therapy is reported under revenue code 940 along with HCPCS code 99183.

c. Payment Requirements for A/B MACs (A)

Payment is as follows:

A/B MAC (A) payment is allowed for HBO therapy for diabetic wounds of the lower extremities when performed as a physician service in a hospital outpatient setting and for inpatients. Payment is allowed for claims with valid diagnosis codes as shown above with dates of service on or after April 1, 2003. Those claims with invalid codes should be denied as not medically necessary.

For hospitals, payment will be based upon the Ambulatory Payment Classification (APC) or the inpatient Diagnosis Related Group (DRG). Deductible and coinsurance apply.

Payment to Critical Access Hospitals (electing Method I) is made under cost reimbursement. For Critical Access Hospitals electing Method II, the technical component is paid under cost reimbursement and the professional component is paid under the Physician Fee Schedule.

II. A/B MAC (B) Billing Requirements

Claims for this service should be submitted using the ASC X12 837 professional claim format or Form CMS-1500.

The following HCPCS code applies:

99183 – Physician attendance and supervision of hyperbaric oxygen therapy, per session.

a. Payment Requirements for A/B MACs (B)

Payment and pricing information will occur through updates to the Medicare Physician Fee Schedule Database (MPFSDB). Pay for this service on the basis of the MPFSDB. Deductible and coinsurance apply. Claims from physicians or other practitioners whose assignment was not taken, are subject to the Medicare limiting charge.

III. Medicare Summary Notices (MSNs)

Use the following MSN Messages where appropriate:

In situations where the claim is being denied on the basis that the condition does not meet our coverage requirements, use one of the following MSN Messages:

"Medicare does not pay for this item or service for this condition." (MSN Message 16.48)

The Spanish version of the MSN message should read:

"Medicare no paga por este articulo o servicio para esta afeccion."

In situations where, based on the above utilization policy, medical review of the claim results in a determination that the service is not medically necessary, use the following MSN message:

"The information provided does not support the need for this service or item." (MSN Message 15.4)

The Spanish version of the MSN message should read:

"La informacion proporcionada no confirma la necesidad para este servicio o articulo."

IV. Remittance Advice Notices

Use appropriate existing remittance advice remark codes and claim adjustment reason codes at the line level to express the specific reason if you deny payment for HBO therapy for the treatment of diabetic wounds of lower extremities.

100-4, 32, 60.4.1

Allowable Covered Diagnosis Codes

Allowable Covered Diagnosis Codes

For services furnished on or after July 1, 2002, the applicable ICD-9-CM diagnosis code for this benefit is V43.3, organ or tissue replaced by other means; heart valve.

For services furnished on or after March 19, 2008, the applicable ICD-9-CM diagnosis codes for this benefit are:

- V43.3 (organ or tissue replaced by other means; heart valve),
- 289.81 (primary hypercoagulable state),
- 451.0-451.9 (includes 451.11, 451.19, 451.2, 451.80-451.84, 451.89) (phlebitis & thrombophlebitis),
- 453.0-453.3 (other venous embolism & thrombosis),
- 453.40-453.49 (includes 453.40-453.42, 453.8-453.9) (venous embolism and thrombosis of the deep vessels of the lower extremity, and other specified veins/unspecified sites)
- 415.11-415.12, 415.19 (pulmonary embolism & infarction) or,
- 427.31 (atrial fibrillation (established) (paroxysmal)).

For services furnished on or after the implementation of ICD-10 the applicable ICD-10-CM diagnosis codes for this benefit are:

Heart Valve Replacement

- Z95.2 - Presence of prosthetic heart valve

Primary Hypercoagulable State

ICD-10-CM	Code Description
D68.51	Activated protein C resistance

ICD-10-CM	Code Description
D68.52	Prothrombin gene mutation
D68.59	Other primary thrombophilia
D68.61	Antiphospholipid syndrome
D68.62	Lupus anticoagulant syndrome

Phlebitis & Thrombophlebitis

ICD-10-CM	Code Description
I80.00	Phlebitis and thrombophlebitis of superficial vessels of unspecified lower extremity
I80.01	Phlebitis and thrombophlebitis of superficial vessels of right lower extremity
I80.02	Phlebitis and thrombophlebitis of superficial vessels of left lower extremity
I80.03	Phlebitis and thrombophlebitis of superficial vessels of lower extremities, bilateral
I80.10	Phlebitis and thrombophlebitis of unspecified femoral vein
I80.11	Phlebitis and thrombophlebitis of right femoral vein
I80.12	Phlebitis and thrombophlebitis of left femoral vein
I80.13	Phlebitis and thrombophlebitis of femoral vein, bilateral
I80.201	Phlebitis and thrombophlebitis of unspecified deep vessels of right lower extremity
I80.202	Phlebitis and thrombophlebitis of unspecified deep vessels of left lower extremity
I80.203	Phlebitis and thrombophlebitis of unspecified deep vessels of lower extremities, bilateral
I80.209	Phlebitis and thrombophlebitis of unspecified deep vessels of unspecified lower extremity
I80.221	Phlebitis and thrombophlebitis of right popliteal vein
I80.222	Phlebitis and thrombophlebitis of left popliteal vein
I80.223	Phlebitis and thrombophlebitis of popliteal vein, bilateral
I80.229	Phlebitis and thrombophlebitis of unspecified popliteal vein
I80.231	Phlebitis and thrombophlebitis of right tibial vein
I80.232	Phlebitis and thrombophlebitis of left tibial vein
I80.233	Phlebitis and thrombophlebitis of tibial vein, bilateral
I80.239	Phlebitis and thrombophlebitis of unspecified tibial vein
I80.291	Phlebitis and thrombophlebitis of other deep vessels of right lower extremity
I80.292	Phlebitis and thrombophlebitis of other deep vessels of left lower extremity
I80.293	Phlebitis and thrombophlebitis of other deep vessels of lower extremity, bilateral
I80.299	Phlebitis and thrombophlebitis of other deep vessels of unspecified lower extremity
I80.3	Phlebitis and thrombophlebitis of lower extremities, unspecified
I80.211	Phlebitis and thrombophlebitis of right iliac vein
I80.212	Phlebitis and thrombophlebitis of left iliac vein
I80.213	Phlebitis and thrombophlebitis of iliac vein, bilateral
I80.219	Phlebitis and thrombophlebitis of unspecified iliac vein
I80.8	Phlebitis and thrombophlebitis of other sites
I80.9	Phlebitis and thrombophlebitis of unspecified site

Other Venous Embolism & Thrombosis

ICD-10-CM	Code Description
I82.0	Budd- Chiari syndrome
I82.1	Thrombophlebitis migrans
I82.211	Chronic embolism and thrombosis of superior vena cava
I82.220	Acute embolism and thrombosis of inferior vena cava
I82.221	Chronic embolism and thrombosis of inferior vena cava
I82.291	Chronic embolism and thrombosis of other thoracic veins
I82.3	Embolism and thrombosis of renal vein

Venous Embolism and thrombosis of the deep vessels of the lower extremity, and other specified veins/unspecified sites

ICD-10-CM	Code Description
I82.401	Acute embolism and thrombosis of unspecified deep veins of right lower extremity
I82.402	Acute embolism and thrombosis of unspecified deep veins of left lower extremity
I82.403	Acute embolism and thrombosis of unspecified deep veins of lower extremity, bilateral
I82.409	Acute embolism and thrombosis of unspecified deep veins of unspecified lower extremity
I82.411	Acute embolism and thrombosis of right femoral vein
I82.412	Acute embolism and thrombosis of left femoral vein
I82.413	Acute embolism and thrombosis of femoral vein, bilateral
I82.419	Acute embolism and thrombosis of unspecified femoral vein
I82.421	Acute embolism and thrombosis of right iliac vein
I82.422	Acute embolism and thrombosis of left iliac vein
I82.423	Acute embolism and thrombosis of iliac vein, bilateral
I82.429	Acute embolism and thrombosis of unspecified iliac vein
I82.431	Acute embolism and thrombosis of right popliteal vein
I82.432	Acute embolism and thrombosis of left popliteal vein
I82.433	Acute embolism and thrombosis of popliteal vein, bilateral
I82.439	Acute embolism and thrombosis of unspecified popliteal vein
I82.4Y1	Acute embolism and thrombosis of unspecified deep veins of right proximal lower extremity
I82.4Y2	Acute embolism and thrombosis of unspecified deep veins of left proximal lower extremity
I82.4Y3	Acute embolism and thrombosis of unspecified deep veins of proximal lower extremity, bilateral
I82.4Y9	Acute embolism and thrombosis of unspecified deep veins of unspecified proximal lower extremity
I82.441	Acute embolism and thrombosis of right tibial vein
I82.442	Acute embolism and thrombosis of left tibial vein
I82.443	Acute embolism and thrombosis of tibial vein, bilateral
I82.449	Acute embolism and thrombosis of unspecified tibial vein
I82.491	Acute embolism and thrombosis of other specified deep vein of right lower extremity
I82.492	Acute embolism and thrombosis of other specified deep vein of left lower extremity
I82.493	Acute embolism and thrombosis of other specified deep vein of lower extremity, bilateral
I82.499	Acute embolism and thrombosis of other specified deep vein of unspecified lower extremity
I82.4Z1	Acute embolism and thrombosis of unspecified deep veins of right distal lower extremity
I82.4Z2	Acute embolism and thrombosis of unspecified deep veins of left distal lower extremity
I82.4Z3	Acute embolism and thrombosis of unspecified deep veins of distal lower extremity, bilateral
I82.4Z9	Acute embolism and thrombosis of unspecified deep veins of unspecified distal lower extremity
I82.501	Chronic embolism and thrombosis of unspecified deep veins of right lower extremity
I82.502	Chronic embolism and thrombosis of unspecified deep veins of left lower extremity
I82.503	Chronic embolism and thrombosis of unspecified deep veins of lower extremity, bilateral
I82.509	Chronic embolism and thrombosis of unspecified deep veins of unspecified lower extremity
I82.591	Chronic embolism and thrombosis of other specified deep vein of right lower extremity

ICD-10-CM	Code Description
I82.592	Chronic embolism and thrombosis of other specified deep vein of left lower extremity
I82.593	Chronic embolism and thrombosis of other specified deep vein of lower extremity, bilateral
I82.599	Chronic embolism and thrombosis of other specified deep vein of unspecified lower extremity
I82.511	Chronic embolism and thrombosis of right femoral vein
I82.512	Chronic embolism and thrombosis of left femoral vein
I82.513	Chronic embolism and thrombosis of femoral vein, bilateral
I82.519	Chronic embolism and thrombosis of unspecified femoral vein
I82.521	Chronic embolism and thrombosis of right iliac vein
I82.522	Chronic embolism and thrombosis of left iliac vein
I82.523	Chronic embolism and thrombosis of iliac vein, bilateral
I82.529	Chronic embolism and thrombosis of unspecified iliac vein
I82.531	Chronic embolism and thrombosis of right popliteal vein
I82.532	Chronic embolism and thrombosis of left popliteal vein
I82.533	Chronic embolism and thrombosis of popliteal vein, bilateral
I82.539	Chronic embolism and thrombosis of unspecified popliteal vein
I82.5Y1	Chronic embolism and thrombosis of unspecified deep veins of right proximal lower extremity
I82.5Y2	Chronic embolism and thrombosis of unspecified deep veins of left proximal lower extremity
I82.5Y3	Chronic embolism and thrombosis of unspecified deep veins of proximal lower extremity, bilateral
I82.5Y9	Chronic embolism and thrombosis of unspecified deep veins of unspecified proximal lower extremity
I82.541	Chronic embolism and thrombosis of right tibial vein
I82.542	Chronic embolism and thrombosis of left tibial vein
I82.543	Chronic embolism and thrombosis of tibial vein, bilateral
I82.549	Chronic embolism and thrombosis of unspecified tibial vein
I82.5Z1	Chronic embolism and thrombosis of unspecified deep veins of right distal lower extremity
I82.5Z2	Chronic embolism and thrombosis of unspecified deep veins of left distal lower extremity
I82.5Z3	Chronic embolism and thrombosis of unspecified deep veins of distal lower extremity, bilateral
I82.5Z9	Chronic embolism and thrombosis of unspecified deep veins of unspecified distal lower extremity
I82.611	Acute embolism and thrombosis of superficial veins of right upper extremity
I82.612	Acute embolism and thrombosis of superficial veins of left upper extremity
I82.613	Acute embolism and thrombosis of superficial veins of upper extremity, bilateral
I82.619	Acute embolism and thrombosis of superficial veins of unspecified upper extremity
I82.621	Acute embolism and thrombosis of deep veins of right upper extremity
I82.622	Acute embolism and thrombosis of deep veins of left upper extremity
I82.623	Acute embolism and thrombosis of deep veins of upper extremity, bilateral
I82.629	Acute embolism and thrombosis of deep veins of unspecified upper extremity
I82.601	Acute embolism and thrombosis of unspecified veins of right upper extremity
I82.602	Acute embolism and thrombosis of unspecified veins of left upper extremity
I82.603	Acute embolism and thrombosis of unspecified veins of upper extremity, bilateral
I82.609	Acute embolism and thrombosis of unspecified veins of unspecified upper extremity
I82.A11	Acute embolism and thrombosis of right axillary vein
I82.A12	Acute embolism and thrombosis of left axillary vein
I82.A13	Acute embolism and thrombosis of axillary vein, bilateral
I82.A19	Acute embolism and thrombosis of unspecified axillary vein
I82.A21	Chronic embolism and thrombosis of right axillary vein
I82.A22	Chronic embolism and thrombosis of left axillary vein
I82.A23	Chronic embolism and thrombosis of axillary vein, bilateral
I82.A29	Chronic embolism and thrombosis of unspecified axillary vein
I82.B11	Acute embolism and thrombosis of right subclavian vein

ICD-10-CM	Code Description
I82.B12	Acute embolism and thrombosis of left subclavian vein
I82.B13	Acute embolism and thrombosis of subclavian vein, bilateral
I82.B19	Acute embolism and thrombosis of unspecified subclavian vein
I82.B21	Chronic embolism and thrombosis of right subclavian vein
I82.B22	Chronic embolism and thrombosis of left subclavian vein
I82.B23	Chronic embolism and thrombosis of subclavian vein, bilateral
I82.B29	Chronic embolism and thrombosis of unspecified subclavian vein
I82.C11	Acute embolism and thrombosis of right internal jugular vein
I82.C12	Acute embolism and thrombosis of left internal jugular vein
I82.C13	Acute embolism and thrombosis of internal jugular vein, bilateral
I82.C19	Acute embolism and thrombosis of unspecified internal jugular vein
I82.C21	Chronic embolism and thrombosis of right internal jugular vein
I82.C22	Chronic embolism and thrombosis of left internal jugular vein
I82.C23	Chronic embolism and thrombosis of internal jugular vein, bilateral
I82.C29	Chronic embolism and thrombosis of unspecified internal jugular vein
I82.210	Acute embolism and thrombosis of superior vena cava
I82.290	Acute embolism and thrombosis of other thoracic veins
I82.701	Chronic embolism and thrombosis of unspecified veins of right upper extremity
I82.702	Chronic embolism and thrombosis of unspecified veins of left upper extremity
I82.703	Chronic embolism and thrombosis of unspecified veins of upper extremity, bilateral
I82.709	Chronic embolism and thrombosis of unspecified veins of unspecified upper extremity
I82.711	Chronic embolism and thrombosis of superficial veins of right upper extremity
I82.712	Chronic embolism and thrombosis of superficial veins of left upper extremity
I82.713	Chronic embolism and thrombosis of superficial veins of upper extremity, bilateral
I82.719	Chronic embolism and thrombosis of superficial veins of unspecified upper extremity
I82.721	Chronic embolism and thrombosis of deep veins of right upper extremity
I82.722	Chronic embolism and thrombosis of deep veins of left upper extremity
I82.723	Chronic embolism and thrombosis of deep veins of upper extremity, bilateral
I82.729	Chronic embolism and thrombosis of deep veins of unspecified upper extremity
I82.811	Embolism and thrombosis of superficial veins of right lower extremities
I82.812	Embolism and thrombosis of superficial veins of left lower extremities
I82.813	Embolism and thrombosis of superficial veins of lower extremities, bilateral
I82.819	Embolism and thrombosis of superficial veins of unspecified lower extremities
I82.890	Acute embolism and thrombosis of other specified veins
I82.891	Chronic embolism and thrombosis of other specified veins
I82.90	Acute embolism and thrombosis of unspecified vein
I82.91	Chronic embolism and thrombosis of unspecified vein

Pulmonary Embolism & Infarction

ICD-10-CM	Code Description
I26.90	Septic pulmonary embolism without acute cor pulmonale
I26.99	Other pulmonary embolism without acute cor pulmonale
I26.01	Septic pulmonary embolism with acute cor pulmonale
I26.90	Septic pulmonary embolism without acute cor pulmonale
I26.09	Other pulmonary embolism with acute cor pulmonale
I26.99	Other pulmonary embolism without acute cor pulmonale

Atrial Fibrillation

ICD-10-CM	Code Description
I48.0	Paroxysmal atrial fibrillation
I48.2	Chronic atrial fibrillation
I48	-91 Unspecified atrial fibrillation Other
I23.6	Thrombosis of atrium, auricular appendage, and ventricle as current complications following acute myocardial infarction

ICD-10-CM	Code Description
I27.82	Chronic pulmonary embolism
I67.6	Nonpyogenic thrombosis of intracranial venous system
O22.50	Cerebral venous thrombosis in pregnancy, unspecified trimester
O22.51	Cerebral venous thrombosis in pregnancy, first trimester
O22.52	Cerebral venous thrombosis in pregnancy, second trimester
O22.53	Cerebral venous thrombosis in pregnancy, third trimester
O87.3	Cerebral venous thrombosis in the puerperium
Z79.01	Long term (current) use of anticoagulants

Coverage policy can be found in Pub. 100-3, Medicare National Coverage Determinations Manual, Chapter 1, section 190.11 PT/INR. (http://www.cms.hhs.gov/manuals/103_cov_determ/ncd103index.asp

100-4, 32, 60.5.2

Applicable Diagnosis Codes for Carriers

Applicable Diagnosis Codes for Carriers

For services furnished on or after July 1, 2002, the applicable ICD-9-CM diagnosis code for this benefit is V43.3, organ or tissue replaced by other means; heart valve.

For services furnished on or after March 19, 2008, the applicable ICD-9-CM diagnosis codes for this benefit are:

- V43.3 (organ or tissue replaced by other means; heart valve),
- 289.81 (primary hypercoagulable state),
- 451.0-451.9 (includes 451.11, 451.19, 451.2, 451.80-451.84, 451.89) (phlebitis & thrombophlebitis),
- 453.0-453.3 (other venous embolism & thrombosis),
- 453.40-453.49 (includes 453.40-453.42, 453.8-453.9) (venous embolism and thrombosis of the deep vessels of the lower extremity, and other specified veins/unspecified sites)
- 415.11-415.12, 415.19 (pulmonary embolism & infarction) or,
- 427.31 (atrial fibrillation (established) (paroxysmal)).

For services furnished on or after implementation of ICD-10 the applicable ICD-10-CM diagnosis codes for this benefit are:

Heart Valve Replacement

- Z95.2 - Presence of prosthetic heart valve

Primary Hypercoagulable State

ICD-10-CM	Code Description
D68.51	Activated protein C resistance
D68.52	Prothrombin gene mutation
D68.59	Other primary thrombophilia
D68.61	Antiphospholipid syndrome
D68.62	Lupus anticoagulant syndrome

Phlebitis & Thrombophlebitis

ICD-10-CM	Code Description
I80.00	Phlebitis and thrombophlebitis of superficial vessels of unspecified lower extremity
I80.01	Phlebitis and thrombophlebitis of superficial vessels of right lower extremity
I80.02	Phlebitis and thrombophlebitis of superficial vessels of left lower extremity
I80.03	Phlebitis and thrombophlebitis of superficial vessels of lower extremities, bilateral
I80.10	Phlebitis and thrombophlebitis of unspecified femoral vein
I80.11	Phlebitis and thrombophlebitis of right femoral vein
I80.12	Phlebitis and thrombophlebitis of left femoral vein
I80.13	Phlebitis and thrombophlebitis of femoral vein, bilateral
I80.201	Phlebitis and thrombophlebitis of unspecified deep vessels of right lower extremity
I80.202	Phlebitis and thrombophlebitis of unspecified deep vessels of left lower extremity
I80.203	Phlebitis and thrombophlebitis of unspecified deep vessels of lower extremities, bilateral
I80.209	Phlebitis and thrombophlebitis of unspecified deep vessels of unspecified lower extremity
I80.221	Phlebitis and thrombophlebitis of right popliteal vein
I80.222	Phlebitis and thrombophlebitis of left popliteal vein
I80.223	Phlebitis and thrombophlebitis of popliteal vein, bilateral
I80.229	Phlebitis and thrombophlebitis of unspecified popliteal vein
I80.231	Phlebitis and thrombophlebitis of right tibial vein

ICD-10-CM	Code Description
I80.232	Phlebitis and thrombophlebitis of left tibial vein
I80.233	Phlebitis and thrombophlebitis of tibial vein, bilateral
I80.239	Phlebitis and thrombophlebitis of unspecified tibial vein
I80.291	Phlebitis and thrombophlebitis of other deep vessels of right lower extremity
I80.292	Phlebitis and thrombophlebitis of other deep vessels of left lower extremity
I80.293	Phlebitis and thrombophlebitis of other deep vessels of lower extremity, bilateral
I80.299	Phlebitis and thrombophlebitis of other deep vessels of unspecified lower extremity
I80.3	Phlebitis and thrombophlebitis of lower extremities, unspecified
I80.211	Phlebitis and thrombophlebitis of right iliac vein
I80.212	Phlebitis and thrombophlebitis of left iliac vein
I80.213	Phlebitis and thrombophlebitis of iliac vein, bilateral
I80.219	Phlebitis and thrombophlebitis of unspecified iliac vein
I80.8	Phlebitis and thrombophlebitis of other sites
I80.9	Phlebitis and thrombophlebitis of unspecified site

Other Venous Embolism & Thrombosis

ICD-10-CM	Code Description
I82.0	Budd- Chiari syndrome
I82.1	Thrombophlebitis migrans
I82.211	Chronic embolism and thrombosis of superior vena cava
I82220	Acute embolism and thrombosis of inferior vena cava
I82.221	Chronic embolism and thrombosis of inferior vena cava
I82.291	Chronic embolism and thrombosis of other thoracic veins
I82.3	Embolism and thrombosis of renal vein

Venous Embolism and thrombosis of the deep vessels of the lower extremity, and other specified veins/unspecified sites

ICD-10-CM	Code Description
I82.401	Acute embolism and thrombosis of unspecified deep veins of right lower extremity
I82.402	Acute embolism and thrombosis of unspecified deep veins of left lower extremity
I82.403	Acute embolism and thrombosis of unspecified deep veins of lower extremity, bilateral
I82. 409	Acute embolism and thrombosis of unspecified deep veins of unspecified lower extremity
I82.411	Acute embolism and thrombosis of right femoral vein
I82.412	Acute embolism and thrombosis of left femoral vein
I82.413	Acute embolism and thrombosis of femoral vein, bilateral
I82.419	Acute embolism and thrombosis of unspecified femoral vein
I82.421	Acute embolism and thrombosis of right iliac vein
I82.422	Acute embolism and thrombosis of left iliac vein
I82.423	Acute embolism and thrombosis of iliac vein, bilateral
I82.429	Acute embolism and thrombosis of unspecified iliac vein
I82.431	Acute embolism and thrombosis of right popliteal vein
I82.432	Acute embolism and thrombosis of left popliteal vein
I82.433	Acute embolism and thrombosis of popliteal vein, bilateral
I82.439	Acute embolism and thrombosis of unspecified popliteal vein
I82.4Y1	Acute embolism and thrombosis of unspecified deep veins of right proximal lower extremity
I82.4Y2	Acute embolism and thrombosis of unspecified deep veins of left proximal lower extremity
I82.4Y3	Acute embolism and thrombosis of unspecified deep veins of proximal lower extremity, bilateral
I82.4Y9	Acute embolism and thrombosis of unspecified deep veins of unspecified proximal lower extremity
I82.441	Acute embolism and thrombosis of right tibial vein
I82.442	Acute embolism and thrombosis of left tibial vein
I82.443	Acute embolism and thrombosis of tibial vein, bilateral
I82.449	Acute embolism and thrombosis of unspecified tibial vein
I82.491	Acute embolism and thrombosis of other specified deep vein of right lower extremity
I82.492	Acute embolism and thrombosis of other specified deep vein of left lower extremity

ICD-10-CM	Code Description
I82.493	Acute embolism and thrombosis of other specified deep vein of lower extremity, bilateral
I82.499	Acute embolism and thrombosis of other specified deep vein of unspecified lower extremity
I82.4Z1	Acute embolism and thrombosis of unspecified deep veins of right distal lower extremity
I82.4Z2	Acute embolism and thrombosis of unspecified deep veins of left distal lower extremity
I82.4Z3	Acute embolism and thrombosis of unspecified deep veins of distal lower extremity, bilateral
I82.4Z9	Acute embolism and thrombosis of unspecified deep veins of unspecified distal lower extremity
I82.501	Chronic embolism and thrombosis of unspecified deep veins of right lower extremity
I82.502	Chronic embolism and thrombosis of unspecified deep veins of left lower extremity
I82.503	Chronic embolism and thrombosis of unspecified deep veins of lower extremity, bilateral
I82.509	Chronic embolism and thrombosis of unspecified deep veins of unspecified lower extremity
I82.591	Chronic embolism and thrombosis of other specified deep vein of right lower extremity
I82.592	Chronic embolism and thrombosis of other specified deep vein of left lower extremity
I82.593	Chronic embolism and thrombosis of other specified deep vein of lower extremity, bilateral
I82.599	Chronic embolism and thrombosis of other specified deep vein of unspecified lower extremity
I82.511	Chronic embolism and thrombosis of right femoral vein
I82.512	Chronic embolism and thrombosis of left femoral vein
I82.513	Chronic embolism and thrombosis of femoral vein, bilateral
I82.519	Chronic embolism and thrombosis of unspecified femoral vein
I82.521	Chronic embolism and thrombosis of right iliac vein
I82.522	Chronic embolism and thrombosis of left iliac vein
I82.523	Chronic embolism and thrombosis of iliac vein, bilateral
I82.529	Chronic embolism and thrombosis of unspecified iliac vein
I82.531	Chronic embolism and thrombosis of right popliteal vein
I82.532	Chronic embolism and thrombosis of left popliteal vein
I82.533	Chronic embolism and thrombosis of popliteal vein, bilateral
I82.539	Chronic embolism and thrombosis of unspecified popliteal vein
I82.5Y1	Chronic embolism and thrombosis of unspecified deep veins of right proximal lower extremity
I82.5Y2	Chronic embolism and thrombosis of unspecified deep veins of left proximal lower extremity
I82.5Y3	Chronic embolism and thrombosis of unspecified deep veins of proximal lower extremity, bilateral
I82.5Y9	Chronic embolism and thrombosis of unspecified deep veins of unspecified proximal lower extremity
I82.541	Chronic embolism and thrombosis of right tibial vein
I82.42	Chronic embolism and thrombosis of left tibial vein
I82.543	Chronic embolism and thrombosis of tibial vein, bilateral
I82.549	Chronic embolism and thrombosis of unspecified tibial vein
I82.5Z1	Chronic embolism and thrombosis of unspecified deep veins of right distal lower extremity
I82.5Z2	Chronic embolism and thrombosis of unspecified deep veins of left distal lower extremity
I82.5Z3	Chronic embolism and thrombosis of unspecified deep veins of distal lower extremity, bilateral
I82.5Z9	Chronic embolism and thrombosis of unspecified deep veins of unspecified distal lower extremity
I82.611	Acute embolism and thrombosis of superficial veins of right upper extremity
I82.612	Acute embolism and thrombosis of superficial veins of left upper extremity
I82.613	Acute embolism and thrombosis of superficial veins of upper extremity, bilateral
I82.619	Acute embolism and thrombosis of superficial veins of unspecified upper extremity
I82.621	Acute embolism and thrombosis of deep veins of right upper extremity
I82.622	Acute embolism and thrombosis of deep veins of left upper extremity

ICD-10-CM	Code Description
I82.623	Acute embolism and thrombosis of deep veins of upper extremity, bilateral
I82.629	Acute embolism and thrombosis of deep veins of unspecified upper extremity
I82.601	Acute embolism and thrombosis of unspecified veins of right upper extremity
I82.602	Acute embolism and thrombosis of unspecified veins of left upper extremity
I82.603	Acute embolism and thrombosis of unspecified veins of upper extremity, bilateral
I82.609	Acute embolism and thrombosis of unspecified veins of unspecified upper extremity
I82.A11	Acute embolism and thrombosis of right axillary vein
I82.A12	Acute embolism and thrombosis of left axillary vein
I82.A13	Acute embolism and thrombosis of axillary vein, bilateral
I82.A19	Acute embolism and thrombosis of unspecified axillary vein
I82.A21	Chronic embolism and thrombosis of right axillary vein
I82.A22	Chronic embolism and thrombosis of left axillary vein
I82.A23	Chronic embolism and thrombosis of axillary vein, bilateral
I82.A29	Chronic embolism and thrombosis of unspecified axillary vein
I82.B11	Acute embolism and thrombosis of right subclavian vein
I82.B12	Acute embolism and thrombosis of left subclavian vein
I82.B13	Acute embolism and thrombosis of subclavian vein, bilateral
I82.B19	Acute embolism and thrombosis of unspecified subclavian vein
I82.B21	Chronic embolism and thrombosis of right subclavian vein
I82.B22	Chronic embolism and thrombosis of left subclavian vein
I82.B23	Chronic embolism and thrombosis of subclavian vein, bilateral
I82.B29	Chronic embolism and thrombosis of unspecified subclavian vein
I82.C11	Acute embolism and thrombosis of right internal jugular vein
I82.C12	Acute embolism and thrombosis of left internal jugular vein
I82.C13	Acute embolism and thrombosis of internal jugular vein, bilateral
I82.C19	Acute embolism and thrombosis of unspecified internal jugular vein
I82.C21	Chronic embolism and thrombosis of right internal jugular vein
I82.C22	Chronic embolism and thrombosis of left internal jugular vein
I82.C23	Chronic embolism and thrombosis of internal jugular vein, bilateral
I82.C29	Chronic embolism and thrombosis of unspecified internal jugular vein
I82.210	Acute embolism and thrombosis of superior vena cava
I82.290	Acute embolism and thrombosis of other thoracic veins
I82.701	Chronic embolism and thrombosis of unspecified veins of right upper extremity
I82.702	Chronic embolism and thrombosis of unspecified veins of left upper extremity
I82.703	Chronic embolism and thrombosis of unspecified veins of upper extremity, bilateral
I82.709	Chronic embolism and thrombosis of unspecified veins of unspecified upper extremity
I82.711	Chronic embolism and thrombosis of superficial veins of right upper extremity
I82.712	Chronic embolism and thrombosis of superficial veins of left upper extremity
I82.713	Chronic embolism and thrombosis of superficial veins of upper extremity, bilateral
I82.719	Chronic embolism and thrombosis of superficial veins of unspecified upper extremity
I82.721	Chronic embolism and thrombosis of deep veins of right upper extremity
I82.722	Chronic embolism and thrombosis of deep veins of left upper extremity
I82.723	Chronic embolism and thrombosis of deep veins of upper extremity, bilateral
I82.729	Chronic embolism and thrombosis of deep veins of unspecified upper extremity
I82.811	Embolism and thrombosis of superficial veins of right lower extremities
I82.812	Embolism and thrombosis of superficial veins of left lower extremities
I82.813	Embolism and thrombosis of superficial veins of lower extremities, bilateral
I82.819	Embolism and thrombosis of superficial veins of unspecified lower extremities
I82.890	Acute embolism and thrombosis of other specified veins

ICD-10-CM	Code Description
I82.891	Chronic embolism and thrombosis of other specified veins
I82.90	Acute embolism and thrombosis of unspecified vein
I82.91	Chronic embolism and thrombosis of unspecified vein

Pulmonary Embolism & Infarction

ICD-10-CM	Code Description
I26.Ø1	Septic pulmonary embolism with acute cor pulmonale
I26.90	Septic pulmonary embolism without acute cor pulmonale
I26.Ø9	Other pulmonary embolism with acute cor pulmonale
I26.99	Other pulmonary embolism without acute cor pulmonale

Atrial Fibrillation

ICD-10-CM	Code Description
I48.Ø	Paroxysmal atrial fibrillation
I48.2	Chronic atrial fibrillation
I48.	-91 Unspecified atrial fibrillation Other
I23.6	Thrombosis of atrium, auricular appendage, and ventricle as current complications following acute myocardial infarction
I27.82	Chronic pulmonary embolism
I67.6	Nonpyogenic thrombosis of intracranial venous system
O22.5Ø	Cerebral venous thrombosis in pregnancy, unspecified trimester
O22.51	Cerebral venous thrombosis in pregnancy, first trimester
O22.52	Cerebral venous thrombosis in pregnancy, second trimester
O22.53	Cerebral venous thrombosis in pregnancy, third trimester
O87.3	Cerebral venous thrombosis in the puerperium
Z79.Ø1	Long term (current) use of anticoagulants
Z86.718	Personal history of other venous thrombosis and embolism
Z95.4	Presence of other heart

Coverage policy can be found in Pub. 100-3, Medicare National Coverage Determinations Manual, Chapter 1, section 190.11 PT/INR. (http://www.cms.hhs.gov/manuals/103_cov_determ/ncd103index.asp

100-4, 32, 80.8
CWF Utilization Edits

Edit 1

Should CWF receive a claim from an FI for G0245 or G0246 and a second claim from a contractor for either G0245 or G0246 (or vice versa) and they are different dates of service and less than 6 months apart, the second claim will reject. CWF will edit to allow G0245 or G0246 to be paid no more than every 6 months for a particular beneficiary, regardless of who furnished the service. If G0245 has been paid, regardless of whether it was posted as a facility or professional claim, it must be 6 months before G0245 can be paid again or G0246 can be paid. If G0246 has been paid, regardless of whether it was posted as a facility or professional claim, it must be 6 months before G0246 can be paid again or G0245 can be paid. CWF will not impose limits on how many times each code can be paid for a beneficiary as long as there has been 6 months between each service.

The CWF will return a specific reject code for this edit to the contractors and FIs that will be identified in the CWF documentation. Based on the CWF reject code, the contractors and FIs must deny the claims and return the following messages:

MSN 18.4 -- This service is being denied because it has not been ___ months since your last examination of this kind (NOTE: Insert 6 as the appropriate number of months.)

RA claim adjustment reason code 96 - Non-covered charges, along with remark code M86 - Service denied because payment already made for same/similar procedure within set time frame.

Edit 2

The CWF will edit to allow G0247 to pay only if either G0245 or G0246 has been submitted and accepted as payable on the same date of service. CWF will return a specific reject code for this edit to the contractors and FIs that will be identified in the CWF documentation. Based on this reject code, contractors and FIs will deny the claims and return the following messages:

MSN 21.21 - This service was denied because Medicare only covers this service under certain circumstances.

RA claim adjustment reason code 107 - The related or qualifying claim/service was not identified on this claim.

Edit 3

Once a beneficiary's condition has progressed to the point where routine foot care becomes a covered service, payment will no longer be made for LOPS evaluation and management services. Those services would be considered to be included in the regular exams and treatments afforded to the beneficiary on a routine basis. The physician or provider must then just bill the routine foot care codes, per Pub 100-2, Chapter 15, Sec. 290.

The CWF will edit to reject LOPS codes G0245, G0246, and/or G0247 when on the beneficiary's record it shows that one of the following routine foot care codes were billed and paid within the prior 6 months: 11055, 11056, 11057, 11719, 11720, and/or 11721.

The CWF will return a specific reject code for this edit to the contractors and FIs that will be identified in the CWF documentation. Based on the CWF reject code, the contractors and FIs must deny the claims and return the following messages:

MSN 21.21 - This service was denied because Medicare only covers this service under certain circumstances.

The RA claim adjustment reason code 96 - Non-covered charges, along with remark code M86 - Service denied because payment already made for same/similar procedure within set time frame.

100-4, 32, 90
Stem Cell Transplantation

Stem cell transplantation is a process in which stem cells are harvested from either a patient's or donor's bone marrow or peripheral blood for intravenous infusion. Autologous stem cell transplantation (AuSCT) must be used to effect hematopoietic reconstitution following severely myelotoxic doses of chemotherapy (HDCT) and/or radiotherapy used to treat various malignancies. Allogeneic stem cell transplant may also be used to restore function in recipients having an inherited or acquired deficiency or defect.

Bone marrow and peripheral blood stem cell transplantation is a process which includes mobilization, harvesting, and transplant of bone marrow or peripheral blood stem cells and the administration of high dose chemotherapy or radiotherapy prior to the actual transplant. When bone marrow or peripheral blood stem cell transplantation is covered, all necessary steps are included in coverage. When bone marrow or peripheral blood stem cell transplantation is non-covered, none of the steps are covered.

Allogeneic and autologous stem cell transplants are covered under Medicare for specific diagnoses. See Pub. 100-3, National Coverage Determinations Manual, section 110.8.1, for a complete description of covered and noncovered conditions. For Part A hospital inpatient claims processing instructions, refer to Pub. 100-4, Chapter 3, section 90.3. The following sections contain claims processing instructions for all other claims.

100-4, 32, 90.2
HCPCS and Diagnosis Coding

Allogeneic Stem Cell Transplantation
- Effective for services performed on or after August 1, 1978:

  - For the treatment of leukemia or leukemia in remission, providers shall use ICD-9-CM codes 204.00 through 208.91 and HCPCS code 38240.

  - For the treatment of aplastic anemia, providers shall use ICD-9-CM codes 284.0 through 284.9 and HCPCS code 38240.

- Effective for services performed on or after June 3, 1985:

  - For the treatment of severe combined immunodeficiency disease, providers shall use ICD-9-CM code 279.2 and HCPCS code 38240.

  - For the treatment of Wiskott-Aldrich syndrome, providers shall use ICD-9-CM code 279.12 and HCPCS code 38240.

- Effective for services performed on or after May 24, 1996:

  - Allogeneic stem cell transplantation, HCPCS code 38240 is not covered as treatment for the diagnosis of multiple myeloma ICD-9-CM codes 203.00 or 203.01.

Autologous Stem Cell Transplantation.--Is covered under the following circumstances effective for services performed on or after April 28, 1989:

- For the treatment of patients with acute leukemia in remission who have a high probability of relapse and who have no human leucocyte antigens (HLA) matched, providers shall use ICD-9-CM code 204.01 lymphoid; ICD-9-CM code 205.01 myeloid; ICD-9-CM code 206.01 monocytic; or ICD-9-CM code 207.01 acute erythremia and erythroleukemia; or ICD-9-CM code 208.01 unspecified cell type and HCPCS code 38241.

- For the treatment of resistant non-Hodgkin's lymphomas for those patients presenting with poor prognostic features following an initial response, providers shall use ICD-9-CM codes 200.00 - 200.08, 200.10-200.18, 200.20-200.28, 200.80-200.88, 202.00-202.08, 202.80-202.88 or 202.90-202.98 and HCPCS code 38241.

- For the treatment of recurrent or refractory neuroblastoma, providers shall use ICD-9-CM codes Neoplasm by site, malignant, the appropriate HCPCS code and HCPCS code 38241.

- For the treatment of advanced Hodgkin's disease for patients who have failed conventional therapy and have no HLA-matched donor, providers shall use ICD-9-CM codes 201.00 - 201.98 and HCPCS code 38241.

Autologous Stem Cell Transplantation.--Is covered under the following circumstances effective for services furnished on or after October 1, 2000:

- For the treatment of multiple myeloma (only for beneficiaries who are less than age 78, have Durie-Salmon stage II or III newly diagnosed or responsive multiple myeloma, and have adequate cardiac, renal, pulmonary and hepatic functioning), providers shall use ICD- 9-CM code 203.00 or 238.6 and HCPCS code 38241.

- For the treatment of recurrent or refractory neuroblastoma, providers shall use appropriate code (see ICD-9-CM neoplasm by site, malignant) and HCPCS code 38241.

- Effective for services performed on or after March 15, 2005, when recognized clinical risk factors are employed to select patients for transplantation, high-dose melphalan (HDM) together with autologous stem cell transplantation (HDM/AuSCT) is reasonable and necessary for Medicare beneficiaries of any age group for the treatment of primary amyloid light chain (AL) amyloidosis, ICD-9-CM code 277.3 who meet the following criteria:

- Amyloid deposition in 2 or fewer organs; and,

- Cardiac left ventricular ejection fraction (EF) greater than 45%.

100-4, 32, 90.2.1

HCPCS and Diagnosis Coding for Stem Cell Transplantation - ICD-10-CM Applicable

ICD-10 is applicable to services on and after the implementation of ICD-.

For services provided use the appropriate code from the ICD-10 CM codes in the table below. See §90.2 for a list of covered conditions.

ICD-10	Description
C91.01	Acute lymphoblastic leukemia, in remission
C91.11	Chronic lymphocytic leukemia of B-cell type in remission
C91.31	Prolymphocytic leukemia of B-cell type, in remission
C91.51	Adult T-cell lymphoma/leukemia (HTLV-1-associated), in remission
C91.61	Prolymphocytic leukemia of T-cell type, in remission
C91.91	Lymphoid leukemia, unspecified, in remission
C91.A1	Mature B-cell leukemia Burkitt-type, in remission
C91.Z1	Other lymphoid leukemia, in remission
C92.01	Acute myeloblastic leukemia, in remission
C92.11	Chronic myeloid leukemia, BCR/ABL-positive, in remission
C92.21	Atypical chronic myeloid leukemia, BCR/ABL-negative, in remission
C92.31	Myeloid sarcoma, in remission
C92.41	Acute promyelocytic leukemia, in remission
C92.51	Acute myelomonocytic leukemia, in remission
C92.61	Acute myeloid leukemia with 11q23-abnormality in remission
C92.91	Myeloid leukemia, unspecified in remission
C92.A1	Acute myeloid leukemia with multilineage dysplasia, in remission
C92.Z1	Other myeloid leukemia, in remission
C93.01	Acute monoblastic/monocytic leukemia, in remission
C93.11	Chronic myelomonocytic leukemia, in remission
C93.31	Juvenile myelomonocytic leukemia, in remission
C93.91	Monocytic leukemia, unspecified in remission
C93.91	Monocytic leukemia, unspecified in remission
C93.Z1	Other monocytic leukemia, in remission
C94.01	Acute erythroid leukemia, in remission
C94.21	Acute megakaryoblastic leukemia, in remission
C94.31	Mast cell leukemia, in remission
C94.81	Other specified leukemias, in remission
C95.01	Acute leukemia of unspecified cell type, in remission
C95.11	Chronic leukemia of unspecified cell type, in remission
C95.91	Leukemia, unspecified, in remission
D45	Polycythemia vera
D61.01	Constitutional (pure) red blood cell aplasia
D61.09	Other constitutional aplastic anemia
D82.0	Wiskott-Aldrich syndrome
D81.0	Severe combined immunodeficiency [SCID] with reticular dysgenesis
D81.1	Severe combined immunodeficiency [SCID] with low T- and B-cell numbers
D81.2	Severe combined immunodeficiency [SCID] with low or normal B-cell numbers
D81.6	Major histocompatibility complex class I deficiency
D81.7	Major histocompatibility complex class II deficiency
D81.89	Other combined immunodeficiencies
D81.9	Combined immunodeficiency, unspecified
D81.2	Severe combined immunodeficiency [SCID] with low or normal B-cell numbers

ICD-10	Description
D81.6	Major histocompatibility complex class I deficiency
D60.0	Chronic acquired pure red cell aplasia
D60.1	Transient acquired pure red cell aplasia
D60.8	Other acquired pure red cell aplasias
D60.9	Acquired pure red cell aplasia, unspecified
D61.01	Constitutional (pure) red blood cell aplasia
D61.09	Other constitutional aplastic anemia
D61.1	Drug-induced aplastic anemia
D61.2	Aplastic anemia due to other external agents
D61.3	Idiopathic aplastic anemia
D61.810	Antineoplastic chemotherapy induced pancytopenia
D61.811	Other drug-induced pancytopenia
D61.818	Other pancytopenia
D61.82	Myelophthisis
D61.89	Other specified aplastic anemias and other bone marrow failure syndromes
D61.9	Aplastic anemia, unspecified

- If ICD-10-CM is applicable, the following ranges of ICD-10-CM codes are also covered for AuSCT: Resistant non-Hodgkin's lymphomas, ICD-10-CM diagnosis codes C82.00-C85.29, C85.80-C86.6, C96.4, and C96.Z-C96.9.

- Tandem transplantation (multiple rounds of autologous stem cell transplantation) for patients with multiple myeloma, ICD-10-CM codes C90.00 and D47.Z9

NOTE: The following conditions are not covered:

- Acute leukemia not in remission

- Chronic granulocytic leukemia

- Solid tumors (other than neuroblastoma)

- Multiple myeloma

- For Medicare beneficiaries age 64 or older, all forms of amyloidosis, primary and non-primary

- Non-primary amyloidosis

Also coverage for conditions other than those specifically designated as covered in §90.2 or specifically designated as non-covered in this section or in §90.3 will be at the discretion of the individual contractor.

100-4, 32, 90.3

Non-Covered Conditions

Autologous stem cell transplantation is not covered for the following conditions:

- Acute leukemia not in remission (If ICD-9-CM is applicable, ICD-9-CM codes 204.00, 205.00, 206.00, 207.00 and 208.00) or (If ICD-10-CM is applicable, ICD-10-CM codes C91.00, C92.00, C93.00, C94.00, and C95.00)

- Chronic granulocytic leukemia (ICD-9-CM codes 205.10 and 205.11 if ICD-9-CM is applicable) or (if ICD-10-CM is applicable, ICD-10-CM codes C92.10 and C92.11);

- Solid tumors (other than neuroblastoma) (ICD-9-CM codes 140.0 through 199.1 if ICD-9-CM is applicable or if ICD-10-CM is applicable, ICD-10-CM codes C00.0 – C80.2 and D00.0 – D09.9.)

- Effective for services rendered on or after May 24, 1996 through September 30, 2000, multiple myeloma (ICD-9-CM code 203.00 and 203.01 if ICD-9-CM is applicable or if ICD-10-CM is applicable, ICD-10-CM codes C90.00 and D47.Z9);

- Effective for services on or after October 1, 2000, through March 14, 2005, for Medicare beneficiaries age 64 or older, all forms of amyloidosis, primary and non-primary

- Effective for services on or after 10/01/00, for all Medicare beneficiaries, non-primary amyloidosis

ICD-9-CM	Description	ICD-10-CM	Description
277.30	Amyloidosis, unspecified	E85.9	Amyloidosis, unspecified
277.31	Familial Mediterranean fever	E85.0	Non-neuropathic heredofamilial amyloidosis
277.39	Other amyloidosis	E85.1	Neuropathic heredofamilial amyloidosis
277.39	Other amyloidosis	E85.2	Heredofamilial amyloidosis, unspecified
277.39	Other amyloidosis	E85.3	Secondary systemic amyloidosis
277.39	Other amyloidosis	E85.4	Organ-limited amyloidosis
277.39	Other amyloidosis	E85.8	Other amyloidosis

NOTE: Coverage for conditions other than those specifically designated as covered in 90.2 or 90.2.1 or specifically designated as non-covered in this section will be at the discretion of the individual A/B MAC (B).

100-4, 32, 90.4

Edits

NOTE: Coverage for conditions other than those specifically designated as covered in 80.2 or specifically designated as non-covered in this section will be at the discretion of the individual A/B MAC (B).

Appropriate diagnosis to procedure code edits should be implemented for the non-covered conditions and services in 90.2 90.2.1, and 90.3 as applicable.

As the ICD-9-CM code 277.3 for amyloidosis does not differentiate between primary and non-primary, A/B MACs (B) should perform prepay reviews on all claims with a diagnosis of ICD-9-CM code 277.3 and a HCPCS procedure code of 38241 to determine whether payment is appropriate.

If ICD-10-CM is applicable, the applicable ICD-10 CM codes are: E85.0, E85.1, E85.2, E85.3, E85.4, E85.8, and E85.9.

100-4, 32, 90.6

Clinical Trials for Allogeneic Hematopoietic Stem Cell Transplantation (HSCT) for Myelodysplastic Syndrome (MDS)

A. Background

Myelodysplastic Syndrome (MDS) refers to a group of diverse blood disorders in which the bone marrow does not produce enough healthy, functioning blood cells. These disorders are varied with regard to clinical characteristics, cytologic and pathologic features, and cytogenetics.

On August 4, 2010, the Centers for Medicare & Medicaid Services (CMS) issued a national coverage determination (NCD) stating that CMS believes that the evidence does not demonstrate that the use of allogeneic hematopoietic stem cell transplantation (HSCT) improves health outcomes in Medicare beneficiaries with MDS. Therefore, allogeneic HSCT for MDS is not reasonable and necessary under §1862(a)(1)(A) of the Social Security Act (the Act). However, allogeneic HSCT for MDS is reasonable and necessary under §1862(a)(1)(E) of the Act and therefore covered by Medicare ONLY if provided pursuant to a Medicare-approved clinical study under Coverage with Evidence Development (CED). Refer to Pub.100-3, NCD Manual, Chapter 1, section 110.8.1, for more information about this policy, and Pub. 100-4, MCP Manual, Chapter 3, section 90.3.1, for information on CED.

B. Adjudication Requirements

Payable Conditions. For claims with dates of service on and after August 4, 2010, contractors shall pay for claims for HSCT for MDS when the service was provided pursuant to a Medicare-approved clinical study under CED; these services are paid only in the inpatient setting (Type of Bill (TOB) 11X), as outpatient Part B (TOB 13X), and in Method II critical access hospitals (TOB 85X). Contractors shall require the following coding in order to pay for these claims:

- Existing Medicare-approved clinical trial coding conventions, as required in Pub. 100-4, MCP Manual, Chapter 32, section 69, and inpatient billing requirements regarding acquisition of stem cells in Pub. 100-4, MCP Manual, Chapter 3, section 90.3.3.

- If ICD-9-CM is applicable, for Inpatient Hospital Claims: ICD-9-CM procedure codes 41.02, 41.03, 41.05, and 41.08 or,

- If ICD-10-CM is applicable, ICD-10-PCS, procedure codes 30230G1, 30230Y1, 3023G1, 30233Y1, 30240G1, 30240Y1, 30243G1, 30243Y1, 30250G1,30250Y1, 30253G1, 30253Y1, 30260G1, 30260Y1, 30263G1, and 30263Y1

- If Outpatient Hospital or Professional Claims: HCPCS procedure code 38240

- If ICD-9-CM is applicable, ICD-9-CM diagnosis code 238.75 or If ICD-10-CM is applicable, ICD-10-CM diagnosis codes D46.9, D46.Z, or Z00.6 Professional claims only: place of service codes 21 or 22.

Denials. Contractors shall deny claims failing to meet any of the above criteria. In addition, contractors shall apply the following requirements:

- Providers shall issue a hospital issued notice of non-coverage (HINN) or advance beneficiary notice (ABN) to the beneficiary if the services performed are not provided in accordance with CED.

- Contractors shall deny claims that do not meet the criteria for coverage with the following messages:

    CARC 50 - These are non-covered services because this is not deemed a 'medical necessity' by the payer.

    NOTE: Refer to the 835 Healthcare Policy Identification Segment (loop 2110 Service Payment Information REF), if present.

    RARC N386 - This decision was based on a National Coverage Determination (NCD). An NCD provides a coverage determination as to whether a particular item or service is covered. A copy of this policy is available at http://www.cms.hhs.gov/mcd/search.asp. If you do not have web access, you may contact the contractor to request a copy of the NCD.

    Group Code – Patient Responsibility (PR) if HINN/ABN issued, otherwise Contractual Obligation (CO)

    MSN 16.77 – This service/item was not covered because it was not provided as part of a qualifying trial/study. (Este servicio/artículo no fue cubierto porque no estaba incluido como parte de un ensayo clínico/estudio calificado.)

100-4, 32, 120.2

Coding and General Billing Requirements

Physicians and hospitals must report one of the following Current Procedural Terminology (CPT) codes on the claim:

66982 Extracapsular cataract removal with insertion of intraocular lens prosthesis (one stage procedure), manual or mechanical technique (e.g., irrigation and aspiration or phacoemulsification), complex requiring devices or techniques not generally used in routine cataract surgery (e.g., iris expansion device, suture support for intraocular lens, or primary posterior capsulorrhexis) or performed on patients in the amblyogenic development stage.

66983 Intracapsular cataract with insertion of intraocular lens prosthesis (one stage procedure)

66984 Extracapsular cataract removal with insertion of intraocular lens prosthesis (one stage procedure), manual or mechanical technique (e.g., irrigation and aspiration or phacoemulsification)

66985 Insertion of intraocular lens prosthesis (secondary implant), not associated with concurrent cataract extraction

66986 Exchange of intraocular lens

In addition, physicians inserting a P-C IOL or A-C IOL in an office setting may bill code V2632 (posterior chamber intraocular lens) for the IOL. Medicare will make payment for the lens based on reasonable cost for a conventional IOL. Place of Service (POS) = 11.

Effective for dates of service on and after January 1, 2006, physician, hospitals and ASCs may also bill the non-covered charges related to the P-C function of the IOL using HCPCS code V2788. Effective for dates of service on and after January 22, 2007 through January 1, 2008, non-covered charges related to A-C function of the IOL can be billed using HCPCS code V2788. The type of service indicator for the non-covered billed charges is Q. (The type of service is applied by the Medicare carrier and not the provider). Effective for A-C IOL insertion services on or after January 1, 2008, physicians, hospitals and ASCs should use V2787 rather than V2788 to report any additional charges that accrue.

When denying the non-payable charges submitted with V2787 or V2788, contractors shall use an appropriate Medical Summary Notice (MSN) such as 16.10 (Medicare does not pay for this item or service) and an appropriate claim adjustment reason code such as 96 (non-covered charges) for claims submitted with the non-payable charges.

Hospitals and physicians may use the proper CPT code(s) to bill Medicare for evaluation and management services usually associated with services following cataract extraction surgery, if appropriate.

A - Applicable Bill Types

The hospital applicable bill types are 12X, 13X, 83X and 85X.

B - Other Special Requirements for Hospitals

Hospitals shall continue to pay CAHs method 2 claims under current payment methodologies for conditional IOLs.

100-4, 32, 130.1

Billing and Payment Requirements

Effective for dates of service on or after January 1, 2000, use HCPCS code G0166 (External counterpulsation, per session) to report ECP services. The codes for external cardiac assist (92971), ECG rhythm strip and report (93040 or 93041), pulse oximetry (94760 or 94761) and plethysmography (93922 or 93923) or other monitoring tests for examining the effects of this treatment are not clinically necessary with this service and should not be paid on the same day, unless they occur in a clinical setting not connected with the delivery of the ECP. Daily evaluation and management service, e.g., 99201-99205, 99211-99215, 99217-99220, 99241-99245, cannot be billed with the ECP treatments. Any evaluation and management service must be justified with adequate documentation of the medical necessity of the visit. Deductible and coinsurance apply.

100-4, 32, 140.2

Cardiac Rehabilitation Program Services Furnished On or After January 1, 2010

As specified at 42 CFR 410.49, Medicare covers cardiac rehabilitation items and services for patients who have experienced one or more of the following:

- An acute myocardial infarction within the preceding 12 months; or
- A coronary artery bypass surgery; or
- Current stable angina pectoris; or
- Heart valve repair or replacement; or
- Percutaneous transluminal coronary angioplasty (PTCA) or coronary stenting; or
- A heart or heart-lung transplant or;
- Stable, chronic heart failure defined as patients with left ventricular ejection fraction of 35% or less and New York Heart Association (NYHA) class II to IV symptoms despite being on optimal heart failure therapy for at least 6 weeks (effective February 18, 2014).

Cardiac rehabilitation programs must include the following components:

- Physician-prescribed exercise each day cardiac rehabilitation items and services are furnished;

- Cardiac risk factor modification, including education, counseling, and behavioral intervention at least once during the program, tailored to patients' individual needs;

- Psychosocial assessment;

- Outcomes assessment; and

- An individualized treatment plan detailing how components are utilized for each patient.

Cardiac rehabilitation items and services must be furnished in a physician's office or a hospital outpatient setting. All settings must have a physician immediately available and accessible for medical consultations and emergencies at all times items and services are being furnished under the program. This provision is satisfied if the physician meets the requirements for the direct supervision of physician's office services as specified at 42 CFR 410.26 and for hospital outpatient therapeutic services as specified at 42 CFR 410.27.

As specified at 42 CFR 410.49(f)(1), cardiac rehabilitation program sessions are limited to a maximum of 2 1-hour sessions per day for up to 36 sessions over up to 36 weeks, with the option for an additional 36 sessions over an extended period of time if approved by the Medicare contractor.

100-4, 32, 140.2.1

Coding Requirements for Cardiac Rehabilitation Services Furnished On or After January 1, 2010

The following are the applicable CPT codes for cardiac rehabilitation services: 93797 - Physician services for outpatient cardiac rehabilitation; without continuous ECG monitoring (per session) and 93798 - Physician services for outpatient cardiac rehabilitation; with continuous ECG monitoring (per session) Effective for dates of service on or after January 1, 2010, hospitals and practitioners may report a maximum of 2 1-hour sessions per day. In order to report one session of cardiac rehabilitation services in a day, the duration of treatment must be at least 31 minutes. Two sessions of cardiac rehabilitation services may only be reported in the same day if the duration of treatment is at least 91 minutes. In other words, the first session would account for 60 minutes and the second session would account for at least 31 minutes if two sessions are reported. If several shorter periods of cardiac rehabilitation services are furnished on a given day, the minutes of service during those periods must be added together for reporting in 1-hour session increments.

Example: If the patient receives 20 minutes of cardiac rehabilitation services in the day, no cardiac rehabilitation session may be reported because less than 31 minutes of services were furnished.

Example: If a patient receives 20 minutes of cardiac rehabilitation services in the morning and 35 minutes of cardiac rehabilitation services in the afternoon of a single day, the hospital or practitioner would report 1 session of cardiac rehabilitation services under 1 unit of the appropriate CPT code for the total duration of 55 minutes of cardiac rehabilitation services on that day.

Example: If the patient receives 70 minutes of cardiac rehabilitation services in the morning and 25 minutes of cardiac rehabilitation services in the afternoon of a single day, the hospital or practitioner would report two sessions of cardiac rehabilitation services under the appropriate CPT code(s) because the total duration of cardiac rehabilitation services on that day of 95 minutes exceeds 90 minutes.

Example: If the patient receives 70 minutes of cardiac rehabilitation services in the morning and 85 minutes of cardiac rehabilitation services in the afternoon of a single day, the hospital or practitioner would report two sessions of cardiac rehabilitation services under the appropriate CPT code(s) for the total duration of cardiac rehabilitation services of 155 minutes. A maximum of two sessions per day may be reported, regardless of the total duration of cardiac rehabilitation services.

100-4, 32, 140.2.2.2

Requirements for CR and ICR Services on Institutional Claims

Effective for claims with dates of service on and after January 1, 2010, contractors shall pay for CR and ICR services when submitted on Types of Bill (TOBs) 13X and 85X only. All other TOBs shall be denied.

The following messages shall be used when contractors deny CR and ICR claims for TOBs 13X and 85X:

Claim Adjustment Reason Code (CARC) 171 – Payment is denied when performed/billed by this type of provider in this type of facility.

Remittance Advice Remark Code (RARC) N428 - Service/procedure not covered when performed in this place of service.

Medicare Summary Notice (MSN) 21.25 - This service was denied because Medicare only covers this service in certain settings.

Group Code PR (Patient Responsibility) – Where a claim is received with the GA modifier indicating that a signed ABN is on file.

Group Code CO (Contractor Responsibility) – Where a claim is received with the GZ modifier indicating that no signed ABN is on file.

100-4, 32, 140.2.2.4

Edits for CR Services Exceeding 36 Sessions

Effective for claims with dates of service on or after January 1, 2010, contractors shall deny all claims with HCPCS 93797 and 93798 (both professional and institutional claims) that exceed 36 CR sessions when a KX modifier is not included on the claim line.

The following messages shall be used when contractors deny CR claims that exceed 36 sessions, when a KX modifier is not included on the claim line:

Claim Adjustment Reason Code (CARC) 119 – Benefit maximum for this period or occurrence has been reached.

RARC N435 - Exceeds number/frequency approved/allowed within time period without support documentation.

MSN 23.17- Medicare won't cover these services because they are not considered medically necessary.

Spanish Version - Medicare no cubrirá estos servicios porque no son considerados necesarios por razones médicas.

Group Code PR (Patient Responsibility) – Where a claim is received with the GA modifier indicating that a signed ABN is on file.

Group Code CO (Contractor Responsibility) – Where a claim is received with the GZ modifier indicating that no signed ABN is on file.

Contractors shall not research and adjust CR claims paid for more than 36 sessions processed prior to the implementation of CWF edits. However, contractors may adjust claims brought to their attention.

100-4, 32, 140.3

Intensive Cardiac Rehabilitation Program Services Furnished On or After January 1, 2010

As specified at 42 CFR 410.49, Medicare covers intensive cardiac rehabilitation items and services for patients who have experienced one or more of the following:

- An acute myocardial infarction within the preceding 12 months; or

- A coronary artery bypass surgery; or

- Current stable angina pectoris; or

- Heart valve repair or replacement; or

- Percutaneous transluminal coronary angioplasty (PTCA) or coronary stenting; or

- A heart or heart-lung transplant or;

- A stable, chronic heart failure defined as patients with left ventricular ejection fraction of 35% or less and New York Heart Association (NYHA) class II to IV symptoms despite being on optimal heart failure therapy for at least 6 weeks (effective February 18, 2014).

Intensive cardiac rehabilitation programs must include the following components:

- Physician-prescribed exercise each day cardiac rehabilitation items and services are furnished;

- Cardiac risk factor modification, including education, counseling, and behavioral intervention at least once during the program, tailored to patients' individual needs;

- Psychosocial assessment;

- Outcomes assessment; and

- An individualized treatment plan detailing how components are utilized for each patient.

Intensive cardiac rehabilitation programs must be approved by Medicare. In order to be approved, a program must demonstrate through peer-reviewed published research that it has accomplished one or more of the following for its patients:

- Positively affected the progression of coronary heart disease;

- Reduced the need for coronary bypass surgery; and

- Reduced the need for percutaneous coronary interventions.

An intensive cardiac rehabilitation program must also demonstrate through peer-reviewed published research that it accomplished a statistically significant reduction in 5 or more of the following measures for patients from their levels before cardiac rehabilitation services to after cardiac rehabilitation services:

- Low density lipoprotein;

- Triglycerides;

- Body mass index;

- Systolic blood pressure;

- Diastolic blood pressure; and

- The need for cholesterol, blood pressure, and diabetes medications.

Intensive cardiac rehabilitation items and services must be furnished in a physician's office or a hospital outpatient setting. All settings must have a physician immediately available and accessible for medical consultations and emergencies at all times items and services are being furnished under the program. This provision is satisfied if the physician meets the requirements for direct supervision of physician office services as specified at 42 CFR 410.26 and for hospital outpatient therapeutic services as specified at 42 CFR 410.27.

As specified at 42 CFR 410.49(f)(2), intensive cardiac rehabilitation program sessions are limited to 72 1-hour sessions, up to 6 sessions per day, over a period of up to 18 weeks.

100-4, 32, 150.1

Bariatric Surgery for Treatment of Co-Morbid Conditions Related to Morbid Obesity

Effective for services on or after February 21, 2006, Medicare has determined that the following bariatric surgery procedures are reasonable and necessary under certain conditions for the treatment of morbid obesity. The patient must have a body-mass index (BMI) =35, have at least one co-morbidity related to obesity, and have been previously unsuccessful with medical treatment for obesity. This medical information must be documented in the patient's medical record. In addition, the procedure must be performed at an approved facility. A list of approved facilities may be found at http://www.cms.gov/Medicare/Medicare-General-Information/MedicareApprovedFa cilitie/Bariatric-Surgery.html

Effective for services performed on and after February 12, 2009, Medicare has determined that Type 2 diabetes mellitus is a co-morbidity for purposes of processing bariatric surgery claims.

Effective for dates of service on and after September 24, 2013, the Centers for Medicare & Medicaid Services (CMS) has removed the certified facility requirements for Bariatric Surgery for Treatment of Co-Morbid Conditions Related to Morbid Obesity.

Please note the additional national coverage determinations related to bariatric surgery will be consolidated and subsumed into Publication 100-3, Chapter 1, section 100.1. These include sections 40.5, 100.8, 100.11 and 100.14.

- Open Roux-en-Y gastric bypass (RYGBP)
- Laparoscopic Roux-en-Y gastric bypass (RYGBP)
- Laparoscopic adjustable gastric banding (LAGB)
- Open biliopancreatic diversion with duodenal switch (BPD/DS) or gastric reduction duodenal switch (BPD/GRDS)
- Laparoscopic biliopancreatic diversion with duodenal switch (BPD/DS) or gastric reduction duodenal switch (BPD/GRDS)
- Laparoscopic sleeve gastrectomy (LSG) (Effective June 27, 2012, covered at Medicare Administrative Contractor (MAC) discretion.

100-4, 32, 150.2

HCPCS Procedure Codes for Bariatric Surgery

A. Covered HCPCS Procedure Codes

For services on or after February 21, 2006, the following HCPCS procedure codes are covered for bariatric surgery:

43770　Laparoscopy, surgical, gastric restrictive procedure; placement of adjustable gastric band (gastric band and subcutaneous port components).

43644　Laparoscopy, surgical, gastric restrictive procedure; with gastric bypass and Roux-en-Y gastroenterostomy (roux limb 150 cm or less).

43645　Laparoscopy with gastric bypass and small intestine reconstruction to limit absorption. (Do not report 43645 in conjunction with 49320, 43847.)

43845　Gastric restrictive procedure with partial gastrectomy, pylorus-preserving duodenoileostomy and ileoieostomy (50 to 100 cm common channel) to limit absorption (biliopancreatic diversion with duodenal switch).

43846　Gastric restrictive procedure, with gastric bypass for morbid obesity; with short limb (150 cm or less Roux-en-Y gastroenterostomy. (For greater than 150 cm, use 43847.) (For laparoscopic procedure, use 43644.)

43847　With small intestine reconstruction to limit absorption.

43775　Laparoscopy, surgical, gastric restrictive procedure; longitudinal gastrectomy (i.e., sleeve gastrectomy) (Effective June 27, 2012, covered at contractor's discretion.)

B. Noncovered HCPCS Procedure Codes

For services on or after February 21, 2006, the following HCPCS procedure codes are non-covered for bariatric surgery:

43842　Gastric restrictive procedure, without gastric bypass, for morbid obesity; vertical banded gastroplasty.

NOC code 43999 used to bill for:

Laparoscopic vertical banded gastroplasty

Open sleeve gastrectomy

Laparoscopic sleeve gastrectomy (for contractor non-covered instances)

Open adjustable gastric banding

100-4, 32, 150.5

ICD-9 Diagnosis Codes for BMI Greater Than or Equal to 35

The following ICD-9 diagnosis codes identify BMI >=35 :

V85.35 - Body Mass Index 35.0-35.9, adult

V85.36 - Body Mass Index 36.0-36.9, adult

V85.37 - Body Mass Index 37.0-37.9, adult

V85.38 - Body Mass Index 38.0-38.9, adult

V85.39 - Body Mass Index 39.0-39.9, adult

V85.41 - Body Mass Index 40.0-44.9, adult

V85.42 - Body Mass Index 45.0-49.9, adult

V85.43 - Body Mass Index 50.0-59.9, adult

V85.44 - Body Mass Index 60.0-69.9, adult

V85.45 - Body Mass Index 70.0 and over, adult

The following ICD-10 diagnosis codes identify BMI >=35:

Z6835 - Body Mass Index 35.0-35.9, adult

Z6836 - Body Mass Index 36.0-36.9, adult.

Z6837 - Body Mass Index 37.0-37.9, adult

Z6838 - Body Mass Index 38.0-38.9, adult

Z6839 - Body Mass Index 39.0-39.9, adult

Z6841 - Body Mass Index 40.0-44.9, adult

Z6842 - Body Mass Index 45.0-49.9, adult

Z6843 - Body Mass Index 50.0-59.9, adult

Z6844 - Body Mass Index 60.0-69.9, adult

Z6845 - Body Mass Index 70.0 and over, adult

100-4, 32, 150.6

Claims Guidance for Payment

Covered Bariatric Surgery Procedures for Treatment of Co-Morbid Conditions Related to Morbid Obesity

Contractors shall process covered bariatric surgery claims as follows:

1.　Identify bariatric surgery claims.

　　Contractors identify inpatient bariatric surgery claims by the presence of ICD-9/ICD-10 diagnosis code 278.01/E66.01as the primary diagnosis (for morbid obesity) and one of the covered ICD-9/ICD-10 procedure codes listed in §150.3.

　　Contractors identify practitioner bariatric surgery claims by the presence of ICD-9/ICD-10 diagnosis code 278.01/E66.01 as the primary diagnosis (for morbid obesity) and one of the covered HCPCS procedure codes listed in §150.2.

2.　Perform facility certification validation for all bariatric surgery claims on a pre-pay basis up to and including date of service September 23, 2013.

　　A list of approved facilities are found at the link noted in section 150.1, section A, above.

3.　Review bariatric surgery claims data and determine whether a pre- or post-pay sample of bariatric surgery claims need further review to assure that the beneficiary has a BMI =35 (V85.35-V85.45/Z68.35-Z68.45) (see ICD-10 equivalents above in section 150.5), and at least one co-morbidity related to obesity

　　The A/B MAC medical director may define the appropriate method for addressing the obesity-related co-morbid requirement.

　　Effective for dates of service on and after September 24, 2013, CMS has removed the certified facility requirements for Bariatric Surgery for Treatment of Co-Morbid Conditions Related to Morbid Obesity.

NOTE: If ICD-9/ICD-10 diagnosis code 278.01/E66.01 is present, but a covered procedure code (listed in §150.2 or §150.3) is/are not present, the claim is not for bariatric surgery and should be processed under normal procedures.

100-4, 32, 161

Intracranial Percutaneous Transluminal Angioplasty (PTA) With Stenting

A. Background

In the past, PTA to treat obstructive lesions of the cerebral arteries was non-covered by Medicare because the safety and efficacy of the procedure had not been established. This national coverage determination (NCD) meant that the procedure was also non-covered for beneficiaries participating in Food and Drug Administration (FDA)-approved investigational device exemption (IDE) clinical trials.

B. Policy

On February 9, 2006, a request for reconsideration of this NCD initiated a national coverage analysis. CMS reviewed the evidence and determined that intracranial PTA with stenting is reasonable and necessary under §1862(a)(1)(A) of the Social Security Act for the treatment of cerebral vessels (as specified in The National Coverage Determinations Manual, Chapter 1, part 1, section 20.7) only when furnished in accordance with FDA-approved protocols governing Category B IDE clinical trials. All other indications for intracranial PTA with stenting remain non-covered.

C. Billing

Providers of covered intracranial PTA with stenting shall use Category B IDE billing requirements, as listed above in section 68.4. In addition to these requirements, providers must bill the appropriate procedure and diagnosis codes for the date of service to receive payment. That is, under Part A, providers must bill intracranial PTA using ICD-9-CM procedure codes 00.62 and 00.65, if ICD-9-CM is applicable, or, if ICD-10-PCS is applicable, ICD-10-PCS procedure codes 037G34Z, 037G3DZ, 037G3ZZ, 037G44Z, 037G4DZ, 037G4ZZ, 03CG3ZZ, 057L3DZ, 057L4DZ and 05CL3ZZ. ICD-9-CM diagnosis code 437.0 or ICD-10-CM diagnosis code 167.2applies, depending on the date of service.

Under Part B, providers must bill HCPCS procedure code 37799. If ICD-9-CM is applicable ICD-9-CM diagnosis code 437.0 or if ICD-10-CM is applicable,ICD-10-CM diagnosis code 167.2 applies.

NOTE: ICD- codes are subject to modification. Providers must always ensure they are using the latest and most appropriate codes.

100-4, 32, 190

Billing Requirements for Extracorporeal Photopheresis

Effective for dates of services on and after December 19, 2006, Medicare has expanded coverage for extracorporeal photopheresis for patients with acute cardiac allograft rejection whose disease is refractory to standard immunosuppresive drug treatment and patients with chronic graft versus host disease whose disease is refractory to standard immunosuppresive drug treatment. (See Pub. 100-3, chapter 1, section 110.4, for complete coverage guidelines).

Effective for claims with dates of service on or after April 30, 2012, CMS has expanded coverage for extracorporeal photopheresis for the treatment of BOS following lung allograft transplantation only when extracorporeal photopheresis is provided under a clinical research study that meets specific requirements to assess the effect of extracorporeal photopheresis for the treatment of BOS following lung allograft transplantation. Further coverage criteria is outlined in Publication 100-3, Section 110.4 of the NCD.

100-4, 32, 190.2

Healthcare Common Procedural Coding System (HCPCS), Applicable Diagnosis Codes and Procedure Code

The following HCPCS procedure code is used for billing extracorporeal photopheresis:

- 36522 - Photopheresis, extracorporeal

The following are the applicable ICD-9-CM diagnosis codes for the new expanded coverage:

- 996.83 - Complications of transplanted heart, or,
- 996.85 - Complications of transplanted bone marrow, or,
- 996.88 – Complications of transplanted organ, stem cell

Effective for services for BOS following lung allograft transplantation the following is a list of applicable ICD-9-CM diagnosis codes:

- 996.84 – Complications of transplanted lung
- 491.9 - Unspecified chronic bronchitis
- 491.20 – Obstructive chronic bronchitis without exacerbation
- 491.21 – Obstructive chronic bronchitis with (acute) exacerbation
- 496 – Chronic airway obstruction, not elsewhere classified

The following is the applicable ICD-9-CM procedure code for the new expanded coverage:

- 99.88 - Therapeutic photopheresis

NOTE: Contractors shall edit for an appropriate oncological and autoimmune disorder diagnosis for payment of extracorporeal photopheresis according to the NCD.

Effective for claims with dates of service on or after April 30, 2012, in addition to HCPCS 36522, the following ICD-9-CM codes are applicable for extracorporeal photopheresis for the treatment of BOS following lung allograft transplantation only when extracorporeal photopheresis is provided under a clinical research study as outlined in Section 190 above:

A reference listing of ICD-9 CM and ICD-10-CM coding and descriptions is listed V70.7 below:

ICD9	Long Description	ICD10	ICD10 Description
491.20	Obstructive chronic	J44.9	Chronic obstructive bronchitis without exacerbation pulmonary disease, unspecified

ICD9	Long Description	ICD10	ICD10 Description
491.21	Obstructive chronic bronchitis with (acute) exacerbation	J44.1	Chronic obstructive pulmonary disease with (acute) exacerbation
491.9	Unspecified chronic bronchitis	J42	Unspecified chronic bronchitis
496	Chronic airway obstruction, not elsewhere classified	J44.9	Chronic obstructive pulmonary disease, unspecified
996.84	Complications of transplanted lung	T86.810	Lung transplant rejection
996.84	Complications of transplanted lung	T86.811	Lung transplant failure
996.84	Complications of transplanted lung	T86.812	Lung transplant infection (not recommended for extracorporeal photopheresis coverage)
996.84	Complications of transplanted lung	T86.818	Other complications of lung transplant
996.84	Complications of transplanted lung	T86.819	Unspecified complication of lung transplant
996.88	Complications of Transplanted organ, Stem cell	T86.5	Complications of Stem Cell Transplant
V70.7	Examination of participant in clinical trial	Z00.6	Encounter for examination for normal comparison and control in clinical research program (needed for CED)

Contractors must also report modifier Q0 - (investigational clinical service provided in a clinical research study that is in an approved research study) or Q1 (routine clinical service provided in a clinical research study that is in an approved clinical research study) as appropriate on these claims. Contractors must use diagnosis code V70.7/Z00.6 and condition code 30 (A/B MAC (A) only), along with value code D4 and the 8-digit clinical identifier number (A/MACs only) for these claims.

100-4, 32, 190.3

Medicare Summary Notices (MSNs), Remittance Advice Remark Codes (RAs) and Claim Adjustment Reason Code

Contractors shall continue to use the appropriate existing messages that they have in place when denying claims submitted that do not meet the Medicare coverage criteria for extracorporeal photopheresis.

Contractors shall deny claims when the service is not rendered to an inpatient or outpatient of a hospital, including critical access hospitals (CAHs) using the following codes:

- Claim Adjustment Reason code: 58 – "Claim/service denied/reduced because treatment was deemed by payer to have been rendered in an inappropriate or invalid place of service."
- MSN 16.2 - "This service cannot be paid when provided in this location/facility." Spanish translation: "Este servicio no se puede pagar cuando es suministrado en esta sitio/facilidad." (Include either MSN 36.1 or 36.2 dependant on liablity.)
- RA MA 30 – "Missing/incomplete/invalid type of bill." (FIs and A/MACs only)
- Group Code - CO (Contractual Obligations) or PR (Patient Responsibility) dependant on liability. Contractors shall return to provider/ return as unprocessable claims for BOS containing HCPCS procedure code 36522 along with one of the following ICD-9-CM diagnosis codes: 996.84, 491.9, 491.20, 491.21, and 496 but is missing Diagnosis code V70.7 (as secondary diagnosis, Institutional only), Condition code 30 Institutional claims only), Clinical trial modifier Q0. Use the following messages:
  — CARC 4 – The procedure code is inconsistent with the modifier used or a required modifier is missing. Note: Refer to the 835 Healthcare Policy Identification Segment (loop 2110 Service Payment Information REF), if present.
  — RARC MA 130 – Your claim contains incomplete and/or invalid information, and no appeal rights are afforded because the claim is unprocessable. Please submit a new claim with the complete/correct information.
  — RARC M16 – Alert: Please see our web site, mailings, or bulletins for more details concerning this policy/procedure/decision.

100-4, 32, 220.1

220.1 - General

Effective for services on or after September 29, 2008, the Center for Medicare & Medicaid Services (CMS) made the decision that Thermal Intradiscal Procedures (TIPS) are not reasonable and necessary for the treatment of low back pain. Therefore, TIPs are non-covered. Refer to Pub.100-3, Medicare National Coverage Determination (NCD) Manual Chapter 1, Part 2, Section 150.11, for further information on the NCD.

100-4, 32, 290.1.1

Coding Requirements for TAVR Services Furnished on or After January 1, 2013

Beginning January 1, 2013, the following are the applicable Current Procedural Terminology (CPT) codes for TAVR:

33361   Transcatheter aortic valve replacement (TAVR/TAVI) with prosthetic valve; percutaneous femoral artery approach

33362   Transcatheter aortic valve replacement (TAVR/TAVI) with prosthetic valve; open femoral approach

33363   Transcatheter aortic valve replacement (TAVR/TAVI) with prosthetic valve; open axillary artery approach

33364   Transcatheter aortic valve replacement (TAVR/TAVI) with prosthetic valve; open iliac artery approach

3336   Transcatheter aortic valve replacement (TAVR/TAVI) with prosthetic valve; transaortic approach (e.g., median sternotomy, mediastinotomy)

0318T   Transcatheter aortic valve replacement (TAVR/TAVI) with prosthetic valve; transapical approach (e.g., left thoracotomy)

Beginning January 1, 2014, temporary CPT code 0318T above is retired. TAVR claims with dates of service on and after January 1, 2014 shall instead use permanent CPT code:

33366   Transcatheter aortic valve replacement (TAVR/TAVI) with prosthetic valve; transapical exposure (e.g., left thoracotomy)

100-4, 32, 290.2

Claims Processing Requirements for TAVR Services on Professional Claims

Place of Service (POS) Professional Claims

Effective for claims with dates of service on and after May 1, 2012, place of service (POS) code 21 shall be used for TAVR services. All other POS codes shall be denied.

The following messages shall be used when Medicare contractors deny TAVR claims for POS:

Claim Adjustment Reason Code (CARC) 58: "Treatment was deemed by the payer to have been rendered in an inappropriate or invalid place of service. NOTE: Refer to the 835 Healthcare Policy Identification Segment (loop 2110 Service Payment Information REF), if present."

Remittance advice remark code (RARC) N428: "Not covered when performed in this place of service."

Medicare Summary Notice (MSN) 21.25: "This service was denied because Medicare only covers this service in certain settings."

Spanish Version: "El servicio fue denegado porque Medicare solamente lo cubre en ciertas situaciones."

Professional Claims Modifier -62

For TAVR claims processed on or after July 1, 2013, contractors shall pay claim lines with 0256T, 0257T, 0258T, 0259T, 33361, 33362, 33363, 33364, 33365 & 0318T only when billed with modifier -62. Claim lines billed without modifier -62 shall be returned as unprocessable.

Beginning January 1, 2014, temporary CPT code 0318T above is retired. TAVR claims with dates of service on and after January 1, 2014 shall instead use permanent CPT code 33366.

The following messages shall be used when Medicare contractors return TAVR claims billed without modifier -62 as unprocessable:

CARC 4: "The procedure code is inconsistent with the modifier used or a required modifier is missing. Note: Refer to the 835 Healthcare Policy Identification Segment (loop 2110 Service Payment Information REF), if present."

RARC N29: "Missing documentation/orders/notes/summary/report/chart."

RARC MA130: "Your claim contains incomplete and/or invalid information, and no appeal rights are afforded because the claim is unprocessable. Please submit a new claim with the complete/correct information."

Professional Claims Modifier -Q0

For claims processed on or after July 1, 2013, contractors shall pay TAVR claim lines for 0256T, 0257T, 0258T, 0259T, 33361, 33362, 33363, 33364, 33365 & 0318T when billed with modifier -Q0. Claim lines billed without modifier -Q0 shall be returned as unprocessable.

Beginning January 1, 2014, temporary CPT code 0318T above is retired. TAVR claims with dates of service on and after January 1, 2014 shall instead use permanent CPT code 33366.

The following messages shall be used when Medicare contractors return TAVR claims billed without modifier -Q0 as unprocessable:

CARC 4: "The procedure code is inconsistent with the modifier used or a required modifier is missing. Note: Refer to the 835 Healthcare Policy Identification Segment (loop 2110 Service Payment Information REF), if present."

RARC N29: "Missing documentation/orders/notes/summary/report/chart."

RARC MA130: "Your claim contains incomplete and/or invalid information, and no appeal rights are afforded because the claim is unprocessable. Please submit a new claim with the complete/correct information."

For claims processed on or after July 1, 2013, contractors shall pay TAVR claim lines for 0256T, 0257T, 0258T, 0259T, 33361, 33362, 33363, 33364, 33365 & 0318T when billed with diagnosis code V70.7 (ICD-10=Z00.6). Claim lines billed without diagnosis code V70.7 (ICD-10=Z00.6) shall be returned as unprocessable.

Beginning January 1, 2014, temporary CPT code 0318T above is retired. TAVR claims with dates of service on and after January 1, 2014 shall instead use permanent CPT code 33366.

The following messages shall be used when Medicare contractors return TAVR claims billed without diagnosis code V70.7 (ICD-10=Z00.6) as unprocessable:

CARC 16: "Claim/service lacks information which is needed for adjudication. At least one Remark Code must be provided (may be comprised of either the NCPDP Reject Reason Code, or Remittance Advice Remark Code that is not an ALERT)."

RARC M76: "Missing/incomplete/invalid diagnosis or condition"

RARC MA130: "Your claim contains incomplete and/or invalid information, and no appeal rights are afforded because the claim is unprocessable. Please submit a new claim with the complete/correct information."

Professional Claims 8-digit ClinicalTrials.gov Identifier Number

For claims processed on or after July 1, 2013, contractors shall pay TAVR claim lines for 0256T, 0257T, 0258T, 0259T, 33361, 33362, 33363, 33364, 33365 & 0318T when billed with the numeric, 8-digit clinicaltrials.gov identifier number preceded by the two alpha characters "CT" when placed in Field 19 of paper Form CMS-1500, or when entered without the "CT" prefix in the electronic 837P in Loop 2300REF02(REF01=P4). Claim lines billed without an 8-digit clinicaltrials.gov identifier number shall be returned as unprocessable.

Beginning January 1, 2014, temporary CPT code 0318T above is retired. TAVR claims with dates of service on and after January 1, 2014 shall instead use permanent CPT code 33366.

The following messages shall be used when Medicare contractors return TAVR claims billed without an 8-digit clinicaltrials.gov identifier number as unprocessable:

CARC 16: "Claim/service lacks information which is needed for adjudication. At least one Remark Code must be provided (may be comprised of either NCPDP Reject Reason Code, or Remittance Advice Remark Code that is not an ALERT)."

RARC MA50: "Missing/incomplete/invalid Investigational Device Exemption number for FDA-approved clinical trial services."

RARC MA130: "Your claim contains incomplete and/or invalid information, and no appeal rights are afforded because the claim is unprocessable. Please submit a new claim with the complete/correct information."

NOTE: Clinicaltrials.gov identifier numbers for TAVR are listed on our website: (http://www.cms.gov/Medicare/Coverage/Coverage-with-Evidence-Development/Transcatheter-Aortic-Valve-Replacement-TAVR-.html)

290.3 - Claims Processing Requirements for TAVR Services on Inpatient Hospital Claims

(Rev.2827. Issued: 11-29-13, Effective: 01-01-14, Implementation: 01-06-14)

Inpatient hospitals shall bill for TAVR on an 11X TOB effective for discharges on or after May 1, 2012. Refer to Section 69 of this chapter for further guidance on billing under CED.

Inpatient hospital discharges for TAVR shall be covered when billed with:

- V70.7 and Condition Code 30.
- An 8-digit clinicaltrials.gov identifier number listed on the CMS website (effective July 1, 2013)

Inpatient hospital discharges for TAVR shall be rejected when billed without:

- V70.7 and Condition Code 30.
- An 8-digit clinicaltrials.gov identifier number listed on the CMS website (effective July 1, 2013)

Claims billed by hospitals not participating in the trial/registry shall be rejected with the following messages:

CARC: 50 -These are non-covered services because this is not deemed a "medical necessity" by the payer.

RARC N386 - This decision was based on a National Coverage Determination (NCD). An NCD provides a coverage determination as to whether a particular item or service is covered. A copy of this policy is available at http://www.cms.hhs.gov/mcd/search.asp. If you do not have web access, you may contact the contractor to request a copy of the NCD.

Group Code –Contractual Obligation (CO)

MSN 16.77 – This service/item was not covered because it was not provided as part of a qualifying trial/study. (Este servicio/artículo no fue cubierto porque no estaba incluido como parte de un ensayo clínico/estudio calificado.)

100-4, 32, 290.3

Claims Processing Requirements for TAVR Services on Inpatient Hospital Claims

Inpatient hospitals shall bill for TAVR on an 11X TOB effective for discharges on or after May 1, 2012. Refer to Section 69 of this chapter for further guidance on billing under CED.

Inpatient hospital discharges for TAVR shall be covered when billed with:

- V70.7 and Condition Code 30.
- An 8-digit clinicaltrials.gov identifier number listed on the CMS website (effective July 1, 2013)

Inpatient hospital discharges for TAVR shall be rejected when billed without:

- V70.7 and Condition Code 30.
- An 8-digit clinicaltrials.gov identifier number listed on the CMS website (effective July 1, 2013)

Claims billed by hospitals not participating in the trial/registry shall be rejected with the following messages:

CARC: 50 -These are non-covered services because this is not deemed a "medical necessity" by the payer.

RARC N386 - This decision was based on a National Coverage Determination (NCD). An NCD provides a coverage determination as to whether a particular item or service is covered. A copy of this policy is available at http://www.cms.hhs.gov/mcd/ search.asp. If you do not have web access, you may contact the contractor to request a copy of the NCD.

Group Code –Contractual Obligation (CO)

MSN 16.77 – This service/item was not covered because it was not provided as part of a qualifying trial/study. (Este servicio/artículo no fue cubierto porque no estaba incluido como parte de un ensayo clínico/estudio calificado.)

100-4, 32, 290.4

Claims Processing Requirements for TAVR Services for Medicare Advantage (MA) Plan Participants

MA plans are responsible for payment of TAVR services for MA plan participants. Medicare coverage for TAVR is included under section 310.1 of the NCD Manual (Routine Costs in Clinical Trials).

100-4, 32, 320.1

Coding Requirements for Artificial Hearts Furnished Before May 1, 2008

Effective for discharges before May 1, 2008, Medicare does not cover the use of artificial hearts, either as a permanent replacement for a human heart or as a temporary life-support system until a human heart becomes available for transplant (often referred to a "bridge to transplant").

100-4, 32, 320.2

Coding Requirements for Artificial Hearts Furnished On or After May 1, 2008

Effective for discharges on or after May 1, 2008, the use of artificial hearts will be covered by Medicare under Coverage with Evidence Development (CED) when beneficiaries are enrolled in a clinical study that meets all of the criteria listed in IOM Pub. 100-3, Medicare NCD Manual, section 20.9.

Claims Coding

For claims with dates of service on or after May 1, 2008, artificial hearts in the context of an approved clinical study for a Category A IDE, refer to section 69 in this manual for more detail on CED billing. Appropriate ICD-10 diagnosis and procedure codes are included below:

ICD-10 Diagnosis Code	Definition	Discharges Effective
I09.81	Rheumatic heart failure	On or After ICD-10 Implementation
I11.0	Hypertensive heart disease with heart failure	
I13.0	Hypertensive heart and chronic kidney disease with heart failure and stage 1 through stage 4 chronic kidney disease, or unspecified chronic kidney disease	
I13.2	Hypertensive heart and chronic kidney disease with heart failure and with stage 5 chronic kidney disease, or end stage renal disease	
I20.0	Unstable angina	
I21.01	ST elevation (STEMI) myocardial infarction involving left main coronary artery	
I21.02	ST elevation (STEMI) myocardial infarction involving left anterior descending coronary artery	
I21.09	ST elevation (STEMI) myocardial infarction involving other coronary artery of anterior wall	
I21.11	ST elevation (STEMI) myocardial infarction involving right coronary artery	
I21.19	ST elevation (STEMI) myocardial infarction involving other coronary artery of inferior wall	
I21.21	ST elevation (STEMI) myocardial infarction involving left circumflex coronary artery	
I21.29	ST elevation (STEMI) myocardial infarction involving other sites	
I21.3	ST elevation (STEMI) myocardial infarction of unspecified site	
I21.4	Non-ST elevation (NSTEMI) myocardial infarction	
I22.0	Subsequent ST elevation (STEMI) myocardial infarction of anterior wall	
I22.1	Subsequent ST elevation (STEMI) myocardial infarction of inferior wall	
I22.2	Subsequent non-ST elevation (NSTEMI) myocardial infarction	
I22.8	Subsequent ST elevation (STEMI) myocardial infarction of other sites	
I22.9	Subsequent ST elevation (STEMI) myocardial infarction of unspecified site	
I24.0	Acute coronary thrombosis not resulting in myocardial infarction	
I24.1	Dressler's syndrome	
I24.8	Other forms of acute ischemic heart disease	
I24.9	Acute ischemic heart disease, unspecified	
I25.10	Atherosclerotic heart disease of native coronary artery without angina pectoris	
I25.110	Atherosclerotic heart disease of native coronary artery with unstable angina pectoris	
I25.111	Atherosclerotic heart disease of native coronary artery with angina pectoris with documented spasm	
I25.118	Atherosclerotic heart disease of native coronary artery with other forms of angina pectoris	
I25.119	Atherosclerotic heart disease of native coronary artery with unspecified angina pectoris	
I25.5	Ischemic cardiomyopathy	
I25.6	Silent myocardial ischemia	
I25.700	Atherosclerosis of coronary artery bypass graft(s), unspecified, with unstable angina pectoris	
I25.701	Atherosclerosis of coronary artery bypass graft(s), unspecified, with angina pectoris with documented spasm	
I25.708	Atherosclerosis of coronary artery bypass graft(s), unspecified, with other forms of angina pectoris	

© 2015 Optum360, LLC

ICD-10 Diagnosis Code	Definition	Discharges Effective
I25.709	Atherosclerosis of coronary artery bypass graft(s), unspecified, with unspecified angina pectoris	On or After ICD-10 Implementation
I25.710	Atherosclerosis of autologous vein coronary artery bypass graft(s) with unstable angina pectoris	
I25.711	Atherosclerosis of autologous vein coronary artery bypass graft(s) with angina pectoris with documented spasm	
I25.718	Atherosclerosis of autologous vein coronary artery bypass graft(s) with other forms of angina pectoris	
I25.719	Atherosclerosis of autologous vein coronary artery bypass graft(s) with unspecified angina pectoris	
I25.720	Atherosclerosis of autologous artery coronary artery bypass graft(s) with unstable angina pectoris	
I25.721	Atherosclerosis of autologous artery coronary artery bypass graft(s) with angina pectoris with documented spasm	
I25.728	Atherosclerosis of autologous artery coronary artery bypass graft(s) with other forms of angina pectoris	
I25.729	Atherosclerosis of autologous artery coronary artery bypass graft(s) with unspecified angina pectoris	
I25.730	Atherosclerosis of nonautologous biological coronary artery bypass graft(s) with unstable angina pectoris	
I25.731	Atherosclerosis of nonautologous biological coronary artery bypass graft(s) with angina pectoris with documented spasm	
I25.738	Atherosclerosis of nonautologous biological coronary artery bypass graft(s) with other forms of angina pectoris	
I25.739	Atherosclerosis of nonautologous biological coronary artery bypass graft(s) with unspecified angina pectoris	
I25.750	Atherosclerosis of native coronary artery of transplanted heart with unstable angina	
I25.751	Atherosclerosis of native coronary artery of transplanted heart with angina pectoris with documented spasm	
I25.758	Atherosclerosis of native coronary artery of transplanted heart with other forms of angina pectoris	
I25.759	Atherosclerosis of native coronary artery of transplanted heart with unspecified angina pectoris	
I25.760	Atherosclerosis of bypass graft of coronary artery of transplanted heart with unstable angina	
I25.761	Atherosclerosis of bypass graft of coronary artery of transplanted heart with angina pectoris with documented spasm	
I25.768	Atherosclerosis of bypass graft of coronary artery of transplanted heart with other forms of angina pectoris	
I25.769	Atherosclerosis of bypass graft of coronary artery of transplanted heart with unspecified angina pectoris	
I25.790	Atherosclerosis of other coronary artery bypass graft(s) with unstable angina pectoris	
I25.791	Atherosclerosis of other coronary artery bypass graft(s) with angina pectoris with documented spasm	
I25.798	Atherosclerosis of other coronary artery bypass graft(s) with other forms of angina pectoris	
I25.799	Atherosclerosis of other coronary artery bypass graft(s) with unspecified angina pectoris	
I25.810	Atherosclerosis of coronary artery bypass graft(s) without angina pectoris	
I25.811	Atherosclerosis of native coronary artery of transplanted heart without angina pectoris	

ICD-10 Diagnosis Code	Definition	Discharges Effective
I25.812	Atherosclerosis of bypass graft of coronary artery of transplanted heart without angina pectoris	On or After ICD-10 Implementation
I25.89	Other forms of chronic ischemic heart disease	
I25.9	Chronic ischemic heart disease, unspecified	
I34.0	Nonrheumatic mitral (valve) insufficiency	
I34.1	Nonrheumatic mitral (valve) prolapse	
I34.2	Nonrheumatic mitral (valve) stenosis	
I34.8	Other nonrheumatic mitral valve disorders	
I34.9	Nonrheumatic mitral valve disorder, unspecified	
I35.0	Nonrheumatic aortic (valve) stenosis	
I35.1	Nonrheumatic aortic (valve) insufficiency	
I35.2	Nonrheumatic aortic (valve) stenosis with insufficiency	
I35.8	Other nonrheumatic aortic valve disorders	
I35.9	Nonrheumatic aortic valve disorder, unspecified	
I36.0	Nonrheumatic tricuspid (valve) stenosis	
I36.1	Nonrheumatic tricuspid (valve) insufficiency	
I36.2	Nonrheumatic tricuspid (valve) stenosis with insufficiency	
I36.8	Other nonrheumatic tricuspid valve disorders	
I36.9	Nonrheumatic tricuspid valve disorder, unspecified	
I37.0	Nonrheumatic pulmonary valve stenosis	
I37.1	Nonrheumatic pulmonary valve insufficiency	
I37.2	Nonrheumatic pulmonary valve stenosis with insufficiency	
I37.8	Other nonrheumatic pulmonary valve disorders	
I37.9	Nonrheumatic pulmonary valve disorder, unspecified	
I38	Endocarditis, valve unspecified	
I39	Endocarditis and heart valve disorders in diseases classified elsewhere	
I42.0	Dilated cardiomyopathy	
I42.2	Other hypertrophic cardiomyopathy	
I42.3	Endomyocardial (eosinophilic) disease	
I42.4	Endocardial fibroelastosis	
I42.5	Other restrictive cardiomyopathy	
I42.6	Alcoholic cardiomyopathy	
I42.7	Cardiomyopathy due to drug and external agent	
I42.8	Other cardiomyopathies	
I42.9	Cardiomyopathy, unspecified	
I43	Cardiomyopathy in diseases classified elsewhere	
I46.2	Cardiac arrest due to underlying cardiac condition	
I46.8	Cardiac arrest due to other underlying condition	
I46.9	Cardiac arrest, cause unspecified	
I47.0	Re-entry ventricular arrhythmia	
I47.1	Supraventricular tachycardia	
I47.2	Ventricular tachycardia	
I47.9	Paroxysmal tachycardia, unspecified	
I48.0	Atrial fibrillation	
I48.1	Atrial flutter	
I49.01	Ventricular fibrillation	
I49.02	Ventricular flutter	
I49.1	Atrial premature depolarization	
I49.2	Junctional premature depolarization	
I49.3	Ventricular premature depolarization	
I49.40	Unspecified premature depolarization	
I49.49	Other premature depolarization	
I49.5	Sick sinus syndrome	
I49.8	Other specified cardiac arrhythmias	

ICD-10 Diagnosis Code	Definition	Discharges Effective
I49.9	Cardiac arrhythmia, unspecified	On or After ICD-10 Implementation
I50.1	Left ventricular failure	
I50.20	Unspecified systolic (congestive) heart failure	
I50.21	Acute systolic (congestive) heart failure	
I50.22	Chronic systolic (congestive) heart failure	
I50.23	Acute on chronic systolic (congestive) heart failure	
I50.30	Unspecified diastolic (congestive) heart failure	
I50.31	Acute diastolic (congestive) heart failure	
I50.32	Chronic diastolic (congestive) heart failure	
I50.33	Acute on chronic diastolic (congestive) heart failure	
I50.40	Unspecified combined systolic (congestive) and diastolic (congestive) heart failure	
I50.41	Acute combined systolic (congestive) and diastolic (congestive) heart failure	
I50.42	Chronic combined systolic (congestive) and diastolic (congestive) heart failure	
I50.43	Acute on chronic combined systolic (congestive) and diastolic (congestive) heart failure	
I50.9	Heart failure, unspecified	
I51.4	Myocarditis, unspecified	
I51.9	Heart disease, unspecified	
I52	Other heart disorders in diseases classified elsewhere	
I97.0	Postcardiotomy syndrome	
I97.110	Postprocedural cardiac insufficiency following cardiac surgery	
I97.111	Postprocedural cardiac insufficiency following other surgery	
I97.120	Postprocedural cardiac arrest following cardiac surgery	
I97.121	Postprocedural cardiac arrest following other surgery	
I97.130	Postprocedural heart failure following cardiac surgery	
I97.131	Postprocedural heart failure following other surgery	
I97.190	Other postprocedural cardiac functional disturbances following cardiac surgery	
I97.191	Other postprocedural cardiac functional disturbances following other surgery	
I97.710	Intraoperative cardiac arrest during cardiac surgery	
I97.711	Intraoperative cardiac arrest during other surgery	
I97.790	Other intraoperative cardiac functional disturbances during cardiac surgery	
I97.791	Other intraoperative cardiac functional disturbances during other surgery	
I97.88	Other intraoperative complications of the circulatory system, not elsewhere classified	
I97.89	Other postprocedural complications and disorders of the circulatory system, not elsewhere classified	
M32.11	Endocarditis in systemic lupus erythematosus	
O90.89	Other complications of the puerperium, not elsewhere classified	
Q20.0	Common arterial trunk	
Q20.1	Double outlet right ventricle	
Q20.2	Double outlet left ventricle	
Q20.3	Discordant ventriculoarterial connection	
Q20.4	Double inlet ventricle	
Q20.5	Discordant atrioventricular connection	
Q20.6	Isomerism of atrial appendages	
Q20.8	Other congenital malformations of cardiac chambers and connections	
Q20.9	Congenital malformation of cardiac chambers and connections, unspecified	

ICD-10 Diagnosis Code	Definition	Discharges Effective
Q21.0	Ventricular septal defect	On or After ICD-10 Implementation
Q21.1	Atrial septal defect	
Q21.2	Atrioventricular septal defect	
Q21.3	Tetralogy of Fallot	
Q21.4	Aortopulmonary septal defect	
Q21.8	Other congenital malformations of cardiac septa	
Q21.9	Congenital malformation of cardiac septum, unspecified	
Q22.0	Pulmonary valve atresia	
Q22.1	Congenital pulmonary valve stenosis	
Q22.2	Congenital pulmonary valve insufficiency	
Q22.3	Other congenital malformations of pulmonary valve	
Q22.4	Congenital tricuspid stenosis	
Q22.5	Ebstein's anomaly	
Q22.6	Hypoplastic right heart syndrome	
Q22.8	Other congenital malformations of tricuspid valve	
Q22.9	Congenital malformation of tricuspid valve, unspecified	
Q23.0	Congenital stenosis of aortic valve	
Q23.1	Congenital insufficiency of aortic valve	
Q23.2	Congenital mitral stenosis	
Q23.3	Congenital mitral insufficiency	
Q23.4	Hypoplastic left heart syndrome	
Q23.8	Other congenital malformations of aortic and mitral valves	
Q23.9	Congenital malformation of aortic and mitral valves, unspecified	
Q24.0	Dextrocardia	
Q24.1	Levocardia	
Q24.2	Cor triatriatum	
Q24.3	Pulmonary infundibular stenosis	
Q24.4	Congenital subaortic stenosis	
Q24.5	Malformation of coronary vessels	
Q24.6	Congenital heart block	
Q24.8	Other specified congenital malformations of heart	
Q24.9	Congenital malformation of heart, unspecified	
R00.1	Bradycardia, unspecified	
R57.0	Cardiogenic shock	
T82.221A	Breakdown (mechanical) of biological heart valve graft, initial encounter	
T82.222A	Displacement of biological heart valve graft, initial encounter	
T82.223A	Leakage of biological heart valve graft, initial encounter	
T82.228A	Other mechanical complication of biological heart valve graft, initial encounter	
T82.512A	Breakdown (mechanical) of artificial heart, initial encounter	
T82.514A	Breakdown (mechanical) of infusion catheter, initial encounter	
T82.518A	Breakdown (mechanical) of other cardiac and vascular devices and implants, initial encounter	
T82.519A	Breakdown (mechanical) of unspecified cardiac and vascular devices and implants, initial encounter	
T82.522A	Displacement of artificial heart, initial encounter	
T82.524A	Displacement of infusion catheter, initial encounter	
T82.528A	Displacement of other cardiac and vascular devices and implants, initial encounter	
T82.529A	Displacement of unspecified cardiac and vascular devices and implants, initial encounter	
T82.532A	Leakage of artificial heart, initial encounter	
T82.534A	Leakage of infusion catheter, initial encounter	

ICD-10 Diagnosis Code	Definition	Discharges Effective
T82.538A	Leakage of other cardiac and vascular devices and implants, initial encounter	On or After ICD-10 Implementation
T82.539A	Leakage of unspecified cardiac and vascular devices and implants, initial encounter	
T82.592A	Other mechanical complication of artificial heart, initial encounter	
T82.594A	Other mechanical complication of infusion catheter, initial encounter	
T82.598A	Other mechanical complication of other cardiac and vascular devices and implants, initial encounter	
T82.599A	Other mechanical complication of unspecified cardiac and vascular devices and implants, initial encounter	
T86.20	Unspecified complication of heart transplant	
T86.21	Heart transplant rejection	
T86.22	Heart transplant failure	
T86.23	Heart transplant infection	
T86.290	Cardiac allograft vasculopathy	
T86.298	Other complications of heart transplant	
T86.30	Unspecified complication of heart-lung transplant	
T86.31	Heart-lung transplant rejection	
T86.32	Heart-lung transplant failure	
T86.33	Heart-lung transplant infection	
T86.39	Other complications of heart-lung transplant	
Z48.21	Encounter for aftercare following heart transplant	
Z48.280	Encounter for aftercare following heart-lung transplant	
Z94.1	Heart transplant status	
Z94.3	Heart and lungs transplant status	
Z95.9	Presence of cardiac and vascular implant and graft, unspecified	
Q24.0	Dextrocardia	
Q24.1	Levocardia	
Q24.2	Cor triatriatum	
Q24.3	Pulmonary infundibular stenosis	
Q24.4	Congenital subaortic stenosis	
Q24.5	Malformation of coronary vessels	
Q24.6	Congenital heart block	
Q24.8	Other specified congenital malformations of heart	
Q24.9	Congenital malformation of heart, unspecified	
R00.1	Bradycardia, unspecified	
R57.0	Cardiogenic shock	
T82.221A	Breakdown (mechanical) of biological heart valve graft, initial encounter	
T82.222A	Displacement of biological heart valve graft, initial encounter	
T82.223A	Leakage of biological heart valve graft, initial encounter	
T82.228A	Other mechanical complication of biological heart valve graft, initial encounter	
T82.512A	Breakdown (mechanical) of artificial heart, initial encounter	
T82.514A	Breakdown (mechanical) of infusion catheter, initial encounter	
T82.518A	Breakdown (mechanical) of other cardiac and vascular devices and implants, initial encounter	
T82.519A	Breakdown (mechanical) of unspecified cardiac and vascular devices and implants, initial encounter	
T82.522A	Displacement of artificial heart, initial encounter	
T82.524A	Displacement of infusion catheter, initial encounter	
T82.528A	Displacement of other cardiac and vascular devices and implants, initial encounter	

ICD-10 Diagnosis Code	Definition	Discharges Effective
T82.529A	Displacement of unspecified cardiac and vascular devices and implants, initial encounter	On or After ICD-10 Implementation
T82.532A	Leakage of artificial heart, initial encounter	
T82.534A	Leakage of infusion catheter, initial encounter	
T82.538A	Leakage of other cardiac and vascular devices and implants, initial encounter	
T82.539A	Leakage of unspecified cardiac and vascular devices and implants, initial encounter	
T82.592A	Other mechanical complication of artificial heart, initial encounter	
T82.594A	Other mechanical complication of infusion catheter, initial encounter	
T82.598A	Other mechanical complication of other cardiac and vascular devices and implants, initial encounter	
T82.599A	Other mechanical complication of unspecified cardiac and vascular devices and implants, initial encounter	
T86.20	Unspecified complication of heart transplant	
T86.21	Heart transplant rejection	
T86.22	Heart transplant failure	
T86.23	Heart transplant infection	
T86.290	Cardiac allograft vasculopathy	
T86.298	Other complications of heart transplant	
T86.30	Unspecified complication of heart-lung transplant	
T86.31	Heart-lung transplant rejection	
T86.32	Heart-lung transplant failure	
T86.33	Heart-lung transplant infection	
T86.39	Other complications of heart-lung transplant	
Z48.21	Encounter for aftercare following heart transplant	
Z48.280	Encounter for aftercare following heart-lung transplant	
Z94.1	Heart transplant status	
Z94.3	Heart and lungs transplant status	
Z95.9	Presence of cardiac and vascular implant and graft, unspecified	

ICD-10 Diagnosis Code	Definition	Discharges Effective
02RK0JZ	Replacement of Right Ventricle with Synthetic Substitute, Open Approach	On or After ICD-10 Implementation
02RL0JZ	Revision of Synthetic Substitute in Heart, Open Approach	
02WA0JZ	Revision of Synthetic Substitute in Heart, Open Approach	

NOTE: Total artificial heart is reported with a "cluster" of 2 codes for open replacement with synthetic substitute of the right and left ventricles- 02RK0JZ + 02RL0JZ

100-4, 32, 320.3

Ventricular Assist Devices

Medicare may cover a Ventricular Assist Device (VAD). A VAD is used to assist a damaged or weakened heart in pumping blood. VADs are used as a bridge to a heart transplant, for support of blood circulation post-cardiotomy or destination therapy. Refer to the IOM Pub. 100-3, NCD Manual, section 20.9.1 for coverage criteria.

100-4, 32, 320.3.1

Post-cardiotomy

Post-cardiotomy is the period following open-heart surgery. VADs used for support of blood circulation post-cardiotomy are covered only if they have received approval from the Food and Drug Administration (FDA) for that purpose, and the VADs are used according to the FDA-approved labeling instructions

100-4, 32, 320.3.2

Bridge- to -Transplantation (BTT)

Coverage for BTT is restricted to patients listed for heart transplantation. The Centers for Medicare & Medicaid Services (CMS) has clearly identified that the patient must be active on the waitlist maintained by the Organ Procurement and Transplantation Network. CMS has also removed the general time requirement that patients receive a transplant as soon as medically reasonable.

100-4, 32, 370

Microvolt T-wave Alternans (MTWA)

On March 21, 2006, the Centers for Medicare & Medicaid Services (CMS) began national coverage of microvolt T-wave Alternans (MTWA) diagnostic testing when it was performed using only the spectral analysis (SA) method for the evaluation of patients at risk for sudden cardiac death (SCD) from ventricular arrhythmias and patients who may be candidates for Medicare coverage of the placement of an implantable cardiac defibrillator (ICD).

Effective for claims with dates of service on and after January 13, 2015, Medicare Administrative Contractors (MACs) may determine coverage of MTWA diagnostic testing when it is performed using methods of analysis other than SA for the evaluation of patients at risk for SCD from ventricular arrhythmias. Further information can be found at Publication 100-3, section 20.30, of the National Coverage Determinations Manual.

100-4, 32, 370.1

Coding and Claims Processing for MTWA

Effective for claims with dates of service on and after March 21, 2006, MACs shall accept CPT 93025 (MTWA for assessment of ventricular arrhythmias) for MTWA diagnostic testing for the evaluation of patients at risk for SCD with the SA method of analysis only. All other methods of analysis for MTWA are non-covered.

Effective for claims with dates of service on and after January 13, 2015, MACs shall at their discretion determine coverage for CPT 93025 for MTWA diagnostic testing for the evaluation of patients at risk for SCD with methods of analysis other than SA. The –KX modifier shall be used as an attestation by the practitioner and/or provider of the service that documentation is on file verifying the MTWA was performed using a method of analysis other than SA for the evaluation of patients at risk for SCD from ventricular arrhythmias and that all other NCD criteria was met.

NOTE: The –KX modifier is NOT required on MTWA claims for the evaluation of patients at risk for SCD if the SA analysis method is used.

NOTE: This diagnosis code list/translation was approved by CMS/Coverage. It may or may not be a complete list of covered indications/diagnosis codes that are covered but should serve as a finite starting point.

As this policy indicates, individual A/B MACs within their respective jurisdictions have the discretion to make coverage determinations they deem reasonable and necessary under section 1862(a)1)(A) of the Social Security Act. Therefore, A/B MACs may have additional covered diagnosis codes in their individual policies where contractor discretion is appropriate.

ICD-9 Codes

410.11	Acute myocardial infarction of other anterior wall, initial episode of care
410.11	Acute myocardial infarction of other anterior wall, initial episode of care
410.01	Acute myocardial infarction of anterolateral wall, initial episode of care
410.11	Acute myocardial infarction of other anterior wall, initial episode of care
410.31	Acute myocardial infarction of inferoposterior wall, initial episode of care
410.21	Acute myocardial infarction of inferolateral wall, initial episode of care
410.41	Acute myocardial infarction of other inferior wall, initial episode of care
410.81	Acute myocardial infarction of other specified sites, initial episode of care
410.51	Acute myocardial infarction of other lateral wall, initial episode of care
410.61	True posterior wall infarction, initial episode of care
410.81	Acute myocardial infarction of other specified sites, initial episode of care
410.91	Acute myocardial infarction of unspecified site, initial episode of care
410.71	Subendocardial infarction, initial episode of care
410.01	Acute myocardial infarction of anterolateral wall, initial episode of care
410.11	Acute myocardial infarction of other anterior wall, initial episode of care
410.21	Acute myocardial infarction of inferolateral wall, initial episode of care
410.31	Acute myocardial infarction of inferoposterior wall, initial episode of care
410.41	Acute myocardial infarction of other inferior wall, initial episode of care
410.71	Subendocardial infarction, initial episode of care
410.51	Acute myocardial infarction of other lateral wall, initial episode of care
410.61	True posterior wall infarction, initial episode of care
410.81	Acute myocardial infarction of other specified sites, initial episode of care
410.91	Acute myocardial infarction of unspecified site, initial episode of care
411.89	Other acute and subacute forms of ischemic heart disease, other
411.89	Other acute and subacute forms of ischemic heart disease, other

427.1	Paroxysmal ventricular tachycardia
427.1	Paroxysmal ventricular tachycardia
427.41	Ventricular fibrillation
427.42	Ventricular flutter
780.2	Syncope and collapse
V45.89	Other postprocedural status

ICD- 10 Codes

I21.01	ST elevation (STEMI) myocardial infarction involving left main coronary artery
I21.02	ST elevation (STEMI) myocardial infarction involving left anterior descending coron
I21.09	ST elevation (STEMI) myocardial infarction involving other coronary artery of anteri
I21.09	ST elevation (STEMI) myocardial infarction involving other coronary artery of anteri
I21.11	ST elevation (STEMI) myocardial infarction involving right coronary artery
I21.19	ST elevation (STEMI) myocardial infarction involving other coronary artery of inferi
I21.19	ST elevation (STEMI) myocardial infarction involving other coronary artery of inferi
I21.21	ST elevation (STEMI) myocardial infarction involving left circumflex coronary artery
I21.29	ST elevation (STEMI) myocardial infarction involving other sites
I21.29	ST elevation (STEMI) myocardial infarction involving other sites
I21.29	ST elevation (STEMI) myocardial infarction involving other sites
I21.3	ST elevation (STEMI) myocardial infarction of unspecified site
I21.4	Non-ST elevation (NSTEMI) myocardial infarction
I22.0	Subsequent ST elevation (STEMI) myocardial infarction of anterior wall
I22.0	Subsequent ST elevation (STEMI) myocardial infarction of anterior wall
I22.1	Subsequent ST elevation (STEMI) myocardial infarction of inferior wall
I22.1	Subsequent ST elevation (STEMI) myocardial infarction of inferior wall
I22.1	Subsequent ST elevation (STEMI) myocardial infarction of inferior wall
I22.2	Subsequent non-ST elevation (NSTEMI) myocardial infarction
I22.8	Subsequent ST elevation (STEMI) myocardial infarction of other sites
I22.8	Subsequent ST elevation (STEMI) myocardial infarction of other sites
I22.8	Subsequent ST elevation (STEMI) myocardial infarction of other sites
I22.9	Subsequent ST elevation (STEMI) myocardial infarction of unspecified site
I24.8	Other forms of acute ischemic heart disease
I24.9	Acute ischemic heart disease, unspecified
I47.0	Re-entry ventricular arrhythmia
I47.2	Ventricular tachycardia
I49.01	Ventricular fibrillation
I49.02	Ventricular flutter
R55	Syncope and collapse
Z98.89	Other specified postprocedural states

100-4, 32, 370.2

Messaging for MTWA

Effective for claims with dates of service on and after January 13, 2015, MACs shall deny claims for MTWA CPT 93025 with methods of analysis other than SA without modifier -KX using the following messages:

CARC 4: "The procedure code is inconsistent with the modifier used or a required modifier is missing. Note: Refer to the 835 Healthcare Policy Identification Segment (loop 2110 Service Payment Information REF), if present."

RARC N657 – This should be billed with the appropriate code for these services.

Group Code: CO (Contractual Obligation) assigning financial liability to the provider

MSN 15.20 - The following policies [NCD 20.30] were used when we made this decision

Spanish Equivalent - 15.20 - Las siguientes políticas [NCD 20.30] fueron utilizadas cuando se tomó esta decisión.

Appendix G — Physician Quality Reporting System (PQRS)

The Physician Quality Reporting System (PQRS) contains a considerable amount of information for the measures and associated numerators and denominators. With the implementation of ICD-10-CM on October 1, 2015, the associated diagnostic denominator information provided in this appendix was removed as it would not fit within the confines of this book. For that reason, this book provides only the following information about PQRS. For all of the 2016 diagnostic and procedure information, see www.OptumCoding.com/Product/Updates/PQRS16. This information will be available online effective February 2016.

Topic Measure	Measure Title	Associated Denominator	Associated Numerator	Associated Modifier
1	Diabetes: Hemoglobin A1c Poor Control	99201, 99203, 99205-99211, 99213, 99215, 99219, 99221-99222, 99231, 99233, 99238, 99282, 99284-99285, 99291, 99304-99315, 99318-99337, 99342, 99345, 99348, 99350, 97802-97803, G0271, G0402, G0438-G0439	3044F-3046F	8P
5	Heart Failure (HF): Angiotensin-Converting Enzyme (ACE) Inhibitor or Angiotensin Receptor Blocker (ARB) Therapy for Left Ventricular Systolic Dysfunction (LVSD)	99201-99205, 99212-99215, 99304-99310, 99324-99337, 99341-99350	3021F, 4010F	1P, 2P, 3P, 8P
5.01	Heart Failure (HF): Angiotensin-Converting Enzyme (ACE) Inhibitor or Angiotensin Receptor Blocker (ARB) Therapy for Left Ventricular Systolic Dysfunction (LVSD) (Option 2)	99238-99239	3021F, 4010F	1P, 2P, 3P, 8P
6	Coronary Artery Disease (CAD): Antiplatelet Therapy	99201-99205, 99212-99215, 99304-99310, 99324-99337, 99341-99350	4086F	1P, 2P, 3P, 8P
7	Coronary Artery Disease (CAD): Beta-Blocker Therapy - Prior Myocardial Infarction (MI) or Left Ventricular Systolic Dysfunction (LVEF < 40%)	99201-99205, 99212-99215, 99304-99310, 99324-99337, 99341-99350, 33140, 33510-33523, 33533-33536, 92920, 92924, 92928, 92933, 92937, 92941-92943, G8694	G9188	
7.01	Coronary Artery Disese (CAD): Beta-Blocker Therapy - Prior Myocardial Infarction (MI) or Left Ventricular Systolic Dysfunction (LVEF < 40%) (Option 2)	99201-99205, 99212-99215, 99304-99310, 99324-99337, 99341-99350, 33140, 33510-33523, 33533-33536, 92920, 92924, 92928, 92933, 92937, 92941-92943	4008F	1P, 2P, 3P, 8P
8	Heart Failure (HF): Beta-blocker Therapy for Left Ventricular Systolic Dysfunction (LVSD)	99201-99205, 99212-99215, 99304-99310, 99324-99337, 99341-99350, G8923	G8450-G8452	
8.01	Heart Failure (HF): Beta-blocker Therapy for Left Ventricular Systolic Dysfunction (LVSD) (Option 2)	99238-99239, 3021F	G8450-G8452	
12	Primary Open-Angle Glaucoma (POAG): Optic Nerve Evaluation	99201-99205, 99212-99215, 99304-99310, 99324-99337, 92002-92014	2027F	1P, 8P
14	Age-Related Macular Degeneration (AMD): Dilated Macular Examination	99201-99205, 99212-99215, 99304-99310, 99324-99337, 92002-92014	2019F	1P, 2P, 8P
19	Diabetic Retinopathy: Communication with the Physician Managing Ongoing Diabetes Care	99201-99205, 99212-99215, 99304-99310, 99324-99337, 92002-92014	5010F, G8397	1P, 2P, 8P

Topic Measure	Measure Title	Associated Denominator	Associated Numerator	Associated Modifier
21	Perioperative Care: Selection of Prophylactic Antibiotic - First OR Second Generation Cephalosporin	15732-15738, 15830-15837, 19260-19272, 19300-19380, 21627, 21632, 21740, 21750, 21825, 22325, 22551, 22554, 22558, 22586, 22600, 22612, 22630, 22633, 22800-22804, 23470-23474, 23616, 24363, 24370-24371, 27080, 27125-27138, 27158, 27202, 27235-27236, 27244-27245, 27269, 27280-27282, 27440-27447, 27702-27704, 27758-27759, 27766, 27769, 27792, 27814, 27880-27888, 28192-28193, 28293, 28415-28420, 28445, 28465, 28485, 28505, 28525, 28531, 28555, 28585, 28615, 28645, 28675-28737, 31400-31420, 31760-31775, 31786, 31805, 32096-32150, 32215-32320, 32440-32491, 32505-32507, 32800-32815, 32900-32940, 33020-33202, 33250-33251, 33256, 33261, 33300-33322, 33335-33366, 33400-33411, 33413, 33416, 33422-33465, 33475, 33496, 33510-33572, 33877-33883, 33886-33891, 34051, 34800-34805, 34812, 34820-34825, 34830-34834, 34841-34900, 35011-35021, 35081-35103, 35131, 35141-35152, 35206, 35211-35216, 35241-35246, 35266-35276, 35301, 35311, 35363-35372, 35460, 35512, 35521-35526, 35533, 35537-35558, 35565-35587, 35601-35671, 36830, 37224-37231, 37616-37617, 38100-38101, 38115-38120, 38381, 38571-38572, 38700-38780, 39000-39220, 39501, 39540-39561, 43020-43135, 43279-43282, 43300-43337, 43340-43425, 43496, 43500-43634, 43640-43645, 43651-43653, 43770-43830, 43832-43840, 43843-43880, 43886-43888, 44005-44010, 44020-44021, 44050-44100, 44120, 44125-44127, 44130-44136, 44140-44202, 44204-44212, 44227, 44300-44346, 44602-44700, 44800-44850, 44900-44970, 45000, 45020, 45110-45172, 45395-45402, 45540-45825, 47100-47130, 47140-47142, 47350, 47370-47371, 47380-47381, 47400-47480, 47562-47570, 47600-47900, 48000-48155, 48500-48548, 48554-48556, 49000-49060, 49203-49250, 49320-49323, 49505-49507, 49568, 50320, 50340-50380, 57267, 58150-58294, 58951, 58953-58956, 60505, 61154, 61312-61313, 61315, 61510-61512, 61518, 61548, 61697, 61700, 61750-61751, 61867, 62223, 62230, 63015, 63020-63030, 63042, 63045-63047, 63056, 63075, 63081, 63267, 63276, 64746, 0236T	G9196-G9198	

Topic Measure	Measure Title	Associated Denominator	Associated Numerator	Associated Modifier
22	Perioperative Care: Discontinuation of Prophylactic Parenteral Antibiotics (Non-Cardiac Procedures)	15732-15738, 15830-15837, 19260-19272, 19300-19380, 21346-21348, 21422-21423, 21432-21436, 21454-21470, 21627, 21632, 21740, 21750, 21825, 22325, 22551, 22554, 22558, 22586, 22600, 22612, 22630, 22633, 22800-22804, 23470-23474, 23616, 24363, 24370-24371, 27080, 27125-27138, 27158, 27202, 27235-27236, 27244-27245, 27269, 27280-27282, 27440-27447, 27702-27704, 27758-27759, 27766, 27769, 27792, 27814, 27880-27888, 28192-28193, 28293, 28415-28420, 28445, 28465, 28485, 28505, 28525, 28531, 28555, 28585, 28615, 28645, 28675-28737, 31360-31420, 31760-31775, 31786, 31805, 32096-32150, 32215-32320, 32440-32491, 32505-32507, 32800-32815, 32900-32940, 33020-33050, 33203-33208, 33212-33213, 33214-33233, 33234-33240, 33241, 33243-33249, 33254-33255, 33300, 33310, 33320, 33361-33364, 33877-33883, 33886-33891, 34051, 34800-34805, 34812, 34820-34825, 34830-34834, 34841-34900, 35011-35021, 35081-35103, 35131, 35141-35152, 35206, 35211-35216, 35241-35246, 35266-35276, 35301, 35311, 35363-35372, 35460, 35512, 35521-35526, 35533, 35537-35558, 35565-35587, 35601-35671, 36830, 37224-37231, 37616-37617, 38100-38101, 38115-38120, 38381, 38571-38572, 38700-38780, 39000-39220, 39501, 39540-39561, 41130-41155, 43020-43135, 43279-43282, 43300-43337, 43340-43425, 43496, 43500-43634, 43640-43645, 43651-43653, 43770-43830, 43832-43840, 43843-43880, 43886-43888, 44005-44010, 44020-44021, 44050-44100, 44120, 44125-44127, 44130-44136, 44140-44202, 44204-44212, 44227, 44300-44346, 44602-44700, 44800-44850, 44900-44970, 45000, 45020, 45108-45190, 45395-45402, 45500-45505, 45540-45825, 47100-47130, 47140-47142, 47350, 47370-47371, 47380-47381, 47400-47480, 47562-47570, 47600-47900, 48000-48155, 48500-48548, 48554-48556, 49000-49060, 49203-49250, 49320-49323, 49505-49507, 49568, 50320, 50340-50380, 57267, 58150-58294, 58951, 58953-58956, 60505, 61154, 61312-61313, 61315, 61510-61512, 61518, 61520, 61526-61530, 61548, 61591, 61595-61596, 61598, 61606, 61616-61619, 61697, 61700, 61750-61751, 61867, 62223, 62230, 63015, 63020-63030, 63042, 63045-63047, 63056, 63075, 63081, 63267, 63276, 64746, 69720, 69930, 69955-69970, 0236T	4042F, 4046F, 4049F	1P, 8P

Topic Measure	Measure Title	Associated Denominator	Associated Numerator	Associated Modifier
23	Perioperative Care: Venous Thromboembolism (VTE) Prophylaxis (When Indicated in ALL Patients)	15734, 15830-15837, 19260-19272, 19300-19324, 19361-19369, 19380, 21346-21348, 21422-21423, 21432-21436, 21454-21470, 21627, 21632, 21740, 21750, 21825, 22551, 22554, 22558, 22600, 22612, 22630, 22633, 27080, 27125-27138, 27158, 27202, 27235-27236, 27244-27245, 27269, 27280-27282, 27440-27447, 27880-27888, 31360-31395, 31760-31775, 31786, 31805, 32096-32150, 32215-32320, 32440-32491, 32505-32507, 32800-32815, 32900-32940, 33020-33050, 33300, 33310, 33320, 33361-33366, 33877-33883, 33886-33891, 34051, 34800-34805, 34812, 34820-34825, 34830-34834, 34841-34900, 35011-35021, 35081-35103, 35131, 35141-35152, 35206, 35211-35216, 35241-35246, 35266-35276, 35301, 35311, 35363-35372, 35460, 35512, 35521-35526, 35533, 35537-35558, 35565-35587, 35601-35671, 36830, 37224-37231, 37616-37617, 38100-38101, 38115-38120, 38381, 38571-38572, 38700-38724, 38746-38780, 39000-39220, 39501, 39540-39561, 41130-41155, 43020-43135, 43279-43282, 43300-43337, 43340-43425, 43496, 43500-43634, 43640-43645, 43651-43653, 43770-43774, 43800-43830, 43832-43840, 43843-43880, 43886-43888, 44005-44010, 44020-44055, 44110-44120, 44125-44127, 44130, 44140-44202, 44204-44212, 44227, 44300-44346, 44602-44700, 44800-44850, 44900-44970, 45000, 45020-45190, 45395-45402, 45500-45505, 45540-45825, 46715-46762, 47010-47130, 47135-47142, 47300-47371, 47380-47382, 47400-47480, 47562-47570, 47600-47900, 48000-48155, 48500-48548, 48554-48556, 49000-49060, 49203-49323, 49505-49507, 49560-49566, 49570, 50020, 50220-50240, 50320, 50340-50380, 50543, 50545-50548, 50715-50728, 50760-50820, 50947-50948, 51550-51597, 51800-51820, 51900-51925, 51960, 55810-55845, 55866, 56630-56640, 57267, 58150-58294, 58951, 58953-58956, 60200-60281, 60500-60505, 60520-60650, 61312-61313, 61315, 61510-61512, 61518, 61520, 61526-61530, 61548, 61591, 61595-61596, 61598, 61606, 61616-61619, 61697, 61700, 62223, 62230, 63015, 63020-63030, 63042, 63045-63047, 63056, 63075, 63081, 63267, 63276, 64746, 69720, 69955-69970, 0236T	4044F	1P, 8P
24	Osteoporosis: Communication with the Physician Managing On-going Care Post-Fracture of Hip, Spine or Distal Radius for Men and Women Aged 50 Years and Older	99201-99205, 99212-99215, 99238-99239, G0402	5015F	1P, 2P, 8P
24.01	Osteoporosis: Communication with the Physician Managing On-going Care Post-Fracture of Hip, Spine or Distal Radius for Men and Women Aged 50 Years and Older (Option 2)	22305-22327, 25600-25609, 27230-27248	5015F	1P, 2P, 8P
32	Stroke and Stroke Rehabilitation: Discharged on Antithrombotic Therapy	99221-99239	G8696	
33	Stroke and Stroke Rehabilitation: Anticoagulant Therapy Prescribed for Atrial Fibrillation (AF) at Discharge	99221-99233, 99238-99239	4075F	1P, 2P, 8P
39	Screening or Therapy for Osteoporosis for Women Aged 65 Years and Older	99201-99205, 99212-99215	G8399-G8401	
40	Osteoporosis: Management Following Fracture of Hip, Spine or Distal Radius for Men and Women Aged 50 Years and Older	99201-99205, 99212-99215, 99238-99239, G0402	3095F-3096F, G8633	1P, 2P, 3P, 8P

　　　　© 2015 Optum360, LLC

Topic Measure	Measure Title	Associated Denominator	Associated Numerator	Associated Modifier
40.01	Osteoporosis: Management Following Fracture of Hip, Spine or Distal Radius for Men and Women Aged 50 Years and Older (Option 2)	22305-22327, 25600-25609, 27230-27248, G8633-G8635	3095F-3096F	1P, 2P, 3P, 8P
41	Osteoporosis: Pharmacologic Therapy for Men and Women Aged 50 Years and Older	99201-99205, 99212-99215, G0402	4005F	1P, 2P, 3P, 8P
43	Coronary Artery Bypass Graft (CABG): Use of Internal Mammary Artery (IMA) in Patients with Isolated CABG Surgery	33510-33523, 33533-33536	4110F	1P, 8P
44	Coronary Artery Bypass Graft (CABG): Preoperative Beta-Blocker in Patients with Isolated CABG Surgery	00566-00567, 33510-33523, 33533-33536	4115F	1P, 8P
44.01	Coronary Artery Bypass Graft (CABG): Preoperative Beta-Blocker in Patients with Isolated CABG Surgery (Option 2)	00562, 33510-33536	4115F	1P, 8P
46	Medication Reconciliation	99201-99215, 99324-99337, 99341-99350, 99495-99496, 90791-90832, 90834, 90837, 90839, 90845, G0402	1111F	8P
47	Advance Care Plan	99201-99205, 99212-99215, 99218-99220, 99221-99236, 99291, 99304-99310, 99324-99337, 99341-99350, G0402	1123F-1124F	8P
48	Urinary Incontinence: Assessment of Presence or Absence of Urinary Incontinence in Women Aged 65 Years and Older	99201-99205, 99212-99215, 99324-99337, 99341-99350, G0402	1090F	1P, 8P
50	Urinary Incontinence: Plan of Care for Urinary Incontinence in Women Aged 65 Years and Older	99201-99205, 99212-99215, 99324-99337, 99341-99350, G0402	0509F	8P
51	Chronic Obstructive Pulmonary Disease (COPD): Spirometry Evaluation	99201-99205, 99212-99215	3023F	1P, 2P, 3P, 8P
52	Chronic Obstructive Pulmonary Disease (COPD): Inhaled Bronchodilator Therapy	99201-99205, 99212-99215	4025F, G8924	1P, 2P, 3P, 8P
53	Asthma: Pharmacologic Therapy for Persistent Asthma - Ambulatory Care Setting	99201-99205, 99212-99215, 99341-99350, 1038F	4140F, 4144F	2P, 8P
54	Emergency Medicine: 12-Lead Electrocardiogram (ECG) Performed for Non-Traumatic Chest Pain	99281-99285, 99291	3120F	1P, 2P, 8P
65	Appropriate Treatment for Children with Upper Respiratory Infection (URI)	99201-99205, 99212-99220, 99281-99285, G0402	G8708	
66	Appropriate Testing for Children with Pharyngitis	99202-99205, 99212-99220, 99281-99285, G0402	3210F	8P
67	Hematology: Myelodysplastic Syndrome (MDS) and Acute Leukemias: Baseline Cytogenetic Testing Performed on Bone Marrow	99201-99205, 99212-99215	3155F	1P, 2P, 3P, 8P
68	Hematology: Myelodysplastic Syndrome (MDS): Documentation of Iron Stores in Patients Receiving Erythropoietin Therapy	99201-99205, 99212-99215, 4090F	3160F	3P, 8P
69	Hematology: Multiple Myeloma: Treatment with Bisphosphonates	99201-99205, 99212-99215	4100F	1P, 2P, 8P
70	Hematology: Chronic Lymphocytic Leukemia (CLL): Baseline Flow Cytometry	99201-99205, 99212-99215	3170F	1P, 2P, 3P, 8P
71	Breast Cancer: Hormonal Therapy for Stage IC - IIIC Estrogen Receptor/Progesterone Receptor (ER/PR) Positive Breast Cancer	99201-99205, 99212-99215	3315F-3316F, 3370F-3380F, 4179F	1P, 2P, 3P, 8P
72	Colon Cancer: Chemotherapy for AJCC Stage III Colon Cancer Patients	99201-99205, 99212-99215	3382F-3390F, G8927	8P
76	Prevention of Central Venous Catheter (CVC) - Related Bloodstream Infections	36555-36571, 36578-36585, 93503	6030F	1P, 8P
81	Adult Kidney Disease: Hemodialysis Adequacy: Solute	90957-90962, 90965-90966, 90969-90970, G8714	G8713, G8717	
82	Adult Kidney Disease: Peritoneal Dialysis Adequacy: Solute	90945-90947, 90957-90962, 90965-90966, 90969-90970	G8718	

Topic Measure	Measure Title	Associated Denominator	Associated Numerator	Associated Modifier
91	Acute Otitis Externa (AOE): Topical Therapy	99201-99205, 99212-99215, 99281-99285, 99304-99310, 99324-99336, 99341-99350	4130F	1P, 2P, 8P
93	Acute Otitis Externa (AOE): Systemic Antimicrobial Therapy - Avoidance of Inappropriate Use	99201-99205, 99212-99215, 99281-99285, 99304-99310, 99324-99336, 99341-99350	4131F-4132F	1P
99	Breast Cancer Resection Pathology Reporting: pT Category (Primary Tumor) and pN Category (Regional Lymph Nodes) with Histologic Grade	88307-88309	3250F-3260F	1P, 8P
100	Colorectal Cancer Resection Pathology Reporting: pT Category (Primary Tumor) and pN Category (Regional Lymph Nodes) with Histologic Grade	88309	G8721	
102	Prostate Cancer: Avoidance of Overuse of Bone Scan for Staging Low Risk Prostate Cancer Patients	55810-55815, 55840-55845, 55866, 55873-55876, 77427, 77778, 3271F	3269F-3270F	1P, 3P
104	Prostate Cancer: Adjuvant Hormonal Therapy for High Risk Prostate Cancer Patients	77427, 77435, G8465	4164F	1P, 2P, 8P
109	Osteoarthritis (OA): Function and Pain Assessment	99201-99205, 99212-99215	1006F	8P
110	Preventive Care and Screening: Influenza Immunization	99201-99205, 99212-99215, 99304-99316, 99324-99337, 99341-99350, 90945-90970, G0438	G8482	
111	Pneumonia Vaccination Status for Older Adults	99201-99215, 99324-99337, 99341-99350, 99356-99357, G0402	4040F	8P
112	Breast Cancer Screening	99201-99205, 99212-99215, G0402	3014F	1P, 8P
113	Colorectal Cancer Screening	99201-99205, 99212-99215, 99304-99310, 99324-99337, G0402	3017F	1P, 8P
116	Avoidance of Antibiotic Treatment in Adults with Acute Bronchitis	99201-99205, 99212-99220, 99281-99285, G0402	4120F-4124F	1P
117	Diabetes: Eye Exam	99201-99220, 99221-99233, 99238-99239, 99281-99285, 99291, 99304-99337, 99341-99350, 92002-92014, G0402, G0438-G0439	2022F-2026F, 3072F	8P
118	Coronary Artery Disease (CAD): Angiotensin-Converting Enzyme (ACE) Inhibitor or Angiotensin Receptor Blocker (ARB) Therapy - Diabetes or Left Ventricular Systolic Dysfunction (LVEF < 40%)	99201-99205, 99212-99215, 99304-99310, 99324-99337, 99341-99350, G8934	G8935-G8937	
118.01	Coronary Artery Disease (CAD): Angiotensin-Converting Enzyme (ACE) Inhibitor or Angiotensin Receptor Blocker (ARB) Therapy - Diabetes or Left Ventricular Systolic Dysfunction (LVEF < 40%) (Option 2)	99201-99205, 99212-99215, 99304-99310, 99324-99337, 99341-99350	G8473	
119	Diabetes: Medical Attention for Nephropathy	99201-99219, 99221-99233, 99238-99239, 99281-99285, 99291, 99304-99337, 99341-99350, G0402	3060F-3066F, G8506	8P
121	Adult Kidney Disease: Laboratory Testing (Lipid Profile)	99201-99205, 99212-99215, 99304-99310, 99324-99337, 99341-99350	G8725	
122	Adult Kidney Disease: Blood Pressure Management	99201-99205, 99212-99215, 99304-99310, 99324-99337, 99341-99350	0513F, G8476-G8478	8P
126	Diabetes Mellitus: Diabetic Foot and Ankle Care, Peripheral Neuropathy - Neurological Evaluation	99201-99205, 99212-99215, 99304-99310, 99324-99337, 99341-99350, 11042, 11043, 11044, 11055-11057, 11719-11730, 11740, 97001-97002, 97597-97598, 97802-97803	G8404-G8405	
127	Diabetes Mellitus: Diabetic Foot and Ankle Care, Ulcer Prevention - Evaluation of Footwear	99201-99205, 99212-99215, 99304-99310, 99324-99337, 99341-99350, 11042, 11043, 11044, 11055-11057, 11719-11730, 11740, 97001-97002, 97597-97598, 97802-97803	G8410-G8416	

Topic Measure	Measure Title	Associated Denominator	Associated Numerator	Associated Modifier
128	Preventive Care and Screening: Body Mass Index (BMI) Screening and Follow-Up Plan	99201-99205, 99212-99215, 90791-90832, 90834, 90837, 90839, 96150-96152, 97001, 97003, 97802-97803, 98960, D7140-D7210, G0101, G0108, G0270-G0271, G0402, G0438-G0439, G0447	G8417-G8422, G8938	
130	Documentation of Current Medications in the Medical Record	99201-99205, 99212-99215, 99221-99223, 99324-99337, 99341-99350, 99495-99496, 90791-90832, 90834, 90837, 90839, 90957-90960, 90962, 90965-90966, 92002-92014, 92507-92508, 92526, 92541-92545, 92547-92548, 92557, 92567-92570, 92585, 92588, 92626, 96116, 96150-96152, 97001-97004, 97532, 97802-97804, 98960-98962, G0101, G0108, G0270, G0402, G0438-G0439	G8427-G8430	
131	Pain Assessment and Follow-up	99201-99205, 99212-99215, 90791-90792, 92002-92014, 92507-92508, 92526, 96116-96118, 96150-96151, 97001-97004, 97532, 98940-98942, D7140-D7210, G0101, G0402, G0438-G0439	G8442, G8509, G8730-G8732, G8939	
134	Preventive Care and Screening: Screening for Clinical Depression and Follow-Up Plan	99201-99205, 99212-99215, 90791-90832, 90834, 90837, 90839, 92625, 96116-96118, 96150-96151, 97003, G0101	G8431	
137	Melanoma: Continuity of Care - Recall System	99201-99205, 99212-99215	7010F	3P, 8P
138	Melanoma: Coordination of Care	11600-11646, 14000-14301, 17311, 17313	5050F	2P, 3P, 8P
138.01	Melanoma: Coordination of Care (Option 2)	99201-99205, 99212-99215	5050F	2P, 3P, 8P
140	Age-Related Macular Degeneration (AMD): Counseling on Antioxidant Supplement	99201-99205, 99212-99215, 99307-99310, 99324-99337, 92002-92014	4177F	8P
141	Primary Open-Angle Glaucoma (POAG): Reduction of Intraocular Pressure (IOP) by 15% OR Documentation of a Plan of Care	99201-99205, 99212-99215, 99307-99310, 99324-99337, 92002-92014	0517F, 3284F-3285F	8P
143	Oncology: Medical and Radiation - Pain Intensity Quantified	99201-99205, 99212-99215, 51720, 77427-77435, 77470, 96401-96409, 96413, 96416, 96420-96422, 96425-96549	1125F-1126F	8P
144	Oncology: Medical and Radiation - Plan of Care for Pain	99201-99205, 99212-99215, 51720, 77427-77435, 77470, 96401-96409, 96413, 96416, 96420-96422, 96425-96549	0521F, 1125F	8P
145	Radiology: Exposure Time Reported for Procedures Using Fluoroscopy	25606, 25651, 26608, 26650, 26676, 26706, 26727, 27235, 27244-27245, 27509, 27756, 27759, 28406, 28436, 28456, 28476, 36147, 36221-36226, 36251-36254, 36598, 37182-37184, 37187-37188, 37211-37215, 37217, 37220-37236, 37238, 37241-37244, 43260-43265, 43275-43278, 43752, 44500, 49440-49465, 50382-50389, 50590, 61623, 61630-61635, 62263-62264, 62280-62282, 63610, 64610, 64620, 70010-70015, 70170, 70332, 70370-70371, 70390, 71023, 71034, 72240-72295, 73040, 73085, 73115, 73525, 73580, 73615, 74190-74260, 74270-74300, 74328-74363, 74425-74485, 74740-74742, 75600-75630, 75658-75756, 75791-75810, 75825-75962, 75966, 75970-75984, 76000-76001, 76080, 76120, 76496, 77001-77003, 92611, 93565-93568, 0075T, 0234T-0238T, 0338T-0339T, G0106	6045F	8P
146	Radiology: Inappropriate Use of "Probably Benign" Assessment Category in Mammography Screening	77057, G0202	3340F-3350F	TC
147	Nuclear Medicine: Correlation with Existing Imaging Studies for All Patients Undergoing Bone Scintigraphy	78300-78320	3570F	TC, 3P, 8P
154	Falls: Risk Assessment	99201-99215, 99304-99310, 99324-99337, 99341-99350, 97001-97004, G0402	1100F-1101F, 3288F	1P, 8P

Topic Measure	Measure Title	Associated Denominator	Associated Numerator	Associated Modifier
155	Falls: Plan of Care	99201-99215, 99304-99310, 99324-99337, 99341-99350, 97001-97004, G0402	0518F, 1100F	1P, 8P
156	Oncology: Radiation Dose Limits to Normal Tissues	77295	0520F	8P
163	Diabetes: Foot Exam	99201-99220, 99221-99233, 99238-99239, 99281-99285, 99291, 99304-99337, 99341-99350, G0402, G0438-G0439	G9225-G9226	
164	Coronary Artery Bypass Graft (CABG): Prolonged Intubation	33510-33523, 33533-33536	G8569	
164.01	Coronary Artery Bypass Graft (CABG): Prolonged Intubation (Option 2)	33510-33536, G8569-G8570		
165	Coronary Artery Bypass Graft (CABG): Deep Sternal Wound Infection Rate	33510-33523, 33533-33536	G8571	
165.01	Coronary Artery Bypass Graft (CABG): Deep Sternal Wound Infection Rate (Option 2)	33510-33536, G8571-G8572		
166	Coronary Artery Bypass Graft (CABG): Stroke	33510-33523, 33533-33536	G8573	
166.01	Coronary Artery Bypass Graft (CABG): Stroke (Option 2)	33510-33536		
167	Coronary Artery Bypass Graft (CABG): Postoperative Renal Failure	33510-33523, 33533-33536	G8575	
167.01	Coronary Artery Bypass Graft (CABG): Postoperative Renal Failure (Option 2)	33510-33536, G8575-G8576		
168	Coronary Artery Bypass Graft (CABG): Surgical Re-Exploration	33510-33523, 33533-33536	G8577	
168.01	Coronary Artery Bypass Graft (CABG): Surgical Re-Exploration (Option 2)	33510-33536, G8577-G8578		
172	Hemodialysis Vascular Access Decision-Making by Surgeon to Maximize Placement of Autogenous Arterial Venous (AV) Fistula	36818-36821, 36825-36830	G8530	
173	Preventive Care and Screening: Unhealthy Alcohol Use - Screening	99201-99205, 99212-99215, 90791-90832, 90834, 90837, 90845, 96150-96152, 97003-97004, 97802-97804, G0270	3016F	1P, 8P
178	Rheumatoid Arthritis (RA): Functional Status Assessment	99201-99205, 99212-99215, 99341-99350, G0402	1170F	8P
181	Elder Maltreatment Screen and Follow-Up Plan	99201-99205, 99212-99215, 99304-99310, 99318-99337, 99341-99350, 90791-90832, 90834, 90837, 96116, 96150-96151, 97003, 97802-97803, G0101, G0270, G0402, G0438-G0439	G8535-G8536, G8733-G8735, G8941	
182	Functional Outcome Assessment	97001-97004, 98940-98942	G8539	
185	Colonoscopy Interval for Patients with a History of Adenomatous Polyps - Avoidance of Inappropriate Use	44388-44389, 44392, 44394, 45378, 45380-45381, 45384-45385, G0105	0529F	52, 53, 73 or 74, 1P, 3P, 8P
187	Stroke and Stroke Rehabilitation: Thrombolytic Therapy	99218-99233, 99281-99285, 99291	G8600	
191	Cataracts: 20/40 or Better Visual Acuity within 90 Days Following Cataract Surgery	66840-66984	4175F	55 or 56, 8P
192	Cataracts: Complications within 30 days Following Cataract Surgery Requiring Additional Surgical Procedures	65235, 65860, 65880-65920, 66030, 66250, 66820, 66825-66984, 66986, 67005-67025, 67028-67110, 67141-67145, 67250-67255	G8627	55 or 56
193	Perioperative Temperature Management	00100-00560, 00566, 00580-01860, 01924-01952, 01961-01966, 01968-01969	4250F-4255F, G9362	1P, 8P
194	Oncology: Cancer Stage Documented	99201-99205, 99212-99215, 77261-77263	3300F-3301F	8P
195	Radiology: Stenosis Measurement in Carotid Imaging Reports	36222, 70498, 70547-70549, 93880-93882	3100F	8P

Topic Measure	Measure Title	Associated Denominator	Associated Numerator	Associated Modifier
204	Ischemic Vascular Disease (IVD): Use of Aspirin or Another Antithrombotic	99201-99215, 99341-99350, 33510-33523, 33533-33536, 92920, 92924, 92928, 92933, 92937, 92941-92943, G0402	G8598-G8599	
205	HIV/AIDS: Sexually Transmitted Disease Screening for Chlamydia, Gonorrhea, and Syphilis	99201-99205, 99212-99215, G0402	G9228-G9230	
217	Functional Deficit: Change in Risk-Adjusted Functional Status for Patients with Knee Impairments	97001-97002, G8980, G8983, G8986, G8989, G8992	G8647-G8650	
217.01	Functional Deficit: Change in Risk-Adjusted Functional Status for Patients with Knee Impairments (Option 2)	97003-97004, G8980, G8983, G8986, G8989, G8992	G8647-G8650	
218	Functional Deficit: Change in Risk-Adjusted Functional Status for Patients with Hip Impairments	97001-97002, G8980, G8983, G8986, G8989, G8992	G8651-G8654	
218.01	Functional Deficit: Change in Risk-Adjusted Functional Status for Patients with Hip Impairments (Option 2)	97003-97004, G8980, G8983, G8986, G8989, G8992	G8651-G8654	
219	Functional Deficit: Change in Risk-Adjusted Functional Status for Patients with Lower Leg, Foot or Ankle Impairments	97001-97002, G8980, G8983, G8986, G8989, G8992	G8655-G8658	
219.01	Functional Deficit: Change in Risk-Adjusted Functional Status for Patients with Lower Leg, Foot or Ankle Impairments (Option 2)	97003-97004, G8980	G8655	
220	Functional Deficit: Change in Risk-Adjusted Functional Status for Patients with Lumbar Spine Impairments	97001-97002, G8980, G8983, G8986, G8989, G8992	G8659-G8662	
220.01	Functional Deficit: Change in Risk-Adjusted Functional Status for Patients with Lumbar Spine Impairments (Option 2)	97003-97004, G8980, G8983, G8986, G8989, G8992	G8659-G8662	
221	Functional Deficit: Change in Risk-Adjusted Functional Status for Patients with Shoulder Impairments	97001-97002, G8980, G8983, G8986, G8989, G8992	G8663-G8666	
221.01	Functional Deficit: Change in Risk-Adjusted Functional Status for Patients with Shoulder Impairments (Option 2)	97003-97004, G8980, G8983, G8986, G8989, G8992	G8663-G8666	
222	Functional Deficit: Change in Risk-Adjusted Functional Status for Patients with Elbow, Wrist or Hand Impairments	97001-97002, G8980, G8983, G8986, G8989, G8992	G8667-G8670	
222.01	Functional Deficit: Change in Risk-Adjusted Functional Status for Patients with Elbow, Wrist or Hand Impairments (Option 2)	97003-97004, G8980, G8983, G8986, G8989, G8992	G8667-G8670	
223	Functional Deficit: Change in Risk-Adjusted Functional Status for Patients with Neck, Cranium, Mandible, Thoracic Spine, Ribs, or Other General Orthopedic Impairments	97001-97002, G8980, G8983, G8986, G8989, G8992	G8671-G8674	
223.01	Functional Deficit: Change in Risk-Adjusted Functional Status for Patients with Neck, Cranium, Mandible, Thoracic Spine, Ribs, or Other General Orthopedic Impairments (Option 2)	97003-97004, G8980	G8671	
224	Melanoma: Overutilization of Imaging Studies in Melanoma	99201-99205, 99212-99215, G8749	3319F-3320F	1P, 3P
224.01	Melanoma: Overutilization of Imaging Studies in Melanoma (Option 2)	99201-99205, 99212-99215, G8749	3319F-3320F	1P, 3P
225	Radiology: Reminder System for Sceening Mammograms	77057, G0202	7025F	8P
226	Preventive Care and Screening: Tobacco Use: Screening and Cessation Intervention	99201-99205, 99212-99215, 99406-99407, 90791-90832, 90834, 90837, 90845, 92002-92014, 96150-96152, 97003-97004, G0438	1036F, 4004F	1P, 8P

Appendix G — Physician Quality Reporting System (PQRS)

Appendix G — Physician Quality Reporting System (PQRS)

Topic Measure	Measure Title	Associated Denominator	Associated Numerator	Associated Modifier
236	Controlling High Blood Pressure	99201-99215, G0402, G0438-G0439	G8752-G8756, G9231	
238	Use of High-Risk Medications in the Elderly - National Quality Strategy Domain: Patient Safety	99201-99205, 99212-99215, 99341-99348, 99350, G0438-G0439	G9365-G9366	
238.01	Use of High-Risk Medications in the Elderly - National Quality Strategy Domain: Patient Safety (Option 2)	99201-99205, 99212-99215, 99341-99350, G0438	G9367	
242	Coronary Artery Disease (CAD): Symptom Management	99201-99205, 99212-99215, 99304-99310, 99324-99337, 99341-99350	0557F, 1010F-1012F	1P, 2P, 3P, 8P
243	Cardiac Rehabilitation Patient Referral From an Outpatient Setting	99201-99205, 99212-99215, 33361-33365, 33400-33417, 33420-33430, 33463-33471, 33475-33476, 33478-33496, 33510-33536, 33572-33602, 33935, 33945, 33999, 35500, 35600, 92920, 92924, 92928, 92933, 92937, 92941-92943, G0438	1460F, 4500F-4510F	1P, 2P, 3P, 8P
249	Barrett's Esophagus	88305	3126F, G8797	1P, 8P
250	Radical Prostatectomy Pathology Reporting	88309	3267F, G8798	1P, 8P
251	Quantitative Immunohistochemical (IHC) Evaluation of Human Epidermal Growth Factor Receptor 2 Testing (HER2) for Breast Cancer Patients	88360-88361	3394F-3395F	8P
254	Ultrasound Determination of Pregnancy Location of Pregnancy Location for Pregnant Patients with Abdominal Pain	99281-99285, 99291	G8806	
254.01	Ultrasound Determination of Pregnancy Location of Pregnancy Location for Pregnant Patients with Abdominal Pain (Option 2)	99281-99285, 99291, G8806-G8808		
255	Rh Immunoglobulin (Rhogam) for Rh-Negative Pregnant Women at Risk of Fetal Blood Exposure	99281-99285, 99291	G8809-G8811	
257	Statin Therapy at Discharge after Lower Extermity Bypass (LEB)	35556, 35566, 35571, 35583-35587, 35656, 35666-35671	G8815	
258	Rate of Open Repair Small or Moderate Non-Ruptured Abdominal Aortic Aneurysms (AAA) without Major Complications (Discharged to Home by Post-Operative Day #7)	35081, 35102	9003F-9004F, G8818	
259	Rate of Endovascular Aneurysm Repair (EVAR) of Small or Moderate Non-Ruptured Abdominal Aortic Aneurysms (AAA) without Major Complications (Discharged to Home by Post Operative Day #2)	34800-34805	9003F-9004F, G8826	
260	Rate of Carotid Endarterectomy (CEA) for Asymptomatic Patients, without Major Complications (Discharged to Home Post-Operative Day #2)	35301	9006F-9007F, G8834-G8838	
261	Referral for Otologic Evaluation for Patients with Acute or Chronic Dizziness	92540-92550, 92557, 92567-92570, 92575	G8856-G8858	
262	Image Confirmation of Successful Excision of Image-Localized Breast Lesion	19125, 19301-19302	G8872-G8874	
263	Preoperative Diagnosis of Breast Cancer	19301-19303, 19307	G8875-G8877, G8946	
264	Sentinel Lymph Node Biopsy for Invasive Breast Cancer	19301-19302, 19307, 38500, 38510-38542, 38740-38745, 38900, G8879	G8878, G8880, G8882	

Topic Measure	Measure Title	Associated Denominator	Associated Numerator	Associated Modifier
265	Biopsy Follow-Up	99201-99205, 11100, 11755, 19081, 19083, 19085, 19100-19101, 19125, 20200-20251, 21550, 21920-21925, 23065-23066, 23100-23101, 24065-24066, 24100-24101, 25065-25066, 25100-25101, 26100-26110, 27040-27041, 27050-27052, 27323-27324, 27330-27331, 27613-27614, 27620, 28050-28054, 29800, 29805, 29830, 29840, 29860, 29870, 29900, 30100, 31050-31051, 31237, 31510, 31576, 31625, 31628-31629, 31632-31633, 31717, 32096-32098, 32400-32405, 32604-32609, 37200, 37609, 38221, 38500-38530, 38570, 38572, 40490, 40808, 41100-41108, 42100, 42400-42405, 42800-42806, 43193, 43197-43198, 43202, 43239, 43261, 43605, 44010, 44020, 44025, 44100, 44322, 44361, 44377, 44382, 44386, 44389, 45100, 45305, 45331, 45380, 45392, 46606, 47000-47001, 47100, 47553, 48100-48102, 49000, 49010, 49180, 49321, 50200-50205, 50555-50557, 50574, 50576, 50955-50957, 50974-50976, 52007, 52204, 52224, 52250, 52354, 53200, 54100-54105, 54500-54505, 54800, 54865, 55700-55706, 55812, 55842, 55862, 56605, 56821, 57100-57105, 57421, 57454-57455, 57460, 57500, 57520, 58100, 58558, 58900, 59015, 60100, 60540-60545, 60650, 61140, 61575-61576, 61750-61751, 62269, 63275-63290, 63615, 64795, 65410, 67346, 67400, 67450, 67810, 68100, 68510, 68525, 69100-69105, 75970, 93505	G8883	
268	Epilespy: Counseling for Women of Childbearing Potential with Epilepsy	99201-99205, 99212-99215, 99304-99309	4340F	1P, 8P
303	Cataracts: Improvement in Patient's Visual Function within 90 Days Following Cataract Surgery	66840-66940, 66983-66984	G0913-G0915	55 or 56
304	Cataracts: Patient Satisfaction within 90 Days Following Cataract Surgery	66840-66940, 66983-66984	G0916-G0918	55 or 56
317	Preventive Care and Screening: Screening for High Blood Pressure and Follow-Up Documented	99201-99205, 99212-99215, 99218-99226, 99234-99236, 99281-99285, 99304-99310, 99318-99337, 99340-99350, 90791-90832, 90834, 90837, 90839, 90845, 90880, 92002-92014, 96118, 97532, D7140-D7210, G0101, G0402, G0438-G0439	G8783-G8785, G8950-G8952	
320	Appropriate Follow-up Interval for Normal Colonoscopy in Average Risk Patients	44388, 45378, G0121	0528F	52, 53, 73 or 74, 1P, 8P
322	Cardiac Stress Imaging Not Meeting Appropriate Use Criteria: Preoperative Evaluation in Low Risk Surgery Patients	75559, 75563, 75571-75574, 78451-78454, 78491-78494, 93350-93351	G8961-G8962	
323	Cardiac Stress Imaging Not Meeting Appropriate Use Criteria: Routine Testing After Percutaneous Coronary Intervention (PCI)	75559, 75563, 75571-75574, 78451-78454, 78491-78494, 93350-93351	G8963-G8964	
324	Cardiac Stress Imaging Not Meeting Appropriate Use Criteria: Testing in Asymptomatic, Low-Risk Patients	75559, 75563, 75571-75574, 78451-78454, 78491-78494, 93350-93351	G8965-G8966	
325	Adult Major Depressive Disorder (MDD): Coordination of Care of Patients with Specific Comorbid Conditions	99201-99205, 99212-99215, 90791-90832, 90834, 90837, 90845	G8959-G8960, G9232	
326	Atrial Fibrillation and Atrial Flutter: Chronic Anticoagulation Therapy	99201-99205, 99212-99215, 99281-99285, 99304-99310, 99324-99337, 99341-99350	G8967-G8972	
327	Pediatric Kidney Disease: Adequacy of Volume Management	90951-90959, 90963-90965, 90967-90969, G8956	G8955, G8958	

Topic Measure	Measure Title	Associated Denominator	Associated Numerator	Associated Modifier
328	Pediatric Kidney Disease: ESRD Patients Receiving Dialysis: Hemoglobin Level < 10g/dL	90945-90959, 90963-90965, 90967-90969	G8973-G8976	
329	Adult Kidney Disease: Catheter Use at Initiation of Hemodialysis	90957-90962, 90966, 90970	G9239	
330	Adult Kidney Disease: Catheter Use for Greater Than or Equal to 90 Days	90957-90962, 90966, 90970, G9240	G9264-G9266	
331	Adult Sinusitis: Antibiotic Prescribed for Acute Sinusitis (Appropriate Use)	99201-99205, 99212-99215, 99281-99285, 99304-99310, 99324-99337, 99341-99350	G9286-G9287	
332	Adult Sinusitis: Appropriate Choice of Antibiotic: Amoxicillin Prescribed for Patients with Acute Bacterial Sinusitis (Appropriate Use)	99201-99205, 99212-99215, 99281-99285, 99304-99310, 99324-99337, 99341-99350, G9364	G9313-G9315	
333	Adult Sinusitis: Computerized Tomography (CT) for Acute Sinusitis (Overuse)	99201-99205, 99212-99215, 99281-99285, 99304-99310, 99324-99337, 99341-99350	G9348-G9350	
334	Adult Sinusitis: More than One Computerized Tomography (CT) Scan Within 90 Days for Chronic Sinusitis (Overuse)	99201-99205, 99212-99215, 99281-99285, 99304-99310, 99324-99337, 99341-99350	G9352-G9354	
335	Maternity Care: Elective Delivery or Early Induction Without Medical Indication at >= 37 and < 39 Weeks	59409, 59514, 59612, 59620	G9355-G9356, G9361	
336	Maternity Care: Post-Partum Follow-Up and Care Coordination	59400, 59410, 59430-59510, 59515, 59610, 59614-59618, 59622, G9361	G9357-G9358	
337	Tuberculosis Prevention for Psoriasis, Psoriatic Arthritis and Rheumatoid Arthritis Patients on a Biological Immune Response Modifier	99201-99205, 99212-99215, G0402	G9359-G9360	
342	Pain Brought Under Control Within 48 Hours	99324-99326, 99337, 99377, G0182	G9250	
343	Screening Colonoscopy Adenoma Detection Rate	45378, 45380-45381, 45384-45385, G0121	3775F-3776F	52, 53, 73 or 74
344	Rate of Carotid Artery Stenting (CAS) for Asymptomatic Patients, Without Major Complications (Discharged to Home by Post-Operative Day #2)	37215, 9006F-9007F	G9254-G9255	
345	Rate of Postoperative Stroke or Death in Asymptomatic Patients Undergoing Carotid Artery Stenting (CAS)	37215, 9006F-9007F	G9256-G9257, G9259	
346	Rate of Postoperative Stroke or Death in Asymptomatic Patients Undergoing Carotid Endarterectomy (CEA)	35301, 9006F-9007F	G9258, G9260-G9261	
347	Rate of Endovascular Aneurysm Repair (EVAR) of Small or Moderate Non-Ruptured Abdominal Aortic Aneurysms (AAA) Who Die While in Hospital	34800-34802, 9003F-9004F	G9262-G9263	
348	HRS-3 Implantable Cardioverter-Defibrillator (ICD) Complications Rate	33216-33220, 33223, 33240, 33241, 33249	G9267, G9269	
348.1	HRS-3 Implantable Cardioverter-Defibrillator (ICD) Complications Rate (Option 2)	33216-33220, 33223, 33240, 33241, 33249	G9268, G9270	
349	Optimal Vascular Care Composite	99201-99215, 99455-99456, G0402	G9273-G9278	
358	Patient-centered Surgical Risk Assessment and Communication	10121-11006, 11010-11011, 11042, 11043, 11044, 11401-11446, 11601-11603, 11960, 14301, 15040, 15150, 15155, 15200, 15220, 15240, 15260, 15570-15770, 15830, 15920-15951, 15953-15958, 19020, 19101, 19110, 19120-19125, 19260-19272, 19296-19380, 19499-20150, 20696, 20900-20910, 20922, 20926, 20938, 20955-20956, 20999, 21011-21026, 21034-21049, 21139, 21154, 21235, 21299, 21360, 21395, 21462-21465, 21499-21510, 21555-21600, 21615-21705, 21740-21750, 21825-22102, 22110-22114, 22206-22207, 22210-22214, 22220-22224, 22318-22327, 22532-22533, 22548-22551,	G9316-G9317	

Topic Measure	Measure Title	Associated Denominator	Associated Numerator	Associated Modifier
358 (continued)	Patient-centered Surgical Risk Assessment and Communication	22554-22558, 22586-22612, 22630, 22800-22830, 22841, 22849-22850, 22852-22856, 22857-23044, 23075-23078, 23101, 23106-23140, 23146-23150, 23156-23170, 23180-23220, 23395-23405, 23410-23472, 23480-23485, 23491, 23515, 23530-23532, 23550-23552, 23585, 23615-23616, 23630, 23660, 23670, 23680, 23800-23920, 23929, 23935-24079, 24102-24105, 24116-24125, 24130-24136, 24140-24145, 24149-24152, 24201, 24301, 24310-24330, 24332-24342, 24344-24346, 24358-24361, 24363-24366, 24400, 24430-24435, 24495-24498, 24515-24516, 24538-24546, 24575, 24579, 24586-24587, 24615, 24635, 24665-24666, 24685-24925, 24999-25025, 25040-25085, 25101-25107, 25110-25118, 25120-25125, 25130-25240, 25248, 25260-25270, 25274-25295, 25301-25315, 25320-25332, 25337-25360, 25375-25392, 25400-25420, 25430-25440, 25442-25443, 25445-25449, 25490, 25515, 25525-25526, 25545, 25574-25575, 25607-25609, 25628, 25645, 25652, 25670, 25676, 25685, 25695, 25900-25905, 25909, 25920, 25927, 25999, 26115-26123, 26130, 26145, 26180, 26350-26410, 26415, 26418-26426, 26433-26471, 26477-26478, 26480-26492, 26496-26498, 26500-26502, 26510, 26520-26548, 26561, 26565-26568, 26587, 26591-26593, 26615, 26650-26665, 26676-26686, 26715, 26727-26735, 26746, 26765, 26776-26785, 26952-27001, 27005-27059, 27054-27066, 27070-27087, 27097, 27110, 27120-27170, 27176-27177, 27179-27181, 27187, 27202, 27226-27228, 27235-27238, 27244-27245, 27248, 27253-27254, 27258-27259, 27267, 27269, 27280, 27290-27305, 27307-27310, 27327-27339, 27331-27357, 27360-27365, 27372-27390, 27392, 27403-27472, 27477, 27485-27499, 27506-27507, 27509, 27511-27514, 27519, 27524, 27535-27536, 27540, 27556-27557, 27566, 27580-27612, 27615-27647, 27650-27687, 27695-27709, 27715-27726, 27745, 27756-27759, 27766, 27769, 27784, 27792, 27814, 27822-27823, 27826-27829, 27832, 27846-27848, 27880-27899, 28002-28003, 28043-28047, 28192-28193, 28293, 28415-28420, 28445-28446, 28465, 28485, 28505, 28525, 28531, 28555, 28585, 28615, 28645, 28675-28737, 28800-28825, 29806-29825, 29827-29828, 29834-29835, 29837-29838, 29844, 29846-29847, 29850, 29855, 29862, 29914-29868, 29871-29891, 29893, 29895-29898, 29904-29999, 31300-31367, 31370-31420, 31580, 31587, 31590, 31599, 31611, 31614, 31750-31760, 31775-31800, 31820-31825, 31899-32036, 32100-32320, 32440-32491, 32503-32505, 32540, 32560, 32650-32666, 32669-32672, 32800-32820, 32900-32940, 32999, 33020-33050, 33300, 33310, 33320, 33875-33883, 33886-33891, 34001-34805, 34812, 34820-34825, 34830-34834, 34900-35021, 35045-35152, 35184, 35189-35236, 35246-35271, 35281-35305, 35311-35372, 35471-35472, 35501-35510, 35512-35571, 35583-35587, 35601-35671, 35691-35695, 35701-35907, 36475, 36478, 36818-36821, 36825-36830, 36838, 37140, 37160-37181, 37215, 37220-37221, 37224-37231, 37500, 37565, 37605, 37607, 37615-37618, 37650-37785, 37799-38101, 38115-38129, 38230, 38305-38382, 38542-38745, 38760-38780, 38999-39220, 39499-39599,	G9316-G9317	

Topic Measure	Measure Title	Associated Denominator	Associated Numerator	Associated Modifier
358 (continued)	Patient-centered Surgical Risk Assessment and Communication	40510-40525, 40530-40652, 40800-40801, 40810-40816, 41000-41009, 41016-41018, 41110-41114, 41116-41155, 41599, 41806-41820, 41822-41826, 41830-41850, 42104-42160, 42210, 42300-42305, 42330-42340, 42408-42507, 42665-42725, 42808, 42810-42815, 42821, 42826, 42831, 42836-42845, 42870-42894, 42950-42962, 42972-43135, 43279-43282, 43289-43313, 43320-43337, 43340-43425, 43496, 43500-43634, 43640-43645, 43651-43652, 43659, 43770-43825, 43832-43840, 43843-43880, 43886-44010, 44020-44055, 44110-44120, 44125-44127, 44130, 44140-44202, 44204-44212, 44227-44238, 44310-44346, 44602-44700, 44800-44950, 44960-45020, 45108-45160, 45190, 45395-45505, 45540-45825, 45905-45910, 45999-46045, 46060, 46080, 46945-46946, 46250-46288, 46700-46706, 46710-46715, 46730-46740, 46744, 46748-46750, 46753, 46760-46947, 46924-46999, 47010-47130, 47300-47382, 47399-47490, 47562-47700, 47711-47800, 47802-48000, 48020-48100, 48105-48155, 48500-48548, 48999-49062, 49203-49255, 49321-49325, 49329, 49402, 49418-49422, 49425-49426, 49505-49566, 49570-49600, 49606, 49650-50020, 50060-50065, 50075, 50120, 50130-50135, 50205-50290, 50389, 50400-50405, 50500, 50540-50546, 50548-50549, 50610, 50630-50660, 50700, 50715, 50725-50900, 50940-50949, 51040-51080, 51500, 51525-51597, 51800-51920, 51960-51999, 52234-52240, 52320, 52341-52342, 52344-52346, 52400-52402, 52450-53010, 53040, 53210-53240, 53260-53265, 53400-53425, 53431-53447, 53449-53460, 53505-53510, 53520, 53852, 53899, 54015-54050, 54057, 54065, 54110-54135, 54300, 54308, 54324-54326, 54340-54360, 54420-54435, 54440, 54520-54550, 54600-54692, 54840-54861, 54901, 55040-55200, 55530-55550, 55600, 55680, 55801-55845, 55862, 55866, 55873, 55876-55899, 56405-56440, 56501-56515, 56620-56640, 56740-56800, 56810, 57000-57010, 57065, 57106-57110, 57120-57135, 57200-57210, 57240-57265, 57268-57285, 57288-57335, 57423-57425, 57522-57540, 57550-57556, 57720, 58120-58294, 58356-58400, 58520-58554, 58570-58579, 58700-58825, 58920-58960, 59120-59130, 59136-59151, 59350, 60200-60281, 60500-60505, 60520-60699, 61304-61315, 61320-61460, 61500-61516, 61518-61541, 61545-61548, 61556-61557, 61566, 61570, 61575, 61590, 61613, 61680-61705, 61710-61711, 61860, 61880-62100, 63001-63030, 63040-63042, 63045-63047, 63050-63056, 63064, 63075, 63077, 63081, 63085, 63087-63090, 63101-63102, 63170-63290, 63300-63307, 63700, 63707-63709, 64702-64708, 64713, 64722, 64727, 64755-64760, 64804-64818, 64856, 64862, 69511-69530, 69601-69604, 69610, 69631-69637, 69642, 69644-69646, 69801, 0184T, 0202T, 0236T, 0238T	G9316-G9317	
383	Adherence to Antipsychotic Medications for Individuals with Schizophrenia	99201-99233, 99238-99239, 99281-99285, 99291-99337, 99341-99350, 90785-90838, 90845, 90847-90853, 90870, 90880, 98960-98962, 99078, G0409	G9369-G9370	
384	Adult Primary Rhegmatogenous Retinal Detachment Repair Success Rate	67113	G9376-G9377	

Topic Measure	Measure Title	Associated Denominator	Associated Numerator	Associated Modifier
385	Adult Primary Rhegmatogenous Retinal Detachment Surgery Success Rate	67113	G9378-G9379	
386	Amytrophic Lateral Sclerosis (ALS) Patient Care Preferences	99201-99205, 99212-99215, 99304-99310, 99318-99337, 99354-99355	G9380-G9382	
387	Annual Hepatitis C Virus (HCS) Screening for Patients Who are Active Injection Drug Users	99201-99205, 99212-99215, 99304-99310, 99324-99337, 99341-99350, G0438-G0439	G9383-G9386	
388	Cataract Surgery with Intra-Operative Complications (Unplanned Rupture of Posterior Capsule Requiring Unplanned Virectomy)	66840-66984	G9389-G9390	55 or 56
389	Cataract Surgery: Difference Between Planned and Final Refraction	66840-66984	G9391-G9392	55 or 56
390	Discussion and Shared Decision Making Surrounding Treatment Options	99201-99205, 99212-99215	G9399-G9401	
391	Follow-Up After Hospitalization for Mental Illness (FUH)	99221-99233, 99238-99239, 99291	G9402-G9404	
391.01	Follow-Up After Hospitalization for Mental Illness (FUH) (Option 2)	99221-99233, 99238-99239, 99291	G9405-G9407	
392	HRS-12: Cardiac Tamponade and/or Pericardiocentesis Following Atrial Fibrillation Ablation	33250-33256, 33265-33266, 93650-93653, 93656	G9408-G9409	
393	HRS-9: Infection within 180 Days of Cardiac Implantable Electronic Device (CIED) Implantation, Replacement, or Revision	33202-33208, 33212-33234, 33240, 33241-33264, 33249, 33282	G9410-G9411	
393.01	HRS-9: Infection within 180 Days of Cardiac Implantable Electronic Device (CIED) Implantation, Replacement, or Revision (Option 2)	33202-33208, 33212-33234, 33240, 33241-33264, 33249, 33282	G9412-G9413	
394	Immunizations for Adolescents	99201-99215, 99324-99337, 99341-99350, G0402	G9414-G9417	
395	Lung Cancer Reporting (Biopsy/Cytology Specimens)	88305-88307	G9418-G9421	
396	Lung Cancer Reporting (Resection Specimens)	88309	G9422-G9425	
397	Melanoma Reporting	88305	G9428-G9431	
398	Optimal Asthma Control	99201-99205, 99212-99215, 99341-99355	G9432-G9434	
399	Post-Procedural Optimal Medical Therapy Composite (Percutaneous Coronary Intervention)	92920, 92924, 92928, 92933	G9435	
400	Hepatitis C: One-Time Screening for Hepatitis C Virus (HCV) for Patients at Risk	99201-99205, 99212-99215, 99304-99310, 99324-99337, 99341-99350, 90951-90970, G0438-G0439, G9448-G9450	G9451-G9454	
401	Screening for Hepatocellular Carcinoma (HCC) in Patients with Hepatitis C Cirrhosis	99201-99205, 99212-99215	G9455-G9457	
402	Tobacco Use and Help with Quitting Among Adolescents	99201-99205, 99212-99215, 99406-99407, 90791-90832, 90834, 90837, 90839, 90845, 92002-92014, 96150-96152, 97003-97004, G0438	G9458	

Appendix H — Medically Unlikely Edits (MUEs)

The Centers for Medicare & Medicaid Services (CMS) began to publish many of the edits used in the medically unlikely edits (MUE) program for the first time effective October 2008. What follows below is a list of the published CPT codes that have MUEs assigned to them and the number of units allowed with each code. CMS publishes the updates on a quarterly basis. Not all MUEs will be published, however. MUEs intended to detect and discourage any questionable payments will not be published as the agency feels the efficacy of these edits would be compromised. CMS added another component to the MUEs—the MUE Adjudication Indicator (MAI). The appropriate MAI can be found in parentheses following the MUE in this table and specify the maximum units of service (UOS) for a CPT/HCPCS code for the service. The MAI designates whether the UOS edit is applied to the line or claim.

The three MAIs are defined as follows:

MAI 1 (Line Edit) This MAI will continue to be adjudicated as the line edit on the claim and is auto-adjudicated by the contractor.

MAI 2 (Date of Service Edit, Policy) This MAI is considered to be the "absolute date of service edit" and is based on policy. The total unit of services (UOS) for that CPT code and that date of service (DOS) are combined for this edit. Medicare contractors are required to review all claims for the same patient, same date of service, and same provider.

MAI 3 (Date of Service Edit: Clinical) This MAI is also a date-of-service edit but is based upon clinical standards. The review takes current and previously submitted claims for the same patient, same date of service, and same provider into account. When medical necessity is clearly documented, the edit may be bypassed or the claim resubmitted.

The quarterly updates are published on the CMS website at http://www.cms.gov/NationalCorrectCodInitEd/08_MUE.asp.

Professional

CPT	MUE	CPT	MUE	CPT	MUE	CPT	MUE	CPT	MUE	CPT	MUE	CPT	MUE	CPT	MUE
01996	1(2)	0182T	3(1)	0244T	1(2)	0302T	1(1)	0362T	1(2)	10121	2(3)	11420	3(3)	11740	3(3)
0019T	1(1)	0184T	1(1)	0249T	1(2)	0303T	1(1)	0363T	3(3)	10140	2(3)	11421	3(3)	11750	6(3)
0042T	1(1)	0190T	2(2)	0253T	1(1)	0304T	1(1)	0364T	1(2)	10160	3(3)	11422	3(3)	11752	3(3)
0051T	1(2)	0191T	2(2)	0254T	2(2)	0305T	1(1)	0366T	1(2)	10180	2(3)	11423	2(3)	11755	4(3)
0052T	1(2)	0195T	1(2)	0255T	2(2)	0306T	1(1)	0368T	1(2)	11000	1(2)	11424	2(3)	11760	4(3)
0053T	1(2)	0196T	1(2)	0262T	1(1)	0307T	1(1)	0370T	1(3)	11001	1(3)	11426	2(3)	11762	2(3)
0054T	2(1)	0198T	2(2)	0263T	1(1)	0308T	1(1)	0371T	1(3)	11004	1(2)	11440	4(3)	11765	4(3)
0055T	2(1)	0200T	1(2)	0264T	1(1)	0309T	1(1)	0372T	1(3)	11005	1(2)	11441	3(3)	11770	1(3)
0058T	1(1)	0201T	1(2)	0265T	1(1)	0310T	1(1)	0373T	1(2)	11006	1(2)	11442	3(3)	11771	1(3)
0071T	1(2)	0202T	1(3)	0266T	1(1)	0311T	1(1)	0375T	1(2)	11008	1(2)	11443	2(3)	11772	1(3)
0072T	1(2)	0206T	1(1)	0267T	1(1)	0312T	1(1)	0376T	2(3)	11010	2(3)	11444	2(3)	11900	1(2)
0075T	1(2)	0207T	2(2)	0268T	1(1)	0313T	1(1)	0377T	1(2)	11011	2(3)	11446	2(3)	11901	1(2)
0076T	2(1)	0208T	1(1)	0269T	1(1)	0314T	1(1)	0378T	1(2)	11012	2(3)	11450	1(2)	11920	1(2)
0095T	1(1)	0209T	1(1)	0270T	1(1)	0315T	1(1)	0379T	1(2)	11042	1(2)	11451	1(2)	11921	1(2)
0098T	1(1)	0210T	1(1)	0271T	1(1)	0316T	1(1)	0380T	1(2)	11043	1(2)	11462	1(2)	11922	1(3)
0099T	2(2)	0211T	1(1)	0272T	1(1)	0317T	1(1)	0381T	1(2)	11044	1(2)	11463	1(2)	11950	1(2)
0100T	2(2)	0212T	1(1)	0273T	1(1)	0329T	1(2)	0382T	1(2)	11055	1(2)	11470	3(2)	11951	1(2)
0101T	1(1)	0213T	1(2)	0274T	1(2)	0330T	1(2)	0383T	1(2)	11056	1(2)	11471	2(3)	11952	1(2)
0102T	2(2)	0214T	1(2)	0275T	1(2)	0331T	1(3)	0384T	1(2)	11057	1(2)	11600	2(3)	11954	1(3)
0103T	1(1)	0215T	1(2)	0278T	1(1)	0332T	1(3)	0385T	1(2)	11100	1(2)	11601	2(3)	11960	2(3)
0106T	4(2)	0216T	1(2)	0281T	1(2)	0333T	1(2)	0386T	1(2)	11101	6(3)	11602	3(3)	11970	2(3)
0107T	4(2)	0217T	1(2)	0282T	1(3)	0335T	2(2)	0387T	1(3)	11200	1(2)	11603	2(3)	11971	2(3)
0108T	4(2)	0218T	1(2)	0283T	1(3)	0336T	1(3)	0388T	1(3)	11201	0(3)	11604	2(3)	11976	1(2)
0109T	4(2)	0219T	1(2)	0284T	1(1)	0337T	1(3)	0389T	1(3)	11300	5(3)	11606	2(3)	11980	1(2)
0110T	4(2)	0220T	1(2)	0285T	1(1)	0338T	1(2)	0390T	1(3)	11301	6(3)	11620	2(3)	11981	1(3)
0111T	1(1)	0221T	1(2)	0286T	1(2)	0339T	1(2)	0391T	1(3)	11302	4(3)	11621	2(3)	11982	1(3)
0123T	2(2)	0222T	1(1)	0287T	2(1)	0347T	1(3)	0001M	1(1)	11303	3(3)	11622	2(3)	11983	1(3)
0126T	1(1)	0223T	1(1)	0288T	1(2)	0348T	1(3)	0002M	1(1)	11305	4(3)	11623	2(3)	12001	1(2)
0159T	2(2)	0224T	1(1)	0289T	2(2)	0349T	1(3)	0003M	1(1)	11306	4(3)	11624	2(3)	12002	1(2)
0163T	2(1)	0225T	1(1)	0290T	1(1)	0350T	1(3)	0006M	1(2)	11307	3(3)	11626	2(3)	12004	1(2)
0164T	4(2)	0228T	1(2)	0291T	1(2)	0351T	5(3)	0007M	1(2)	11308	4(3)	11640	2(3)	12005	1(2)
0165T	4(2)	0230T	1(2)	0292T	1(2)	0352T	5(3)	0008M	1(3)	11310	4(3)	11641	2(3)	12006	1(2)
0169T	1(1)	0232T	1(1)	0293T	1(2)	0353T	2(3)	10021	4(3)	11311	4(3)	11642	3(3)	12007	1(2)
0171T	1(2)	0233T	1(1)	0294T	1(1)	0354T	2(3)	10022	4(3)	11312	3(3)	11643	2(3)	12011	1(2)
0172T	3(1)	0234T	2(2)	0295T	1(2)	0355T	1(2)	10030	2(3)	11313	3(3)	11644	2(3)	12013	1(2)
0174T	1(1)	0235T	2(1)	0296T	1(2)	0356T	4(2)	10040	1(2)	11400	3(3)	11646	2(3)	12014	1(2)
0175T	1(1)	0236T	1(2)	0297T	1(2)	0357T	1(2)	10060	1(2)	11401	3(3)	11719	1(2)	12015	1(2)
0178T	1(1)	0237T	2(1)	0298T	1(2)	0358T	1(2)	10061	1(2)	11402	3(3)	11720	1(2)	12016	1(2)
0179T	1(1)	0240T	1(1)	0299T	1(2)	0359T	1(2)	10080	1(3)	11403	2(3)	11721	1(2)	12017	1(2)
0180T	1(1)	0241T	1(1)	0300T	1(1)	0360T	1(2)	10081	1(3)	11404	2(3)	11730	1(2)	12018	1(2)
		0243T	1(2)	0301T	1(1)	0361T	3(3)	10120	3(3)	11406	2(3)	11732	9(3)	12020	2(3)

CPT	MUE	CPT	MUE	CPT	MUE	CPT	MUE	CPT	MUE	CPT	MUE	CPT	MUE	CPT	MUE
12021	3(3)	15155	1(2)	15835	1(3)	17282	5(3)	19366	1(2)	20900	2(3)	21116	1(2)	21296	1(2)
12031	1(2)	15156	1(2)	15836	1(2)	17283	4(3)	19367	1(2)	20902	2(3)	21120	1(2)	21310	1(2)
12032	1(2)	15157	1(3)	15837	2(3)	17284	3(3)	19368	1(2)	20910	1(3)	21121	1(2)	21315	1(2)
12034	1(2)	15200	1(2)	15838	1(2)	17286	3(3)	19369	1(2)	20912	1(3)	21122	1(2)	21320	1(2)
12035	1(2)	15201	9(3)	15839	2(3)	17311	4(3)	19370	1(2)	20920	1(3)	21123	1(2)	21325	1(2)
12036	1(2)	15220	1(2)	15840	1(3)	17312	6(3)	19371	1(2)	20922	1(3)	21125	2(2)	21330	1(2)
12037	1(2)	15221	9(3)	15841	2(3)	17313	3(3)	19380	1(2)	20924	2(3)	21127	2(3)	21335	1(2)
12041	1(2)	15240	1(2)	15842	2(3)	17314	4(3)	19396	1(2)	20926	2(3)	21137	1(2)	21336	1(2)
12042	1(2)	15241	9(3)	15845	2(3)	17315	15(3)	20005	4(3)	20931	1(2)	21138	1(2)	21337	1(2)
12044	1(2)	15260	1(2)	15847	1(2)	17340	1(2)	20100	2(3)	20937	1(2)	21139	1(2)	21338	1(2)
12045	1(2)	15261	6(3)	15851	1(2)	17360	1(2)	20101	2(3)	20938	1(2)	21141	1(2)	21339	1(2)
12046	1(2)	15271	1(2)	15852	1(3)	17380	1(3)	20102	3(3)	20950	2(3)	21142	1(2)	21340	1(2)
12047	1(2)	15272	3(3)	15860	1(3)	19000	2(3)	20103	4(3)	20955	1(3)	21143	1(2)	21343	1(2)
12051	1(2)	15273	1(2)	15876	1(2)	19001	5(3)	20150	2(3)	20956	1(3)	21145	1(2)	21344	1(2)
12052	1(2)	15275	1(2)	15877	1(2)	19020	2(3)	20200	2(3)	20957	1(3)	21146	1(2)	21345	1(2)
12053	1(2)	15276	3(2)	15878	1(2)	19030	1(2)	20205	4(3)	20962	1(3)	21147	1(2)	21346	1(2)
12054	1(2)	15277	1(2)	15879	1(2)	19081	1(2)	20206	3(3)	20969	2(3)	21150	1(2)	21347	1(2)
12055	1(2)	15570	2(3)	15920	1(3)	19082	2(3)	20220	4(3)	20970	1(3)	21151	1(2)	21348	1(2)
12056	1(2)	15572	2(3)	15922	1(3)	19083	1(2)	20225	4(3)	20972	2(3)	21154	1(2)	21355	1(2)
12057	1(2)	15574	2(3)	15931	1(3)	19084	2(3)	20240	4(3)	20973	1(2)	21155	1(2)	21356	1(2)
13100	1(2)	15576	2(3)	15933	1(3)	19085	1(2)	20245	4(3)	20974	1(3)	21159	1(2)	21360	1(2)
13101	1(2)	15600	2(3)	15934	1(3)	19086	2(3)	20250	3(3)	20975	1(3)	21160	1(2)	21365	1(2)
13102	9(3)	15610	2(3)	15935	1(3)	19100	4(3)	20251	3(3)	20979	1(3)	21172	1(3)	21366	1(2)
13120	1(2)	15620	2(3)	15936	1(3)	19101	3(3)	20500	2(3)	20982	1(2)	21175	1(2)	21385	1(2)
13121	1(2)	15630	2(3)	15937	1(3)	19105	2(3)	20501	2(3)	20983	1(2)	21179	1(2)	21386	1(2)
13122	9(3)	15650	1(3)	15940	2(3)	19110	1(3)	20520	4(3)	20985	2(3)	21180	1(2)	21387	1(2)
13131	1(2)	15731	1(3)	15941	2(3)	19112	2(3)	20525	4(3)	21010	1(2)	21181	1(3)	21390	1(2)
13132	1(2)	15732	3(3)	15944	2(3)	19120	1(2)	20526	1(2)	21011	4(3)	21182	1(2)	21395	1(2)
13133	7(3)	15734	4(3)	15945	2(3)	19125	1(2)	20527	2(3)	21012	3(3)	21183	1(2)	21400	1(2)
13151	1(2)	15736	2(3)	15946	2(3)	19126	3(3)	20550	5(3)	21013	4(3)	21184	1(2)	21401	1(2)
13152	1(2)	15738	4(3)	15950	2(3)	19260	2(3)	20551	5(3)	21014	3(3)	21188	1(2)	21406	1(2)
13153	2(3)	15740	3(3)	15951	2(3)	19271	1(3)	20552	1(2)	21015	2(3)	21193	1(2)	21407	1(2)
13160	2(3)	15750	2(3)	15952	2(3)	19272	1(3)	20553	1(2)	21016	2(3)	21194	1(2)	21408	1(2)
14000	2(3)	15756	2(3)	15953	2(3)	19281	1(2)	20555	1(3)	21025	2(3)	21195	1(2)	21421	1(2)
14001	2(3)	15757	2(3)	15956	2(3)	19282	2(3)	20600	6(3)	21026	2(3)	21196	1(2)	21422	1(2)
14020	4(3)	15758	2(3)	15958	2(3)	19283	1(2)	20604	4(3)	21029	1(3)	21198	1(3)	21423	1(2)
14021	3(3)	15760	2(3)	16000	1(2)	19284	2(3)	20605	4(3)	21030	1(3)	21199	1(2)	21431	1(2)
14040	4(3)	15770	2(3)	16020	1(3)	19285	1(2)	20606	4(3)	21031	2(3)	21206	1(3)	21432	1(2)
14041	3(3)	15775	1(2)	16025	1(3)	19286	2(3)	20610	4(3)	21032	1(3)	21208	1(3)	21433	1(2)
14060	4(3)	15776	1(2)	16030	1(3)	19287	1(2)	20611	4(3)	21034	1(3)	21209	1(3)	21435	1(2)
14061	2(3)	15777	1(3)	16035	1(2)	19288	2(3)	20612	2(3)	21040	2(3)	21210	2(3)	21436	1(2)
14301	2(3)	15780	1(2)	16036	8(3)	19296	1(3)	20615	1(3)	21044	1(3)	21215	2(3)	21440	2(2)
14302	8(3)	15781	1(3)	17000	1(2)	19297	2(3)	20650	4(3)	21045	1(3)	21230	2(3)	21445	2(2)
14350	2(3)	15782	1(3)	17003	13(2)	19298	1(2)	20660	1(2)	21046	2(3)	21235	2(3)	21450	1(2)
15002	1(2)	15783	1(3)	17004	1(2)	19300	1(2)	20661	1(2)	21047	2(3)	21240	1(2)	21451	1(2)
15003	60(3)	15786	1(2)	17106	1(2)	19301	1(2)	20662	1(2)	21048	2(3)	21242	1(2)	21452	1(2)
15004	1(2)	15787	2(3)	17107	1(2)	19302	1(2)	20663	1(2)	21049	1(3)	21243	1(2)	21453	1(2)
15005	19(3)	15788	1(2)	17108	1(2)	19303	1(2)	20664	1(2)	21050	1(2)	21244	1(2)	21454	1(2)
15040	1(2)	15789	1(2)	17110	1(2)	19304	1(2)	20665	1(2)	21060	1(2)	21245	2(2)	21461	1(2)
15050	1(3)	15792	1(3)	17111	1(2)	19305	1(2)	20670	3(3)	21070	1(2)	21246	2(2)	21462	1(2)
15100	1(2)	15793	1(3)	17250	4(3)	19306	1(2)	20680	3(3)	21073	1(2)	21247	1(2)	21465	1(2)
15101	40(3)	15819	1(2)	17260	7(3)	19307	1(2)	20690	2(3)	21076	1(2)	21248	2(3)	21470	1(2)
15110	1(2)	15820	1(2)	17261	7(3)	19316	1(2)	20692	2(3)	21077	1(2)	21249	2(3)	21480	1(2)
15111	5(3)	15821	1(2)	17262	6(3)	19318	1(2)	20693	2(3)	21079	1(2)	21255	1(2)	21485	1(2)
15115	1(2)	15822	1(2)	17263	5(3)	19324	1(2)	20694	2(3)	21080	1(2)	21256	1(2)	21490	1(2)
15116	2(3)	15823	1(2)	17264	3(3)	19325	1(2)	20696	2(3)	21081	1(2)	21260	1(2)	21495	1(2)
15120	1(2)	15824	1(2)	17266	2(3)	19328	1(2)	20697	4(3)	21082	1(2)	21261	1(2)	21497	1(2)
15121	8(3)	15825	1(2)	17270	6(3)	19330	1(2)	20802	1(2)	21083	1(2)	21263	1(2)	21501	3(3)
15130	1(2)	15826	1(2)	17271	4(3)	19340	1(2)	20805	1(2)	21084	1(2)	21267	1(2)	21502	1(3)
15131	2(3)	15828	1(2)	17272	5(3)	19342	1(2)	20808	1(2)	21085	1(3)	21268	1(2)	21510	1(3)
15135	1(2)	15829	1(2)	17273	4(3)	19350	1(2)	20816	3(3)	21086	1(2)	21270	1(2)	21550	3(3)
15136	1(3)	15830	1(2)	17274	4(3)	19355	1(2)	20822	3(3)	21087	1(2)	21275	1(2)	21552	4(3)
15150	1(2)	15832	1(2)	17276	3(3)	19357	1(2)	20824	1(2)	21088	1(2)	21280	1(2)	21554	2(3)
15151	1(2)	15833	1(2)	17280	6(3)	19361	1(2)	20827	1(2)	21100	1(2)	21282	1(2)	21555	4(3)
15152	2(3)	15834	1(2)	17281	6(3)	19364	1(2)	20838	1(2)	21110	2(3)	21295	1(2)	21556	3(3)

CPT	MUE	CPT	MUE	CPT	MUE	CPT	MUE	CPT	MUE	CPT	MUE	CPT	MUE	CPT	MUE
21557	1(3)	22511	1(3)	23035	1(3)	23491	1(2)	24149	1(2)	24620	1(2)	25248	3(3)	25545	1(2)
21558	1(3)	22512	5(3)	23040	1(3)	23500	1(2)	24150	1(3)	24635	1(2)	25250	1(2)	25560	1(2)
21600	5(3)	22513	1(2)	23044	1(3)	23505	1(2)	24152	1(3)	24640	1(2)	25251	1(2)	25565	1(2)
21610	1(3)	22514	1(2)	23065	2(3)	23515	1(2)	24155	1(2)	24650	1(2)	25259	1(2)	25574	1(2)
21615	1(2)	22515	5(3)	23066	2(3)	23520	1(2)	24160	1(2)	24655	1(2)	25260	9(3)	25575	1(2)
21616	1(2)	22532	1(2)	23071	2(3)	23525	1(2)	24164	1(2)	24665	1(2)	25263	4(3)	25600	1(2)
21620	1(2)	22533	1(2)	23073	2(3)	23530	1(2)	24200	3(3)	24666	1(2)	25265	4(3)	25605	1(2)
21627	1(2)	22534	3(3)	23075	3(3)	23532	1(2)	24201	3(3)	24670	1(2)	25270	8(3)	25606	1(2)
21630	1(2)	22548	1(2)	23076	2(3)	23540	1(2)	24220	1(2)	24675	1(2)	25272	4(3)	25607	1(2)
21632	1(2)	22551	1(2)	23077	1(3)	23545	1(2)	24300	1(2)	24685	1(2)	25274	4(3)	25608	1(2)
21685	1(2)	22552	5(3)	23078	1(3)	23550	1(2)	24301	2(3)	24800	1(2)	25275	2(3)	25609	1(2)
21700	1(2)	22554	1(2)	23100	1(2)	23552	1(2)	24305	4(3)	24802	1(2)	25280	9(3)	25622	1(2)
21705	1(2)	22556	1(2)	23101	2(2)	23570	1(2)	24310	3(3)	24900	1(2)	25290	12(3)	25624	1(2)
21720	1(3)	22558	1(2)	23105	1(2)	23575	1(2)	24320	2(3)	24920	1(2)	25295	9(3)	25628	1(2)
21725	1(3)	22585	7(3)	23106	1(2)	23585	1(2)	24330	1(3)	24925	1(2)	25300	1(2)	25630	1(3)
21740	1(2)	22586	1(2)	23107	1(2)	23600	1(2)	24331	1(3)	24930	1(2)	25301	1(2)	25635	1(3)
21742	1(2)	22590	1(2)	23120	1(2)	23605	1(2)	24332	1(2)	24931	1(2)	25310	5(3)	25645	1(3)
21743	1(2)	22595	1(2)	23125	1(2)	23615	1(2)	24340	1(2)	24935	1(2)	25312	5(3)	25650	1(2)
21750	1(2)	22600	1(2)	23130	1(2)	23616	1(2)	24341	2(3)	24940	1(2)	25315	1(3)	25651	1(2)
21805	3(3)	22610	1(2)	23140	1(3)	23620	1(2)	24342	2(3)	25000	2(3)	25316	1(3)	25652	1(2)
21811	1(2)	22612	1(2)	23145	1(3)	23625	1(2)	24343	1(2)	25001	1(3)	25320	1(2)	25660	1(2)
21812	1(2)	22614	13(3)	23146	1(3)	23630	1(2)	24344	1(2)	25020	1(2)	25332	1(2)	25670	1(2)
21813	1(2)	22630	1(2)	23150	1(3)	23650	1(2)	24345	1(2)	25023	1(2)	25335	1(2)	25671	1(2)
21820	1(2)	22632	4(2)	23155	1(3)	23655	1(2)	24346	1(2)	25024	1(2)	25337	1(2)	25675	1(2)
21825	1(2)	22633	1(2)	23156	1(3)	23660	1(2)	24357	2(3)	25025	1(2)	25350	1(3)	25676	1(2)
21920	3(3)	22634	4(2)	23170	1(3)	23665	1(2)	24358	2(3)	25028	4(3)	25355	1(3)	25680	1(2)
21925	3(3)	22800	1(2)	23172	1(3)	23670	1(2)	24359	2(3)	25031	1(2)	25360	1(3)	25685	1(2)
21930	5(3)	22802	1(2)	23174	1(3)	23675	1(2)	24360	1(2)	25035	2(3)	25365	1(3)	25690	1(2)
21931	3(3)	22804	1(2)	23180	1(3)	23680	1(2)	24361	1(2)	25040	1(3)	25370	1(2)	25695	1(2)
21932	4(3)	22808	1(2)	23182	1(3)	23700	1(2)	24362	1(2)	25065	3(3)	25375	1(2)	25800	1(2)
21933	3(3)	22810	1(2)	23184	1(3)	23800	1(2)	24363	1(2)	25066	2(3)	25390	1(2)	25805	1(2)
21935	1(3)	22812	1(2)	23190	1(3)	23802	1(2)	24365	1(2)	25071	3(3)	25391	1(2)	25810	1(2)
21936	1(3)	22818	1(2)	23195	1(2)	23900	1(2)	24366	1(2)	25073	3(3)	25392	1(2)	25820	1(2)
22010	2(3)	22819	1(2)	23200	1(3)	23920	1(2)	24370	1(2)	25075	6(3)	25393	1(2)	25825	1(2)
22015	2(3)	22830	1(2)	23210	1(3)	23921	1(2)	24371	1(2)	25076	5(3)	25394	1(3)	25830	1(2)
22100	1(2)	22840	1(2)	23220	1(3)	23930	2(3)	24400	1(3)	25077	1(3)	25400	1(2)	25900	1(2)
22101	1(2)	22842	1(2)	23330	2(3)	23931	2(3)	24410	1(2)	25078	1(3)	25405	1(2)	25905	1(2)
22102	1(2)	22843	1(2)	23333	1(3)	23935	2(3)	24420	1(2)	25085	1(2)	25415	1(2)	25907	1(2)
22103	3(3)	22844	1(2)	23334	1(2)	24000	1(2)	24430	1(3)	25100	1(2)	25420	1(2)	25909	1(2)
22110	1(2)	22845	1(2)	23335	1(2)	24006	1(2)	24435	1(3)	25101	1(2)	25425	1(2)	25915	1(2)
22112	1(2)	22846	1(2)	23350	1(2)	24065	2(3)	24470	1(2)	25105	1(2)	25426	1(2)	25920	1(2)
22114	1(2)	22847	1(2)	23395	1(2)	24066	2(3)	24495	1(2)	25107	1(2)	25430	1(3)	25922	1(2)
22116	3(3)	22848	1(2)	23397	1(3)	24071	3(3)	24498	1(2)	25109	4(3)	25431	1(3)	25924	1(2)
22206	1(2)	22849	1(2)	23400	1(2)	24073	3(3)	24500	1(2)	25110	3(3)	25440	1(2)	25927	1(2)
22207	1(2)	22850	1(2)	23405	2(3)	24075	5(3)	24505	1(2)	25111	1(3)	25441	1(2)	25929	1(2)
22208	6(3)	22851	5(3)	23406	1(3)	24076	4(3)	24515	1(2)	25112	1(3)	25442	1(2)	25931	1(2)
22210	1(2)	22852	1(2)	23410	1(2)	24077	1(3)	24516	1(2)	25115	1(3)	25443	1(2)	26010	2(3)
22212	1(2)	22855	1(2)	23412	1(2)	24079	1(3)	24530	1(2)	25116	1(3)	25444	1(2)	26011	3(3)
22214	1(2)	22856	1(2)	23415	1(2)	24100	1(2)	24535	1(2)	25118	5(3)	25445	1(2)	26020	4(3)
22216	6(3)	22857	1(2)	23420	1(2)	24101	1(2)	24538	1(2)	25119	1(2)	25446	1(2)	26025	1(2)
22220	1(2)	22858	1(2)	23430	1(2)	24102	1(2)	24545	1(2)	25120	1(3)	25447	4(3)	26030	1(2)
22222	1(2)	22861	1(2)	23440	1(2)	24105	1(2)	24546	1(2)	25125	1(3)	25449	1(2)	26034	2(3)
22224	1(2)	22862	1(2)	23450	1(2)	24110	1(3)	24560	1(3)	25126	1(3)	25450	1(2)	26035	1(3)
22226	4(3)	22864	1(2)	23455	1(2)	24115	1(3)	24565	1(3)	25130	1(3)	25455	1(2)	26037	1(3)
22305	1(2)	22865	1(2)	23460	1(2)	24116	1(3)	24566	1(3)	25135	1(3)	25490	1(2)	26040	1(2)
22310	1(2)	22900	3(3)	23462	1(2)	24120	1(3)	24575	1(3)	25136	1(3)	25491	1(2)	26045	1(2)
22315	1(2)	22901	2(3)	23465	1(2)	24125	1(3)	24576	1(3)	25145	1(3)	25492	1(2)	26055	5(3)
22318	1(2)	22902	4(3)	23466	1(2)	24126	1(3)	24577	1(3)	25150	1(3)	25500	1(2)	26060	5(3)
22319	1(2)	22903	3(3)	23470	1(2)	24130	1(2)	24579	1(3)	25151	1(3)	25505	1(2)	26070	2(3)
22325	1(2)	22904	1(3)	23472	1(2)	24134	1(3)	24582	1(3)	25170	1(3)	25515	1(2)	26075	4(3)
22326	1(2)	22905	1(3)	23473	1(2)	24136	1(3)	24586	1(3)	25210	2(1)	25520	1(2)	26080	4(3)
22327	1(2)	23000	1(2)	23474	1(2)	24138	1(3)	24587	1(2)	25215	1(2)	25525	1(2)	26100	1(3)
22328	6(3)	23020	1(2)	23480	1(2)	24140	1(3)	24600	1(2)	25230	1(2)	25526	1(2)	26105	2(3)
22505	1(2)	23030	2(3)	23485	1(2)	24145	1(3)	24605	1(2)	25240	1(2)	25530	1(2)	26110	3(3)
22510	1(2)	23031	1(3)	23490	1(2)	24147	1(2)	24615	1(2)	25246	1(2)	25535	1(2)	26111	4(3)

Appendix H — Medically Unlikely Edits (MUEs) — Professional

CPT	MUE	CPT	MUE	CPT	MUE	CPT	MUE	CPT	MUE	CPT	MUE	CPT	MUE	CPT	MUE
26113	4(3)	26483	4(3)	26720	4(3)	27078	1(2)	27258	1(2)	27409	1(2)	27536	1(2)	27690	2(3)
26115	4(3)	26485	4(3)	26725	4(3)	27080	1(2)	27259	1(2)	27412	1(2)	27538	1(2)	27691	2(3)
26116	2(3)	26489	3(3)	26727	4(3)	27086	1(3)	27265	1(2)	27415	1(2)	27540	1(2)	27692	4(3)
26117	2(3)	26490	3(3)	26735	4(3)	27087	1(3)	27266	1(2)	27416	1(2)	27550	1(2)	27695	1(2)
26118	1(3)	26492	2(3)	26740	3(3)	27090	1(2)	27267	1(2)	27418	1(2)	27552	1(2)	27696	1(2)
26121	1(2)	26494	1(3)	26742	3(3)	27091	1(2)	27268	1(2)	27420	1(2)	27556	1(2)	27698	2(2)
26123	1(2)	26496	1(3)	26746	3(3)	27093	1(2)	27269	1(2)	27422	1(2)	27557	1(2)	27700	1(2)
26125	4(3)	26497	2(3)	26750	3(3)	27095	1(2)	27275	2(2)	27424	1(2)	27558	1(2)	27702	1(2)
26130	1(3)	26498	1(3)	26755	3(3)	27096	1(2)	27279	1(2)	27425	1(2)	27560	1(2)	27703	1(2)
26135	4(3)	26499	2(3)	26756	3(3)	27097	1(3)	27280	1(2)	27427	1(2)	27562	1(2)	27704	1(2)
26140	3(3)	26500	4(3)	26765	5(3)	27098	1(2)	27282	1(2)	27428	1(2)	27566	1(2)	27705	1(3)
26145	6(3)	26502	3(3)	26770	3(3)	27100	1(2)	27284	1(2)	27429	1(2)	27570	1(2)	27707	1(3)
26160	5(3)	26508	1(2)	26775	4(3)	27105	1(3)	27286	1(2)	27430	1(2)	27580	1(2)	27709	1(3)
26170	5(3)	26510	4(3)	26776	4(3)	27110	1(2)	27290	1(2)	27435	1(2)	27590	1(2)	27712	1(2)
26180	4(3)	26516	1(2)	26785	3(3)	27111	1(2)	27295	1(2)	27437	1(2)	27591	1(2)	27715	1(2)
26185	1(3)	26517	1(2)	26820	1(2)	27120	1(2)	27301	3(3)	27438	1(2)	27592	1(2)	27720	1(2)
26200	2(3)	26518	1(2)	26841	1(2)	27122	1(2)	27303	2(3)	27440	1(2)	27594	1(2)	27722	1(2)
26205	1(3)	26520	4(3)	26842	1(2)	27125	1(2)	27305	1(2)	27441	1(2)	27596	1(2)	27724	1(2)
26210	2(3)	26525	4(3)	26843	2(3)	27130	1(2)	27306	1(2)	27442	1(2)	27598	1(2)	27725	1(2)
26215	2(3)	26530	4(3)	26844	2(3)	27132	1(2)	27307	1(2)	27443	1(2)	27600	1(2)	27726	1(2)
26230	2(3)	26531	4(3)	26850	5(3)	27134	1(2)	27310	1(2)	27445	1(2)	27601	1(2)	27727	1(2)
26235	2(3)	26535	4(3)	26852	2(3)	27137	1(2)	27323	2(3)	27446	1(2)	27602	1(2)	27730	1(2)
26236	2(3)	26536	4(3)	26860	1(2)	27138	1(2)	27324	3(3)	27447	1(2)	27603	2(3)	27732	1(2)
26250	2(3)	26540	4(3)	26861	4(3)	27140	1(2)	27325	1(2)	27448	1(3)	27604	2(3)	27734	1(2)
26260	1(3)	26541	4(3)	26862	1(2)	27146	1(3)	27326	1(2)	27450	1(3)	27605	1(2)	27740	1(2)
26262	1(3)	26542	4(3)	26863	3(3)	27147	1(3)	27327	5(3)	27454	1(2)	27606	1(2)	27742	1(2)
26320	4(3)	26545	4(3)	26910	4(3)	27151	1(3)	27328	4(3)	27455	1(3)	27607	2(3)	27745	1(2)
26340	4(3)	26546	2(3)	26951	8(3)	27156	1(2)	27329	1(3)	27457	1(3)	27610	1(2)	27750	1(2)
26341	2(3)	26548	3(3)	26952	5(3)	27158	1(2)	27330	1(2)	27465	1(2)	27612	1(2)	27752	1(2)
26350	6(3)	26550	1(2)	26990	2(3)	27161	1(2)	27331	1(2)	27466	1(2)	27613	4(3)	27756	1(2)
26352	2(3)	26551	1(2)	26991	1(3)	27165	1(2)	27332	1(2)	27468	1(2)	27614	3(3)	27758	1(2)
26356	4(3)	26553	1(3)	26992	2(3)	27170	1(2)	27333	1(2)	27470	1(2)	27615	1(3)	27759	1(2)
26357	2(3)	26554	1(3)	27000	1(3)	27175	1(2)	27334	1(2)	27472	1(2)	27616	1(3)	27760	1(2)
26358	2(3)	26555	2(3)	27001	1(3)	27176	1(2)	27335	1(2)	27475	1(2)	27618	4(3)	27762	1(2)
26370	3(3)	26556	2(3)	27003	1(2)	27177	1(2)	27337	4(3)	27477	1(2)	27619	4(3)	27766	1(2)
26372	1(3)	26560	2(3)	27005	1(2)	27178	1(2)	27339	4(3)	27479	1(2)	27620	1(2)	27767	1(2)
26373	2(3)	26561	2(3)	27006	1(2)	27179	1(2)	27340	1(2)	27485	1(2)	27625	1(2)	27768	1(2)
26390	2(3)	26562	2(3)	27025	1(3)	27181	1(2)	27345	1(2)	27486	1(2)	27626	1(2)	27769	1(2)
26392	2(3)	26565	3(3)	27027	1(2)	27185	1(2)	27347	1(2)	27487	1(2)	27630	2(3)	27780	1(2)
26410	4(3)	26567	3(3)	27030	1(2)	27187	1(2)	27350	1(2)	27488	1(2)	27632	4(3)	27781	1(2)
26412	3(3)	26568	2(3)	27033	1(2)	27193	1(2)	27355	1(3)	27495	1(2)	27634	2(3)	27784	1(2)
26415	2(3)	26580	1(2)	27035	1(2)	27194	1(2)	27356	1(3)	27496	1(2)	27635	1(3)	27786	1(2)
26416	2(3)	26587	2(3)	27036	1(2)	27200	1(2)	27357	1(3)	27497	1(2)	27637	1(3)	27788	1(2)
26418	4(3)	26590	2(3)	27040	2(3)	27202	1(2)	27358	1(3)	27498	1(2)	27638	1(3)	27792	1(2)
26420	4(3)	26591	4(3)	27041	3(3)	27220	1(2)	27360	2(3)	27499	1(2)	27640	1(3)	27808	1(2)
26426	4(3)	26593	9(3)	27043	3(3)	27222	1(2)	27364	1(3)	27500	1(2)	27641	1(3)	27810	1(2)
26428	2(3)	26596	1(3)	27045	3(3)	27226	1(2)	27365	1(3)	27501	1(2)	27645	1(3)	27814	1(2)
26432	2(3)	26600	2(3)	27047	4(3)	27227	1(2)	27370	1(2)	27502	1(2)	27646	1(3)	27816	1(2)
26433	2(3)	26605	3(3)	27048	2(3)	27228	1(2)	27372	2(3)	27503	1(2)	27647	1(3)	27818	1(2)
26434	2(3)	26607	2(3)	27049	1(3)	27230	1(2)	27380	2(2)	27506	1(2)	27648	1(2)	27822	1(2)
26437	4(3)	26608	5(3)	27050	1(2)	27232	1(2)	27381	2(2)	27507	1(2)	27650	1(2)	27823	1(2)
26440	6(3)	26615	4(3)	27052	1(2)	27235	1(2)	27385	2(3)	27508	1(2)	27652	1(2)	27824	1(2)
26442	5(3)	26641	1(2)	27054	1(2)	27236	1(2)	27386	2(3)	27509	1(2)	27654	1(2)	27825	1(2)
26445	5(3)	26645	1(2)	27057	1(2)	27238	1(2)	27390	1(2)	27510	1(2)	27656	1(3)	27826	1(2)
26449	5(3)	26650	1(2)	27059	1(3)	27240	1(2)	27391	1(2)	27511	1(2)	27658	2(3)	27827	1(2)
26450	6(3)	26665	1(2)	27060	1(2)	27244	1(2)	27392	1(2)	27513	1(2)	27659	2(3)	27828	1(2)
26455	6(3)	26670	2(3)	27062	1(2)	27245	1(2)	27393	1(2)	27514	1(2)	27664	2(3)	27829	1(2)
26460	4(3)	26675	1(3)	27065	1(3)	27246	1(2)	27394	1(2)	27516	1(2)	27665	2(3)	27830	1(2)
26471	4(3)	26676	3(3)	27066	1(3)	27248	1(2)	27395	1(2)	27517	1(2)	27675	1(2)	27831	1(2)
26474	4(3)	26685	3(3)	27067	1(3)	27250	1(2)	27396	1(2)	27519	1(2)	27676	1(2)	27832	1(2)
26476	4(3)	26686	3(3)	27070	1(3)	27252	1(2)	27397	1(2)	27520	1(2)	27680	3(3)	27840	1(2)
26477	4(3)	26700	3(3)	27071	1(3)	27253	1(2)	27400	1(2)	27524	1(2)	27681	1(2)	27842	1(2)
26478	6(3)	26705	3(3)	27075	1(3)	27254	1(2)	27403	1(3)	27530	1(2)	27685	2(3)	27846	1(2)
26479	4(3)	26706	4(3)	27076	1(2)	27256	1(2)	27405	2(2)	27532	1(2)	27686	3(3)	27848	1(2)
26480	4(3)	26715	4(3)	27077	1(2)	27257	1(2)	27407	2(2)	27535	1(2)	27687	1(2)	27860	1(2)

CPT	MUE	CPT	MUE	CPT	MUE	CPT	MUE	CPT	MUE	CPT	MUE	CPT	MUE	CPT	MUE
27870	1(2)	28173	2(3)	28445	1(2)	29065	1(3)	29843	1(2)	30150	1(2)	31256	1(2)	31600	1(2)
27871	1(3)	28175	2(3)	28446	1(2)	29075	1(3)	29844	1(2)	30160	1(2)	31267	1(2)	31601	1(2)
27880	1(2)	28190	3(3)	28450	2(3)	29085	1(3)	29845	1(2)	30200	1(2)	31276	1(2)	31603	1(2)
27881	1(2)	28192	2(3)	28455	3(3)	29086	2(3)	29846	1(2)	30210	1(3)	31287	1(2)	31605	1(2)
27882	1(2)	28193	2(3)	28456	2(3)	29105	1(2)	29847	1(2)	30220	1(2)	31288	1(2)	31610	1(2)
27884	1(2)	28200	4(3)	28465	3(3)	29125	1(2)	29848	1(2)	30300	1(3)	31290	1(2)	31611	1(2)
27886	1(2)	28202	2(3)	28470	2(3)	29126	1(2)	29850	1(2)	30310	1(3)	31291	1(2)	31612	1(3)
27888	1(2)	28208	4(3)	28475	5(3)	29130	3(3)	29851	1(2)	30320	1(3)	31292	1(2)	31613	1(2)
27889	1(2)	28210	2(3)	28476	4(3)	29131	2(3)	29855	1(2)	30400	1(2)	31293	1(2)	31614	1(2)
27892	1(2)	28220	1(2)	28485	5(3)	29200	1(2)	29856	1(2)	30410	1(2)	31294	1(2)	31615	1(3)
27893	1(2)	28222	1(2)	28490	1(2)	29240	1(2)	29860	1(2)	30420	1(2)	31295	1(2)	31620	1(3)
27894	1(2)	28225	1(2)	28495	1(2)	29260	1(3)	29861	1(2)	30430	1(2)	31296	1(2)	31622	1(3)
28001	2(3)	28226	1(2)	28496	1(2)	29280	2(3)	29862	1(2)	30435	1(2)	31297	1(2)	31623	1(3)
28002	3(3)	28230	1(2)	28505	1(2)	29305	1(3)	29863	1(2)	30450	1(2)	31300	1(2)	31624	1(3)
28003	2(3)	28232	6(3)	28510	4(3)	29325	1(3)	29866	1(2)	30460	1(2)	31320	1(2)	31625	1(2)
28005	3(3)	28234	6(3)	28515	4(3)	29345	1(3)	29867	1(2)	30462	1(2)	31360	1(2)	31626	1(2)
28008	2(3)	28238	1(2)	28525	4(3)	29355	1(3)	29868	1(3)	30465	1(2)	31365	1(2)	31627	1(3)
28020	2(3)	28240	1(2)	28530	1(2)	29358	1(3)	29870	1(2)	30520	1(2)	31367	1(2)	31628	1(2)
28022	4(3)	28250	1(2)	28531	1(2)	29365	1(3)	29871	1(2)	30540	1(2)	31368	1(2)	31629	1(2)
28024	4(3)	28260	1(2)	28540	1(3)	29405	1(3)	29873	1(2)	30545	1(2)	31370	1(2)	31630	1(3)
28035	1(2)	28261	1(3)	28545	1(3)	29425	1(3)	29874	1(2)	30560	1(2)	31375	1(2)	31631	1(2)
28039	3(3)	28262	1(2)	28546	1(3)	29435	1(3)	29875	1(2)	30580	2(3)	31380	1(2)	31632	2(3)
28041	3(3)	28264	1(2)	28555	1(3)	29440	1(2)	29876	1(2)	30600	1(3)	31382	1(2)	31633	2(3)
28043	4(3)	28270	6(3)	28570	1(2)	29445	1(3)	29877	1(2)	30620	1(2)	31390	1(2)	31634	1(2)
28045	4(3)	28272	6(3)	28575	1(2)	29450	1(3)	29879	1(2)	30630	1(2)	31395	1(2)	31635	1(3)
28046	1(3)	28280	1(2)	28576	1(2)	29505	1(2)	29880	1(2)	30801	1(2)	31400	1(3)	31636	1(2)
28047	1(3)	28285	4(3)	28585	1(3)	29515	1(2)	29881	1(2)	30802	1(2)	31420	1(2)	31637	2(3)
28050	2(3)	28286	1(2)	28600	2(3)	29520	1(2)	29882	1(2)	30901	1(3)	31500	2(3)	31638	1(3)
28052	2(3)	28288	5(3)	28605	2(3)	29530	1(2)	29883	1(2)	30903	1(3)	31502	1(3)	31640	1(3)
28054	2(3)	28289	1(2)	28606	3(3)	29540	1(2)	29884	1(2)	30905	1(2)	31505	1(3)	31641	1(3)
28055	1(3)	28290	1(2)	28615	5(3)	29550	1(2)	29885	1(2)	30906	1(3)	31510	1(2)	31643	1(2)
28060	1(2)	28292	1(2)	28630	2(3)	29580	1(2)	29886	1(2)	30915	1(3)	31511	1(3)	31645	1(2)
28062	1(2)	28293	1(2)	28635	2(3)	29581	1(2)	29887	1(2)	30920	1(3)	31512	1(3)	31646	2(3)
28070	2(3)	28294	1(2)	28636	4(3)	29582	1(2)	29888	1(2)	30930	1(2)	31513	1(3)	31647	1(2)
28072	4(3)	28296	1(2)	28645	4(3)	29583	1(2)	29889	1(2)	31000	1(2)	31515	1(3)	31648	1(2)
28080	4(3)	28297	1(2)	28660	4(3)	29584	1(2)	29891	1(2)	31002	1(2)	31520	1(3)	31649	2(3)
28086	2(3)	28298	1(2)	28665	4(3)	29700	2(3)	29892	1(2)	31020	1(2)	31525	1(3)	31651	3(3)
28088	2(3)	28299	1(2)	28666	4(3)	29705	1(3)	29893	1(2)	31030	1(2)	31526	1(3)	31660	1(2)
28090	2(3)	28300	1(2)	28675	4(3)	29710	1(2)	29894	1(2)	31032	1(2)	31527	1(2)	31661	1(2)
28092	2(3)	28302	1(2)	28705	1(2)	29720	1(2)	29895	1(2)	31040	1(2)	31528	1(2)	31717	1(3)
28100	1(3)	28304	1(3)	28715	1(2)	29730	1(3)	29897	1(2)	31050	1(2)	31529	1(3)	31720	1(3)
28102	1(3)	28305	1(3)	28725	1(2)	29740	1(3)	29898	1(2)	31051	1(2)	31530	1(3)	31725	1(3)
28103	1(3)	28306	1(2)	28730	1(2)	29750	1(3)	29899	1(2)	31070	1(2)	31531	1(3)	31730	1(3)
28104	2(3)	28307	1(2)	28735	1(2)	29800	1(2)	29900	2(3)	31075	1(2)	31535	1(3)	31750	1(2)
28106	1(3)	28308	4(3)	28737	1(2)	29804	1(2)	29901	2(3)	31080	1(2)	31536	1(3)	31755	1(2)
28107	1(3)	28309	1(2)	28740	5(3)	29805	1(2)	29902	2(3)	31081	1(2)	31540	1(3)	31760	1(2)
28108	2(3)	28310	1(2)	28750	1(2)	29806	1(2)	29904	1(2)	31084	1(2)	31541	1(3)	31766	1(2)
28110	1(2)	28312	4(3)	28755	1(2)	29807	1(2)	29905	1(2)	31085	1(2)	31545	1(2)	31770	2(3)
28111	1(2)	28313	4(3)	28760	1(2)	29819	1(2)	29906	1(2)	31086	1(2)	31546	1(2)	31775	1(3)
28112	4(3)	28315	1(2)	28800	1(2)	29820	1(2)	29907	1(2)	31087	1(2)	31560	1(2)	31780	1(2)
28113	1(2)	28320	1(2)	28805	1(2)	29821	1(2)	29914	1(2)	31090	1(2)	31561	1(2)	31781	1(2)
28114	1(2)	28322	2(3)	28810	6(3)	29822	1(2)	29915	1(2)	31200	1(2)	31570	1(2)	31785	1(3)
28116	1(2)	28340	2(3)	28820	6(3)	29823	1(2)	29916	1(2)	31201	1(2)	31571	1(2)	31786	1(3)
28118	1(2)	28341	2(3)	28825	10(2)	29824	1(2)	30000	1(3)	31205	1(2)	31575	1(3)	31800	1(3)
28119	1(2)	28344	1(2)	28890	1(2)	29825	1(2)	30020	1(3)	31225	1(2)	31576	1(3)	31805	1(3)
28120	2(3)	28345	2(3)	29000	1(3)	29826	1(2)	30100	2(3)	31230	1(2)	31577	1(3)	31820	1(2)
28122	4(3)	28360	1(2)	29010	1(3)	29827	1(2)	30110	1(2)	31231	1(2)	31578	1(3)	31825	1(2)
28124	4(3)	28400	1(2)	29015	1(3)	29828	1(2)	30115	1(2)	31233	1(2)	31579	1(2)	31830	1(2)
28126	4(3)	28405	1(2)	29035	1(3)	29830	1(2)	30117	2(3)	31235	1(2)	31580	1(2)	32035	1(2)
28130	1(2)	28406	1(2)	29040	1(3)	29834	1(2)	30118	1(3)	31237	1(2)	31582	1(2)	32036	1(3)
28140	4(3)	28415	1(2)	29044	1(3)	29835	1(2)	30120	1(2)	31238	1(3)	31584	1(2)	32096	1(3)
28150	4(3)	28420	1(2)	29046	1(3)	29836	1(2)	30124	2(3)	31239	1(2)	31587	1(2)	32097	1(3)
28153	6(3)	28430	1(2)	29049	1(3)	29837	1(2)	30125	1(3)	31240	1(2)	31588	1(2)	32098	1(2)
28160	5(3)	28435	1(2)	29055	1(3)	29838	1(2)	30130	1(2)	31254	1(2)	31590	1(2)	32100	1(3)
28171	1(3)	28436	1(2)	29058	1(3)	29840	1(2)	30140	1(2)	31255	1(2)	31595	1(2)	32110	1(3)

CPT	MUE	CPT	MUE	CPT	MUE	CPT	MUE	CPT	MUE	CPT	MUE	CPT	MUE	CPT	MUE
32120	1(3)	32669	2(3)	33235	1(2)	33425	1(2)	33675	1(2)	33886	1(2)	34111	2(3)	35180	2(3)
32124	1(3)	32670	1(2)	33236	1(2)	33426	1(2)	33676	1(2)	33889	1(2)	34151	2(3)	35182	2(3)
32140	1(3)	32671	1(2)	33237	1(2)	33427	1(2)	33677	1(2)	33891	1(2)	34201	1(3)	35184	2(3)
32141	1(3)	32672	1(3)	33238	1(2)	33430	1(2)	33681	1(2)	33910	1(3)	34203	1(2)	35188	2(3)
32150	1(3)	32673	1(2)	33240	1(3)	33460	1(2)	33684	1(2)	33915	1(3)	34401	1(3)	35189	1(3)
32151	1(3)	32674	1(2)	33241	1(2)	33463	1(2)	33688	1(2)	33916	1(3)	34421	1(3)	35190	2(3)
32160	1(3)	32701	1(2)	33243	1(2)	33464	1(2)	33690	1(2)	33917	1(2)	34451	1(3)	35201	2(3)
32200	2(3)	32800	1(3)	33244	1(2)	33465	1(2)	33692	1(2)	33920	1(2)	34471	1(2)	35206	2(3)
32215	1(2)	32810	1(3)	33249	1(3)	33468	1(2)	33694	1(2)	33922	1(2)	34490	1(2)	35207	3(3)
32220	1(2)	32815	1(3)	33250	1(2)	33470	1(2)	33697	1(2)	33924	1(2)	34501	1(2)	35211	3(3)
32225	1(2)	32820	1(2)	33251	1(2)	33471	1(2)	33702	1(2)	33925	1(2)	34502	1(2)	35216	2(3)
32310	1(3)	32850	1(2)	33254	1(2)	33474	1(2)	33710	1(2)	33926	1(2)	34510	2(3)	35221	3(3)
32320	1(3)	32851	1(2)	33255	1(2)	33475	1(2)	33720	1(2)	33930	1(2)	34520	1(3)	35226	3(3)
32400	2(3)	32852	1(2)	33256	1(2)	33476	1(2)	33722	1(3)	33933	1(2)	34530	1(2)	35231	2(3)
32405	2(3)	32853	1(2)	33257	1(2)	33478	1(2)	33724	1(2)	33935	1(2)	34800	1(2)	35236	2(3)
32440	1(2)	32854	1(2)	33258	1(2)	33496	1(3)	33726	1(2)	33940	1(2)	34802	1(2)	35241	2(3)
32442	1(2)	32855	1(2)	33259	1(2)	33500	1(3)	33730	1(2)	33944	1(2)	34803	1(2)	35246	2(3)
32445	1(2)	32856	1(2)	33261	1(2)	33501	1(3)	33732	1(2)	33945	1(2)	34804	1(2)	35251	2(3)
32480	1(2)	32900	1(3)	33262	1(3)	33502	1(3)	33735	1(2)	33946	1(2)	34805	1(2)	35256	2(3)
32482	1(2)	32905	1(2)	33263	1(3)	33503	1(3)	33736	1(2)	33947	1(2)	34806	1(2)	35261	1(3)
32484	2(3)	32906	1(2)	33264	1(3)	33504	1(3)	33737	1(2)	33948	1(2)	34808	1(3)	35266	2(3)
32486	1(3)	32940	1(3)	33265	1(2)	33505	1(3)	33750	1(3)	33949	1(2)	34812	1(2)	35271	2(3)
32488	1(2)	32960	1(2)	33266	1(2)	33506	1(2)	33755	1(2)	33951	1(1)	34813	1(2)	35276	2(3)
32491	1(2)	32997	1(2)	33270	1(3)	33507	1(3)	33762	1(2)	33952	1(1)	34820	1(2)	35281	2(3)
32501	1(3)	32998	1(2)	33271	1(3)	33508	1(2)	33764	1(3)	33953	1(1)	34825	2(2)	35286	2(3)
32503	1(2)	33010	1(2)	33272	1(3)	33510	1(2)	33766	1(2)	33954	1(1)	34826	4(3)	35301	2(3)
32504	1(2)	33011	1(3)	33273	1(3)	33511	1(2)	33767	1(2)	33955	1(3)	34830	1(2)	35302	1(2)
32505	1(2)	33015	1(3)	33282	1(2)	33512	1(2)	33768	1(2)	33956	1(3)	34831	1(2)	35303	1(2)
32506	3(3)	33020	1(3)	33284	1(2)	33513	1(2)	33770	1(2)	33957	1(3)	34832	1(2)	35304	1(2)
32507	2(3)	33025	1(2)	33300	1(3)	33514	1(2)	33771	1(2)	33958	1(3)	34833	1(2)	35305	1(2)
32540	1(3)	33030	1(2)	33305	1(3)	33516	1(2)	33774	1(2)	33959	1(3)	34834	1(2)	35306	2(3)
32550	2(3)	33031	1(2)	33310	1(2)	33517	1(2)	33775	1(2)	33962	1(3)	34839	1(2)	35311	1(2)
32551	2(3)	33050	1(2)	33315	1(2)	33518	1(2)	33776	1(2)	33963	1(3)	34841	1(2)	35321	1(2)
32552	2(2)	33120	1(3)	33320	1(3)	33519	1(2)	33777	1(2)	33964	1(3)	34842	1(2)	35331	1(2)
32553	1(2)	33130	1(3)	33321	1(3)	33521	1(2)	33778	1(2)	33965	1(3)	34843	1(2)	35341	3(3)
32554	2(3)	33140	1(2)	33322	1(3)	33522	1(2)	33779	1(2)	33966	1(3)	34844	1(2)	35351	1(3)
32555	2(3)	33141	1(2)	33330	1(3)	33523	1(2)	33780	1(2)	33967	1(3)	34845	1(2)	35355	1(2)
32556	2(3)	33202	1(2)	33335	1(3)	33530	1(2)	33781	1(2)	33968	1(3)	34846	1(2)	35361	1(2)
32557	2(3)	33203	1(2)	33361	1(2)	33533	1(2)	33782	1(2)	33969	1(3)	34847	1(2)	35363	1(2)
32560	1(3)	33206	1(3)	33362	1(2)	33534	1(2)	33783	1(2)	33970	1(3)	34848	1(2)	35371	1(2)
32561	1(2)	33207	1(3)	33363	1(2)	33535	1(2)	33786	1(2)	33971	1(3)	34900	1(2)	35372	1(2)
32562	1(2)	33208	1(3)	33364	1(2)	33536	1(2)	33788	1(2)	33973	1(3)	35001	1(2)	35390	1(3)
32601	1(3)	33210	1(3)	33365	1(2)	33542	1(2)	33800	1(2)	33974	1(3)	35002	1(3)	35400	1(3)
32604	1(3)	33211	1(3)	33366	1(2)	33545	1(2)	33802	1(3)	33975	1(3)	35005	1(2)	35450	2(3)
32606	1(3)	33212	1(3)	33367	1(2)	33548	1(2)	33803	1(3)	33976	1(3)	35011	1(2)	35452	1(2)
32607	1(3)	33213	1(3)	33368	1(2)	33572	3(2)	33813	1(3)	33977	1(3)	35013	1(2)	35458	2(3)
32608	1(3)	33214	1(3)	33369	1(2)	33600	1(3)	33814	1(2)	33978	1(3)	35021	1(2)	35460	2(3)
32609	1(3)	33215	2(3)	33400	1(2)	33602	1(3)	33820	1(2)	33979	1(3)	35022	1(2)	35471	3(3)
32650	1(2)	33216	1(3)	33401	1(2)	33606	1(2)	33822	1(2)	33980	1(3)	35045	2(3)	35472	1(2)
32651	1(2)	33217	1(3)	33403	1(2)	33608	1(2)	33824	1(2)	33981	1(3)	35081	1(2)	35475	4(3)
32652	1(2)	33218	1(3)	33404	1(2)	33610	1(2)	33840	1(2)	33982	1(3)	35082	1(2)	35476	5(3)
32653	1(3)	33220	1(3)	33405	1(2)	33611	1(2)	33845	1(2)	33983	1(3)	35091	1(2)	35500	2(3)
32654	1(3)	33221	1(3)	33406	1(2)	33612	1(2)	33851	1(2)	33984	1(3)	35092	1(2)	35501	1(3)
32655	1(3)	33222	1(3)	33410	1(2)	33615	1(2)	33852	1(2)	33985	1(3)	35102	1(2)	35506	1(3)
32656	1(2)	33223	1(3)	33411	1(2)	33617	1(2)	33853	1(2)	33986	1(3)	35103	1(2)	35508	1(3)
32658	1(3)	33224	1(3)	33412	1(2)	33619	1(2)	33860	1(2)	33987	1(3)	35111	1(2)	35509	1(3)
32659	1(2)	33225	1(3)	33413	1(2)	33620	1(2)	33863	1(2)	33988	1(3)	35112	1(2)	35510	1(3)
32661	1(3)	33226	1(3)	33414	1(2)	33621	1(3)	33864	1(2)	33989	1(3)	35121	1(3)	35511	1(3)
32662	1(3)	33227	1(3)	33415	1(2)	33622	1(2)	33870	1(2)	33990	1(3)	35122	1(3)	35512	1(3)
32663	1(3)	33228	1(3)	33416	1(2)	33641	1(2)	33875	1(2)	33991	1(3)	35131	1(2)	35515	1(3)
32664	1(2)	33229	1(3)	33417	1(2)	33645	1(2)	33877	1(2)	33992	1(2)	35132	1(2)	35516	1(3)
32665	1(2)	33230	1(3)	33418	1(3)	33647	1(2)	33880	1(2)	33993	1(3)	35141	1(2)	35518	1(3)
32666	1(3)	33231	1(3)	33419	1(3)	33660	1(2)	33881	1(2)	34001	1(3)	35142	1(2)	35521	1(3)
32667	3(3)	33233	1(2)	33420	1(2)	33665	1(2)	33883	1(2)	34051	1(3)	35151	1(2)	35522	1(3)
32668	2(3)	33234	1(2)	33422	1(2)	33670	1(2)	33884	2(3)	34101	1(3)	35152	1(2)	35523	1(3)

CPT	MUE	CPT	MUE	CPT	MUE	CPT	MUE	CPT	MUE	CPT	MUE	CPT	MUE	CPT	MUE
35525	1(3)	35820	2(3)	36468	1(3)	36832	2(3)	37615	2(3)	38724	1(2)	41009	2(3)	42226	1(2)
35526	1(3)	35840	2(3)	36470	1(3)	36833	1(3)	37616	1(3)	38740	1(2)	41010	1(2)	42227	1(2)
35531	2(3)	35860	2(3)	36471	1(2)	36835	1(3)	37617	3(3)	38745	1(2)	41015	2(3)	42235	1(2)
35533	1(3)	35870	1(3)	36475	1(3)	36838	1(3)	37618	2(3)	38746	1(2)	41016	2(3)	42260	1(3)
35535	1(3)	35875	2(3)	36476	2(3)	36860	2(3)	37619	1(2)	38747	1(2)	41017	2(3)	42280	1(2)
35536	1(3)	35876	2(3)	36478	1(3)	36861	2(3)	37650	1(2)	38760	1(2)	41018	2(3)	42281	1(2)
35537	1(3)	35879	2(3)	36479	2(3)	36870	2(3)	37660	1(2)	38765	1(2)	41019	1(2)	42300	2(3)
35538	1(3)	35881	2(3)	36481	1(3)	37140	1(2)	37700	1(2)	38770	1(2)	41100	3(3)	42305	2(3)
35539	1(3)	35883	1(3)	36500	4(3)	37145	1(3)	37718	1(2)	38780	1(2)	41105	3(3)	42310	2(3)
35540	1(3)	35884	1(3)	36510	1(3)	37160	1(3)	37722	1(2)	38790	1(2)	41108	2(3)	42320	2(3)
35556	1(3)	35901	1(3)	36511	1(3)	37180	1(2)	37735	1(2)	38792	1(3)	41110	2(3)	42330	2(3)
35558	1(3)	35903	2(3)	36512	1(3)	37181	1(2)	37760	1(2)	38794	1(2)	41112	2(3)	42335	2(2)
35560	1(3)	35905	1(3)	36513	1(3)	37182	1(2)	37761	1(2)	38900	1(3)	41113	2(3)	42340	1(2)
35563	1(3)	35907	1(3)	36514	1(3)	37183	1(2)	37765	1(2)	39000	1(2)	41114	2(3)	42400	2(3)
35565	1(3)	36000	4(3)	36515	1(3)	37184	1(2)	37766	1(2)	39010	1(2)	41115	1(2)	42405	2(3)
35566	1(3)	36002	2(3)	36516	1(3)	37185	2(3)	37780	1(2)	39200	1(2)	41116	2(3)	42408	1(3)
35570	1(3)	36005	2(3)	36522	1(3)	37186	2(3)	37785	1(2)	39220	1(2)	41120	1(2)	42409	1(3)
35571	2(3)	36010	2(3)	36555	2(3)	37187	1(3)	37788	1(2)	39400	1(2)	41130	1(2)	42410	1(2)
35572	2(3)	36011	4(3)	36556	2(3)	37188	1(3)	37790	1(2)	39501	1(3)	41135	1(2)	42415	1(2)
35583	1(2)	36012	4(3)	36557	2(3)	37191	1(3)	38100	1(2)	39503	1(2)	41140	1(2)	42420	1(2)
35585	2(3)	36013	2(3)	36558	2(3)	37192	1(3)	38101	1(3)	39540	1(2)	41145	1(2)	42425	1(2)
35587	2(2)	36014	2(3)	36560	2(3)	37193	1(3)	38102	1(3)	39541	1(2)	41150	1(2)	42426	1(2)
35600	2(3)	36015	4(3)	36561	2(3)	37195	1(3)	38115	1(3)	39545	1(2)	41153	1(2)	42440	1(2)
35601	1(3)	36100	2(3)	36563	1(3)	37197	2(3)	38120	1(3)	39560	1(3)	41155	1(2)	42450	2(3)
35606	1(3)	36120	2(3)	36565	1(3)	37200	2(3)	38200	1(3)	39561	1(3)	41250	2(3)	42500	2(3)
35612	1(3)	36140	3(3)	36566	1(3)	37202	4(3)	38205	1(3)	40490	3(3)	41251	2(3)	42505	2(3)
35616	1(3)	36147	2(3)	36568	2(3)	37211	1(2)	38206	1(3)	40500	2(3)	41252	2(3)	42507	1(2)
35621	1(3)	36148	1(3)	36569	2(3)	37212	1(2)	38208	0(3)	40510	2(3)	41500	1(2)	42509	1(2)
35623	1(3)	36160	2(3)	36570	2(3)	37213	1(2)	38209	0(3)	40520	2(3)	41510	1(2)	42510	1(2)
35626	3(3)	36200	2(3)	36571	2(3)	37214	1(2)	38210	0(3)	40525	2(3)	41512	1(2)	42550	2(3)
35631	4(3)	36215	6(3)	36575	2(3)	37215	1(2)	38211	0(3)	40527	2(3)	41520	1(3)	42600	2(3)
35632	1(3)	36216	4(3)	36576	2(3)	37217	1(2)	38212	0(3)	40530	2(3)	41530	1(3)	42650	2(3)
35633	1(3)	36217	2(3)	36578	2(3)	37218	1(2)	38213	0(3)	40650	2(3)	41800	2(3)	42660	2(3)
35634	1(3)	36218	6(3)	36580	2(3)	37220	2(2)	38214	0(3)	40652	2(3)	41805	3(3)	42665	2(3)
35636	1(3)	36221	1(3)	36581	2(3)	37221	2(2)	38215	0(3)	40654	2(3)	41806	3(3)	42700	2(3)
35637	1(3)	36222	1(3)	36582	2(3)	37222	2(3)	38220	1(3)	40700	1(2)	41820	4(2)	42720	1(3)
35638	1(3)	36223	1(3)	36583	2(3)	37223	2(3)	38221	1(3)	40701	1(2)	41821	2(3)	42725	1(3)
35642	1(3)	36224	1(3)	36584	2(3)	37224	2(2)	38230	1(2)	40702	1(2)	41822	1(2)	42800	3(3)
35645	1(3)	36225	1(3)	36585	2(3)	37225	2(2)	38232	1(2)	40720	1(2)	41823	1(2)	42804	3(3)
35646	1(3)	36226	1(3)	36589	2(3)	37226	2(2)	38240	1(3)	40761	1(2)	41825	2(3)	42806	1(3)
35647	1(3)	36227	1(3)	36590	2(3)	37227	2(2)	38241	1(2)	40800	2(3)	41826	2(3)	42808	2(3)
35650	1(3)	36228	4(3)	36591	2(3)	37228	2(2)	38242	1(2)	40801	2(3)	41827	2(3)	42809	1(3)
35654	1(3)	36245	6(3)	36592	1(3)	37229	2(2)	38243	1(3)	40804	2(3)	41828	4(2)	42810	1(3)
35656	1(3)	36246	4(3)	36593	2(3)	37230	2(2)	38300	1(3)	40805	2(3)	41830	2(3)	42815	1(3)
35661	1(3)	36247	3(3)	36595	2(3)	37231	2(2)	38305	1(3)	40806	2(2)	41850	2(3)	42820	1(2)
35663	1(3)	36248	6(3)	36596	2(3)	37232	2(3)	38308	1(3)	40808	4(3)	41870	2(3)	42821	1(2)
35665	1(3)	36251	1(3)	36597	2(3)	37233	2(3)	38380	1(2)	40810	4(3)	41872	4(2)	42825	1(2)
35666	2(3)	36252	1(3)	36598	2(3)	37234	2(3)	38381	1(2)	40812	4(3)	41874	4(2)	42826	1(2)
35671	2(3)	36253	1(3)	36600	4(3)	37235	2(3)	38382	1(2)	40814	4(3)	42000	1(3)	42830	1(2)
35681	1(3)	36254	1(3)	36620	3(3)	37236	1(2)	38500	2(3)	40816	2(3)	42100	3(3)	42831	1(2)
35682	1(2)	36260	1(2)	36625	2(3)	37237	2(3)	38505	3(3)	40818	2(3)	42104	3(3)	42835	1(2)
35683	1(2)	36261	1(2)	36640	1(3)	37238	1(2)	38510	1(2)	40819	2(2)	42106	2(3)	42836	1(2)
35685	2(3)	36262	1(2)	36660	1(3)	37239	2(3)	38520	1(2)	40820	5(3)	42107	2(3)	42842	1(3)
35686	1(3)	36400	1(3)	36680	1(3)	37241	2(3)	38525	1(2)	40830	2(3)	42120	1(2)	42844	1(3)
35691	1(3)	36405	1(3)	36800	1(3)	37242	2(3)	38530	1(2)	40831	2(3)	42140	1(2)	42845	1(3)
35693	1(3)	36406	1(3)	36810	1(3)	37243	1(3)	38542	1(2)	40840	1(2)	42145	1(2)	42860	1(3)
35694	1(3)	36410	3(3)	36815	1(3)	37244	2(3)	38550	1(3)	40842	1(2)	42160	2(3)	42870	1(3)
35695	1(3)	36415	4(3)	36818	1(3)	37250	1(2)	38555	1(3)	40843	1(2)	42180	1(3)	42890	1(2)
35697	2(3)	36420	2(3)	36819	1(3)	37500	1(3)	38562	1(2)	40844	1(2)	42182	1(3)	42892	1(3)
35700	2(3)	36425	2(3)	36820	1(3)	37565	1(2)	38564	1(2)	40845	1(3)	42200	1(2)	42894	1(3)
35701	1(2)	36430	1(2)	36821	2(3)	37600	1(3)	38570	1(2)	41000	2(3)	42205	1(2)	42900	1(3)
35721	1(2)	36440	1(3)	36823	1(3)	37605	1(3)	38571	1(2)	41005	2(3)	42210	1(2)	42950	1(2)
35741	1(2)	36450	1(3)	36825	1(3)	37606	1(3)	38572	1(2)	41006	2(3)	42215	1(2)	42953	1(3)
35761	2(3)	36455	1(3)	36830	2(3)	37607	1(3)	38700	1(2)	41007	2(3)	42220	1(2)	42955	1(2)
35800	2(3)	36460	2(3)	36831	1(3)	37609	1(2)	38720	1(2)	41008	2(3)	42225	1(2)	42960	1(3)

CPT	MUE	CPT	MUE	CPT	MUE	CPT	MUE	CPT	MUE	CPT	MUE	CPT	MUE	CPT	MUE
42961	1(3)	43248	1(3)	43500	1(2)	44005	1(2)	44364	1(2)	45130	1(2)	46045	2(3)	46945	1(2)
42962	1(3)	43249	1(3)	43501	1(3)	44010	1(2)	44365	1(2)	45135	1(2)	46050	2(3)	46946	1(2)
42970	1(3)	43250	1(2)	43502	1(2)	44015	1(2)	44366	1(3)	45136	1(2)	46060	2(3)	46947	1(2)
42971	1(3)	43251	1(2)	43510	1(2)	44020	2(3)	44369	1(2)	45150	1(2)	46070	1(2)	47000	3(3)
42972	1(3)	43252	1(2)	43520	1(2)	44021	1(3)	44370	1(2)	45160	1(3)	46080	1(2)	47001	3(3)
43020	1(2)	43253	1(3)	43605	1(2)	44025	1(3)	44372	1(2)	45171	2(3)	46083	2(3)	47010	3(3)
43030	1(2)	43254	1(3)	43610	2(3)	44050	1(2)	44373	1(2)	45172	2(3)	46200	1(3)	47015	1(2)
43045	1(2)	43255	2(3)	43611	2(3)	44055	1(2)	44376	1(3)	45190	1(3)	46220	1(2)	47100	3(3)
43100	1(3)	43257	1(2)	43620	1(2)	44100	1(2)	44377	1(2)	45300	1(3)	46221	1(2)	47120	2(3)
43101	1(3)	43259	1(2)	43621	1(2)	44110	1(2)	44378	1(3)	45303	1(3)	46230	1(2)	47122	1(2)
43107	1(2)	43260	1(3)	43622	1(2)	44111	1(2)	44379	1(2)	45305	1(2)	46250	1(2)	47125	1(2)
43108	1(2)	43261	1(2)	43631	1(2)	44120	1(2)	44380	1(3)	45307	1(3)	46255	1(2)	47130	1(2)
43112	1(2)	43262	2(2)	43632	1(2)	44121	4(3)	44382	1(2)	45308	1(2)	46257	1(2)	47133	1(2)
43113	1(2)	43263	1(2)	43633	1(2)	44125	1(2)	44385	1(3)	45309	1(2)	46258	1(2)	47135	1(2)
43116	1(2)	43264	1(2)	43634	1(2)	44126	1(2)	44386	1(2)	45315	1(2)	46260	1(2)	47136	1(2)
43117	1(2)	43265	1(2)	43635	1(2)	44127	1(2)	44388	1(3)	45317	1(3)	46261	1(2)	47140	1(2)
43118	1(2)	43266	1(3)	43640	1(2)	44128	2(3)	44389	1(2)	45320	1(2)	46262	1(2)	47141	1(2)
43121	1(2)	43270	1(3)	43641	1(2)	44130	3(3)	44390	1(3)	45321	1(2)	46270	1(3)	47142	1(2)
43122	1(2)	43273	1(2)	43644	1(2)	44132	1(2)	44391	1(3)	45327	1(2)	46275	1(3)	47143	1(2)
43123	1(2)	43274	2(3)	43645	1(2)	44133	1(2)	44392	1(2)	45330	1(3)	46280	1(2)	47144	1(2)
43124	1(2)	43275	1(3)	43647	1(2)	44135	1(2)	44394	1(2)	45331	1(2)	46285	1(3)	47145	1(2)
43130	1(3)	43276	2(3)	43648	1(2)	44136	1(2)	44500	1(3)	45332	1(3)	46288	1(3)	47146	3(3)
43135	1(3)	43277	3(3)	43651	1(2)	44137	1(2)	44602	1(2)	45333	1(2)	46320	2(3)	47147	2(3)
43180	1(2)	43278	1(3)	43652	1(2)	44139	1(2)	44603	1(2)	45334	1(3)	46500	1(2)	47300	2(3)
43191	1(3)	43279	1(2)	43653	1(2)	44140	2(3)	44604	1(2)	45335	1(2)	46505	1(2)	47350	1(3)
43192	1(3)	43280	1(2)	43752	2(3)	44141	1(3)	44605	1(2)	45337	1(2)	46600	1(3)	47360	1(3)
43193	1(3)	43281	1(2)	43753	1(3)	44143	1(2)	44615	4(3)	45338	1(2)	46604	1(2)	47361	1(3)
43194	1(3)	43282	1(2)	43754	1(3)	44144	1(3)	44620	2(3)	45340	1(2)	46606	1(2)	47362	1(3)
43195	1(3)	43283	1(2)	43755	1(3)	44145	1(2)	44625	1(3)	45341	1(2)	46608	1(3)	47370	1(2)
43196	1(3)	43300	1(2)	43756	1(2)	44146	1(2)	44626	1(3)	45342	1(2)	46610	1(2)	47371	1(2)
43197	1(3)	43305	1(2)	43757	1(2)	44147	1(3)	44640	2(3)	45378	1(3)	46611	1(2)	47380	1(2)
43198	1(3)	43310	1(2)	43760	2(3)	44150	1(2)	44650	2(3)	45379	1(3)	46612	1(2)	47381	1(2)
43200	1(3)	43312	1(2)	43761	2(3)	44151	1(2)	44660	1(3)	45380	1(2)	46614	1(3)	47382	1(2)
43201	1(2)	43313	1(2)	43770	1(2)	44155	1(2)	44661	1(3)	45381	1(2)	46615	1(2)	47383	1(2)
43202	1(2)	43314	1(2)	43771	1(2)	44156	1(2)	44680	1(3)	45382	1(3)	46700	1(2)	47400	1(3)
43204	1(2)	43320	1(2)	43772	1(2)	44157	1(2)	44700	1(2)	45384	1(2)	46705	1(2)	47420	1(2)
43205	1(2)	43325	1(2)	43773	1(2)	44158	1(2)	44701	1(2)	45385	1(2)	46706	1(3)	47425	1(2)
43206	1(2)	43327	1(2)	43774	1(2)	44160	1(2)	44705	1(3)	45386	1(2)	46707	1(3)	47460	1(2)
43211	1(3)	43328	1(2)	43775	1(2)	44180	1(2)	44715	1(2)	45391	1(2)	46710	1(3)	47480	1(2)
43212	1(3)	43330	1(2)	43800	1(2)	44186	1(2)	44720	2(3)	45392	1(2)	46712	1(3)	47490	1(2)
43213	1(2)	43331	1(2)	43810	1(2)	44187	1(3)	44721	2(3)	45395	1(2)	46715	1(2)	47500	2(3)
43214	1(3)	43332	1(2)	43820	1(2)	44188	1(3)	44800	1(3)	45397	1(2)	46716	1(2)	47505	2(3)
43215	1(2)	43333	1(2)	43825	1(2)	44202	1(2)	44820	1(3)	45400	1(2)	46730	1(2)	47510	2(3)
43216	1(2)	43334	1(2)	43830	1(2)	44203	2(3)	44850	1(3)	45402	1(2)	46735	1(2)	47511	2(3)
43217	1(2)	43335	1(2)	43831	1(2)	44204	2(3)	44900	1(2)	45500	1(2)	46740	1(2)	47525	3(3)
43220	1(3)	43336	1(2)	43832	1(2)	44205	1(2)	44950	1(2)	45505	1(2)	46742	1(2)	47530	2(3)
43226	1(3)	43337	1(2)	43840	2(3)	44206	1(2)	44955	1(2)	45520	1(2)	46744	1(2)	47550	1(3)
43227	1(3)	43338	1(2)	43843	1(2)	44207	1(2)	44960	1(2)	45540	1(2)	46746	1(2)	47552	1(3)
43229	1(3)	43340	1(2)	43845	1(2)	44208	1(2)	44970	1(2)	45541	1(2)	46748	1(2)	47553	1(2)
43231	1(2)	43341	1(2)	43846	1(2)	44210	1(2)	45000	1(3)	45550	1(2)	46750	1(2)	47554	1(3)
43232	1(2)	43351	1(2)	43847	1(2)	44211	1(2)	45005	1(3)	45560	1(2)	46751	1(2)	47555	1(2)
43233	1(3)	43352	1(2)	43848	1(2)	44212	1(2)	45020	1(3)	45562	1(2)	46753	1(2)	47556	1(2)
43235	1(3)	43360	1(2)	43850	1(2)	44213	1(2)	45100	2(3)	45563	1(2)	46754	1(3)	47560	1(3)
43236	1(2)	43361	1(2)	43855	1(2)	44227	1(3)	45108	1(2)	45800	1(3)	46760	1(2)	47561	1(3)
43237	1(2)	43400	1(2)	43860	1(2)	44300	1(3)	45110	1(2)	45805	1(3)	46761	1(2)	47562	1(2)
43238	1(2)	43401	1(2)	43865	1(2)	44310	2(3)	45111	1(2)	45820	1(3)	46762	1(2)	47563	1(2)
43239	1(2)	43405	1(2)	43870	1(2)	44312	1(2)	45112	1(2)	45825	1(3)	46900	1(2)	47564	1(2)
43240	1(2)	43410	1(3)	43880	1(3)	44314	1(2)	45113	1(2)	45900	1(2)	46910	1(2)	47570	1(2)
43241	1(3)	43415	1(3)	43881	1(3)	44316	1(2)	45114	1(2)	45905	1(2)	46916	1(2)	47600	1(2)
43242	1(2)	43420	1(3)	43882	1(3)	44320	1(2)	45116	1(2)	45910	1(2)	46917	1(2)	47605	1(2)
43243	1(2)	43425	1(3)	43886	1(2)	44322	1(2)	45119	1(2)	45915	1(2)	46922	1(2)	47610	1(2)
43244	1(2)	43450	1(3)	43887	1(2)	44340	1(2)	45120	1(2)	45990	1(2)	46924	1(2)	47612	1(2)
43245	1(2)	43453	1(3)	43888	1(2)	44345	1(2)	45121	1(2)	46020	2(3)	46930	1(2)	47620	1(2)
43246	1(2)	43460	1(3)	44005	1(2)	44346	1(2)	45123	1(2)	46030	1(3)	46940	1(2)	47630	1(3)
43247	1(2)	43496	1(3)	44010	1(2)	44360	1(3)	45126	1(2)	46040	2(3)	46942	1(3)	47700	1(2)

Appendix H — Medically Unlikely Edits (MUEs) — Professional

CPT	MUE	CPT	MUE	CPT	MUE	CPT	MUE	CPT	MUE	CPT	MUE	CPT	MUE	CPT	MUE
47701	1(2)	49322	1(2)	49606	1(2)	50396	1(3)	50860	1(2)	51792	1(3)	52354	1(3)	53660	1(2)
47711	1(2)	49323	1(2)	49610	1(2)	50398	1(3)	50900	1(3)	51797	1(3)	52355	1(3)	53661	1(3)
47712	1(2)	49324	1(2)	49611	1(2)	50400	1(2)	50920	2(3)	51798	1(3)	52356	1(2)	53665	1(3)
47715	1(2)	49325	1(2)	49650	1(2)	50405	1(2)	50930	2(3)	51800	1(2)	52400	1(2)	53850	1(2)
47720	1(2)	49326	1(2)	49651	1(2)	50500	1(3)	50940	1(2)	51820	1(2)	52402	1(2)	53852	1(2)
47721	1(2)	49327	1(2)	49652	2(3)	50520	1(3)	50945	1(2)	51840	1(2)	52441	1(2)	53855	1(2)
47740	1(2)	49400	1(3)	49653	2(3)	50525	1(3)	50947	1(2)	51841	1(2)	52442	5(1)	53860	1(2)
47741	1(2)	49402	1(3)	49654	2(3)	50526	1(3)	50948	1(2)	51845	1(2)	52450	1(2)	54000	1(2)
47760	1(2)	49405	2(3)	49655	2(3)	50540	1(2)	50951	1(3)	51860	1(3)	52500	1(2)	54001	1(2)
47765	1(2)	49406	2(3)	49656	2(3)	50541	1(2)	50953	1(3)	51865	1(3)	52601	1(2)	54015	1(3)
47780	1(2)	49407	1(3)	49657	2(3)	50542	1(2)	50955	1(2)	51880	1(2)	52630	1(2)	54050	1(2)
47785	1(2)	49411	1(2)	49900	1(3)	50543	1(2)	50957	1(2)	51900	1(3)	52640	1(2)	54055	1(2)
47800	1(2)	49412	1(2)	49904	1(3)	50544	1(2)	50961	1(2)	51920	1(3)	52647	1(2)	54056	1(2)
47801	1(3)	49418	1(3)	49905	1(3)	50545	1(2)	50970	1(3)	51925	1(2)	52648	1(2)	54057	1(2)
47802	1(2)	49419	1(2)	49906	1(3)	50546	1(2)	50972	1(3)	51940	1(2)	52649	1(2)	54060	1(2)
47900	1(2)	49421	1(2)	50010	1(2)	50547	1(2)	50974	1(2)	51960	1(2)	52700	1(3)	54065	1(2)
48000	1(2)	49422	1(2)	50020	1(3)	50548	1(2)	50976	1(2)	51980	1(2)	53000	1(2)	54100	2(3)
48001	1(2)	49423	2(3)	50040	1(2)	50551	1(3)	50980	1(2)	51990	1(2)	53010	1(2)	54105	2(3)
48020	1(3)	49424	3(3)	50045	1(2)	50553	1(3)	51020	1(2)	51992	1(2)	53020	1(2)	54110	1(2)
48100	1(3)	49425	1(2)	50060	1(2)	50555	1(2)	51030	1(2)	52000	1(3)	53025	1(2)	54111	1(2)
48102	1(3)	49426	1(3)	50065	1(2)	50557	1(2)	51040	1(3)	52001	1(3)	53040	1(3)	54112	1(3)
48105	1(2)	49427	1(3)	50070	1(2)	50561	1(2)	51045	2(3)	52005	2(3)	53060	1(3)	54115	1(3)
48120	1(3)	49428	1(2)	50075	1(2)	50562	1(3)	51050	1(2)	52007	1(2)	53080	1(3)	54120	1(2)
48140	1(2)	49429	1(2)	50080	1(2)	50570	1(3)	51060	1(3)	52010	1(2)	53085	1(3)	54125	1(2)
48145	1(2)	49435	1(2)	50081	1(2)	50572	1(2)	51065	1(3)	52204	1(2)	53200	1(3)	54130	1(2)
48146	1(2)	49436	1(2)	50100	1(2)	50574	1(2)	51080	1(3)	52214	1(2)	53210	1(2)	54135	1(2)
48148	1(2)	49440	1(3)	50120	1(2)	50575	1(2)	51100	1(3)	52224	1(2)	53215	1(2)	54150	1(2)
48150	1(2)	49441	1(3)	50125	1(2)	50576	1(2)	51101	1(3)	52234	1(2)	53220	1(3)	54160	1(2)
48152	1(2)	49442	1(3)	50130	1(2)	50580	1(2)	51102	1(3)	52235	1(2)	53230	1(3)	54161	1(2)
48153	1(2)	49446	1(2)	50135	1(2)	50590	1(2)	51500	1(2)	52240	1(2)	53235	1(3)	54162	1(2)
48154	1(2)	49450	1(3)	50200	1(3)	50592	1(2)	51520	1(2)	52250	1(2)	53240	1(3)	54163	1(2)
48155	1(2)	49451	1(3)	50205	1(3)	50593	1(2)	51525	1(2)	52260	1(2)	53250	1(3)	54164	1(2)
48400	1(3)	49452	1(3)	50220	1(2)	50600	1(3)	51530	1(2)	52265	1(2)	53260	1(2)	54200	1(2)
48500	1(3)	49460	1(3)	50225	1(2)	50605	1(3)	51535	1(2)	52270	1(2)	53265	1(3)	54205	1(2)
48510	1(3)	49465	1(3)	50230	1(2)	50610	1(2)	51550	1(2)	52275	1(2)	53270	1(2)	54220	1(3)
48520	1(3)	49491	1(2)	50234	1(2)	50620	1(2)	51555	1(2)	52276	1(2)	53275	1(2)	54230	1(3)
48540	1(3)	49492	1(2)	50236	1(2)	50630	1(2)	51565	1(2)	52277	1(2)	53400	1(2)	54231	1(3)
48545	1(3)	49495	1(2)	50240	1(2)	50650	1(2)	51570	1(2)	52281	1(2)	53405	1(2)	54235	1(3)
48547	1(2)	49496	1(2)	50250	1(3)	50660	1(3)	51575	1(2)	52282	1(2)	53410	1(2)	54240	1(2)
48548	1(2)	49500	1(2)	50280	1(2)	50684	1(3)	51580	1(2)	52283	1(2)	53415	1(2)	54250	1(2)
48550	1(2)	49501	1(2)	50290	1(3)	50686	2(3)	51585	1(2)	52285	1(2)	53420	1(2)	54300	1(2)
48551	1(2)	49505	1(2)	50300	1(2)	50688	2(3)	51590	1(2)	52287	1(2)	53425	1(2)	54304	1(2)
48552	2(3)	49507	1(2)	50320	1(2)	50690	2(3)	51595	1(2)	52290	1(2)	53430	1(2)	54308	1(2)
48554	1(2)	49520	1(2)	50323	1(2)	50700	1(2)	51596	1(2)	52300	1(2)	53431	1(2)	54312	1(2)
48556	1(2)	49521	1(2)	50325	1(2)	50715	1(2)	51597	1(2)	52301	1(2)	53440	1(2)	54316	1(2)
49000	1(2)	49525	1(2)	50327	1(3)	50722	1(2)	51600	1(3)	52305	1(2)	53442	1(2)	54318	1(2)
49002	1(3)	49540	1(2)	50328	1(3)	50725	1(3)	51605	1(3)	52310	1(2)	53444	1(3)	54322	1(2)
49010	1(3)	49550	1(2)	50329	1(3)	50727	1(3)	51610	1(3)	52315	2(3)	53445	1(2)	54324	1(2)
49020	2(3)	49553	1(2)	50340	1(2)	50728	1(3)	51700	1(3)	52317	1(3)	53446	1(2)	54326	1(2)
49040	2(3)	49555	1(2)	50360	1(2)	50740	1(2)	51701	2(3)	52318	1(3)	53447	1(2)	54328	1(2)
49060	2(3)	49557	1(2)	50365	1(2)	50750	1(2)	51702	2(3)	52320	1(2)	53448	1(2)	54332	1(2)
49062	1(3)	49560	2(3)	50370	1(2)	50760	1(2)	51703	2(3)	52325	1(3)	53449	1(2)	54336	1(2)
49082	1(3)	49561	2(3)	50380	1(2)	50770	1(2)	51705	1(3)	52327	1(2)	53450	1(2)	54340	1(2)
49083	2(3)	49565	2(3)	50382	1(3)	50780	1(2)	51710	1(3)	52330	1(2)	53460	1(2)	54344	1(2)
49084	1(3)	49566	2(3)	50384	1(3)	50782	1(2)	51715	1(2)	52332	1(2)	53500	1(2)	54348	1(2)
49180	2(3)	49568	2(3)	50385	1(3)	50783	1(2)	51720	1(3)	52334	1(2)	53502	1(3)	54352	1(2)
49203	1(2)	49570	1(3)	50386	1(3)	50785	1(2)	51725	1(3)	52341	1(2)	53505	1(3)	54360	1(2)
49204	1(2)	49572	1(3)	50387	1(3)	50800	1(2)	51726	1(3)	52342	1(2)	53510	1(3)	54380	1(2)
49205	1(2)	49580	1(2)	50389	1(3)	50810	1(3)	51727	1(3)	52343	1(2)	53515	1(3)	54385	1(2)
49215	1(2)	49582	1(2)	50390	2(3)	50815	1(2)	51728	1(3)	52344	1(2)	53520	1(3)	54390	1(2)
49220	1(2)	49585	1(2)	50391	1(3)	50820	1(2)	51729	1(3)	52345	1(2)	53600	1(3)	54400	1(2)
49250	1(2)	49587	1(2)	50392	1(3)	50825	1(3)	51736	1(3)	52346	1(2)	53601	1(3)	54401	1(2)
49255	1(2)	49590	1(2)	50393	1(3)	50830	1(3)	51741	1(3)	52351	1(3)	53605	1(3)	54405	1(2)
49320	1(3)	49600	1(2)	50394	1(3)	50840	1(2)	51784	1(3)	52352	1(2)	53620	1(2)	54406	1(2)
49321	1(2)	49605	1(2)	50395	1(2)	50845	1(2)	51785	1(3)	52353	1(2)	53621	1(3)	54408	1(2)

CPT	MUE	CPT	MUE	CPT	MUE	CPT	MUE	CPT	MUE	CPT	MUE	CPT	MUE	CPT	MUE
54410	1(2)	55720	1(3)	57156	1(3)	57700	1(3)	58600	1(2)	59320	1(2)	61001	1(2)	61543	1(2)
54411	1(2)	55725	1(3)	57160	1(2)	57720	1(3)	58605	1(2)	59325	1(2)	61020	2(3)	61544	1(3)
54415	1(2)	55801	1(2)	57170	1(2)	57800	1(3)	58611	1(2)	59350	1(2)	61026	2(3)	61545	1(2)
54416	1(2)	55810	1(2)	57180	1(3)	58100	1(3)	58615	1(2)	59400	1(2)	61050	1(3)	61546	1(2)
54417	1(2)	55812	1(2)	57200	1(3)	58110	1(3)	58660	1(2)	59409	2(3)	61055	1(3)	61548	1(2)
54420	1(2)	55815	1(2)	57210	1(3)	58120	1(3)	58661	1(2)	59410	1(2)	61070	2(3)	61550	1(2)
54430	1(2)	55821	1(2)	57220	1(2)	58140	1(3)	58662	1(2)	59412	1(3)	61105	1(3)	61552	1(2)
54435	1(2)	55831	1(2)	57230	1(2)	58145	1(3)	58670	1(2)	59414	1(3)	61107	1(3)	61556	1(3)
54440	1(2)	55840	1(2)	57240	1(2)	58146	1(3)	58671	1(2)	59425	1(2)	61108	1(3)	61557	1(2)
54450	1(2)	55842	1(2)	57250	1(2)	58150	1(3)	58672	1(2)	59426	1(2)	61120	1(3)	61558	1(3)
54500	1(3)	55845	1(2)	57260	1(2)	58152	1(2)	58673	1(2)	59430	1(2)	61140	1(3)	61559	1(3)
54505	1(3)	55860	1(2)	57265	1(2)	58180	1(3)	58700	1(2)	59510	1(2)	61150	1(3)	61563	2(3)
54512	1(3)	55862	1(2)	57267	2(3)	58200	1(2)	58720	1(2)	59514	1(3)	61151	1(3)	61564	1(2)
54520	1(2)	55865	1(2)	57268	1(2)	58210	1(2)	58740	1(2)	59515	1(2)	61154	1(3)	61566	1(3)
54522	1(2)	55866	1(2)	57270	1(2)	58240	1(2)	58750	1(2)	59525	1(2)	61156	1(3)	61567	1(2)
54530	1(2)	55870	1(2)	57280	1(2)	58260	1(3)	58752	1(2)	59610	1(2)	61210	1(3)	61570	1(3)
54535	1(2)	55873	1(2)	57282	1(2)	58262	1(3)	58760	1(2)	59612	2(3)	61215	1(3)	61571	1(3)
54550	1(2)	55875	1(2)	57283	1(2)	58263	1(2)	58770	1(2)	59614	1(2)	61250	1(3)	61575	1(2)
54560	1(2)	55876	1(2)	57284	1(2)	58267	1(2)	58800	1(2)	59618	1(2)	61253	1(3)	61576	1(2)
54600	1(2)	55920	1(2)	57285	1(2)	58270	1(2)	58805	1(2)	59620	1(2)	61304	1(3)	61580	1(2)
54620	1(2)	56405	2(3)	57287	1(2)	58275	1(2)	58820	1(3)	59622	1(2)	61305	1(3)	61581	1(2)
54640	1(2)	56420	1(3)	57288	1(2)	58280	1(2)	58822	1(3)	59812	1(2)	61312	2(3)	61582	1(2)
54650	1(2)	56440	1(3)	57289	1(2)	58285	1(3)	58825	1(2)	59820	1(2)	61313	2(3)	61583	1(2)
54660	1(2)	56441	1(2)	57291	1(2)	58290	1(3)	58900	1(2)	59821	1(2)	61314	2(3)	61584	1(2)
54670	1(3)	56442	1(2)	57292	1(2)	58291	1(2)	58920	1(2)	59830	1(2)	61315	1(3)	61585	1(2)
54680	1(2)	56501	1(2)	57295	1(2)	58292	1(2)	58925	1(2)	59840	1(2)	61316	1(3)	61586	1(3)
54690	1(2)	56515	1(2)	57296	1(2)	58293	1(2)	58940	1(2)	59841	1(2)	61320	2(3)	61590	1(2)
54692	1(2)	56605	1(2)	57300	1(3)	58294	1(2)	58943	1(2)	59850	1(2)	61321	1(3)	61591	1(2)
54700	1(3)	56606	6(3)	57305	1(3)	58301	1(3)	58950	1(2)	59851	1(2)	61322	1(3)	61592	1(2)
54800	1(2)	56620	1(2)	57307	1(3)	58321	1(2)	58951	1(2)	59852	1(2)	61323	1(3)	61595	1(2)
54830	1(2)	56625	1(2)	57308	1(3)	58322	1(2)	58952	1(2)	59855	1(2)	61330	1(2)	61596	1(2)
54840	1(2)	56630	1(2)	57310	1(3)	58323	1(2)	58953	1(2)	59856	1(2)	61332	1(2)	61597	1(2)
54860	1(2)	56631	1(2)	57311	1(3)	58340	1(3)	58954	1(2)	59857	1(2)	61333	1(2)	61598	1(3)
54861	1(2)	56632	1(2)	57320	1(3)	58345	1(3)	58956	1(2)	59866	1(2)	61340	1(2)	61600	1(3)
54865	1(3)	56633	1(2)	57330	1(3)	58346	1(2)	58957	1(2)	59870	1(2)	61343	1(2)	61601	1(3)
54900	1(2)	56634	1(2)	57335	1(2)	58350	1(2)	58958	1(2)	59871	1(2)	61345	1(3)	61605	1(3)
54901	1(2)	56637	1(2)	57400	1(2)	58353	1(3)	58960	1(2)	60000	1(3)	61450	1(3)	61606	1(3)
55000	1(3)	56640	1(2)	57410	1(2)	58356	1(3)	58970	1(3)	60100	3(3)	61458	1(2)	61607	1(3)
55040	1(2)	56700	1(2)	57415	1(3)	58400	1(3)	58974	1(3)	60200	2(3)	61460	1(2)	61608	1(3)
55041	1(2)	56740	1(3)	57420	1(3)	58410	1(2)	58976	2(3)	60210	1(2)	61480	1(2)	61610	1(3)
55060	1(2)	56800	1(2)	57421	1(3)	58520	1(2)	59000	1(3)	60212	1(2)	61500	1(3)	61611	1(3)
55100	2(3)	56805	1(2)	57423	1(2)	58540	1(3)	59001	1(3)	60220	1(3)	61501	1(3)	61612	1(3)
55110	1(2)	56810	1(2)	57425	1(2)	58541	1(3)	59012	1(3)	60225	1(2)	61510	1(3)	61613	1(3)
55120	1(3)	56820	1(2)	57426	1(2)	58542	1(2)	59015	1(3)	60240	1(2)	61512	1(3)	61615	1(3)
55150	1(2)	56821	1(2)	57452	1(3)	58543	1(3)	59020	2(3)	60252	1(2)	61514	2(3)	61616	1(3)
55175	1(2)	57000	1(3)	57454	1(3)	58544	1(2)	59025	3(3)	60254	1(2)	61516	1(3)	61618	2(3)
55180	1(2)	57010	1(3)	57455	1(3)	58545	1(2)	59030	4(3)	60260	1(2)	61517	1(3)	61619	2(3)
55200	1(2)	57020	1(3)	57456	1(3)	58546	1(2)	59050	1(3)	60270	1(2)	61518	1(3)	61623	2(3)
55250	1(2)	57022	1(3)	57460	1(3)	58548	1(2)	59051	1(3)	60271	1(2)	61519	1(3)	61624	2(3)
55300	1(2)	57023	1(3)	57461	1(3)	58550	1(3)	59070	2(3)	60280	1(3)	61520	1(3)	61626	2(3)
55400	1(2)	57061	1(2)	57500	1(3)	58552	1(3)	59072	2(3)	60281	1(3)	61521	1(3)	61630	1(3)
55450	1(2)	57065	1(2)	57505	1(3)	58553	1(3)	59074	1(3)	60300	2(3)	61522	1(3)	61635	2(3)
55500	1(2)	57100	3(3)	57510	1(3)	58554	1(2)	59076	1(3)	60500	1(2)	61524	2(3)	61680	1(3)
55520	1(2)	57105	2(3)	57511	1(3)	58555	1(3)	59100	1(2)	60502	1(3)	61526	1(3)	61682	1(3)
55530	1(2)	57106	1(2)	57513	1(3)	58558	1(3)	59120	1(3)	60505	1(3)	61530	1(3)	61684	1(3)
55535	1(2)	57107	1(2)	57520	1(3)	58559	1(3)	59121	1(3)	60512	1(3)	61531	1(2)	61686	1(3)
55540	1(2)	57109	1(2)	57522	1(3)	58560	1(3)	59130	1(3)	60520	1(2)	61533	2(3)	61690	1(3)
55550	1(2)	57110	1(2)	57530	1(3)	58561	1(3)	59135	1(3)	60521	1(2)	61534	1(3)	61692	1(3)
55600	1(2)	57111	1(2)	57531	1(2)	58562	1(3)	59136	1(3)	60522	1(2)	61535	2(3)	61697	2(3)
55605	1(2)	57112	1(2)	57540	1(2)	58563	1(3)	59140	1(2)	60540	1(2)	61536	1(3)	61698	1(3)
55650	1(2)	57120	1(2)	57545	1(3)	58565	1(2)	59150	1(3)	60545	1(2)	61537	1(3)	61700	2(3)
55680	1(3)	57130	1(2)	57550	1(3)	58570	1(3)	59151	1(3)	60600	1(3)	61538	1(2)	61702	1(3)
55700	1(2)	57135	2(3)	57555	1(2)	58571	1(2)	59160	1(2)	60605	1(3)	61539	1(3)	61703	1(3)
55705	1(2)	57150	1(3)	57556	1(2)	58572	1(3)	59200	1(3)	60650	1(2)	61540	1(3)	61705	1(3)
55706	1(2)	57155	1(3)	57558	1(3)	58573	1(2)	59300	1(2)	61000	1(2)	61541	1(2)	61708	1(3)

CPT	MUE	CPT	MUE	CPT	MUE	CPT	MUE	CPT	MUE	CPT	MUE	CPT	MUE
61710	1(3)	62264	1(2)	63081	1(2)	63655	1(3)	64565	2(3)	64776	1(2)	65135	1(2)	66174	1(2)
61711	1(3)	62267	2(3)	63082	6(2)	63661	1(2)	64566	1(3)	64778	1(3)	65140	1(2)	66175	1(2)
61720	1(3)	62268	1(3)	63085	1(2)	63662	1(2)	64568	1(3)	64782	2(2)	65150	1(2)	66179	1(2)
61735	1(3)	62269	2(3)	63086	2(3)	63663	1(3)	64569	1(3)	64783	2(3)	65155	1(2)	66180	1(2)
61750	2(3)	62270	2(3)	63087	1(2)	63664	1(3)	64570	1(3)	64784	3(3)	65175	1(2)	66183	1(3)
61751	2(3)	62272	1(3)	63088	4(3)	63685	1(3)	64575	2(3)	64786	1(3)	65205	1(3)	66184	1(2)
61760	1(2)	62273	2(3)	63090	1(2)	63688	1(3)	64580	2(3)	64787	4(3)	65210	1(3)	66185	1(3)
61770	1(2)	62280	1(3)	63091	3(3)	63700	1(3)	64581	2(3)	64788	5(3)	65220	1(3)	66220	1(2)
61781	1(3)	62281	1(3)	63101	1(2)	63702	1(3)	64585	2(3)	64790	1(3)	65222	1(3)	66225	1(2)
61782	1(3)	62282	1(3)	63102	1(2)	63704	1(3)	64590	1(3)	64792	2(3)	65235	1(3)	66250	1(2)
61783	1(3)	62284	1(3)	63103	3(3)	63706	1(3)	64595	1(3)	64795	2(3)	65260	1(3)	66500	1(2)
61790	1(2)	62287	1(2)	63170	1(3)	63707	1(3)	64600	2(3)	64802	1(2)	65265	1(3)	66505	1(2)
61791	1(2)	62290	5(2)	63172	1(3)	63709	1(3)	64605	1(2)	64804	1(2)	65270	1(3)	66600	1(2)
61796	1(2)	62291	4(3)	63173	1(3)	63710	1(3)	64610	1(2)	64809	1(2)	65272	1(3)	66605	1(2)
61797	4(3)	62292	1(2)	63180	1(2)	63740	1(3)	64611	1(2)	64818	1(2)	65273	1(3)	66625	1(2)
61798	1(2)	62294	1(3)	63182	1(2)	63741	1(3)	64612	1(2)	64820	4(3)	65275	1(3)	66630	1(2)
61799	4(3)	62302	1(3)	63185	1(2)	63744	1(3)	64615	1(2)	64821	1(2)	65280	1(3)	66635	1(2)
61800	1(2)	62303	1(3)	63190	1(2)	63746	1(2)	64616	1(2)	64822	1(2)	65285	1(3)	66680	1(2)
61850	1(3)	62304	1(3)	63191	1(2)	64400	4(3)	64617	1(2)	64823	1(2)	65286	1(3)	66682	1(2)
61860	1(3)	62305	1(3)	63194	1(2)	64402	1(3)	64620	5(3)	64831	1(2)	65290	1(3)	66700	1(2)
61863	1(2)	62310	1(3)	63195	1(2)	64405	1(3)	64630	1(3)	64832	3(3)	65400	1(3)	66710	1(2)
61864	1(3)	62311	1(3)	63196	1(2)	64408	1(3)	64632	1(2)	64834	1(2)	65410	1(3)	66711	1(2)
61867	1(2)	62318	1(3)	63197	1(2)	64410	1(3)	64633	1(2)	64835	1(2)	65420	1(2)	66720	1(2)
61868	2(3)	62319	1(3)	63198	1(2)	64412	1(3)	64634	4(3)	64836	1(2)	65426	1(2)	66740	1(2)
61870	1(3)	62350	1(3)	63199	1(2)	64413	1(3)	64635	1(2)	64837	2(3)	65430	1(2)	66761	1(2)
61880	1(2)	62351	1(3)	63200	1(2)	64415	1(3)	64636	4(2)	64840	1(2)	65435	1(2)	66762	1(2)
61885	1(3)	62355	1(3)	63250	1(3)	64416	1(2)	64640	5(3)	64856	2(3)	65436	1(2)	66770	1(3)
61886	1(3)	62360	1(2)	63251	1(3)	64417	1(3)	64642	1(2)	64857	2(3)	65450	1(3)	66820	1(2)
61888	1(3)	62361	1(2)	63252	1(3)	64418	1(3)	64643	3(2)	64858	1(2)	65600	1(2)	66821	1(2)
62000	1(3)	62362	1(2)	63265	1(3)	64420	3(3)	64644	1(2)	64859	2(3)	65710	1(2)	66825	1(2)
62005	1(3)	62365	1(2)	63266	1(3)	64421	3(3)	64645	3(2)	64861	1(2)	65730	1(2)	66830	1(2)
62010	1(3)	62367	1(3)	63267	1(3)	64425	1(3)	64646	1(2)	64862	1(2)	65750	1(2)	66840	1(2)
62100	1(3)	62368	1(3)	63268	1(3)	64430	1(3)	64647	1(2)	64864	2(3)	65755	1(2)	66850	1(2)
62115	1(2)	62369	1(3)	63270	1(3)	64435	1(3)	64650	1(2)	64865	1(3)	65756	1(2)	66852	1(2)
62117	1(2)	62370	1(3)	63271	1(3)	64445	1(3)	64653	1(2)	64866	1(3)	65757	1(3)	66920	1(2)
62120	1(2)	63001	1(2)	63272	1(3)	64446	1(2)	64680	1(2)	64868	1(3)	65770	1(2)	66930	1(2)
62121	1(2)	63003	1(2)	63273	1(3)	64447	1(3)	64681	1(2)	64872	1(3)	65772	1(2)	66940	1(2)
62140	1(3)	63005	1(2)	63275	1(3)	64448	1(2)	64702	2(3)	64874	1(3)	65775	1(2)	66982	1(2)
62141	1(3)	63011	1(2)	63276	1(3)	64449	1(2)	64704	4(3)	64876	1(3)	65778	1(2)	66983	1(2)
62142	2(3)	63012	1(2)	63277	1(3)	64450	10(3)	64708	3(3)	64885	1(3)	65779	1(2)	66984	1(2)
62143	2(3)	63015	1(2)	63278	1(3)	64455	1(2)	64712	1(2)	64886	1(3)	65780	1(2)	66985	1(2)
62145	2(3)	63016	1(2)	63280	1(3)	64479	1(2)	64713	1(2)	64890	2(3)	65781	1(2)	66986	1(2)
62146	2(3)	63017	1(2)	63281	1(3)	64480	4(3)	64714	1(2)	64891	2(3)	65782	1(2)	66990	1(3)
62147	1(3)	63020	1(2)	63282	1(3)	64483	1(2)	64716	2(3)	64892	2(3)	65800	1(2)	67005	1(2)
62148	1(3)	63030	1(2)	63283	1(3)	64484	4(3)	64718	1(2)	64893	2(3)	65810	1(2)	67010	1(2)
62160	1(3)	63035	4(3)	63285	1(3)	64486	1(3)	64719	1(2)	64895	2(3)	65815	1(3)	67015	1(2)
62161	1(3)	63040	1(2)	63286	1(3)	64487	1(2)	64721	1(2)	64896	2(3)	65820	1(2)	67025	1(2)
62162	1(3)	63042	1(2)	63287	1(3)	64488	1(3)	64722	4(3)	64897	2(3)	65850	1(2)	67027	1(2)
62163	1(3)	63043	4(3)	63290	1(3)	64489	1(2)	64726	2(3)	64898	2(3)	65855	1(2)	67028	1(3)
62164	1(3)	63044	4(2)	63295	1(2)	64490	1(2)	64727	2(3)	64901	2(3)	65860	1(2)	67030	1(2)
62165	1(2)	63045	1(2)	63300	1(2)	64491	1(2)	64732	1(2)	64902	1(3)	65865	1(2)	67031	1(2)
62180	1(3)	63046	1(2)	63301	1(2)	64492	1(2)	64734	1(2)	64905	1(3)	65870	1(2)	67036	1(2)
62190	1(3)	63047	1(2)	63302	1(2)	64493	1(2)	64736	1(2)	64907	1(3)	65875	1(2)	67039	1(2)
62192	1(3)	63048	5(3)	63303	1(2)	64494	1(2)	64738	1(2)	64910	3(3)	65880	1(2)	67040	1(2)
62194	1(3)	63050	1(2)	63304	1(2)	64495	1(2)	64740	1(2)	64911	2(3)	65900	1(3)	67041	1(2)
62200	1(2)	63051	1(2)	63305	1(2)	64505	1(3)	64742	1(2)	65091	1(2)	65920	1(2)	67042	1(2)
62201	1(2)	63055	1(2)	63306	1(2)	64508	1(3)	64744	1(2)	65093	1(2)	65930	1(3)	67043	1(2)
62220	1(3)	63056	1(2)	63307	1(2)	64510	1(3)	64746	1(2)	65101	1(2)	66020	1(3)	67101	1(2)
62223	1(3)	63057	3(3)	63308	3(3)	64517	1(3)	64755	1(2)	65103	1(2)	66030	1(3)	67105	1(2)
62225	2(3)	63064	1(2)	63600	2(3)	64520	1(3)	64760	1(2)	65105	1(2)	66130	1(3)	67107	1(2)
62230	2(3)	63066	1(3)	63610	1(3)	64530	1(3)	64763	1(2)	65110	1(2)	66150	1(2)	67108	1(2)
62252	2(3)	63075	1(2)	63615	1(3)	64550	1(3)	64766	1(2)	65112	1(2)	66155	1(2)	67110	1(2)
62256	1(3)	63076	3(3)	63620	1(2)	64553	1(3)	64771	2(3)	65114	1(2)	66160	1(2)	67112	1(2)
62258	1(3)	63077	1(2)	63621	2(2)	64555	2(3)	64772	2(3)	65125	1(2)	66170	1(2)	67113	1(2)
62263	1(2)	63078	3(3)	63650	2(3)	64561	1(3)	64774	2(3)	65130	1(2)	66172	1(2)	67115	1(2)

CPT	MUE	CPT	MUE	CPT	MUE	CPT	MUE	CPT	MUE	CPT	MUE	CPT	MUE	CPT	MUE
67120	1(2)	67902	1(2)	68811	1(2)	69667	1(2)	70481	1(1)	72127	1(1)	73525	2(2)	74300	1(1)
67121	1(2)	67903	1(2)	68815	1(2)	69670	1(2)	70482	1(1)	72128	1(1)	73530	2(3)	74301	2(1)
67141	1(2)	67904	1(2)	68816	1(2)	69676	1(2)	70486	1(1)	72129	1(1)	73540	1(1)	74305	1(1)
67145	1(2)	67906	1(2)	68840	1(2)	69700	1(3)	70487	1(1)	72130	1(1)	73550	2(1)	74320	1(1)
67208	1(2)	67908	1(2)	68850	1(3)	69711	1(2)	70488	1(1)	72131	1(1)	73560	2(1)	74327	1(3)
67210	1(2)	67909	1(2)	69000	1(3)	69714	1(2)	70490	1(1)	72132	1(1)	73562	2(1)	74328	1(1)
67218	1(2)	67911	4(2)	69005	1(3)	69715	1(3)	70491	1(1)	72133	1(1)	73564	2(1)	74329	1(1)
67220	1(2)	67912	1(2)	69020	1(3)	69717	1(2)	70492	1(1)	72141	1(1)	73565	1(1)	74330	1(1)
67221	1(2)	67914	1(3)	69100	3(3)	69718	1(2)	70496	1(1)	72142	1(1)	73580	2(2)	74340	1(1)
67225	1(2)	67915	1(3)	69105	1(3)	69720	1(2)	70498	1(1)	72146	1(1)	73590	2(1)	74355	1(3)
67227	1(2)	67916	1(3)	69110	1(2)	69725	1(2)	70540	1(1)	72147	1(1)	73592	2(1)	74360	1(1)
67228	1(2)	67917	1(3)	69120	1(3)	69740	1(2)	70542	1(1)	72148	1(1)	73600	2(1)	74363	2(1)
67229	1(2)	67921	1(3)	69140	1(2)	69745	1(2)	70543	1(1)	72149	1(1)	73610	2(1)	74400	1(1)
67250	1(2)	67922	1(3)	69145	1(3)	69801	1(3)	70544	1(1)	72156	1(1)	73615	2(2)	74410	1(1)
67255	1(2)	67923	1(3)	69150	1(3)	69805	1(3)	70545	1(1)	72157	1(1)	73620	2(1)	74415	1(1)
67311	1(2)	67924	1(3)	69155	1(3)	69806	1(3)	70546	1(1)	72158	1(1)	73630	2(1)	74420	2(1)
67312	1(2)	67930	2(3)	69200	1(2)	69820	1(2)	70547	1(1)	72170	1(1)	73650	2(1)	74425	1(1)
67314	1(2)	67935	2(3)	69205	1(3)	69840	1(3)	70548	1(1)	72190	1(1)	73660	2(1)	74430	1(1)
67316	1(2)	67938	2(3)	69210	1(2)	69905	1(2)	70549	1(1)	72191	1(1)	73700	2(1)	74440	1(2)
67318	1(2)	67950	2(2)	69220	1(2)	69910	1(2)	70551	1(1)	72192	1(1)	73701	2(1)	74445	1(2)
67320	2(3)	67961	4(2)	69222	1(2)	69915	1(2)	70552	1(1)	72193	1(1)	73702	2(1)	74450	1(1)
67331	1(2)	67966	4(2)	69300	1(2)	69930	1(2)	70553	1(1)	72194	1(1)	73706	2(1)	74455	1(1)
67332	1(2)	67971	1(2)	69310	1(2)	69950	1(2)	70554	1(3)	72195	1(1)	73718	2(1)	74470	2(2)
67334	1(2)	67973	1(2)	69320	1(2)	69955	1(2)	70555	1(3)	72196	1(1)	73719	2(1)	74475	2(1)
67335	1(2)	67974	1(2)	69420	1(2)	69960	1(2)	70557	1(3)	72197	1(1)	73720	2(1)	74480	2(1)
67340	2(2)	67975	1(2)	69421	1(2)	69970	1(3)	70558	1(3)	72198	1(1)	73721	4(1)	74485	2(1)
67343	1(2)	68020	1(3)	69424	1(2)	69990	1(3)	70559	1(3)	72200	1(1)	73722	2(1)	74710	1(3)
67345	1(3)	68040	1(2)	69433	1(2)	70010	1(3)	71015	2(1)	72202	1(1)	73723	4(1)	74740	1(3)
67346	1(3)	68100	1(3)	69436	1(2)	70015	1(1)	71021	1(1)	72220	1(1)	73725	2(1)	74742	2(2)
67400	1(2)	68110	1(3)	69440	1(2)	70030	2(2)	71022	1(1)	72240	1(2)	74000	3(1)	74775	1(2)
67405	1(2)	68115	1(3)	69450	1(2)	70100	1(1)	71023	2(1)	72255	1(2)	74010	2(1)	75557	1(3)
67412	1(2)	68130	1(3)	69501	1(3)	70110	1(1)	71030	2(1)	72265	1(2)	74020	2(1)	75559	1(3)
67413	1(2)	68135	1(3)	69502	1(2)	70120	2(1)	71034	1(1)	72270	1(2)	74022	2(1)	75561	1(1)
67414	1(2)	68200	1(3)	69505	1(2)	70130	2(1)	71035	2(1)	72275	3(1)	74150	1(1)	75563	1(3)
67415	1(3)	68320	1(2)	69511	1(2)	70134	1(3)	71100	1(1)	73000	2(1)	74160	1(1)	75565	1(1)
67420	1(2)	68325	1(2)	69530	1(2)	70140	1(1)	71101	1(1)	73010	2(1)	74170	1(1)	75571	1(1)
67430	1(2)	68326	2(2)	69535	1(2)	70150	1(1)	71110	1(1)	73020	2(1)	74174	1(1)	75572	1(1)
67440	1(2)	68328	2(2)	69540	1(3)	70160	1(1)	71111	1(1)	73030	2(1)	74175	1(1)	75573	1(3)
67445	1(2)	68330	1(3)	69550	1(3)	70170	2(2)	71120	1(1)	73040	2(2)	74176	1(1)	75574	1(1)
67450	1(2)	68335	1(3)	69552	1(2)	70190	1(2)	71130	1(1)	73050	1(1)	74177	1(1)	75600	1(3)
67500	1(3)	68340	1(3)	69554	1(2)	70200	1(1)	71250	1(1)	73060	2(1)	74178	1(1)	75605	1(1)
67505	1(3)	68360	1(3)	69601	1(2)	70210	1(1)	71260	1(1)	73070	2(1)	74181	1(1)	75625	1(1)
67515	1(3)	68362	1(3)	69602	1(2)	70220	1(1)	71270	1(1)	73080	2(1)	74182	1(1)	75630	1(1)
67550	1(2)	68371	1(3)	69603	1(2)	70240	1(2)	71275	1(1)	73085	2(2)	74183	1(1)	75635	1(1)
67560	1(2)	68400	1(2)	69604	1(2)	70250	1(1)	71550	1(1)	73090	2(1)	74185	1(1)	75658	2(1)
67570	1(2)	68420	1(2)	69605	1(2)	70260	1(1)	71551	1(3)	73092	2(1)	74190	1(1)	75710	1(1)
67700	2(3)	68440	2(2)	69610	1(2)	70300	1(1)	71552	1(1)	73100	2(1)	74210	1(3)	75716	1(1)
67710	1(2)	68500	1(2)	69620	1(2)	70310	1(3)	71555	1(1)	73110	2(1)	74220	1(1)	75726	3(1)
67715	1(3)	68505	1(2)	69631	1(2)	70320	1(1)	72010	1(2)	73115	2(2)	74230	1(1)	75731	1(3)
67800	1(2)	68510	1(2)	69632	1(3)	70328	1(1)	72020	4(1)	73120	2(1)	74235	1(3)	75733	1(3)
67801	1(2)	68520	1(2)	69633	1(2)	70330	1(1)	72040	3(1)	73130	2(1)	74240	1(1)	75736	2(1)
67805	1(2)	68525	1(2)	69635	1(3)	70332	2(1)	72050	1(1)	73140	2(1)	74241	1(1)	75741	1(3)
67808	1(2)	68530	1(2)	69636	1(3)	70336	1(1)	72052	1(1)	73200	2(1)	74245	1(1)	75743	1(1)
67810	2(3)	68540	1(2)	69637	1(3)	70350	1(1)	72069	1(2)	73201	2(1)	74246	1(1)	75746	1(1)
67820	1(2)	68550	1(2)	69641	1(2)	70355	1(1)	72070	1(1)	73202	2(1)	74247	1(1)	75756	2(1)
67825	1(2)	68700	1(2)	69642	1(2)	70360	1(1)	72072	1(1)	73206	2(1)	74249	1(1)	75791	1(1)
67830	1(2)	68705	2(2)	69643	1(2)	70370	1(3)	72074	1(1)	73218	2(1)	74250	1(1)	75801	1(1)
67835	1(2)	68720	1(2)	69644	1(2)	70371	1(2)	72080	1(1)	73219	2(1)	74251	1(3)	75803	1(3)
67840	4(3)	68745	1(2)	69645	1(2)	70373	1(3)	72090	1(1)	73220	2(1)	74260	1(2)	75805	1(2)
67850	3(3)	68750	1(2)	69646	1(2)	70380	2(3)	72100	1(1)	73221	2(1)	74261	1(2)	75807	1(2)
67875	1(2)	68760	4(2)	69650	1(2)	70390	2(3)	72110	1(1)	73222	2(1)	74262	1(2)	75809	1(3)
67880	1(2)	68761	4(2)	69660	1(2)	70450	3(1)	72114	1(1)	73223	2(1)	74270	1(1)	75810	1(3)
67882	1(2)	68770	1(3)	69661	1(2)	70460	1(1)	72120	1(1)	73500	1(1)	74280	1(1)	75820	1(1)
67900	1(2)	68801	4(2)	69662	1(2)	70470	2(1)	72125	1(1)	73510	2(1)	74283	1(3)	75822	1(1)
67901	1(2)	68810	1(2)	69666	1(2)	70480	1(1)	72126	1(1)	73520	2(1)	74290	1(3)	75825	1(1)

CPT	MUE	CPT	MUE	CPT	MUE	CPT	MUE	CPT	MUE	CPT	MUE	CPT	MUE	CPT	MUE
75827	1(1)	76801	1(2)	77085	1(2)	78014	1(2)	78468	1(3)	80069	1(3)	81000	2(3)	81280	1(3)
75831	1(1)	76802	3(1)	77086	1(2)	78015	1(3)	78469	1(3)	80074	1(2)	81001	2(3)	81281	1(3)
75833	1(1)	76805	1(2)	77261	1(3)	78016	1(3)	78472	1(2)	80076	1(3)	81002	2(3)	81282	1(3)
75840	1(3)	76810	3(1)	77262	1(3)	78018	1(3)	78473	1(2)	80150	2(3)	81003	2(3)	81287	1(3)
75842	1(3)	76811	1(2)	77263	1(3)	78020	1(3)	78481	1(2)	80155	1(3)	81005	2(1)	81288	1(3)
75860	2(1)	76812	3(1)	77280	2(3)	78070	1(2)	78483	1(2)	80156	2(3)	81007	1(3)	81290	1(3)
75870	1(1)	76813	1(2)	77285	1(3)	78071	1(3)	78491	1(3)	80157	2(3)	81015	2(3)	81291	1(3)
75872	1(3)	76814	3(1)	77290	1(3)	78072	1(3)	78492	1(2)	80158	2(1)	81020	1(3)	81292	1(2)
75880	2(1)	76815	1(2)	77293	1(3)	78075	1(2)	78494	1(3)	80159	2(3)	81025	1(3)	81293	1(3)
75885	1(3)	76817	1(1)	77295	1(3)	78102	1(2)	78496	1(3)	80162	2(3)	81050	2(1)	81294	1(3)
75887	1(3)	76830	1(1)	77300	10(3)	78103	1(2)	78579	1(3)	80163	2(3)	81161	1(3)	81295	1(2)
75889	1(1)	76831	1(3)	77301	1(3)	78104	1(2)	78580	1(3)	80164	2(3)	81200	1(2)	81296	1(3)
75891	1(1)	76856	1(1)	77306	1(3)	78110	1(2)	78582	1(3)	80165	2(3)	81201	1(2)	81297	1(3)
75896	3(1)	76857	1(1)	77307	1(3)	78111	1(2)	78597	1(3)	80168	2(3)	81202	1(3)	81298	1(2)
75898	1(1)	76870	1(2)	77316	1(3)	78120	1(2)	78598	1(3)	80169	1(3)	81203	1(3)	81299	1(3)
75901	1(1)	76872	1(1)	77317	1(3)	78121	1(2)	78600	1(3)	80170	2(3)	81205	1(3)	81300	1(3)
75902	2(1)	76873	1(2)	77318	1(3)	78122	1(2)	78601	1(3)	80171	1(3)	81206	1(3)	81301	1(3)
75945	1(3)	76881	2(1)	77321	1(2)	78130	1(2)	78605	1(3)	80173	2(3)	81207	1(3)	81302	1(3)
75952	1(2)	76882	2(1)	77331	3(3)	78135	1(3)	78606	1(3)	80175	1(3)	81208	1(3)	81303	1(3)
75953	4(1)	76885	1(2)	77332	4(3)	78140	1(3)	78607	1(3)	80176	1(3)	81209	1(3)	81304	1(3)
75954	2(3)	76886	1(2)	77333	2(3)	78185	1(2)	78608	1(3)	80177	1(3)	81210	1(3)	81310	1(3)
75956	1(2)	76930	1(1)	77336	1(2)	78190	1(2)	78610	1(3)	80178	2(3)	81211	1(2)	81313	1(3)
75957	1(2)	76932	1(2)	77338	1(3)	78191	1(2)	78630	1(3)	80180	1(3)	81212	1(3)	81315	1(3)
75958	2(1)	76936	2(1)	77370	1(3)	78195	1(2)	78635	1(3)	80183	1(3)	81213	1(2)	81316	1(2)
75959	1(2)	76937	2(1)	77371	1(2)	78201	1(3)	78645	1(3)	80184	2(3)	81214	1(2)	81317	1(3)
75962	1(1)	76940	1(1)	77372	1(2)	78202	1(3)	78647	1(3)	80185	2(3)	81215	1(2)	81318	1(3)
75964	4(1)	76942	1(3)	77373	1(3)	78205	1(3)	78650	1(3)	80186	2(3)	81216	1(2)	81319	1(2)
75966	1(1)	76945	1(3)	77401	1(2)	78206	1(3)	78660	1(2)	80188	2(3)	81217	1(2)	81321	1(3)
75968	2(1)	76946	1(3)	77402	2(3)	78215	1(3)	78700	1(3)	80190	2(3)	81220	1(3)	81322	1(3)
75970	2(1)	76948	1(2)	77407	2(3)	78216	1(3)	78701	1(3)	80192	2(3)	81221	1(3)	81323	1(3)
75980	1(1)	76965	2(1)	77412	2(3)	78226	1(3)	78707	1(2)	80194	2(3)	81222	1(3)	81324	1(3)
75982	2(1)	76970	1(1)	77417	1(2)	78227	1(3)	78708	1(2)	80195	2(3)	81223	1(2)	81325	1(3)
75984	2(1)	76975	1(3)	77422	1(3)	78230	1(3)	78709	1(2)	80197	2(3)	81224	1(3)	81326	1(3)
75989	2(1)	76977	1(2)	77423	1(3)	78231	1(3)	78710	1(3)	80198	2(3)	81225	1(3)	81330	1(3)
76000	3(1)	76998	1(1)	77424	1(2)	78232	1(3)	78725	1(3)	80199	1(3)	81226	1(3)	81331	1(3)
76001	2(1)	77001	1(1)	77425	1(3)	78258	1(2)	78730	1(2)	80200	2(3)	81227	1(3)	81332	1(3)
76010	2(1)	77002	1(3)	77427	1(2)	78261	1(2)	78740	1(2)	80201	2(3)	81228	1(3)	81340	1(3)
76080	2(1)	77003	1(3)	77431	1(2)	78262	1(2)	78761	1(2)	80202	2(3)	81229	1(3)	81341	1(3)
76100	2(1)	77011	1(1)	77432	1(2)	78264	1(2)	78800	1(2)	80203	1(3)	81235	1(3)	81342	1(3)
76101	1(1)	77012	1(3)	77435	1(2)	78267	1(2)	78801	1(2)	80299	3(3)	81240	1(2)	81350	1(3)
76102	1(3)	77013	1(1)	77469	1(2)	78268	1(2)	78802	1(2)	80400	1(3)	81241	1(2)	81355	1(3)
76120	1(1)	77014	2(1)	77470	1(2)	78270	1(2)	78803	1(2)	80402	1(3)	81242	1(3)	81370	1(2)
76125	1(1)	77021	1(3)	77520	1(3)	78271	1(2)	78804	1(2)	80406	1(3)	81243	1(3)	81371	1(2)
76376	2(1)	77022	1(3)	77522	1(3)	78272	1(2)	78805	1(3)	80408	1(3)	81244	1(3)	81372	1(2)
76377	2(1)	77051	1(1)	77523	1(3)	78278	2(3)	78806	1(2)	80410	1(3)	81245	1(3)	81373	2(2)
76380	1(1)	77052	1(2)	77525	1(3)	78282	1(2)	78807	1(3)	80412	1(3)	81246	1(3)	81374	1(3)
76506	1(2)	77053	2(2)	77600	1(3)	78290	1(3)	78808	1(2)	80414	1(3)	81250	1(3)	81375	1(2)
76510	2(2)	77054	2(2)	77605	1(3)	78291	1(3)	78811	1(2)	80415	1(3)	81251	1(3)	81376	5(3)
76511	2(2)	77055	1(1)	77610	1(3)	78300	1(3)	78812	1(2)	80416	1(3)	81252	1(3)	81377	2(3)
76512	2(2)	77056	1(1)	77615	1(3)	78305	1(2)	78813	1(2)	80417	1(3)	81253	1(3)	81378	1(3)
76513	2(2)	77057	1(2)	77620	1(3)	78306	1(2)	78814	1(2)	80418	1(3)	81254	1(3)	81379	1(2)
76514	1(2)	77058	1(2)	77750	1(3)	78315	1(2)	78815	1(2)	80420	1(2)	81255	1(3)	81380	2(2)
76516	1(2)	77059	1(2)	77761	1(3)	78320	1(2)	78816	1(2)	80422	1(3)	81256	1(2)	81381	3(3)
76519	2(2)	77063	1(2)	77762	1(3)	78414	1(2)	79005	1(3)	80424	1(3)	81257	1(2)	81382	6(3)
76529	2(2)	77071	1(3)	77763	1(3)	78428	1(3)	79101	1(3)	80426	1(3)	81260	1(3)	81383	2(3)
76536	1(1)	77072	1(2)	77776	1(3)	78445	1(3)	79200	1(3)	80428	1(3)	81261	1(3)	81400	2(3)
76604	1(1)	77073	1(2)	77777	1(3)	78451	1(2)	79300	1(3)	80430	1(3)	81262	1(3)	81401	2(3)
76641	2(2)	77074	1(2)	77778	1(3)	78452	1(2)	79403	1(3)	80432	1(3)	81263	1(3)	81402	1(3)
76642	2(2)	77075	1(2)	77785	2(3)	78453	1(2)	79440	1(3)	80434	1(3)	81264	1(3)	81403	4(3)
76700	1(1)	77076	1(2)	77786	3(3)	78454	1(2)	79445	1(3)	80435	1(3)	81265	1(3)	81404	5(3)
76705	2(1)	77077	1(2)	77787	3(3)	78456	1(3)	80047	2(3)	80436	1(3)	81266	2(3)	81405	2(3)
76770	1(1)	77078	1(2)	77789	2(3)	78457	1(2)	80048	2(3)	80438	1(3)	81267	1(3)	81406	2(3)
76775	2(1)	77080	1(2)	77790	2(1)	78458	1(2)	80051	2(3)	80439	1(3)	81268	4(3)	81407	1(3)
76776	1(1)	77081	1(2)	78012	1(3)	78459	1(3)	80053	1(3)	80500	1(3)	81270	1(2)	81408	2(3)
76800	1(1)	77084	1(2)	78013	1(3)	78466	1(3)	80061	1(3)	80502	1(3)	81275	1(3)	81410	1(3)

CPT	MUE	CPT	MUE	CPT	MUE	CPT	MUE	CPT	MUE	CPT	MUE	CPT	MUE	CPT	MUE
81411	1(3)	82163	1(3)	82541	4(3)	82947	5(3)	83631	1(3)	84106	1(2)	84432	1(2)	85060	1(3)
81415	1(1)	82164	1(3)	82542	6(3)	82950	3(3)	83632	1(3)	84110	1(3)	84436	1(2)	85097	2(3)
81416	2(1)	82172	3(3)	82543	2(3)	82951	1(2)	83633	1(3)	84112	1(3)	84437	1(2)	85130	1(3)
81417	1(1)	82175	2(3)	82544	2(3)	82952	3(3)	83655	2(3)	84119	1(2)	84439	1(2)	85170	1(3)
81420	1(3)	82180	1(2)	82550	3(3)	82955	1(2)	83661	3(3)	84120	1(3)	84442	1(2)	85175	1(3)
81425	1(1)	82190	2(3)	82552	3(3)	82960	1(2)	83662	4(3)	84126	1(3)	84443	4(2)	85210	2(3)
81426	2(1)	82232	2(3)	82553	3(3)	82963	1(3)	83663	3(3)	84132	2(3)	84445	1(2)	85220	2(3)
81427	1(1)	82239	1(3)	82554	1(3)	82965	1(3)	83664	3(3)	84133	2(3)	84446	1(2)	85230	2(3)
81430	1(2)	82240	1(3)	82565	2(1)	82977	1(3)	83670	1(3)	84134	1(3)	84449	1(3)	85240	2(3)
81431	1(2)	82247	2(3)	82570	3(3)	82978	1(3)	83690	2(3)	84135	1(3)	84450	1(3)	85244	1(3)
81435	1(2)	82248	2(3)	82575	1(3)	82979	1(3)	83695	1(3)	84138	1(3)	84460	1(3)	85245	2(3)
81436	1(2)	82252	1(3)	82585	1(2)	82985	1(3)	83698	1(3)	84140	1(3)	84466	1(3)	85246	2(3)
81440	1(2)	82261	1(3)	82595	1(3)	83001	1(3)	83700	1(2)	84143	2(3)	84478	1(3)	85247	2(3)
81445	1(2)	82270	1(3)	82600	1(3)	83002	1(3)	83701	1(3)	84144	1(3)	84479	1(2)	85250	2(3)
81450	1(2)	82271	1(3)	82607	1(2)	83003	5(3)	83704	1(3)	84145	1(3)	84480	1(2)	85260	2(3)
81455	1(2)	82272	1(3)	82608	1(2)	83006	1(2)	83718	1(3)	84146	3(3)	84481	1(2)	85270	2(3)
81460	1(2)	82274	1(3)	82610	1(3)	83009	1(3)	83719	1(3)	84150	2(3)	84482	1(2)	85280	2(3)
81465	1(2)	82286	1(3)	82615	1(3)	83010	1(3)	83721	1(3)	84152	1(2)	84484	2(3)	85290	2(3)
81470	1(2)	82300	1(3)	82626	1(3)	83012	1(2)	83727	1(3)	84153	1(2)	84485	1(3)	85291	1(3)
81471	1(2)	82306	1(2)	82627	1(3)	83013	1(3)	83735	4(3)	84154	1(2)	84488	1(3)	85292	1(3)
81500	1(3)	82308	1(3)	82633	1(3)	83014	1(2)	83775	1(3)	84155	1(3)	84490	1(2)	85293	1(3)
81503	1(3)	82310	2(3)	82634	1(3)	83015	1(2)	83785	1(3)	84156	1(3)	84510	1(3)	85300	2(3)
81504	1(3)	82330	2(3)	82638	1(3)	83018	4(3)	83788	3(3)	84157	2(3)	84512	1(3)	85301	1(3)
81506	1(3)	82331	1(3)	82652	1(2)	83020	2(3)	83789	4(3)	84160	2(3)	84520	4(1)	85302	1(3)
81507	1(3)	82340	1(3)	82656	1(3)	83021	2(3)	83825	2(3)	84163	1(3)	84525	1(3)	85303	2(3)
81508	1(3)	82355	2(3)	82657	3(3)	83026	1(3)	83835	2(3)	84165	1(2)	84540	2(3)	85305	2(3)
81509	1(3)	82360	2(3)	82658	2(3)	83030	1(3)	83857	1(3)	84166	2(3)	84545	1(3)	85306	2(3)
81510	1(3)	82365	2(3)	82664	2(3)	83033	1(3)	83861	2(2)	84181	3(3)	84550	1(3)	85307	1(3)
81511	1(3)	82370	2(3)	82668	1(3)	83036	1(2)	83864	1(2)	84182	6(3)	84560	2(3)	85335	2(3)
81512	1(3)	82373	1(3)	82670	2(3)	83037	1(2)	83872	2(3)	84202	1(2)	84577	1(3)	85337	1(3)
81519	1(2)	82374	2(1)	82671	1(3)	83045	1(3)	83873	1(3)	84203	1(2)	84578	1(3)	85345	1(3)
82009	1(3)	82375	1(3)	82672	1(3)	83050	1(3)	83874	2(3)	84206	1(2)	84580	1(3)	85347	5(3)
82010	1(3)	82376	1(1)	82677	1(3)	83051	1(3)	83876	1(3)	84207	1(2)	84583	1(3)	85348	1(3)
82013	1(3)	82378	1(3)	82679	1(3)	83060	1(3)	83880	1(3)	84210	1(3)	84585	1(2)	85360	1(3)
82016	1(3)	82379	1(3)	82693	2(3)	83065	1(2)	83883	6(3)	84220	1(3)	84586	1(2)	85362	2(3)
82017	1(3)	82380	1(3)	82696	1(3)	83068	1(2)	83885	2(3)	84228	1(3)	84588	1(3)	85366	1(3)
82024	4(3)	82382	1(2)	82705	1(3)	83069	1(3)	83915	1(3)	84233	1(3)	84590	1(2)	85370	1(3)
82030	1(3)	82383	1(3)	82710	1(3)	83070	1(2)	83916	2(3)	84234	1(3)	84591	1(3)	85378	1(3)
82040	1(3)	82384	2(3)	82715	3(3)	83080	2(3)	83918	2(3)	84235	1(3)	84597	1(3)	85379	2(3)
82042	2(3)	82387	1(3)	82725	1(3)	83088	1(3)	83919	1(3)	84238	3(3)	84600	2(3)	85380	1(3)
82043	1(3)	82390	1(2)	82726	1(3)	83090	2(3)	83921	2(1)	84244	2(3)	84620	1(2)	85384	2(3)
82044	1(3)	82397	3(3)	82728	1(3)	83150	1(3)	83930	2(3)	84252	1(2)	84630	2(3)	85385	1(3)
82045	1(3)	82415	1(3)	82731	1(3)	83491	1(3)	83935	2(3)	84255	2(3)	84681	1(3)	85390	3(3)
82075	2(3)	82435	2(1)	82735	1(3)	83497	1(3)	83937	1(3)	84260	1(3)	84702	2(3)	85396	1(2)
82085	1(3)	82436	1(3)	82746	1(2)	83498	2(3)	83945	2(3)	84270	1(3)	84703	1(3)	85397	3(3)
82088	2(3)	82438	1(3)	82747	1(2)	83499	1(3)	83950	1(2)	84275	1(3)	84704	1(3)	85400	1(3)
82103	1(3)	82441	1(2)	82757	1(2)	83500	1(3)	83951	1(2)	84285	1(3)	84830	1(2)	85410	1(3)
82104	1(2)	82465	1(3)	82759	1(3)	83505	1(3)	83970	2(3)	84295	3(1)	85002	1(3)	85415	2(3)
82105	1(3)	82480	2(3)	82760	1(2)	83516	4(3)	83986	2(3)	84300	2(3)	85004	1(3)	85420	2(3)
82106	2(3)	82482	1(3)	82775	1(3)	83518	1(3)	83987	1(3)	84302	1(1)	85007	1(3)	85421	1(3)
82107	1(3)	82485	1(3)	82776	1(2)	83519	5(3)	83992	2(3)	84305	1(3)	85008	1(3)	85441	1(2)
82108	1(3)	82486	2(3)	82777	1(3)	83520	8(3)	83993	1(3)	84307	1(3)	85009	1(3)	85445	1(2)
82120	1(3)	82487	1(3)	82784	6(3)	83525	4(3)	84030	1(2)	84311	2(3)	85013	1(3)	85460	1(3)
82127	1(3)	82488	1(3)	82785	1(3)	83527	1(3)	84035	1(2)	84315	1(3)	85014	2(3)	85461	1(2)
82128	2(3)	82489	2(3)	82787	4(3)	83528	1(3)	84060	1(3)	84375	1(3)	85018	2(3)	85475	1(3)
82131	2(3)	82491	4(3)	82800	1(1)	83540	2(3)	84061	1(3)	84376	1(3)	85025	2(3)	85520	1(3)
82135	1(3)	82492	2(3)	82805	2(1)	83550	1(3)	84066	1(3)	84377	1(3)	85027	2(3)	85525	2(3)
82136	2(3)	82495	1(3)	82810	2(3)	83570	1(3)	84075	2(3)	84378	2(3)	85032	1(3)	85530	1(3)
82139	2(3)	82507	1(3)	82820	1(3)	83582	1(3)	84078	1(2)	84379	1(3)	85041	1(3)	85536	1(2)
82140	2(3)	82523	1(3)	82930	1(1)	83586	1(3)	84080	1(3)	84392	1(3)	85044	1(2)	85540	1(2)
82143	2(3)	82525	2(3)	82938	1(3)	83593	1(3)	84081	1(3)	84402	1(3)	85045	1(2)	85547	1(2)
82150	2(3)	82528	1(3)	82941	1(3)	83605	3(1)	84085	1(2)	84403	2(3)	85046	1(2)	85549	1(3)
82154	1(3)	82530	4(3)	82943	1(3)	83615	2(3)	84087	1(3)	84425	1(2)	85048	2(3)	85555	1(2)
82157	1(3)	82533	5(3)	82945	4(3)	83625	1(3)	84100	2(3)	84430	1(3)	85049	2(3)	85557	1(2)
82160	1(3)	82540	1(3)	82946	1(2)	83630	1(3)	84105	1(3)	84431	1(3)	85055	1(3)	85576	7(3)

CPT	MUE	CPT	MUE	CPT	MUE	CPT	MUE	CPT	MUE	CPT	MUE	CPT	MUE	CPT	MUE
85597	1(3)	86327	1(3)	86664	2(3)	86812	1(2)	87086	3(3)	87301	1(3)	87525	1(3)	87902	1(2)
85598	1(3)	86329	3(3)	86665	2(3)	86813	1(2)	87088	6(3)	87305	1(3)	87526	1(3)	87903	1(2)
85610	4(3)	86331	12(3)	86666	4(3)	86816	1(2)	87101	4(3)	87320	1(3)	87527	1(3)	87904	14(3)
85611	2(3)	86332	1(3)	86668	2(3)	86817	1(2)	87102	4(3)	87324	2(3)	87528	1(3)	87905	2(3)
85612	1(3)	86334	1(2)	86671	3(3)	86821	1(3)	87103	2(3)	87327	1(3)	87529	2(3)	87906	2(3)
85613	1(3)	86335	2(3)	86674	3(3)	86822	1(3)	87106	4(3)	87328	2(3)	87530	2(3)	87910	1(3)
85635	1(3)	86336	1(3)	86677	3(3)	86825	1(3)	87107	4(3)	87329	2(3)	87531	1(3)	87912	1(3)
85651	1(2)	86337	1(2)	86682	2(3)	86826	2(3)	87109	2(3)	87332	1(3)	87532	1(3)	88104	5(3)
85652	1(2)	86340	1(2)	86684	2(3)	86828	2(1)	87110	2(3)	87335	1(3)	87533	1(3)	88106	5(3)
85660	1(2)	86341	1(3)	86687	1(3)	86829	2(1)	87116	2(1)	87336	1(3)	87534	1(3)	88108	6(3)
85670	2(3)	86343	1(3)	86688	1(3)	86830	2(3)	87118	3(3)	87337	1(3)	87535	1(3)	88112	6(3)
85675	1(3)	86344	1(2)	86689	2(3)	86831	2(3)	87140	3(3)	87338	1(1)	87536	1(3)	88120	2(3)
85705	1(3)	86352	1(3)	86692	2(3)	86832	2(3)	87143	2(3)	87339	1(3)	87537	1(3)	88121	2(3)
85730	4(3)	86353	7(3)	86694	2(3)	86833	1(3)	87149	4(3)	87340	1(2)	87538	1(3)	88125	1(3)
85732	4(3)	86355	1(2)	86695	2(3)	86834	1(3)	87150	12(3)	87341	1(2)	87539	1(3)	88130	1(2)
85810	2(3)	86356	7(3)	86696	2(3)	86835	1(3)	87152	1(3)	87350	1(2)	87540	1(3)	88140	1(2)
86000	6(3)	86357	1(2)	86698	3(3)	86850	3(3)	87153	3(3)	87380	1(2)	87541	1(3)	88141	1(3)
86005	2(3)	86359	1(2)	86701	1(3)	86860	2(3)	87158	1(1)	87385	2(3)	87542	1(3)	88142	1(3)
86021	1(2)	86360	1(2)	86702	2(3)	86870	2(3)	87164	2(3)	87389	1(3)	87550	1(3)	88143	1(3)
86022	1(2)	86361	1(2)	86703	1(2)	86880	4(3)	87166	2(3)	87390	1(3)	87551	2(3)	88147	1(3)
86023	3(3)	86367	1(3)	86704	1(2)	86885	2(3)	87168	2(3)	87391	1(3)	87552	1(3)	88148	1(3)
86038	1(3)	86376	2(3)	86705	1(2)	86886	3(1)	87169	2(3)	87400	2(3)	87555	1(1)	88150	1(3)
86039	1(3)	86378	1(3)	86706	2(3)	86890	1(1)	87172	1(3)	87420	1(3)	87556	1(1)	88152	1(3)
86060	1(3)	86382	3(3)	86707	1(3)	86891	1(1)	87176	2(3)	87425	1(3)	87557	1(3)	88153	1(3)
86063	1(3)	86384	1(3)	86708	1(2)	86900	1(3)	87177	3(3)	87427	2(3)	87560	1(3)	88154	1(3)
86077	1(2)	86386	1(2)	86709	1(2)	86901	1(3)	87181	12(3)	87430	1(3)	87561	1(3)	88155	1(3)
86078	1(3)	86406	2(3)	86710	4(3)	86902	6(3)	87184	8(3)	87449	3(3)	87562	1(3)	88160	4(3)
86079	1(3)	86430	2(3)	86711	2(3)	86904	2(1)	87185	4(3)	87450	2(3)	87580	1(3)	88161	4(3)
86140	1(2)	86431	2(3)	86713	3(3)	86905	8(3)	87187	3(3)	87451	2(3)	87581	1(3)	88162	3(3)
86141	1(2)	86480	1(3)	86717	8(3)	86906	1(2)	87188	6(3)	87470	1(3)	87582	1(3)	88164	1(3)
86146	3(3)	86481	1(3)	86720	2(3)	86920	9(3)	87190	9(3)	87471	1(3)	87590	1(3)	88165	1(3)
86147	4(3)	86485	1(2)	86723	2(3)	86921	2(1)	87197	1(3)	87472	1(3)	87591	2(3)	88166	1(3)
86148	3(3)	86486	2(3)	86727	2(3)	86922	5(3)	87205	3(1)	87475	1(3)	87592	1(3)	88167	1(3)
86152	1(3)	86490	1(2)	86729	0(2)	86923	10(3)	87206	6(3)	87476	1(3)	87623	1(2)	88172	5(3)
86153	1(3)	86510	1(2)	86732	2(3)	86927	2(1)	87207	3(3)	87477	1(3)	87624	1(2)	88173	5(3)
86155	1(3)	86580	1(2)	86735	2(3)	86930	0(3)	87209	4(3)	87480	1(3)	87625	1(2)	88174	1(3)
86156	1(2)	86590	1(3)	86738	2(3)	86931	1(3)	87210	4(3)	87481	1(1)	87631	1(3)	88175	1(3)
86157	1(2)	86592	2(3)	86741	2(3)	86932	2(1)	87220	3(3)	87482	1(3)	87632	1(3)	88177	6(3)
86160	4(3)	86593	2(3)	86744	2(3)	86940	1(3)	87230	3(3)	87485	1(3)	87633	1(3)	88182	2(1)
86161	2(3)	86602	3(3)	86747	2(3)	86941	1(3)	87250	1(3)	87486	1(3)	87640	1(3)	88184	2(3)
86162	1(2)	86603	2(3)	86750	4(3)	86945	2(3)	87252	2(3)	87487	1(3)	87641	1(3)	88187	2(3)
86171	2(3)	86609	14(3)	86753	3(3)	86950	1(3)	87253	2(3)	87490	1(3)	87650	1(3)	88188	2(3)
86185	1(3)	86611	4(3)	86756	2(3)	86960	1(3)	87254	7(3)	87491	2(3)	87651	1(3)	88189	2(3)
86200	1(3)	86612	2(3)	86757	6(3)	86965	1(3)	87255	2(3)	87492	1(3)	87652	1(3)	88230	2(1)
86215	1(3)	86615	6(3)	86759	2(3)	86970	1(1)	87260	1(3)	87493	2(3)	87653	1(3)	88233	3(1)
86225	1(3)	86617	2(3)	86762	2(3)	86971	1(3)	87265	1(3)	87495	1(3)	87660	1(3)	88239	3(1)
86226	1(3)	86618	2(3)	86765	2(3)	86972	1(3)	87267	1(3)	87496	1(3)	87661	1(1)	88240	3(1)
86235	10(3)	86619	2(3)	86768	5(3)	86975	1(3)	87269	1(3)	87497	2(3)	87797	3(3)	88241	3(1)
86243	1(3)	86622	2(3)	86771	2(3)	86976	1(3)	87270	1(3)	87498	1(3)	87798	13(3)	88245	1(2)
86255	5(3)	86625	1(3)	86774	2(3)	86977	1(3)	87271	1(3)	87500	1(3)	87799	3(3)	88248	1(2)
86256	9(3)	86628	3(3)	86777	2(3)	86978	1(1)	87272	1(3)	87501	1(3)	87800	2(3)	88249	1(2)
86277	1(3)	86631	6(3)	86778	2(3)	86985	1(1)	87273	1(3)	87502	1(3)	87801	3(3)	88261	2(1)
86280	1(3)	86632	3(3)	86780	2(3)	87003	1(3)	87274	1(3)	87503	1(3)	87802	2(3)	88262	2(1)
86294	1(3)	86635	4(3)	86784	1(3)	87015	4(3)	87275	1(3)	87505	1(2)	87803	3(3)	88263	1(3)
86300	2(3)	86638	6(3)	86787	2(3)	87040	2(1)	87276	1(3)	87506	1(2)	87804	3(3)	88264	2(1)
86301	1(2)	86641	2(3)	86788	2(3)	87045	3(3)	87277	1(3)	87507	1(3)	87806	1(2)	88267	2(1)
86304	1(2)	86644	2(3)	86789	2(3)	87046	6(3)	87278	1(3)	87510	1(3)	87807	2(3)	88269	2(1)
86305	1(2)	86645	1(3)	86790	4(3)	87070	3(1)	87279	1(3)	87511	1(3)	87808	1(3)	88273	3(1)
86308	1(2)	86648	2(3)	86793	2(3)	87071	4(3)	87280	1(3)	87512	1(3)	87809	2(3)	88283	2(1)
86309	1(2)	86651	2(3)	86800	1(3)	87073	3(3)	87281	1(3)	87515	1(3)	87810	2(3)	88289	1(3)
86310	1(2)	86652	2(3)	86803	1(3)	87075	6(3)	87283	1(3)	87516	1(3)	87850	1(3)	88291	1(1)
86316	2(3)	86653	2(3)	86804	1(2)	87076	6(3)	87285	1(3)	87517	1(3)	87880	2(3)	88300	2(1)
86318	2(3)	86654	2(3)	86805	2(3)	87077	10(3)	87290	1(3)	87520	1(3)	87899	4(3)	88302	2(1)
86320	1(2)	86658	12(3)	86807	2(3)	87081	6(3)	87299	1(3)	87521	1(3)	87900	1(2)	88309	3(1)
86325	2(3)	86663	2(3)	86808	1(3)	87084	1(3)	87300	2(3)	87522	1(3)	87901	1(2)	88311	4(1)

Appendix H — Medically Unlikely Edits (MUEs) — Professional

CPT	MUE	CPT	MUE	CPT	MUE	CPT	MUE	CPT	MUE	CPT	MUE	CPT	MUE	CPT	MUE
88321	1(2)	89310	1(2)	90675	1(2)	90868	1(3)	92060	1(2)	92544	1(3)	92975	1(1)	93316	1(3)
88323	1(2)	89320	1(2)	90676	1(2)	90869	1(3)	92065	1(2)	92545	1(3)	92977	1(3)	93317	1(3)
88325	1(2)	89321	1(2)	90680	1(2)	90870	2(3)	92071	2(2)	92546	1(3)	92978	1(3)	93318	1(3)
88329	4(1)	89322	1(2)	90681	1(2)	90880	1(3)	92072	1(2)	92547	1(3)	92979	2(1)	93320	1(3)
88331	11(1)	89325	1(2)	90685	1(2)	90885	0(3)	92081	1(2)	92548	1(3)	92986	1(2)	93321	1(3)
88333	4(1)	89329	1(2)	90686	1(2)	90887	0(3)	92082	1(2)	92550	1(2)	92987	1(2)	93325	1(3)
88342	3(3)	89330	1(2)	90687	1(2)	90889	0(3)	92083	1(2)	92552	1(2)	92990	1(2)	93350	1(2)
88344	1(1)	89331	1(2)	90688	1(2)	90901	1(3)	92100	1(2)	92553	1(2)	92992	1(2)	93351	1(2)
88347	4(1)	89335	1(3)	90690	1(2)	90911	1(3)	92132	1(2)	92555	1(2)	92993	1(2)	93352	1(3)
88348	1(3)	89337	1(2)	90691	1(2)	90935	1(3)	92133	1(2)	92556	1(2)	92997	1(2)	93355	1(3)
88355	1(3)	89342	1(2)	90692	1(2)	90937	1(3)	92134	1(2)	92557	1(2)	92998	2(1)	93451	1(3)
88356	1(1)	89343	1(2)	90693	1(2)	90940	2(1)	92136	2(2)	92558	0(3)	93000	3(1)	93452	1(3)
88358	2(1)	89344	1(2)	90696	1(2)	90945	1(3)	92140	1(2)	92561	1(2)	93005	3(1)	93453	1(3)
88360	6(3)	89346	1(2)	90697	1(2)	90947	1(3)	92145	1(2)	92562	1(2)	93015	1(3)	93454	1(3)
88361	6(3)	89352	1(2)	90698	1(2)	90951	1(2)	92225	2(2)	92563	1(2)	93016	1(3)	93455	1(3)
88362	1(3)	89353	1(3)	90700	1(2)	90952	1(2)	92226	2(2)	92564	1(2)	93017	1(3)	93456	1(3)
88363	2(3)	89354	1(3)	90702	1(2)	90953	1(2)	92227	1(2)	92565	1(2)	93018	1(3)	93457	1(3)
88364	3(3)	89356	2(3)	90703	1(2)	90954	1(2)	92228	1(2)	92567	1(2)	93024	1(3)	93458	1(3)
88365	2(1)	90284	1(1)	90704	1(2)	90955	1(2)	92230	2(2)	92568	1(2)	93025	1(2)	93459	1(3)
88366	1(1)	90296	1(1)	90705	1(2)	90956	1(2)	92235	2(2)	92570	1(2)	93040	3(1)	93460	1(3)
88367	2(1)	90375	20(1)	90706	1(2)	90957	1(2)	92240	2(2)	92571	1(2)	93041	2(1)	93461	1(3)
88368	2(1)	90376	20(1)	90707	1(2)	90958	1(2)	92250	1(2)	92572	1(2)	93042	3(1)	93462	1(3)
88369	3(1)	90385	1(2)	90708	1(2)	90959	1(2)	92260	1(2)	92575	1(2)	93224	1(2)	93463	1(3)
88371	1(3)	90393	1(1)	90710	1(2)	90960	1(2)	92265	1(2)	92576	1(2)	93225	1(2)	93464	1(3)
88372	1(3)	90396	1(1)	90712	1(2)	90961	1(2)	92270	1(2)	92577	1(2)	93226	1(2)	93503	2(1)
88373	3(1)	90460	6(3)	90713	1(2)	90962	1(2)	92275	1(2)	92579	1(2)	93227	1(2)	93505	1(2)
88374	1(1)	90471	1(3)	90714	1(2)	90963	1(2)	92283	1(2)	92582	1(2)	93228	1(2)	93530	1(3)
88375	1(3)	90472	4(1)	90715	1(2)	90964	1(2)	92284	1(2)	92583	1(2)	93229	1(2)	93531	1(3)
88377	1(1)	90473	1(2)	90716	1(2)	90965	1(2)	92285	1(2)	92584	1(2)	93260	1(2)	93532	1(3)
88380	1(1)	90474	1(1)	90717	1(2)	90966	1(2)	92286	1(2)	92585	1(2)	93261	1(3)	93533	1(3)
88381	1(1)	90476	1(2)	90719	1(2)	90967	1(2)	92287	1(2)	92586	1(2)	93268	1(2)	93561	1(3)
88387	3(1)	90477	1(2)	90720	1(2)	90968	1(2)	92311	1(2)	92587	1(2)	93270	1(2)	93562	1(3)
88388	3(1)	90581	1(2)	90721	1(2)	90969	1(2)	92312	1(2)	92588	1(2)	93271	1(2)	93563	1(3)
88720	1(3)	90585	1(2)	90725	1(2)	90970	1(2)	92313	1(3)	92596	1(2)	93272	1(2)	93564	1(3)
88738	1(1)	90586	1(2)	90727	1(2)	90989	1(2)	92315	1(2)	92601	1(3)	93278	1(3)	93565	1(3)
88740	1(2)	90630	1(2)	90732	1(2)	90993	1(3)	92316	1(2)	92602	1(3)	93279	1(3)	93566	1(3)
88741	1(2)	90632	1(2)	90733	1(2)	90997	1(3)	92317	1(3)	92603	1(3)	93280	1(3)	93567	1(3)
89049	1(3)	90633	1(2)	90734	1(2)	91010	1(2)	92325	1(3)	92604	1(3)	93281	1(3)	93568	1(3)
89050	2(1)	90634	1(2)	90735	1(2)	91013	1(3)	92326	2(2)	92605	0(3)	93282	1(3)	93571	1(3)
89051	2(1)	90636	1(2)	90736	1(2)	91020	1(2)	92352	0(3)	92609	1(3)	93283	1(3)	93572	2(1)
89055	2(1)	90644	1(2)	90738	1(2)	91022	1(2)	92353	0(3)	92610	1(2)	93284	1(3)	93580	1(3)
89060	2(1)	90645	1(2)	90739	1(2)	91030	1(2)	92354	0(3)	92613	1(2)	93285	1(3)	93581	1(3)
89125	2(1)	90646	1(2)	90740	1(2)	91034	1(2)	92355	0(3)	92615	1(2)	93286	2(3)	93582	1(2)
89160	1(3)	90647	1(2)	90743	1(2)	91035	1(2)	92358	0(3)	92617	1(2)	93287	2(3)	93583	1(2)
89190	1(3)	90648	1(2)	90744	1(2)	91037	1(2)	92371	0(3)	92618	0(1)	93288	1(3)	93600	1(3)
89220	1(1)	90649	1(2)	90746	1(2)	91038	1(2)	92502	1(3)	92620	1(2)	93289	1(3)	93602	1(3)
89230	1(2)	90650	1(2)	90747	1(2)	91040	1(2)	92504	1(3)	92625	1(2)	93290	1(3)	93603	1(3)
89250	1(2)	90651	1(2)	90785	1(1)	91065	2(2)	92507	1(3)	92626	1(2)	93291	1(3)	93609	1(3)
89251	1(2)	90653	1(2)	90791	1(1)	91110	1(2)	92508	1(3)	92920	1(1)	93292	1(3)	93610	1(3)
89253	1(3)	90654	1(2)	90792	1(1)	91111	1(2)	92511	1(3)	92924	1(1)	93293	1(2)	93612	1(3)
89254	1(3)	90655	1(2)	90832	1(3)	91112	1(1)	92512	1(2)	92928	1(1)	93294	1(2)	93613	1(3)
89255	1(3)	90656	1(2)	90833	1(1)	91117	1(2)	92516	1(3)	92933	1(1)	93295	1(2)	93615	1(3)
89257	1(3)	90657	1(2)	90834	1(3)	91120	1(2)	92520	1(2)	92937	3(1)	93296	1(2)	93616	1(3)
89258	1(2)	90658	1(2)	90836	1(1)	91122	1(2)	92521	1(2)	92938	3(1)	93297	1(2)	93618	1(3)
89259	1(2)	90660	1(2)	90837	1(3)	91132	1(3)	92522	1(2)	92941	1(1)	93298	1(2)	93619	1(3)
89260	1(2)	90661	1(2)	90838	1(1)	91133	1(3)	92523	1(2)	92943	1(1)	93299	1(2)	93620	1(3)
89261	1(2)	90662	1(2)	90839	1(1)	91200	1(3)	92524	1(2)	92944	1(1)	93303	1(3)	93621	1(3)
89264	1(3)	90664	1(2)	90845	1(2)	92002	1(2)	92526	1(2)	92950	3(1)	93304	1(1)	93622	1(3)
89268	1(2)	90666	1(2)	90846	1(3)	92004	1(2)	92531	0(3)	92953	2(3)	93306	1(3)	93623	1(3)
89272	1(2)	90667	1(2)	90847	1(3)	92012	1(3)	92532	0(3)	92960	2(3)	93307	1(3)	93624	1(3)
89280	1(2)	90668	1(2)	90849	1(3)	92014	1(3)	92534	0(3)	92961	1(3)	93308	1(3)	93631	1(3)
89281	1(2)	90669	1(2)	90853	1(3)	92018	1(2)	92540	1(3)	92970	1(3)	93312	1(3)	93640	1(3)
89290	1(2)	90670	1(2)	90863	1(1)	92019	1(2)	92541	1(3)	92971	1(3)	93313	1(3)	93641	1(2)
89291	1(2)	90672	1(1)	90865	1(3)	92020	1(2)	92542	1(3)	92973	2(1)	93314	1(3)	93642	1(3)
89300	1(2)	90673	1(2)	90867	1(2)	92025	1(2)	92543	4(2)	92974	1(1)	93315	1(3)	93644	1(2)

CPT	MUE	CPT	MUE	CPT	MUE	CPT	MUE	CPT	MUE	CPT	MUE	CPT	MUE	CPT	MUE
93650	1(2)	94453	1(2)	95831	5(2)	95992	1(2)	97607	1(3)	99236	1(3)	99478	1(2)	A4562	1(1)
93653	1(3)	94610	2(3)	95832	1(3)	96000	1(2)	97608	1(3)	99238	1(2)	99479	1(2)	A4565	2(3)
93654	1(3)	94620	1(3)	95851	3(1)	96001	1(2)	97610	1(2)	99239	1(2)	99480	1(2)	A4606	0(3)
93655	2(3)	94621	1(3)	95852	1(3)	96002	1(3)	98925	1(2)	99281	1(3)	99485	1(1)	A4611	0(3)
93656	1(3)	94640	4(3)	95857	1(2)	96003	1(3)	98926	1(2)	99282	1(3)	99487	1(1)	A4614	1(1)
93657	1(3)	94642	1(3)	95860	1(3)	96004	1(2)	98927	1(2)	99283	1(3)	99490	1(2)	A4625	30(3)
93660	1(3)	94644	1(2)	95861	1(3)	96020	1(2)	98928	1(2)	99284	1(3)	99495	1(1)	A4633	0(3)
93662	1(3)	94645	2(1)	95863	1(3)	96103	1(2)	98929	1(2)	99285	1(3)	99496	1(1)	A4635	0(3)
93701	1(2)	94660	1(2)	95864	1(3)	96105	3(1)	98940	1(2)	99288	0(3)	99605	0(2)	A4638	0(3)
93702	1(2)	94662	1(2)	95865	1(3)	96120	1(2)	98941	1(2)	99291	1(2)	99606	0(3)	A4640	0(3)
93724	1(3)	94664	1(3)	95866	1(3)	96125	2(1)	98942	1(2)	99304	1(2)	99607	0(3)	A4642	1(1)
93740	0(3)	94667	1(2)	95867	1(3)	96127	2(1)	99002	0(3)	99305	1(2)	A0021	0(3)	A4648	5(3)
93745	1(2)	94669	4(3)	95868	1(3)	96360	1(1)	99024	0(3)	99306	1(2)	A0080	0(3)	A4650	3(1)
93750	4(3)	94680	1(3)	95869	1(3)	96365	1(1)	99050	0(3)	99307	1(2)	A0090	0(3)	A5056	90(3)
93770	0(3)	94681	1(3)	95873	1(2)	96368	1(2)	99051	0(3)	99308	1(2)	A0100	0(3)	A5057	90(3)
93784	1(2)	94690	1(3)	95874	1(2)	96369	1(2)	99053	0(3)	99309	1(2)	A0110	0(3)	A5120	150(3)
93786	1(2)	94726	1(3)	95875	2(3)	96370	3(1)	99056	0(3)	99310	1(2)	A0120	0(3)	A5500	0(3)
93788	1(2)	94727	1(3)	95885	4(2)	96371	1(3)	99058	0(3)	99315	1(2)	A0130	0(3)	A5501	0(3)
93790	1(2)	94728	1(3)	95886	4(2)	96373	2(1)	99060	0(3)	99316	1(2)	A0140	0(3)	A5503	0(3)
93797	2(2)	94729	1(3)	95887	1(2)	96374	1(3)	99070	0(3)	99318	1(2)	A0160	0(3)	A5504	0(3)
93798	2(2)	94750	1(3)	95905	2(3)	96376	0(3)	99071	0(3)	99324	1(2)	A0170	0(3)	A5505	0(3)
93880	1(3)	94760	1(3)	95907	1(2)	96402	2(3)	99078	0(3)	99325	1(2)	A0180	0(3)	A5506	0(3)
93882	1(3)	94761	1(2)	95908	1(2)	96405	1(2)	99080	0(3)	99326	1(2)	A0190	0(3)	A5507	0(3)
93886	1(3)	94762	1(2)	95909	1(2)	96406	1(2)	99082	1(1)	99327	1(2)	A0200	0(3)	A5508	0(3)
93888	1(3)	94770	1(3)	95910	1(2)	96409	1(3)	99090	0(3)	99328	1(2)	A0210	0(3)	A5510	0(3)
93890	1(3)	94772	1(2)	95911	1(2)	96413	1(3)	99091	0(3)	99334	1(3)	A0225	0(3)	A5512	0(3)
93892	1(3)	94774	1(2)	95912	1(2)	96416	1(3)	99116	0(3)	99335	1(3)	A0380	0(3)	A5513	0(3)
93893	1(3)	94775	1(2)	95913	1(2)	96420	2(1)	99135	0(3)	99336	1(3)	A0382	0(3)	A6501	2(1)
93922	1(1)	94776	1(2)	95921	1(3)	96422	2(3)	99140	0(3)	99337	1(3)	A0384	0(3)	A6502	2(1)
93923	1(1)	94777	1(2)	95922	1(3)	96425	1(3)	99143	2(3)	99341	1(2)	A0390	0(3)	A6503	2(1)
93924	1(2)	94780	1(2)	95923	1(3)	96440	1(3)	99144	2(3)	99342	1(2)	A0392	0(3)	A6504	4(1)
93925	1(3)	94781	1(1)	95924	1(1)	96446	1(3)	99148	2(3)	99343	1(2)	A0394	0(3)	A6505	4(1)
93926	1(3)	95012	2(3)	95925	1(3)	96450	1(3)	99149	2(3)	99344	1(2)	A0396	0(3)	A6506	4(1)
93930	1(3)	95018	19(3)	95926	1(3)	96521	2(3)	99170	1(3)	99345	1(2)	A0398	0(3)	A6507	4(1)
93931	1(3)	95056	1(2)	95927	1(3)	96522	1(3)	99175	1(3)	99347	1(3)	A0420	0(3)	A6508	4(1)
93965	1(3)	95060	1(2)	95928	1(3)	96523	1(3)	99183	1(3)	99348	1(3)	A0422	0(3)	A6509	2(1)
93970	1(3)	95065	1(3)	95929	1(3)	96542	1(3)	99184	1(2)	99349	1(3)	A0424	0(3)	A6510	2(1)
93971	1(3)	95070	1(3)	95930	1(3)	96567	1(3)	99191	1(3)	99350	1(3)	A0426	2(3)	A6511	2(1)
93975	1(3)	95071	1(2)	95933	1(3)	96570	1(2)	99192	1(3)	99354	1(2)	A0427	2(3)	A6513	0(3)
93976	1(3)	95076	1(1)	95938	1(3)	96571	3(1)	99195	2(1)	99356	1(2)	A0428	4(3)	A6531	0(3)
93978	1(3)	95079	2(1)	95939	1(3)	96900	1(3)	99201	1(2)	99366	0(3)	A0429	2(3)	A6532	0(3)
93979	1(3)	95115	1(2)	95943	1(3)	96902	0(3)	99202	1(2)	99367	0(3)	A0430	1(3)	A6545	0(3)
93980	1(3)	95117	1(2)	95950	1(2)	96904	1(2)	99203	1(2)	99368	0(3)	A0431	1(3)	A7000	0(3)
93981	1(3)	95250	1(2)	95951	1(2)	96910	1(3)	99204	1(2)	99406	1(2)	A0432	1(3)	A7003	0(3)
93982	1(3)	95251	1(2)	95953	1(2)	96912	1(3)	99205	1(2)	99407	1(2)	A0433	1(3)	A7005	0(3)
93990	2(3)	95782	1(2)	95954	1(3)	96913	1(3)	99211	1(3)	99446	1(2)	A0434	2(3)	A7006	0(3)
94002	1(2)	95783	1(2)	95955	1(3)	96920	1(2)	99212	2(3)	99447	1(2)	A0435	999(3)	A7013	0(3)
94003	1(2)	95800	1(2)	95956	1(2)	96921	1(2)	99213	2(3)	99448	1(2)	A0436	300(3)	A7014	0(3)
94004	1(2)	95801	1(2)	95957	1(3)	96922	1(2)	99214	2(3)	99449	1(2)	A0888	0(3)	A7016	0(3)
94010	1(3)	95803	1(2)	95958	1(3)	97010	0(3)	99215	1(3)	99455	1(3)	A0998	0(3)	A7017	0(3)
94011	1(3)	95805	1(2)	95961	1(2)	97012	1(3)	99217	1(2)	99456	1(3)	A4221	0(3)	A7020	0(3)
94012	1(3)	95806	1(2)	95965	1(3)	97014	0(3)	99218	1(2)	99460	1(2)	A4235	2(1)	A7025	0(3)
94013	1(3)	95807	1(2)	95966	1(3)	97016	1(3)	99219	1(2)	99461	1(2)	A4253	0(3)	A7026	0(3)
94014	1(2)	95808	1(2)	95967	3(1)	97018	1(3)	99220	1(2)	99462	1(2)	A4255	0(3)	A7027	0(3)
94015	1(2)	95810	1(2)	95970	1(3)	97022	1(3)	99221	1(3)	99463	1(2)	A4257	0(3)	A7028	0(3)
94016	1(2)	95811	1(2)	95971	1(3)	97024	1(3)	99222	1(3)	99464	1(2)	A4258	0(3)	A7029	0(3)
94060	1(3)	95812	1(3)	95972	1(2)	97026	1(3)	99223	1(3)	99465	1(2)	A4259	0(3)	A7032	0(3)
94070	1(2)	95813	1(3)	95974	1(2)	97028	1(3)	99224	1(2)	99466	1(2)	A4301	1(2)	A7035	0(3)
94150	0(3)	95816	1(3)	95975	2(1)	97150	1(3)	99225	1(2)	99468	1(2)	A4356	1(1)	A7036	0(3)
94200	1(3)	95819	1(3)	95978	1(2)	97545	1(2)	99226	1(2)	99469	1(2)	A4459	0(3)	A7037	0(3)
94250	1(3)	95822	1(3)	95980	1(3)	97546	2(1)	99231	1(3)	99471	1(2)	A4470	1(1)	A7039	0(3)
94375	1(3)	95824	1(3)	95981	1(3)	97597	1(3)	99232	1(3)	99472	1(2)	A4480	1(1)	A7040	2(1)
94400	1(3)	95827	1(2)	95982	1(3)	97602	0(3)	99233	1(3)	99475	1(2)	A4555	0(3)	A7041	2(1)
94450	1(3)	95829	1(3)	95990	2(1)	97605	1(3)	99234	1(3)	99476	1(2)	A4557	2(1)	A7044	0(3)
94452	1(2)	95830	1(3)	95991	2(1)	97606	1(3)	99235	1(3)	99477	1(2)	A4561	1(1)	A7047	0(3)

CPT	MUE	CPT	MUE	CPT	MUE	CPT	MUE	CPT	MUE	CPT	MUE	CPT	MUE	CPT	MUE
A7048	10(3)	A9586	1(1)	C2641	150(3)	C9364	600(3)	E0185	0(3)	E0302	0(3)	E0601	0(3)	E0761	0(3)
A7501	0(3)	A9599	1(3)	C2642	120(3)	C9442	300(3)	E0186	0(3)	E0303	0(3)	E0602	0(3)	E0762	0(3)
A7504	0(3)	A9600	7(3)	C2643	120(3)	C9443	100(3)	E0187	0(3)	E0304	0(3)	E0603	0(3)	E0764	0(3)
A7507	0(3)	A9604	1(3)	C5271	1(2)	C9444	120(3)	E0188	0(3)	E0305	0(3)	E0604	0(3)	E0765	0(3)
A7520	0(3)	A9700	2(1)	C5272	3(2)	C9446	200(3)	E0189	0(3)	E0310	0(3)	E0605	0(3)	E0766	0(3)
A7524	0(3)	B4081	0(3)	C5273	1(2)	C9497	1(3)	E0190	0(3)	E0315	0(3)	E0606	0(3)	E0769	0(3)
A7527	0(3)	B4082	0(3)	C5274	35(3)	C9600	3(3)	E0191	0(3)	E0316	0(3)	E0607	0(3)	E0770	1(3)
A9272	0(1)	B4083	0(3)	C5275	1(2)	C9601	2(3)	E0193	0(3)	E0325	0(3)	E0610	0(3)	E0776	0(3)
A9284	0(3)	B4087	0(3)	C5276	3(2)	C9602	3(3)	E0194	0(3)	E0326	0(3)	E0615	0(3)	E0779	0(3)
A9500	3(1)	B4088	0(3)	C5277	1(2)	C9603	2(3)	E0196	0(3)	E0328	0(3)	E0616	1(2)	E0780	0(3)
A9501	3(1)	B4149	0(3)	C5278	15(3)	C9604	3(3)	E0197	0(3)	E0329	0(3)	E0617	0(3)	E0781	1(2)
A9502	3(1)	B4153	0(3)	C8900	1(3)	C9605	3(3)	E0198	0(3)	E0350	0(3)	E0618	0(3)	E0782	1(2)
A9503	1(1)	B4157	0(3)	C8901	1(3)	C9606	2(3)	E0199	0(3)	E0352	0(3)	E0619	0(3)	E0783	1(2)
A9504	1(1)	B4160	0(3)	C8902	1(3)	C9607	1(2)	E0200	0(3)	E0370	0(3)	E0620	0(3)	E0784	0(3)
A9505	4(3)	B4164	0(3)	C8903	1(3)	C9608	2(3)	E0202	0(3)	E0371	0(3)	E0621	0(3)	E0785	1(2)
A9507	1(1)	B4168	0(3)	C8904	1(3)	C9724	1(2)	E0203	0(3)	E0372	0(3)	E0625	0(3)	E0786	1(2)
A9508	2(3)	B4172	0(3)	C8905	1(3)	C9725	1(3)	E0205	0(3)	E0373	0(3)	E0627	0(3)	E0791	0(3)
A9510	1(1)	B4176	0(3)	C8906	1(3)	C9727	1(2)	E0210	0(3)	E0424	0(3)	E0628	0(3)	E0830	0(3)
A9512	30(3)	B4178	0(3)	C8907	1(3)	C9728	1(2)	E0215	0(3)	E0425	0(3)	E0629	0(3)	E0840	0(3)
A9516	4(3)	B4180	0(3)	C8908	1(3)	C9733	1(3)	E0217	0(3)	E0430	0(3)	E0630	0(3)	E0849	0(3)
A9520	1(3)	B4189	0(3)	C8909	1(3)	C9734	1(3)	E0218	0(3)	E0431	0(3)	E0635	0(3)	E0850	0(3)
A9521	2(1)	B4199	0(3)	C8910	1(3)	C9739	1(2)	E0221	0(3)	E0434	0(3)	E0636	0(3)	E0855	0(3)
A9524	10(3)	B5000	0(3)	C8911	1(3)	C9740	1(2)	E0225	0(3)	E0435	0(3)	E0637	0(3)	E0856	0(3)
A9526	2(1)	B5100	0(3)	C8912	1(3)	C9741	1(3)	E0231	0(3)	E0439	0(3)	E0638	0(3)	E0860	0(3)
A9536	1(1)	B5200	0(3)	C8913	1(3)	C9742	1(2)	E0232	0(3)	E0440	0(3)	E0639	0(3)	E0870	0(3)
A9537	1(1)	C1716	4(3)	C8914	1(3)	E0100	0(3)	E0235	0(3)	E0441	0(3)	E0640	0(3)	E0880	0(3)
A9538	1(1)	C1717	10(3)	C8918	1(3)	E0105	0(3)	E0236	0(3)	E0442	0(3)	E0641	0(3)	E0890	0(3)
A9539	2(1)	C1719	99(3)	C8919	1(3)	E0110	0(3)	E0239	0(3)	E0443	0(3)	E0642	0(3)	E0900	0(3)
A9540	2(1)	C1721	1(3)	C8920	1(3)	E0111	0(3)	E0240	0(3)	E0444	0(3)	E0650	0(3)	E0910	0(3)
A9541	1(1)	C1722	1(3)	C8921	1(3)	E0112	0(3)	E0241	0(3)	E0445	0(3)	E0651	0(3)	E0911	0(3)
A9542	1(1)	C1749	1(3)	C8922	1(3)	E0113	0(3)	E0242	0(3)	E0446	0(3)	E0652	0(3)	E0912	0(3)
A9543	1(1)	C1764	1(3)	C8923	1(3)	E0114	0(3)	E0243	0(3)	E0450	0(3)	E0655	0(3)	E0920	0(3)
A9544	1(1)	C1767	2(3)	C8924	1(3)	E0116	0(3)	E0244	0(3)	E0455	0(3)	E0656	0(3)	E0930	0(3)
A9545	1(1)	C1771	1(3)	C8925	1(3)	E0117	0(3)	E0245	0(3)	E0457	0(3)	E0657	0(3)	E0935	0(3)
A9546	1(1)	C1772	1(3)	C8926	1(3)	E0118	0(3)	E0246	0(3)	E0459	0(3)	E0660	0(3)	E0936	0(3)
A9547	2(3)	C1776	10(3)	C8927	1(3)	E0130	0(3)	E0247	0(3)	E0460	0(3)	E0665	0(3)	E0940	0(3)
A9548	2(3)	C1778	4(3)	C8928	1(2)	E0135	0(3)	E0248	0(3)	E0461	0(3)	E0666	0(3)	E0941	0(3)
A9550	1(1)	C1782	1(3)	C8929	1(3)	E0140	0(3)	E0249	0(3)	E0462	0(3)	E0667	0(3)	E0942	0(3)
A9551	1(1)	C1785	1(3)	C8930	1(2)	E0141	0(3)	E0250	0(3)	E0463	0(3)	E0668	0(3)	E0944	0(3)
A9552	1(1)	C1786	1(3)	C8931	1(3)	E0143	0(3)	E0251	0(3)	E0464	0(3)	E0669	0(3)	E0945	0(3)
A9553	1(1)	C1813	1(3)	C8932	1(3)	E0144	0(3)	E0255	0(3)	E0470	0(3)	E0670	0(3)	E0946	0(3)
A9554	1(1)	C1815	1(3)	C8933	1(3)	E0147	0(3)	E0256	0(3)	E0471	0(3)	E0671	0(3)	E0947	0(3)
A9555	3(1)	C1817	1(3)	C8957	2(3)	E0148	0(3)	E0260	0(3)	E0472	0(3)	E0672	0(3)	E0948	0(3)
A9556	10(3)	C1820	2(3)	C9025	300(3)	E0149	0(3)	E0261	0(3)	E0480	0(3)	E0673	0(3)	E0950	0(3)
A9557	2(1)	C1830	2(3)	C9026	300(3)	E0153	0(3)	E0265	0(3)	E0481	0(3)	E0675	0(3)	E0951	0(3)
A9558	7(3)	C1840	1(3)	C9027	300(3)	E0154	0(3)	E0266	0(3)	E0482	0(3)	E0676	1(3)	E0952	0(3)
A9559	1(1)	C1841	1(3)	C9132	5500(3)	E0155	0(3)	E0270	0(3)	E0483	0(3)	E0691	0(3)	E0955	0(3)
A9560	2(1)	C1882	1(3)	C9250	1(3)	E0156	0(3)	E0271	0(3)	E0484	0(3)	E0692	0(3)	E0956	0(3)
A9561	1(1)	C1886	1(3)	C9254	0(3)	E0157	0(3)	E0272	0(3)	E0485	0(3)	E0693	0(3)	E0957	0(3)
A9562	2(1)	C1900	1(3)	C9257	5(3)	E0158	0(3)	E0273	0(3)	E0486	0(3)	E0694	0(3)	E0958	0(3)
A9564	20(3)	C2616	1(3)	C9275	1(3)	E0159	2(2)	E0274	0(3)	E0487	0(3)	E0700	0(3)	E0959	0(3)
A9566	1(1)	C2619	1(3)	C9285	2(3)	E0160	0(3)	E0275	0(3)	E0500	0(3)	E0705	0(3)	E0960	0(3)
A9567	2(1)	C2620	1(3)	C9290	266(3)	E0161	0(3)	E0276	0(3)	E0550	0(3)	E0710	0(3)	E0961	0(3)
A9568	0(3)	C2621	1(3)	C9293	700(3)	E0162	0(3)	E0277	0(3)	E0555	0(3)	E0720	0(3)	E0966	0(3)
A9569	1(1)	C2622	1(3)	C9352	3(3)	E0163	0(3)	E0280	0(3)	E0560	0(3)	E0730	0(3)	E0967	0(3)
A9570	1(1)	C2624	1(3)	C9353	4(3)	E0165	0(3)	E0290	0(3)	E0561	0(3)	E0731	0(3)	E0968	0(3)
A9571	1(1)	C2626	1(3)	C9354	300(3)	E0167	0(3)	E0291	0(3)	E0562	0(3)	E0740	0(3)	E0970	0(3)
A9572	1(3)	C2631	1(3)	C9355	3(3)	E0168	0(3)	E0292	0(3)	E0565	0(3)	E0744	0(3)	E0971	0(3)
A9575	200(3)	C2634	24(3)	C9356	125(3)	E0170	0(3)	E0293	0(3)	E0570	0(3)	E0745	0(3)	E0973	0(3)
A9579	100(3)	C2635	124(3)	C9358	800(3)	E0171	0(3)	E0294	0(3)	E0572	0(3)	E0746	1(3)	E0974	0(3)
A9580	1(1)	C2636	150(3)	C9359	30(3)	E0172	0(3)	E0295	0(3)	E0574	0(3)	E0747	0(3)	E0978	0(3)
A9582	1(3)	C2637	0(3)	C9360	300(3)	E0175	0(3)	E0296	0(3)	E0575	0(3)	E0748	0(3)	E0981	0(3)
A9583	18(3)	C2638	150(3)	C9361	10(3)	E0181	0(3)	E0297	0(3)	E0580	0(3)	E0749	1(3)	E0982	0(3)
A9584	1(1)	C2639	150(3)	C9362	60(3)	E0182	0(3)	E0300	0(3)	E0585	0(3)	E0755	0(3)	E0983	0(3)
A9585	300(3)	C2640	150(3)	C9363	500(3)	E0184	0(3)	E0301	0(3)	E0600	0(3)	E0760	0(3)	E0984	0(3)

CPT	MUE	CPT	MUE	CPT	MUE	CPT	MUE	CPT	MUE	CPT	MUE	CPT	MUE	CPT	MUE
E0985	0(3)	E1228	0(3)	E1805	0(3)	E2327	0(3)	E2615	0(3)	G0249	3(3)	G0432	1(2)	G6045	1(3)
E0986	0(3)	E1229	0(3)	E1806	0(3)	E2328	0(3)	E2616	0(3)	G0250	1(2)	G0433	1(2)	G6046	1(3)
E0988	0(3)	E1230	0(3)	E1810	0(3)	E2329	0(3)	E2617	0(3)	G0257	0(3)	G0434	1(2)	G6047	1(3)
E0990	0(3)	E1231	0(3)	E1811	0(3)	E2330	0(3)	E2619	0(3)	G0259	2(3)	G0435	1(2)	G6048	1(3)
E0992	0(3)	E1232	0(3)	E1812	0(3)	E2331	0(3)	E2620	0(3)	G0260	2(3)	G0436	1(2)	G6049	1(3)
E0994	0(3)	E1233	0(3)	E1815	0(3)	E2340	0(3)	E2621	0(3)	G0268	1(2)	G0437	1(2)	G6050	1(3)
E0995	0(3)	E1234	0(3)	E1816	0(3)	E2341	0(3)	E2622	0(3)	G0270	8(3)	G0438	1(2)	G6051	1(3)
E1002	0(3)	E1235	0(3)	E1818	0(3)	E2342	0(3)	E2623	0(3)	G0271	4(3)	G0439	1(2)	G6052	2(3)
E1003	0(3)	E1236	0(3)	E1820	0(3)	E2343	0(3)	E2624	0(3)	G0277	5(3)	G0442	1(2)	G6053	2(3)
E1004	0(3)	E1237	0(3)	E1821	0(3)	E2351	0(3)	E2625	0(3)	G0278	1(2)	G0443	1(2)	G6054	1(3)
E1005	0(3)	E1238	0(3)	E1825	0(3)	E2358	0(3)	E2626	0(3)	G0281	1(3)	G0444	1(2)	G6055	2(3)
E1006	0(3)	E1240	0(3)	E1830	0(3)	E2359	0(3)	E2627	0(3)	G0283	1(3)	G0445	1(2)	G6056	4(3)
E1007	0(3)	E1250	0(3)	E1831	0(3)	E2361	0(3)	E2628	0(3)	G0288	1(2)	G0446	1(3)	G6057	2(3)
E1008	0(3)	E1260	0(3)	E1840	0(3)	E2363	0(3)	E2629	0(3)	G0289	1(2)	G0447	2(3)	G6058	10(3)
E1009	0(3)	E1270	0(3)	E1841	0(3)	E2365	0(3)	E2630	0(3)	G0293	1(2)	G0448	1(3)	G9143	1(2)
E1010	0(3)	E1280	0(3)	E1902	0(3)	E2366	0(3)	E2631	0(3)	G0294	1(2)	G0452	6(3)	G9156	1(2)
E1011	0(3)	E1285	0(3)	E2000	0(3)	E2367	0(3)	E2632	0(3)	G0302	1(2)	G0453	40(3)	G9157	1(2)
E1014	0(3)	E1290	0(3)	E2100	0(3)	E2368	0(3)	E2633	0(3)	G0303	1(2)	G0454	1(2)	G9187	1(3)
E1015	0(3)	E1295	0(3)	E2101	0(3)	E2369	0(3)	G0008	1(2)	G0304	1(2)	G0455	1(2)	J0129	100(3)
E1016	0(3)	E1300	0(3)	E2120	0(3)	E2370	0(3)	G0009	1(2)	G0305	1(2)	G0458	1(1)	J0130	6(3)
E1017	0(3)	E1310	0(3)	E2201	0(3)	E2371	0(3)	G0010	1(3)	G0306	1(3)	G0459	1(2)	J0131	400(3)
E1018	0(3)	E1352	0(3)	E2202	0(3)	E2373	0(3)	G0027	1(2)	G0307	1(3)	G0460	1(3)	J0133	1200(3)
E1020	0(3)	E1353	0(3)	E2203	0(3)	E2374	0(3)	G0101	1(2)	G0328	1(2)	G0463	0(3)	J0135	8(3)
E1028	0(3)	E1354	0(3)	E2204	0(3)	E2375	0(3)	G0102	1(2)	G0329	1(3)	G0464	1(2)	J0153	180(3)
E1029	0(3)	E1355	0(3)	E2205	0(3)	E2376	0(3)	G0103	1(2)	G0333	0(3)	G0472	1(2)	J0178	4(3)
E1030	0(3)	E1356	0(3)	E2206	0(3)	E2377	0(3)	G0104	1(2)	G0337	1(2)	G3001	1(2)	J0180	150(3)
E1031	0(3)	E1357	0(3)	E2207	0(3)	E2378	0(3)	G0105	1(2)	G0339	1(2)	G6001	1(2)	J0210	4(3)
E1035	0(3)	E1358	0(3)	E2208	0(3)	E2381	0(3)	G0106	1(2)	G0340	2(3)	G6002	2(3)	J0215	30(3)
E1037	0(3)	E1372	0(3)	E2209	0(3)	E2382	0(3)	G0108	6(3)	G0341	1(2)	G6003	2(3)	J0220	1(3)
E1038	0(3)	E1390	0(3)	E2210	0(3)	E2383	0(3)	G0109	12(3)	G0342	1(2)	G6004	2(3)	J0221	300(3)
E1039	0(3)	E1391	0(3)	E2211	0(3)	E2384	0(3)	G0117	1(2)	G0343	1(2)	G6005	2(3)	J0256	3500(3)
E1050	0(3)	E1392	0(3)	E2212	0(3)	E2385	0(3)	G0118	1(2)	G0364	2(3)	G6006	2(3)	J0257	1400(3)
E1060	0(3)	E1405	0(3)	E2213	0(3)	E2386	0(3)	G0120	1(2)	G0365	2(3)	G6007	2(3)	J0275	1(3)
E1070	0(3)	E1406	0(3)	E2214	0(3)	E2387	0(3)	G0121	1(2)	G0372	1(2)	G6008	2(3)	J0278	15(3)
E1083	0(3)	E1500	0(3)	E2215	0(3)	E2388	0(3)	G0123	1(3)	G0379	0(3)	G6009	2(3)	J0280	7(3)
E1084	0(3)	E1510	0(3)	E2216	0(3)	E2389	0(3)	G0124	1(3)	G0389	1(2)	G6010	2(3)	J0289	50(3)
E1085	0(3)	E1520	0(3)	E2217	0(3)	E2390	0(3)	G0127	1(2)	G0396	1(2)	G6011	2(3)	J0300	8(3)
E1086	0(3)	E1530	0(3)	E2218	0(3)	E2391	0(3)	G0128	1(1)	G0397	1(2)	G6012	2(3)	J0348	200(3)
E1087	0(3)	E1540	0(3)	E2219	0(3)	E2392	0(3)	G0130	1(2)	G0398	1(2)	G6013	2(3)	J0350	0(3)
E1088	0(3)	E1550	0(3)	E2220	0(3)	E2394	0(3)	G0141	1(3)	G0399	1(2)	G6014	2(3)	J0360	2(3)
E1089	0(3)	E1560	0(3)	E2221	0(3)	E2395	0(3)	G0143	1(3)	G0400	1(2)	G6015	2(3)	J0364	6(3)
E1090	0(3)	E1570	0(3)	E2222	0(3)	E2396	0(3)	G0144	1(3)	G0402	1(2)	G6016	2(1)	J0400	39(3)
E1092	0(3)	E1575	0(3)	E2224	0(3)	E2397	0(3)	G0145	1(3)	G0403	1(2)	G6017	2(3)	J0401	400(3)
E1093	0(3)	E1580	0(3)	E2225	0(3)	E2402	0(3)	G0147	1(3)	G0404	1(2)	G6018	1(2)	J0456	4(3)
E1100	0(3)	E1590	0(3)	E2226	0(3)	E2500	0(3)	G0148	1(3)	G0405	1(2)	G6019	1(2)	J0475	8(3)
E1110	0(3)	E1592	0(3)	E2227	0(3)	E2502	0(3)	G0166	2(3)	G0406	1(2)	G6020	1(2)	J0476	2(3)
E1130	0(3)	E1594	0(3)	E2228	0(3)	E2504	0(3)	G0168	2(3)	G0407	1(2)	G6022	1(2)	J0480	1(3)
E1140	0(3)	E1600	0(3)	E2231	0(3)	E2506	0(3)	G0175	1(3)	G0408	1(2)	G6023	1(2)	J0485	1500(3)
E1150	0(3)	E1610	0(3)	E2291	1(2)	E2508	0(3)	G0177	0(3)	G0410	1(3)	G6024	1(2)	J0490	160(3)
E1160	0(3)	E1615	0(3)	E2292	1(2)	E2510	0(3)	G0179	1(2)	G0411	1(3)	G6025	1(2)	J0500	4(3)
E1161	0(3)	E1620	0(3)	E2293	1(2)	E2511	0(3)	G0180	1(2)	G0412	1(2)	G6027	1(3)	J0558	24(3)
E1170	0(3)	E1625	0(3)	E2294	1(2)	E2512	0(3)	G0181	1(2)	G0413	1(2)	G6028	1(2)	J0561	24(3)
E1171	0(3)	E1630	0(3)	E2295	0(3)	E2601	0(3)	G0182	1(2)	G0414	1(2)	G6030	2(3)	J0571	0(3)
E1172	0(3)	E1632	0(3)	E2300	0(3)	E2602	0(3)	G0186	1(2)	G0415	1(2)	G6031	2(3)	J0572	0(3)
E1180	0(3)	E1634	0(3)	E2301	0(3)	E2603	0(3)	G0202	1(2)	G0416	1(2)	G6032	2(3)	J0573	0(3)
E1190	0(3)	E1635	0(3)	E2310	0(3)	E2604	0(3)	G0204	2(3)	G0420	2(3)	G6034	2(3)	J0574	0(3)
E1195	0(3)	E1636	0(3)	E2311	0(3)	E2605	0(3)	G0206	2(3)	G0421	4(3)	G6035	2(1)	J0575	0(3)
E1200	0(3)	E1637	0(3)	E2312	0(3)	E2606	0(3)	G0235	1(3)	G0422	6(2)	G6036	2(3)	J0586	300(3)
E1220	0(3)	E1639	0(3)	E2313	0(3)	E2607	0(3)	G0237	8(3)	G0423	6(2)	G6037	2(3)	J0594	320(3)
E1221	0(3)	E1700	0(3)	E2321	0(3)	E2608	0(3)	G0238	8(3)	G0424	2(2)	G6039	2(1)	J0597	250(3)
E1222	0(3)	E1701	0(3)	E2322	0(3)	E2609	0(3)	G0239	1(3)	G0425	1(3)	G6040	2(3)	J0598	100(3)
E1223	0(3)	E1702	0(3)	E2323	0(3)	E2611	0(3)	G0245	1(2)	G0426	1(3)	G6041	1(1)	J0600	3(3)
E1224	0(3)	E1800	0(3)	E2324	0(3)	E2612	0(3)	G0246	1(2)	G0427	1(3)	G6042	2(3)	J0610	15(3)
E1225	0(3)	E1801	0(3)	E2325	0(3)	E2613	0(3)	G0247	1(2)	G0429	1(2)	G6043	2(3)	J0620	1(3)
E1226	0(3)	E1802	0(3)	E2326	0(3)	E2614	0(3)	G0248	1(2)	G0431	1(2)	G6044	2(3)	J0637	20(3)

CPT	MUE	CPT	MUE	CPT	MUE	CPT	MUE	CPT	MUE	CPT	MUE	CPT	MUE	CPT	MUE
J0638	150(3)	J1561	300(3)	J2597	45(3)	J7321	2(2)	J9171	240(3)	K0053	0(3)	K0854	0(3)	L0492	0(3)
J0640	24(3)	J1568	300(3)	J2675	1(3)	J7323	2(2)	J9179	50(3)	K0056	0(3)	K0855	0(3)	L0621	0(3)
J0690	12(3)	J1569	300(3)	J2680	4(3)	J7324	2(2)	J9190	20(3)	K0065	0(3)	K0856	0(3)	L0622	0(3)
J0692	12(3)	J1570	4(3)	J2690	4(3)	J7326	2(2)	J9202	3(3)	K0069	0(3)	K0857	0(3)	L0623	0(3)
J0694	8(3)	J1571	20(3)	J2720	5(3)	J7327	2(2)	J9206	42(3)	K0070	0(3)	K0858	0(3)	L0624	0(3)
J0696	16(3)	J1572	300(3)	J2724	4000(3)	J7336	1120(3)	J9211	6(3)	K0071	0(3)	K0859	0(3)	L0625	0(3)
J0697	4(3)	J1580	9(3)	J2730	2(3)	J7504	15(3)	J9213	12(3)	K0072	0(3)	K0860	0(3)	L0626	0(3)
J0698	10(3)	J1599	300(3)	J2760	2(3)	J7508	0(3)	J9216	2(3)	K0073	0(3)	K0861	0(3)	L0627	0(3)
J0706	1(3)	J1600	2(3)	J2770	6(3)	J7511	9(3)	J9217	6(3)	K0077	0(3)	K0862	0(3)	L0628	0(3)
J0712	120(3)	J1602	300(3)	J2778	10(3)	J7516	1(3)	J9219	1(3)	K0105	0(3)	K0863	0(3)	L0629	0(3)
J0713	12(3)	J1610	2(3)	J2780	16(3)	J7525	2(3)	J9225	1(3)	K0195	0(3)	K0864	0(3)	L0630	0(3)
J0717	400(3)	J1631	9(3)	J2783	60(3)	J7527	0(3)	J9228	450(3)	K0455	0(3)	K0868	0(3)	L0631	0(3)
J0720	15(3)	J1645	10(3)	J2785	4(3)	J7604	0(3)	J9230	5(3)	K0462	0(3)	K0869	0(3)	L0632	0(3)
J0735	50(3)	J1650	30(3)	J2788	1(3)	J7607	0(3)	J9261	80(3)	K0602	0(3)	K0870	0(3)	L0633	0(3)
J0740	2(3)	J1652	20(3)	J2791	50(3)	J7609	0(3)	J9262	700(3)	K0605	0(3)	K0871	0(3)	L0634	0(3)
J0743	16(3)	J1725	250(3)	J2793	320(3)	J7610	0(3)	J9266	2(3)	K0606	0(3)	K0877	0(3)	L0635	0(3)
J0744	6(3)	J1740	3(3)	J2794	100(3)	J7615	0(3)	J9267	750(3)	K0607	0(3)	K0878	0(3)	L0636	0(3)
J0745	2(3)	J1741	8(3)	J2795	200(3)	J7622	0(3)	J9268	1(3)	K0608	0(3)	K0879	0(3)	L0637	0(3)
J0760	4(3)	J1742	2(3)	J2796	150(3)	J7624	0(3)	J9280	12(3)	K0609	0(3)	K0880	0(3)	L0638	0(3)
J0770	5(3)	J1743	66(3)	J2800	3(3)	J7627	0(3)	J9293	8(3)	K0672	0(3)	K0884	0(3)	L0639	0(3)
J0775	180(3)	J1744	30(3)	J2805	3(3)	J7628	0(3)	J9300	0(3)	K0730	0(3)	K0885	0(3)	L0640	0(3)
J0780	4(3)	J1745	150(3)	J2941	8(3)	J7629	0(3)	J9301	100(3)	K0733	0(3)	K0886	0(3)	L0641	0(3)
J0800	3(3)	J1786	900(3)	J2993	2(3)	J7632	0(3)	J9303	100(3)	K0738	0(3)	K0890	0(3)	L0642	0(3)
J0833	3(3)	J1790	2(3)	J2995	0(3)	J7634	0(3)	J9305	150(3)	K0743	0(3)	K0891	0(3)	L0643	0(3)
J0834	3(3)	J1817	0(3)	J2997	8(3)	J7635	0(3)	J9306	840(3)	K0744	0(3)	K0898	1(2)	L0648	0(3)
J0840	6(3)	J1830	1(3)	J3000	2(3)	J7636	0(3)	J9307	80(3)	K0745	0(3)	K0900	0(3)	L0649	0(3)
J0886	40(3)	J1840	3(3)	J3010	100(3)	J7637	0(3)	J9310	12(3)	K0746	0(3)	K0901	0(3)	L0650	0(3)
J0890	0(2)	J1885	8(3)	J3030	1(3)	J7638	0(3)	J9315	40(3)	K0800	0(3)	K0902	0(3)	L0651	0(3)
J0895	12(3)	J1930	120(3)	J3060	900(3)	J7640	0(3)	J9320	4(3)	K0801	0(3)	L0112	0(3)	L0700	0(3)
J0897	120(3)	J1931	760(3)	J3095	150(3)	J7641	0(3)	J9354	600(3)	K0802	0(3)	L0113	0(3)	L0710	0(3)
J0945	4(3)	J1953	300(3)	J3101	50(3)	J7642	0(3)	J9355	100(3)	K0806	0(3)	L0120	0(3)	L0810	0(3)
J1000	1(3)	J1955	11(3)	J3121	400(3)	J7643	0(3)	J9360	45(3)	K0807	0(3)	L0130	0(3)	L0820	0(3)
J1050	1000(3)	J1956	4(3)	J3145	750(3)	J7645	0(3)	J9370	4(3)	K0808	0(3)	L0140	0(3)	L0830	0(3)
J1071	400(3)	J2001	60(3)	J3240	1(3)	J7647	0(3)	J9371	5(3)	K0812	0(3)	L0150	0(3)	L0859	0(3)
J1110	3(3)	J2020	6(3)	J3243	150(3)	J7650	0(3)	J9390	36(3)	K0813	0(3)	L0160	0(3)	L0861	0(3)
J1120	2(3)	J2150	8(3)	J3246	1(3)	J7657	0(3)	J9395	20(3)	K0814	0(3)	L0170	0(3)	L0970	0(3)
J1160	2(3)	J2175	4(3)	J3250	2(3)	J7660	0(3)	J9400	600(3)	K0815	0(3)	L0172	0(3)	L0972	0(3)
J1162	1(3)	J2185	30(3)	J3262	800(3)	J7665	127(2)	J9600	4(3)	K0816	0(3)	L0174	0(3)	L0974	0(3)
J1165	50(3)	J2212	240(3)	J3285	1(3)	J7667	0(3)	K0001	0(3)	K0820	0(3)	L0180	0(3)	L0976	0(3)
J1180	2(3)	J2248	150(3)	J3300	160(3)	J7670	0(3)	K0002	0(3)	K0821	0(3)	L0190	0(3)	L0978	0(3)
J1190	8(3)	J2265	400(3)	J3301	16(3)	J7676	0(3)	K0003	0(3)	K0822	0(3)	L0200	0(3)	L0980	0(3)
J1200	8(3)	J2280	4(3)	J3302	0(3)	J7680	0(3)	K0004	0(3)	K0823	0(3)	L0220	0(3)	L0982	0(3)
J1205	4(3)	J2300	4(3)	J3315	6(3)	J7681	0(3)	K0005	0(3)	K0824	0(3)	L0450	0(3)	L0984	0(3)
J1212	1(3)	J2310	4(3)	J3357	90(3)	J7683	0(3)	K0006	0(3)	K0825	0(3)	L0452	0(3)	L1000	0(3)
J1240	6(3)	J2315	380(3)	J3360	6(3)	J7684	0(3)	K0007	0(3)	K0826	0(3)	L0454	0(3)	L1001	0(3)
J1245	6(3)	J2320	4(3)	J3370	12(3)	J7685	0(3)	K0009	0(3)	K0827	0(3)	L0455	0(3)	L1005	0(3)
J1260	2(3)	J2323	300(3)	J3396	150(3)	J8510	0(3)	K0015	0(3)	K0828	0(3)	L0456	0(3)	L1010	0(3)
J1267	150(3)	J2354	60(3)	J3410	8(3)	J9010	3(3)	K0017	0(3)	K0829	0(3)	L0457	0(3)	L1020	0(3)
J1300	120(3)	J2355	2(3)	J3415	6(3)	J9019	60(3)	K0018	0(3)	K0830	0(3)	L0458	0(3)	L1025	0(3)
J1327	1(3)	J2358	405(3)	J3420	1(3)	J9025	300(3)	K0019	0(3)	K0831	0(3)	L0460	0(3)	L1030	0(3)
J1335	2(3)	J2360	2(3)	J3430	25(3)	J9031	1(3)	K0020	0(3)	K0835	0(3)	L0462	0(3)	L1040	0(3)
J1364	2(3)	J2405	64(3)	J3465	40(3)	J9033	300(3)	K0037	0(3)	K0836	0(3)	L0464	0(3)	L1050	0(3)
J1380	4(3)	J2426	234(3)	J3473	450(3)	J9040	4(3)	K0038	0(3)	K0837	0(3)	L0466	0(3)	L1060	0(3)
J1430	10(3)	J2430	3(3)	J3486	4(3)	J9042	200(3)	K0039	0(3)	K0838	0(3)	L0467	0(3)	L1070	0(3)
J1435	1(3)	J2469	10(3)	J3489	5(3)	J9043	60(3)	K0040	0(3)	K0839	0(3)	L0468	0(3)	L1080	0(3)
J1438	2(3)	J2503	2(3)	J7100	2(3)	J9045	22(3)	K0041	0(3)	K0840	0(3)	L0469	0(3)	L1085	0(3)
J1439	750(3)	J2504	15(3)	J7110	2(3)	J9047	120(3)	K0042	0(3)	K0841	0(3)	L0470	0(3)	L1090	0(3)
J1442	3360(3)	J2505	1(3)	J7131	500(3)	J9050	6(3)	K0043	0(3)	K0842	0(3)	L0472	0(3)	L1100	0(3)
J1446	192(3)	J2507	8(3)	J7196	175(3)	J9055	120(3)	K0044	0(3)	K0843	0(3)	L0480	0(3)	L1110	0(3)
J1450	4(3)	J2510	4(3)	J7301	0(3)	J9060	24(3)	K0045	0(3)	K0848	0(3)	L0482	0(3)	L1120	0(3)
J1451	1(3)	J2540	75(3)	J7310	2(2)	J9065	20(3)	K0046	0(3)	K0849	0(3)	L0484	0(3)	L1200	0(3)
J1453	150(3)	J2543	16(3)	J7311	1(3)	J9098	5(3)	K0047	0(3)	K0850	0(3)	L0486	0(3)	L1210	0(3)
J1457	500(3)	J2545	1(3)	J7312	14(3)	J9130	24(3)	K0050	0(3)	K0851	0(3)	L0488	0(3)	L1220	0(3)
J1556	300(3)	J2550	3(3)	J7315	2(3)	J9155	240(3)	K0051	0(3)	K0852	0(3)	L0490	0(3)	L1230	0(3)
J1557	300(3)	J2590	3(3)	J7316	4(2)	J9160	7(3)	K0052	0(3)	K0853	0(3)	L0491	0(3)	L1240	0(3)

CPT	MUE	CPT	MUE	CPT	MUE	CPT	MUE	CPT	MUE	CPT	MUE	CPT	MUE	CPT	MUE
L1250	0(3)	L2030	0(3)	L2525	0(3)	L3330	0(3)	L3908	0(3)	L5020	0(3)	L5646	0(3)	L5811	0(3)
L1260	0(3)	L2034	0(3)	L2526	0(3)	L3332	0(3)	L3912	0(3)	L5050	0(3)	L5647	0(3)	L5812	0(3)
L1270	0(3)	L2035	0(3)	L2530	0(3)	L3334	0(3)	L3913	0(3)	L5060	0(3)	L5648	0(3)	L5814	0(3)
L1280	0(3)	L2036	0(3)	L2540	0(3)	L3340	0(3)	L3915	0(3)	L5100	0(3)	L5649	0(3)	L5816	0(3)
L1290	0(3)	L2037	0(3)	L2550	0(3)	L3350	0(3)	L3916	0(3)	L5105	0(3)	L5650	0(3)	L5818	0(3)
L1300	0(3)	L2038	0(3)	L2570	0(3)	L3360	0(3)	L3917	0(3)	L5150	0(3)	L5651	0(3)	L5822	0(3)
L1310	0(3)	L2040	0(3)	L2580	0(3)	L3370	0(3)	L3918	0(3)	L5160	0(3)	L5652	0(3)	L5824	0(3)
L1499	1(3)	L2050	0(3)	L2600	0(3)	L3380	0(3)	L3919	0(3)	L5200	0(3)	L5653	0(3)	L5826	0(3)
L1600	0(3)	L2060	0(3)	L2610	0(3)	L3390	0(3)	L3921	0(3)	L5210	0(3)	L5654	0(3)	L5828	0(3)
L1610	0(3)	L2070	0(3)	L2620	0(3)	L3400	0(3)	L3923	0(3)	L5220	0(3)	L5655	0(3)	L5830	0(3)
L1620	0(3)	L2080	0(3)	L2622	0(3)	L3410	0(3)	L3924	0(3)	L5230	0(3)	L5656	0(3)	L5840	0(3)
L1630	0(3)	L2090	0(3)	L2624	0(3)	L3420	0(3)	L3925	0(3)	L5250	0(3)	L5658	0(3)	L5845	0(3)
L1640	0(3)	L2106	0(3)	L2627	0(3)	L3430	0(3)	L3927	0(3)	L5270	0(3)	L5661	0(3)	L5848	0(3)
L1650	0(3)	L2108	0(3)	L2628	0(3)	L3440	0(3)	L3929	0(3)	L5280	0(3)	L5665	0(3)	L5850	0(3)
L1652	0(3)	L2112	0(3)	L2630	0(3)	L3450	0(3)	L3930	0(3)	L5301	0(3)	L5666	0(3)	L5855	0(3)
L1660	0(3)	L2114	0(3)	L2640	0(3)	L3455	0(3)	L3931	0(3)	L5312	0(3)	L5668	0(3)	L5856	0(3)
L1680	0(3)	L2116	0(3)	L2650	0(3)	L3460	0(3)	L3933	0(3)	L5321	0(3)	L5670	0(3)	L5857	0(3)
L1685	0(3)	L2126	0(3)	L2660	0(3)	L3465	0(3)	L3935	0(3)	L5331	0(3)	L5671	0(3)	L5858	0(3)
L1686	0(3)	L2128	0(3)	L2670	0(3)	L3470	0(3)	L3956	0(3)	L5341	0(3)	L5672	0(3)	L5859	0(3)
L1690	0(3)	L2132	0(3)	L2680	0(3)	L3480	0(3)	L3960	0(3)	L5400	0(3)	L5673	0(3)	L5910	0(3)
L1700	0(3)	L2134	0(3)	L2750	0(3)	L3485	0(3)	L3961	0(3)	L5410	0(3)	L5676	0(3)	L5920	0(3)
L1710	0(3)	L2136	0(3)	L2755	0(3)	L3500	0(3)	L3962	0(3)	L5420	0(3)	L5677	0(3)	L5925	0(3)
L1720	0(3)	L2180	0(3)	L2760	0(3)	L3510	0(3)	L3967	0(3)	L5430	0(3)	L5678	0(3)	L5930	0(3)
L1730	0(3)	L2182	0(3)	L2768	0(3)	L3520	0(3)	L3971	0(3)	L5450	0(3)	L5679	0(3)	L5940	0(3)
L1755	0(3)	L2184	0(3)	L2780	0(3)	L3530	0(3)	L3973	0(3)	L5460	0(3)	L5680	0(3)	L5950	0(3)
L1810	0(3)	L2186	0(3)	L2785	0(3)	L3540	0(3)	L3975	0(3)	L5500	0(3)	L5681	0(3)	L5960	0(3)
L1812	0(3)	L2188	0(3)	L2795	0(3)	L3550	0(3)	L3976	0(3)	L5505	0(3)	L5682	0(3)	L5961	0(3)
L1820	0(3)	L2190	0(3)	L2800	0(3)	L3560	0(3)	L3977	0(3)	L5510	0(3)	L5683	0(3)	L5962	0(3)
L1830	0(3)	L2192	0(3)	L2810	0(3)	L3570	0(3)	L3978	0(3)	L5520	0(3)	L5684	0(3)	L5964	0(3)
L1831	0(3)	L2200	0(3)	L2820	0(3)	L3580	0(3)	L3980	0(3)	L5530	0(3)	L5685	0(3)	L5966	0(3)
L1832	0(3)	L2210	0(3)	L2830	0(3)	L3590	0(3)	L3981	0(3)	L5535	0(3)	L5686	0(3)	L5968	0(3)
L1833	0(3)	L2220	0(3)	L3000	0(3)	L3595	0(3)	L3982	0(3)	L5540	0(3)	L5688	0(3)	L5969	0(3)
L1834	0(3)	L2230	0(3)	L3001	0(3)	L3600	0(3)	L3984	0(3)	L5560	0(3)	L5690	0(3)	L5970	0(3)
L1836	0(3)	L2232	0(3)	L3002	0(3)	L3610	0(3)	L4000	0(3)	L5570	0(3)	L5692	0(3)	L5971	0(3)
L1840	0(3)	L2240	0(3)	L3003	0(3)	L3620	0(3)	L4002	0(3)	L5580	0(3)	L5694	0(3)	L5972	0(3)
L1843	0(3)	L2250	0(3)	L3010	0(3)	L3630	0(3)	L4010	0(3)	L5585	0(3)	L5695	0(3)	L5974	0(3)
L1844	0(3)	L2260	0(3)	L3020	0(3)	L3640	0(3)	L4020	0(3)	L5590	0(3)	L5696	0(3)	L5975	0(3)
L1845	0(3)	L2265	0(3)	L3030	0(3)	L3650	0(3)	L4030	0(3)	L5595	0(3)	L5697	0(3)	L5976	0(3)
L1846	0(3)	L2270	0(3)	L3031	0(3)	L3660	0(3)	L4040	0(3)	L5600	0(3)	L5698	0(3)	L5978	0(3)
L1847	0(3)	L2275	0(3)	L3040	0(3)	L3670	0(3)	L4045	0(3)	L5610	0(3)	L5699	0(3)	L5979	0(3)
L1848	0(3)	L2280	0(3)	L3050	0(3)	L3671	0(3)	L4050	0(3)	L5611	0(3)	L5700	0(3)	L5980	0(3)
L1850	0(3)	L2300	0(3)	L3060	0(3)	L3674	0(3)	L4055	0(3)	L5613	0(3)	L5701	0(3)	L5981	0(3)
L1860	0(3)	L2310	0(3)	L3070	0(3)	L3675	0(3)	L4060	0(3)	L5614	0(3)	L5702	0(3)	L5982	0(3)
L1900	0(3)	L2320	0(3)	L3080	0(3)	L3677	0(3)	L4070	0(3)	L5616	0(3)	L5703	0(3)	L5984	0(3)
L1902	0(3)	L2330	0(3)	L3090	0(3)	L3678	0(3)	L4080	0(3)	L5617	0(3)	L5704	0(3)	L5985	0(3)
L1904	0(3)	L2335	0(3)	L3100	0(3)	L3702	0(3)	L4090	0(3)	L5618	0(3)	L5705	0(3)	L5986	0(3)
L1906	0(3)	L2340	0(3)	L3140	0(3)	L3710	0(3)	L4100	0(3)	L5620	0(3)	L5706	0(3)	L5987	0(3)
L1907	0(3)	L2350	0(3)	L3150	0(3)	L3720	0(3)	L4110	0(3)	L5622	0(3)	L5707	0(3)	L5988	0(3)
L1910	0(3)	L2360	0(3)	L3160	0(3)	L3730	0(3)	L4130	0(3)	L5624	0(3)	L5710	0(3)	L5990	0(3)
L1920	0(3)	L2370	0(3)	L3170	0(3)	L3740	0(3)	L4205	0(3)	L5626	0(3)	L5711	0(3)	L6000	0(3)
L1930	0(3)	L2375	0(3)	L3215	0(3)	L3760	0(3)	L4210	0(3)	L5628	0(3)	L5712	0(3)	L6010	0(3)
L1932	0(3)	L2380	0(3)	L3216	0(3)	L3762	0(3)	L4350	0(3)	L5629	0(3)	L5714	0(3)	L6020	0(3)
L1940	0(3)	L2385	0(3)	L3217	0(3)	L3763	0(3)	L4360	0(3)	L5630	0(3)	L5716	0(3)	L6026	0(3)
L1945	0(3)	L2387	0(3)	L3219	0(3)	L3764	0(3)	L4361	0(3)	L5631	0(3)	L5718	0(3)	L6050	0(3)
L1950	0(3)	L2390	0(3)	L3221	0(3)	L3765	0(3)	L4370	0(3)	L5632	0(3)	L5722	0(3)	L6055	0(3)
L1951	0(3)	L2395	0(3)	L3222	0(3)	L3766	0(3)	L4386	0(3)	L5634	0(3)	L5724	0(3)	L6100	0(3)
L1960	0(3)	L2397	0(3)	L3224	0(3)	L3806	0(3)	L4387	0(3)	L5636	0(3)	L5726	0(3)	L6110	0(3)
L1970	0(3)	L2405	0(3)	L3225	0(3)	L3807	0(3)	L4392	0(3)	L5637	0(3)	L5728	0(3)	L6120	0(3)
L1971	0(3)	L2415	0(3)	L3230	0(3)	L3808	0(3)	L4394	0(3)	L5638	0(3)	L5780	0(3)	L6130	0(3)
L1980	0(3)	L2425	0(3)	L3250	0(3)	L3809	0(3)	L4396	0(3)	L5639	0(3)	L5781	0(3)	L6200	0(3)
L1990	0(3)	L2430	0(3)	L3251	0(3)	L3900	0(3)	L4397	0(3)	L5640	0(3)	L5782	0(3)	L6205	0(3)
L2000	0(3)	L2492	0(3)	L3252	0(3)	L3901	0(3)	L4398	0(3)	L5642	0(3)	L5785	0(3)	L6250	0(3)
L2005	0(3)	L2500	0(3)	L3253	0(3)	L3904	0(3)	L4631	0(3)	L5643	0(3)	L5790	0(3)	L6300	0(3)
L2010	0(3)	L2510	0(3)	L3300	0(3)	L3905	0(3)	L5000	0(3)	L5644	0(3)	L5795	0(3)	L6310	0(3)
L2020	0(3)	L2520	0(3)	L3310	0(3)	L3906	0(3)	L5010	0(3)	L5645	0(3)	L5810	0(3)	L6320	0(3)

CPT	MUE	CPT	MUE	CPT	MUE	CPT	MUE	CPT	MUE	CPT	MUE	CPT	MUE	CPT	MUE
L6350	0(3)	L6691	0(3)	L7362	0(3)	L8605	4(3)	Q0161	0(3)	Q4101	88(3)	V2110	0(3)	V2513	0(3)
L6360	0(3)	L6692	0(3)	L7364	0(3)	L8606	5(3)	Q0478	1(1)	Q4102	21(3)	V2111	0(3)	V2520	2(1)
L6370	0(3)	L6693	0(3)	L7366	0(3)	L8609	1(1)	Q0479	1(1)	Q4103	0(3)	V2112	0(3)	V2521	2(1)
L6380	0(3)	L6694	0(3)	L7367	0(3)	L8610	2(1)	Q0480	1(1)	Q4104	50(3)	V2113	0(3)	V2522	2(1)
L6382	0(3)	L6695	0(3)	L7368	0(3)	L8612	2(1)	Q0481	1(2)	Q4105	250(3)	V2114	0(3)	V2523	2(1)
L6384	0(3)	L6696	0(3)	L7400	0(3)	L8613	2(1)	Q0482	1(1)	Q4106	76(3)	V2115	0(3)	V2530	0(3)
L6386	0(3)	L6697	0(3)	L7401	0(3)	L8614	2(1)	Q0483	1(1)	Q4107	50(3)	V2118	0(3)	V2531	0(3)
L6388	0(3)	L6698	0(3)	L7402	0(3)	L8615	2(1)	Q0484	1(1)	Q4108	250(3)	V2121	0(3)	V2599	2(3)
L6400	0(3)	L6703	0(3)	L7403	0(3)	L8616	2(1)	Q0485	1(1)	Q4110	250(3)	V2199	2(3)	V2600	0(3)
L6450	0(3)	L6704	0(3)	L7404	0(3)	L8617	2(1)	Q0486	1(1)	Q4111	56(3)	V2200	0(3)	V2610	0(3)
L6500	0(3)	L6706	0(3)	L7405	0(3)	L8618	2(1)	Q0487	1(1)	Q4112	2(3)	V2201	0(3)	V2615	0(3)
L6550	0(3)	L6707	0(3)	L7510	4(3)	L8619	2(1)	Q0488	1(1)	Q4113	4(3)	V2202	0(3)	V2623	0(3)
L6570	0(3)	L6708	0(3)	L7900	0(3)	L8621	600(3)	Q0489	1(1)	Q4114	6(3)	V2203	0(3)	V2624	0(3)
L6580	0(3)	L6709	0(3)	L7902	0(3)	L8622	2(1)	Q0490	1(1)	Q4115	240(3)	V2204	0(3)	V2625	0(3)
L6582	0(3)	L6711	0(3)	L8000	0(3)	L8627	2(2)	Q0491	1(1)	Q4116	192(3)	V2205	0(3)	V2626	0(3)
L6584	0(3)	L6712	0(3)	L8001	0(3)	L8628	2(2)	Q0492	1(1)	Q4117	0(3)	V2206	0(3)	V2627	0(3)
L6586	0(3)	L6713	0(3)	L8002	0(3)	L8629	2(2)	Q0493	1(1)	Q4118	1000(3)	V2207	0(3)	V2628	0(3)
L6588	0(3)	L6714	0(3)	L8015	0(3)	L8631	4(1)	Q0494	1(1)	Q4119	150(3)	V2208	0(3)	V2629	0(3)
L6590	0(3)	L6715	0(3)	L8020	0(3)	L8641	4(1)	Q0495	1(1)	Q4120	50(3)	V2209	0(3)	V2630	2(1)
L6600	0(3)	L6721	0(3)	L8030	0(3)	L8642	2(1)	Q0497	2(1)	Q4121	78(3)	V2210	0(3)	V2631	2(1)
L6605	0(3)	L6722	0(3)	L8031	0(3)	L8658	4(1)	Q0498	1(1)	Q4122	96(3)	V2211	0(3)	V2632	2(1)
L6610	0(3)	L6805	0(3)	L8032	0(3)	L8659	4(1)	Q0499	1(1)	Q4123	160(3)	V2212	0(3)	V2700	0(3)
L6611	0(3)	L6810	0(3)	L8035	0(3)	L8670	4(1)	Q0501	1(1)	Q4124	140(3)	V2213	0(3)	V2702	0(3)
L6615	0(3)	L6880	0(3)	L8039	0(3)	L8679	3(3)	Q0502	1(1)	Q4125	28(3)	V2214	0(3)	V2710	0(3)
L6616	0(3)	L6881	0(3)	L8040	0(3)	L8681	1(1)	Q0503	3(1)	Q4126	32(3)	V2215	0(3)	V2715	0(3)
L6620	0(3)	L6882	0(3)	L8041	0(3)	L8682	2(1)	Q0504	1(1)	Q4127	100(3)	V2218	0(3)	V2718	0(3)
L6621	0(3)	L6883	0(3)	L8042	0(3)	L8683	1(1)	Q0506	8(3)	Q4128	128(3)	V2219	0(3)	V2730	0(3)
L6623	0(3)	L6884	0(3)	L8043	0(3)	L8684	1(1)	Q0507	1(3)	Q4129	81(3)	V2220	0(3)	V2744	0(3)
L6624	0(3)	L6885	0(3)	L8044	0(3)	L8685	1(1)	Q0508	1(3)	Q4130	100(3)	V2221	0(3)	V2745	0(3)
L6625	0(3)	L6890	0(3)	L8045	0(3)	L8686	2(1)	Q0509	1(3)	Q4131	60(3)	V2299	0(3)	V2750	0(3)
L6628	0(3)	L6895	0(3)	L8046	0(3)	L8687	1(1)	Q0510	0(3)	Q4132	50(3)	V2300	0(3)	V2755	0(3)
L6629	0(3)	L6900	0(3)	L8047	0(3)	L8688	1(1)	Q0511	0(3)	Q4133	113(3)	V2301	0(3)	V2756	0(3)
L6630	0(3)	L6905	0(3)	L8048	1(3)	L8689	1(1)	Q0512	0(3)	Q4134	160(3)	V2302	0(3)	V2760	0(3)
L6632	0(3)	L6910	0(3)	L8049	0(3)	L8690	2(2)	Q0513	0(3)	Q4135	900(3)	V2303	0(3)	V2761	0(3)
L6635	0(3)	L6915	0(3)	L8300	0(3)	L8691	1(3)	Q0514	0(3)	Q4136	900(3)	V2304	0(3)	V2762	0(3)
L6637	0(3)	L6920	0(3)	L8310	0(3)	L8692	0(3)	Q1004	2(1)	Q4139	2(3)	V2305	0(3)	V2770	0(3)
L6638	0(3)	L6925	0(3)	L8320	0(3)	L8693	1(3)	Q1005	2(1)	Q9953	10(3)	V2306	0(3)	V2780	0(3)
L6640	0(3)	L6930	0(3)	L8330	0(3)	L8695	1(1)	Q2004	1(3)	Q9955	10(2)	V2307	0(3)	V2781	0(3)
L6641	0(3)	L6935	0(3)	L8400	0(3)	L8696	1(3)	Q2026	45(3)	Q9956	9(3)	V2308	0(3)	V2782	0(3)
L6642	0(3)	L6940	0(3)	L8410	0(3)	P2028	1(1)	Q2028	1470(3)	Q9957	3(3)	V2309	0(3)	V2783	0(3)
L6645	0(3)	L6945	0(3)	L8415	0(3)	P2029	1(1)	Q2034	1(1)	Q9958	300(3)	V2310	0(3)	V2784	0(3)
L6646	0(3)	L6950	0(3)	L8417	0(3)	P2033	1(1)	Q2035	1(2)	Q9960	250(3)	V2311	0(3)	V2785	2(1)
L6647	0(3)	L6955	0(3)	L8420	0(3)	P2038	1(1)	Q2036	1(2)	Q9961	200(3)	V2312	0(3)	V2786	0(3)
L6648	0(3)	L6960	0(3)	L8430	0(3)	P3000	1(3)	Q2037	1(2)	Q9962	150(3)	V2313	0(3)	V2790	1(1)
L6650	0(3)	L6965	0(3)	L8435	0(3)	P3001	1(3)	Q2038	1(2)	Q9963	240(3)	V2314	0(3)	V2797	0(3)
L6655	0(3)	L6970	0(3)	L8440	0(3)	P9041	5(3)	Q2039	1(2)	Q9966	250(3)	V2315	0(3)	V5008	0(1)
L6660	0(3)	L6975	0(3)	L8460	0(3)	P9043	5(3)	Q2043	1(1)	Q9967	300(3)	V2318	0(3)	V5010	0(1)
L6665	0(3)	L7007	0(3)	L8465	0(3)	P9045	20(3)	Q2050	14(3)	R0070	2(3)	V2319	0(3)	V5011	0(1)
L6670	0(3)	L7008	0(3)	L8470	0(3)	P9046	25(3)	Q2052	1(3)	R0075	2(3)	V2320	0(3)	V5274	0(3)
L6672	0(3)	L7009	0(3)	L8480	0(3)	P9047	20(3)	Q3014	1(3)	V2020	0(3)	V2321	0(3)	V5281	0(1)
L6675	0(3)	L7040	0(3)	L8485	0(3)	P9048	1(3)	Q3027	30(3)	V2025	0(3)	V2399	0(3)	V5282	0(1)
L6676	0(3)	L7045	0(3)	L8500	0(3)	P9612	1(3)	Q3028	0(3)	V2100	0(3)	V2410	0(3)	V5284	0(1)
L6677	0(3)	L7170	0(3)	L8501	0(3)	P9615	1(3)	Q4001	1(1)	V2101	0(3)	V2430	0(3)	V5285	0(1)
L6680	0(3)	L7180	0(3)	L8507	0(3)	Q0035	1(1)	Q4002	1(1)	V2102	0(3)	V2499	2(3)	V5286	0(1)
L6682	0(3)	L7181	0(3)	L8509	1(1)	Q0091	1(1)	Q4003	2(1)	V2103	0(3)	V2500	0(3)	V5287	0(1)
L6684	0(3)	L7185	0(3)	L8510	0(3)	Q0111	2(1)	Q4004	2(1)	V2104	0(3)	V2501	0(3)	V5288	0(1)
L6686	0(3)	L7186	0(3)	L8511	1(1)	Q0112	3(1)	Q4025	1(1)	V2105	0(3)	V2502	0(3)	V5289	0(1)
L6687	0(3)	L7190	0(3)	L8514	1(1)	Q0113	2(1)	Q4026	1(1)	V2106	0(3)	V2503	0(3)		
L6688	0(3)	L7191	0(3)	L8515	1(1)	Q0114	1(1)	Q4027	1(1)	V2107	0(3)	V2510	0(3)		
L6689	0(3)	L7259	0(3)	L8600	2(1)	Q0115	1(1)	Q4028	1(1)	V2108	0(3)	V2511	0(3)		
L6690	0(3)	L7360	0(3)	L8604	3(3)	Q0144	0(3)	Q4074	3(3)	V2109	0(3)	V2512	0(3)		

OPPS

CPT	MUE	CPT	MUE	CPT	MUE	CPT	MUE	CPT	MUE	CPT	MUE	CPT	MUE	CPT	MUE
0019T	1(1)	0222T	1(1)	0310T	1(1)	0008M	1(3)	11451	1(2)	12015	1(2)	15131	2(3)	15826	1(2)
0042T	1(1)	0223T	1(1)	0311T	1(1)	10021	4(3)	11462	1(2)	12016	1(2)	15135	1(2)	15828	1(2)
0051T	1(2)	0224T	1(1)	0312T	1(1)	10022	4(3)	11463	1(2)	12017	1(2)	15136	1(3)	15829	1(2)
0052T	1(2)	0225T	1(1)	0313T	1(1)	10030	2(3)	11470	3(2)	12018	1(2)	15150	1(2)	15830	1(2)
0053T	1(2)	0228T	1(2)	0314T	1(1)	10040	1(2)	11471	2(3)	12020	2(3)	15151	1(2)	15832	1(2)
0054T	2(1)	0230T	1(2)	0315T	1(1)	10060	1(2)	11600	2(3)	12021	3(3)	15152	2(3)	15833	1(2)
0055T	2(1)	0232T	1(1)	0316T	1(1)	10061	1(2)	11601	2(3)	12031	1(2)	15155	1(2)	15834	1(2)
0058T	1(1)	0233T	1(1)	0317T	1(1)	10080	1(3)	11602	3(3)	12032	1(2)	15156	1(2)	15835	1(3)
0071T	1(2)	0234T	2(2)	0329T	1(2)	10081	1(3)	11603	2(3)	12034	1(2)	15157	1(3)	15836	1(2)
0072T	1(2)	0235T	2(1)	0330T	1(2)	10120	3(3)	11604	2(3)	12035	1(2)	15200	1(2)	15837	2(3)
0075T	1(2)	0236T	1(2)	0331T	1(3)	10121	2(3)	11606	2(3)	12036	1(2)	15201	9(3)	15838	1(2)
0076T	2(1)	0237T	2(1)	0332T	1(3)	10140	2(3)	11620	2(3)	12037	1(2)	15220	1(2)	15839	2(3)
0095T	1(1)	0240T	1(1)	0333T	1(2)	10160	3(3)	11621	2(3)	12041	1(2)	15221	9(3)	15840	1(3)
0098T	1(1)	0241T	1(1)	0335T	2(2)	10180	2(3)	11622	2(3)	12042	1(2)	15240	1(2)	15841	2(3)
0099T	2(2)	0243T	1(2)	0336T	1(3)	11000	1(2)	11623	2(3)	12044	1(2)	15241	9(3)	15842	2(3)
0100T	2(2)	0244T	1(2)	0337T	1(3)	11001	1(3)	11624	2(3)	12045	1(2)	15260	1(2)	15845	2(3)
0101T	1(1)	0249T	1(2)	0338T	1(2)	11004	1(2)	11626	2(3)	12046	1(2)	15261	6(3)	15847	1(2)
0102T	2(2)	0253T	1(1)	0339T	1(2)	11005	1(2)	11640	2(3)	12047	1(2)	15271	1(2)	15850	1(2)
0103T	1(1)	0254T	2(2)	0347T	1(3)	11006	1(2)	11641	2(3)	12051	1(2)	15272	3(3)	15851	1(2)
0106T	4(2)	0255T	2(2)	0348T	1(3)	11008	1(2)	11642	3(3)	12052	1(2)	15273	1(2)	15852	1(3)
0107T	4(2)	0262T	1(1)	0349T	1(3)	11010	2(3)	11643	2(3)	12053	1(2)	15275	1(2)	15860	1(3)
0108T	4(2)	0263T	1(1)	0350T	1(3)	11011	2(3)	11644	2(3)	12054	1(2)	15276	3(2)	15876	1(2)
0109T	4(2)	0264T	1(1)	0351T	5(3)	11012	2(3)	11646	2(3)	12055	1(2)	15277	1(2)	15877	1(2)
0110T	4(2)	0265T	1(1)	0352T	5(3)	11042	1(2)	11719	1(2)	12056	1(2)	15570	2(3)	15878	1(2)
0111T	1(1)	0266T	1(1)	0353T	2(3)	11043	1(2)	11720	1(2)	12057	1(2)	15572	2(3)	15879	1(2)
0123T	2(2)	0267T	1(1)	0354T	2(3)	11044	1(2)	11721	1(2)	13100	1(2)	15574	2(3)	15920	1(3)
0159T	2(2)	0268T	1(1)	0355T	1(2)	11055	1(2)	11730	1(2)	13101	1(2)	15576	2(3)	15922	1(3)
0163T	2(1)	0269T	1(1)	0356T	4(2)	11056	1(2)	11732	9(3)	13102	9(3)	15600	2(3)	15931	1(3)
0164T	4(2)	0270T	1(1)	0357T	1(2)	11057	1(2)	11740	3(3)	13120	1(2)	15610	2(3)	15933	1(3)
0165T	4(2)	0271T	1(1)	0358T	1(2)	11100	1(2)	11750	6(3)	13121	1(2)	15620	2(3)	15934	1(3)
0169T	1(1)	0272T	1(1)	0359T	1(2)	11101	6(3)	11752	3(3)	13122	9(3)	15630	2(3)	15935	1(3)
0171T	1(2)	0273T	1(1)	0360T	1(2)	11200	1(2)	11755	4(3)	13131	1(2)	15650	1(3)	15936	1(3)
0172T	3(1)	0274T	1(2)	0361T	3(3)	11201	0(3)	11760	4(3)	13132	1(2)	15731	1(3)	15937	1(3)
0174T	1(1)	0275T	1(2)	0362T	1(2)	11300	5(3)	11762	2(3)	13133	7(3)	15732	3(3)	15940	2(3)
0175T	1(2)	0278T	1(1)	0363T	3(3)	11301	6(3)	11765	4(3)	13151	1(2)	15734	4(3)	15941	2(3)
0178T	1(1)	0281T	1(2)	0364T	1(2)	11302	4(3)	11770	1(3)	13152	1(2)	15736	2(3)	15944	2(3)
0179T	1(1)	0282T	1(3)	0366T	1(2)	11303	3(3)	11771	1(3)	13153	2(3)	15738	4(3)	15945	2(3)
0180T	1(1)	0283T	1(3)	0368T	1(2)	11305	4(3)	11772	1(3)	13160	2(3)	15740	3(3)	15946	2(3)
0182T	3(1)	0284T	1(1)	0370T	1(3)	11306	4(3)	11900	1(2)	14000	2(3)	15750	2(3)	15950	2(3)
0190T	2(2)	0285T	1(1)	0371T	1(3)	11307	3(3)	11901	1(2)	14001	2(3)	15756	2(3)	15951	2(3)
0191T	2(2)	0286T	1(2)	0372T	1(3)	11308	4(3)	11920	1(2)	14020	4(3)	15757	2(3)	15952	2(3)
0195T	1(2)	0287T	2(1)	0373T	1(2)	11310	4(3)	11921	1(2)	14021	3(3)	15758	2(3)	15953	2(3)
0196T	1(2)	0288T	1(2)	0375T	1(2)	11311	4(3)	11922	1(3)	14040	4(3)	15760	2(3)	15956	2(3)
0198T	2(2)	0289T	2(2)	0376T	2(3)	11312	3(3)	11950	1(2)	14041	3(3)	15770	2(3)	15958	2(3)
0200T	1(2)	0290T	1(1)	0377T	1(2)	11313	3(3)	11951	1(2)	14060	4(3)	15775	1(2)	16000	1(2)
0201T	1(2)	0291T	1(2)	0378T	1(2)	11400	3(3)	11952	1(2)	14061	2(3)	15776	1(2)	16020	1(3)
0202T	1(3)	0292T	1(1)	0379T	1(2)	11401	3(3)	11954	1(3)	14301	2(3)	15777	1(3)	16025	1(3)
0206T	1(1)	0293T	1(2)	0380T	1(2)	11402	3(3)	11960	2(3)	14302	8(3)	15780	1(2)	16030	1(3)
0207T	2(2)	0294T	1(1)	0381T	1(2)	11403	2(3)	11970	2(3)	14350	2(3)	15781	1(3)	16035	1(2)
0208T	1(1)	0295T	1(2)	0382T	1(2)	11404	2(3)	11971	2(3)	15002	1(2)	15782	1(3)	16036	2(3)
0209T	1(1)	0296T	1(2)	0383T	1(2)	11406	2(3)	11976	1(2)	15003	9(3)	15783	1(3)	17000	1(2)
0210T	1(1)	0297T	1(2)	0384T	1(2)	11420	3(3)	11980	1(2)	15004	1(2)	15786	1(2)	17003	13(2)
0211T	1(1)	0298T	1(2)	0385T	1(2)	11421	3(3)	11981	1(3)	15005	2(3)	15787	2(3)	17004	1(2)
0212T	1(1)	0299T	1(2)	0386T	1(2)	11422	3(3)	11982	1(3)	15040	1(2)	15788	1(2)	17106	1(2)
0213T	1(2)	0300T	1(1)	0387T	1(3)	11423	2(3)	11983	1(3)	15050	1(3)	15789	1(2)	17107	1(2)
0214T	1(2)	0301T	1(1)	0388T	1(3)	11424	2(3)	12001	1(2)	15100	1(2)	15792	1(3)	17108	1(2)
0215T	1(2)	0302T	1(1)	0389T	1(3)	11426	2(3)	12002	1(2)	15101	9(3)	15793	1(3)	17110	1(2)
0216T	1(2)	0303T	1(1)	0390T	1(3)	11440	4(3)	12004	1(2)	15110	1(2)	15819	1(2)	17111	1(2)
0217T	1(2)	0304T	1(1)	0391T	1(3)	11441	3(3)	12005	1(2)	15111	2(3)	15820	1(2)	17250	4(3)
0218T	1(2)	0305T	1(1)	0001M	1(1)	11442	3(3)	12006	1(2)	15115	1(2)	15821	1(2)	17260	7(3)
0219T	1(2)	0306T	1(1)	0002M	1(1)	11443	2(3)	12007	1(2)	15116	2(3)	15822	1(2)	17261	7(3)
0220T	1(2)	0307T	1(1)	0003M	1(1)	11444	2(3)	12011	1(2)	15120	1(2)	15823	1(2)	17262	6(3)
0221T	1(2)	0308T	1(1)	0006M	1(2)	11446	2(3)	12013	1(2)	15121	5(3)	15824	1(2)	17263	5(3)
		0309T	1(1)	0007M	1(2)	11450	1(2)	12014	1(2)	15130	1(2)	15825	1(2)	17264	3(3)

CPT	MUE	CPT	MUE	CPT	MUE	CPT	MUE	CPT	MUE	CPT	MUE	CPT	MUE	CPT	MUE
17266	2(3)	19328	1(2)	20697	4(3)	21082	1(2)	21263	1(2)	21501	3(3)	22318	1(2)	22902	4(3)
17270	6(3)	19330	1(2)	20802	1(2)	21083	1(2)	21267	1(2)	21502	1(3)	22319	1(2)	22903	3(3)
17271	4(3)	19340	1(2)	20805	1(2)	21084	1(2)	21268	1(2)	21510	1(3)	22325	1(2)	22904	1(3)
17272	5(3)	19342	1(2)	20808	1(2)	21085	1(3)	21270	1(2)	21550	3(3)	22326	1(2)	22905	1(3)
17273	4(3)	19350	1(2)	20816	3(3)	21086	1(2)	21275	1(2)	21552	4(3)	22327	1(2)	23000	1(2)
17274	4(3)	19355	1(2)	20822	3(3)	21087	1(2)	21280	1(2)	21554	2(3)	22328	6(3)	23020	1(2)
17276	3(3)	19357	1(2)	20824	1(2)	21088	1(2)	21282	1(2)	21555	4(3)	22505	1(2)	23030	2(3)
17280	6(3)	19361	1(2)	20827	1(2)	21100	1(2)	21295	1(2)	21556	3(3)	22510	1(2)	23031	1(3)
17281	6(3)	19364	1(2)	20838	1(2)	21110	2(3)	21296	1(2)	21557	1(3)	22511	1(2)	23035	1(3)
17282	5(3)	19366	1(2)	20900	2(3)	21116	1(2)	21310	1(2)	21558	1(3)	22512	5(3)	23040	1(2)
17283	4(3)	19367	1(2)	20902	2(3)	21120	1(2)	21315	1(2)	21600	5(3)	22513	1(2)	23044	1(3)
17284	3(3)	19368	1(2)	20910	1(3)	21121	1(2)	21320	1(2)	21610	1(3)	22514	1(2)	23065	2(3)
17286	3(3)	19369	1(2)	20912	1(3)	21122	1(2)	21325	1(2)	21615	1(2)	22515	5(3)	23066	2(3)
17311	4(3)	19370	1(2)	20920	1(3)	21123	1(2)	21330	1(2)	21616	1(2)	22532	1(2)	23071	2(3)
17312	6(3)	19371	1(2)	20922	1(3)	21125	2(2)	21335	1(2)	21620	1(2)	22533	1(2)	23073	2(3)
17313	3(3)	19380	1(2)	20924	2(3)	21127	2(3)	21336	1(2)	21627	1(2)	22534	3(3)	23075	3(3)
17314	4(3)	19396	1(2)	20926	2(3)	21137	1(2)	21337	1(2)	21630	1(2)	22548	1(2)	23076	2(3)
17315	15(3)	20005	4(3)	20931	1(2)	21138	1(2)	21338	1(2)	21632	1(2)	22551	1(2)	23077	1(3)
17340	1(2)	20100	2(3)	20937	1(2)	21139	1(2)	21339	1(2)	21685	1(2)	22552	5(3)	23078	1(3)
17360	1(2)	20101	2(3)	20938	1(2)	21141	1(2)	21340	1(2)	21700	1(2)	22554	1(2)	23100	1(2)
17380	1(3)	20102	3(3)	20950	2(3)	21142	1(2)	21343	1(2)	21705	1(2)	22556	1(2)	23101	2(2)
19000	2(3)	20103	4(3)	20955	1(3)	21143	1(2)	21344	1(2)	21720	1(3)	22558	1(2)	23105	1(2)
19001	5(3)	20150	2(3)	20956	1(3)	21145	1(2)	21345	1(2)	21725	1(3)	22585	7(3)	23106	1(2)
19020	2(3)	20200	2(3)	20957	1(3)	21146	1(2)	21346	1(2)	21740	1(2)	22586	1(2)	23107	1(2)
19030	1(2)	20205	4(3)	20962	1(3)	21147	1(2)	21347	1(2)	21742	1(2)	22590	1(2)	23120	1(2)
19081	1(2)	20206	3(3)	20969	2(3)	21150	1(2)	21348	1(2)	21743	1(2)	22595	1(2)	23125	1(2)
19082	2(3)	20220	4(3)	20970	1(3)	21151	1(2)	21355	1(2)	21750	1(2)	22600	1(2)	23130	1(2)
19083	1(2)	20225	4(3)	20972	2(3)	21154	1(2)	21356	1(2)	21805	3(3)	22610	1(2)	23140	1(3)
19084	2(3)	20240	4(3)	20973	1(2)	21155	1(2)	21360	1(2)	21811	1(2)	22612	1(2)	23145	1(3)
19085	1(2)	20245	4(3)	20974	1(3)	21159	1(2)	21365	1(2)	21812	1(2)	22614	13(3)	23146	1(3)
19086	2(3)	20250	3(3)	20975	1(3)	21160	1(2)	21366	1(2)	21813	1(2)	22630	1(2)	23150	1(3)
19100	4(3)	20251	3(3)	20979	1(3)	21175	1(2)	21385	1(2)	21820	1(2)	22632	4(2)	23155	1(3)
19101	3(3)	20500	2(3)	20982	1(2)	21179	1(2)	21386	1(2)	21825	1(2)	22633	1(2)	23156	1(3)
19105	2(3)	20501	2(3)	20983	1(2)	21180	1(2)	21387	1(2)	21920	3(3)	22634	4(2)	23170	1(3)
19110	1(3)	20520	4(3)	20985	2(3)	21181	1(3)	21390	1(2)	21925	3(3)	22800	1(2)	23172	1(3)
19112	2(3)	20525	4(3)	21010	1(2)	21182	1(2)	21395	1(2)	21930	5(3)	22802	1(2)	23174	1(3)
19120	1(2)	20526	1(2)	21011	4(3)	21183	1(2)	21400	1(2)	21931	3(3)	22804	1(2)	23180	1(3)
19125	1(2)	20527	2(3)	21012	3(3)	21184	1(2)	21401	1(2)	21932	4(3)	22808	1(2)	23182	1(3)
19126	3(3)	20550	5(3)	21013	4(3)	21188	1(2)	21406	1(2)	21933	3(3)	22810	1(2)	23184	1(3)
19260	2(3)	20551	5(3)	21014	3(3)	21193	1(2)	21407	1(2)	21935	1(3)	22812	1(2)	23190	1(3)
19271	1(3)	20552	1(2)	21015	1(3)	21194	1(2)	21408	1(2)	21936	1(3)	22818	1(2)	23195	1(2)
19272	1(3)	20553	1(2)	21016	2(3)	21195	1(2)	21421	1(2)	22010	2(3)	22819	1(2)	23200	1(3)
19281	1(2)	20555	1(3)	21025	2(3)	21196	1(2)	21422	1(2)	22015	2(3)	22830	1(2)	23210	1(3)
19282	2(3)	20600	6(3)	21026	2(3)	21198	1(3)	21423	1(2)	22100	1(2)	22840	1(2)	23220	1(3)
19283	1(2)	20604	4(3)	21029	1(3)	21199	1(2)	21431	1(2)	22101	1(2)	22842	1(2)	23330	2(3)
19284	2(3)	20605	4(3)	21030	1(3)	21206	1(3)	21432	1(2)	22102	1(2)	22843	1(2)	23333	1(3)
19285	1(2)	20606	4(3)	21031	2(3)	21208	1(3)	21433	1(2)	22103	3(3)	22844	1(2)	23334	1(2)
19286	2(3)	20610	4(3)	21032	1(3)	21209	1(3)	21435	1(2)	22110	1(2)	22845	1(2)	23335	1(2)
19287	1(2)	20611	4(3)	21034	1(3)	21210	2(3)	21436	1(2)	22112	1(2)	22846	1(2)	23350	1(2)
19288	2(3)	20612	2(3)	21040	2(3)	21215	2(3)	21440	2(2)	22114	1(2)	22847	1(2)	23395	1(2)
19296	1(3)	20615	1(3)	21044	1(3)	21230	2(3)	21445	2(2)	22116	3(3)	22848	1(2)	23397	1(3)
19297	2(3)	20650	4(3)	21045	1(3)	21235	2(3)	21450	1(2)	22206	1(2)	22849	1(2)	23400	1(2)
19298	1(2)	20660	1(2)	21046	2(3)	21240	1(2)	21451	1(2)	22207	1(2)	22850	1(2)	23405	2(3)
19300	1(2)	20661	1(2)	21047	2(3)	21242	1(2)	21452	1(2)	22208	6(3)	22851	5(3)	23406	1(3)
19301	1(2)	20662	1(2)	21048	2(3)	21243	1(2)	21453	1(2)	22210	1(2)	22852	1(2)	23410	1(2)
19302	1(2)	20663	1(2)	21049	1(3)	21244	1(2)	21454	1(2)	22212	1(2)	22855	1(2)	23412	1(2)
19303	1(2)	20664	1(2)	21050	1(2)	21245	2(2)	21461	1(2)	22214	1(2)	22856	1(2)	23415	1(2)
19304	1(2)	20665	1(2)	21060	1(2)	21246	2(2)	21462	1(2)	22216	6(3)	22857	1(2)	23420	1(2)
19305	1(2)	20670	3(3)	21070	1(2)	21247	1(2)	21465	1(2)	22220	1(2)	22858	1(2)	23430	1(2)
19306	1(2)	20680	3(3)	21073	1(2)	21248	2(3)	21470	1(2)	22222	1(2)	22861	1(2)	23440	1(2)
19307	1(2)	20690	2(3)	21076	1(2)	21249	2(3)	21480	1(2)	22224	1(2)	22862	1(2)	23450	1(2)
19316	1(2)	20692	3(3)	21077	1(2)	21255	1(2)	21485	1(2)	22226	4(3)	22864	1(2)	23455	1(2)
19318	1(2)	20693	2(3)	21079	1(2)	21256	1(2)	21490	1(2)	22305	1(2)	22865	1(2)	23460	1(2)
19324	1(2)	20694	2(3)	21080	1(2)	21260	1(2)	21495	1(2)	22310	1(2)	22900	3(3)	23462	1(2)
19325	1(2)	20696	2(3)	21081	1(2)	21261	1(2)	21497	1(2)	22315	1(2)	22901	2(3)	23465	1(2)

CPT	MUE	CPT	MUE	CPT	MUE	CPT	MUE	CPT	MUE	CPT	MUE	CPT	MUE	CPT	MUE
23466	1(2)	24126	1(3)	24577	1(3)	25150	1(3)	25500	1(2)	26060	5(3)	26460	4(3)	26675	1(3)
23470	1(2)	24130	1(2)	24579	1(3)	25151	1(3)	25505	1(2)	26070	2(3)	26471	4(3)	26676	3(3)
23472	1(2)	24134	1(3)	24582	1(3)	25170	1(3)	25515	1(2)	26075	4(3)	26474	4(3)	26685	3(3)
23473	1(2)	24136	1(3)	24586	1(3)	25210	2(1)	25520	1(2)	26080	4(3)	26476	4(3)	26686	3(3)
23474	1(2)	24138	1(3)	24587	1(2)	25215	1(2)	25525	1(2)	26100	1(3)	26477	4(3)	26700	3(3)
23480	1(2)	24140	1(3)	24600	1(2)	25230	1(2)	25526	1(2)	26105	2(3)	26478	6(3)	26705	3(3)
23485	1(2)	24145	1(3)	24605	1(2)	25240	1(2)	25530	1(2)	26110	3(3)	26479	4(3)	26706	4(3)
23490	1(2)	24147	1(2)	24615	1(2)	25246	1(2)	25535	1(2)	26111	4(3)	26480	4(3)	26715	4(3)
23491	1(2)	24149	1(2)	24620	1(2)	25248	3(3)	25545	1(2)	26113	4(3)	26483	4(3)	26720	4(3)
23500	1(2)	24150	1(3)	24635	1(2)	25250	1(2)	25560	1(2)	26115	4(3)	26485	4(3)	26725	4(3)
23505	1(2)	24152	1(3)	24640	1(2)	25251	1(2)	25565	1(2)	26116	2(3)	26489	3(3)	26727	4(3)
23515	1(2)	24155	1(2)	24650	1(2)	25259	1(2)	25574	1(2)	26117	2(3)	26490	3(3)	26735	4(3)
23520	1(2)	24160	1(2)	24655	1(2)	25260	7(3)	25575	1(2)	26118	1(3)	26492	2(3)	26740	3(3)
23525	1(2)	24164	1(2)	24665	1(2)	25263	4(3)	25600	1(2)	26121	1(2)	26494	1(3)	26742	3(3)
23530	1(2)	24200	3(3)	24666	1(2)	25265	4(3)	25605	1(2)	26123	1(2)	26496	1(3)	26746	3(3)
23532	1(2)	24201	3(3)	24670	1(2)	25270	8(3)	25606	1(2)	26125	4(3)	26497	2(3)	26750	3(3)
23540	1(2)	24220	1(2)	24675	1(2)	25272	4(3)	25607	1(2)	26130	1(3)	26498	1(3)	26755	3(3)
23545	1(2)	24300	1(2)	24685	1(2)	25274	4(3)	25608	1(2)	26135	4(3)	26499	2(3)	26756	3(3)
23550	1(2)	24301	2(3)	24800	1(2)	25275	2(3)	25609	1(2)	26140	3(3)	26500	4(3)	26765	5(3)
23552	1(2)	24305	4(3)	24802	1(2)	25280	9(3)	25622	1(2)	26145	6(3)	26502	3(3)	26770	3(3)
23570	1(2)	24310	3(3)	24900	1(2)	25290	12(3)	25624	1(2)	26160	5(3)	26508	1(2)	26775	4(3)
23575	1(2)	24320	2(3)	24920	1(2)	25295	9(3)	25628	1(2)	26170	5(3)	26510	4(3)	26776	4(3)
23585	1(2)	24330	1(3)	24925	1(2)	25300	1(2)	25630	1(3)	26180	4(3)	26516	1(2)	26785	3(3)
23600	1(2)	24331	1(3)	24930	1(2)	25301	1(2)	25635	1(3)	26185	1(3)	26517	1(2)	26820	1(2)
23605	1(2)	24332	1(2)	24931	1(2)	25310	5(3)	25645	1(3)	26200	2(3)	26518	1(2)	26841	1(2)
23615	1(2)	24340	1(2)	24935	1(2)	25312	5(3)	25650	1(2)	26205	1(3)	26520	4(3)	26842	1(2)
23616	1(2)	24341	2(3)	24940	1(2)	25315	1(3)	25651	1(2)	26210	2(3)	26525	4(3)	26843	2(3)
23620	1(2)	24342	2(3)	25000	2(3)	25316	1(3)	25652	1(2)	26215	2(3)	26530	4(3)	26844	2(3)
23625	1(2)	24343	1(2)	25001	1(3)	25320	1(2)	25660	1(2)	26230	2(3)	26531	4(3)	26850	5(3)
23630	1(2)	24344	1(2)	25020	1(2)	25332	1(2)	25670	1(2)	26235	2(3)	26535	4(3)	26852	2(3)
23650	1(2)	24345	1(2)	25023	1(2)	25335	1(2)	25671	1(2)	26236	2(3)	26536	4(3)	26860	1(2)
23655	1(2)	24346	1(2)	25024	1(2)	25337	1(2)	25675	1(2)	26250	2(3)	26540	4(3)	26861	4(3)
23660	1(2)	24357	2(3)	25025	1(2)	25350	1(3)	25676	1(2)	26260	1(3)	26541	4(3)	26862	1(2)
23665	1(2)	24358	2(3)	25028	4(3)	25355	1(3)	25680	1(2)	26262	1(3)	26542	4(3)	26863	3(3)
23670	1(2)	24359	2(3)	25031	2(3)	25360	1(3)	25685	1(2)	26320	4(3)	26545	4(3)	26910	4(3)
23675	1(2)	24360	1(2)	25035	2(3)	25365	1(3)	25690	1(2)	26340	4(3)	26546	2(3)	26951	8(3)
23680	1(2)	24361	1(2)	25040	1(3)	25370	1(2)	25695	1(2)	26341	2(3)	26548	3(3)	26952	5(3)
23700	1(2)	24362	1(2)	25065	3(3)	25375	1(2)	25800	1(2)	26350	6(3)	26550	1(2)	26990	2(3)
23800	1(2)	24363	1(2)	25066	2(3)	25390	1(2)	25805	1(2)	26352	2(3)	26551	1(2)	26991	2(3)
23802	1(2)	24365	1(2)	25071	3(3)	25391	1(2)	25810	1(2)	26356	4(3)	26553	1(3)	26992	2(3)
23900	1(2)	24366	1(2)	25073	1(3)	25392	1(2)	25820	1(2)	26357	2(3)	26554	1(3)	27000	1(3)
23920	1(2)	24370	1(2)	25075	6(3)	25393	1(2)	25825	1(2)	26358	2(3)	26555	2(3)	27001	1(3)
23921	1(2)	24371	1(2)	25076	5(3)	25394	1(3)	25830	1(2)	26370	3(3)	26556	2(3)	27003	1(2)
23930	2(3)	24400	1(3)	25077	1(3)	25400	1(2)	25900	1(2)	26372	1(3)	26560	2(3)	27005	1(2)
23931	2(3)	24410	1(2)	25078	1(3)	25405	1(2)	25905	1(2)	26373	2(3)	26561	2(3)	27006	1(2)
23935	2(3)	24420	1(2)	25085	1(2)	25415	1(2)	25907	1(2)	26390	2(3)	26562	2(3)	27025	1(3)
24000	1(2)	24430	1(3)	25100	1(2)	25420	1(2)	25909	1(2)	26392	2(3)	26565	3(3)	27027	1(2)
24006	1(2)	24435	1(3)	25101	1(2)	25425	1(2)	25915	1(2)	26410	4(3)	26567	3(3)	27030	1(2)
24065	2(3)	24470	1(2)	25105	1(2)	25426	1(2)	25920	1(2)	26412	3(3)	26568	2(3)	27033	1(2)
24066	2(3)	24495	1(2)	25107	1(2)	25430	1(3)	25922	1(2)	26415	2(3)	26580	1(2)	27035	1(2)
24071	3(3)	24498	1(2)	25109	4(3)	25431	1(3)	25924	1(2)	26416	2(3)	26587	2(3)	27036	1(2)
24073	3(3)	24500	1(2)	25110	3(3)	25440	1(2)	25927	1(2)	26418	4(3)	26590	2(3)	27040	2(3)
24075	5(3)	24505	1(2)	25111	1(3)	25441	1(2)	25929	1(2)	26420	4(3)	26591	4(3)	27041	3(3)
24076	4(3)	24515	1(2)	25112	1(3)	25442	1(2)	25931	1(2)	26426	4(3)	26593	9(3)	27043	3(3)
24077	1(3)	24516	1(2)	25115	1(3)	25443	1(2)	26010	2(3)	26428	2(3)	26596	1(3)	27045	3(3)
24079	1(3)	24530	1(2)	25116	1(3)	25444	1(2)	26011	3(3)	26432	2(3)	26600	2(3)	27047	4(3)
24100	1(2)	24535	1(2)	25118	5(3)	25445	1(2)	26020	4(3)	26433	2(3)	26605	3(3)	27048	2(3)
24101	1(2)	24538	1(2)	25119	1(2)	25446	1(2)	26025	1(2)	26434	2(3)	26607	2(3)	27049	1(3)
24102	1(2)	24545	1(2)	25120	1(3)	25447	4(3)	26030	1(2)	26437	4(3)	26608	5(3)	27050	1(2)
24105	1(2)	24546	1(2)	25125	1(3)	25449	1(2)	26034	2(3)	26440	6(3)	26615	4(3)	27052	1(2)
24110	1(3)	24560	1(3)	25126	1(3)	25450	1(2)	26035	1(3)	26442	5(3)	26641	1(2)	27054	1(2)
24115	1(3)	24565	1(3)	25130	1(3)	25455	1(2)	26037	1(3)	26445	5(3)	26645	1(2)	27057	1(2)
24116	1(3)	24566	1(3)	25135	1(3)	25490	1(2)	26040	1(2)	26449	5(3)	26650	1(2)	27059	1(3)
24120	1(3)	24575	1(3)	25136	1(3)	25491	1(2)	26045	1(2)	26450	6(3)	26665	1(2)	27060	1(2)
24125	1(3)	24576	1(3)	25145	1(3)	25492	1(2)	26055	5(3)	26455	6(3)	26670	2(3)	27062	1(2)

CPT	MUE	CPT	MUE	CPT	MUE	CPT	MUE	CPT	MUE	CPT	MUE	CPT	MUE	CPT	MUE
27065	1(3)	27246	1(2)	27394	1(2)	27516	1(2)	27665	2(3)	27830	1(2)	28124	4(3)	28400	1(2)
27066	1(3)	27248	1(2)	27395	1(2)	27517	1(2)	27675	1(2)	27831	1(2)	28126	4(3)	28405	1(2)
27067	1(3)	27250	1(2)	27396	1(2)	27519	1(2)	27676	1(2)	27832	1(2)	28130	1(2)	28406	1(2)
27070	1(3)	27252	1(2)	27397	1(2)	27520	1(2)	27680	3(3)	27840	1(2)	28140	4(3)	28415	1(2)
27071	1(3)	27253	1(2)	27400	1(2)	27524	1(2)	27681	1(2)	27842	1(2)	28150	4(3)	28420	1(2)
27075	1(3)	27254	1(2)	27403	1(3)	27530	1(2)	27685	2(3)	27846	1(2)	28153	6(3)	28430	1(2)
27076	1(2)	27256	1(2)	27405	2(2)	27532	1(2)	27686	3(3)	27848	1(2)	28160	5(3)	28435	1(2)
27077	1(2)	27257	1(2)	27407	2(2)	27535	1(2)	27687	1(2)	27860	1(2)	28171	1(3)	28436	1(2)
27078	1(2)	27258	1(2)	27409	1(2)	27536	1(2)	27690	2(3)	27870	1(2)	28173	2(3)	28445	1(2)
27080	1(2)	27259	1(2)	27412	1(2)	27538	1(2)	27691	2(3)	27871	1(3)	28175	2(3)	28446	1(2)
27086	1(3)	27265	1(2)	27415	1(2)	27540	1(2)	27692	4(3)	27880	1(2)	28190	3(3)	28450	2(3)
27087	1(3)	27266	1(2)	27416	1(2)	27550	1(2)	27695	1(2)	27881	1(2)	28192	2(3)	28455	3(3)
27090	1(2)	27267	1(2)	27418	1(2)	27552	1(2)	27696	1(2)	27882	1(2)	28193	2(3)	28456	2(3)
27091	1(2)	27268	1(2)	27420	1(2)	27556	1(2)	27698	2(2)	27884	1(2)	28200	4(3)	28465	3(3)
27093	1(2)	27269	1(2)	27422	1(2)	27557	1(2)	27700	1(2)	27886	1(2)	28202	2(3)	28470	2(3)
27095	1(2)	27275	2(2)	27424	1(2)	27558	1(2)	27702	1(2)	27888	1(2)	28208	4(3)	28475	5(3)
27096	1(2)	27279	1(2)	27425	1(2)	27560	1(2)	27703	1(2)	27889	1(2)	28210	2(3)	28476	4(3)
27097	1(3)	27280	1(2)	27427	1(2)	27562	1(2)	27704	1(2)	27892	1(2)	28220	1(2)	28485	5(3)
27098	1(2)	27282	1(2)	27428	1(2)	27566	1(2)	27705	1(3)	27893	1(2)	28222	1(2)	28490	1(2)
27100	1(2)	27284	1(2)	27429	1(2)	27570	1(2)	27707	1(3)	27894	1(2)	28225	1(2)	28495	1(2)
27105	1(3)	27286	1(2)	27430	1(2)	27580	1(2)	27709	1(3)	28001	2(3)	28226	1(2)	28496	1(2)
27110	1(2)	27290	1(2)	27435	1(2)	27590	1(2)	27712	1(2)	28002	3(3)	28230	1(2)	28505	1(2)
27111	1(2)	27295	1(2)	27437	1(2)	27591	1(2)	27715	1(2)	28003	2(3)	28232	6(3)	28510	4(3)
27120	1(2)	27301	3(3)	27438	1(2)	27592	1(2)	27720	1(2)	28005	3(3)	28234	6(3)	28515	4(3)
27122	1(2)	27303	2(3)	27440	1(2)	27594	1(2)	27722	1(2)	28008	2(3)	28238	1(2)	28525	4(3)
27125	1(2)	27305	1(2)	27441	1(2)	27596	1(2)	27724	1(2)	28020	2(3)	28240	1(2)	28530	1(2)
27130	1(2)	27306	1(2)	27442	1(2)	27598	1(2)	27725	1(2)	28022	4(3)	28250	1(2)	28531	1(2)
27132	1(2)	27307	1(2)	27443	1(2)	27600	1(2)	27726	1(2)	28024	4(3)	28260	1(2)	28540	1(3)
27134	1(2)	27310	1(2)	27445	1(2)	27601	1(2)	27727	1(2)	28035	1(2)	28261	1(3)	28545	1(3)
27137	1(2)	27323	2(3)	27446	1(2)	27602	1(2)	27730	1(2)	28039	3(3)	28262	1(2)	28546	1(3)
27138	1(2)	27324	3(3)	27447	1(2)	27603	2(3)	27732	1(2)	28041	3(3)	28264	1(2)	28555	1(3)
27140	1(2)	27325	1(2)	27448	1(3)	27604	2(3)	27734	1(2)	28043	4(3)	28270	6(3)	28570	1(2)
27146	1(3)	27326	1(2)	27450	1(3)	27605	1(2)	27740	1(2)	28045	4(3)	28272	6(3)	28575	1(2)
27147	1(3)	27327	5(3)	27454	1(2)	27606	1(2)	27742	1(2)	28046	1(3)	28280	1(2)	28576	1(2)
27151	1(3)	27328	4(3)	27455	1(3)	27607	2(3)	27745	1(2)	28047	1(3)	28285	4(3)	28585	1(3)
27156	1(2)	27329	1(3)	27457	1(3)	27610	1(2)	27750	1(2)	28050	2(3)	28286	1(2)	28600	2(3)
27158	1(2)	27330	1(2)	27465	1(2)	27612	1(2)	27752	1(2)	28052	2(3)	28288	5(3)	28605	2(3)
27161	1(2)	27331	1(2)	27466	1(2)	27613	4(3)	27756	1(2)	28054	2(3)	28289	1(2)	28606	3(3)
27165	1(2)	27332	1(2)	27468	1(2)	27614	3(3)	27758	1(2)	28055	1(3)	28290	1(2)	28615	5(3)
27170	1(2)	27333	1(2)	27470	1(2)	27615	1(3)	27759	1(2)	28060	1(2)	28292	1(2)	28630	2(3)
27175	1(2)	27334	1(2)	27472	1(2)	27616	1(3)	27760	1(2)	28062	1(2)	28293	1(2)	28635	2(3)
27176	1(2)	27335	1(2)	27475	1(2)	27618	4(3)	27762	1(2)	28070	2(3)	28294	1(2)	28636	4(3)
27177	1(2)	27337	4(3)	27477	1(2)	27619	4(3)	27766	1(2)	28072	4(3)	28296	1(2)	28645	4(3)
27178	1(2)	27339	4(3)	27479	1(2)	27620	1(2)	27767	1(2)	28080	4(3)	28297	1(2)	28660	4(3)
27179	1(2)	27340	1(2)	27485	1(2)	27625	1(2)	27768	1(2)	28086	2(3)	28298	1(2)	28665	4(3)
27181	1(2)	27345	1(2)	27486	1(2)	27626	1(2)	27769	1(2)	28088	2(3)	28299	1(2)	28666	4(3)
27185	1(2)	27347	1(2)	27487	1(2)	27630	2(3)	27780	1(2)	28090	2(3)	28300	1(2)	28675	4(3)
27187	1(2)	27350	1(2)	27488	1(2)	27632	4(3)	27781	1(2)	28092	2(3)	28302	1(2)	28705	1(2)
27193	1(2)	27355	1(3)	27495	1(2)	27634	2(3)	27784	1(2)	28100	1(3)	28304	1(3)	28715	1(2)
27194	1(2)	27356	1(3)	27496	1(2)	27635	1(3)	27786	1(2)	28102	1(3)	28305	1(3)	28725	1(2)
27200	1(2)	27357	1(3)	27497	1(2)	27637	1(3)	27788	1(2)	28103	1(3)	28306	1(2)	28730	1(2)
27202	1(2)	27358	1(3)	27498	1(2)	27638	1(3)	27792	1(2)	28104	2(3)	28307	1(2)	28735	1(2)
27220	1(2)	27360	2(3)	27499	1(2)	27640	1(3)	27808	1(2)	28106	1(3)	28308	4(3)	28737	1(2)
27222	1(2)	27364	1(3)	27500	1(2)	27641	1(3)	27810	1(2)	28107	1(3)	28309	1(2)	28740	5(3)
27226	1(2)	27365	1(3)	27501	1(2)	27645	1(3)	27814	1(2)	28108	2(3)	28310	1(2)	28750	1(2)
27227	1(2)	27370	1(2)	27502	1(2)	27646	1(3)	27816	1(2)	28110	1(2)	28312	4(3)	28755	1(2)
27228	1(2)	27372	2(3)	27503	1(2)	27647	1(3)	27818	1(2)	28111	1(2)	28313	4(3)	28760	1(2)
27230	1(2)	27380	2(2)	27506	1(2)	27648	1(2)	27822	1(2)	28112	4(3)	28315	1(2)	28800	1(2)
27232	1(2)	27381	2(2)	27507	1(2)	27650	1(2)	27823	1(2)	28113	1(2)	28320	1(2)	28805	1(2)
27235	1(2)	27385	2(3)	27508	1(2)	27652	1(2)	27824	1(2)	28114	1(2)	28322	2(3)	28810	6(3)
27236	1(2)	27386	2(3)	27509	1(2)	27654	1(2)	27825	1(2)	28116	1(2)	28340	2(3)	28820	6(3)
27238	1(2)	27390	1(2)	27510	1(2)	27656	1(3)	27826	1(2)	28118	1(2)	28341	2(3)	28825	10(2)
27240	1(2)	27391	1(2)	27511	1(2)	27658	2(3)	27827	1(2)	28119	1(2)	28344	1(2)	28890	1(2)
27244	1(2)	27392	1(2)	27513	1(2)	27659	2(3)	27828	1(2)	28120	2(3)	28345	2(3)	29000	1(3)
27245	1(2)	27393	1(2)	27514	1(2)	27664	2(3)	27829	1(2)	28122	4(3)	28360	1(2)	29010	1(3)

CPT	MUE	CPT	MUE	CPT	MUE	CPT	MUE	CPT	MUE	CPT	MUE	CPT	MUE	CPT	MUE
29015	1(3)	29828	1(2)	30115	1(2)	31233	1(2)	31579	1(2)	31830	1(2)	32661	1(3)	33226	1(3)
29035	1(3)	29830	1(2)	30117	2(3)	31235	1(2)	31580	1(2)	32035	1(2)	32662	1(3)	33227	1(3)
29040	1(3)	29834	1(2)	30118	1(3)	31237	1(2)	31582	1(2)	32036	1(3)	32663	1(3)	33228	1(3)
29044	1(3)	29835	1(2)	30120	1(2)	31238	1(3)	31584	1(2)	32096	1(3)	32664	1(2)	33229	1(3)
29046	1(3)	29836	1(2)	30124	2(3)	31239	1(2)	31587	1(2)	32097	1(3)	32665	1(2)	33230	1(3)
29049	1(3)	29837	1(2)	30125	1(3)	31240	1(2)	31588	1(2)	32098	1(2)	32666	1(3)	33231	1(3)
29055	1(3)	29838	1(2)	30130	1(2)	31254	1(2)	31590	1(2)	32100	1(3)	32667	3(3)	33233	1(2)
29058	1(3)	29840	1(2)	30140	1(2)	31255	1(2)	31595	1(2)	32110	1(3)	32668	2(3)	33234	1(2)
29065	1(3)	29843	1(2)	30150	1(2)	31256	1(2)	31600	1(2)	32120	1(3)	32669	2(3)	33235	1(2)
29075	1(3)	29844	1(2)	30160	1(2)	31267	1(2)	31601	1(2)	32124	1(3)	32670	1(2)	33236	1(2)
29085	1(3)	29845	1(2)	30200	1(2)	31276	1(2)	31603	1(2)	32140	1(3)	32671	1(2)	33237	1(2)
29086	2(3)	29846	1(2)	30210	1(3)	31287	1(2)	31605	1(2)	32141	1(3)	32672	1(3)	33238	1(2)
29105	1(2)	29847	1(2)	30220	1(2)	31288	1(2)	31610	1(2)	32150	1(3)	32673	1(2)	33240	1(3)
29125	1(2)	29848	1(2)	30300	1(3)	31290	1(2)	31611	1(2)	32151	1(3)	32674	1(2)	33241	1(2)
29126	1(2)	29850	1(2)	30310	1(3)	31291	1(2)	31612	1(3)	32160	1(3)	32701	1(2)	33243	1(2)
29130	3(3)	29851	1(2)	30320	1(3)	31292	1(2)	31613	1(2)	32200	2(3)	32800	1(3)	33244	1(2)
29131	2(3)	29855	1(2)	30400	1(2)	31293	1(2)	31614	1(2)	32215	1(2)	32810	1(3)	33249	1(3)
29200	1(2)	29856	1(2)	30410	1(2)	31294	1(2)	31615	1(3)	32220	1(2)	32815	1(3)	33250	1(2)
29240	1(2)	29860	1(2)	30420	1(2)	31295	1(2)	31620	1(3)	32225	1(2)	32820	1(2)	33251	1(2)
29260	1(3)	29861	1(2)	30430	1(2)	31296	1(2)	31622	1(3)	32310	1(3)	32850	1(2)	33254	1(2)
29280	2(3)	29862	1(2)	30435	1(2)	31297	1(2)	31623	1(3)	32320	1(3)	32851	1(2)	33255	1(2)
29305	1(3)	29863	1(2)	30450	1(2)	31300	1(2)	31624	1(3)	32400	2(3)	32852	1(2)	33256	1(2)
29325	1(3)	29866	1(2)	30460	1(2)	31320	1(2)	31625	1(2)	32405	2(3)	32853	1(2)	33257	1(2)
29345	1(3)	29867	1(2)	30462	1(2)	31360	1(2)	31626	1(2)	32440	1(2)	32854	1(2)	33258	1(2)
29355	1(3)	29868	1(3)	30465	1(2)	31365	1(2)	31627	1(2)	32442	1(2)	32855	1(2)	33259	1(2)
29358	1(3)	29870	1(2)	30520	1(2)	31367	1(2)	31628	1(2)	32445	1(2)	32856	1(2)	33261	1(2)
29365	1(3)	29871	1(2)	30540	1(2)	31368	1(2)	31629	1(2)	32480	1(2)	32900	1(2)	33262	1(3)
29405	1(3)	29873	1(2)	30545	1(2)	31370	1(2)	31630	1(3)	32482	1(2)	32905	1(2)	33263	1(3)
29425	1(3)	29874	1(2)	30560	1(2)	31375	1(2)	31631	1(2)	32484	2(3)	32906	1(2)	33264	1(3)
29435	1(3)	29875	1(2)	30580	2(3)	31380	1(2)	31632	2(3)	32486	1(3)	32940	1(3)	33265	1(2)
29440	1(2)	29876	1(2)	30600	1(3)	31382	1(2)	31633	2(3)	32488	1(2)	32960	1(2)	33266	1(2)
29445	1(3)	29877	1(2)	30620	1(2)	31390	1(2)	31634	1(3)	32491	1(2)	32997	1(2)	33270	1(3)
29450	1(3)	29879	1(2)	30630	1(2)	31395	1(2)	31635	1(3)	32501	1(3)	32998	1(2)	33271	1(3)
29505	1(2)	29880	1(2)	30801	1(2)	31400	1(3)	31636	1(2)	32503	1(2)	33010	1(2)	33272	1(3)
29515	1(2)	29881	1(2)	30802	1(2)	31420	1(2)	31637	2(3)	32504	1(2)	33011	1(3)	33273	1(3)
29520	1(2)	29882	1(2)	30901	1(3)	31500	2(3)	31638	1(3)	32505	1(2)	33015	1(3)	33282	1(2)
29530	1(2)	29883	1(2)	30903	1(3)	31502	1(3)	31640	1(3)	32506	3(3)	33020	1(3)	33284	1(2)
29540	1(2)	29884	1(2)	30905	1(2)	31505	1(3)	31641	1(3)	32507	2(3)	33025	1(2)	33300	1(3)
29550	1(2)	29885	1(2)	30906	1(3)	31510	1(2)	31643	1(2)	32540	1(3)	33030	1(2)	33305	1(3)
29580	1(2)	29886	1(2)	30915	1(3)	31511	1(3)	31645	1(2)	32550	2(3)	33031	1(2)	33310	1(2)
29581	1(2)	29887	1(2)	30920	1(3)	31512	1(3)	31646	2(3)	32551	2(3)	33050	1(2)	33315	1(2)
29582	1(2)	29888	1(2)	30930	1(2)	31513	1(3)	31647	1(2)	32552	2(2)	33120	1(3)	33320	1(3)
29583	1(2)	29889	1(2)	31000	1(2)	31515	1(3)	31648	1(2)	32553	1(2)	33130	1(3)	33321	1(3)
29584	1(2)	29891	1(2)	31002	1(2)	31520	1(3)	31649	2(3)	32554	2(3)	33140	1(2)	33322	1(3)
29700	2(3)	29892	1(2)	31020	1(2)	31525	1(3)	31651	3(3)	32555	2(3)	33141	1(2)	33330	1(3)
29705	1(3)	29893	1(2)	31030	1(2)	31526	1(3)	31660	1(2)	32556	2(3)	33202	1(2)	33335	1(3)
29710	1(2)	29894	1(2)	31032	1(2)	31527	1(2)	31661	1(2)	32557	2(3)	33203	1(2)	33361	1(2)
29720	1(2)	29895	1(2)	31040	1(2)	31528	1(2)	31717	1(3)	32560	1(3)	33206	1(3)	33362	1(2)
29730	1(3)	29897	1(2)	31050	1(2)	31529	1(3)	31720	3(3)	32561	1(2)	33207	1(3)	33363	1(2)
29740	1(3)	29898	1(2)	31051	1(2)	31530	1(3)	31725	1(3)	32562	1(2)	33208	1(3)	33364	1(2)
29750	1(3)	29899	1(2)	31070	1(2)	31531	1(3)	31730	1(3)	32601	1(3)	33210	1(3)	33365	1(2)
29800	1(2)	29900	2(3)	31075	1(2)	31535	1(3)	31750	1(2)	32604	1(3)	33211	1(3)	33366	1(2)
29804	1(2)	29901	2(3)	31080	1(2)	31536	1(3)	31755	1(2)	32606	1(3)	33212	1(3)	33367	1(2)
29805	1(2)	29902	2(3)	31081	1(2)	31540	1(3)	31760	1(2)	32607	1(3)	33213	1(3)	33368	1(2)
29806	1(2)	29904	1(2)	31084	1(2)	31541	1(3)	31766	1(2)	32608	1(3)	33214	1(3)	33369	1(2)
29807	1(2)	29905	1(2)	31085	1(2)	31545	1(2)	31770	2(3)	32609	1(3)	33215	2(3)	33400	1(2)
29819	1(2)	29906	1(2)	31086	1(2)	31546	1(2)	31775	1(3)	32650	1(2)	33216	1(3)	33401	1(2)
29820	1(2)	29907	1(2)	31087	1(2)	31560	1(2)	31780	1(2)	32651	1(2)	33217	1(3)	33403	1(2)
29821	1(2)	29914	1(2)	31090	1(2)	31561	1(2)	31781	1(2)	32652	1(2)	33218	1(3)	33404	1(2)
29822	1(2)	29915	1(2)	31200	1(2)	31570	1(2)	31785	1(3)	32653	1(3)	33220	1(3)	33405	1(2)
29823	1(2)	29916	1(2)	31201	1(2)	31571	1(2)	31786	1(3)	32654	1(3)	33221	1(3)	33406	1(2)
29824	1(2)	30000	1(3)	31205	1(2)	31575	1(3)	31800	1(3)	32655	1(3)	33222	1(3)	33410	1(2)
29825	1(2)	30020	1(3)	31225	1(2)	31576	1(3)	31805	1(3)	32656	1(2)	33223	1(3)	33411	1(2)
29826	1(2)	30100	2(3)	31230	1(2)	31577	1(3)	31820	1(2)	32658	1(3)	33224	1(3)	33412	1(2)
29827	1(2)	30110	1(2)	31231	1(2)	31578	1(3)	31825	1(2)	32659	1(2)	33225	1(3)	33413	1(2)

Appendix H — Medically Unlikely Edits (MUEs) — OPPS

CPT	MUE	CPT	MUE	CPT	MUE	CPT	MUE	CPT	MUE	CPT	MUE	CPT	MUE	CPT	MUE
33414	1(2)	33621	1(3)	33864	1(2)	33989	1(3)	35121	1(3)	35511	1(3)	35695	1(3)	36415	5(3)
33415	1(2)	33622	1(2)	33870	1(2)	33990	1(3)	35122	1(3)	35512	1(3)	35697	2(3)	36416	6(3)
33416	1(2)	33641	1(2)	33875	1(2)	33991	1(3)	35131	1(2)	35515	1(3)	35700	2(3)	36420	2(3)
33417	1(2)	33645	1(2)	33877	1(2)	33992	1(2)	35132	1(2)	35516	1(3)	35701	1(2)	36425	2(3)
33418	1(3)	33647	1(2)	33880	1(2)	33993	1(3)	35141	1(2)	35518	1(3)	35721	1(2)	36430	1(2)
33419	1(3)	33660	1(2)	33881	1(2)	34001	1(3)	35142	1(2)	35521	1(3)	35741	1(2)	36440	1(3)
33420	1(2)	33665	1(2)	33883	1(2)	34051	1(3)	35151	1(2)	35522	1(3)	35761	2(3)	36450	1(3)
33422	1(2)	33670	1(2)	33884	2(3)	34101	1(3)	35152	1(2)	35523	1(3)	35800	2(3)	36455	1(3)
33425	1(2)	33675	1(2)	33886	1(2)	34111	2(3)	35180	2(3)	35525	1(3)	35820	2(3)	36460	2(3)
33426	1(2)	33676	1(2)	33889	1(2)	34151	2(3)	35182	2(3)	35526	1(3)	35840	2(3)	36468	1(3)
33427	1(2)	33677	1(2)	33891	1(2)	34201	1(3)	35184	2(3)	35531	2(3)	35860	2(3)	36470	1(3)
33430	1(2)	33681	1(2)	33910	1(3)	34203	1(2)	35188	2(3)	35533	1(3)	35870	1(3)	36471	1(2)
33460	1(2)	33684	1(2)	33915	1(3)	34401	1(3)	35189	1(3)	35535	1(3)	35875	2(3)	36475	1(3)
33463	1(2)	33688	1(2)	33916	1(3)	34421	1(3)	35190	2(3)	35536	1(3)	35876	2(3)	36476	2(3)
33464	1(2)	33690	1(2)	33917	1(2)	34451	1(3)	35201	2(3)	35537	1(3)	35879	2(3)	36478	1(3)
33465	1(2)	33692	1(2)	33920	1(2)	34471	1(2)	35206	2(3)	35538	1(3)	35881	2(3)	36479	2(3)
33468	1(2)	33694	1(2)	33922	1(2)	34490	1(2)	35207	3(3)	35539	1(3)	35883	1(3)	36481	1(3)
33470	1(2)	33697	1(2)	33924	1(2)	34501	1(2)	35211	3(3)	35540	1(3)	35884	1(3)	36500	4(3)
33471	1(2)	33702	1(2)	33925	1(2)	34502	1(2)	35216	2(3)	35556	1(3)	35901	1(3)	36510	1(3)
33474	1(2)	33710	1(2)	33926	1(2)	34510	2(3)	35221	3(3)	35558	1(3)	35903	2(3)	36511	1(3)
33475	1(2)	33720	1(2)	33930	1(2)	34520	1(3)	35226	3(3)	35560	1(3)	35905	1(3)	36512	1(3)
33476	1(2)	33722	1(3)	33933	1(2)	34530	1(3)	35231	2(3)	35563	1(3)	35907	1(3)	36513	1(3)
33478	1(2)	33724	1(2)	33935	1(2)	34800	1(3)	35236	2(3)	35565	1(3)	36000	4(3)	36514	1(3)
33496	1(3)	33726	1(2)	33940	1(2)	34802	1(2)	35241	2(3)	35566	1(3)	36002	2(3)	36515	1(3)
33500	1(3)	33730	1(2)	33944	1(2)	34803	1(2)	35246	2(3)	35570	1(3)	36005	2(3)	36516	1(3)
33501	1(3)	33732	1(2)	33945	1(2)	34804	1(2)	35251	2(3)	35571	2(3)	36010	2(3)	36522	1(3)
33502	1(3)	33735	1(2)	33946	1(2)	34805	1(2)	35256	2(3)	35572	2(3)	36011	4(3)	36555	2(3)
33503	1(3)	33736	1(2)	33947	1(2)	34806	1(2)	35261	1(3)	35583	1(2)	36012	4(3)	36556	2(3)
33504	1(3)	33737	1(2)	33948	1(2)	34808	1(3)	35266	2(3)	35585	2(3)	36013	2(3)	36557	2(3)
33505	1(3)	33750	1(3)	33949	1(2)	34812	1(2)	35271	2(3)	35587	2(2)	36014	2(3)	36558	2(3)
33506	1(3)	33755	1(2)	33951	1(1)	34813	1(2)	35276	2(3)	35600	2(3)	36015	4(3)	36560	2(3)
33507	1(3)	33762	1(2)	33952	1(1)	34820	1(2)	35281	2(3)	35601	1(3)	36100	2(3)	36561	2(3)
33508	1(2)	33764	1(3)	33953	1(1)	34825	2(2)	35286	2(3)	35606	1(3)	36120	2(3)	36563	1(3)
33510	1(2)	33766	1(2)	33954	1(1)	34826	4(3)	35301	2(3)	35612	1(3)	36140	3(3)	36565	1(3)
33511	1(2)	33767	1(2)	33955	1(3)	34830	1(2)	35302	1(2)	35616	1(3)	36147	2(3)	36566	1(3)
33512	1(2)	33768	1(2)	33956	1(3)	34831	1(2)	35303	1(2)	35621	1(3)	36148	1(3)	36568	2(3)
33513	1(2)	33770	1(2)	33957	1(3)	34832	1(2)	35304	1(2)	35623	1(3)	36160	2(3)	36569	2(3)
33514	1(2)	33771	1(2)	33958	1(3)	34833	1(2)	35305	1(2)	35626	3(3)	36200	2(3)	36570	2(3)
33516	1(2)	33774	1(2)	33959	1(3)	34834	1(2)	35306	2(3)	35631	4(3)	36215	2(3)	36571	2(3)
33517	1(2)	33775	1(2)	33962	1(3)	34839	1(2)	35311	1(2)	35632	1(3)	36216	2(3)	36575	2(3)
33518	1(2)	33776	1(2)	33963	1(3)	34841	1(2)	35321	1(2)	35633	1(3)	36217	2(3)	36576	2(3)
33519	1(2)	33777	1(2)	33964	1(3)	34842	1(2)	35331	1(2)	35634	1(3)	36218	2(3)	36578	2(3)
33521	1(2)	33778	1(2)	33965	1(3)	34843	1(2)	35341	3(3)	35636	1(3)	36221	1(3)	36580	2(3)
33522	1(2)	33779	1(2)	33966	1(3)	34844	1(2)	35351	1(3)	35637	1(3)	36222	1(3)	36581	2(3)
33523	1(2)	33780	1(2)	33967	1(3)	34845	1(2)	35355	1(3)	35638	1(3)	36223	1(3)	36582	2(3)
33530	1(2)	33781	1(2)	33968	1(3)	34846	1(2)	35361	1(2)	35642	1(3)	36224	1(3)	36583	2(3)
33533	1(2)	33782	1(2)	33969	1(3)	34847	1(2)	35363	1(2)	35645	1(3)	36225	1(3)	36584	2(3)
33534	1(2)	33783	1(2)	33970	1(3)	34848	1(2)	35371	1(2)	35646	1(3)	36226	1(3)	36585	2(3)
33535	1(2)	33786	1(2)	33971	1(3)	34900	1(2)	35372	1(2)	35647	1(3)	36227	1(3)	36589	2(3)
33536	1(2)	33788	1(2)	33973	1(3)	35001	1(2)	35390	1(3)	35650	1(3)	36228	2(3)	36590	2(3)
33542	1(2)	33800	1(2)	33974	1(3)	35002	1(2)	35400	1(3)	35654	1(3)	36245	2(3)	36591	2(3)
33545	1(2)	33802	1(3)	33975	1(3)	35005	1(2)	35450	2(3)	35656	1(3)	36246	4(3)	36592	1(3)
33548	1(2)	33803	1(3)	33976	1(3)	35011	1(2)	35452	1(2)	35661	1(3)	36247	2(3)	36593	2(3)
33572	3(2)	33813	1(2)	33977	1(3)	35013	1(2)	35458	2(3)	35663	1(3)	36248	2(3)	36595	2(3)
33600	1(3)	33814	1(2)	33978	1(3)	35021	1(2)	35460	2(3)	35665	1(3)	36251	1(3)	36596	2(3)
33602	1(3)	33820	1(2)	33979	1(3)	35022	1(2)	35471	3(3)	35666	2(3)	36252	1(3)	36597	2(3)
33606	1(2)	33822	1(2)	33980	1(3)	35045	2(3)	35472	1(2)	35671	2(3)	36253	1(3)	36598	2(3)
33608	1(2)	33824	1(2)	33981	1(3)	35081	1(2)	35475	4(3)	35681	1(3)	36254	1(3)	36600	4(3)
33610	1(2)	33840	1(2)	33982	1(3)	35082	1(2)	35476	5(3)	35682	1(2)	36260	1(2)	36620	3(3)
33611	1(2)	33845	1(2)	33983	1(3)	35091	1(2)	35500	2(3)	35683	1(2)	36261	1(2)	36625	2(3)
33612	1(2)	33851	1(2)	33984	1(3)	35092	1(2)	35501	1(3)	35685	2(3)	36262	1(2)	36640	1(3)
33615	1(2)	33852	1(2)	33985	1(3)	35102	1(2)	35506	1(3)	35686	1(3)	36400	1(3)	36660	1(3)
33617	1(2)	33853	1(2)	33986	1(3)	35103	1(2)	35508	1(3)	35691	1(3)	36405	1(3)	36680	1(3)
33619	1(2)	33860	1(2)	33987	1(3)	35111	1(2)	35509	1(3)	35693	1(3)	36406	1(3)	36800	1(3)
33620	1(2)	33863	1(2)	33988	1(3)	35112	1(2)	35510	1(3)	35694	1(3)	36410	3(3)	36810	1(3)

　© 2015 American Medical Association. All Rights Reserved.　© 2015 Optum360, LLC

CPT	MUE	CPT	MUE	CPT	MUE	CPT	MUE	CPT	MUE	CPT	MUE	CPT	MUE	CPT	MUE
36815	1(3)	37244	2(3)	38530	1(2)	40831	2(3)	42140	1(2)	42845	1(3)	43237	1(2)	43401	1(2)
36818	1(3)	37250	1(2)	38542	1(2)	40840	1(2)	42145	1(2)	42860	1(3)	43238	1(2)	43405	1(2)
36819	1(3)	37500	1(3)	38550	1(3)	40842	1(2)	42160	2(3)	42870	1(3)	43239	1(2)	43410	1(3)
36820	1(3)	37565	1(2)	38555	1(3)	40843	1(2)	42180	1(3)	42890	1(2)	43240	1(2)	43415	1(3)
36821	2(3)	37600	1(3)	38562	1(2)	40844	1(2)	42182	1(3)	42892	1(3)	43241	1(3)	43420	1(3)
36823	1(3)	37605	1(3)	38564	1(2)	40845	1(3)	42200	1(2)	42894	1(3)	43242	1(2)	43425	1(3)
36825	1(3)	37606	1(3)	38570	1(2)	41000	2(3)	42205	1(2)	42900	1(3)	43243	1(2)	43450	1(3)
36830	2(3)	37607	1(3)	38571	1(2)	41005	2(3)	42210	1(2)	42950	1(3)	43244	1(2)	43453	1(3)
36831	1(3)	37609	1(2)	38572	1(2)	41006	2(3)	42215	1(2)	42953	1(3)	43245	1(2)	43460	1(3)
36832	2(3)	37615	2(3)	38700	1(2)	41007	2(3)	42220	1(2)	42955	1(3)	43246	1(2)	43496	1(3)
36833	1(3)	37616	1(3)	38720	1(2)	41008	2(3)	42225	1(2)	42960	1(3)	43247	1(2)	43500	1(2)
36835	1(3)	37617	3(3)	38724	1(2)	41009	2(3)	42226	1(2)	42961	1(3)	43248	1(3)	43501	1(3)
36838	1(3)	37618	2(3)	38740	1(2)	41010	1(2)	42227	1(2)	42962	1(3)	43249	1(3)	43502	1(2)
36860	2(3)	37619	1(2)	38745	1(2)	41015	2(3)	42235	1(2)	42970	1(3)	43250	1(2)	43510	1(2)
36861	2(3)	37650	1(2)	38746	1(2)	41016	2(3)	42260	1(3)	42971	1(3)	43251	1(2)	43520	1(2)
36870	2(3)	37660	1(2)	38747	1(2)	41017	2(3)	42280	1(2)	42972	1(3)	43252	1(2)	43605	1(2)
37140	1(2)	37700	1(2)	38760	1(2)	41018	2(3)	42281	1(2)	43020	1(2)	43253	1(3)	43610	2(3)
37145	1(3)	37718	1(2)	38765	1(2)	41019	1(2)	42300	2(3)	43030	1(2)	43254	1(3)	43611	2(3)
37160	1(3)	37722	1(2)	38770	1(2)	41100	3(3)	42305	2(3)	43045	1(2)	43255	2(3)	43620	1(2)
37180	1(2)	37735	1(2)	38780	1(2)	41105	3(3)	42310	2(3)	43100	1(3)	43257	1(2)	43621	1(2)
37181	1(2)	37760	1(2)	38790	1(2)	41108	2(3)	42320	2(3)	43101	1(3)	43259	1(2)	43622	1(2)
37182	1(2)	37761	1(2)	38792	1(3)	41110	2(3)	42330	2(3)	43107	1(2)	43260	1(3)	43631	1(2)
37183	1(2)	37765	1(2)	38794	1(2)	41112	2(3)	42335	2(2)	43108	1(2)	43261	1(2)	43632	1(2)
37184	1(2)	37766	1(2)	38900	1(3)	41113	2(3)	42340	1(2)	43112	1(2)	43262	2(2)	43633	1(2)
37185	2(3)	37780	1(2)	39000	1(2)	41114	2(3)	42400	2(3)	43113	1(2)	43263	1(2)	43634	1(2)
37186	2(3)	37785	1(2)	39010	1(2)	41115	1(2)	42405	2(3)	43116	1(2)	43264	1(2)	43635	1(2)
37187	1(3)	37788	1(2)	39200	1(2)	41116	2(3)	42408	1(3)	43117	1(2)	43265	1(2)	43640	1(2)
37188	1(3)	37790	1(2)	39220	1(2)	41120	1(2)	42409	1(3)	43118	1(2)	43266	1(3)	43641	1(2)
37191	1(3)	38100	1(2)	39400	1(2)	41130	1(2)	42410	1(2)	43121	1(2)	43270	1(3)	43644	1(2)
37192	1(3)	38101	1(3)	39501	1(3)	41135	1(2)	42415	1(2)	43122	1(2)	43273	1(2)	43645	1(2)
37193	1(3)	38102	1(2)	39503	1(2)	41140	1(2)	42420	1(2)	43123	1(2)	43274	2(3)	43647	1(2)
37195	1(3)	38115	1(3)	39540	1(2)	41145	1(2)	42425	1(2)	43124	1(2)	43275	1(3)	43648	1(2)
37197	2(3)	38120	1(2)	39541	1(2)	41150	1(2)	42426	1(2)	43130	1(3)	43276	2(3)	43651	1(2)
37200	2(3)	38200	1(3)	39545	1(2)	41153	1(2)	42440	1(2)	43135	1(3)	43277	3(3)	43652	1(2)
37202	4(3)	38204	1(2)	39560	1(3)	41155	1(2)	42450	2(3)	43180	1(2)	43278	1(3)	43653	1(2)
37211	1(2)	38205	1(3)	39561	1(3)	41250	2(3)	42500	2(3)	43191	1(3)	43279	1(2)	43752	2(3)
37212	1(2)	38206	1(3)	40490	3(3)	41251	2(3)	42505	2(3)	43192	1(3)	43280	1(2)	43753	1(3)
37213	1(2)	38207	1(3)	40500	2(3)	41252	2(3)	42507	1(2)	43193	1(3)	43282	1(2)	43754	1(3)
37214	1(2)	38208	1(3)	40510	2(3)	41500	1(2)	42509	1(2)	43194	1(3)	43283	1(2)	43755	1(3)
37215	1(2)	38209	1(3)	40520	2(3)	41510	1(2)	42510	1(2)	43195	1(3)	43300	1(2)	43756	1(2)
37217	1(2)	38210	1(3)	40525	2(3)	41512	1(2)	42550	2(3)	43196	1(3)	43305	1(2)	43757	1(2)
37218	1(2)	38211	1(3)	40527	2(3)	41520	1(3)	42600	2(3)	43197	1(3)	43310	1(2)	43760	2(3)
37220	2(2)	38212	1(3)	40530	2(3)	41530	1(3)	42650	2(3)	43198	1(3)	43312	1(2)	43761	2(3)
37221	2(2)	38213	1(3)	40650	2(3)	41800	2(3)	42660	2(3)	43200	1(3)	43313	1(2)	43770	1(2)
37222	2(3)	38214	1(3)	40652	2(3)	41805	3(3)	42665	2(3)	43201	1(2)	43314	1(2)	43771	1(2)
37223	2(3)	38215	1(3)	40654	2(3)	41806	3(3)	42700	2(3)	43202	1(2)	43320	1(2)	43772	1(2)
37224	2(2)	38220	1(3)	40700	1(2)	41820	4(2)	42720	1(3)	43204	1(2)	43325	1(2)	43773	1(2)
37225	2(2)	38221	1(3)	40701	1(2)	41821	2(3)	42725	1(3)	43205	1(2)	43327	1(2)	43774	1(2)
37226	2(2)	38230	1(2)	40702	1(2)	41822	1(2)	42800	3(3)	43206	1(2)	43328	1(2)	43775	1(2)
37227	2(2)	38232	1(2)	40720	1(2)	41823	1(2)	42804	3(3)	43211	1(3)	43330	1(2)	43800	1(2)
37228	2(2)	38240	1(3)	40761	1(2)	41825	2(3)	42806	1(3)	43212	1(3)	43331	1(2)	43810	1(2)
37229	2(2)	38241	1(2)	40800	2(3)	41826	2(3)	42808	2(3)	43213	1(2)	43332	1(2)	43820	1(2)
37230	2(2)	38242	1(2)	40801	2(3)	41827	2(3)	42809	1(3)	43214	1(3)	43333	1(2)	43825	1(2)
37231	2(2)	38243	1(3)	40804	2(3)	41828	4(2)	42810	1(3)	43215	1(3)	43334	1(2)	43830	1(2)
37232	2(3)	38300	1(3)	40805	2(3)	41830	2(3)	42815	1(3)	43216	1(2)	43335	1(2)	43831	1(2)
37233	2(3)	38305	1(3)	40806	2(3)	41850	2(3)	42820	1(2)	43217	1(2)	43336	1(2)	43832	1(2)
37234	2(3)	38308	1(3)	40808	4(3)	41870	2(3)	42821	1(2)	43220	1(3)	43337	1(2)	43840	2(3)
37235	2(3)	38380	1(2)	40810	4(3)	41872	4(2)	42825	1(2)	43226	1(3)	43338	1(2)	43843	1(2)
37236	1(2)	38381	1(2)	40812	4(3)	41874	4(2)	42826	1(2)	43227	1(3)	43340	1(2)	43845	1(2)
37237	2(3)	38382	1(2)	40814	4(3)	42000	1(3)	42830	1(2)	43229	1(3)	43341	1(2)	43846	1(2)
37238	1(2)	38500	2(3)	40816	2(3)	42100	3(3)	42831	1(2)	43231	1(2)	43351	1(2)	43847	1(2)
37239	2(3)	38505	3(3)	40818	2(3)	42104	3(3)	42835	1(2)	43232	1(2)	43352	1(2)	43848	1(2)
37241	2(3)	38510	1(2)	40819	2(2)	42106	2(3)	42836	1(2)	43233	1(3)	43360	1(2)	43850	1(2)
37242	2(3)	38520	1(2)	40820	5(3)	42107	2(3)	42842	1(3)	43235	1(3)	43361	1(2)	43855	1(2)
37243	1(3)	38525	1(2)	40830	2(3)	42120	1(2)	42844	1(3)	43236	1(2)	43400	1(2)	43860	1(2)

CPT	MUE	CPT	MUE	CPT	MUE	CPT	MUE	CPT	MUE	CPT	MUE	CPT	MUE	CPT	MUE
43865	1(2)	44314	1(2)	44950	1(2)	45391	1(2)	46700	1(2)	47400	1(3)	48510	1(3)	49465	1(3)
43870	1(2)	44316	1(2)	44955	1(2)	45392	1(2)	46705	1(2)	47420	1(2)	48520	1(3)	49491	1(2)
43880	1(3)	44320	1(2)	44960	1(2)	45393	1(3)	46706	1(3)	47425	1(2)	48540	1(3)	49492	1(2)
43881	1(3)	44322	1(2)	44970	1(2)	45395	1(2)	46707	1(3)	47460	1(2)	48545	1(3)	49495	1(2)
43882	1(3)	44340	1(2)	45000	1(3)	45397	1(2)	46710	1(3)	47480	1(2)	48547	1(2)	49496	1(2)
43886	1(2)	44345	1(2)	45005	1(3)	45398	1(2)	46712	1(3)	47490	1(2)	48548	1(2)	49500	1(2)
43887	1(2)	44346	1(2)	45020	1(3)	45400	1(2)	46715	1(2)	47500	2(3)	48550	1(2)	49501	1(2)
43888	1(2)	44360	1(3)	45100	2(3)	45402	1(2)	46716	1(2)	47505	2(3)	48551	1(2)	49505	1(2)
44005	1(2)	44361	1(2)	45108	1(2)	45500	1(2)	46730	1(2)	47510	2(3)	48552	1(2)	49507	1(2)
44010	1(2)	44363	1(3)	45110	1(2)	45505	1(2)	46735	1(2)	47511	2(3)	48554	1(2)	49520	1(2)
44015	1(2)	44364	1(2)	45111	1(2)	45520	1(2)	46740	1(2)	47525	3(3)	48556	1(2)	49521	1(2)
44020	2(3)	44365	1(2)	45112	1(2)	45540	1(2)	46742	1(2)	47530	2(3)	49000	1(2)	49525	1(2)
44021	1(3)	44366	1(3)	45113	1(2)	45541	1(2)	46744	1(2)	47550	1(3)	49002	1(3)	49540	1(2)
44025	1(3)	44369	1(2)	45114	1(2)	45550	1(2)	46746	1(2)	47552	1(3)	49010	1(3)	49550	1(2)
44050	1(2)	44370	1(2)	45116	1(2)	45560	1(2)	46748	1(2)	47553	1(2)	49020	2(3)	49553	1(2)
44055	1(2)	44372	1(2)	45119	1(2)	45562	1(2)	46750	1(2)	47554	1(3)	49040	2(3)	49555	1(2)
44100	1(2)	44373	1(2)	45120	1(2)	45563	1(2)	46751	1(2)	47555	1(2)	49060	2(3)	49557	1(2)
44110	1(2)	44376	1(3)	45121	1(2)	45800	1(3)	46753	1(2)	47556	1(2)	49062	1(3)	49560	2(3)
44111	1(2)	44377	1(2)	45123	1(2)	45805	1(3)	46754	1(3)	47560	1(3)	49082	1(3)	49561	2(3)
44120	1(2)	44378	1(3)	45126	1(2)	45820	1(3)	46760	1(2)	47561	1(3)	49083	2(3)	49565	2(3)
44121	4(3)	44379	1(2)	45130	1(2)	45825	1(3)	46761	1(2)	47562	1(2)	49084	1(3)	49566	2(3)
44125	1(2)	44380	1(3)	45135	1(2)	45900	1(2)	46762	1(2)	47563	1(2)	49180	2(3)	49568	2(3)
44126	1(2)	44381	1(3)	45136	1(2)	45905	1(2)	46900	1(2)	47564	1(2)	49203	1(2)	49570	1(3)
44127	1(2)	44382	1(2)	45150	1(2)	45910	1(2)	46910	1(2)	47570	1(2)	49204	1(2)	49572	1(3)
44128	2(3)	44384	1(3)	45160	1(3)	45915	1(2)	46916	1(2)	47600	1(2)	49205	1(2)	49580	1(2)
44130	3(3)	44385	1(3)	45171	2(3)	45990	1(2)	46917	1(2)	47605	1(2)	49215	1(2)	49582	1(2)
44132	1(2)	44386	1(2)	45172	2(3)	46020	2(3)	46922	1(2)	47610	1(2)	49220	1(2)	49585	1(2)
44133	1(2)	44388	1(3)	45190	1(3)	46030	1(3)	46924	1(2)	47612	1(2)	49250	1(2)	49587	1(2)
44135	1(2)	44389	1(2)	45300	1(3)	46040	2(3)	46930	1(2)	47620	1(2)	49255	1(2)	49590	1(2)
44136	1(2)	44390	1(3)	45303	1(3)	46045	2(3)	46940	1(2)	47630	1(3)	49320	1(3)	49600	1(2)
44137	1(2)	44391	1(3)	45305	1(2)	46050	2(3)	46942	1(3)	47700	1(2)	49321	1(2)	49605	1(2)
44139	1(2)	44392	1(2)	45307	1(3)	46060	2(3)	46945	1(2)	47701	1(2)	49322	1(2)	49606	1(2)
44140	2(3)	44394	1(2)	45308	1(2)	46070	1(2)	46946	1(2)	47711	1(2)	49323	1(2)	49610	1(2)
44141	1(3)	44401	1(2)	45309	1(2)	46080	1(2)	46947	1(2)	47712	1(2)	49324	1(2)	49611	1(2)
44143	1(2)	44402	1(3)	45315	1(2)	46083	2(3)	47000	3(3)	47715	1(2)	49325	1(2)	49650	1(2)
44144	1(3)	44403	1(3)	45317	1(3)	46200	1(3)	47001	3(3)	47720	1(2)	49326	1(2)	49651	1(2)
44145	1(2)	44404	1(3)	45320	1(2)	46220	1(2)	47010	3(3)	47721	1(2)	49327	1(2)	49652	2(3)
44146	1(2)	44405	1(3)	45321	1(2)	46221	1(2)	47015	1(2)	47740	1(2)	49400	1(3)	49653	2(3)
44147	1(3)	44406	1(3)	45327	1(2)	46230	1(2)	47100	3(3)	47741	1(2)	49402	1(3)	49654	2(3)
44150	1(2)	44407	1(2)	45330	1(3)	46250	1(2)	47120	2(3)	47760	1(2)	49405	2(3)	49655	2(3)
44151	1(2)	44408	1(3)	45331	1(2)	46255	1(2)	47122	1(2)	47765	1(2)	49406	2(3)	49656	2(3)
44155	1(2)	44500	1(3)	45332	1(3)	46257	1(2)	47125	1(2)	47780	1(2)	49407	1(3)	49657	2(3)
44156	1(2)	44602	1(2)	45333	1(2)	46258	1(2)	47130	1(2)	47785	1(2)	49411	1(2)	49900	1(3)
44157	1(2)	44603	1(2)	45334	1(3)	46260	1(2)	47133	1(2)	47800	1(2)	49412	1(2)	49904	1(3)
44158	1(2)	44604	1(2)	45335	1(2)	46261	1(2)	47135	1(2)	47801	1(3)	49418	1(3)	49905	1(3)
44160	1(2)	44605	1(2)	45337	1(2)	46262	1(2)	47136	1(2)	47802	1(2)	49419	1(2)	49906	1(3)
44180	1(2)	44615	4(3)	45338	1(2)	46270	1(3)	47140	1(2)	47900	1(2)	49421	1(2)	50010	1(2)
44186	1(2)	44620	2(3)	45340	1(2)	46275	1(3)	47141	1(2)	48000	1(2)	49422	1(2)	50020	1(3)
44187	1(3)	44625	1(3)	45341	1(2)	46280	1(2)	47142	1(2)	48001	1(2)	49423	2(3)	50040	1(2)
44188	1(3)	44626	1(3)	45342	1(2)	46285	1(3)	47143	1(2)	48020	1(3)	49424	3(3)	50045	1(2)
44202	1(2)	44640	2(3)	45346	1(2)	46288	1(3)	47144	1(2)	48100	1(3)	49425	1(2)	50060	1(2)
44203	2(3)	44650	2(3)	45347	1(3)	46320	2(3)	47145	1(2)	48102	1(3)	49426	1(3)	50065	1(2)
44204	2(3)	44660	1(3)	45349	1(3)	46500	1(2)	47146	3(3)	48105	1(2)	49427	1(2)	50070	1(2)
44205	1(2)	44661	1(3)	45350	1(2)	46505	1(2)	47147	2(3)	48120	1(3)	49428	1(2)	50075	1(2)
44206	1(2)	44680	1(3)	45378	1(3)	46600	1(3)	47300	2(3)	48140	1(2)	49429	1(2)	50080	1(2)
44207	1(2)	44700	1(2)	45379	1(3)	46601	1(3)	47350	1(3)	48145	1(2)	49435	1(2)	50081	1(2)
44208	1(2)	44701	1(2)	45380	1(2)	46604	1(2)	47360	1(3)	48146	1(2)	49436	1(2)	50100	1(2)
44210	1(2)	44705	1(3)	45381	1(2)	46606	1(2)	47361	1(3)	48148	1(2)	49440	1(3)	50120	1(2)
44211	1(2)	44715	1(2)	45382	1(3)	46607	1(2)	47362	1(3)	48150	1(2)	49441	1(3)	50125	1(2)
44212	1(2)	44720	2(3)	45384	1(2)	46608	1(3)	47370	1(2)	48152	1(2)	49442	1(3)	50130	1(2)
44213	1(2)	44721	2(3)	45385	1(2)	46610	1(2)	47371	1(2)	48153	1(2)	49446	1(2)	50135	1(2)
44227	1(3)	44800	1(3)	45386	1(2)	46611	1(2)	47380	1(2)	48154	1(2)	49450	1(3)	50200	1(3)
44300	1(3)	44820	1(3)	45388	1(2)	46612	1(2)	47381	1(2)	48155	1(2)	49451	1(3)	50205	1(3)
44310	2(3)	44850	1(3)	45389	1(3)	46614	1(3)	47382	1(2)	48400	1(3)	49452	1(3)	50220	1(2)
44312	1(2)	44900	1(2)	45390	1(3)	46615	1(2)	47383	1(2)	48500	1(3)	49460	1(3)	50225	1(2)

　© 2015 Optum360, LLC

CPT	MUE	CPT	MUE	CPT	MUE	CPT	MUE	CPT	MUE	CPT	MUE	CPT	MUE	CPT	MUE
50230	1(2)	50610	1(2)	51555	1(2)	52276	1(2)	53275	1(2)	54230	1(3)	54900	1(2)	56634	1(2)
50234	1(2)	50620	1(2)	51565	1(2)	52277	1(2)	53400	1(2)	54231	1(3)	54901	1(2)	56637	1(2)
50236	1(2)	50630	1(2)	51570	1(2)	52281	1(2)	53405	1(2)	54235	1(3)	55000	1(3)	56640	1(2)
50240	1(2)	50650	1(2)	51575	1(2)	52282	1(2)	53410	1(2)	54240	1(2)	55040	1(2)	56700	1(2)
50250	1(3)	50660	1(3)	51580	1(2)	52283	1(2)	53415	1(2)	54250	1(2)	55041	1(2)	56740	1(3)
50280	1(2)	50684	1(3)	51585	1(2)	52285	1(2)	53420	1(2)	54300	1(2)	55060	1(2)	56800	1(2)
50290	1(3)	50686	2(3)	51590	1(2)	52287	1(2)	53425	1(2)	54304	1(2)	55100	2(3)	56805	1(2)
50300	1(2)	50688	2(3)	51595	1(2)	52290	1(2)	53430	1(2)	54308	1(2)	55110	1(2)	56810	1(2)
50320	1(2)	50690	2(3)	51596	1(2)	52300	1(2)	53431	1(2)	54312	1(2)	55120	1(3)	56820	1(2)
50323	1(2)	50700	1(2)	51597	1(2)	52301	1(2)	53440	1(2)	54316	1(2)	55150	1(2)	56821	1(2)
50325	1(2)	50715	1(2)	51600	1(3)	52305	1(2)	53442	1(2)	54318	1(2)	55175	1(2)	57000	1(3)
50327	1(3)	50722	1(2)	51605	1(3)	52310	1(3)	53444	1(3)	54322	1(2)	55180	1(2)	57010	1(3)
50328	1(3)	50725	1(3)	51610	1(3)	52315	2(3)	53445	1(2)	54324	1(2)	55200	1(2)	57020	1(3)
50329	1(3)	50727	1(3)	51700	1(3)	52317	1(3)	53446	1(2)	54326	1(2)	55250	1(2)	57022	1(3)
50340	1(2)	50728	1(3)	51701	2(3)	52318	1(3)	53447	1(2)	54328	1(2)	55300	1(2)	57023	1(3)
50360	1(2)	50740	1(2)	51702	2(3)	52320	1(2)	53448	1(2)	54332	1(2)	55400	1(2)	57061	1(2)
50365	1(2)	50750	1(2)	51703	2(3)	52325	1(3)	53449	1(2)	54336	1(2)	55450	1(2)	57065	1(2)
50370	1(2)	50760	1(2)	51705	2(3)	52327	1(2)	53450	1(2)	54340	1(2)	55500	1(2)	57100	3(3)
50380	1(2)	50770	1(2)	51710	1(3)	52330	1(2)	53460	1(2)	54344	1(2)	55520	1(2)	57105	2(3)
50382	1(3)	50780	1(2)	51715	1(2)	52332	1(2)	53500	1(2)	54348	1(2)	55530	1(2)	57106	1(2)
50384	1(3)	50782	1(2)	51720	1(2)	52334	1(2)	53502	1(3)	54352	1(2)	55535	1(2)	57107	1(2)
50385	1(3)	50783	1(2)	51725	1(3)	52341	1(2)	53505	1(3)	54360	1(2)	55540	1(2)	57109	1(2)
50386	1(3)	50785	1(2)	51726	1(3)	52342	1(2)	53510	1(3)	54380	1(2)	55550	1(2)	57110	1(2)
50387	1(3)	50810	1(3)	51727	1(3)	52343	1(2)	53515	1(3)	54385	1(2)	55600	1(2)	57111	1(2)
50389	1(3)	50815	1(2)	51728	1(3)	52344	1(2)	53520	1(3)	54390	1(2)	55605	1(2)	57112	1(2)
50390	2(3)	50820	1(2)	51729	1(3)	52345	1(2)	53600	1(3)	54400	1(2)	55650	1(2)	57120	1(2)
50391	1(3)	50825	1(3)	51736	1(3)	52346	1(2)	53601	1(3)	54401	1(2)	55680	1(3)	57130	1(2)
50392	1(3)	50830	1(3)	51741	1(3)	52351	1(3)	53605	1(3)	54405	1(2)	55700	1(2)	57135	2(3)
50393	1(3)	50840	1(2)	51784	1(3)	52352	1(2)	53620	1(2)	54406	1(2)	55705	1(2)	57150	1(3)
50394	1(3)	50845	1(2)	51785	1(3)	52353	1(2)	53621	1(3)	54408	1(2)	55706	1(2)	57155	1(3)
50395	1(2)	50860	1(2)	51792	1(3)	52354	1(3)	53660	1(2)	54410	1(2)	55720	1(3)	57156	1(3)
50396	1(3)	50900	1(3)	51797	1(3)	52355	1(3)	53661	1(3)	54411	1(2)	55725	1(3)	57160	1(2)
50398	1(3)	50920	2(3)	51798	1(3)	52356	1(2)	53665	1(3)	54415	1(2)	55801	1(2)	57170	1(2)
50400	1(2)	50930	2(3)	51800	1(2)	52400	1(2)	53850	1(2)	54416	1(2)	55810	1(2)	57180	1(3)
50405	1(2)	50940	1(2)	51820	1(2)	52402	1(2)	53852	1(2)	54417	1(2)	55812	1(2)	57200	1(3)
50500	1(3)	50945	1(2)	51840	1(2)	52441	1(2)	53855	1(2)	54420	1(2)	55815	1(2)	57210	1(3)
50520	1(3)	50947	1(2)	51841	1(2)	52442	5(1)	53860	1(2)	54430	1(2)	55821	1(2)	57220	1(2)
50525	1(3)	50948	1(2)	51845	1(2)	52450	1(2)	54000	1(2)	54435	1(2)	55831	1(2)	57230	1(2)
50526	1(3)	50951	1(3)	51860	1(3)	52500	1(2)	54001	1(2)	54440	1(2)	55840	1(2)	57240	1(2)
50540	1(2)	50953	1(3)	51865	1(3)	52601	1(2)	54015	1(3)	54450	1(2)	55842	1(2)	57250	1(2)
50541	1(2)	50955	1(2)	51880	1(2)	52630	1(2)	54050	1(2)	54500	1(3)	55845	1(2)	57260	1(2)
50542	1(2)	50957	1(2)	51900	1(3)	52640	1(2)	54055	1(2)	54505	1(3)	55860	1(2)	57265	1(2)
50543	1(2)	50961	1(2)	51920	1(3)	52647	1(2)	54056	1(2)	54512	1(3)	55862	1(2)	57267	2(3)
50544	1(2)	50970	1(3)	51925	1(2)	52648	1(2)	54057	1(2)	54520	1(2)	55865	1(2)	57268	1(2)
50545	1(2)	50972	1(3)	51940	1(2)	52649	1(2)	54060	1(2)	54522	1(2)	55866	1(2)	57270	1(2)
50546	1(2)	50974	1(2)	51960	1(2)	52700	1(3)	54065	1(2)	54530	1(2)	55870	1(2)	57280	1(2)
50547	1(2)	50976	1(2)	51980	1(2)	53000	1(2)	54100	2(3)	54535	1(2)	55873	1(2)	57282	1(2)
50548	1(2)	50980	1(2)	51990	1(2)	53010	1(2)	54105	2(3)	54550	1(2)	55875	1(2)	57283	1(2)
50551	1(3)	51020	1(2)	51992	1(2)	53020	1(2)	54110	1(2)	54560	1(2)	55876	1(2)	57284	1(2)
50553	1(3)	51030	1(2)	52000	1(3)	53025	1(2)	54111	1(2)	54600	1(2)	55920	1(2)	57285	1(2)
50555	1(2)	51040	1(3)	52001	1(3)	53040	1(3)	54112	1(3)	54620	1(2)	56405	2(3)	57287	1(2)
50557	1(2)	51045	2(3)	52005	2(3)	53060	1(3)	54115	1(3)	54640	1(2)	56420	1(3)	57288	1(2)
50561	1(2)	51050	1(3)	52007	1(2)	53080	1(3)	54120	1(2)	54650	1(2)	56440	1(3)	57289	1(2)
50562	1(3)	51060	1(3)	52010	1(2)	53085	1(3)	54125	1(2)	54660	1(2)	56441	1(2)	57291	1(2)
50570	1(3)	51065	1(3)	52204	1(2)	53200	1(3)	54130	1(2)	54670	1(3)	56442	1(2)	57292	1(2)
50572	1(3)	51080	1(3)	52214	1(2)	53210	1(2)	54135	1(3)	54680	1(2)	56501	1(2)	57295	1(2)
50574	1(2)	51100	1(3)	52224	1(2)	53215	1(2)	54150	1(2)	54690	1(2)	56515	1(2)	57296	1(2)
50575	1(2)	51101	1(3)	52234	1(2)	53220	1(3)	54160	1(2)	54692	1(2)	56605	1(2)	57300	1(3)
50576	1(2)	51102	1(3)	52235	1(2)	53230	1(2)	54161	1(2)	54700	1(3)	56606	6(3)	57305	1(3)
50580	1(2)	51500	1(2)	52240	1(2)	53235	1(3)	54162	1(2)	54800	1(2)	56620	1(2)	57307	1(3)
50590	1(2)	51520	1(2)	52250	1(2)	53240	1(3)	54163	1(2)	54830	1(2)	56625	1(2)	57308	1(3)
50592	1(2)	51525	1(2)	52260	1(2)	53250	1(3)	54164	1(2)	54840	1(2)	56630	1(2)	57310	1(3)
50593	1(2)	51530	1(2)	52265	1(2)	53260	1(2)	54200	1(2)	54860	1(2)	56631	1(2)	57311	1(3)
50600	1(3)	51535	1(2)	52270	1(2)	53265	1(3)	54205	1(2)	54861	1(2)	56632	1(2)	57320	1(3)
50605	1(3)	51550	1(2)	52275	1(2)	53270	1(2)	54220	1(3)	54865	1(3)	56633	1(2)	57330	1(3)

CPT	MUE	CPT	MUE	CPT	MUE	CPT	MUE	CPT	MUE	CPT	MUE	CPT	MUE	CPT	MUE
57335	1(2)	58350	1(2)	58958	1(2)	59871	1(2)	61345	1(3)	61605	1(3)	62120	1(2)	63001	1(2)
57400	1(2)	58353	1(3)	58960	1(2)	60000	1(3)	61450	1(3)	61606	1(3)	62121	1(2)	63003	1(2)
57410	1(2)	58356	1(3)	58970	1(3)	60100	3(3)	61458	1(2)	61607	1(3)	62140	1(3)	63005	1(2)
57415	1(3)	58400	1(3)	58974	1(3)	60200	2(3)	61460	1(2)	61608	1(3)	62141	1(3)	63011	1(2)
57420	1(3)	58410	1(2)	58976	2(3)	60210	1(2)	61480	1(2)	61610	1(3)	62142	2(3)	63012	1(2)
57421	1(3)	58520	1(2)	59000	1(3)	60212	1(2)	61500	1(3)	61611	1(3)	62143	2(3)	63015	1(2)
57423	1(2)	58540	1(3)	59001	1(3)	60220	1(3)	61501	1(3)	61612	1(3)	62145	2(3)	63016	1(2)
57425	1(2)	58541	1(3)	59012	1(3)	60225	1(2)	61510	1(3)	61613	1(3)	62146	2(3)	63017	1(2)
57426	1(2)	58542	1(2)	59015	1(3)	60240	1(2)	61512	1(3)	61615	1(3)	62147	1(3)	63020	1(2)
57452	1(3)	58543	1(3)	59020	2(3)	60252	1(2)	61514	2(3)	61616	1(3)	62148	1(3)	63030	1(2)
57454	1(3)	58544	1(2)	59025	3(3)	60254	1(2)	61516	1(3)	61618	2(3)	62160	1(3)	63035	4(3)
57455	1(3)	58545	1(2)	59030	4(3)	60260	1(2)	61517	1(3)	61619	2(3)	62161	1(3)	63040	1(2)
57456	1(3)	58546	1(2)	59050	1(3)	60270	1(2)	61518	1(3)	61623	2(3)	62162	1(3)	63042	1(2)
57460	1(3)	58548	1(2)	59051	1(3)	60271	1(2)	61519	1(3)	61624	2(3)	62163	1(3)	63043	4(3)
57461	1(3)	58550	1(3)	59070	2(3)	60280	1(3)	61520	1(3)	61626	2(3)	62164	1(3)	63044	4(2)
57500	1(3)	58552	1(3)	59072	2(3)	60281	1(3)	61521	1(3)	61630	1(3)	62165	1(2)	63045	1(2)
57505	1(3)	58553	1(3)	59074	1(3)	60300	2(3)	61522	1(3)	61635	2(3)	62180	1(3)	63046	1(2)
57510	1(3)	58554	1(2)	59076	1(3)	60500	1(2)	61524	2(3)	61680	1(3)	62190	1(3)	63047	1(2)
57511	1(3)	58555	1(3)	59100	1(2)	60502	1(3)	61526	1(3)	61682	1(3)	62192	1(3)	63048	5(3)
57513	1(3)	58558	1(3)	59120	1(3)	60505	1(3)	61530	1(3)	61684	1(3)	62194	1(3)	63050	1(2)
57520	1(3)	58559	1(3)	59121	1(3)	60512	1(2)	61531	1(2)	61686	1(3)	62200	1(2)	63051	1(2)
57522	1(3)	58560	1(3)	59130	1(3)	60520	1(2)	61533	2(3)	61690	1(3)	62201	1(2)	63055	1(2)
57530	1(3)	58561	1(3)	59135	1(3)	60521	1(2)	61534	1(3)	61692	1(3)	62220	1(3)	63056	1(2)
57531	1(2)	58562	1(3)	59136	1(3)	60522	1(2)	61535	2(3)	61697	2(3)	62223	1(3)	63057	3(3)
57540	1(2)	58563	1(3)	59140	1(2)	60540	1(2)	61536	1(3)	61698	1(3)	62225	2(3)	63064	1(2)
57545	1(3)	58565	1(2)	59150	1(3)	60545	1(2)	61537	1(3)	61700	2(3)	62230	2(3)	63066	1(3)
57550	1(3)	58570	1(3)	59151	1(3)	60600	1(3)	61538	1(2)	61702	1(3)	62252	2(3)	63075	1(2)
57555	1(2)	58571	1(2)	59160	1(2)	60605	1(3)	61539	1(3)	61703	1(3)	62256	1(3)	63076	3(3)
57556	1(2)	58572	1(3)	59200	1(3)	60650	1(2)	61540	1(3)	61705	1(3)	62258	1(3)	63077	1(2)
57558	1(3)	58573	1(2)	59300	1(2)	61000	1(2)	61541	1(2)	61708	1(3)	62263	1(2)	63078	3(3)
57700	1(3)	58600	1(2)	59320	1(2)	61001	1(2)	61543	1(2)	61710	1(3)	62264	1(2)	63081	1(2)
57720	1(3)	58605	1(2)	59325	1(2)	61020	2(3)	61544	1(3)	61711	1(3)	62267	2(3)	63082	6(2)
57800	1(3)	58611	1(2)	59350	1(2)	61026	2(3)	61545	1(2)	61720	1(3)	62268	1(3)	63085	1(2)
58100	1(3)	58615	1(2)	59400	1(2)	61050	1(3)	61546	1(2)	61735	1(3)	62269	2(3)	63086	2(3)
58110	1(3)	58660	1(2)	59409	2(3)	61055	1(3)	61548	1(2)	61750	2(3)	62270	2(3)	63087	1(2)
58120	1(3)	58661	1(2)	59410	1(2)	61070	2(3)	61550	1(2)	61751	2(3)	62272	2(3)	63088	4(3)
58140	1(3)	58662	1(2)	59412	1(3)	61105	1(3)	61552	1(2)	61760	1(2)	62273	2(3)	63090	1(2)
58145	1(3)	58670	1(2)	59414	1(3)	61107	1(3)	61556	1(3)	61770	1(2)	62280	1(3)	63091	3(3)
58146	1(3)	58671	1(2)	59425	1(2)	61108	1(3)	61557	1(2)	61781	1(3)	62281	1(3)	63101	1(2)
58150	1(3)	58672	1(2)	59426	1(2)	61120	1(3)	61558	1(3)	61782	1(3)	62282	1(3)	63102	1(2)
58152	1(2)	58673	1(2)	59430	1(2)	61140	1(3)	61559	1(3)	61783	1(3)	62284	1(3)	63103	3(3)
58180	1(3)	58700	1(2)	59510	1(3)	61150	1(3)	61563	2(3)	61790	1(2)	62287	1(2)	63170	1(3)
58200	1(2)	58720	1(2)	59514	1(3)	61151	1(3)	61564	1(2)	61791	1(2)	62290	5(2)	63172	1(3)
58210	1(2)	58740	1(2)	59515	1(2)	61154	1(3)	61566	1(3)	61796	1(3)	62291	4(3)	63173	1(3)
58240	1(2)	58750	1(2)	59525	1(2)	61156	1(3)	61567	1(2)	61797	4(3)	62292	1(2)	63180	1(2)
58260	1(3)	58752	1(2)	59610	1(2)	61210	1(3)	61570	1(3)	61798	1(2)	62294	1(3)	63182	1(2)
58262	1(3)	58760	1(2)	59612	2(3)	61215	1(3)	61571	1(3)	61799	4(3)	62302	1(3)	63185	1(2)
58263	1(2)	58770	1(2)	59614	1(2)	61250	1(3)	61575	1(2)	61800	1(2)	62303	1(3)	63190	1(2)
58267	1(2)	58800	1(2)	59618	1(2)	61253	1(3)	61576	1(2)	61850	1(3)	62304	1(3)	63191	1(2)
58270	1(2)	58805	1(2)	59620	1(2)	61304	1(3)	61580	1(2)	61860	1(3)	62305	1(3)	63194	1(2)
58275	1(2)	58820	1(3)	59622	1(2)	61305	1(3)	61581	1(2)	61863	1(3)	62310	1(3)	63195	1(2)
58280	1(2)	58822	1(3)	59812	1(2)	61312	2(3)	61582	1(2)	61864	1(3)	62311	1(3)	63196	1(2)
58285	1(3)	58825	1(2)	59820	1(2)	61313	2(3)	61583	1(2)	61867	1(2)	62318	1(3)	63197	1(2)
58290	1(3)	58900	1(2)	59821	1(2)	61314	2(3)	61584	1(2)	61868	2(3)	62319	1(3)	63198	1(2)
58291	1(2)	58920	1(2)	59830	1(2)	61315	1(3)	61585	1(2)	61870	1(3)	62350	1(3)	63199	1(2)
58292	1(2)	58925	1(3)	59840	1(2)	61316	1(3)	61586	1(3)	61880	1(2)	62351	1(3)	63200	1(2)
58293	1(2)	58940	1(2)	59841	1(2)	61320	2(3)	61590	1(2)	61885	1(3)	62355	1(3)	63250	1(3)
58294	1(2)	58943	1(2)	59850	1(2)	61321	1(3)	61591	1(2)	61886	1(3)	62360	1(2)	63251	1(3)
58301	1(3)	58950	1(2)	59851	1(2)	61322	1(3)	61592	1(2)	61888	1(3)	62361	1(2)	63252	1(3)
58321	1(2)	58951	1(2)	59852	1(2)	61323	1(3)	61595	1(2)	62000	1(3)	62362	1(2)	63265	1(3)
58322	1(2)	58952	1(2)	59855	1(2)	61330	1(2)	61596	1(2)	62005	1(3)	62365	1(2)	63266	1(3)
58323	1(3)	58953	1(2)	59856	1(2)	61332	1(2)	61597	1(2)	62010	1(3)	62367	1(3)	63267	1(3)
58340	1(3)	58954	1(2)	59857	1(2)	61333	1(2)	61598	1(3)	62100	1(3)	62368	1(3)	63268	1(3)
58345	1(3)	58956	1(2)	59866	1(2)	61340	1(2)	61600	1(3)	62115	1(2)	62369	1(3)	63270	1(3)
58346	1(2)	58957	1(2)	59870	1(2)	61343	1(2)	61601	1(3)	62117	1(2)	62370	1(3)	63271	1(3)

CPT	MUE	CPT	MUE	CPT	MUE	CPT	MUE	CPT	MUE	CPT	MUE	CPT	MUE	CPT	MUE
63272	1(3)	64446	1(2)	64680	1(2)	64868	1(3)	65770	1(2)	66930	1(2)	67420	1(2)	68325	1(2)
63273	1(3)	64447	1(3)	64681	1(2)	64872	1(3)	65772	1(2)	66940	1(2)	67430	1(2)	68326	2(2)
63275	1(3)	64448	1(2)	64702	2(3)	64874	1(3)	65775	1(2)	66982	1(2)	67440	1(2)	68328	2(2)
63276	1(3)	64449	1(2)	64704	4(3)	64876	1(3)	65778	1(2)	66983	1(2)	67445	1(2)	68330	1(3)
63277	1(3)	64450	10(3)	64708	3(3)	64885	1(3)	65779	1(2)	66984	1(2)	67450	1(2)	68335	1(3)
63278	1(3)	64455	1(2)	64712	1(2)	64886	1(3)	65780	1(2)	66985	1(2)	67500	1(3)	68340	1(3)
63280	1(3)	64479	1(2)	64713	1(2)	64890	2(3)	65781	1(2)	66986	1(2)	67505	1(3)	68360	1(3)
63281	1(3)	64480	4(3)	64714	1(2)	64891	2(3)	65782	1(2)	66990	1(3)	67515	1(3)	68362	1(3)
63282	1(3)	64483	1(2)	64716	2(3)	64892	2(3)	65800	1(2)	67005	1(2)	67550	1(2)	68371	1(3)
63283	1(3)	64484	4(3)	64718	1(2)	64893	2(3)	65810	1(2)	67010	1(2)	67560	1(2)	68400	1(2)
63285	1(3)	64486	1(3)	64719	1(2)	64895	2(3)	65815	1(3)	67015	1(2)	67570	1(2)	68420	1(2)
63286	1(3)	64487	1(2)	64721	1(2)	64896	2(3)	65820	1(2)	67025	1(2)	67700	2(3)	68440	2(2)
63287	1(3)	64488	1(3)	64722	4(3)	64897	2(3)	65850	1(2)	67027	1(2)	67710	1(2)	68500	1(2)
63290	1(3)	64489	1(2)	64726	2(3)	64898	2(3)	65855	1(2)	67028	1(3)	67715	1(3)	68505	1(2)
63295	1(2)	64490	1(2)	64727	2(3)	64901	2(3)	65860	1(2)	67030	1(2)	67800	1(2)	68510	1(2)
63300	1(2)	64491	1(2)	64732	1(2)	64902	1(3)	65865	1(2)	67031	1(2)	67801	1(2)	68520	1(2)
63301	1(2)	64492	1(2)	64734	1(2)	64905	1(3)	65870	1(2)	67036	1(2)	67805	1(2)	68525	1(2)
63302	1(2)	64493	1(2)	64736	1(2)	64907	1(3)	65875	1(2)	67039	1(2)	67808	1(2)	68530	1(2)
63303	1(2)	64494	1(2)	64738	1(2)	64910	3(3)	65880	1(2)	67040	1(2)	67810	2(3)	68540	1(2)
63304	1(2)	64495	1(2)	64740	1(2)	64911	2(3)	65900	1(3)	67041	1(2)	67820	1(2)	68550	1(2)
63305	1(2)	64505	1(3)	64742	1(2)	65091	1(2)	65920	1(2)	67042	1(2)	67825	1(2)	68700	1(2)
63306	1(2)	64508	1(3)	64744	1(2)	65093	1(2)	65930	1(3)	67043	1(2)	67830	1(2)	68705	2(2)
63307	1(2)	64510	1(3)	64746	1(2)	65101	1(2)	66020	1(3)	67101	1(2)	67835	1(2)	68720	1(2)
63308	3(3)	64517	1(3)	64755	1(2)	65103	1(2)	66030	1(3)	67105	1(2)	67840	4(3)	68745	1(2)
63600	2(3)	64520	1(3)	64760	1(2)	65105	1(2)	66130	1(3)	67107	1(2)	67850	3(3)	68750	1(2)
63610	1(3)	64530	1(3)	64763	1(2)	65110	1(2)	66150	1(2)	67108	1(2)	67875	1(2)	68760	4(2)
63615	1(3)	64550	1(3)	64766	1(2)	65112	1(2)	66155	1(2)	67110	1(2)	67880	1(2)	68761	4(2)
63620	1(2)	64553	1(3)	64771	2(3)	65114	1(2)	66160	1(2)	67112	1(2)	67882	1(2)	68770	1(3)
63621	2(2)	64555	2(3)	64772	2(3)	65125	1(2)	66170	1(2)	67113	1(2)	67900	1(2)	68801	4(2)
63650	2(3)	64561	1(3)	64774	2(3)	65130	1(2)	66172	1(2)	67115	1(2)	67901	1(2)	68810	1(2)
63655	1(3)	64565	2(3)	64776	1(2)	65135	1(2)	66174	1(2)	67120	1(2)	67902	1(2)	68811	1(2)
63661	1(2)	64566	1(3)	64778	1(3)	65140	1(2)	66175	1(2)	67121	1(2)	67903	1(2)	68815	1(2)
63662	1(2)	64568	1(3)	64782	2(2)	65150	1(2)	66179	1(2)	67141	1(2)	67904	1(2)	68816	1(2)
63663	1(3)	64569	1(3)	64783	2(3)	65155	1(2)	66180	1(2)	67145	1(2)	67906	1(2)	68840	1(2)
63664	1(3)	64570	1(3)	64784	3(3)	65175	1(2)	66183	1(3)	67208	1(2)	67908	1(2)	68850	1(3)
63685	1(3)	64575	2(3)	64786	1(3)	65205	1(3)	66184	1(2)	67210	1(2)	67909	1(2)	69000	1(3)
63688	1(3)	64580	2(3)	64787	4(3)	65210	1(3)	66185	1(3)	67218	1(2)	67911	4(2)	69005	1(3)
63700	1(3)	64581	2(3)	64788	5(3)	65220	1(3)	66220	1(2)	67220	1(2)	67912	1(2)	69020	1(3)
63702	1(3)	64585	2(3)	64790	1(3)	65222	1(3)	66225	1(2)	67221	1(2)	67914	1(3)	69100	3(3)
63704	1(3)	64590	1(3)	64792	2(3)	65235	1(3)	66250	1(2)	67225	1(2)	67915	1(3)	69105	1(3)
63706	1(3)	64595	1(3)	64795	2(3)	65260	1(3)	66500	1(2)	67227	1(2)	67916	1(3)	69110	1(2)
63707	1(3)	64600	2(3)	64802	1(2)	65265	1(3)	66505	1(2)	67228	1(2)	67917	1(3)	69120	1(3)
63709	1(3)	64605	1(2)	64804	1(2)	65270	1(3)	66600	1(2)	67229	1(2)	67921	1(3)	69140	1(2)
63710	1(3)	64610	1(2)	64809	1(2)	65272	1(3)	66605	1(2)	67250	1(2)	67922	1(3)	69145	1(3)
63740	1(3)	64611	1(2)	64818	1(2)	65273	1(3)	66625	1(2)	67255	1(2)	67923	1(3)	69150	1(3)
63741	1(3)	64612	1(2)	64820	4(3)	65275	1(3)	66630	1(2)	67311	1(2)	67924	1(3)	69155	1(3)
63744	1(3)	64615	1(2)	64821	1(2)	65280	1(3)	66635	1(2)	67312	1(2)	67930	2(3)	69200	1(2)
63746	1(2)	64616	1(2)	64822	1(2)	65285	1(3)	66680	1(2)	67314	1(2)	67935	2(3)	69205	1(3)
64400	4(3)	64617	1(2)	64823	1(2)	65286	1(3)	66682	1(2)	67316	1(2)	67938	2(3)	69210	1(2)
64402	1(3)	64620	5(3)	64831	1(2)	65290	1(3)	66700	1(2)	67318	1(2)	67950	2(2)	69220	1(2)
64405	1(3)	64630	1(3)	64832	3(3)	65400	1(3)	66710	1(2)	67320	2(3)	67961	4(2)	69222	1(2)
64408	1(3)	64632	1(2)	64834	1(2)	65410	1(3)	66711	1(2)	67331	1(2)	67966	4(2)	69300	1(2)
64410	1(3)	64633	1(2)	64835	1(2)	65420	1(2)	66720	1(2)	67332	1(2)	67971	1(2)	69310	1(2)
64412	1(3)	64634	4(3)	64836	1(2)	65426	1(2)	66740	1(2)	67334	1(2)	67973	1(2)	69320	1(2)
64413	1(3)	64635	1(2)	64837	2(3)	65430	1(2)	66761	1(2)	67335	1(2)	67974	1(2)	69420	1(2)
64415	1(3)	64636	4(2)	64840	1(2)	65435	1(2)	66762	1(2)	67340	2(2)	67975	1(2)	69421	1(2)
64416	1(2)	64640	5(3)	64856	2(3)	65436	1(2)	66770	1(3)	67343	1(2)	68020	1(3)	69424	1(2)
64417	1(3)	64642	1(2)	64857	2(3)	65450	1(3)	66820	1(2)	67345	1(3)	68040	1(2)	69433	1(2)
64418	1(3)	64643	3(2)	64858	1(2)	65600	1(2)	66821	1(2)	67346	1(3)	68100	1(3)	69436	1(2)
64420	3(3)	64644	1(2)	64859	2(3)	65710	1(2)	66825	1(2)	67400	1(2)	68110	1(3)	69440	1(2)
64421	3(3)	64645	3(2)	64861	1(2)	65730	1(2)	66830	1(2)	67405	1(2)	68115	1(3)	69450	1(2)
64425	1(3)	64646	1(2)	64862	1(2)	65750	1(2)	66840	1(2)	67412	1(2)	68130	1(3)	69501	1(3)
64430	1(3)	64647	1(2)	64864	2(3)	65755	1(2)	66850	1(2)	67413	1(2)	68135	1(3)	69502	1(2)
64435	1(3)	64650	1(2)	64865	1(3)	65756	1(2)	66852	1(2)	67414	1(2)	68200	1(3)	69505	1(2)
64445	1(3)	64653	1(2)	64866	1(3)	65757	1(3)	66920	1(2)	67415	1(3)	68320	1(2)	69511	1(2)

CPT	MUE	CPT	MUE	CPT	MUE	CPT	MUE	CPT	MUE	CPT	MUE	CPT	MUE	CPT	MUE
69530	1(2)	70140	1(1)	71101	1(1)	73010	2(1)	74170	1(1)	75571	1(1)	76001	2(1)	77001	2(1)
69535	1(2)	70150	1(1)	71110	1(1)	73020	2(1)	74174	1(1)	75572	1(1)	76010	2(1)	77002	1(3)
69540	1(3)	70160	1(1)	71111	1(1)	73030	2(1)	74175	1(1)	75573	1(3)	76080	2(1)	77003	1(3)
69550	1(3)	70170	2(2)	71120	1(1)	73040	2(2)	74176	1(1)	75574	1(1)	76100	2(1)	77011	1(1)
69552	1(2)	70190	1(2)	71130	1(1)	73050	1(1)	74177	1(1)	75600	1(3)	76101	1(1)	77012	1(3)
69554	1(2)	70200	1(1)	71250	1(1)	73060	2(1)	74178	1(1)	75605	1(1)	76102	1(3)	77013	1(1)
69601	1(2)	70210	1(1)	71260	1(1)	73070	2(1)	74181	1(1)	75625	1(1)	76120	1(1)	77014	2(1)
69602	1(2)	70220	1(1)	71270	1(1)	73080	2(1)	74182	1(1)	75630	1(1)	76125	1(1)	77021	1(3)
69603	1(2)	70240	1(2)	71275	1(1)	73085	2(2)	74183	1(1)	75635	1(1)	76376	2(1)	77022	1(3)
69604	1(2)	70250	1(1)	71550	1(1)	73090	2(1)	74185	1(1)	75658	2(1)	76377	2(1)	77051	1(1)
69605	1(2)	70260	1(1)	71551	1(3)	73092	2(1)	74190	1(1)	75710	1(1)	76380	2(1)	77052	1(2)
69610	1(2)	70300	1(1)	71552	1(1)	73100	2(1)	74210	1(3)	75716	1(1)	76506	1(2)	77053	2(2)
69620	1(2)	70310	1(3)	71555	1(1)	73110	2(1)	74220	1(1)	75726	3(1)	76510	2(2)	77054	2(2)
69631	1(2)	70320	1(1)	72010	1(2)	73115	2(2)	74230	1(1)	75731	1(3)	76511	2(2)	77055	1(1)
69632	1(3)	70328	1(1)	72020	4(1)	73120	2(1)	74235	1(3)	75733	1(3)	76512	2(2)	77056	1(1)
69633	1(2)	70330	1(1)	72040	3(1)	73130	2(1)	74240	1(1)	75736	2(1)	76513	2(2)	77057	1(2)
69635	1(3)	70332	2(1)	72050	1(1)	73140	2(1)	74241	1(1)	75741	1(3)	76514	1(2)	77058	1(2)
69636	1(3)	70336	1(1)	72052	1(1)	73200	2(1)	74245	1(1)	75743	1(1)	76516	1(2)	77059	1(2)
69637	1(3)	70350	1(1)	72069	1(2)	73201	2(1)	74246	1(1)	75746	1(1)	76519	2(2)	77061	1(2)
69641	1(2)	70355	1(1)	72070	1(1)	73202	2(1)	74247	1(1)	75756	2(1)	76529	2(2)	77062	1(2)
69642	1(2)	70360	1(1)	72072	1(1)	73206	2(1)	74249	1(1)	75791	1(1)	76536	1(1)	77063	1(2)
69643	1(2)	70370	1(3)	72074	1(1)	73218	2(1)	74250	1(1)	75801	1(1)	76604	1(1)	77071	1(3)
69644	1(2)	70371	1(2)	72080	1(1)	73219	2(1)	74251	1(3)	75803	1(3)	76641	2(2)	77072	1(2)
69645	1(2)	70373	1(3)	72090	1(1)	73220	2(1)	74260	1(2)	75805	1(2)	76642	2(2)	77073	1(2)
69646	1(2)	70380	2(3)	72100	1(1)	73221	2(1)	74261	1(2)	75807	1(2)	76700	1(1)	77074	1(2)
69650	1(2)	70390	2(3)	72110	1(1)	73222	2(1)	74262	1(2)	75809	1(3)	76705	2(1)	77075	1(2)
69660	1(2)	70450	3(1)	72114	1(1)	73223	2(1)	74270	1(1)	75810	1(3)	76770	1(1)	77076	1(2)
69661	1(2)	70460	1(1)	72120	1(1)	73500	1(1)	74280	1(1)	75820	1(1)	76775	2(1)	77077	1(2)
69662	1(2)	70470	2(1)	72125	1(1)	73510	2(1)	74283	1(3)	75822	1(1)	76776	1(1)	77078	1(2)
69666	1(2)	70480	1(1)	72126	1(1)	73520	2(1)	74290	1(3)	75825	1(1)	76800	1(1)	77080	1(2)
69667	1(2)	70481	1(1)	72127	1(1)	73525	2(2)	74300	1(1)	75827	1(1)	76801	1(2)	77081	1(2)
69670	1(2)	70482	1(1)	72128	1(1)	73530	2(3)	74301	2(1)	75831	1(1)	76802	3(1)	77084	1(2)
69676	1(2)	70486	1(1)	72129	1(1)	73540	1(1)	74305	1(1)	75833	1(1)	76805	1(2)	77085	1(2)
69700	1(3)	70487	1(1)	72130	1(1)	73550	2(1)	74320	1(1)	75840	1(3)	76810	3(1)	77086	1(2)
69711	1(2)	70488	1(1)	72131	1(1)	73560	2(1)	74327	1(3)	75842	1(3)	76811	1(2)	77261	1(3)
69714	1(2)	70490	1(1)	72132	1(1)	73562	2(1)	74328	1(1)	75860	2(1)	76812	3(1)	77262	1(3)
69715	1(3)	70491	1(1)	72133	1(1)	73564	2(1)	74329	1(1)	75870	1(1)	76813	1(2)	77263	1(3)
69717	1(2)	70492	1(1)	72141	1(1)	73565	1(1)	74330	1(1)	75872	1(3)	76814	3(1)	77280	2(3)
69718	1(2)	70496	1(1)	72142	1(1)	73580	2(2)	74340	1(1)	75880	2(1)	76815	1(2)	77285	1(3)
69720	1(2)	70498	1(1)	72146	1(1)	73590	2(1)	74355	1(3)	75885	1(3)	76817	1(1)	77290	1(3)
69725	1(2)	70540	1(1)	72147	1(1)	73592	2(1)	74360	1(1)	75887	1(3)	76830	1(1)	77293	1(3)
69740	1(2)	70542	1(1)	72148	1(1)	73600	2(1)	74363	2(1)	75889	1(1)	76831	1(3)	77295	1(3)
69745	1(2)	70543	1(1)	72149	1(1)	73610	2(1)	74400	1(1)	75891	1(1)	76856	1(1)	77300	10(3)
69801	1(3)	70544	1(1)	72156	1(1)	73615	2(2)	74410	1(1)	75896	3(1)	76857	1(1)	77301	1(3)
69805	1(3)	70545	1(1)	72157	1(1)	73620	2(1)	74415	1(1)	75898	1(1)	76870	1(2)	77306	1(3)
69806	1(3)	70546	1(1)	72158	1(1)	73630	2(1)	74420	2(1)	75901	1(1)	76872	1(1)	77307	1(3)
69820	1(2)	70547	1(1)	72170	1(1)	73650	2(1)	74425	1(1)	75902	2(1)	76873	1(2)	77316	1(3)
69840	1(3)	70548	1(1)	72190	1(1)	73660	2(1)	74430	1(1)	75945	1(3)	76881	2(1)	77317	1(3)
69905	1(2)	70549	1(1)	72191	1(1)	73700	2(1)	74440	1(2)	75952	1(2)	76882	2(1)	77318	1(3)
69910	1(2)	70551	1(1)	72192	1(1)	73701	2(1)	74445	1(2)	75953	4(1)	76885	1(2)	77321	1(2)
69915	1(3)	70552	1(1)	72193	1(1)	73702	2(1)	74450	1(1)	75954	2(3)	76886	1(2)	77331	3(3)
69930	1(2)	70553	1(1)	72194	1(1)	73706	2(1)	74455	1(1)	75956	1(2)	76930	1(1)	77332	4(3)
69950	1(2)	70554	1(3)	72195	1(1)	73718	2(1)	74470	2(2)	75957	1(2)	76932	1(2)	77333	2(3)
69955	1(2)	70555	1(3)	72196	1(1)	73719	2(1)	74475	2(1)	75958	2(1)	76936	2(1)	77336	1(2)
69960	1(2)	70557	1(3)	72197	1(1)	73720	2(1)	74480	2(1)	75959	1(2)	76937	2(1)	77338	1(3)
69970	1(3)	70558	1(3)	72198	1(1)	73721	4(1)	74485	2(1)	75962	1(1)	76940	1(1)	77370	1(3)
69990	1(3)	70559	1(3)	72200	1(1)	73722	2(1)	74710	1(3)	75964	4(1)	76942	1(3)	77371	1(2)
70010	1(3)	71015	2(1)	72202	1(1)	73723	4(1)	74740	1(3)	75966	1(1)	76945	1(3)	77372	1(2)
70015	1(1)	71021	1(1)	72220	1(1)	73725	2(1)	74742	2(2)	75968	2(1)	76946	1(3)	77373	1(3)
70030	2(2)	71022	1(1)	72240	1(2)	74000	3(1)	74775	1(2)	75970	2(1)	76948	1(2)	77385	2(3)
70100	1(1)	71023	2(1)	72255	1(2)	74010	2(1)	75557	1(3)	75980	1(1)	76965	2(1)	77386	2(3)
70110	1(1)	71030	2(1)	72265	1(2)	74020	2(1)	75559	1(3)	75982	2(1)	76970	1(1)	77387	2(3)
70120	2(1)	71034	1(1)	72270	1(2)	74022	2(1)	75561	1(1)	75984	2(1)	76975	1(3)	77401	1(2)
70130	2(1)	71035	2(1)	72275	3(1)	74150	1(1)	75563	1(3)	75989	2(1)	76977	1(2)	77402	2(3)
70134	1(3)	71100	1(1)	73000	2(1)	74160	1(1)	75565	1(1)	76000	3(1)	76998	1(1)	77407	2(3)

© 2015 Optum360, LLC

CPT	MUE	CPT	MUE	CPT	MUE	CPT	MUE	CPT	MUE	CPT	MUE	CPT	MUE	CPT	MUE
77412	2(3)	78226	1(3)	78707	1(2)	80194	2(3)	81222	1(3)	81324	1(3)	81519	1(2)	82374	3(1)
77417	1(2)	78227	1(3)	78708	1(2)	80195	2(3)	81223	1(2)	81325	1(3)	82009	3(3)	82375	4(3)
77422	1(3)	78230	1(3)	78709	1(2)	80197	2(3)	81224	1(3)	81326	1(3)	82010	3(3)	82376	2(1)
77423	1(3)	78231	1(3)	78710	1(3)	80198	2(3)	81225	1(3)	81330	1(3)	82013	1(3)	82378	1(3)
77424	1(2)	78232	1(3)	78725	1(3)	80199	1(3)	81226	1(3)	81331	1(3)	82016	1(3)	82379	1(3)
77425	1(3)	78258	1(2)	78730	1(2)	80200	2(3)	81227	1(3)	81332	1(3)	82017	1(3)	82380	1(3)
77427	1(2)	78261	1(2)	78740	1(2)	80201	2(3)	81228	1(3)	81340	1(3)	82024	4(3)	82382	1(2)
77431	1(2)	78262	1(2)	78761	1(2)	80202	2(3)	81229	1(3)	81341	1(3)	82030	1(3)	82383	1(3)
77432	1(2)	78264	1(2)	78800	1(2)	80203	1(3)	81235	1(3)	81342	1(3)	82040	1(3)	82384	2(3)
77435	1(2)	78267	1(2)	78801	1(2)	80299	3(3)	81240	1(2)	81350	1(3)	82042	2(3)	82387	1(3)
77469	1(2)	78268	1(2)	78802	1(2)	80400	1(3)	81241	1(2)	81355	1(3)	82043	1(3)	82390	1(2)
77470	1(2)	78270	1(2)	78803	1(2)	80402	1(3)	81242	1(3)	81370	1(2)	82044	1(3)	82397	4(3)
77520	1(3)	78271	1(2)	78804	1(2)	80406	1(3)	81243	1(3)	81371	1(2)	82045	1(3)	82415	1(3)
77522	1(3)	78272	1(2)	78805	1(3)	80408	1(3)	81244	1(3)	81372	1(2)	82075	2(3)	82435	3(1)
77523	1(3)	78278	2(3)	78806	1(2)	80410	1(3)	81245	1(3)	81373	2(2)	82085	1(3)	82436	1(3)
77525	1(3)	78282	1(2)	78807	1(3)	80412	1(3)	81246	1(3)	81374	1(3)	82088	2(3)	82438	1(3)
77600	1(3)	78290	1(3)	78808	1(2)	80414	1(3)	81250	1(3)	81375	1(2)	82103	1(3)	82441	1(2)
77605	1(3)	78291	1(3)	78811	1(2)	80415	1(3)	81251	1(3)	81376	5(3)	82104	1(2)	82465	1(3)
77610	1(3)	78300	1(2)	78812	1(2)	80416	1(3)	81252	1(3)	81377	2(3)	82105	1(3)	82480	2(3)
77615	1(3)	78305	1(2)	78813	1(2)	80417	1(3)	81253	1(3)	81378	1(2)	82106	2(3)	82482	1(3)
77750	1(3)	78306	1(2)	78814	1(2)	80418	1(3)	81254	1(3)	81379	1(2)	82107	1(3)	82485	1(3)
77761	1(3)	78315	1(2)	78815	1(2)	80420	1(2)	81255	1(3)	81380	2(2)	82108	1(3)	82486	2(3)
77762	1(3)	78320	1(2)	78816	1(2)	80422	1(3)	81256	1(2)	81381	3(3)	82120	1(3)	82487	1(3)
77763	1(3)	78414	1(2)	79005	1(3)	80424	1(3)	81257	1(2)	81382	6(3)	82127	1(3)	82488	1(3)
77776	1(3)	78428	1(3)	79101	1(3)	80426	1(3)	81260	1(3)	81383	2(3)	82128	2(3)	82489	2(3)
77777	1(3)	78445	1(3)	79200	1(3)	80428	1(3)	81261	1(3)	81400	2(3)	82131	2(3)	82491	4(3)
77778	1(3)	78451	1(2)	79300	1(3)	80430	1(3)	81262	1(3)	81401	3(3)	82135	1(3)	82492	2(3)
77785	2(3)	78452	1(2)	79403	1(3)	80432	1(3)	81263	1(3)	81402	1(3)	82136	2(3)	82495	1(3)
77786	3(3)	78453	1(2)	79440	1(3)	80434	1(3)	81264	1(3)	81403	3(3)	82139	2(3)	82507	1(3)
77787	3(3)	78454	1(2)	79445	1(3)	80435	1(3)	81265	1(3)	81404	3(3)	82140	2(3)	82523	1(3)
77789	2(3)	78456	1(3)	80047	2(3)	80436	1(3)	81266	2(3)	81405	2(3)	82143	2(3)	82525	2(3)
77790	2(1)	78457	1(2)	80048	2(3)	80438	1(3)	81267	1(3)	81406	3(3)	82150	4(3)	82528	1(3)
78012	1(3)	78458	1(2)	80051	4(3)	80439	1(3)	81268	4(3)	81407	1(3)	82154	1(3)	82530	4(3)
78013	1(3)	78459	1(3)	80053	1(3)	80500	1(3)	81270	1(2)	81408	1(3)	82157	1(3)	82533	5(3)
78014	1(2)	78466	1(3)	80061	1(3)	80502	1(3)	81275	1(3)	81410	1(3)	82160	1(3)	82540	1(3)
78015	1(3)	78468	1(3)	80069	1(3)	81000	2(3)	81280	1(3)	81411	1(3)	82163	1(3)	82541	4(3)
78016	1(3)	78469	1(3)	80074	1(2)	81001	2(3)	81281	1(3)	81415	1(1)	82164	1(3)	82542	6(3)
78018	1(2)	78472	1(2)	80076	1(3)	81002	2(3)	81282	1(3)	81416	2(1)	82172	3(3)	82543	2(3)
78020	1(3)	78473	1(2)	80150	2(3)	81003	2(3)	81287	1(3)	81417	1(1)	82175	2(3)	82544	2(3)
78070	1(2)	78481	1(2)	80155	1(3)	81005	2(1)	81288	1(3)	81420	1(3)	82180	1(2)	82550	3(3)
78071	1(3)	78483	1(2)	80156	2(3)	81007	1(3)	81290	1(3)	81425	1(1)	82190	2(3)	82552	3(3)
78072	1(3)	78491	1(3)	80157	2(3)	81015	2(3)	81291	1(3)	81426	2(1)	82232	2(3)	82553	3(3)
78075	1(2)	78492	1(2)	80158	3(1)	81020	1(3)	81292	1(2)	81427	1(1)	82239	2(3)	82554	2(3)
78102	1(2)	78494	1(3)	80159	2(3)	81025	1(3)	81293	1(3)	81430	1(2)	82240	1(3)	82565	3(1)
78103	1(2)	78496	1(3)	80162	2(3)	81050	2(1)	81294	1(3)	81431	1(2)	82247	2(3)	82570	3(3)
78104	1(2)	78579	1(3)	80163	2(3)	81161	1(3)	81295	1(2)	81435	1(2)	82248	2(3)	82575	1(3)
78110	1(2)	78580	1(3)	80164	2(3)	81200	1(2)	81296	1(3)	81436	1(2)	82252	1(3)	82585	1(2)
78111	1(2)	78582	1(3)	80165	2(3)	81201	1(2)	81297	1(3)	81440	1(2)	82261	1(3)	82595	1(3)
78120	1(2)	78597	1(3)	80168	2(3)	81202	1(3)	81298	1(2)	81445	1(2)	82270	1(3)	82600	1(3)
78121	1(2)	78598	1(3)	80169	2(3)	81203	1(3)	81299	1(3)	81450	1(2)	82271	3(3)	82607	1(2)
78122	1(2)	78600	1(3)	80170	2(3)	81205	1(3)	81300	1(3)	81455	1(2)	82272	1(3)	82608	1(2)
78130	1(2)	78601	1(3)	80171	1(3)	81206	1(3)	81301	1(3)	81460	1(2)	82274	1(3)	82610	1(3)
78135	1(3)	78605	1(3)	80173	2(3)	81207	1(3)	81302	1(3)	81465	1(2)	82286	1(3)	82615	1(3)
78140	1(3)	78606	1(3)	80175	1(3)	81208	1(3)	81303	1(3)	81470	1(2)	82300	1(3)	82626	1(3)
78185	1(2)	78607	1(3)	80176	1(3)	81209	1(3)	81304	1(3)	81471	1(2)	82306	1(2)	82627	1(3)
78190	1(2)	78608	1(3)	80177	1(3)	81210	1(3)	81310	1(3)	81500	1(3)	82308	1(3)	82633	1(3)
78191	1(2)	78610	1(3)	80178	2(3)	81211	1(2)	81313	1(3)	81503	1(3)	82310	4(3)	82634	1(3)
78195	1(2)	78630	1(3)	80180	1(3)	81212	1(2)	81315	1(3)	81504	1(3)	82330	4(3)	82638	1(3)
78201	1(3)	78635	1(3)	80183	1(3)	81213	1(2)	81316	1(3)	81506	1(3)	82331	1(3)	82652	1(2)
78202	1(3)	78645	1(3)	80184	2(3)	81214	1(2)	81317	1(3)	81507	1(3)	82340	1(3)	82656	1(3)
78205	1(3)	78647	1(3)	80185	2(3)	81215	1(2)	81318	1(3)	81508	1(3)	82355	2(3)	82657	3(3)
78206	1(3)	78650	1(3)	80186	2(3)	81216	1(2)	81319	1(2)	81509	1(3)	82360	2(3)	82658	2(3)
78215	1(3)	78660	1(2)	80188	2(3)	81217	1(2)	81321	1(3)	81510	1(3)	82365	2(3)	82664	2(3)
78216	1(3)	78700	1(3)	80190	2(3)	81220	1(3)	81322	1(3)	81511	1(3)	82370	2(3)	82668	1(3)
		78701	1(3)	80192	2(3)	81221	1(3)	81323	1(3)	81512	1(3)	82373	1(3)	82670	2(3)

CPT	MUE	CPT	MUE	CPT	MUE	CPT	MUE	CPT	MUE	CPT	MUE	CPT	MUE	CPT	MUE
82671	1(3)	83050	2(3)	83874	4(3)	84206	1(2)	84580	1(3)	85347	9(3)	86147	4(3)	86485	1(2)
82672	1(3)	83051	1(3)	83876	1(3)	84207	1(2)	84583	1(3)	85348	4(3)	86148	3(3)	86486	2(3)
82677	1(3)	83060	1(3)	83880	1(3)	84210	1(3)	84585	1(2)	85360	1(3)	86152	1(3)	86490	1(2)
82679	1(3)	83065	1(2)	83883	6(3)	84220	1(3)	84586	1(2)	85362	2(3)	86153	1(3)	86510	1(2)
82693	2(3)	83068	1(2)	83885	2(3)	84228	1(3)	84588	1(3)	85366	1(3)	86155	1(3)	86580	1(2)
82696	1(3)	83069	1(3)	83915	1(3)	84233	1(3)	84590	1(2)	85370	1(3)	86156	1(2)	86590	1(3)
82705	1(3)	83070	1(2)	83916	2(3)	84234	1(3)	84591	1(3)	85378	2(3)	86157	1(2)	86592	2(3)
82710	1(3)	83080	2(3)	83918	2(3)	84235	1(3)	84597	1(3)	85379	2(3)	86160	4(3)	86593	2(3)
82715	3(3)	83088	1(3)	83919	1(3)	84238	3(3)	84600	2(3)	85380	2(3)	86161	2(3)	86602	3(3)
82725	1(3)	83090	2(3)	83921	2(1)	84244	2(3)	84620	1(2)	85384	2(3)	86162	1(2)	86603	2(3)
82726	1(3)	83150	1(3)	83930	2(3)	84252	1(2)	84630	2(3)	85385	1(3)	86171	2(3)	86609	14(3)
82728	1(3)	83491	1(3)	83935	2(3)	84255	2(3)	84681	1(3)	85390	3(3)	86185	1(3)	86611	4(3)
82731	1(3)	83497	1(3)	83937	1(3)	84260	1(3)	84702	2(3)	85396	1(2)	86200	1(3)	86612	2(3)
82735	1(3)	83498	2(3)	83945	2(3)	84270	1(3)	84703	1(3)	85397	3(3)	86215	1(3)	86615	6(3)
82746	1(2)	83499	1(3)	83950	1(2)	84275	1(3)	84704	1(3)	85400	1(3)	86225	1(3)	86617	2(3)
82747	1(2)	83500	1(3)	83951	1(2)	84285	1(3)	84830	1(2)	85410	1(3)	86226	1(3)	86618	2(3)
82757	1(2)	83505	1(3)	83970	4(3)	84295	4(1)	85002	1(3)	85415	2(3)	86235	10(3)	86619	2(3)
82759	1(3)	83516	5(3)	83986	2(3)	84300	2(3)	85004	2(3)	85420	2(3)	86243	1(3)	86622	2(3)
82760	1(3)	83518	1(3)	83987	1(3)	84302	3(1)	85007	1(3)	85421	1(3)	86255	5(3)	86625	1(3)
82775	1(3)	83519	5(3)	83992	2(3)	84305	1(3)	85008	1(3)	85441	1(2)	86256	9(3)	86628	3(3)
82776	1(2)	83520	8(3)	83993	1(3)	84307	1(3)	85009	1(3)	85445	1(2)	86277	1(3)	86631	6(3)
82777	1(3)	83525	4(3)	84030	1(2)	84311	2(3)	85013	1(3)	85460	1(3)	86280	1(3)	86632	3(3)
82784	6(3)	83527	1(3)	84035	1(2)	84315	1(3)	85014	4(3)	85461	1(2)	86294	1(3)	86635	4(3)
82785	1(3)	83528	1(3)	84060	1(3)	84375	1(3)	85018	4(3)	85475	1(3)	86300	2(3)	86638	6(3)
82787	4(3)	83540	2(3)	84061	1(3)	84376	1(3)	85025	4(3)	85520	3(3)	86301	1(2)	86641	2(3)
82800	2(1)	83550	1(3)	84066	1(3)	84377	1(3)	85027	4(3)	85525	2(3)	86304	1(2)	86644	2(3)
82810	4(3)	83570	1(3)	84075	2(3)	84378	2(3)	85032	2(3)	85530	1(3)	86305	1(2)	86645	1(3)
82820	1(3)	83582	1(3)	84078	1(2)	84379	1(3)	85041	1(3)	85536	1(2)	86308	1(2)	86648	2(3)
82930	1(1)	83586	1(3)	84080	1(3)	84392	1(3)	85044	1(2)	85540	1(2)	86309	1(2)	86651	2(3)
82938	1(3)	83593	1(3)	84081	1(3)	84402	1(3)	85045	1(2)	85547	1(2)	86310	1(2)	86652	2(3)
82941	1(3)	83605	3(1)	84085	1(2)	84403	2(3)	85046	1(2)	85549	1(3)	86316	2(3)	86653	2(3)
82943	1(3)	83615	3(3)	84087	1(3)	84425	1(2)	85048	2(3)	85555	1(2)	86318	2(3)	86654	2(3)
82945	4(3)	83625	1(3)	84100	2(3)	84430	1(3)	85049	2(3)	85557	1(2)	86320	1(2)	86658	12(3)
82946	1(2)	83630	1(3)	84105	1(3)	84431	1(3)	85055	1(3)	85576	7(3)	86325	2(3)	86663	2(3)
82947	5(3)	83631	1(3)	84106	1(2)	84432	1(2)	85060	1(3)	85597	1(3)	86327	1(3)	86664	2(3)
82950	3(3)	83632	1(3)	84110	1(3)	84436	1(2)	85097	2(3)	85598	1(3)	86329	3(3)	86665	2(3)
82951	1(2)	83633	1(3)	84112	1(3)	84437	1(2)	85130	1(3)	85610	4(3)	86331	12(3)	86666	4(3)
82952	3(3)	83655	2(3)	84119	1(2)	84439	1(2)	85170	1(3)	85611	2(3)	86332	1(3)	86668	2(3)
82955	1(2)	83661	3(3)	84120	1(3)	84442	1(2)	85175	1(3)	85612	1(3)	86334	1(2)	86671	3(3)
82960	1(2)	83662	4(3)	84126	1(3)	84443	4(2)	85210	2(3)	85613	1(3)	86335	2(3)	86674	3(3)
82963	1(3)	83663	3(3)	84132	3(3)	84445	1(2)	85220	2(3)	85635	1(3)	86336	1(3)	86677	3(3)
82965	1(3)	83664	3(3)	84133	2(3)	84446	1(2)	85230	2(3)	85651	1(2)	86337	1(2)	86682	2(3)
82977	1(3)	83670	1(3)	84134	1(3)	84449	1(3)	85240	2(3)	85652	1(2)	86340	1(2)	86684	2(3)
82978	1(3)	83690	2(3)	84135	1(3)	84450	1(3)	85244	1(3)	85660	1(2)	86341	1(3)	86687	1(3)
82979	1(3)	83695	1(3)	84138	1(3)	84460	1(3)	85245	2(3)	85670	2(3)	86343	1(3)	86688	1(3)
82985	1(3)	83698	1(3)	84140	1(3)	84466	1(3)	85246	2(3)	85675	1(3)	86344	1(2)	86689	2(3)
83001	1(3)	83700	1(2)	84143	2(3)	84478	1(3)	85247	2(3)	85705	1(3)	86352	1(3)	86692	2(3)
83002	1(3)	83701	1(3)	84144	1(3)	84479	1(3)	85250	2(3)	85730	4(3)	86353	7(3)	86694	2(3)
83003	5(3)	83704	1(3)	84145	1(3)	84480	1(2)	85260	2(3)	85732	4(3)	86355	1(2)	86695	2(3)
83006	1(2)	83718	1(3)	84146	3(3)	84481	1(2)	85270	2(3)	85810	2(3)	86356	7(3)	86696	2(3)
83009	1(3)	83719	1(3)	84150	2(3)	84482	1(2)	85280	2(3)	86000	6(3)	86357	1(2)	86698	3(3)
83010	1(3)	83721	1(3)	84152	1(2)	84484	4(3)	85290	2(3)	86005	6(3)	86359	1(2)	86701	1(3)
83012	1(2)	83727	1(3)	84153	1(2)	84485	1(3)	85291	1(3)	86021	1(2)	86360	1(2)	86702	2(3)
83013	1(3)	83735	4(3)	84154	1(2)	84488	1(3)	85292	1(3)	86022	1(2)	86361	1(2)	86703	1(2)
83014	1(2)	83775	1(3)	84155	1(3)	84490	1(2)	85293	1(3)	86023	3(3)	86367	2(3)	86704	1(2)
83015	1(2)	83785	1(3)	84156	1(3)	84510	1(3)	85300	2(3)	86038	1(3)	86376	2(3)	86705	1(2)
83018	4(3)	83788	3(3)	84157	2(3)	84512	3(3)	85301	1(3)	86039	1(3)	86378	1(3)	86706	2(3)
83020	2(3)	83789	4(3)	84160	2(3)	84520	4(1)	85302	1(3)	86060	1(3)	86382	3(3)	86707	1(3)
83021	2(3)	83825	2(3)	84163	1(3)	84525	1(3)	85303	2(3)	86063	1(3)	86384	1(3)	86708	1(2)
83026	1(3)	83835	2(3)	84165	1(2)	84540	2(3)	85305	2(3)	86077	1(2)	86386	1(2)	86709	1(2)
83030	1(3)	83857	1(3)	84166	2(3)	84545	1(3)	85306	2(3)	86078	1(3)	86406	2(3)	86710	4(3)
83033	1(3)	83861	2(2)	84181	3(3)	84550	1(3)	85307	2(3)	86079	1(3)	86430	2(3)	86711	2(3)
83036	1(2)	83864	1(2)	84182	6(3)	84560	2(3)	85335	2(3)	86140	1(2)	86431	2(3)	86713	3(3)
83037	1(2)	83872	2(3)	84202	1(2)	84577	1(3)	85337	1(3)	86141	1(2)	86480	1(3)	86717	8(3)
83045	1(3)	83873	1(3)	84203	1(2)	84578	1(3)	85345	1(3)	86146	3(3)	86481	1(3)	86720	2(3)

© 2015 Optum360, LLC

CPT	MUE	CPT	MUE	CPT	MUE	CPT	MUE	CPT	MUE	CPT	MUE	CPT	MUE	CPT	MUE
86723	2(3)	86923	10(3)	87255	2(3)	87492	1(3)	87652	1(3)	88230	2(1)	89160	1(3)	90646	1(2)
86727	2(3)	86930	3(3)	87260	1(3)	87493	2(3)	87653	1(3)	88233	2(1)	89190	1(3)	90647	1(2)
86729	0(2)	86931	4(3)	87265	1(3)	87495	1(3)	87660	1(3)	88239	3(1)	89220	2(1)	90648	1(2)
86732	2(3)	86940	3(3)	87267	1(3)	87496	1(3)	87661	1(1)	88240	3(1)	89230	1(2)	90649	1(2)
86735	2(3)	86941	3(3)	87269	1(3)	87497	2(3)	87797	3(3)	88241	3(1)	89240	2(1)	90650	1(2)
86738	2(3)	86945	5(3)	87270	1(3)	87498	1(3)	87798	21(3)	88245	1(2)	89250	1(2)	90651	1(2)
86741	2(3)	86950	1(3)	87271	1(3)	87500	1(3)	87799	3(3)	88248	1(2)	89251	1(2)	90653	1(2)
86744	2(3)	86960	3(3)	87272	1(3)	87501	1(3)	87800	2(3)	88249	1(2)	89253	1(3)	90654	1(2)
86747	2(3)	86965	4(3)	87273	1(3)	87502	1(3)	87801	3(3)	88261	2(1)	89254	1(3)	90655	1(2)
86750	4(3)	86971	6(3)	87274	1(3)	87503	1(3)	87802	2(3)	88262	2(1)	89255	1(3)	90656	1(2)
86753	3(3)	86972	2(3)	87275	1(3)	87505	1(2)	87803	3(3)	88263	1(3)	89257	1(3)	90657	1(2)
86756	2(3)	86975	2(3)	87276	1(3)	87506	1(2)	87804	3(3)	88264	2(3)	89258	1(2)	90658	1(2)
86757	6(3)	86976	2(3)	87277	1(3)	87507	1(3)	87806	1(2)	88267	2(1)	89259	1(2)	90660	1(2)
86759	2(3)	86977	2(3)	87278	1(3)	87510	1(3)	87807	2(3)	88269	2(1)	89260	1(2)	90661	1(2)
86762	2(3)	87003	1(3)	87279	1(3)	87511	1(3)	87808	1(3)	88273	3(1)	89261	1(2)	90662	1(2)
86765	2(3)	87015	6(3)	87280	1(3)	87512	1(3)	87809	2(3)	88283	2(1)	89264	1(3)	90664	1(2)
86768	5(3)	87045	3(3)	87281	1(3)	87515	1(3)	87810	2(3)	88289	1(3)	89268	1(2)	90666	1(2)
86771	2(3)	87046	6(3)	87283	1(3)	87516	1(3)	87850	1(3)	88291	1(1)	89272	1(2)	90667	1(2)
86774	2(3)	87071	4(3)	87285	1(3)	87517	1(3)	87880	2(3)	88300	2(1)	89280	1(2)	90668	1(2)
86777	2(3)	87073	3(3)	87290	1(3)	87520	1(3)	87899	6(3)	88302	2(1)	89281	1(2)	90669	1(2)
86778	2(3)	87075	6(3)	87299	1(3)	87521	1(3)	87900	1(2)	88309	3(1)	89290	1(2)	90670	1(2)
86780	2(3)	87076	6(3)	87300	2(3)	87522	1(3)	87901	2(3)	88311	4(1)	89291	1(2)	90672	1(1)
86784	1(3)	87077	10(3)	87301	1(3)	87525	1(3)	87902	1(2)	88321	1(2)	89300	1(2)	90673	1(2)
86787	2(3)	87081	6(3)	87305	1(3)	87526	1(3)	87903	1(2)	88323	1(2)	89310	1(2)	90675	1(2)
86788	2(3)	87084	1(3)	87320	1(3)	87527	1(3)	87904	14(3)	88325	1(2)	89320	1(2)	90676	1(2)
86789	2(3)	87086	3(3)	87324	2(3)	87528	1(3)	87905	2(3)	88329	4(1)	89321	1(2)	90680	1(2)
86790	4(3)	87088	6(3)	87327	1(3)	87529	2(3)	87906	2(3)	88331	11(1)	89322	1(2)	90681	1(2)
86793	2(3)	87101	4(3)	87328	2(3)	87530	2(3)	87910	1(3)	88333	4(1)	89325	1(2)	90685	1(2)
86800	1(3)	87102	4(3)	87329	2(3)	87531	1(3)	87912	1(3)	88342	3(3)	89329	1(2)	90686	1(2)
86803	1(3)	87103	2(3)	87332	1(3)	87532	1(3)	88104	5(3)	88344	1(1)	89330	1(2)	90687	1(2)
86804	1(2)	87106	4(3)	87335	1(3)	87533	1(3)	88106	5(3)	88347	4(1)	89331	1(2)	90688	1(2)
86805	12(3)	87107	4(3)	87336	1(3)	87534	1(3)	88108	6(3)	88348	1(3)	89335	1(3)	90690	1(2)
86807	2(3)	87109	2(3)	87337	1(3)	87535	1(3)	88112	6(3)	88355	1(3)	89337	1(2)	90691	1(2)
86808	1(3)	87110	2(3)	87338	1(1)	87536	1(3)	88120	2(3)	88356	1(1)	89342	1(2)	90692	1(2)
86812	1(2)	87118	3(3)	87339	1(3)	87537	1(3)	88121	2(3)	88358	2(1)	89343	1(2)	90693	1(2)
86813	1(2)	87140	3(3)	87340	1(2)	87538	1(3)	88125	1(3)	88360	6(3)	89344	1(2)	90696	1(2)
86816	1(2)	87143	2(3)	87341	1(2)	87539	1(3)	88130	1(2)	88361	6(3)	89346	1(2)	90697	1(2)
86817	1(2)	87149	11(3)	87350	1(2)	87540	1(3)	88140	1(2)	88362	1(3)	89352	1(2)	90698	1(2)
86821	1(3)	87150	12(3)	87380	1(2)	87541	1(3)	88141	1(3)	88363	2(3)	89353	1(3)	90700	1(2)
86822	1(3)	87152	1(3)	87385	2(3)	87542	1(3)	88142	1(3)	88364	3(3)	89354	1(3)	90702	1(2)
86825	1(3)	87153	3(3)	87389	1(3)	87550	1(3)	88143	1(3)	88365	2(1)	89356	2(3)	90703	1(2)
86826	8(3)	87164	2(3)	87390	1(3)	87551	2(3)	88147	1(3)	88366	1(1)			90704	1(2)
86828	2(1)	87166	2(3)	87391	1(3)	87552	1(3)	88148	1(3)	88367	2(1)			90705	1(2)
86829	2(1)	87168	2(3)	87400	2(3)	87555	1(1)	88150	1(3)	88368	2(1)			90706	1(2)
86830	2(3)	87169	2(3)	87420	1(3)	87556	1(1)	88152	1(3)	88369	3(1)			90707	1(2)
86831	2(3)	87172	1(3)	87425	1(3)	87557	1(3)	88153	1(3)	88371	6(3)			90708	1(2)
86832	2(3)	87176	3(3)	87427	2(3)	87560	1(3)	88154	1(3)	88372	1(3)			90710	1(2)
86833	1(3)	87177	3(3)	87430	1(3)	87561	1(3)	88155	1(3)	88373	3(1)			90712	1(2)
86834	1(3)	87181	12(3)	87449	3(3)	87562	1(3)	88160	4(3)	88374	1(1)			90713	1(2)
86835	1(3)	87184	8(3)	87450	2(3)	87580	1(3)	88161	4(3)	88375	1(3)			90714	1(2)
86850	3(3)	87185	4(3)	87451	2(3)	87581	1(3)	88162	3(3)	88377	1(1)			90715	1(2)
86860	2(3)	87187	3(3)	87470	1(3)	87582	1(3)	88164	1(3)	88380	1(1)			90716	1(2)
86870	6(3)	87188	14(3)	87471	1(3)	87590	1(3)	88165	1(3)	88381	1(1)			90717	1(2)
86880	4(3)	87190	10(3)	87472	1(3)	87591	2(3)	88166	1(3)	88387	3(1)			90719	1(2)
86885	3(3)	87197	1(3)	87475	1(3)	87592	1(3)	88167	1(3)	88388	3(1)			90720	1(2)
86886	3(1)	87206	6(3)	87476	1(3)	87623	1(2)	88172	7(3)	88720	1(3)			90721	1(2)
86890	2(1)	87207	3(3)	87477	1(3)	87624	1(2)	88173	7(3)	88738	2(1)			90725	1(2)
86891	2(1)	87209	4(3)	87480	1(3)	87625	1(2)	88174	1(3)	88740	1(2)			90727	1(2)
86900	3(3)	87210	4(3)	87481	1(1)	87631	1(3)	88175	1(3)	88741	1(2)			90732	1(2)
86901	3(3)	87220	3(3)	87482	1(3)	87632	1(3)	88177	6(3)	89049	1(3)			90733	1(2)
86902	40(3)	87230	3(3)	87485	1(3)	87633	1(3)	88182	2(1)	89050	2(1)			90734	1(2)
86905	28(3)	87250	1(3)	87486	1(3)	87640	1(3)	88184	2(3)	89051	2(1)			90735	1(2)
86906	1(2)	87252	4(3)	87487	1(3)	87641	1(3)	88187	2(3)	89055	1(2)			90736	1(2)
86920	19(3)	87253	3(3)	87490	1(3)	87650	1(3)	88188	2(3)	89060	2(1)			90738	1(2)
86922	10(3)	87254	10(3)	87491	2(3)	87651	1(3)	88189	2(3)	89125	2(1)			90739	1(2)

CPT	MUE	CPT	MUE	CPT	MUE	CPT	MUE	CPT	MUE	CPT	MUE	CPT	MUE	CPT	MUE
90740	1(2)	91034	1(2)	92355	1(3)	92610	1(2)	93284	1(3)	93580	1(3)	93976	1(3)	95076	1(1)
90743	1(2)	91035	1(2)	92358	1(3)	92613	1(2)	93285	1(3)	93581	1(3)	93978	1(3)	95079	2(1)
90744	1(2)	91037	1(2)	92371	1(3)	92615	1(2)	93286	2(3)	93582	1(2)	93979	1(3)	95115	1(2)
90746	1(2)	91038	1(2)	92502	1(3)	92617	1(2)	93287	2(3)	93583	1(2)	93980	1(3)	95117	1(2)
90747	1(2)	91040	1(2)	92504	1(3)	92618	1(1)	93288	1(3)	93600	1(3)	93981	1(3)	95250	1(2)
90785	2(1)	91065	2(2)	92507	1(3)	92620	1(2)	93289	1(3)	93602	1(3)	93982	1(3)	95251	1(2)
90791	1(1)	91110	1(2)	92508	1(3)	92625	1(2)	93290	1(3)	93603	1(3)	93990	2(3)	95782	1(2)
90792	2(1)	91111	1(2)	92511	1(3)	92626	1(2)	93291	1(3)	93609	1(3)	94002	1(2)	95783	1(2)
90832	2(3)	91112	1(1)	92512	1(2)	92920	1(1)	93292	1(3)	93610	1(3)	94003	1(2)	95800	1(2)
90833	2(1)	91117	1(2)	92516	1(3)	92924	1(1)	93293	1(2)	93612	1(3)	94004	1(2)	95801	1(2)
90834	2(3)	91120	1(2)	92520	1(2)	92928	1(1)	93294	1(2)	93613	1(3)	94010	1(3)	95803	1(2)
90836	2(1)	91122	1(2)	92521	1(2)	92933	1(1)	93295	1(2)	93615	1(3)	94011	1(3)	95805	1(2)
90837	2(3)	91132	1(3)	92522	1(2)	92937	3(1)	93296	1(2)	93616	1(3)	94012	1(3)	95806	1(2)
90838	2(1)	91133	1(3)	92523	1(2)	92938	3(1)	93297	1(2)	93618	1(3)	94013	1(3)	95807	1(2)
90839	1(1)	91200	1(3)	92524	1(2)	92941	1(1)	93298	1(2)	93619	1(3)	94014	1(2)	95808	1(2)
90845	1(2)	92002	1(2)	92526	1(2)	92943	1(1)	93299	1(2)	93620	1(3)	94015	1(2)	95810	1(2)
90846	2(3)	92004	1(2)	92531	1(3)	92944	1(1)	93303	1(3)	93621	1(3)	94016	1(2)	95811	1(2)
90847	2(3)	92012	1(3)	92532	1(3)	92950	4(1)	93304	1(1)	93622	1(3)	94060	1(3)	95812	1(3)
90849	2(3)	92014	1(3)	92533	4(2)	92953	2(3)	93306	1(3)	93623	1(3)	94070	1(2)	95813	1(3)
90853	5(3)	92018	1(2)	92534	1(3)	92960	2(3)	93307	1(3)	93624	1(3)	94150	2(3)	95816	1(3)
90863	1(1)	92019	1(2)	92540	1(3)	92961	1(3)	93308	1(3)	93631	1(3)	94200	1(3)	95819	1(3)
90865	1(3)	92020	1(2)	92541	1(3)	92970	1(3)	93312	1(3)	93640	1(3)	94250	1(3)	95822	1(3)
90867	1(2)	92025	1(2)	92542	1(3)	92971	1(3)	93313	1(3)	93641	1(2)	94375	1(3)	95824	1(3)
90868	1(3)	92060	1(2)	92543	4(2)	92973	2(1)	93314	1(3)	93642	1(3)	94400	1(3)	95827	1(2)
90869	1(3)	92065	1(2)	92544	1(3)	92974	1(1)	93315	1(3)	93644	1(2)	94450	1(3)	95829	1(3)
90870	2(3)	92071	2(2)	92545	1(3)	92975	1(1)	93316	1(3)	93650	1(2)	94452	1(2)	95830	1(3)
90880	1(3)	92072	1(2)	92546	1(3)	92977	1(3)	93317	1(3)	93653	1(3)	94453	1(2)	95831	5(2)
90885	1(3)	92081	1(2)	92547	1(3)	92978	1(3)	93318	1(3)	93654	1(3)	94610	2(3)	95832	1(3)
90887	1(3)	92082	1(2)	92548	1(3)	92979	2(1)	93320	1(3)	93655	2(3)	94620	1(3)	95851	3(1)
90889	1(3)	92083	1(2)	92550	1(2)	92986	1(2)	93321	1(3)	93656	1(3)	94621	1(3)	95852	1(3)
90901	1(3)	92100	1(2)	92552	1(2)	92987	1(2)	93325	1(3)	93657	1(3)	94640	10(3)	95857	1(2)
90911	1(3)	92132	1(2)	92553	1(2)	92990	1(2)	93350	1(2)	93660	1(3)	94642	1(3)	95860	1(3)
90935	1(3)	92133	1(2)	92555	1(2)	92992	1(2)	93351	1(2)	93662	1(3)	94644	1(2)	95861	1(3)
90937	1(3)	92134	1(2)	92556	1(2)	92993	1(2)	93352	1(3)	93701	1(2)	94645	2(1)	95863	1(3)
90940	2(1)	92136	1(2)	92557	1(2)	92997	1(2)	93355	1(3)	93702	1(2)	94660	1(2)	95864	1(3)
90945	1(3)	92140	1(2)	92558	0(3)	92998	2(1)	93451	1(3)	93724	1(3)	94662	1(2)	95865	1(3)
90947	1(3)	92145	1(2)	92561	1(2)	93000	3(1)	93452	1(3)	93740	1(3)	94664	1(3)	95866	1(3)
90951	1(2)	92225	2(2)	92562	1(2)	93005	3(1)	93453	1(3)	93745	1(2)	94667	1(2)	95867	1(3)
90952	1(2)	92226	2(2)	92563	1(2)	93015	1(3)	93454	1(3)	93750	1(3)	94669	4(3)	95868	1(3)
90953	1(2)	92227	1(2)	92564	1(2)	93016	1(3)	93455	1(3)	93770	1(3)	94680	1(3)	95869	1(3)
90954	1(2)	92228	1(2)	92565	1(2)	93017	1(3)	93456	1(3)	93784	1(2)	94681	1(3)	95873	1(2)
90955	1(2)	92230	2(2)	92567	1(2)	93018	1(3)	93457	1(3)	93786	1(2)	94690	1(3)	95874	1(2)
90956	1(2)	92235	2(2)	92568	1(2)	93024	1(3)	93458	1(3)	93788	1(2)	94726	1(3)	95875	2(3)
90957	1(2)	92240	2(2)	92570	1(2)	93025	1(2)	93459	1(3)	93790	1(2)	94727	1(3)	95885	4(2)
90958	1(2)	92250	1(2)	92571	1(2)	93040	3(1)	93460	1(3)	93797	2(2)	94728	1(3)	95886	4(2)
90959	1(2)	92260	1(2)	92572	1(2)	93041	3(1)	93461	1(3)	93798	2(2)	94729	1(3)	95887	1(2)
90960	1(2)	92265	1(2)	92575	1(2)	93042	3(1)	93462	1(3)	93880	1(3)	94750	1(3)	95905	2(3)
90961	1(2)	92270	1(2)	92576	1(2)	93224	1(2)	93463	1(3)	93882	1(3)	94760	1(3)	95907	1(2)
90962	1(2)	92275	1(2)	92577	1(2)	93225	1(2)	93464	1(3)	93886	1(3)	94761	1(2)	95908	1(2)
90963	1(2)	92283	1(2)	92579	1(2)	93226	1(2)	93503	2(1)	93888	1(3)	94762	1(2)	95909	1(2)
90964	1(2)	92284	1(2)	92582	1(2)	93227	1(2)	93505	1(2)	93890	1(3)	94770	1(3)	95910	1(2)
90965	1(2)	92285	1(2)	92583	1(2)	93228	1(2)	93530	1(3)	93892	1(3)	94772	1(2)	95911	1(2)
90966	1(2)	92286	1(2)	92584	1(2)	93229	1(2)	93531	1(3)	93893	1(3)	94774	1(2)	95912	1(2)
90967	1(2)	92287	1(2)	92585	1(2)	93260	1(2)	93532	1(3)	93895	1(2)	94775	1(2)	95913	1(2)
90968	1(2)	92311	1(2)	92586	1(2)	93261	1(3)	93533	1(3)	93922	1(1)	94776	1(2)	95921	1(3)
90969	1(2)	92312	1(2)	92587	1(2)	93268	1(2)	93561	1(3)	93923	1(1)	94777	1(2)	95922	1(3)
90970	1(2)	92313	1(3)	92588	1(2)	93270	1(2)	93562	1(3)	93924	1(2)	94780	1(2)	95923	1(3)
90989	1(2)	92315	1(2)	92596	1(2)	93271	1(2)	93563	1(3)	93925	1(3)	94781	1(1)	95924	1(1)
90993	1(3)	92316	1(2)	92601	1(3)	93272	1(2)	93564	1(3)	93926	1(3)	95012	2(3)	95925	1(3)
90997	1(3)	92317	1(3)	92602	1(3)	93278	1(3)	93565	1(3)	93930	1(3)	95018	19(3)	95926	1(3)
91010	1(2)	92325	1(3)	92603	1(3)	93279	1(3)	93566	1(3)	93931	1(3)	95056	1(2)	95927	1(3)
91013	1(3)	92326	2(2)	92604	1(3)	93280	1(3)	93567	1(3)	93965	1(3)	95060	1(2)	95928	1(3)
91020	1(2)	92352	1(3)	92605	1(2)	93281	1(3)	93568	1(3)	93970	1(3)	95065	1(3)	95929	1(3)
91022	1(2)	92353	1(3)	92606	1(2)	93282	1(3)	93571	1(3)	93971	1(3)	95070	1(3)	95930	1(3)
91030	1(2)	92354	1(3)	92609	1(3)	93283	1(3)	93572	2(1)	93975	1(3)	95071	1(2)	95933	1(3)

CPT	MUE	CPT	MUE	CPT	MUE	CPT	MUE	CPT	MUE	CPT	MUE	CPT	MUE	CPT	MUE
95938	1(3)	96570	1(2)	99188	1(2)	99347	1(3)	A0210	0(3)	A4623	90(3)	A7029	0(3)	A9557	2(1)
95939	1(3)	96571	3(1)	99191	1(3)	99348	1(3)	A0225	0(3)	A4624	0(3)	A7030	0(3)	A9558	7(3)
95943	1(3)	96900	1(3)	99192	1(3)	99349	1(3)	A0380	0(3)	A4625	30(3)	A7031	0(3)	A9559	1(1)
95950	1(2)	96902	1(3)	99195	2(1)	99350	1(3)	A0382	0(3)	A4628	0(3)	A7032	0(3)	A9560	2(1)
95951	1(2)	96904	1(2)	99201	1(2)	99354	1(2)	A0384	0(3)	A4633	0(3)	A7033	0(3)	A9561	1(1)
95953	1(2)	96910	1(3)	99202	1(2)	99356	1(2)	A0390	0(3)	A4635	0(3)	A7034	0(3)	A9562	2(1)
95954	1(3)	96912	1(3)	99203	1(2)	99358	1(2)	A0392	0(3)	A4636	0(3)	A7035	0(3)	A9564	20(3)
95955	1(3)	96913	1(3)	99204	1(2)	99359	1(1)	A0394	0(3)	A4637	0(3)	A7036	0(3)	A9566	1(1)
95956	1(2)	96920	1(2)	99205	1(2)	99363	1(2)	A0396	0(3)	A4638	0(3)	A7037	0(3)	A9567	2(1)
95957	1(3)	96921	1(2)	99211	2(3)	99364	1(2)	A0398	0(3)	A4640	0(3)	A7038	0(3)	A9568	0(3)
95958	1(3)	96922	1(2)	99212	2(3)	99366	3(3)	A0420	0(3)	A4642	1(1)	A7039	0(3)	A9569	1(1)
95961	1(2)	97010	1(3)	99213	2(3)	99367	1(3)	A0422	0(3)	A4648	3(3)	A7040	2(1)	A9570	1(1)
95962	3(1)	97012	1(3)	99214	2(3)	99368	3(3)	A0424	0(3)	A4650	3(1)	A7041	2(1)	A9571	1(1)
95965	1(3)	97014	0(3)	99215	2(3)	99374	1(2)	A0426	2(3)	A4670	0(3)	A7044	0(3)	A9572	1(3)
95966	1(3)	97016	1(3)	99217	1(2)	99377	1(2)	A0427	2(3)	A4932	0(3)	A7045	0(3)	A9575	200(3)
95967	3(1)	97018	1(3)	99218	1(2)	99379	1(2)	A0428	4(3)	A5056	90(3)	A7046	0(3)	A9579	100(3)
95970	1(3)	97022	1(3)	99219	1(2)	99380	1(2)	A0429	2(3)	A5057	90(3)	A7047	0(3)	A9580	1(1)
95971	1(3)	97024	1(3)	99220	1(2)	99406	1(2)	A0430	1(3)	A5102	1(1)	A7048	10(3)	A9582	1(3)
95972	1(2)	97026	1(3)	99221	0(3)	99407	1(2)	A0431	1(3)	A5120	150(3)	A7502	3(1)	A9583	18(3)
95974	1(2)	97028	1(3)	99222	0(3)	99446	1(2)	A0432	1(3)	A5500	0(3)	A7503	1(1)	A9584	1(1)
95975	2(1)	97150	2(3)	99223	0(3)	99447	1(2)	A0433	1(3)	A5501	0(3)	A7504	180(3)	A9585	300(3)
95978	1(2)	97545	1(2)	99224	1(2)	99448	1(2)	A0434	2(3)	A5503	0(3)	A7506	90(3)	A9586	1(1)
95980	1(3)	97546	2(1)	99225	1(2)	99449	1(2)	A0435	999(3)	A5504	0(3)	A7507	200(3)	A9599	1(3)
95981	1(3)	97597	1(3)	99226	1(2)	99455	1(3)	A0436	300(3)	A5505	0(3)	A7508	200(3)	A9600	7(3)
95982	1(3)	97602	1(3)	99231	0(3)	99456	1(3)	A0888	0(3)	A5506	0(3)	A7509	300(3)	A9604	1(3)
95990	2(1)	97605	1(3)	99232	0(3)	99460	1(2)	A0998	0(3)	A5507	0(3)	A7522	1(2)	A9700	2(1)
95991	2(1)	97606	1(3)	99233	0(3)	99461	1(2)	A4221	0(3)	A5508	0(3)	A7524	2(1)	B4034	0(3)
95992	1(2)	97607	1(3)	99234	1(3)	99462	1(2)	A4222	0(3)	A5510	0(3)	A7526	36(3)	B4035	0(3)
96000	1(2)	97608	1(3)	99235	1(3)	99463	1(2)	A4233	0(3)	A5512	0(3)	A9272	0(1)	B4036	0(3)
96001	1(2)	97610	1(2)	99236	1(3)	99464	1(2)	A4234	0(3)	A5513	0(3)	A9284	1(1)	B4081	0(3)
96002	1(3)	98925	1(2)	99238	0(3)	99465	1(2)	A4235	0(3)	A6501	2(1)	A9500	3(1)	B4082	0(3)
96003	1(3)	98926	1(2)	99239	0(3)	99466	1(2)	A4236	0(3)	A6502	2(1)	A9501	3(1)	B4083	0(3)
96004	1(2)	98927	1(2)	99281	2(3)	99468	1(2)	A4253	0(3)	A6503	2(1)	A9502	3(1)	B4087	1(3)
96020	1(2)	98928	1(2)	99282	2(3)	99469	1(2)	A4255	0(3)	A6504	4(1)	A9503	1(1)	B4088	1(3)
96103	1(2)	98929	1(2)	99283	2(3)	99471	1(2)	A4256	0(3)	A6505	4(1)	A9504	1(1)	B4149	0(3)
96105	3(1)	98940	1(2)	99284	2(3)	99472	1(2)	A4257	0(3)	A6506	4(1)	A9505	4(3)	B4150	0(3)
96120	1(2)	98941	1(2)	99285	2(3)	99475	1(2)	A4258	0(3)	A6507	4(1)	A9507	1(1)	B4152	0(3)
96125	2(1)	98942	1(2)	99288	1(3)	99476	1(2)	A4259	0(3)	A6508	4(1)	A9508	2(3)	B4153	0(3)
96127	2(1)	99002	1(3)	99291	1(2)	99477	1(2)	A4262	4(2)	A6509	2(1)	A9510	1(1)	B4154	0(3)
96360	1(1)	99024	1(3)	99304	1(2)	99478	1(2)	A4263	4(2)	A6510	2(1)	A9512	30(3)	B4155	0(3)
96365	1(1)	99050	1(3)	99305	1(2)	99479	1(2)	A4270	4(3)	A6511	2(1)	A9516	1(3)	B4157	0(3)
96368	1(2)	99051	1(3)	99306	1(2)	99480	1(2)	A4300	0(3)	A6513	2(1)	A9520	1(3)	B4158	0(3)
96369	1(2)	99053	1(3)	99307	1(2)	99485	1(1)	A4301	1(2)	A6545	2(1)	A9521	2(1)	B4159	0(3)
96370	3(1)	99056	1(3)	99308	1(2)	99487	1(1)	A4356	1(1)	A6550	0(3)	A9524	10(3)	B4160	0(3)
96371	1(3)	99058	1(3)	99309	1(2)	99490	1(2)	A4396	3(1)	A7000	0(3)	A9526	2(1)	B4161	0(3)
96373	3(1)	99060	1(3)	99310	1(2)	99495	1(1)	A4399	2(1)	A7001	0(3)	A9536	1(1)	B4162	0(3)
96374	1(3)	99070	1(3)	99315	1(2)	99496	1(1)	A4459	1(3)	A7002	0(3)	A9537	1(1)	B4164	0(3)
96376	10(3)	99071	1(3)	99316	1(2)	99497	1(2)	A4463	3(1)	A7003	0(3)	A9538	1(1)	B4168	0(3)
96402	2(3)	99078	3(3)	99318	1(2)	99498	3(3)	A4470	1(1)	A7004	0(3)	A9539	2(1)	B4172	0(3)
96405	1(2)	99080	1(3)	99324	1(2)	99605	0(2)	A4480	1(1)	A7005	0(3)	A9540	2(1)	B4176	0(3)
96406	1(2)	99082	1(1)	99325	1(2)	99606	0(3)	A4550	3(3)	A7006	0(3)	A9541	1(1)	B4178	0(3)
96409	1(3)	99090	1(3)	99326	1(2)	99607	0(3)	A4555	0(3)	A7007	0(3)	A9542	1(1)	B4180	0(3)
96413	1(3)	99091	1(3)	99327	1(2)	A0021	0(3)	A4557	0(3)	A7010	0(3)	A9543	1(1)	B4189	0(3)
96416	1(3)	99100	3(1)	99328	1(2)	A0080	0(3)	A4561	1(1)	A7012	0(3)	A9544	1(1)	B4193	0(3)
96420	2(1)	99116	1(3)	99334	1(3)	A0090	0(3)	A4562	1(1)	A7013	0(3)	A9545	1(1)	B4197	0(3)
96422	2(3)	99135	1(3)	99335	1(3)	A0100	0(3)	A4565	2(3)	A7014	0(3)	A9546	1(1)	B4199	0(3)
96425	1(3)	99140	2(3)	99336	1(3)	A0110	0(3)	A4595	0(3)	A7015	0(3)	A9547	2(3)	B4216	0(3)
96440	1(3)	99143	2(3)	99337	1(3)	A0120	0(3)	A4604	0(3)	A7016	0(3)	A9548	2(3)	B4220	0(3)
96446	1(3)	99144	2(3)	99339	1(2)	A0130	0(3)	A4605	0(3)	A7017	0(3)	A9550	1(1)	B4222	0(3)
96450	1(3)	99148	2(3)	99340	1(2)	A0140	0(3)	A4606	1(3)	A7018	0(3)	A9551	1(1)	B5000	0(3)
96521	2(3)	99149	2(3)	99341	1(2)	A0160	0(3)	A4611	0(3)	A7020	0(3)	A9552	1(1)	B5100	0(3)
96522	1(3)	99170	1(3)	99342	1(2)	A0170	0(3)	A4612	0(3)	A7025	0(3)	A9553	1(1)	B5200	0(3)
96523	2(3)	99175	1(3)	99343	1(2)	A0180	0(3)	A4613	0(3)	A7026	0(3)	A9554	1(1)	B9000	0(3)
96542	1(3)	99183	1(3)	99344	1(2)	A0190	0(3)	A4614	0(3)	A7027	0(3)	A9555	3(1)	B9002	0(3)
96567	1(3)	99184	1(2)	99345	1(2)	A0200	0(3)	A4618	0(3)	A7028	0(3)	A9556	10(3)		

CPT	MUE	CPT	MUE	CPT	MUE	CPT	MUE	CPT	MUE	CPT	MUE	CPT	MUE	CPT	MUE
B9004	0(3)	C1820	2(3)	C8901	1(3)	C9603	2(3)	E0191	0(3)	E0316	0(3)	E0606	0(3)	E0769	0(3)
B9006	0(3)	C1821	4(3)	C8902	1(3)	C9604	3(3)	E0193	0(3)	E0325	0(3)	E0607	0(3)	E0770	1(3)
C1713	20(3)	C1830	2(3)	C8903	1(3)	C9605	3(3)	E0194	0(3)	E0326	0(3)	E0610	0(3)	E0776	0(3)
C1714	4(3)	C1840	1(3)	C8904	1(3)	C9606	2(3)	E0196	0(3)	E0328	0(3)	E0615	0(3)	E0779	0(3)
C1715	45(3)	C1841	1(3)	C8905	1(3)	C9607	1(2)	E0197	0(3)	E0329	0(3)	E0616	1(2)	E0780	0(3)
C1716	4(3)	C1874	5(3)	C8906	1(3)	C9608	2(3)	E0198	0(3)	E0350	0(3)	E0617	0(3)	E0781	0(3)
C1717	10(3)	C1875	5(3)	C8907	1(3)	C9724	1(3)	E0199	0(3)	E0352	0(3)	E0618	0(3)	E0782	1(2)
C1719	99(3)	C1876	5(3)	C8908	1(3)	C9725	1(3)	E0200	0(3)	E0370	0(3)	E0619	0(3)	E0783	1(2)
C1721	1(3)	C1877	5(3)	C8909	1(3)	C9726	2(3)	E0202	0(3)	E0371	0(3)	E0620	0(3)	E0784	0(3)
C1722	1(3)	C1878	2(3)	C8910	1(3)	C9727	1(2)	E0203	0(3)	E0372	0(3)	E0621	0(3)	E0785	1(2)
C1724	5(3)	C1880	2(3)	C8911	1(3)	C9728	1(2)	E0205	0(3)	E0373	0(3)	E0625	0(3)	E0786	1(2)
C1725	9(3)	C1881	2(3)	C8912	1(3)	C9733	1(3)	E0210	0(3)	E0424	0(3)	E0627	0(3)	E0791	0(3)
C1726	5(3)	C1882	1(3)	C8913	1(3)	C9734	1(3)	E0215	0(3)	E0425	0(3)	E0628	0(3)	E0830	0(3)
C1727	4(3)	C1883	4(3)	C8914	1(3)	C9739	1(2)	E0217	0(3)	E0430	0(3)	E0629	0(3)	E0840	0(3)
C1728	5(3)	C1884	4(3)	C8918	1(3)	C9740	1(2)	E0218	0(3)	E0431	0(3)	E0630	0(3)	E0849	0(3)
C1729	6(3)	C1885	2(3)	C8919	1(3)	C9741	1(3)	E0221	0(3)	E0433	0(3)	E0635	0(3)	E0850	0(3)
C1730	4(3)	C1886	1(3)	C8920	1(3)	C9742	1(2)	E0225	0(3)	E0434	0(3)	E0636	0(3)	E0855	0(3)
C1731	2(3)	C1887	7(3)	C8921	1(3)	C9800	1(1)	E0231	0(3)	E0435	0(3)	E0637	0(3)	E0856	0(3)
C1732	3(3)	C1888	2(3)	C8922	1(3)	C9898	1(3)	E0232	0(3)	E0439	0(3)	E0638	0(3)	E0860	0(3)
C1733	3(3)	C1891	1(1)	C8923	1(3)	E0100	0(3)	E0235	0(3)	E0440	0(3)	E0639	0(3)	E0870	0(3)
C1749	1(3)	C1892	6(3)	C8924	1(3)	E0105	0(3)	E0236	0(3)	E0441	0(3)	E0640	0(3)	E0880	0(3)
C1750	2(3)	C1893	6(3)	C8925	1(3)	E0110	0(3)	E0239	0(3)	E0442	0(3)	E0641	0(3)	E0890	0(3)
C1751	3(3)	C1894	6(3)	C8926	1(3)	E0111	0(3)	E0240	0(3)	E0443	0(3)	E0642	0(3)	E0900	0(3)
C1752	2(3)	C1895	2(3)	C8927	1(3)	E0112	0(3)	E0241	0(3)	E0444	0(3)	E0650	0(3)	E0910	0(3)
C1753	2(3)	C1896	2(3)	C8928	1(2)	E0113	0(3)	E0242	0(3)	E0445	0(3)	E0651	0(3)	E0911	0(3)
C1754	2(3)	C1897	2(3)	C8929	1(3)	E0114	0(3)	E0243	0(3)	E0446	0(3)	E0652	0(3)	E0912	0(3)
C1755	2(3)	C1898	2(3)	C8930	1(2)	E0116	0(3)	E0244	0(3)	E0450	0(3)	E0655	0(3)	E0920	0(3)
C1756	2(3)	C1899	2(3)	C8931	1(3)	E0117	0(3)	E0245	0(3)	E0455	0(3)	E0656	0(3)	E0930	0(3)
C1757	6(3)	C1900	1(3)	C8932	1(3)	E0118	0(3)	E0246	0(3)	E0457	0(3)	E0657	0(3)	E0935	0(3)
C1758	2(3)	C2614	3(3)	C8933	1(3)	E0130	0(3)	E0247	0(3)	E0459	0(3)	E0660	0(3)	E0936	0(3)
C1759	2(3)	C2615	2(3)	C8934	2(3)	E0135	0(3)	E0248	0(3)	E0460	0(3)	E0665	0(3)	E0940	0(3)
C1760	4(3)	C2616	1(3)	C8935	2(3)	E0140	0(3)	E0249	0(3)	E0461	0(3)	E0666	0(3)	E0941	0(3)
C1762	4(3)	C2617	4(3)	C8936	2(3)	E0141	0(3)	E0250	0(3)	E0462	0(3)	E0667	0(3)	E0942	0(3)
C1763	4(3)	C2618	4(3)	C8957	2(3)	E0143	0(3)	E0251	0(3)	E0463	0(3)	E0668	0(3)	E0944	0(3)
C1764	1(3)	C2619	1(3)	C9025	300(3)	E0144	0(3)	E0255	0(3)	E0464	0(3)	E0669	0(3)	E0945	0(3)
C1765	4(3)	C2620	1(3)	C9026	300(3)	E0147	0(3)	E0256	0(3)	E0470	0(3)	E0670	0(3)	E0946	0(3)
C1766	4(3)	C2621	1(3)	C9027	300(3)	E0148	0(3)	E0260	0(3)	E0471	0(3)	E0671	0(3)	E0947	0(3)
C1767	2(3)	C2622	1(3)	C9132	5500(3)	E0149	0(3)	E0261	0(3)	E0472	0(3)	E0672	0(3)	E0948	0(3)
C1768	3(3)	C2624	1(3)	C9250	5(3)	E0153	0(3)	E0265	0(3)	E0480	0(3)	E0673	0(3)	E0950	0(3)
C1769	9(3)	C2625	4(3)	C9254	400(3)	E0154	0(3)	E0266	0(3)	E0481	0(3)	E0675	0(3)	E0951	0(3)
C1770	3(3)	C2626	1(3)	C9257	8000(3)	E0155	0(3)	E0270	0(3)	E0482	0(3)	E0676	1(3)	E0952	0(3)
C1771	1(3)	C2627	2(3)	C9275	1(3)	E0156	0(3)	E0271	0(3)	E0483	0(3)	E0691	0(3)	E0955	0(3)
C1772	1(3)	C2628	4(3)	C9285	2(3)	E0157	0(3)	E0272	0(3)	E0484	0(3)	E0692	0(3)	E0956	0(3)
C1773	3(3)	C2629	4(3)	C9290	266(3)	E0158	0(3)	E0273	0(3)	E0485	0(3)	E0693	0(3)	E0957	0(3)
C1776	10(3)	C2630	4(3)	C9293	700(3)	E0159	0(3)	E0274	0(3)	E0486	0(3)	E0694	0(3)	E0958	0(3)
C1777	2(3)	C2631	1(3)	C9352	3(3)	E0160	0(3)	E0275	0(3)	E0487	0(3)	E0700	0(3)	E0959	2(1)
C1778	4(3)	C2634	24(3)	C9353	4(3)	E0161	0(3)	E0276	0(3)	E0500	0(3)	E0705	1(2)	E0960	0(3)
C1779	2(3)	C2635	124(3)	C9354	300(3)	E0162	0(3)	E0277	0(3)	E0550	0(3)	E0710	0(3)	E0961	2(1)
C1780	2(3)	C2636	150(3)	C9355	3(3)	E0163	0(3)	E0280	0(3)	E0555	0(3)	E0720	0(3)	E0966	1(1)
C1781	4(3)	C2637	0(3)	C9356	125(3)	E0165	0(3)	E0290	0(3)	E0560	0(3)	E0730	0(3)	E0967	0(3)
C1782	1(3)	C2638	150(3)	C9358	800(3)	E0167	0(3)	E0291	0(3)	E0561	0(3)	E0731	0(3)	E0968	0(3)
C1783	2(3)	C2639	150(3)	C9359	30(3)	E0168	0(3)	E0292	0(3)	E0562	0(3)	E0740	0(3)	E0970	0(3)
C1784	2(3)	C2640	150(3)	C9360	300(3)	E0170	0(3)	E0293	0(3)	E0565	0(3)	E0744	0(3)	E0971	2(1)
C1785	1(3)	C2641	150(3)	C9361	10(3)	E0171	0(3)	E0294	0(3)	E0570	0(3)	E0745	0(3)	E0973	2(1)
C1786	1(3)	C2642	120(3)	C9362	60(3)	E0172	0(3)	E0295	0(3)	E0572	0(3)	E0746	1(3)	E0974	2(1)
C1787	2(3)	C2643	120(3)	C9363	500(3)	E0175	0(3)	E0296	0(3)	E0574	0(3)	E0747	0(3)	E0978	1(1)
C1788	2(3)	C5271	1(2)	C9364	600(3)	E0181	0(3)	E0297	0(3)	E0575	0(3)	E0748	0(3)	E0981	0(3)
C1789	2(3)	C5272	3(2)	C9442	300(3)	E0182	0(3)	E0300	0(3)	E0580	0(3)	E0749	1(3)	E0982	0(3)
C1813	1(3)	C5273	1(2)	C9443	100(3)	E0184	0(3)	E0301	0(3)	E0585	0(3)	E0755	0(3)	E0983	0(3)
C1814	2(3)	C5274	35(3)	C9444	120(3)	E0185	0(3)	E0302	0(3)	E0600	0(3)	E0760	0(3)	E0984	0(3)
C1815	1(3)	C5275	1(2)	C9446	200(3)	E0186	0(3)	E0303	0(3)	E0601	0(3)	E0761	0(3)	E0985	0(3)
C1816	2(3)	C5276	3(2)	C9497	1(3)	E0187	0(3)	E0304	0(3)	E0602	0(3)	E0762	1(3)	E0986	0(3)
C1817	1(3)	C5277	1(2)	C9600	3(3)	E0188	0(3)	E0305	0(3)	E0603	0(3)	E0764	0(3)	E0988	0(3)
C1818	2(3)	C5278	15(3)	C9601	2(3)	E0189	0(3)	E0310	0(3)	E0604	0(3)	E0765	0(3)	E0990	2(1)
C1819	4(3)	C8900	1(3)	C9602	3(3)	E0190	0(3)	E0315	0(3)	E0605	0(3)	E0766	0(3)	E0992	1(1)

CPT	MUE	CPT	MUE	CPT	MUE	CPT	MUE	CPT	MUE	CPT	MUE	CPT	MUE	CPT	MUE
E0994	0(3)	E1232	0(3)	E1811	0(3)	E2330	0(3)	E2619	0(3)	G0250	1(2)	G0423	6(2)	G6037	2(3)
E0995	2(1)	E1233	0(3)	E1812	0(3)	E2331	0(3)	E2620	0(3)	G0257	1(3)	G0424	2(2)	G6039	3(1)
E1002	0(3)	E1234	0(3)	E1815	0(3)	E2340	0(3)	E2621	0(3)	G0259	2(3)	G0425	1(3)	G6040	3(3)
E1003	0(3)	E1235	0(3)	E1816	0(3)	E2341	0(3)	E2622	0(3)	G0260	2(3)	G0426	0(3)	G6041	1(1)
E1004	0(3)	E1236	0(3)	E1818	0(3)	E2342	0(3)	E2623	0(3)	G0268	1(2)	G0427	0(3)	G6042	2(3)
E1005	0(3)	E1237	0(3)	E1820	0(3)	E2343	0(3)	E2624	0(3)	G0269	2(3)	G0429	1(2)	G6043	2(3)
E1006	0(3)	E1238	0(3)	E1821	0(3)	E2351	0(3)	E2625	0(3)	G0270	8(3)	G0431	1(2)	G6044	2(3)
E1007	0(3)	E1239	0(3)	E1825	0(3)	E2358	0(3)	E2626	0(3)	G0271	4(3)	G0432	1(2)	G6045	1(3)
E1008	0(3)	E1240	0(3)	E1830	0(3)	E2359	0(3)	E2627	0(3)	G0277	5(3)	G0433	1(2)	G6046	1(3)
E1009	0(3)	E1250	0(3)	E1831	0(3)	E2361	0(3)	E2628	0(3)	G0278	1(2)	G0434	1(2)	G6047	1(3)
E1010	0(3)	E1260	0(3)	E1840	0(3)	E2363	0(3)	E2629	0(3)	G0281	1(3)	G0435	1(2)	G6048	1(3)
E1011	0(3)	E1270	0(3)	E1841	0(3)	E2365	0(3)	E2630	0(3)	G0283	1(3)	G0436	1(2)	G6049	1(3)
E1014	0(3)	E1280	0(3)	E1902	0(3)	E2366	0(3)	E2631	0(3)	G0288	1(2)	G0437	1(2)	G6050	1(3)
E1015	0(3)	E1285	0(3)	E2000	0(3)	E2367	0(3)	E2632	0(3)	G0289	1(2)	G0438	1(2)	G6051	1(3)
E1016	0(3)	E1290	0(3)	E2100	0(3)	E2368	0(3)	E2633	0(3)	G0293	1(2)	G0439	1(2)	G6052	2(3)
E1017	0(3)	E1295	0(3)	E2101	0(3)	E2369	0(3)	G0008	1(2)	G0294	1(2)	G0442	1(2)	G6053	2(3)
E1018	0(3)	E1300	0(3)	E2120	0(3)	E2370	0(3)	G0009	1(2)	G0302	1(2)	G0443	1(2)	G6054	1(3)
E1020	0(3)	E1310	0(3)	E2201	0(3)	E2371	0(3)	G0010	1(3)	G0303	1(2)	G0444	1(2)	G6055	2(3)
E1028	0(3)	E1352	0(3)	E2202	0(3)	E2373	0(3)	G0027	1(2)	G0304	1(2)	G0445	1(2)	G6056	4(3)
E1029	0(3)	E1353	0(3)	E2203	0(3)	E2374	0(3)	G0101	1(2)	G0305	1(2)	G0446	1(2)	G6057	2(3)
E1030	0(3)	E1354	0(3)	E2204	0(3)	E2375	0(3)	G0102	1(2)	G0306	4(3)	G0447	2(3)	G6058	10(3)
E1031	0(3)	E1355	0(3)	E2205	0(3)	E2376	0(3)	G0103	1(2)	G0307	4(3)	G0448	1(3)	G9143	1(2)
E1035	0(3)	E1356	0(3)	E2206	0(3)	E2377	0(3)	G0104	1(2)	G0328	1(2)	G0452	1(3)	G9156	1(2)
E1036	0(3)	E1357	0(3)	E2207	0(3)	E2378	0(3)	G0105	1(2)	G0329	1(3)	G0453	10(3)	G9157	1(2)
E1037	0(3)	E1358	0(3)	E2208	0(3)	E2381	0(3)	G0106	1(2)	G0333	0(3)	G0454	1(2)	G9187	0(3)
E1038	0(3)	E1372	0(3)	E2209	0(3)	E2382	0(3)	G0108	8(3)	G0337	1(2)	G0455	1(2)	J0129	100(3)
E1039	0(3)	E1390	0(3)	E2210	0(3)	E2383	0(3)	G0109	12(3)	G0339	1(2)	G0458	1(1)	J0130	6(3)
E1050	0(3)	E1391	0(3)	E2211	0(3)	E2384	0(3)	G0117	1(2)	G0340	2(3)	G0459	0(3)	J0131	400(3)
E1060	0(3)	E1392	0(3)	E2212	0(3)	E2385	0(3)	G0118	1(2)	G0341	1(2)	G0460	1(3)	J0133	1200(3)
E1070	0(3)	E1405	0(3)	E2213	0(3)	E2386	0(3)	G0120	1(2)	G0342	1(2)	G0463	6(3)	J0135	8(3)
E1083	0(3)	E1406	0(3)	E2214	0(3)	E2387	0(3)	G0121	1(2)	G0343	1(2)	G0464	1(2)	J0153	180(3)
E1084	0(3)	E1500	0(3)	E2215	0(3)	E2388	0(3)	G0123	1(3)	G0364	2(3)	G0472	1(2)	J0178	4(3)
E1085	0(3)	E1510	0(3)	E2216	0(3)	E2389	0(3)	G0124	1(3)	G0365	2(3)	G3001	1(2)	J0180	150(3)
E1086	0(3)	E1520	0(3)	E2217	0(3)	E2390	0(3)	G0127	1(2)	G0372	1(2)	G6001	1(2)	J0210	16(3)
E1087	0(3)	E1530	0(3)	E2218	0(3)	E2391	0(3)	G0128	1(1)	G0378	72(3)	G6002	2(3)	J0215	30(3)
E1088	0(3)	E1540	0(3)	E2219	0(3)	E2392	0(3)	G0129	3(3)	G0379	1(2)	G6003	2(3)	J0220	20(3)
E1089	0(3)	E1550	0(3)	E2220	0(3)	E2394	0(3)	G0130	1(2)	G0380	2(3)	G6004	2(3)	J0221	300(3)
E1090	0(3)	E1560	0(3)	E2221	0(3)	E2395	0(3)	G0141	1(3)	G0381	2(3)	G6005	2(3)	J0256	3500(3)
E1092	0(3)	E1570	0(3)	E2222	0(3)	E2396	0(3)	G0143	1(3)	G0382	2(3)	G6006	2(3)	J0257	1400(3)
E1093	0(3)	E1575	0(3)	E2224	0(3)	E2397	0(3)	G0144	1(3)	G0383	2(3)	G6007	2(3)	J0275	1(3)
E1100	0(3)	E1580	0(3)	E2225	0(3)	E2402	0(3)	G0145	1(3)	G0384	2(3)	G6008	2(3)	J0278	15(3)
E1110	0(3)	E1590	0(3)	E2226	0(3)	E2500	0(3)	G0147	1(3)	G0389	1(2)	G6009	2(3)	J0280	10(3)
E1130	0(3)	E1592	0(3)	E2227	0(3)	E2502	0(3)	G0148	1(3)	G0390	1(2)	G6010	2(3)	J0289	115(3)
E1140	0(3)	E1594	0(3)	E2228	0(3)	E2504	0(3)	G0166	2(3)	G0396	1(2)	G6011	2(3)	J0300	8(3)
E1150	0(3)	E1600	0(3)	E2231	0(3)	E2506	0(3)	G0168	2(3)	G0397	1(2)	G6012	2(3)	J0348	200(3)
E1160	0(3)	E1610	0(3)	E2291	1(2)	E2508	0(3)	G0175	1(3)	G0398	1(2)	G6013	2(3)	J0350	0(3)
E1161	0(3)	E1615	0(3)	E2292	1(2)	E2510	0(3)	G0176	5(3)	G0399	1(2)	G6014	2(3)	J0360	6(3)
E1170	0(3)	E1620	0(3)	E2293	1(2)	E2511	0(3)	G0177	3(3)	G0400	1(2)	G6015	2(3)	J0364	6(3)
E1171	0(3)	E1625	0(3)	E2294	1(2)	E2512	0(3)	G0179	1(2)	G0402	1(2)	G6016	2(1)	J0400	120(3)
E1172	0(3)	E1630	0(3)	E2295	0(3)	E2601	0(3)	G0180	1(2)	G0403	1(2)	G6017	2(3)	J0401	400(3)
E1180	0(3)	E1632	0(3)	E2300	0(3)	E2602	0(3)	G0181	1(2)	G0404	1(2)	G6018	1(2)	J0456	4(3)
E1190	0(3)	E1634	0(3)	E2301	0(3)	E2603	0(3)	G0182	1(2)	G0405	1(2)	G6019	1(2)	J0475	8(3)
E1195	0(3)	E1635	0(3)	E2310	0(3)	E2604	0(3)	G0186	1(2)	G0406	0(3)	G6020	1(2)	J0476	2(3)
E1200	0(3)	E1636	0(3)	E2311	0(3)	E2605	0(3)	G0202	1(2)	G0407	0(3)	G6022	1(2)	J0480	1(3)
E1220	0(3)	E1637	0(3)	E2312	0(3)	E2606	0(3)	G0204	2(3)	G0408	0(3)	G6023	1(2)	J0485	1500(3)
E1221	0(3)	E1639	0(3)	E2313	0(3)	E2607	0(3)	G0206	2(3)	G0410	6(3)	G6024	1(2)	J0490	160(3)
E1222	0(3)	E1700	0(3)	E2321	0(3)	E2608	0(3)	G0235	1(3)	G0411	6(3)	G6025	1(2)	J0500	4(3)
E1223	0(3)	E1701	0(3)	E2322	0(3)	E2609	0(3)	G0237	8(3)	G0412	1(2)	G6027	1(3)	J0558	24(3)
E1224	0(3)	E1702	0(3)	E2323	0(3)	E2611	0(3)	G0238	8(3)	G0413	1(2)	G6028	1(2)	J0561	24(3)
E1225	0(3)	E1800	0(3)	E2324	0(3)	E2612	0(3)	G0239	2(3)	G0414	1(2)	G6030	2(3)	J0571	0(3)
E1226	1(1)	E1801	0(3)	E2325	0(3)	E2613	0(3)	G0245	1(2)	G0415	1(2)	G6031	2(3)	J0572	0(3)
E1228	0(3)	E1802	0(3)	E2326	0(3)	E2614	0(3)	G0246	1(2)	G0416	1(2)	G6032	2(3)	J0573	0(3)
E1229	0(3)	E1805	0(3)	E2327	0(3)	E2615	0(3)	G0247	1(2)	G0420	2(3)	G6034	2(3)	J0574	0(3)
E1230	0(3)	E1806	0(3)	E2328	0(3)	E2616	0(3)	G0248	1(2)	G0421	4(3)	G6035	2(1)	J0575	0(3)
E1231	0(3)	E1810	0(3)	E2329	0(3)	E2617	0(3)	G0249	3(3)	G0422	6(2)	G6036	2(3)	J0586	300(3)

CPT	MUE	CPT	MUE	CPT	MUE	CPT	MUE	CPT	MUE	CPT	MUE	CPT	MUE
J0594	320(3)	J1446	192(3)	J2507	8(3)	J7196	175(3)	J9055	120(3)	K0042	0(3)	K0841	0(3)	L0470	1(2)
J0597	250(3)	J1450	4(3)	J2510	4(3)	J7301	0(3)	J9060	24(3)	K0043	0(3)	K0842	0(3)	L0472	1(2)
J0598	100(3)	J1451	200(3)	J2540	75(3)	J7310	2(2)	J9065	20(3)	K0044	0(3)	K0843	0(3)	L0480	1(2)
J0600	3(3)	J1453	150(3)	J2543	20(3)	J7311	1(3)	J9098	5(3)	K0045	0(3)	K0848	0(3)	L0482	1(2)
J0610	15(3)	J1457	500(3)	J2545	1(3)	J7312	14(3)	J9130	24(3)	K0046	0(3)	K0849	0(3)	L0484	1(2)
J0620	1(3)	J1556	300(3)	J2550	3(3)	J7315	2(3)	J9155	240(3)	K0047	0(3)	K0850	0(3)	L0486	1(2)
J0637	20(3)	J1557	300(3)	J2590	15(3)	J7316	4(2)	J9160	0(3)	K0050	0(3)	K0851	0(3)	L0488	1(2)
J0638	150(3)	J1561	300(3)	J2597	45(3)	J7321	2(2)	J9171	240(3)	K0051	0(3)	K0852	0(3)	L0490	1(2)
J0640	24(3)	J1568	300(3)	J2675	1(3)	J7323	2(2)	J9179	50(3)	K0052	0(3)	K0853	0(3)	L0491	1(2)
J0690	16(3)	J1569	300(3)	J2680	4(3)	J7324	2(2)	J9190	20(3)	K0053	0(3)	K0854	0(3)	L0492	1(2)
J0692	12(3)	J1570	4(3)	J2690	4(3)	J7326	2(2)	J9202	3(3)	K0056	0(3)	K0855	0(3)	L0621	1(2)
J0694	12(3)	J1571	20(3)	J2720	10(3)	J7327	2(2)	J9206	42(3)	K0065	0(3)	K0856	0(3)	L0622	1(2)
J0696	16(3)	J1572	300(3)	J2724	4000(3)	J7336	1120(3)	J9211	6(3)	K0069	0(3)	K0857	0(3)	L0623	1(2)
J0697	12(3)	J1580	9(3)	J2730	2(3)	J7504	15(3)	J9213	12(3)	K0070	0(3)	K0858	0(3)	L0624	1(2)
J0698	12(3)	J1599	300(3)	J2760	2(3)	J7508	300(3)	J9216	2(3)	K0071	0(3)	K0859	0(3)	L0625	1(2)
J0706	16(3)	J1600	2(3)	J2770	7(3)	J7511	9(3)	J9217	6(3)	K0072	0(3)	K0860	0(3)	L0626	1(2)
J0712	180(3)	J1602	300(3)	J2778	10(3)	J7516	4(3)	J9219	1(3)	K0073	0(3)	K0861	0(3)	L0627	1(2)
J0713	12(3)	J1610	3(3)	J2780	16(3)	J7525	2(3)	J9225	1(3)	K0077	0(3)	K0862	0(3)	L0628	1(2)
J0717	400(3)	J1631	9(3)	J2783	60(3)	J7527	20(3)	J9228	450(3)	K0105	0(3)	K0863	0(3)	L0629	1(2)
J0720	15(3)	J1645	10(3)	J2785	4(3)	J7604	0(3)	J9230	5(3)	K0195	0(3)	K0864	0(3)	L0630	1(2)
J0735	50(3)	J1650	30(3)	J2788	1(3)	J7607	0(3)	J9261	80(3)	K0455	0(3)	K0868	0(3)	L0631	1(2)
J0740	2(3)	J1652	20(3)	J2791	275(3)	J7609	0(3)	J9262	700(3)	K0462	0(3)	K0869	0(3)	L0632	1(2)
J0743	16(3)	J1725	250(3)	J2793	320(3)	J7610	0(3)	J9266	2(3)	K0552	0(3)	K0870	0(3)	L0633	1(2)
J0744	8(3)	J1740	3(3)	J2794	100(3)	J7615	0(3)	J9267	750(3)	K0601	0(3)	K0871	0(3)	L0634	1(2)
J0745	8(3)	J1741	32(3)	J2795	2400(3)	J7622	0(3)	J9268	1(3)	K0602	0(3)	K0877	0(3)	L0635	1(2)
J0760	4(3)	J1742	4(3)	J2796	150(3)	J7624	0(3)	J9280	12(3)	K0603	0(3)	K0878	0(3)	L0636	1(2)
J0770	5(3)	J1743	66(3)	J2800	3(3)	J7627	0(3)	J9293	8(3)	K0604	0(3)	K0879	0(3)	L0637	1(2)
J0775	180(3)	J1744	90(3)	J2805	3(3)	J7628	0(3)	J9300	0(3)	K0605	0(3)	K0880	0(3)	L0638	1(2)
J0780	10(3)	J1745	150(3)	J2941	8(3)	J7629	0(3)	J9301	100(3)	K0606	0(3)	K0884	0(3)	L0639	1(2)
J0800	3(3)	J1786	900(3)	J2993	2(3)	J7632	0(3)	J9303	100(3)	K0607	0(3)	K0885	0(3)	L0640	1(2)
J0833	3(3)	J1790	2(3)	J2995	0(3)	J7634	0(3)	J9305	150(3)	K0608	0(3)	K0886	0(3)	L0641	1(2)
J0834	3(3)	J1817	0(3)	J2997	100(3)	J7635	0(3)	J9306	840(3)	K0609	0(3)	K0890	0(3)	L0642	1(2)
J0840	18(3)	J1830	1(3)	J3000	2(3)	J7636	0(3)	J9307	80(3)	K0730	0(3)	K0891	0(3)	L0643	1(2)
J0886	40(3)	J1840	3(3)	J3010	100(3)	J7637	0(3)	J9310	12(3)	K0733	0(3)	K0898	1(2)	L0648	1(2)
J0890	0(3)	J1885	8(3)	J3030	2(3)	J7638	0(3)	J9315	40(3)	K0738	0(3)	K0900	0(3)	L0649	1(2)
J0895	12(3)	J1930	120(3)	J3060	900(3)	J7640	0(3)	J9320	4(3)	K0743	0(3)	K0901	2(2)	L0650	1(2)
J0897	120(3)	J1931	760(3)	J3095	150(3)	J7641	0(3)	J9354	600(3)	K0800	0(3)	K0902	2(2)	L0651	1(2)
J0945	4(3)	J1953	300(3)	J3101	50(3)	J7642	0(3)	J9355	100(3)	K0801	0(3)	L0112	1(2)	L0700	1(2)
J1000	1(3)	J1955	11(3)	J3121	400(3)	J7643	0(3)	J9360	45(3)	K0802	0(3)	L0113	1(2)	L0710	1(2)
J1050	1000(3)	J1956	4(3)	J3145	750(3)	J7645	0(3)	J9370	4(3)	K0806	0(3)	L0120	1(2)	L0810	1(2)
J1071	400(3)	J2001	400(3)	J3240	1(3)	J7647	0(3)	J9371	5(3)	K0807	0(3)	L0130	1(2)	L0820	1(2)
J1110	3(3)	J2020	6(3)	J3243	200(3)	J7650	0(3)	J9390	36(3)	K0808	0(3)	L0140	1(2)	L0830	1(2)
J1120	2(3)	J2150	8(3)	J3246	100(3)	J7657	0(3)	J9395	20(3)	K0812	0(3)	L0150	1(2)	L0859	1(2)
J1160	3(3)	J2175	6(3)	J3250	4(3)	J7660	0(3)	J9400	600(3)	K0813	0(3)	L0160	1(2)	L0861	1(2)
J1162	10(3)	J2185	60(3)	J3262	800(3)	J7665	127(2)	J9600	4(3)	K0814	0(3)	L0170	1(2)	L0970	1(2)
J1165	50(3)	J2212	240(3)	J3285	9(3)	J7667	0(3)	K0001	0(3)	K0815	0(3)	L0172	1(2)	L0972	1(2)
J1180	0(3)	J2248	300(3)	J3300	160(3)	J7670	0(3)	K0002	0(3)	K0816	0(3)	L0174	1(2)	L0974	1(2)
J1190	8(3)	J2265	400(3)	J3301	16(3)	J7676	0(3)	K0003	0(3)	K0820	0(3)	L0180	1(2)	L0976	1(2)
J1200	8(3)	J2280	8(3)	J3302	0(3)	J7680	0(3)	K0004	0(3)	K0821	0(3)	L0190	1(2)	L0978	2(3)
J1205	4(3)	J2300	10(3)	J3315	6(3)	J7681	0(3)	K0005	0(3)	K0822	0(3)	L0200	1(2)	L0980	1(2)
J1212	1(3)	J2310	10(3)	J3357	90(3)	J7683	0(3)	K0006	0(3)	K0823	0(3)	L0220	1(3)	L0982	1(3)
J1240	6(3)	J2315	380(3)	J3360	6(3)	J7684	0(3)	K0007	0(3)	K0824	0(3)	L0450	1(2)	L0984	3(3)
J1245	6(3)	J2320	4(3)	J3370	12(3)	J7685	0(3)	K0008	0(3)	K0825	0(3)	L0452	1(2)	L1000	1(2)
J1260	2(3)	J2323	300(3)	J3396	150(3)	J8510	5(3)	K0009	0(3)	K0826	0(3)	L0454	1(2)	L1001	1(2)
J1267	150(3)	J2354	60(3)	J3410	16(3)	J9010	3(3)	K0013	0(3)	K0827	0(3)	L0455	1(2)	L1005	1(2)
J1300	120(3)	J2355	2(3)	J3415	6(3)	J9019	60(3)	K0015	0(3)	K0828	0(3)	L0456	1(2)	L1010	2(2)
J1327	99(3)	J2358	405(3)	J3420	1(3)	J9025	300(3)	K0017	0(3)	K0829	0(3)	L0457	1(2)	L1020	2(3)
J1335	2(3)	J2360	3(3)	J3430	50(3)	J9031	1(3)	K0018	0(3)	K0830	0(3)	L0458	1(2)	L1025	1(3)
J1364	8(3)	J2405	64(3)	J3465	120(3)	J9033	300(3)	K0019	0(3)	K0831	0(3)	L0460	1(2)	L1030	1(3)
J1380	4(3)	J2426	234(3)	J3473	450(3)	J9040	4(3)	K0020	0(3)	K0835	0(3)	L0462	1(2)	L1040	1(3)
J1430	10(3)	J2430	3(3)	J3486	4(3)	J9042	200(3)	K0037	0(3)	K0836	0(3)	L0464	1(2)	L1050	1(3)
J1435	1(3)	J2469	10(3)	J3489	5(3)	J9043	60(3)	K0038	0(3)	K0837	0(3)	L0466	1(2)	L1060	1(3)
J1438	2(3)	J2503	2(3)	J7100	5(3)	J9045	22(3)	K0039	0(3)	K0838	0(3)	L0467	1(2)	L1070	2(2)
J1439	750(3)	J2504	15(3)	J7110	3(3)	J9047	120(3)	K0040	0(3)	K0839	0(3)	L0468	1(2)	L1080	2(2)
J1442	3360(3)	J2505	1(3)	J7131	500(3)	J9050	6(3)	K0041	0(3)	K0840	0(3)	L0469	1(2)	L1085	1(2)

　　　© 2015 American Medical Association. All Rights Reserved.　　　© 2015 Optum360, LLC

CPT	MUE	CPT	MUE	CPT	MUE	CPT	MUE	CPT	MUE	CPT	MUE	CPT	MUE	CPT	MUE
L1090	1(3)	L1960	2(2)	L2526	2(1)	L3420	2(1)	L3925	4(3)	L5321	2(2)	L5678	2(1)	L5950	2(1)
L1100	2(2)	L1970	2(2)	L2530	2(1)	L3430	2(1)	L3927	4(3)	L5331	2(2)	L5680	2(1)	L5960	2(1)
L1110	2(2)	L1971	2(2)	L2540	2(1)	L3440	2(1)	L3929	2(2)	L5341	2(2)	L5681	2(1)	L5961	1(1)
L1120	3(3)	L1980	2(2)	L2550	2(1)	L3450	2(1)	L3930	2(2)	L5400	2(2)	L5682	2(1)	L5962	2(1)
L1200	1(2)	L1990	2(2)	L2570	2(1)	L3455	2(1)	L3931	2(2)	L5410	2(2)	L5683	2(1)	L5964	2(1)
L1210	2(3)	L2000	2(2)	L2580	2(1)	L3460	2(1)	L3933	3(3)	L5420	2(2)	L5684	2(1)	L5966	2(1)
L1220	1(3)	L2005	2(2)	L2600	2(1)	L3465	2(1)	L3935	3(3)	L5430	2(2)	L5686	2(1)	L5968	2(1)
L1230	1(2)	L2010	2(2)	L2610	2(1)	L3470	2(1)	L3960	1(3)	L5450	2(2)	L5688	2(1)	L5969	0(3)
L1240	1(3)	L2020	2(2)	L2620	2(1)	L3480	2(1)	L3961	1(3)	L5460	2(2)	L5690	2(1)	L5970	2(1)
L1250	2(3)	L2030	2(2)	L2622	2(1)	L3485	2(1)	L3962	1(3)	L5500	2(2)	L5692	2(1)	L5971	2(1)
L1260	1(3)	L2034	2(2)	L2624	2(1)	L3500	2(1)	L3967	1(3)	L5505	2(2)	L5694	2(1)	L5972	2(1)
L1270	3(3)	L2035	2(2)	L2627	1(1)	L3510	2(1)	L3971	1(3)	L5510	2(2)	L5695	2(1)	L5973	2(1)
L1280	2(3)	L2036	2(2)	L2628	1(1)	L3520	2(1)	L3973	1(3)	L5520	2(2)	L5696	2(1)	L5974	2(1)
L1290	2(3)	L2037	2(2)	L2630	1(1)	L3530	2(1)	L3975	1(3)	L5530	2(2)	L5697	2(1)	L5975	2(1)
L1300	1(2)	L2038	2(2)	L2640	1(1)	L3540	2(1)	L3976	1(3)	L5535	2(2)	L5698	2(1)	L5976	2(1)
L1310	1(2)	L2040	1(2)	L2650	2(1)	L3550	2(1)	L3977	1(3)	L5540	2(2)	L5699	2(1)	L5978	2(1)
L1499	1(3)	L2050	1(2)	L2660	1(1)	L3560	2(1)	L3978	1(3)	L5560	2(2)	L5700	2(1)	L5979	2(1)
L1600	1(2)	L2060	1(2)	L2670	2(1)	L3570	2(1)	L3980	2(2)	L5570	2(2)	L5701	2(1)	L5980	2(1)
L1610	1(2)	L2070	1(2)	L2680	2(1)	L3580	2(1)	L3981	2(2)	L5580	2(2)	L5702	2(1)	L5981	2(1)
L1620	1(2)	L2080	1(2)	L2795	2(1)	L3590	2(1)	L3982	2(2)	L5585	2(2)	L5703	2(1)	L5982	2(1)
L1630	1(2)	L2090	1(2)	L2800	2(1)	L3595	2(1)	L3984	2(2)	L5590	2(2)	L5704	2(1)	L5984	2(1)
L1640	1(2)	L2106	2(2)	L2820	2(1)	L3600	2(1)	L4000	1(1)	L5595	2(2)	L5705	2(1)	L5985	2(1)
L1650	1(2)	L2108	2(2)	L2830	2(1)	L3610	2(1)	L4010	2(1)	L5600	2(2)	L5706	2(1)	L5986	2(1)
L1652	1(2)	L2112	2(2)	L3000	2(1)	L3620	2(1)	L4020	2(1)	L5610	2(1)	L5707	2(1)	L5987	2(1)
L1660	1(2)	L2114	2(2)	L3001	2(1)	L3630	2(1)	L4030	2(1)	L5611	2(1)	L5710	2(1)	L5988	2(1)
L1680	1(2)	L2116	2(2)	L3002	2(1)	L3640	1(1)	L4040	2(1)	L5613	2(1)	L5711	2(1)	L5990	2(1)
L1685	1(2)	L2126	2(2)	L3003	2(1)	L3650	1(2)	L4045	2(1)	L5614	2(1)	L5712	2(1)	L6000	2(2)
L1686	1(3)	L2128	2(2)	L3010	2(1)	L3660	1(2)	L4050	2(1)	L5616	2(1)	L5714	2(1)	L6010	2(2)
L1690	1(2)	L2132	2(2)	L3020	2(1)	L3670	1(3)	L4055	2(1)	L5617	2(1)	L5716	2(1)	L6020	2(2)
L1700	1(2)	L2134	2(2)	L3030	2(1)	L3671	1(3)	L4060	2(1)	L5628	2(1)	L5718	2(1)	L6026	2(2)
L1710	1(2)	L2136	2(2)	L3031	2(1)	L3674	1(3)	L4070	2(1)	L5629	2(1)	L5722	2(1)	L6050	2(2)
L1720	2(2)	L2180	2(2)	L3040	2(1)	L3675	1(2)	L4080	2(1)	L5630	2(1)	L5724	2(1)	L6055	2(2)
L1730	1(2)	L2182	4(2)	L3050	2(1)	L3677	1(2)	L4100	2(1)	L5631	2(1)	L5726	2(1)	L6100	2(2)
L1755	2(2)	L2184	4(2)	L3060	2(1)	L3678	1(2)	L4130	2(1)	L5632	2(1)	L5728	2(1)	L6110	2(2)
L1810	2(2)	L2186	4(2)	L3070	2(1)	L3702	2(2)	L4210	4(3)	L5634	2(1)	L5780	2(1)	L6120	2(2)
L1812	2(2)	L2188	2(2)	L3080	2(1)	L3710	2(2)	L4350	2(2)	L5636	2(1)	L5781	2(1)	L6130	2(2)
L1820	2(2)	L2190	2(2)	L3090	2(1)	L3720	2(2)	L4360	2(2)	L5637	2(1)	L5782	2(1)	L6200	2(2)
L1830	2(2)	L2192	2(2)	L3100	2(1)	L3730	2(2)	L4361	2(2)	L5638	2(1)	L5785	2(1)	L6205	2(2)
L1831	2(2)	L2200	4(2)	L3140	1(1)	L3740	2(2)	L4370	2(2)	L5639	2(1)	L5790	2(1)	L6250	2(2)
L1832	2(2)	L2210	4(2)	L3150	1(1)	L3760	2(2)	L4386	2(2)	L5640	2(1)	L5795	2(1)	L6300	2(2)
L1833	2(2)	L2220	4(2)	L3160	2(1)	L3762	2(2)	L4387	2(2)	L5642	2(1)	L5810	2(1)	L6310	2(2)
L1834	2(2)	L2230	2(2)	L3170	2(1)	L3763	2(2)	L4392	2(1)	L5643	2(1)	L5811	2(1)	L6320	2(2)
L1836	2(2)	L2232	2(2)	L3215	0(3)	L3764	2(2)	L4394	2(1)	L5644	2(1)	L5812	2(1)	L6350	2(2)
L1840	2(2)	L2240	2(2)	L3216	0(3)	L3765	2(2)	L4396	2(2)	L5645	2(1)	L5814	2(1)	L6360	2(2)
L1843	2(2)	L2250	2(2)	L3217	0(3)	L3766	2(2)	L4397	2(2)	L5646	2(1)	L5816	2(1)	L6370	2(2)
L1844	2(2)	L2260	2(2)	L3219	0(3)	L3806	2(2)	L4398	2(2)	L5647	2(1)	L5818	2(1)	L6380	2(2)
L1845	2(2)	L2265	2(2)	L3221	0(3)	L3807	2(2)	L4631	2(2)	L5648	2(1)	L5822	2(1)	L6382	2(2)
L1846	2(2)	L2270	2(3)	L3222	0(3)	L3808	2(2)	L5000	2(3)	L5649	2(1)	L5824	2(1)	L6384	2(2)
L1847	2(2)	L2275	2(3)	L3224	2(1)	L3809	2(2)	L5010	2(2)	L5650	2(1)	L5826	2(1)	L6386	2(2)
L1848	2(2)	L2280	2(2)	L3225	2(1)	L3900	2(2)	L5020	2(2)	L5651	2(1)	L5828	2(1)	L6388	2(2)
L1850	2(2)	L2300	1(2)	L3230	2(1)	L3901	2(2)	L5050	2(2)	L5652	2(1)	L5830	2(1)	L6400	2(2)
L1860	2(2)	L2310	1(2)	L3250	2(1)	L3904	2(2)	L5060	2(2)	L5653	2(1)	L5840	2(1)	L6450	2(2)
L1900	2(2)	L2320	2(1)	L3251	2(1)	L3905	2(2)	L5100	2(2)	L5654	2(1)	L5845	2(1)	L6500	2(2)
L1902	2(2)	L2330	2(1)	L3252	2(1)	L3906	2(2)	L5105	2(2)	L5655	2(1)	L5848	2(1)	L6550	2(2)
L1904	2(2)	L2335	2(1)	L3253	2(1)	L3908	2(2)	L5150	2(2)	L5656	2(1)	L5850	2(1)	L6570	2(2)
L1906	2(2)	L2340	2(1)	L3330	2(1)	L3912	2(3)	L5160	2(2)	L5658	2(1)	L5855	2(1)	L6580	2(2)
L1907	2(2)	L2350	2(1)	L3332	2(1)	L3913	2(2)	L5200	2(2)	L5661	2(1)	L5856	2(1)	L6582	2(2)
L1910	2(2)	L2360	2(1)	L3340	2(1)	L3915	2(2)	L5210	2(2)	L5665	2(1)	L5857	2(1)	L6584	2(2)
L1920	2(2)	L2370	2(1)	L3350	2(1)	L3916	2(2)	L5220	2(2)	L5666	2(1)	L5858	2(1)	L6586	2(2)
L1930	2(2)	L2375	2(1)	L3360	2(1)	L3917	2(2)	L5230	2(2)	L5668	2(1)	L5859	2(1)	L6588	2(2)
L1932	2(2)	L2380	2(1)	L3370	2(1)	L3918	2(2)	L5250	2(2)	L5670	2(1)	L5910	2(1)	L6590	2(2)
L1940	2(2)	L2500	2(1)	L3380	2(1)	L3919	2(2)	L5270	2(2)	L5671	2(1)	L5920	2(1)	L6600	2(1)
L1945	2(2)	L2510	2(1)	L3390	2(1)	L3921	2(2)	L5280	2(2)	L5672	2(1)	L5925	2(1)	L6605	2(1)
L1950	2(2)	L2520	2(1)	L3400	2(1)	L3923	2(2)	L5301	2(2)	L5676	2(1)	L5930	2(1)	L6610	2(1)
L1951	2(2)	L2525	2(1)	L3410	2(1)	L3924	2(2)	L5312	2(2)	L5677	2(1)	L5940	2(1)	L6611	2(1)

CPT	MUE	CPT	MUE	CPT	MUE	CPT	MUE	CPT	MUE	CPT	MUE	CPT	MUE	CPT	MUE
L6615	2(1)	L6884	2(1)	L8046	1(1)	L8696	1(3)	Q0509	1(3)	Q4125	28(3)	V2208	2(1)	V2624	2(1)
L6616	2(1)	L6885	2(1)	L8047	1(1)	P2028	1(1)	Q0510	1(2)	Q4126	0(3)	V2209	2(1)	V2625	2(1)
L6620	2(1)	L6890	2(1)	L8048	1(3)	P2029	1(1)	Q0511	1(2)	Q4127	100(3)	V2210	2(1)	V2626	2(1)
L6621	2(1)	L6895	2(1)	L8300	1(1)	P2033	1(1)	Q0512	4(3)	Q4128	128(3)	V2211	2(1)	V2627	2(1)
L6623	2(1)	L6900	2(1)	L8310	1(1)	P2038	1(1)	Q0513	1(2)	Q4129	81(3)	V2212	2(1)	V2628	2(1)
L6624	2(1)	L6905	2(1)	L8320	2(1)	P3000	1(3)	Q0514	1(2)	Q4130	100(3)	V2213	2(1)	V2629	2(1)
L6625	2(1)	L6910	2(1)	L8330	2(1)	P3001	1(3)	Q1004	2(1)	Q4131	98(3)	V2214	2(1)	V2630	2(1)
L6628	2(1)	L6915	2(1)	L8500	1(1)	P9041	100(3)	Q1005	2(1)	Q4132	50(3)	V2215	2(1)	V2631	2(1)
L6629	2(1)	L6920	2(2)	L8501	2(1)	P9043	10(3)	Q2004	1(3)	Q4133	113(3)	V2218	2(1)	V2632	2(1)
L6630	2(1)	L6925	2(2)	L8507	3(1)	P9045	20(3)	Q2026	45(3)	Q4134	160(3)	V2219	2(1)	V2700	2(1)
L6635	2(1)	L6930	2(2)	L8509	1(1)	P9046	40(3)	Q2028	1470(3)	Q4135	900(3)	V2220	2(1)	V2702	0(3)
L6637	2(1)	L6935	2(2)	L8510	1(1)	P9047	20(3)	Q2034	1(1)	Q4136	900(3)	V2221	2(1)	V2710	2(1)
L6638	2(1)	L6940	2(2)	L8511	1(1)	P9048	2(3)	Q2035	1(2)	Q4139	2(3)	V2299	2(1)	V2715	4(3)
L6640	2(1)	L6945	2(2)	L8514	1(1)	P9612	1(3)	Q2036	1(2)	Q9953	10(3)	V2300	2(1)	V2718	2(1)
L6641	2(1)	L6950	2(2)	L8515	1(1)	P9615	1(3)	Q2037	1(2)	Q9955	10(2)	V2301	2(1)	V2730	2(1)
L6642	2(1)	L6955	2(2)	L8600	2(1)	Q0035	1(1)	Q2038	1(2)	Q9956	9(3)	V2302	2(1)	V2744	2(3)
L6645	2(1)	L6960	2(2)	L8604	3(3)	Q0081	2(3)	Q2039	1(2)	Q9957	3(3)	V2303	2(1)	V2745	2(3)
L6646	2(1)	L6965	2(2)	L8605	4(3)	Q0083	2(3)	Q2043	1(1)	Q9958	600(3)	V2304	2(1)	V2750	2(3)
L6647	2(1)	L6970	2(2)	L8606	5(3)	Q0084	2(3)	Q2050	20(3)	Q9960	250(3)	V2305	2(1)	V2755	2(3)
L6648	2(1)	L6975	2(2)	L8609	1(1)	Q0085	2(3)	Q2052	0(3)	Q9961	200(3)	V2306	2(1)	V2756	0(3)
L6650	2(1)	L7007	2(1)	L8610	2(1)	Q0091	1(1)	Q3014	2(3)	Q9962	200(3)	V2307	2(1)	V2760	0(3)
L6670	2(1)	L7008	2(1)	L8612	2(1)	Q0111	2(1)	Q3027	30(3)	Q9963	240(3)	V2308	2(1)	V2761	2(1)
L6672	2(1)	L7009	2(1)	L8613	2(1)	Q0112	3(1)	Q3028	0(3)	Q9966	250(3)	V2309	2(1)	V2762	0(3)
L6675	2(1)	L7040	2(1)	L8614	2(1)	Q0113	2(1)	Q3031	1(1)	Q9967	300(3)	V2310	2(1)	V2770	2(1)
L6676	2(1)	L7045	2(1)	L8615	2(1)	Q0114	1(1)	Q4001	1(1)	R0070	2(3)	V2311	2(1)	V2780	2(1)
L6677	2(1)	L7170	2(1)	L8616	2(1)	Q0115	1(1)	Q4002	1(1)	R0075	2(3)	V2312	2(1)	V2781	2(1)
L6686	2(1)	L7180	2(1)	L8617	2(1)	Q0144	0(3)	Q4003	2(1)	R0076	1(1)	V2313	2(1)	V2782	2(1)
L6687	2(1)	L7181	2(1)	L8618	2(1)	Q0161	30(3)	Q4004	2(1)	V2020	1(1)	V2314	2(1)	V2783	2(1)
L6688	2(1)	L7185	2(1)	L8619	2(1)	Q0478	1(1)	Q4025	1(1)	V2025	0(3)	V2315	2(1)	V2784	2(3)
L6689	2(1)	L7186	2(1)	L8621	600(3)	Q0479	1(1)	Q4026	1(1)	V2100	2(3)	V2318	2(1)	V2785	2(1)
L6690	2(1)	L7190	2(1)	L8622	2(1)	Q0480	1(1)	Q4027	1(1)	V2101	2(1)	V2319	2(1)	V2786	0(3)
L6693	2(1)	L7191	2(1)	L8627	2(2)	Q0481	1(2)	Q4028	1(1)	V2102	2(1)	V2320	2(1)	V2790	1(1)
L6694	2(1)	L7259	2(2)	L8628	2(2)	Q0482	1(1)	Q4074	0(3)	V2103	2(3)	V2321	2(1)	V2797	0(3)
L6695	2(1)	L7362	1(1)	L8629	2(2)	Q0483	1(1)	Q4101	176(3)	V2104	2(1)	V2399	2(3)	V5008	0(1)
L6696	2(1)	L7366	1(1)	L8631	4(1)	Q0484	1(1)	Q4102	140(3)	V2105	2(1)	V2410	2(1)	V5010	0(1)
L6697	2(1)	L7368	1(1)	L8641	4(1)	Q0485	1(1)	Q4103	0(3)	V2106	2(1)	V2430	2(1)	V5011	0(1)
L6698	2(1)	L7400	2(1)	L8642	2(1)	Q0486	1(1)	Q4104	250(3)	V2107	2(1)	V2499	2(3)	V5274	0(3)
L6703	2(1)	L7401	2(1)	L8658	4(1)	Q0487	1(1)	Q4105	250(3)	V2108	2(1)	V2500	2(1)	V5281	0(1)
L6704	2(1)	L7402	2(1)	L8659	4(1)	Q0488	1(1)	Q4106	152(3)	V2109	2(1)	V2501	2(1)	V5282	0(1)
L6706	2(1)	L7403	2(1)	L8670	4(1)	Q0489	1(1)	Q4107	128(3)	V2110	2(1)	V2502	2(1)	V5284	0(1)
L6707	2(1)	L7404	2(1)	L8679	3(3)	Q0490	1(1)	Q4108	250(3)	V2111	2(1)	V2503	2(1)	V5285	0(1)
L6708	2(1)	L7405	2(1)	L8680	0(3)	Q0491	1(1)	Q4110	250(3)	V2112	2(1)	V2510	2(1)	V5286	0(1)
L6709	2(1)	L7510	4(3)	L8681	1(1)	Q0492	1(1)	Q4111	112(3)	V2113	2(1)	V2511	2(1)	V5287	0(1)
L6711	2(1)	L7900	1(1)	L8682	2(1)	Q0493	1(1)	Q4112	2(3)	V2114	2(1)	V2512	2(1)	V5288	0(1)
L6712	2(1)	L7902	1(1)	L8683	1(1)	Q0494	1(1)	Q4113	4(3)	V2115	2(1)	V2513	2(1)	V5289	0(1)
L6713	2(1)	L8030	2(1)	L8684	1(1)	Q0495	1(1)	Q4114	6(3)	V2118	2(1)	V2520	2(1)		
L6714	2(1)	L8031	2(1)	L8685	1(1)	Q0497	2(1)	Q4115	240(3)	V2121	2(1)	V2521	2(1)		
L6715	4(3)	L8032	2(1)	L8686	2(1)	Q0498	1(1)	Q4116	320(3)	V2199	2(3)	V2522	2(1)		
L6721	2(1)	L8035	2(1)	L8687	1(1)	Q0499	1(1)	Q4117	0(3)	V2200	2(1)	V2523	2(1)		
L6722	2(1)	L8039	2(1)	L8688	1(1)	Q0501	1(1)	Q4118	1000(3)	V2201	2(1)	V2530	2(1)		
L6805	2(1)	L8040	1(1)	L8689	1(1)	Q0502	1(1)	Q4119	300(3)	V2202	2(1)	V2531	2(1)		
L6810	2(1)	L8041	2(1)	L8690	2(2)	Q0503	3(1)	Q4120	300(3)	V2203	2(1)	V2599	2(3)		
L6880	2(1)	L8042	2(1)	L8691	1(3)	Q0504	1(1)	Q4121	156(3)	V2204	2(1)	V2600	1(1)		
L6881	2(1)	L8043	1(1)	L8692	0(3)	Q0506	8(3)	Q4122	96(3)	V2205	2(1)	V2610	1(1)		
L6882	2(1)	L8044	1(1)	L8693	1(3)	Q0507	1(3)	Q4123	160(3)	V2206	2(1)	V2615	2(1)		
L6883	2(1)	L8045	2(1)	L8695	1(1)	Q0508	1(3)	Q4124	280(3)	V2207	2(1)	V2623	2(1)		

Appendix I — Inpatient Only Procedures

Inpatient Only Procedures—This appendix identifies services with the status indicator C. Medicare will not pay an OPPS hospital or ASC when they are performed on a Medicare patient as an outpatient. Physicians should refer to this list when scheduling Medicare patients for surgical procedures. CMS updates this list quarterly.

0169T Place stereo cath brain	21141 Lefort i-1 piece w/o graft	22207 Incis spine 3 column lumbar
01756 Anesth radical humerus surg	21142 Lefort i-2 piece w/o graft	22208 Incis spine 3 column adl seg
0195T Prescrl fuse w/o instr l5/s1	21143 Lefort i-3/> piece w/o graft	22210 Incis 1 vertebral seg cerv
0196T Prescrl fuse w/o instr l4/l5	21145 Lefort i-1 piece w/ graft	22212 Incis 1 vertebral seg thorac
01990 Support for organ donor	21146 Lefort i-2 piece w/ graft	22214 Incis 1 vertebral seg lumbar
0202T Post vert arthrplst 1 lumbar	21147 Lefort i-3/> piece w/ graft	22216 Incis addl spine segment
0219T Plmt post facet implt cerv	21151 Lefort ii w/bone grafts	22220 Incis w/discectomy cervical
0220T Plmt post facet implt thor	21154 Lefort iii w/o lefort i	22222 Incis w/discectomy thoracic
0235T Trluml perip athrc visceral	21155 Lefort iii w/ lefort i	22224 Incis w/discectomy lumbar
0254T Evasc rpr iliac art bifur	21159 Lefort iii w/fhdw/o lefort i	22226 Revise extra spine segment
0255T Evasc rpr iliac art bifr s&i	21160 Lefort iii w/fhd w/ lefort i	22318 Treat odontoid fx w/o graft
0262T Impltj pulm vlv evasc appr	21179 Reconstruct entire forehead	22319 Treat odontoid fx w/graft
0266T Implt/rpl crtd sns dev total	21180 Reconstruct entire forehead	22325 Treat spine fracture
0281T Laa closure w/implant	21182 Reconstruct cranial bone	22326 Treat neck spine fracture
0293T Ins lt atrl press monitor	21183 Reconstruct cranial bone	22327 Treat thorax spine fracture
0294T Ins lt atrl mont pres lead	21184 Reconstruct cranial bone	22328 Treat each add spine fx
0309T Prescrl fuse w/ instr l4/l5	21188 Reconstruction of midface	22532 Lat thorax spine fusion
0345T Transcath mtral vlve repair	21194 Reconst lwr jaw w/graft	22533 Lat lumbar spine fusion
0375T Total disc arthrp ant appr	21196 Reconst lwr jaw w/fixation	22534 Lat thor/lumb addl seg
11004 Debride genitalia & perineum	21247 Reconstruct lower jaw bone	22548 Neck spine fusion
11005 Debride abdom wall	21255 Reconstruct lower jaw bone	22556 Thorax spine fusion
11006 Debride genit/per/abdom wall	21268 Revise eye sockets	22558 Lumbar spine fusion
11008 Remove mesh from abd wall	21343 Open tx dprsd front sinus fx	22585 Additional spinal fusion
15756 Free myo/skin flap microvasc	21344 Open tx compl front sinus fx	22586 Prescrl fuse w/ instr l5-s1
15757 Free skin flap microvasc	21347 Opn tx nasomax fx multple	22590 Spine & skull spinal fusion
15758 Free fascial flap microvasc	21348 Opn tx nasomax fx w/graft	22595 Neck spinal fusion
16036 Escharotomy addl incision	21366 Opn tx complx malar w/grft	22600 Neck spine fusion
19271 Revision of chest wall	21422 Treat mouth roof fracture	22610 Thorax spine fusion
19272 Extensive chest wall surgery	21423 Treat mouth roof fracture	22630 Lumbar spine fusion
19305 Mast radical	21431 Treat craniofacial fracture	22632 Spine fusion extra segment
19306 Mast rad urban type	21432 Treat craniofacial fracture	22633 Lumbar spine fusion combined
19361 Breast reconstr w/lat flap	21433 Treat craniofacial fracture	22634 Spine fusion extra segment
19364 Breast reconstruction	21435 Treat craniofacial fracture	22800 Post fusion </6 vert seg
19367 Breast reconstruction	21436 Treat craniofacial fracture	22802 Post fusion 7-12 vert seg
19368 Breast reconstruction	21510 Drainage of bone lesion	22804 Post fusion 13/> vert seg
19369 Breast reconstruction	21615 Removal of rib	22808 Ant fusion 2-3 vert seg
20661 Application of head brace	21616 Removal of rib and nerves	22810 Ant fusion 4-7 vert seg
20664 Application of halo	21620 Partial removal of sternum	22812 Ant fusion 8/> vert seg
20802 Replantation arm complete	21627 Sternal debridement	22818 Kyphectomy 1-2 segments
20805 Replant forearm complete	21630 Extensive sternum surgery	22819 Kyphectomy 3 or more
20808 Replantation hand complete	21632 Extensive sternum surgery	22830 Exploration of spinal fusion
20816 Replantation digit complete	21705 Revision of neck muscle/rib	22840 Insert spine fixation device
20824 Replantation thumb complete	21740 Reconstruction of sternum	22841 Insert spine fixation device
20827 Replantation thumb complete	21750 Repair of sternum separation	22842 Insert spine fixation device
20838 Replantation foot complete	21825 Treat sternum fracture	22843 Insert spine fixation device
20955 Fibula bone graft microvasc	22010 I&d p-spine c/t/cerv-thor	22844 Insert spine fixation device
20956 Iliac bone graft microvasc	22015 I&d abscess p-spine l/s/ls	22845 Insert spine fixation device
20957 Mt bone graft microvasc	22110 Remove part of neck vertebra	22846 Insert spine fixation device
20962 Other bone graft microvasc	22112 Remove part thorax vertebra	22847 Insert spine fixation device
20969 Bone/skin graft microvasc	22114 Remove part lumbar vertebra	22848 Insert pelv fixation device
20970 Bone/skin graft iliac crest	22116 Remove extra spine segment	22849 Reinsert spinal fixation
21045 Extensive jaw surgery	22206 Incis spine 3 column thorac	22850 Remove spine fixation device

22852	Remove spine fixation device	27158	Revision of pelvis	27536	Treat knee fracture
22855	Remove spine fixation device	27161	Incision of neck of femur	27540	Treat knee fracture
22857	Lumbar artif diskectomy	27165	Incision/fixation of femur	27556	Treat knee dislocation
22858	Second level cer diskectomy	27170	Repair/graft femur head/neck	27557	Treat knee dislocation
22861	Revise cerv artific disc	27175	Treat slipped epiphysis	27558	Treat knee dislocation
22862	Revise lumbar artif disc	27176	Treat slipped epiphysis	27580	Fusion of knee
22864	Remove cerv artif disc	27177	Treat slipped epiphysis	27590	Amputate leg at thigh
22865	Remove lumb artif disc	27178	Treat slipped epiphysis	27591	Amputate leg at thigh
23200	Resect clavicle tumor	27181	Treat slipped epiphysis	27592	Amputate leg at thigh
23210	Resect scapula tumor	27185	Revision of femur epiphysis	27596	Amputation follow-up surgery
23220	Resect prox humerus tumor	27187	Reinforce hip bones	27598	Amputate lower leg at knee
23335	Shoulder prosthesis removal	27222	Treat hip socket fracture	27645	Resect tibia tumor
23472	Reconstruct shoulder joint	27226	Treat hip wall fracture	27646	Resect fibula tumor
23474	Revis reconst shoulder joint	27227	Treat hip fracture(s)	27702	Reconstruct ankle joint
23900	Amputation of arm & girdle	27228	Treat hip fracture(s)	27703	Reconstruction ankle joint
23920	Amputation at shoulder joint	27232	Treat thigh fracture	27712	Realignment of lower leg
24900	Amputation of upper arm	27236	Treat thigh fracture	27715	Revision of lower leg
24920	Amputation of upper arm	27240	Treat thigh fracture	27724	Repair/graft of tibia
24930	Amputation follow-up surgery	27244	Treat thigh fracture	27725	Repair of lower leg
24931	Amputate upper arm & implant	27245	Treat thigh fracture	27727	Repair of lower leg
24940	Revision of upper arm	27248	Treat thigh fracture	27880	Amputation of lower leg
25900	Amputation of forearm	27253	Treat hip dislocation	27881	Amputation of lower leg
25905	Amputation of forearm	27254	Treat hip dislocation	27882	Amputation of lower leg
25915	Amputation of forearm	27258	Treat hip dislocation	27886	Amputation follow-up surgery
25920	Amputate hand at wrist	27259	Treat hip dislocation	27888	Amputation of foot at ankle
25924	Amputation follow-up surgery	27268	Cltx thigh fx w/mnpj	28800	Amputation of midfoot
25927	Amputation of hand	27269	Optx thigh fx	31225	Removal of upper jaw
26551	Great toe-hand transfer	27280	Fusion of sacroiliac joint	31230	Removal of upper jaw
26553	Single transfer toe-hand	27282	Fusion of pubic bones	31290	Nasal/sinus endoscopy surg
26554	Double transfer toe-hand	27284	Fusion of hip joint	31291	Nasal/sinus endoscopy surg
26556	Toe joint transfer	27286	Fusion of hip joint	31360	Removal of larynx
26992	Drainage of bone lesion	27290	Amputation of leg at hip	31365	Removal of larynx
27005	Incision of hip tendon	27295	Amputation of leg at hip	31367	Partial removal of larynx
27025	Incision of hip/thigh fascia	27303	Drainage of bone lesion	31368	Partial removal of larynx
27030	Drainage of hip joint	27365	Resect femur/knee tumor	31370	Partial removal of larynx
27036	Excision of hip joint/muscle	27445	Revision of knee joint	31375	Partial removal of larynx
27054	Removal of hip joint lining	27447	Total knee arthroplasty	31380	Partial removal of larynx
27070	Part remove hip bone super	27448	Incision of thigh	31382	Partial removal of larynx
27071	Part removal hip bone deep	27450	Incision of thigh	31390	Removal of larynx & pharynx
27075	Resect hip tumor	27454	Realignment of thigh bone	31395	Reconstruct larynx & pharynx
27076	Resect hip tum incl acetabul	27455	Realignment of knee	31584	Treat larynx fracture
27077	Resect hip tum w/innom bone	27457	Realignment of knee	31587	Revision of larynx
27078	Rsect hip tum incl femur	27465	Shortening of thigh bone	31725	Clearance of airways
27090	Removal of hip prosthesis	27466	Lengthening of thigh bone	31760	Repair of windpipe
27091	Removal of hip prosthesis	27468	Shorten/lengthen thighs	31766	Reconstruction of windpipe
27120	Reconstruction of hip socket	27470	Repair of thigh	31770	Repair/graft of bronchus
27122	Reconstruction of hip socket	27472	Repair/graft of thigh	31775	Reconstruct bronchus
27125	Partial hip replacement	27486	Revise/replace knee joint	31780	Reconstruct windpipe
27130	Total hip arthroplasty	27487	Revise/replace knee joint	31781	Reconstruct windpipe
27132	Total hip arthroplasty	27488	Removal of knee prosthesis	31786	Remove windpipe lesion
27134	Revise hip joint replacement	27495	Reinforce thigh	31800	Repair of windpipe injury
27137	Revise hip joint replacement	27506	Treatment of thigh fracture	31805	Repair of windpipe injury
27138	Revise hip joint replacement	27507	Treatment of thigh fracture	32035	Thoracostomy w/rib resection
27140	Transplant femur ridge	27511	Treatment of thigh fracture	32036	Thoracostomy w/flap drainage
27146	Incision of hip bone	27513	Treatment of thigh fracture	32096	Open wedge/bx lung infiltr
27147	Revision of hip bone	27514	Treatment of thigh fracture	32097	Open wedge/bx lung nodule
27151	Incision of hip bones	27519	Treat thigh fx growth plate	32098	Open biopsy of lung pleura
27156	Revision of hip bones	27535	Treat knee fracture	32100	Exploration of chest

32110 Explore/repair chest	32851 Lung transplant single	33403 Valvuloplasty w/cp bypass
32120 Re-exploration of chest	32852 Lung transplant with bypass	33404 Prepare heart-aorta conduit
32124 Explore chest free adhesions	32853 Lung transplant double	33405 Replacement of aortic valve
32140 Removal of lung lesion(s)	32854 Lung transplant with bypass	33406 Replacement of aortic valve
32141 Remove/treat lung lesions	32855 Prepare donor lung single	33410 Replacement of aortic valve
32150 Removal of lung lesion(s)	32856 Prepare donor lung double	33411 Replacement of aortic valve
32151 Remove lung foreign body	32900 Removal of rib(s)	33412 Replacement of aortic valve
32160 Open chest heart massage	32905 Revise & repair chest wall	33413 Replacement of aortic valve
32200 Drain open lung lesion	32906 Revise & repair chest wall	33414 Repair of aortic valve
32215 Treat chest lining	32940 Revision of lung	33415 Revision subvalvular tissue
32220 Release of lung	32997 Total lung lavage	33416 Revise ventricle muscle
32225 Partial release of lung	33015 Incision of heart sac	33417 Repair of aortic valve
32310 Removal of chest lining	33020 Incision of heart sac	33418 Repair tcat mitral valve
32320 Free/remove chest lining	33025 Incision of heart sac	33420 Revision of mitral valve
32440 Remove lung pneumonectomy	33030 Partial removal of heart sac	33422 Revision of mitral valve
32442 Sleeve pneumonectomy	33031 Partial removal of heart sac	33425 Repair of mitral valve
32445 Removal of lung extrapleural	33050 Resect heart sac lesion	33426 Repair of mitral valve
32480 Partial removal of lung	33120 Removal of heart lesion	33427 Repair of mitral valve
32482 Bilobectomy	33130 Removal of heart lesion	33430 Replacement of mitral valve
32484 Segmentectomy	33140 Heart revascularize (tmr)	33460 Revision of tricuspid valve
32486 Sleeve lobectomy	33141 Heart tmr w/other procedure	33463 Valvuloplasty tricuspid
32488 Completion pneumonectomy	33202 Insert epicard eltrd open	33464 Valvuloplasty tricuspid
32491 Lung volume reduction	33203 Insert epicard eltrd endo	33465 Replace tricuspid valve
32501 Repair bronchus add-on	33236 Remove electrode/thoracotomy	33468 Revision of tricuspid valve
32503 Resect apical lung tumor	33237 Remove electrode/thoracotomy	33470 Revision of pulmonary valve
32504 Resect apical lung tum/chest	33238 Remove electrode/thoracotomy	33471 Valvotomy pulmonary valve
32505 Wedge resect of lung initial	33243 Remove eltrd/thoracotomy	33474 Revision of pulmonary valve
32506 Wedge resect of lung add-on	33250 Ablate heart dysrhythm focus	33475 Replacement pulmonary valve
32507 Wedge resect of lung diag	33251 Ablate heart dysrhythm focus	33476 Revision of heart chamber
32540 Removal of lung lesion	33254 Ablate atria lmtd	33478 Revision of heart chamber
32650 Thoracoscopy w/pleurodesis	33255 Ablate atria w/o bypass ext	33496 Repair prosth valve clot
32651 Thoracoscopy remove cortex	33256 Ablate atria w/bypass exten	33500 Repair heart vessel fistula
32652 Thoracoscopy rem totl cortex	33257 Ablate atria lmtd add-on	33501 Repair heart vessel fistula
32653 Thoracoscopy remov fb/fibrin	33258 Ablate atria x10sv add-on	33502 Coronary artery correction
32654 Thoracoscopy contrl bleeding	33259 Ablate atria w/bypass add-on	33503 Coronary artery graft
32655 Thoracoscopy resect bullae	33261 Ablate heart dysrhythm focus	33504 Coronary artery graft
32656 Thoracoscopy w/pleurectomy	33265 Ablate atria lmtd endo	33505 Repair artery w/tunnel
32658 Thoracoscopy w/sac fb remove	33266 Ablate atria x10sv endo	33506 Repair artery translocation
32659 Thoracoscopy w/sac drainage	33300 Repair of heart wound	33507 Repair art intramural
32661 Thoracoscopy w/pericard exc	33305 Repair of heart wound	33510 Cabg vein single
32662 Thoracoscopy w/mediast exc	33310 Exploratory heart surgery	33511 Cabg vein two
32663 Thoracoscopy w/lobectomy	33315 Exploratory heart surgery	33512 Cabg vein three
32664 Thoracoscopy w/ th nrv exc	33320 Repair major blood vessel(s)	33513 Cabg vein four
32665 Thoracoscop w/esoph musc exc	33321 Repair major vessel	33514 Cabg vein five
32666 Thoracoscopy w/wedge resect	33322 Repair major blood vessel(s)	33516 Cabg vein six or more
32667 Thoracoscopy w/w resect addl	33330 Insert major vessel graft	33517 Cabg artery-vein single
32668 Thoracoscopy w/w resect diag	33335 Insert major vessel graft	33518 Cabg artery-vein two
32669 Thoracoscopy remove segment	33361 Replace aortic valve perq	33519 Cabg artery-vein three
32670 Thoracoscopy bilobectomy	33362 Replace aortic valve open	33521 Cabg artery-vein four
32671 Thoracoscopy pneumonectomy	33363 Replace aortic valve open	33522 Cabg artery-vein five
32672 Thoracoscopy for lvrs	33364 Replace aortic valve open	33523 Cabg art-vein six or more
32673 Thoracoscopy w/thymus resect	33365 Replace aortic valve open	33530 Coronary artery bypass/reop
32674 Thoracoscopy lymph node exc	33366 Trcath replace aortic valve	33533 Cabg arterial single
32800 Repair lung hernia	33367 Replace aortic valve w/byp	33534 Cabg arterial two
32810 Close chest after drainage	33368 Replace aortic valve w/byp	33535 Cabg arterial three
32815 Close bronchial fistula	33369 Replace aortic valve w/byp	33536 Cabg arterial four or more
32820 Reconstruct injured chest	33400 Repair of aortic valve	33542 Removal of heart lesion
32850 Donor pneumonectomy	33401 Valvuloplasty open	33545 Repair of heart damage

33548	Restore/remodel ventricle
33572	Open coronary endarterectomy
33600	Closure of valve
33602	Closure of valve
33606	Anastomosis/artery-aorta
33608	Repair anomaly w/conduit
33610	Repair by enlargement
33611	Repair double ventricle
33612	Repair double ventricle
33615	Repair modified fontan
33617	Repair single ventricle
33619	Repair single ventricle
33620	Apply r&l pulm art bands
33621	Transthor cath for stent
33622	Redo compl cardiac anomaly
33641	Repair heart septum defect
33645	Revision of heart veins
33647	Repair heart septum defects
33660	Repair of heart defects
33665	Repair of heart defects
33670	Repair of heart chambers
33675	Close mult vsd
33676	Close mult vsd w/resection
33677	Cl mult vsd w/rem pul band
33681	Repair heart septum defect
33684	Repair heart septum defect
33688	Repair heart septum defect
33690	Reinforce pulmonary artery
33692	Repair of heart defects
33694	Repair of heart defects
33697	Repair of heart defects
33702	Repair of heart defects
33710	Repair of heart defects
33720	Repair of heart defect
33722	Repair of heart defect
33724	Repair venous anomaly
33726	Repair pul venous stenosis
33730	Repair heart-vein defect(s)
33732	Repair heart-vein defect
33735	Revision of heart chamber
33736	Revision of heart chamber
33737	Revision of heart chamber
33750	Major vessel shunt
33755	Major vessel shunt
33762	Major vessel shunt
33764	Major vessel shunt & graft
33766	Major vessel shunt
33767	Major vessel shunt
33768	Cavopulmonary shunting
33770	Repair great vessels defect
33771	Repair great vessels defect
33774	Repair great vessels defect
33775	Repair great vessels defect
33776	Repair great vessels defect
33777	Repair great vessels defect
33778	Repair great vessels defect
33779	Repair great vessels defect
33780	Repair great vessels defect
33781	Repair great vessels defect
33782	Nikaidoh proc
33783	Nikaidoh proc w/ostia implt
33786	Repair arterial trunk
33788	Revision of pulmonary artery
33800	Aortic suspension
33802	Repair vessel defect
33803	Repair vessel defect
33813	Repair septal defect
33814	Repair septal defect
33820	Revise major vessel
33822	Revise major vessel
33824	Revise major vessel
33840	Remove aorta constriction
33845	Remove aorta constriction
33851	Remove aorta constriction
33852	Repair septal defect
33853	Repair septal defect
33860	Ascending aortic graft
33863	Ascending aortic graft
33864	Ascending aortic graft
33870	Transverse aortic arch graft
33875	Thoracic aortic graft
33877	Thoracoabdominal graft
33880	Endovasc taa repr incl subcl
33881	Endovasc taa repr w/o subcl
33883	Insert endovasc prosth taa
33884	Endovasc prosth taa add-on
33886	Endovasc prosth delayed
33889	Artery transpose/endovas taa
33891	Car-car bp grft/endovas taa
33910	Remove lung artery emboli
33915	Remove lung artery emboli
33916	Surgery of great vessel
33917	Repair pulmonary artery
33920	Repair pulmonary atresia
33922	Transect pulmonary artery
33924	Remove pulmonary shunt
33925	Rpr pul art unifocal w/o cpb
33926	Repr pul art unifocal w/cpb
33930	Removal of donor heart/lung
33933	Prepare donor heart/lung
33935	Transplantation heart/lung
33940	Removal of donor heart
33944	Prepare donor heart
33945	Transplantation of heart
33946	Ecmo/ecls initiation venous
33947	Ecmo/ecls initiation artery
33948	Ecmo/ecls daily mgmt-venous
33949	Ecmo/ecls daily mgmt artery
33951	Ecmo/ecls insj prph cannula
33952	Ecmo/ecls insj prph cannula
33953	Ecmo/ecls insj prph cannula
33954	Ecmo/ecls insj prph cannula
33955	Ecmo/ecls insj ctr cannula
33956	Ecmo/ecls insj ctr cannula
33957	Ecmo/ecls repos perph cnula
33958	Ecmo/ecls repos perph cnula
33959	Ecmo/ecls repos perph cnula
33962	Ecmo/ecls repos perph cnula
33963	Ecmo/ecls repos perph cnula
33964	Ecmo/ecls repos perph cnula
33965	Ecmo/ecls rmvl perph cannula
33966	Ecmo/ecls rmvl prph cannula
33967	Insert i-aort percut device
33968	Remove aortic assist device
33969	Ecmo/ecls rmvl perph cannula
33970	Aortic circulation assist
33971	Aortic circulation assist
33973	Insert balloon device
33974	Remove intra-aortic balloon
33975	Implant ventricular device
33976	Implant ventricular device
33977	Remove ventricular device
33978	Remove ventricular device
33979	Insert intracorporeal device
33980	Remove intracorporeal device
33981	Replace vad pump ext
33982	Replace vad intra w/o bp
33983	Replace vad intra w/bp
33984	Ecmo/ecls rmvl prph cannula
33985	Ecmo/ecls rmvl ctr cannula
33986	Ecmo/ecls rmvl ctr cannula
33987	Artery expos/graft artery
33988	Insertion of left heart vent
33989	Removal of left heart vent
33990	Insert vad artery access
33991	Insert vad art&vein access
33992	Remove vad different session
33993	Reposition vad diff session
34001	Removal of artery clot
34051	Removal of artery clot
34151	Removal of artery clot
34401	Removal of vein clot
34451	Removal of vein clot
34502	Reconstruct vena cava
34800	Endovas aaa repr w/sm tube
34802	Endovas aaa repr w/2-p part
34803	Endovas aaa repr w/3-p part
34804	Endovas aaa repr w/1-p part
34805	Endovas aaa repr w/long tube
34806	Aneurysm press sensor add-on
34808	Endovas iliac a device addon
34812	Xpose for endoprosth femorl
34813	Femoral endovas graft add-on
34820	Xpose for endoprosth iliac
34825	Endovasc extend prosth init
34826	Endovasc exten prosth addl
34830	Open aortic tube prosth repr
34831	Open aortoiliac prosth repr
34832	Open aortofemor prosth repr
34833	Xpose for endoprosth iliac
34834	Xpose endoprosth brachial
34841	Endovasc visc aorta 1 graft
34842	Endovasc visc aorta 2 graft
34843	Endovasc visc aorta 3 graft

34844 Endovasc visc aorta 4 graft	35501 Art byp grft ipsilat carotid	35665 Art byp iliofemoral
34845 Visc & infraren abd 1 prosth	35506 Art byp grft subclav-carotid	35666 Art byp fem-ant-post tib/prl
34846 Visc & infraren abd 2 prosth	35508 Art byp grft carotid-vertbrl	35671 Art byp pop-tibl-prl-other
34847 Visc & infraren abd 3 prosth	35509 Art byp grft contral carotid	35681 Composite byp grft pros&vein
34848 Visc & infraren abd 4+ prost	35510 Art byp grft carotid-brchial	35682 Composite byp grft 2 veins
34900 Endovasc iliac repr w/graft	35511 Art byp grft subclav-subclav	35683 Composite byp grft 3/> segmt
35001 Repair defect of artery	35512 Art byp grft subclav-brchial	35691 Art trnsposj vertbrl carotid
35002 Repair artery rupture neck	35515 Art byp grft subclav-vertbrl	35693 Art trnsposj subclavian
35005 Repair defect of artery	35516 Art byp grft subclav-axilary	35694 Art trnsposj subclav carotid
35013 Repair artery rupture arm	35518 Art byp grft axillary-axilry	35695 Art trnsposj carotid subclav
35021 Repair defect of artery	35521 Art byp grft axill-femoral	35697 Reimplant artery each
35022 Repair artery rupture chest	35522 Art byp grft axill-brachial	35700 Reoperation bypass graft
35081 Repair defect of artery	35523 Art byp grft brchl-ulnr-rdl	35701 Exploration carotid artery
35082 Repair artery rupture aorta	35525 Art byp grft brachial-brchl	35721 Exploration femoral artery
35091 Repair defect of artery	35526 Art byp grft aor/carot/innom	35741 Exploration popliteal artery
35092 Repair artery rupture aorta	35531 Art byp grft aorcel/aormesen	35800 Explore neck vessels
35102 Repair defect of artery	35533 Art byp grft axill/fem/fem	35820 Explore chest vessels
35103 Repair artery rupture aorta	35535 Art byp grft hepatorenal	35840 Explore abdominal vessels
35111 Repair defect of artery	35536 Art byp grft splenorenal	35870 Repair vessel graft defect
35112 Repair artery rupture spleen	35537 Art byp grft aortoiliac	35901 Excision graft neck
35121 Repair defect of artery	35538 Art byp grft aortobi-iliac	35905 Excision graft thorax
35122 Repair artery rupture belly	35539 Art byp grft aortofemoral	35907 Excision graft abdomen
35131 Repair defect of artery	35540 Art byp grft aortbifemoral	36660 Insertion catheter artery
35132 Repair artery rupture groin	35556 Art byp grft fem-popliteal	36823 Insertion of cannula(s)
35141 Repair defect of artery	35558 Art byp grft fem-femoral	37140 Revision of circulation
35142 Repair artery rupture thigh	35560 Art byp grft aortorenal	37145 Revision of circulation
35151 Repair defect of artery	35563 Art byp grft ilioiliac	37160 Revision of circulation
35152 Repair ruptd popliteal art	35565 Art byp grft iliofemoral	37180 Revision of circulation
35182 Repair blood vessel lesion	35566 Art byp fem-ant-post tib/prl	37181 Splice spleen/kidney veins
35189 Repair blood vessel lesion	35570 Art byp tibial-tib/peroneal	37182 Insert hepatic shunt (tips)
35211 Repair blood vessel lesion	35571 Art byp pop-tibl-prl-other	37215 Transcath stent cca w/eps
35216 Repair blood vessel lesion	35583 Vein byp grft fem-popliteal	37217 Stent placemt retro carotid
35221 Repair blood vessel lesion	35585 Vein byp fem-tibial peroneal	37218 Stent placemt ante carotid
35241 Repair blood vessel lesion	35587 Vein byp pop-tibl peroneal	37616 Ligation of chest artery
35246 Repair blood vessel lesion	35600 Harvest art for cabg add-on	37617 Ligation of abdomen artery
35251 Repair blood vessel lesion	35601 Art byp common ipsi carotid	37618 Ligation of extremity artery
35271 Repair blood vessel lesion	35606 Art byp carotid-subclavian	37660 Revision of major vein
35276 Repair blood vessel lesion	35612 Art byp subclav-subclavian	37788 Revascularization penis
35281 Repair blood vessel lesion	35616 Art byp subclav-axillary	38100 Removal of spleen total
35301 Rechanneling of artery	35621 Art byp axillary-femoral	38101 Removal of spleen partial
35302 Rechanneling of artery	35623 Art byp axillary-pop-tibial	38102 Removal of spleen total
35303 Rechanneling of artery	35626 Art byp aorsubcl/carot/innom	38115 Repair of ruptured spleen
35304 Rechanneling of artery	35631 Art byp aor-celiac-msn-renal	38380 Thoracic duct procedure
35305 Rechanneling of artery	35632 Art byp ilio-celiac	38381 Thoracic duct procedure
35306 Rechanneling of artery	35633 Art byp ilio-mesenteric	38382 Thoracic duct procedure
35311 Rechanneling of artery	35634 Art byp iliorenal	38562 Removal pelvic lymph nodes
35331 Rechanneling of artery	35636 Art byp spenorenal	38564 Removal abdomen lymph nodes
35341 Rechanneling of artery	35637 Art byp aortoiliac	38724 Removal of lymph nodes neck
35351 Rechanneling of artery	35638 Art byp aortobi-iliac	38746 Remove thoracic lymph nodes
35355 Rechanneling of artery	35642 Art byp carotid-vertebral	38747 Remove abdominal lymph nodes
35361 Rechanneling of artery	35645 Art byp subclav-vertebrl	38765 Remove groin lymph nodes
35363 Rechanneling of artery	35646 Art byp aortobifemoral	38770 Remove pelvis lymph nodes
35371 Rechanneling of artery	35647 Art byp aortofemoral	38780 Remove abdomen lymph nodes
35372 Rechanneling of artery	35650 Art byp axillary-axillary	39000 Exploration of chest
35390 Reoperation carotid add-on	35654 Art byp axill-fem-femoral	39010 Exploration of chest
35400 Angioscopy	35656 Art byp femoral-popliteal	39200 Resect mediastinal cyst
35450 Repair arterial blockage	35661 Art byp femoral-femoral	39220 Resect mediastinal tumor
35452 Repair arterial blockage	35663 Art byp ilioiliac	39499 Chest procedure

39501	Repair diaphragm laceration
39503	Repair of diaphragm hernia
39540	Repair of diaphragm hernia
39541	Repair of diaphragm hernia
39545	Revision of diaphragm
39560	Resect diaphragm simple
39561	Resect diaphragm complex
39599	Diaphragm surgery procedure
41130	Partial removal of tongue
41135	Tongue and neck surgery
41140	Removal of tongue
41145	Tongue removal neck surgery
41150	Tongue mouth jaw surgery
41153	Tongue mouth neck surgery
41155	Tongue jaw & neck surgery
42426	Excise parotid gland/lesion
42845	Extensive surgery of throat
42894	Revision of pharyngeal walls
42953	Repair throat esophagus
42961	Control throat bleeding
42971	Control nose/throat bleeding
43045	Incision of esophagus
43100	Excision of esophagus lesion
43101	Excision of esophagus lesion
43107	Removal of esophagus
43108	Removal of esophagus
43112	Removal of esophagus
43113	Removal of esophagus
43116	Partial removal of esophagus
43117	Partial removal of esophagus
43118	Partial removal of esophagus
43121	Partial removal of esophagus
43122	Partial removal of esophagus
43123	Partial removal of esophagus
43124	Removal of esophagus
43135	Removal of esophagus pouch
43279	Lap myotomy heller
43282	Lap paraesoph her rpr w/mesh
43283	Lap esoph lengthening
43300	Repair of esophagus
43305	Repair esophagus and fistula
43310	Repair of esophagus
43312	Repair esophagus and fistula
43313	Esophagoplasty congenital
43314	Tracheo-esophagoplasty cong
43320	Fuse esophagus & stomach
43325	Revise esophagus & stomach
43327	Esoph fundoplasty lap
43328	Esoph fundoplasty thor
43330	Esophagomyotomy abdominal
43331	Esophagomyotomy thoracic
43332	Transab esoph hiat hern rpr
43333	Transab esoph hiat hern rpr
43334	Transthor diaphrag hern rpr
43335	Transthor diaphrag hern rpr
43336	Thorabd diaphr hern repair
43337	Thorabd diaphr hern repair
43338	Esoph lengthening

43340	Fuse esophagus & intestine
43341	Fuse esophagus & intestine
43351	Surgical opening esophagus
43352	Surgical opening esophagus
43360	Gastrointestinal repair
43361	Gastrointestinal repair
43400	Ligate esophagus veins
43401	Esophagus surgery for veins
43405	Ligate/staple esophagus
43410	Repair esophagus wound
43415	Repair esophagus wound
43425	Repair esophagus opening
43460	Pressure treatment esophagus
43496	Free jejunum flap microvasc
43500	Surgical opening of stomach
43501	Surgical repair of stomach
43502	Surgical repair of stomach
43520	Incision of pyloric muscle
43605	Biopsy of stomach
43610	Excision of stomach lesion
43611	Excision of stomach lesion
43620	Removal of stomach
43621	Removal of stomach
43622	Removal of stomach
43631	Removal of stomach partial
43632	Removal of stomach partial
43633	Removal of stomach partial
43634	Removal of stomach partial
43635	Removal of stomach partial
43640	Vagotomy & pylorus repair
43641	Vagotomy & pylorus repair
43644	Lap gastric bypass/roux-en-y
43645	Lap gastr bypass incl smll i
43771	Lap revise gastr adj device
43772	Lap rmvl gastr adj device
43773	Lap replace gastr adj device
43774	Lap rmvl gastr adj all parts
43775	Lap sleeve gastrectomy
43800	Reconstruction of pylorus
43810	Fusion of stomach and bowel
43820	Fusion of stomach and bowel
43825	Fusion of stomach and bowel
43832	Place gastrostomy tube
43840	Repair of stomach lesion
43843	Gastroplasty w/o v-band
43845	Gastroplasty duodenal switch
43846	Gastric bypass for obesity
43847	Gastric bypass incl small i
43848	Revision gastroplasty
43850	Revise stomach-bowel fusion
43855	Revise stomach-bowel fusion
43860	Revise stomach-bowel fusion
43865	Revise stomach-bowel fusion
43880	Repair stomach-bowel fistula
43881	Impl/redo electrd antrum
43882	Revise/remove electrd antrum
44005	Freeing of bowel adhesion
44010	Incision of small bowel

44015	Insert needle cath bowel
44020	Explore small intestine
44021	Decompress small bowel
44025	Incision of large bowel
44050	Reduce bowel obstruction
44055	Correct malrotation of bowel
44110	Excise intestine lesion(s)
44111	Excision of bowel lesion(s)
44120	Removal of small intestine
44121	Removal of small intestine
44125	Removal of small intestine
44126	Enterectomy w/o taper cong
44127	Enterectomy w/taper cong
44128	Enterectomy cong add-on
44130	Bowel to bowel fusion
44132	Enterectomy cadaver donor
44133	Enterectomy live donor
44135	Intestine transplnt cadaver
44136	Intestine transplant live
44137	Remove intestinal allograft
44139	Mobilization of colon
44140	Partial removal of colon
44141	Partial removal of colon
44143	Partial removal of colon
44144	Partial removal of colon
44145	Partial removal of colon
44146	Partial removal of colon
44147	Partial removal of colon
44150	Removal of colon
44151	Removal of colon/ileostomy
44155	Removal of colon/ileostomy
44156	Removal of colon/ileostomy
44157	Colectomy w/ileoanal anast
44158	Colectomy w/neo-rectum pouch
44160	Removal of colon
44187	Lap ileo/jejuno-stomy
44188	Lap colostomy
44202	Lap enterectomy
44203	Lap resect s/intestine addl
44204	Laparo partial colectomy
44205	Lap colectomy part w/ileum
44206	Lap part colectomy w/stoma
44207	L colectomy/coloproctostomy
44208	L colectomy/coloproctostomy
44210	Laparo total proctocolectomy
44211	Lap colectomy w/proctectomy
44212	Laparo total proctocolectomy
44213	Lap mobil splenic fl add-on
44227	Lap close enterostomy
44300	Open bowel to skin
44310	Ileostomy/jejunostomy
44314	Revision of ileostomy
44316	Devise bowel pouch
44320	Colostomy
44322	Colostomy with biopsies
44345	Revision of colostomy
44346	Revision of colostomy
44602	Suture small intestine

44603	Suture small intestine	46746	Repair of cloacal anomaly	48001	Placement of drain pancreas
44604	Suture large intestine	46748	Repair of cloacal anomaly	48020	Removal of pancreatic stone
44605	Repair of bowel lesion	46751	Repair of anal sphincter	48100	Biopsy of pancreas open
44615	Intestinal stricturoplasty	47010	Open drainage liver lesion	48105	Resect/debride pancreas
44620	Repair bowel opening	47015	Inject/aspirate liver cyst	48120	Removal of pancreas lesion
44625	Repair bowel opening	47100	Wedge biopsy of liver	48140	Partial removal of pancreas
44626	Repair bowel opening	47120	Partial removal of liver	48145	Partial removal of pancreas
44640	Repair bowel-skin fistula	47122	Extensive removal of liver	48146	Pancreatectomy
44650	Repair bowel fistula	47125	Partial removal of liver	48148	Removal of pancreatic duct
44660	Repair bowel-bladder fistula	47130	Partial removal of liver	48150	Partial removal of pancreas
44661	Repair bowel-bladder fistula	47133	Removal of donor liver	48152	Pancreatectomy
44680	Surgical revision intestine	47135	Transplantation of liver	48153	Pancreatectomy
44700	Suspend bowel w/prosthesis	47136	Transplantation of liver	48154	Pancreatectomy
44715	Prepare donor intestine	47140	Partial removal donor liver	48155	Removal of pancreas
44720	Prep donor intestine/venous	47141	Partial removal donor liver	48400	Injection intraop add-on
44721	Prep donor intestine/artery	47142	Partial removal donor liver	48500	Surgery of pancreatic cyst
44800	Excision of bowel pouch	47143	Prep donor liver whole	48510	Drain pancreatic pseudocyst
44820	Excision of mesentery lesion	47144	Prep donor liver 3-segment	48520	Fuse pancreas cyst and bowel
44850	Repair of mesentery	47145	Prep donor liver lobe split	48540	Fuse pancreas cyst and bowel
44899	Bowel surgery procedure	47146	Prep donor liver/venous	48545	Pancreatorrhaphy
44900	Drain appendix abscess open	47147	Prep donor liver/arterial	48547	Duodenal exclusion
44960	Appendectomy	47300	Surgery for liver lesion	48548	Fuse pancreas and bowel
45110	Removal of rectum	47350	Repair liver wound	48551	Prep donor pancreas
45111	Partial removal of rectum	47360	Repair liver wound	48552	Prep donor pancreas/venous
45112	Removal of rectum	47361	Repair liver wound	48554	Transpl allograft pancreas
45113	Partial proctectomy	47362	Repair liver wound	48556	Removal allograft pancreas
45114	Partial removal of rectum	47380	Open ablate liver tumor rf	49000	Exploration of abdomen
45116	Partial removal of rectum	47381	Open ablate liver tumor cryo	49002	Reopening of abdomen
45119	Remove rectum w/reservoir	47400	Incision of liver duct	49010	Exploration behind abdomen
45120	Removal of rectum	47420	Incision of bile duct	49020	Drainage abdom abscess open
45121	Removal of rectum and colon	47425	Incision of bile duct	49040	Drain open abdom abscess
45123	Partial proctectomy	47460	Incise bile duct sphincter	49060	Drain open retroperi abscess
45126	Pelvic exenteration	47480	Incision of gallbladder	49062	Drain to peritoneal cavity
45130	Excision of rectal prolapse	47550	Bile duct endoscopy add-on	49203	Exc abd tum 5 cm or less
45135	Excision of rectal prolapse	47570	Laparo cholecystoenterostomy	49204	Exc abd tum over 5 cm
45136	Excise ileoanal reservoir	47600	Removal of gallbladder	49205	Exc abd tum over 10 cm
45395	Lap removal of rectum	47605	Removal of gallbladder	49215	Excise sacral spine tumor
45397	Lap remove rectum w/pouch	47610	Removal of gallbladder	49220	Multiple surgery abdomen
45400	Laparoscopic proc	47612	Removal of gallbladder	49255	Removal of omentum
45402	Lap proctopexy w/sig resect	47620	Removal of gallbladder	49412	Ins device for rt guide open
45540	Correct rectal prolapse	47700	Exploration of bile ducts	49425	Insert abdomen-venous drain
45550	Repair rectum/remove sigmoid	47701	Bile duct revision	49428	Ligation of shunt
45562	Exploration/repair of rectum	47711	Excision of bile duct tumor	49605	Repair umbilical lesion
45563	Exploration/repair of rectum	47712	Excision of bile duct tumor	49606	Repair umbilical lesion
45800	Repair rect/bladder fistula	47715	Excision of bile duct cyst	49610	Repair umbilical lesion
45805	Repair fistula w/colostomy	47720	Fuse gallbladder & bowel	49611	Repair umbilical lesion
45820	Repair rectourethral fistula	47721	Fuse upper gi structures	49900	Repair of abdominal wall
45825	Repair fistula w/colostomy	47740	Fuse gallbladder & bowel	49904	Omental flap extra-abdom
46705	Repair of anal stricture	47741	Fuse gallbladder & bowel	49905	Omental flap intra-abdom
46710	Repr per/vag pouch sngl proc	47760	Fuse bile ducts and bowel	49906	Free omental flap microvasc
46712	Repr per/vag pouch dbl proc	47765	Fuse liver ducts & bowel	50010	Exploration of kidney
46715	Rep perf anoper fistu	47780	Fuse bile ducts and bowel	50040	Drainage of kidney
46716	Rep perf anoper/vestib fistu	47785	Fuse bile ducts and bowel	50045	Exploration of kidney
46730	Construction of absent anus	47800	Reconstruction of bile ducts	50060	Removal of kidney stone
46735	Construction of absent anus	47801	Placement bile duct support	50065	Incision of kidney
46740	Construction of absent anus	47802	Fuse liver duct & intestine	50070	Incision of kidney
46742	Repair of imperforated anus	47900	Suture bile duct injury	50075	Removal of kidney stone
46744	Repair of cloacal anomaly	48000	Drainage of abdomen	50100	Revise kidney blood vessels

50120	Exploration of kidney	50810	Fusion of ureter & bowel	56631	Extensive vulva surgery
50125	Explore and drain kidney	50815	Urine shunt to intestine	56632	Extensive vulva surgery
50130	Removal of kidney stone	50820	Construct bowel bladder	56633	Extensive vulva surgery
50135	Exploration of kidney	50825	Construct bowel bladder	56634	Extensive vulva surgery
50205	Renal biopsy open	50830	Revise urine flow	56637	Extensive vulva surgery
50220	Remove kidney open	50840	Replace ureter by bowel	56640	Extensive vulva surgery
50225	Removal kidney open complex	50845	Appendico-vesicostomy	57110	Remove vagina wall complete
50230	Removal kidney open radical	50860	Transplant ureter to skin	57111	Remove vagina tissue compl
50234	Removal of kidney & ureter	50900	Repair of ureter	57112	Vaginectomy w/nodes compl
50236	Removal of kidney & ureter	50920	Closure ureter/skin fistula	57270	Repair of bowel pouch
50240	Partial removal of kidney	50930	Closure ureter/bowel fistula	57280	Suspension of vagina
50250	Cryoablate renal mass open	50940	Release of ureter	57296	Revise vag graft open abd
50280	Removal of kidney lesion	51525	Removal of bladder lesion	57305	Repair rectum-vagina fistula
50290	Removal of kidney lesion	51530	Removal of bladder lesion	57307	Fistula repair & colostomy
50300	Remove cadaver donor kidney	51550	Partial removal of bladder	57308	Fistula repair transperine
50320	Remove kidney living donor	51555	Partial removal of bladder	57311	Repair urethrovaginal lesion
50323	Prep cadaver renal allograft	51565	Revise bladder & ureter(s)	57531	Removal of cervix radical
50325	Prep donor renal graft	51570	Removal of bladder	57540	Removal of residual cervix
50327	Prep renal graft/venous	51575	Removal of bladder & nodes	57545	Remove cervix/repair pelvis
50328	Prep renal graft/arterial	51580	Remove bladder/revise tract	58140	Myomectomy abdom method
50329	Prep renal graft/ureteral	51585	Removal of bladder & nodes	58146	Myomectomy abdom complex
50340	Removal of kidney	51590	Remove bladder/revise tract	58150	Total hysterectomy
50360	Transplantation of kidney	51595	Remove bladder/revise tract	58152	Total hysterectomy
50365	Transplantation of kidney	51596	Remove bladder/create pouch	58180	Partial hysterectomy
50370	Remove transplanted kidney	51597	Removal of pelvic structures	58200	Extensive hysterectomy
50380	Reimplantation of kidney	51800	Revision of bladder/urethra	58210	Extensive hysterectomy
50400	Revision of kidney/ureter	51820	Revision of urinary tract	58240	Removal of pelvis contents
50405	Revision of kidney/ureter	51840	Attach bladder/urethra	58267	Vag hyst w/urinary repair
50500	Repair of kidney wound	51841	Attach bladder/urethra	58275	Hysterectomy/revise vagina
50520	Close kidney-skin fistula	51865	Repair of bladder wound	58280	Hysterectomy/revise vagina
50525	Repair renal-abdomen fistula	51900	Repair bladder/vagina lesion	58285	Extensive hysterectomy
50526	Repair renal-abdomen fistula	51920	Close bladder-uterus fistula	58293	Vag hyst w/uro repair compl
50540	Revision of horseshoe kidney	51925	Hysterectomy/bladder repair	58400	Suspension of uterus
50545	Laparo radical nephrectomy	51940	Correction of bladder defect	58410	Suspension of uterus
50546	Laparoscopic nephrectomy	51960	Revision of bladder & bowel	58520	Repair of ruptured uterus
50547	Laparo removal donor kidney	51980	Construct bladder opening	58540	Revision of uterus
50548	Laparo remove w/ureter	53415	Reconstruction of urethra	58548	Lap radical hyst
50600	Exploration of ureter	53448	Remov/replc ur sphinctr comp	58605	Division of fallopian tube
50605	Insert ureteral support	54125	Removal of penis	58611	Ligate oviduct(s) add-on
50610	Removal of ureter stone	54130	Remove penis & nodes	58700	Removal of fallopian tube
50620	Removal of ureter stone	54135	Remove penis & nodes	58720	Removal of ovary/tube(s)
50630	Removal of ureter stone	54390	Repair penis and bladder	58740	Adhesiolysis tube ovary
50650	Removal of ureter	54430	Revision of penis	58750	Repair oviduct
50660	Removal of ureter	55605	Incise sperm duct pouch	58752	Revise ovarian tube(s)
50700	Revision of ureter	55650	Remove sperm duct pouch	58760	Fimbrioplasty
50715	Release of ureter	55801	Removal of prostate	58822	Drain ovary abscess percut
50722	Release of ureter	55810	Extensive prostate surgery	58825	Transposition ovary(s)
50725	Release/revise ureter	55812	Extensive prostate surgery	58940	Removal of ovary(s)
50728	Revise ureter	55815	Extensive prostate surgery	58943	Removal of ovary(s)
50740	Fusion of ureter & kidney	55821	Removal of prostate	58950	Resect ovarian malignancy
50750	Fusion of ureter & kidney	55831	Removal of prostate	58951	Resect ovarian malignancy
50760	Fusion of ureters	55840	Extensive prostate surgery	58952	Resect ovarian malignancy
50770	Splicing of ureters	55842	Extensive prostate surgery	58953	Tah rad dissect for debulk
50780	Reimplant ureter in bladder	55845	Extensive prostate surgery	58954	Tah rad debulk/lymph remove
50782	Reimplant ureter in bladder	55862	Extensive prostate surgery	58956	Bso omentectomy w/tah
50783	Reimplant ureter in bladder	55865	Extensive prostate surgery	58957	Resect recurrent gyn mal
50785	Reimplant ureter in bladder	55866	Laparo radical prostatectomy	58958	Resect recur gyn mal w/lym
50800	Implant ureter in bowel	56630	Extensive vulva surgery	58960	Exploration of abdomen

59120 Treat ectopic pregnancy	61460 Incise skull for surgery	61597 Transcondylar approach/skull
59121 Treat ectopic pregnancy	61480 Incise skull for surgery	61598 Transpetrosal approach/skull
59130 Treat ectopic pregnancy	61500 Removal of skull lesion	61600 Resect/excise cranial lesion
59135 Treat ectopic pregnancy	61501 Remove infected skull bone	61601 Resect/excise cranial lesion
59136 Treat ectopic pregnancy	61510 Removal of brain lesion	61605 Resect/excise cranial lesion
59140 Treat ectopic pregnancy	61512 Remove brain lining lesion	61606 Resect/excise cranial lesion
59325 Revision of cervix	61514 Removal of brain abscess	61607 Resect/excise cranial lesion
59350 Repair of uterus	61516 Removal of brain lesion	61608 Resect/excise cranial lesion
59514 Cesarean delivery only	61517 Implt brain chemotx add-on	61610 Transect artery sinus
59525 Remove uterus after cesarean	61518 Removal of brain lesion	61611 Transect artery sinus
59620 Attempted vbac delivery only	61519 Remove brain lining lesion	61612 Transect artery sinus
59830 Treat uterus infection	61520 Removal of brain lesion	61613 Remove aneurysm sinus
59850 Abortion	61521 Removal of brain lesion	61615 Resect/excise lesion skull
59851 Abortion	61522 Removal of brain abscess	61616 Resect/excise lesion skull
59852 Abortion	61524 Removal of brain lesion	61618 Repair dura
59855 Abortion	61526 Removal of brain lesion	61619 Repair dura
59856 Abortion	61530 Removal of brain lesion	61624 Transcath occlusion cns
59857 Abortion	61531 Implant brain electrodes	61630 Intracranial angioplasty
60254 Extensive thyroid surgery	61533 Implant brain electrodes	61635 Intracran angioplsty w/stent
60270 Removal of thyroid	61534 Removal of brain lesion	61680 Intracranial vessel surgery
60505 Explore parathyroid glands	61535 Remove brain electrodes	61682 Intracranial vessel surgery
60521 Removal of thymus gland	61536 Removal of brain lesion	61684 Intracranial vessel surgery
60522 Removal of thymus gland	61537 Removal of brain tissue	61686 Intracranial vessel surgery
60540 Explore adrenal gland	61538 Removal of brain tissue	61690 Intracranial vessel surgery
60545 Explore adrenal gland	61539 Removal of brain tissue	61692 Intracranial vessel surgery
60600 Remove carotid body lesion	61540 Removal of brain tissue	61697 Brain aneurysm repr complx
60605 Remove carotid body lesion	61541 Incision of brain tissue	61698 Brain aneurysm repr complx
60650 Laparoscopy adrenalectomy	61543 Removal of brain tissue	61700 Brain aneurysm repr simple
61105 Twist drill hole	61544 Remove & treat brain lesion	61702 Inner skull vessel surgery
61107 Drill skull for implantation	61545 Excision of brain tumor	61703 Clamp neck artery
61108 Drill skull for drainage	61546 Removal of pituitary gland	61705 Revise circulation to head
61120 Burr hole for puncture	61548 Removal of pituitary gland	61708 Revise circulation to head
61140 Pierce skull for biopsy	61550 Release of skull seams	61710 Revise circulation to head
61150 Pierce skull for drainage	61552 Release of skull seams	61711 Fusion of skull arteries
61151 Pierce skull for drainage	61556 Incise skull/sutures	61735 Incise skull/brain surgery
61154 Pierce skull & remove clot	61557 Incise skull/sutures	61750 Incise skull/brain biopsy
61156 Pierce skull for drainage	61558 Excision of skull/sutures	61751 Brain biopsy w/ct/mr guide
61210 Pierce skull implant device	61559 Excision of skull/sutures	61760 Implant brain electrodes
61250 Pierce skull & explore	61563 Excision of skull tumor	61850 Implant neuroelectrodes
61253 Pierce skull & explore	61564 Excision of skull tumor	61860 Implant neuroelectrodes
61304 Open skull for exploration	61566 Removal of brain tissue	61863 Implant neuroelectrode
61305 Open skull for exploration	61567 Incision of brain tissue	61864 Implant neuroelectrde addl
61312 Open skull for drainage	61570 Remove foreign body brain	61867 Implant neuroelectrode
61313 Open skull for drainage	61571 Incise skull for brain wound	61868 Implant neuroelectrde addl
61314 Open skull for drainage	61575 Skull base/brainstem surgery	61870 Implant neuroelectrodes
61315 Open skull for drainage	61576 Skull base/brainstem surgery	62005 Treat skull fracture
61316 Implt cran bone flap to abdo	61580 Craniofacial approach skull	62010 Treatment of head injury
61320 Open skull for drainage	61581 Craniofacial approach skull	62100 Repair brain fluid leakage
61321 Open skull for drainage	61582 Craniofacial approach skull	62115 Reduction of skull defect
61322 Decompressive craniotomy	61583 Craniofacial approach skull	62117 Reduction of skull defect
61323 Decompressive lobectomy	61584 Orbitocranial approach/skull	62120 Repair skull cavity lesion
61332 Explore/biopsy eye socket	61585 Orbitocranial approach/skull	62121 Incise skull repair
61333 Explore orbit/remove lesion	61586 Resect nasopharynx skull	62140 Repair of skull defect
61340 Subtemporal decompression	61590 Infratemporal approach/skull	62141 Repair of skull defect
61343 Incise skull (press relief)	61591 Infratemporal approach/skull	62142 Remove skull plate/flap
61345 Relieve cranial pressure	61592 Orbitocranial approach/skull	62143 Replace skull plate/flap
61450 Incise skull for surgery	61595 Transtemporal approach/skull	62145 Repair of skull & brain
61458 Incise skull for brain wound	61596 Transcochlear approach/skull	62146 Repair of skull with graft

62147	Repair of skull with graft	63200	Release spinal cord lumbar	64818	Remove sympathetic nerves
62148	Retr bone flap to fix skull	63250	Revise spinal cord vsls crvl	64866	Fusion of facial/other nerve
62161	Dissect brain w/scope	63251	Revise spinal cord vsls thrc	64868	Fusion of facial/other nerve
62162	Remove colloid cyst w/scope	63252	Revise spine cord vsl thrlmb	65273	Repair of eye wound
62163	Zneuroendoscopy w/fb removal	63265	Excise intraspinl lesion crv	69155	Extensive ear/neck surgery
62164	Remove brain tumor w/scope	63266	Excise intrspinl lesion thrc	69535	Remove part of temporal bone
62165	Remove pituit tumor w/scope	63267	Excise intrspinl lesion lmbr	69554	Remove ear lesion
62180	Establish brain cavity shunt	63268	Excise intrspinl lesion scrl	69950	Incise inner ear nerve
62190	Establish brain cavity shunt	63270	Excise intrspinl lesion crvl	75952	Endovasc repair abdom aorta
62192	Establish brain cavity shunt	63271	Excise intrspinl lesion thrc	75953	Abdom aneurysm endovas rpr
62200	Establish brain cavity shunt	63272	Excise intrspinl lesion lmbr	75954	Iliac aneurysm endovas rpr
62201	Brain cavity shunt w/scope	63273	Excise intrspinl lesion scrl	75956	Xray endovasc thor ao repr
62220	Establish brain cavity shunt	63275	Bx/exc xdrl spine lesn crvl	75957	Xray endovasc thor ao repr
62223	Establish brain cavity shunt	63276	Bx/exc xdrl spine lesn thrc	75958	Xray place prox ext thor ao
62256	Remove brain cavity shunt	63277	Bx/exc xdrl spine lesn lmbr	75959	Xray place dist ext thor ao
62258	Replace brain cavity shunt	63278	Bx/exc xdrl spine lesn scrl	92970	Cardioassist internal
63050	Cervical laminoplsty 2/> seg	63280	Bx/exc idrl spine lesn crvl	92971	Cardioassist external
63051	C-laminoplasty w/graft/plate	63281	Bx/exc idrl spine lesn thrc	92975	Dissolve clot heart vessel
63077	Spine disk surgery thorax	63282	Bx/exc idrl spine lesn lmbr	92992	Revision of heart chamber
63078	Spine disk surgery thorax	63283	Bx/exc idrl spine lesn scrl	92993	Revision of heart chamber
63081	Remove vert body dcmprn crvl	63285	Bx/exc idrl imed lesn cervl	93583	Perq transcath septal reduxn
63082	Remove vertebral body add-on	63286	Bx/exc idrl imed lesn thrc	99184	Hypothermia ill neonate
63085	Remove vert body dcmprn thrc	63287	Bx/exc idrl imed lesn thrlmb	99190	Special pump services
63086	Remove vertebral body add-on	63290	Bx/exc xdrl/idrl lsn any lvl	99191	Special pump services
63087	Remov vertbr dcmprn thrclmbr	63295	Repair laminectomy defect	99192	Special pump services
63088	Remove vertebral body add-on	63300	Remove vert xdrl body crvcl	99356	Prolonged service inpatient
63090	Remove vert body dcmprn lmbr	63301	Remove vert xdrl body thrc	99357	Prolonged service inpatient
63091	Remove vertebral body add-on	63302	Remove vert xdrl body thrlmb	99462	Sbsq nb em per day hosp
63101	Remove vert body dcmprn thrc	63303	Remov vert xdrl bdy lmbr/sac	99468	Neonate crit care initial
63102	Remove vert body dcmprn lmbr	63304	Remove vert idrl body crvcl	99469	Neonate crit care subsq
63103	Remove vertebral body add-on	63305	Remove vert idrl body thrc	99471	Ped critical care initial
63170	Incise spinal cord tract(s)	63306	Remov vert idrl bdy thrclmbr	99472	Ped critical care subsq
63172	Drainage of spinal cyst	63307	Remov vert idrl bdy lmbr/sac	99475	Ped crit care age 2-5 init
63173	Drainage of spinal cyst	63308	Remove vertebral body add-on	99476	Ped crit care age 2-5 subsq
63180	Revise spinal cord ligaments	63700	Repair of spinal herniation	99477	Init day hosp neonate care
63182	Revise spinal cord ligaments	63702	Repair of spinal herniation	99478	Ic lbw inf < 1500 gm subsq
63185	Incise spine nrv half segmnt	63704	Repair of spinal herniation	99479	Ic lbw inf 1500-2500 g subsq
63190	Incise spine nrv >2 segmnts	63706	Repair of spinal herniation	99480	Ic inf pbw 2501-5000 g subsq
63191	Incise spine accessory nerve	63707	Repair spinal fluid leakage	G0341	Percutaneous islet celltrans
63194	Incise spine & cord cervical	63709	Repair spinal fluid leakage	G0342	Laparoscopy islet cell trans
63195	Incise spine & cord thoracic	63710	Graft repair of spine defect	G0343	Laparotomy islet cell transp
63196/tlIncise spine&cord 2 trx crvl		63740	Install spinal shunt	G0412	Open tx iliac spine uni/bil
63197	Incise spine&cord 2 trx thrc	64755	Incision of stomach nerves	G0414	Pelvic ring fx treat int fix
63198	Incise spin&cord 2 stgs crvl	64760	Incision of vagus nerve	G0415	Open tx post pelvic fxcture
63199	Incise spin&cord 2 stgs thrc	64809	Remove sympathetic nerves		

Appendix J — Place of Service and Type of Service

Place-of-Service Codes for Professional Claims

Listed below are place of service codes and descriptions. These codes should be used on professional claims to specify the entity where service(s) were rendered. Check with individual payers (e.g., Medicare, Medicaid, other private insurance) for reimbursement policies regarding these codes. To comment on a code(s) or description(s), please send your request to posinfo@cms.gov.

01 Pharmacy — A facility or location where drugs and other medically related items and services are sold, dispensed, or otherwise provided directly to patients.

02 Unassigned — N/A

03 School — A facility whose primary purpose is education.

04 Homeless shelter — A facility or location whose primary purpose is to provide temporary housing to homeless individuals (e.g., emergency shelters, individual or family shelters).

05 Indian Health Service freestanding facility — A facility or location, owned and operated by the Indian Health Service, which provides diagnostic, therapeutic (surgical and non-surgical), and rehabilitation services to American Indians and Alaska natives who do not require hospitalization.

06 Indian Health Service provider-based facility — A facility or location, owned and operated by the Indian Health Service, which provides diagnostic, therapeutic (surgical and nonsurgical), and rehabilitation services rendered by, or under the supervision of, physicians to American Indians and Alaska natives admitted as inpatients or outpatients.

07 Tribal 638 freestanding facility — A facility or location owned and operated by a federally recognized American Indian or Alaska native tribe or tribal organization under a 638 agreement, which provides diagnostic, therapeutic (surgical and nonsurgical), and rehabilitation services to tribal members who do not require hospitalization.

08 Tribal 638 provider-based Facility — A facility or location owned and operated by a federally recognized American Indian or Alaska native tribe or tribal organization under a 638 agreement, which provides diagnostic, therapeutic (surgical and nonsurgical), and rehabilitation services to tribal members admitted as inpatients or outpatients.

09 Prison/correctional facility — A prison, jail, reformatory, work farm, detention center, or any other similar facility maintained by either federal, state or local authorities for the purpose of confinement or rehabilitation of adult or juvenile criminal offenders.

10 Unassigned — N/A

11 Office — Location, other than a hospital, skilled nursing facility (SNF), military treatment facility, community health center, State or local public health clinic, or intermediate care facility (ICF), where the health professional routinely provides health examinations, diagnosis, and treatment of illness or injury on an ambulatory basis.

12 Home — Location, other than a hospital or other facility, where the patient receives care in a private residence.

13 Assisted living facility — Congregate residential facility with self-contained living units providing assessment of each resident's needs and on-site support 24 hours a day, 7 days a week, with the capacity to deliver or arrange for services including some health care and other services.

14 Group home — A residence, with shared living areas, where clients receive supervision and other services such as social and/or behavioral services, custodial service, and minimal services (e.g., medication administration).

15 Mobile unit — A facility/unit that moves from place-to-place equipped to provide preventive, screening, diagnostic, and/or treatment services.

16 Temporary lodging — A short-term accommodation such as a hotel, campground, hostel, cruise ship or resort where the patient receives care, and which is not identified by any other POS code.

17 Walk-in retail health clinic — A walk-in health clinic, other than an office, urgent care facility, pharmacy, or independent clinic and not described by any other place of service code, that is located within a retail operation and provides preventive and primary care services on an ambulatory basis.

18 Place of employment/worksite — A location, not described by any other POS code, owned or operated by a public or private entity where the patient is employed, and where a health professional provides on-going or episodic occupational medical, therapeutic or rehabilitative services to the individual.

19 Off campus-outpatient hospital — A portion of an off-campus hospital provider based department which provides diagnostic, therapeutic (both surgical and nonsurgical), and rehabilitation services to sick or injured persons who do not require hospitalization or institutionalization. (Effective January 1, 2016)

20 Urgent care facility — Location, distinct from a hospital emergency room, an office, or a clinic, whose purpose is to diagnose and treat illness or injury for unscheduled, ambulatory patients seeking immediate medical attention.

21	Inpatient hospital	A facility, other than psychiatric, which primarily provides diagnostic, therapeutic (both surgical and nonsurgical), and rehabilitation services by, or under, the supervision of physicians to patients admitted for a variety of medical conditions.
22	On campus-outpatient hospital	A portion of a hospital's main campus which provides diagnostic, therapeutic (both surgical and nonsurgical), and rehabilitation services to sick or injured persons who do not require hospitalization or institutionalization. (Description change effective January 1, 2016)
23	Emergency room—hospital	A portion of a hospital where emergency diagnosis and treatment of illness or injury is provided.
24	Ambulatory surgical center	A freestanding facility, other than a physician's office, where surgical and diagnostic services are provided on an ambulatory basis.
25	Birthing center	A facility, other than a hospital's maternity facilities or a physician's office, which provides a setting for labor, delivery, and immediate post-partum care as well as immediate care of new born infants.
26	Military treatment facility	A medical facility operated by one or more of the uniformed services. Military treatment facility (MTF) also refers to certain former U.S. Public Health Service (USPHS) facilities now designated as uniformed service treatment facilities (USTF).
27-30	Unassigned	N/A
31	Skilled nursing facility	A facility which primarily provides inpatient skilled nursing care and related services to patients who require medical, nursing, or rehabilitative services but does not provide the level of care or treatment available in a hospital.
32	Nursing facility	A facility which primarily provides to residents skilled nursing care and related services for the rehabilitation of injured, disabled, or sick persons, or, on a regular basis, health-related care services above the level of custodial care to other than mentally retarded individuals.
33	Custodial care facility	A facility which provides room, board, and other personal assistance services, generally on a long-term basis, and which does not include a medical component.
34	Hospice	A facility, other than a patient's home, in which palliative and supportive care for terminally ill patients and their families are provided.
35-40	Unassigned	N/A
41	Ambulance—land	A land vehicle specifically designed, equipped and staffed for lifesaving and transporting the sick or injured.
42	Ambulance—air or water	An air or water vehicle specifically designed, equipped and staffed for lifesaving and transporting the sick or injured.
43-48	Unassigned	N/A
49	Independent clinic	A location, not part of a hospital and not described by any other place-of-service code, that is organized and operated to provide preventive, diagnostic, therapeutic, rehabilitative, or palliative services to outpatients only.
50	Federally qualified health center	A facility located in a medically underserved area that provides Medicare beneficiaries preventive primary medical care under the general direction of a physician.
51	Inpatient psychiatric facility	A facility that provides inpatient psychiatric services for the diagnosis and treatment of mental illness on a 24-hour basis, by or under the supervision of a physician.
52	Psychiatric facility-partial hospitalization	A facility for the diagnosis and treatment of mental illness that provides a planned therapeutic program for patients who do not require full time hospitalization, but who need broader programs than are possible from outpatient visits to a hospital-based or hospital-affiliated facility.
53	Community mental health center	A facility that provides the following services: outpatient services, including specialized outpatient services for children, the elderly, individuals who are chronically ill, and residents of the CMHC's mental health services area who have been discharged from inpatient treatment at a mental health facility; 24 hour a day emergency care services; day treatment, other partial hospitalization services, or psychosocial rehabilitation services; screening for patients being considered for admission to state mental health facilities to determine the appropriateness of such admission; and consultation and education services.
54	Intermediate care facility/individuals with intellectual disabilities	A facility which primarily provides health-related care and services above the level of custodial care to individuals with Intellectual Disabilities but does not provide the level of care or treatment available in a hospital or SNF.
55	Residential substance abuse treatment facility	A facility which provides treatment for substance (alcohol and drug) abuse to live-in residents who do not require acute medical care. Services include individual and group therapy and counseling, family counseling, laboratory tests, drugs and supplies, psychological testing, and room and board.
56	Psychiatric residential treatment center	A facility or distinct part of a facility for psychiatric care which provides a total 24-hour therapeutically planned and professionally staffed group living and learning environment.
57	Non-residential substance abuse treatment facility	A location which provides treatment for substance (alcohol and drug) abuse on an ambulatory basis. Services include individual and group therapy and counseling, family counseling, laboratory tests, drugs and supplies, and psychological testing.
58-59	Unassigned	N/A

© 2015 Optum360, LLC

60	Mass immunization center	A location where providers administer pneumococcal pneumonia and influenza virus vaccinations and submit these services as electronic media claims, paper claims, or using the roster billing method. This generally takes place in a mass immunization setting, such as, a public health center, pharmacy, or mall but may include a physician office setting.
61	Comprehensive inpatient rehabilitation facility	A facility that provides comprehensive rehabilitation services under the supervision of a physician to inpatients with physical disabilities. Services include physical therapy, occupational therapy, speech pathology, social or psychological services, and orthotics and prosthetics services.
62	Comprehensive outpatient rehabilitation facility	A facility that provides comprehensive rehabilitation services under the supervision of a physician to outpatients with physical disabilities. Services include physical therapy, occupational therapy, and speech pathology services.
63-64	Unassigned	N/A
65	End-stage renal disease treatment facility	A facility other than a hospital, which provides dialysis treatment, maintenance, and/or training to patients or caregivers on an ambulatory or home-care basis.
66-70	Unassigned	N/A
71	State or local public health clinic	A facility maintained by either state or local health departments that provides ambulatory primary medical care under the general direction of a physician.
72	Rural health clinic	A certified facility which is located in a rural medically underserved area that provides ambulatory primary medical care under the general direction of a physician.
73-80	Unassigned	N/A
81	Independent laboratory	A laboratory certified to perform diagnostic and/or clinical tests independent of an institution or a physician's office.
82-98	Unassigned	N/A
99	Other place of service	Other place of service not identified above.

Type of Service

Common Working File Type of Service (TOS) Indicators

For submitting a claim to the Common Working File (CWF), use the following table to assign the proper TOS. Some procedures may have more than one applicable TOS. CWF will reject alerts on codes with incorrect TOS designations. CWF will produce alerts on codes with incorrect TOS designations.

The only exceptions to this annual update are:

- Surgical services billed for dates of service through December 31, 2007, containing the ASC facility service modifier SG must be reported as TOS F. Effective for services on or after January 1, 2008, the SG modifier is no longer applicable for Medicare services. ASC providers should discontinue applying the SG modifier on ASC facility claims. The indicator F does not appear in the TOS table because its use depends upon claims submitted with POS 24 (ASC facility) from an ASC (specialty 49). This became effective for dates of service January 1, 2008, or after.

- Surgical services billed with an assistant-at-surgery modifier (80-82, AS,) must be reported with TOS 8. The 8 indicator does not appear on the TOS table because its use is dependent upon the use of the appropriate modifier. (See Pub. 100-4 *Medicare Claims Processing*

Manual, chapter 12, "Physician/Practitioner Billing," for instructions on when assistant-at-surgery is allowable.)

- Psychiatric treatment services that are subject to the outpatient mental health treatment limitation should be reported with TOS T.

- TOS H appears in the list of descriptors. However, it does not appear in the table. In CWF, "H" is used only as an indicator for hospice. The contractor should not submit TOS H to CWF at this time.

- For outpatient services, when a transfusion medicine code appears on a claim that also contains a blood product, the service is paid under reasonable charge at 80 percent; coinsurance and deductible apply. When transfusion medicine codes are paid under the clinical laboratory fee schedule they are paid at 100 percent; coinsurance and deductible do not apply.

Note: For injection codes with more than one possible TOS designation, use the following guidelines when assigning the TOS:

When the choice is L or 1:

- Use TOS L when the drug is used related to ESRD; or

- Use TOS 1 when the drug is not related to ESRD and is administered in the office.

When the choice is G or 1:

- Use TOS G when the drug is an immunosuppressive drug; or

- Use TOS 1 when the drug is used for other than immunosuppression.

When the choice is P or 1:

- Use TOS P if the drug is administered through durable medical equipment (DME); or

- Use TOS 1 if the drug is administered in the office.

The place of service or diagnosis may be considered when determining the appropriate TOS. The descriptors for each of the TOS codes listed in the annual HCPCS update are:

0	Whole blood
1	Medical care
2	Surgery
3	Consultation
4	Diagnostic radiology
5	Diagnostic laboratory
6	Therapeutic radiology
7	Anesthesia
8	Assistant at surgery
9	Other medical items or services
A	Used DME
D	Ambulance
E	Enteral/parenteral nutrients/supplies
F	Ambulatory surgical center (facility usage for surgical services)
G	Immunosuppressive drugs
J	Diabetic shoes
K	Hearing items and services
L	ESRD supplies
M	Monthly capitation payment for dialysis
N	Kidney donor
P	Lump sum purchase of DME, prosthetics, orthotics
Q	Vision items or services
R	Rental of DME
S	Surgical dressings or other medical supplies
U	Occupational therapy
V	Pneumococcal/flu vaccine
W	Physical therapy

Berenson-Eggers Type of Service (BETOS) Codes

The BETOS coding system was developed primarily for analyzing the growth in Medicare expenditures. The coding system covers all HCPCS codes; assigns a HCPCS code to only one BETOS code; consists of readily understood clinical categories (as opposed to statistical or financial categories); consists of categories that permit objective assignment; is stable over time; and is relatively immune to minor changes in technology or practice patterns.

BETOS Codes and Descriptions:

1. Evaluation and Management
1. M1A — Office visits—new
2. M1B — Office visits—established
3. M2A — Hospital visit—initial
4. M2B — Hospital visit—subsequent
5. M2C — Hospital visit—critical care
6. M3 — Emergency room visit
7. M4A — Home visit
8. M4B — Nursing home visit
9. M5A — Specialist—pathology
10. M5B — Specialist—psychiatry
11. M5C — Specialist—ophthalmology
12. M5D — Specialist—other
13. M6 — Consultations

2. Procedures
1. P0 — Anesthesia
2. P1A — Major procedure—breast
3. P1B — Major procedure—colectomy
4. P1C — Major procedure—cholecystectomy
5. P1D — Major procedure—TURP
6. P1E — Major procedure—hysterectomy
7. P1F — Major procedure—explor/decompr/excis disc
8. P1G — Major procedure—other
9. P2A — Major procedure, cardiovascular—CABG
10. P2B — Major procedure, cardiovascular—aneurysm repair
11. P2C — Major procedure, cardiovascular—thromboendarterectomy
12. P2D — Major procedure, cardiovascular—coronary angioplasty (PTCA)
13. P2E — Major procedure, cardiovascular—pacemaker insertion
14. P2F — Major procedure, cardiovascular—other
15. P3A — Major procedure, orthopedic—hip fracture repair
16. P3B — Major procedure, orthopedic—hip replacement
17. P3C — Major procedure, orthopedic—knee replacement
18. P3D — Major procedure, orthopedic—other
19. P4A — Eye procedure—corneal transplant
20. P4B — Eye procedure—cataract removal/lens insertion
21. P4C — Eye procedure—retinal detachment
22. P4D — Eye procedure—treatment of retinal lesions
23. P4E — Eye procedure—other
24. P5A — Ambulatory procedures—skin
25. P5B — Ambulatory procedures—musculoskeletal
26. P5C — Ambulatory procedures—inguinal hernia repair
27. P5D — Ambulatory procedures—lithotripsy
28. P5E — Ambulatory procedures—other
29. P6A — Minor procedures—skin
30. P6B — Minor procedures—musculoskeletal
31. P6C — Minor procedures—other (Medicare fee schedule)
32. P6D — Minor procedures—other (non-Medicare fee schedule)
33. P7A — Oncology—radiation therapy
34. P7B — Oncology—other
35. P8A — Endoscopy—arthroscopy
36. P8B — Endoscopy—upper gastrointestinal
37. P8C — Endoscopy—sigmoidoscopy
38. P8D — Endoscopy—colonoscopy
39. P8E — Endoscopy—cystoscopy
40. P8F — Endoscopy—bronchoscopy
41. P8G — Endoscopy—laparoscopic cholecystectomy
42. P8H — Endoscopy—laryngoscopy
43. P8I — Endoscopy—other
44. P9A — Dialysis services (Medicare fee schedule)
45. P9B — Dialysis services (non-Medicare fee schedule)

3. Imaging
1. I1A — Standard imaging—chest
2. I1B — Standard imaging—musculoskeletal
3. I1C — Standard imaging—breast
4. I1D — Standard imaging—contrast gastrointestinal
5. I1E — Standard imaging—nuclear medicine
6. I1F — Standard imaging—other
7. I2A — Advanced imaging—CAT/CT/CTA; brain/head/neck
8. I2B — Advanced imaging—CAT/CT/CTA; other
9. I2C — Advanced imaging—MRI/MRA; brain/head/neck
10. I2D — Advanced imaging—MRI/MRA; other
11. I3A — Echography/ultrasonography—eye
12. I3B — Echography/ultrasonography—abdomen/pelvis
13. I3C — Echography/ultrasonography—heart
14. I3D — Echography/ultrasonography—carotid arteries
15. I3E — Echography/ultrasonography—prostate, transrectal
16. I3F — Echography/ultrasonography—other
17. I4A — Imaging/procedure—heart, including cardiac catheterization
18. I4B — Imaging/procedure—other

4. Tests
1. T1A — Lab tests—routine venipuncture (non-Medicare fee schedule)
2. T1B — Lab tests—automated general profiles
3. T1C — Lab tests—urinalysis
4. T1D — Lab tests—blood counts
5. T1E — Lab tests—glucose
6. T1F — Lab tests—bacterial cultures
7. T1G — Lab tests—other (Medicare fee schedule)
8. T1H — Lab tests—other (non-Medicare fee schedule)
9. T2A — Other tests—electrocardiograms
10. T2B — Other tests—cardiovascular stress tests
11. T2C — Other tests—EKG monitoring
12. T2D — Other tests—other

5. Durable Medical Equipment
1. D1A — Medical/surgical supplies
1. D1B — Hospital beds
1. D1C — Oxygen and supplies
1. D1D — Wheelchairs
1. D1E — Other DME
1. D1F — Prosthetic/orthotic devices
1. D1G — Drugs administered through DME

6. Other
1. O1A — Ambulance
2. O1B — Chiropractic
3. O1C — Enteral and parenteral
4. O1D — Chemotherapy
5. O1E — Other drugs
6. O1F — Hearing and speech services
7. O1G — Immunizations/vaccinations

7. Exceptions/Unclassified
1. Y1 — Other—Medicare fee schedule
2. Y2 — Other—Non-Medicare fee schedule
3. Z1 — Local codes
4. Z2 — Undefined codes

Appendix K — Multianalyte Assays with Algorithmic Analyses

The following is a list of administrative codes for multianalyte assays with algorithmic analysis (MAAA) procedures that are usually exclusive to one single clinical laboratory or manufacturer. These tests use the results from several different assays, including molecular pathology assays, fluorescent in situ hybridization assays, and nonnucleic acid-based assays (e.g., proteins, polypeptides, lipids, and carbohydrates) to perform an algorithmic analysis that is reported as a numeric score or probability. Although the laboratory report may list results of individual component tests of the MAAAs, these assays are not separately reportable.

The following list includes the proprietary name and clinical laboratory/manufacturer, an alphanumeric code, and the code descriptor.

The format for the code descriptor usually includes:

- Type of disease (e.g., oncology, autoimmune, tissue rejection)
- Chemical(s) analyzed (e.g., DNA, RNA, protein, antibody)
- Number of markers (e.g., number of genes, number of proteins)

- Methodology(s) (e.g., microarray, real-time [RT]-PCR, in situ hybridization [ISH], enzyme linked immunosorbent assays [ELISA])
- Number of functional domains (when indicated)
- Type of specimen (e.g., blood, fresh tissue, formalin-fixed paraffin embedded)
- Type of algorithm result (e.g., prognostic, diagnostic)
- Report (e.g., probability index, risk score)

MAAA procedures with a Category I code are noted on the following list and can also be found in code range 81500–81599 in the pathology and laboratory chapter. If a specific MAAA test does not have a Category I code, it is denoted with a four-digit number and the letter M. Use code 81599 if an MAAA test is not included on the following list or in the Category I codes. The codes on the list are exclusive to the assays identified by proprietary name. Report code 81599 also when an analysis is performed that may possibly fall within a specific descriptor but the proprietary name is not included in the list. The list does not contain all MAAA procedures.

Proprietary Name/Clinical Laboratory/Manufacturer	Code	Descriptor
Administrative Codes for Multianalyte Assays with Algorithmic Analyses (MAAA)		
HCV FibroSURE™, LabCorp FibroTest™, Quest Diagnostics/BioPredictive	▲ 0001M	Infectious disease, HCV, six biochemical assays (ALT, A2-macroglobulin, apolipoprotein A-1, total bilirubin, GGT, and haptoglobin) utilizing serum, prognostic algorithm reported as scores for fibrosis and necroinflammatory activity in liver
ASH FibroSURE™, LabCorp	0002M	Liver disease, 10 biochemical assays (ALT, A2-macroglobulin, apolipoprotein A-1, total bilirubin, GGT, haptoglobin, AST, glucose, total cholesterol, and triglycerides) utilizing serum, prognostic algorithm reported as quantitative scores for fibrosis, steatosis, and alcoholic steatohepatitis (ASH)
NASH FibroSURE™, LabCorp	0003M	Liver disease, 10 biochemical assays (ALT, A2-macroglobulin, apolipoprotein A-1, total bilirubin, GGT, haptoglobin, AST, glucose, total cholesterol, and triglycerides) utilizing serum, prognostic algorithm reported as quantitative scores for fibrosis, steatosis, and nonalcoholic steatohepatitis (NASH)
ScoliScore™ Transgenomic	0004M	Scoliosis, DNA analysis of 53 single nucleotide polymorphisms (SNPs), using saliva, prognostic algorithm reported as a risk score
HeproDX™, GoPath Laboratories, LLC	0006M	Oncology (hepatic), mRNA expression levels of 161 genes, utilizing fresh hepatocellular carcinoma tumor tissue, with alpha-fetoprotein level, algorithm reported as a risk classifier
NETest (Wren Laboratories, LLC)	0007M	Oncology (gastrointestinal neuroendocrine tumors), real-time PCR expression analysis of 51 genes, utilizing whole peripheral blood, algorithm reported as a nomogram of tumor disease index
Prosigna Breast Cancer Assay (NanoString Technologies)	0008M	Oncology (breast), mRNA analysis of 58 genes using hybrid capture, on formalin-fixed paraffin-embedded (FFPE) tissue, prognostic algorithm reported as a risk score
VisibiliT™ test, Sequenom Center for Molecular Medicine, LLC	0009M	Fetal aneuploidy (trisomy 21, and 18) DNA sequence analysis of selected regions using maternal plasma, algorithm reported as a risk score for each trisomy
4Kscore™ test, OPKO Diagnostics, LLC	0010M	Oncology (High-Grade Prostate Cancer), biochemical assay of four proteins (Total PSA, Free PSA, Intact PSA and human kallikrein 2 [hK2]) plus patient age, digital rectal examination status, and no history of positive prostate biopsy, utilizing plasma, prognostic algorithm reported as a probability score
Category I Codes for Multianalyte Assays with Algorithmic Analyses (MAAA)		
Vectra® DA, Crescendo Bioscience, Inc	● 81490	Autoimmune (rheumatoid arthritis), analysis of 12 biomarkers using immunoassays, utilizing serum, prognostic algorithm reported as a disease activity score (Do not report 81490 with 86140)
Corus® CAD, CardioDx, Inc.	● 81493	Coronary artery disease, mRNA, gene expression profiling by real-time RT-PCR of 23 genes, utilizing whole peripheral blood, algorithm reported as a risk score
Risk of Ovarian Malignancy Algorithm (ROMA)™, Fujirebio Diagnostics	81500	Oncology (ovarian), biochemical assays of two proteins (CA-125 and HE4), utilizing serum, with menopausal status, algorithm reported as a risk score

Appendix K — Multianalyte Assays with Algorithmic Analyses

Proprietary Name/Clinical Laboratory/Manufacturer	Code	Descriptor
OVA1™, Vermillion, Inc.	81503	Oncology (ovarian), biochemical assays of five proteins (CA-125, apolipoprotein A1, beta-2 microglobulin, transferrin, and pre-albumin), utilizing serum, algorithm reported as a risk score
Pathwork® Tissue of Origin Test, Pathwork Diagnostics	81504	Oncology (tissue of origin), microarray gene expression profiling of >2000 genes, utilizing formalin-fixed paraffin embedded tissue, algorithm reported as tissue similarity scores
PreDx Diabetes Risk Score™, Tethys Clinical Laboratory	81506	Endocrinology (type 2 diabetes), biochemical assays of seven analytes (glucose, HbA1c, insulin, hs-CRP, adiponectin, ferritin, interleukin 2-receptor alpha), utilizing serum or plasma, algorithm reporting a risk score
Harmony™ Prenatal Test, Ariosa Diagnostics	81507	Fetal aneuploidy (trisomy 21, 18, and 13) DNA sequence analysis of selected regions using maternal plasma, algorithm reported as a risk score for each trisomy
No proprietary name and clinical laboratory or manufacturer. Maternal serum screening procedures are performed by many labs and are not exclusive to a single facility.	81508	Fetal congenital abnormalities, biochemical assays of two proteins (PAPP-A, hCG [any form]), utilizing maternal serum, algorithm reported as a risk score
	81509	Fetal congenital abnormalities, biochemical assays of three proteins (PAPP-A, hCG [any form], DIA), utilizing maternal serum, algorithm reported as a risk score
	81510	Fetal congenital abnormalities, biochemical assays of three analytes (AFP, uE3, hCG (any form)), utilizing maternal serum, algorithm reported as a risk score
	81511	Fetal congenital abnormalities, biochemical assays of four analytes (AFP, uE3, hCG (any form), DIA) utilizing maternal serum, algorithm reported as a risk score (may include additional results from previous biochemical testing)
	81512	Fetal congenital abnormalities, biochemical assays of five analytes (AFP, uE3, total hCG, hyperglycosylated hCG, DIA) utilizing maternal serum, algorithm reported as a risk score
Oncotype DX® (Genomic Health)	81519	Oncology (breast), mRNA, gene expression profiling by real-time RT-PCR of 21 genes, utilizing formalin-fixed paraffin embedded tissue, algorithm reported as recurrence score
Oncotype DX® Colon Cancer Assay, Genomic Health	● 81525	Oncology (colon), mRNA, gene expression profiling by real-time RT-PCR of 12 genes (7 content and 5 housekeeping), utilizing formalin-fixed paraffin-embedded tissue, algorithm reported as a recurrence score
Cologuard™, Exact Sciences, Inc.	● 81528	Oncology (colorectal) screening, quantitative real-time target and signal amplification of 10 DNA markers (KRAS mutations, promoter methylation of NDRG4 and BMP3) and fecal hemoglobin, utilizing stool, algorithm reported as a positive or negative result (Do not report 81528 with 81275, 82274)
ChemoFX®, Helomics, Corp.	● 81535	Oncology (gynecologic), live tumor cell culture and chemotherapeutic response by DAPI stain and morphology, predictive algorithm reported as a drug response score; first single drug or drug combination
ChemoFX®, Helomics, Corp.	● + 81536	Oncology (gynecologic), live tumor cell culture and chemotherapeutic response by DAPI stain and morphology, predictive algorithm reported as a drug response score; each additional single drug or drug combination (List separately in addition to code for primary procedure) (Code first 81535)
VeriStrat, Biodesix, Inc.	● 81538	Oncology (lung), mass spectrometric 8-protein signature, including amyloid A, utilizing serum, prognostic and predictive algorithm reported as good versus poor overall survival
CancerTYPE ID, bioTheranostics, Inc.	● 81540	Oncology (tumor of unknown origin), mRNA, gene expression profiling by real-time RT-PCR of 92 genes (87 content and 5 housekeeping) to classify tumor into main cancer type and subtype, utilizing formalin-fixed paraffin-embedded tissue, algorithm reported as a probability of a predicted main cancer type and subtype
Afirma® Gene Expression Classifier, Veracyte, Inc.	● 81545	Oncology (thyroid), gene expression analysis of 142 genes, utilizing fine needle aspirate, algorithm reported as a categorical result (eg, benign or suspicious)
AlloMap®, CareDx, Inc	● 81595	Cardiology (heart transplant, mRNA gene expression profiling by real-time qualitative PCR of 20 genes (11 content and 9 housekeeping), utilizing subfraction of peripheral blood, algorithm reported as a rejection risk score
	81599	Unlisted multianalyte assay with algorithmic analysis

Appendix L — Glossary

-centesis. Puncture, as with a needle, trocar, or aspirator; often done for withdrawing fluid from a cavity.

-ectomy. Excision, removal.

-orrhaphy. Suturing.

-ostomy. Indicates a surgically created artificial opening.

-otomy. Making an incision or opening.

-plasty. Indicates surgically formed or molded.

abdominal lymphadenectomy. Surgical removal of the abdominal lymph nodes grouping, with or without para-aortic and vena cava nodes.

ablation. Removal or destruction of a body part or tissue or its function. Ablation may be performed by surgical means, hormones, drugs, radiofrequency, heat, chemical application, or other methods.

abnormal alleles. Form of gene that includes disease-related variations.

absorbable sutures. Strands prepared from collagen or a synthetic polymer and capable of being absorbed by tissue over time. Examples include surgical gut and collagen sutures; or synthetics like polydioxanone (PDS), polyglactin 910 (Vicryl), poliglecaprone 25 (Monocryl), polyglyconate (Maxon), and polyglycolic acid (Dexon).

acetabuloplasty. Surgical repair or reconstruction of the large cup-shaped socket in the hipbone (acetabulum) with which the head of the femur articulates.

Achilles tendon. Tendon attached to the back of the heel bone (calcaneus) that flexes the foot downward.

acromioclavicular joint. Junction between the clavicle and the scapula. The acromion is the projection from the back of the scapula that forms the highest point of the shoulder and connects with the clavicle. Trauma or injury to the acromioclavicular joint is often referred to as a dislocation of the shoulder. This is not correct, however, as a dislocation of the shoulder is a disruption of the glenohumeral joint.

acromionectomy. Surgical treatment for acromioclavicular arthritis in which the distal portion of the acromion process is removed.

acromioplasty. Repair of the part of the shoulder blade that connects to the deltoid muscles and clavicle.

actigraphy. Science of monitoring activity levels, particularly during sleep. In most cases, the patient wears a wristband that records motion while sleeping. The data are recorded, analyzed, and interpreted to study sleep/wake patterns and circadian rhythms.

air conduction. Transportation of sound from the air, through the external auditory canal, to the tympanic membrane and ossicular chain. Air conduction hearing is tested by presenting an acoustic stimulus through earphones or a loudspeaker to the ear.

air puff device. Instrument that measures intraocular pressure by evaluating the force of a reflected amount of air blown against the cornea.

alleles. Form of gene usually arising from a mutation responsible for a hereditary variation.

allogeneic collection. Collection of blood or blood components from one person for the use of another. Allogeneic collection was formerly termed homologous collection.

allograft. Graft from one individual to another of the same species.

amniocentesis. Surgical puncture through the abdominal wall, with a specialized needle and under ultrasonic guidance, into the interior of the pregnant uterus and directly into the amniotic sac to collect fluid for diagnostic analysis or therapeutic reduction of fluid levels.

anastomosis. Surgically created connection between ducts, blood vessels, or bowel segments to allow flow from one to the other.

anesthesia time. Time period factored into anesthesia procedures beginning with the anesthesiologist preparing the patient for surgery and ending when the patient is turned over to the recovery department.

Angelman syndrome. Early childhood emergence of a pattern of interrupted development, stiff, jerky gait, absence or impairment of speech, excessive laughter, and seizures.

angioplasty. Reconstruction or repair of a diseased or damaged blood vessel.

annuloplasty. Surgical plicaton of weakened tissue of the heart, to improve its muscular function. Annuli are thick, fibrous rings and one is found surrounding each of the cardiac chambers. The atrial and ventricular muscle fibers attach to the annuli. In annuloplasty, weakened annuli may be surgically plicated, or tucked, to improve muscular functions.

anorectal anometry. Measurement of pressure generated by anal sphincter to diagnose incontinence.

anterior chamber lenses. Lenses inserted into the anterior chamber following intracapsular cataract extraction.

applanation tonometer. Instrument that measures intraocular pressure by recording the force required to flatten an area of the cornea.

appropriateness of care. Proper setting of medical care that best meets the patient's care or diagnosis, as defined by a health care plan or other legal entity.

aqueous humor. Fluid within the anterior and posterior chambers of the eye that is continually replenished as it diffuses out into the blood. When the flow of aqueous is blocked, a build-up of fluid in the eye causes increased intraocular pressure and leads to glaucoma and blindness.

arteriogram. Radiograph of arteries.

arteriovenous fistula. Connecting passage between an artery and a vein.

arteriovenous malformation. Connecting passage between an artery and a vein.

arthrotomy. Surgical incision into a joint that may include exploration, drainage, or removal of a foreign body.

ASA. 1) Acetylsalicylic acid. Synonym: aspirin. 2) American Society of Anesthesiologists. National organization for anesthesiology that maintains and publishes the guidelines and relative values for anesthesia coding.

aspirate. To withdraw fluid or air from a body cavity by suction.

assay. Chemical analysis of a substance to establish the presence and strength of its components. A therapeutic drug assay is used to determine if a drug is within the expected therapeutic range for a patient.

atrial septal defect. Cardiac anomaly consisting of a patent opening in the atrial septum due to a fusion failure, classified as ostium secundum type, ostium primum defect, or endocardial cushion defect.

attended surveillance. Ability of a technician at a remote surveillance center or location to respond immediately to patient transmissions regarding rhythm or device alerts as they are produced and received at the remote location. These transmissions may originate from wearable or implanted therapy or monitoring devices.

auricle. External ear, which is a single elastic cartilage covered in skin and normal adnexal features (hair follicles, sweat glands, and sebaceous glands), shaped to channel sound waves into the acoustic meatus.

autogenous transplant. Tissue, such as bone, that is harvested from the patient and used for transplantation back into the same patient.

autograft. Any tissue harvested from one anatomical site of a person and grafted to another anatomical site of the same person. Most commonly, blood vessels, skin, tendons, fascia, and bone are used as autografts.

AVF. Arteriovenous fistula.

AVM. Arteriovenous malformation. Clusters of abnormal blood vessels that grow in the brain comprised of a blood vessel "nidus" or nest through which arteries and veins connect directly without going through the capillaries. As time passes, the nidus may enlarge resulting in the formation of a mass that may bleed. AVMs are more prone to bleeding in patients ages 10 to 55. Once older than age 55, the possibility of bleeding is reduced dramatically.

backbench preparation. Procedures performed on a donor organ following procurement to prepare the organ for transplant into the recipient. Excess fat and other tissue may be removed, the organ may be perfused, and vital arteries may be sized, repaired, or modified to fit the patient. These procedures are done on a back table in the operating room before transplantation can begin.

Bartholin's gland. Mucous-producing gland found in the vestibular bulbs on either side of the vaginal orifice and connected to the mucosal membrane at the opening by a duct.

Bartholin's gland abscess. Pocket of pus and surrounding cellulitis caused by infection of the Bartholin's gland and causing localized swelling and pain in the posterior labia majora that may extend into the lower vagina.

basic value. Relative weighted value based upon the usual anesthesia services and the relative work or cost of the specific anesthesia service assigned to each anesthesia-specific procedure code.

Berman locator. Small, sensitive tool used to detect the location of a metallic foreign body in the eye.

bifurcated. Having two branches or divisions, such as the left pulmonary veins that split off from the left atrium to carry oxygenated blood away from the heart.

Billroth's operation. Anastomosis of the stomach to the duodenum or jejunum.

bioprosthetic heart valve. Replacement cardiac valve made of biological tissue. Allograft, xenograft or engineered tissue.

biopsy. Tissue or fluid removed for diagnostic purposes through analysis of the cells in the biopsy material.

Blalock-Hanlon procedure. Excision of a segment of the right atrium, creating an atrial septal defect.

Blalock-Taussig procedure. Anastomosis of the left subclavian artery to the left pulmonary artery or the right subclavian artery to the right pulmonary artery in order to shunt some of the blood flow from the systemic to the pulmonary circulation.

blepharochalasis. Loss of elasticity and relaxation of skin of the eyelid, thickened or indurated skin on the eyelid associated with recurrent episodes of edema, and intracellular atrophy.

blepharoplasty. Plastic surgery of the eyelids to remove excess fat and redundant skin weighting down the lid. The eyelid is pulled tight and sutured to support sagging muscles.

blepharoptosis. Droop or displacement of the upper eyelid, caused by paralysis, muscle problems, or outside mechanical forces.

blepharorrhaphy. Suture of a portion or all of the opposing eyelids to shorten the palpebral fissure or close it entirely.

bone conduction. Transportation of sound through the bones of the skull to the inner ear.

bone mass measurement. Radiologic or radioisotopic procedure or other procedure approved by the FDA for identifying bone mass, detecting bone loss, or determining bone quality. The procedure includes a physician's interpretation of the results. Qualifying individuals must be an estrogen-deficient woman at clinical risk for osteoporosis with vertebral abnormalities.

brachytherapy. Form of radiation therapy in which radioactive pellets or seeds are implanted directly into the tissue being treated to deliver their dose of radiation in a more directed fashion. Brachytherapy provides radiation to the prescribed body area while minimizing exposure to normal tissue.

breakpoint. Point at which a chromosome breaks.

Bristow procedure. Anterior capsulorrhaphy prevents chronic separation of the shoulder. In this procedure, the bone block is affixed to the anterior glenoid rim with a screw.

buccal mucosa. Tissue from the mucous membrane on the inside of the cheek.

bundle of His. Bundle of modified cardiac fibers that begins at the atrioventricular node and passes through the right atrioventricular fibrous ring to the interventricular septum, where it divides into two branches. Bundle of His recordings are taken for intracardiac electrograms.

Caldwell-Luc operation. Intraoral antrostomy approach into the maxillary sinus for the removal of tooth roots or tissue, or for packing the sinus to reduce zygomatic fractures by creating a window above the teeth in the canine fossa area.

canthorrhaphy. Suturing of the palpebral fissure, the juncture between the eyelids, at either end of the eye.

canthotomy. Horizontal incision at the canthus (junction of upper and lower eyelids) to divide the outer canthus and enlarge lid margin separation.

cardio-. Relating to the heart.

cardiopulmonary bypass. Venous blood is diverted to a heart-lung machine, which mechanically pumps and oxygenates the blood temporarily so the heart can be bypassed while an open procedure on the heart or coronary arteries is performed. During bypass, the lungs are deflated and immobile.

cardioverter-defibrillator. Device that uses both low energy cardioversion or defibrillating shocks and antitachycardia pacing to treat ventricular tachycardia or ventricular fibrillation.

care plan oversight services. Physician's ongoing review and revision of a patient's care plan involving complex or multidisciplinary care modalities.

case management services. Physician case management is a process of involving direct patient care as well as coordinating and controlling access to the patient or initiating and/or supervising other necessary health care services.

cataract extraction. Surgical removal of the cataract or cloudy lens. Anterior chamber lenses are inserted in conjunction with intracapsular cataract extraction and posterior chamber lenses are inserted in conjunction with extracapsular cataract extraction.

catheter. Flexible tube inserted into an area of the body for introducing or withdrawing fluid.

Centers for Medicare and Medicaid Services. Federal agency that oversees the administration of the public health programs such as Medicare, Medicaid, and State Children's Insurance Program.

certified nurse midwife. Registered nurse who has successfully completed a program of study and clinical experience or has been certified by a recognized organization for the care of pregnant or delivering patients.

CFR. Code of Federal Regulations.

CHAMPUS. Civilian Health and Medical Program of the Uniformed Services. See Tricare.

CHAMPVA. Civilian Health and Medical Program of the Department of Veterans Affairs.

chemodenervation. Chemical destruction of nerves. A substance, for example, Botox, is used to temporarily inhibit the transfer of chemicals at the presynaptic membrane, blocking the neuromuscular junctions.

chemoembolization. Administration of chemotherapeutic agents directly to a tumor in combination with the percutaneous administration of an occlusive substance into a vessel to deprive the tumor of its blood supply. This ensures a prolonged level of therapy directed at the tumor. Chemoembolization is primarily being used for cancers of the liver and endocrine system.

chemosurgery. Application of chemical agents to destroy tissue, originally referring to the in situ chemical fixation of premalignant or malignant lesions to facilitate surgical excision.

Chiari osteotomy. Top of the femur is altered to correct a dislocated hip caused by congenital conditions or cerebral palsy. Plate and screws are often used.

chimera. Organ or anatomic structure consisting of tissues of diverse genetic constitution.

choanal atresia. Congenital, membranous, or bony closure of one or both posterior nostrils due to failure of the embryonic bucconasal membrane to rupture and open up the nasal passageway.

chondromalacia. Condition in which the articular cartilage softens, seen in various body sites but most often in the patella, and may be congenital or acquired.

chorionic villus sampling. Aspiration of a placental sample through a catheter, under ultrasonic guidance. The specialized needle is placed transvaginally through the cervix or transabdominally into the uterine cavity.

chronic pain management services. Distinct services frequently performed by anesthesiologists who have additional training in pain management procedures. Pain management services include initial and subsequent evaluation and management (E/M) services, trigger point injections, spine and spinal cord injections, and nerve blocks.

cineplastic amputation. Amputation in which muscles and tendons of the remaining portion of the extremity are arranged so that they may be utilized for motor functions. Following this type of amputation, a specially constructed prosthetic device allows the individual to execute more complex movements because the muscles and tendons are able to communicate independent movements to the device.

circadian. Relating to a cyclic, 24-hour period.

clinical social worker. Individual who possesses a master's or doctor's degree in social work and, after obtaining the degree, has performed at least two years of supervised clinical social work. A clinical social worker must be licensed by the state or, in the case of states without licensure, must completed at least two years or 3,000 hours of post-master's degree supervised clinical social work practice under the supervision of a master's level social worker.

clinical staff. Someone who works for, or under, the direction of a physician or qualified health care professional and does not bill services separately. The person may be licensed or regulated to help the physician perform specific duties.

clonal. Originating from one cell.

CMS. Centers for Medicare and Medicaid Services. Federal agency that administers the public health programs.

CO₂ laser. Carbon dioxide laser that emits an invisible beam and vaporizes water-rich tissue. The vapor is suctioned from the site.

codons. Series of three adjoining bases in one polynucleotide chain of a DNA or RNA molecule that provides the codes for a specific amino acid.

cognitive. Being aware by drawing from knowledge, such as judgment, reason, perception, and memory.

colostomy. Artificial surgical opening anywhere along the length of the colon to the skin surface for the diversion of feces.

commissurotomy. Surgical division or disruption of any two parts that are joined to form a commissure in order to increase the opening. The procedure most often refers to opening the adherent leaflet bands of fibrous tissue in a stenosed mitral valve.

common variants. Nucleotide sequence differences associated with abnormal gene function. Tests are usually performed in a single series of laboratory testing (in a single, typically multiplex, assay arrangement or using more than one assay to include all variants to be examined). Variants are representative of a mutation that mainly causes a single disease, such as cystic fibrosis. Other uncommon variants could provide additional information. Tests may be performed based on society recommendations and guidelines.

community mental health center. Facility providing outpatient mental health day treatment, assessments, and education as appropriate to community members.

computerized corneal topography. Digital imaging and analysis by computer of the shape of the corneal.

conjunctiva. Mucous membrane lining of the eyelids and covering of the exposed, anterior sclera.

conjunctivodacryocystostomy. Surgical connection of the lacrimal sac directly to the conjunctival sac.

conjunctivorhinostomy. Correction of an obstruction of the lacrimal canal achieved by suturing the posterior flaps and removing any lacrimal obstruction, preserving the conjunctiva.

constitutional. Cells containing genetic code that may be passed down to future generations. May also be referred to as germline.

consultation. Advice or opinion regarding diagnosis and treatment or determination to accept transfer of care of a patient rendered by a medical professional at the request of the primary care provider.

continuous positive airway pressure device. Pressurized device used to maintain the patient's airway for spontaneous or mechanically aided breathing. Often used for patients with mild to moderate sleep apnea.

core needle biopsy. Large-bore biopsy needle inserted into a mass and a core of tissue is removed for diagnostic study.

corpectomy. Removal of the body of a bone, such as a vertebra.

costochondral. Pertaining to the ribs and the scapula.

CPT. Current Procedural Terminology. Definitive procedural coding system developed by the American Medical Association that lists descriptive terms and identifying codes to provide a uniform language that describes medical, surgical, and diagnostic services for nationwide communication among physicians, patients, and third parties, used to report professional and outpatient services.

craniosynostosis. Congenital condition in which one or more of the cranial sutures fuse prematurely, creating a deformed or aberrant head shape.

craterization. Excision of a portion of bone creating a crater-like depression to facilitate drainage from infected areas of bone.

cricoid. Circular cartilage around the trachea.

CRNA. Certified registered nurse anesthetist. Nurse trained and specializing in the administration of anesthesia.

cryolathe. Tool used for reshaping a button of corneal tissue.

cryosurgery. Application of intense cold, usually produced using liquid nitrogen, to locally freeze diseased or unwanted tissue and induce tissue necrosis without causing harm to adjacent tissue.

CT. Computed tomography.

cutdown. Small, incised opening in the skin to expose a blood vessel, especially over a vein (venous cutdown) to allow venipuncture and permit a needle or cannula to be inserted for the withdrawal of blood or administration of fluids.

cytogenetic studies. Procedures in CPT that are related to the branch of genetics that studies cellular (cyto) structure and function as it relates to heredity (genetics). White blood cells, specifically T-lymphocytes, are the most commonly used specimen for chromosome analysis.

cytogenomic. Chromosomic evaluation using molecular methods.

dacryocystotome. Instrument used for incising the lacrimal duct strictures.

debride. To remove all foreign objects and devitalized or infected tissue from a burn or wound to prevent infection and promote healing.

definitive drug testing. Drug tests used to further analyze or confirm the presence or absence of specific drugs or classes of drugs used by the patient. These tests are able to provide more conclusive information regarding the concentration of the drug and their metabolites. May be used for medical, workplace, or legal purposes.

definitive identification. Identification of microorganisms using additional tests to specify the genus or species (e.g., slide cultures or biochemical panels).

dentoalveolar structure. Area of alveolar bone surrounding the teeth and adjacent tissue.

Department of Health and Human Services. Cabinet department that oversees the operating divisions of the federal government responsible for health and welfare. HHS oversees the Centers for Medicare and Medicaid Services, Food and Drug Administration, Public Health Service, and other such entities.

Department of Justice. Attorneys from the DOJ and the United States Attorney's Office have, under the memorandum of understanding, the same direct access to contractor data and records as the OIG and the Federal Bureau of Investigation (FBI). DOJ is responsible for prosecution of fraud and civil or criminal cases presented.

dermis. Skin layer found under the epidermis that contains a papillary upper layer and the deep reticular layer of collagen, vascular bed, and nerves.

dermis graft. Skin graft that has been separated from the epidermal tissue and the underlying subcutaneous fat, used primarily as a substitute for fascia grafts in plastic surgery.

desensitization. 1) Administration of extracts of allergens periodically to build immunity in the patient. 2) Application of medication to decrease the symptoms, usually pain, associated with a dental condition or disease.

destruction. Ablation or eradication of a structure or tissue.

diabetes outpatient self-management training services. Educational and training services furnished by a certified provider in an outpatient setting. The physician managing the individual's diabetic condition must certify that the services are needed under a comprehensive plan of care and provide the patient with the skills and knowledge necessary for therapeutic program compliance (including skills related to the self-administration of injectable drugs). The provider must meet applicable standards established by the National Diabetes Advisory or be recognized by an organization that represents individuals with diabetes as meeting standards for furnishing the services.

diagnostic procedures. Procedure performed on a patient to obtain information to assess the medical condition of the patient or to identify a disease and to determine the nature and severity of an illness or injury.

diaphragm. 1) Muscular wall separating the thorax and its structures from the abdomen. 2) Flexible disk inserted into the vagina and against the cervix as a method of birth control.

diaphysectomy. Surgical removal of a portion of the shaft of a long bone, often done to facilitate drainage from infected bone.

diathermy. Applying heat to body tissues by various methods for therapeutic treatment or surgical purposes to coagulate and seal tissue.

dilation. Artificial increase in the diameter of an opening or lumen made by medication or by instrumentation.

dissect. Cut apart or separate tissue for surgical purposes or for visual or microscopic study.

DNA. Deoxyribonucleic acid. Chemical containing the genetic information necessary to produce and propagate living organisms. Molecules are comprised of two twisting paired strands, called a double helix.

DNA marker. Specific gene sequence within a chromosome indicating the inheritance of a certain trait.

dorsal. Pertaining to the back or posterior aspect.

drugs and biologicals. Drugs and biologicals included - or approved for inclusion - in the United States Pharmacopoeia, the National Formulary, the United States Homeopathic Pharmacopoeia, in New Drugs or Accepted Dental Remedies, or approved by the pharmacy and drug therapeutics committee of the medical staff of the hospital. Also included are medically

accepted and FDA approved drugs used in an anticancer chemotherapeutic regimen. The carrier determines medical acceptance based on supportive clinical evidence.

dual-lead device. Implantable cardiac device (pacemaker or implantable cardioverter-defibrillator [ICD]) in which pacing and sensing components are placed in only two chambers of the heart.

duplex scan. Noninvasive vascular diagnostic technique that uses ultrasonic scanning to identify the pattern and direction of blood flow within arteries or veins displayed in real time images. Duplex scanning combines B-mode two-dimensional pictures of the vessel structure with spectra and/or color flow Doppler mapping or imaging of the blood as it moves through the vessels.

duplication/deletion (DUP/DEL). Term used in molecular testing which examines genomic regions to determine if there are extra chromosomes (duplication) or missing chromosomes (deletions). Normal gene dosage is two copies per cell except for the sex chromosomes which have one per cell.

DuToit staple capsulorrhaphy. Reattachment of the capsule of the shoulder and glenoid labrum to the glenoid lip using staples to anchor the avulsed capsule and glenoid labrum.

Dx. Diagnosis.

DXA. Dual energy x-ray absorptiometry. Radiological technique for bone density measurement using a two-dimensional projection system in which two x-ray beams with different levels of energy are pulsed alternately and the results are given in two scores, reported as standard deviations from peak bone mass density.

dynamic mutation. Unstable or changing polynucleotides resulting in repeats related to genes that can undergo disease-producing increases or decreases in the repeats that differ within tissues or over generations.

ECMO. Extracorporeal membrane oxygenation.

ectropion. Drooping of the lower eyelid away from the eye or outward turning or eversion of the edge of the eyelid, exposing the palpebral conjunctiva and causing irritation.

Eden-Hybinette procedure. Anterior shoulder repair using an anterior bone block to augment the bony anterior glenoid lip.

EDTA. Drug used to inhibit damage to the cornea by collagenase. EDTA is especially effective in alkali burns as it neutralizes soluble alkali, including lye.

effusion. Escape of fluid from within a body cavity.

electrocardiographic rhythm derived. Analysis of data obtained from readings of the heart's electrical activation, including heart rate and rhythm, variability of heart rate, ST analysis, and T-wave alternans. Other data may also be assessed when warranted.

electrocautery. Division or cutting of tissue using high-frequency electrical current to produce heat, which destroys cells.

electrode array. Electronic device containing more than one contact whose function can be adjusted during programming services. Electrodes are specialized for a particular electrochemical reaction that acts as a medium between a body surface and another instrument.

electromyography. Test that measures muscle response to nerve stimulation determining if muscle weakness is present and if it is related to the muscles themselves or a problem with the nerves that supply the muscles.

electrooculogram (EOG). Record of electrical activity associated with eye movements.

electrophysiologic studies. Electrical stimulation and monitoring to diagnose heart conduction abnormalities that predispose patients to bradyarrhythmias and to determine a patient's chance for developing ventricular and supraventricular tachyarrhythmias.

embolization. Placement of a clotting agent, such as a coil, plastic particles, gel, foam, etc., into an area of hemorrhage to stop the bleeding or to block blood flow to a problem area, such as an aneurysm or a tumor.

emergency. Serious medical condition or symptom (including severe pain) resulting from injury, sickness, or mental illness that arises suddenly and requires immediate care and treatment, generally received within 24 hours of onset, to avoid jeopardy to the life, limb, or health of a covered person.

empyema. Accumulation of pus within the respiratory, or pleural, cavity.

EMTALA. Emergency Medical Treatment and Active Labor Act.

end-stage renal disease. Chronic, advanced kidney disease requiring renal dialysis or a kidney transplant to prevent imminent death.

endarterectomy. Removal of the thickened, endothelial lining of a diseased or damaged artery.

endomicroscopy. Diagnostic technology that allows for the examination of tissue at the cellular level during endoscopy. The technology decreases the need for biopsy with histological examination for some types of lesions.

endovascular embolization. Procedure whereby vessels are occluded by a variety of therapeutic substances for the treatment of abnormal blood vessels by inhibiting the flow of blood to a tumor, arteriovenous malformations, lymphatic malformation, and to prevent or stop hemorrhage.

entropion. Inversion of the eyelid, turning the edge in toward the eyeball and causing irritation from contact of the lashes with the surface of the eye.

enucleation. Removal of a growth or organ cleanly so as to extract it in one piece.

epidermis. Outermost, nonvascular layer of skin that contains four to five differentiated layers depending on its body location: stratum corneum, lucidum, granulosum, spinosum, and basale.

epiphysiodesis. Surgical fusion of an epiphysis performed to prematurely stop further bone growth.

escharotomy. Surgical incision into the scab or crust resulting from a severe burn in order to relieve constriction and allow blood flow to the distal unburned tissue.

established patient. 1) Patient who has received professional services in a face-to-face setting within the last three years from the same physician/qualified health care professional or another physician/qualified health care professional of the exact same specialty and subspecialty who belongs to the same group practice. 2) For OPPS hospitals, patient who has been registered as an inpatient or outpatient in a hospital's provider-based clinic or emergency department within the past three years.

evacuation. Removal or purging of waste material.

evaluation and management codes. Assessment and management of a patient's health care.

evaluation and management service components. Key components of history, examination, and medical decision making that are key to selecting the correct E/M codes. Other non-key components include counseling, coordination of care, nature of presenting problem, and time.

event recorder. Portable, ambulatory heart monitor worn by the patient that makes electrocardiographic recordings of the length and frequency of aberrant cardiac rhythm to help diagnose heart conditions and to assess pacemaker functioning or programming.

exenteration. Surgical removal of the entire contents of a body cavity, such as the pelvis or orbit.

exon. One of multiple nucleic acid sequences used to encode information for a gene polypeptide or protein. Exons are separated from other exons by non-protein-coding sequences known as introns.

extended care services. Items and services provided to an inpatient of a skilled nursing facility, including nursing care, physical or occupational therapy, speech pathology, drugs and supplies, and medical social services.

external electrical capacitor device. External electrical stimulation device designed to promote bone healing. This device may also promote neural regeneration, revascularization, epiphyseal growth, and ligament maturation.

external pulsating electromagnetic field. External stimulation device designed to promote bone healing. This device may also promote neural regeneration, revascularization, epiphyseal growth, and ligament maturation.

extracorporeal. Located or taking place outside the body.

Eyre-Brook capsulorrhaphy. Reattachment of the capsule of the shoulder and glenoid labrum to the glenoid lip.

False Claims Act. Governs civil actions for filing false claims. Liability under this act pertains to any person who knowingly presents or causes to be presented a false or fraudulent claim to the government for payment or approval.

fascia. Fibrous sheet or band of tissue that envelops organs, muscles, and groupings of muscles.

fasciectomy. Excision of fascia or strips of fascial tissue.

fasciotomy. Incision or transection of fascial tissue.

fat graft. Graft composed of fatty tissue completely freed from surrounding tissue that is used primarily to fill in depressions.

FDA. Food and Drug Administration. Federal agency responsible for protecting public health by substantiating the safety, efficacy, and security of human and veterinary drugs, biological products, medical devices, national food supply, cosmetics, and items that give off radiation.

filtered speech test. Test most commonly used to identify central auditory dysfunction in which the patient is presented monosyllabic words that are low pass filtered, allowing only the parts of each word below a certain pitch to be presented. A score is given on the number of correct responses. This may be a subset of a standard battery of tests provided during a single encounter.

fissure. Deep furrow, groove, or cleft in tissue structures.

fistulization. Creation of a communication between two structures that were not previously connected.

flexor digitorum profundus tendon. Tendon originating in the proximal forearm and extending to the index finger and wrist. A thickened FDP sheath, usually caused by age, illness, or injury, can fill the carpal canal and lead to impingement of the median nerve.

fluoroscopy. Radiology technique that allows visual examination of part of the body or a function of an organ using a device that projects an x-ray image on a fluorescent screen.

focal length. Distance between the object in focus and the lens.

focused medical review. Process of targeting and directing medical review efforts on Medicare claims where the greatest risk of inappropriate program payment exists. The goal is to reduce the number of noncovered claims or unnecessary services. CMS analyzes national data such as internal billing, utilization, and payment data and provides its findings to the FI. Local medical review policies are developed identifying aberrances, abuse, and overutilized services. Providers are responsible for knowing national Medicare coverage and billing guidelines and local medical review policies, and for determining whether the services provided to Medicare beneficiaries are covered by Medicare.

fragile X syndrome. Intellectual disabilities, enlarged testes, big jaw, high forehead, and long ears in males. In females, fragile X presents with mild intellectual disabilities and heterozygous sexual structures. In some families, males have shown no symptoms but carry the gene.

free flap. Tissue that is completely detached from the donor site and transplanted to the recipient site, receiving its blood supply from capillary ingrowth at the recipient site.

free microvascular flap. Tissue that is completely detached from the donor site following careful dissection and preservation of the blood vessels, then attached to the recipient site with the transferred blood vessels anastomosed to the vessels in the recipient bed.

fulguration. Destruction of living tissue by using sparks from a high-frequency electric current.

gas tamponade. Absorbable gas may be injected to force the retina against the choroid. Common gases include room air, short-acting sulfahexafluoride, intermediate-acting perfluoroethane, or long-acting perfluorooctane.

Gaucher disease. Genetic metabolic disorder in which fat deposits may accumulate in the spleen, liver, lungs, bone marrow, and brain.

gene. Basic unit of heredity that contains nucleic acid. Genes are arranged in different and unique sequences or strings that determine the gene's function. Human genes usually include multiple protein coding regions such as exons separated by introns which are nonprotein coding sections.

genome. Complete set of DNA of an organism. Each cell in the human body is comprised of a complete copy of the approximately three billion DNA base pairs that constitute the human genome.

HCPCS. Healthcare Common Procedure Coding System.

HCPCS Level I. Healthcare Common Procedure Coding System Level I. Numeric coding system used by physicians, facility outpatient departments, and ambulatory surgery centers (ASC) to code ambulatory, laboratory, radiology, and other diagnostic services for Medicare billing. This coding system contains only the American Medical Association's Physicians' Current Procedural Terminology (CPT) codes. The AMA updates codes annually.

HCPCS Level II. Healthcare Common Procedure Coding System Level II. National coding system, developed by CMS, that contains alphanumeric codes for physician and nonphysician services not included in the CPT coding system. HCPCS Level II covers such things as ambulance services, durable medical equipment, and orthotic and prosthetic devices.

HCPCS modifiers. Two-character code (AA-ZZ) that identifies circumstances that alter or enhance the description of a service or supply. They are recognized by carriers nationally and are updated annually by CMS.

Hct. Hematocrit.

health care provider. Entity that administers diagnostic and therapeutic services.

hemilaminectomy. Excision of a portion of the vertebral lamina.

hemodialysis. Cleansing of wastes and contaminating elements from the blood by virtue of different diffusion rates through a semipermeable membrane, which separates blood from a filtration solution that diffuses other elements out of the blood.

hemoperitoneum. Effusion of blood into the peritoneal cavity, the space between the continuous membrane lining the abdominopelvic walls and encasing the visceral organs.

heterograft. Surgical graft of tissue from one animal species to a different animal species. A common type of heterograft is porcine (pig) tissue, used for temporary wound closure.

heterotopic transplant. Tissue transplanted from a different anatomical site for usage as is natural for that tissue, for example, buccal mucosa to a conjunctival site.

HGNC. HUGO gene nomenclature committee.

HGVS. Human genome variation society.

Hickman catheter. Central venous catheter used for long-term delivery of medications, such as antibiotics, nutritional substances, or chemotherapeutic agents.

HLA. Human leukocyte antigen.

home health services. Services furnished to patients in their homes under the care of physicians. These services include part-time or intermittent skilled nursing care, physical therapy, medical social services, medical supplies, and some rehabilitation equipment. Home health supplies and services must be prescribed by a physician, and the beneficiary must be confined at home in order for Medicare to pay the benefits in full.

homograft. Graft from one individual to another of the same species.

hospice care. Items and services provided to a terminally ill individual by a hospice program under a written plan established and periodically reviewed by the individual's attending physician and by the medical

director: Nursing care provided by or under the supervision of a registered professional nurse; Physical or occupational therapy or speech-language pathology services; Medical social services under the direction of a physician; Services of a home health aide who has successfully completed a training program; Medical supplies (including drugs and biologicals) and the use of medical appliances; Physicians' services; Short-term inpatient care (including both respite care and procedures necessary for pain control and acute and chronic symptom management) in an inpatient facility on an intermittent basis and not consecutively over longer than five days; Counseling (including dietary counseling) with respect to care of the terminally ill individual and adjustment to his death; Any item or service which is specified in the plan and for which payment may be made.

hospital. Institution that provides, under the supervision of physicians, diagnostic, therapeutic, and rehabilitation services for medical diagnosis, treatment, and care of patients. Hospitals receiving federal funds must maintain clinical records on all patients, provide 24-hour nursing services, and have a discharge planning process in place. The term "hospital" also includes religious nonmedical health care institutions and facilities of 50 beds or less located in rural areas.

HUGO. Human genome organization

IA. Intra-arterial.

ICD. Implantable cardioverter defibrillator.

ICD-10-CM. International Classification of Diseases, 10th Revision, Clinical Modification. Clinical modification of the alphanumeric classification of diseases used by the World Health Organization, already in use in much of the world, and used for mortality reporting in the United States. The implementation date for ICD-10-CM diagnostic coding system to replace ICD-9-CM in the United States is October 1, 2015.

ICD-10-PCS. International Classification of Diseases, 10th Revision, Procedure Coding System. Beginning October 1, 2015, inpatient hospital services and surgical procedures must be coded using ICD-10-PCS codes, replacing the current ICD-9-CM, Volume 3 for procedures.

ICM. Implantable cardiovascular monitor.

ileostomy. Artificial surgical opening that brings the end of the ileum out through the abdominal wall to the skin surface for the diversion of feces through a stoma.

iliopsoas tendon. Fibrous tissue that connects muscle to bone in the pelvic region, common to the iliacus and psoas major.

ILR. Implantable loop recorder.

IM. 1) Infectious mononucleosis. 2) Internal medicine. 3) Intramuscular.

immunotherapy. Therapeutic use of serum or gamma globulin.

implant. Material or device inserted or placed within the body for therapeutic, reconstructive, or diagnostic purposes.

implantable cardiovascular monitor. Implantable electronic device that stores cardiovascular physiologic data such as intracardiac pressure waveforms collected from internal sensors or data such as weight and blood pressure collected from external sensors. The information stored in these devices is used as an aid in managing patients with heart failure and other cardiac conditions that are non-rhythm related. The data may be transmitted via local telemetry or remotely to a surveillance technician or an internet-based file server.

implantable cardioverter-defibrillator. Implantable electronic cardiac device used to control rhythm abnormalities such as tachycardia, fibrillation, or bradycardia by producing high- or low-energy stimulation and pacemaker functions. It may also have the capability to provide the functions of an implantable loop recorder or implantable cardiovascular monitor.

implantable loop recorder. Implantable electronic cardiac device that constantly monitors and records electrocardiographic rhythm. It may be triggered by the patient when a symptomatic episode occurs or activated automatically by rapid or slow heart rates. This may be the sole purpose of the device or it may be a component of another cardiac device, such as a pacemaker or implantable cardioverter-defibrillator. The data can be transmitted via local telemetry or remotely to a surveillance technician or an internet-based file server.

implantable venous access device. Catheter implanted for continuous access to the venous system for long-term parenteral feeding or for the administration of fluids or medications.

IMRT. Intensity modulated radiation therapy. External beam radiation therapy delivery using computer planning to specify the target dose and to modulate the radiation intensity, usually as a treatment for a malignancy. The delivery system approaches the patient from multiple angles, minimizing damage to normal tissue.

in situ. Located in the natural position or contained within the origin site, not spread into neighboring tissue.

incontinence. Inability to control urination or defecation.

infundibulectomy. Excision of the anterosuperior portion of the right ventricle of the heart.

internal direct current stimulator. Electrostimulation device placed directly into the surgical site designed to promote bone regeneration by encouraging cellular healing response in bone and ligaments.

interrogation device evaluation. Assessment of an implantable cardiac device (pacemaker, cardioverter-defibrillator, cardiovascular monitor, or loop recorder) in which collected data about the patient's heart rate and rhythm, battery and pulse generator function, and any leads or sensors present, are retrieved and evaluated. Determinations regarding device programming and appropriate treatment settings are made based on the findings. CPT provides required components for evaluation of the various types of devices.

intramedullary implants. Nail, rod, or pin placed into the intramedullary canal at the fracture site. Intramedullary implants not only provide a method of aligning the fracture, they also act as a splint and may reduce fracture pain. Implants may be rigid or flexible. Rigid implants are preferred for prophylactic treatment of diseased bone, while flexible implants are preferred for traumatic injuries.

intraocular lens. Artificial lens implanted into the eye to replace a damaged natural lens or cataract.

intravenous. Within a vein or veins.

introducer. Instrument, such as a catheter, needle, or tube, through which another instrument or device is introduced into the body.

intron. Nonprotein section of a gene that separates exons in human genes. Contains vital sequences that allow splicing of exons to produce a functional protein from a gene. Sometimes referred to as intervening sequences (IVS).

IP. 1) Interphalangeal. 2) Intraperitoneal.

irrigation. To wash out or cleanse a body cavity, wound, or tissue with water or other fluid.

Kayser-Fleischer ring. Condition found in Wilson's disease in which deposits of copper cause a pigmented ring around the cornea's outer border in the deep epithelial layers.

keratoprosthesis. Surgical procedure in which the physician creates a new anterior chamber with a plastic optical implant to replace a severely damaged cornea that cannot be repaired.

keratotomy. Surgical incision of the cornea.

krypton laser. Laser light energy that uses ionized krypton by electric current as the active source, has a radiation beam between the visible yellow-red spectrum, and is effective in photocoagulation of retinal bleeding, macular lesions, and vessel aberrations of the choroid.

lacrimal. Tear-producing gland or ducts that provides lubrication and flushing of the eyes and nasal cavities.

lacrimal punctum. Opening of the lacrimal papilla of the eyelid through which tears flow to the canaliculi to the lacrimal sac.

lacrimotome. Knife for cutting the lacrimal sac or duct.

lacrimotomy. Incision of the lacrimal sac or duct.

laparotomy. Incision through the flank or abdomen for therapeutic or diagnostic purposes.

laryngoscopy. Examination of the hypopharynx, larynx, and tongue base with an endoscope.

larynx. Musculocartilaginous structure between the trachea and the pharynx that functions as the valve preventing food and other particles from entering the respiratory tract, as well as the voice mechanism. Also called the voicebox, the larynx is composed of three single cartilages: cricoid, epiglottis, and thyroid; and three paired cartilages: arytenoid, corniculate, and cuneiform.

laser surgery. Use of concentrated, sharply defined light beams to cut, cauterize, coagulate, seal, or vaporize tissue.

LEEP. Loop electrode excision procedure. Biopsy specimen or cone shaped wedge of cervical tissue is removed using a hot cautery wire loop with an electrical current running through it.

levonorgestrel. Drug inhibiting ovulation and preventing sperm from penetrating cervical mucus. It is delivered subcutaneously in polysiloxone capsules. The capsules can be effective for up to five years, and provide a cumulative pregnancy rate of less than 2 percent. The capsules are not biodegradable, and therefore must be removed. Removal is more difficult than insertion of levonorgestrel capsules because fibrosis develops around the capsules. Normal hormonal activity and a return to fertility begins immediately upon removal.

ligament. Band or sheet of fibrous tissue that connects the articular surfaces of bones or supports visceral organs.

ligation. Tying off a blood vessel or duct with a suture or a soft, thin wire.

lymphadenectomy. Dissection of lymph nodes free from the vessels and removal for examination by frozen section in a separate procedure to detect early-stage metastases.

lysis. Destruction, breakdown, dissolution, or decomposition of cells or substances by a specific catalyzing agent.

Magnuson-Stack procedure. Treatment for recurrent anterior dislocation of the shoulder that involves tightening and realigning the subscapularis tendon.

maintenance of wakefulness test. Attended study determining the patient's ability to stay awake.

Manchester operation. Preservation of the uterus following prolapse by amputating the vaginal portion of the cervix, shortening the cardinal ligaments, and performing a colpoperineorrhaphy posteriorly.

mapping. Multidimensional depiction of a tachycardia that identifies its site of origin and its electrical conduction pathway after tachycardia has been induced. The recording is made from multiple catheter sites within the heart, obtaining electrograms simultaneously or sequentially.

marsupialization. Creation of a pouch in surgical treatment of a cyst in which one wall is resected and the remaining cut edges are sutured to adjacent tissue creating an open pouch of the previously enclosed cyst.

mastectomy. Surgical removal of one or both breasts.

McDonald procedure. Polyester tape is placed around the cervix with a running stitch to assist in the prevention of pre-term delivery. Tape is removed at term for vaginal delivery.

MCP. Metacarpophalangeal.

medial. Middle or midline.

mediastinotomy. Incision into the mediastinum for purposes of exploration, foreign body removal, drainage, or biopsy.

medical review. Review by a Medicare administrative contractor, carrier, and/or quality improvement organization (QIO) of services and items provided by physicians, other health care practitioners, and providers of health care services under Medicare. The review determines if the items and services are reasonable and necessary and meet Medicare coverage requirements, whether the quality meets professionally recognized standards of health care, and whether the services are medically

appropriate in an inpatient, outpatient, or other setting as supported by documentation.

Medicare contractor. Medicare Part A fiscal intermediary, Medicare Part B carrier, Medicare administrative contractor (MAC), or a durable medical equipment Medicare administrative contractor (DME MAC).

Medicare physician fee schedule. List of payments Medicare allows by procedure or service. Payments may vary through geographic adjustments. The MPFS is based on the resource-based relative value scale (RBRVS). A national total relative value unit (RVU) is given to each procedure (HCPCS Level I CPT, Level II national codes). Each total RVU has three components: physician work, practice expense, and malpractice insurance.

metabolite. Chemical compound resulting from the natural process of metabolism. In drug testing, the metabolite of the drug may endure in a higher concentration or for a longer duration than the initial "parent" drug.

methylation. Mechanism used to regulate genes and protect DNA from some types of cleavage.

microarray. Small surface onto which multiple specific nucleic acid sequences can be attached to be used for analysis. Microarray may also be known as a gene chip or DNA chip. Tests can be run on the sequences for any variants that may be present.

mitral valve. Valve with two cusps that is between the left atrium and left ventricle of the heart.

moderate sedation. Medically controlled state of depressed consciousness, with or without analgesia, while maintaining the patient's airway, protective reflexes, and ability to respond to stimulation or verbal commands.

Mohs micrographic surgery. Special technique used to treat complex or ill-defined skin cancer and requires a single physician to provide two distinct services. The first service is surgical and involves the destruction of the lesion by a combination of chemosurgery and excision. The second service is that of a pathologist and includes mapping, color coding of specimens, microscopic examination of specimens, and complete histopathologic preparation.

monitored anesthesia care. Sedation, with or without analgesia, used to achieve a medically controlled state of depressed consciousness while maintaining the patient's airway, protective reflexes, and ability to respond to stimulation or verbal commands. In dental conscious sedation, the patient is rendered free of fear, apprehension, and anxiety through the use of pharmacological agents.

monoclonal. Relating to a single clone of cells.

multiple sleep latency test (MSLT). Attended study to determine the tendency of the patient to fall asleep.

multiple-lead device. Implantable cardiac device (pacemaker or implantable cardioverter-defibrillator [ICD]) in which pacing and sensing components are placed in at least three chambers of the heart.

Mustard procedure. Corrective measure for transposition of great vessels involves an intra-atrial baffle made of pericardial tissue or synthetic material. The baffle is secured between pulmonary veins and mitral valve and between mitral and tricuspid valves. The baffle directs systemic venous flow into the left ventricle and lungs and pulmonary venous flow into the right ventricle and aorta.

mutation. Alteration in gene function that results in changes to a gene or chromosome. Can cause deficits or disease that can be inherited, can have beneficial effects, or result in no noticeable change.

mutation scanning. Process normally used on multiple polymerase chain reaction (PCR) amplicons to determine DNA sequence variants by differences in characteristics compared to normal. Specific DNA variants can then be studied further.

myasthenia gravis. Autoimmune neuromuscular disorder caused by antibodies to the acetylcholine receptors at the neuromuscular junction, interfering with proper binding of the neurotransmitter from the neuron to the target muscle, causing muscle weakness, fatigue, and exhaustion, without pain or atrophy.

myotomy. Surgical cutting of a muscle to gain access to underlying tissues or for therapeutic reasons.

myringotomy. Incision in the eardrum done to prevent spontaneous rupture precipitated by fluid pressure build-up behind the tympanic membrane and to prevent stagnant infection and erosion of the ossicles.

nasal polyp. Fleshy outgrowth projecting from the mucous membrane of the nose or nasal sinus cavity that may obstruct ventilation or affect the sense of smell.

nasal sinus. Air-filled cavities in the cranial bones lined with mucous membrane and continuous with the nasal cavity, draining fluids through the nose.

nasogastric tube. Long, hollow, cylindrical catheter made of soft rubber or plastic that is inserted through the nose down into the stomach, and is used for feeding, instilling medication, or withdrawing gastric contents.

nasolacrimal punctum. Opening of the lacrimal duct near the nose.

nasopharynx. Membranous passage above the level of the soft palate.

Nd:YAG laser. Laser light energy that uses an yttrium, aluminum, and garnet crystal doped with neodymium ions as the active source, has a radiation beam nearing the infrared spectrum, and is effective in photocoagulation, photoablation, cataract extraction, and lysis of vitreous strands.

nebulizer. Latin for mist, a device that converts liquid into a fine spray and is commonly used to deliver medicine to the upper respiratory, bronchial, and lung areas.

nerve conduction study. Diagnostic test performed to assess muscle or nerve damage. Nerves are stimulated with electric shocks along the course of the muscle. Sensors are utilized to measure and record nerve functions, including conduction and velocity.

neurectomy. Excision of all or a portion of a nerve.

neuromuscular junction. Nerve synapse at the meeting point between the terminal end of a nerve (motor neuron) and a muscle fiber.

neuropsychological testing. Evaluation of a patient's behavioral abilities wherein a physician or other health care professional administers a series of tests in thinking, reasoning, and judgment.

new patient. Patient who is receiving face-to-face care from a provider/qualified health care professional or another physician/qualified health care professional of the exact same specialty and subspecialty who belongs to the same group practice for the first time in three years. For OPPS hospitals, a patient who has not been registered as an inpatient or outpatient, including off-campus provider based clinic or emergency department, within the past three years.

Niemann-Pick syndrome. Accumulation of phospholipid in histiocytes in the bone marrow, liver, lymph nodes, and spleen, cerebral involvement, and red macular spots similar to Tay-Sachs disease. Most commonly found in Jewish infants.

Nissen fundoplasty. Surgical repair technique that involves the fundus of the stomach being wrapped around the lower end of the esophagus to treat reflux esophagitis.

nonabsorbable sutures. Strands of natural or synthetic material that resist absorption into living tissue and are removed once healing is under way. Nonabsorbable sutures are commonly used to close skin wounds and repair tendons or collagenous tissue.

obturator. Prosthesis used to close an acquired or congenital opening in the palate that aids in speech and chewing.

obturator nerve. Lumbar plexus nerve with anterior and posterior divisions that innervate the adductor muscles (e.g., adductor longus, adductor brevis) of the leg and the skin over the medial area of the thigh or a sacral plexus nerve with anterior and posterior divisions that innervate the superior gemellus muscles.

occult blood test. Chemical or microscopic test to determine the presence of blood in a specimen.

ocular implant. Implant inside muscular cone.

oophorectomy. Surgical removal of all or part of one or both ovaries, either as open procedure or laparoscopically. Menstruation and childbearing ability continues when one ovary is removed.

orthosis. Derived from a Greek word meaning "to make straight," it is an artificial appliance that supports, aligns, or corrects an anatomical deformity or improves the use of a moveable body part. Unlike a prosthesis, an orthotic device is always functional in nature.

osteo-. Having to do with bone.

osteogenesis stimulator. Device used to stimulate the growth of bone by electrical impulses or ultrasound.

osteotomy. Surgical cutting of a bone.

ostomy. Artificial (surgical) opening in the body used for drainage or for delivery of medications or nutrients.

pacemaker. Implantable cardiac device that controls the heart's rhythm and maintains regular beats by artificial electric discharges. This device consists of the pulse generator with a battery and the electrodes, or leads, which are placed in single or dual chambers of the heart, usually transvenously.

palmaris longus tendon. Tendon located in the hand that flexes the wrist joint.

paratenon graft. Graft composed of the fatty tissue found between a tendon and its sheath.

passive mobilization. Pressure, movement, or pulling of a limb or body part utilizing an apparatus or device.

pedicle flap. Full-thickness skin and subcutaneous tissue for grafting that remains partially attached to the donor site by a pedicle or stem in which the blood vessels supplying the flap remain intact.

Pemberton osteotomy. Osteotomy is performed to position triradiate cartilage as a hinge for rotating the acetabular roof in cases of dysplasia of the hip in children.

penetrance. Being formed by, or pertaining to, a single clone.

percutaneous intradiscal electrothermal annuloplasty. Procedure corrects tears in the vertebral annulus by applying heat to the collagen disc walls percutaneously through a catheter. The heat contracts and thickens the wall, which may contract and close any annular tears.

percutaneous skeletal fixation. Treatment that is neither open nor closed and the injury site is not directly visualized. Fixation devices (pins, screws) are placed through the skin to stabilize the dislocation using x-ray guidance.

pericardium. Thin and slippery case in which the heart lies that is lined with fluid so that the heart is free to pulse and move as it beats.

peripheral arterial tonometry (PAT). Pulsatile volume changes in a digit are measured to determine activity in the sympathetic nervous system for respiratory analysis.

peritoneal. Space between the lining of the abdominal wall, or parietal peritoneum, and the surface layer of the abdominal organs, or visceral peritoneum. It contains a thin, watery fluid that keeps the peritoneal surfaces moist.

peritoneal dialysis. Dialysis that filters waste from blood inside the body using the peritoneum, the natural lining of the abdomen, as the semipermeable membrane across which ultrafiltration is accomplished. A special catheter is inserted into the abdomen and a dialysis solution is drained into the abdomen. This solution extracts fluids and wastes, which are then discarded when the fluid is drained. Various forms of peritoneal dialysis include CAPD, CCPD, and NIDP.

peritoneal effusion. Persistent escape of fluid within the peritoneal cavity.

pessary. Device placed in the vagina to support and reposition a prolapsing or retropositioned uterus, rectum, or vagina.

phenotype. Physical expression of a trait or characteristic as determined by an individual's genetic makeup or genotype.

photocoagulation. Application of an intense laser beam of light to disrupt tissue and condense protein material to a residual mass, used especially for treating ocular conditions.

physical status modifiers. Alphanumeric modifier used to identify the patient's health status as it affects the work related to providing the anesthesia service.

physical therapy modality. Therapeutic agent or regimen applied or used to provide appropriate treatment of the musculoskeletal system.

physician. Legally authorized practitioners including a doctor of medicine or osteopathy, a doctor of dental surgery or of dental medicine, a doctor of podiatric medicine, a doctor of optometry, and a chiropractor only with respect to treatment by means of manual manipulation of the spine (to correct a subluxation).

PICC. Peripherally inserted central catheter. PICC is inserted into one of the large veins of the arm and threaded through the vein until the tip sits in a large vein just above the heart.

PKR. Photorefractive therapy. Procedure involving the removal of the surface layer of the cornea (epithelium) by gentle scraping and use of a computer-controlled excimer laser to reshape the stroma.

pleurodesis. Injection of a sclerosing agent into the pleural space for creating adhesions between the parietal and the visceral pleura to treat a collapsed lung caused by air trapped in the pleural cavity, or severe cases of pleural effusion.

plication. Surgical technique involving folding, tucking, or pleating to reduce the size of a hollow structure or organ.

polyclonal. Containing one or more cells.

polymorphism. Genetic variation in the same species that does not harm the gene function or create disease.

polypeptide. Chain of amino acids held together by covalent bonds. Proteins are made up of amino acids.

polysomnography. Test involving monitoring of respiratory, cardiac, muscle, brain, and ocular function during sleep.

Potts-Smith-Gibson procedure. Side-to-side anastomosis of the aorta and left pulmonary artery creating a shunt that enlarges as the child grows.

Prader-Willi syndrome. Rounded face, almond-shaped eyes, strabismus, low forehead, hypogonadism, hypotonia, intellectual disabilities, and an insatiable appetite.

presumptive drug testing. Drug screening tests to identify the presence or absence of drugs in a patient's system. Tests are usually able to identify low concentrations of the drug. These tests may be used for medical, workplace, or legal purposes.

presumptive identification. Identification of microorganisms using media growth, colony morphology, gram stains, or up to three specific tests (e.g., catalase, indole, oxidase, urease).

professional component. Portion of a charge for health care services that represents the physician's (or other practitioner's) work in providing the service, including interpretation and report of the procedure. This component of the service usually is charged for and billed separately from the inpatient hospital charges.

profunda. Denotes a part of a structure that is deeper from the surface of the body than the rest of the structure.

prolonged physician services. Extended pre- or post-service care provided to a patient whose condition requires services beyond the usual.

prostate. Male gland surrounding the bladder neck and urethra that secretes a substance into the seminal fluid.

prosthetic. Device that replaces all or part of an internal body organ or body part, or that replaces part of the function of a permanently inoperable or malfunctioning internal body organ or body part.

provider of services. Institution, individual, or organization that provides health care.

proximal. Located closest to a specified reference point, usually the midline or trunk.

psychiatric hospital. Specialized institution that provides, under the supervision of physicians, services for the diagnosis and treatment of mentally ill persons.

pterygium. Benign, wedge-shaped, conjunctival thickening that advances from the inner corner of the eye toward the cornea.

pterygomaxillary fossa. Wide depression on the external surface of the maxilla above and to the side of the canine tooth socket.

pulmonary artery banding. Surgical constriction of the pulmonary artery to prevent irreversible pulmonary vascular obstructive changes and overflow into the left ventricle.

Putti-Platt procedure. Realignment of the subscapularis tendon to treat recurrent anterior dislocation, thereby partially eliminating external rotation. The anterior capsule is also tightened and reinforced.

pyloroplasty. Enlargement and reconstruction of the lower portion of the stomach opening into the duodenum performed after vagotomy to speed gastric emptying and treat duodenal ulcers.

qualified health care professional. Educated, licensed or certified, and regulated professional operating under a specified scope of practice to provide patient services that are separate and distinct from other clinical staff. Services may be billed independently or under the facility's services.

RAC. Recovery audit contractor. National program using CMS-affiliated contractors to review claims prior to payment as well as for payments on claims already processed, including overpayments and underpayments.

radiation therapy simulation. Radiation therapy simulation. Procedure by which the specific body area to be treated with radiation is defined and marked. A CT scan is performed to define the body contours and these images are used to create a plan customized treatment for the patient, targeting the area to be treated while sparing adjacent tissue. The center of the area to be treated is marked and an immobilization device (e.g., cradle, mold) is created to make sure the patient is in the same position each time for treatment. Complexity of treatment depends on the number of treatment areas and the use of tools to isolate the area of treatment.

radioactive substances. Materials used in the diagnosis and treatment of disease that emit high-speed particles and energy-containing rays.

radiology services. Services that include diagnostic and therapeutic radiology, nuclear medicine, CT scan procedures, magnetic resonance imaging services, ultrasound, and other imaging procedures.

radiotherapy afterloading. Part of the radiation therapy process in which the chemotherapy agent is actually instilled into the tumor area subsequent to surgery and placement of an expandable catheter into the void remaining after tumor excision. The specialized catheter remains in place and the patient may come in for multiple treatments with radioisotope placed to treat the margin of tissue surrounding the excision. After the radiotherapy is completed, the patient returns to have the catheter emptied and removed. This is a new therapy in breast cancer treatment.

Rashkind procedure. Transvenous balloon atrial septectomy or septostomy performed by cardiac catheterization. A balloon catheter is inserted into the heart either to create or enlarge an opening in the interatrial septal wall.

repair. Surgical closure of a wound. The wound may be a result of injury/trauma or it may be a surgically created defect. Repairs are divided into three categories: simple, intermediate, and complex. Simple repair is performed when the wound is superficial and only requires simple, one layer, primary suturing. Intermediate repair is performed for wounds and lacerations in which one or more of the deeper layers of subcutaneous tissue and non-muscle fascia are repaired in addition to the skin and subcutaneous tissue. Complex repair includes repair of wounds requiring more than layered closure.

respiratory airflow (ventilation). Assessment of air movement during inhalation and exhalation as measured by nasal pressure sensors and thermistor.

respiratory analysis. Assessment of components of respiration obtained by other methods such as airflow or peripheral arterial tone.

respiratory effort. Measurement of diaphragm and/or intercostal muscle for airflow using transducers to estimate thoracic and abdominal motion.

respiratory movement. Measurement of chest and abdomen movement during respiration.

ribbons. In oncology, small plastic tubes containing radioactive sources for interstitial placement that may be cut into specific lengths tailored to the size of the area receiving ionizing radiation treatment.

Ridell sinusotomy. Frontal sinus tissue is destroyed to eliminate tumors.

RNA. Ribonucleic acid.

rural health clinic. Clinic in an area where there is a shortage of health services staffed by a nurse practitioner, physician assistant, or certified nurse midwife under physician direction that provides routine diagnostic services, including clinical laboratory services, drugs, and biologicals and that has prompt access to additional diagnostic services from facilities meeting federal requirements.

Salter osteotomy. Innominate bone of the hip is cut, removed, and repositioned to repair a congenital dislocation, subluxation, or deformity.

saucerization. Creation of a shallow, saucer-like depression in the bone to facilitate drainage of infected areas.

Schiotz tonometer. Instrument that measures intraocular pressure by recording the depth of an indentation on the cornea by a plunger of known weight.

screening mammography. Radiologic images taken of the female breast for the early detection of breast cancer.

screening pap smear. Diagnostic laboratory test consisting of a routine exfoliative cytology test (Papanicolaou test) provided to a woman for the early detection of cervical or vaginal cancer. The exam includes a clinical breast examination and a physician's interpretation of the results.

seeds. Small (1 mm or less) sources of radioactive material that are permanently placed directly into tumors.

senning procedure. Flaps of intra-atrial septum and right atrial wall are used to create two interatrial channels to divert the systemic and pulmonary venous circulation.

sensitivity tests. Number of methods of applying selective suspected allergens to the skin or mucous.

sensorineural conduction. Transportation of sound from the cochlea to the acoustic nerve and central auditory pathway to the brain.

sentinel lymph node. First node to which lymph drainage and metastasis from a cancer can occur.

separate procedures. Services commonly carried out as a fundamental part of a total service and, as such, do not usually warrant separate identification. These services are identified in CPT with the parenthetical phrase (separate procedure) at the end of the description and are payable only when performed alone.

septectomy. 1) Surgical removal of all or part of the nasal septum. 2) Submucosal resection of the nasal septum.

Shirodkar procedure. Treatment of an incompetent cervical os by placing nonabsorbent suture material in purse-string sutures as a cerclage to support the cervix.

short tandem repeat (STR). Short sequences of a DNA pattern that are repeated. Can be used as genetic markers for human identity testing.

sialodochoplasty. Surgical repair of a salivary gland duct.

single-lead device. Implantable cardiac device (pacemaker or implantable cardioverter-defibrillator [ICD]) in which pacing and sensing components are placed in only one chamber of the heart.

single-nucleotide polymorphism (SNP). Single nucleotide (A, T, C, or G that is different in a DNA sequence. This difference occurs at a significant frequency in the population.

sinus of Valsalva. Any of three sinuses corresponding to the individual cusps of the aortic valve, located in the most proximal part of the aorta just above the cusps. These structures are contained within the pericardium and appear as distinct but subtle outpouchings or dilations of the aortic wall between each of the semilunar cusps of the valve.

sleep apnea. Intermittent cessation of breathing during sleep that may cause hypoxemia and pulmonary arterial hypertension.

sleep latency. Time period between lying down in bed and the onset of sleep.

sleep staging. Determination of the separate levels of sleep according to physiological measurements.

somatic. 1) Pertaining to the body or trunk. 2) In genetics acquired or occurring after birth.

speculoscopy. Viewing the cervix utilizing a magnifier and a special wavelength of light, allowing detection of abnormalities that may not be discovered on a routine Pap smear.

speech-language pathology services. Speech, language, and related function assessment and rehabilitation service furnished by a qualified speech-language pathologist. Audiology services include hearing and balance assessment services furnished by a qualified audiologist. A qualified speech pathologist and audiologist must have a master's or doctoral degree in their respective fields and be licensed to serve in the state. Speech pathologists and audiologists practicing in states without licensure must complete 350 hours of supervised clinical work and perform at least nine months of supervised full-time service after earning their degrees.

sphincteroplasty. Surgical repair done to correct, augment, or improve the muscular function of a sphincter, such as the anus or intestines.

spirometry. Measurement of the lungs' breathing capacity.

splint. Brace or support. 1) dynamic splint: brace that permits movement of an anatomical structure such as a hand, wrist, foot, or other part of the body after surgery or injury. 2) static splint: brace that prevents movement and maintains support and position for an anatomical structure after surgery or injury.

stent. Tube to provide support in a body cavity or lumen.

stereotactic radiosurgery. Delivery of externally-generated ionizing radiation to specific targets for destruction or inactivation. Most often utilized in the treatment of brain or spinal tumors, high-resolution stereotactic imaging is used to identify the target and then deliver the treatment. Computer-assisted planning may also be employed. Simple and complex cranial lesions and spinal lesions are typically treated in a single planning and treatment session, although a maximum of five sessions may be required. No incision is made for stereotactic radiosurgery procedures.

stereotaxis. Three-dimensional method for precisely locating structures.

Stoffel rhizotomy. Nerve roots are sectioned to relieve pain or spastic paralysis.

strabismus. Misalignment of the eyes due to an imbalance in extraocular muscles.

surgical package. Normal, uncomplicated performance of specific surgical services, with the assumption that, on average, all surgical procedures of a given type are similar with respect to skill level, duration, and length of normal follow-up care.

symblepharopterygium. Adhesion in which the eyelid is adhered to the eyeball by a band that resembles a pterygium.

sympathectomy. Surgical interruption or transection of a sympathetic nervous system pathway.

tarso-. 1) Relating to the foot. 2) Relating to the margin of the eyelid.

tarsocheiloplasty. Plastic operation upon the edge of the eyelid for the treatment of trichiasis.

tarsorrhaphy. Suture of a portion or all of the opposing eyelids together for the purpose of shortening the palpebral fissure or closing it entirely.

technical component. Portion of a health care service that identifies the provision of the equipment, supplies, technical personnel, and costs attendant to the performance of the procedure other than the professional services.

tendon. Fibrous tissue that connects muscle to bone, consisting primarily of collagen and containing little vasculature.

tendon allograft. Allografts are tissues obtained from another individual of the same species. Tendon allografts are usually obtained from cadavers and frozen or freeze dried for later use in soft tissue repairs where the physician elects not to obtain an autogenous graft (a graft obtained from the individual on whom the surgery is being performed).

tendon suture material. Tendons are composed of fibrous tissue consisting primarily of collagen and containing few cells or blood vessels. This tissue heals more slowly than tissues with more vascularization. Because of this, tendons are usually repaired with nonabsorbable suture material. Examples include surgical silk, surgical cotton, linen, stainless steel, surgical nylon, polyester fiber, polybutester (Novafil), polyethylene (Dermalene), and polypropylene (Prolene, Surilene).

tendon transplant. Replacement of a tendon with another tendon.

tenon's capsule. Connective tissue that forms the capsule enclosing the posterior eyeball, extending from the conjunctival fornix and continuous with the muscular fascia of the eye.

tenonectomy. Excision of a portion of a tendon to make it shorter.

tenotomy. Cutting into a tendon.

TENS. Transcutaneous electrical nerve stimulator. TENS is applied by placing electrode pads over the area to be stimulated and connecting the electrodes to a transmitter box, which sends a current through the skin to sensory nerve fibers to help decrease pain in that nerve distribution.

tensilon. Edrophonium chloride. Agent used for evaluation and treatment of myasthenia gravis.

terminally ill. Individual whose medical prognosis for life expectancy is six months or less.

tetralogy of Fallot. Specific combination of congenital cardiac defects: obstruction of the right ventricular outflow tract with pulmonary stenosis, interventricular septal defect, malposition of the aorta, overriding the interventricular septum and receiving blood from both the venous and arterial systems, and enlargement of the right ventricle.

therapeutic services. Services performed for treatment of a specific diagnosis. These services include performance of the procedure, various incidental elements, and normal, related follow-up care.

thoracentesis. Surgical puncture of the chest cavity with a specialized needle or hollow tubing to aspirate fluid from within the pleural space for diagnostic or therapeutic reasons.

thoracic lymphadenectomy. Procedure to cut out the lymph nodes near the lungs, around the heart, and behind the trachea.

thoracostomy. Creation of an opening in the chest wall for drainage.

thyroglossal duct. Embryonic duct at the front of the neck, which becomes the pyramidal lobe of the thyroid gland with obliteration of the remaining duct, but may form a cyst or sinus in adulthood if it persists.

total disc arthroplasty with artificial disc. Removal of an intravertebral disc and its replacement with an implant. The implant is an artificial disc consisting of two metal plates with a weight-bearing surface of polyethylene between the plates. The plates are anchored to the vertebral immediately above and below the affected disc.

total shoulder replacement. Prosthetic replacement of the entire shoulder joint, including the humeral head and the glenoid fossa.

trabeculae carneae cordis. Bands of muscular tissue that line the walls of the ventricles in the heart.

trabeculectomy. Surgical incision between the anterior portion of the eye and the canal of Schlemm to drain the aqueous humor.

tracheostomy. Formation of a tracheal opening on the neck surface with tube insertion to allow for respiration in cases of obstruction or decreased patency. A tracheostomy may be planned or performed on an emergency basis for temporary or long-term use.

tracheotomy. Formation of a tracheal opening on the neck surface with tube insertion to allow for respiration in cases of obstruction or decreased patency. A tracheotomy may be planned or performed on an emergency basis for temporary or long-term use.

traction. Drawing out or holding tension on an area by applying a direct therapeutic pulling force.

transcranial magnetic stimulation. Application of electromagnetic energy to the brain through a coil placed on the scalp. The procedure stimulates cortical neurons and is intended to activate and normalize their processes.

transcription. Process by which messenger RNA is synthesized from a DNA template resulting in the transfer of genetic information from the DNA molecule to the messenger RNA.

translocation. Disconnection of all or part of a chromosome that reattaches to another position in the DNA sequence of the same or another chromosome. Often results in a reciprocal exchange of DNA sequences between two differently numbered chromosomes. May or may not result in a clinically significant loss of DNA.

trephine. 1) Specialized round saw for cutting circular holes in bone, especially the skull. 2) Instrument that removes small disc-shaped buttons of corneal tissue for transplanting.

tricuspid atresia. Congenital absence of the valve that may occur with other defects, such as atrial septal defect, pulmonary atresia, and transposition of great vessels.

turbinates. Scroll or shell-shaped elevations from the wall of the nasal cavity, the inferior turbinate being a separate bone, while the superior and middle turbinates are of the ethmoid bone.

tympanic membrane. Thin, sensitive membrane across the entrance to the middle ear that vibrates in response to sound waves, allowing the waves to be transmitted via the ossicular chain to the internal ear.

tympanoplasty. Surgical repair of the structures of the middle ear, including the eardrum and the three small bones, or ossicles.

unlisted procedure. Procedural descriptions used when the overall procedure and outcome of the procedure are not adequately described by an existing procedure code. Such codes are used as a last resort and only when there is not a more appropriate procedure code.

ureterorrhaphy. Surgical repair using sutures to close an open wound or injury of the ureter.

vagotomy. Division of the vagus nerves, interrupting impulses resulting in lower gastric acid production and hastening gastric emptying. Used in the treatment of chronic gastric, pyloric, and duodenal ulcers that can cause severe pain and difficulties in eating and sleeping.

variant. Nucleotide deviation from the normal sequence of a region. Variations are usually either substitutions or deletions. Substitution variations are the result of one nucleotide taking the place of another. A deletion occurs when one or more nucleotides are left out. In some cases, several in a reasonably close proximity on the same chromosome in a DNA strand. These variations result in amino acid changes in the protein made by the gene. However, the term variant does not itself imply a functional change. Intron variations are usually described in one of two ways: 1) the changed nucleotide is defined by a plus or a minus sign indicating the position relative to the first or last nucleotide to the intron, or 2) the second variant description is indicated relative to the last nucleotide of the preceding exon or first nucleotide of the following exon.

vascular family. Group of vessels (family) that branch from the aorta or vena cava. At each branching, the vascular order increases by one. The first order vessel is the primary branch off the aorta or vena cava. The second order vessel branches from the first order, the third order branches from the second order, and any further branching is beyond the third order. For example, for the inferior vena cava, the common iliac artery is a first order vessel. The internal and external iliac arteries are second order vessels, as they each originate from the first order common iliac artery. The external iliac artery extends directly from the common iliac artery and the internal iliac artery bifurcates from the common iliac artery. A third order vessel from the external iliac artery is the inferior epigastric artery and a third order vessel from the internal iliac artery is the obturator artery. Note orders are not always identical bilaterally (e.g., the left common carotid artery is a first order and the right common carotid is a second order). Synonym: vascular origins and distributions.

vasectomy. Surgical procedure involving the removal of all or part of the vas deferens, usually performed for sterilization or in conjunction with a prostatectomy.

vena cava interruption. Procedure that places a filter device, called an umbrella or sieve, within the large vein returning deoxygenated blood to the heart to prevent pulmonary embolism caused by clots.

ventricular assist device. Temporary measure used to support the heart by substituting for left and/or right heart function. The device replaces the work of the left and/or right ventricle when a patient has a damaged or weakened heart. A left ventricular assist device (VAD) helps the heart pump blood through the rest of the body. A right VAD helps the heart pump blood to the lungs to become oxygenated again. Catheters are inserted to circulate the blood through external tubing to a pump machine located outside of the body and back to the correct artery.

ventricular septal defect. Congenital cardiac anomaly resulting in a continual opening in the septum between the ventricles that, in severe cases, causes oxygenated blood to flow back into the lungs, resulting in pulmonary hypertension.

vertebral interspace. Non-bony space between two adjacent vertebral bodies that contains the cushioning intervertebral disk.

volar. Palm of the hand (palmar) or sole of the foot (plantar).

Waterston procedure. Type of aortopulmonary shunting done to increase pulmonary blood flow where the ascending aorta is anastomosed to the right pulmonary artery.

Wharton's ducts. Salivary ducts below the mandible.

wick catheter. Device used to monitor interstitial fluid pressure, and sometimes used intraoperatively during fasciotomy procedures to evaluate the effectiveness of the decompression.

xenograft. Tissue that is nonhuman and harvested from one species and grafted to another. Pigskin is the most common xenograft for human skin and is applied to a wound as a temporary closure until a permanent option is performed.

z-plasty. Plastic surgery technique used primarily to release tension or elongate contracted scar tissue in which a Z-shaped incision is made with the middle line of the Z crossing the area of greatest tension. The triangular flaps are then rotated so that they cross the incision line in the opposite direction, creating a reversed Z.

ZPIC. Zone Program Integrity Contractor. CMS contractor that replaced the existing Program Safeguard Contractors (PSC). Contractors are responsible for ensuring the integrity of all Medicare-related claims under Parts A and B (hospital, skilled nursing, home health, provider, and durable medical equipment claims), Part C (Medicare Advantage health plans), Part D (prescription drug plans), and coordination of Medicare-Medicaid data matches (Medi-Medi).

Appendix M — Listing of Sensory, Motor, and Mixed Nerves

This list contains the sensory, motor, and mixed nerves assigned to each nerve conduction study to improve coding accuracy. Each nerve makes up one single unit of service.

Motor Nerves Assigned to Codes 95900 and 95907-95913

I. Upper extremity, cervical plexus, and brachial plexus motor nerves

   A. Axillary motor nerve to the deltoid

   B. Long thoracic motor nerve to the serratus anterior

   C. Median nerve

      1. Median motor nerve to the abductor pollicis brevis

      2. Median motor nerve, anterior interosseous branch, to the flexor pollicis longus

      3. Median motor nerve, anterior interosseous branch, to the pronator quadratus

      4. Median motor nerve to the first lumbrical

      5. Median motor nerve to the second lumbrical

   D. Musculocutaneous motor nerve to the biceps brachii

   E. Radial nerve

      1. Radial motor nerve to the extensor carpi ulnaris

      2. Radial motor nerve to the extensor digitorum communis

      3. Radial motor nerve to the extensor indicis proprius

      4. Radial motor nerve to the brachioradialis

   F. Suprascapular nerve

      1. Suprascapular motor nerve to the supraspinatus

      2. Suprascapular motor nerve to the infraspinatus

   G. Thoracodorsal motor nerve to the latissimus dorsi

   H. Ulnar nerve

      1. Ulnar motor nerve to the abductor digiti minimi

      2. Ulnar motor nerve to the palmar interosseous

      3. Ulnar motor nerve to the first dorsal interosseous

      4. Ulnar motor nerve to the flexor carpi ulnaris

   I. Other

II. Lower extremity motor nerves

   A. Femoral motor nerve to the quadriceps

      1. Femoral motor nerve to vastus medialis

      2. Femoral motor nerve to vastus lateralis

      3. Femoral motor nerve to vastus intermedialis

      4. Femoral motor nerve to rectus femoris

   B. Ilioinguinal motor nerve

   C. Peroneal (fibular) nerve

      1. Peroneal motor nerve to the extensor digitorum brevis

      2. Peroneal motor nerve to the peroneus brevis

      3. Peroneal motor nerve to the peroneus longus

      4. Peroneal motor nerve to the tibialis anterior

   D. Plantar motor nerve

   E. Sciatic nerve

   F. Tibial nerve

      1. Tibial motor nerve, inferior calcaneal branch, to the abductor digiti minimi

      2. Tibial motor nerve, medial plantar branch, to the abductor hallucis

      3. Tibial motor nerve, lateral plantar branch, to the flexor digiti minimi brevis

   G. Other

III. Cranial nerves and trunk

   A. Cranial nerve VII (facial motor nerve)

      1. Facial nerve to the frontalis

      2. Facial nerve to the nasalis

      3. Facial nerve to the orbicularis oculi

      4. Facial nerve to the orbicularis oris

   B. Cranial nerve XI (spinal accessory motor nerve)

   C. Cranial nerve XII (hypoglossal motor nerve)

   D. Intercostal motor nerve

   E. Phrenic motor nerve to the diaphragm

   F. Recurrent laryngeal nerve

   G. Other

IV. Nerve Roots

   A. Cervical nerve root stimulation

      1. Cervical level 5 (C5)

      2. Cervical level 6 (C6)

      3. Cervical level 7 (C7)

      4. Cervical level 8 (C8)

   B. Thoracic nerve root stimulation

      1. Thoracic level 1 (T1)

      2. Thoracic level 2 (T2)

      3. Thoracic level 3 (T3)

      4. Thoracic level 4 (T4)

      5. Thoracic level 5 (T5)

      6. Thoracic level 6 (T6)

      7. Thoracic level 7 (T7)

      8. Thoracic level 8 (T8)

      9. Thoracic level 9 (T9)

      10. Thoracic level 10 (T10)

      11. Thoracic level 11 (T11)

      12. Thoracic level 12 (T12)

   C. Lumbar nerve root stimulation

      1. Lumbar level 1 (L1)

      2. Lumbar level 2 (L2)

      3. Lumbar level 3 (L3)

      4. Lumbar level 4 (L4)

      5. Lumbar level 5 (L5)

   D. Sacral nerve root stimulation

      1. Sacral level 1 (S1)

      2. Sacral level 2 (S2)

3.   Sacral level 3 (S3)

4.   Sacral level 4 (S4)

Sensory and Mixed Nerves Assigned to Codes 95907–95913

I.   Upper extremity sensory and mixed nerves

   A.   Lateral antebrachial cutaneous sensory nerve

   B.   Medial antebrachial cutaneous sensory nerve

   C.   Medial brachial cutaneous sensory nerve

   D.   Median nerve

      1.   Median sensory nerve to the first digit

      2.   Median sensory nerve to the second digit

      3.   Median sensory nerve to the third digit

      4.   Median sensory nerve to the fourth digit

      5.   Median palmar cutaneous sensory nerve

      6.   Median palmar mixed nerve

   E.   Posterior antebrachial cutaneous sensory nerve

   F.   Radial sensory nerve

      1.   Radial sensory nerve to the base of the thumb

      2.   Radial sensory nerve to digit 1

   G.   Ulnar nerve

      1.   Ulnar dorsal cutaneous sensory nerve

      2.   Ulnar sensory nerve to the fourth digit

      3.   Ulnar sensory nerve to the fifth digit

      4.   Ulnar palmar mixed nerve

   H.   Intercostal sensory nerve

   I.   Other

II.   Lower extremity sensory and mixed nerves

   A.   Lateral femoral cutaneous sensory nerve

   B.   Medical calcaneal sensory nerve

   C.   Medial femoral cutaneous sensory nerve

   D.   Peroneal nerve

      1.   Deep peroneal sensory nerve

      2.   Superficial peroneal sensory nerve, medial dorsal cutaneous branch

      3.   Superficial peroneal sensory nerve, intermediate dorsal cutaneous branch

   E.   Posterior femoral cutaneous sensory nerve

   F.   Saphenous nerve

      1.   Saphenous sensory nerve (distal technique)

      2.   Saphenous sensory nerve (proximal technique)

   G.   Sural nerve

      1.   Sural sensory nerve, lateral dorsal cutaneous branch

      2.   Sural sensory nerve

   H.   Tibial sensory nerve (digital nerve to toe 1)

   I.   Tibial sensory nerve (medial plantar nerve)

   J.   Tibial sensory nerve (lateral plantar nerve)

   K.   Other

III.   Head and trunk sensory nerves

   A.   Dorsal nerve of the penis

   B.   Greater auricular nerve

   C.   Ophthalmic branch of the trigeminal nerve

   D.   Pudendal sensory nerve

   E.   Suprascapular sensory nerves

   F.   Other

In the following table, the reasonable maximum number of studies per diagnostic category is listed that allows for a physician or other qualified health care professional to obtain a diagnosis for 90 percent of patients with that same final diagnosis. The numbers denote the suggested number of studies, although the decision is up to the provider.

Type of Study/Maximum Number of Studies

Indication	Limbs Studied by Needle EMG (95860–95864, 95867–95870, 95885–95887)	Nerve Conduction Studies (Total nerves studied, 95907-95913)	Neuromuscular Junction Testing (Repetitive Stimulation 95937)
Carpal Tunnel (Unilateral)	1	7	—
Carpal Tunnel (Bilateral)	2	10	—
Radiculopathy	2	7	—
Mononeuropathy	1	8	—
Polyneuropathy/Mononeuropathy Multiplex	3	10	—
Myopathy	2	4	2
Motor Neuronopathy (e.g., ALS)	4	6	2
Plexopathy	2	12	—
Neuromuscular Junction	2	4	3
Tarsal Tunnel Syndrome (Unilateral)	1	8	—
Tarsal Tunnel Syndrome (Bilateral)	2	11	—
Weakness, Fatigue, Cramps, or Twitching (Focal)	2	7	2
Weakness, Fatigue, Cramps, or Twitching (General)	4	8	2
Pain, Numbness, or Tingling (Unilateral)	1	9	—
Pain, Numbness, or Tingling (Bilateral)	2	12	—

Appendix N — Vascular Families

This table assumes that the starting point is aortic catheterization. This categorization would not be accurate, for instance, if a femoral or carotid artery were catheterized with the blood's flow. The names of the arteries appearing in bold face type in the following table indicate those arteries that are most often the subject of arteriographic procedures.

First Order	Second Order Branch	Third Order Branch	Beyond Third Order Branches
Innominate	**Right Common Carotid**	**Right Internal Carotid**	Right Ophthalmic Right Posterior Communicating Right Middle Cerebral Right Anterior Cerebral
		Right External Carotid	Right Superior Thyroid Right Ascending Pharyngeal Right Facial Right Lingual Right Occipital Right Posterior Auricular Right Superficial Temporal Right Internal Maxillary Right Middle Meningeal
	Right Subclavian and Axillary	**Right Vertebral**	Basilar
		Right Internal Thoracic (Internal Mammary)	
		Right Thyrocervical Trunk	Right Inferior Thyroid Right Suprascapular Right Transverse Cervical
		Right Costocervical Trunk	Right Highest Intercostal Right Deep Cervical
		Right Lateral Thoracic Right Thoracromial Right Humeral Circumflex (A/P)	
		Right Subscapular	Right Circumflex Scapular
		Right Brachial	
		Right Deep Brachial	Right Ulnar Right Radial Right Interosseous Right Deep Palmar Arch Right Superficial Palmar Arch Right Metacarpals and Digitals
Left Common Carotid	**Left Internal Carotid**	Left Ophthalmic Left Posterior Communicating Left Middle Cerebral Left Anterior Cerebral	
	Left External Carotid	Left Superior Thyroid Left Ascending Pharyngeal Left Facial Left Lingual Left Occipital Left Posterior Auricular Left Superficial Temporal	
		Left Internal Maxillary	Left Middle Meningeal

First Order	Second Order Branch	Third Order Branch	Beyond Third Order Branches

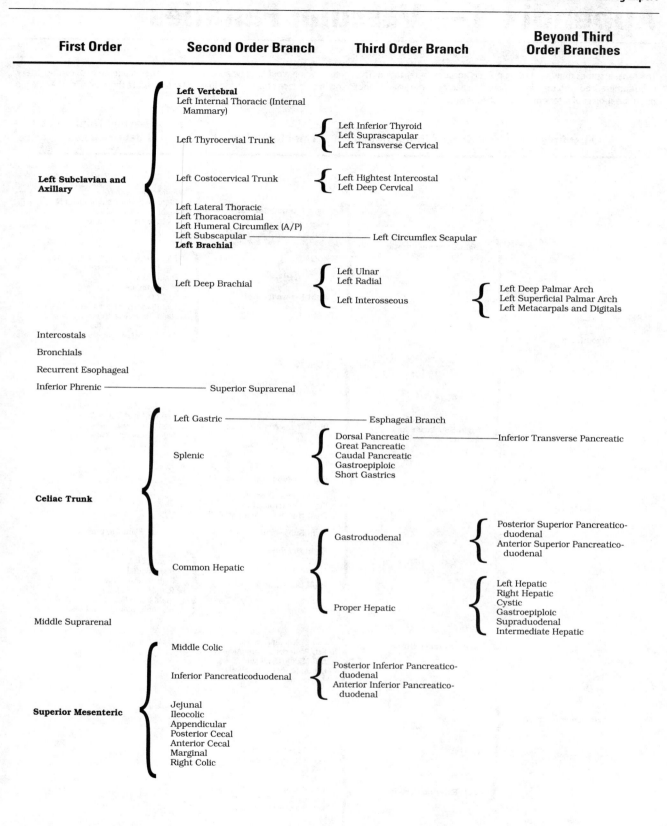

Left Subclavian and Axillary
- **Left Vertebral**
- Left Internal Thoracic (Internal Mammary)
- Left Thyrocervial Trunk
  - Left Inferior Thyroid
  - Left Suprascapular
  - Left Transverse Cervical
- Left Costocervical Trunk
  - Left Hightest Intercostal
  - Left Deep Cervical
- Left Lateral Thoracic
- Left Thoracoacromial
- Left Humeral Circumflex (A/P)
- Left Subscapular —— Left Circumflex Scapular
- **Left Brachial**
- Left Deep Brachial
  - Left Ulnar
  - Left Radial
  - Left Interosseous
    - Left Deep Palmar Arch
    - Left Superficial Palmar Arch
    - Left Metacarpals and Digitals

Intercostals

Bronchials

Recurrent Esophageal

Inferior Phrenic —————— Superior Suprarenal

Celiac Trunk
- Left Gastric ——————— Esphageal Branch
- Splenic
  - Dorsal Pancreatic ————— Inferior Transverse Pancreatic
  - Great Pancreatic
  - Caudal Pancreatic
  - Gastroepiploic
  - Short Gastrics
- Common Hepatic
  - Gastroduodenal
    - Posterior Superior Pancreatico-duodenal
    - Anterior Superior Pancreatico-duodenal
  - Proper Hepatic
    - Left Hepatic
    - Right Hepatic
    - Cystic
    - Gastroepiploic
    - Supraduodenal
    - Intermediate Hepatic

Middle Suprarenal

Superior Mesenteric
- Middle Colic
- Inferior Pancreaticoduodenal
  - Posterior Inferior Pancreatico-duodenal
  - Anterior Inferior Pancreatico-duodenal
- Jejunal
- Ileocolic
- Appendicular
- Posterior Cecal
- Anterior Cecal
- Marginal
- Right Colic

First Order	Second Order Branch	Third Order Branch	Beyond Third Order Branches

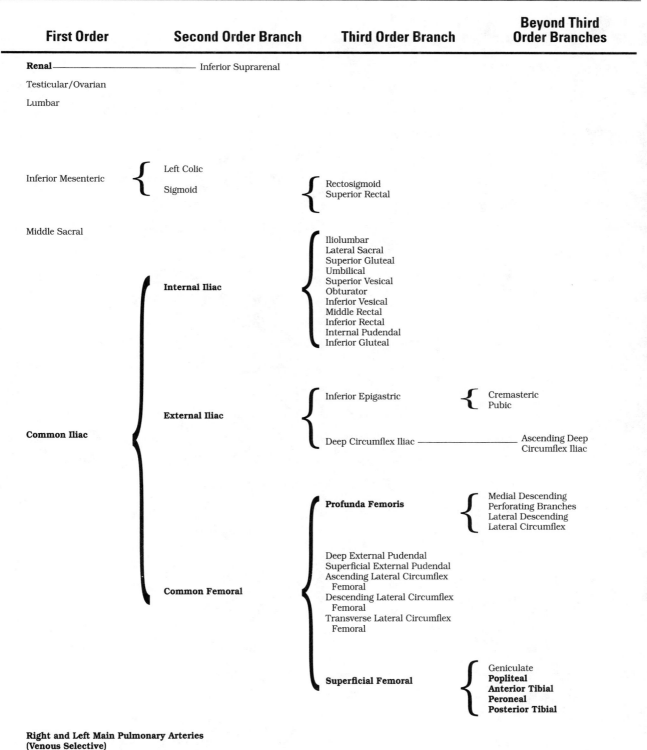

Renal————————————————— Inferior Suprarenal

Testicular/Ovarian

Lumbar

Inferior Mesenteric { Left Colic

Sigmoid { Rectosigmoid
Superior Rectal

Middle Sacral

Internal Iliac { Iliolumbar
Lateral Sacral
Superior Gluteal
Umbilical
Superior Vesical
Obturator
Inferior Vesical
Middle Rectal
Inferior Rectal
Internal Pudendal
Inferior Gluteal

External Iliac { Inferior Epigastric { Cremasteric
Pubic

Deep Circumflex Iliac ——————————— Ascending Deep
Circumflex Iliac

Common Iliac

Profunda Femoris { Medial Descending
Perforating Branches
Lateral Descending
Lateral Circumflex

Common Femoral { Deep External Pudendal
Superficial External Pudendal
Ascending Lateral Circumflex
    Femoral
Descending Lateral Circumflex
    Femoral
Transverse Lateral Circumflex
    Femoral

Superficial Femoral { Geniculate
Popliteal
Anterior Tibial
Peroneal
Posterior Tibial

Right and Left Main Pulmonary Arteries
(Venous Selective)

Reference: Kadir S. *Atlas of Normal and Variant Angiographic Anatomy.* Philadelphia, Pa: WB Saunders Co; 1991

Appendix O — Interventional Radiology Illustrations

Normal Aortic Arch and Branch Anatomy—Transfemoral Approach

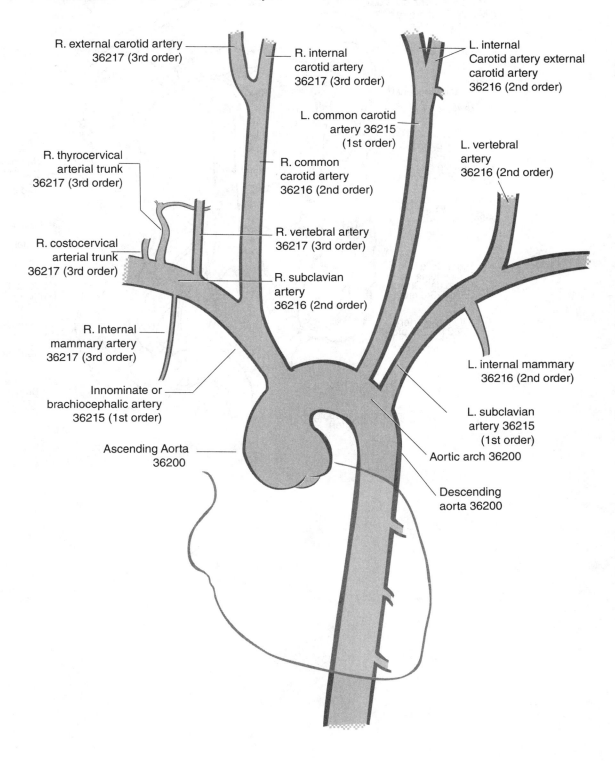

R. external carotid artery
36217 (3rd order)

R. internal carotid artery
36217 (3rd order)

L. internal Carotid artery external carotid artery
36216 (2nd order)

L. common carotid artery 36215 (1st order)

R. thyrocervical arterial trunk
36217 (3rd order)

R. common carotid artery
36216 (2nd order)

L. vertebral artery
36216 (2nd order)

R. costocervical arterial trunk
36217 (3rd order)

R. vertebral artery
36217 (3rd order)

R. subclavian artery
36216 (2nd order)

R. Internal mammary artery
36217 (3rd order)

L. internal mammary
36216 (2nd order)

Innominate or brachiocephalic artery
36215 (1st order)

L. subclavian artery 36215 (1st order)

Aortic arch 36200

Ascending Aorta
36200

Descending aorta 36200

Superior and Inferior Mesenteric Arteries and Branches

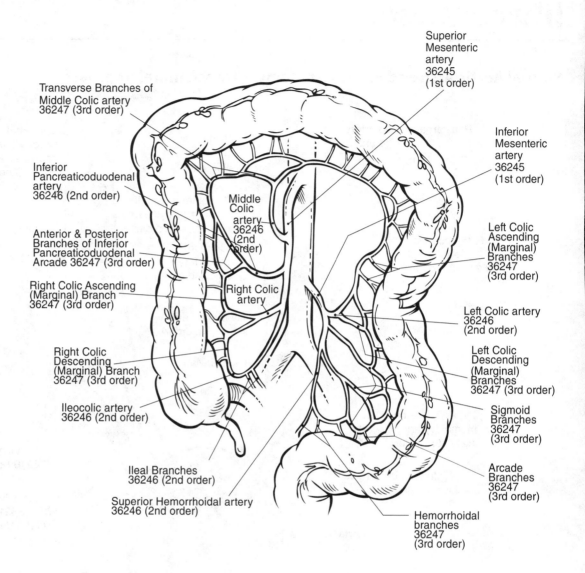

Transverse Branches of
Middle Colic artery
36247 (3rd order)

Inferior
Pancreaticoduodenal
artery
36246 (2nd order)

Anterior & Posterior
Branches of Inferior
Pancreaticoduodenal
Arcade 36247 (3rd order)

Right Colic Ascending
(Marginal) Branch
36247 (3rd order)

Right Colic
Descending
(Marginal) Branch
36247 (3rd order)

Ileocolic artery
36246 (2nd order)

Ileal Branches
36246 (2nd order)

Superior Hemorrhoidal artery
36246 (2nd order)

Middle
Colic
artery
36246
(2nd
order)

Right Colic
artery

Superior
Mesenteric
artery
36245
(1st order)

Inferior
Mesenteric
artery
36245
(1st order)

Left Colic
Ascending
(Marginal)
Branches
36247
(3rd order)

Left Colic artery
36246
(2nd order)

Left Colic
Descending
(Marginal)
Branches
36247 (3rd order)

Sigmoid
Branches
36247
(3rd order)

Arcade
Branches
36247
(3rd order)

Hemorrhoidal
branches
36247
(3rd order)

Portal System

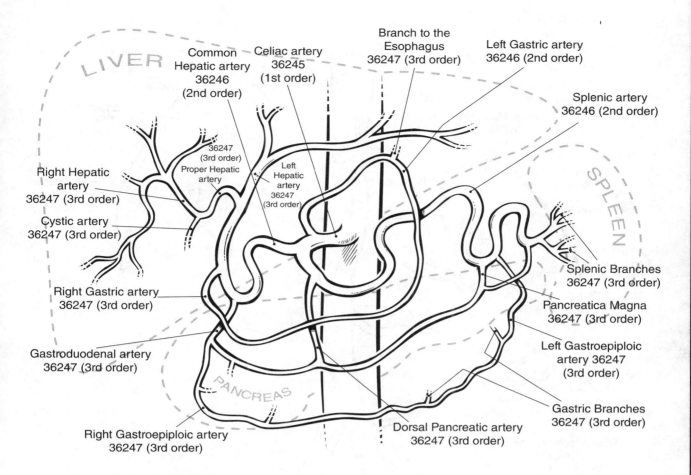

Renal Artery Anatomy—Femoral Approach

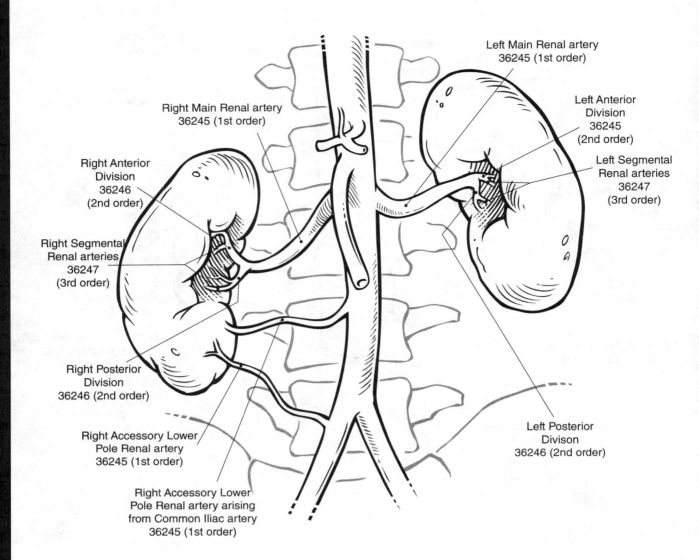

Left Main Renal artery
36245 (1st order)

Right Main Renal artery
36245 (1st order)

Left Anterior
Division
36245
(2nd order)

Right Anterior
Division
36246
(2nd order)

Left Segmental
Renal arteries
36247
(3rd order)

Right Segmental
Renal arteries
36247
(3rd order)

Right Posterior
Division
36246 (2nd order)

Left Posterior
Divison
36246 (2nd order)

Right Accessory Lower
Pole Renal artery
36245 (1st order)

Right Accessory Lower
Pole Renal artery arising
from Common Iliac artery
36245 (1st order)

Upper Extremity Arterial Anatomy—Transfemoral or Contralateral Approach

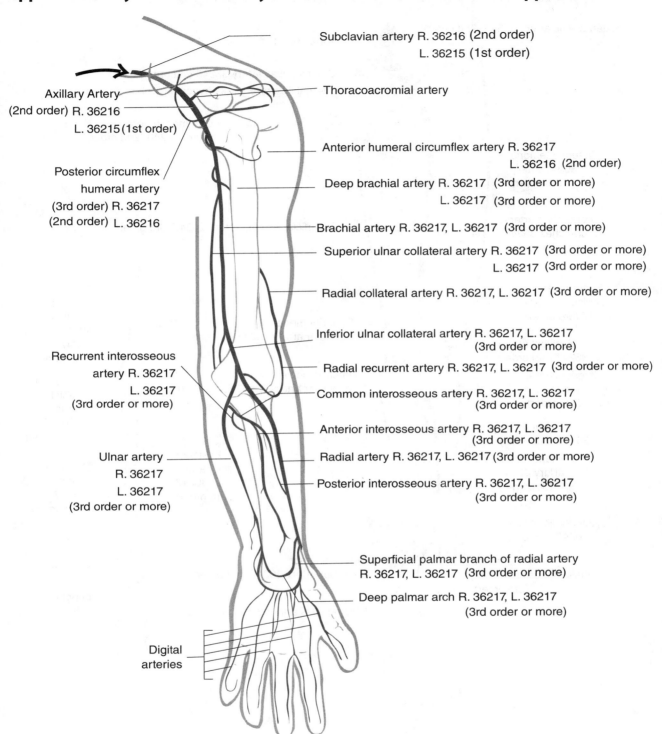

Subclavian artery R. 36216 (2nd order)
L. 36215 (1st order)

Thoracoacromial artery

Axillary Artery
(2nd order) R. 36216
L. 36215 (1st order)

Anterior humeral circumflex artery R. 36217
L. 36216 (2nd order)

Deep brachial artery R. 36217 (3rd order or more)
L. 36217 (3rd order or more)

Posterior circumflex
humeral artery
(3rd order) R. 36217
(2nd order) L. 36216

Brachial artery R. 36217, L. 36217 (3rd order or more)

Superior ulnar collateral artery R. 36217 (3rd order or more)
L. 36217 (3rd order or more)

Radial collateral artery R. 36217, L. 36217 (3rd order or more)

Inferior ulnar collateral artery R. 36217, L. 36217
(3rd order or more)

Recurrent interosseous
artery R. 36217
L. 36217
(3rd order or more)

Radial recurrent artery R. 36217, L. 36217 (3rd order or more)

Common interosseous artery R. 36217, L. 36217
(3rd order or more)

Anterior interosseous artery R. 36217, L. 36217
(3rd order or more)

Ulnar artery
R. 36217
L. 36217
(3rd order or more)

Radial artery R. 36217, L. 36217 (3rd order or more)

Posterior interosseous artery R. 36217, L. 36217
(3rd order or more)

Superficial palmar branch of radial artery
R. 36217, L. 36217 (3rd order or more)

Deep palmar arch R. 36217, L. 36217
(3rd order or more)

Digital
arteries

Lower Extremity Arterial Anatomy—Contralateral, Axillary or Brachial Approach

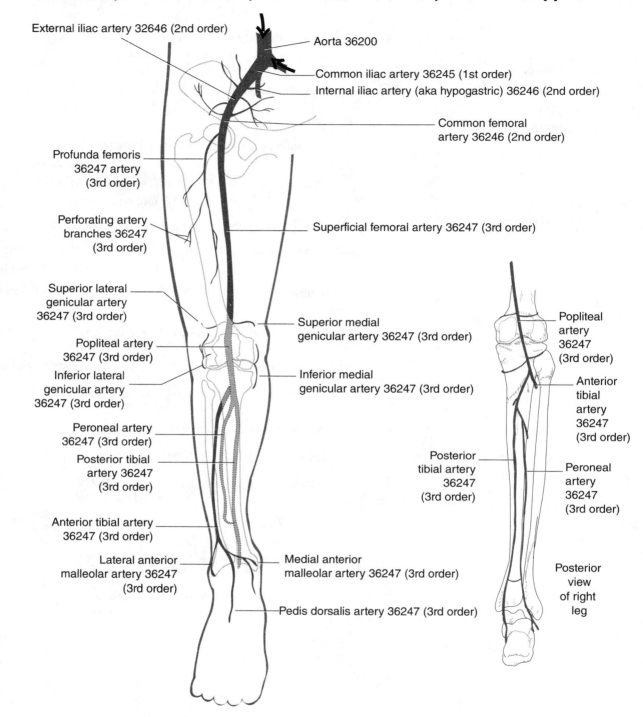

External iliac artery 32646 (2nd order)

Aorta 36200

Common iliac artery 36245 (1st order)

Internal iliac artery (aka hypogastric) 36246 (2nd order)

Common femoral artery 36246 (2nd order)

Profunda femoris 36247 artery (3rd order)

Superficial femoral artery 36247 (3rd order)

Perforating artery branches 36247 (3rd order)

Superior lateral genicular artery 36247 (3rd order)

Superior medial genicular artery 36247 (3rd order)

Popliteal artery 36247 (3rd order)

Inferior lateral genicular artery 36247 (3rd order)

Inferior medial genicular artery 36247 (3rd order)

Peroneal artery 36247 (3rd order)

Posterior tibial artery 36247 (3rd order)

Anterior tibial artery 36247 (3rd order)

Lateral anterior malleolar artery 36247 (3rd order)

Medial anterior malleolar artery 36247 (3rd order)

Pedis dorsalis artery 36247 (3rd order)

Popliteal artery 36247 (3rd order)

Anterior tibial artery 36247 (3rd order)

Posterior tibial artery 36247 (3rd order)

Peroneal artery 36247 (3rd order)

Posterior view of right leg

Portal System

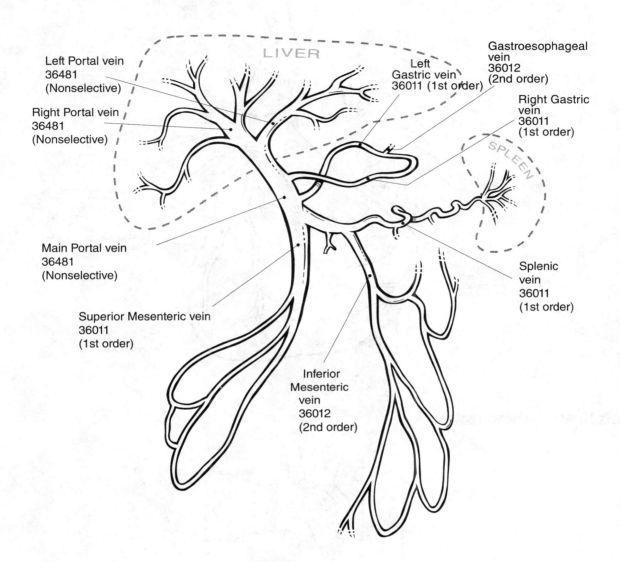

Left Portal vein
36481
(Nonselective)

Right Portal vein
36481
(Nonselective)

LIVER

Left
Gastric vein
36011 (1st order)

Gastroesophageal
vein
36012
(2nd order)

Right Gastric
vein
36011
(1st order)

SPLEEN

Main Portal vein
36481
(Nonselective)

Superior Mesenteric vein
36011
(1st order)

Inferior
Mesenteric
vein
36012
(2nd order)

Splenic
vein
36011
(1st order)

Coronary Arteries Anterior View

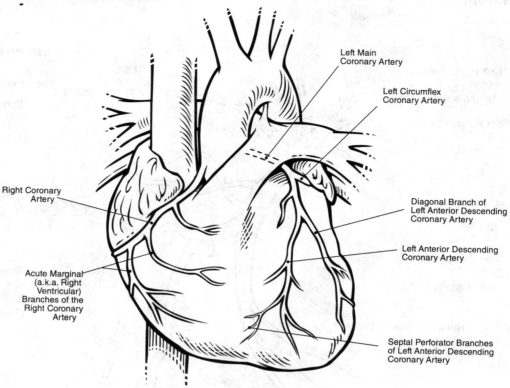

Left Main Coronary Artery

Left Circumflex Coronary Artery

Right Coronary Artery

Diagonal Branch of Left Anterior Descending Coronary Artery

Left Anterior Descending Coronary Artery

Acute Marginal (a.k.a. Right Ventricular) Branches of the Right Coronary Artery

Septal Perforator Branches of Left Anterior Descending Coronary Artery

Left Heart Catheterization

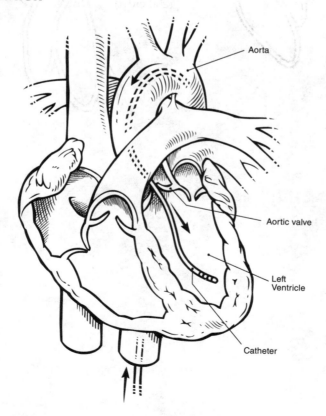

Aorta

Aortic valve

Left Ventricle

Catheter

Heart Conduction System

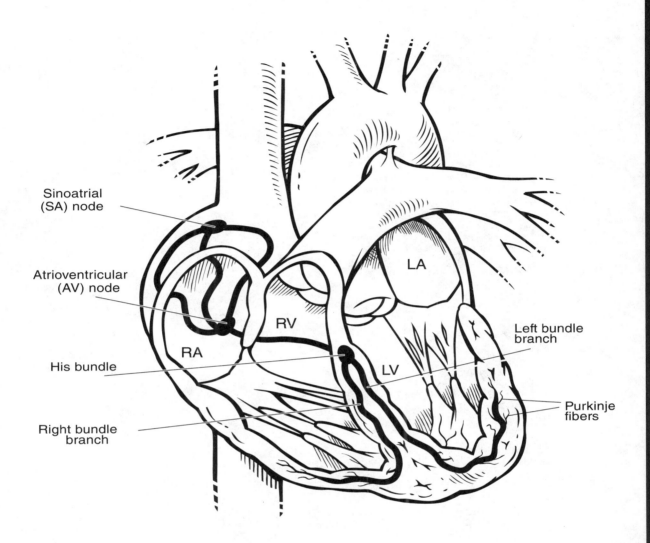

Sinoatrial (SA) node

Atrioventricular (AV) node

His bundle

Right bundle branch

LA

RV

RA

LV

Left bundle branch

Purkinje fibers